Dietary Reference Intakes (DRIs): **Recommended Intakes for Individuals, Minerals**
Food and Nutrition Board, Institute of Medicine, National Academies

Life-Stage Group	Calcium (mg/d)	Chromium (μg/d)	Copper (μg/d)	Fluoride (mg/d)	Iodine (μg/d)	Iron (mg/d)	Magnesium (mg/d)	Mang (mg	Moly (μg/	Pho (mg	Sele (μg	Zinc (mg/d)
Infants												
0-6 mo	210*	0.2*	200*	0.01*	110*	0.27*	30*	0.003*	2*	100*	15*	2*
7-12 mo	270*	5.5*	220*	0.5*	130*	**11**	75*	0.6*	3*	275*	20*	**3**
Children												
1-3 yr	500*	11*	**340**	0.7*	**90**	**7**	**80**	1.2*	**17**	**460**	**20**	**3**
4-8 yr	800*	15*	**440**	1*	**90**	**10**	**130**	1.5*	**22**	**500**	**30**	**5**
Males												
9-13 yr	1300*	25*	**700**	2*	**120**	**8**	**240**	1.9*	**34**	**1250**	**40**	**8**
14-18 yr	1300*	35*	**890**	3*	**150**	**11**	**410**	2.2*	**43**	**1250**	**55**	**11**
19-30 yr	1000*	35*	**900**	4*	**150**	**8**	**400**	2.3*	**45**	**700**	**55**	**11**
31-50 yr	1000*	35*	**900**	4*	**150**	**8**	**420**	2.3*	**45**	**700**	**55**	**11**
51-70 yr	1200*	30*	**900**	4*	**150**	**8**	**420**	2.3*	**45**	**700**	**55**	**11**
>70 yr	1200*	30*	**900**	4*	**150**	**8**	**420**	2.3*	**45**	**700**	**55**	**11**
Females												
9-13 yr	1300*	21*	**700**	2*	**120**	**8**	**240**	1.6*	**34**	**1250**	**40**	**8**
14-18 yr	1300*	24*	**890**	3*	**150**	**15**	**360**	1.6*	**43**	**1250**	**55**	**9**
19-30 yr	1000*	25*	**900**	3*	**150**	**18**	**310**	1.8*	**45**	**700**	**55**	**8**
31-50 yr	1000*	25*	**900**	3*	**150**	**18**	**320**	1.8*	**45**	**700**	**55**	**8**
51-70 yr	1200*	20*	**900**	3*	**150**	**8**	**320**	1.8*	**45**	**700**	**55**	**8**
>70 yr	1200*	20*	**900**	3*	**150**	**8**	**320**	1.8*	**45**	**700**	**55**	**8**
Pregnancy												
≤18 yr	1300*	29*	**1000**	3*	**220**	**27**	**400**	2.0*	**50**	**1250**	**60**	**13**
19-30 yr	1000*	30*	**1000**	3*	**220**	**27**	**350**	2.0*	**50**	**700**	**60**	**11**
31-50 yr	1000*	30*	**1000**	3*	**220**	**27**	**360**	2.0*	**50**	**700**	**60**	**11**
Lactation												
≤18 yr	1300*	44*	**1300**	3*	**290**	**10**	**360**	2.6*	**50**	**1250**	**70**	**14**
19-30 yr	1000*	45*	**1300**	3*	**290**	**9**	**310**	2.6*	**50**	**700**	**70**	**12**
31-50 yr	1000*	45*	**1300**	3*	**290**	**9**	**320**	2.6*	**50**	**700**	**70**	**12**

SOURCES: Dietary Reference Intakes for Calcium, Phosphorus, Magnesium, Vitamin D, and Fluoride (1997); Dietary Reference Intakes for Thiamin, Riboflavin, Niacin, Vitamin B_6, Folate, Vitamin B_{12}, Pantothenic Acid, Biotin, and Choline (1998); Dietary Reference Intakes for Vitamin C, Vitamin E, Selenium, and Carotenoids (2000); and Dietary Reference Intakes for Vitamin A, Vitamin K, Arsenic, Boron, Chromium, Copper, Iodine, Iron, Manganese, Molybdenum, Nickel, Silicon, Vanadium, and Zinc (2001).

NOTE: This table presents Recommended Dietary Allowances (RDAs) in **bold type** and Adequate Intakes (AIs) in ordinary type followed by an asterisk (*). RDAs and AIs may both be used as goals for individual intake. RDAs are set to meet the needs of almost all (97%-98%) individuals in a group. For healthy breastfed infants, the AI is the mean intake. The AI for other life-stage and gender groups is believed to cover needs of all individuals in the group, but lack of data or uncertainty in the data prevent being able to specify with confidence the percentage of individuals covered by this intake.

Dietary Reference Intakes (DRIs): **Tolerable Upper Intake Levels (UL[a]), Minerals**
Food and Nutrition Board, Institute of Medicine, National Academies

Life-Stage Group	Arsenic[b]	Boron (mg/d)	Calcium (g/d)	Chromium	Copper (μg/d)	Fluoride (mg/d)	Iodine (μg/d)	Iron (mg/d)	Magnesium (mg/d)[c]	Manganese (mg/d)	Molybdenum (μg/d)	Nickel (mg/d)	Phosphorus (g/d)	Selenium (μg/d)	Silicon[d]	Vanadium (mg/d)[e]	Zinc (mg/d)
Infants																	
0-6 mo	ND[f]	ND	ND	ND	ND	0.7	ND	40	ND	ND	ND	ND	ND	45	ND	ND	4
7-12 mo	ND	ND	ND	ND	ND	0.9	ND	40	ND	ND	ND	ND	ND	60	ND	ND	5
Children																	
1-3 yr	ND	3	2.5	ND	1000	1.3	200	40	65	2	300	0.2	3	90	ND	ND	7
4-8 yr	ND	6	2.5	ND	3000	2.2	300	40	110	3	600	0.3	3	150	ND	ND	12
Males, Females																	
9-13 yr	ND	11	2.5	ND	5000	10	600	40	350	6	1100	0.6	4	280	ND	ND	23
14-18 yr	ND	17	2.5	ND	8000	10	900	45	350	9	1700	1.0	4	400	ND	ND	34
19-70 yr	ND	20	2.5	ND	10,000	10	1100	45	350	11	2000	1.0	4	400	ND	1.8	40
>70 yr	ND	20	2.5	ND	10,000	10	1100	45	350	11	2000	1.0	3	400	ND	1.8	40
Pregnancy																	
≤18 yr	ND	17	2.5	ND	8000	10	900	45	350	9	1700	1.0	3.5	400	ND	ND	34
19-50 yr	ND	20	2.5	ND	10,000	10	1100	45	350	11	2000	1.0	3.5	400	ND	ND	40
Lactation																	
≤18 yr	ND	17	2.5	ND	8000	10	900	45	350	9	1700	1.0	4	400	ND	ND	34
19-50 yr	ND	20	2.5	ND	10,000	10	1100	45	350	11	2000	1.0	4	400	ND	ND	40

SOURCES: Dietary Reference Intakes for Calcium, Phosphorous, Magnesium, Vitamin D, and Fluoride (1997); Dietary Reference Intakes for Thiamin, Riboflavin, Niacin, Vitamin B_6, Folate, Vitamin B_{12}, Pantothenic Acid, Biotin, and Choline (1998); Dietary Reference Intakes for Vitamin C, Vitamin E, Selenium, and Carotenoids (2000); and Dietary Reference Intakes for Vitamin A, Vitamin K, Arsenic, Boron, Chromium, Copper, Iodine, Iron, Manganese, Molybdenum, Nickel, Silicon, Vanadium, and Zinc (2001). These reports may be accessed via www.nap.edu.

[a]UL = The maximum level of daily nutrient intake that is likely to pose no risk of adverse effects. Unless otherwise specified, the UL represents total intake from food, water, and supplements. Due to lack of suitable data, ULs could not be established for arsenic, chromium, and silicon. In the absence of ULs, extra caution may be warranted in consuming levels above recommended intakes.

[b]Although the UL was not determined for arsenic, there is no justification for adding arsenic to food or supplements.

[c]The ULs for magnesium represent intake from a pharmacologic agent only and do not include intake from food and water.

[d]Although silicon has not been shown to cause adverse effects in humans, there is no justification for adding silicon to supplements.

[e]Although vanadium in food has not been shown to cause adverse effects in humans, there is no justification for adding vanadium to food, and vanadium supplements should be used with caution. The UL is based on adverse effects in laboratory animals, and this data could be used to set a UL for adults but not children and adolescents.

[f]ND = Not determinable due to lack of data of adverse effects in this age group and concern with regard to lack of ability to handle excess amounts. Source of intake should be from food only to prevent high levels of intake.

Dietary Reference Intake Values for Energy for Active Individuals*
Food and Nutrition Board, Institute of Medicine, National Academies

LIFE-STAGE GROUP	CRITERION	ACTIVE PAL EER (kcal/day)† MALE	ACTIVE PAL EER (kcal/day)† FEMALE
Infants			
0-6 mo	Energy expenditure + Energy deposition	570	520 (3 mo)
7-12 mo	Energy expenditure + Energy deposition	743	676 (9 mo)
Children			
1-2 yr	Energy expenditure + Energy deposition	1046	992 (24 mo)
3-8 yr	Energy expenditure + Energy deposition	1742	1642 (6 yr)
9-13 yr	Energy expenditure + Energy deposition	2279	2071 (11 yr)
14-18 yr	Energy expenditure + Energy deposition	3152	2368 (16 yr)
Adults			
>18 yr	Energy expenditure	3067‡	2403‡ (19 yr)
Pregnant Women			
14-18 yr	Adolescent female EER + Change in TEE + Pregnancy energy deposition		
First trimester			2368 (16 yr)
Second trimester			2708 (16 yr)
Third trimester			2820 (16 yr)
19-50 yr	Adult female EER + Change in TEE + Pregnancy energy deposition		
First trimester			2403‡ (19 yr)
Second trimester			2743‡ (19 yr)
Third trimester			2855‡ (19 yr)
Lactating Women			
14-18 yr	Adolescent female EER + Milk energy output − Weight loss		
First 6 mo			2698 (16 yr)
Second 6 mo			2768 (16 yr)
19-50 yr	Adult female EER + Milk energy output − Weight loss		
First 6 mo			2733‡ (19 yr)
Second 6 mo			2803‡ (19 yr)

From Institute of Medicine of The National Academies: *Dietary reference intakes for energy, carbohydrate, fiber, fat, fatty acids, cholesterol, protein, and amino acids,* Washington, DC, 2002, The National Academies Press.
*For healthy active Americans and Canadians at the reference height and weight.
†*PAL,* Physical activity level; *EER,* estimated energy requirement; *TEE,* total energy expenditure.
‡Subtract 10 kcal/day for men and 7 kcal/day for women for each year of age above 19 years.

Dietary Reference Intakes (DRIs): **Recommended Intakes for Individuals, Macronutrients**
Food and Nutrition Board, Institute of Medicine, National Academies

LIFE-STAGE GROUP	PROTEIN RDA/AI g/day[a]	PROTEIN AMDR[b]	CARBOHYDRATE RDA/AI g/day	CARBOHYDRATE AMDR	FIBER RDA/AI g/day	FIBER AMDR	FAT RDA/AI g/day	FAT AMDR	*n-6* POLYUNSATURATED FATTY ACIDS (LINOLEIC ACID) RDA/AI g/day	*n-6* AMDR	*n-3* POLYUNSATURATED FATTY ACIDS (α-LINOLENIC ACID) RDA/AI g/day	*n-3* AMDR[d]	SATURATED AND *TRANS* FATTY ACIDS AND CHOLESTEROL RDA/AI g/day	SATURATED AND *TRANS* FATTY ACIDS AND CHOLESTEROL AMDR
Infants														
0-6 mo	9.1	ND[c]	60	ND	ND		31		4.4	ND	0.5	ND		
7-12 mo	**13.5**	ND	95	ND	ND		30		4.6	ND	0.5	ND		
Children														
1-3 yr	**13**	**5-20**	**130**	45-65	19			30-40	7	5-10	0.7	0.6-1.2		
4-8 yr	**19**	**10-30**	**130**	45-65	25			25-35	10	5-10	0.9	0.6-1.2		
Males														
9-13 yr	**34**	**10-30**	**130**	45-65	31			25-35	12	5-10	1.2	0.6-1.2		
14-18 yr	**52**	**10-30**	**130**	45-65	38			25-35	16	5-10	1.6	0.6-1.2		
19-30 yr	**56**	**10-35**	**130**	45-65	38			20-35	17	5-10	1.6	0.6-1.2		
31-50 yr	**56**	**10-35**	**130**	45-65	38			20-35	17	5-10	1.6	0.6-1.2		
50-70 yr	**56**	**10-35**	**130**	45-65	30			20-35	14	5-10	1.6	0.6-1.2		
>70 yr	**56**	**10-35**	**130**	45-65	30			20-35	14	5-10	1.6	0.6-1.2		
Females														
9-13 yr	**34**	**10-30**	**130**	45-65	26			25-35	10	5-10	1.0	0.6-1.2		
14-18 yr	**46**	**10-30**	**130**	45-65	26			25-35	11	5-10	1.1	0.6-1.2		
19-30 yr	**46**	**10-35**	**130**	45-65	25			20-35	12	5-10	1.1	0.6-1.2		
31-50 yr	**46**	**10-35**	**130**	45-65	25			20-35	12	5-10	1.1	0.6-1.2		
50-70 yr	**46**	**10-35**	**130**	45-65	21			20-35	11	5-10	1.1	0.6-1.2		
>70 yr	**46**	**10-35**	**130**	45-65	21			20-35	11	5-10	1.1	0.6-1.2		
Pregnant														
≤18 yr	**71**	**10-35**	**175**	45-65	28			20-35	13	5-10	1.4	0.6-1.2		
19-30 yr	**71**	**10-35**	**175**	45-65	28			20-35	13	5-10	1.4	0.6-1.2		
31-50 yr	**71**	**10-35**		45-65	28			20-35	13	5-10	1.4	0.6-1.2		
Lactating														
≤18 yr	**71**	**10-35**	**210**	45-65	29			20-35	13	5-10	1.3	0.6-1.2		
19-30 yr	**71**	**10-35**	**210**	45-65	29			20-35	13	5-10	1.3	0.6-1.2		
31-50 yr	**71**	**10-35**	**210**	45-65	29			20-35	13	5-10	1.3	0.6-1.2		

Data from *Dietary reference intakes for energy, carbohydrate, fiber, fat, fatty acids, cholesterol, protein, and amino acids,* Washington, DC, 2002, The National Academies Press.
NOTE: This table represents Recommended Dietary Allowances (RDAs) in **bold type** and Adequate Intakes (AIs) in ordinary type. RDAs and AIs may both be used as goals for individual intake. RDAs are set to meet the needs of almost all (97%-98%) individuals in a group. For healthy breastfed infants, the AI is the mean intake. The AI for other life-stage and gender groups is believed to cover the needs of all individuals in the group, but lack of data prevents being able to specify with confidence the percentage of individuals covered by this intake.
[a]Based on 1.5 g/kg/day for infants, 1.1 g/kg/day for 1-3 yr, 0.95 g/kg/day for 4-13 yr, 0.85 g/kg/day for 14-18 yr, 0.8 g/kg/day for adults, and 1.1 g/kg/day for pregnant (using prepregnancy weight) and lactating women.
[b]Acceptable Macronutrient Distribution Range (AMDR) is the range of intake for a particular energy source that is associated with reduced risk of chronic disease while providing intakes of essential nutrients. If an individual has consumed in excess of the AMDR, there is a potential of increasing the risk of chronic diseases and insufficient intakes of essential nutrients.
[c]ND = Not determinable due to lack of data of adverse effects in this age group and concern with regard to lack of ability to handle excess amounts. Source of intake should be from food only to prevent high levels of intake.
[d]Approximately 10% of the total can come from longer-chain, *n*-3 fatty acids.

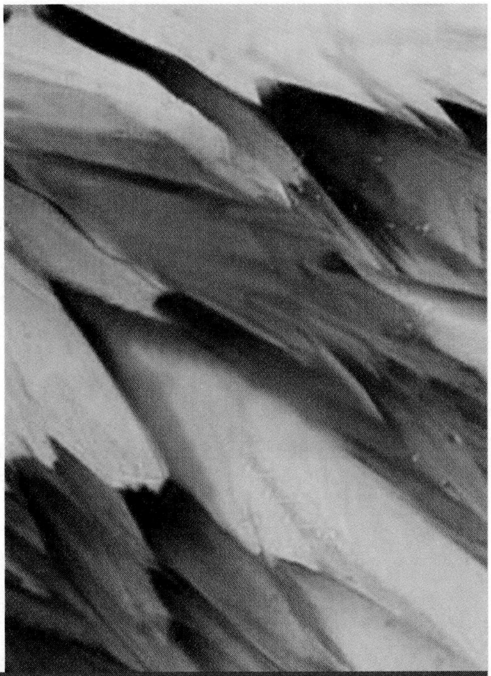

Krause's

Food, Nutrition, & Diet Therapy

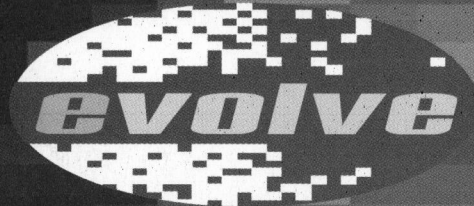

Krause's

Food, Nutrition, & Diet Therapy

11th Edition

L. Kathleen Mahan, MS, RD, CDE
Clinical Associate
Department of Pediatrics
School of Medicine
University of Washington
Seattle, Washington

Nutrition Counselor
Nutrition by Design
Seattle, Washington

Sylvia Escott-Stump, MA, RD, LDN
Dietetic Programs Director
Department of Nutrition & Hospitality Management
East Carolina University
Greenville, North Carolina

Consulting Nutritionist
Nutritional Balance
Winterville, North Carolina

SAUNDERS
An Imprint of Elsevier

The Curtis Center
Independence Square West
Philadelphia, Pennsylvania 19106

KRAUSE'S FOOD, NUTRITION, & DIET THERAPY ISBN: 0-7216-9784-4

NOTICE

Nutrition is an ever-changing field. Standard safety precautions must be followed, but as new research and clinical experience broaden our knowledge, changes in treatment and drug therapy may become necessary or appropriate. Readers are advised to check the most current product information provided by the manufacturer of each drug to be administered to verify the recommended dose, the method and duration of administration, and contraindications. It is the responsibility of the licensed health care provider, relying on experience and knowledge of the patient, to determine dosages and the best treatment for each individual patient. Neither the publisher nor the editor assumes any liability for any injury and/or damage to persons or property arising from this publication.

Previous editions copyrighted 1952, 1957, 1961, 1966, 1972, 1979, 1984, 1992, 1996, 2000.

International Standard Book Number 0-7216-9784-4

Vice President and Publishing Director: Sally Schrefer
Senior Editor: Yvonne Alexopoulos
Senior Developmental Editor: Melissa K. Boyle
Associate Developmental Editor: Kristin Hebberd
Publishing Services Manager: John Rogers
Senior Project Manager: Cheryl A. Abbott
Designer: Mark Bernard
Cover Image: The book's cover image is a crystallized cholesterol molecule.

Printed in The United States of America.

Last digit is print number: 9 8 7 6 5 4 3 2

CONTRIBUTORS

John J.B. Anderson, PhD
Professor
Nutrition Department
University of North Carolina at Chapel Hill
Chapel Hill, North Carolina

Diane M. Anderson, PhD, RD, CSP, FADA
Associate Professor
Department of Pediatrics
Section of Neonatology
Baylor College of Medicine
Houston, Texas

Cynthia Taft Bayerl, MS, RD, LDN
Director, Perinatal and Pediatric Nutrition Programs
Nutrition and Physical Activity Initiative
Bureau of Family and Community Health
Massachusetts Department of Public Health
Boston, Massachusetts

Jacqueline R. Berning, PhD, RD
Assistant Professor
Department of Biology
University of Colorado at Colorado Springs
Colorado Springs, Colorado

Peter L. Beyer, MS, RD, LD
Associate Professor
Department of Dietetics and Nutrition
University of Kansas Medical Center
Kansas City, Kansas

Abby S. Bloch, PhD, RD, FADA
Nutrition Consultant
New York, New York

Cynthia M. Brylinsky, MS, RD, LDN
Director, Guest Services
Geisinger Health System
Danville, Pennsylvania

Timothy H. Carlson, PhD, RD, NRCC
Laboratory Director
Pacific Biometrics, Inc.
Seattle, Washington

Sr. Jeanne P. Crowe, PharmD, RPH
Pharmacist
Camilla Hall
Immaculata, Pennsylvania

Ruth M. DeBusk, PhD, RD
Owner
DeBusk Communications, LC
Tallahassee, Florida

Judith L. Dodd, MS, RD, FADA, LD
Adjunct Assistant Professor
Department of Clinical Dietetics and Nutrition
School of Health and Rehabilitation Sciences
University of Pittsburgh
Pittsburgh, Pennsylvania;
Nutrition Consultant
Allison Park, Pennsylvania

Lisa Dorfman, MS, RD, LMHC
Director, Sports Nutrition
Food and Fitness International, Inc.
Miami, Florida

Robert Earl, MPH, RD
Senior Director, Nutrition Policy
National Food Processors Association
Washington, District of Columbia

Barbara Eldridge, MS, RD, LD
Clinical Research Associate
Cancer Treatment Center
Saint Alphonsus Regional Medical Center
Boise, Idaho

Susan Ettinger, PhD, RD
Associate Professor and Chair
Clinical Nutrition Department
New York Institute of Technology
Old Westbury, New York

Marcy Fenton, MS, RD
Nutritionist
Treatment, Education, Nutrition, and HIV Program
AIDS Project Los Angeles
Los Angeles, California

Marion J. Franz, MS, RD, LD, CDE
Nutrition/Health Consultant
Nutrition Concepts by Franz
Minneapolis, Minnesota

Carol D. Frary, MS, RD
Clinical Research Coordinator
Dean's Office
College of Agriculture and Life Sciences
University of Vermont
Burlington, Vermont

Margie Lee Gallagher, PhD, RD, MS
Associate Dean, College of Human Ecology
Professor and Senior Scientist
Department of Nutrition & Hospitality Management
East Carolina University
Greenville, North Carolina

Kathleen A. Hammond, MS, RD, LD, CNSD, RN, BSN, CNSN
Coordinator, Continuing Education
Clinical Nutrition Specialist
Chartwell Management Company
Atlanta, Georgia;
Adjunct Assistant Professor
Department of Foods and Nutrition
University of Georgia
Athens, Georgia

Nancy G. Harris, MS, RD, LDN, FADA
Faculty Member
Department of Nutrition & Hospitality Management
East Carolina University
Greenville, North Carolina

Jeanette M. Hasse, PhD, RD, LD, CNSD, FADA
Transplant Nutrition Specialist
Transplant Services
Baylor University Medical Center
Dallas, Texas

Sherry K. Hubbard, RD, LD
Manager and Clinical Dietitian
Nutrition Department
Oklahoma Allergy and Asthma Clinic
Oklahoma City, Oklahoma

Rachel K. Johnson, PhD, MPH, RD
Professor and Dean
College of Agriculture and Life Sciences
University of Vermont
Burlington, Vermont

Veena Juneja, MSc, RD
Senior Renal Dietitian
Nutrition Services
St. Joseph's Healthcare
Hamilton, Ontario, Canada

Debra A. Krummel, PhD, RD, LD
Assistant Professor
Department of Community Medicine
West Virginia University
Morgantown, West Virginia

Idamarie Laquatra, PhD, RD
Nutrition Consultant
Pittsburgh, Pennsylvania

Betty L. Lucas, MPH, RD, CD
Nutritionist
Center of Human Development & Disablility
University of Washington
Seattle, Washington

Ainsley M. Malone, MS, RD, CNSD
Nutrition Support Team Dietitian
Pharmacy Department
Mount Carmel West Hospital
Columbus, Ohio

Laura E. Matarese, MS, RD, LD, CNSD, FADA
Director, Nutrition Intestinal Rehabilitation
Department of Nutrition Support & Vascular Access
The Cleveland Clinic Foundation
Cleveland, Ohio

Kimberly Mathai, MS, RD, CN
Nutrition Counselor
Nutrition by Design
Seattle, Washington

Charles Mueller, PhD, MS, RD, CNSD, CDN
Nutrition Research Manager
General Clinical Research Center
Weill Medical College
Department of Medicine
Cornell University
New York, New York

Donna H. Mueller, PhD, RD, FADA
Associate Professor
Department of Bioscience and Biotechnology
Drexel University
Philadelphia, Pennsylvania

Zaneta M. Pronsky, MS, RD, LDN, FADA
Author, Speaker, Consultant Dietitian
Food Medications Interactions
Birchrunville, Pennsylvania

Pamela Reichert-Anderson, MA, RD
Nutritionist
Department of Pediatrics
Schneider Children's Hospital
New Hyde Park, New York

Valentina M. Remig, PhD, RD, LD, FADA
Assistant Professor
Department of Human Nutrition
College of Human Ecology
Kansas State University
Manhattan, Kansas

Cecilia Romero, MD
Assistant Dean of Student Affairs
School of Medicine
University of Texas Medical Branch
Galveston, Texas

Janet E. Schebendach, MA, RD
Nutritionist, Eating Disorders Research
New York State Psychiatric Institute
New York, New York

Judith K. Shabert, MD, RD, MPH
Instructor
Department of Obstetrics, Gynecology, and Reproductive Biology
Harvard Medical School
Boston, Massachusetts

Ellyn Silverman, MPH, RD
President
ECS Nutrition Services
Long Beach, California

Linda G. Snetselaar, BS, MS, PhD, RD
Associate Professor
College of Public Health, Epidemiology
University of Iowa
Iowa City, Iowa

Bonnie A. Spear, PhD, RD
Associate Professor
Department of Pediatrics
General Pediatrics and Adolescent Medicine
University of Alabama at Birmingham
Birmingham, Alabama

Tracy Stopler, MS, RD
President, Nutrition E.T.C., Inc.
Plainview, New York;
Associate Professor
Department of Nutrition and Human Performance
Adelphi University
Garden City, New York

Riva Touger-Decker, PhD, RD, FADA
Associate Professor and Program Director
Primary Care
School of Health-Related Professions
University of Medicine & Dentistry of New Jersey
Newark, New Jersey

Cristine M. Trahms, MS, RD, CD, FADA
Lecturer, Department of Pediatrics
Director, Nutrition Services
Center on Human Development and Disability
University of Washington
Seattle, Washington

Susan J. Whitmire, RD, LDN, CNSD
Nutrition Support Dietitian
Department of Gastroenterology and Nutrition
Geisinger Medical Center
Danville, Pennsylvania

Katy G. Wilkens, MS, RD
Manager, Department of Nutrition & Fitness Services
Northwest Kidney Centers
Seattle, Washington

Marion F. Winkler, MS, RD, LDN, CNSD
Surgical Nutrition Specialist
Surgery/Nutritional Support Service
Rhode Island Hospital
Providence, Rhode Island

REVIEWERS

Mary Babcock, MS, RD
Medical Nutrition Therapist
Wilkes-Barre Veterans Administration Medical Center
Wilkes-Barre, Pennsylvania;
Adjunct Professor
Marywood University
Scranton, Pennsylvania

Hope Barkouris, PhD, RD, LD
Department of Nutrition
Case Western Reserve University
Cleveland, Ohio

Leila T. Beker, PhD, RD
Director, Bionutrition Care
Clinical Research Center, Children's Research Institute
Assistant Clinical Professor of Pediatrics
The George Washington University School of Medicine
Children's National Medical Center
Washington, District of Columbia

Carmen Boyd, MS, RD, LPC
Southwest Missouri State University Biomedical Sciences
Springfield, Missouri

Kathryn Camp, MS, RD, CSP
Pediatric Nutritionist
Walter Reed Army Medical Center
Washington, District of Columbia

Margaret M. Cicirella, MS, MA, RD, LD
Instructor in Nutrition
Department of Nutrition
Case Western Reserve University
Cleveland, Ohio

Harriet H. Cloud, MS, RD
Owner, Nutrition Matters—Pediatric Consulting
Professor Emeritus, Department of Nutrition Sciences
University of Alabama at Birmingham
Birmingham, Alabama

Dorice M. Czajka-Narins, PhD
Former Professor and Chair
Department of Nutrition and Food Science
Texas Women's University
Denton, Texas

Michele DeBiasse-Fortin, MS, RD, LDN, CNSD
Clinical Nutrition Manager/Nutrition Support Dietitian
Quincy Medical Center
Department of Food and Nutrition Services
Quincy, Massachusetts

Judith L. Dodd, MS, RD, FADA, LD
Adjunct Assistant Professor
Department of Clinical Dietetics and Nutrition
School of Health and Rehabilitation Sciences
University of Pittsburgh
Pittsburgh, Pennsylvania;
Nutrition Consultant
Allison Park, Pennsylvania

Julie C. Duffy, RD, LDN
Pediatric Nutritionist
Brenner Children's Hospital
Wake Forest University Baptist Medical Center
Winston-Salem, North Carolina

Robert Earl, MPH, RD
Senior Director, Nutrition Policy
National Food Processors Association
Washington, District of Columbia

Patti G. Eisenberg, MSN, RN, CS
Clinical Nurse Specialist
Community Health Network
Department Clinical Practice, Education and Research
Indianapolis, Indiana

Rachel M. Fournet, PhD, RD, LDN
Dietetic Internship Director
Assistant Professor
University of Louisiana at Lafayette
Lafayette, Louisiana

Valerie A. George, PhD, LD
Research Associate Professor
Department of Dietetics and Nutrition
College of Health and Urban Affairs
Florida International University
Miami, Florida

Dawn Goodholm, RD, LD
Clinical Nutrition Manager, Food and Nutrition Services
Brooks Rehabilitation Center
Jacksonville, Florida

Rachel Griehs, MS, RD
Bariatric Clinical Specialist
Bariatric Surgery Program
University of Pennsylvania Medical Center
Department of Surgery
Philadelphia, Pennsylvania

Kathy Hammond, MS, RD, LD, CNSD, RN, BSN, CNSN
Coordinator, Continuing Education
Clinical Nutrition Specialist
Chartwell Management Company
Atlanta, Georgia;
Adjunct Assistant Professor
Department of Foods and Nutrition
University of Georgia
Athens, Georgia

Sharon M. Herr, RD, CDN
Author, *Herb-Drug Interactions Handbook*
Nassau, New York

Dorothy G. Herron, PhD, RN, CS
Assistant Professor, Department of Adult Health Nursing
University of Maryland
Baltimore, Maryland

Debra A. Indorato, RD
Owner, Approach Nutrition and Fitness
Chesapeake, Virginia

Mary Jacob, PhD
Department of Family and Consumer Sciences
California State University
Long Beach, California

Kessey J. Kieselhorst, MPA, RD, CDE, LDN
Manager, Clinical Nutrition Services
Geisinger Health System
Danville, Pennsylvania

Kelly J. Kohls, PhD, RD, LD
Owner, Able Weight and Wellness Services
Lebanon, Ohio

Cynthia Kupper, RD, CD
Executive Director, Gluten Intolerance Group
Seattle, Washington
Chairman, Dietitians in Gluten Intolerance Diseases
Board of Digestive Diseases National Coalition
National Digestive Diseases Information Clearinghouse Coordinating Committee

Edith Lerner, PhD, LD
Associate Professor and Vice-Chair
Department of Nutrition
Case Western Reserve University
Cleveland, Ohio

Barbara D. Liles, MEd, RD, LDN
Instructor, Department of Nutrition
University of North Carolina at Greensboro
Greensboro, North Carolina

Alice K. Lindeman, PhD, RD
Associate Professor
Department of Applied Health Sciences
Indiana University
Bloomington, Indiana

Dena McDowell, RD, CD
Clinical Dietitian
Froedtert Hospital
Milwaukee, Wisconsin

Pat McGinty, RD, LD
Assistant Director, Clinical Nutrition Services
Department of Nutrition and Dietetics
The Ohio State University Hospitals
Columbus, Ohio

Michael Edward Mayo, MBBS, FRCS
Professor of Urology
Department of Urology
University of Washington
Seattle, Washington

Laurie J. Moyer-Mileur, PhD, RD
Research Associate Professor, Pediatrics
Director, Center for Pediatric Nutrition Research
University of Utah
Salt Lake City, Utah

Jesse Pavlinac, MS, RD, CSR, LD
Oregon Health & Science University
Clinical Nutrition Manager
Senior Instructor, School of Medicine
Portland, Oregon

Rena Quinton, MS, RD
Assistant Professor/Lecturer II
Marywood University
Nutrition and Dietetics
Scranton, Pennsylvania

Anita K. Reed, MSN, RN
Instructor of Nursing
St. Elizabeth School of Nursing
Lafayette, Indiana

Tracey Ryan, RD, CNSD
Chief Clinical Dietitian
Froedtert Hospital
Milwaukee, Wisconsin

Vivian Sun, MS, RD, CNSD, CDN
Associate Director
New York City Health and Hospital Corporation
Bellevue Hospital
New York, New York

Jennifer Zesdorn Weber, RD, CNSD
Clinical Dietitian
Clinical Nutrition Support Services
Hospital of the University of Pennsylvania
Philadelphia, Pennsylvania

Jennifer M. Williams, MS, RD, CNSD
Senior Clinical Dietitian Specialist
Clinical Nutrition Support Service
University of Pennsylvania Health System
Philadelphia, Pennsylvania

Fiona Wolf, RD
Nutrition and Fitness Services
Northwest Kidney Centers
Seattle, Washington

Linda O. Young, MS, RD, LMNT
Director, Didactic Program in Dietetics
Department of Nutritional Science and Dietetics
University of Nebraska-Lincoln
Lincoln, Nebraska

We would like to dedicate this edition to the memory of Elsa Lundell Mahan, who recently passed away and who was a constant and loving support to Kathleen through her many writings of this text over the past 25 years, and to our supportive families.

—The Authors, 11th Edition

Foreword

I remember when I first learned about the *Krause* textbook. At that time, 1975, it was in its 5th edition. I was preparing for the RD exam and was told to study from this textbook. I did, and I passed! From then on my connection with this text has been fond and continuous. As a clinical practitioner, I always had a copy of the latest edition of *Krause* on my desk as a reference. Now, as a dietetic educator, I rely on this text again. I use *Krause's Food, Nutrition, & Diet Therapy* as a foundation for the didactic component of my classes to prepare students for supervised practice in the clinical arena. I am thrilled to be asked to write a few words about this text, which has served me so well professionally throughout all these years.

Medical nutrition therapy, or maintenance of proper nutrition, has been documented as a cornerstone of patient care since the time of Hippocrates. However, many illnesses, as well as trauma and infection, can alter function of the gastrointestinal tract, decrease appetite, and intensify metabolic demands, all of which can result in poor nutritional status leading to increased morbidity. Consequently, nutrition and the metabolic processes of the body are intimately linked and interacting. Naturally, it follows that medical nutrition therapy should support or modify metabolic events in a beneficial way to decrease morbidity and mortality.

Medical nutrition therapy has changed significantly since the first edition of *Krause's Food, Nutrition, & Diet Therapy* was published in 1952, but this text has always remained current. The editors of this 11th edition of *Krause's Food, Nutrition, & Diet Therapy* have been successful in compiling a single volume sharply focused on medical nutrition therapy, with fitting reference to relevant physiologic and metabolic background. As a valuable resource for practitioners caring for today's patients, it contains chapters written by experts who provide theoretical and practical information in specific areas of nutrition and metabolism. Educators and students will find this text effective in promoting learning in students preparing to practice tomorrow's patient care.

Each chapter of *Krause* includes simple clinical scenarios to help link clinical experiences with the material presented. Transferring knowledge into practice in a didactic setting is often difficult. One way to use the classroom as a bridge between integration of knowledge from previously learned information and the clinical setting is through the use of case studies. These practice scenarios require students to integrate knowledge from many sources, support the use of previously learned information, put students into decision-making roles, and nurture critical thinking (Nelms MN, Anderson SL: *Medical nutrition therapy: a case study approach,* Florence, Ky, 2003, Wadsworth/Thomson Learning).

I have come to rely on the integration of this text with my case study approach and am pleased to know that there is a new edition of the same quality and reliability of the past editions.

Sara Long, PhD, RD

Professor and Director
Didactic Program in Dietetics
Southern Illinois University
Carbondale, Illinois

PREFACE

The 11th edition of this classic text recognizes that the emerging field of nutritional genomics will play a major role in the management of health, fitness, and medical nutrition therapy in the future. The text furnishes theoretical knowledge and clinical information in a form that is useful to students in nursing, dietetics, and other allied health professions, many of whom are receiving education and training in an interdisciplinary clinical setting. It is valuable as an ancillary text for use in other disciplines such as medicine, dentistry, child development, and health education.

As always, with its extensive appendixes, tables, illustrations, and clinical insight boxes providing practical hands-on procedures and clinical tools, it continues to be the textbook that can accompany the graduating student into clinical practice as a treasured reference source. All of the popular features have been retained in this edition, and material has been updated and referenced extensively to reflect the most current information available.

A few new guest authors join those who are back by popular demand. Many new reviewers also joined the preparation process. The contributions of these reputable authors and reviewers, all experts in their fields, reflect the effort of this text to cover the increasing sophistication of nutritional care and education.

Organization and Content

This edition is organized into five parts. Part 1, Nutrition Basics, and Part 2, Nutrition in the Life Cycle, are appropriate for use as the text for a basic nutrition course. Although Parts 3, 4, and 5 are progressively more clinical in content, sections of Part 4, Nutrition for Health and Fitness, fit very well into a basic nutrition course. Part 3, Nutrition Care, and Part 5, Medical Nutrition Therapy, provide the basis for training in medical nutrition therapy and add the background information and hands-on tools necessary for successful clinical practice.

Part 1–Nutrition Basics–continues to furnish material appropriate for teaching basic nutrition. Practical information is provided by many tables with useful clinical applications, such as calculation of energy requirements and expenditure, and the best food sources for each vitamin and mineral. The vitamin chapter has been simplified and reflects the role that vitamins play in gene expression.

Part 2–Nutrition in the Life Cycle–presents in-depth information by expert guest authors on the importance of nutrition from pregnancy to the aging process. These chapters discuss the nutrition issues in each life stage.

Part 3–Nutrition Care–covers the concepts of the individual's nutritional status as a reflection of eating habits, pharmacological and nutritional treatment, and the nutrition resources in the community. A new chapter, Nutritional Genomics, highlights the essential nature of nutrition and gene interaction at the cellular level in health and disease management. The Nutrition Care Process chapter has been updated to reflect the new procedures that have been adopted by the profession of dietetics. Nutrition diagnosis is underway, and standardized language will be added in the next edition.

Part 4–Nutrition for Health and Fitness–continues to bring together nutrition concepts that have particular meaning in the achievement and maintenance of health and fitness and the prevention of chronic disease. Chapters on dental health, bone health, and athletic training and sports focus on the role of nutrition in the prevention of problems in these areas.

Part 5–Medical Nutrition Therapy–continues to reflect the current knowledge and trends in nutrition therapy. All of the chapters are written and reviewed by specialists in the nutritional aspects of conditions such as diabetes, renal disease, and pulmonary disease. The chronic diseases of atherosclerosis and hypertension have been moved to this section to reflect the necessary medical nutrition therapy.

Features New to the 11th Edition

One of the continuing emphases in this edition is pathophysiology as it relates to nutrition care. Algorithms that illustrate pathophysiology and signs of disease, and present appropriate medical and nutritional management, continue to equip students with an understanding of the illness process as a background for providing optimal nutritional care.

Throughout the text we have incorporated the new Dietary Reference Intakes (DRIs), including Recommended Dietary Allowances (RDAs), Adequate Intakes (AIs), and Tolerable Upper Levels of Intake (ULs).

Rather than list Web site addresses throughout the text, we have created a Relevant Web Sites section at the end of every chapter. These Web site references give the student additional resources for study and continue to make this text current, practical, and comprehensive.

In the extensive Appendixes the reader will still find, all in one place, the clinical references and tools that have always been a valued feature of this text. There are several new appendixes. Appendix 53 provides the new 2003 Exchange Lists for Meal Planning, and Appendix 54 now includes not only the Glycemic Index but also the glycemic load for various carbohydrates. Appendix 55 is the new National Dysphagia Diet, and Appendix 56 has been added to include the specific definitions and procedures that are to be used in the nutrition care process for dietetics professionals.

"Focus On," "Clinical Insights," and "New Directions" boxes in each chapter continue to provide the student and teacher with expanded information and suggested areas for further discussion, study, or research.

Ancillary Materials

Continuing with this edition is the Instructor's Resource on CD-ROM and—new to this edition—the Instructor's Resource and Student's Resource on line. The Instructor's Resource materials—both on CD-ROM and on line—include PowerPoint presentations for each chapter that contain both images and tables from the text and lecture slides for instruction, as well as a thorough Test Bank with more than 800 questions separated by chapter and presented in ExamView. The Student's Resource on line contains Study Exercises—multiple-choice and matching questions—for self-assessment via the Elsevier Web site for those programs adopting the text.

Our goal with each new edition has always been to maintain a premier text in the field of dietetics that students and educators will turn to and that clinicians will continue to use with ease and confidence in providing nutrition care.

L. Kathleen Mahan

L. Kathleen Mahan, MS, RD, CDE

Sylvia Escott-Stump

Sylvia Escott-Stump, MA, RD, LDN

ACKNOWLEDGMENTS

We wish to acknowledge the hard work and support of Yvonne Alexopoulos, Senior Editor; Melissa Boyle and Kristin Hebberd, Developmental Editors; Cheryl Abbott, Senior Project Manager; Emily Porterfield, who assisted with the Instructor and Student ancillaries; and all of the reviewers. We would also like to thank the contributors of this edition; they are amazingly committed to the accuracy and reliability of this book!

Most important is the continuing encouragement and support from our families, without whom this work would not be possible. Kathleen thanks Robert, Carly, and Ana Raab and Jim Mahan and his family. Sylvia would like to thank Russ, Matthew, and Lindsay Stump; Clara Escott Florianne Stump; and Joyce Stanley and her family.

Krause's

Food, Nutrition, & Diet Therapy

11th Edition

CONTENTS

APPENDIXES

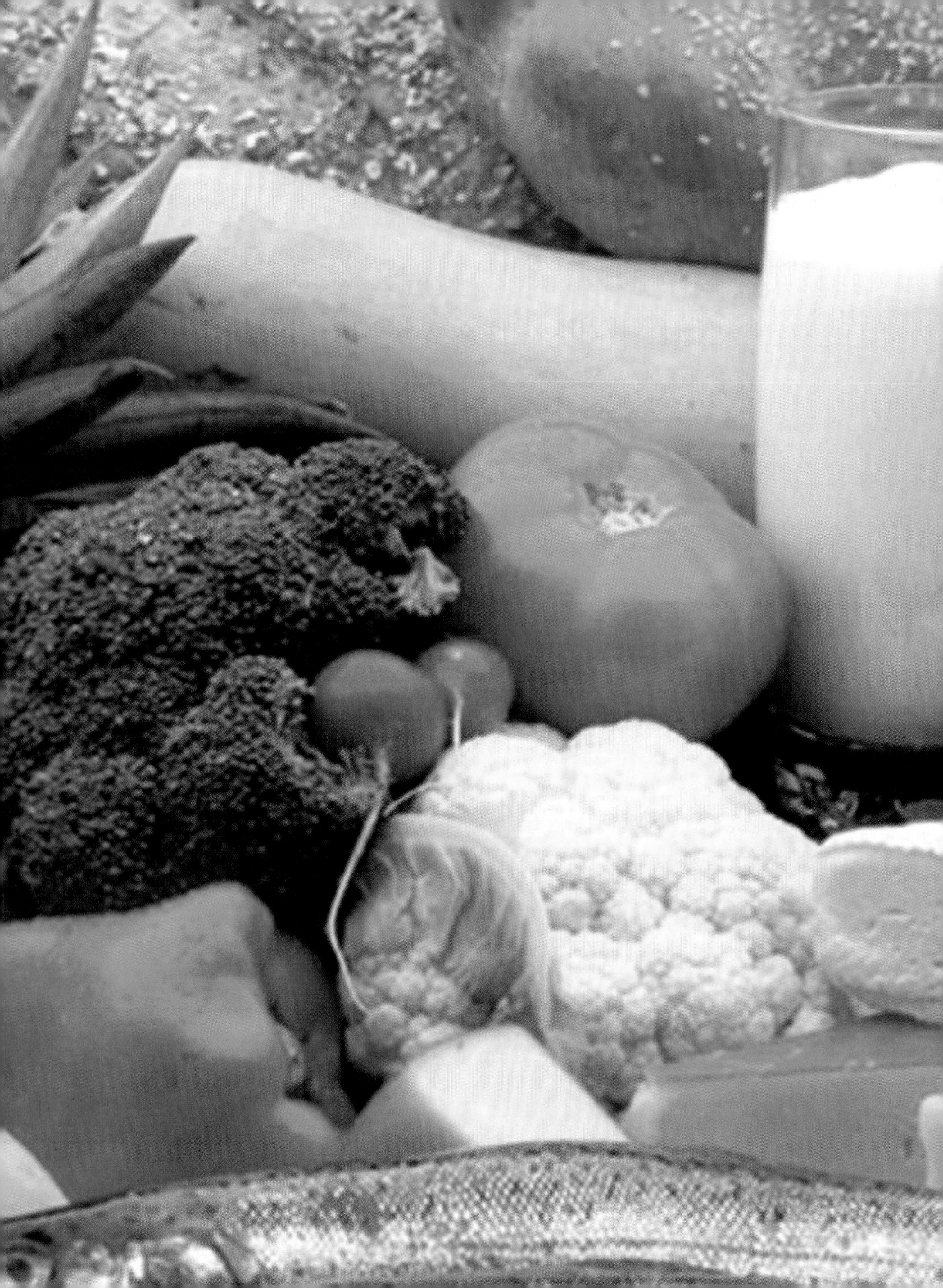

PART 1

NUTRITION BASICS

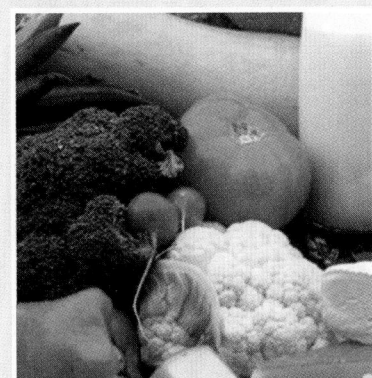

Food provides the energy and building materials for the countless substances that are essential for the growth and survival of living things. The way nutrients become integral parts of the body and contribute to its function depends on the physiologic and biochemical processes that govern their actions.

This section opens with an overview of the processes of digestion, absorption, transportation, and excretion because they are needed for food to enter the body to be metabolized. Different foods invite consumption for various reasons, including form, texture, and flavor, as well as a host of psychosocial factors. However, once inside the alimentary tract, their appeal is no longer relevant because processes of digestion reduce them all to the same common denominators in a size and form capable of absorption and transportation to individual cells.

Proteins, fats, and carbohydrates all contribute to the total energy pool, but the energy they yield is all in the same form. Utilization and conservation of this energy to build and maintain the body requires the involvement of vitamins and minerals, which function as coenzymes, co-catalysts, and buffers in the miraculous, watery arena of metabolism.

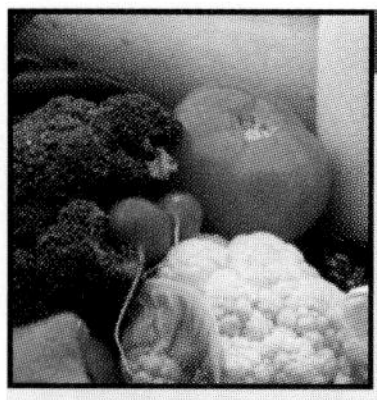

CHAPTER 1

Digestion, Absorption, Transport, and Excretion of Nutrients

PETER L. BEYER, MS, RD

CHAPTER OUTLINE

- The Gastrointestinal Tract
- Overview of Digestive and Absorptive Processes
- The Small Intestine: Primary Site of Nutrient Absorption
- The Large Intestine

KEY TERMS

active transport–the movement of particles via a carrier protein across cell membranes and epithelial layers; requires expenditure of energy

amylase–an enzyme that is secreted in saliva and from the pancreas and catalyzes the hydrolysis of starch

brush border–the microvilli that greatly increase the surface area of intestinal mucosal cells

chelation–the process by which a mineral is bound to a ligand—usually an acid, an organic acid, or a sugar—so that it is in a form capable of being absorbed into intestinal cells

cholecystokinin (CCK)–a hormone that is secreted by the proximal small bowel and stimulates the pancreas to secrete enzymes (and to a lesser extent, bicarbonate and water), stimulates gallbladder contraction, slows gastric emptying, stimulates colonic activity, and may regulate appetite

chyme–the semifluid, gruel-like material produced by the gastric digestion of food

colonic salvage–the process of fermenting and absorbing end products of dietary carbohydrates, fiber, and amino acids from the large intestine

enterogastrone–a hormone secreted by the duodenal mucosa in response to the presence of fat in the duodenum; inhibits gastric secretion and motility, slowing the delivery of additional lipids into the duodenum

facilitated diffusion–the movement of particles across a membrane via a carrier protein

gastric inhibitory polypeptide (GIP)–a hormone that is released from the intestinal mucosa in the presence of fat and glucose and inhibits gastric acid secretion and stimulates insulin release

gastrin–a hormone that is produced by the antral mucosa of the stomach and stimulates gastric secretions and motility

glucagon-like peptide 1 (GLP-1), glucagon-like peptide 2 (GLP-2)–hormones released from the intestinal mucosa that slow gastric emptying, lower glucagon concentration, stimulate proinsulin synthesis, and increase insulin sensitivity

lactase–an intestinal enzyme that hydrolyzes lactose into glucose and galactose

maltase–an intestinal enzyme that hydrolyzes maltose into glucose

micelle–a complex of primarily free fatty acids, monoglycerides, and bile salts that allows lipids to be absorbed into intestinal mucosal cells

microvilli–minute cylindrical processes that are found on the surface of the intestinal cells and greatly increase their absorptive surface area

motilin–a polypeptide GI hormone that promotes gastric emptying and intestinal motility.

pancreatic lipase–an enzyme in pancreatic juice that hydrolyzes the ester linkages between fatty acids and glycerol

parietal cells–large cells that are scattered along the walls of the stomach and secrete the hydrochloric acid in gastric juice

passive diffusion–the random movement of particles through openings in cellular membranes according to electrochemical and concentration gradients

peristalsis–the movement by which the alimentary canal propels its contents

proteolytic enzymes–the enzymes trypsin, chymotrypsin, and carboxypeptidase, all of which break down protein into proteoses, peptones, peptides, and amino acids

secretin–a hormone released from the duodenal wall into the bloodstream that stimulates the pancreas to secrete water and bicarbonate and inhibits gastrin secretion

somatostatin–a polypeptide hormone secreted from the stomach, small intestine and pancreas that tends to inhibit other GI secretions and inhibit motility

sucrase–the intestinal enzyme that hydrolyzes sucrose into glucose and fructose

villi–the numerous fingerlike projections that cover the surface of the small intestine mucosa

Most of the major nutrients in foods must be made smaller, unbound, or made more soluble before they can be absorbed from the intestine. The digestive system is responsible for reducing these large particles and molecules into smaller, more readily absorbed units and converting the insoluble molecules into soluble forms. Proper functioning of the absorptive and transport mechanisms is crucial in the delivery of the products of digestion to individual cells. Malfunctions in any of these systems can result in malnutrition, even when an adequate diet is being consumed.

THE GASTROINTESTINAL TRACT

The primary roles of the gastrointestinal (GI) tract are to (1) extract macronutrients, protein, carbohydrates, lipids, water, and ethanol from ingested foods and beverages; (2) absorb necessary micronutrients and trace elements; and (3) serve as a physical and immunologic barrier to microorganisms, foreign material, and potential antigens consumed with food or formed during the passage of food through the GI tract. In addition to its primary roles, the GI tract also participates in many other regulatory, metabolic, and immunologic functions that affect the entire body.

The human GI tract is well suited for digesting and absorbing nutrients from a wide variety of foods, including meats, dairy products, fruits, vegetables, grains, complex starches, sugars, fats, and oils. Depending on the nature of the diet consumed, about 92% to 97% of it is digested and absorbed; most of the unabsorbed material is of plant origin. Compared with ruminants and animals with a very large cecum, humans are considerably less efficient at extracting energy from grasses, stems, seeds, and other coarse fibrous materials. Humans lack the enzymes to hydrolyze the chemical bonds that link the molecules of sugars that make up plant fibers. Fibrous foods are fermented to varying degrees by bacteria in the human colon, but only 5% to 10% of the energy needed by humans can be derived from this process (Bjorck et al 1994, Stevens and Hume, 1998). (See Chapter 3.)

The GI tract extends from the mouth to the anus and includes the oropharyngeal structures, esophagus, stomach, liver and gallbladder, pancreas, and small and large intestine. It is one of the largest organs in the body (Figure 1-1). In addition to having a large surface area, the GI tract is extremely active in carrying out the physiologic and metabolic functions of secretion, digestion, absorption, and cellular reproduction. The human intestine is about 7 m long and configured in a pattern of folds, pits, and fingerlike projections called villi. The villi are lined with epithelial cells and even smaller, cylindrical extensions called microvilli. The result is a tremendous increase in surface area compared with that expected from a smooth, hollow cylinder. The cells lining the intestinal tract have a life span of approximately 3 to 5 days, and then they are sloughed into the lumen and "recycled." They are fully functional only for the last 2 to 3 days as they migrate from the crypts to the distal third of the villi.

It is becoming increasingly apparent that the health of the body depends on a healthy and functional GI tract (see Chapter 12). Because of the unusually high metabolic activity and requirements of the GI tract, it is more susceptible than most tissues to micronutrient deficiencies, protein calorie malnutrition, and damage resulting from toxins, drugs, irradiation, or interruption of its blood supply. Approximately 45% of the energy requirement of the small intestine and 70% of the energy requirement of cells lining the colon are supplied by nutrients passing through its lumen. After only a few days of starvation, the GI tract atrophies; that is, the surface area decreases markedly and secretions, synthetic functions, blood flow, and absorptive capacity are all reduced. Resumption of food intake, even with less than adequate calories, results in cellular proliferation and return of normal GI function after only a few days. Optimum function of the human GI tract seems to depend on frequent consumption of healthy foods rather than food consumption interspersed with prolonged fasts (Bengmark and Jeppsson, 1995; Spiller, 1994).

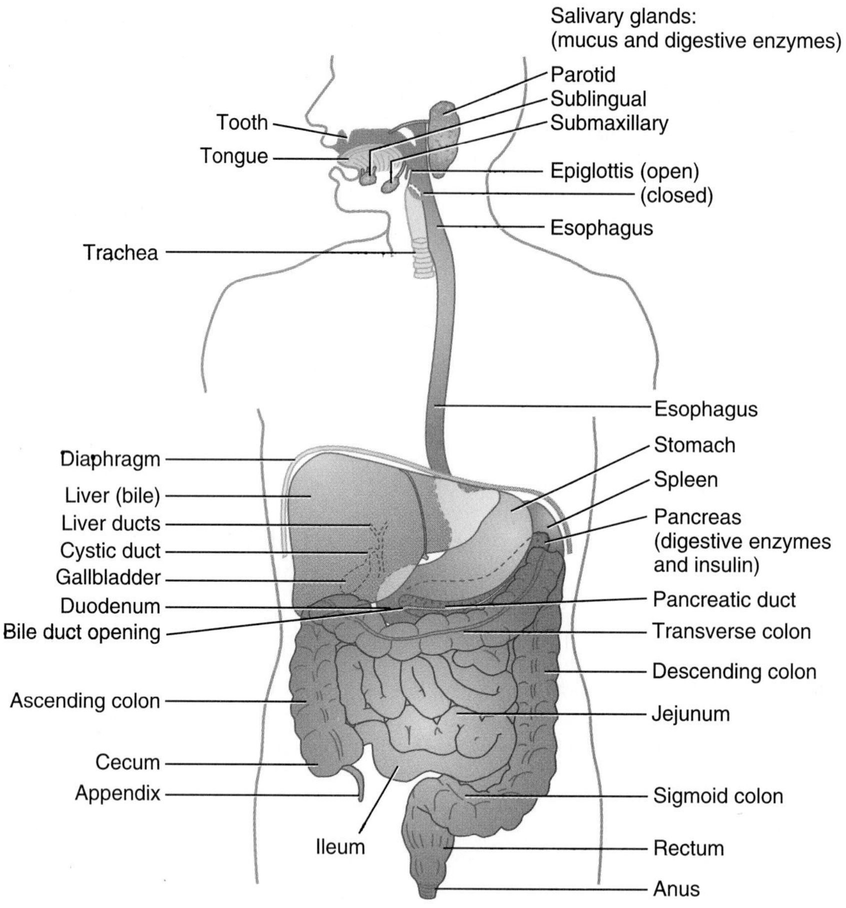

FIGURE 1-1 • The digestive system.

OVERVIEW OF DIGESTIVE AND ABSORPTIVE PROCESSES

In the mouth, chewing reduces the size of food particles, which are mixed with salivary secretions that prepare them for swallowing. The esophagus transports food and liquid from the oral cavity and pharynx to the stomach. In the stomach, food is mixed with acidic fluid and proteolytic and lipolytic enzymes. Until this point, only limited starch and lipid digestion have taken place, and protein digestion has just begun. When food reaches the appropriate consistency and concentration, the stomach allows its contents to pass into the small intestine, where most digestion takes place. In the first 100 cm of small intestine, a flurry of activity occurs, resulting in the digestion and absorption of most of the food ingested. Starches are exposed to powerful enzymes from the pancreas and reduced to simple sugars. Enzymes from the pancreas and brush border of the small intestine complete the digestion of proteins, converting them into small peptides and amino acids. Fats are reduced from visible droplets to microscopic emulsions that pancreatic lipase can attack, reducing the fats to mixtures of smaller molecules, primarily fatty acids and monoglycerides (Caspary 1992; Chang et al, 1996). In addition to secretions from the mouth and stomach, the secretions from the pancreas, small intestine, and gallbladder also contribute a considerable amount of fluid. In all, about three to four times more fluid is secreted from the alimentary tract than is normally consumed orally, and more than 98% of fluid is reabsorbed. The movement of GI contents and secretions into the GI tract is regulated primarily by peptide hormones, nerves, and enteric muscles (Kuemmerle, 2000; Rehfeld, 1998). Along the remaining length of the small intestine, macronutrients, minerals, vitamins, trace elements, and most of the remaining water are absorbed before reaching the colon, or large intestine.

The colon and rectum absorb most of the remaining liter or so of fluid delivered from the small intestine; the colon absorbs electrolytes and to some extent some of the final products of digestion. Most of the nutrients absorbed from the GI tract enter the liver by

CLINICAL INSIGHT

The Gastrointestinal Tract—The Ultimate Food Processor

Each day an assortment of foods enters the GI tract, and with remarkable efficiency, the GI tract goes about its tasks of secretion, digestion, and absorption. All are started, regulated, and stopped automatically.

Sight, aroma, even sounds and thoughts of food. Presence and nature of food in the mouth.

Perception of hunger from the GI tract. Hypothalamic signals after sampling substrates and hormones in blood.

Presence of food in stomach.

All start the secretion of hormones, acid, and enzymes from the GI tract.

Presence of partially digested food and acid from the stomach reaching the small intestine:

Increases GI secretions, motility, blood flow, cell growth, gastric emptying, and promotes feeding.

Presence of digesta in the intestine and colon:

Stimulates bile secretion, alkali, enzymes, from pancreas and small intestine.

Provides fuel for host and cells lining GI tract. Promotes growth of intestinal flora.

Slows gastric emptying, limits gastric acid and enzyme secretion, increases satiety, promotes satiety

Presence of digesta in distal colon and rectum: Stimulates peristalsis and relaxation of anal sphincter

Tract is also remarkable because:

- The degree and type of hormonal, motor, and secretory response is appropriate for amount and type of foods consumed.
- Despite tremendous variations in types and mixtures of foods, the GI tract is efficient in the digestion and absorption of foods and fluids.
- It is the organ with the largest surface area, the greatest number of immune cells, and the most hormones produced.
- It protects the host tissues from strong acids, potent digestive enzymes, and potentially toxic compounds, and prevents tremendous numbers of microbes from entering the circulation.

way of the portal vein, where they may be stored, transformed into other substances, or released into circulation. Most fats enter lymphatic circulation. The colonic flora play an essential role in fermentation of part of the remaining fiber, resistant starch, sugar, and amino acids. Fermentation of the remaining carbohydrates results in the production of short-chain fatty acids (SCFAs) and gas. SCFAs help maintain normal mucosal function, salvage some of the residual energy substrates, and facilitate the absorption of the remaining salt and water (Stevens and Hume, 1998). The large intestine also provides temporary storage for waste products, and the distal colon, rectum, and anus control defecation (see *Clinical Insight:* The Gastrointestinal Tract—The Ultimate Food Processor).

Enzymes in Digestion

Digestion of food is accomplished by hydrolysis under the direction of enzymes. Cofactors such as hydrochloric acid, bile, and sodium bicarbonate support the digestive and absorptive processes. Most digestive enzymes are synthesized in specialized cells in the mouth, stomach, pancreas, and small intestine and are released into the lumen. Some enzymes are localized in the lipoprotein membranes of the mucosal cells and attach to their substrates as they enter the cell. Table 1-1 summarizes the GI enzymes and their functions in the small intestine. No additional digestive enzymes are secreted from the large intestine. Digestion and absorption are completed by the time material reaches the colon. Primarily, water, salt, some vitamins, and minerals are absorbed thereafter.

Water, monosaccharides, vitamins, minerals, and alcohol are usually absorbed in their basic form. For the most part, the disaccharides and polysaccharides, lipids, and proteins must be converted to their simple constituents by digestive enzymes before they are absorbed. (See Chapter 3.)

Regulators of GI Activity: Nerves, Neurotransmitters, and Neuropeptide Hormones

Neural Mechanisms

GI movements including contraction, mixing, and propulsion of luminal contents are the results of the coordinated activity of enteric nerves, extrinsic nerves, endocrine cells, and smooth muscle. The neural mechanisms include (1) an intrinsic system consisting of two layers of nerves embedded in the gut

TABLE 1-1 Summary of Enzymatic Digestion and Absorption

SECRETION AND SOURCE	ENZYMES	SUBSTRATE	ACTION AND RESULTING PRODUCTS	FINAL PRODUCTS ABSORBED
Saliva from salivary glands in mouth	Ptyalin (salivary amylase)	Starch	Hydrolysis to form dextrins and branched oligosaccharides	—
Gastric juice from gastric glands in stomach mucosa	Pepsin	Protein (in presence of hydrochloric acid)	Hydrolysis of peptide bonds to form polypeptides and amino acids	—
	Gastric lipase	Fat, especially shorter chain	Hydrolysis to form free fatty acids	—
Exocrine secretions from pancreas	Lipase	Fat (in presence of bile salts)	Hydrolysis to form monoglycerides and fatty acids; incorporated into micelles	Fatty acids into mucosal cells; reesterified as triglycerides
	Cholesterol esterase	Cholesterol	Hydrolysis to form esters of cholesterol and fatty acids; incorporated into micelles	Cholesterol into mucosal cells; transferred to chylomicrons
	α-Amylase	Starch and dextrins	Hydrolysis to form dextrins and maltose	—
	Trypsin (activated trypsinogen)	Proteins and polypeptides	Hydrolysis of interior peptide bonds to form polypeptides	—
	Chymotrypsin (activated chymotrypsinogen)	Proteins and peptides	Hydrolysis of interior peptide bonds to form polypeptides	—
	Carboxypeptidase	Polypeptides	Hydrolysis of terminal peptide bonds (carboxyl end) to form amino acids	Amino acids
	Ribonuclease and deoxyribonuclease	Ribonucleic acids and deoxyribonucleic acids	Hydrolysis to form mononucleotides	Mononucleotides
	Elastase	Fibrous protein	Hydrolysis to form peptides and amino acids	—
Small intestine enzymes (primarily in brush border)	Carboxypeptidase, aminopeptidase, and dipeptidase	Polypeptides	Hydrolysis of carboxyl terminus, amino terminus, or internal peptide bonds	Amino acids
	Enterokinase	Trypsinogen	Activates trypsin	Dipeptides and tripeptides
	Sucrase	Sucrose	Hydrolysis to form glucose and fructose	Glucose and fructose
	α-Dextrinase (isomaltase)	Dextrin (isomaltose)	Hydrolysis to form glucose	Glucose
	Maltase	Maltose	Hydrolysis to form glucose	Glucose
	Lactase	Lactose	Hydrolysis to form glucose and galactose	Glucose and galactose
	Nucleotidases	Nucleic acids	Hydrolysis to form nucleotides and phosphates	Nucleotides
	Nucleosidase and phosphorylase	Nucleosides	Hydrolysis to form purines, pyrimidines, and pentose phosphate	Purine and pyrimidine bases

wall and (2) an external system of nerve fibers running to and from the central and autonomic nervous systems. Mucosal receptors in the gut wall are appropriately sensitive to the composition of the chyme (a semiliquid substance of acid, fatty acids, and amino acids) and lumen distention (i.e., fullness) and send impulses through submucosal and mysenteric nerves. Neurotransmitters and neuropeptides with small molecular weights signal nerves to contract or relax muscles, increase or decrease fluid secretions, or change blood flow. The GI tract then largely regulates its own motility and secretory activity. However, signals from the central nervous system can override the enteric system and affect GI function (Furness and Clerc, 2000; Kuemmerle, 2000). Numerous hormones, neuropeptides, and neurotransmitters in the GI tract not only affect GI function but also have an impact on other nerves and tissues in many parts of the body. Some examples of neurotransmitters released from enteric nerve endings and their actions are listed in Table 1-2. In people with GI disease (e.g., infections, inflammatory bowel disease, irritable bowel syndrome), the enteric nervous system may be overstimulated, resulting in abnormal secretion, altered blood flow, increased permeability, and altered immune function.

Autonomic innervation is supplied by the sympathetic fibers that run along blood vessels and by the parasympathetic fibers in the vagal and pelvic nerves. In general, sympathetic neurons, which are activated by fear, anger, and stress, tend to slow transit of GI contents by inhibiting neurons affecting muscle contraction and inhibiting secretions. The parasympathetic nerves innervate specific areas of the alimentary tract. For example, the sight or smell of food stimulates vagal activity and subsequent secretion of acid from parietal cells scattered along the walls of the stomach. The GI tract also sends signals that are perceived as colicky pain, sharp pain, nausea, urgency or gastric fullness, or gastric emptiness by way of the vagal and spinal nerves. Inflammation, dysmotility, and various types of intestinal damage may intensify these perceptions.

Neuropeptide Hormones

Regulation of the GI system also involves numerous peptide hormones that can act locally or distally. Many of these regulators can act locally in an autocrine or a paracrine role and as endocrine hormones by traveling through the blood to their target organs. More than 100 peptide hormones and hormonelike growth factors secreted by more than 30 different types of neuroendocrine cells have been identified. Their actions are often complex and extend well beyond the GI tract. Some of the hormones (e.g., of the cholecystokinin [CCK] and somatostatin family) also serve as neurotransmitters between neurons (see *Focus On:* Roles of GI Neuropeptide Hormones and Neurotransmitters). The digestive and secretory functions of several GI hormones have been well described, but the complete actions of these and many other peptide hormones that affect GI cell growth, secretion, movement, or metabolism have not been fully evaluated (Holst et al, 1996; Rehfeld 1998). Some of the classic hormones involved in digestive and absorptive processes are reviewed in the following paragraphs and summarized in Table 1-3. Knowledge of major hormone functions becomes especially important when the sites of their secretion or action are diseased or removed in surgical procedures or when hormones and their analogues are used to suppress or enhance some aspect of GI function.

Gastrin, a hormone that stimulates gastric secretions and motility, is secreted primarily from cells in the antral mucosa of the stomach. Secretion is initiated by (1) distention of the antrum after a meal, (2) impulses from the vagus nerve such as those triggered by the smell or sight of food, and (3) the presence in the antrum of secretagogues such as partially digested proteins, fermented alcoholic beverages (e.g., wine), caffeine, or food extracts (e.g., bouillon). When the lumen gets more acidic, feedback involving other hormones inhibits gastrin release.

Secretin, a hormone released from the duodenal wall into the bloodstream, opposes the action and se-

TABLE 1-2 Examples of Neurotransmitters and Their Actions

NEUROTRANSMITTER	SITE OF RELEASE	PRIMARY ACTIONS
α-Aminobutyric acid (GABA)	Central nervous system	Relaxes lower esophageal sphincter
Norepinephrine	Central nervous system, spinal cord, sympathetic nerves	Decreases motility, increases contraction of sphincters, inhibits secretions
Acetylcholine	Central nervous system, autonomic system, other tissues	Increases motility, relaxes sphincters, stimulates secretions
Neurotensin	GI tract, central nervous system	Inhibits release of gastric emptying and acid secretion
Neuropeptide Y	Central nervous system, autonomic system	Stimulates feeding behavior
Serotonin (5-HT)	GI tract, spinal cord	Facilitates secretion and peristalsis
Nitric oxide	Central nervous system, GI tract	Regulates blood flow, maintains muscle tone, maintains gastric motor activity
Substance P	Gut, central nervous system, skin	Increases sensory awareness (mainly pain), and peristalsis

FOCUS ON

Role of GI Neuropeptide Hormones and Neurotransmitters

Scientists continue to discover more GI neuropeptide hormones that affect not only digestive activity but participate in many other regulatory functions within and beyond the GI tract. The GI tract secretes more than 30 families of neuropeptide hormones, which makes it the largest endocrine organ in the body (Ahlman and Nilsson, 2001; Rehfeld, 1998). GI hormones are involved in initiating and terminating feeding, bringing on sensations of hunger and satiety, increasing or decreasing movements of the GI tract, enhancing or retarding esophageal and gastric emptying, regulating blood flow and permeability, regulating immune functions, and stimulating the growth of cells (within and beyond the GI tract). *Ghrelin,* a relatively newly identified neuropeptide that is secreted from the stomach, sends a "hungry" message to the brain, whereas PYY 3-36, another recently identified hormone that is produced by the digestive tract, seems to signal appetite suppression. Cholecystokinin, gastric inhibitory polypeptide (GIP), glucagon-like polypeptide-1 (GLP-1), pancreatic polypeptide, and gastrin-releasing polypeptide *(bombesin)* also tend to decrease hunger and increase satiety (Havel, 2001; Hellstrom and Naslund, 2001).

Some of the GI hormones (including some of those that affect satiety), seem to slow gastric emptying and decrease secretions (e.g., somatostatin). Other GI hormones (e.g., motilin) increase motility. These signaling agents of the GI tract are also involved in several metabolic functions. The neuropeptides GIP and GLP-1 are called *incretin hormones* because they help lower blood sugar by facilitating insulin secretion, decreasing gastric emptying, and increasing satiety.

Several of these neuropeptide hormones and analogues are already being used in clinical practice or being tested in the management of clinical problems such as obesity, anorexia, cachexia, delayed or rapid gastrointestinal transit, inflammatory bowel disease, irritable bowel syndrome, diarrhea and constipation, diabetes, GI malignancies, and a host of others.

TABLE 1-3 Functions of Major Gastrointestinal Hormones

HORMONE	SITE OF RELEASE	STIMULANTS FOR RELEASE	ORGANS AFFECTED	EFFECTS ON ORGANS
Gastrin	Gastric mucosa duodenum	Peptides and amino acids, caffeine, distention of antrum, some alcoholic beverages, vagus nerve	Stomach, esophagus, and entire GI tract	Stimulates secretion of hydrochloric acid and pepsinogen, increases gastric antral motility, and increases lower esophageal sphincter tone
			Gallbladder	Weakly stimulates contraction of gallbladder
			Pancreas	Weakly stimulates pancreatic secretion of bicarbonate
Secretin	Duodenal mucosa	Acid in small intestine	Pancreas	Stimulates output of water and bicarbonate and increases release of insulin and some pancreatic enzyme secretions
			Duodenum	Decreases motility and increases mucus output
Cholecystokinin (CCK)	Proximal small bowel	Peptides, amino acids, fat, and hydrochloric acid	Pancreas	Stimulates secretion of pancreatic enzymes
			Gallbladder	Causes contraction of gallbladder
			Stomach	Slows gastric emptying
			Colon	Increases motility
				Increases satiety
Gastric inhibitory polypeptide (GIP)	Small intestine	Glucose and fat	Stomach and pancreas	Inhibits gastrin-stimulated gastric acid secretion
			Small intestine	Inhibits motility
Motilin	Stomach and small and large intestine	Biliary and pancreatic secretions	Stomach, small and large intestines	Promotes gastric emptying and increases GI motility
Somatostatin	Stomach, pancreas, and upper small intestine	Gastric and duodenal acidity and products of protein and fat digestion	Stomach, pancreas, small intestine, and gallbladder	Inhibits release of gastrin, motilin, and pancreatic secretions; decreases motility and contractions of GI tract

cretion of gastrin. Secreted in response to acidic chyme emptied into the duodenum, it stimulates the pancreas to secrete water and bicarbonate into the duodenum. Neutralization of the acidity protects the duodenal mucosa from prolonged exposure to acid and provides the appropriate environment for the activity of intestinal and pancreatic enzymes.

Other cells of the small bowel mucosa secrete cholecystokinin (CCK), an important multifunctional hormone released during protein and fat digestion (Liddle, 1997). The major GI functions of CCK are to (1) stimulate the pancreas to secrete enzymes (and to a lesser extent bicarbonate and water), (2) stimulate gallbladder contraction, (3) increase colonic and rectal motility, (4) slow gastric emptying, and (5) possibly reduce food intake to a limited degree (see Chapter 24).

Gastric inhibitory polypeptide (GIP), which is released from the intestinal mucosa in the presence of fat and glucose, inhibits gastric acid secretion and stimulates insulin release. Glucagon-like peptide 1 (GLP-1) and glucagon-like peptide 2 (GLP-2) slow gastric emptying, decrease glucagon concentrations, stimulate (pro)insulin synthesis, increase insulin sensitivity, and may help control food intake. As a result of GIP, GLP-1, and GLP-2 (all of which are incretin hormones, which help control blood glucose changes after a meal), a glucose load received enterally results in less of an increase in blood glucose than when an equal amount of glucose is received intravenously (L'Heureux and Brubaker, 2001; Nauck, 1999).

Motilin, which is released by the cells of the upper small intestine in response to bile and pancreatic secretions into the duodenum, increases the rate of gastric emptying and stimulates gut motility. Erythromycin, an antibiotic, has been shown to bind to motilin receptors, so analogues of erythromycin and motilin are being evaluated as therapeutic agents to treat delayed gastric emptying (Feighner et al, 1999; Sarna, Gonzalez, and Ryan, 2000).

Somatostatin is a hormone with far-reaching actions. Its general actions seem to be inhibitory and antisecretory, but it also regulates numerous other hormones. Somatostatin and its analogue octreotide are being used to treat certain malignant diseases (Farthing, 1996; Tulassay, 1998), as well as numerous GI disorders such as diarrhea, short bowel syndrome, pancreatitis, dumping syndrome, and gastric hypersecretion.

Digestion in the Mouth

In the mouth the teeth grind and crush food into small particles. The food mass is simultaneously moistened and lubricated by saliva. Three pairs of salivary glands—the parotid, submaxillary, and sublingual glands—produce about 1.5 L of saliva daily. A serous secretion containing amylase (ptyalin) begins the digestion of starch. The starch digestion is minimal, and the amylase becomes inactive when it reaches the acidic contents of the stomach. Another type of saliva contains mucus, a protein that causes particles of food to stick together and lubricates the mass for swallowing. The oropharyngeal secretions also contain a lipase that is capable of digesting some fats. Because fatty materials are still mixed with whole foods, not extensively processed, and not retained in the mouth or esophagus for any length of time, the contribution of this lipase to overall fat digestion is usually minimal.

The masticated food mass, or *bolus,* is passed back to the pharynx under voluntary control, but throughout the esophagus the process of swallowing *(deglutition)* is involuntary. Peristalsis then moves the food rapidly into the stomach. (See Chapter 43 for a more detailed discussion of swallowing.)

Digestion in the Stomach

Food particles are propelled forward and mixed with gastric secretions by wavelike contractions that progress forward from the upper portion of the stomach—the fundus—to the antrum and pylorus. In the stomach, gastric secretions are mixed with food and beverages. An average of 2000 to 2500 ml of gastric juice is secreted daily. The gastric secretions contain hydrochloric acid (secreted by the parietal cells in the walls of the stomach), a protease, gastric lipase, mucus, intrinsic factor (a glycoprotein that facilitates vitamin B_{12} absorption in the ileum), and the GI hormone gastrin. In the process of gastric digestion, most of the food becomes semiliquid (chyme), containing approximately 50% water. Digestion of protein begins in the stomach, primarily through the action of pepsin. Pepsin is secreted in an inactive form *(pepsinogen),* which is converted by hydrochloric acid to its active form. Pepsin is active only in the acid environment of the stomach and serves primarily to change the shape and size of some of the proteins in a normal meal.

An acid-stable lipase is secreted into the stomach by *chief cells* (Canaan et al, 1999). Although this lipase is considerably less active than pancreatic lipase, it contributes to the overall processing of dietary triglycerides. Gastric lipase is more specific for triglycerides composed of medium- and short-chain fatty acids, but the normal diet contains few of these fats. Lipases secreted in the upper portions of the GI tract may have a relatively important role in the liquid diet of infants, but when pancreatic insufficiency occurs in adults, lingual and gastric lipases are not potent enough to prevent lipid malabsorption (Layer and Keller, 1999).

When food is consumed, significant numbers of microorganisms are also consumed. The acid in the stomach is quite strong, with a pH ranging from about 1 to 4. The combined actions of hydrochloric acid and proteolytic enzymes from the stomach result in a significant reduction in the concentration of microorganisms ingested. Some microbes may escape and enter the intestine if consumed in sufficient concentrations. Achlorhydria, gastrectomy, GI dysfunction or disease, or poor nutrition may increase the risk of bacterial overgrowth in the intestine.

The stomach continuously mixes and churns food and normally releases the mixture in small quantities into the small intestine. The amount emptied with each contraction of the antrum and pylorus varies with the volume and type of food consumed but is only a few milliliters at a time. Most of a liquid meal empties in 1 to 2 hours, and most of a solid meal empties within 2 to 3 hours. When eaten alone, carbohydrates leave the stomach the most rapidly, followed by protein, fat, and fibrous food. In a meal with mixed types of foods, emptying of the stomach depends on the overall volume and characteristics of the foods. Liquids empty more rapidly than solids, large particles empty more slowly than small particles, and concentrated food tends to empty more slowly than low-calorie meals (Collins et al, 1996). These factors are important considerations for practitioners who counsel patients with nausea, vomiting, diabetic gastroparesis, or partial obstruction or practitioners monitoring patients after GI surgery or who are malnourished.

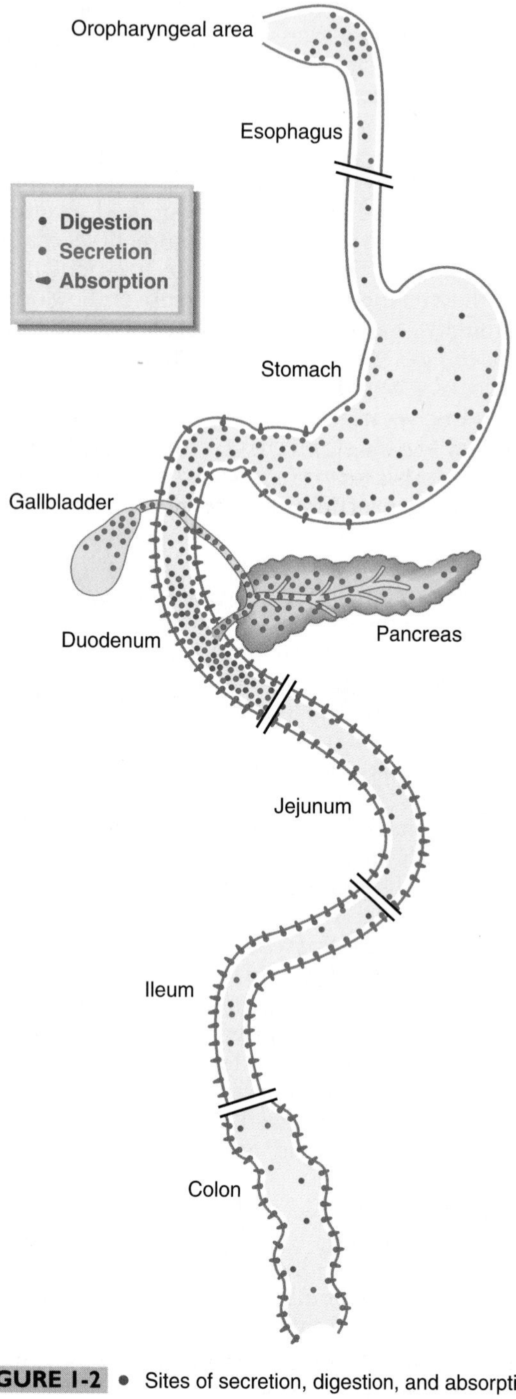

FIGURE 1-2 • Sites of secretion, digestion, and absorption.

The lower esophageal sphincter above the entrance to the stomach prevents reflux of gastric contents into the esophagus, and the pyloric sphincter in the distal portion of the stomach helps regulate exit of gastric contents and prevents backflow of chyme from the duodenum into the stomach. Emotional changes, food, and GI regulators can affect the activity of these sphincters. Irritation from nearby ulcers may also alter the performance of strictures. Certain foods and beverages may also alter the lower esophageal sphincter pressure, permitting reflux of the GI contents into the esophagus. Food in the intestine and hormone regulators provide feedback to slow gastric emptying (see Chapters 29 and 30).

Digestion in the Small Intestine

The small intestine is the primary site for digestion of foods and nutrients. The small intestine is divided into the duodenum, the jejunum, and the ileum (Figure 1-2). The duodenum is about 0.5 m long, the jejunum is 2 to 3 m, and the ileum is 3 to 4 m. Most of the digestive process is completed in the duodenum and upper jejunum, and the absorption of nutrients is largely complete by the time the material reaches the middle of the jejunum. The acidic chyme from the stomach enters the duodenum, where it is mixed with duodenal juices and the secretions from the pancreas and biliary tract. As a result of the secretion of bicarbonate-containing fluid from the pancreas and dilution from other secretions, acid chyme is neutralized. Enzymes of the small intestine and pancreas operate more effectively in a more neutral pH.

The entry of partially digested foods, primarily fats and protein, stimulates the release of several hormones that in turn stimulate the secretion of enzymes and fluids and affect GI motility and satiety. Bile, which is predominantly a mixture of water, bile salts, and small amounts of pigments and cholesterol, is secreted from the liver and gallbladder. Through their emulsifying properties, the bile salts facilitate the digestion and absorption of lipids. The pancreas secretes enzymes capable of digesting all of the major nutrients, and enzymes from the small intestine help complete the process. Lipid-digesting enzymes secreted by the pancreas and small intestine include lipase, colipase, phospholipase, and cholesterol esterase. Proteolytic enzymes include trypsin and chymotrypsin, carboxypeptidase, aminopeptidase, ribonuclease, and deoxyribonuclease. Trypsin and chymotrypsin are secreted in their inactive forms and are activated by enterokinase (also known as *enteropeptidase*), which is secreted when chyme contacts the intestinal mucosa. Pancreatic amylase is secreted to hydrolyze starch. Most of the ingested starches are digested into oligosaccharides and disaccharides by pancreatic amylase. Enzymes lining the brush border of the villi further break down the carbohydrate molecules into monosaccharides before absorption. Varying amounts of resistant starches and most ingested dietary fiber escape digestion in the small intestine and may add to fibrous material available for fermentation by colonic microbes (Cummings and Englyst, 1995; Levin, 1994).

Intestinal contents move along the small intestine at a rate of 1 cm per minute, taking from 3 to 8 hours to travel through the entire intestine to the ileocecal valve (Guyton and Hall, 1996). The ileocecal valve, like the pyloric valve, serves as a "brake" to regulate the movement of intestinal material passed into the colon. A damaged or nonfunctional ileocecal valve results in the entry of significant amounts of fluid and substrate into the colon and increased chance for microbial overgrowth in the distal small intestine (see Chapter 30).

THE SMALL INTESTINE: PRIMARY SITE OF NUTRIENT ABSORPTION

Structure and Function

The primary organ of absorption is the small intestine, which is characterized by its expansive absorptive area. This is attributable to its extensive length, as well as to the organization of the mucosal lining into *convolutions (valvulae conniventes).* These folds are covered with the fingerlike projections called villi (Figure 1-3), which in turn are covered by microvilli, or the brush border. The combination of folds, villous projections, and microvillous border creates an enormous absorptive surface of about 200 to 250 m^2. The villi rest on a supporting structure called the *lamina propria.* In the lamina propria, which is composed of connective tissue, the blood and lymph vessels receive the products of digestion. Each day the small intestine absorbs 200 to 300 g of monosaccharides, 60 to 100 g of fatty acids, 60 to 120 g of amino acids and peptides, and 50 to 100 g of ions. The capacity for absorption in the healthy individual far exceeds the normal macronutrient and caloric requirements. All but 1 to 1.5 L of the 7 or 8 L of fluid secreted from the upper portions of the GI tract in addition to 1.5 to 3 L of dietary fluids is absorbed when the material reaches the end of the small intestine. About 95% of the secreted bile salts are reabsorbed as bile acids in the distal ileum. Without this recycling of bile acids from the GI tract *(enterohepatic circulation),* de novo synthesis of bile acids in the liver would not keep pace with needs for adequate lipid digestion. Bile salt insufficiency becomes clinically important in patients who have resections of the small bowel and diseases affecting the small intestine, such as Crohn's disease, radiation enteritis, and cystic fibrosis. The distal ileum is also the site for vitamin B_{12} (with intrinsic factor) absorption.

Emulsification of fats in the small intestine is followed by their digestion, primarily by pancreatic lipase, into free fatty acids and β-monoglycerides (in which one fatty acid is attached to the middle glycerol carbon). When the concentration of bile salts reaches a certain level, they combine to form micelles—complexes of free fatty acids, monoglycerides, and bile salts—which are organized with the polar ends of the molecules oriented toward the watery lumen of the intestine. The products of lipid digestion are rapidly solubilized in the central portion of the micelles and carried to the area of the brush border (Figure 1-4).

At the surface of the *unstirred water layer (UWL)*—the slightly acidic and watery plate that forms a boundary between the intestinal lumen and the brush border membranes—the lipids detach from the micelles and the micelles return to the lumen for further

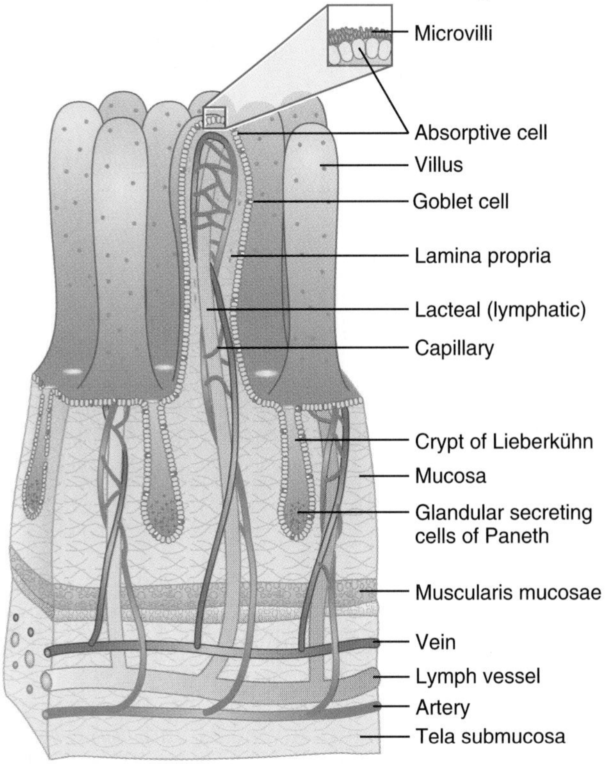

FIGURE 1-3 • Structure of the villi of the human intestine, showing blood and lymph vessels.

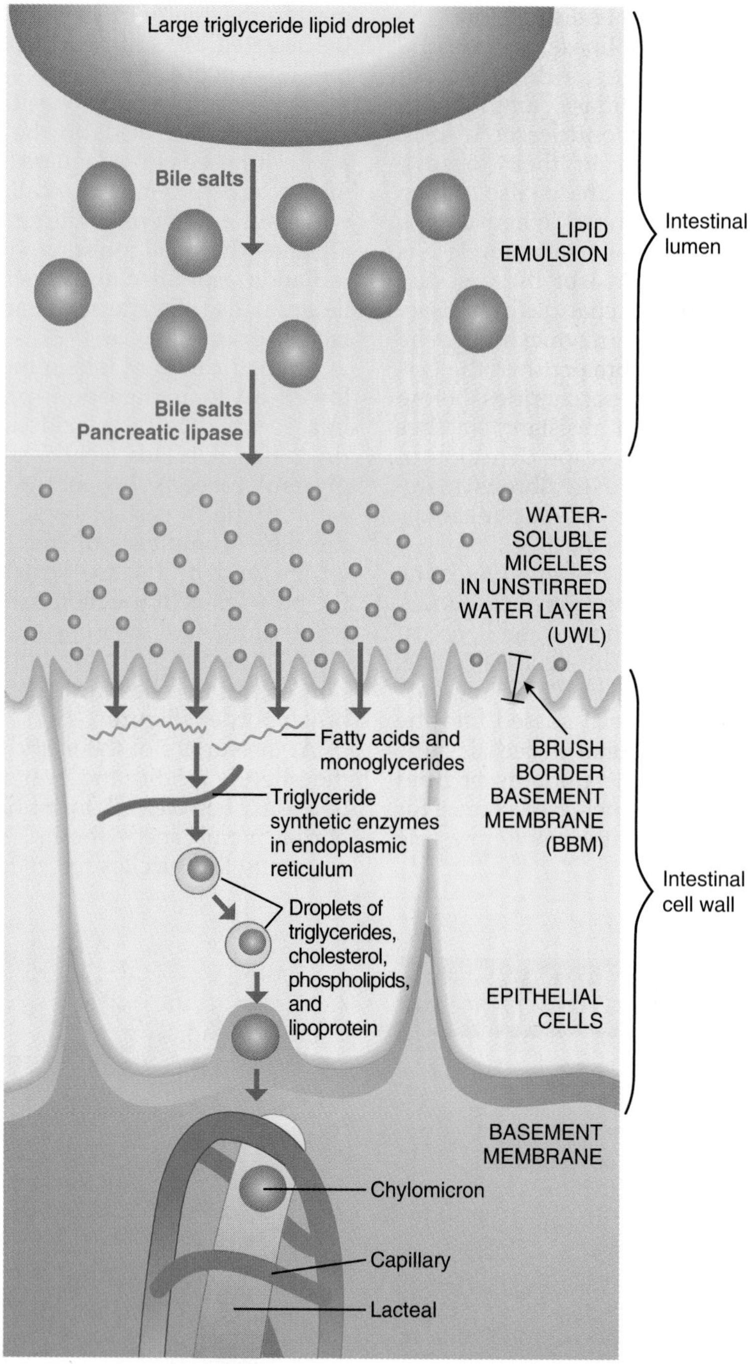

FIGURE 1-4 • Summary of fat absorption.

transport. The monoglycerides and fatty acids are thus left to make their way across the lipophobic UWL to the more lipid-friendly membrane cells of the brush border. When they arrive, they are rapidly taken up for processing and entry into the transport system. For long-chain fatty acids and cholesterol, passage through the UWL is the rate-limiting step for absorption (Thompson et al, 1993).

Absorptive Mechanisms

Absorption is an extremely complex process, combining the more intricate process of *active transport* and the relatively simple process of passive diffusion, in which nutrients pass through the intestinal mucosal cells (enterocytes or colonocytes) into the bloodstream. Diffusion involves random movement

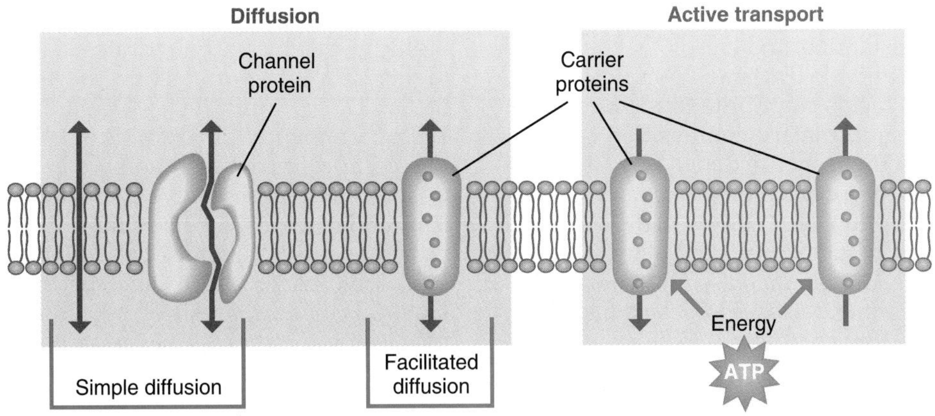

FIGURE 1-5 • Transport pathways through the cell membrane, as well as basic transport mechanisms.

through openings in the membranes of the mucosal cell walls using channel proteins *(simple diffusion)* or carrier proteins (facilitated diffusion) (Figure 1-5).

Active transport involves the input of energy to move ions or other substances, in combination with a carrier protein, across a membrane against an energy gradient. Some nutrients may share the same carrier and thus compete for absorption. Carrier systems can also become saturated, slowing the absorption of the nutrient. A notable example of such a carrier is the previously mentioned intrinsic factor, which is responsible for the absorption of vitamin B_{12} (see Chapters 4 and 34).

Some molecules are moved from the intestinal lumen into mucosal cells by means of pumps, which require a carrier and energy from adenosine triphosphate (ATP). The absorption of glucose, sodium, galactose, potassium, magnesium, phosphate, iodide, calcium, iron, and amino acids is thought to occur in this way.

Pinocytosis has been described as the "drinking in," or engulfing, by the epithelial cell membrane of a small drop of intestinal contents. Pinocytosis allows large particles, such as whole proteins, to be absorbed in small quantities. The movement of foreign proteins across the GI tract into the bloodstream, where they cause allergic reactions, may be the result of pinocytosis. The immunoglobulins from breast milk are probably absorbed through pinocytosis.

THE LARGE INTESTINE

The large intestine is the site of absorption of the remaining water and salts, as well as the vitamins synthesized in this organ by bacterial action. The large intestine is approximately 1.5 m long and consists of the cecum, colon, and rectum. Most of the water contained in the 500 to 1000 ml of chyme entering the colon each day is absorbed, leaving 50 to 200 ml to be excreted in the feces. Colonic contents move forward slowly at a rate of 5 cm/hr, and some remaining nutrients may be absorbed.

Large amounts of mucus secreted by the mucosa of the large intestine protect the intestinal wall from excoriation and bacterial activity and provide the medium for binding the feces together. Bicarbonate ions secreted in exchange for absorbed chloride ions help to neutralize the acidic end products produced from bacterial action.

Bacterial Action

The gut microflora make up a complex community in which hundreds of species have been identified (MacFarlane and MacFarlane, 1997). At birth the GI tract is essentially sterile, but implantation of various microorganisms soon takes place. *Lactobacillus* organisms are the chief component of the GI tract flora until an infant begins to eat solid foods. *Escherichia coli* then become predominant in the distal ileum, and the primary colonic flora are anaerobic, with species of the genus *Bacteroides* occurring most frequently. Lactobacilli are also present in the stools of most people who consume an ordinary mixed diet.

Normally, very little bacterial action occurs in the stomach because the hydrochloric acid is a germicidal agent. However, conditions marked by decreased secretion of hydrochloric acid may lower resistance to bacterial action, occasionally leading to inflammation of the gastric mucosa *(gastritis)* or an increased risk of overgrowth in the small intestine, which is usually relatively sterile.

Bacterial action is most intense in the large intestine. Colonic bacteria contribute to the formation of gases (e.g., hydrogen, carbon dioxide, nitrogen, and in some individuals, methane) and organic acids (e.g., acetic, propionic, butyric, and lactic acids). Bacterial action also may result in the formation of potentially toxic substances, such as ammonia, indoles, amines, and phenolic compounds such as indolacetate, tyramine, histamine, and cresol (Geypens et al, 1997; MacFarlane and MacFarlane, 1997). Some of the gases and organic acids contribute to the odor of feces. Major changes in dietary composition can alter the fecal flora, but the response depends on the original host flora and the nature of the dietary change. Increased consumption of prebiotic material, which may include certain sugars, resistant starch, and dietary fiber, may lead to an increased microbial mass, as well as more bifidobacteria and lactobacilli, indigenous bacteria that are thought to be beneficial. A low-fiber diet based primarily on meat, fat, and highly digestible carbohydrates is said to result in a higher ratio of "putrefactive" bacteria such as clostridia, *E. coli,* and *Proteus* organisms (Roberfroid, 2001; Salminen et al, 1998). Probiotic foods containing significant concentrations of bacteria considered to be healthy or protective against pathogenic organisms and disease may also change the colonic flora to varying degrees (Dunne et al, 2001).

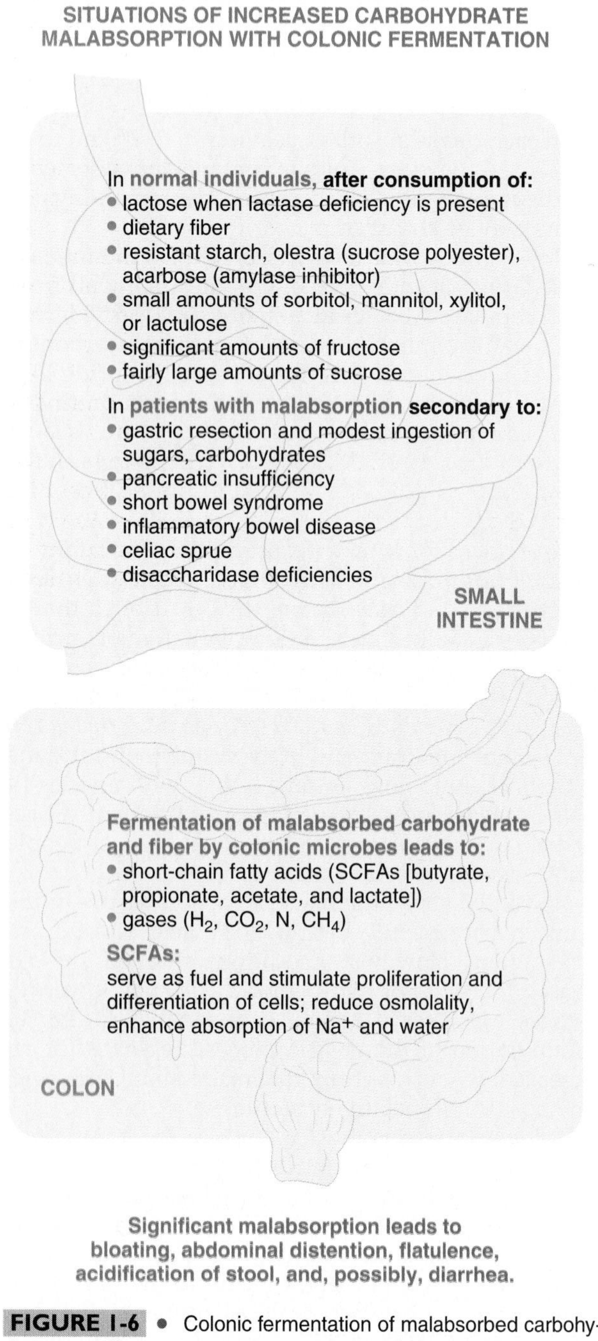
SITUATIONS OF INCREASED CARBOHYDRATE MALABSORPTION WITH COLONIC FERMENTATION
In normal individuals, after consumption of:
• lactose when lactase deficiency is present
• dietary fiber
• resistant starch, olestra (sucrose polyester), acarbose (amylase inhibitor)
• small amounts of sorbitol, mannitol, xylitol, or lactulose
• significant amounts of fructose
• fairly large amounts of sucrose
In patients with malabsorption secondary to:
• gastric resection and modest ingestion of sugars, carbohydrates
• pancreatic insufficiency
• short bowel syndrome
• inflammatory bowel disease
• celiac sprue
• disaccharidase deficiencies
SMALL INTESTINE
Fermentation of malabsorbed carbohydrate and fiber by colonic microbes leads to:
• short-chain fatty acids (SCFAs [butyrate, propionate, acetate, and lactate])
• gases (H_2, CO_2, N, CH_4)
SCFAs:
serve as fuel and stimulate proliferation and differentiation of cells; reduce osmolality, enhance absorption of Na^+ and water
COLON
Significant malabsorption leads to bloating, abdominal distention, flatulence, acidification of stool, and, possibly, diarrhea.

FIGURE 1-6 • Colonic fermentation of malabsorbed carbohydrates and fiber.

Colonic bacteria continue the digestion of some materials that have resisted previous digestive activity. During the process, several nutrients are formed by bacterial synthesis (Hill, 1997; Salminen et al, 1998; Stevens and Hume, 1998). The nutrients are used to varying degrees by GI mucosal cells but contribute little to meeting the nutrient requirements of the human host. Examples of nutrients produced include vitamin K, vitamin B_{12}, thiamin, and riboflavin.

Intestinal flora help to ferment any carbohydrate that is malabsorbed or resistant to digestion and help to convert dietary fiber into SCFAs and gases. Rapid absorption of SCFAs enhances absorption of sodium and water and helps reduce the osmotic load of accumulating carbohydrate. The process of fermenting and using end products of dietary carbohydrates is called colonic salvage (Figure 1-6). Fermentation of residual carbohydrates, most types of fiber, and some amino acids (1) salvages a small amount of residual energy substrate; (2) increases the production of SCFAs, which provide fuel for the colonocytes; (3) stimulates colonocyte proliferation and differentiation; (4) reduces the osmotic load of malabsorbed sugars; and (5) enhances the absorption of electrolytes and water (Bengmark and Jeppsson, 1995; Mortensen and Clausen 1996). The ability to salvage carbohydrates is limited in humans, and colonic fermentation normally disposes of about 20 to 25 g of carbohydrate in 24 hours. Excess amounts of carbohydrate and fermentable fiber in the colon can cause abdominal (colonic) distention, bloating, pain, increased flatulence, and occasionally loose stools, especially if the individual consumes a large amount at once. Adaptation seems to occur in individuals consuming diets high in carbohydrates and fiber that are resistant to human digestive enzymes.

Current research indicates that consumption of about 20 to 35 g of dietary fiber from fruits, vegetables, and whole grains is valuable for (1) maintaining the health of the cells lining the colon, (2) preventing excessive intracolonic pressure, and (3) preventing constipation and possibly other colonic disorders.

The feces generally consist of 75% water and 25% solids, but the proportions vary greatly. About one third of the solid matter consists of dead bacteria. Inorganic materials and fat make up 20% to 40%, and protein constitutes approximately 2% to 3%. The remainder includes undigested dietary fiber, sloughed epithelial cells, and components of digestive juices, such as bile pigments.

Defecation, or expulsion of feces through the anus, occurs with varying frequency, ranging from three times daily to once every 3 days or more. Normal stool weight is in the range of 100 to 200 g, and mouth-to-anus transit time may vary from 18 to 72 hours. A diet that includes abundant fruits, vegetables, and whole grains typically results in a shorter overall GI transit time, more frequent defecation, and larger and softer stools.

Digestion and Absorption of Specific Types of Nutrients

Carbohydrates and Fiber

Most dietary carbohydrates are consumed in the form of starches, disaccharides, and monosaccharides. Starches, or polysaccharides, usually make up the greatest proportion of carbohydrates. Starches are large molecules composed of straight or branched chains of sugar molecules that are joined together, primarily in α 1-4 and 1-6 linkages. Cellulose is also composed of a chain of sugar molecules, but in this case the two hydrogens are positioned on the opposite (beta) side of the oxygen in the link instead of the alpha. That humans have significant ability to digest starch and not cellulose is an example of the stereospecificity of enzymes. Most of the dietary starches are *amylopectins,* the branching polysaccharides, and *amylose,* the straight-chain–type polymers.

In the mouth, the enzyme salivary amylase (ptyalin), which operates at a neutral or slightly alkaline pH, starts the digestive action by hydrolyzing a small amount of the starch molecules into smaller fragments (Figure 1-7). Amylase deactivates after contact with hydrochloric acid. If digestible carbohydrates remained in the stomach long enough, acid hydrolysis would eventually reduce much of it into monosaccharides. However, the stomach usually empties itself before significant digestion can take place, and carbohydrate digestion occurs almost entirely in the proximal small intestine.

Pancreatic amylase breaks the large starch molecules at α 1-4 linkages to create maltose, maltotriose, and "alpha-limit" dextrins remaining from the amylopectin branches. Enzymes from the brush border of the enterocytes further break the disaccharides and oligosaccharides into monosaccharides. For example, maltase from the mucosal cells breaks down the disaccharide maltose into two molecules of glucose. These outer cell membranes also contain the enzymes sucrase, lactase, and isomaltase (or *α-dextrinase*), which act on sucrose, lactose, and isomaltose, respectively (Figure 1-8).

The resultant monosaccharides—glucose, galactose, and fructose—pass through the mucosal cells and into the bloodstream via the capillaries of the villi, where they are carried by the portal vein to the liver. Glucose and galactose are absorbed by active transport, primarily by a sodium-dependent carrier; fructose is more slowly absorbed by facilitated diffusion that is probably also sodium dependent (Levin, 1994). The sodium-dependent transport of monosaccharides is the reason why sodium-glucose drinks are used to rehydrate infants with diarrhea or athletes who have lost too much fluid. Glucose is transported from the liver to the tissues, although some glucose is stored in the liver and muscles as glycogen. A small amount of fructose may be converted to glucose before it passes

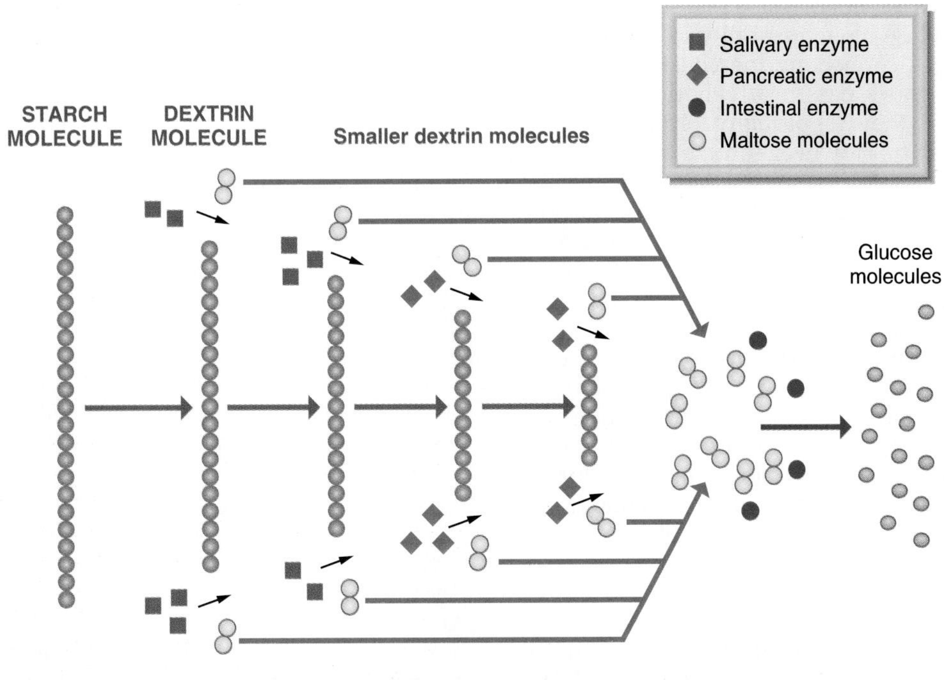

FIGURE 1-7 • The gradual breakdown of large starch molecules into glucose by digestion enzymes.

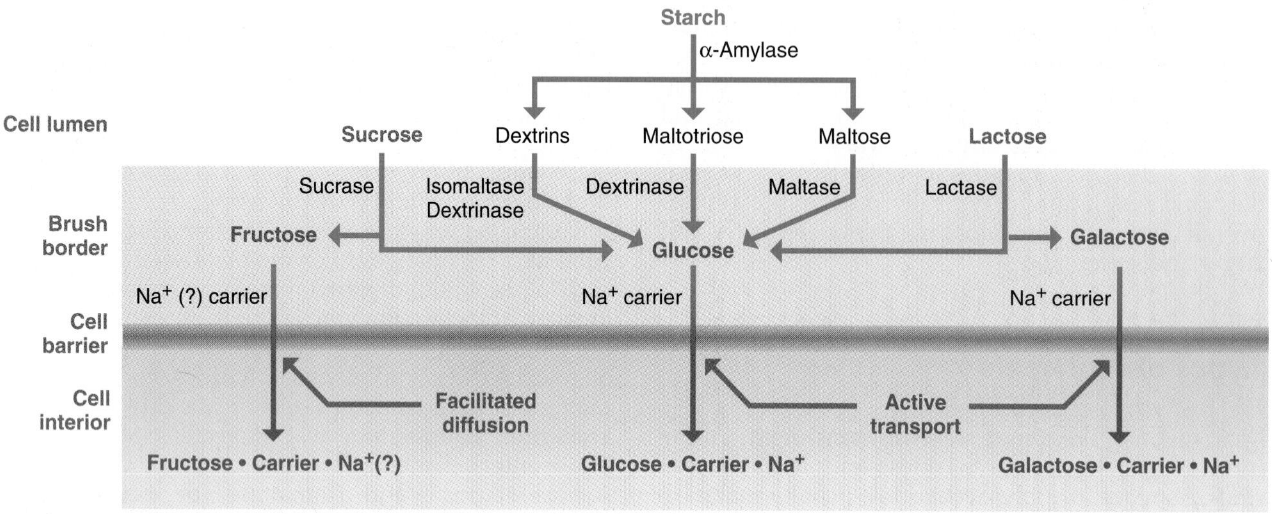

FIGURE I-8 • Digestion and absorption of carbohydrates. Sodium, in addition to glucose or galactose, combines with the carrier. The sugar-carrier-sodium ion complex is transported across the cell membrane into the cell interior. Once inside the cell, the glucose diffuses passively across the serosal membrane, and the sodium is actively pumped back out of the cell. The driving force for glucose transport against a concentration gradient is the sodium ion gradient across the membrane that contains a glucose carrier.

from the intestinal cell into the blood, but most is transported as fructose to the liver where, like galactose, it is converted to glucose. Consumption of large amounts of lactose (especially in individuals with a lactase deficiency), fructose, stachyose, raffinose, and alcohol sugars (e.g., sorbitol, mannitol, or xylitol) can result in considerable amounts of these sugars passing unabsorbed into the colon (Levin, 1994; Rumessen and Gudmand-Hoyer, 1988) and may cause increased gas and loose stools.

Some forms of carbohydrate—cellulose, hemicellulose, pectin, gum, and other forms of fiber—cannot be digested by humans because neither salivary nor pancreatic amylase have the ability to split the β 1-2 and 1-4 linkages connecting the constituent sugars. These carbohydrates pass relatively unchanged into the colon, where they are partially fermented by bacteria in the colon. However, unlike humans, cows and other ruminants can subsist on high-fiber food because of the bacterial digestion of these carbohydrates that takes place in the rumen. Other resistant starches and sugars are also less well digested or absorbed by humans, so their consumption may result in significant amounts of starch and sugar in the colon. The resistant starches and some types of dietary fiber are fermented into SCFAs and gases. Starches resistant to digestion tend to include plant foods with a high protein and fiber content, such as those from legumes and whole grains. One form of dietary fiber, lignin, is made of cyclopentane units and is not readily soluble or fermentable.

Proteins

Protein digestion begins in the stomach, where proteins are split into proteoses, peptones, and large polypeptides. Inactive pepsinogen is converted into the enzyme pepsin when it contacts hydrochloric acid and other pepsin molecules. Unlike any of the other proteolytic enzymes, pepsin digests collagen, the major protein of connective tissue. However, most protein digestion takes place in the duodenum, and the contribution of the stomach to the total digestion process is small.

Contact between chyme and the intestinal mucosa stimulates release of *enterokinase,* an enzyme that transforms inactive pancreatic trypsinogen into active trypsin, which in turn activates the other pancreatic proteolytic enzymes. Pancreatic trypsin, chymotrypsin, and carboxypeptidase break down intact protein and continue the breakdown started in the stomach until small polypeptides and amino acids are formed.

Proteolytic peptidases located on the brush border also act on polypeptides, breaking them down into amino acids, dipeptides, and tripeptides. Usually, many small peptides are efficiently absorbed intact. The final phase of protein digestion takes place in the brush border, where dipeptides and tripeptides are hydrolyzed into their constituent amino acids by peptide hydrolases. The presence of antibodies to many food proteins in the circulation of healthy individuals indicates that immunologically significant amounts of large intact peptides escape hydrolysis and can enter the portal circulation (see Chapter 32).

Amino acids are absorbed through four distinct active transport systems: one each for the neutral, basic, and acidic amino acids and one for proline and hydroxyproline. Amino acid transport is controlled by the same type of sodium cotransport mechanism used for glucose. Absorbed peptides and amino acids are transported to the liver via the portal vein for metabolism by the liver and release into the general circulation.

Almost all protein is absorbed by the time it reaches the end of the jejunum, and only 1% of ingested protein is found in the feces. Some amino acids may remain in the epithelial cells and are used for synthesis of new proteins, including intestinal enzymes and new cells. Most of the endogenous protein from intestinal secretions and desquamated epithelial cells is also digested, recycled, and absorbed from the small intestine.

Lipids

About 97% of dietary lipids are in the form of triglycerides and the rest are in the form of phospholipids and cholesterol. Small amounts of fat are digested in the mouth with lingual lipase and in the stomach from the action of gastric lipase *(tributyrinase).* Gastric lipase hydrolyzes some triglycerides, especially short-chain triglycerides (such as those found in butter), into fatty acids and glycerol. However, most fat digestion takes place in the small intestine through pancreatic lipase.

Entrance of fat stimulates the release of CCK and enterogastrone, which inhibit gastric secretions and motility, thus slowing the delivery of lipids. As a result, a portion of a large, fatty meal may remain in the stomach for 4 hours or longer. CCK, in addition to its many other functions, stimulates biliary and pancreatic secretions. The peristaltic action of the small intestine breaks large fat globules into smaller particles, and the emulsifying action of the bile keeps them separated and thus more accessible to digestion by the more potent lipid enzyme, pancreatic lipase.

Bile is a liver secretion composed of bile acids (primarily conjugates of cholic and chenodeoxycholic acids with glycine or taurine), bile pigments (which color the feces), inorganic salts, some protein, cholesterol, lecithin, and many compounds such as detoxified drugs that are metabolized and secreted by the liver. From its storage organ, the gallbladder, about 1 L of bile is secreted daily in response to the stimulus of food in the duodenum and stomach.

The free fatty acids and monoglycerides produced by digestion form complexes with bile salts called micelles. The micelles facilitate passage of the lipids through the watery environment of the intestinal lumen to the brush border (see Figure 1-4). The micelles release the lipid components and are returned to the gut lumen. Most of the bile salts are actively reabsorbed in the terminal ileum and returned to the liver to reenter the gut in bile secretions. This efficient recycling process is known as the *enterohepatic circulation.* The pool of bile acids may circulate from 3 to 15 times per day, depending on the amount of food ingested.

In the mucosal cells, the fatty acids and monoglycerides are reassembled into new triglycerides. A few are further digested into free fatty acids and glycerol and then reassembled to form triglycerides. These triglycerides, along with cholesterol and phospholipids, are surrounded by a β-lipoprotein coat, forming chylomicrons (see Figure 1-4). The globules pass into the lacteals of the villi by a process of exocytosis. Chylomicrons are transported by the lymphatic vessels to the thoracic duct and emptied into the systemic circulation at the junction of the left internal jugular and left subclavian veins. The chylomicrons are then carried through the bloodstream to several tissues, including adipose, liver, and muscle. In the liver the triglycerides from the chylomicrons are repackaged into very-low-density lipoproteins (VLDLs) and transported primarily to the adipose tissue for metabolism and storage.

Cholesterol is absorbed in a similar way after being hydrolyzed from the ester form by pancreatic cholesterol esterase. The fat-soluble vitamins A, D, E, and K are also absorbed in a micellar fashion, although water-soluble forms of vitamins A, E, and K supplements and carotene can be absorbed in the absence of bile acids.

Under normal conditions, approximately 95% to 97% of ingested fat is absorbed into lymph vessels. Because of their shorter length and thus increased solubility, fatty acids of 8 to 12 carbons—medium-chain fatty acids (MCFAs)—can be absorbed directly into mucosal cells without the presence of bile and micelle formation. After entering mucosal cells, they are able to go directly without esterification into the portal vein, which carries them to the liver.

Use of medium-chain triglycerides (which have fatty acids of 8 to 12 carbons) is clinically valuable for individuals who lack necessary bile salts for emulsification and micellar formation required for long-chain fatty acid transport (see Chapter 30) or lack the ability to transport triglycerides from the intestinal epithelial cells into the lymphatics, as occurs in abetalipoproteinemia. Supplements for clinical use are normally provided in the form of oil or a dietary beverage with other macronutrients and micronutrients.

Increased motility, intestinal mucosal changes, pancreatic insufficiency, or the absence of bile can decrease absorption of fat. When undigested fat appears in the feces, the condition is known as *steatorrhea* (see Chapter 30).

Vitamins and Minerals

Vitamins, minerals, and fluids are absorbed simultaneously through the intestinal mucosa (Figure 1-9). Various factors affect the bioavailability of vitamins and minerals in this process, including the presence or absence of other specific nutrients. Each day, about 8 to 9 L of fluid from the body pass back and forth across the gut membrane to keep the nutrients in solution.

Most vitamins and water pass unchanged from the small intestine into the blood by passive diffusion. Drugs are primarily absorbed by passive diffusion. The drugs absorbed by active transport may compete with nutrients at the cell membrane, possibly decreasing or increasing the actual absorption of either the medication or the nutrient.

Mineral absorption is more complex and proceeds in three stages. The *intraluminal stage* consists of the chemical reactions and interactions that take place in the stomach and intestines. These reactions, which are predominantly determined by the pH of the luminal contents and the composition of the food entering from the stomach, primarily affect the cations. Small anions such as fluoride are not influenced by either pH or the composition of the diet and are absorbed quite freely. Cations, which are soluble in the acidic pH of the stomach, form insoluble hydroxides when the chyme passes into the higher pH of the small intestine. These cations are made available for absorption by *ligands* (molecules that bind to other molecules), such as amino acids and other organic acids and sugars, with which they form combination, or chelation, compounds.

The *translocation stage* involves passage across the membrane into intestinal mucosal cells. Transport of small anions may be by simple diffusion. For most cationic elements, the mechanism is either facilitated diffusion or active transport. For many minerals,

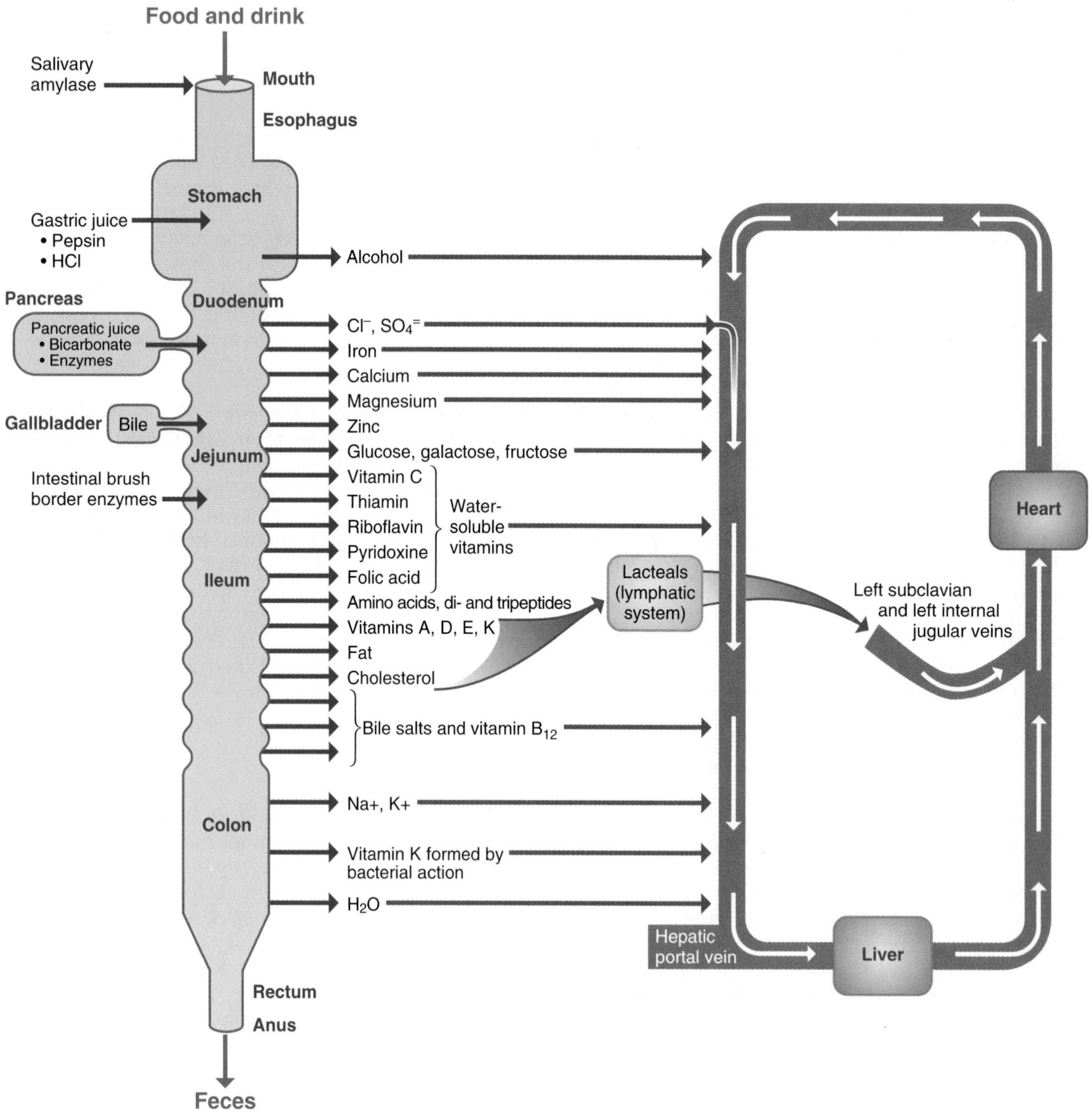

FIGURE 1-9 • Sites of secretion and absorption in the gastrointestinal tract.

more than one method of translocation may be possible, depending on the concentration of a particular trace element in the intestinal contents.

During the *mobilization stage,* minerals are either transported across the serosal surfaces of the intestinal cells into the bloodstream or are sequestered within the cell. For example, iron and zinc are either bound to proteins within the intestinal cell or added to the intracellular pool. The ions in the pool are then mobilized and transported across the serosal surface, whereas the protein-bound ions are either released to become part of the pool or remain bound, in which case they are lost with the cell during desquamation.

The GI tract is the site of important interactions among minerals. Supplementation with large amounts of iron or zinc may decrease the absorption of copper. In turn, copper may lower iron and molybdenum absorption. Cobalt absorption is increased in patients with iron deficiency, but cobalt and iron compete and inhibit one another's absorption. These interactions are probably the result of an overlap of mineral absorption mechanisms.

Minerals are transported bound to protein carriers. The protein binding is either specific (e.g., transferrin, which binds with iron) or general (e.g., albumin, which binds a variety of minerals). A fraction of each mineral is also carried in the serum in the form of amino acid or peptide complexes. Specific protein carriers are usually not completely saturated; the reserve capacity may serve as a buffer against excessive exposure. Toxicity from minerals usually results only after this buffering capacity is exceeded.

Factors Affecting Digestion

Psychologic Factors

The appearance, smell, and taste of food, in addition to emotional states, have an impact on digestion. The sight, smell, taste, and even thought of food increase secretion of GI hormones, fluids, and enzymes and increase the muscular activity of the GI tract. After ingestion of food, digestive products then trigger feedback mechanisms to inhibit GI activity and limit food intake. Fear, anger, and worry stimulate the hypothalamus to activate the autonomic nervous system, which then depresses secretions, inhibits peristalsis, and slows propulsion of food by increasing sphincter tone (Bray, 2000; Katschinski, 2000; Mattes, 1997). Strong odors, noxious stimuli, and very strong emotions may induce nausea and vomiting. Strong signals from the GI tract as a result of disease, inflammation, distention, or dysmotility may send signals to the central nervous system, resulting in the perception of nausea or abdominal comfort.

Food Processing

Cooking food, especially at high temperatures for prolonged periods can destroy several nutrients such as ascorbic acid and folate, but in general, properly cooked food is more digestible than raw food. For example, cooking meat loosens its connective tissue, facilitates chewing, and makes the meat more accessible to digestive juices. Cooking softens dietary fiber, makes certain fiber more fermentable, and may make the digestible nutrients attached to fiber more available. Claims have been made that fruits and vegetables should be consumed raw because their inherent carbohydrate- or protein-digesting enzymes facilitate digestion of foods and are destroyed with cooking. Enzymes from a few raw fruits and vegetables may still have some activity in the GI tract, but their contribution to the digestion of foods is miniscule and pales compared with the powerful human digestive enzymes. During grain refinement for breads and cereals, many of the nutrients, phytochemicals, and fibrous materials are lost. Enrichment replaces several of the lost nutrients but not the dietary fiber or phytochemicals.

With some types of cooking, chemical reactions between food and the secretions of the digestive system affect digestion. For example, *acrolein,* a decomposition product produced by frying foods at excessively high temperatures, retards the flow of digestive juices. In contrast, meat extracts stimulate secretion of digestive secretions, hormones, and enzymes.

SUMMARY

With few exceptions the human GI tract is remarkably efficient. Humans can consume a wide variety of foods in random combinations without significantly affecting digestion. The GI tract has remarkable self-regulating mechanisms for coordinating digestive, immunologic, secretory, and absorptive functions. A transient disruption of these homeostatic mechanisms may occur as a result of dietary extremes, and more long-term dysfunction can result from malnutrition, disease, or trauma.

Clinical Scenario I

After reading about the benefits of a powdered fiber supplement in a magazine one day, Mary consumed a 20-g dose of a soluble fiber source and increased her dietary fiber intake from her average 10 g per day to 25 g. Later that day, she had abdominal cramping and distention, increased flatulence, and loose stools.

1. What is the likely explanation for her symptoms?
2. How could she have increased her fiber without causing such severe symptoms?
3. Is her new fiber intake reasonable?

Clinical Scenario 2

Joseph, who had a long history of pancreatitis, came to his physician because of weight loss and more frequent defecation. After several tests, Joseph's physician told him his pancreas had lost the ability to secrete enough enzymes to be able to digest foods properly and prescribed enzyme tablets to take with meals and snacks.

1. Which enzymes does the pancreas produce?
2. To what extent must the pancreas have been damaged to result in Joseph's inability to digest foods sufficiently?
3. Are any of the pancreatic enzymes more important, or irreplaceable, than others?

Relevant Web Sites

American Gastroenterological Association
www.gastro.org/public/digestinfo.html
NIH Digestive Diseases
www.niddk.nih.gov/health/digest/digest.htm

Cited References

Allman H, Nilsson O: The gut as the largest endocrine organ in the body, *Ann Oncol* 12(suppl 2):63, 2001.

Bengmark S, Jeppsson B: Gastrointestinal surface protection and mucosal reconditioning, *J Parent Ent Nutr* 19:410, 1995.

Bjorck I et al: Food properties affecting digestion and absorption of carbohydrates, *Am J Clin Nutr* 59(suppl):699-705, 1994.

Bray GA: Afferent signals regulating food intake, *Proc Nutr Soc* 59:373, 2000.

Canaan S et al: Gastric lipase: crystal structure and activity, *Biochim Biophysica Acta* 1441:197, 1999.

Caspary WF: Physiology and pathophysiology of intestinal absorption *Am J Clin Nutr* 55S:299, 1992.

Chang EB et al: *Gastrointestinal, hepatobiliary, and nutritional physiology,* Philadelphia, 1996, Lippincott-Raven.

Collins PJ et al: Effects of increasing solid component size of a mixed solid/liquid meal on solid and liquid gastric emptying, *Am J Physiol* 271:G539, 1996.

Cummings JH, Englyst HN: Gastrointestinal effects of food carbohydrate, *Am J Clin Nutr* 61(suppl):938, 1995.

Dunne C et al: In vitro selection criteria for probiotic bacteria of human origin: correlation with in vivo findings, *Am J Clin Nutr* 73S:386, 2001.

Farthing MJ: The role of somatostatin analogues in the treatment of refractory diarrhea, *Digestion* 57(suppl):107, 1996.

Feighner SD et al: Receptor for motilin identified in the human gastrointestinal system, *Science* 284:2184, 1999.

Furness JB, Clerc N: Responses of afferent neurons to the contents of the digestive tract, and their relation to endocrine and immune responses, *Prog Brain Res* 122:159, 2000.

Geypens B et al: Influence of dietary protein supplements on the formation of bacterial metabolites in the colon, *Gut* 41:70 1997.

Guyton AC, Hall JE: *Textbook of medical physiology,* ed 9, Philadelphia, 1996, WB Saunders.

Havel PJ: Peripheral signals conveying metabolic information to the brain: short-term and long-term regulation of food intake and energy homeostasis, *Exp Biol Med* 226:963, 2001.

Hellstrom PM, Naslund E: Interactions between gastric emptying and satiety, with special reference to glucagon-like peptide-1, *Physiol Behav* 74:735, 2001.

Hill MJ: Intestinal flora and endogenous vitamin synthesis, *Eur J Cancer Prev* S1:43 1997.

Holst JJ et al: Gastrointestinal endocrinology, *Scand J Gastroenterol* 216(suppl):27, 1996.

Katschinski M: Nutritional implications of cephalic phase gastrointestinal responses, *Appetite* 34:189, 2000.

Kuemmerle JF: Motility disorders of the small intestine: new insights into old problems, *J Clin Gastroenterol* 31:276, 2000.

Layer P, Keller J: Pancreatic enzymes: secretion and luminal nutrient digestion in health and disease, *J Clin Gastroenterol* 28: 3, 1999.

Levin RJ: Digestion and absorption of carbohydrates—from molecules and membranes to humans, *Am J Clin Nutr* 59(suppl): 690, 1994.

L'Heureux MC, Brubaker PL: Therapeutic potential of the intestinotropic hormone, glucagon-like peptide-2, *Ann Med* 33: 229, 2001.

Liddle RA: Cholecystokinin cells, *Annu Rev Physiol* 59:221, 1997.

MacFarlane GT, MacFarlane S: Human colonic microbiota: ecology physiology and metabolic potential of intestinal bacteria, *Scand J Gastroenterol* 222(suppl):3-9, 1997.

Mattes RD: Physiologic responses to sensory stimulation by food: Nutritional implications, *J Am Diet Assoc* 97:406, 1997.

Mortensen PB, Clausen MR: Short-chain fatty acids in the human colon: relation to gastrointestinal health and disease, *Scand J Gastroenterol* 216:132, 1996.

Nauck MA: Is glucagon-like peptide-1 an incretin hormone? *Diabetologia* 42:373, 1999.

Rehfeld JF: The new biology of gastrointestinal hormones, *Physiol Rev* 78:1087, 1998.

Roberfroid MB: Prebiotics: preferential substrates for specific germs? *Am J Clin Nutr* 73(suppl):406, 2001.

Rumessen JJ, Gudmand-Hoyer E: Functional bowel disease: malabsorption and abdominal distress after ingestion of fructose, sorbitol, and fructose-sorbitol mixtures, *Gastroenterology* 95: 694, 1988.

Salminen S et al: Functional food science and gastrointestinal physiology and function, *Br J Nutr* 80S:147, 1998.

Sarna SK, Gonzalez A, Ryan RP: Enteric locus of prokinetics: ABT-229, motilin, and erythromycin, *Am J Physiol Gastrointest Liver Physiol* 278:G744, 2000.

Spiller RC: Intestinal absorptive function, *Gut* 31(suppl):5, 1994.

Stevens EC, Hume ID: Contributions of microbes in vertebrate gastrointestinal tract to production and conservation of nutrients, *Physiol Rev* 78:393, 1998.

Thompson ABR et al: Lipid absorption: passing through the unstirred layers, brush border membrane, and beyond, *Can J Physiol Pharmacol* 71:531, 1993

Tulassay Z: Somatostatin and the gastrointestinal tract, *Scand J Gastroenterol* 228:115, 1998.

Additional References

Furness JB: Types of neurons in the enteric nervous system, *J Auton Nerv Syst* 81:87, 2000.

Johnson LR et al: *Physiology of the gastrointestinal tract,* ed 3, vols 1 and 2, New York, 1994, Raven Press.

Olsson C, Holmgren S: The control of gut motility, *Comp Biochem Physiol A Mol Integr Physiol* 128:481, 2001.

Tougas G et al: Assessment of gastric emptying using a low-fat meal: establishment of international control values, *Am J Gastroenterol* 95:1456, 2000.

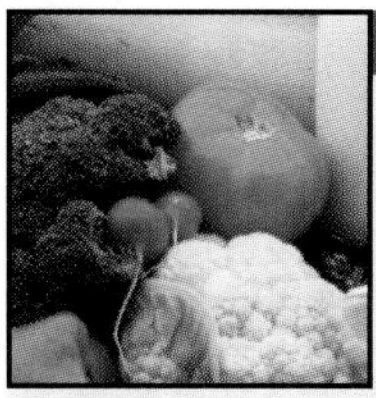

CHAPTER 2

Energy

CAROL D. FRARY, MS, RD
RACHEL K. JOHNSON, PhD, MPH, RD

CHAPTER OUTLINE

- Components of Energy Expenditure
- Measurement of Energy Expenditure
- Estimating Energy Requirements
- Calculating Food Energy

KEY TERMS

basal energy expenditure (BEE)–the measurement of the basal metabolic rate; usually expressed as kilocalories per 24 hours (kcal/24 hr)

basal metabolic rate (BMR)–the energy needed to sustain the metabolic activities of cells and tissues and to maintain circulatory, respiratory, gastrointestinal, and renal processes

calorie–the amount of energy required to raise the temperature of 1 ml of water at 15° C by 1° C

direct calorimetry–a method for measuring the amount of energy expended by monitoring the rate at which a person loses heat from the body to the environment when placed inside a structure large enough to permit moderate amounts of activity

doubly labeled water (DLW)–used to measure total energy expenditure in free-living people using two stable isotopes of water (deuterium [^2H_2O] and oxygen-18 [$H_2{}^{18}O$]); the difference in the turnover rates of the two isotopes measures the carbon dioxide production rate, from which total energy expenditure can be calculated

energy expended in physical activity (EEPA)–the energy expended during voluntary exercise and involuntary activities such as shivering and fidgeting; the most variable component of total energy expenditure

estimated energy requirement (EER)–the average dietary energy intake that is predicted to maintain energy balance in a healthy adult of a defined age, gender, weight, height, and level of physical activity consistent with good health. In children and pregnant and lactating women, the EER is taken to include the energy needs associated with the deposition of tissues or the secretion of milk at rates consistent with good health

facultative thermogenesis–a portion of the thermic effect of food; "excess" energy expended in addition to the obligatory thermogenesis—thought to be partially mediated by sympathetic nervous system activity

indirect calorimetry–a method for estimating energy production by measuring oxygen consumption and carbon dioxide production rather than by directly measuring heat transfer; typically takes 30 minutes to 1 hour to complete

joule–the measure of energy in terms of mechanical work; the amount of energy required to accelerate 1 Newton (N) a distance of 1 m; 1 kcal = 4.184 kJ

kilocalorie (kcal or cal)–1000 calories; sometimes written as *Calorie*

metabolic equivalents (METs)–the measure of caloric expenditure by the amount of oxygen consumed per minute per kilogram of body weight; 1 MET = ~3.5 ml oxygen consumed per kilogram of body weight per minute in adults

obligatory thermogenesis–a portion of the thermic effect of food; the energy required to digest, absorb, and metabolize nutrients

physical activity level (PAL)–the ratio of total energy expenditure (TEE) to basal energy expenditure (BEE); PAL = TEE/BEE

resting energy expenditure (REE)–a measurement of the resting metabolic rate; usually expressed as kilocalories per 24 hours (kcal/24 hr)

KEY TERMS—Continued

resting metabolic rate (RMR)–the energy expended for the maintenance of normal body functions and homeostasis; represents the largest portion of total energy expenditure; may be as much as 10% to 20% higher than the basal energy expenditure, allowing for the energy spent as a result of the thermic effect of food or excess postexercise oxygen consumption

respiratory quotient (RQ)–the ratio of moles of carbon dioxide produced to the moles of oxygen consumed

thermic effect of food (TEF)–the increase in energy expenditure associated with the processes of digestion, absorption, and metabolism of food; represents approximately 10% of the sum of the resting metabolic rate and the energy expended in physical activity and includes facultative thermogenesis and obligatory thermogenesis; often called *diet-induced thermogenesis (DIT), specific dynamic action (SDA)*, or the *specific effect of food (SEF)*

total energy expenditure (TEE)–the sum of the resting energy expenditure, energy expended in physical activity, and the thermic effect of food; the energy expended by an individual in 24 hours

Energy is defined as "the capacity to do work." The ultimate source of all energy in living organisms is the sun. Through the process of photosynthesis, green plants intercept a portion of the sunlight reaching their leaves and capture it within the chemical bonds of glucose. Proteins, fats, and other carbohydrates are synthesized from this basic carbohydrate to meet the needs of the plant. Animals and humans obtain these nutrients and the energy they contain by consuming plants and the flesh of other animals. The body makes use of the energy from carbohydrates, proteins, fats, and alcohol in the diet. Energy provided from the macronutrients is locked in chemical bonds within food and is released when food is metabolized. Energy must be supplied regularly to meet the energy needs for the body's survival. Although all energy eventually takes the form of heat, which dissipates into the atmosphere, unique cellular processes first make possible its use for all of the tasks required to maintain life. Among these processes are chemical reactions that accomplish synthesis and maintenance of body tissues, electrical conduction of nerve activity, the mechanical work of muscles, and heat production to maintain body temperature.

The Food and Agriculture Organization/World Health Organization/United Nations University (FAO/WHO/UNU) Expert Consultation on Energy and Protein requirements defines energy requirements as follows (WHO, 1985):

> The energy requirement of an individual is the level of energy intake from food that will balance energy expenditure when the individual has a body size and composition, and level of physical activity, consistent with long-term good health; and that will allow for the maintenance of economically necessary and socially desirable physical activity. In children and pregnant or lactating women the energy requirement includes the energy needs associated with the deposition of tissues or the secretion of milk at rates consistent with good health.

Unlike with other nutrient requirements, body weight is an indicator of energy adequacy or inadequacy. The body has the unique ability to shift the fuel mixture of carbohydrates, proteins, and fats to accommodate energy needs. However, consuming too much or too little over time results in body weight changes. Hence, body weight reflects adequacy of energy intake but it is not a reliable indicator of macronutrient or micronutrient adequacy.

COMPONENTS OF ENERGY EXPENDITURE

Energy is expended by the human body in the form of resting energy expenditure (REE), the thermic effect of food (TEF), and energy expended in physical activity (EEPA). These three components make up a person's daily total energy expenditure (TEE) (Figure 2-1). Except in extremely active individuals, the REE constitutes the largest portion (60% to 75%) of the TEE (Poehlman, 1993). The TEF represents approximately 10% of the total daily energy expenditure. The contribution of physical activity is the most variable component of TEE, which may be as low as 100 kilocalories (kcal) per day in sedentary people or as high as 3000 kcal per day in very active people.

Resting and Basal Energy Expenditure

Definition

Resting energy expenditure (REE) is the energy expended in the activities necessary to sustain normal body functions and homeostasis. These activities include respiration and circulation, the synthesis of organic compounds, the pumping of ions across membranes, the energy required by the central nervous system, and maintenance of body temperature. Of the total, 29% is used by the liver, much of which is involved in synthesizing glucose and ketone bodies as fuels for the brain (Table 2-1).

Basal energy expenditure (BEE) can be simply defined as the minimal amount of energy expended that is compatible with life. A person's BEE reflects the amount of energy used over 24 hours while physically (i.e., lying down) and mentally resting in a thermoneutral environment that prevents the activation of heat-generating processes such as shivering. Basal metabolic rate (BMR) measurements are made early in the morning, before the person has engaged in any physical activity and 10 to 12 hours after the ingestion of any food, drink, or nicotine. The BMR remains remarkably constant on a daily basis (Durnin, 1996) and typically represents approximately 60% to 70% of the TEE (Shetty et al, 1996). If any of the conditions for the BMR are not met, energy expenditure should be referred to as the resting metabolic rate (RMR). For practical reasons the BMR is now rarely measured. RMR measurements are used in its place, which in most cases are higher than the BMR.

Factors Affecting Resting Energy Expenditure

Numerous factors cause the REE to vary among individuals. Major variables include body size and composition, yet age, sex, and hormonal status affect REE as well.

Body Size

Larger people generally have higher metabolic rates than smaller people, yet tall, thin people have higher metabolic rates than short, wide people. For example, if two people weigh the same but one person is taller, the taller person with the larger body surface area has the higher metabolic rate (Whitney and Rolfes, 2002). Hence those with the greater surface area have the higher metabolic rate.

The amount of lean body mass is highly correlated with total body size. For example, obese children have higher RMRs than lean children, yet when RMR is adjusted for body weight no RMR differences are found (Laessle et al, 1997).

Body Composition

The major single determinant of REE is fat-free mass (FFM) or lean body mass (LBM) (Poehlman and Horton, 1998). FFM is the metabolically active tissue in the body; therefore most of the variation in REE among people can be accounted for by the variation in their FFM. Because of their greater FFM, athletes with greater muscular development have approximately a 5% higher basal metabolism than nonathletic individuals.

FFM can be measured most accurately by using reference body composition methods. These methods include underwater weighing *(hydrodensitometry)*, dual x-ray absorptiometry *(DEXA* or *DXA)*, and air-displacement plethysmography (e.g., the Bod Pod). Underwater weighing determines body fat by measuring a person's body density and is considered the gold standard for measuring body composition. Body density is the difference between the dry weight before underwater weighing and the underwater weight. Because fat is less dense and more buoyant in water than FFM, the less a person weighs underwater the higher the body fat. (The underwater procedure can be viewed at http://nutrition.uvm.edu/bodycomp [Pintauro and Buzzell, 1999]). The Bod Pod (Figure 2-2) is based on the same principle as underwater weighing except that it uses air displacement technology (Callahan, 2002). DXA is a novel scanning technique that accurately estimates bone mineral, fat, and fat-free soft tissue. Radiation exposure is minimal—approximately a single day's background radiation—for a whole-body composition analysis (Figure 2-3).

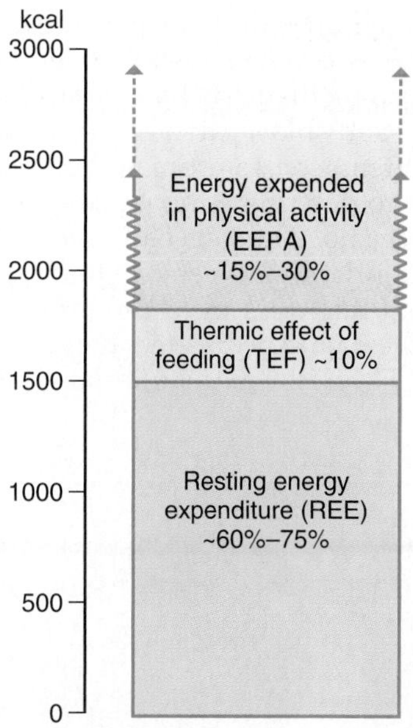

FIGURE 2-1 • The components of total energy expenditure (TEE). (From Poehlman ET, Horton ES: Energy needs: assessment and requirements in humans. In Bloch AS, Shils ME, eds: *Modern nutrition in health and disease*, Baltimore, 1988, Williams & Wilkins.)

TABLE 2-1 Approximate Energy Expenditure of Organs in Human Adults

ORGAN	PERCENTAGE OF REE*
Liver	29
Brain	19
Heart	10
Kidney	7
Skeletal muscles (at rest)	18
Remainder	17
TOTAL	100

Modified from Grande F: Energy expenditure of organs and tissues. In Kinney JM, eds: *Assessment of energy metabolism in health and disease,* Columbus, Ohio, 1980, Ross Laboratories.
**REE,* Resting energy expenditure.

However, because of the expense and impractical nature of these reference methods, less accurate but more practical methods such as skinfold anthropometry (SFA) and bioelectrical impedance analysis (BIA), are often used to estimate body composition. SFA is used to determine the percentage of body fat by measuring subcutaneous fat tissue with a skinfold caliper. A highly trained person should perform and read skinfold-thickness measurements to obtain the most accurate data. The BIA technique can be used to determine FFM in the extremities and involves placing electrodes on the wrist and ankle. BIA electrical measurements are used to estimate a person's total body water (TBW). From TBW measurements, FFM can be estimated because FFM is primarily composed of water. Subsequently, an approximation of fat mass can be calculated as the difference between body weight and FFM (Pintauro and Buzzell, 1999).

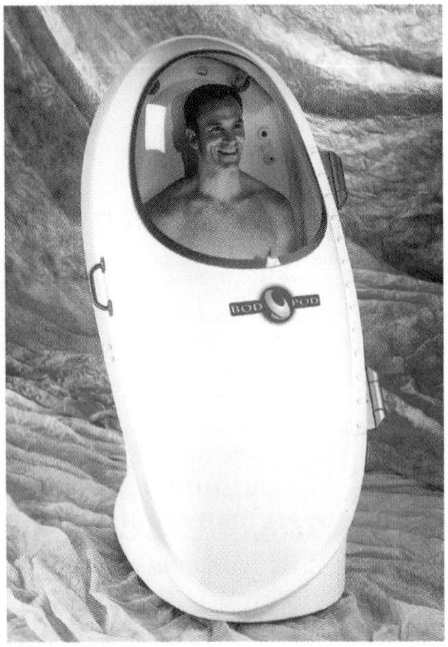

FIGURE 2-2 • The Bod Pod uses air displacement technology to measure body composition. (Courtesy Life Measurement, Inc., Concord, Calif.)

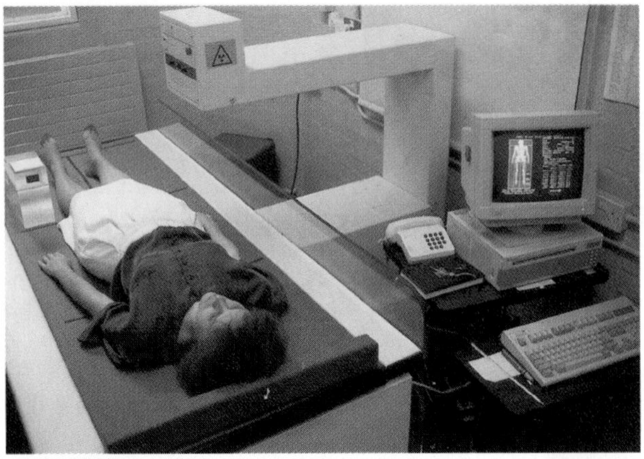

FIGURE 2-3 • Dual-energy x-ray absorptiometry (DXA) is a scanning technique that accurately estimates bone mineral, fat, and fat-free soft tissue. Radiation exposure for a whole-body analysis is minimal, being approximately equivalent to the x-ray associated with a dental x-ray. (Courtesy The Dunn Nutrition Centre, University of Cambridge, Cambridge, England.)

Age

Because it is determined by the FFM, the REE is highest during periods of rapid growth, chiefly during the first and second years of life, and reaches a lesser peak throughout puberty and adolescence (Torun et al, 1996). The additional energy required for synthesizing and depositing body tissue is about 5 kcal per gram of tissue gained (Roberts and Young, 1988). Growing infants may store as much as 12% to 15% of the energy value of their food in the form of new tissue. As a child becomes older, the caloric requirement for growth is reduced to about 1% of the total energy requirement.

The loss of FFM with aging is associated with a decline in RMR, amounting to about a 2% to 3% decline per decade after early adulthood. These changes in body composition can be attenuated by exercise; exercise can help maintain a higher lean body mass and thus a higher RMR (Poehlman, 1993).

Sex

Sex differences in metabolic rates are primarily attributable to differences in body size and composition. Women, who generally have more fat in proportion to muscle than men, have metabolic rates that are approximately 5% to 10% lower than men of the same weight and height.

Hormonal Status

Hormonal status can affect metabolic rate, particularly in those with endocrine disorders such as hyperthyroidism and hypothyroidism, which increase or decrease energy expenditure, respectively. Stimulation of the sympathetic nervous system (e.g., during periods of emotional excitement or stress) causes the release of epinephrine, which directly promotes glycogenolysis and increases cellular activity. Endogenous growth hormone (GH) levels among healthy adults were determined to have no association with RMR (Jorgensen et al, 1998).

The metabolic rate of women fluctuates with the menstrual cycle. An average of 359 kcal/day difference in the BMR has been measured between the low point, about 1 week before ovulation on day 14, and the high point, just before the onset of menstruation. The mean increase in energy expenditure is about 150 kcal/day during the second half of the menstrual cycle (Webb, 1986). During pregnancy, RMR seems to decrease in the early stages, whereas later in pregnancy the metabolic rate increases because of uterine, placental, and fetal growth and the mother's increased cardiac workload (Goldberg et al, 1993).

Other Factors

Fevers increase the metabolic rate by about 7% for each degree increase in body temperature above 98.6° Fahrenheit (i.e., 13% for each degree above 37° Centigrade).

RMR is also affected by extremes in environmental temperature. People living in tropical climates usually have RMRs that are 5% to 20% higher than those living in temperate areas. Exercise in temperatures greater than 86° F also imposes a small additional metabolic load of about 5% from increased sweat gland activity. The extent to which energy metabolism increases in extremely cold environments depends on the insulation available from body fat and protective clothing.

Thermic Effect of Food

Definition

The thermic effect of food (TEF) is the increase in energy expenditure associated with the consumption of food. The TEF accounts for approximately 10% of the TEE (Poehlman and Horton, 1998). The TEF is also referred to as *diet-induced thermogenesis (DIT), specific dynamic action (SDA),* and the *specific effect of food (SEF).* TEF can be separated into obligatory and facultative (or adaptive) subcomponents. Obligatory thermogenesis is the energy required to digest, absorb, and metabolize nutrients, including the synthesis and storage of protein, fat, and carbohydrates. Adaptive, or facultative, thermogenesis is the "excess" energy expended in addition to the obligatory thermogenesis and is thought to be attributable to the metabolic inefficiency of the system stimulated by sympathetic nervous activity.

Factors Affecting the Thermic Effect of Food

The TEF varies with the composition of the diet and is greater after consumption of carbohydrates and proteins than after fat. Fat is metabolized efficiently, with only 4% wastage, compared with 25% wastage when carbohydrate is converted to fat for storage. These factors are thought to contribute to the obesity-promoting characteristics of fat (Prentice, 1995). The role of TEF in weight management is discussed in more detail in Chapter 24.

Spicy foods enhance and prolong the effect of the TEF. Meals with chili and mustard may increase the metabolic rate as much as 33% more than unspiced meals, and this effect may last for more than 3 hours (McCrory et al, 1994). Caffeine and nicotine also stimulate the TEF. When ingested every 2 hours for 12 hours, the amount of caffeine in one cup of coffee (100 mg) has been shown to increase the TEF by 8% to 11% (Dulloo et al, 1989). Nicotine has a similar effect (Hofstetter, 1986).

Energy Expended in Physical Activity

Definition

The energy expended in physical activity (EEPA) is the most variable component of TEE. It may range from as little as 10% in a person who is bedridden to as much as 50% of TEE in an athlete. EEPA includes energy expended in voluntary exercise and during involuntary activities such as shivering, fidgeting, and maintaining postural control.

Factors Affecting the Energy Expended in Physical Activity

EEPA varies considerably depending on body size and the efficiency of individual habits of motion. The level of fitness also affects the energy expenditure of voluntary activity, probably because of variations in muscle mass.

EEPA tends to decrease with age, a trend that is associated with a decline in FFM and an increase in fat mass. Men generally have a higher EEPA than women, primarily because of their larger body size and greater FFM.

Excess postexercise oxygen consumption (EPOC) affects energy expenditure. The duration (Bahr et al, 1987) and magnitude (Bahr et al, 1992) of physical activity have been shown to increase EPOC, resulting in an elevated metabolic rate even after exercise has ceased. Habitual exercise does not cause a significantly prolonged increase in metabolic rate per unit of active tissue, but it does cause an 8% to 14% higher metabolic rate in men who are moderately and highly active, respectively, because of their increased FFM (Horton and Geissler, 1994). These differences seem to be related to the individual, not to the activity.

MEASUREMENT OF ENERGY EXPENDITURE

Units of Measurement

The standard unit for measuring energy is the calorie, which is the amount of heat energy required to raise the temperature of 1 ml of water at 15° C by 1° C. Because the amount of energy involved in the metabolism of food is fairly large, the kilocalorie (1000 calories) is commonly used to measure it. A popular convention is to designate kilocalorie by *Calorie* (with a capital "C"). In this text, *kilocalorie* is abbreviated *kcal.*

The joule (J) measures energy in terms of mechanical work and is the amount of energy required to accelerate with a force of 1 Newton (N) for a distance of 1 m; this measurement is widely used in countries

CLINICAL INSIGHT

The Joule

The *joule,* a unit of energy based on mechanical energy, is defined as the work done by a force of 1 N acting for a distance of 1 m. The International Organization for Standardization has recommended the adoption of the joule (J) as the preferred unit for energy measurement in all branches of science. This recommendation was adopted by the U.S. National Bureau of Standards in 1964; in 1970 the Committee on Nomenclature of the American Institute of Nutrition recommended that it be used as soon as the mechanics of the transition could be established. Although the joule has been in use internationally for numerous years, currently the United States and Canada have not made the change.

The multiplier recommended by the Committee on Nomenclature, International Union of Nutritional Sciences, to convert kilocalories to kilojoules is 4.184 (although 4.2 may be used). Energy values per gram of each nutrient expressed in kilojoules (kJ) are as follows: carbohydrate, 17 kJ; protein, 17 kJ; and fat, 38 kJ. Because the energy value of diets is usually greater than 1000 kJ, the megajoule (mJ), equivalent to 1000 kJ, is often used.

other than the United States. One kcal is equivalent to 4.184 kilojoules (kJ) (see *Clinical Insight:* The Joule).

Measuring Human Energy Expenditure

Various methods are available to measure human energy expenditure. It is important to gain an understanding of the differences in these methods and how they can be applied in practical and research settings.

Direct Calorimetry

Direct calorimetry monitors the amount of heat produced by a person placed inside a structure large enough to permit moderate amounts of activity. These structures are referred to as *whole-room calorimeters.* Direct calorimetry provides a measure of energy expended in the form of heat but provides no information on the kind of fuel being oxidized. The method is also limited by the confined nature of the testing conditions. Hence the measurement of TEE using this method is not representative of a free-living (i.e., engaged in normal daily activities) individual in a normal environment because physical activity within the chamber is limited. Its high cost and complex engineering and the scarcity of appropriate facilities around the world also limit the use of this method.

Indirect Calorimetry

Indirect calorimetry estimates energy expenditure by determining the oxygen consumption and carbon dioxide production of the body over a given period. The equipment varies, but the person usually breathes into a mouthpiece or ventilated hood through which his or her expired gases are collected. Indirect calorimetry has the advantage of mobility and low equipment cost. The most widely used form of indirect calorimetry is the measurement of RMR through a respirator gas-exchange canopy (Figure 2-4). These ventilated hoods are useful for short- and long-term measurements. Although less advantageous in measuring EEPA, indirect calorimetry can be used to measure EEPA during various activities in a laboratory setting. In the clinical setting, metabolic carts are often used at the hospital bedside to assess patients' energy requirements.

Data are obtained from indirect calorimetry in a form that permits calculation of the respiratory quotient (RQ):

$$RQ = \text{Moles } CO_2 \text{ expired/Moles } O_2 \text{ consumed}$$

This determination is converted into kilocalories of heat produced per square meter of body surface per hour and is extrapolated to energy expenditure in 24 hours.

The RQ depends on the fuel mixture being metabolized. The RQ for carbohydrate is 1, because the number of carbon dioxide molecules produced is equal to the number of oxygen molecules consumed.

$$RQ = 1 \text{ for carbohydrate, } 0.85 \text{ for a mixed diet, } 0.82 \text{ for protein, and } 0.7 \text{ for fat.}$$

Doubly Labeled Water

The doubly labeled water (DLW) technique for measuring TEE revolutionized the understanding of energy requirements and energy balance in humans. The method was first applied to humans in 1982 and since that time, scientists developed a database that was used to develop recommendations for energy intake (Institute of Medicine, 2002). The DLW method is based on the principle that carbon dioxide production can be estimated from the difference in the elimination rates of body hydrogen and oxygen. After administering an oral loading dose of water labeled with deuterium oxide (^2H_2O) and oxygen-18 ($H_2{}^{18}O$)—hence the term *doubly labeled water*—the deuterium is eliminated from the body as water, and the oxygen-18 is eliminated as water and carbon dioxide. The elimi-

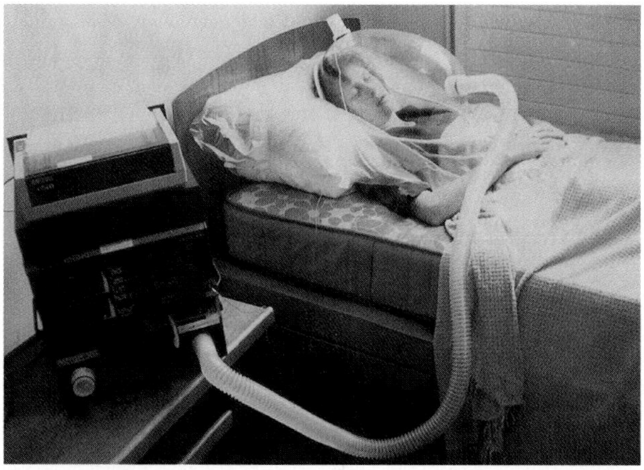

FIGURE 2-4 • Measuring resting metabolic rate (RMR) using a ventilated hood system. (Courtesy The Dunn Nutrition Centre, University of Cambridge, Cambridge, England.)

nation rates of the two isotopes are measured for 10 to 14 days by periodic sampling of body water from urine, saliva, or plasma. The difference between the two elimination rates is a measure of carbon dioxide production. Carbon dioxide production can then be equated to TEE using standard indirect calorimetric techniques for the calculation of energy expenditure.

The DLW technique has numerous advantages, which make it the ideal method for measuring TEE in various populations. First, it provides a measure of energy expenditure that incorporates all the components of TEE, REE, TEF, and EEPA. The administration is easy, and the person is able to engage in typical daily living activities throughout the measurement period. Therefore the technique provides a measure of the person's usual daily TEE, which is beneficial for those such as infants, young children, older adults, and disabled individuals, who cannot easily withstand the rigorous testing involved in the measurement of oxygen consumption during various activities. DLW also provides a method by which more subjective estimates of energy intakes (e.g., diet recalls and records) and energy expenditure (e.g., physical activity logs) can be validated (Schoeller, 1990). Most important, the method is accurate and has a precision of 2% to 8% (Schoeller, 1988).

However, the DLW technique also has drawbacks—namely, the expense of the stable isotopes and the expertise required to operate the highly sophisticated and costly mass spectrometer for the analysis of the isotope enrichments. These disadvantages make the DLW technique impractical for daily use by clinicians. However, DLW research studies have provided the data used to develop prediction equations to estimate total energy requirements (Institute of Medicine, 2002). These equations should be used only as a guide or starting point, after which the person must be monitored closely and interventions developed to promote optimal nutrition status.

Thermic Effect of Food

Actual measurement of the TEF is appropriate only for research purposes. For practical purposes, it is calculated as 10% of the sum of the RMR and the EEPA. The TEF, also referred as *postprandial thermogenesis,* is the increase in heat produced after the ingestion of a meal. Increases in heat produced after the consumption of food may last at least 5 hours (Reed and Hill, 1996) to support the metabolic processes involved in the digestion, absorption, transport, metabolism, and storage of energy from foods. Because the TEF concomitantly increases the BMR, the TEF is the energy expended in excess of BMR after a meal. Hence to measure the TEF, it is necessary to determine a baseline BMR and the energy expended in excess of BMR every 30 minutes for at least 5 hours after a meal.

Energy Expended in Physical Activity

Doubly Labeled Water

The caloric value of EEPA can be estimated using the DLW method in conjunction with indirect calorimetry. After the postprandial RMR (which includes a measure of the TEF) has been measured using indirect calorimetry, an estimated EEPA can be determined by subtracting the postprandial RMR from the TEE that was measured using DLW (Goran et al, 1995). This method is generally only used in research settings but can be used to validate other, more practical and easily administered methods of measuring physical activity.

Caltrac Monitor

Uniaxial monitors measure the degree and intensity of movement in a vertical plane. Resembling a pager worn on the hip, the uniaxial monitor is a portable device designed for children and adults to use to estimate EEPA. The accuracy of the Caltrac accelerometer (Muscle Dynamic Fitness Network, Torrance, Calif.) was found to be effective in measuring EEPA among school-age children within a supervised setting (Sallis et al, 1989). However, the Caltrac was not useful in assessing EEPA in free-living children (Johnson et al, 1998). Among adults, the Caltrac accelerometer was found to be an effective tool for measuring energy expenditure when compared with the DLW technique (Gretebeck et al, 1991, 1992). It may be acceptable for estimates of EEPA in groups of people, but it has limited use with individuals.

Tracmor Monitor

Because human movement is multidirectional, studies that measure movements on three different planes may be superior to those relying on one-plane measurements. A triaxial accelerometer monitor has three uniaxial accelerometers. The Tracmor (Philips Research, Eindhoven, The Netherlands) is a triaxial monitor with a data unit. Determined by DLW, the measurement of EEPA was found to be more accurate using the triaxial monitors than the uniaxial monitors (Bouten et al, 1996).

Heart Rate Monitor

A heart rate monitor is a simple to use and inexpensive device that estimates energy expenditure. In the past the validity of the equipment for monitoring sedentary intervals was questionable because of the uncertain relationship between heart rate and oxygen consumption. However, the use of a minute-by-minute heart rate monitor has been found to be a reliable method for estimating habitual TEE and physical activity level (PAL) in groups of free-living, healthy children but not for individuals (Livingstone et al, 1992).

Physical Activity Questionnaire

Physical activity questionnaires are easily used, inexpensive tools for gaining information about a person's activity level (Kriska and Caspersen, 1997; Philippaerts et al, 1999). DLW allows researchers to determine the validity of questionnaires. The Seven Day Recall and the Yale Physical Activity Survey are two questionnaires that have been shown to be valid (Bonnefoy et al, 2001). The Baecke questionnaire and an adapted version of the Tecumseh Community Health Study questionnaire have been shown to be useful for determining whether a group or an individual is active or inactive (Philippaerts et al, 1999).

ESTIMATING ENERGY REQUIREMENTS

Knowledge of energy requirements throughout the life cycle, to meet various physiologic conditions such as pregnancy and lactation, and for those with various diseases is essential for the promotion of optimal health. In the past the measurement of energy intake served as an important tool from which recommendations for energy requirements for all age groups were derived (World Health Organization [WHO], 1985). However, since the advent of the DLW technique, scientists have established energy requirements based on the actual measurement of TEE in free-living individuals.

Measuring Energy Intake

Traditionally, recommendations for energy requirements have been based on self-recorded estimates (e.g., diet records) or self-reported estimates (e.g., 24-hour recalls) of food intake. However, it is now well-accepted that these methods do not provide accurate or unbiased estimates of a person's energy intake and that underestimation of food intake is pervasive (Johnson, 2000). The percentage of people who underestimate, or underreport, their food intake ranges from 10% to 45%, depending on the person's age, sex, and body composition. Underestimating tends to increase as children age, is worse among women than men, and is more prevalent and severe among the obese in comparison with the lean (Johnson, 2000). This conclusion is confirmed by studies using the DLW technique, which measures TEE to assess the accuracy of estimates of energy intake (Schoeller, 1990).

Determining who is likely to underestimate energy intake is important. It is also necessary to identify the foods and food groups that are frequently underreported such as beer, chips, popcorn, pizza, pretzels, cookies and brownies, pancakes and waffles, cakes and pies, frozen dairy desserts, ready-to-eat cereals (and milk on cereal), meat mixtures, and condiments. Diet soft drinks are more likely to be recorded than nondiet (Krebs-Smith et al, 2000).

Until methods of determining energy intake are developed that minimize the problem of underreporting, it is no longer acceptable to base recommendations for energy requirements on estimates of energy intake (Black and Cole, 2000; Black et al, 1993; Livingstone, 1995). The World Health Organization (WHO, 1985) stated that "as a matter of principle, we believe the estimates of energy requirements should, as far as possible, be based on estimates of energy expenditure."

Measuring Basal and Resting Metabolic Rate

Over the years, several equations have been developed to measure the RMR. The Harris-Benedict equations, developed in 1919, are some of the most widely used equations in the United States (Harris and Benedict, 1919). The Harris-Benedict formulas have been found to overestimate REE by 7% to 24% (Daly et al, 1985; Owen et al, 1986, 1987). Recently, new BEE predictive equations have been formulated (Henry, 2000; Schofield, 1985).

Estimations of Energy Expenditure

The National Academy of Sciences, Institute of Medicine (IOM), and Food and Nutrition Board in partnership with Health Canada, developed the estimated energy requirement (EER) for men, women, children, and infants and for pregnant and lactating women (Institute of Medicine, 2002). Table 2-2 lists average Dietary Reference Intake (DRI) values for energy in healthy, active people of reference height, weight, and age for each life-stage group (Institute of Medicine, 2002). Supported by DLW studies, new prediction equations have been developed to estimate energy requirements for people according to their life-stage group. Box 2-1 lists the EER prediction equations for people of normal weight in the various life-stage groups. TEE prediction equations are also listed for various overweight and obese groups, as well as for weight maintenance in obese girls and boys. All equations have been developed to maintain current body weight and current levels of physical activity for all subsets of the population; they are not intended to promote weight loss (Institute of Medicine, 2002).

The EER incorporates age, weight, height, gender, and level of physical activity for people ages 3 years and older. Although variables such as age, gender, and feeding type (i.e., breast milk, formula) can impact TEE among infants and young children, weight has been determined as the sole predictor of TEE needs (Institute of Medicine, 2002). Beyond TEE requirements, additional calories to support the deposition of tissues needed for growth are required for infants and young children, children ages 3 through 18, and pregnant and lactating females; hence, the EER among these subsets of the population is the sum of TEE plus the caloric requirements for energy deposition. The prediction equations include a physical activity coefficient (PA) for all groups except infants and young children (see Box 2-1). PA coefficients correspond to a person's physical activity level (PAL). Four lifestyle categories of physical activity levels have been identified as *sedentary, low active, active,* and *very active.* The sedentary lifestyle category reflects the energy spent during activities of daily living. Lifestyle categories that include activity levels beyond sedentary living were determined according to the energy spent by an adult walking at a set pace (Institute of Medicine, 2002). Table 2-3 lists the PAL value ranges that correspond to the walking equivalents for each PAL lifestyle category. Thus low-active, active, and very active lifestyles correspond with an average weight adult walking, on average, 2, 7, and 17 miles per day (at 3 to 4 mph) respectively (Institute of Medicine, 2002).

TABLE 2-2 Dietary Reference Intake Values for Energy for Active Individuals*

		ACTIVE PAL EER (kcal/day)†	
LIFE-STAGE GROUP	**CRITERION**	**MALE**	**FEMALE**
Infants			
0-6 mo	Energy expenditure + Energy deposition	570	520 (3 mo)
7-12 mo	Energy expenditure + Energy deposition	743	676 (9 mo)
Children			
1-2 yr	Energy expenditure + Energy deposition	1046	992 (24 mo)
3-8 yr	Energy expenditure + Energy deposition	1742	1642 (6 yr)
9-13 yr	Energy expenditure + Energy deposition	2279	2071 (11 yr)
14-18 yr	Energy expenditure + Energy deposition	3152	2368 (16 yr)
Adults			
>18 yr	Energy expenditure	3067‡	2403‡ (19 yr)
Pregnant Women			
14-18 yr	Adolescent female EER + Change in TEE + Pregnancy energy deposition		
First trimester			2368 (16 yr)
Second trimester			2708 (16 yr)
Third trimester			2820 (16 yr)
19-50 yr	Adult female EER + Change in TEE + Pregnancy energy deposition		
First trimester			2403‡ (19 yr)
Second trimester			2743‡ (19 yr)
Third trimester			2855‡ (19 yr)
Lactating Women			
14-18 yr	Adolescent female EER + Milk energy output − Weight loss		
First 6 mo			2698 (16 yr)
Second 6 mo			2768 (16 yr)
19-50 yr	Adult female EER + Milk energy output − Weight loss		
First 6 mo			2733‡ (19 yr)
Second 6 mo			2803‡ (19 yr)

From Institute of Medicine of The National Academies: *Dietary reference intakes for energy, carbohydrate, fiber, fat, fatty acids, cholesterol, protein, and amino acids,* Washington, DC, 2002, The National Academies Press.
*For healthy active Americans and Canadians at the reference height and weight.
†*PAL,* Physical activity level; *EER,* estimated energy requirement; *TEE,* total energy expenditure.
‡Subtract 10 kcal/day for men and 7 kcal/day for women for each year of age above 19 years.

Box 2-1. Estimated Energy Expenditure* Prediction Equations at Four Physical Activity Levels†

EER for Infants and Young Children 0-2 Years (Within the 3rd-97th Percentile for Weight-for-Height)

EER = TEE‡ + Energy deposition

0-3 months	(89 × Weight of infant [kg] − 100) + 175 (kcal for energy deposition)
4-6 months	(89 × Weight of infant [kg] − 100) + 56 (kcal for energy deposition)
7-12 months	(89 × Weight of infant [kg] − 100) + 22 (kcal for energy deposition)
13-35 months	(89 × Weight of child [kg] − 100) + 20 (kcal for energy deposition)

EER for Boys 3-8 Years (Within the 5th-85th Percentile for BMI§)

EER = TEE + Energy deposition
EER = 88.5 − 61.9 × Age (yr) + PA × (26.7 × Weight [kg] + 903 × Height [m]) + 20 (kcal for energy deposition)

EER for Boys 9-18 Years (Within the 5th-85th Percentile for BMI)

EER = TEE + Energy deposition
EER = 88.5 − 61.9 × Age (yr) + PA × (26.7 × Weight [kg] + 903 × Height [m]) + 25 (kcal for energy deposition)

where

PA = Physical activity coefficient for boys 3-18 years:
PA = 1.0 if PAL is estimated to be ≥ 1.0 < 1.4 (Sedentary)
PA = 1.13 if PAL is estimated to be ≥ 1.4 < 1.6 (Low active)
PA = 1.26 if PAL is estimated to be ≥ 1.6 < 1.9 (Active)
PA = 1.42 if PAL is estimated to be ≥ 1.9 < 2.5 (Very active)

EER for Girls 3-8 Years (Within the 5th-85th Percentile for BMI)

EER = TEE + Energy deposition
EER = 135.3 − 30.8 × Age (yr) + PA × (10 × Weight [kg] + 934 × Height [m]) + 20 (kcal for energy deposition)

EER for Girls 9-18 Years (Within the 5th-85th Percentile for BMI)

EER = TEE + Energy deposition
EER = 135.3 − 30.8 × Age (yr) + PA × (10 × Weight [kg] + 934 × Height [m]) + 25 (kcal for energy deposition)

where

PA = Physical activity coefficient for girls 3-18 years:
PA = 1.0 if PAL is estimated to be ≥ 1.0 < 1.4 (Sedentary)
PA = 1.16 if PAL is estimated to be ≥ 1.4 < 1.6 (Low active)
PA = 1.31 if PAL is estimated to be ≥ 1.6 < 1.9 (Active)
PA = 1.56 if PAL is estimated to be ≥ 1.9 < 2.5 (Very active)

EER for Men 19 Years and Older (BMI 18.5-25 kg/m^2)

EER = TEE
EER = 662 − 9.53 × Age (yr) + PA × (15.91 × Weight [kg] + 539.6 × Height [m])

where

PA = Physical activity coefficient:
PA = 1.0 if PAL is estimated to be ≥ 1.0 < 1.4 (Sedentary)
PA = 1.11 if PAL is estimated to be ≥ 1.4 < 1.6 (Low active)
PA = 1.25 if PAL is estimated to be ≥ 1.6 < 1.9 (Active)
PA = 1.48 if PAL is estimated to be ≥ 1.9 < 2.5 (Very active)

From Institute of Medicine, Food and Nutrition Board: *Dietary reference intakes for energy, carbohydrate, fiber, fat, fatty acids, cholesterol, protein, and amino acids,* Washington, DC, 2002, The National Academies Press, www.nap.edu.

*Estimated energy expenditure (EER) is the average dietary energy intake that is predicted to maintain energy balance in a healthy adult of a defined age, gender, weight, height, and level of physical activity consistent with good health. In children and pregnant and lactating women, the EER includes the needs associated with the deposition of tissues or the secretion of milk at rates consistent with good health.

†Physical activity level (PAL) is the physical activity level that is the ratio of the total energy expenditure to the basal energy expenditure.

‡Total energy expenditure (TEE) is the sum of the resting energy expenditure, energy expended in physical activity, and the thermic effect of food.

§Body mass index (BMI) is determined by dividing the weight (in kilograms) by the square of the height (in meters).

Box 2-1. Estimated Energy Expenditure* Prediction Equations at Four Physical Activity Levels†—cont'd

EER for Women 19 Years and Older (BMI 18.5-25 kg/m^2)

EER = TEE
EER = 354 − 6.91 × Age (yr) + PA × (9.36 × Weight [kg] + 726 × Height [m])
where
PA = Physical activity coefficient:
PA = 1.0 if PAL is estimated to be ≥ 1.0 < 1.4 (Sedentary)
PA = 1.12 if PAL is estimated to be ≥ 1.4 < 1.6 (Low active)
PA = 1.27 if PAL is estimated to be ≥ 1.6 < 1.9 (Active)
PA = 1.45 if PAL is estimated to be ≥ 1.9 < 2.5 (Very active)

EER for Pregnant Women

14-18 years: EER = Adolescent EER + Pregnancy energy deposition
First trimester = Adolescent EER + 0 (Pregnancy energy deposition)
Second trimester = Adolescent EER + 160 kcal (8 kcal/wk × 20 wk) + 180 kcal
Third trimester = Adolescent EER + 272 kcal (8 kcal/wk × 34 wk) + 180 kcal

19-50 years: EER = Adult EER + Pregnancy energy deposition
First trimester = Adult EER + 0 (Pregnancy energy deposition)
Second trimester = Adult EER + 160 kcal (8 kcal/wk × 20 wk) + 180 kcal
Third trimester = Adult EER + 272 kcal (8 kcal/wk × 34 wk) + 180 kcal

EER for Lactating Women

14-18 years: EER = Adolescent EER + Milk energy output − Weight loss
First 6 months = Adolescent EER + 500 − 170 (Milk energy output − Weight loss)
Second 6 months = Adolescent EER + 400 − 0 (Milk energy output − Weight loss)

19-50 years: EAR = Adult EER + Milk energy output − Weight loss
First 6 months = Adult EER + 500 − 170 (Milk energy output − Weight loss)
Second 6 months = Adult EER + 400 − 0 (Milk energy output − Weight loss)

Weight Maintenance TEE for Overweight and At-Risk for Overweight Boys 3-18 Years (BMI >85th Percentile for Overweight)

TEE = 114 − 50.9 × Age (yr) + PA × (19.5 × Weight [kg] + 1161.4 × Height [m])
where
PA = Physical activity coefficient:
PA = 1.0 if PAL is estimated to be ≥ 1.0 < 1.4 (Sedentary)
PA = 1.12 if PAL is estimated to be ≥ 1.4 < 1.6 (Low active)
PA = 1.24 if PAL is estimated to be ≥ 1.6 < 1.9 (Active)
PA = 1.45 if PAL is estimated to be ≥ 1.9 < 2.5 (Very active)

Weight Maintenance TEE for Overweight and At-Risk for Overweight Girls 3-18 Years (BMI >85th Percentile for Overweight)

TEE = 389 − 41.2 × Age (yr) + PA × (15 × Weight [kg] + 701.6 × Height [m])
where
PA = Physical activity coefficient:
PA = 1.0 if PAL is estimated to be ≥ 1.0 < 1.4 (Sedentary)
PA = 1.18 if PAL is estimated to be ≥ 1.4 < 1.6 (Low active)
PA = 1.35 if PAL is estimated to be ≥ 1.6 < 1.9 (Active)
PA = 1.60 if PAL is estimated to be ≥ 1.9 < 2.5 (Very active)

Overweight and Obese Men 19 Years and Older (BMI ≥25 kg/m^2)

TEE = 1086 − 10.1 × Age (yr) + PA × (13.7 × Weight [kg] + 416 × Height [m])
where
PA = Physical activity coefficient:
PA = 1.0 if PAL is estimated to be ≥ 1.0 < 1.4 (Sedentary)
PA = 1.12 if PAL is estimated to be ≥ 1.4 < 1.6 (Low active)
PA = 1.29 if PAL is estimated to be ≥ 1.6 < 1.9 (Active)
PA = 1.59 if PAL is estimated to be ≥ 1.9 < 2.5 (Very active)

Continued

Box 2-1. Estimated Energy Expenditure* Prediction Equations at Four Physical Activity Levels†—cont'd

Overweight and Obese Women 19 Years and Older (BMI ≥25 kg/m²)

TEE = 448 − 7.95 × Age (yr) + PA × (11.4 × Weight [kg] + 619 × Height [m])
where
PA = Physical activity coefficient:
PA = 1.0 if PAL is estimated to be ≥ 1.0 < 1.4 (Sedentary)
PA = 1.16 if PAL is estimated to be ≥ 1.4 < 1.6 (Low active)
PA = 1.27 if PAL is estimated to be ≥ 1.6 < 1.9 (Active)
PA = 1.44 if PAL is estimated to be ≥ 1.9 < 2.5 (Very active)

Normal and Overweight or Obese Men 19 Years and Older (BMI ≥18.5 kg/m²)

TEE = 864 − 9.72 × Age (yr) + PA × (14.2 × Weight [kg] + 503 × Height [m])
where
PA = Physical activity coefficient:
PA = 1.0 if PAL is estimated to be ≥ 1.0 < 1.4 (Sedentary)
PA = 1.12 if PAL is estimated to be ≥ 1.4 < 1.6 (Low active)
PA = 1.27 if PAL is estimated to be ≥ 1.6 < 1.9 (Active)
PA = 1.54 if PAL is estimated to be ≥ 1.9 < 2.5 (Very active)

Normal and Overweight or Obese Women 19 Years and Older (BMI ≥18.5 kg/m²)

TEE = 387 − 7.31 × Age (yr) + PA × (10.9 × Weight [kg] + 660.7 × Height [m])
where
PA = Physical activity coefficient:
PA = 1.0 if PAL is estimated to be ≥ 1.0 < 1.4 (Sedentary)
PA = 1.14 if PAL is estimated to be ≥ 1.4 < 1.6 (Low active)
PA = 1.27 if PAL is estimated to be ≥ 1.6 < 1.9 (Active)
PA = 1.45 if PAL is estimated to be ≥ 1.9 < 2.5 (Very active)

*Estimated energy expenditure (EER) is the average dietary energy intake that is predicted to maintain energy balance in a healthy adult of a defined age, gender, weight, height, and level of physical activity consistent with good health. In children and pregnant and lactating women, the EER includes the needs associated with the deposition of tissues or the secretion of milk at rates consistent with good health.
†Physical activity level (PAL) is the physical activity level that is the ratio of the total energy expenditure to the basal energy expenditure.

TABLE 2-3 Physical Activity Level Categories and Walking Equivalence

PAL CATEGORY	PAL VALUES	WALKING EQUIVALENCE (miles/day at 3-4 mph)*
Sedentary	1-1.39	
Low active	1.4-1.59	1.5, 2.2, 2.9 for PAL = 1.5
Active	1.6-1.89	3, 4.4, 5.8 for PAL = 1.6
		5.3, 7.3, 9.9 for PAL = 1.75
Very active	1.9-2.5	7.5, 10.3, 14 for PAL = 1.9
		12.3, 16.7, 22.5 for PAL = 2.2
		17, 23, 31 for PAL = 2.5

From Institute of Medicine of The National Academies: *Dietary reference intakes for energy, carbohydrate, fiber, fat, fatty acids, cholesterol, protein, and amino acids,* Washington, DC, 2002, The National Academies Press.
*In addition to energy spent for the generally unscheduled activities that are part of a normal daily life. The low, middle, and high miles/day values apply to relatively heavyweight (120-kg), midweight (70-kg), and lightweight (44-kg) individuals, respectively.

Estimated Energy Expended in Physical Activity

A nutrition professional can determine EEPA with two methods: (1) the method shown in Appendix 52, which represents energy spent during common activities and incorporates body weight and the duration of time for each activity as variables, and (2) the method shown in Table 2-4, which represents energy spent by adults during various *intensities* of physical activity—energy that is expressed as metabolic equivalents (METs) (Institute of Medicine, 2002).

Estimating Energy Expenditure of Selected Activities Using Metabolic Equivalents

Energy expenditure (EE) is determined by the amount of oxygen metabolized by the body. Metabolic equivalents (METs) are units of measure that correspond to a person's metabolic rate during selected physical activities of varying intensities and are expressed as multiples of RMR (see Table 2-4) (Institute of Medicine, 2002). A MET value of 1 is the oxygen metabolized at rest (3.5 ml of oxygen per kilogram of body weight per minute in adults) and can be expressed as 1 kcal per kilogram body weight per hour (1 kcal × Body weight (kg) × Hour) (Ainsworth et al, 1993). Thus the EE of adults can be estimated using MET values by multiplying body weight in kilograms by the MET value and the duration of the activity. For example, an adult who weighs 65 kg and is walking moderately at a pace of 4 mph (which is a MET value

TABLE 2-4 Intensity and Impact of Various Activities on Physical Activity Level in Adults*

PHYSICAL ACTIVITY	METs†	Δ PAL/10 MIN‡	Δ PAL/HR‡
Daily Activities			
Lying quietly	1	0	0
Riding in a car	1	0	0
Light activity while sitting	1.5	0.005	0.03
Watering plants	2.5	0.014	0.09
Walking the dog	3	0.019	0.11
Vacuuming	3.5	0.024	0.14
Doing household tasks (moderate effort)	3.5	0.024	0.14
Gardening (no lifting)	4.4	0.032	0.19
Mowing lawn (power mower)	4.5	0.033	0.20
Leisure Activities: Mild			
Walking (2 mph)	2.5	0.014	0.09
Canoeing (leisurely)	2.5	0.014	0.09
Golfing (with cart)	2.5	0.014	0.09
Dancing (ballroom)	2.9	0.018	0.11
Leisure Activities: Moderate			
Walking (3 mph)	3.3	0.022	0.13
Cycling (leisurely)	3.5	0.024	0.14
Performing calisthenics (no weight)	4	0.029	0.17
Walking (4 mph)	4.5	0.033	0.20
Leisure Activities: Vigorous			
Chopping wood	4.9	0.037	0.22
Playing tennis (doubles)	5	0.038	0.23
Ice skating	5.5	0.043	0.26
Cycling (moderate)	5.7	0.045	0.27
Skiing (downhill or water)	6.8	0.055	0.33
Swimming	7	0.057	0.34
Climbing hills (5-kg load)	7.4	0.061	0.37
Walking (5 mph)	8	0.067	0.40
Jogging (10-minute mile)	10.2	0.088	0.53
Skipping rope	12	0.105	0.63

Modified from Institute of Medicine of The National Academies: *Dietary reference intakes for energy, carbohydrate, fiber, fat, fatty acids, protein, and amino acids,* Washington, DC, 2002, The National Academies Press.
*Physical activity level (PAL) is the physical activity level that is the ratio of the total energy expenditure (TEE) to the basal energy expenditure (BEE).
†*METs,* Metabolic equivalents. METs are multiples of an individual's resting oxygen uptakes, defined as the rate of oxygen (O_2) consumption of 3.5 ml of O_2/min/kg body weight in adults.
‡The Δ PAL is the allowance made to include the delayed effect of physical activity in causing excess postexercise oxygen consumption (EPOC) and the dissipation of some of the food energy consumed through the thermic effect of food (TEF).

of 4.5) for 1 hour would expend 293 calories (65 kg × 4.5 × 1 = 293).

In addition, the *impact* of various activities on an adult's physical activity level (PAL), also referred to as *the change in a physical activity level (Δ PAL),* is given in Table 2-4 (Institute of Medicine, 2002). The PAL value for various activities performed throughout the day can be determined by adding the Δ PAL for each activity. Because PAL is the ratio of TEE to BEE, it is necessary to include the TEF when calculating PAL (Institute of Medicine, 2002). To determine the PAL value for an adult walking for 1 hour at 4 mph and then skiing for 1 hour, take the sum of the activities (0.20 + 0.33 [from Table 2-4]) plus the BEE (1.0) adjusted for the 10% TEF (1.1) so that the final formula would be .53 + 1.1 = 1.63. The PAL value of 1.6 represents the energy spent for the described activities in addition to the energy needs of daily living and consequently corresponds to an *active* lifestyle (see Table 2-3). The PA coefficient that corresponds to an *active* lifestyle PAL can then be included when determining EER. For example, the EER for a 30-year-old woman who weighs 65 kg and is 1.77 m tall and has an active lifestyle can be estimated by using the EER equation for women 19 years and older (see Box 2-1) (Institute of Medicine, 2002) with the PA coefficient that corresponds with an active lifestyle.

$$EER = 354 - 6.91 \times Age\ (yr) + PA \times (9.36 \times Weight\ [kg] + 726 \times Height\ [m])$$
$$EER = 354 - (6.91 \times 30) + 1.27 \times ([9.36 \times 65] + [726 \times 1.77])$$
$$EER = 2551\ kcal$$

Physical Activity in Children

Energy spent during various activities and the intensity and impact of selected activities can also be determined for children and teens (Institute of Medicine, 2002).

CALCULATING FOOD ENERGY

The total energy available from a food is measured with a bomb calorimeter. This device consists of a

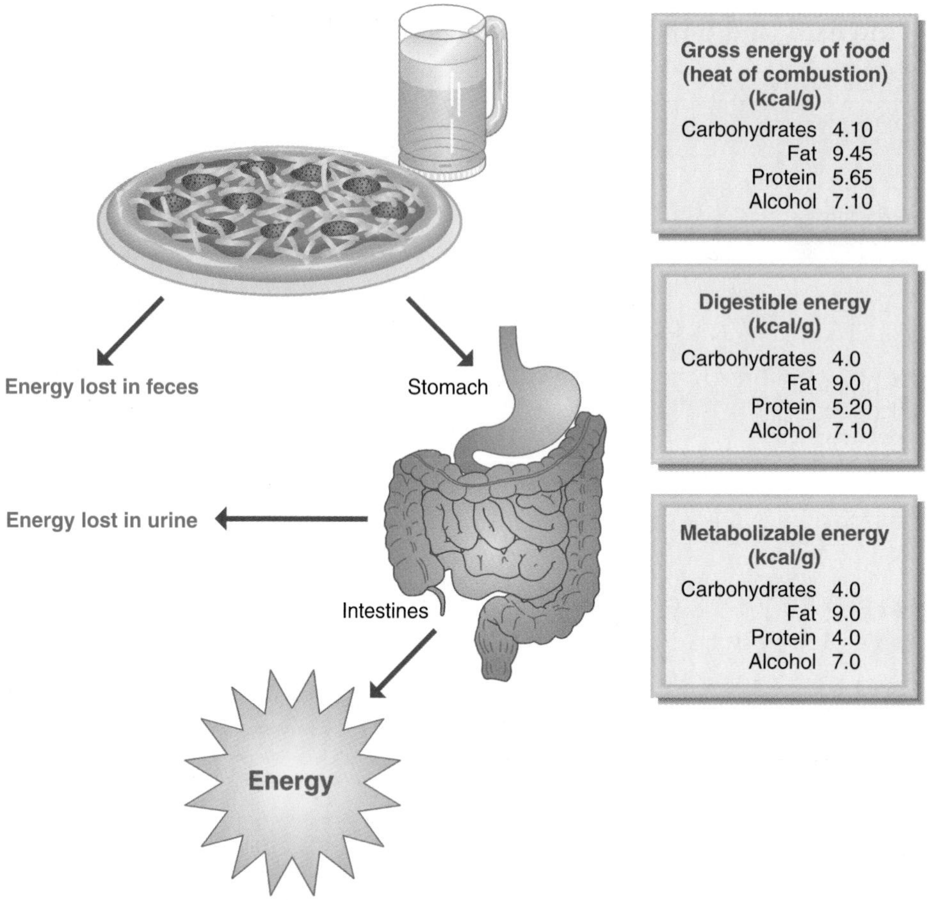

FIGURE 2-5 • Energy value of food.

closed container in which a weighed food sample, ignited with an electric spark, is burned in an oxygenated atmosphere. The container is immersed in a known volume of water, and the rise in the temperature of the water after igniting the food is used to calculate the heat energy generated.

Not all of the energy in foods and alcohol is available to the body's cells. The processes of digestion and absorption are not completely efficient, and the nitrogenous portion of amino acids is not oxidized but is excreted in the form of urea. Therefore the biologically available energy from foods and alcohol is expressed in values rounded off slightly below those obtained using the calorimeter. These values for protein, fat, carbohydrate, and alcohol (Figure 2-5) are 4, 9, 4, and 7 kcal/g, respectively. The figure of 2 kcal/g has been proposed for fiber because of the "unavailable carbohydrate" that resists digestion and absorption (Guenther and Jensen, 2000).

Although the energy value of each nutrient is known precisely, only a few foods such as oils and sugars are made up of a single nutrient. More commonly, foods contain a mixture of protein, fat, and carbohydrate. For example, the energy value of one medium-size (50-g) egg calculated in terms of weight is derived from protein (13%), fat (12%), and carbohydrate (1%) as follows:

Protein: 13% × 50 g = 6.5 g × 4 kcal/g = 26 kcal
Fat: 12% × 50 g = 6 g × 9 kcal/g = 54 kcal
Carbohydrate:
1% × 50 g = 0.5 g × 4 kcal/g = 2 kcal
TOTAL = 82 kcal

Energy values of foods based on chemical analyses may be obtained from the U.S. Department of Agriculture's (USDA's) Nutrient Data Laboratory Web site: http://www.nal.usda.gov/fnic/foodcomp. Another source of nutrient values for common serving sizes of foods is Bowes and Church's *Food Values of Portions Commonly Used* (Pennington, 1998). Many computer software programs that use the USDA nutrient database as the standard reference are also available. In addition, the diet analysis program of the Department of Nutrition and Food Sciences at the University of Vermont, is available at their Web site: http://nutrition.uvm.edu/htm/fs_inter.htm.

Kilocalories in alcoholic beverages may be calculated as shown in *Clinical Insight:* Calculation of Energy Value of Alcoholic Beverages and Mixes; see also Appendix 44.

CLINICAL INSIGHT

Calculation of Energy Value of Alcoholic Beverages and Mixes

The energy value of alcoholic beverages, which is expressed in kilocalories, can be determined by the following equation (Gastineau, 1976):

Kilocalories = Amount of beverage (oz) × Proof × 0.8 kcal/proof/1 oz

where

Proof = The proportion of alcohol to water or other liquids in an alcoholic beverage. (The standard in the United States defines 100-proof as being equal to 50% of ethyl alcohol by volume.)

To determine the percentage of ethyl alcohol in a beverage, divide the proof value by 2. For example, 86-proof whiskey contains 43% ethyl alcohol.

The latter part of the equation—0.8 kcal/proof/1 oz—is the factor that accounts for the caloric density of alcohol (7 kcal/g) and the fact that not all of the alcohol in liquor is available for energy. For example, the number of kilocalories in 1½ oz of 86-proof whiskey would be determined as follows:

1½ oz × 86-proof × 0.8 kcal/proof/1 oz = 103 kcal

Clinical Scenario

Allen has been active all of his life because of his work. Now at the age of 54, he wants to start a structured exercise program that includes walking three times a week at a moderate pace of 3 mph and swimming twice a week. After obtaining his physician's approval for this increase in activity, Allen schedules an appointment to see you, the nutrition counselor. He is 5 ft, 8 in tall, weighs 175 lb, and has no prior medical conditions that are a factor in his health care treatment. He is a landscape architect who has a moderate physical activity level during the workday.

1. What information is needed to give Allen appropriate nutritional guidance?
2. What specific nutrition advice may be useful to Allen on days that he is more active than usual?
3. Allen thinks he should double his energy intake because of his increase in activity. Estimate Allen's energy requirements (EER) for a typical workday and for days that include the selected physical activities.

Relevant Web Sites

Centers for Disease Control
www.cdc.gov/needphp/dnpa
National Academy Press—Publisher of Institute of Medicine DRIs for Energy
www.nal.usda.gov/fnic/foodcomp/
National Institutes of Health—Bioelectrical Impedance Analysis
http://consensus.nih.gov/ta/015/015_statement.htm
U.S. Department of Agriculture Food Composition Tables
www.nal.usda.gov/fnic/foodcomp/www.nap.edu/books/0309085373/html/
University of Vermont Body Composition and Diet Analysis
http://nutrition.uvm.edu/bodycomp
http://nutrition.uvm.edu/htm/fs_inter.htm

Cited References

Ainsworth BE et al: Compendium of physical activities: classification of energy costs of human physical activities, *Med Sci Sports Exerc* 25:71, 1993.

Bahr R et al: Effect of duration of exercise on excess postexercise O_2 consumption, *J Appl Physiol* 62:485, 1987.

Bahr R et al: Effect of supramaximal exercise on excess postexercise O_2 consumption, *Med Sci Sports Exerc* 24:66, 1992.

Black AE, Cole TJ: Within- and between-subject variation in energy expenditure measured by the doubly labeled water technique: implications for validating reported dietary energy intake, *Eur J Clin Nutr* 54:386, 2000.

Black AE et al: Measurements of total energy expenditure provide insights into the validity of dietary measurements of energy intake, *J Am Diet Assoc* 93:572, 1993.

Bonnefoy M et al: Simultaneous validation of ten physical activity questionnaires in older men: a doubly labeled water study, *JAGS* 49:28, 2001.

Bouten C et al: Daily physical activity assessment: comparison between movement registration and doubly labeled water, *J Appl Physiol* 81:1019, 1996.

Callahan T: Personal communication, May 29, 2002.

Daly JM et al: Human energy requirements: overestimation by widely used prediction equation, *Am J Clin Nutr* 42:1170, 1985.

Dulloo AG et al: Normal caffeine consumption: influence on thermogenesis and daily energy expenditure in lean and postobese human volunteers, *Am J Clin Nutr* 49:44, 1989.

Durnin JVGA: Energy requirements: general principles, *Eur J Clin Nutr* 50(suppl 1):2, 1996.

Gastineau CF: Alcohol and calories. *Mayo Clin Proc* 51(2):88, 1976.

Goldberg GR et al: Longitudinal assessment of energy expenditure in pregnancy by the doubly labeled water method, *Am J Clin Nutr* 57:494, 1993.

Goran MI et al: Energy requirements across the life span: new findings based on measurement of total energy expenditure with doubly labeled water, *Nutr Res* 15:115, 1995.

Gretebeck R et al: Comparison of the doubly labeled water method for measuring energy expenditure with Caltrac Accelerometer recordings, *Med Sci Sports Exerc* 23(suppl):60, 1991.

Gretebeck R et al: Assessment of energy expenditure in active older women using doubly labeled water and Caltrac recordings, *Med Sci Sports Exerc* 23(suppl):68, 1992.

Guenther PM, Jensen HH: Estimating energy contributed by fiber using a general factor of 2 vs. 4 kcal/g, *J Am Diet Assoc* 100:944, 2000.

Harris JA, Benedict FG: *A biometric study of basal metabolism in man*, Pub No. 279, Washington, DC, 1919, Carnegie Institute of Washington.

Henry CJK: Mechanisms of changes in basal metabolism during ageing, *Eur J Clin Nutr* 54(suppl 3):77, 2000.
Hofstetter A: Increased 24-hour energy expenditure in cigarette smokers, *N Engl J Med* 314:79, 1986.
Horton T, Geissler C: Effect of habitual exercise on daily energy expenditure and metabolic rate during standardized activity, *Am J Clin Nutr* 59:13, 1994.
Institute of Medicine, Food and Nutrition Board: *Dietary reference intakes: for energy, carbohydrate, fiber, fat, fatty acids, cholesterol, protein, and amino acids,* Washington, DC, 2002, The National Academies Press.
Johnson RK: What are people *really* eating, and why does it matter? *Nutr Today* 35:40, 2000.
Johnson RK et al: Physical activity related energy expenditure in children by doubly labeled water as compared with the Caltrac accelerometer, *Int J Obes Relat Metab Disord* 22:1046, 1998.
Jorgensen J et al: Resting metabolic rate in healthy adults: relation to growth hormone status and leptin levels, *Metabolism* 47:1134, 1998.
Krebs-Smith SM et al: Low energy reporters vs. others: a comparison of reported food intakes, *Eur J Clin Nutr* 54:281, 2000.
Kriska A, Caspersen C: Introduction to a collection of physical activity questionnaires, *Med Sci Sports Exerc* 29:3-201, 1997.
Laessle RG et al: A comparison of resting metabolic rate, self-rated food intake, growth hormone, and insulin levels in obese and nonobese preadolescents, *Physiol Behav* 61:725, 1997.
Livingstone MBE: Assessment of food intake: are we measuring what people eat? *Br J Biomed Sci* 52:58, 1995.
Livingstone MBE et al: Daily energy expenditure in free-living children: comparison of heart-rate monitoring with the doubly labeled water method, *Am J Clin Nutr* 56:343, 1992.
McCrory P et al: Energy balance, food intake and obesity. In Hills AP, Wahlqvist ML, eds: *Exercise and obesity,* London, 1994, Smith-Gordon.
Owen OE et al: A reappraisal of caloric requirements in healthy women, *Am J Clin Nutr* 44:1, 1986.
Owen OE et al: A reappraisal of the caloric requirements of men, *Am J Clin Nutr* 46:875, 1987.
Pennington JA: *Bowes and Church's food values of portions commonly used,* ed 17, Philadelphia, 1998, Lippincott.
Philippaerts RM et al: Doubly labeled water validation of three physical activity questionnaires, *Int J Sports Med* 20:284, 1999.
Pintauro S, Buzzell P: *Methods of body composition analysis tutorials,* 1999. http://nutrition.uvm.edu/bodycomp.
Poehlman ET: Regulation of energy expenditure in aging humans, *Geriatr Biosci* 41:552, 1993.
Poehlman ET, Horton ES: Energy needs: assessment and requirements in humans. In Bloch AS, Shils ME, eds: *Modern nutrition in health and disease,* Baltimore, 1998, Williams & Wilkins.
Prentice AM: All calories are not equal, *International dialogue on carbohydrates* 5(4):1, 1995.
Reed GW, Hill JO: Measuring the thermic effect of food, *Am J Clin Nutr* 63:164, 1996.
Roberts SB, Young VR: Energy costs of fat and protein deposition in the human infant, *Am J Clin Nutr* 48:951, 1988.
Sallis JF et al: The Caltrac accelerometer as a physical activity monitor for school-age children, *Med Sci Sports Exerc* 22:698-703, 1989.
Schoeller DA: Measurement of energy expenditure in free-living humans by using doubly labeled water, *J Nutr* 118:1278, 1988.
Schoeller DA: How accurate is self-reported dietary energy intake? *Nutr Rev* 48:373, 1990.
Schofield WN: Predicting basal metabolic rate, new standards and review of previous work, *Hum Nutr Clin Nutr* 39(suppl 1):5-41, 1985.
Shetty PS et al: Energy requirements of adults: an update on basal metabolic rates (BMRs) and physical activity levels (PALs), *Eur J Clin Nutr* 50(suppl 1):11, 1996.
Torun B et al: Energy requirements and dietary energy recommendations for children and adolescents 1 to 18 years old, *Eur J Clin Nutr* 50(suppl 1):37, 1996.
Webb P: 24-hour energy expenditure and the menstrual cycle, *Am J Clin Nutr* 44:614, 1986.
Whitney EN, Rolfes SR: *Understanding nutrition,* ed 9, Belmont, Calif, 2002, Wadsworth-Thomson Learning.
World Health Organization: *Energy and protein requirements.* Report of a Joint Food and Agriculture Organization/World Health Organization/United Nations University (FAO/WHO/UNU) Expert Consultation, Technical Report Series 724, Geneva, 1985, WHO.

Additional References

Defining energy for a new millennium: Proceedings of a symposium. Washington, DC, USA. April 4-5, 2000, *Nutr Rev* 59(1 pt 2):S1-39, 2001.
Friedman A, Johnson RK: Doubly labeled water: new advances and applications for the practitioner, *Nutr Today* 37:243-249, 2002.
Johnson RK: Dietary intake—how do we measure what people are really eating? *Obes Res* 10(suppl 1):63, 2002.

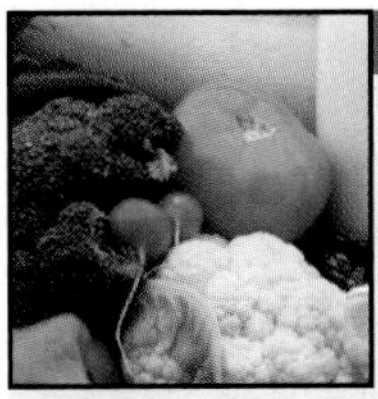

CHAPTER 3

Macronutrients: Carbohydrates, Proteins, and Lipids

SUSAN ETTINGER, PhD, RD

CHAPTER OUTLINE

- Carbohydrates
- Fats and Lipids
- Amino Acids and Protein
- Macronutrient Use and Storage in the Fed State
- Macronutrient Catabolism in the Fasted State

KEY TERMS

acetyl coenzyme a (acetyl CoA)–a molecule produced by fatty acid oxidation

amino acid–an organic compound containing an amino (NH_2) group and a carboxyl (COOH) group; links with other amino acids to form proteins

amino acid score–a method of protein evaluation in which the milligrams of the limiting essential amino acid in the test protein are divided by the milligrams of the same essential amino acid in the reference protein

amylopectin–a form of starch made up of highly branched glucose polymers

amylose–a form of starch made up of long, straight chains of glucose units

carnitine–a required cofactor derived from the essential amino acids methionine and lysine; facilitates transfer of long-chain fatty acids across the mitochondrial membranes for use as an energy source

cellulose–a carbohydrate made of long, straight glucose polymers in β linkage that resists hydrolysis in the human digestive tract; a dietary fiber

chitin–a homopolymer of *N*-acetylglucosamine in the exoskeleton of invertebrates; sometimes included in food products as *chitosan,* a fiber component

cholesterol–a sterol found in cell membranes of all animal tissues that is also necessary for production of bile and steroid hormones

chylomicrons–lipoprotein particles formed in the intestine after lipid absorption to transport dietary triglycerides and cholesterol through the lymph and into the systemic circulation

deamination–removal of nitrogen groups from organic molecules

denaturation–"unraveling," or breaking down, of the tertiary structure of proteins by mechanical agitation, heat, cold, acidity, or alkalinity

dextrin–an intermediate product of starch hydrolysis

dextrose–glucose produced by the hydrolysis of cornstarch

dietary fiber–the amount of plant material remaining after treatment with digestive enzymes and reduction with acid and alkali; may be soluble or insoluble

diacylglycerols (diglycerides)–lipids with only two fatty acids attached to the glycerol molecule

disaccharides–sugars capable of being hydrolyzed into two monosaccharide molecules

essential amino acids–amino acids for which bodily synthesis is inadequate to meet metabolic needs and that must be supplied in the diet: threonine, tryptophan, histidine, lysine, leucine, isoleucine, methionine, valine, and phenylalanine; formerly called an "indispensable amino acid"

essential fatty acid–a fatty acid the body needs but cannot synthesize; the primary EFAs are linoleic and α-linolenic acids

fructooligosaccharides–nonabsorbed polymers of fructose; support the growth of beneficial colonic bacteria

fructose–a monosaccharide in fruit, honey, and some vegetables; the sweetest of the monosaccharides

galactose–a monosaccharide produced by the hydrolysis of lactose by digestive enzymes

KEY TERMS—Continued

glucose–the main monosaccharide in blood and an important source of energy for living organisms; usually found as a disaccharide linked to fructose (sucrose), galactose (lactose), or glucose (maltose).

glycemic index–the ranking of different dietary carbohydrates on their ability to raise blood glucose levels as compared with a reference food

glycogen–a branched-chain glucose polymer used for glucose storage in animals

glycolipids–membrane lipids with one or more sugar molecules attached to the polar head group; high concentrations in the brain

hydrogenation–the process of adding hydrogen across the unsaturated fatty acid double bond; commercial hydrogenation of oils increases saturation and makes the oil more solid at room temperature

isoprenoids–members of a large family of lipids with a carbon skeleton based on five-carbon isoprene units with alternating single- and double-bond structure (conjugated double bonds); long isoprenoid structures function as antioxidants by quenching free radicals; examples include fat-soluble vitamins, carotenoids, and other phytochemicals—lycopene and limonene—as well as steroid hormones

ketosis–a metabolic condition in which ketone bodies are produced more rapidly than they are used

ketone bodies–three compounds (acetoacetic acid, acetone, and β-hydroxybutyric acid) formed by linking two acetyl coenzyme A (acetyl CoA) groups

lactose–the principal sugar in mammalian milk; a disaccharide composed of glucose and galactose

lecithin (phosphatidylcholine)–a phospholipid containing choline; found in the membranes of biologic organisms; is part of bile, where it emulsifies fats, and is part of lipoproteins, where it transports triglyceride and cholesterol

lignin–a woody fiber found in the stems and seeds of fruits and vegetables and in the bran layer of cereals; because of conjugated double bonds, is an excellent antioxidant; some, such as that found in flaxseed, have phytoestrogen activity

limiting amino acid–an amino acid in short supply as a precursor for protein synthesis; lack of a specific limiting amino acid restricts the level of protein synthesis in the body

macronutrients–macromolecules in plant and animal structures that can be digested, absorbed, and used by another organism as energy sources and as substrates for synthesis of the carbohydrates, fats, and proteins required to maintain cell and system integrity

medium-chain triglyceride (MCT)–a fat with fatty acid chain lengths of between 6 and 12 carbons, which are short enough to be water soluble; requires less bile salt for solubilization, is not reesterified in the enterocyte, and is transported as free fatty acid bound to albumin through the portal system

monoacylglycerols (monoglycerides)–lipids with only one fatty acid attached to the glycerol molecule

monosaccharides–the simplest sugar units with the formula $(CH_2O)n$

monounsaturated fatty acids (MFAs)–fatty acids containing one double bond

nonessential amino acids–amino acids with a carbon skeleton made in the body; if needed, the body can add an amino group to endogenous intermediates to form the nonessential amino acids

omega-3 fatty acid–a fatty acid with the first double bond located at the third carbon from the methyl end (e.g., eicosapentaenoic acid [C20:5 ω-3])

omega-6 fatty acid–a fatty acid with the first double bond located at the sixth carbon from the methyl end (e.g., linoleic acid [C18:2 ω-6])

peptide bond–a chemical bond between two amino acids; links amino acids into proteins

phospholipid–a lipid molecule used to construct biologic membranes; composed of two fatty acids and one of several polar groups linked to glycerol phosphate

polysaccharide–a carbohydrate polymer with more than 10 monosaccharide units

polyunsaturated fatty acids (PUFAs)–fatty acids containing at least two double bonds

proteins–complex nitrogenous compounds made up of amino acids in peptide linkages

protein digestibility corrected amino acid score (PDCAAS)–the official assay for evaluating protein quality

resistant starch–starch that resists digestive enzyme action and reaches the colon; a starch encased in a nondigestible plant seed coat or modified by cooking or processing can be resistant

saturated fatty acid (SFA)–a fatty acid in which all available carbon binding sites are saturated with hydrogen

short-chain fatty acids (SCFAS)–fatty acids with 4 to 6 carbons; the fatty acids acetate (2 carbons), butyrate (4 carbons), and proprionate (3 carbons), which account for 85% of all SCFAs produced in the human colon; are readily absorbed by the intestinal and colonic mucosa

sorbitol–a sugar alcohol occurring naturally in fruits; in mammals, sorbitol is found in some tissues such as the lens of the eye

structured lipid–a synthetic triglyceride with medium-chain fatty acids and long-chain fatty acids esterified to glycerol; used in parenteral nutrition formulas

sucrose–a disaccharide composed of one glucose unit and one fructose unit; the major form in which glucose is transported between plant cells; ordinary table sugar

transamination–reversible transfer of an amino group between an amino acid and a keto acid

***trans*-fatty acid**–a stereoisomer of the naturally occurring *cis*-fatty acid in which hydrogen is added back across the double bond; results from a hydrogenation process and is naturally occurring to a limited extent in milk and in meat from ruminants, where microflora convert *cis*- to *trans*-fatty acids

triglyceride (triacylglycerol)–a lipid consisting of three fatty acid chains esterified to a glycerol phosphate molecule

urea–product of the urea cycle containing two nitrogen atoms and carbon dioxide; the chief form in which nitrogenous end products are excreted in terrestrial animals

All *organotrophic* organisms (derived from the Greek word *trophe,* meaning "food") ultimately obtain energy from the sun. Photosynthesis describes the sequential process through which green plants transduce light energy into chemical energy. The plant stores energy within carbon bonds by linking energy-poor carbon dioxide molecules with the addition of hydrogen. During this process, the plant forms the first stable carbohydrate, the three-carbon triose. Trioses are converted into glucose and fructose and then into sucrose.

In contrast to animals, plants use sucrose as their major fuel transport vehicle. Sucrose is transported from the photosynthesizing (green) parts of a plant to nonphotosynthesizing tissues such as roots, tubers, and seeds. In these tissues, sucrose is used for energy, for the creation of structural cellulose and other fibrous elements, or stored as starch polysaccharide in specialized storage granules. Although plants use carbohydrates primarily for energy and as a basis for structural tissues, they also use carbohydrate precursors to synthesize specialized fats and amino acids for growth and reproduction. Seeds, nuts, and dried legumes are rich sources of protein and lipids not only for the developing plant embryo but also for the organotrophic (i.e., humans) organisms that consume them.

Thus *phototrophic* organisms and plants (i.e., those that feed on light) use light energy, carbon dioxide, water, and minerals to form all macronutrients required for animals and humans to survive. It is true that microscopic *lithotrophic* organisms (i.e., those that feed on rock) obtain energy from geochemical sources deep in the oceans and other inhospitable areas and comprise an important part of the living world. Nonetheless, virtually all living things—human or animal, omnivore or carnivore—derive their nutrition from the sun via phototrophic organisms and plants.

This chapter discusses the structure, properties, food sources, and clinical implications of the three classes of macronutrients—carbohydrate, lipids, and proteins. Macronutrients often play a protective role in human health. Active phytochemicals in plants include carbohydrate, lignins (Craig, 1999), and antioxidants that may include lipid structures (see Chapter 12). Figure 3-1 illustrates the ability of the cell to use all macronutrient substrates for energy and synthetic processes.

CARBOHYDRATES

Plant carbohydrates vary widely in sweetness, texture, rate of digestion, and degree to which they are absorbed after passage through the human gastrointestinal (GI) tract. The diversity, physiologic properties, and potential health benefits of carbohydrate

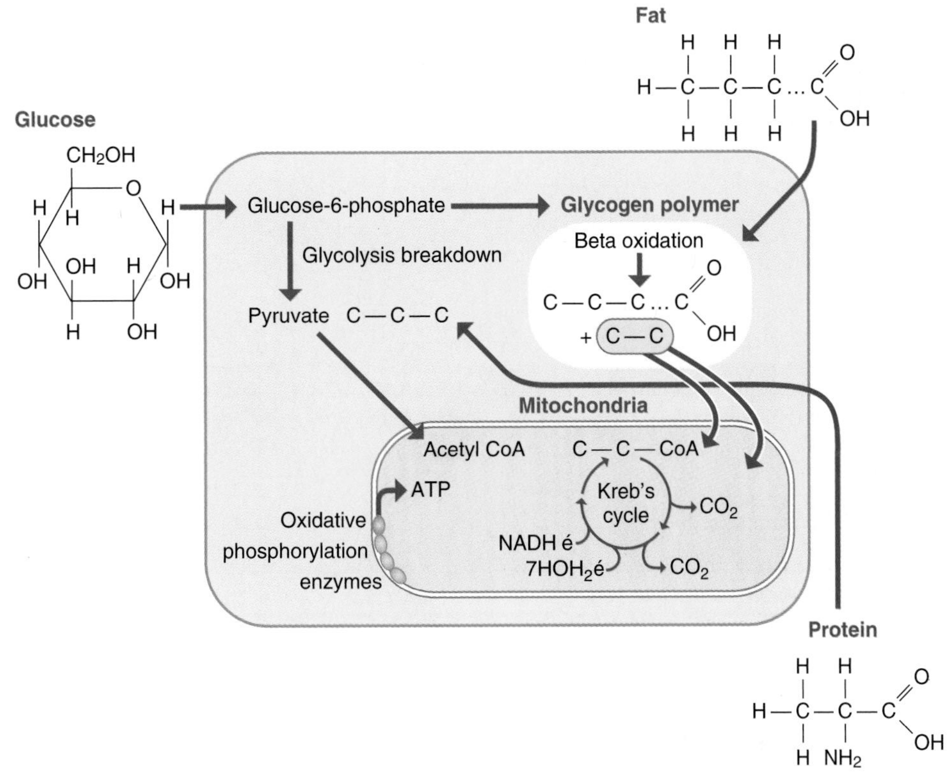

FIGURE 3-1 • Typical cell use of macronutrients for energy.

TABLE 3-1 Types, Sources, and End Products of Carbohydrates

CARBOHYDRATES	FOOD SOURCES	END PRODUCTS OF DIGESTION	REMARKS
Polysaccharides			
Indigestible			
Celluloses Hemicelluloses	Stalks and leaves of vegetables, outer covering of seeds	—	These polysaccharides may be partially split to glucose by bacterial action in large bowel; they have an affinity for water, form bulk, slow gastric emptying time, and may bind bile acids.
Pectins	Fruits	—	
Gums and mucilages	Plant secretions and seeds	—	
Algal substances	Seaweeds and algae	—	
Partially digestible			
Inulin	Jerusalem artichokes, onions, garlic, mushrooms	Fructose	Digestion is incomplete, and further splitting by bacteria may occur in the large bowel. Flatus may result from raffinose and stachyose.
Galactogens	Snails	Galactose	
Mannosans	Legumes	Mannose	
Raffinose	Sugar beets, kidney beans, lentils, and navy beans	Glucose, fructose, and galactose	
Stachyose	Beans	Pentoses	
Pentosans	Fruits and gums		
Digestible			
Starch and dextrins	Grains, vegetables (especially tubers and legumes)	Glucose	These substances comprise the most important group quantitatively and are usually accompanied by some maltose
Glycogen	Meat products and seafood	Glucose	
Disaccharides and Oligosaccharides			
Sucrose	Cane and beet sugars, molasses, and maple syrup	Glucose and fructose	
Lactose	Milk and milk products	Glucose and galactose	
Maltose and maltotriose	Malt products, some breakfast cereals	Glucose	
Lactulose	Synthetic products	Not metabolized	Lactulose does not appear in foods and is synthetic. It is not digested and is used as a laxative.
Trehalose	Mushrooms, insects, yeast	Glucose	
Sucralose	Splenda	—	Sweetener
Monosaccharides			
Hexoses			
Glucose	Fruits, honey, corn syrup	Glucose	In fruits and vegetables the amount of glucose and fructose depends on species ripeness and state of preservation.
Sorbitol*	Fruits, vegetables, dietetic products		
Fructose	Fruits, honey	Fructose	These monosaccharides do not exist in free form in foods.
Galactose		Galactose	
Mannose		Mannose	
Mannitol*	Pineapples, olives, asparagus, sweet potatoes, carrots, dietetic products		
Pentoses			
Ribose	—	Ribose	Ribose, xylose, and arabinose do not exist in free form in foods. They are derived from pentosans of fruits and from the nucleic acids of meat products and seafood.
Xylose	Fruits, vegetables, cereals, mushrooms, seaweed, dietetic chewing gum, other dietetic products	Xylose	
Xylitol*			
Arabinose	—	Arabinose	
Carbohydrate Derivatives			
Ethyl alcohol	Fermented liquors		
Lactic acid	Milk and milk products	Absorbed as same	These substances are the products of natural or induced carbohydrate breakdown.
Malic acid	Fruits		

*Sugar alcohol forms of the designated sugars.

sources in the food supply can best be appreciated by examining the chemical properties of each major carbohydrate type. Carbohydrates can be categorized as (1) monosaccharides, (2) disaccharides and oligosaccharides, or (3) polysaccharides—starch and fibers (Table 3-1).

Monosaccharides

General Properties

Monosaccharides are seldom found free in nature and are typically linked into disaccharide and polysaccharide forms. Only a fraction of the many monosaccharide structures formed in nature can be absorbed and used by humans. It is likely that the sweet taste of edible sugars, especially fructose and sucrose, was a great evolutionary advantage because their sweetness would have guided the first humans to select plant foods providing the greatest energy value. Table 3-2 lists the sweetness values of common sugars and artificial sweeteners. Artificial sweeteners are described in more detail in Chapter 33.

The smallest carbohydrate unit has the formula $(CH_2O)n$, in which *n* can be any integer from 3 to 8. Although 12 hexose (6-carbon) and 6 pentose (5-carbon) isomers can be formed in nature, only three hexoses—glucose, galactose, and fructose—can be absorbed by humans. The edible hexoses all have the same chemical formula but differ in chemical behavior, taste, sweetness, and dietary sources. These differences result from slight but significant differences in their chemical structure. As illustrated in Figure 3-2, glucose and galactose contain an aldehyde group on carbon 1 (C-1), whereas fructose has a ketone at C-2. The active aldehyde and ketone carbons perform two special functions: (1) they can react with the hydroxyl group (OH) of C-5 to form a ring structure as illustrated, and (2) once the ring is formed, the active carbons can link to other sugars by forming a glycosidic linkage with another hydroxyl group. Because the hydroxyl group on C-1 can *reduce* (donate a hydrogen to) metals such as copper and iron, glucose and galactose are called *reducing sugars.* Note that the active ketone at C-2 in fructose reacts with the hydroxyl at C-5 to form a five-membered ring, compared with the six-membered ring formed by the aldoses glucose and galactose.

Specific Monosaccharides

Glucose is the most widely distributed sugar in nature, although it is seldom consumed in its monosaccharide form. In its polymer form, glucose is present as starch and cellulose and found in all edible disaccharides. Glucose, both as a monomer and linked with fructose to form the disaccharide sucrose, makes up a large fraction of the total solid content of fruits and vegetables. "Blood sugar" refers to glucose, and the brain is highly dependent on a regular, predictable supply. Many physiologic functions are required to provide glucose to the bloodstream to maintain adequate blood glucose levels.

Fructose (also known as *levulose* and *fruit sugar*) is the sweetest of all monosaccharides, although its sweetness varies. When tasted in its crystalline form, it is about twice as sweet as sucrose. If it is dissolved in liquid, its sweetness rapidly diminishes, possibly because dissolved fructose is free to assume less sweet configurations (Shallenberger, 1976). Most fruits contain from 1% to 7% fructose, with some containing considerably greater concentrations. As might be expected from the differences in sweetness, fructose makes up about 3% of the dry weight in vegetables and about 40% of honey. As fruit ripens, enzymes

TABLE 3-2 Sweetness of Sugars and Artificial Sweeteners

SUBSTANCE	SWEETNESS VALUE
Sugar or Sugar Product	
Levulose, fructose	173
Invert sugar	130
Sucrose	100
Glucose	74
Sorbitol	60
Mannitol	50
Galactose	32
Maltose	32
Lactose	16
Artificial Sweeteners	
Cyclamate (banned in United States)	30
Aspartame (NutraSweet)*	180
Acesulfame-K (Sunette)	200
Saccharin (Sweet'N Low)	300
Sucralose (Splenda)	600
Alitame (approval pending)	2000

*Nutritive (has calories).

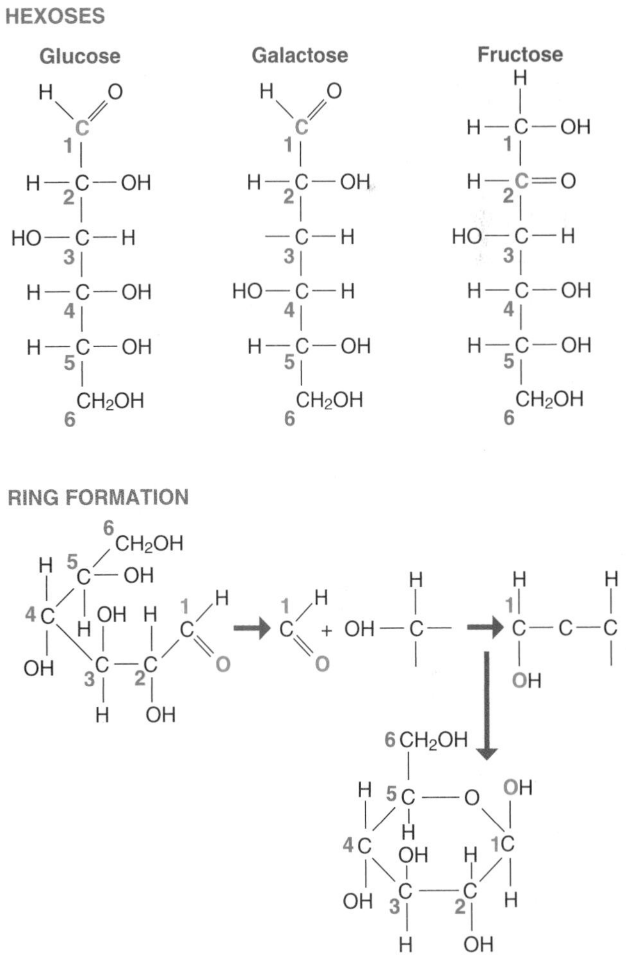

FIGURE 3-2 • Edible hexoses differ in chemical behavior, taste, sweetness, and the type of food in which they are found. These differences result from slight but significant differences in chemical structure.

cleave sucrose into glucose and fructose, resulting in a sweeter taste.

Galactose is rarely free in nature. Most dietary galactose is produced from lactose (milk sugar) by hydrolysis during the digestive process. Some infants are born with an inability to metabolize galactose, a condition called *galactosemia* (see Chapter 45).

Disaccharides and Oligosaccharides

General Properties

Monosaccharide units are joined by a glycosidic linkage between the active aldehyde or ketone carbon and any hydroxyl on any other sugar (Figure 3-3). In monosaccharide form the hydroxyl group on the active carbon can rapidly change position from *above* the ring (the β position) to *below* the ring (the α position). Once two sugars form a glycosidic linkage, the position is frozen as it is in the edible disaccharides sucrose, lactose, and maltose. Each hexose has six hydroxyl groups, each of which is in the β position (above the ring) or the α position (below the ring). Random linkages between hydroxyl groups of different sugars creates a bewildering variety of disaccharide and oligosaccharide configurations in nature. For example, one glucose molecule can form glycosidic links between the six carbons on a second glucose, in α or β positions, to form 11 different configurations.

The most common configurations formed by two glucose units are maltose, which uses α linkages to form starch, and cellobiose, which uses β linkages to form cellulose. Only the α link in maltose can be cleaved by α-amylase, allowing glucose to be absorbed. As described in a later section, dietary fiber is composed of an enormously diverse range of monosaccharides other than glucose.

The human absorptive capacity for carbohydrates is limited to only a few of the many possible disaccharide and oligosaccharide configurations in the food supply. Amylase, secreted by the salivary glands and the pancreas, cleaves only the α bond between two glucose molecules. Enzymes in the brush border of the intestinal mucosal cells hydrolyze only the following four glycosidic bonds:

Sucrase: Cleaves the α bond between glucose C-1 and fructose C-2 (Glcα1-2Fru)

Maltase: Cleaves the α bond between glucose C-1 and glucose C-4 (Glcα1-4Glc)

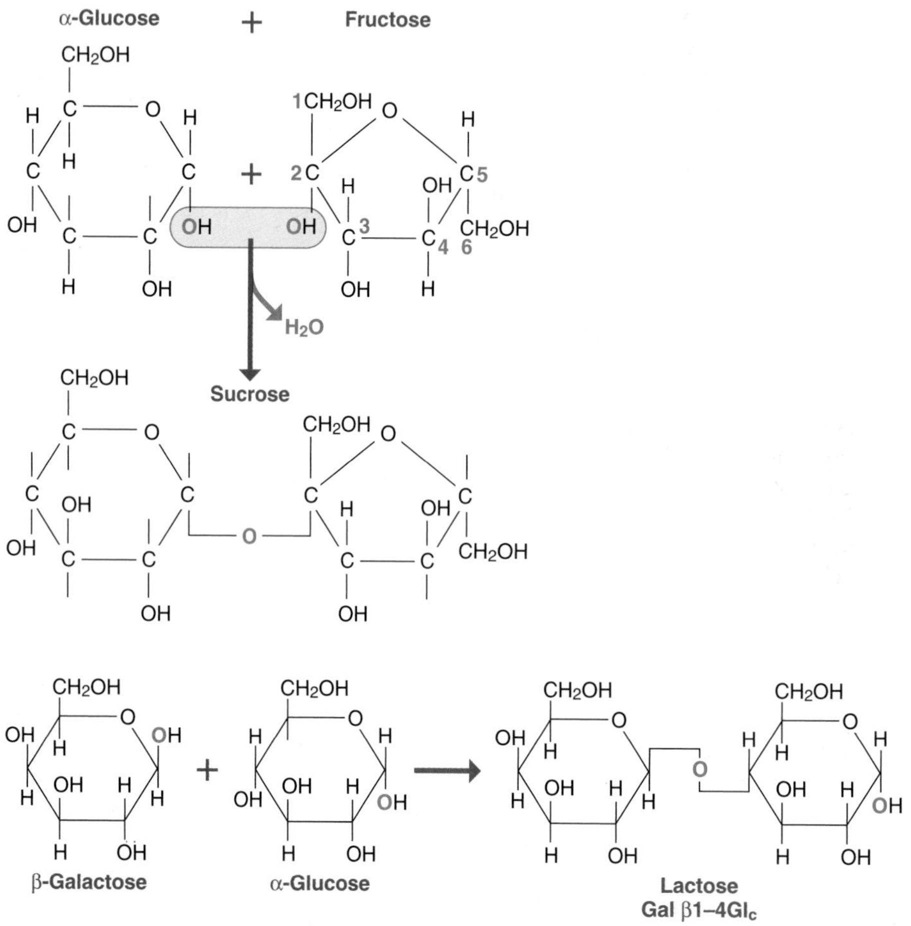

FIGURE 3-3 • Disaccharide formation. Glycosidic links between active *(red)* oxygen molecules and free hydroxyl groups.

Isomaltase: Cleaves the α bond between glucose C-1 and glucose C-6 (Glcα1-6Glc)
Lactase: Cleaves the β bond between galactose C-1 and glucose C-4 (Galβ1-4Glc)

Carbohydrates containing any other linkages cannot be digested and are classified as dietary fiber.

Oligosaccharides are low–molecular-weight polymers containing 2 to 20 sugar molecules. Because they are small, they are readily water soluble and often quite sweet (Roberfroid et al, 1993). Nondigestible oligosaccharides (NDOs) are resistant to stomach acid and the action of amylase and intestinal hydrolytic enzymes. They enter the large intestine intact and can be fermented by indigenous bacteria. *Raffinose,* found in sugar beets, is a trisaccharide made from galactose, glucose, and fructose. *Stachyose* is a tetrasaccharide composed of two galactoses, one glucose, and one fructose and is found in vegetables such as legumes and squash. Because oligosaccharides are fermented by gut bacteria, their ingestion often causes gas and bloating.

Specific Disaccharides and Oligosaccharides

Sucrose (e.g., table sugar, cane sugar, beet sugar, grape sugar) is formed by glucose and fructose linked together by their active carbons (Glcα1–2Fru). Dietary sucrose can be hydrolyzed into glucose and fructose monomers in dilute acid or in the presence of the enzyme *invertase.* When sucrose is used in the preparation of acidic foods (e.g., to sweeten fruit drinks), it becomes inverted within a few hours. Sucrose occurs naturally in many foods and is also an additive in commercially processed items; it is consumed in large amounts by most Americans.

Invert sugar is a form of sugar used commercially because it is sweeter than equal concentrations of sucrose. Sucrose is inverted to glucose and fructose, with smaller crystals than sucrose; thus invert sugar is preferred to sucrose in the preparation of delicate candies and icings. Honey is an invert sugar.

Lactose, or milk sugar, is made almost exclusively in the mammary glands of lactating animals and accounts for 7.5% and 4.5% of the composition of human and cow's milk, respectively. It is less soluble than the other disaccharides and is only about one sixth as sweet as glucose. The β linkage (Galcβ1–4Glc) in lactose is hydrolyzed by lactase in the intestinal cells. Although the sucrase and maltase enzymes are expressed as soon as the intestinal cell is formed at the base of the villus, the lactase enzyme is only expressed by the intestinal cell toward the end of its migration to the tip of the villus. For this reason, GI diseases that injure the intestinal cells and cause sloughing are often associated with lactase deficiency and lactose intolerance.

Most mammals do not consume milk after weaning. It has been estimated that the vast majority of the world's human populations have a limited ability to express the lactase enzyme after weaning. In contrast, a small minority of human populations, largely of Northern European origin, continue to express large amounts of the enzyme throughout life. It is hypothesized that a genetic mutation resulting in enhanced lactase expression throughout life provided a survival advantage. Individuals with such a mutation, which permitted them to absorb and utilize the lactose in milk from their herd animals, would have survived the severe winters of Northern Europe and transmitted the altered gene to their offspring. It follows that descendants with the mutated gene should have the ability to consume large amounts of lactose-containing milk without difficulty. Lactose intolerance, although uncomfortable, does not seem to damage the GI tract or be associated with any long-term pathologic conditions (see Chapter 30).

Maltose (malt sugar) is formed by hydrolysis of starch polymers. Maltose in its disaccharide form is seldom found naturally in the food supply but is consumed as an additive in numerous food products. Germinating seeds produce *diastase,* an enzyme that hydrolyzes starch into maltose for use by the new plant. Therefore sprouting grains contain maltose. Diastase is also used commercially to hydrolyze starch to the maltose (i.e., malt) used in beer making. Because maltose in its disaccharide form is sweeter than its starch polymer, barley malt is also used as a sweetener. It is often found in commercial products that are marketed as "sugar free," even though maltose and sucrose have the same caloric value.

Dextrose is glucose that is produced after the hydrolysis of cornstarch and is commonly used in food production. *Dextran* and *levan* are structural bacterial products derived from various sugars including sucrose and maltose. Some bacteria produce dextran, a linear polymer containing isomaltose (glucose with an α 1,6 branch) as a repeating unit. Levan is a repeating polymer of fructose units in 2,6-fructoside linkage formed from sucrose. Dental plaque consists of levan-producing bacteria embedded in the sticky, adherent matrix they produce. Individuals whose mouth flora include levan-producing bacteria are prone to dental plaque, especially when they consume large amounts of sucrose (see Chapter 28).

Honey, which is made from plant nectar, contains sucrose and small amounts of starch that are harvested by the honeybee. The honeybee secretes *sucrase* (also known as *invertase*) and *amylase,* which together hydrolyze sucrose and starch into glucose and fructose, increasing the sweetness of the product. As indicated previously, approximately 40% of the sugar in mature honey is free fructose. Because the molecular configuration of fructose determines its relative sweetness, the degree of crystallization influences the sweetness of honey.

Honey is calorie dense because monosaccharides pack more closely than disaccharides. One tablespoon of honey contains 64 kcal, whereas an equal amount of sugar contains 46 kcal. It also contains vitamins and minerals, as well as flavonoids and other phytochemicals in trace amounts, but they are inconsequential in terms of daily needs. Commercial honey is heated to 150°F to 160°F to prevent crystallization and growth of unwanted yeasts; "organic," or "raw," honey has not been heat treated.

Honey has important microbiologic actions. Since ancient times, honey has been used as a topical antimicrobial agent, largely because of its high osmolarity and ability to minimize water availability to bacteria (Bowler et al, 2001). Honeybees also produce *glucose oxidase*, an enzyme that converts glucose to gluconic acid and hydrogen peroxide. Together, these products account for the slightly acidic, antiseptic action of honey (Ohashi et al, 1999).

Honey has been reported to contain spores of the ubiquitous *Clostridium botulinum*. Heat treatment is insufficient to destroy spores, but the high sugar content of honey prevents spore germination and risk for deadly botulism. Although honey consumption by normal adults is presumed safe, premature and very young infants may be at risk when consuming honey because the higher pH and sparse flora of their immature GI tracts can promote spore germination. To be safe, it is recommended that caregivers refrain from sweetening pacifiers with honey or feeding honey to infants younger than 1 year of age (see Chapter 8).

High-fructose corn syrup is intensely sweet and inexpensive. It is manufactured enzymatically by changing the glucose in cornstarch to fructose. High-fructose corn syrup is added to canned and frozen fruits to preserve the structure of the fruit. It penetrates the fruit easily and preserves the natural form, flavor, and color. Corn sweetener is added to soft drinks and fruit beverages and adds body without affecting or masking flavors.

During the past few decades, high-fructose corn sweetener consumption increased dramatically. During the same period, consumption of honey and edible syrups remained relatively constant, and that of cane and beet sugar declined. Thus the overall 23% increase in sugar consumption in recent years is largely a result of an increase in corn sweetener intake. The Kantor report (1998) analyzed the distribution of added sweetener in the food supply and reported that 45% goes into beverages, 18% into cereal and bakery products, and 11% into confectionary products. Guthrie and Morton (2000) reported that regular soft drinks accounted for about one third of the approximately 82 g of added sweeteners per day consumed by Americans 2 years and older. Putnam (1999) comments that "sugar is the number one food additive" because it is so ubiquitous and unnoticed. Today 75% of the sugar consumed is in the commercial food supply. In the 1950s, most sugar was purchased for use in preparing food in the home.

Polysaccharides: Starch

General Properties

Plants store carbohydrates as starch granules formed by linking α-glucans (glucose polymers in α-1,4 straight chains with α-1,6 branches) into a complex granular structure. The more carbohydrate the plant makes during photosynthesis, the greater the rate of starch formation. Starch is stored in *plastids* (storage vesicles) called *leucoplasts* adapted for starch storage *(amyloplasts)*. (*Leukos* is a Greek word meaning "white.") Some amyloplasts can grow quite large; for example, the amyloplasts in the potato can be as large as an average animal cell.

Edible plants make two types of starch, amylose and amylopectin. Amylose is a smaller, linear molecule (10^5 to 10^6 daltons) that is less than 1% branched. Amylopectin is highly branched, containing up to 5% α-1,6 branches, with a very–high-molecular weight (10^7 to 10^8 daltons). Because of its larger size, amylopectin is more abundant in the food supply and makes up a greater fraction of the starch in grains and starchy tubers.

Specific Starches

Plants encase starch granules in plastids within rigid cellulose walls. In whole foods, raw starch is poorly digested by digestive enzymes; note the poor digestibility of raw potato and grains. Moist cooking causes the granules to swell, gelatinizes the starch, softens and ruptures the cell wall, and makes the starch more digestible. Some starch remains intact throughout the cooking process or otherwise resists enzyme breakdown. This resistant starch yields limited amounts of glucose for absorption. Starches from different plant sources such as corn, arrowroot, rice, potato, tapioca, and other plants are all glucose polymers with the same chemical composition. Their unique character, including their taste, texture, and absorbability, is determined by the relative numbers of glucose units in straight and branched configurations and the degree of accessibility to digestive enzymes.

Waxy starch is obtained from corn and rice strains bred to contain a greater percentage of branched amylopectin chains. When dissolved in water, waxy starch forms a smooth paste that does not gel until the concentration becomes very high. Once a gel forms, the product remains thick during freezing and thawing, making it an ideal thickener for commercially frozen fruit pies, sauces, and gravies.

Modified food starch is chemically or physically modified to change its hot paste viscosity, ability to gel, and other texture properties. Pregelatinized starch, dried on hot rolls or drums and made into powder, is porous and rapidly rehydrated with cold liquid. This starch rapidly thickens, making it useful for instant puddings, salad dressings, pie fillings, gravies, and baby food. Because it is purified to remove protein, fiber, and other structural constituents usually present in flour, smaller amounts of modified starch are required for thickening.

Dextrins are large, linear glucose polysaccharides of intermediate lengths cleaved from high amylose starch by α-amylase. *Limit dextrins* are cleaved from amylopectin containing branch points not cleaved by amylase; they can subsequently be digested into glucose by the mucosal enzyme isomaltase.

Animal Carbohydrates: Glycogen

Plants use carbohydrates, especially cellulose, for their structural components. In contrast, animal structures are made predominately from the protein collagen. In the animal, carbohydrates are used primarily to support blood glucose concentrations between feedings. To ensure a readily available supply, all cells store carbohydrate in the easily mobilized glycogen polymer (Figure 3-4).

Because it is a carbohydrate, glycogen forms hydrogen bonds with water molecules. The adsorbed water makes glycogen a large and cumbersome molecule, unsuitable for long-term energy storage. The 70-kg "average man" stores only an 18-hour fuel supply as glycogen, compared with a 2-month supply stored as fat. It has been estimated that if all human energy stores were glycogen, humans would need to weigh 60 additional pounds (Alberts et al, 2002). About 150 g of glycogen is stored in muscle; this amount can be increased fivefold with physical training (see Chapter 26).

Despite its presence in animal tissue, meat and other animal products do not contain appreciable amounts of glycogen. In response to epinephrine and other stress hormones released at slaughter, glycogen stores are largely depleted. Glucose released is converted to lactic acid after death. The glycogen store in the human liver is about 90 g and is involved in the hormonal control of blood sugar (see *Clinical Insight:* Hormonal Control of Blood Sugar).

Nondigestible Carbohydrate Homopolymers: Cellulose

Cellulose is the most abundant organic compound in the world, constituting 50% or more of all the carbon in vegetation. Some 10^{15} kg of cellulose, from cellulose in the giant redwood to the delicate flower, are synthesized and degraded on earth each year. The simple polymer of glucose units in β (1-4) glycosidic linkage is ideal for a support molecule because the β linkage allows formation of very long straight chains. The long cellulose molecule folds back on itself like a ribbon and is held in place by hydrogen bonds formed between the hydroxyls on adjacent loops (Figure 3-5). The ribbon structure gives cellulose fibrils great mechanical strength but limited flexibility.

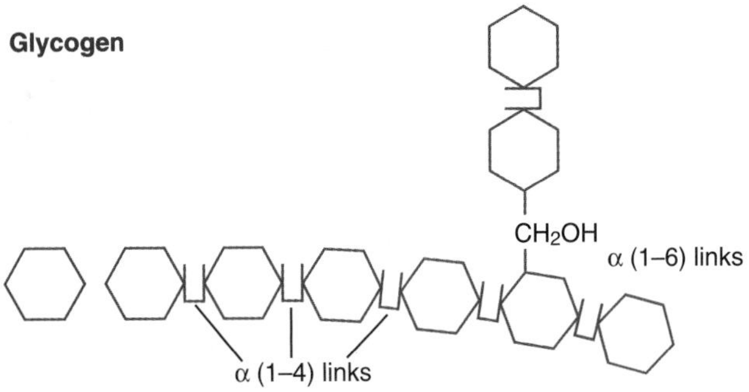

FIGURE 3-4 • Glycogen is a branched glucose polymer similar to amylopectin, but the branches in glycogen are shorter and more numerous.

This strength of cellulose fibrils allows trees to grow to great heights and gives vegetables their unique textures. Cellulose is found in carrots, celery, broccoli, and many other vegetables.

Nondigestible Carbohydrate Heteropolymers: Hemicellulose and Gums

Plant cell walls consist of rigid cellulose microfibrils embedded in a gel-like matrix. The matrix is made by modifying the basic cellulose structure to form heteropolysaccharides of differing water solubilities. One modification is to change the glycosidic linkage. Remember that both amylopectin and cellulose consist of glucose polymers—but cellulose is straight and rigid, whereas amylopectin is highly branched. Matrix polymers include β-*glucans* with repeated β (1–4) links interspersed with β (1–3) bonds, making the molecule less linear than cellulose and therefore more soluble. Soluble fiber sources such as oats and barley are rich in β-glucans (Box 3-1).

Hemicellulose is a glucose polymer substituted with other sugars; different sugar molecules have different water solubilities (Table 3-3). The predominant sugar is used to name the hemicellulose (e.g., xylan, galactan, mannan, arabinose, galactose.)

Pectins and *gums* contain sugars and sugar alcohols that make these molecules even more water soluble than hemicellulose. Gel-forming fibers are composed of a galacturonic acid backbone that have rhamnose units inserted at intervals and side chains of arabinose and galactose. Pectin is found in apples, citrus fruit, strawberries, and other fruits. Gums and mucilages (e.g., guar gum) are similar in structure to pectin except that their galactose units are combined with other sugars (e.g., glucose) and polysaccharides. Gums are found in plant secretions and seeds.

The galacturonic acid structure of pectin absorbs water and forms a gel, so it is widely used for making jams and jellies. Pectin gel cooked with sugar and fruit juice or pulp is stable for months at room temperature. Such jams and jellies are often sealed

CLINICAL INSIGHT

Hormonal Control of Blood Sugar

In the body, blood glucose must be maintained at a minimal level (70 to 100 mg/100 ml) to provide fuel for the brain, central nervous system, and other obligate consumers of glucose. If blood glucose is chronically higher than this range, damage to cells and systems takes place, as it does in patients with diabetes. Glucose *homeostasis* (equilibrium) is controlled in the fed and fasted states through actions of hormones that store, release, or oxidize glucose as needed.

In the fed state, *insulin* is the principal anabolic hormone and is responsible for fuel storage and use. It is produced by the β cells of the islets of Langerhans in the pancreas and released into the bloodstream in response to the postprandial increase in blood glucose. Insulin release can also be stimulated, although to a lesser extent, by the ingestion of protein or infusion of amino acids or ketone bodies. Insulin release is also stimulated by GI hormones, vagus nerve activity, and certain drugs (e.g., glucotrol, an oral hypoglycemic agent). Insulin binds to receptors on muscle and adipose cells and facilitates glucose entry through specialized GLUT 4 transporters. In the liver, insulin facilitates glucose oxidation and glycogen synthesis. If food intake is excessive, insulin also facilitates fatty acid synthesis and storage in the adipose cells, thereby reducing the glucose concentration in the bloodstream.

In the fasted state, *glucagon* is secreted by the α cells of the islets of Langerhans. This hormone acts primarily on the liver to stimulate glycogen breakdown to maintain blood glucose levels. In the absence of insulin, glucagon inhibits hepatic glucose oxidation and enhances gluconeogenesis. The net result of these activities is return of blood glucose levels to the normal range. Fasting also stimulates the release of *epinephrine* from the adrenal medulla and *norepinephrine* from peripheral nerve endings. These catabolic hormones act primarily on the muscle to mobilize glycogen and on adipocytes to release triglycerides.

Epinephrine and norepinephrine levels increase when a person is angry or afraid, resulting in the "fight-or-flight" response. Under these conditions, glucose is needed to provide extra energy for crisis response. *Glucocorticoids* such as cortisol are steroid hormones elaborated by the adrenal cortex in the fasting or stressed state. As the name suggests, glucocorticoids increase blood glucose levels, largely by stimulating gluconeogenesis. Cortisol also enhances the release of fat and amino acids from adipose and muscle tissue, thereby providing a substrate for adenosine triphosphate (ATP) synthesis and gluconeogenesis. *Growth hormone*, produced by the anterior pituitary gland, increases the blood glucose level by antagonizing insulin action and diminishing cellular uptake of glucose. It also increases amino acid uptake and protein synthesis by all cells and increases the mobilization of fat for energy. Finally, in the absence of insulin binding, muscle and adipose tissues cannot take up glucose. The net actions of these counter-regulatory hormones maintain the blood glucose concentration within the range required for optimal cell function.

with wax to prevent bacterial or fungal growth. Pectin is added to fat-free yogurt and other products to provide texture and stability. The specific textural qualities of gums and mucilages are commercially useful when added to processed foods such as ice cream.

The fructooligosaccharides (FOSs) *inulin* and *fructans* are composed of fructose polymers, often linked with an initial glucose. Inulin comprises a diverse group of fructose polymers widely distributed in plants as a storage carbohydrate. Oligofructose is a subgroup of inulin, containing less than 10 fructose units. FOSs are poorly digested in the upper GI tract and thus supply only about 1 kcal/g (Roberfroid et al, 1993). Because they contain fructose, FOSs have a sweet, clean flavor and are half as sweet as sucrose.

FOSs are found in more than 36,000 plant species; diets that contain more fruits and vegetables are naturally higher in these compounds. Americans ingest an average of 1 to 4 g of FOS per day, whereas Europeans consume 3 to 10 g. Major sources of FOS include wheat, onions, garlic, bananas, and chicory; other sources include tomatoes, barley, rye, asparagus, and Jerusalem artichokes.

Inulin and related FOSs are used widely in the commercial formulation of innovative food products because of their sweet, clean flavor and unabsorbable nature. When used as an ingredient, FOS is either synthesized from sucrose by adding fructose monomers to an initial sucrose molecule or extracted from chicory roots (Niness, 1999). The sweetness derived from its fructose content has been used to improve the flavor of low-calorie foods and improve the stability and acceptability of fat-reduced foods. Because it is not absorbed in the proximal intestine, FOS has been used as a sugar replacement for diabetic patients. Mixed with milk, FOS can form microcrystals that give table spreads and dairy products a creamy, fatlike feel in the mouth. FOS adds fiber to food without increasing viscosity.

A high-performance product with longer polymers (about 25 fructose units per molecule) and low sugar content has been formulated with almost twice the fat mimetic characteristics of standard inulin and no sweetness contribution. Extensive testing revealed that naturally occurring and commercially produced FOSs (marketed under the brand name Nutraflora) are safe and have no significant adverse effects at doses up to 2170 mg/kg/day (Spiegel et al, 1994). FOSs also increase colonic bacterial growth and have been added to yogurts containing live bacterial cultures and marketed as prebiotics to enhance colonic flora (see Chapter 12).

Although FOSs are poorly digested in the small intestine and enter the colon intact, once they reach the colon, they are hydrolyzed by intestinal bacteria into short-chain volatile fatty acids and gases such as methane and carbon dioxide. These volatile substances have many physiologic effects (see Chapter 30).

Lignin is a woody fiber found in the stems and seeds of fruits and vegetables and the bran layer of cereals. It is actually not a carbohydrate but is a polymer composed of phenylopropyl alcohols and acids, some of which have a net positive or negative charge. The phenyl groups contain conjugated double bonds, which make them excellent antioxidants. Flaxseed lignin also has phytoestrogen activity and can mimic estrogen at its receptors on reproductive organs and bone; the role of flaxseed in the prevention of cancer and other chronic diseases is under investigation (Stark and Madar, 2002).

Algal polysaccharides (e.g., carrageenan) are extracted from seaweed and algae and used as thickening and stabilizing agents in many processed foods. *Carrageenan* is a sulfated polygalactant algal polysaccharide extracted from macroalgae or seaweed (Evans, 1989). In nature the mucilaginous polysaccharide confers structural integrity to sea plants. In the cell wall, alginate, carrageenan, and agar prevent desiccation, provide for selective adsorption of ions, and facilitate bioadhesion of the plant to rocks and other anchors. Algal polysaccharides are used commercially because they form weak gels with proteins and stabilize food mixtures, preventing suspended ingredients from settling. Carrageenan is an ingredient in pudding and used commercially to add body to infant formulas, ice cream, milk pudding, and sour cream products.

Carrageenan at high doses has also been reported to induce mucosal thymidine kinase activity in rats (Calvert and Satchithanandam, 1992), resulting in excess proliferation of the colonic mucosa and increased cancer risk. Concern for its safety remains (Tobacman, 2001).

Carrageenan damages human cells in culture and destroys human mammary myoepithelial cells at concentrations as low as 0.00014% (Tobacman, 1997). With its wide use in commercial food preparation and uncertainty about the extent of human sensitivity, further investigation of carrageenan is needed.

Chitin, a homopolymer of *N*-acetyl-β-D-glucosamine, is a polysaccharide produced by lower animal forms for structural support. This polymer is folded like cellulose except that the hydroxyl on C-2 of each residue is replaced by acetylated amino groups. Chitin is widely distributed among various organisms, including algae, fungi, and yeasts. It is best known as the major component in the exoskeleton of arthropod, mollusk, and marine invertebrates, including lobster and shrimp. Chitin forms a matrix on which minerals are deposited, much as collagen forms a matrix for vertebrate bone mineralization.

Chitosan is a polymer of glucosamine obtained by the deacetylation of chitin (Shiau and Yu, 1998). Chitin and chitosan have been studied for their hypocholesterolemic effect. The strong positive charge on chitosan binds negatively charged lipids, blocking their absorption. Hypercholesterolemic mice given chitosan for 20 weeks had significantly lower blood

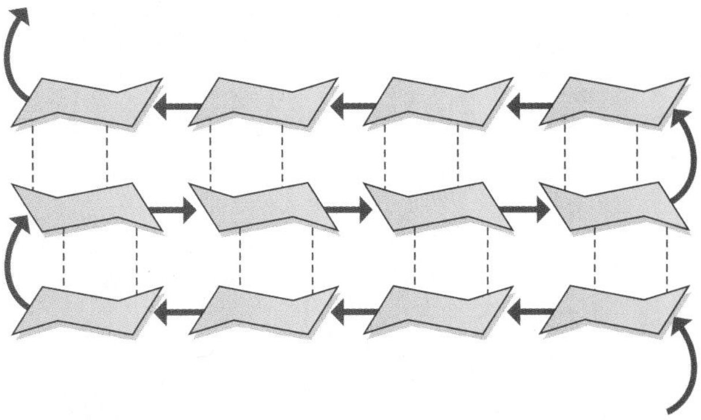

FIGURE 3-5 • The ribbonlike structure of cellulose. Note the cross-links between adjacent molecules.

Box 3-1. Sources of Fiber Components

Insoluble

Cellulose	**Hemicellulose**	**Lignin**
Whole-wheat flour	Bran	Mature vegetables
Bran	Whole grains	Wheat
Vegetables		Fruits and edible seeds, such as flaxseeds and strawberries

Soluble

Gums	**Pectin**
Oats	Apples
Legumes	Citrus fruits
Guar	Strawberries
Barley	Carrots

TABLE 3-3 Dietary Fiber Content of Foods in Commonly Served Portions

FOOD GROUP	<1 g	1-1.9 g	2-2.9 g	3-3.9 g	4-4.9 g	5-5.9 g	>6 g
Breads (1 slice)	Bagel White French	Whole wheat	Bran muffin (1)	NA*	NA	NA	NA
Cereals (1 oz)	Rice Krispies Special K Cornflakes	Oatmeal Nutri-Grain Cheerios	Wheaties Shredded Wheat	Most Honey Bran	Bran Chex 40% Bran Flakes Raisin Bran	Corn Bran	All-Bran Bran Buds 100% Bran
Pasta (1 cup)	NA	Macaroni Spaghetti	NA	Whole-wheat spaghetti	NA	NA	NA
Rice (½ cup)	White	Brown	NA	NA	NA	NA	NA
Legumes (½ cup) cooked	NA	NA	NA	Lentils	Lima beans Dried peas	NA	Kidney beans Baked beans Navy beans
Vegetables (½ cup unless stated)	Cucumber Lettuce (1 cup) Green pepper	Asparagus Green beans Cabbage Cauliflower Potato, without skin (1) Celery	Broccoli Brussels sprouts Carrots Corn Potato, with skin (1) Spinach	Peas	NA	NA	NA
Fruits (1 medium unless stated)	Grapes (20) Watermelon (1 cup)	Apricots (3) Grapefruit (½) Peach, with skin Pineapple (½ cup)	Apple, without skin Banana Orange	Apple, with skin Pear, with skin Raspberries (½ cup)	NA	NA	NA

From Slavin JL: Dietary fiber: classification, chemical analyses, and food sources, *J Am Diet Assoc* 87:1164, 1987.
*Not applicable.

cholesterol levels (64% of controls) and highly significant inhibition of atherogenesis in the aorta (Ormrod et al, 1998). In contrast, chitosan feeding resulted in severe malabsorption of fat-soluble vitamins and bone minerals in rats (Deuchi et al, 1995). More research is needed to assess the safety of this substance for long-term human consumption.

The Impact of Carbohydrates on Metabolism

A growing body of evidence suggests that dietary carbohydrates, especially nonabsorbable oligosaccharides, and fibers have a significant impact on human physiology. It is now recognized that specific carbohydrates not only modulate whole-body energy dynamics but also affect disease processes.

Glucose Absorption and the Glycemic Index

Dietary carbohydrates are digested into glucose, fructose, and galactose through the actions of α-amylase and brush border digestive enzymes in the upper GI tract. The ability to digest carbohydrate is modified by (1) the relative availability (or resistance) of the starch to enzyme action; (2) the activity of digestive enzymes, especially lactase, at the mucosal brush border; and (3) the presence of other dietary factors such as fat that slow stomach emptying, nonabsorbable oligosaccharides, and viscous dietary fibers such as pectins, β-glucans, and gums that dilute enzyme concentration. Thus a diet rich in whole foods such as fruits, vegetables, legumes, nuts, and minimally processed grains tends to slow down the pace of glucose absorption.

Once digested, glucose is actively absorbed across the intestinal cell and transferred to the portal blood for transport to the liver as described in Chapter 1. The liver removes about 50% of absorbed glucose for oxidation and for storage as glycogen. Galactose and fructose are modified and used as intermediates in these pathways. Glucose exits the liver and enters the systemic circulation. Only then is glucose available for insulin-dependent uptake by peripheral tissues. Thus the major regulators of blood glucose concentration after a meal are (1) the amount and digestibility of ingested carbohydrate, (2) the absorption and degree of liver uptake, and (3) insulin secretion and the sensitivity of peripheral tissues to insulin action.

In 1981, Jenkins defined a glycemic index to rank different dietary carbohydrates as compared with a reference food on their ability to raise blood glucose levels (Jenkins, 1981). It was assumed that under test conditions, intestinal absorptive capacity, liver metabolism, pancreatic insulin secretion and other regulatory systems behave similarly, but that dietary carbohydrate sources release glucose differently. Since then, studies suggest that the glycemic index is reproducible and may have use in the dietary management of diabetes and hyperlipidemia (Brand-Miller, 1994). Published data on the glycemic indexes of individual foods, using white bread and glucose as reference foods, have been consolidated for the convenience of users. Use of the glycemic index to modify diets and prevent and control chronic disease is under intense investigation (see Appendix 54 and Chapter 12).

It is possible that genetic links exist and some high-risk individuals have subtle genetic changes that impair their ability to tolerate dietary carbohydrates (Salas et al, 1998). Observations from the Third National Health and Nutrition Examination Survey (NANES III) clearly demonstrate prevalence of this as the metabolic syndrome in various age groups (Ford, 2002). Prevalence rises from less than 10% for individuals in the 20- to 29-year age group to 45% in the 60- to 69-year age group, suggesting possible interactions between the process of aging and the cumulative effect of increased sugar consumption. For more details about the metabolic syndrome (which is also called *insulin resistance* and *syndrome X*, see Chapters 12, 33, and 35).

Regulation of Blood Lipids

Carbohydrate-induced hypertriglyceridemia can result from consuming a high-carbohydrate diet. It is important to remember that fat intake does not translate directly into blood lipid changes because the body regulates macronutrient levels to provide adequate supplies of fuel to body tissues. For example, the brain uses the major portion of the approximately 200 g of glucose required per day. If the blood glucose level falls below 40 mg/dl, counter-regulatory hormones release macronutrients from stores; if the blood glucose level rises above 180 mg/dl, glucose is spilled into the urine. High intakes of carbohydrate can trigger large releases of insulin. This anabolic hormone stimulates compensatory responses, including insulin-dependent glucose uptake by muscle and fat and active glycogen and fat synthesis, thereby lowering the blood glucose level to a normal range. About 2 hours after a meal, intestinal absorption is complete, but insulin effects persist and the blood glucose level falls, sometimes below the normal range. The body interprets this hypoglycemic state as starvation and secretes counter-regulatory hormones that release free fatty acids from fat cells (Ludwig, 2002). Fatty acids are packed into transport lipoproteins (very–low-density lipoproteins [VLDLs]) in the liver, thereby elevating serum triglycerides.

Parks and Hellerstein (2000) reviewed evidence for the paradoxical rise in serum lipid levels and fall in high-density lipoprotein (HDL) levels after consumption of a diet higher than usual in carbohydrates. Although conclusive human studies have not yet been done, researchers are focusing on the increase in Americans' obesity coupled with their higher sugar consumption as the cause and calling for additional studies to clearly define the way the macronutrient composition of the diet can influence health.

Serum lipid concentrations can be modified by insoluble fibers such as cellulose, lignin, chitin, and more soluble fibers because (1) fibers bind fecal bile acids and increase excretion of bile-acid–derived cholesterol, (2) fibers prevent dietary fat and cholesterol absorption by binding bile acids or fat and lipids, and (3) fermentable oligosaccharides and dietary fiber are converted by intestinal bacteria to short-chain fatty acids (SCFAs) and lower blood lipids by mechanisms that are currently unclear. Evidence for the hypocholesterolemic effect of soluble fibers, including FOS, viscous pectin, guar gum, oat bran, psyllium husk, beans, legumes, and fruits and vegetables, is conflicting. Cholesterol-lowering effects have been reported, but the effect varies with the type and amount of fiber (Trautwein et al, 1998). Jenkins et al (1991) reported that inulin actually raised low-density lipoprotein (LDL) concentrations in humans, possibly because of production of the cholesterol acetate by gut fermentation. Other studies reported a mild lipid-lowering action of FOS in humans, possibly involving changes in hepatic triglyceride synthesis, VLDL secretion, or reabsorption of bile acids (Davidson and Maki, 1999).

Vitamin and Mineral Absorption

Nonnutrient components of plants, including tannins, saponins, lectins, and phytates, interact with dietary macronutrients, vitamins, and minerals and can reduce macronutrient and micronutrient absorption. *Phytate,* a six-carbon ring with phosphate bound to each carbon, is found in the seed coat of grains and legumes and has the ability to bind metal ions, especially calcium, copper, iron, and zinc (Couzy et al, 1998). Because calcium catalyzes the action of amylase, which hydrolyzes starch, excess phytate also reduces starch hydrolysis.

Constituents other than phytate also bind nutrients and prevent their absorption, as shown in studies of dephytinized insoluble fiber from oat, wheat, or rice bran (Bergman et al, 1997) (see Chapter 5).

In contrast, some non-digestible oligosaccharides (NDOs) may increase mineral absorption (Scholz-Ahrens, 2001). Calcium, magnesium, iron, and zinc absorption are increased by oligosaccharides in experimental animals, possibly because of the minerals' increased solubility in the cecum and colon as a consequence of increased microbial fermentation and lower luminal pH. Results of the few human trials reported are less consistent. After adding soluble fiber to the diets of nine healthy human adults, Coudray et al (1997) reported enhanced calcium absorption without adverse effect on other metals. The European Project on Nondigestible Oligosaccharides issued a consensus statement claiming a positive effect of NDOs on mineral, especially calcium, absorption in humans (Van Loo et al, 1999). More studies on NDOs and their effects on mineral absorption are needed. Table 3-4 describes foods that contain carbohydrates.

Role of Nonabsorbable Carbohydrates and Short-Chain Fatty Acid Production

Gibson and Roberfroid (1995) first introduced the concept of *prebiotics* as nondigestible food substances that selectively stimulate the growth, activity, or both of beneficial bacterial species already resident in the colon *(probiotics)*, beneficial to the host. Various prebiotics, especially FOSs, variably stimulate the growth of intestinal bacteria, principally *bifidobacteria.* In a healthy person, 80% to 90% of nonabsorbable carbohydrate is fermented by colonic bacteria into carbon dioxide, hydrogen, methane, and SCFAs (Cummings et al, 2001).

A possible mechanism for prebiotic modulation of metabolic pathways is by their fermentation into the short-chain fatty acids (acetate, butyrate, and proprionate), which account for 85% of all SCFAs produced in the human colon. SCFAs are readily absorbed by the intestinal and colonic mucosa; they (1) enhance sodium and water absorption, (2) increase colonocyte proliferation, (3) increase metabolic energy production, (4) enhance colonic blood flow, (5) stimulate the autonomic nervous system, and (6) increase GI hormone production (Compher et al, 1997).

More than 70% of the fuel for colonocytes is the SCFA butyrate (4C), which is actually produced more from starch than from fat. The preference of colonocytes for butyrate was found even in the neonatal rat in the immediate postnatal period before butyrate is available from bacterial fermentation (Krishnan et al, 1998). Proprionate (3C) is absorbed and cleared by the liver and may be important in hepatic lipid or glucose metabolism. Acetate (2C) is produced in the greatest quantities from undigested carbohydrate. It is rapidly metabolized into carbon dioxide by peripheral tissues and can serve as substrate for lipid and cholesterol synthesis (Cummings et al, 2001).

In summary, carbohydrates have the general formula, $(CH_2O)n$ and provide 4 kcal/g. They are formed by plants in a bewildering array of possible single-unit and polymer structures. Humans have the ability to digest only a few of the many possible bonds linking carbohydrate units with each other and other types of organic molecules. More than 80% of edible carbohydrates are absorbed as single glucose units. Depending on their structure, nondigestible carbohydrates pass to a greater or lesser degree through the intestine and enter the colon, where they are metabolized by gut bacteria and can have a significant impact on the prevention and control of disease.

TABLE 3-4 Carbohydrate Content of Foods

FOOD	CARBOHYDRATE (PERCENTAGE OF WEIGHT)
Sugar	
Concentrated sweets	
Sugar: Cane, beet, powdered,	99.5
brown, maple	90-96
Candies	70-95
Honey (extracted)	82
Syrup: Table blends, molasses	55-75
Jams, jellies, marmalades	70
Carbonated, sweetened beverages	10-12
Fruits	
Prunes, apricots, figs (cooked, unsweet)	12-31
Bananas, grapes, cherries, apples, pears	15-23
Fresh: Pineapples, grapefruits, oranges, apricots, strawberries	8-14
Milk	
Skim	6
Whole	5
Starch	
Grain products	
Starches: Corn, tapioca, arrowroot	86-88
Cereals (dry): Corn, wheat, oat, bran	68-85
Flour: Corn, wheat (sifted)	70-80
Popcorn (popped)	77
Cookies: Plain, assorted	71
Crackers, saltines	72
Cakes: Plain, without icing	56
Bread: White, rye, whole wheat	48-52
Macaroni, spaghetti, noodles, rice (cooked)	23-30
Cereals (cooked): Oat, wheat, grits	10-16
Vegetables	
Boiled: Corn, white and sweet potatoes, lima and dried beans, peas	15-26
Beets, carrots, onions, tomatoes	5-7
Leafy: Lettuce, asparagus, cabbage, greens, spinach	3-4

FATS AND LIPIDS

Lipid Structures and Functions

Fats and lipids constitute approximately 34% of the energy in the human diet. Because fat is energy rich and provides 9 kcal/g of energy, humans are able to obtain adequate energy with a reasonable daily consumption of fat-containing food items. Dietary fat is stored in *adipose* (fat) cells located in depots on the human frame. The ability to store and use large amounts of fat enables humans to survive without food for weeks and sometimes months. This ability is thought to have contributed to survival of primitive humans in times of famine. If sufficient fat is unavailable, an organism cannot adapt to starvation, and malnutrition results.

Some fat deposits are not used during a fast and are classified as *structural fat.* Structural fat pads hold the body organs and nerves in position and protect them against traumatic injury and shock. Fat pads on the palms and buttocks protect the bones from mechanical pressure. Humans also have a subcutaneous layer of fat that insulates the body, preserving body heat and maintaining body temperature.

Dietary fat is also essential for the digestion, absorption, and transport of the fat-soluble vitamins and fat-soluble phytochemicals such as carotenoids and lycopenes. As described in Chapter 1, dietary fat depresses gastric secretions, slows gastric emptying, and stimulates biliary and pancreatic flow, thereby facilitating the digestive process.

Possibly because fat is essential for survival, humans and other animals seem to have a "hard-wired" taste for fat. Consider that humans prefer the taste and texture of high-fat chocolate compared with the intense, somewhat unpleasant sweetness of fat-free chocolate. Food manufacturers use fat for its textural properties; fat in ice cream contributes to its smoothness, and fat in baked goods increases the tenderness of the product by "shortening" the strands of gluten in batters and doughs (Vail, 1978). Great chefs know that a judicious amount of fat adds to the palatability of the meal and produces a feeling of satiety after a meal. Box 3-2 shows the fat content of common foods.

Unlike carbohydrates, lipids are not polymers; they are small molecules extracted from animal and plant tissues. Lipids comprise a heterogeneous group of compounds characterized by their insolubility in water, and they can be classified into three major

Box 3-2. Fat Content of Some Common Foods

0 g

Most fruits and vegetables
Nonfat milk
Nonfat yogurt
Plain pasta and rice
Angel food cake
Popcorn, air popped, unbuttered
Soft drinks
Jam or jelly

1 to 3 g

Popcorn, oil popped, unbuttered, 1 cup
Low-calorie salad dressing, 1 tbsp
Baked beans, ½ cup
Soup, chicken noodle, canned, 1 cup
Whole-wheat bread, 1 slice
Dinner roll, 1
Waffle, frozen, 4 inch, 1
Coleslaw, ½ cup
Flounder or sole, baked, 3 oz
Chicken, without skin, roasted, 3 oz
Tuna, canned in water, 3 oz
Cheese, cottage, 2% fat, ½ cup
Ice milk, soft serve, ½ cup

4 to 6 g

Low-fat yogurt, 1 cup
Cheese, mozarella, part skim, 1 oz
Chicken, roasted with skin, 3 oz
Egg, scrambled, 1
Turkey, roasted, 3 oz
Granola, 1 oz
Muffin, bran, 1 small
Pizza, cheese, ¼ of 12 inch
Burrito, bean, 1
Brownie, with nuts, 1 small
Margarine or butter, 1 tsp
Popcorn, oil popped, buttered, 1 cup
French dressing, regular, 1 tbsp

7 to 10 g

Cheese, cheddar, 1 oz
Milk, whole, 1 cup
Bologna, beef, 1 slice
Sausage, 1 patty
Steak, sirloin, broiled, 3 oz
Potatoes, French fried, 10
Chow mein, chicken, 1 cup
Chocolate candy bar, 1 oz
Corn chips, 1 oz
Doughnut, cake type, plain, 1
Mayonnaise, 1 tbsp

15 g

Hot dog, beef, 2 oz
McDonald's Chicken McNuggets, 6 pieces
Peanut butter, 2 tbsp
Pork chop, broiled, 3 oz
Sunflower seeds, dry roasted, ¼ cup
Avocado, ½ medium
Chop suey, beef and pork, 1 cup
Cinnamon roll, 1

20 g

Cheesecake, 1/12 cake
Lasagna with meat, 1 medium piece
Macaroni and cheese, homemade, 1 cup
Peanuts, dry roasted, ¼ cup
Ground beef, broiled, 3 oz

25+ g

Polish sausage, 3 oz
Cheeseburger, large
Pie, pecan, ⅛ of 9 inch
Chicken pot pie, frozen, baked, 1 pie
Quiche, bacon, ⅛ pie

Data from Healthy Dividends, Rosemont, Ill., 1990, National Dairy Council.

Box 3-3. Classification of Lipids

Simple Lipids

Fatty acids
Neutral fats: Esters of fatty acids with glycerol
Monoglycerides, diglycerides, triglycerides
Waxes: Esters of fatty acids with high–molecular-weight alcohols
Sterol esters (e.g., cholesterol ester)
Nonsterol esters (e.g., retinyl palmitate [vitamin A esters])

Compound Lipids

Phospholipids: Compounds of phosphoric acid, fatty acids, and a nitrogenous base
Glycerophospholipids (e.g., lecithins, cephalins, plasmologens)
Glycosphingolipids (e.g., sphingomyelins)
Glycolipids: Compounds of fatty acids, monosaccharides, and a nitrogenous base (e.g., cerebrosides, gangliosides, ceramide)
Lipoproteins: Particles of lipid and protein

Miscellaneous Lipids

Sterols (e.g., cholesterol, vitamin D, bile salts)
Vitamins A, E, K

From Examples of current and proposed ingredients for fats, *J Am Diet Assoc* 92:472, 1992.

groups (Box 3-3). Figure 3-6 shows some of the more important lipid structures.

Fatty Acids

Fatty acids are rarely free in nature and almost always are linked to other molecules by their *hydrophilic* (i.e., "water-loving") carboxylic acid head group (Figure 3-6, *1*). They exist primarily as unbranched hydrocarbon chains with an even number of carbons that are variably saturated with hydrogen. Fatty acids are classified according to the number of carbons, the number of double bonds, and the position of the first double bond in the chain. Chain length and extent of saturation contribute to the melting temperature of a fat. In general, fats with shorter fatty acid chains or more double bonds are liquid at room temperature. Saturated fats, especially those with long chains (e.g., beef tallow, which has 18 carbons), are solid at room temperature.

Because triglycerides in natural foods are mixtures of fatty acids of different melting points, the fatty acids solidify at different rates during cooling. Some manufacturers cool oil and filter out solidified particles before sale; the resultant "winterized" oil remains clear when refrigerated. Olive oil is about 75% monounsaturated fatty acids. Its long, 18-carbon chains make it cloudy and viscous when cooled, even with their single double bond. In contrast, coconut oil is highly saturated but semiliquid at room temperature because the predominant fatty acids are short, between 8 and 14 carbons long.

Chain Length

Each individual plant and animal species makes fatty acids of specific chain lengths and saturation for its unique structural and metabolic needs. Organisms have evolved the capacity to synthesize and elongate available fatty acids to meet these needs. For this reason, food from different plants and animals differ in the length of their fatty acid chains. In general, butter and milk fat contain SCFAs with 4 to 6 carbons, coconut oil contains fatty acids with 12 to 14 carbons, and animal fat contains long-chain fatty acids (LCFAs) with 16 to 20 carbons (Table 3-5).

Saturation

Each carbon in a fatty acid chain has four binding sites. In a saturated fatty acid (SFA), all binding sites not linked to carbon are "saturated" with (bound to) hydrogen. Monounsaturated fatty acids (MFAs) contain only one double bond, and polyunsaturated fatty acids (PUFAs) contain two or more double bonds. In MFAs and PUFAs, one or more pairs of hydrogen have been removed, and double bonds form between adjacent carbons. As they have for fatty acid chain length, each organism has evolved its own optimal fatty acid composition. Because fatty acids with double bonds are vulnerable to oxidative damage, humans and other warm-blooded organisms store fat predominantly as saturated palmitic fatty acid ($C_{16}H_{32}O_2$ = C16:0) and stearic fatty acid ($C_{18}H_{36}O_2$ = C18:0). On the other hand, the biomembrane must be stable and flexible for optimal function. To achieve this requirement, biomembrane phospholipids contain one saturated and one highly polyunsaturated fatty acid, the most abundant of which is arachidonic acid (C20:4). The most abundant MFA in human blood is monounsaturated oleic acid ($C_{18}H_{34}O_2$ = C18:1). Food sources of fatty acids are found in Table 3-6.

Location of Double Bonds

Fatty acids are also characterized by the location of their double bonds. Two conventions are used to describe the location of the double bonds. With one convention, the Greek capital letter *delta* (Δ) refers to the carbon preceding the double bond. For example, *Δ9* refers to the double bond between carbons 9 and 10. With another convention, lowercase Greek letters are used to refer to the placement of the carbons within the fatty acid. *Alpha* (α) refers to the first carbon adjacent to the carboxyl group, *beta* (β) to the second car-

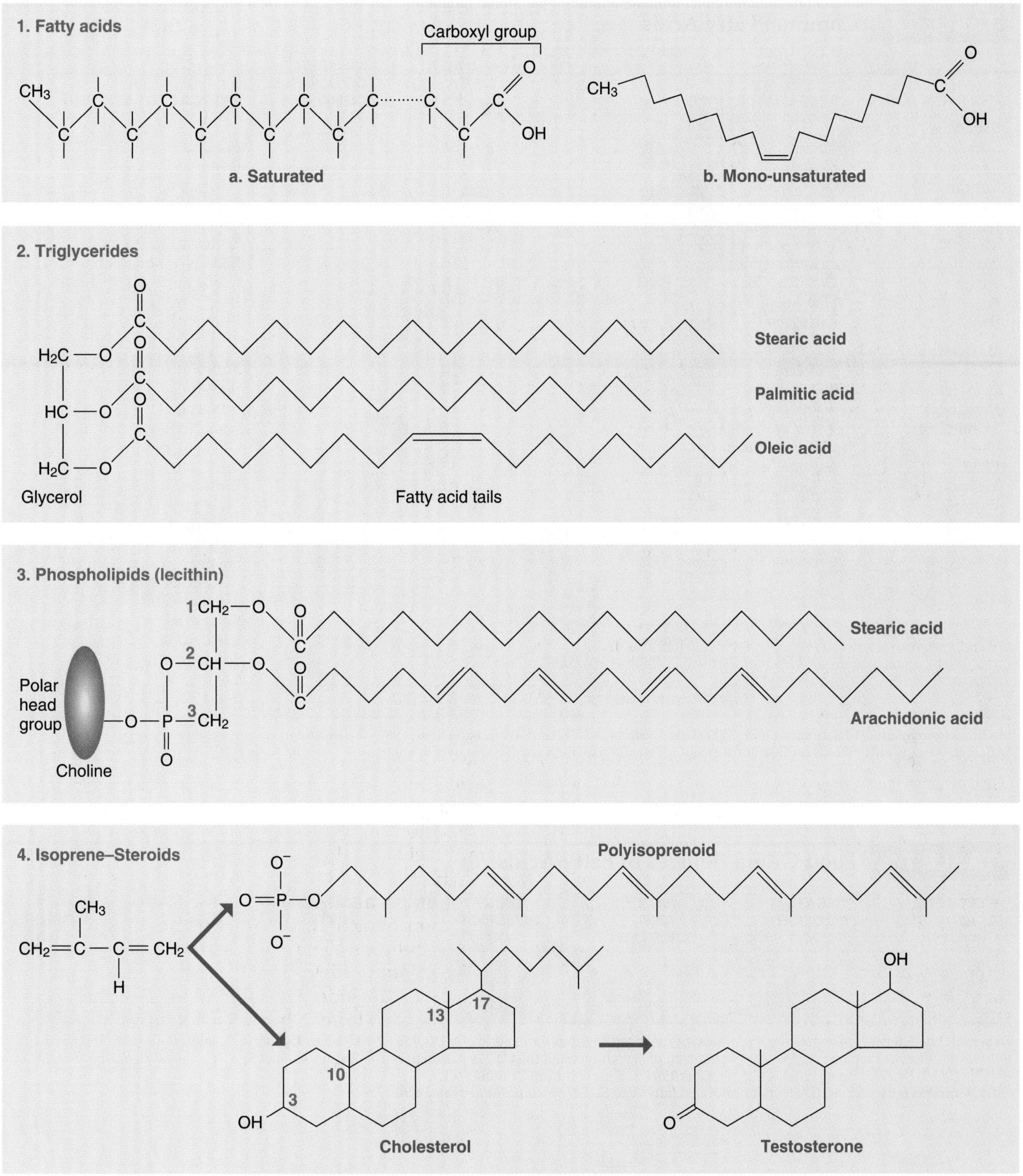

FIGURE 3-6 • Structures of physiologically important fats and lipids.

bon, and *omega* (ω) to the last carbon (which is referred to as the fatty acid's **omega number**). Double bonds labeled with ω are counted from the terminal methyl carbon. Thus arachidonic acid (20:4 ω-6), the major highly polyunsaturated fat in the membranes of land animals, is an omega-6 fatty acid. It has four double bonds, the first of which is six carbons from the terminal methyl group. Eicosapentaenoic acid (EPA) (eicosa = 20, pent = 5; 20:5 ω-3) is found in marine organisms and is an omega-3 fatty acid. It has

TABLE 3-5 Common Fatty Acids

COMMON NAME	SYSTEMATIC NAME	NUMBER OF CARBON ATOMS*	NUMBER OF DOUBLE BONDS	TYPICAL FAT SOURCE
Saturated Fatty Acids				
Butyric	Butanoic	4	0	Butterfat
Caproic	Hexanoic	6	0	Butterfat
Caprylic	Octanolic	8	0	Coconut oil
Capric	Decanoic	10	0	Coconut oil
Lauric	Dodecanoic	12	0	Coconut oil, palm kernel oil
Myristic	Tetradecanoic	14	0	Butterfat, coconut oil
Palmitic	Hexadecanoic	16	0	Palm oil, animal fat
Stearic	Octadecanoic	18	0	Cocoa butter, animal fat
Arachidic	Elcosanoic	20	0	Peanut oil
Behenic	Docosanoic	22	0	Peanut oil
Unsaturated Fatty Acids				
Caproleic	9-Decenoic	10	1	Butterfat
Lauroleic	9-Dodecenoic	12	1	Butterfat
Myristoleic	9-Tetradecenoic	14	1	Butterfat
Palmitoleic	9-Hexadecenoic	16	1	Some fish oils, beef fat
Oleic	9-Octadecenoic	18	1	Olive oil, canola oil
Elaidic	9-Octadecenoic	18	1	Butterfat
Vacceric	11-Octadecenoic	18	1	Butterfat
Linoleic	9, 12-Octadecadienoic	18	2	Most vegetable oils, especially safflower, corn, soybean, cottonseed
Linolenic	9, 12, 15-Octadecatrienoic	18	3	Soybean oil, canola oil, walnuts, wheat germ oil, flaxseed oil
Gadoleic	9-Eicosenoic	20	1	Some fish oils
Arachidonic	5, 8, 11, 14-Eicosatetraenoic	20	4	Lard, meats
—	5, 8, 11, 14, 17-Eicosapentaenoic (EPA)	20	5	Some fish oils, shellfish
Erucic	13-Docosenoic	22	1	Canola oil
—	4, 7, 10, 13, 16, 19-Docosahexaenoic (DHA)	22	6	Some fish oils, shellfish

Modified from Institute of Shortening and Edible Oils: *Food fats and oils*, ed 6, Washington, DC, 1988, The Institute.
*All double bonds are in the *cis* configuration except for elaidic acid and vaccenic acid, which are *trans*.

TABLE 3-6 Food Group Sources of Fatty Acids

FATTY ACID GROUP*	MEATS, POULTRY, FISH (%)	FATS AND OILS (%)	DAIRY PRODUCT (%)	LEGUMES, NUTS (%)	EGGS (%)	OTHER (%)
SFA	39	34	20	2	2	3
MUFA	35	48	8	4	2	3
PUFA	18	68	2	6	2	6

Data from Life Science Research Office, Federation of American Societies for Experimental Biology: *Nutrition monitoring in the United States—an update report on nutrition monitoring*. Prepared for the U.S. Department of Agriculture and the U.S. Department of Health and Human Services, Public Health Service, DHHS Pub No (PHA) 89-1255, Washington, DC, September 1989, U.S. Government Printing Office.
**SFA*, Saturated fatty acid; *MUFA*, monounsaturated fatty acid; *PUFA*, polyunsaturated fatty acid.

five double bonds, the first of which is three carbons from the terminal methyl group. Plants make oils of omega-6 fatty acid and omega-3 fatty acid types. Linoleic acid (C18:2 ω-6) has 18 carbons and 2 double bonds, and α-linolenic acid (ALA; C18:3 ω-3) has 18 carbons and 3 double bonds and is an omega-3 fatty acid. MFAs, such as oleic acid (C18:1 ω-9) in olive and canola oils, has a double bond nine carbons from the methyl group and is classed as an omega-9 fatty acid.

Sources of Fatty Acids

The percentages of saturated, monounsaturated, and polyunsaturated fatty acids typically obtained from various food groups are shown in Table 3-6. Sources of omega-3 fatty acids from selected marine sources are listed in Table 3-7. The fatty acid content in the diet of an organism determines the proportion of that fatty acid in the animal product. For example, eggs from chickens that are fed fish meal or linseed

TABLE 3-7 Sources of Omega-3 Fatty Acids

FOOD SOURCE (100 g EDIBLE PORTION, RAW)	TOTAL FAT (GRAMS)	OMEGA-3 FAT DHA (22:6 ω-3)* EPA (20:5 ω-3)
Sardines, in sardine oil	15.5	3.3
Mackerel, Atlantic	13.9	2.5
Herring, Atlantic	9	1.6
Salmon, Chinook	10.4	1.4
Anchovy	4.8	1.4
Salmon, Atlantic	5.4	1.2
Bluefish	6.5	1.2
Salmon, pink	3.4	1
Pompano, Florida	9.5	0.6
Tuna	2.5	0.5
Trout, brook	2.7	0.4
Shrimp	1.1	0.3
Catfish, channel	4.3	0.3
Lobster, northern	0.9	0.2
Haddock	0.7	0.2
Flounder	1	0.2

Modified from Conner SL, Conner WE: Are fish oils beneficial in the prevention and treatment of coronary artery disease? *Am J Clin Nutr* (suppl 4):1020-1031, 1997.
**DNA,* Docosahexenoic acid; *EPA,* eicosapentaenoic acid.

(flaxseed) oil are higher in omega-3 fatty acids (Farrell, 1998). Similarly, the omega-3 fatty acid content of fish differs by species (e.g., Atlantic versus Chinook salmon) and origin (e.g., farm raised versus wild [being higher]). Thus values given in Table 3-7 and other nutrient databases should be used as a rough estimate rather than a precise calculation of omega-3 fatty acid content.

The Omega-6/Omega-3 Ratio

It has been postulated that humans evolved by consuming a diet lower in saturated fat and higher in omega-3 fatty acids than is consumed today (Crawford, 1992). Ancient humans either lived by the oceans and subsisted primarily on fish or lived inland and consumed large quantities of green plants high in ALA (C18:3 ω-3). Humans can convert ALA to EPA (C20:5 ω-3) and the longer docosahexaenoic acid (DHA; C22:6 ω-3). The Paleolithic diet is thought to have been richer in marine and plant sources of omega-3 fatty acids and lower in omega-6 fatty acid sources, resulting in an omega-6/omega-3 ratio that approximated 1:1 (Eaton, 1985). In contrast, the modern diet is richer in omega-6 fatty acids from animal protein and especially from oils extracted from grains, such as corn and safflower oils, with an estimated omega-6/omega-3 ratio of 8:1 to 12:1.

Dietary precursors for the synthesis omega-3 and omega-6 fatty acids are made by the chloroplasts of marine phytoplankton and land plants, respectively. Plants make omega-3 and omega-6 oils; however, omega-6 is more widely distributed in plants compared with omega-3. Animals higher on the evolutionary scale cannot introduce double bonds closer to the terminal than C-7, nor can mammalian cells convert omega-3 to omega-6. Humans can desaturate and elongate ALA (C18:3 ω-3) into EPA (C20:5 ω-3) and DHA (C22:6 ω-3) but only when the omega-6/omega-3 ratio is low. Excess omega-6 fatty acids in the diet saturates the enzymes and prevents conversion of ALA into longer EPA and DHA forms (Kris-Etherton, 2000).

Because the optimal omega-6/omega-3 ratio has been estimated to be 2:1 to 3:1, four times lower than the current intake, it is recommended that humans consume more omega-3 fatty acids from vegetable and marine sources. ALA can be obtained from flaxseed (57%), canola (8%), and soybean (7%) oils and green leaves in a few plants such as purslane. Sources of the longer EPA and DHA omega-3 fatty acids are primarily marine: cod liver oil, mackerel, salmon, and sardines, as well as crab, shrimp, and oysters.

Commercial attempts have been made to supplement livestock, including chickens and fish, with sources of omega-3 fatty acids. At this time, eggs are the only supplemented product commercially available. Eggland's Best eggs have 100 mg of omega-3 fatty acid per egg, Wilcox Farms eggs have 350 mg per egg, Country Hen has 240 mg per egg, and other eggs claim to have various amounts.

Trans-Fatty Acids

General Properties

In natural unsaturated fatty acids, the two carbons participating in a double bond each bind a hydrogen on the *same* side of the bond (the *cis*-isomer form). Because the two remaining hydrogens take up space, the *cis* configuration causes the fatty acid to crimp, or bend, toward the empty side (see Figure 3-6, *1*). The more double bonds per fatty acid, the more bends in the molecule. Hydrogenation of unsaturated fat can occur during anaerobic fermentation in the rumen of cows and sheep and by chemical methods that add hydrogen to liquid oils to form a stable, solid fat such as margarine. Hydrogen can be added both in the natural *cis* position (with two hydrogens on the same side of the double bond) and in the *trans* position (with one hydrogen on opposite sides of the double bond). Major sources of *trans*-fatty acids in the U.S. diet are partially hydrogenated margarine, shortening, commercial frying fats, high-fat baked goods, and salty snacks containing these fats. Butter and animal fat can also contain *trans*-fatty acids from bacterial fermentation, as discussed previously.

Membrane Function

Membrane function depends on the three-dimensional configuration of membrane fatty acids. The *cis* double bonds in membrane PUFAs form kinks and allow the fatty acids to pack more loosely, an arrangement that makes the membrane less stiff and rigid. Because proteins embedded in a biomembrane float or sink depending on the membrane's fluidity, biomembrane viscosity is important for membrane protein function. Because *trans*-fatty acids do not kink, they pack into the biomembrane as tightly as if they were fully saturated. Clinical and epidemiologic studies suggest that higher intakes of *trans*-fatty acids are associated with increased risk for coronary heart disease, cancer, and other chronic diseases, possibly because of their potential to influence membrane fluidity. *Trans*-fatty acids have also been shown to inhibit the desaturation and elongation of linoleic and ALA to form long-chain essential fatty acids, as discussed previously. Long-chain PUFAs are critical for fetal brain and organ development. Until more is known about the extent of their risk, it is recommended that dietary consumption of hydrogenated and saturated fatty acids be reduced. The role of *trans*-fatty acids in atherosclerosis is discussed in Chapter 35, and its role in pregnancy and child development is discussed in Chapters 7 through 10 (see *Clinical Insight:* Essential Fatty Acid Deficiency).

Triglycerides

The body forms triglycerides (formally, **triacylglycerols**) by joining three fatty acids to a glycerol side chain (see Figure 3-6, 2), thereby neutralizing reactive fatty acids. Free fatty acids are potentially dangerous because they contain a carboxylic (COOH) acid head group that reacts readily with other molecules. To avoid tissue damage, biologic organisms form triglycerides by binding three fatty acids to glycerol. As indicated in Figure 3-6, 2, the hydroxyl group on each fatty acid is bound to a hydroxyl group on glycerol. At each site a molecule of water is released, and an ester (—O—) linkage is formed. Fatty acids linked to glycerol are neutral and have no free hydroxyl groups, making triglycerides water insoluble *(hydrophobic).* Neutral fats can be safely transported in the blood and stored in fat cells (adipocytes) as an energy reserve. More than 95% of lipids in the food supply are in the triglyceride storage form.

The fatty acids that make up triglycerides reflect the fatty acid constituents of the plant or animal. Fatty acids in a food source can vary in length and saturation, and different fatty acids can comprise a single triglyceride. SFAs are relatively inert and not susceptible to oxidative damage during storage. Thus storage triglycerides from land animals are predominately saturated. Cold-water creatures must maintain their fatty acids in liquid form even at low temperatures; triglycerides in fish oils and marine-derived fats contain even longer (20C and 22C) but highly unsaturated fatty acids.

CLINICAL INSIGHT

Essential Fatty Acid Deficiency

The consequences of reduced availability of omega-3 fatty acids are just now beginning to be understood. The human brain, central nervous system, and membranes throughout the body require omega-3 fatty acids, especially EPA and DHA, for optimal function. Connor et al (1992) proposed that greater availability of long-chain omega-3 fatty acids allowed humans to develop their complex brain and neural system. An animal deficient in omega-3 fatty acids grows and reproduces normally but is at risk for developing learning problems, impaired vision, and polydipsia.

The impact of omega-3 fatty acids on cardiovascular disease, arthritis, cancer, and other chronic diseases, as well as on altered immune and mental states, including attention deficit hyperactivity disorder, is under intense study. Abnormal omega-6/omega-3 ratios have been linked to changes in vascular membrane lipid composition and increased incidence of atherosclerosis and inflammatory disorders (see Chapters 35 and 44). Deficiencies of omega-6 essential fatty acids also have clinical implications, including growth retardation, skin lesions, reproductive failure, fatty liver, and polydipsia. Fat-free diets may lead to essential fatty acid deficiencies and eventually death if missing nutrient is not provided.

Phospholipids

Phospholipids are derivatives of phosphatidic acid, a triglyceride modified to contain a phosphate group at the third position (see Figure 3-6, *3*). Phosphatidic acid is esterified into a nitrogen-containing molecule, usually a choline, serine, inositol, or ethanolamine, and named for its nitrogenous base (e.g., phosphatidylcholine, phosphatidylserine). Membrane phospholipids usually contain one SFA (C16 to C18) at C-1 and a highly polyunsaturated fatty acid (C16 to C20) at C-2. The SFA is relatively inert; the PUFA is bent because of the double bonds. ALA (C18:3 ω-3), arachidonic acid (C20:4 ω-6), and omega-3 substitutes can be cleaved from the lipid bilayer and provide substrate for synthesis of prostaglandins and other local mediators of cell activity.

Because it is polar at physiologic pH, the phosphate-containing portion of the molecule forms hydrogen bonds with water, whereas the two fatty acids have hydrophobic interactions with fats (Figure 3-7). Because of their dual water- and fat-loving affinity, phospholipids are called *biologic amphiphiles* (derived from the Greek words *ampho* meaning "both" and *philos* meaning "fond"). The polar head groups face outward into the aqueous external and cytoplasmic fluids, whereas the centrally placed fatty acid tails participate in hydrophobic interactions at the membrane center. The barrier formed by this lipid bilayer can only be crossed by very small lipid soluble molecules (e.g., oxygen, carbon dioxide, and nitrogen) and to a limited extent by small, uncharged polar molecules such as water and urea.

In the duodenum a single amphiphilic layer of phospholipids incorporates bile acids to create mixed micelles; the hydrophilic heads form an aqueous sphere, and the hydrophobic fatty acid tail binds dietary fats and oils. In this way, fats are emulsified in digestive secretions and made available for digestion by pancreatic lipases. Single layers of phospholipids also form lipoprotein vehicles that transport fats through the bloodstream.

Lecithin

Lecithin (phosphatidylcholine) contains choline and is the major phospholipid components in the biomembrane's outer leaflet. Lecithin is also a major component of lipoproteins used to transport fats and cholesterol. HDLs contain a copper-dependent enzyme, *lecithin-cholesterol acyltransferase,* used to transfer a fatty acid from lecithin to free cholesterol taken from the cell membrane. The resultant neutral cholesterol ester is stored in the HDL lipid center for safe transport to the liver.

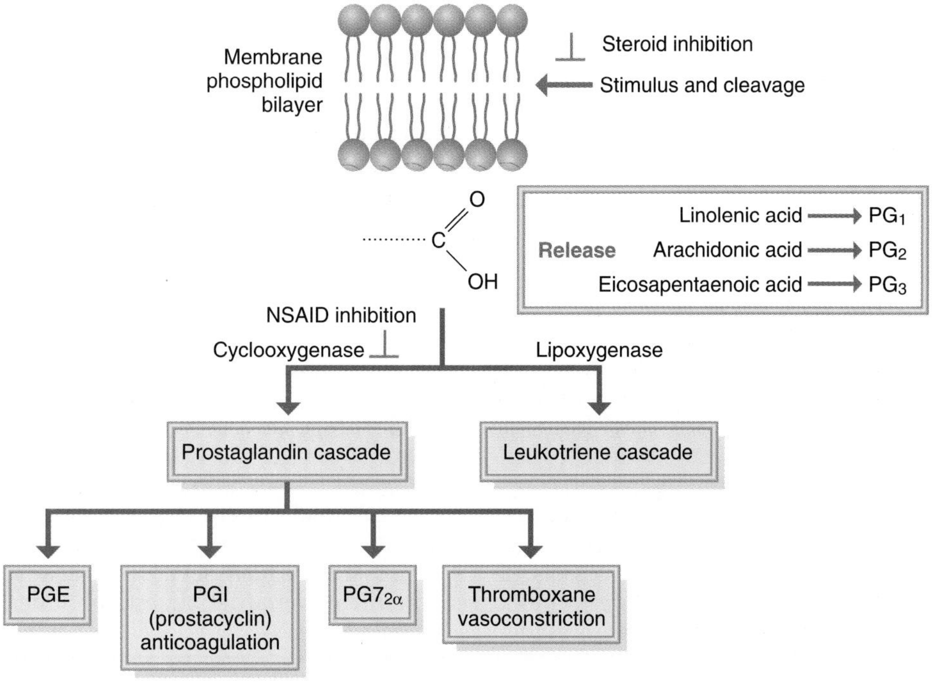

FIGURE 3-7 • Eicosanoid synthesis after phospholipid cleavage in the biomembrane. Injury, inflammation, and other stimuli cleave the highly unsaturated fatty acid at the C-2 position of the membrane phospholipid. Arachidonic acid (AA) or eicosapentaenoic acid (EPA) is the major fatty acid released; the pathway entered depends on the degree to which the target tissue expresses the enzyme. The cyclooxygenase pathway leads to prostaglandin (PG), thromboxane, and prostacyclin synthesis. The lipoxygenase pathway, which is common in the lungs and bronchi, leads to leukotriene synthesis and subsequent bronchoconstriction. Note the point at which steroidal and nonsteroidal antiinflammatory drugs (NSAIDs) act.

CLINICAL INSIGHT

Bleeding Tendency

Arachidonic acid (C20:4 ω-6) is a precursor of the prostaglandin thromboxane A2 (TXA2), a strong activator of platelet aggregation, vasoconstriction, and clot formation (Connor and Connor, 1997). Marine fish and oils in the diet increase the number of EPA (C20:5 ω-3) molecules in the platelet biomembrane. If EPA, rather than arachidonic acid, is cleaved from the membrane, the prostaglandin TXA3 is formed. This hormone is a much weaker vasoconstrictor than TXA2, and platelets are less likely to aggregate. Fish oil also reduces fibrinogen and other clotting proteins, increases platelet survival, and decreases the risk that a clot will form. At the same time, fish oil ingestion causes vascular endothelial cells to produce more prostacyclin (PGI3) and secrete more endothelial cell-derived relaxation factor. These mediators counter vasoconstriction and inhibit the tendency to clot. Omega-3 fatty acids inhibit the desaturase enzyme, thereby reducing the amount of arachidonic acid formed from ALA. Thus eicosanoids made from EPA inhibit the tendency to clot, whereas eicosanoids from arachidonic acid (i.e., animal fat) increase clotting. The omega-6/omega-3 fatty acid ratio in the membrane seems to be of utmost importance, and the ratio is largely determined by the type of dietary fatty acids ingested.

Lecithin is made by the body de novo and in biomembranes and is widely distributed in the food supply. Because all cells contain lecithin as a lipid bilayer component, animal products, especially liver and egg yolks, are rich sources of lecithin. Plant products such as soybeans, peanuts, legumes, spinach, and wheat germ are also rich sources. Its amphiphilic quality makes lecithin an ideal additive to bind water and fat together to form a stable emulsion that does not separate over time. Lecithin is added to food products such as margarine, ice cream, snack crackers, and confections. Lecithin is a fat and contains 9 kcal/g.

Eicosanoids and Paracrine Mediators

Long-chain PUFAs in membrane phospholipids are cleaved in response to injury and inflammation (see Figure 3-7). Fatty acids are classified by the number of their double bonds: linoleic (three), arachidonic (four), and eicosapentaenoic (five). Depending on the tissue involved, fatty acids enter either the prostaglandin or leukotriene cascade, leading to the production of eicosanoid hormones. Because these hormones are made and used in nearby tissues, they are designated *paracrine mediators* (with *para,* from the Greek, meaning "alongside"), in contrast to endocrine hormones made by distant organs and transported in the blood (see Chapter 1). These paracrine hormones have multiple local functions. They can alter the size and permeability of the blood vessels, alter the activity of platelets and contribute to blood clotting, and modify the processes of inflammation (see *Clinical Insight:* Bleeding Tendency).

In addition to eicosanoids, a bewildering variety of mediators exist, including interleukins, cytokines, chemokines, clotting factors, growth factors, adhesion factors, and other molecules that are influenced by dietary lipid consumption. Too little is known yet to make more than a few basic recommendations about the amount and type of dietary lipids that provide optimal biomembrane substrate. Roles for omega-3 fatty acids in cardiovascular disease are discussed in Chapter 35; arthritis and inflammatory conditions are discussed in Chapter 44.

Sphingolipids, Alcohols, Waxes, Isoprenoids, and Steroids

All organisms produce small amounts of complex lipids with specialized, critical functions. Many of these lipids do not contain glycerol and are built from two-carbon acetyl coenzyme A (acetyl CoA) units.

Sphingolipids are lipid esters attached to a sphingosine base rather than a glycerol. They are widely distributed in the nervous systems of animals and the membranes of plants and lower eukaryotes such as yeast. *Sphingomyelin* includes the nitrogenous base choline and makes up more than 25% of the myelin sheath, the lipid-rich structure that protects and insulates cells of the central nervous system. In addition to phosphatidylcholine, sphingomyelin is found in the outer leaflet of all biomembranes. Sphingolipids are constantly synthesized and degraded in the lysosome. *Sphingolipidoses* comprise a group of genetic lipid storage diseases in which sphingolipid degradation through the lysosomal pathway is blocked. Tay-Sachs disease is an example of a lipid storage disease in which an enzyme deficiency results in accumulation of the lipid metabolite, especially in the brain. Patients have severe nervous system degeneration, mental retardation, and blindness and then die, usually by age 4.

Long-chain alcohols are metabolic by-products. The feces contain cetyl alcohol, a by-product of palmitic acid. Beeswax is rich in the alcohol myricyl palmitate. Waxes consist of LCFAs bound to long-chain alcohols. These molecules are almost completely water insoluble and often used as water repellants, as they are in the feathers of birds and on the leaves of plants.

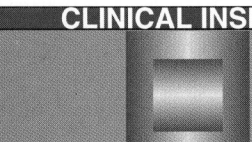

FOCUS ON

Reductase Inhibitors and Cholesterol-Reducing Drugs

The first step in cholesterol biosynthesis is the formation of six-carbon mevalonate using the enzyme 3-hydroxy-3-methylglutaryl-CoA reductase (HMG CoA reductase). By reducing the precursor for cholesterol synthesis, drugs such as reductase inhibitors and statins (e.g., lovastatin, pravastatin) reduce cholesterol biosynthesis, especially in the liver. They are now considered drugs of choice for high-risk patients with hyperlipidemia (Clark, 2003). Statins have recently been reported to reduce cardiovascular risk by acting on blood-clotting systems and endothelial cells. On the other hand, mevalonate is also used as precursor for complex lipids and their derivatives, including coenzyme Q. Statins do not reduce triglyceride synthesis and thus are not used to treat hypertriglyceridemia. Statins inhibit this pathway and may decrease coenzyme Q levels.

Isoprenoids, activated derivatives of isoprene, are an extraordinarily large and diverse group of lipids built from one or more five-carbon units (see Figure 3-6). Isoprene contains alternating single and double (conjugated) bonds, an arrangement that can quench free radicals by accepting or donating electrons. *Terpene* is a generic term for all compounds synthesized from isoprene precursors and includes essential oils of plants (e.g., turpentine from trees and limonene from lemons). Plant pigments that transfer electrons in photosynthesis are also isoprenoids and include lycopene (the red pigment in tomatoes), carotenoids (the yellow and orange pigments in squash and carrots), and the yellow/green chlorophyll group. Fat-soluble vitamins A, D, E, and K and the electron transducer coenzyme Q have isoprenoid structures. Vitamin E, lycopene, and β-carotene are effective antioxidants. Nonnutritive phytochemicals with antioxidant function usually have an isoprenoid structure (see Chapter 12).

Steroids constitute a class of lipids derived from a four-membered saturated ring (see Figure 3-6, *4*). Several important steroid derivatives are made in the body. Glucocorticoids (cortisone) and mineralocorticoids (aldosterone) are made in the adrenal gland, androgens (testosterone) and estrogens (estradiol) are made in the testes and ovaries, respectively, and bile acids are made in the liver. Vitamin D hormone is made when ultraviolet rays from the sun cleave cholesterol in subcutaneous fat to form cholecalciferol (D_3). Synthetic vitamin D is made by irradiating the plant steroid ergosterol to form ergocalciferol (D_2).

Cholesterol is the basis for all steroid derivatives made in the body and plays an important role in membrane function. The rigid, four-ringed cholesterol molecule is bound into the hydrophobic membrane by its hydroxyl group (see Figure 3-6). The stiff, planar rings spread apart and partially immobilize the fatty acid chains near the polar region. At the same time, the nonpolar hydrocarbon tail contributes to greater fluidity in the interior of the membrane. Plasma membranes contain large amounts of cholesterol—up to one molecule for every phospholipid molecule (Alberts et al, 1994) (see *Focus On:* Reductase Inhibitors and Cholesterol-Reducing Drugs).

Glycolipids include the cerebrosides and gangliosides, which are composed of a sphingosine base and very–long-chain (22C) fatty acids. Cerebrosides contain galactose; gangliosides also contain glucose and a complex compound containing an amino sugar. Structurally, both compounds are components of nerve tissue and certain cell membranes, where they play a role in lipid transport.

Synthetic Lipids

Synthetic lipids are commercially synthesized for specific purposes. Examples include medium-chain triglycerides, structured lipids, and fat replacers. Medium-chain triglycerides (MCTs) are SFAs with a chain length of between 6 and 12 carbons. They are short enough to be water soluble, require less bile salt for solubilization, are not reesterified in the enterocyte, and are transported as free fatty acids, bound to albumin, through the portal system. Because the portal blood flow rate is about 250 times faster than the lymph flow, MCTs are digested quickly and not likely to be affected by intestinal factors that inhibit fat absorption (Linscheer and Vergroesen, 1994). They are not stored in adipose tissue but are oxidized to acetic acid.

Natural MCTs are found in milk fat, coconut oil, and palm kernel oil. Commercial MCT oil is a by-product of margarine production. It contains approximately 65% caprylic acid (C8:0) and 25% caproic acid (C10:0), and its remaining fatty acids are less than 6 carbons and greater than 10 carbons in length. MCT oils provide 8.25 kcal/g. Clinically, MCT oil is used for patients with fat malabsorption or with catabolic states, such those with acquired immunodeficiency syndrome (AIDS) or cancer or those needing a ketogenic diet. Specific uses of MCT oil are discussed in Chapters 23 and 43.

Structured lipids include MCT oil esterified with a desired fatty acid such as linoleic acid or an omega-3 lipid. The combined product is absorbed faster than the long-chain triglyceride alone. Clinically, structured lipids are being studied for their role in parenteral and enteral formulas in specific situations (e.g., to enhance immune function or athletic performance).

Fat replacers (Table 3-8) are structurally different from fats and do not provide readily absorbable nutrients. Their commercial importance is that they imitate the texture and other sensations of fat, especially in the mouth. Fat replacers differ in their macronutrient base and the extent to which they mimic the characteristics of fat. The caloric value of these substitutes

TABLE 3-8 Examples of Fat Replacers and Their Functions and Properties

CLASS OF FAT REPLACERS	TRADE NAMES	APPLICATIONS	FUNCTIONAL PROPERTIES
Carbohydrate Based			
Polydextrose	Litesse,[a] Sta-Lite[b]	Dairy products, sauces, frozen desserts, salad dressings, baked goods, confections, gelatins, puddings, meat products, chewing gum, dry cake and cookie mixes, frostings and icings	Moisture retention, bulking agent, texturizer
Starch (modified food starch)	Amalean I & II,[c] N-Lite,[d] Instant Stellar,[e] Sta-Slim,[b] OptaGrade,[e] Pure-gel[f]	Processed meats, salad dressings, baked goods, fillings and frostings, condiments, frozen desserts, dairy products	Gelling, thickening, stabilizing, texturizer
Maltodextrins	CrystaLean,[e] Maltrin,[f] Lycadex,[g] Star-Dri,[b] Paselli Excell,[h] Rice-Trim[i]	Baked goods, dairy products, salad dressings, spreads, sauces, fillings and frostings, processed meat, frozen desserts, extruded products	Gelling, thickening, stabilizing, texturizer
Grain based (fiber)	Betatrim,[j] Opta[e] Oat Fibere,[k] Snowite[k] TrimChoice,[b] Fibrim[l]	Baked goods, meats, extruded products, spreads	Gelling, thickening, stabilizing, texturizer
Dextrins	N-Oil,[d] Stadex[b]	Salad dressings, puddings, spreads, dairy products, frozen desserts, chips, baked goods, meat products, frostings, soups	Gelling, thickening, stabilizing, texturizer
Gums (xanthan, guar, locust bean carrageenan, alginates)	Kelcogel,[m] Keltrol,[n] Viscarin,[o] Gel-carin,[o] Fibrex,[p] Novagel,[q] Rohodi-gel,[j] Jaguar[r]	Salad dressings, processed meats, formulated foods (e.g., desserts, processed meats)	Water retention, texturizer, thickener, mouth texture, stabilizer
Pectin	Grindsted,[s] Slendid,[t] Splendid[t]	Baked goods, soups, sauces, dressings	Gelling, thickening, mouth texture
Cellulose (carboxymethyl cellulose, microcrystalline cellulose)	Avicel,[q] cellulose gel, Methocel,[u] Solka-Floc,[v] Just Fiber[w]	Dairy products, sauces, frozen desserts, salad dressings	Water retention, texturizer, stablizer, mouth texture
Fruit based (fiber)	Prune paste, dried plum paste, Lighter Bake,[x] WonderSlim,[y] fruit powder	Baked goods, candy, dairy products	Moisturizer, mouth texture
Protein Based	Simplesse,[z] K-Blazer,[aa] Dairy-lo,[bb] Veri-lo,[bb] Ultra-Bake,[b] Powerpro,[cc] Proplus,[dd] Supro[dd]	Cheese, mayonnaise, butter, salad dressing, sour cream, spreads, bakery products	Mouth texture
Fat Based	Caprenin,[ee] Olean,[ee] Benefat,[bb] Dur-Em[w] Dur-Lo[w]	Chocolate, confections, bakery products, savory snacks	Mouth texture
Combinations	Prolestra,[ff] Nutrifat,[ff] Finesse[ff]	Ice cream, salad oils, mayonnaise, spreads, sauces, bakery products	Mouth texture

From American Dietetic Association: Position of the American Dietetic Association: fat replacers, *J Am Diet Assoc* 98:463, 1998.
[a]Cultor Food Science, Inc, Ardsley, NY.
[b]AE Staley Manufacturing Co, Decatur, Ill.
[c]Cerestar USA, Inc, Hammond, Ind.
[d]National Starch and Chemical Co. Bridgewater, NJ.
[e]Opta Food Ingredients, Bedford, Mass.
[f]Grain Processing Corp, Muscatine, Iowa
[g]Roquette America, Inc, Keokuk, Iowa
[h]AVEBE America Inc, Princeton, NJ.
[i]Zumbro, Inc, Hayfield, Minn.
[j]Rhone-Poulenc, Inc, Cranbury, NJ.
[k]Canadian Harvest USA, Cambridge, Minn.
[l]Protein Technologies International, Pryor, Okla.
[m]Monsanto, Chicago, Ill.
[n]Kelco, Division of Merck, Clark, NJ.
[o]FMC Corp, Rockland, Me.
[p]Purity Foods, Okemos, Mich.
[q]FMC Corp, Philadelphia, Pa.
[r]Aston Chemicals, Aylesbury, Buckinghamshire, England.
[s]Danisco, New Century, KY.
[t]Hercules Inc, Wilmington, Del.
[u]Dow Chemical, Midland, Mich.
[v]Fiber Sales and Development Corp, Green Brook, NJ.
[w]Loders Croklaan, Glen Ellyn, Ill.
[x]Sunsweet Growers, Yuba City, Calif.
[y]The Heart Garden Corporation, Los Angeles, Calif.
[z]Nutrasweet, San Diego, Calif.
[aa]Kraft Food Ingredients, Memphis, Ind.
[bb]Cultor Food Science, Ardsley, NY.
[cc]Land O'Lakes Food Division, Arden Hill, Minn.
[dd]Protein Technologies International, St Louis, Mo.
[ee]Procter and Gamble, Cincinnati, Ohio.
[ff]Reach Associates, South Orange, NJ.

varies between 5 kcal/g (e.g., caprenin) and 0 kcal/g (e.g., olestra, carrageenan).

The largest group of fat replacers is derived from plant polysaccharides such as gums, cellulose, dextrins, fiber, maltodextrins, starches, and polydextrose. Some products can be digested and provide 4 kcal/g. If the carbohydrate is hydrated (i.e., contains more water), the energy in the molecule can be as little as 1 to 2 kcal/g. Cellulose and nonabsorbable fibers provide no energy. Alcohols of carbohydrates (e.g., polyols such as sorbitol) are not fully absorbed and metabolized and provide less than 4 kcal/g.

Protein-based fat replacers alter the texture of a product in various ways. Microparticulated proteins can act like small ball bearings, providing a fatlike feeling in the mouth. These replacers contribute between 1.3 and 4 kcal/g and augment the protein content of the food. Note that some proteins can stimulate an allergic or antigenic response in susceptible individuals.

Fat sources can be modified to reduce GI absorption, thereby reducing caloric availability. Monoglycerols and diacylglycerols (diglycerides) are used as emulsifiers and contribute the sensory properties of fat but have fewer calories (approximately 5 kcal/g). Salatrim (a short- and long-chain fatty acid triglyceride molecule) also contains approximately 5 kcal/g because of reduced absorbability.

The need for reducing GI fat absorption prompted creation of a new synthetic fat replacer, a sucrose polyester with the generic name *olestra.* Sucrose is esterified with six to eight fatty acids to form esters. The fatty acid chains range in length from 12 to 24 carbons and are derived from edible oils such as soybean, cottonseed, and corn oils. The product has the physical properties of natural dietary fats. Because they are nonabsorbable, sucrose polyesters do not contribute calories to the diet.

Some have raised concerns about the long-term effects of fat substitutes. In particular, if fat substitutes are not absorbed, can they bind essential fatty acids and fat-soluble vitamins and contribute to their malabsorption (Gershoff, 1995)? On the other hand, sufficient research has been done for the Food and Drug Administration (FDA) to grant most fat substitutes the status of "generally recognized as safe." In the case of sucrose polyester, the FDA determined that it had not previously been found in food, classified it as a food additive, and required extensive data on its safety before allowing it to be added to food (Clydesdale, 1997). The American Dietetic Association (1998) reviewed fat replacers and concluded that "fat replacers may offer a safe, feasible, and effective means to maintain the palatability of diets with controlled amounts of fat and/or energy."

Food Sources of Fat and Reasonable Recommendations

The vast array of fat types in the diet, coupled with the growing realization that the type of dietary fat consumed may have important consequences in the body, suggests that recommendations about dietary fat consumption must consider fat type as well as fat amount. The following guidelines have been suggested, with the understanding that fat metabolism is a dynamic and ever-changing field.

Types of Fat in the Diet

All naturally occurring fats are mixtures of PUFAs, SFAs, and MFAs, although one type predominates in most foods. Animals maintain their storage fats in as saturated a state as possible but still liquid at body temperature; thus storage fat depots in foods of land animal origin are primarily saturated (SFAs). Marine animals, especially those from cold waters, must maintain their fat in liquid form as unsaturated oils (PUFAs). Plants that grow in temperate climates, for example, corn and soybeans, form PUFA oils, mainly linoleic acid (C18:2 ω-6) stored in their seeds. Some tropical plants, such as coconut, cocoa, and palm, store saturated fats, possibly because their growing temperature is higher. MFAs are found in olive oil, canola oil, peanut oil, peanuts, pecans, almonds, and avocados. Omega-3 PUFAs come primarily from marine sources (see Table 3-7), although vegetable precursors can be obtained from flaxseed and canola oils, walnuts, and green leafy sources.

Saturated fatty acids are known to increase LDLs and HDLs, whereas PUFAs decrease the "bad" and "good" lipoproteins. Thus a judicious mix of SFAs, MFAs, and PUFAs has been recommended. On the other hand, too much PUFA can be dangerous. Double bonds are highly reactive and bind oxygen to form peroxides when exposed to air or heat. Oxidized fats produce the bad flavors and odors characteristic of *rancidity.* Saturated fat and partially hydrogenated oils have fewer oxygen-binding sites and thereby have increased stability and a longer shelf life. PUFA-rich oils are also reactive in cooking. When subjected to routine frying or cooking, PUFAs can generate high levels of toxic aldehyde products that promote cardiovascular disease and cancer. To prevent toxic product formation, PUFAs are often fortified with vitamin E or synthetic antioxidants such as butylated hydroxyanisole (BHA) and butylated hydroxytoluene (BHT). However, toxic products are produced during cooking, even in the presence of antioxidants such as vitamin E. Saturated and monounsaturated fatty acids, especially those in olive oil, that were similarly thermally stressed did not produce these toxic products (Grootveld et al, 1998).

Dietary Cholesterol

The association between high serum cholesterol concentrations and risk for heart disease has led to dietary restrictions of cholesterol-rich foods such as eggs, each of which has 250 mg of cholesterol. However, serum cholesterol levels are homeostatically controlled, and individual responses to dietary cholesterol are highly variable. For example, eggs are an inexpensive source of high-biologic-value protein and also contain omega-3 fatty acids and lecithin, substances associated with reduced risk for hyperlipidemia and heart disease. Dietary cholesterol may have negative effects on some people's lipid levels, so limits may be necessary.

In summary, lipids play a major role in cell biology. As energy stores in adipocytes, they provide a concentrated source of fuel, especially in the fasting state. As structural fat pads, they protect organs and bones from injury. Phospholipids are integral to all biomembranes, where they function as lipid barriers, insulators, and substrates for paracrine hormones and complex lipids. Fat-soluble vitamins regulate metabolic functions in diverse ways. Vitamin E protects membranes from oxidative damage, whereas vitamins A and D regulate gene expression. Nutrition science is in its infancy, as researchers begin to probe the full extent of lipid action at the molecular and cellular level and examine the precise interactions between dietary and endogenous lipids on lipid homeostasis. In view of the well-described mammalian preference for fat, which is apparently an innate part of the human physiology, scientists can conclude that humans require fat in the diet. Until more is known, the recommendation to consume various SFAs, PUFAs, and MFAs in the diet and avoid rapid and high heat harsh cooking practices seems justified. In short, moderation and diversity are critical.

AMINO ACIDS AND PROTEIN

Protein: The Nitrogen Cycle and Dietary Protein Sources

In a never-ending "nitrogen cycle," plants incorporate inorganic nitrogen from nitrogen-fixing bacteria to form amino acids and proteins. Animals eat the plants and convert the amino acids to proteins according to their needs. Humans eat animals and plants and again rearrange the nitrogen to make the pattern of amino acids required. Finally, everybody dies; organic molecules are degraded by microorganisms, nitrogen goes back into the soil to be used by nitrogen-fixing bacteria, and the cycle starts again.

Nitrogen contained in all amino acids originates as nitrogen gas (N_2) in the biosphere. Certain microorganisms, *Rhizobium* bacteria in soil, cyanobacteria in fresh water, and blue-green algae in sea water have the capacity to use inorganic nitrogen and "fix" (or incorporate) it into organic molecules such as glutamate. Soil bacteria attach to the roots of plants such as soybean, clover, and alfalfa. A symbiotic relationship is formed in which the bacteria provide organic nitrogen in exchange for sugars and other nutrients from the plant. This process accounts for the high nitrogen content in legumes such as soybeans and beans. Agricultural practices take advantage of this phenomenon; farmers rotate legume crops with corn and wheat to provide added nitrogen to the soil.

Whereas plant structures are primarily composed of carbohydrates, the body structure of humans and animals is built on protein. Protein is also an energy source. Nitrogen can be removed from amino acids in a process called deamination, and the resulting carbohydrate can be used for energy at the rate of 4 kcal/g. Protein in muscles and body tissue is in constant turnover. Tissue protein is degraded and nitrogen excreted in the urine. New protein is required daily to maintain the body in a steady state.

According to current recommendations, a healthy adult human requires 0.8 g of protein per kilogram of healthy body weight. To obtain this quantity of protein, humans benefit when dietary protein makes up approximately 10% to 15% of total energy intake. Protein requirements increase during times of stress and disease (see Chapter 42). Protein-rich foods are obtained primarily from animal flesh or animal products such as eggs and milk. Most plant foods are relatively poor sources of protein, with the exception of legumes and beans.

Amino Acid Structure

Amino acids are carbohydrates with an amino (NH_2) group added to the α-carbon, which is the carbon next to the carboxyl group (Figure 3-8). Some carbohydrate skeletons can be made in the body (e.g., from intermediates in metabolic pathways). Because these carbon skeletons can be made and an amino group added, the resulting amino acids are called nonessential amino acids. For example, *pyruvate* is a carbohydrate intermediate formed during glycolysis. Add an amino group, and it becomes the amino acid alanine.

Essential amino acids have carbon skeletons that humans cannot make and can obtain only from the diet (see Figure 3-8). Humans can transfer nitrogen between amino acids and carbohydrates through a process called transamination. This process requires vitamin B_6 and is carried out by multiple forms of aminotransaminase enzymes using the following format:

$$\text{Carbohydrate} + \text{Amino acid} \Longleftrightarrow \text{Amino acid} + \text{Carbohydrate}$$

In this way, a carbohydrate can be converted into an amino acid and vice versa, for example, pyruvate to alanine. The ability to transaminate carbohydrates increases the likelihood that all 20 amino acids are available for protein synthesis.

Figure 3-8 illustrates the general structure of the 20 amino acids necessary for human protein synthesis. Each amino acid contains a carboxyl group (COOH); an α-carbon, to which a hydrogen and the amino group are attached; and a side chain *(R group)*. The general structure of the 20 amino acids is the same; only the R group differs. The R group dictates the identity and function of the amino acid. The three-

All amino acids have the same general structure 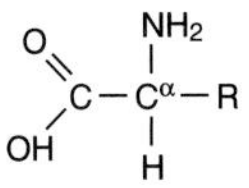 in which R is different for each.

FUNCTIONAL TYPE	AMINO ACID (abbr.)	R GROUP	CHARACTERISTICS OF THE AMINO ACID
Aliphatic	Glycine (Gly) G	H	Tiny R group (H), which allows hairpin bends in the peptide chains
	Alanine (Ala) A	CH_3	Can be deaminated to pyruvate and used for glucose synthesis
	Valine (Val) V*	$-CH(CH_3)_2$	Branched-chain amino acids; metabolized in muscle
	Leucine (Leu) L*	$-CH_2-CH(CH_3)_2$	Branched-chain amino acids more hydophobic; muscle metabolism
	Isoleucine (Ile) I*	$-CH(CH_3)-CH_2-CH_3$	Branched-chain amino acids most hydophobic; muscle metabolism
Sulfur	Cysteine (Cys) C**	$-CH_2-SH$	Essential for glutatione synthesis; synthesis limited in chronic diseases
	Methionine (Met) M*	$-CH_2-CH_2-S-CH_2$	Converted to S-adenosylmethionine (SAM), the universal methyl donor, and cysteine
Hydroxyl	Serine (Ser) S	$-CH_2-OH$	Hydroxyl group phosphorylated to activate and inactivate protein
	Threonine (Thr) T	$-CH_2-CH_2-S-CH_3$	Also site for regulatory phosphorylation
Aromatic	Phenylalanine (Phe) F*	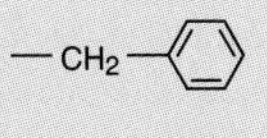	Converted to tyrosine for synthesis of norepinephrine, epinephrine, and dopamine
	Tyrosine (Tyr) Y	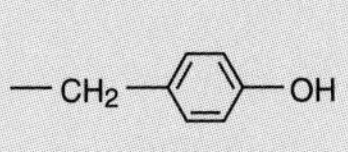	Converted to neurotransmitters norepinephrine, epinephrine, and dopamine
	Tryptophan (Trp) W*	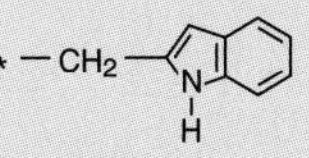	Converted to neurotransmitter serotonin and to niacin
Cyclic	Proline (Pro) P*	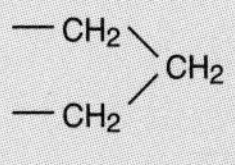	Allows triple helix; proline in collagen to be hydroxylated for cross-linkage
Basic	Lysine (Lys) K	$-CH_2-CH_2-CH_2-CH_2-\overset{+}{N}H_3$	Site for hydroxylation in proteins; hydrophylic; used in signaling
	Histidine (His) H**	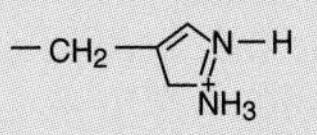	Hydrophilic, binds zinc in signaling proteins
	Arginine (Arg) R	$-CH_2-CH_2-CH_2-NH-C(=\overset{+}{N}H_2)-NH_2$	Formed in the urea cycle; essential for synthesis of nitric oxide signaling pathway
Acidic	Aspartic acid (Asp) D	$-CH_2-C(=O)O^-$	Takes a second nitrogen to form asparagine (Asn) $N-CH_2-C(=O)NH_2$
	Glutamic acid (Glu) E	$-CH_2-CH_2-C(=O)O^-$	Takes a second nitrogen to form glutamine (Gln) Q $-CH_2-CH_2-C(=O)NH_2$

FIGURE 3-8 • Structures and functions of the 20 amino acids required by humans. All amino acids have the same general structure, but the R group is different for each. Amino acids are abbreviated using a three-letter and single-letter code. Amino acids marked with an asterisk *(*)* are essential; those marked with double asterisks *(**)* are essential for infants and those with certain chronic diseases.

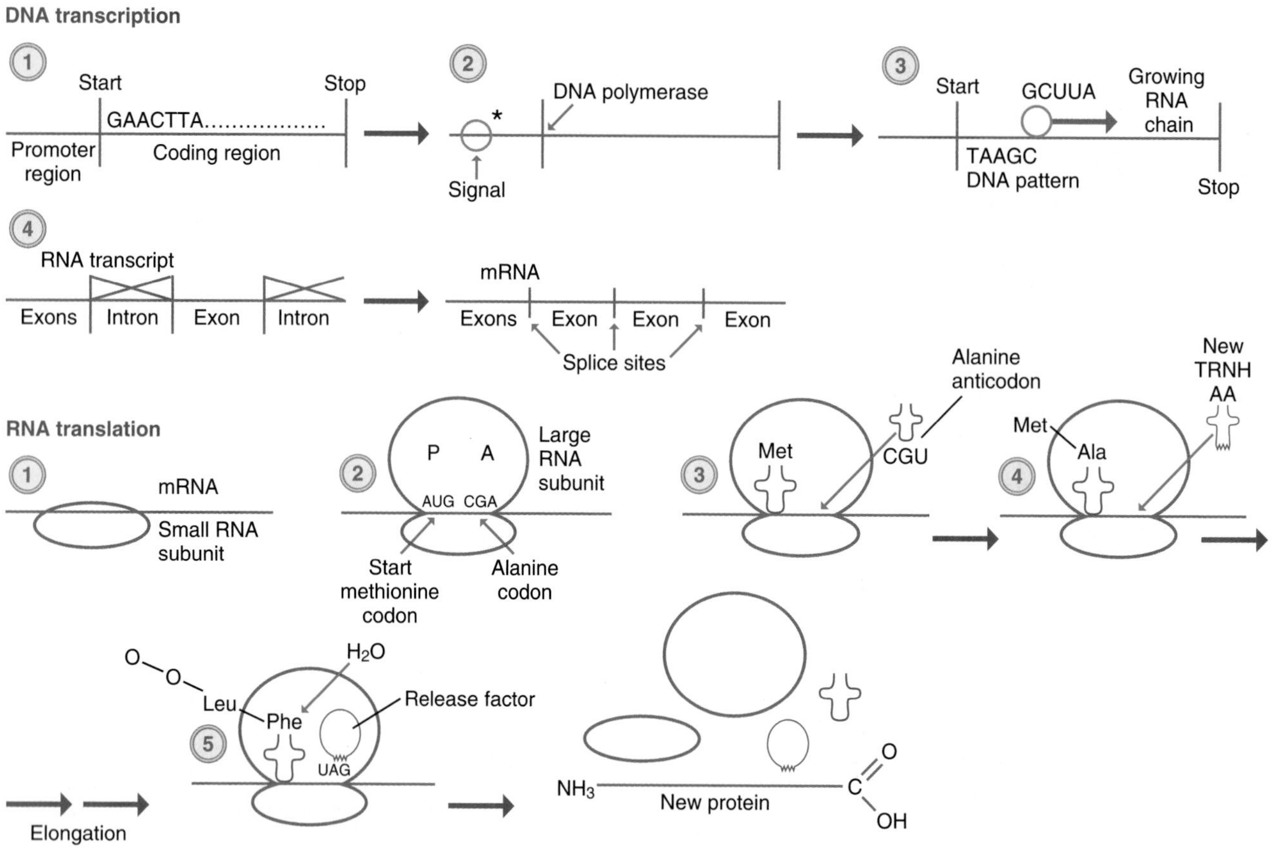

FIGURE 3-9 • Summary of DNA transcription and RNA translation in the eukaryotic cell.

letter and single-letter abbreviations shown in Figure 3-8 are commonly used to describe the amino acid sequence of a protein.

Protein Synthesis

Amino acids are important because they are used as substrates for protein synthesis. The patterns for all proteins are contained in the deoxyribonucleic acid (DNA) of each organism (see Chapter 16). As illustrated in Figure 3-9, protein synthesis is a complex process through which the protein pattern is copied from DNA to ribonucleic acid (RNA). The RNA message is taken to the cytoplasm, where the amino acids are attached in a precise, linear sequence. Specific details of protein synthesis can be obtained from current biochemistry and cell biology texts.

Figure 3-10 illustrates the end product of protein synthesis—the formation of the peptide bond. The peptide bond is formed between the carboxyl group of the first amino acid and the amine group of the next.

The pattern for protein synthesis is contained on messenger RNA (mRNA) and is directly copied from DNA. New proteins are built by attaching amino acids as dictated by the mRNA. When the protein has been built, it detaches from the message and is ready to be used (see *Focus On:* DNA Transcription and RNA Translation).

Protein Folding: Three-Dimensional Structure

Proper folding of the completed linear amino acid chain is essential for a protein to perform its unique functions. The linear sequence of individual amino acids dictates the configuration of the mature protein. As indicated in Figure 3-10, R groups protrude from the newly synthesized peptide chain and are in position to react with each other. Folding is accomplished through hydrogen bonding, ionic bonding, and hydrophobic and other interactions between individual R groups on each amino acid. For example, a negative charge on one amino acid R group forms an attraction with a positive charge on another. This allows the protein to form a precise, three-dimensional structure. Proteins have four levels of structure, as indicated below (see Figure 3-10):

1. *Primary structure:* Peptide bonds are formed between sequential amino acids according to directions on mRNA. The completed protein is a linear chain of amino acids.
2. *Secondary structure:* Attractions between R groups of amino acids create helices and pleated sheet structures.
3. *Tertiary structure:* Helices and pleated sheets are folded into compact domains. Small proteins have

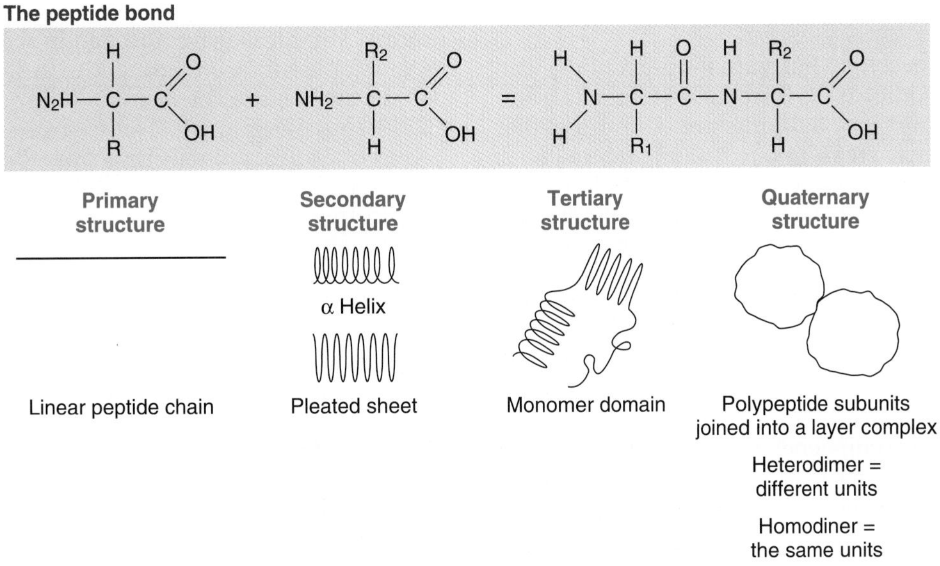

FIGURE 3-10 • The peptide bond and protein folding.

FOCUS ON

DNA Transcription and RNA Translation

DNA Transcription

1. All cells have the ability to make all proteins needed by the body. The linear sequence of each protein is dictated by the linear sequence of nucleotide bases: *thymine, adenine, guanine,* and *cytosine.* A linear sequence of three bases, or *codon,* codes for each of the 20 amino acids. Because the four bases can be combined in 64 ways, more than one three-base codon can code for a single amino acid.
2. As they differentiate, cells inactivate various regions of the DNA that codes for specific proteins. For example, only the precursor to the red blood cell makes hemoglobin. The gene for hemoglobin is inactivated in all other differentiated cells.
3. In front of each coding region is a *promoter region.* The promoter region receives a signal that the protein is needed. Nutrients, including vitamins A and D and minerals such as zinc, play major roles in regulating gene expression in the promoter region.
4. When nutrients and other molecules bind to the promoter region, *RNA polymerase* binds to the start code in the coding region, opens the DNA double helix, and builds a new RNA chain complementary to the DNA coding region.
5. When the RNA polymerase reaches the stop code at the end of the protein coding region, polymerase detaches, releasing the completed RNA transcript. The DNA helix re-forms, and the RNA transcript is modified to remove *introns,* which are intervening, noncoding sequences that are not part of the final protein pattern. The modified RNA transcript is called *messenger RNA (mRNA).*
6. At the same time, in another region of the DNA, RNA polymerase molecules make copies of *ribosomal RNA (rRNA)* and *transfer RNA (tRNA).*
7. The mRNA, rRNA, and tRNA leave the nucleus and enter the cytoplasm (see Figure 3-9).

RNA Translation

1. Small rRNA subunits are activated and bind mRNA. Large rRNA subunits bind and hold the mRNA firmly. The mRNA is sandwiched between the two rRNA subunits, and two three-base codons are available for binding tRNA.
2. Each of 20 tRNA types binds the amino acid that matches its anticodon region. The tRNA, with its attached amino acid and matching anticodon, recognizes its mRNA codon. This process ensures that the linear amino acid sequence is an exact representation of the original DNA code.
3. After each tRNA binds the A site, its amino acid is linked to the growing peptide chain by an enzyme, *peptidyl transferase,* which forms a peptide bond between the end carboxyl and the amino group of the incoming amino acid.
4. The ribosome moves forward. The tRNA, now attached to the peptide chain in the P (peptide) site, and another tRNA enters.
5. The stop codon, UAG, signals the end of the protein. A release factor binds at the A site and attaches a water molecule to the peptide chain, creating the carboxyl (COOH) terminus. The newly formed peptide chain detaches, and the tRNA and rRNA units separate.

one domain, and large proteins have multiple domains.

4. *Quaternary structure:* Individual polypeptides can serve as subunits in the formation of larger assemblies, or complexes. Subunits are bound together by numerous weak, noncovalent interactions; sometimes they are stabilized by disulfide bonds. For example, four hemoglobin monomers are joined to form the tetramer hemoglobin molecule.

Protein structure is a critical component of protein function. The active and catalytic sites at which protein action occurs are formed by juxtaposing functional groups from nearby but occasionally distant R groups. If the linear protein sequence is altered, as it is in those with certain genetic diseases, the protein is unable to form active sites and its activity may be reduced or eliminated entirely.

Dietary Protein Quality

As discussed, linear proteins are formed on the basis of DNA instructions and are composed of specific amino acids. Each organism makes only those proteins required to carry out its specific required tasks. As a result, each source of dietary protein contains its own unique proportion of the 20 common amino acids. More than 50 years ago, it was proposed that the nutritional quality of a protein depended on its amino acid profile. It was also suggested that a protein's biologic value could be determined by the essential amino acid present in the least concentration compared with human requirements (Block and Mitchel, 1946). This essential amino acid is the most limiting amino acid from which a "chemical score" of protein quality is calculated. Table 3-9 indicates requirements by age group.

Protein quality is also determined by measuring the amount of protein actually used by an organism; *net protein utilization (NPU)* is the simplest method of doing so. Dietary protein is equated with its metabolic products by measuring nitrogen in the diet and biologic samples and converting it to the amount of protein on the basis of the formula [Nitrogen (grams) $\times$ 6.25 $=$ Protein (grams)]. The nitrogen content in the bodies of control animals is compared with the nitrogen in the carcasses of an experimental group fed a protein-free diet for the same length of time. The gain in nitrogen is compared with the nitrogen intake, and the proportion of nitrogen retained in the body is computed to obtain the NPU. The NPU ranges from approximately 40 to 94, with protein from animal products scoring higher and protein from vegetables scoring lower (Crim and Munro, 1994).

Soy protein originally received a low NPU score when tested with rats until it was recognized that methionine, which is low in soy protein, is a limiting amino acid for rats. Rats require approximately 50% more methionine than humans (Sarwar et al, 1985). The World Health Organization (WHO) and the U.S. FDA adopted a corrected protein digestibility corrected amino acid score (PDCAAS) as the official assay for evaluating protein quality in the human. The PDCAAS is based on amino acid requirements of children ages 2 to 5 years and represents the amino acid score after correcting for digestibility (Messina, 1995). After being corrected for digestibility, proteins that provide amino acids equal to or in excess of requirements receive a PDCAAS of 1. Soy protein has a PDCAAS of 1 and meets protein needs of human adults when consumed as a sole source of protein at the rate of at least 0.6 g per kilogram of body weight (Young, 1991).

Protein Processing and Digestibility

The digestibility of protein sources is affected by multiple factors. Meat preparation procedures often involve wine or vinegar marinades and moist heat to tenderize tough cuts of meat through denaturation.

TABLE 3-9 Estimates of Amino Acid Requirements

	REQUIREMENTS (mg/kg/day) BY AGE GROUP			
AMINO ACID	INFANTS, AGE 3-4 mo*	CHILDREN, AGE ~2 yr†	CHILDREN, AGE 10-12 yr‡	ADULTS§
Histidine	28	Not determined	Not determined	8-12
Isoleucine	70	31	28	10
Leucine	161	73	44	14
Lysine	103	64	44	12
Methionine plus cystine	58	27	22	13
Phenylalanine plus tyrosine	125	69	22	14
Threonine	87	37	28	7
Tryptophan	17	12.5	3.3	3.5
Valine	93	38	25	10
Total without histidine	714	352	216	84

Modified from World Health Organization: *Energy and protein requirements report of a joint FAO/WHO/UNU expert consultation,* Technical Report Series 724, p. 65, Geneva, 1985, WHO.

*Based on amounts of amino acids in human milk or cow's milk formulas fed at levels that supported good growth.

†Based on achievement of nitrogen balance sufficient to support adequate lean tissue gain (16 mg nitrogen/kg/day).

‡Based on upper range of requirement for positive nitrogen balance.

§Based on highest estimate of requirement to achieve nitrogen balance.

Proteins are kept in the proper configuration by their hydrogen and ionic interactions; these bonds loosen in the presence of acid, salt, and heat. Because they denature proteins, these methods also soften gristle, or connective tissue proteins, and release muscle proteins from their attachments, thereby making all proteins more available to digestive enzymes.

Vegetable protein is less well digested than animal protein, partly because it is encased in carbohydrate cell walls and is less available to digestive enzymes. Some plants also contain enzymes that interfere with protein digestion, so the enzymes must be heat inactivated before consumption. For example, soybeans contain a trypsinase that inactivates trypsin, the major protein-digesting enzyme in the intestine.

Food processing can also damage amino acids and reduce their digestive availability in several ways (Crim and Munro, 1994). Mild heat treatment in the presence of reducing sugars (e.g., glucose and galactose), a procedure used in milk processing, causes a loss of available lysine. Lactose reacts with lysine side chains and renders them unavailable. This reaction, which is called *browning*, or the *Maillard reaction*, can cause significant lysine loss at high temperatures. Under severe heating conditions in the presence (or even absence) of sugars or oxidized lipids, all amino acids in food proteins become resistant to digestion. When protein is exposed to severe treatment with alkali, the amino acids lysine and cysteine can react together and form a potentially toxic lysinoalanine. Exposure to sulfur dioxide and other oxidative conditions can result in loss of methionine. Thermal processing and low-moisture storage of proteins can also result in reductive binding of vitamin B_6 to lysine residues, thereby inactivating the vitamin (Williams and Erdman, 1994). Therefore proper handling of protein foods is necessary to maintain their integrity and usefulness.

Protein Complementarity

Closely related species tend to make proteins with a similar spectrum of amino acids. In contrast, very different species (e.g., plants and humans) have quite different amino acid needs. Although nonessential amino acids can be formed from carbohydrate intermediates in the body, essential amino acids must be obtained from food. If a food's amino acid profile does not match human needs, the amino acids that are in short supply are considered *limiting*. Diets based on a single plant food staple do not foster optimal growth because the diet does not have enough of the limiting amino acid to provide substrates for protein synthesis. If a plant protein that contains an excess of the limiting amino acid is added to the diet, the protein combination is *complemented*. In other words, the plant combination provides adequate amounts of essential amino acids to adequately support human protein synthesis.

Throughout history, humans have thrived because they have been able to develop traditional dishes containing a mixture of vegetable proteins that compensated for amino acid deficiencies by including vegetables with excess amino acids. The concept of protein complementarity is primarily important for populations at risk for consuming insufficiently diverse mixed foods that contain various amino acids. Certain foods, when eaten together, provide all of the essential amino acids (Table 3-10).

It is now considered unnecessary to eat complementary amino acids during a single meal, but they should be eaten within the same day (American Dietetic Association, 1997). Children, pregnant women, and nursing mothers who have vegetarian diets need to plan their diets carefully to include a mixture of amino acid–containing foods.

As discussed previously, the NPU score of vegetable protein may not accurately reflect its available protein. If a person's vegetarian diet is otherwise healthy and the overall protein intake above the minimal requirements, the source of amino acids is probably not of concern. The amino acid compositions of selected foods are listed in Table 3-11.

TABLE 3-10 Food Combinations Providing All Essential Amino Acids

EXCELLENT COMBINATIONS*	EXAMPLES
Grains and legumes	Rice and beans, pea soup and toast, lentil curry and rice
Grains and dairy	Pasta and cheese, rice pudding, cheese sandwich
Legumes and seeds	Garbanzo beans and sesame seeds; hummus as dip, falafel, or soup

*Other combinations, such as dairy and seeds, dairy and legumes, grains and seeds, are less effective because the chemical scores are similar and not effectively complementary.

Protein Use and Nitrogen Balance

Products of protein digestion and protein secreted into the gut lumen (e.g., enzymes, sloughed cells) are available for absorption and transported in the portal vein to the liver. Homeostatic regulations control the concentrations of specific amino acids in the amino acid pool and the rate at which muscle and plasma proteins are synthesized and broken down. Body protein synthesis and breakdown, or turnover, is regulated. In healthy individuals the amount of protein taken in is exactly balanced by protein used for body maintenance and excreted in feces, in urine, and from skin.

Nitrogen balance studies have demonstrated that the nitrogen in the protein eaten by a healthy adult is exactly balanced by the nitrogen excreted, resulting in a zero protein balance (Figure 3-11). A patient with an infection or a traumatic injury excretes more nitrogen than is ingested. Inflammatory cytokines and other mediators are thought to cause nitrogen loss and negative nitrogen balance under these conditions. The pregnant woman and her growing child use ingested protein for growth and maintain a positive nitrogen balance.

TABLE 3-11 Amino Acid Composition of Some Foods

ESSENTIAL AMINO ACID	CHEESE, EGGS, MILK, AND MEAT	CORN	CEREAL	LEGUMES	WHOLE GRAINS (WITH GERM)	NUTS, SEED OILS, AND SOYBEANS	SESAME AND SUNFLOWER SEEDS	PEANUTS	GREEN, LEAFY VEGETABLES	GELATIN	YEAST
Methionine			X	—	X	—	X	—	—	—	X
Isoleucine	X										
Leucine	X										
Lysine	X	—	—	X	X	X	—	—		—	
Phenylalanine											—
Threonine	X	—	—	X	—	X		—			X
Tryptophan		—		—			X			—	
Valine	X										

Modified from Erhard D: Nutrition education for the "now" generation, *J Nutr Educ* 3:135, 1971.
X, High amount of amino acid; —, low amount of amino acid; *blank spaces,* a general good balance of amino acids.

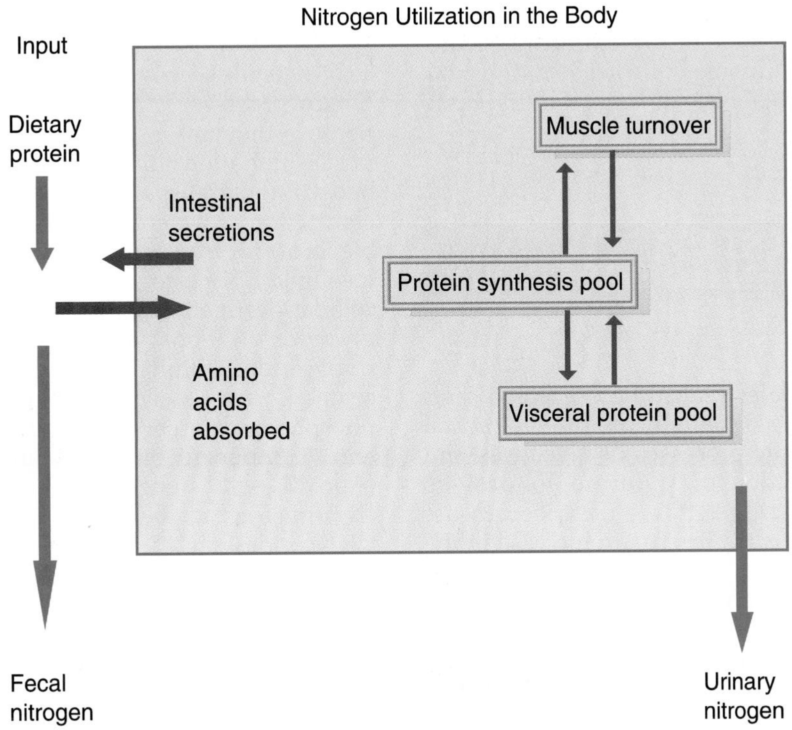

FIGURE 3-11 • Nitrogen use in the body. Protein supplies nitrogen in the form of amino acids, according to the formula [Nitrogen (grams) = Protein (grams) ÷ 6.25]. Dietary protein and protein from endogenous secretions is available for absorption across the GI tract. More than 95% of protein is normally absorbed and enters the synthetic pool. Muscle proteins and visceral (i.e., plasma) proteins are broken down and built up daily. Nitrogen is converted to urea and excreted in the urine. Minor amounts of nitrogen are lost in the menstrual flow and the normal secretions and turnover of skin and its appendages. In a healthy individual, nitrogen intake equals nitrogen losses; the person is in zero protein balance. (Modified from Crim MC, Munro HN: Proteins and amino acids. In Shils ME et al, eds: *Modern nutrition in health and disease*, Philadelphia, 1994, Lea & Febiger.)

Muscle mass, often described as *somatic protein*, is equilibrated with the circulating amino acid pool such that similar quantities of muscle protein are destroyed and rebuilt daily. Muscle mass can be estimated using the creatinine/height index and the midarm muscle circumference (see Chapter 17). Amino acids are also required for synthesis of visceral proteins by the liver and other tissues (see Chapter 18).

Nitrogen Excretion: The Urea Cycle

Nitrogen in the form of ammonia (NH_3) is highly toxic, easily crosses biomembranes, and cannot be allowed to travel unbound throughout the body. In the fed state, pyruvate and other carbon skeletons take up nitrogen and transport it to the liver as nonessential amino acids, usually alanine and glutamic acid (from α-ketoglutarate). When the amino acids reach the liver, they are deaminated into carbohydrate. The ammonia ion is combined with carbon dioxide in the presence of high-energy phosphate and magnesium by the enzyme *carbamoyl phosphate synthase* to form the first intermediate of the urea cycle. Details of the urea cycle can be found in any biochemistry text, as well as in Chapter 45.

Urea makes up 90% of urinary nitrogen in the fed state. Arginine, one of the basic amino acids (see Figure 3-8), is a by-product of the urea cycle. Recent research has found that arginine is required for formation of nitric oxide and other mediators of the inflammatory response (Abcouwer and Souba, 1998). Although classified as a nonessential amino acid, arginine may be essential for critically ill individuals (see Chapter 42).

In summary, protein is essential for maintaining animal structure, routine bodily housekeeping activities, fighting infections, and other important physiologic processes. Protein can also be used as an energy source, at 4 kcal/g, by removing the nitrogen and oxidizing the carbon skeleton. Protein consists of linear chains of amino acids that are precisely linked according to protein coding regions in the DNA of all cells. The final protein configuration depends on interactions between the amino acid R groups. Genetic mutations that change the linear sequence of amino acids can change the final protein structure and drastically alter protein function, possibly with lethal results.

Dietary protein is digested, and amino acids are absorbed and enter the circulating amino acid pool. This pool provides amino acids for synthesis of all body proteins. All body proteins are replaced at different rates; the net rate of protein turnover dictates the protein requirement for each individual. In the fed state, nitrogen is excreted from the body as urea.

MACRONUTRIENT USE AND STORAGE IN THE FED STATE

Carbohydrates

As discussed in Chapter 1, absorbed carbohydrates are transported as plasma glucose in the portal vein. (The cytoplasmic processes of glycolysis and mitochondrial oxidation of pyruvate to provide adenosine triphosphate [ATP] are described in detail in biochemistry texts.) Briefly, an increase in the glucose level in the portal vein stimulates preformed insulin secretion from the pancreas. The liver is the first organ to receive portal blood glucose. The liver does not require insulin to take up approximately 50% of absorbed glucose via receptors or to phosphorylate glucose into glucose-6-phosphate, thereby retaining glucose in the cell. Insulin is required to enhance the oxidation of glucose in the cytosol through the glycolytic pathway. Insulin also stimulates *pyruvate dehydrogenase,* a thiamine-requiring mitochondrial enzyme that removes a carbon from pyruvate with the formation of acetate. Energy-rich bonds in the acetate molecule (bound to coenzyme A) are broken, the energy is transported to the oxidative phosphorylation enzymes on the inner mitochondrial membrane, and ATP is generated.

If carbohydrate intake exceeds the body's oxidative and storage capacities, the cells can convert carbohydrate into fat. Carbohydrate-induced lipogenesis in the rat model has been well described (Kibir et al, 1998). Well-absorbed carbohydrates increase the synthesis of fatty acid synthetase, an insulin-dependent enzyme that regulates fatty acid synthesis, and was recently confirmed in human subjects maintained on moderate fat intake (30% kcal) and very low fat (10% kcal) diets (Hudgins et al, 2000).

Glucose is stored as highly branched glycogen polymers. Cells add glucose residues (as glucose-6-phosphate) to the growing end of preformed glycogen clusters. In the presence of insulin, glucose is added to the polymer in an α (1–4) or α (1–6) linkage by the enzyme *glycogen synthetase.* Muscle glycogen is used within the muscle cell to provide ATP for muscle contraction. Its concentration in the muscle depends on the physical activity of the individual and can be greatly increased by physical training. Liver glycogen serves as a reservoir, providing a readily available supply of glucose to maintain blood glucose levels during the fasting state.

Lipid Transport and Storage

Triglycerides From Gut to Adipocyte: Chylomicrons

Because they are fat soluble, lipids cannot be transported unbound through the aqueous media of the body. Lipid transport can best be understood as a conversion of water-insoluble lipids into water-soluble forms for transport; lipids revert back into water-insoluble lipid esters when they have reached their cellular destination. Absorbed fatty acids and monoglycerides (monoacylglycerols) are reesterified into triglycerides within mucosal cells, and the fat-soluble center is covered with a thin layer of protein and phospholipid to get it ready for transport. The protein component includes markers—apoproteins (Apo) B, A, C, and E on the surface. The resulting chylomicrons contain only 2% protein; the rest is triglycerides (84%), cholesterol, and phospholipid. The lipid-rich particles leave the mucosal cells and travel through lymphatic channels to the thoracic duct that empties into the right side of the heart. Rapid blood flow in the heart prevents the large, lipid-rich chylomicrons from forming clumps and fat emboli. Chylomicrons transport dietary fat and are usually found in serum only after meals. High concentrations of chylomicrons make the plasma appear milky after a high-fat meal.

Chylomicrons leave the heart through the aorta and are transported to the adipocytes (fat cells). An enzyme, *lipoprotein lipase (LPL),* is expressed on the membrane of endothelial cells lining capillaries in the region of the adipocytes and elsewhere. LPL is activated by lipoprotein-bound apoprotein C (Apo C) to bind chylomicrons and cleave triglycerides, releasing fatty acids and monoglycerides that cross the fatty lipid membrane, enter the adipocytes, and become reesterified into triglyceride for safe and hydrophobic storage. Note that insulin, the predominant hormone in the fed state, activates LDL and facilitates fat storage. The chylomicron remnant, relieved of some of its triglyceride content, is bound to liver receptors through its surface markers Apo B and Apo E and recycled.

Triglycerides From Liver to Adipocyte: Very-Low-Density Lipoproteins

The liver receives fat from numerous sources: (1) chylomicron remnants, (2) circulating fatty acids, (3) uptake of intermediate lipoproteins and other lipoproteins, and (4) endogenous body synthesis. The liver reesterifies fat from all sources and wraps it in a heavier coat of protein and phospholipid to form VLDLs. These lipoproteins are relatively richer in cholesterol compared with chylomicrons but still contain a large proportion of triglyceride. VLDLs also contain apoproteins B, E, and C and adsorb Apo A as they circulate. In the fed state, numerous VLDLs are formed and transported to the adipocytes, where triglycerides are again hydrolyzed, reesterified, and stored. Even in the fasted state, VLDLs are formed to carry endogenous lipids.

Cholesterol From Diet and Liver to All Cells: Low-Density Lipoproteins

All cells require cholesterol for their membranes. Cholesterol is a substrate for steroid hormones such as cortisone and estrogens; glands that produce steroid hormones require additional cholesterol biosynthesis. The liver uses cholesterol for synthesis of bile acids. Dietary cholesterol is transported via chylomicrons and VLDLs but is not removed by LPL activity. After LPL has cleaved the maximal triglyceride from VLDL, the remnant remaining is called an *intermediate-density lipoprotein (IDL)* if triglycerides are largely depleted. LDLs primarily carry cholesterol. Although LDL can be taken up by the liver on receptors for Apo B and Apo E, it is first taken up by specific LDL receptors that bind these cholesterol-rich particles. After uptake, endocytic vesicles containing LDL fuse with a lysosome. The digestive enzymes in the lysosome break down the protein and phospholipids, leaving free cholesterol for use by the cell. Free cholesterol is inserted into the plasma membrane and stored as cholesterol ester for biosynthesis.

Each cell regulates its uptake and use of cholesterol by downregulating cellular synthesis of the LDL receptor, reducing receptor expression on the membrane, or both or downregulating endogenous cholesterol synthesis by inhibiting HMG CoA reductase, the rate-limiting enzyme.

Cholesterol From Cells to the Liver and Excretion: High-Density Lipoproteins

Cholesterol is removed from the cell membrane and other lipoproteins by HDLs. HDL particles are formed in the liver as protein-phospholipid disks. They circulate in the bloodstream and accumulate free cholesterol, which they esterify with fatty acid from their phosphatidylcholine (lecithin) phospholipid structure. The ability of HDL to function as a cholesterol transporter depends on the activity of its copper-dependent enzyme *lecithin-cholesterol acyltransferase,* which esterifies cholesterol and stores it in its hydrophobic center. When it has accumulated sufficient lipid to become spherical, HDL is taken up by the liver and recycled. Recycled cholesterol is used for bile acid synthesis and stored in subcutaneous tissue, where it can be formed into vitamin D or secreted as VLDL.

Oxidized Lipid to Macrophages: Low-Density Lipoprotein Scavenger Pathway

Macrophages—large cells that "eat," or engulf, other particles—are distributed throughout the body, play a major role in immune defense, and inhabit the arteries, where they serve as a surveillance mechanism against foreign and microbial agents in the blood. Although macrophages do not recognize and ingest normal lipoproteins, they do recognize lipoproteins that have undergone oxidation as foreign. Macrophages ingest oxidized LDL and accumulate ingested fat within their cytoplasm, giving them a foamy appearance (thus the name *foam cells*). LDL ingestion activates macrophages and stimulates them to secrete mediators that trigger multiple inflammatory and proliferative cascades, some of which lead to atherosclerosis. Evidence now supports the proposal that the macrophage plays a role in the pathogenesis of atherosclerosis (Chisolm and Penn, 1996) (see Chapter 35).

MACRONUTRIENT CATABOLISM IN THE FASTED STATE

The body has a remarkable ability to withstand food deprivation. Adaptive changes allow it to access stored macronutrients to provide for routine activities of the body. Adaptation to starvation has an evolutionary connection; it allowed primitive humans to survive cycles of feast and famine.

Individuals with *protein energy,* or *protein-calorie, malnutrition* can have varying symptoms determined by the cause of the malnutrition. Simple starvation (the absolute deprivation of food) leads to *marasmus* and represents one end of the protein-energy malnutrition continuum. At the opposite end of the continuum is protein deprivation that occurs in individuals who are consuming carbohydrates. This condition is called *kwashiorkor,* from an African word meaning "the disease of the displaced child" (Williams, 1933). Kwashiorkor develops when a mother's first child is weaned from protein-rich breast milk to a protein-poor carbohydrate food source. As mentioned, individuals with malnutrition can display symptoms at multiple points on the protein-calorie malnutrition continuum.

Adapted Starvation: Marasmus

Glucose is an obligate nutrient for the brain and nervous system, red blood cells, white blood cells, and other glucose-requiring tissues. To maintain function, the blood glucose level must be maintained within a normal range at all times. Glucose can be obtained from glycogen, but stores last only about 24 hours. This means that glucose must be synthesized de novo using protein as a substrate. During fasting and in the absence of insulin, catabolic hormones epinephrine, thyroxine, and glucagon are released. These hormones stimulate glycogen breakdown and the release of muscle protein and other available substrates for gluconeogenesis (see previous *Clinical Insight:* Hormonal Control of Blood Sugar).

The most common amino acid substrate for gluconeogenesis is alanine because when its nitrogen is removed, alanine becomes pyruvate. Note that glycogen is never totally depleted, even during long-term starvation. A small amount of preformed glycogen is carefully guarded as a primer for glycogen resynthesis. As starvation proceeds and the body adapts, liver gluconeogenesis decreases from producing 90% of the glucose to less than 50%, with the remainder being supplied by the kidney.

Muscle and the brain are unable to release free glucose, but muscle can release pyruvate and lactate for gluconeogenesis in a process called the *Cori cycle.* Muscle also can release glutamine. During prolonged fasting, the kidney requires ammonia to excrete acidic metabolic products. Muscle-derived glutamine is used for this purpose; the glutamate product can be deaminated into carbohydrate and converted into glucose. Thus during starvation, glucose production by the kidney increases, and production by the liver decreases.

In addition to glucose a reliable energy source is required during fasting. The best source is fat that is stored in adipocytes and used primarily by muscles, including the heart muscle, to make ATP. Fatty acid release and use requires insulin levels to be kept low and an increase of the antiinsulin hormones glucagon, cortisone, epinephrine, and growth hormone. Antiinsulin hormones activate the hormone-sensitive lipase enzyme on the adipocyte membrane. This enzyme cleaves stored triglycerides, releasing fatty acids and glycerol from fat cells. Fatty acids travel to the liver bound to serum albumin and easily enter the liver cells. Fatty acids cannot enter the liver mitochondria for use as an energy source unless they are bound to carnitine. Via the transport system carnitine acyltransferase, fatty acid carnitine esters can cross the mitochondrial membrane. Once inside the mitochondria, two carbon (acetate) segments are sequentially cleaved from LCFAs via the process of beta oxidation. Acetate binds to coenzyme A to form acetyl CoA and is oxidized through the citric acid cycle. Excess acetyl CoA molecules, when not required for hepatocyte use, are joined to form four-carbon, energy-rich fragments called **ketones.**

Adaptation to starvation depends on ketone production. As the blood ketone level rises during fasting, the brain and nervous system, although obligate glucose consumers, begin to use ketones as an energy source. Because the brain is using a fuel other than glucose, the demand on muscle protein for gluconeogenesis declines, thereby reducing the rate of muscle catabolism. Reduced muscle catabolism reduces the amount of ammonia received by the liver. Liver synthesis of urea decreases precipitously, reflecting the slower rate of muscle protein deamination. If the fast extends for weeks, the rate of urea synthesis and excretion is minimized. As discussed previously, in an individual who has adapted to starvation, urea is excreted at approximately the same rate as uric acid produced by the kidney.

Thus in an individual who is adapting to starvation, protein losses are minimized and lean body mass spared. Although fat cannot be converted into glucose, fat does provide fuel for the muscle and brain in the form of ketones. As long as water is available, a normal-weight individual can fast for a month. Relatively normal nutritional indices, immune function, and other system function are maintained. When fat stores are exhausted, protein is used and the patient dies.

Nonadapted Starvation

Trauma and Sepsis

If an individual who is fasting develops an infection, inflammatory mediators such as *interleukin-1* and *tumor necrosis factor* stimulate insulin secretion and prevent the development of mild ketosis. Without ketones, the brain and other tissues continue to depend on glucose, thereby limiting the person's ability to adapt to starvation. Muscle mass erodes to provide glucose substrates. A fasting person with an infection rapidly develops a negative nitrogen balance. When 50% of the protein stores are exhausted, the person's ability to recover from the infection is poor; the person may die if the respiratory muscles cannot support breathing.

Kwashiorkor

Adaptation to starvation is also not possible for those with kwashiorkor because the carbohydrate intake stimulates insulin production. Insulin is a storage hormone that prevents fat stores from being accessed for fuel. It also inhibits fat from being formed into ketones, thereby limiting adaptation to starvation. Insulin secretion inhibits muscle breakdown. Protein cannot be used to make albumin and other visceral proteins. Edema results because albumin exerts osmotic pressure in the vessels. If the albumin concentration is low, fluid remains in the extracellular spaces and causes edema. Compromised neural function and GI absorption, decreased cardiac output, immune function, fatigue, and other symptoms of protein-calorie malnutrition result from inadequate protein synthesis, inadequate ATP production, and fluid accumulation in the tissues.

Nonadapted protein-calorie malnutrition is dangerous. Not only can unremitting protein loss become life threatening by compromising the muscles of the heart and respiratory system, it can compromise the immune system. By limiting a person's immune defenses, it makes the individual susceptible to a vicious cycle of infections, diarrhea, additional nutrient loss, an even weaker immune system, and finally, opportunistic infections and death. Iatrogenic, or "physician-induced," malnutrition was recognized long ago as a danger for hospitalized patients (Butterworth, 1974) and remains so to this day (Souba and Wilmore, 1998).

SUMMARY

Macronutrients in food have vastly varied forms and quality. Biologic organisms have a remarkable ability to use extremely diverse plant and animal foods for growth and maintenance. If an organism is deprived of food, alternate adaptive mechanisms parcel stored macronutrients to maintain body integrity. When adaptation mechanisms are compromised, serious disease and death can result.

Clinical Scenario

Joe is a 38-year-old man who recently began to increase his fiber intake as recommended by his physician because he has hyperlipidemia and is 50 pounds overweight. From a diet history taken at the office, it has been determined that Joe normally consumed 15 g of fiber per day before this change. He is now consuming 45 g on an average day. He is complaining about increased gas and flatulence from this change in his routine.

1. Which changes would you suggest Joe make in his fiber intake? His fat intake?
2. Which types and amounts of fiber would you recommend if Joe began to show signs of carbohydrate intolerance?
3. Calculate the fiber and protein content of your own diet for 3 days. How many grams of fiber do you eat? Which foods would you add to your diet to change your intake to the recommended intake of 25 to 35 g daily? How much protein do you eat?
4. Joe's wife asks you about the benefits of a vegetarian diet. What will you discuss?

Relevant Web Sites

American Society for Nutrition Sciences
www. nutrition.org/
National Academy of Sciences: DRI Tables for Macronutrients
www4.nas.edu/iom/iomhome.nsf/WFiles/FNBMacronutrientTable/$file/FNBMacronutrient Table.pdf

Cited References

Abcouwer SF, Souba WW: Glutamine and arginine. In Shils ME et al, eds: *Modern nutrition in health and disease,* ed 9, Baltimore, 1998, Williams & Wilkins.

Alberts B et al: Cell chemistry and biosynthesis (Chapter 2); Membrane structure (Chapter 11); Energy conversion, mitochondria and chloroplasts (Chapter 14). In *Molecular biology of the cell,* ed 4, New York, 2002, Garland Science; Taylor and Francis Group.

American Dietetic Association: Position of the American Dietetic Association: fat replacers, *J Am Diet Assoc* 98:463, 1998.

American Dietetic Association: Position of the American Dietetic Association: vegetarian diets, *J Am Diet Assoc* 97:1317, 1997.

Autio JT: Effect of xylitol chewing gum on salivary Streptococcus mutans in preschool children, *ASCD J Dent Child* 69:81-86, 2002.

Bergman CJ et al: Mineral binding capacity of dephytinized insoluble fiber from extruded wheat, oat and rice brans, *Plant Foods Hum Nutr* 51:295, 1997.

Block RJ, Mitchel HH: *Nutr Abstr Rev* 16:249, 1946.

Bowler PG et al: Wound microbiology and associated approaches to wound management, *Clin Microbiol Rev* 14:244, 2001.

Brand-Miller JC et al: Glycemic index and obesity, *Am J Clin Nutr* 76:281S-5S, 2002.

Butterworth CE: The skeleton in the hospital closet, *Nutrition* 10:435, 1974.

Calvert RJ, Satchithanandam S: Effects of graded levels of high-molecular-weight carrageenan on colonic mucosal thymidine kinase activity, *Nutrition* 8:252, 1992.

Chisolm GM III, Penn MS: Oxidized lipoproteins and atherosclerosis. In Fuster V et al, eds: *Atherosclerosis and coronary artery disease,* Philadelphia, 1996, Lippincott-Raven.

Clark LT: Treating dyslipidemia with statins: the risk benefit profile, *Am Heart J* 145:387-396, 2003.

Clydesdale FM: Olestra: the approval process in letter and spirit, *Food Technol* 51:104, 1997.

Compher C et al: Dietary fiber and its clinical applications to enteral nutrition. In Rombeau JL, Rolandelli RH, eds: *Enteral and tube feeding,* ed 3, Philadelphia, 1997, WB Saunders.

Connor SL, Connor WE: Are fish oils beneficial in the prevention and treatment of coronary artery disease? *Am J Clin Nutr* 66(suppl 4):1020, 1997.

Connor WE et al: Essential fatty acids: the importance of n-3 fatty acids in the retina and brain, *Nutr Rev* 50:21, 1992.

Coudray C et al: Effect of soluble or partly soluble dietary fibres supplementation on absorption and balance of calcium, magnesium, iron and zinc in healthy young men, *Eur J Clin Nutr* 51:375, 1997.

Couzy F et al: Effect of dietary phytic acid on zinc absorption in the healthy elderly, as assessed by serum concentration curve tests, *Br J Nutr* 80:177, 1998.

Craig WJ: Health-promoting properties of common herbs, *Am J Clin Nutr* 70:491, 1999.

Crawford MA: The role of dietary fatty acids in biology: their place in the evolution of the human brain *Nutr Rev* 50:3, 1992.

Crim MC, Munro HN: Proteins and amino acids. In Shils ME et al, eds: *Modern nutrition in health and disease,* Philadelphia, 1994, Lea & Febiger.

Cummings JH et al: Prebiotic digestion and fermentation, *Am J Clin Nutr* 73:415S, 2001.

Davidson MH, Maki KC: Effects of dietary inulin on serum lipids, *J Nutr* 129:1474S, 1999.

DePinieux G et al: Lipid-lowering drugs and mitochondrial function: effects of HMG-CoA reductase inhibitors on serum ubiquinone and blood lactate/pyruvate ratio, *Br J Clin Pharmacol* 42:333-337, 1996.

Deuchi K et al: Continuous and massive intake of chitosan affects mineral and fat-soluble vitamin status in rats fed on a high-fat diet, *Biosci Biotechnol Biochem* 59:1211, 1995.

Eaton SB, Konner M: Paleolithic nutrition: a consideration of its nature and current implications, *N Engl J Med* 312:283, 1985.

Evans LV: Mucilaginous substances from macroalgae: an overview, *Symp Soc Exp Biol* 43:455, 1989.

Farrell DJ: Enrichment of hen eggs with n-3 long chain fatty acids and evaluation of enriched eggs in humans, *Am J Clin Nutr* 68:538, 1998.

Ford ES et al: Prevalence of the metabolic syndrome among US adults: findings from the Third National Health and Nutrition Examination Survey, *JAMA* 287:356, 2002.

Garg A: Efficacy of dietary fiber in lowering serum cholesterol, *Am J Med* 97:501, 1994.

Gershoff SN: Nutrition evaluation of dietary fat substitutes, *Nutr Rev* 53:305, 1995.

Gibson GR, Roberfroid MB: Dietary modulation of the human colonic microbiota: introducing the concept of prebiotics, *J Nutr* 125:1401, 1995

Grootveld M et al: In vivo absorption, metabolism and urinary excretion of a,b-unsaturated aldehydes in experimental animals:

relevance to the development of cardiovascular diseases by the dietary ingestion of thermally stressed polyunsaturate-rich culinary oils, *J Clin Invest* 101:1210, 1998.
Guthrie JF, Morton JF: Food sources of added sweeteners in the diets of Americans, *Am Diet Assoc,* 100:43-51, 2000.
Harris PJ et al: The effects of soluble-fiber polysaccharides on the adsorption of a hydrophobic carcinogen to an insoluble dietary fiber, *Nutr Cancer* 19:43, 1993.
Hegsted DM: Serum-cholesterol response to dietary cholesterol: a re-evaluation, *Am J Clin Nutr* 44:299, 1986.
Jenkins DJA et al: Glycemic index of foods: a physiological basis for carbohydrate exchange, *Am J Clin Nutr* 34:362, 1981.
Jenkins DJA et al: Specific types of colonic fermentation may raise low-density lipoprotein cholesterol concentrations, *Am J Clin Nutr* 54:141, 1991.
Kantor LS: *A dietary assessment of the U.S. food supply: comparing per capita food consumption with Food Guide Pyramid serving recommendations,* Food and Rural Economics Division, Economics Research Service, U.S. Department of Agriculture Agricultural Economic Report No 772, 1998.
Kazuaki SN et al: Epidemiology of soy and cancer: perspectives and directions, *J Nutr* 125:709S, 1995.
Kibir M et al: A high glycemic index starch diet affects lipid storage-related enzymes in normal, and to a lesser extent in diabetic, rats, *J Nutr* 128:1878, 1998.
Kris-Etherton PM et al: Polyunsaturated fatty acids in the food chain in the United States, *Am J Clin Nutr* 71:179, 2000.
Krishnan S et al: The ability of enteric diarrheal pathogens to ferment starch to short-chain fatty acids in vitro, *Scand J Gastroenterol* 33:242, 1998.
Linscheer WG, Vergroesen AJ: Lipids. In Shils ME et al, eds: Modern *nutrition in health and disease,* ed 8, Philadelphia, 1994, Lea & Febiger.
Ludwig DS: The glycemic index: physiological mechanisms relating to obesity, diabetes and cardiovascular disease, *JAMA* 287:2414-2423, 2002.
Messina M: Modern applications for an ancient bean: soybeans and the prevention and treatment of chronic disease, *J Nutr* 125:567S, 1995.
Molteni A et al: In vitro hormonal effects of soybean isoflavones, *J Nutr* 125:751S, 1995.
National Institutes of Health Consensus Conference: Coronary heart disease, *JAMA* 209:505, 1993.
Niness KR: Inulin and oligofructose: what are they? *J Nutr* 129:1402S, 1999.
Ohashi K et al: Expression of amylase and glucose oxidase in the hypopharyngeal gland with an age-dependent role change of the worker honeybee *(Apis mellifera L.), Eur J Biochem* 265:127-133, 1999.
Ormrod DJ et al: Dietary chitosan inhibits hypercholesterolemia and atherogenesis in the apolipoprotein E-deficient mouse model of atherosclerosis, *Atherosclerosis* 138:329, 1998.
Pamuk ON, Sonsuz A: The effect of mannitol infusion on the response to diuretic therapy in cirrhotic patients with ascites, *J Clin Gastroenterol* 35(5):403, 2002.
Parks EJ, Hellerstein MK: Carbohydrate-induced hypertriacylglycerolemia: historical perspective and review of biological mechanisms, *Am J Clin Nutr* 71:412-433. 2000.
Putnam J: US food supply providing more food and calories, *Food Rev* 22:2-12, 1999.
Roberfroid M et al: The biochemistry of oligofructose, a nondigestible fiber: an approach to calculate its caloric value, *Nutr Rev* 51:137, 1993.
Salas J et al: The SstI polymorphism of the apolipoprotein C-III gene determines the insulin response to an oral-glucose-tolerance test after consumption of a diet rich in saturated fats, *Am J Clin Nutr* 68:396, 1998.
Sarwar G et al: Corrected relative net protein ratio (CRNPR) method based on differences in rats and human requirements for sulfur amino acids, *J Am Oil Chem Soc* 68:689, 1985.
Scholz-Ahrens KE et al: Effects of prebiotics on mineral metabolism, *Am J Clin Nutr* 73:459S-464S, 2001.
Shallenberger RS: Taste and bioavailability of sugars as related to structure. In, *Carbohydrate metabolism: regulation and physiological role,* 1976, John Wiley & Sons.
Shiau SY, Yu YP: Chitin but not chitosan supplementation enhances growth of grass shrimp, *Penaeus monodon, J Nutr* 128:908, 1998.
Souba WW, Wilmore D: Diet and nutrition in the care of the patient with surgery, trauma and sepsis. In Shils ME et al, eds: *Modern nutrition in health and disease,* ed 9, Baltimore, 1998, Williams & Wilkins.
Spiegel S et al: Safety and benefits of fructooligosaccharides as food ingredients, *Food Technol,* 48:85, 1994.
Stark A, Madar Z: Phytoestrogens: a review of recent findings, *J Pediatr Endocrinol Metab* 15:561, 2002.
Stipanuk MH: Homocysteine, cysteine and taurine. In Shils ME et al, eds: *Modern nutrition in health and disease,* ed 9, Baltimore, 1999, Williams & Wilkins.
Tobacman JK: Filament disassembly and loss of mammary myoepithelial cells after exposure to lambda-carrageenan, *Cancer Res* 57:2823, 1997.
Tobacman JK: Review of harmful gastrointestinal effects of carrageenan in animal experiments, *Environ Health Perspect* 109:983, 2001.
Trautwein EA et al: Dietary inulin lowers plasma cholesterol and triacylglycerol and alters bile acid profile in hamsters, *J Nutr* 128:1937, 1998.
Vail GE et al: *Foods,* ed 7, Boston, 1978, Houghton Mifflin Company.
Van Loo J et al: Functional food properties of nondigestible oligosaccharides: a consensus report from the ENDO project, *Br J Nutr* 81:121, 1999.
Williams AW, Erdman JW Jr: Food processing: nutrition, safety and quality balances. In Shils ME et al, eds: *Modern nutrition in health and disease,* Philadelphia, 1994, Lea & Febiger.
Williams CD: A nutritional disease of childhood associated with a maize diet, *Arch Dis Child* 8:423-433, 1933.
Young VR: Soy protein in relation to human protein and amino acid nutrition, *J Am Diet Assoc* 91:828, 1991.

Additional References

Bolton-Smith C et al: Evidence for age-related differences in the fatty acid composition of human adipose tissue, independent of diet, *Eur J Clin Nutr* 51:619, 1997.
Hunt JR et al: Zinc absorption, mineral balance, and blood lipids in women consuming controlled lactoovovegetarian and omnivorous diets for 8 weeks, *Am J Clin Nutr* 67:421, 1998.
Katan MB: Impact of low-fat diets on plasma high-density lipoprotein concentrations, *Am J Clin Nutr* 67(suppl):573, 1998.
Krebs-Smith SM: Choose beverages and foods to moderate your intake of sugars: measurement requires quantification, *J Nutr* 131:527S, 2001.

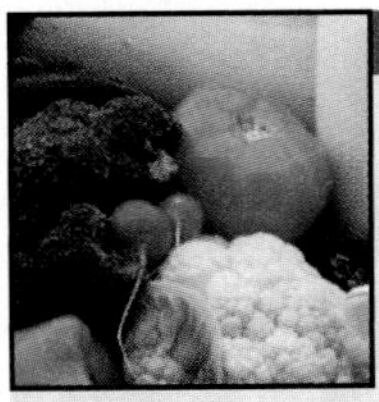

CHAPTER 4

Vitamins

MARGIE LEE GALLAGHER, PhD, RD, MS

CHAPTER OUTLINE

- The Fat-Soluble Vitamins
- The Water-Soluble Vitamins
- Other Vitamin-Like Factors

KEY TERMS

antioxidant–a substance that can inhibit reactions of free radicals such as reactive species of oxygen; used to describe vitamins C and E, some carotenoids, ubiquinones, and bioflavonoids

ascorbic acid–vitamin C, a water-soluble vitamin that plays essential roles in mineral metabolism and intracellular antioxidant functions; biosynthesized from glucose by most nonprimate species

beriberi–a neuropathy caused by thiamin deficiency

bioflavonoids–a group of vitamin-like substances found in plants with antioxidant activities

biotin–a sulfur-containing vitamin synthesized by microorganisms in the lower gastrointestinal tract

calcitriol–hormonally active form of vitamin D produced by the kidney; 1,25-dihydroxycholecalciferol (1,25-$[OH]_2D_3$)

carnitine–a vitamin-like factor essential for the oxidation of fatty acids; can be biosynthesized from the amino acid lysine

carotenoids–yellow or red pigments found in carrots, sweet potatoes, leafy vegetables, milk fat, and egg yolk, which can be converted into vitamin A (retinol) in the body

cholecalciferol–the form of the fat-soluble vitamin D_3, produced when 7-dehydrocholesterol in the skin is photolysed by ultraviolet irradiation

choline–a metabolic precursor of the key structural element of membranes, phosphatidylcholine, and the neurotransmitter acetylcholine

cobalamin–vitamin B_{12}, a B-complex vitamin that has essential roles in the metabolism of single-carbon units and propionate

coenzyme Q_{10} (CoQ_{10})–a ubiquinone that exists naturally in the body and is an essential component of the mitochondrial electron transport system

folic acid (folate)–a specific folic acid folate vitamer also called pteroylglutamic acid, a deficiency of which results in macrocytic anemia

hypercarotenodermia–an accumulation of carotenoids in the skin, causing skin yellowing

menadione–a fat-soluble synthetic form of vitamin K

menaquinones–the form of vitamin K produced by bacteria and found in animal tissue

***myo*-inositol**–a vitamin-like factor synthesized from glucose that plays important metabolic roles as a constituent of phospholipids and mediator of cellular responses to external stimuli

niacin–vitamin B_3; the general term for the antipellagra vitamers nicotinamide (also niacinamide) and nicotinic acid, which play essential roles as cofactors for numerous enzymes involved in the metabolism of carbohydrates, protein, and energy

night blindness–impaired dark adaptation caused by loss of visual pigments from vitamin A deficiency; also called *nyctalopia*

pantothenic acid–a B-complex vitamin that plays essential roles in the synthesis and oxidation of fatty acids

pellagra–a dermatitis caused by niacin deficiency in humans

pyridoxine (PN)–a B-complex vitamin (B_6) that plays essential roles in the metabolism of amino acids

retinol–a form of vitamin A that is essential to the visual process and cell differentiation

KEY TERMS—Continued

retinol activity equivalents (RAE)–the measure of the vitamin A activity in foods

riboflavin–a B-complex vitamin, vitamin B_2, that plays essential roles as a cofactor of enzymes involved in many cell oxidation-reduction reactions

rickets–a disease of infants and young animals characterized by impaired mineralization of growing bone caused by deficiencies of vitamin D, calcium, or phosphorus

scurvy–a disease characterized by impaired maturation of connective tissues caused by a vitamin C deficiency

thiamin–a B-complex vitamin (B_1) that plays an essential role as a cofactor of enzymes involved in dehydrogenase and transketolase reactions

tocopherols–a form of the fat-soluble antioxidant vitamin, vitamin E

tryptophan–an amino acid that serves as the metabolic precursor of niacin

ubiquinones–vitamin-like metabolites such as coenzyme Q_{10} that play essential roles in processes such as respiratory energy metabolism and have antioxidant functions that may spare vitamin E in cells

vitamer–one of multiple forms (all isomers and active analogues) of a vitamin

vitamin–an organic compound, essential in very small amounts in supporting normal physiologic function, that cannot generally be biosynthesized quickly enough to meet the needs of the body

vitamin K–a fat-soluble vitamin that plays essential roles in the biosynthesis of several proteins involved in blood clotting and bone mineralization

xerophthalmia–a disease caused by vitamin A deficiency; characterized by dryness and eventual ulceration of the cornea

The discovery of vitamins gave birth to the field of nutrition. The elucidation of the compounds is an exciting and convoluted story (see *Focus On:* Pellegra, Politics, and the Poor). Eventually the term vitamin came to describe a group of essential micronutrients that generally satisfy the following criteria:

- Organic compounds (or class of compounds) distinct from fats, carbohydrates, and proteins
- Natural components of foods; usually present in minute amounts
- Not synthesized by the body in amounts adequate to meet normal physiologic needs
- Essential, also usually in minute amounts, for normal physiologic function (i.e., maintenance, growth, development, and reproduction)
- Cause a specific deficiency syndrome by their absence or insufficient use

Vitamers are the multiple forms (all isomers and active analogues) of vitamins (See Table 4-1). Although the vitamins have few close chemical similarities, their metabolic functions can be classified into four general groups: (1) membrane stabilizers, (2) hydrogen (H+) and electron (e−) donors and acceptors, (3) hormones, and (4) coenzymes.

The vitamins are usually classified into two groups based on their solubilities: the *fat-soluble vitamins* (A, D, E, and K) and the *water-soluble vitamins* (ascorbic acid, thiamin, riboflavin, niacin, pyridoxine, biotin, pantothenic acid, folate, and cobalamin). The fat-soluble vitamins are usually absorbed passively and must be transported with dietary lipid. They tend to be found in the lipid portions of the cell such as membranes and lipid droplets. The water-soluble vitamins are absorbed by passive and active mechanisms, transported by carriers, and not stored in appreciable amounts in the body. Fat-soluble vitamins are generally excreted with the feces via enterohepatic circulation, whereas water-soluble vitamins or their metabolites are excreted in the urine.

THE FAT-SOLUBLE VITAMINS

Vitamin A

Vitamin A (or the retinoids) refers to three preformed compounds that exhibit metabolic activity: the alcohol (retinol), the aldehyde (retinal or retinaldehyde), and the acid (retinoic acid) (Figure 4-1). Stored retinol is often esterified to a fatty acid (usually palmitate) and is called *retinyl-palmitate.* These retinyl esters are also usually found complexed with proteins in foods. These active forms of vitamin A exist in only animal products.

In addition to preformed vitamin A found in animal products, plants contain a group of compounds known collectively as carotenoids, which can yield retinoids when metabolized in the body. Although several hundred carotenoids exist in foods naturally, only a few have significant vitamin A activity. The most important of these is β-*carotene* (see Figure 4-1). The amount of vitamin A available from dietary carotenoids depends on how well they are absorbed and how efficiently they are converted to retinol.

The absorption of carotenoids varies greatly (from 5% to 50%) and is affected by other dietary factors such as the digestibility of the proteins complexed with the carotenoids and the level and type of fat in the diet. (Fat-soluble vitamins need fat for proper absorption.)

FOCUS ON

Pellagra, Politics, and the Poor

The history of niacin and pellagra is an example of the long and often convoluted search for the vitamins. Even though oranges and lemons were used as early as 1601 on the ships of the East India Company to prevent scurvy, the idea that a chemical in the diet could prevent certain diseases eluded the scientific and medical communities for hundreds of years. Pellagra was among these diseases. In 1915, 11,000 deaths from pellagra were reported in the southern United States. By 1917, more than 170,000 cases developed in the southern United States. The situation was so grave that the Public Health Service sent Joseph Goldberger to the South to investigate the deaths. He determined a nutrient deficiency to be the cause of the disease and that it could be cured by a diet containing high-quality protein. In fact, he showed that he could eliminate the disease simply by improving the diet. In 1918, Goldberger published these findings. Considering these facts, why in 1927 were 120,000 cases reported in the South? Between 1927 and 1930 27,103 deaths were recorded (Harris, 1955). Why were there so many deaths from a disease that was entirely preventable?

Several factors contributed to the situation. First, Pasteur's germ theory of disease was sweeping the scientific community. In fact, it was accepted that scurvy, beriberi, and rickets were each caused by a microbe rather than by the lack of a nutrient. The antiberiberi actions of whole-grain rice were thought to be caused by a pharmacologic substance that acted against an unknown bacterium, rather than a substance that served as a nutrient (thiamin). Even after Goldberger showed that pellagra was not contagious, doubts persisted. The problem was further complicated, as is now known, because (1) high-quality protein does not contain niacin—it contains the tryptophan precursor, and (2) the isolation of individual vitamins from the B-complex isolate took many years of painstaking laboratory research (Elvehjem et al, 1938). Many more years passed before tryptophan was recognized as an important precursor of niacin.

Perhaps the most significant factors contributing to the numerous deaths from pellagra—factors that affected the southern United States into the 1940s (with more than 2000 deaths per year) and early 1950s (with more than 500 deaths per year)—were economic and social. All of those who died from pellagra were poor and got poorer as the Great Depression of the late 1920s and 1930s deepened. The deaths primarily affected black Americans. In the South, people died from a lack of food, whereas in other parts of the country, farmers burned or threw away food because they could not sell the excess (Harris, 1955).

TABLE 4-1 Vitamins, Vitamers, and Their Functions

GROUP	VITAMERS	PROVITAMINS	PHYSIOLOGIC FUNCTIONS
Vitamin A	Retinol Retinal Retinoic acid	β-carotene Cryptoxanthin	Visual pigments; cell differentiation; gene regulation
Vitamin D	Cholecalciferol (D_3) Ergocalciferol (D_2)		Ca homeostasis; bone metabolism
Vitamin E	α-tocopherol γ-tocopherol Tocotrienols		Membrane antioxidant
Vitamin K	Phylloquinones (K_1) Menaquinones (K_2) Menadione (K_3)		Blood clotting; Ca metabolism
Vitamin C	Ascorbic acid Dehydroascorbic acid		Reductant in hydroxylations in biosynthesis of collagen and carnitine and in the metabolism of drugs and steroids
Vitamin B_1	Thiamin		Coenzyme for decarboxylations of 2-keto acids and transketolations
Vitamin B_2	Riboflavin		Coenzyme in redox reactions of fatty acids and the TCA cycle
Niacin	Nicotinic acid Nicotinamide		Coenzymes for several dehydrogenases
Vitamin B_6	Pyridoxol Pyridoxal Pyridoxamine		Coenzymes in amino acid metabolism
Folic acid	Folic acid Polyglutamyl folacins		Coenzymes in single-carbon metabolism
Biotin	Biotin		Coenzyme for carboxylations
Pantothenic acid	Pantothenic acid		Coenzyme in fatty acid metabolism
Vitamin B_{12}	Cobalamin		Coenzyme in metabolism of propionate, amino acids, and single carbon fragments

TCA, Tricarboxylic acid.

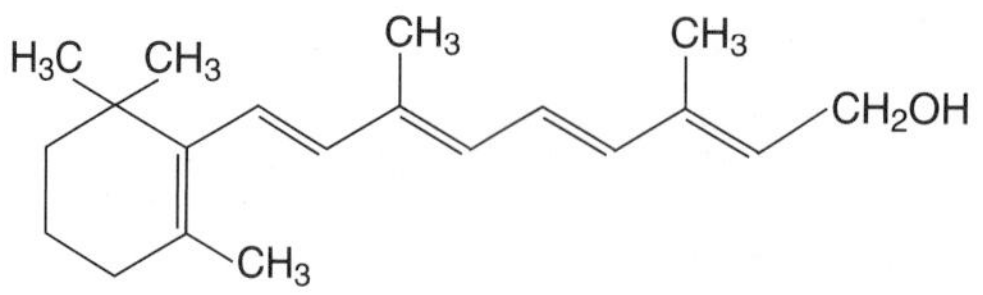

All-*trans*-retinal

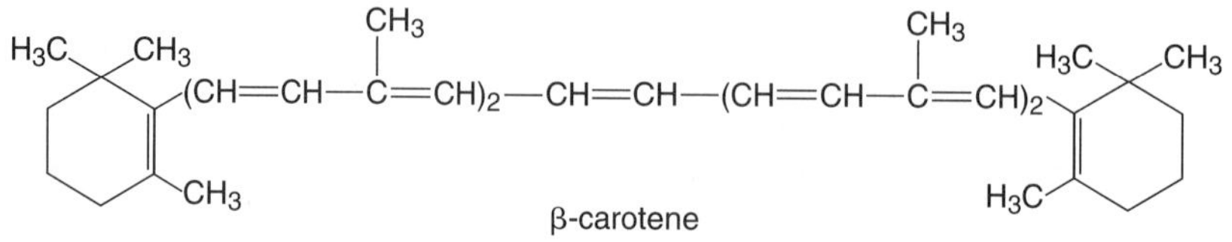

β-carotene

FIGURE 4-1 • Structure of vitamin A and β-carotene.

Absorption, Transport, and Storage

Before either vitamin A or its carotenoid provitamins can be absorbed, proteases in the stomach and small intestine must hydrolyze proteins that are usually complexed with these compounds. In addition, retinyl esters must be hydrolyzed in the small intestine by lipases to retinol and free fatty acids (Figure 4-2, *A*). Retinoids and carotenoids are incorporated into micelles along with other lipids for passive absorption into the mucosal cells of the small intestine. Once in the intestinal mucosal cells, retinol is bound to a cellular retinol-binding protein (CRBP) and reesterified (primarily by lecithin retinol acyl transferase [LRAT]) into retinyl esters. Carotenoids and retinyl esters are incorporated into chylomicrons for transport into the lymph and eventually the bloodstream or may be cleaved into retinal, which is then reduced to retinol and reesterified into retinyl esters. These retinyl esters, like those produced from absorbed retinol, are also incorporated into chylomicrons (Figure 4-2, *B*).

The liver plays an important role in vitamin A transport and storage (Figure 4-2, *C*). Chylomicron remnants deliver retinyl esters to the liver. These esters are immediately hydrolyzed into retinol and free fatty acids. Retinol in the liver has three major metabolic fates. First, retinol may be bound to CRBP, which controls free retinol concentrations that can be toxic in the cell. Second, retinol may be reesterified to form retinyl esters, mostly retinyl palmitate, for storage. Some 50% to 80% of the vitamin A in the body is stored in the liver, although other tissues such as the adipose tissue, lungs, and kidneys also store retinyl esters in specialized cells called *stellate cells*. This storage capacity buffers the effects of highly variable patterns of vitamin A intake and is particularly important during periods of low intake when a person is at risk for developing a deficiency (Li and Norris, 1996).

Finally, retinol may be bound to retinol-binding protein (RBP). Retinol bound to RBP leaves the liver and enters the blood, where another protein—transthyretin (TTR)—attaches, forming a complex that is used to transport retinol in the blood to the peripheral tissues. Hepatic RBP synthesis depends on adequate protein. Therefore blood levels of retinol can be affected by protein deficiency as well as by chronic vitamin A deficiency. Thus children with protein-calorie malnutrition typically have low circulating retinol levels that may not respond to vitamin A supplementation unless the protein deficiency is also corrected.

The retinol-RBP-TTR complex delivers retinol to other tissues via cell surface receptors. Retinol is transferred from RBP to CRBP with the subsequent release of apo retinol-binding protein (apo RBP) into BP and TTR to the blood. Apo RBP is eventually metabolized and excreted by the kidney. In addition to CRBPs, cellular retinoic acid–binding proteins (CRABPs) bind retinoic acid in the cell and serve to control retinoic acid concentrations similar to the way CRBPs control retinol concentrations.

Metabolism

In addition to being esterified for storage, the transport form of retinol can also be oxidized into retinal and then into retinoic acid or conjugated into retinyl glucuronide or retinyl phosphate. After retinoic acid is formed, it is converted to forms that are readily excreted. Chain-shortened and oxidized forms of vitamin A are excreted in the urine; intact forms are excreted in the bile and feces. The metabolism of retinoids seems to be regulated by the CRBPs, which channel their ligands via protein-protein interactions among the various enzymes involved in their metabolism.

Functions

Vitamin A has essential but separate roles in vision and various systemic functions, including normal cell differentiation and cell surface function (e.g., cell recognition), growth and development, immune functions, and reproduction.

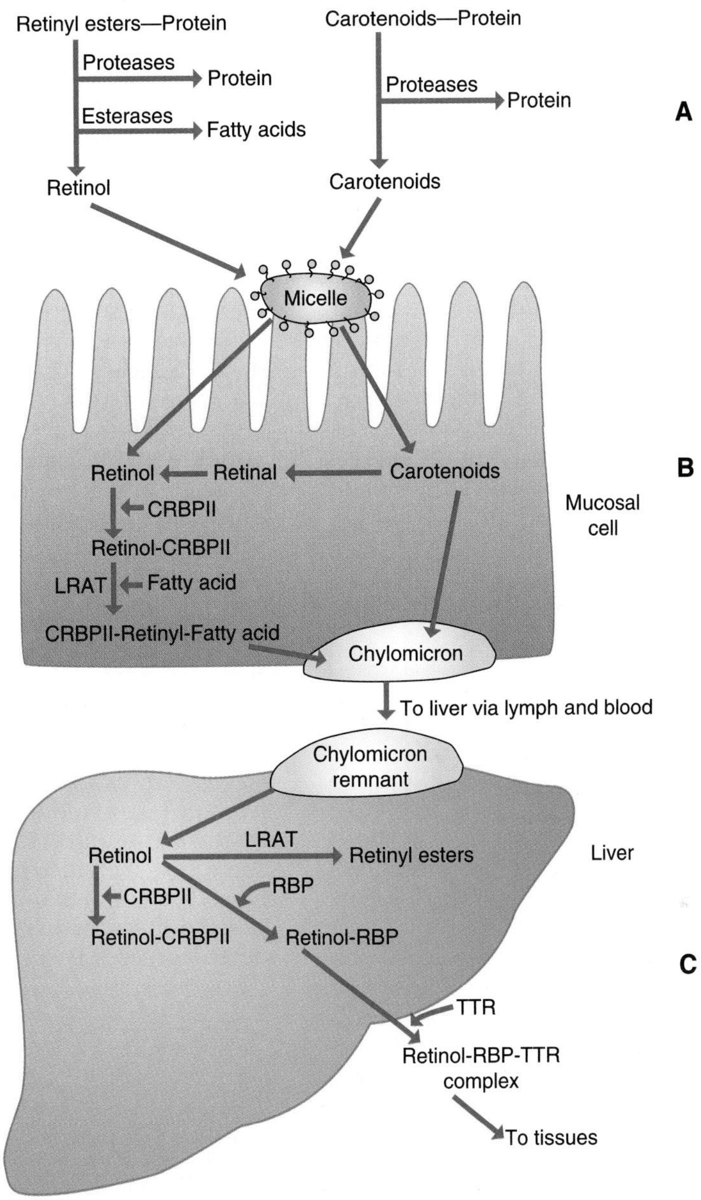

CRBPII, Cellular Retinol-Binding Protein II
RBP, Retinol-Binding Protein
LRAT, Lecithin Retinol Acyl Transferase
TRR, Transthyretin

FIGURE 4-2 • Retinol and carotenoids. **A,** Digestion. **B,** Absorption. **C,** Transport.

Retinal is a structural component of the visual pigments of the rod and cone cells of the retina and as such is essential to photoreception. The 11-*cis* isomer, 11-*cis*-retinal, constitutes the photosensitive group of various visual pigment proteins (i.e., the *opsins*—rhodopsin in the rods and iodopsin in the cones). Photoreception results from light-induced isomerization of 11-*cis*-retinal to the completely all-*trans* form. For example, in the rod, rhodopsin progresses though a series of reactions leading to the dissociation of "bleached" rhodopsin into all-*trans*-retinal and opsin, a reaction that is coupled to nervous stimulation of the visual centers of the brain. All-*trans*-retinal can then be converted back enzymatically to 11-*cis*-retinal for subsequent binding to opsin (Figure 4-3). The movement of retinal into designated sites in the retina is controlled by the proteins, and interphotoreceptor retinal-binding protein (IRBP), which, although distinct from other retinal–retinal-binding proteins, serves a similar function.

Although the systemic functions of vitamin A are far from being completely understood, they can be separated into two major categories. First, vitamin A (specifically, retinoic acid) acts as a hormone to affect gene expression. Within the cell, CRABP transports retinoic acid to the nucleus. In the nucleus, retinoic acid and 9-*cis*-retinoic acid bind to retinoic acid receptors (RARs) or retinoid receptors (RXRs) on the gene (Figure 4-4). Subsequent interactions allow stimulation or inhibition of transcription of specific genes, thus affecting protein synthesis and many body processes. Only a few of these processes are known, and they include morphogenesis in embryonic development and epithelial cell function (including differentiation and production of keratin proteins). The second major role of vitamin A in systemic functions involves glycoprotein synthesis. In a series of reactions, retinol forms retinyl-phosphomannose and then transfers the mannose to the glycoprotein. Glycoproteins are important for normal cell surface functions such as cell aggregation and cell recognition. This role in glycoprotein synthesis may also account for the importance of vitamin A in cell growth because it may increase glycoprotein synthesis for cell receptors that respond to growth factors.

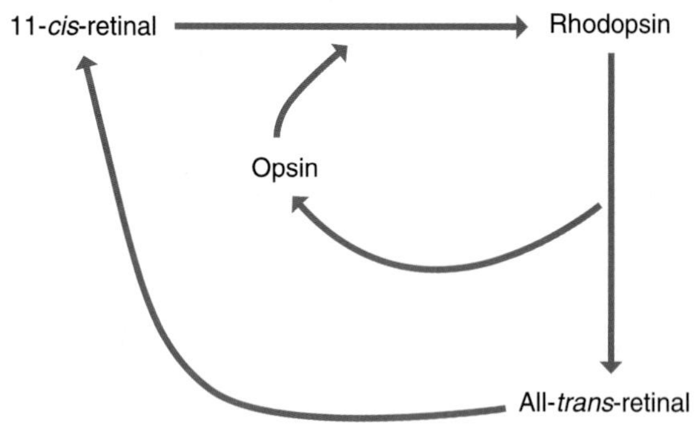

FIGURE 4-3 • The visual cycle.

Vitamin A is also essential for normal reproduction (retinol), bone development and function, and immune system function, although its actions in these roles are currently unclear.

Although a consistent body of epidemiologic evidence indicates that higher blood levels of carotenoids reduce the risk of several chronic diseases, the only clear function of the carotenoids is as provitamin A (Institute of Medicine, 2001). β-Carotene can act as an antioxidant, but its other properties that are unrelated to antioxidant actions, such as retinoid-dependent signaling, gap junction communications, regulation of cell growth, and induction of enzymes, may be more important properties (Stahl, Ale-Agha, and Polidori, 2002).

Dietary Reference Intakes Measurement

The vitamin A content of foods is measured as retinol activity equivalents (RAE). One RAE equals the activity of 1 μg of retinol. (1 μg of retinol is equal to 3.33 international units [IU]) (Box 4-1). Because new data show that the efficiency of β-carotene absorption is much less (14%) than that previously believed (33%), 12 μg of β-carotene is equal to 1 RAE, and 24 μg of other carotenoids equal 1 RAE. In other words, ap-

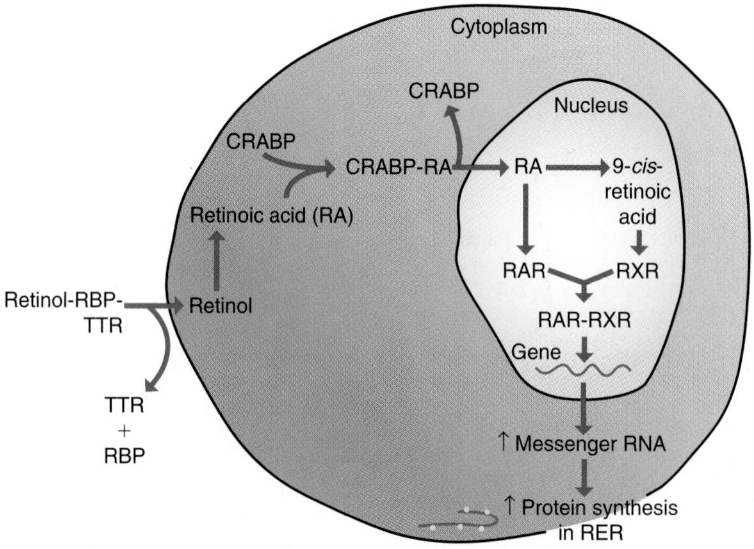

RBP, Retinol-Binding Protein
TTR, Transthyretin
CRABP, Cellular Retinoic Acid–Binding Protein
RAR, Retinoic Acid Receptor
RXR, Retinoid X Receptor

FIGURE 4-4 • Role of vitamin A in gene expression.

proximately twice as much carotenoid is needed in the diet as was previously believed.

Dietary reference intakes (DRIs) have been determined for vitamin A and are expressed in micrograms per day (μg/day) (Table 4-2). The adequate intake (AI) for infants is based on the amount of retinol in human milk. The DRIs for adults are based on levels that provide adequate blood levels and liver stores and are adjusted for differences in average body size. Increased amounts of the vitamin during pregnancy and lactation allow for fetal storage and the vitamin A in breast milk.

No DRIs have been established for the carotenoids. Indeed, supplementation has not been shown to be beneficial and may be harmful. However, increased consumption of fruits and vegetables with carotenoids is clearly beneficial (Institute of Medicine, 2001). (For a complete explanation of the DRIs, see Chapter 15.)

Sources

Preformed vitamin A exists only in foods of animal origin, either in storage areas such as the liver or in the fat of milk and eggs. Very high concentrations of vitamin A are found in cod and halibut liver oils. Nonfat milk in the United States, which by U.S. law can contain 0.1% fat, is routinely fortified with retinol. Provitamin A carotenoids are found in dark green leafy and yellow-orange vegetables and fruit; deeper colors are associated with higher carotenoid levels. In much of the world, carotenoids supply most of the dietary vitamin A. The American food supply provides roughly equal amounts of preformed vitamin A and provitamin A carotenoids. Carrots, greens, spinach, orange juice, sweet potatoes, and cantaloupe are rich sources of provitamin A. In many of these foods, vitamin A bioavailability is limited by binding of carotenoids to proteins, but this can be overcome by cooking, which disrupts the protein association and frees the carotenoid. Table 4-3 lists the vitamin A content of selected foods.

Deficiency

Primary deficiencies of vitamin A result from inadequate intakes of preformed vitamin A or provitamin A carotenoids. Secondary deficiencies can result from malabsorption caused by insufficient dietary fat, biliary or pancreatic insufficiency, and impaired transport from abetalipoproteinemia, liver disease, protein-energy malnutrition, or zinc deficiency.

Vitamin A deficiency is the most significant cause of blindness in the developing world, and an estimated 250 million children are at risk. Between 250,000 and 500,000 cases of blindness from vitamin A deficiency occur annually. In 1991, nearly 14 million preschool children, most from South Asia, had clinical eye disease (xerophthalmia) caused by vitamin A deficiency. Two thirds of those newly diag-

Box 4-1. Vitamin A Activity

1 RAE (retinol activity equivalent) =
- 1 μg of retinol
- 12 mg of β-carotene (from food)
- 3.33 IU of vitamin A activity (on a label)*

5000 IU vitamin A (supplement or food label) =
- 1500 RAE = 1500 μg of retinol

Data from Institute of Medicine, Food and Nutrition Board: *Dietary reference intakes for vitamin A, vitamin K, arsenic, boron, chromium, copper, iodine, iron, manganese, molybdenum, nickel, silicon, vanadium, and zinc*, Washington, DC, 2001, National Academy Press.

*The vitamin A activity on a food or supplement label is stated in international units (IU), a term outdated scientifically but still required legally on labels.

TABLE 4-2 Dietary Reference Intakes for Vitamin A

LIFE-STAGE GROUP	RDA (μg RAE/day)*	UL (mg RAE/day)*
Infants		
0-0.5	400†	600
0.5-1	400†	600
Children		
1-3	300	600
4-8	400	900
Males		
9-13	600	1700
14-18	900	2800
19-30	900	3000
31-50	900	3000
51-70	900	3000
≥70	900	3000
Females		
9-13	600	1700
14-18	700	2500
19-30	700	3000
31-50	700	3000
51-70	700	3000
≥70	700	3000
Pregnant		
≤18	750	2800
19-30	770	3000
31-50	770	3000
Lactating		
≤18	1200	2800
19-30	1300	3000
31-50	1300	3000

From Institute of Medicine, Food and Nutrition Board: *Dietary reference intakes for vitamin A, vitamin K, arsenic, boron, chromium, copper, iodine, iron, manganese, molybdenum, nickel, silicon, vanadium, and zinc*, Washington, DC, 2001, National Academy Press.

**RAE*, Retinol activity equivalents; *RDA*, recommended dietary allowance; *UL*, tolerable upper intake level.

†Adequate intake (AI).

TABLE 4-3 Vitamin A Content of Selected Foods

FOOD*	RAE†
Turkey, 1 cup	2628
Sweet potato, baked, 1 small	797
Carrots, raw, 1 cup	774
Spinach, cooked, 1 cup	368
Squash, butternut, 1 cup	200
Mixed vegetables, frozen, 1 cup	194
Apricots, canned, 1 cup	103
Cantaloupe, 1 cup	129
Broccoli, cooked, 1 cup	87
Brussel sprouts, 1 cup	28
Tomatoes, 1 cup	28
Peaches, canned, 1 cup	23

From U.S. Department of Agriculture, Agricultural Research Service: *USDA nutrient database for standard reference,* Release 14, 2001, Data laboratory home page, http://www.nal.usda.gov/fnic/foodcomp. (This site provides an easily accessible list of nutrients in foods sorted alphabetically or by content of nutrients.)

*100-g edible portion.

†*RAE,* Retinol activity equivalents, 1 IU = 0.3 mg retinol; RAE from plant sources calculated based on 12 mg β-carotene = 1 RAE.

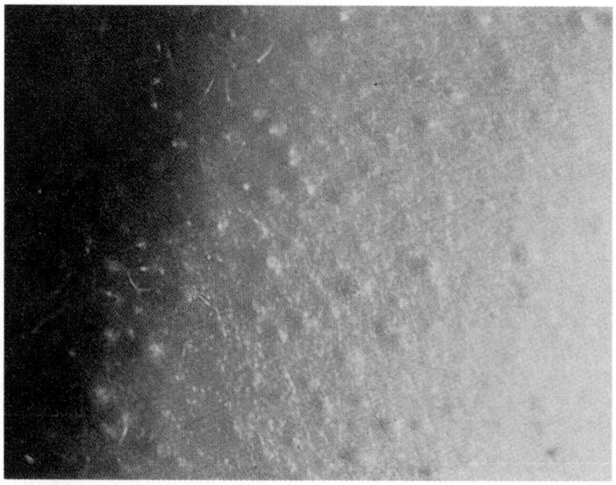

FIGURE 4-5 • Follicular hyperkeratosis. Dry, bumpy skin associated with vitamin A or linoleic acid (essential fatty acid) deficiency. Linoleic acid deficiency may also result in eczematous skin, especially in infants. (From Taylor KB, Anthony LE: *Clinical nutrition,* New York, 1983, McGraw-Hill.)

nosed die within months of going blind because enhanced susceptibility to infections. Even subclinical vitamin A deficiency increases childhood morbidity and mortality (Olson, 1996).

One of the first signs of vitamin A deficiency is impaired vision from the loss of visual pigments. This manifests clinically as night blindness, or nyctalopia. This impairment of dark adaptation (the ability to adapt from being in a bright light or glare to being in darkness [e.g., while driving at night or moving from a brightly lighted to a dark room]), results from the failure of the retina to regenerate rhodopsin. Individuals with night blindness have poor visual discriminatory abilities and may not be able to see in dim light or at twilight. In addition to measuring plasma retinol levels, dark adaptation testing is one of the recommended methods for testing for vitamin A adequacy (Institute of Medicine, 2001).

Subsequently, vitamin A deficiency leads to failures in its systemic functions, which are characterized by impaired embryonic development, impaired spermatogenesis or spontaneous abortion, anemia, impaired immunocompetence (reduced numbers and mitogenic responsiveness of circulating T lymphocytes), and fewer osteoclasts, with subsequent excessive deposition of periosteal bone. Vitamin A deficiency also leads to the keratinization of the mucous membranes that line the respiratory tract, alimentary canal, urinary tract, skin, and epithelium of the eye. Clinically, these conditions manifest as poor growth, blindness caused by xerophthalmia, corneal ulceration, or occlusion of the optic foramina from periosteal overgrowth of the cranium. Xerophthalmia involves atrophy of the periocular glands, hyperkeratosis of the conjunctiva, and finally, involvement of the cornea, leading to softening (keratomalacia) and blindness. Although the condition is now rare in the United States (where it is usually associated with malabsorption), it is more common in developing countries, where it is a major source of blindness among children.

Vitamin A deficiency produces characteristic changes in skin texture involving follicular hyperkeratosis (phrynoderma). Blockage of the hair follicles with plugs of keratin causes the distinctive "goose flesh" or "toad skin," and the skin becomes dry, scaly, and rough. At first the forearms and thighs are affected, but in advanced stages the whole body is affected (Figure 4-5). Loss of mucous membrane integrity as a result of vitamin A deficiency increases host susceptibility to bacterial, viral, or parasitic infections. The deficiency also leads to impairments in certain aspects of cell-mediated immunity, ultimately increasing the risk for infection, particularly for respiratory infections.

Acute vitamin A deficiency is treated with large doses of vitamin A given orally. When the deficiency is part of concomitant protein-energy malnutrition, the malnutrition must be treated for the patient to benefit from vitamin A treatment. The signs and symptoms of deficiency respond to vitamin A supplementation in about the same order as they appear; night blindness responds very quickly, whereas the skin abnormalities may take several weeks to resolve. Massive, intermittent dosing with large doses of vitamin A has been used in developing countries. Treatments with single doses of 60,000 RAE of vitamin A have reduced child mortality by 35% to 70% (Institute of Medicine, 2001). This approach is very costly, which has stimulated interest in increasing the vitamin A content of local food systems as a more sustainable approach to preventing the deficiency.

Box 4-2. Signs of Vitamin A Toxicity

Serum vitamin A of 75-2000 RAE/100 ml
Bone pain and fragility
Hydrocephalus and vomiting (infants and children)
Dry, fissured skin
Brittle nails
Hair loss (alopecia)
Gingivitis
Cheilosis
Anorexia
Irritability
Fatigue
Hepatomegaly and abnormal liver function
Ascites and portal hypertension

Toxicity

Persistent, large doses of vitamin A (more than 100 times the required amount) overcome the capacity of the liver to store the vitamin and can produce intoxication and eventually lead to liver disease. This intoxication is marked by high plasma levels of retinyl esters associated with lipoproteins. Hypervitaminosis A in humans is characterized by changes in the skin and mucous membranes (Box 4-2). Dry lips *(cheilitis)* is a common initial sign, followed by dryness of the nasal mucosa and eyes; more advanced signs include dryness, erythema, scaling and peeling of the skin, hair loss, and nail fragility. Headache, nausea, and vomiting have also been reported. Animals with hypervitaminosis A frequently have bone abnormalities involving overgrowth of periosteal bone (Hathcock et al, 1990); recently, an increased incidence of hip fractures was found in women with intakes of 2000 μg/day of retinol compared with those who consumed 500 μg. Women who took supplements had a 40% increase in risk of hip fracture (Feskanick et al, 2002).

Hypervitaminosis A can be induced by single doses of retinol greater than 200 mg (200,000 RAE) in adults or greater than 100 mg (100,000 RAE) in children. Chronic hypervitaminosis A can result from chronic intakes (usually from misuse of supplements) greater than at least 10 times the AI—or 4000 RAE for an infant or 7000 RAE for an adult (Olson, 1996). Dramatic stories in the literature describe reddening and exfoliation of the skin of Arctic explorers and fishermen who feasted on polar bear liver (which has 3 million RAE) or halibut liver.

Retinoids can be toxic to embryos exposed in the womb (Maden, 1994). This is particularly true for 13-*cis*-retinoic acid (Accutane), a form very effective in treating severe cystic acne but that can cause craniofacial, central nervous system, cardiovascular, and thymic malformations in the fetus. Fetal malformations have also been linked to daily exposures of 6000 to 7500 RAE of vitamin A from supplements, and pregnant women are advised against exceeding 3000 RAE/day of vitamin A.

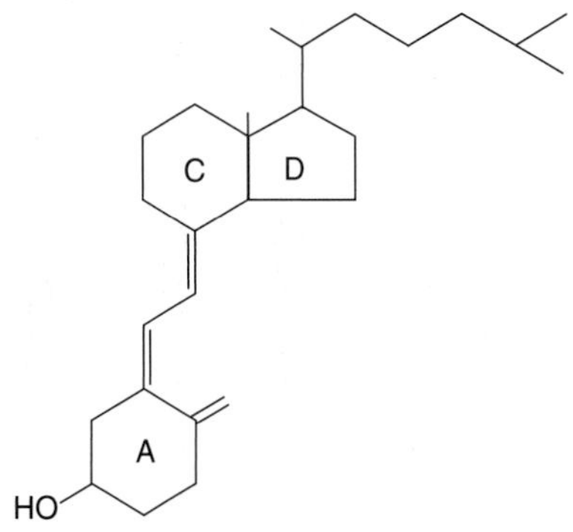

Vitamin D_3
(cholecalciferol)

FIGURE 4-6 • Structure of vitamin D.

The toxicities of carotenoids are low, and daily intakes of as much as 30 mg of β-carotene have no side effects other than the accumulation of the carotenoid in the skin and consequent yellowing. Hypercarotenodermia can be differentiated from jaundice in that the former affects only the skin, leaving the sclera (white) of the eye clear. Hypercarotenodermia is reversible if excessive carotene intake is decreased. However, high doses of β-carotene have been implicated as playing a role in some types of lung cancer, especially in smokers (Caution, 1994) (see Chapter 40).

Vitamin D (Calciferol)

Vitamin D is known as the *sunshine vitamin* because modest exposure to sunlight is usually sufficient for most people to produce their own vitamin D using ultraviolet light and cholesterol in the skin. Because the vitamin can be produced in the body, has specific target tissues, and does not have to be supplied in the diet, it meets the definition of a hormone and usually acts as a steroid hormone.

Two sterols—one in the lipids of animals (7-dehydrocholesterol) and one in plants (ergosterol)—can serve as precursors of vitamin D. Each of these can undergo photolytic ring opening when exposed to ultraviolet irradiation. Ring opening of 7-dehydrocholesterol yields a provitamin form of 7-dehydrocholesterol, which yields cholecalciferol, or vitamin D_3 (Figure 4-6). Ergosterol ring opening yields ergocalciferol, or vitamin D_2. Vitamins D_2 and D_3 require further metabolism to yield the metabolically active forms of 1,25-dihydroxyvitamin D_2 and D_3 (calcitriol) (Figure 4-7). In this way, vitamin D plays an important role, in addition to calcium and phosphorus, in the maintenance of calcium homeostasis and healthy bones and teeth.

Absorption, Transport, and Storage

Dietary vitamin D is incorporated with other lipids into micelles and absorbed with lipids into the intestine by passive diffusion. Inside the absorptive cells the vitamin is incorporated into chylomicrons, enters the lymphatic system, and subsequently enters the plasma, where it is delivered to the liver by chylomicron remnants or to the specific carrier vitamin D–binding protein (DBP), or *transcalciferin.* The efficiency of this absorption process seems to be about

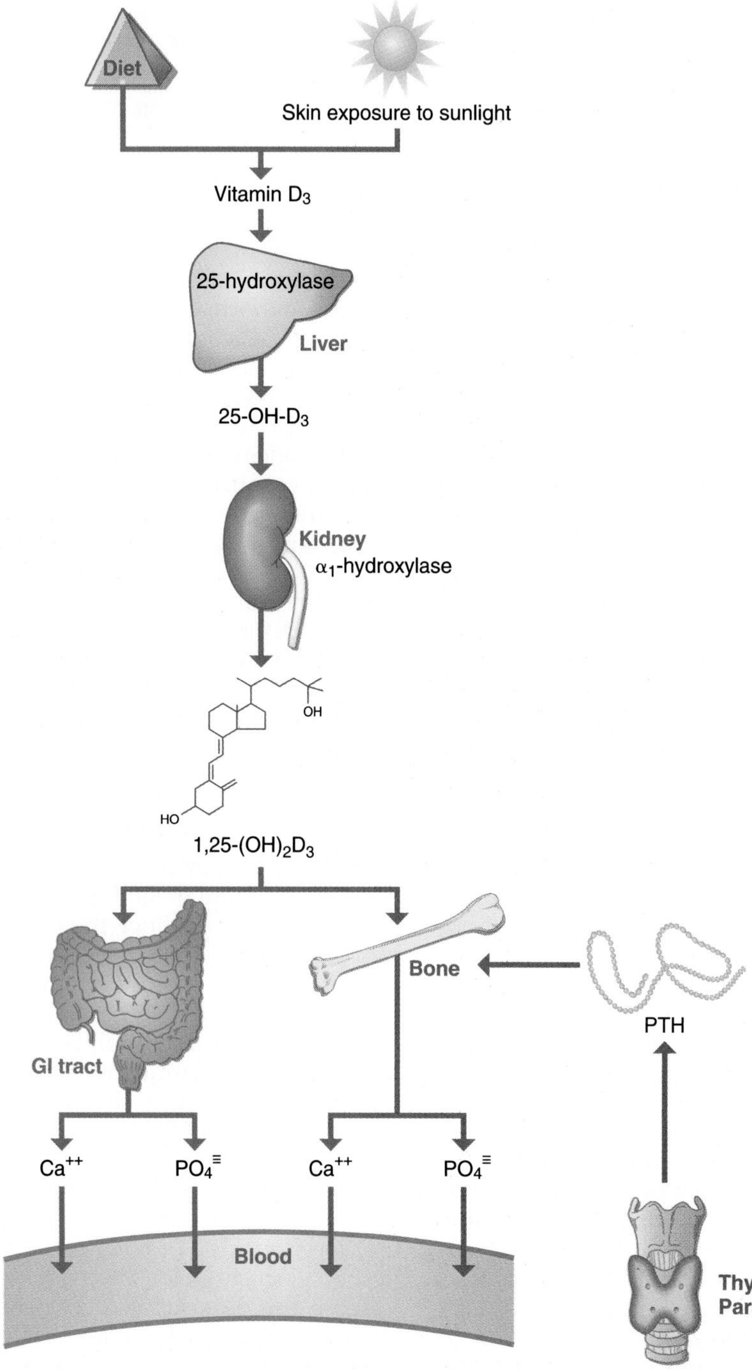

FIGURE 4-7 • Metabolism and function of vitamin D. Vitamin D_3 (cholecalciferol) changes into its biologically active forms: 25-(OH)D_3 and 1,25-$(OH)_2D_3$ (calcitriol). Calcitriol increases calcium and phosphate absorption in the intestine, increases calcium and phosphate resorption in bone, and acts on the kidney to decrease calcium loss in urine.

50%. Vitamin D synthesized in the skin from cholesterol enters the capillary system and is transported by DBP. Vitamin D attached to DBP is delivered to the peripheral tissues. Little vitamin D is stored in the liver.

Metabolism

Vitamin D must be activated by two sequential hydroxylations. The first occurs in the liver and yields 25-hydroxyvitamin D (25-hydroxycholecalciferol). This metabolite is the predominant circulating form of the vitamin. The second hydroxylation is carried out by the enzyme α-1-hydroxylase in the kidney and yields 1,25-dihydroxyvitamin D, the most active form of the vitamin. The activity of α-1-hydroxylase is increased by parathyroid hormone (PTH) in the presence of low plasma concentrations of calcium, yielding increased production of 1,25-dihydroxyvitamin D (calcitriol). The activity of the enzyme decreases when calcitriol levels are increasing (see Figure 4-7).

Functions

Calcitriol (1,25-dihydroxyvitamin D_3) functions primarily like a steroid hormone. Its major actions involve interaction with cell membrane receptors and nuclear vitamin D receptor (VDR) proteins to affect gene transcription in a wide variety of tissues. When calcitriol binds to VDR proteins in the nucleus, the affinity of the VDR proteins for specific promoter regions of the genes—*vitamin D response elements (VDRE)*—increases, allowing the VDR-calcitriol complex to bind to the VDRE. Once the VDR-calcitriol complex is attached to the VDRE region, transcription for specific messenger ribonucleic acids (mRNAs) for specific proteins is enhanced (promoted) or inhibited (Figure 4-8). More than 50 genes are known to be regulated by vitamin D (Omdahl, Morris, and May, 2002), including the gene for the calcium-binding protein *calbindin;* however, most of the genes regulated by vitamin D are not involved in mineral metabolism.

The most well understood functions of vitamin D are in the maintenance of calcium and phosphorus homeostasis, which it can affect in three major ways. First, through gene expression, calcitriol in the small intestine enhances the active transport of calcium across the gut, which stimulates synthesis of calcium-binding proteins (including calbindin) in the mucosal brush border. These proteins then increase calcium absorption. (Vitamin D may also increase calcium absorption in a separate mechanism unrelated to gene expression. This mechanism apparently operates by opening voltage-gated calcium channels [Brown, Finch, and Slatopolsky 2002].) Phosphate absorption is also increased by enhancing acid phosphatase activity, which cleaves phosphate esters and allows increased phosphorus absorption. Second, in the bone, PTH alone or with calcitriol, estrogen, or both, moves calcium and phosphorus from the bone to maintain normal blood levels. The process most probably involves increased osteoclast activity, increased numbers of new osteoclasts through cell differentiation, or both. Finally, in the kidney, calcitriol increases renal tubular reabsorption of calcium and phosphate. These activities are coordinated with the purpose of maintaining plasma calcium concentrations within a narrow range. Calcitonin secreted by the thyroid counters the activity of calcitriol and PTH by suppression of bone mobilization and increases the renal excretion of calcium and phosphate (see Chapters 5 and 27).

Calcitriol plays roles—that are not well understood—in cell differentiation, proliferation, and growth in many tissues, including skin, muscles, the pancreas, nerves, the parathyroid gland, and the immune system. For example, as mentioned previously, it stimulates differentiation of intestinal epithelial cells and osteoblasts; however, it seems to inhibit cell proliferation and growth.

Dietary Reference Intakes

The preferred units for quantification of vitamin D are micrograms (μg) of vitamin D_3. For nonavian species, vitamins D_2 and D_3 have equivalent biologic activities; thus both are used to quantify total vitamin D. International units (IU) are still occasionally used. One IU of vitamin D_3 equals 0.025 μg, and 1 μg of vitamin D_3 equals 40 IU of vitamin D_3.

DRIs for vitamin D are AIs set to meet the body's needs when a person has inadequate exposure to sunlight and the tolerable upper intake levels (ULs)

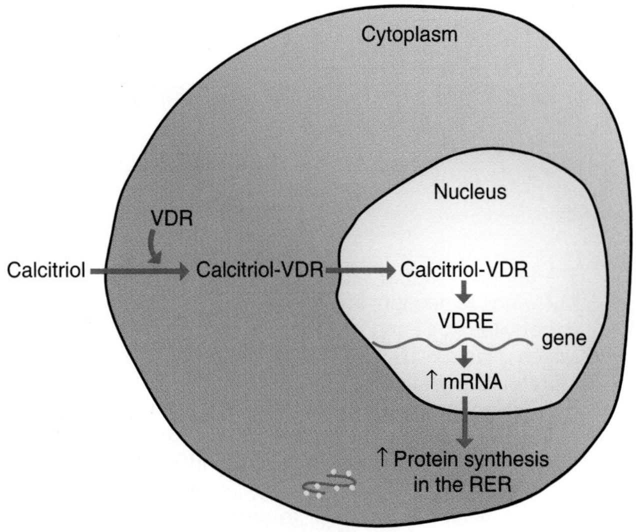

VDR, Vitamin D Receptor Protein
VDRE, Vitamin D Response Elements
RER, Rough Endoplasmic Reticulum

FIGURE 4-8 • Role of vitamin D in gene expression.

are set at those considered to pose no risk of adverse effects. Although 2.5 μg (100 IU) of vitamin D daily is sufficient to prevent vitamin D–deficiency rickets, higher levels (AI of 5 μg/day) are recommended for infants and children throughout the period of skeletal development. Continued intake of the vitamin at this level during adulthood is necessary to support the normal process of continual bone remodeling and adequate calcium and phosphorus homeostasis. The AI increases to 10 μg/day for adults age 51 years and older and increases even more to 15 μg/day (600 IU) for adults 71 years and older. The UL for vitamin D for infants is 25 μg/day (1000 IU) and for children and adults is 50 μg/day (2000 IU) (Table 4-4) (Food and Nutrition Board, 1989).

The normal adult is presumed to obtain sufficient vitamin D from exposure to sunlight and incidental ingestion through small amounts in foods (see *Focus On:* Sunshine, Vitamin D, and Fortification). However, increasing evidence suggests that vitamin D intake in the United States is low (Thomas et al, 1998), and increasing sources of vitamin D in the diet has been recommended (Utiger, 1998). Supplemental vitamin D is appropriate for individuals consistently shielded from sunlight, such as those who are housebound, live in northern latitudes or areas with high atmospheric pollution, wear clothing that completely covers the body, or work at night and stay indoors during the day.

TABLE 4-4 Dietary Reference Intakes for Vitamin D

LIFE-STAGE GROUP	AI (μg/day)*	UL (μg/day)*
Infants		
0-6 mo	5	25
7-12 mo	5	25
Children		
1-3 yr	5	50
4-8 yr	5	50
Males		
9-13 yr	5	50
14-18 yr	5	50
19-30 yr	5	50
31-50 yr	5	50
51-70 yr	10	50
>70 yr	15	50
Females		
9-13 yr	5	50
14-18 yr	5	50
19-30 yr	5	50
31-50 yr	5	50
51-70 yr	10	50
>70 yr	15	50
Pregnant, lactating		
≤18 yr	5	50
19-50 yr	5	50

From Institute of Medicine, Food and Nutrition Board: *Dietary reference intakes for calcium, phosphorus, magnesium, vitamin D, and fluoride,* Washington, DC, 1997, National Academy Press.
**AI,* Adequate intake (as cholecalciferol: 1 μg cholecalciferol = 40 IU vitamin D; in the absence of adequate exposure to sunlight); *UL,* tolerable upper intake level.

Sources

Vitamin D_3 exists naturally in animal products, and the richest sources are fish-liver oils. It is found in only small and highly variable amounts in butter, cream, egg yolk, and liver. Human milk and unfortified cow's milk tend to be poor sources of vitamin D_3, providing only 0.4 to 1 μg/L. However, approximately 98% of all fluid milk sold in the United States is fortified with vitamin D_2 (usually 10 μg [400 IU]/qt), as are most dried whole milk and evaporated milk and some margarines, butters, soy milks, certain cereals, and all infant formula products. Vitamin D is

FOCUS ON

Sunshine, Vitamin D, and Fortification

Brief and casual exposure of the face, arms, and hands to sunlight is thought to equal about 5 μg (200 IU) of vitamin D, and prolonged exposure with erythema raises plasma 25-(OH)D_3 concentrations as much as long-term ingestion of 250 μg (10,000 IU) of vitamin D daily (Haddad, 1992). Ultraviolet light penetration depends on the amount of melanin in the skin, clothing type, blockage of effective rays by window glass, and the use of sunscreens. Casual exposure now seems to provide sufficient vitamin D to last through the winter months except in those unable or unwilling to go outside. Fortification of foods with vitamin D seems to be adequate for these types of individuals (who reside in the United States), because vitamin D deficiency is unusual in this country. Milk continues to be a food of choice for vitamin D fortification because of its calcium. Soy milks and other nondairy milks are now often fortified with the same amount of vitamin D and calcium found in cow's milk. However, milk and infant formulas may not always contain the amount of vitamin D stated on the label (Holick et al, 1992). Eight cases of hypervitaminosis D resulting from drinking incorrectly and excessively fortified milk have been reported. Fortification must be carefully regulated to prevent this problem (Jacobus et al, 1992). Overfortification and underfortification are dangerous, so a unified fortification monitoring program is needed (Chen et al, 1993).

very stable and does not deteriorate when foods are heated or stored for long periods (Table 4-5).

Deficiency

Vitamin D deficiency manifests as rickets in children and growing animals and as osteomalacia in adults.

Rickets

Rickets is a disease involving impaired mineralization of growing bones. It can not only result from deprivation of vitamin D but also from deficiencies of calcium and phosphorus. Rickets is characterized by structural abnormalities of the weight-bearing bones (e.g., tibia, ribs, humerus, radius, ulna) (Figure 4-9) and is associated with accompanying bone pain, muscular tenderness, and hypocalcemic tetany. Soft, pliable, rachitic bones cannot withstand ordinary stresses and strains, resulting in bowed legs, "knock knees," beaded ribs (the rachitic rosary), pigeon breast, and frontal bossing of the skull. Radiography reveals enlarged epiphyseal growth plates manifested as enlarged wrists and ankles resulting from their failure to mineralize and continue growth. Patients have increased plasma and serum levels of alkaline phosphatase, which is released by the affected osteoblasts.

Historically, those with rickets have been poor children in industrialized cities where exposure to sunlight is limited. In North America, the vitamin D supplementation of foods has virtually eliminated the disease. However, the incidence of vitamin D–dependent rickets is increasing in American children. The children most at risk have dark skin and breast-feed for long periods without exposure to sunlight or vitamin D supplements (Fitzpatrick et al, 2000; Sills, 2001). Rickets can also develop in children with chronic problems of lipid malabsorption and in those undergoing long-term anticonvulsant therapy (which reduces the circulating levels of 1,25-dihydroxyvitamin D_3).

TABLE 4-5 Vitamin D Content of Selected Foods

FOOD	CONTENT (μg)*
Herring, fresh, raw, 1 oz	6.6
Salmon, cooked, 1 oz	3.5
Milk, cow's fortified, 1 cup	2.5
Sardines, canned, 1 oz	2.1
Liver, chicken, cooked, 3 oz	1.1
Shrimp, canned, 1 oz	0.7
Egg yolk	0.6
Milk, human, 1 cup	0-0.6
Liver, calf, cooked, 3 oz	0.4

From U.S. Department of Agriculture: *Composition of foods,* Handbook No. 8 Series, Washington, DC, 1976-1986, Agricultural Research Service, USDA.
*Recalculated in micrograms of D3; IU = 0.025 μg.

Rickets caused strictly by vitamin D deprivation can be treated effectively with oral preparations of the vitamin or natural sources rich in the vitamin. For example, vitamin D concentrates of fish-liver oil have been prescribed; 1 teaspoon (4 ml) of cod-liver oil contains 9 μg (360 IU) of vitamin D. For those with calcium deficiency–related or hypophosphatemic vitamin D–refractory rickets, vitamin D treatment alone may not be effective, and active vitamin D metabolites, such as 25-(OH)D_3 or 1,25(OH)2D_3, or a synthetic analogue become necessary.

Osteomalacia

Osteomalacia develops in adults whose epiphyseal closures make that portion of the bone resistant to vitamin D deficiency. Therefore the disease involves generalized reductions in bone density and the presence of pseudofractures, especially of the

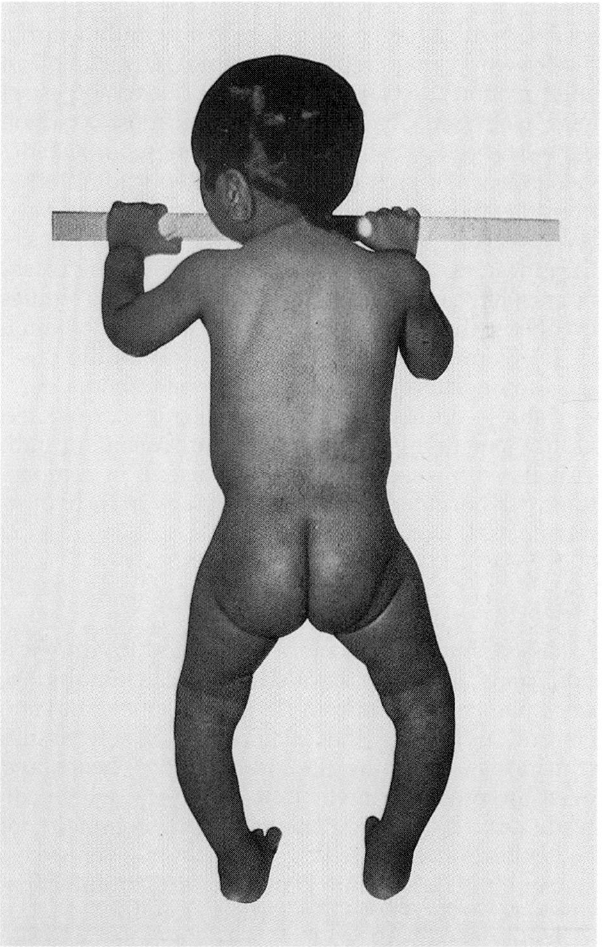

FIGURE 4-9 • Severely bowed legs caused by rickets, an indication of vitamin D and calcium deficiencies in children (rickets is a disorder of cartilage cell growth, and enlargement of epiphyseal growth plates). (From Latham MC et al: *Scope manual on nutrition,* Kalamazoo, Mich, 1980, The Upjohn Company. Copyright by Rose Lee Nemir, MD.)

spine, femur, and humerus. Patients experience muscular weakness and bone tenderness and have a greater risk of fractures, particularly of the wrist and pelvis.

Prevention of osteomalacia is usually possible with an adequate consumption of vitamin D, calcium, and phosphorus in the diet. It has been estimated that as little as 10 to 15 minutes of sun exposure on a clear summer day, two or three times a week, is sufficient to prevent osteomalacia among most older adults. Osteomalacia can be treated effectively with vitamin D_3 in doses of 25 to 125 μg/day; in those whose conditions are complicated by lipid malabsorption, daily doses as large as 1250 μg have been used.

Osteoporosis

Osteoporosis is frequently confused with osteomalacia; however, it is a very different bone disease, one that involves diminished bone mass but the retention of a normal histologic appearance. Osteoporosis is associated with aging; it is thought to be a multifactorial disease involving impaired vitamin D metabolism and function associated with low or decreasing estrogen levels (see Chapter 27). It is the most common bone disease of postmenopausal women but also develops in older men. A study of patients admitted to hospitals showed that an alarmingly high number had low levels of vitamin D (Thomas et al, 1998). Studies of the efficacies of various vitamers D in treating osteoporosis have been inconsistent, but two large studies involving the chronic use of 1,25-dihydroxyvitamin D_3 by women showed significant delay of the onset (and some reversal) of the signs and symptoms. A recent study concluded that neither calcium nor vitamin D supplements alone are sufficient treatment for individuals with osteoporosis but are useful in conjunction with hormone replacement therapy in early postmenopausal women (Delmas, 2002).

Toxicity

Excessive intake of vitamin D can produce intoxication characterized by elevated serum calcium (hypercalcemia) and phosphorus (hyperphosphatemia) levels and ultimately the calcification of soft tissues (calcinosis), including the kidney, lungs, heart, and even the tympanic membrane of the ear, which can result in deafness. Patients often complain of headache and nausea (Box 4-3). Infants given excessive amounts of vitamin D may have gastrointestinal upset, bone fragility, and retarded growth.

Hypervitaminosis D is a progressive intoxication, and individuals seem to vary in their susceptibility to the condition. The UL for vitamin D is 25 μg/day for infants and 50 μg/day for children and adults. It is clear that infants and small children are most susceptible to hypervitaminosis D.

Box 4-3. Signs of Vitamin D Toxicity

Excessive calcification of bone
Kidney stones
Metastatic calcification of soft tissues (kidney, heart, lung, and tympanic membrane)
Hypercalcemia
Headache
Weakness
Nausea and vomiting
Constipation
Polyuria
Polydipsia

Vitamin E

Vitamin E has a fundamental role in protecting the body against the damaging effects of reactive oxygen species that are formed metabolically or encountered in the environment. Vitamin E includes two classes of biologically active substances: (1) the tocopherols and (2) the related but much less biologically active compounds, the *tocotrienols.* The vitamers of each series are named according to the position and number of methyl groups on their ring systems. The most important of these is α-tocopherol (Figure 4-10) in the natural D-isomer form or the 50% less active synthetic forms (Horwitt, 1999).

Absorption, Transport, and Storage

Vitamin E is absorbed in the upper small intestine by micelle-dependent diffusion, and like the other fat-soluble vitamins, its use depends on the presence of dietary fat and adequate biliary and pancreatic function. The esterified forms of vitamin E found in supplements (which are more stable) can only be absorbed after hydrolysis by esterases at the duodenal mucosa. However, esters of natural and synthetic α-tocopherol are digested equally well (Institute of Medicine, 2000b). The absorption of vitamin E is highly variable, and efficiencies range from 20% to 70%. Absorbed vitamin E is incorporated into chylomicrons and transported into the general circulation via lymph. Vitamin E delivered to the liver is incorporated into very–low-density lipoproteins (VLDLs) using a transport protein specific for vitamin E. In the plasma, tocopherol is also partitioned into low-density lipoproteins (LDLs) and high-density lipoproteins (HDLs), where it may protect the lipoproteins from oxidation.

The cellular uptake of vitamin E can occur either as a receptor-mediated process (in which LDLs deliver the vitamin into the cell) or as a process mediated by lipoprotein lipase (LP) as vitamin E is released from chylomicrons and VLDLs by the action of LP. Within the cell, intracellular transport of the tocopherol requires an intracellular tocopherol-binding protein (TBP). In most nonadipose cells, vitamin E is located almost exclusively in membranes from which it can be mobilized; in adipose tissues, it is partitioned primarily in the bulk lipid phase, from which it is not readily mobilized.

Metabolism

The metabolism of vitamin E is limited. It is primarily oxidized into the biologically inactive tocopheryl quinone, which can be reduced to tocopheryl hydroquinone. Glucuronic acid conjugates of the hydroquinone are secreted in the bile, making excretion in the feces the major route of elimination of the vitamin. With usual intakes of vitamin E, a very small portion is excreted in the urine as water-soluble, side-chain metabolites (tocopheronic acid and tocopheronolactone).

Functions

Vitamin E is the most important lipid-soluble antioxidant in the cell. Located in the lipid portion of cell membranes, it protects unsaturated phospholipids of the membrane from oxidative degradation from highly reactive oxygen species and other free radicals. Vitamin E performs this function through its ability to reduce such radicals into harmless metabolites by donating a hydrogen to them (see Figure 4-10). This process is called free radical *scavenging*.

As a membrane free radical scavenger, vitamin E is now understood to be an important component of the cellular antioxidant defense system, which involves other enzymes (e.g., superoxide dismutases [SODs], glutathione peroxidases [GPXs], glutathione reductase [GR], catalase, thioredoxin reductase [TR]) and nonenzymatic factors (e.g., glutathione, uric acid), many of which depend on other essential nutrients. For example, the expressions of the GPXs and TR depend on adequate selenium status; the expressions of the SODs depend on adequate copper, zinc, and manganese statuses; and the activity of GR depends on adequate riboflavin status. Therefore the antioxidant function of vitamin E can be affected by the levels of one or more nutrients. This phenomenon is involved in several deficiency diseases of animals (e.g., myopathies, vascular disorders) in which vitamin E can seem to be interchangeable with selenium—a phenomenon referred to as *nutritional sparing*.

This antioxidant function suggests that vitamin E and related nutrients may collectively be important in protecting the body against and treating conditions related to oxidative stress, such as aging, arthritis (Can et al, 2002), cancer (Malmberg et al, 2002), cardiovascular disease (Fairfield and Fletcher, 2002),

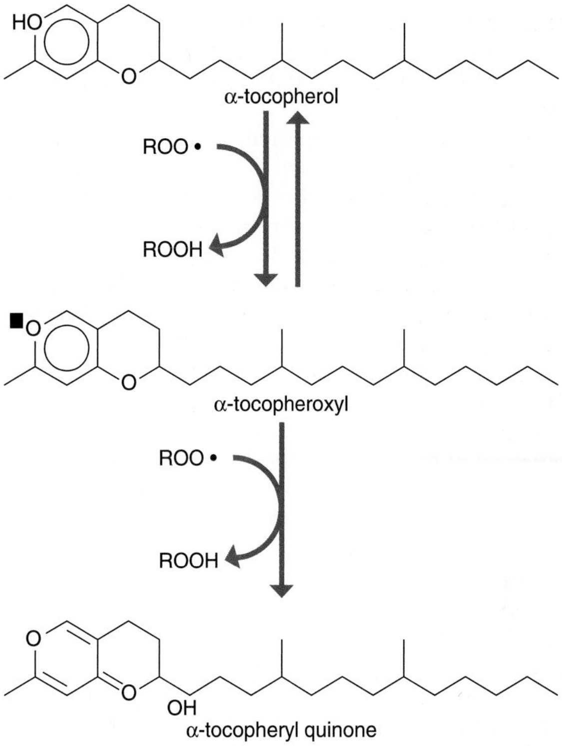

FIGURE 4-10 • Mechanism of vitamin E scavenging oxygen-centered free radicals *(ROO·)*. (From Combs GF: *The vitamins: fundamental aspects in nutrition and health,* ed 2, Orlando, 1998, Academic Press.)

cataracts, diabetes, and infection and in some cases of Alzheimer's disease (Morris et al, 2002) (see *Focus On:* Topical Application of Vitamins).

Dietary Reference Intakes

Vitamin E is quantified in terms of α-tocopherol equivalents (α-TE); 1 mg of R,R,R-α-tocopherol is defined as 1 α-TE, and 1 mg of the synthetic all-*rac*-α-tocopherol is defined as 0.5 α-TE. Although outdated, IU of vitamin E are still found on some food labels. An IU of vitamin E is equal to 0.67 mg of RRR-α-tocopherol and 1 mg of all-*rac*-α-tocopherol (Institute of Medicine, 2000b). The DRIs for vitamin E have been established (Institute of Medicine, 2000b), with AIs for infants and recommended dietary allowances (RDAs) for children and adults based solely on the α-tocopherol form of the vitamin because other forms are not converted to α-tocopherol in humans; they are generally higher than the previous RDAs (Institute of Medicine, 1998) (Table 4-6). The need for vitamin E depends in part on the amount of polyunsaturated fatty acids (PUFAs) consumed. For Americans, typical intakes are about 0.4 mg α-TE/mg PUFA; because the United States does not have significant vitamin E deficiency problems, this ratio is thought to be adequate.

Sources

Because tocopherols and tocotrienols are synthesized only by plants, plant products—especially the oils—are the best sources of them, with α- and γ-tocopherols being predominant compounds in most common foods. Nearly two thirds of the vitamin E in the typical American diet is supplied by salad oils, margarines, and shortenings; about 11% by fruits and vegetables; and about 7% by grains and grain products. Table 4-7 lists the vitamin E content of selected foods (Institute of Medicine, 2000b).

The free alcohol forms of vitamin E (e.g., tocopherols) are fairly stable but can be destroyed by oxidation. Vitamin E esters (e.g., tocopheryl acetate) are very stable, even in oxidizing conditions. Because the vitamers E are insoluble in water, they are not lost by cooking in water but can be destroyed by deep-fat frying.

Deficiency

The clinical manifestations of vitamin E deficiency vary considerably among species. In general, the targets are the neuromuscular, vascular, and reproductive systems. In the neuromuscular system, vitamin E deficiency, which may take 5 to 10 years to develop, manifests clinically as loss of deep tendon reflexes, impaired vibratory and position sensation, changes in balance and coordination, muscle weakness, and visual disturbances (Sokol, 2001). Symptoms in humans are uncommon and have occurred only in those with lipid malabsorption (e.g., biliary atresia, exocrine pancreatic insufficiency) or lipid transport abnormalities (e.g., abetalipoproteinemia).

At the cellular level, a deficiency of vitamin E is accompanied by an increase in lipid peroxidation of the cell membrane. Because of this, vitamin E–deficient cells exposed to an oxidant stress experience more rapid injury and necrosis.

The limited transplacental movement of vitamin E results in newborn infants having low tissue concentrations of vitamin E. Premature infants may therefore be at risk for vitamin E deficiency because they typically have a limited lipid absorptive capacity for some time (see Chapter 9).

Toxicity

Vitamin E is one of the least toxic of the vitamins. Humans and animals seem to be able to tolerate relatively high intakes—at least 100 times the nutritional requirement. The UL for vitamin E in adults is 1000 mg/day; see Table 4-6). However, in very high doses, vitamin E can decrease the body's ability to use other fat-soluble vitamins. For example, animals fed excessive amounts of vitamin E have developed impaired bone mineralization, impaired hepatic vitamin A storage, and prolonged blood coagulation. The latter effect on vitamin K status may be a concern for patients receiving anticoagulant therapy because a regular daily intake of 800 TE of vitamin E was found to exacerbate the effect of a coumarin drug.

FOCUS ON

Topical Application of Vitamins

Although topical retinoic acid and other vitamin A derivatives have been used to treat acne for 3 decades (Bershad, 2001), Dreher and Maibach (2001) and Krol, Kramer-Ktickland, and Liebler (2000) recently suggested that regular use of skin care products, such as sunscreens containing antioxidants (including vitamins A, E, and C), may protect skin from oxidative stress, such as the stress induced by ultraviolet light (UV) light. Topical application of α-tocopherol, retinol, and retinal causes an increase in these vitamins in the epidermis, which is where they also exist naturally; application of these vitamins apparently confers sustained antioxidant ability to the skin and causes pigment darkening after exposure to UV light to occur more quickly. The effects of topical application of vitamin E seem to be related to its antioxidant properties and its UV absorptive properties. (Sorg, Tran, and Saurat, 2001). Vitamins E and A absorb UV light because of their physical properties. In these topical preparations. vitamin C apparently prevents the oxidation of other antioxidants (i.e., vitamins A and E in the preparation itself). Vitamins C and E in topical applications also prevented the peroxidation of eicosapentaenoic acid (EPA) in pig skin, where EPA protects the skin against UV damage (Moison and Beijersbergen van Henegouwen, 2002).

Vitamin E used orally and topically reduced acute and chronic skin damage and incidence of skin cancer in mice (Budiyanto et al, 2000; Burke et al, 2000). However, the form of the vitamin being used is important. Gensler et al (1996) found that stable esters of vitamin E not only failed to prevent photocarcinogenesis in mice, but it may have enhanced it. McVean and Liebler (1999) note that only the α-tocopherols conferred photodamage protection in mice.

Although human studies have shown the photoprotective effects of natural and synthetic antioxidants, their role in cancer prevention is less clear. Caution should be used in the topical application of vitamin E for wound healing and improving the outcome of scarring; in one study, it was found that topical vitamin E not only failed to improve the cosmetic appearance of scars, but it also led to a high incidence of contact dermatitis (Baumann and Spencer, 1999).

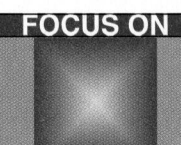

Vitamin K

In addition to playing an essential role in blood clotting, scientists now know that vitamin K plays a role in bone formation (Heaney, 1993). Naturally occurring forms of vitamin K are the phylloquinones (the vitamin K_1 series), which are synthesized by green plants, and the menaquinones (the vitamin K_2 series), which are synthesized by bacteria. Both of these natural forms have a 2-methyl-1,4-napthoquinone ring and alkylated side chains (Figure 4-11). The synthetic compound menadione (vitamin K_3) has no side chain but can be alkylated in the liver to produce menaquinones. Menadione is twice as potent biologically as the naturally occurring forms vitamins K_1 and K_2 (Suttie, 1995).

Absorption, Transport, and Storage

The phylloquinones (K_1) are absorbed by an energy-dependent process in the small intestine. However, the menaquinones (K_2) and menadione (K_3) are absorbed in the small intestine and colon by passive diffusion. Like the other fat-soluble vitamins, absorption depends on a minimum amount of dietary fat and on bile salts and pancreatic juices. The absorbed vitamers K are incorporated into chylomicrons in the lymph and taken to the liver, where they are incorporated into VLDLs and subsequently delivered to the peripheral tissues by low-density lipoproteins.

Vitamin K is found in low concentrations in many tissues, where it is localized in cellular membranes. Because of the metabolism of the vitamin, tissues show mixtures of vitamers K even when a single form is consumed. Most tissues contain phylloquinones and menaquinones.

Metabolism

Phylloquinones can be converted to menaquinones by successive bacterial dealkylation and realkylation before absorption. Side-chain shortening and oxidation produce metabolites that are excreted in the feces via the bile, frequently as glucuronic acid conjugates, and catabolize phylloquinones and menaquinones. Menadione is metabolized more rapidly; it is excreted primarily in the urine as a phosphate, sulfate, or glucuronide derivative.

Functions

Vitamin K is essential for the posttranslational carboxylation of glutamic acid residues in proteins to form carboxyglutamate (GLA) residues (Ferland, 1998); the residues bind calcium (Vermeer et al, 1996). In the process of generating residues, vitamin K is oxidized (i.e., donates a hydrogen) to an epoxide. It is restored to its hydroquinone form by the enzyme expoxide reductase (Figure 4-12). This process is known as the *vitamin K cycle.* The vitamin K cycle can be disrupted by inhibitors of the regeneration of reduced vitamin K, including coumarin-type drugs such as

TABLE 4-6 Dietary Reference Intakes for Vitamin E

LIFE-STAGE GROUP	RDA (mg α-TE/day)*	UL (mg/day)*
Infants		
0-0.5	4	ND
0.5-1	5	ND
Children		
1-3	6	200
4-8	7	300
Males		
9-13	11	600
14-18	15	800
19-30	15	1000
31-50	15	1000
51-70	15	1000
≥70	15	1000
Females		
9-13	11	600
14-18	15	800
19-30	15	1000
31-50	15	1000
51-70	15	1000
≥70	15	1000
Pregnant		
≤18	15	800
19-30	15	1000
31-50	15	1000
Lactating		
≤18	19	800
19-30	19	1000
31-50	19	1000

From Institute of Medicine, Food and Nutrition Board: *Dietary reference intakes for vitamin C, vitamin E, selenium, and carotenoids,* Washington, DC, 2000, National Academy Press.

**RDA,* Recommended dietary allowance; *α-TE,* α-tocopherol equivalents; *UL,* tolerable upper intake level; *ND,* not determinable.

TABLE 4-7 Vitamin E Content of Selected Foods

FOOD	α-TE (mg)*
Raisin bran, 1 cup	29.97
Almonds, 1 oz	7.42
Sunflower oil, 1 tbsp	6.88
Canola oil, 1 tbsp	2.93
Corn oil, 1 tbsp	2.87
Soybean oil, 1 tbsp	2.47
Asparagus, 1 cup	2.25
Peanuts, 1 oz	2.101
Margarine, 1 tbsp	1.80
Olive oil, 1 tbsp	1.67
Flounder, 3 oz	1.60
Baked beans, canned with pork, 1 cup	1.37
Apricots, canned, sweetened, ½ cup	1.15

From U.S. Department of Agriculture, Agricultural Research Service: *USDA nutrient database for standard reference,* Release 14, 2001, Data laboratory home page, http://www.nal.usda.gov/fnic/foodcomp.

*α-*TE,* α-Tocopherol equivalents.

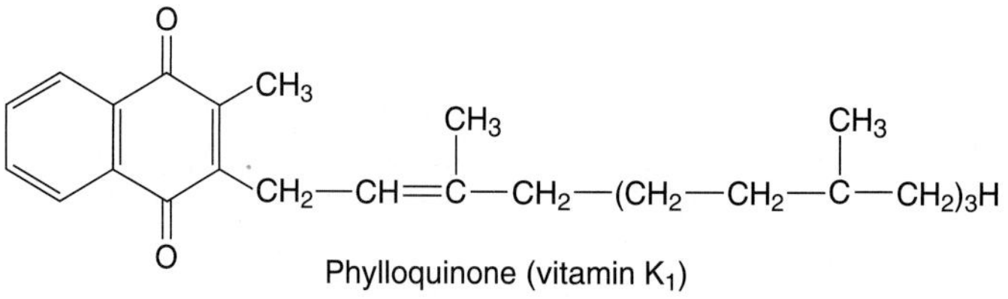

FIGURE 4-11 • Structure of vitamin K.

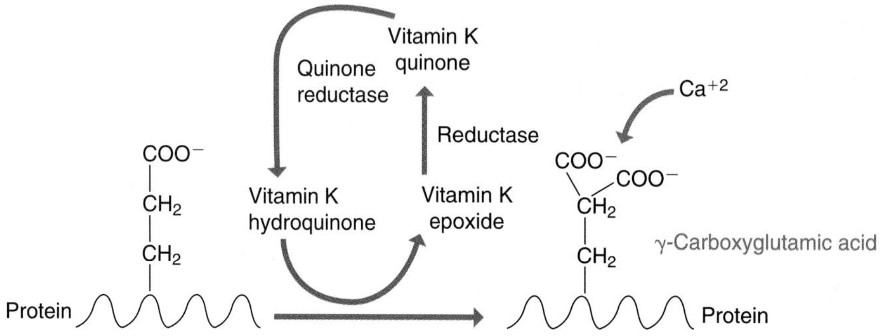

FIGURE 4-12 • Function and regeneration of vitamin K in the production of γ-carboxyglutamic acid.

warfarin and dicumarol (which is the basis for their anticoagulant activities).

Four plasma-clotting GLA proteins have been identified, including thrombin, which is necessary for the conversion of fibrinogen to fibrin in blood clotting. In addition, at least three proteins found in calcified tissues (including osteocalcin; see Chapter 27) and at least one protein found in calcified atherosclerotic tissue (atherocalcin; see Chapter 35) have been identified.

Dietary Reference Intakes

Although the various vitamers K vary widely in their biopotencies, no standardization of means exists for accommodating these differences when quantifying the amounts of the vitamin K in foods or diets. Each vitamer is expressed in terms of its mass in micrograms of vitamin K.

The DRIs for vitamin K are given as AIs, and no UL has been determined (Table 4-8). However, it should not be assumed that high vitamin K consumption has adverse effects because data on such effects are very limited.

Sources

Vitamin K is found in large amounts in green leafy vegetables, especially broccoli, cabbage, turnip greens, and dark lettuces, usually at levels greater than 100 μg/100 g. The amounts of the vitamin in dairy products, meats, and eggs tend to vary, ranging from 1 to 50 μg/g, and fruits and cereals usually contain about 15 μg/g. Breast milk tends to be low in vi-

TABLE 4-8 Dietary Reference Intakes for Vitamin K

LIFE-STAGE GROUP	AI (μg/day)*
Infants	
0-0.5	2
0.5-1	2.5
Children	
1-3	30
4-8	55
Males	
9-13	60
14-18	75
19-30	120
31-50	120
51-70	120
≥70	120
Females	
9-13	60
14-18	75
19-30	90
31-50	90
51-70	90
≥70	90
Pregnant	
≤18	75
19-30	90
31-50	90
Lactating	
≤18	75
19-30	90
31-50	90

From Institute of Medicine, Food and Nutrition Board: *Dietary reference intakes for vitamin A, vitamin K, arsenic, boron, chromium, copper, iodine, iron, manganese, molybdenum, nickel, silicon, vanadium, and zinc,* Washington, DC, 2001, National Academy Press.

**AI,* Adequate intake; tolerable upper intake levels (ULs) not determined.

TABLE 4-9 Vitamin K Content of Selected Foods

FOOD	CONTENT (μg)
Spinach, raw, 1 cup	400
Lettuce, iceberg, 1 cup	210
Broccoli, raw, 1 cup	205
Cabbage, raw, 1 cup	145
Green beans, raw, 1 cup	47
Asparagus, raw, 1 cup	40
Avocado, raw, 1 cup	40
Carrot, raw, 1 cup	4
Potato, baked, 1 medium	4
Ground beef, raw, 3 oz	≤0.5
Orange, raw, 1 medium	≤0.1
Turkey, raw, 3 oz	≤0.02

From U.S. Department of Agriculture, Agricultural Research Service: *Provisional table on the vitamin K content of foods,* HNIS/PT-104, 1994, Data laboratory home page, http://www.nal.usda.gov/fnic/foodcomp.

tamin K and does not provide enough of the vitamin for infants less than 6 months of age (see Chapters 8 and 9). Table 4-9 shows the provisional vitamin K contents of some selected foods. An extensive list of vitamin K sources is available for practitioners working with patients who are taking anticoagulants (Booth, 1999).

The analytic task of determining the vitamers K in foods is formidable, therefore it is understandable that tabulated vitamin K values for food are often inaccurate. Nevertheless, the absence of evidence of a significant vitamin K deficiency in the general population indicates that adequate amounts of the vitamin can normally be obtained by foods or produced by enteric microflora. Vitamin K is fairly stable; it is not destroyed by ordinary cooking methods, nor is it lost in cooking water. However, it is sensitive to light and alkalis.

Deficiency

The predominant sign of vitamin K deficiency is hemorrhage, which in severe cases can cause fatal anemia. The underlying condition is hypoprothrombinemia, which is characterized by prolonged clotting time. Vitamin K deficiencies are rare among humans but have been associated with lipid malabsorption, destruction of intestinal flora in those receiving chronic antibiotic therapy, and liver disease. Newborn infants, particularly those who are premature or exclusively breast-fed, are susceptible to hypoprothrombinemia during the first few days of life as the result of poor placental transfer of vitamin K and failure to establish a vitamin K-producing intestinal microflora. Hemorrhagic disease in the newborn is treated prophylactically by administering menadione intramuscularly at birth. Low intakes of vitamin K have been associated with increased incidence of hip fractures in older adults (U.S. Department of Agriculture, 2000).

Toxicity

Neither the phylloquinones nor the menaquinones have shown any adverse effects by any route of administration. However, menadione can be toxic; excessive doses have produced hemolytic anemia in rats and severe jaundice in infants.

THE WATER-SOLUBLE VITAMINS

Thiamin, riboflavin, niacin, vitamin B_6, pantothenic acid, biotin, folic acid, vitamin B_{12}, and vitamin C are usually referred to as the *water-soluble vitamins,* and solubility in water is one of the only characteristics that they share. Because they are water soluble, these vitamins tend to be absorbed by simple diffusion when ingested in large amounts and by carrier-mediated processes when ingested in smaller amounts. They are distributed in the aqueous phases of the cell (i.e., the cytoplasm and mitochondrial matrix space) and are essential cofactors or cosubstrates of enzymes involved in various aspects of metabolism (Combs, 1998). Most are not stored in appreciable amounts, making their regular consumption a necessity.

Thiamin

Thiamin (Figure 4-13) plays essential roles in carbohydrate metabolism and neural function. The vitamin must be activated by phosphorylation into *thiamin triphosphate (TTP),* or *cocarboxylase,* which serves as a coenzyme in energy metabolism and the synthesis of pentoses. Thiamin's role in neural function is unclear, but it probably does not act as a coenzyme (Groff and Gropper, 1999).

Absorption, Transport, and Storage

Thiamin is absorbed from the proximal small intestine by active transport (in low doses) and passive diffusion (in high doses—i.e., >5 mg/day). Active transport is inhibited by alcohol consumption, which interferes with transport of the vitamin, and by folate deficiency, which interferes with the replication of enterocytes. The mucosal uptake of thiamin is coupled to its phosphorylation into thiamin pyrophosphate (TPP). The activated TPP is carried to the liver by the portal circulation.

Most (approximately 90%) of circulating thiamin is carried as TPP by erythrocytes, although small amounts exist primarily as free thiamin and *thiamin monophosphate (TMP)* bound chiefly to albumin. Uptake by cells of peripheral tissues occurs by passive diffusion and active transport. Tissues retain thiamin as phosphate esters, most of which are bound to proteins. Tissue levels of thiamin vary, with no appreciable storage of the vitamin.

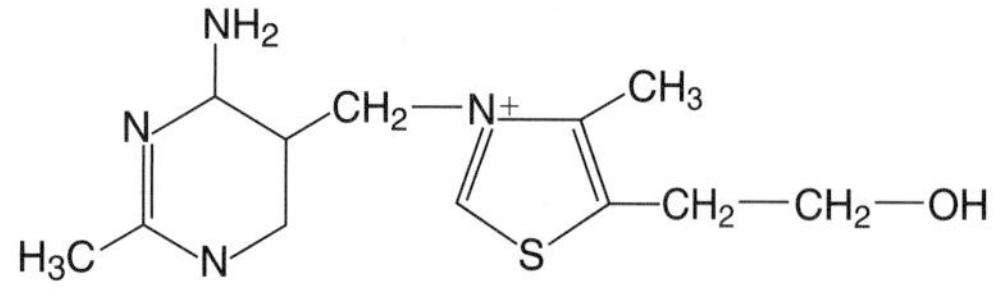

Thiamin

FIGURE 4-13 • Structure of thiamin.

Metabolism

Thiamin is phosphorylated in many tissues by specific kinases into the diphosphate and triphosphate esters. Each of these esters can be catabolized by a phosphorylase to yield TMP. Small amounts of some 20 other excretory metabolites are also produced and excreted in the urine.

Functions

The functional form of thiamin is TPP, which is a coenzyme for several dehydrogenase enzyme complexes essential in the metabolism of pyruvate and other α-keto acids. Thiamin is essential for the oxidative decarboxylation of α-keto acids, including for the oxidative conversion of pyruvate to acetyl coenzyme A (acetyl CoA), which enters the *tricarboxylic acid (TCA)*, or *Krebs, cycle* to generate energy. It is also required for the conversion of α-ketoglutarate and the 2-ketocarboxylates derived from the amino acids methionine, threonine, leucine, isoleucine, and valine. TPP also serves as the coenzyme for transketolase, which catalyzes 2-carbon fragment exchange reactions in the oxidation of glucose by the hexose monophosphate shunt (see Chapter 3).

TABLE 4-10 Dietary Reference Intakes for Thiamin

LIFE-STAGE GROUP	RDA (mg/day)*
Infants	
0-6 mo	0.2†
7-12 mo	0.3†
Children	
1-3 yr	0.5
4-8 yr	0.6
Males	
9-13 yr	0.9
14-18 yr	1.2
19-30 yr	1.2
31-50 yr	1.2
51-70 yr	1.2
>70 yr	1.2
Females	
9-13 yr	0.9
14-18 yr	1.0
19-30 yr	1.1
31-50 yr	1.1
51-70 yr	1.1
>70 yr	1.1
Pregnant	
≤18 yr	1.4
19-30 yr	1.4
31-50 yr	1.4
Lactating	
≤18 yr	1.5
19-30 yr	1.5
31-50 yr	1.5

From Institute of Medicine, Food and Nutrition Board: *Dietary reference intakes for thiamin, riboflavin, niacin, vitamin B_6, folate, vitamin B_{12}, pantothenic acid, biotin, and choline,* Washington, DC, 1998, National Academy Press.
**RDA,* Recommended daily allowance; tolerable upper intake levels (ULs) not determined.
†Adequate intake (AI).

Dietary Reference Intakes

Thiamin is expressed quantitatively in terms of its mass, usually in milligrams. The DRIs for thiamin include AIs for infants and the newly defined RDAs. In general, the RDAs are based on levels of energy intake because of the direct role of thiamin in energy metabolism, whereas the AIs for infants are based on the thiamin levels typically found in human milk (Table 4-10).

Sources

Thiamin is widely distributed in many foods, most of which contain only low concentrations. The richest sources are yeasts and liver; however, cereal grains comprise the most important source of the vitamin in most human diets. Although whole grains are typically rich in thiamin, most of it is removed during milling and refining. However, in the United States, most refined grain products are supplemented with thiamin and other B vitamins. Plant foods contain thiamin predominantly in the free form, whereas almost all of the thiamin in animal products exists as the more efficiently used TPP (Table 4-11).

Thiamin can be destroyed by heat, oxidation, and ionizing radiation, but it is stable when frozen. Cooking losses of the vitamin tend to vary widely, depending on cooking time, pH, temperature, quantity of water used and discarded, and whether the water is chlorinated. Thiamin can be destroyed by several sulfites added in processing; by thiamin-degrading enzymes (thiaminases) in raw fish, shellfish, and some bacteria; and by certain heat-stable factors in several plants (e.g., ferns, tea, betel nuts).

Deficiency

Thiamin deficiency is characterized by anorexia and weight loss as well as cardiac and neurologic signs. In humans, thiamin deficiency eventually results in beriberi, the symptoms of which include mental confusion, muscular wasting, edema (in those with *wet beriberi*), peripheral neuropathy, tachycardia, and cardiomegaly. The nonedematous (or *dry*) form of the disease is usually associated with energy deprivation

TABLE 4-11 Thiamin Content of Selected Foods

FOOD	CONTENT (mg)
Fortified dry cereal, 1 cup	1.5
Pork chop, lean, 3 oz	1.06
Ham, lean, 3 oz	0.82
Sunflower seeds, shelled, 1 oz	0.59
Bagel, plain, 4 inch	0.479
Tuna sushi, 6-inch roll	0.46
Green peas, 1 cup	0.45
Beans, baked, 1 cup	0.39
Pasta, spaghetti, cooked, 1 cup	0.29
Rice, white, enriched, cooked, 1 cup	0.26
Potato, mashed, 1 cup	0.23
Doughnut, yeast, 1	0.22
Orange juice, from frozen concentrate, 1 cup	0.2

From U.S. Department of Agriculture, Agricultural Research Service: *USDA nutrient database for standard reference,* Release 14, 2001, Data Laboratory home page, http://www.nal.usda.gov/fnic/foodcomp.

TABLE 4-12 Clinical Features of Thiamin Deficiency

DEFICIENCY TYPE	FEATURES
Early stage of deficiency	Anorexia Indigestion Constipation Malaise Heaviness and weakness of legs Tender calf muscles "Pins and needles" and numbness in legs Anesthesia of skin, particularly at the tibia Increased pulse rate and palpitations
Wet beriberi	Edema of legs, face, trunk, and serous cavities Tense calf muscles Fast pulse Distended neck veins High blood pressure Decreased urine volume
Dry beriberi	Worsening of early-stage polyneuritis Difficulty walking *Wernicke-Korsakoff syndrome:* possible encephalopathy • Loss of immediate memory • Disorientation • Nystagmus (jerky movements of eyes) • Ataxia (staggering gait)
Infantile beriberi (2-5 mo of age)	*Acute:* • Decreased urine output • Excessive crying; thin and plaintive whining • Cardiac failure *Chronic:* • Constipation and vomiting • Fretfulness • Soft, toneless muscles • Pallor of skin with cyanosis

and inactivity, whereas the wet form is usually associated with a high carbohydrate intake along with strenuous physical exertion. The latter is characterized by edema caused by biventricular heart failure with pulmonary congestion. Without TPP, pyruvate cannot be converted to acetyl CoA and enter the TCA cycle, and energy deprivation of the heart muscle results in heart failure. Beriberi has been reported in infants (infantile beriberi) who were fed formulated diets that were not supplemented with thiamin; deterioration was sudden and characterized by cardiac failure and cyanosis. Beriberi responds to thiamin treatment, particularly if neural damage and cardiac involvement are not great.

Historically, beriberi has been endemic among the poor in areas of the world where polished white rice is the major staple food and particularly where people also consume raw fish or other sources of thiaminase. Such conditions usually produce not only beriberi but also multiple nutritional deficiencies.

Frank thiamin deficiency is not common in the United States because of the thiamin supplementation of rice and other refined cereal products. Subclinical thiamin deficiency develops in those with alcoholism who tend to have inadequate thiamin intake and impaired absorption of the vitamin. In addition thiamin is required for the metabolism and detoxification of alcohol, so those with alcoholism need more. Some older Americans are at risk for thiamin deficiency because of their poor diet and long-term use of diuretics. Affected individuals have a type of encephalopathy called *Wernicke-Korsakoff syndrome,* the signs of which range from mild confusion to coma. Many have an apparently inherited abnormal transketolase incapable of normal TPP binding. Table 4-12 summarizes the symptoms of thiamin deficiency. Biochemical changes that reflect thiamin status occur well before the appearance of overt symptoms. Thus thiamin status can be assessed by determining erythrocyte transketolase activity, measuring blood or serum levels of thiamin, or measuring urinary thiamin excretions levels.

Toxicity

Little information exists about the toxic potential of thiamin, although massive doses (i.e., 1000 times greater than nutritional needs) of the commercial form, thiamin hydrochloride, have suppressed the respiratory center, causing death (Institute of Medicine, 2000a). Parenteral doses of thiamin at 100 times the recommended levels have produced headache, convulsions, muscular weakness, cardiac arrhythmia, and allergic reactions.

Riboflavin

Riboflavin (Figure 4-14) is essential for the metabolism of carbohydrates, amino acids, and lipids and supports antioxidant protection. It carries out these functions as the coenzymes *flavin adenine dinucleotide*

(FAD) and *flavin adenine mononucleotide (FMN)*. Because of its fundamental roles in metabolism, riboflavin deficiencies are first evident in tissues that have rapid cellular turnover, such as the skin and epithelia.

Absorption, Transport, and Storage

Riboflavin is absorbed in the free form by a carrier-mediated process in the proximal small intestine. Because most foods contain the vitamin in its coenzyme forms, FMN and FAD, absorption occurs only after the hydrolytic cleavage of free riboflavin from its various flavoprotein complexes by various phosphatases. Riboflavin absorption is a carrier-mediated process that requires adenosine triphosphate (ATP). The mucosal uptake of free riboflavin depends on its phosphorylation into FMN.

Riboflavin is transported in the plasma as free riboflavin and FMN, both of which are mainly bound to plasma proteins, primarily albumin. A specific *riboflavin-binding protein (RfBP)* has also been identified and is thought to function in the transplacental movement of the vitamin. Riboflavin is transported in its free form into cells by a carrier-mediated process. It is then converted to FMN or FAD; because both are primarily protein bound, it prevents their diffusion out of the cell and makes them resistant to catabolism. Although small amounts of the vitamin are found in the liver and kidney, it is not stored in any useful amount and must therefore be supplied in the diet regularly.

Metabolism

Riboflavin is converted to its coenzyme forms by ATP-dependent phosphorylation to yield *riboflavin-5′-phosphate*, or FMN, by the enzyme *flavokinase*. Most FMN is then converted to FAD by FAD-pyrophosphorylase. Both steps are regulated by the thyroid hormones *adrenocorticotropic hormone (ACTH)* and aldosterone.

Most excess riboflavin is excreted as such in the urine. However, free riboflavin can be glycosylated in the liver and the glycosylated metabolite excreted.

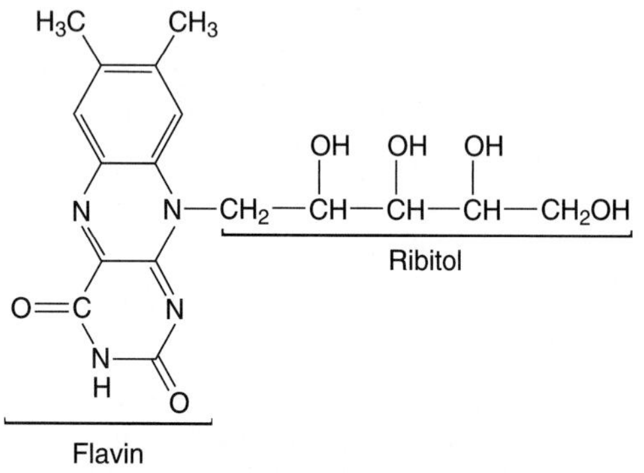

FIGURE 4-14 • Structure of riboflavin.

Riboflavin may also have a direct metabolic function. It can also be catabolized by oxidation, demethylation, and hydroxylation of its ring system to yield products that are excreted in the urine with free riboflavin.

Functions

The flavin coenzymes FMN and FAD are versatile redox cofactors because they can accept pairs of hydrogen atoms forming $FMNH_2$ or $FADH_2$. As such they can participate in either one- or two-electron redox reactions. FMN and FAD serve as prosthetic groups of several flavoprotein enzymes that catalyze oxidation-reduction reactions in the cells and function as hydrogen carriers in the mitochondrial electron transport system. In other cellular roles, mechanisms dependent on riboflavin and nicotinamide adenine dinucleotide phosphate (NADP) seem to combat oxidative damage to the cell. In one study, riboflavin was administered during experimental ischemia and seemed to decrease the negative consequences (Christensen, 1993). A cataract study in Linxian, China, suggested that nutritional supplements (including riboflavin) helped improve cataracts, at least in those who were marginally nourished (Kuzniarz et al, 2000; Sanchez-Castillo et al, 2001).

FMN and FAD are also coenzymes of dehydrogenases that catalyze the initial oxidations of fatty acids and several intermediates in glucose metabolism. FMN is also required for the conversion of pyridoxine (vitamin B_6) to its functional form, pyridoxal phosphate. FAD is also required for the biosynthesis of the vitamin niacin from the amino acid tryptophan.

Dietary Reference Intakes

The DRIs for riboflavin include AIs for infants and newly defined RDAs (Table 4-13). In general, the RDAs are based on the amount required to maintain normal tissue reserves based on urinary excretion, red blood cell riboflavin contents, and erythrocyte glutathione reductase activity. Riboflavin requirements are higher during pregnancy and lactation so that they can meet the needs of increased tissue synthesis and the losses of riboflavin secreted in breast milk.

Sources

Riboflavin, measured in milligrams in foods, is widely distributed in foods in a form bound to proteins as FMN and FAD. Rapidly growing, green leafy vegetables are rich in the vitamin; however, meats and dairy products are the most important contributors to the American diet (Table 4-14). More than half of the vitamin is lost when flour is milled; however, most breads and cereals are enriched with riboflavin and contribute appreciably to the total daily intake.

Riboflavin is stable when heated but can be readily destroyed by alkali and exposure to ultraviolet irradiation. Very little of the vitamin is destroyed during the cooking and processing of foods; however, because of its sensitivity to alkali, the practice of adding baking soda to soften dried peas or beans destroys much of their riboflavin content. Wax-lined paper containers protect milk against riboflavin loss from exposure to sunlight.

Deficiency

Riboflavin deficiency becomes manifest after several months of deprivation of the vitamin. The initial symptoms include photophobia, tearing, burning and itching of the eyes, loss of visual acuity, and soreness and burning of lips, mouth, and tongue. More advanced symptoms include cheilosis (fissuring of the lips); angular stomatitis (cracks in the skin at the corners of the mouth); a greasy eruption of the skin in the nasolabial folds, scrotum, or vulva; a purple, swollen tongue (Figure 4-15); capillary overgrowth around the cornea of the eye; and peripheral neuropathy (Box 4-4). Riboflavin has also been implicated in cataract formation when multiple vitamin deficiencies are also present (Kuzniarz et al, 2001).

TABLE 4-13 Dietary Reference Intakes for Riboflavin

LIFE-STAGE GROUP	RDA (mg/day)*
Infants	
0-6 mo	0.3†
7-12 mo	0.4†
Children	
1-3 yr	0.5
4-8 yr	0.6
Males	
9-13 yr	0.9
14-18 yr	1.3
19-30 yr	1.3
31-50 yr	1.3
51-70 yr	1.3
>70 yr	1.3
Females	
9-13 yr	0.9
14-18 yr	1.0
19-30 yr	1.1
31-50 yr	1.1
51-70 yr	1.1
>70 yr	1.1
Pregnant	
≤18 yr	1.4
19-30 yr	1.4
31-50 yr	1.4
Lactating	
≤18 yr	1.6
19-30 yr	1.6
31-50 yr	1.6

From Institute of Medicine, Food and Nutrition Board: *Dietary reference intakes for thiamin, riboflavin, niacin, vitamin B_6, folate, vitamin B_{12}, pantothenic acid, biotin, and choline*, Washington, DC, 1998, National Academy Press.
**RDA*, Recommended daily allowance; tolerable upper intake levels (ULs) not determined.
†Adequate intake (AI).

Phototherapy for infants with hyperbilirubinemia often leads to riboflavin deficiency (by photodestruction of the vitamin) if the therapy does not also include riboflavin supplementation. Otherwise, riboflavin deficiencies occur usually in combination with deficiencies of other water-soluble vitamins, such as thiamin and niacin in those who are malnourished. Riboflavin status is measured by assessment of the activity of *erythrocyte glutathione reductase*. This enzyme requires FAD and converts oxidized glutathione to reduced glutathione.

Toxicity

Riboflavin is not known to be toxic; high oral doses are considered essentially nontoxic. However, high doses are not beneficial.

TABLE 4-14 Riboflavin Content of Selected Foods

FOOD	CONTENT (mg)
Liver, beef, 3 oz	3.77
Fortified dry cereal, 1 cup	1.70
Milk, 2% fat, 1 cup	0.40
Yogurt, fruit flavored, low fat, 1 cup	0.37
Clams, canned, 3 oz	0.36
Cheese, cottage, 1 cup	0.34
Egg, 1	0.25
Custard, baked, ½ cup	0.25
Pork, roast loin, 3 oz	0.24
Bagel, plain, 1	0.22
Hamburger, lean, broiled medium, 3.5 oz	0.21
Spinach, fresh, cooked, ½ cup	0.21
Chicken, dark meat, 3 oz	0.21
Broccoli, 1 cup	0.11
Cheese, American, 1 oz	0.10

From U.S. Department of Agriculture, Agricultural Research Service: *USDA nutrient database for standard reference*, Release 14, 2001, Data laboratory home page, http://www.nal.usda.gov/fnic/foodcomp.

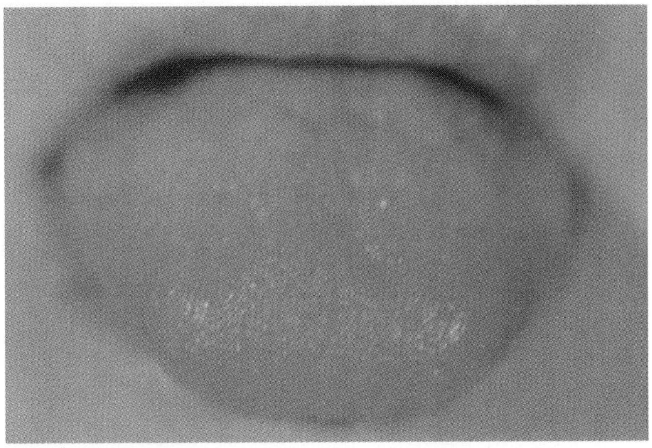

FIGURE 4-15 • Magenta tongue, a sign of riboflavin deficiency. In contrast, a person with an iron deficiency often has a pale tongue, and vitamin B-complex deficiency results in a beefy, red-colored tongue. (From McLaren DS: *Colour atlas of nutritional diseases*, England, 1981, Yearbook Medical Publishers.)

Niacin

Niacin is the generic term for nicotinamide and nicotinic acid (Figure 4-16). It functions as a component of the pyridine nucleotide coenzymes *nicotinamide adenine dinucleotide (NADH)* and *nicotinamide adenine dinucleotide phosphate (NADPH),* which are essential in all cells for energy production and metabolism. Recall that NADH and NADPH are the reduced forms of NAD and NADP (i.e., they carry a hydrogen ion).

Niacin was identified as a result of the search for the cause and cure of pellagra, a disease common in Spain and Italy in the eighteenth century and that devastated the southern United States in the early twentieth century (See *Focus On:* Pellegra, Politics, and the Poor).

Biosynthesis, Absorption, Transport, and Storage

Niacin can be synthesized from the essential amino acid tryptophan. Even though this process is not very efficient, dietary tryptophan intake is important to the overall niacin economy of the body (Figure 4-17).

Niacin in many foods, particularly those from animal sources, consists mostly of the coenzyme forms, NADH and NADPH, each of which must be digested to release the absorbed forms, nicotinamide (Nam) and nicotinic acid (NA). Many foods derived from plants, particularly grains, contain niacin in covalently bound complexes with small peptides and carbohydrates that are not released during digestion. These forms, collectively referred to as *niacytin,* are not biologically available but can become bioavailable through alkaline hydrolysis. Thus the Central American tradition of soaking maize in lime water before preparing tortillas effectively increases the bioavailability of niacin in what otherwise would be considered a low-niacin food.

Ultimately, Nam and NA are absorbed in the stomach and small intestine by carrier-mediated facilitated diffusion. Both are transported in the plasma in free solution, and each is taken up by most tissues through passive diffusion, although some tissues (e.g., erythrocytes, kidney, brain) also have a transport system for NA. Niacin is retained in tissues by being converted primarily to NADH but is also converted to NADPH.

Metabolism

The de novo synthesis of NADH and NADPH occurs from quinolinic acid, a metabolite of the indispensable amino acid tryptophan (see Figure 4-17). This interconversion involves steps dependent on FAD and

Box 4-4. Signs of Possible Riboflavin Deficiency

Soreness and burning of lips, mouth, and tongue*
Cheilosis*
Angular stomatitis*
Glossitis*
Purplish or magenta tongue*
Hypertrophy or atrophy of tongue papillae*
Seborrheic dermatitis of nasolabial folds, vestibule of nose, and sometimes the ears and eyelids, scrotum, and vulva
Ocular pathologic conditions (sometimes)
- Inflammation of conjunctiva
- Superficial vascularization of cornea
- Ulcerations of cornea
- Photophobia

Anemia—normocytic and normochronic
Neuropathy

Modified from Goldsmith GA: Riboflavin deficiency. In Rivlin RS, ed: *Riboflavin,* New York, 1975, Plenum Press.
*Tongue and mouth changes are difficult to differentiate from those caused by niacin, folic acid, thiamin, vitamin B_6, or vitamin B_{12} deficiency.

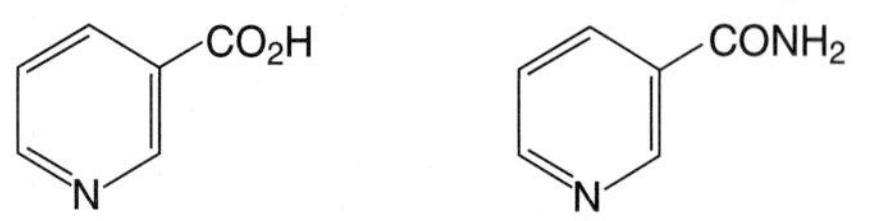

Nicotinic acid (niacin) Nicotinamide (niacinamide)

FIGURE 4-16 • Structure of niacin.

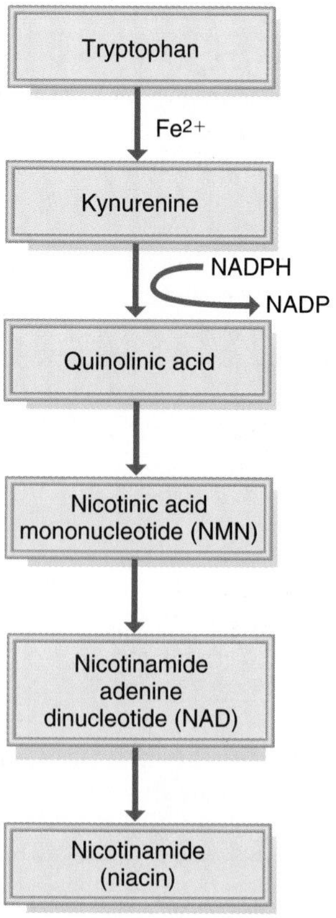

NADPH, Nicotinamide adenine dinucleotide phosphate in the reduced form.

FIGURE 4-17 • Synthesis of niacin from tryptophan.

pyridoxal phosphate, and therefore the body must have adequate levels of riboflavin and to a lesser extent vitamin B_6. The rate-limiting enzymes in this pathway are 3-hydroxyanthranilic acid oxidase (3-HAAO) and picolinic acid carboxylase (PAC). Species with low 3-HAAO/PAC ratios (e.g., ducks, cats) cannot efficiently convert tryptophan to niacin and thus have relatively high requirements for the preformed niacin. Humans seem to be moderately efficient at this conversion; about 60 mg of tryptophan is required to produce 1 mg of niacin. This aspect of tryptophan metabolism yields *nicotinic acid mononucleotide (NMN)*, which is phosphoradenylated to form NAD.

NADH and NADPH can be produced from NA and Nam obtained from the diet. Nam is deaminated to yield NA. Then, two ribose phosphates are attached to the nitrogen in the pyridine ring. Next, adenosine is attached to the ribose. Finally, an amino group is added to the acid group, forming an amide, yielding NADH. NADH can be phosphorylated in the hexose monophosphate shunt to yield NADPH.

NADH and NADPH are catabolized by hydrolysis to yield Nam, which can be deaminated into NA or methylated to yield 1-methylnicotinamide (mNAm). Dietary protein deficiency changes the profile of urinary metabolites, presumably because of changes in the amount of tryptophan converted to niacin.

Functions

The coenzymes NADH and NADPH are the most central electron carriers of cells, playing essential roles as cosubstrates of more than 200 enzymes involved in the metabolism of carbohydrates, fatty acids, and amino acids. In general, NADH and NADPH facilitate hydrogen transport by two-electron transfers, which use the hydride ion (H^+) as the carrier but play very different roles in metabolism. The NADH-dependent reactions are involved in intracellular respiration (e.g., beta-oxidation, TCA cycle function, and the electron transport system. NADPH, on the other hand, is important for biosynthetic (e.g., fatty acid, sterol) pathways.

Dietary Reference Intakes

Niacin is expressed in total milligrams of niacin or niacin equivalents (NE), which are calculated from the preformed niacin content plus 1/60 of the tryptophan content. The DRIs established for niacin include AIs for infants, RDAs, and the tolerable UL (Table 4-15). Requirements are directly related to energy intake because of niacin's role in energy-producing reactions in metabolism. They are expressed as niacin equivalents from preformed niacin and tryptophan.

Sources

Significant amounts of niacin are found in many foods; lean meats, poultry, fish, peanuts, and yeasts are particularly rich sources. Niacin exists predominantly as protein-bound NA in plant tissues and as Nam, NADH, and NADPH in animal tissues. Milk and eggs contain small amounts of niacin, but they are excellent sources of tryptophan, giving them significant niacin equivalent contents. The amount of niacin in foods depends up the total milligrams of niacin (NA and Nam) plus 1/60 of the tryptophan content. Although the conversion of tryptophan to niacin depends on such factors as the amount of tryptophan and niacin ingested and pyridoxine status, 60 mg of tryptophan is considered equal to 1 mg of niacin. Table 4-16 lists the preformed niacin content of various foods. Most tables of food nutrient composition list only preformed niacin, thus underestimating the total niacin equivalencies of many foods.

Deficiency

Niacin deficiency symptoms initially include muscular weakness, anorexia, indigestion, and skin eruptions. Severe deficiency of niacin leads to pellagra, which is characterized by dermatitis, dementia, and

TABLE 4-15 Dietary Reference Intakes for Niacin

LIFE-STAGE GROUP	RDA* (mg NE/day)†	UL* (mg NE/day)†
Infants		
0-6 mo	2‡	ND
7-12 mo	4‡	ND
Children		
1-3 yr	6	10
4-8 yr	8	15
Males		
9-13 yr	12	20
14-18 yr	16	30
19-30 yr	16	35
31-50 yr	16	35
51-70 yr	16	35
>70 yr	16	35
Females		
9-13 yr	12	20
14-18 yr	14	30
19-30 yr	14	35
31-50 yr	14	35
51-70 yr	14	35
>70 yr	14	35
Pregnant		
≤18 yr	18	30
19-30 yr	18	35
31-50 yr	18	35
Lactating		
≤18 yr	17	30
19-30 yr	17	35
31-50 yr	17	35

From Institute of Medicine, Food and Nutrition Board: *Dietary reference intakes for thiamin, riboflavin, niacin, vitamin B_6, folate, vitamin B_{12}, pantothenic acid, biotin, and choline*, Washington, DC, 1998, National Academy Press.
**RDA*, Recommended dietary intake; *UL*, tolerable upper intake level; *ND*, not determinable because of lack of data.
†As niacin equivalents (NE: 1 mg niacin = 60 mg tryptophan, 0 to 6 mo = preformed niacin not NE).
‡Adequate intake (AI).

diarrhea ("the 3 Ds"); tremors; and sore tongue (or "beef tongue"). The dermatologic changes are usually the most prominent. Skin that has been exposed to the sun develops cracked, pigmented, scaly dermatitis (Figure 4-18). Central nervous system involvement symptoms include confusion, disorientation, and neuritis. Digestive abnormalities cause irritation and inflammation of the mucous membranes of the mouth and the gastrointestinal tract.

TABLE 4-16 Preformed Niacin Content of Selected Foods*

FOOD	CONTENT (mg)
Chicken, ½ breast	13.47
Tuna, canned in water, 3 oz	11.29
Rice, white, 1 cup	7.75
Mushrooms, cooked, 1 cup	6.96
Fortified dry cereal, 1 cup	5.55
Beef, ground regular, cooked	4.55
Ham, canned, 3 oz	4.28
Peanuts, dry roasted, 1 oz	3.83
Coffee, 2 fl oz	3.12
Egg bagel, 4 inch	3.06
Pizza with pepperoni	3.05
Noodles, 1 cup	2.68

From U.S. Department of Agriculture, Agricultural Research Service: *USDA nutrient database for standard reference,* Release 14, 2001, Data laboratory home page, http://www.nal.usda.gov/fnic/foodcomp.
*These data do not take into account niacin available from food via synthesis from tryptophan.

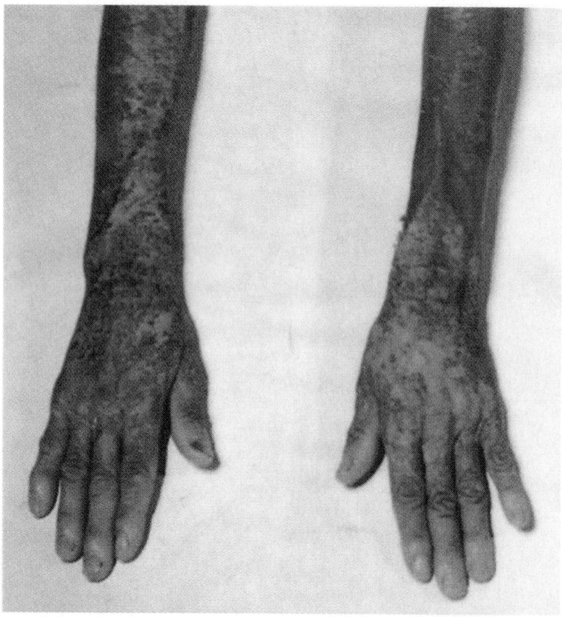

FIGURE 4-18 • Pellagra. Pigmented keratotic scaling lesions caused by niacin deficiency. The lesions are especially prominent in areas exposed to the sun, such as the hands, forearms, neck, and legs. (From Latham MC et al: *Scope manual on nutrition,* Kalamazoo, Mich, 1980, The Upjohn Company. Copyright by Thomas Spies, MD.)

Untreated pellagra can cause death (which is often referred to as "the fourth D").

Patients with pellagra can also show clinical signs of riboflavin deficiency, highlighting the metabolic interrelationships of these vitamins. Patients with pellagra are likely to have very poor diets that not only provide very little niacin but also lack protein and other nutrients. The most reliable method for assessing niacin status is measuring the urinary excretion of the methylated metabolites methylnicotinomide and methylpyridone carboxamide.

Toxicity

In general, niacin toxicity is low. However, high doses of 1 to 2 g of NA three times per day—dosages that have been used in attempts to lower blood cholesterol concentrations—can have side effects (see Chapter 35). The main side effect is a histamine release that causes flushing and may be harmful to those with asthma or peptic ulcer disease. (Nam does not have this effect.) High doses of niacin can also be toxic to the liver, and risks are greater with time-released forms of the vitamin (Reimund and Ramos, 1994). Megavitamin use should be monitored carefully because high doses act as drugs, not nutritional supplements.

Pantothenic Acid

As its name suggests, pantothenic acid is widely distributed in foods; cases of clinical deficiency are rare. The vitamin has critical roles in metabolism. It is an integral part of CoA, which is essential in energy production from the macronutrients, and acyl-carrier protein (ACP), which is used in synthesis reactions (Figure 4-19).

Absorption, Transport, and Storage

Pantothenic acid exists in foods mostly as CoA and ACP. Therefore absorption requires hydrolysis to phosphopantetheine and then conversion to pantothenic acid. Pantothenic acid is absorbed by passive diffusion and active transport in the jejunum. It is then transported in the free acid form in solution in the plasma and taken up by diffusion into erythrocytes, which carry most of the vitamin in the blood. Pantothenic acid is taken up by cells of peripheral tissues by a sodium-dependent active transport process in some tissues and by facilitated diffusion in others. Within the cell the vitamin is converted to CoA, which

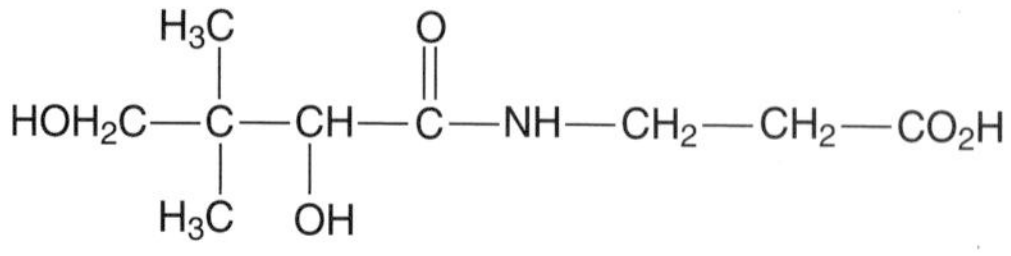

Pantothenic acid

FIGURE 4-19 • Structure of pantothenic acid.

is its predominant form in most tissues, particularly the liver, adrenals, kidney, brain, heart, and testes.

Metabolism

All tissues are capable of synthesizing CoA from pantothenic acid. This multienzyme process takes place in four steps. First pantothenic acid is phosphorylated to yield 4′-phosphopantothenic acid. Then it is condensed with cysteine to yield 4′-phosphopantothenoylcysteine. Next phosphopantothenoylcysteine is decarboxylated to yield 4′-phosphopantetheine, which is finally converted to CoA. ACP contains 4′-phosphopantetheine that is transferred from CoA to bind to the apo acetyl carrier protein forming ACP.

CoA and ACP are degraded to yield free pantothenic acid and other metabolites. The vitamin is excreted mainly in the urine as free pantothenic acid but also as 4′-phosphopantothenate. An appreciable amount (some 15% of the daily intake) is oxidized completely and excreted through the lungs as carbon dioxide.

Functions

CoA and ACP function metabolically as carriers of acyl groups. CoA is critical in the formation of acetyl CoA, which condenses with oxaloacetate and enters the TCA cycle to release energy. It is also the compound in the first steps of the synthesis of fatty acids or cholesterol, or in the acetylation of alcohols, amines, and amino acids. It also activates fatty acids before their incorporation into triglycerides and acts as an acyl donor for proteins. ACP is a component of the multienzyme complex fatty acid synthase, which is necessary for fatty acid synthesis.

Dietary Reference Intakes

Pantothenic acid is measured in milligrams. DRIs are expressed as AIs. No estimated average requirements (EARs) or RDAs have been established (Table 4-17).

Sources

Pantothenic acid is present in all plant and animal tissues. The most important sources in mixed diets are meats (particularly liver and heart), but mushrooms, avocados, broccoli, egg yolks, yeast, skim milk, and sweet potatoes are also good sources of the vitamin (Table 4-18). Pantothenic acid is fairly stable during ordinary cooking and storage, although the vitamin can be lost in frozen meats during thawing. Because it is localized in the outer layers of grains, about half of the vitamin is lost in the milling of flour.

Deficiency

Pantothenic acid deficiency results in impairments in lipid synthesis and energy production. Because the vitamin is so widely distributed in foods, deficiencies are rare. However, pantothenic acid deficiency has been observed among severely malnourished humans. Symptoms include paresthesia in the toes and soles of the feet, burning sensations in the feet, depression, fatigue, insomnia, and weakness (Institute of Medicine, 2000a).

Toxicity

The toxicity of pantothenic acid is negligible; no adverse effects after ingestion of large doses of the vitamin have been reported in any species. Massive doses (e.g., 10 g/day) administered to humans have produced only mild intestinal distress and diarrhea.

Vitamin B_6

Vitamin B_6 (Figure 4-20) is the general term for numerous 2-methyl-3,5-dihydroxymethylpyridine derivatives exhibiting the biologic activity of pyridoxine (PN), the alcohol derivate. The biologically active analogues are the aldehyde *pyridoxal (PL)* and the amine *pyridoxamine (PM).* All three compounds are converted to the metabolically active coenzyme form *pydridoxal phosphate (PLP),* which is primarily involved in metabolism of amino acids.

TABLE 4-17 Dietary Reference Intakes for Pantothenic Acid

LIFE-STAGE GROUP	AI (mg/day)*
Infants	
0-6 mo	1.7
7-12 mo	1.8
Children	
1-3 yr	2
4-8 yr	3
Males	
9-13 yr	4
14-18 yr	5
19-30 yr	5
31-50 yr	5
51-70 yr	5
>70 yr	5
Females	
9-13 yr	4
14-18 yr	5
19-30 yr	5
31-50 yr	5
51-70 yr	5
>70 yr	5
Pregnant	
≤18 yr	6
19-30 yr	6
31-50 yr	6
Lactating	
≤18 yr	7
19-30 yr	7
31-50 yr	7

From Institute of Medicine, Food and Nutrition Board: *Dietary reference intakes for thiamin, riboflavin, niacin, vitamin B_6, folate, vitamin B_{12}, pantothenic acid, biotin, and choline,* Washington, DC, 1998, National Academy Press.
**AI,* Adequate intake; tolerable upper intake levels (ULs) not determined.

Absorption, Transport, and Storage

Vitamin B_6 is absorbed by passive diffusion of the dephosphorylated forms PN, PL, or PM—primarily in the jejunum and ileum. Absorption is driven by phosphorylation to form PLP and *pyridoxamine phosphate (PMP)* and then by protein binding of each of these metabolites in the intestinal mucosa and blood.

The predominant form of the vitamin in the blood is PLP, most of which is derived from the liver after metabolism by hepatic flavoenzymes. Small amounts of free PN are also found in the circulation, but most is as PLP bound to albumin. However, PLP must be dephosphorylated to PL to be taken up by the cells. On uptake, PL is again phosphorylated to PLP and PMP, with the greatest levels being found in liver, brain, kidney, spleen, and muscle, where they are bound to proteins. Muscle is the largest depot, containing 80% to 90% of the total body vitamin stores in the form of PLP bound to glycogen phosphorylase.

Metabolism

The vitamers B_6 are readily metabolically interconverted by phosphorylation-dephosphorylation, oxidation-reduction, and amination-deamination reactions. The limiting step during this metabolism is catalyzed by the FMN enzyme pyridoxal phosphate oxidase. Thus riboflavin deficiency can reduce the conversions of PN and PM to the active coenzyme PLP. In the liver, PLP is dephosphorylated and oxidized by FAD- and NAD-dependent enzymes to yield 4-pyridoxic acid and other inactive metabolites that are excreted in the urine.

TABLE 4-18 Pantothenic Acid Content of Selected Foods

FOOD	CONTENT (mg)
Fortified dry cereal, 1 cup	11.77
Mushrooms, cooked, 1 cup	3.37
Rice, white, 1 cup	1.88
Tropical trail mix, 1 cup	1.70
Corn, sweet, canned, 1 cup	1.45
Yogurt, plain, 8 oz	1.45
Vanilla shake, 16 fl oz	1.39
Potatoes, mashed, 1 cup	1.20
Chicken breast, ½ breast	1.15
Milk, 2% fat, 1 cup	0.78
Salmon, pink, canned, 3 oz	0.47
Oatmeal, regular, cooked, 1 cup	0.47

From U.S. Department of Agriculture, Agricultural Research Service: *USDA nutrient database for standard reference*, Release 14, 2001, Data laboratory home page, http://www.nal.usda.gov/fnic/foodcomp.

Functions

The metabolically active form of vitamin B_6 is PLP, which is a coenzyme for numerous enzymes involved in practically all reactions in the metabolism of amino acids and in several aspects of the metabolism of neurotransmitters, glycogen, sphingolipids, heme, and steroids. These roles relate to the ability of the PLP aldehyde group to react with α-amino groups of the amino acid and thus to stabilize the other bonds on the bound carbon. Thus vitamin B_6 is essential for various amino acid transaminases, decarboxylases, racemases, and isomerases. It is needed for the biosynthesis of the neurotransmitters serotonin, epinephrine, norepinephrine, and γ-aminobutyric acid, the vasodilator and gastric secretagogue histamine, and the porphyrin precursors of heme. The vitamin is also required for the metabolic conversion of tryptophan to niacin, the release of glucose from glycogen, the biosynthesis of sphingolipids in the myelin sheaths of nerve cells, and in the modulation of steroid hormone receptors.

Dietary Reference Intakes

The DRIs for vitamin B_6 include AIs for infants, the redefined RDAs, and the UL for children and adults (Table 4-19) In general, needs for vitamin B_6 increase with increasing intake of protein; adequate vitamin B_6 status seems to be maintained when the vitamin is consumed in an approximate ratio of 0.016 mg per gram of protein (Driskell, 1994).

Sources

Vitamin B_6 is widely distributed in foods, occurring in greatest concentrations in meats, whole grain products (especially wheat), vegetables, and nuts (Table 4-20). Much of the vitamin B_6 in many foods is bound covalently to proteins or glycosylated, the digestibilities of which result in much of the vitamin B_6 content of foods having relatively low bioavailabili-

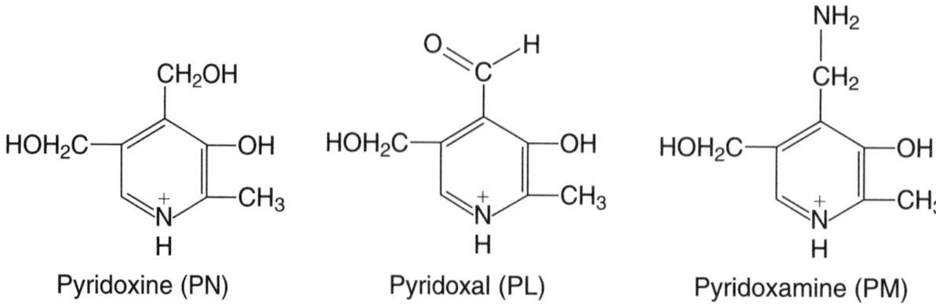

FIGURE 4-20 • Structure of pyridoxine.

ties. PN in some plants (e.g., potatoes, spinach, beans, and other legumes) is often glycosylated and has a low bioavailablity. Vitamin B_6 derived from animal sources tends to have superior bioavailability.

Deficiency

Deprivation of vitamin B_6 leads to metabolic abnormalities resulting from insufficient production of PLP. These manifest clinically as dermatologic and neurologic changes in most species. Humans show symptoms of weakness, sleeplessness, peripheral neuropathies, cheilosis, glossitis, stomatitis, and impaired cell-mediated immunity. Because of the widespread distribution of the vitamin in foods, cases of vitamin B_6 deficiency are relatively rare. However, deficiency may be precipitated by medications (e.g., the antitubercular drug isoniazid) that interfere with the metabolism of the vitamin (see Chapter 19). Infants fed a milk-based formula in which much of vitamin B_6 was unknowingly destroyed in processing developed irritability and convulsions but recovered rapidly after an injection with the vitamin (Coursin, 1954).

TABLE 4-19 Dietary Reference Intakes for Vitamin B_6

LIFE-STAGE GROUP	RDA (mg/day)*	UL (mg/day)*
Infants		
0-6 mo	0.1†	ND
7-12 mo	0.3†	ND
Children		
1-3 yr	0.5	30
4-8 yr	0.6	40
Males		
9-13 yr	1.0	60
14-18 yr	1.3	80
19-30 yr	1.3	100
31-50 yr	1.3	100
51-70 yr	1.7	100
>70 yr	1.7	100
Females		
9-13 yr	1.0	60
14-18 yr	1.2	80
19-30 yr	1.3	100
31-50 yr	1.3	100
51-70 yr	1.5	100
>70 yr	1.5	100
Pregnant		
≤18 yr	1.9	80
19-30 yr	1.9	100
31-50 yr	1.9	100
Lactating		
≤18 yr	2.0	80
19-30 yr	2.0	100
31-50 yr	2.0	100

From Institute of Medicine, Food and Nutrition Board: *Dietary reference intakes for thiamin, riboflavin, niacin, vitamin B_6, folate, vitamin B_{12}, pantothenic acid, biotin, and choline,* Washington, DC, 1998, National Academy Press.
**RDA,* Recommended dietary intake; *UL,* tolerable upper intake level; *ND,* not determinable because of lack of data.
†Adequate intake (AI).

Toxicity

The toxicity of vitamin B_6 seems to be relatively low, although high dosages (several grams per day) have produced sensory neuropathy marked by changes in gait and peripheral sensation (Schaumberg et al, 1983). Many of the signs of vitamin B_6 toxicity resemble those of vitamin B_6 deficiency.

Folate

Folate refers generally to pteroylmonoglutamic acid and its derived compounds (Figure 4-21). The reduced compound, tetrahydrofolic acid (FH_4), functions metabolically as a carrier for single-carbon moieties. Each carrier form is named according to the moiety it carries, and each of these moieties can be used in single-carbon synthesis reactions (Figure 4-22).

Absorption, Transport, and Storage

Dietary folates are absorbed only as the monoglutamate forms of folic acid, 5-methyltetrahydrofolic acid and 5-formyltetrahydrofolic acid. Absorption occurs by active transport mainly in the jejunum, but the vitamin can also be absorbed by passive diffusion when ingested in large amounts.

TABLE 4-20 Pyridoxine Content of Selected Foods

FOOD	mg
Potato, baked, 1	0.70
Banana, 1	0.68
Rice, white, cooked, 1 cup	0.65
Chicken, light meat, fried, 3 oz	0.53
Pork chop, baked, 3 oz	0.44
Baked beans, vegetarian, 1 cup	0.34
Beef, hamburger, broiled, 3 oz	0.32
Chicken, dark meat, fried, 3 oz	0.31
Tuna, canned, 3 oz	0.30
Sunflower seeds, kernels, ¼ cup	0.26
Avocado, California, 1 oz	0.08
Whole wheat bread, 1 slice	0.05

From U.S. Department of Agriculture, Agricultural Research Service: *USDA nutrient database for standard reference,* Release 14, 2001, Data laboratory home page, http://www.nal.usda.gov/fnic/foodcomp.

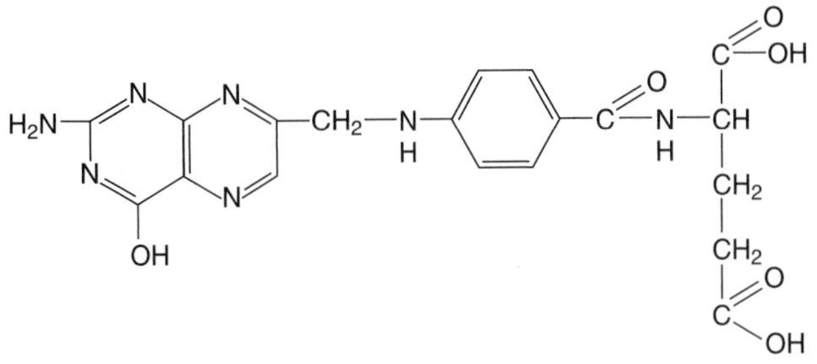

FIGURE 4-21 • Structure of folate.

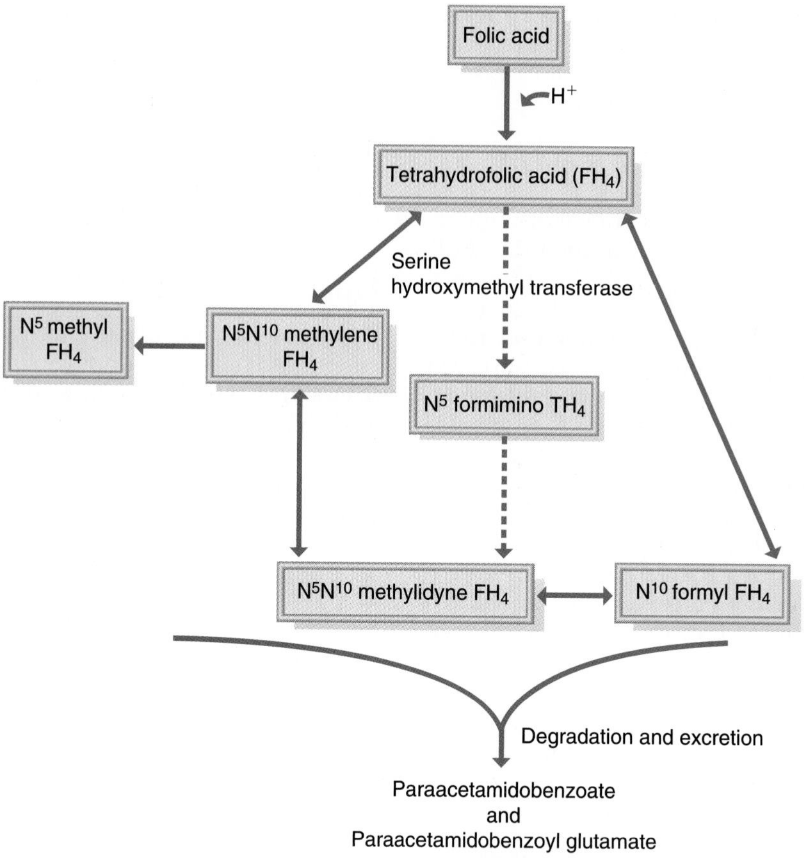

FIGURE 4-22 • Metabolism of folates.

Because most folate in foods is present in polyglutamate forms (forms with more than one glutamate residue attached), absorption requires hydrolysis to monoglutamate forms by conjugases in the brush border and intracellular mucosa. Because hydrolysis is inefficient, the bioavailability of folate in food is about half that of the purified vitamin (Gregory, 2001).

Folate taken up by the intestinal mucosal cell is reduced to FH_4, which can either be transferred to the portal circulation or converted to 5-methyl-FH_4 before entering the circulation. Only monoglutamate derivatives found in plasma are taken up by the cells using an energy-dependent process with a specific folate-binding protein or a carrier-mediated anion-exchange process. Within cells, FH_4 is methylated to 5-methyl-FH_4, which is retained intracellularly by binding to intracellular macromolecules and additional conversion to folyl polyglutamates (Wagner, 1996). The liver is the most important depot for folate, containing about half of the total body store as polyglutamates of 5-methyl-FH_4 and 10-formyl-FH_4. Tissues with high rates of cell division (e.g., intestinal mucosa) tend to have low concentrations of 5-methyl-FH_4 and high concentrations of 10-formyl-FH_4, whereas 5-methyl-FH_4 predominates in tissues with low rates of cell division.

Metabolism

Folates are metabolized in three ways: (1) reduction of the pterin ring by the enzyme reductase in the kidney and liver (and in quickly growing tumors), (2) reactions of the polyglutamyl side chain by the enzyme polyglutamate synthetase, which add the amino acid glutamate, and (3) acquisition of single-carbon moieties at certain positions on the pterin ring.

Folate is metabolically activated by conversion to one of several derivatives with single-carbon units substituted at the N-5 or N-10 (or both) positions of the pterin ring. The main source of the single-carbon fragments is via serine hydroxymethyltransferase, which uses the dispensable amino acid serine and the single-carbon donor to produce 5,10-methylene-FH_4. Other enzymes also yield other single-carbon metabolites: 5-methyl-FH_4, 5,10-methenyl-FH_4, 5-formimino-FH_4, 5-formyl-FH_4, and 10-formyl-FH_4.

Tissue folates turn over by cleavage of their pteridine and para-aminobenzoyl polyglutamate moieties. The latter are further degraded to a variety of water-soluble side-chain metabolites that are excreted in the urine and bile (see Figure 4-22).

Functions

FH_4, with its moieties attached, functions as an enzyme cosubstrate in many synthesis reactions in the metabolism of amino acids and nucleotides by donating or accepting single carbon units. For example, it functions in the de novo synthesis of deoxyribonucleic acid (DNA) by transferring formate (as 5,10-methenyl-FH_4) for purine synthesis and formaldehyde (as 5,10-methylene-FH_4) for thymidylate synthesis. It donates formate (as 10-formyl-FH_4) in purine synthesis. It is required for the conversion of histidine to glutamic acid, impairments of which result in accumulation of the intermediary product, *formiminoglutamic acid (FIGLU)*, which is excreted in the urine. It provides labile methyl groups (as 5-methyl-FH_4) for the synthesis of methionine from homocysteine. This conversion also requires vitamin B_{12}, which passes the methyl group from 5-methyl-FH_4 to homocysteine; therefore deficiencies of either folate or vitamin B_{12} can lead to elevated serum homocysteine levels, or homocysteinemia (see Chapters 34 and 35). Because of this interrelationship, deprivation of vitamin B_{12} alone can produce a functional secondary folate deficiency by interrupting the regeneration of FH_4, effectively trapping the vitamin as 5-methyl-FH_4—a process called the *methyl-folate trap* (see Figure 34-5).

Folate is essential for the formation of red and white blood cells in the bone marrow and for their maturation and is a single-carbon carrier in the formation of heme.

Dietary Reference Intakes

DRIs for folate are expressed as *dietary folate equivalents (DFE)*, which is an attempt to account for known differences in the bioavailability of folates noted previously. One DFE equals 1 μg of food folate, which is equal to 0.6 μg of folic acid consumed with food or 0.5 μg of synthetic folic acid taken as a supplement on an empty stomach. The DRIs for folate include AIs for infants and RDAs for children and adults, which are almost double the previous RDAs in most cases (Table 4-21). The new DRIs for women include increased amounts for women who could become pregnant (see Chapter 7). Although low folate stores are found in approximately 10% of the population, they are not accompanied by signs of deficiency.

TABLE 4-21 Dietary Reference Intakes for Folate[a]

LIFE-STAGE GROUP	RDA (μg/day)[b]	UL (μg/day)[b,e]
Infants		
0-6 mo	65[b]	ND
7-12 mo	80[b]	ND
Children		
1-3 yr	150	300
4-8 yr	200	400
Males		
9-13 yr	300	600
14-18 yr	400	800
19-30 yr	400	1000
31-50 yr	400	1000
51-70 yr	400	1000
>70 yr	400	1000
Females		
9-13 yr	300	600
14-18 yr	400[c]	800
19-30 yr	400[c]	1000
31-50 yr	400[c]	1000
51-70 yr	400	1000
>70 yr	400	1000
Pregnant		
≤18 yr	600[d]	800
19-30 yr	600[d]	1000
31-50 yr	600[d]	1000
Lactating		
≤18 yr	500	800
19-30 yr	500	1000
31-50 yr	500	1000

From Institute of Medicine, Food and Nutrition Board: *Dietary reference intakes for thiamin, riboflavin, niacin, vitamin B_6, folate, vitamin B_{12}, pantothenic acid, biotin, and choline,* Washington, DC, 1998, National Academy Press.

[a]As dietary folate equivalent (DFE). 1 DFE = 1 μg food folate = 0.6 μg folic acid (from fortified food or supplement consumed with food) = 0.5 μg synthetic (supplemental) folic acid taken on an empty stomach.

[b]*RDA*, Recommended dietary intake; *UL*, tolerable upper intake levels; *ND*, not determinable.

[c]In view of evidence linking folate intake with neural tube defects in the fetus, it is recommended that all women capable of becoming pregnant consume 400 μg synthetic folic acid from fortified foods and/or supplements in addition to intake of food folate from a varied diet.

[d]It is assumed that women will continue consuming 400 μg folic acid until their pregnancy is confirmed and they enter prenatal care, which ordinarily occurs after the end of the periconceptional period—the critical time for formation of the neural tube.

[e]The ULs for synthetic folic acid apply to forms obtained from supplements, fortified foods, or a combination of the two.

Sources

Folates exist as reduced folyl polyglutamates (of mostly 5-methyl-FH_4 and 10-formyl-FH_4) in various foods of plant and animal origin. Liver, mushrooms, and green leafy vegetables (especially spinach, asparagus, and broccoli) are rich sources. Lean beef, potatoes, whole wheat bread, orange juice, and dried beans are good sources (Table 4-22). Analysis of foods for their folate content is complex and difficult, and values in tables of food composition may be too low. Folate exists in 150 different forms. The reduced forms in foods are easily oxidized, and losses of 50% to 90% typically occur during storage, cooking, or processing at high temperatures.

The bioavailability of folate in foods varies considerably because of inherent differences among forms of the vitamin, the presence or absence of conjugase inhibitors and folate binders, and the nutritional status of the host; for example, deficiencies of iron and vitamin C can impair folate use. Thus the bioavailabilities of folates in foods vary widely—from 25% to 50%.

TABLE 4-22 Folate Content of Selected Foods

FOOD	CONTENT (μg)
Fortified dry cereal, 1 cup	672
Blackeyed peas, boiled, 1 cup	357
Lentils, boiled, 1 cup	358
Beans, white, boiled, ½ cup	170
Spinach, cooked, ½ cup	131
Asparagus, cooked, ½ cup	121
Broccoli, cooked, 1 cup	103
Cabbage, Chinese, 1 cup	70
Fresh orange juice, 1 cup	75
Cabbage, raw, 1 cup	30
Egg yolk, 1	25
Banana, 1	22

From U.S. Department of Agriculture, Agricultural Research Service: *USDA nutrient database for standard reference,* Release 14, 2001, Data laboratory home page, http://www.nal.usda.gov/fnic/foodcomp.

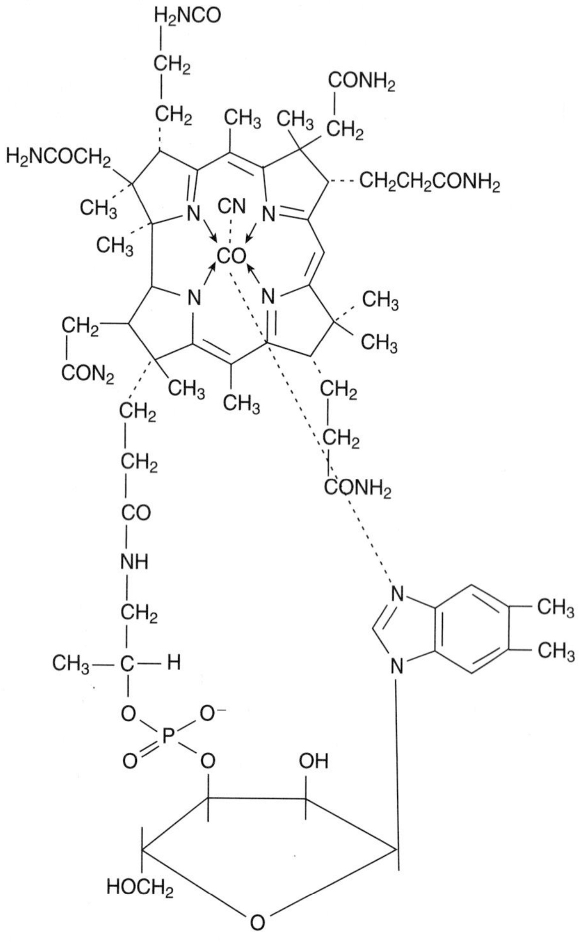

FIGURE 4-23 • Structure of cobalamin.

Deficiency

Deficiencies of folate result in impaired biosynthesis of DNA and RNA, thus reducing cell division, which is most apparent in rapidly multiplying cells such as red blood cells, leukocytes, and epithelial cells of the stomach, intestine, vagina, and uterine cervix. In blood, this is characterized by megaloblastic, macrocytic anemia with large, immature erythrocytes that have excessive amounts of hemoglobin (see Chapter 34). Initial signs of deficiency in humans include nuclear hypersegmentation of circulating polymorphonuclear leukocytes followed by megaloblastic anemia and then general weakness, depression, and polyneuropathy. Dermatologic lesions and poor growth are also symptoms.

Folate-responsive homocysteinemia (which is related to folate's role in regeneration of methionine from homocysteine) is a condition associated with elevated risk for occlusive vascular disease and is prevalent among apparently healthy Americans, suggesting that subclinical folate deficiencies may be common. The role of folate in normal cell division makes it particularly important in embryogenesis (Butterworth and Bendich, 1996) (see Chapter 7). Thus the finding that periconceptual folate supplementation can reduce the risk of serious birth defects (including neural tube defects) by as much as half, combined with the findings regarding subclinical folate deficiencies, stimulated the U.S. government to regulate the addition of folate to wheat flour (see Chapter 14). However, increased dietary methionine is also associated with decreased risk of neural tube defects (Shoob et al, 2001). Folate status is assessed by measuring the erythrocyte folate concentration, sometimes in conjunction with plasma homocysteine concentrations.

Toxicity

No adverse effects of high oral doses of folate have been reported in animals, although parenteral administration of amounts some 1000 times the dietary requirement produce epileptiform seizures in the rat. It has been suggested that high levels of folate may render zinc unavailable through the formation of nonabsorbable complexes in the gut, and studies have shown that folate treatment can exacerbate the teratogenic effects of nutritional zinc deficiency in animals.

Vitamin B_{12}

The term *vitamin B_{12}* (Figure 4-23) refers to a family of cobalamin compounds containing the porphyrin-like, cobalt-centered corrin nucleus. This family includes analogues containing cobalt-bound methyl groups (methylcobalamin), 5′-deoxyadenosyl groups (adenosylcobalamin), hydroxl (OH−) groups (hydroxocobalamin), nitrito groups (nitritocobalamin), or water (aquacobalamin). Of the several cobalamin compounds that exhibit vitamin B_{12} activity, *cyanocobalamin* and *hydroxycobalamin* are the most active.

Absorption, Transport, and Storage

Vitamin B_{12} is bound to protein in food and must be released from it by pepsin digestion in the stomach. The vitamin then combines with R proteins (cobalophilins) in the stomach and moves into the small intestine, where the R proteins are hydrolyzed and *intrinsic factor (IF)*, a specific binding protein for B_{12} produced in the stomach, binds the cobalamin. The majority of vitamin B_{12} is absorbed by this active transport, and IF is essential to the process. Only about 1% can be absorbed by simple diffusion even in high amounts. IF can bind any of the four cobalamins in an IF–vitamin B_{12} complex by which the vitamin is taken into the enterocyte by a process involving binding to a specific membrane receptor on the ileal brush border. IF then drops away (Figure 4-24) (see Chapter 34).

After absorption, cobalamin binds to the plasma R proteins known as *transcobalamins* (*TCs:* TCI, TCII, and TC III). TCII is the main transporter protein for newly absorbed cobalamins as they circulate to peripheral tissues (Groff and Gropper, 1999).

Cellular uptake of vitamin B_{12} seems to be mediated by a specific TC receptor that internalizes the TC-vitamin complex. After lysosomal degradation of TC, the free vitamin is released for binding to vitamin B_{12}–dependent enzymes.

In adequately nourished individuals, vitamin B_{12} is stored in appreciable amounts (~2000 μg) mainly in the liver, which typically accumulates a substantial store—some 5 to 7 years worth—most of which is in the form of adenosylcobalamin. Enterohepatic circulation of the vitamin also contributes to these stores.

Metabolism

Vitamin B_{12} is metabolically active only as derivatives that have either a 5′-deoxyadenosine or a methyl group attached covalently to the corrin ring cobalt atom. These conversions are accomplished by vitamin B_{12} coenzyme synthetase and 5-methyl-FH_4:homocysteine methyltransferase, respectively. Little if any metabolism of the corrinoid ring system occurs, and the vitamin is excreted intact by renal and biliary routes. Apparently, only the free cobalamins (not the adenosylated or methylated forms) in plasma are available for excretion.

Functions

Vitamin B_{12} functions in two coenzyme forms: adenosylcobalamin (with methylcalonyl-CoA mutase and leucine mutase) and methylcobalamin (with methionine synthetase). In these reactions, these forms of the vitamin play important roles in the metabolism of propionate, amino acids, and single carbons, respectively. These steps are essential for normal metabolism of all cells, especially for those of the gastrointestinal (GI) tract, bone marrow, and nervous tissue.

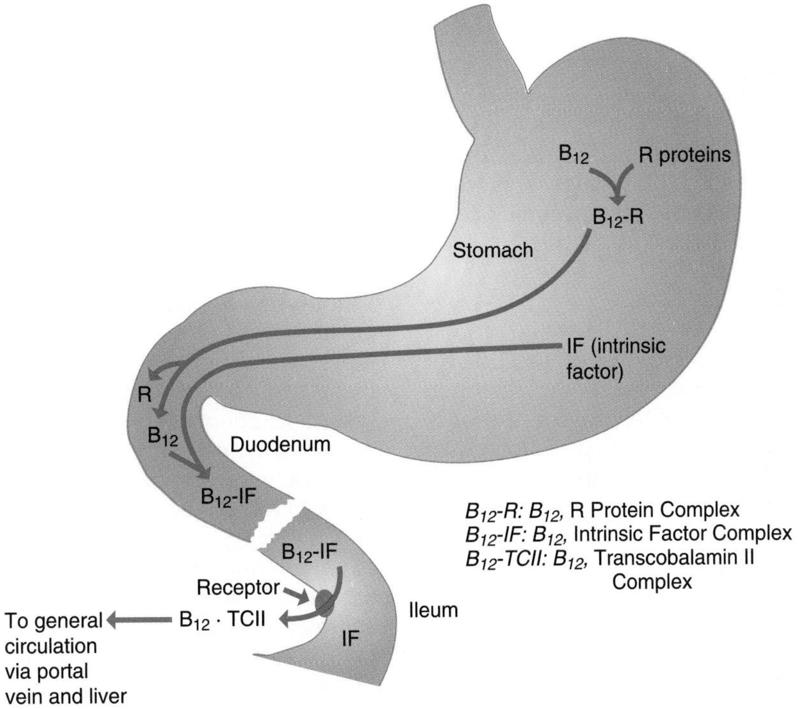

FIGURE 4-24 • Digestion and absorption of B_{12}.

TABLE 4-23 Dietary Reference Intakes for Vitamin B_{12}

LIFE-STAGE GROUP	RDA (μg/day)*
Infants	
0-6 mo	0.4†
7-12 mo	0.5†
Children	
1-3 yr	0.9
4-8 yr	1.2
Males	
9-13 yr	1.8
14-18 yr	2.4
19-30 yr	2.4
31-50 yr	2.4
51-70 yr	2.4†
>70 yr	2.4†
Females	
9-13 yr	1.8
14-18 yr	2.4
19-30 yr	2.4
31-50 yr	2.4
51-70 yr	2.4‡
>70 yr	2.4‡
Pregnant	
≤18 yr	2.6
19-30 yr	2.6
31-50 yr	2.6
Lactating	
≤18 yr	2.8
19-30 yr	2.8
31-50 yr	2.8

From Institute of Medicine, Food and Nutrition Board: *Dietary reference intakes for thiamin, riboflavin, niacin, vitamin B_6, folate, vitamin B_{12}, pantothenic acid, biotin, and choline,* Washington, DC, 1998, National Academy Press.

**RDA,* Recommended dietary allowance; tolerable upper intake levels (ULs) not determined.

†Adequate intake (AI).

‡Because 10% to 30% of older people may malabsorb food-bound vitamin B_{12}, it is advisable for those older than 50 years to meet their RDA mainly by consuming foods fortified with vitamin B_{12} or a supplement containing vitamin B_{12}.

A deficiency of the vitamin therefore is marked by increases in plasma and urinary levels of methylmalonic acid, aminoisocaproate, and homocysteine and losses of FH_4 (via the methyl folate trap).

Dietary Reference Intakes

Vitamin B_{12} is expressed in micrograms. The DRIs for vitamin B_{12} include AIs for infants and newly defined RDAs (Table 4-23). The adult RDA provides for substantial body stores because of the prevalences of achlorhydria and atrophic gastritis associated with losses of IF production and of pernicious anemia in those older than 60 years of age.

Sources

Vitamin B_{12} is synthesized by bacteria, but the vitamin produced from the microflora in the colon is not absorbed. The richest sources of the vitamin are liver and kidney, milk, eggs, fish, cheese, and muscle meats (Table 4-24).

TABLE 4-24 Vitamin B_{12} Content of Selected Foods

FOOD	μg
Liver, beef, 3.5 oz	95.03
Clams, canned, 3 oz	84.06
Oysters, raw, Pacific, 6 medium	13.29
Crab, Alaskan king, raw, 3 oz	9.78
Tuna, light, canned, in water, 3 oz	2.54
Beef, hamburger, lean, broiled, 3.5 oz	2.49
Halibut, baked, ½ filet	2.18
Cottage cheese, 1 cup	1.61
Yogurt with fruit, 8 oz	1.07
Pork chop, boiled, 3.5 oz	0.93
Skim milk, 1 cup	0.93
Bologna, beef and pork, 2 slices	0.75

From U.S. Department of Agriculture, Agricultural Research Service: *USDA nutrient database for standard reference,* Release 14, 2001, Data laboratory home page, http://www.nal.usda.gov/fnic/foodcomp.

Foods of plant origin contain the vitamin only through contamination or bacterial synthesis. Many people believe that fermented foods contain sufficient vitamin B_{12} to meet their needs; however, this theory is not supported by analysis (Specker et al, 1988). Six samples of tempeh (a fermented soybean product) were analyzed, and the vitamin B_{12} concentrations were negligible. In contrast, some cooked sea vegetables contained vitamin B_{12} in the same amounts as beef liver. Individuals consuming strictly vegetarian diets, particularly after 5 to 6 years, typically have lower circulating levels of vitamin B_{12} unless they supplement with the vitamin. This is not true for ovolacto vegetarians whose diets include food sources of vitamin B_{12} (Thorogood, 1995).

Because the vitamin is found in food bound to protein, approximately 70% of its activity is retained during the cooking of most foods; however, appreciable amounts of the vitamin can be lost when milk is pasteurized or evaporated.

Deficiency

Vitamin B_{12} deficiency causes impaired cell division, particularly in the rapidly dividing cells of the bone marrow and intestinal mucosa, through arrested synthesis of DNA. The ensuing reduction in mitotic rate results in abnormally large cells and a characteristic *megaloblastic anemia* (see Chapter 34). The anemia of B_{12} deficiency is related to the fact that inadequate B_{12} leads to a secondary folate deficiency because of the methyl folate trap (see previous discussion). Folate supplementation alleviates the anemia caused by B_{12} deficiency; however, other symptoms progress. Cobalamin deficiency also produces neurologic abnormalities that develop much later than the anemia. These abnormalities involve progressive neuropathy with nerve demyelination commencing peripherally and proceeding centrally. Symptoms include numbness, tingling and burning of the feet, and stiffness and generalized weakness of the legs.

Perhaps the most common cause of vitamin B_{12} deficiency is malabsorption of the vitamin because of inadequate production and secretion of IF. Clinically this condition is called *pernicious anemia,* which can result from aging associated with atrophy of gastric parietal cells, hereditary deficiencies in IF synthesis, or autoimmune incapacitation of IF. Although it is true that the long-term (i.e., for years several years) consumption of strict vegan diets without supplemental vitamin B_{12} typically leads to very low circulating levels of the vitamin, clinical signs among such individuals seem rare and may not be manifest for several years, except among breast-fed infants.

Vitamin B_{12} deficiency may be a common disorder in older adults (Carethers, 1988). Its symptoms often include (1) a lemon-yellow tint to the skin and eyes resulting from concurrent anemia and jaundice from ineffective erythropoeisis; (2) a smooth, beefy, red tongue; and (3) neurologic disorders. Psychiatric manifestations such as impaired mentation and depression may be present. Although the methods are expensive, vitamin B_{12} status is best assessed by measuring blood levels of the metabolites methylmalonic acid and homocysteine, which are B_{12} dependent. B_{12} serum level is not a good indicator of status.

Toxicity

Vitamin B_{12} has no appreciable toxicity.

Biotin

Biotin consists of a ureido ring joined to a thiophene ring with a valeric acid side chain and is necessary for critical carboxylations in metabolism (Figure 4-25).

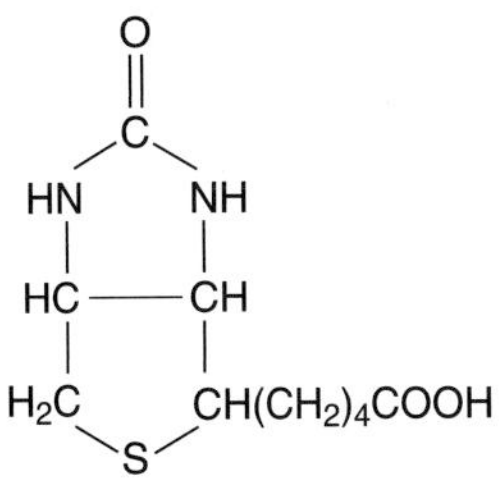

FIGURE 4-25 • Structure of biotin.

Absorption, Transport, and Storage

Biotin in foods is largely protein bound. It is released by proteolytic digestion to yield free biotin, biocytin, or biotiny peptide. Intestinal biotinidase releases free biotin from the latter two compounds. Free biotin is absorbed in the proximal small intestine primarily by carrier-mediated diffusion. Smaller amounts of biotin can also be absorbed from the colon, which facilitates the use of the vitamin produced by hind gut microflora.

Biotin is transported in the plasma primarily as free biotin, but approximately 12% is also bound to protein and biotinidase. Biotin is taken into cells by a specific carrier-mediated process. Appreciable amounts of the vitamin are stored in the liver; however, these stores do not seem to be mobilized well when the body is deprived of the vitamin.

Metabolism

Little catabolism of biotin occurs, but some of the vitamin is oxidized to biotin sulfoxides. The vitamin is rapidly excreted in the urine (95% of an oral dose is excreted within 24 hours)—half as free biotin and the balance as bisnorbiotin, biotin sulfoxides, and various side-chain metabolites.

Functions

Biotin is a carboxyl carrier covalently bound to the carboxylase enzymes pyruvate carboxylase (which converts pyruvate to oxaloacetate in gluconeogenesis), acetyl CoA carboxylase (which synthesizes malonyl CoA for fatty acid formation), propionyl CoA carboxylase (which allows the use of odd-chain fatty acids by converting propionate to succinate), and 3-methylcrotonyl-CoA carboxylase (which catabolizes leucine). These roles of biotin link it to the metabolic roles of folic acid, pantothenic acid, and vitamin B_{12}.

Dietary Reference Intakes

AIs for biotin have been established (Table 4-25). However, because of uncertainty about the amount of biotin provided by intestinal flora and differences in bioavailability of biotin from foods, the establishment of EARs and RDAs is problematic.

Sources

Biotin is widely distributed in foods, but its content varies significantly and has been determined for relatively few foods. Biotin content is not usually reported in food composition tables (Institute of Medicine, 2000a). Marshall (1987) reported that the biotin content of liver is as high as 100 μg per 100 g and the biotin content of milk products is 2 to 24 μg per 100 g. Milk, liver, egg yolk, and a few vegetables are the most important sources of the vitamin in human diets, and intestinal bacteria can also contribute appreciable amounts. Fecal and urinary excretion are considerably higher than dietary intake, reflecting the magnitude of the microfloral synthesis of biotin.

The bioavailability of biotin varies considerably among different foods because of differences in the digestibility of various biotin-protein complexes. Biotin is unstable in oxidizing conditions and is destroyed by heat, especially in the presence of lipid peroxidation.

Deficiency

Because biotin can be obtained from many foods and gut microbial metabolism, simple biotin deficiency in animals is rare. Biotin deficiency has been induced by feeding raw egg white or its active component—the heat-labile, biotin-binding protein *avidin.* Avidin impairs biotin absorption, causing such symptoms as seborrheic dermatitis, alopecia, and paralysis. Impaired biotin absorption can also occur in such GI tract disorders as inflammatory bowel diseases or achlorhydria. The few cases of biotin deficiency that have been described in humans have involved patients receiving incomplete parenteral nutrition and nursing infants whose mothers' milk contained very low amounts of the vitamin. In each case the signs included dermatitis, glossitis, anorexia, nausea, depression, hepatic steatosis, and hypercholesterolemia. Inherited defects in all of the known biotin enzymes have been identified in humans, but they are rare and usually have serious neurologic consequences. Blood levels of biotin are most often used to assess biotin status.

TABLE 4-25 Dietary Reference Intakes for Biotin

LIFE-STAGE GROUP	AI (μg/day)*
Infants	
0-6 mo	5
7-12 mo	6
Children	
1-3 yr	8
4-8 yr	12
Males	
9-13 yr	20
14-18 yr	25
19-30 yr	30
31-50 yr	30
51-70 yr	30
>70 yr	30
Females	
9-13 yr	20
14-18 yr	25
19-30 yr	30
31-50 yr	30
51-70 yr	30
>70 yr	30
Pregnant	
≤18 yr	30
19-30 yr	30
31-50 yr	30
Lactating	
≤18 yr	35
19-30 yr	35
31-50 yr	35

From Institute of Medicine, Food and Nutrition Board: *Dietary reference intakes for thiamin, riboflavin, niacin, vitamin B_6, folate, vitamin B_{12}, pantothenic acid, biotin, and choline,* Washington, DC, 1998, National Academy Press.
**AI,* Adequate intake; tolerable upper intake levels (ULs) not determined.

Toxicity

Biotin has no known toxic effects, even in very large doses.

Ascorbic Acid

Vitamin C, or ascorbic acid (Figure 4-26), functions in oxidation-reduction reactions and is synthesized by plants and most animals from glucose and galactose. However, humans, other primates, guinea pigs, some bats, and a few species of birds, lack the enzyme *l-gulonolactone oxidase* and thus cannot biosynthesize the factor, which for them is consequently a vitamin.

Absorption, Transport, and Storage

Species that cannot biosynthesize ascorbic acid absorb it from the diet by active transport and passive diffusion. The oxidized form of the vitamin, *dehydroascorbic acid,* is better absorbed than the reduced form, *ascorbate,* or ascorbic acid. The efficiency of enteric absorption of the vitamin is high (80% to 90%) at low intakes but declines markedly at intakes greater than about 1 g/day.

Vitamin C is transported in the plasma in the reduced form (ascorbic acid) in free solution. It is taken

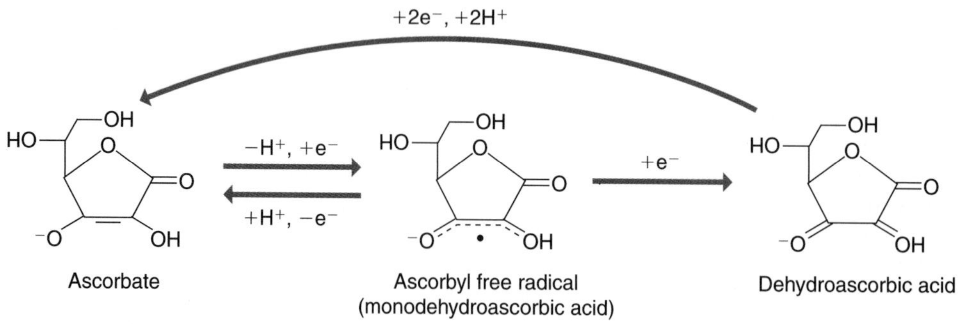

FIGURE 4-26 • Oxidation-reduction reaction of vitamin C. (From Combs GF: *The vitamins: fundamental aspects in nutrition and health,* ed 2, Orlando, 1998, Academic Press.)

up by cells through a glucose transporter and a specific active transport system. Each system moves dehydroascorbic acid into cells, where it is readily reduced to ascorbate. The glucose transporter-based system of uptake is not as fast as the specific system, but it is stimulated by insulin and inhibited by glucose. Thus diabetic patients with high glucose levels typically have high plasma levels and low cellular levels of dehydroascorbic acid. The vitamin is concentrated primarily as dehydroascorbic acid in many vital organs, particularly the adrenals, brain, and eye. It has been suggested that hyperglycemia-induced cellular vitamin C deficiency may lead to oxidative stress in cells and contribute to an increased risk of atherosclerotic disease (Price, Price, and Reynolds, 2001).

Metabolism

Ascorbic acid is oxidized in vivo by two successive losses of single electrons forming the free radical (monodehydroascorbic acid). This intermediate can be further oxidized to dehydroascorbic acid (see Figure 4-26). Subsequently, the oxidized product undergoes irreversible hydrolysis to yield 2,3-diketo-l-gulonic acid, which can be decarboxylated to yield carbon dioxide and several five-carbon fragments (e.g., xylose, xylonic acid) or oxidized to yield oxalic acid and several four-carbon fragments (e.g., threonic acid). In addition, the vitamin can be converted to ascorbic acid 2-sulfate.

It has been suggested that ascorbic acid may also react with tocopheroxyl or urate radicals to regenerate the reduced species of each. Such reactions would extend the known antioxidant roles of vitamin C to the metabolic recycling of other antioxidants.

Functions

Because ascorbic acid easily loses electrons and is reversibly converted to dehydroascorbic acid, it serves as a biochemical redox system involved in many electron transport reactions, including those involved in the synthesis of collagen and carnitine and other metabolic reactions. During collagen and carnitine synthesis, vitamin C acts as a reducing agent to keep iron in its ferrous state, thus enabling hydroxylation enzymes to function. For example, collagen, the major protein of fibrous tissues (connective tissue, cartilage, bone matrix, tooth dentin, skin, and tendons) depends on the posttranslational hydroxylation of proline residues in procollagen to form hydroxyproline, resulting in collagen. Ascorbic acid also participates in the hydroxylation of certain steroids synthesized in adrenal tissue. Vitamin C concentration decreases in periods of stress when adrenal cortical hormone activity is high. During periods of emotional, psychologic, or physiologic stress, the urinary excretion of ascorbic acid increases.

Ascorbic acid also acts as an antioxidant as it undergoes single-electron oxidation to the ascorbyl radical and dehydroascorbate (see Figure 4-26). By reacting with potentially toxic reactive oxygen species, such as the superoxide or hydroxyl radical, the vitamin can prevent oxidative damage. Vitamin C is essential for the oxidation of phenylalanine and tyrosine, the conversion of folate to tetrahydrofolic acid, the conversion of tryptophan to 5-hydroxytryptophan and the neurotransmitter serotonin, and the formation of norepinephrine from dopamine. It also reduces ferric to ferrous iron in the intestinal tract to facilitate iron absorption and is involved in the transfer of iron from plasma transferrin to liver ferritin.

Vitamin C promotes resistance to infection through its involvement with the immunologic activity of leukocytes, the production of interferon, the process of inflammatory reaction, and the integrity of the mucous membranes (Packer and Fuchs, 1997). The value of large amounts of ascorbic acid to prevent and cure the common cold has been reported, but conclusions from these studies are controversial. A number of studies in the 1970s demonstrated a positive effect on cold symptoms (Anderson, 1975; Anderson et al, 1972; Bouhuys, 1974; Coulehan et al, 1974, 1976; Miller et al, 1977; Wilson and Loh, 1973). Carr et al (1981) showed that a strong placebo effect developed when participants believed themselves to be receiving a high dose of vitamin C. Marshall (1992) cautioned that most people taking large doses (12,000 to 40,000 mg/day) would develop chronic diarrhea and possibly kidney stones. It is generally accepted that taking high doses of vitamin C for colds reduces the severity of the symptoms but does not prevent them. Vitamin C maintains proper lung function, as was described by the first National Health and Nutrition Examination Survey (NHANES 1) after a study of 2256 adults. After controlling for other risk and demographic factors, a positive significant correlation was found between pulmonary function and vitamin C intake (Schwartz and Weiss, 1994). The relationship of vitamin C to cancer is discussed in Chapter 40 (see *Clinical Insight:* Vitamin Supplements: To Take or Not to Take).

Dietary Reference Intakes

Vitamin C is expressed quantitatively in milligrams. The DRIs are presented in Table 4-26. Although as little as 10 mg vitamin C can prevent scurvy, this level does not provide acceptable reserves of the vitamin. Because of the lower concentrations of ascorbic acid in the serum of cigarette smokers, it has been recommended that smokers increase their intake to at least 100 mg/day (Food and Nutrition Board, 1989; Lykkesfeldt et al, 2000).

Sources

Vitamin C is found in plants and animal tissues as ascorbic acid and dehydroascorbic acid. The best sources are fruits, vegetables, and organ meats, but the actual ascorbic acid contents of foods can vary with the conditions of growth and degree of ripeness when harvested. Refrigeration and quick freezing help retain the vitamin. Most commercially frozen foods are processed so close to the source of supply that their ascorbic acid content is often higher than that of fresh foods that have been shipped across the country and spent time in storage and on supermarket shelves. Table 4-27 lists the vitamin C content of selected fruits and vegetables. Citrus fruits and juices are very important sources of the vitamin for many Americans, who tend not to eat many servings of other fruits and vegetables.

Ascorbic acid is easily destroyed by oxidation, and because it is soluble in water, it is often extracted and discarded in cooking water. Sodium bicarbonate, added to preserve and improve the color of cooked vegetables, destroys vitamin C. The cumulative losses of the vitamin from prepared vegetables refrigerated for 24 hours can be as high as 45% in fresh products and 52% in frozen products. Because consumers are eating out more frequently and more foods are being supplied to restaurants or institutions partially prepared (e.g., shredded lettuce, peeled and diced vegetables) or served from open salad bars, this vitamin loss must be considered when evaluating dietary intake (Carlson and Tabacchi, 1988).

Deficiency

Acute vitamin C deficiency results in scurvy in individuals unable to synthesize the vitamin. In human adults, signs are manifest after 45 to 80 days of vitamin C deprivation. In children the syndrome is called Moeller-Barlow disease; it can also develop in infants fed formulas not enriched with vitamin C. In both cases, lesions occur in mesenchymal tissues and result in impaired wound healing, edema, hemorrhages, and weakness in bone, cartilage, teeth, and connective tissues (Figure 4-27). Adults with scurvy may have swollen, bleeding gums and eventual tooth loss, lethargy, fatigue, rheumatic pains in the legs, muscular atrophy, skin lesions (Figure 4-28), and various psychologic changes (e.g., hysteria, hypochondria, depression).

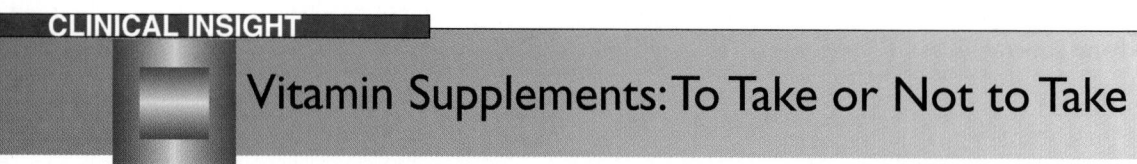

CLINICAL INSIGHT

Vitamin Supplements: To Take or Not to Take

In a recent address to the American Dietetic Association (2001), Dr. David Eisenberg expressed his concern that Americans believe supplements would not be for sale if they were not safe. In fact, the Dietary Supplements Health Education Act of 1994 severely limits the jurisdiction of the Food and Drug Administration (FDA) with regard to supplements (see Chapter 20). By law a supplement contains a vitamin, mineral, herb, or other botanical or amino acid. A supplement is intended for ingestion in a tablet, capsule, powder, soft gel, gel cap, or liquid form and must be labeled as a supplement and not be represented as a conventional food or an item of a meal or diet. The manufacturers of dietary supplements are responsible for ensuring that the label information is truthful and not misleading and that all ingredients in the supplements are safe. The FDA only evaluates a product after it is on the market and when documentation shows that it is unsafe. The consumer is clearly mistaken in thinking that supplements undergo the same scrutiny as drugs or even foods.

Who should take vitamin supplements? How much should they take? Are they safe?

Willett and Stampfer (2001) have recently addressed this question. Although in the past it was generally accepted that nutritional needs could be met by a healthy diet alone, they point out that recent studies—such as those showing that folic acid supplements in early pregnancy can dramatically reduce the incidence of neural tube defects—contradict current teachings (at least in some circumstances). Another example involves vitamin D and bone status. Clearly, certain older adults and younger people who are not exposed to the sun need and benefit from vitamin D supplementation because it maintains their bone health.

Alternatively, not only did carotene supplements fail to reduce the risk of lung cancer in those who smoke, it may have increased it. In addition, persistent use of more than 6600 IU of vitamin A supplements (as the preformed retinol or retinyl palmitate) may be detrimental to the long-term bone health of women (Feskanick et al, 2002). Much larger amounts are found in many multivitamin and mineral supplements.

Evaluation of evidence regarding specific vitamin supplements is complicated by a lack of clinical trials with measurable outcomes and often does not (or cannot) take into account the effect of diets (i.e., good versus poor). Some trials focus on high-risk groups, so the results may not apply to the general population.

Decisions regarding vitamin supplements should be made using a process that evaluates all available evidence and weighs the likelihood of harm against the likelihood of benefit. Using this process, it is reasonable to conclude that a daily multivitamin with component vitamins that do not exceed the DRI is sensible for most adults—especially for women who might become pregnant, older adults, those who drink one or more alcoholic beverages per day, and those who live in poverty and whose diets may be poor (Willett and Stampfer, 2001).

Toxicity

The only consistent adverse effects of high doses of vitamin C in humans are gastrointestinal disturbances and diarrhea. This is fortunate because vitamin C is the most commonly used supplement in the United States, taken by 8% of younger people and 44% of older adults (Johnston and Luo, 1994). However, because the catabolism of vitamin C yields oxalate (among other metabolites), it is reasonable to be concerned about the possibility of high doses of the vitamin increasing the risk of forming renal oxalate stones. However, clinical studies have shown that subjects given multiple daily doses of the vitamin developed only slight oxaluria (Sauberlich, 1994). Nevertheless, prudence dictates that individuals with histories of forming renal stones should avoid consuming too much vitamin C. Excess ascorbic acid excreted in the urine can give a false-positive urinary glucose test.

Table 4-28 summarizes the preceding information on the known vitamins.

TABLE 4-26 Dietary Reference Intakes for Vitamin C

LIFE-STAGE GROUP	RDA (mg/day)*	UL (mg/day)*
Infants		
0.0-0.5	30†	ND
0.5-1	35†	ND
Children		
1-3	15	400
4-8	25	650
Males		
9-13	45	1200
14-18	75	1800
19-30	90	2000
31-50	90	2000
51-70	90	2000
≥70	90	2000
Females		
9-13	45	1200
14-18	65	1800
19-30	75	2000
31-50	75	2000
51-70	75	2000
≥70	75	2000
Pregnant		
≤18	80	1800
19-30	85	2000
31-50	85	2000
Lactating		
≤18	115	1800
19-30	120	2000
31-50	120	2000

From Institute of Medicine, Food and Nutrition Board: *Dietary reference intakes for vitamin C, vitamin E, selenium, and carotenoids,* 2000, Washington, DC, National Academy Press.
**UL,* Tolerable upper intake level; *ND,* not determined.
†Adequate intake (AI).

TABLE 4-27 Vitamin C Content of Selected Foods

FOOD	AMOUNT	CONTENT (mg)
Pepper, sweet, yellow	1 cup	283
Orange juice		
Fresh	1 cup	124
Frozen, diluted, canned	1 cup	97
Canned	1 cup	86
Broccoli		
Fresh, boiled	1 cup	116
Frozen, chopped, boiled	1 cup	74
Brussels sprouts, cooked	1 cup	97
Strawberries	1 cup	106
Grapefruit juice, from frozen concentrate, unsweetened	1 cup	83
Cantaloupe	1 cup	68
Mango	1	57
Kale, from raw, cooked	1 cup	53
Tomato juice	1 cup	45

From U.S. Department of Agriculture, Agricultural Research Service: *USDA nutrient database for standard reference,* Release 14, 2001, Data laboratory home page, http://www.nal.usda.gov/fnic/foodcomp.

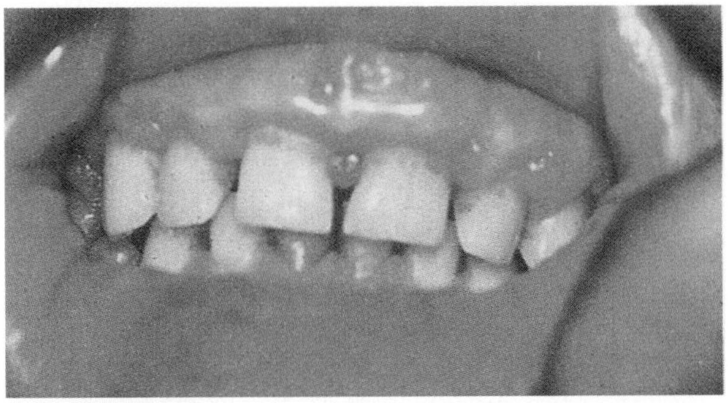

FIGURE 4-27 • Scorbutic gums in vitamin C deficiency. Gums are swollen, ulcerated, and bleeding because of vitamin C–induced defects in oral epithelial basement membrane and periodontal collagen fiber synthesis. (From Taylor KB, Anthony LE: *Clinical nutrition,* New York, 1983, McGraw-Hill.)

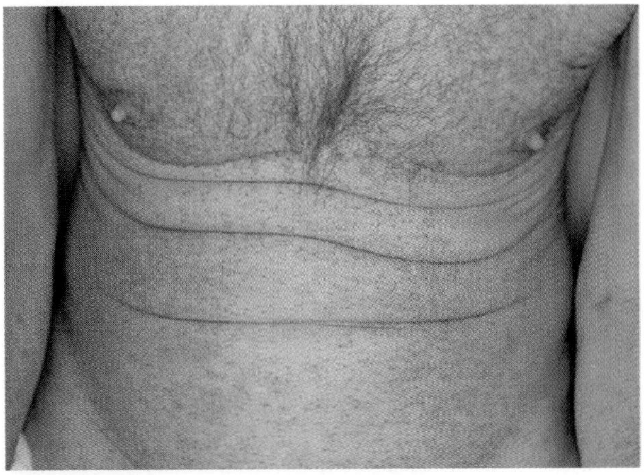

FIGURE 4-28 • Scurvy. (From Callen WBS et al: *Color atlas of dermatology,* Philadelphia, 1993, Saunders.)

TABLE 4-28 Summary of Vitamins

NAME	RDA FOR ADULTS*	SOURCES	STABILITY	COMMENTS
Fat-Soluble Vitamins				
Vitamin A (retinol; α-, β-, γ-carotene)	M: 900 RAE F: 700 RAE	Liver, kidney, milk fat, fortified margarine, egg yolk, yellow and dark-green leafy vegetables, apricots, cantaloupe, peaches.	Stable in presence of light, heat, and usual cooking methods. Destroyed by oxidation, drying, very high temperature, ultraviolet light.	Essential for normal growth, development, and maintenance of epithelial tissue. Essential for the integrity of night vision. Helps promote normal bone development and influences normal tooth formation. Functions as antioxidant. Toxic in large quantities.
Vitamin D (calciferol)	M: 5-15 μg F: 5-15 μg Adequate intake	Vitamin D–fortified milk, irradiated foods, some in milk fat, liver, egg yolk, salmon, tuna fish, sardines. Sunlight converts 7-dehydrocholesterol to cholecalciferol.	Stable in presence of heat and oxidation.	Is a prohormone. Essential for normal growth and development; important for formation and maintenance of normal bones and teeth. Influences absorption and metabolism of phosphorus and calcium. Toxic in large quantities.
Vitamin E (tocopherols and tocotrienols)	M: 15 α-TE F: 15 α-TE	Wheat germ, vegetable oils, green leafy vegetables, milk fat, egg yolk, nuts.	Stable in presence of heat and acids. Destroyed by rancid fats, alkali, oxygen, lead, iron salts, and ultraviolet irradiation.	Is a strong antioxidant. May help prevent oxidation of unsaturated fatty acids and vitamin A in intestinal tract and body tissues. Protects red blood cells from hemolysis. Role in reproduction (in animals). Role in epithelial tissue maintenance and prostaglandin synthesis.
Vitamin K (phylloquinone and menaquinone)	M: 120 μg F: 120 μg Adequate intake	Liver, soybean oil, other vegetable oils, green leafy vegetables, wheat bran. Synthesized by intestinal tract bacteria.	Resistant to heat, oxygen, and moisture. Destroyed by alkali and ultraviolet light.	Aids in production of prothrombin, a compound required for normal clotting of blood. Involved in bone metabolism. Toxic in large amounts.
Water-Soluble Vitamins				
Thiamin	M: 1.2 mg F: 1.1 mg	Pork liver, organ meats, legumes, whole-grain and enriched cereals and breads, wheat germ, potatoes.	Unstable in presence of heat, alkali, or oxygen. Heat stable in acid solution.	As part of cocarboxylase, aids in removal of CO_2 from α-keto acids during oxidation of carbohydrates. Essential for growth, normal appetite, digestion, and healthy nerves.
Riboflavin	M: 1.3 mg F: 1.1 mg	Milk and dairy foods, organ meats, green leafy vegetables, enriched cereals and breads, eggs.	Stable in presence of heat, oxygen, and acid. Unstable in presence of light (especially ultraviolet) or alkali.	Essential for growth. Plays enzymatic role in tissue respiration and acts as a transporter of hydrogen ions. Coenzyme forms FMN and FAD.
Niacin (nicotinic acid and nicotinamide)	M: 16 mg NE F: 14 mg NE	Fish, liver, meat, poultry, many grains, eggs, peanuts, milk, legumes, enriched grains.	Stable in presence of heat, light, oxidation, acid, and alkali.	As part of enzyme system, aids in transfer of hydrogen and acts in metabolism of carbohydrates and amino acids. Involved in glycolysis, fat synthesis, and tissue respiration.
Pantothenic acid	5 mg Adequate intake	All plant and animal foods. Eggs, kidney, liver, salmon, and yeast are best sources. Possibly synthesized by intestinal bacteria.	Unstable in presence of acid, alkali, heat, and certain salts.	As part of coenzyme A, functions in the synthesis and breakdown of many vital body compounds. Essential in the intermediary metabolism of carbohydrate, fat, and protein.

*M, Male; F, female; RAE, retinol activity equivalents; α-TE, α-tocopherol equivalents; NE, niacin equivalents; FMN, flavin adenine mononucleotide; FAD, flavin adenine dinucleotide.

TABLE 4-28 Summary of Vitamins—cont'd

NAME	RDA FOR ADULTS*	SOURCES	STABILITY	COMMENTS
Water-Soluble Vitamins—cont'd				
Vitamin B_6 (pyridoxine, pyridoxal, and pyridoxamine)	M: 1.3-1.7 mg F: 1.3-1.5 mg	Pork, glandular meats, cereal bran and germ, milk, egg yolk, oatmeal, legumes.	Stable in presence of heat, light, and oxidation.	As a coenzyme, aids in the synthesis and breakdown of amino acids and of unsaturated fatty acids from essential fatty acids. Essential for conversion of tryptophan to niacin. Essential for normal growth.
Folate (folic acid, folacin)	400 μg	Green leafy vegetables, organ meats (liver), lean beef, wheat, eggs, fish, dry beans, lentils, cowpeas, asparagus, broccoli, collards, yeast.	Stable in presence of sunlight when in solution. Unstable in presence of heat in acid media.	Essential for biosynthesis of nucleic acids—especially important in early fetal development. Essential for normal maturation of red blood cells. Functions as a coenzyme—tetrahydrofolic acid.
Vitamin B_{12} (cobalamin)	30 μg	Liver, kidney, milk and dairy foods, meat, eggs. Vegans require supplement.	Slowly destroyed by acid, alkali, light, and oxidation.	Involved in the metabolism of single-carbon fragments. Essential for biosynthesis of nucleic acids and nucleoproteins. Role in metabolism of nervous tissue. Involved with folate metabolism. Related to growth.
Biotin	30 μg Adequate intake	Liver, mushrooms, peanuts, yeast, milk, meat, egg yolk, most vegetables, banana, grapefruit, tomato, watermelon, strawberries. Synthesized by intestinal bacteria.	Stable under most conditions.	Essential component of enzymes. Involved in synthesis and breakdown of fatty acids and amino acids through aiding the addition and removal of CO_2 to or from active compounds and the removal of NH_2 from amino acids.
Vitamin C (ascorbic acid)	M: 90 mg F: 75 mg	Acerola (West Indian cherry-like fruit), citrus fruit, tomato, melon, peppers, greens, raw cabbage, guava, strawberries, pineapple, potato, kiwi.	Unstable in presence of heat, alkali, and oxidation, except in acids. Destroyed by storage.	Maintains intracellular cement substance with preservation of capillary integrity. Cosubstrate in hydroxylations requiring molecular oxygen. Important in immune responses, wound healing, and allergic reactions. Increases absorption of nonheme iron.

OTHER VITAMIN-LIKE FACTORS

Other food factors have vitamin characteristics but do not meet the criteria of vitamin status. These quasivitamins include those that can be biosynthesized but may be beneficial as supplements (e.g., choline, carnitine) and those yet to be proven to be essential (e.g., *myo*-inositol, the ubiquinones, the bioflavonoids). Some, such as choline, may need to be provided in the diet only at certain stages of life.

Choline

Choline (2-hydroxy-*N,N,N*-trimethylenthanolamine) is an essential component of animal tissues, where it is a structural component of *phosphatidylcholine (lecithin)* in membrane phospholipids and the neurotransmitter acetylcholine. Choline can be biosynthesized from ethanolamine by sequential methylations using S-adenosylmethionine, but most humans obtain it from dietary phosphatides. Choline is widely distributed in fat, existing predominantly in the form of lecithin in eggs, liver, soybeans, beef, milk, and peanuts. Free choline is present in liver, oatmeal, soybeans, iceberg lettuce, cauliflower, kale, and cabbage. Choline is released by the hydrolysis of lecithin by pancreatic and intestinal lipases and is absorbed by a carrier-mediated process and passive diffusion. Absorbed choline is transported via chylomicrons in the lymphatic circulation primarily in the form of lecithin; it is transferred to lipoproteins in this form for distribution to peripheral tissues.

Choline has several functions in metabolism (Zeisel and Blusztajn, 1994). As phosphatidylcholine, it is a structural element of membranes, a precursor to the sphingolipids, and a promoter of lipid transport. As acetylcholine, it is a neurotransmitter and a component of platelet-activating factor. Choline deficiency can occur in young poultry unable to synthesize it as quickly as needed. Choline-deficient animals have fatty deposition in the liver, hemorrhagic kidney disease, and deformations of the bone organic matrix. Clear cases of choline deficiency have not been found in humans. However, supplemental choline has been used with some success to diminish the short-term memory loss associated with Alzheimer's disease, and very high doses (up to 20 g/day) have been reported to alleviate symptoms of tardive dyskinesia and Huntington's disease (Canty and Zeisel, 1994). AIs were established for choline as part of the 1998 DRIs (Table 4-29).

TABLE 4-29 Dietary Reference Intakes for Choline

LIFE-STAGE GROUP	AI* (mg/day)†	UL* (mg/day)†
Infants		
0-6 mo	125	ND
7-12 mo	150	ND
Children		
1-3 yr	200	1000
4-8 yr	250	1000
Males		
9-13 yr	375	2000
14-18 yr	550	3000
19-30 yr	550	3500
31-50 yr	550	3500
51-70 yr	550	3500
>70 yr	550	3500
Females		
9-13 yr	375	2000
14-18 yr	400	3000
19-30 yr	425	3500
31-50 yr	425	3500
51-70 yr	425	3500
>70 yr	425	3500
Pregnant		
≤18 yr	450	3000
19-30 yr	450	3500
31-50 yr	450	3500
Lactating		
≤18 yr	550	3000
19-30 yr	550	3500
31-50 yr	550	3500

From Institute of Medicine, Food and Nutrition Board: *Dietary reference intakes for thiamin, riboflavin, niacin, vitamin B_6, folate, vitamin B_{12}, pantothenic acid, biotin, and choline,* Washington, DC, 1998, National Academy Press.

**AI,* Adequate intake; *UL,* tolerable upper intake level; *ND,* not determinable because of lack of data of adverse effects.

†Although AIs have been set for choline, few data assess whether a dietary supply of choline is needed at all stages of the life cycle, and it may be that the choline requirement can be met by endogenous synthesis at some of these stages.

Carnitine

Carnitine (β-hydroxy-γ-*N*-trimethylaminobutyrate) helps transport long-chain fatty acids into the mitochondria for oxidation as sources of energy, a process called the *carnitine transport shuttle.* Mammals and birds can synthesize carnitine from the amino acid lysine using a process that requires vitamin C. Little data exists on the carnitine biosynthetic capacities of humans, but the low tissue levels typical in neonates fed diets low in carnitine (e.g., nonsupplemented, soy-based formulas) suggest that they may have limited capacities for synthesizing the factor (Atkins and Clandinin, 1990). In some instances, carnitine may be a *conditionally essential nutrient* (Broquist, 1994).

Foods of plant origin are generally low in carnitine, but meats and dairy products in particular are good sources. Carnitine is efficiently absorbed across the gut by active transport and simple diffusion. About half of carnitine is acetylated during absorption; free and acetylated forms are found in circulation in plasma and erythrocytes. Carnitine is taken up primarily by skeletal peripheral tissues, which contain approximately 90% of the body stores.

Tissue depletion of carnitine has been reported in adults undergoing hemodialysis, adults with liver disease, and preterm infants. Supplemental carnitine has been found to correct the hypertriglyceridemia in such patients (Combs, 1998). Muscle weakness and hypoglycemia have also been described as clinical manifestations of carnitine deficiency (Metabolic, 1990).

myo-Inositol

myo-Inositol (*cis*-1,2,3,5-*trans*-4,6-cyclohexanehexol) functions in metabolism as *phosphatidylinositol (PI),* which provides structural support in membranes and serves as an anchor for membrane proteins by covalent bonding. It is a source of arachidonic acid for the biosynthesis of eicosanoids. In addition, PI is the source of important intracellular signals and secondary cell messengers in response to hormonal stimuli. For example, hormone-sensitive phospholipase C can act on phosphorylated PI, producing free *inositol triphosphate (IP_3)* and a *diacylglycerol (DAG).* IP_3 activates the release of calcium ions, which in turn stimulate calcium-dependent enzymes. DAG initiates a process that results in the alteration of some cellular enzyme activities (Groff and Gropper, 1999). IP is concentrated in the brain and cerebrospinal fluid but also exists in other tissues (Combs, 1998).

Mammals synthesize *myo*-inositol from glucose, but it is also obtained from fruits, grains, vegetables, nuts, legumes, and organ meats such as liver and heart. Dietary sources include various inositol phospholipids in animal products and phytic acid *(inositol hexaphosphate)* in plant materials. Because humans and most other mammals lack an intestinal phytase, phytic acid is not a useful source of *myo*-inositol.

myo-Inositol is efficiently absorbed in its free form by an active transport process. It is transported in the blood primarily in its free form, with some as PI associated with lipoproteins. Free *myo*-inositol is converted in the tissue to PI, which is metabolized by sequential phosphorylations to the monophosphate and diphosphate forms. Only female gerbils and certain fish have been shown to have a clear dietary need for preformed *myo*-inositol. In these animals, deprivation of the factor produced anorexia, dermatologic lesions, and intestinal lipodystrophy. A requirement for humans has yet to be defined.

Ubiquinones

The ubiquinones are a group of substituted 1,4-benzoquinone derivatives with varying lengths of isopentyl side chains. The principal species has 10 such side-chain units and is referred to as coenzyme Q_{10} (CoQ_{10}), which was first isolated in 1957. The ubiquinones are essential components of the mitochondrial electron transport chain, in which they undergo reversible reduction-oxidation reactions to pass electrons from flavoproteins (NADH or succinic dehydrogenases) to the cytochromes via cytochrome b_5. In addition, the redox properties of CoQ_{10} enable it to function as a fat-soluble antioxidant, much like α-tocopherol. Relatively high concentrations of the ubiquinones are maintained in tissues, apparently by biosynthesis from endogenous precursors. It has been suggested that limited ubiquinone synthesis may play a role in the etiology of heart disease (Rosenfeldt et al, 2002) and diabetes (Watts et al, 2002). Indeed, supplemental CoQ_{10} has been found to be useful in treating cardiomyopathy and congestive heart failure (Tran et al, 2001). The use of CoQ_{10} in clinical situations has been extensively reviewed (Jones et al, 2002). CoQ_{10} is concentrated in various foods, notably fish oils, nuts, fish, and meats.

Bioflavonoids

The bioflavonoids (phenolic derivatives of 2-phenyl-1,4-benzopyrone) have no known immediate metabolic function; however, they have been shown to reduce capillary fragility and potentiate the antiscorbutic activity of ascorbic acid, both of which may involve their chelation of divalent metal ions (Cu^{++}, Fe^{++}) and their intrinsic antioxidant properties (Manach et al, 1996). Epidemiologic studies have shown an association between diets high in bioflavonoids and reduced risks for cardiovascular disease and several cancers. The bioflavonoids are ubiquitous in foods of plant origin; more than 800 different bioflavonoids such as quercitin, rutin, and hesperidin have been isolated from plants in which they are the major sources of noncarotenoid red, blue, and yellow pigments (see Chapter 12).

Clinical Scenario

JoAnne is a 40-year-old black executive. She leads an active life and uses oral contraceptives. She works out regularly and eats a very–low-fat diet to manage her weight. She and her husband want to start a family. Her blood tests indicate that she has a low folate level. She has a light breakfast of fruit, a lunch of a sandwich and coffee, and a dinner of a green salad, pasta, fruit, and milk. She comes into your office for advice on how to improve her diet.

What recommendations do you have for her as her nutritional counselor?

1. What are your concerns about her diet?
2. What additional information do you need?
3. In what way could she improve her vitamin intake?
4. Would a supplement be useful?

Relevant Web Sites

National Academy of Sciences, Institute of Medicine
www.iom.edu/iom/
U.S. Department of Agriculture, Agriculture Research Service, Nutrient Database
www.nal.usda.gov/fnic/foodcomp
U.S. Department of Agriculture, Food and Nutrition Service
www.fns.usda.gov/fns/

Cited References

Anderson TW: Large scale trials of vitamin C, *Ann N Y Acad Sci* 258:498, 1975.

Anderson TW et al: Vitamin C and the common cold: a double-blind trial, *Can Med Assoc J* 107:503, 1972.

Atkins J, Clandinin MT: Nutritional significance of factors affecting carnitine-dependent transport of fatty acids in neonates: a review, *Nutr Res* 10:117, 1990.

Baumann LS, Spencer J: The effects of topical vitamin E on the cosmetic appearance of scars, *Dermatol Surg* 25:311, 1999.

Bershad S: Developments in topical retinoid therapy for acne, *Semin Cutan Med Surg* 20:154, 2001.

Booth SL, Centurelli MA: Vitamin K: a practical guide to the dietary management of patients on warfarin, *Nutr Rev* 57:288, 1999.

Bouhuys A: Colds and antihistamine effects of vitamin C, *N Engl J Med* 290:633, 1974.

Broquist HP: Carnitine. In Shils ME et al, eds: *Modern nutrition in health and disease,* ed 8, vol 1, Philadelphia, 1994, Lea & Febiger.

Brown AJ, Finch J, Slatopolsky E: Differential effects of 19-nor-1,25-dihydroxyvitamin D(2) and 1,25-dihydroxyvitamin D(3) on intestinal calcium and phosphate transport, *J Lab Clin Med* 139:279, 2002.

Budiyanto A et al: Protective effect of topically applied olive oil against photocarcinogenesis following UVB exposure of mice, *Carcinogenesis* 21:2085, 2000.

Burke KE et al: Effects of topical and oral vitamin E on pigmentation and skin cancer induced by ultraviolet irradiation in Skh:2 hairless mice, *Nutr Cancer* 38:87, 2000.

Butterworth C Jr, Bendich A: Folic acid and the prevention of birth defects, *Annu Rev Nutr* 16:73, 1996.

Can C et al: Vascular endothelial dysfunction associated with elevated serum homocysteine levels in rat adjuvant arthritis: effect of vitamin E administration, *Life Sci* 71:401, 2002.

Canty DJ, Zeisel SJ: Lecithin and choline in human health and disease, *Nutr Rev* 52:327, 1994.

Carethers M: Diagnosing vitamin B_{12} deficiency, a common geriatric disorder, *Geriatrics* 43:89, 1988.
Carlson BL, Tabacchi MH: Loss of vitamin C in vegetables during the food service cycle, *J Am Diet Assoc* 88:65, 1988.
Carr AB et al: Vitamin C and the common cold: a second MZ cotwin control study, *Acta Genet Med Cemellol* 30:249, 1981.
Caution on use of antioxidants, *Nutrition Today* 29(2):4, 1994.
Chen T et al: An update on the vitamin D content of fortified milk from the United States and Canada, letter, *N Engl J Med* 329:1507, 1993.
Christensen H: Riboflavin can protect tissues from oxidative injury, *Nutr Rev* 51:149, 1993.
Combs GF Jr: *The vitamins: fundamental aspects in nutrition and health,* ed 2, Orlando, 1998, Academic Press.
Coulehan JL et al: Vitamin C and acute illness in Navaho children, *N Engl J Med* 295:973, 1976.
Coulehan JL et al: Vitamin C prophylaxis in a boarding school, *N Engl J Med* 290:6, 1974.
Coursin DB: Convulsive seizures in infants with pyridoxine deficient diet, *JAMA* 154:406, 1954.
Delmas PD: Treatment of postmenopausal osteoporosis, *Lancet* 359:2018, 2002.
Dreher F, Maibach H: Protective effect of topical antioxidants in humans, *Curr Probl Dermatol* 29:157, 2001.
Driskell JA: Vitamin B-6 requirements of humans, *Nutr Res* 14:293, 1994.
Elvehjem CA et al: The isolation and identification of anti-black tongue factor, *J Biol Chem* 123: 137, 1938.
Fairfield KM, Fletcher RH: Vitamins for chronic disease prevention in adults: scientific review, *JAMA* 287: 3116, 2002.
Ferland G: The vitamin K–dependent proteins: an update, *Nutr Rev* 56:223, 1998.
Feskanick et al: Vitamin A intake and hip fracture among postmenopausal women, *JAMA* 287:47, 2002.
Fitzpatrick S et al: Vitamin D–deficient rickets: a multifactorial disease, *Nutr Rev* 58:218, 2000.
Food and Nutrition Board, National Research Council, National Academy of Science: *Recommended dietary allowances,* ed 10, Washington, DC, 1989, National Academy Press.
Gensler HL et al: Importance of the form of typical vitamin E for prevention of photocarcinogenesis, *Nutr Cancer* 26:183, 1996.
Goldberger J et al: A study of the diet of nonpellagrous and pellagrous households, *JAMA* 71:944, 1918.
Gregory, J III: Case study: folate bioavailability, *J Nutr* 131(suppl 4):1376, 2001.
Groff JL, Gropper SS: *Advanced nutrition and human metabolism,* p 584, ed 3, Stamford, Conn, 1999, Wadsworth.
Haddad J: Vitamin D: solar rays, the Milky Way, or both? *N Engl J Med* 326:1213, 1992.
Harris LJ: *Vitamins in theory and practice,* Cambridge, 1955, Cambridge University Press.
Hathcock JN et al: Evaluation of vitamin A toxicity, *Am J Clin Nutr* 52:183, 1990.
Heaney RP: Bone mass, nutrition and other lifestyle factors, *Am J Med* 95:29S, 1993.
Holick M et al: The vitamin D content of fortified milk and infant formula, *N Engl J Med* 326:1178, 1992.
Horwitt MK: My valedictory on the differences in biological potency between *RRR*-alpha-tocopheryl and all-*rac*-alpha-tocopheryl acetate, *Am J Clin Nutr* 69:341, 1999.
Institute of Medicine, Food and Nutrition Board: *Dietary reference intakes. Proposed definition and plan for review of dietary antioxidants and related compounds,* Washington, DC, 1998, National Academy Press.
Institute of Medicine, Food and Nutrition Board: *Dietary reference intakes for thiamin, riboflavin, niacin, vitamin B_6, folate, vitamin B_{12}, pantothenic acid, biotin, and choline,* Washington, DC, 2000a, National Academy Press.
Institute of Medicine, Food and Nutrition Board: *Dietary reference intakes for vitamin C, vitamin E, selenium, and carotenoids,* Washington, DC, 2000b, National Academy Press.
Institute of Medicine, Food and Nutrition Board: *Dietary reference intakes for vitamin A, vitamin K, arsenic, boron, chromium, copper, iodine, iron, manganese, molybdenum, nickel, silicon, vanadium, and zinc,* Washington, DC, 2001, National Academy Press.
Jacobus C et al: Hypervitaminosis D associated with drinking milk, *N Engl J Med* 326:1173, 1992.
Johnston C, Luo B: Comparison of the absorption and excretion of three commercially available sources of vitamin C, *J Am Diet Assoc* 94:779, 1994.
Jones K et al: Coenzyme Q_{10}: efficacy, safety, and use, *Int J Integrative Med* 4:28, 2002.
Kuzniarz M et al: Use of vitamin supplements and cataracts: the Blue Mountain eye study, *Am J Opthamol* 132:19, 2001.
Krol ES, Kramer-Ktickland KA, Liebler DC: Photoprotective actions of topically applied vitamin E, *Drug Metab Rev* 32:413, 2000.
Li E, Norris AW: Structure/function of cytosolic vitamin A–binding proteins, *Annu Rev Nutr* 16:205, 1996.
Lykkesfeldt J et al: Ascorbate is depleted by smoking and repleted by moderate supplementation: a study in male smokers and nonsmokers with matched dietary antioxidant intakes, *Am J Clin Nutr* 71:530, 2000.
Maden M: Vitamin A in embryonic development, *Nutr Rev* 52(suppl):3, 1994.
Malmberg KJ et al: A short term dietary supplementation of high doses of vitamin E increases T helper 1 cytokine production in patients with advanced colorectal cancer, *Clin Cancer Res* 8:1772, 2002.
Manach C et al: Bioavailability, metabolism and physiological impact of 4-oxo-flavonoids, *Nutr Res* 16:517, 1996.
Marshall C: Can megadoses of vitamin C help against colds? *Nutr Forum* 9(5):33, 1992.
Marshall MW: The nutritional importance of biotin—an update, *Nutr Today* 22:26, 1987.
McVean M, Liebler DC: Prevention of DNA photodamage by vitamin E compounds and sunscreens: roles of ultraviolet absorbance and cellular uptake, *Mol Carcinog* 24:169, 1999.
Metabolic effects of carnitine supplementation in subjects with low plasma carnitine levels, *Nutr Rev* 48:159, 1990.
Meydani SN et al: Vitamin E supplementation and in vivo immune response in healthy elderly subjects: a randomized controlled trial, *JAMA* 277:1380, 1997.
Miller JZ et al: Therapeutic effect of vitamin C: a cotwin control study, *JAMA* 237:248, 1977.
Moison RM, Beijersbergen van Henegouwen GM: Topical antioxidant vitamins C and E prevent UVB-radiation-induced peroxidation of eicosapentaenoic acid in pig skin, *Radiat Res* 157:402, 2002.
Morris MC et al: Dietary intake of antioxidant nutrients and the risk of incident Alzheimer disease in a biracial community study, *JAMA* 287:3261, 2002.
Olson JA: Vitamin A. In Zeigler EE, Filer LJ, eds: *Present knowledge in nutrition,* ed 7, Washington, DC, 1996, ILSI Press.
Omdahl JL, Morris HA, May BK: Hydroxylase enzymes of the vitamin D pathway: expression, function, and regulation, *Ann Rev Nutr* 22:139, 2002.
Packer L, Fuchs J, eds: *Vitamin C in health and disease,* New York, 1997, Marcel Dekker.
Price KD, Price CS, Reynolds RD: Hyperglycemia induced ascorbic acid deficiency promotes endothelial dysfunction and the development of atherosclerosis, *Atherosclerosis* 158:1, 2001.
Reimund E, Ramos A: Niacin-induced hepatitis and thrombocytopenia after 10 years of niacin use, *J Clin Gastroenterol* 18:270, 1994.
Rosenfeldt et al: Coenzyme Q10 protects the aging heart against stress: studies in rats, human tissues, and patients, *Ann N Y Acad Sci* 959:355, 2002.
Sanchez-Castillo et al: Nutrition and cataract in low-income Mexicans: experience in an eye camp, *Arch Latinoam Nutr* 51:113, 2001.
Sauberlich HE: Pharmacology of vitamin C, *Annu Rev Nutr* 14:371, 1994.
Schaumberg HJ et al: Sensory neuropathy from pyridoxine abuse, *N Engl J Med* 309:445, 1983.
Schwartz J, Weiss S: Relationship between dietary vitamin C intake and pulmonary function in the first National Health and Nutrition Examination Survey (NHANES 1), *Am J Clin Nutr* 59:110, 1994.
Sills IN: Nutritional rickets: a preventable disease, *Top Clin Nutr* 17:36, 2001.
Shoob et al: Dietary methionine is involved in the etiology of neural tube defect–affected pregnancies in humans, *J Nutr* 131:2653, 2001.

Sokol, RJ: Antioxidant defenses in metal-induced liver damage, *Semin Liver Dis* 16:39, 2001

Sorg O, Tran C, Saurat JH: Cutaneous vitamins A and E in the context of ultraviolet- or chemically-induced oxidative stress, *Skin Pharmacol Appl Skin Physiol* 14:363, 2001.

Specker BL et al: Increased urinary methylmalonic acid excretion in breast-fed infants of vegetarian mothers and identification of and acceptable dietary source of vitamin B_{12}, *Am J Clin Nutr* 47:89, 1988.

Stahl W, Ale-Agha N, Polidori MC: Non-antioxidant properties of carotenoids, *Biol Chem* 383:553, 2002

Suttie JW: The importance of menaquinones in human nutrition, *Annu Rev Nutr* 15:399, 1995.

Thomas MK et al: Hypovitaminosis D in medical patients, *N Engl J Med* 338:777, 1998.

Thorogood M: The epidemiology of vegetarianism and health, *Nutr Res Rev* 8:179, 1995.

Tran MT et al: Role of coenzyme Q_{10} in chronic heart failure, angina, and hypertension, *Pharmacotherapy* 21:797, 2001.

U.S. Department of Agriculture: Agriculture Research Service Quarterly Report, *Human nutrition,* 2000, www.ars.usda.gov/is/qtr.

Utiger RD: The need for more vitamin D, *N Engl J Med* 338:828, 1998.

Vermeer C et al: Effects of vitamin K on bone mass and bone metabolism, *J Nutr* 126:1187, 1996.

Wagner C: Symposium on the subcellular compartmentalization of folate metabolism, *J Nutr* 126:1228, 1996.

Watts et al: Coenzyme Q_{10} improves endothelial dysfunction of the brachial artery in Type II diabetes mellitus, *Diabetologia* 45:420, 2002.

Wilson CW, Loh HS: Common cold and vitamin C, *Lancet* 1:638, 1973.

Willett WC, Stampfer MJ: What vitamin should I be taking, doctor? *N Engl J Med* 345:1819, 2001.

Zeisel SH, Blusztajn JK: Choline and human nutrition, *Annu Rev Nutr* 14:269, 1994.

Additional References

Vitamin A

Goldberg J: Vitamin A and eyesight, *Am J Epidemiol* 128:700, 1988.

Krinsky NI: Carotenoids and cancer: basic research studies. In Frei B, ed: Natural antioxidants in human health and disease, New York, 1994, Academic Press.

Mijewski S et al: Decreased levels of vitamin A in serum of patients with psoriasis, *Arch Dermatol Res* 280:499, 1989.

Palozza P: Prooxidant actions of carotenoids in biologic systems, *Nutr Rev* 56:257, 1998.

Vitamin D

Abrams S. Nutritional rickets: an old disease returns, *Nutr Rev* 60:79, 2002.

Bonner F, Stein W: Calcium homeostasis—an old problem revisited, *J Nutr* 125:1987S, 1995.

Burckhardt P: Calcium and vitamin D in osteoporosis: supplementation or treatment? *Calcif Tissue Int* 70:74, 2002.

Looker AC, Gunter EW: Hypovitaminosis D in medical patients, Letter, *N Engl J Med* 339:344, 1998.

Prentice A: What are the dietary requirements of calcium and vitamin D? *Calcif Tissue Int* 70:83, 2002.

Season, latitude, and ability of sunlight to promote synthesis of vitamin D_3 in skin, *Nutr Rev* 47:252, 1989.

Vitamin E

Allen RG: Oxygen-reactive species and antioxidant responses during development: the metabolic paradox of cellular differentiation, *Proc Soc Exp Biol Med* 196:117, 1991.

Azzi A, Ricciarelli R, Zingg JM: Non-antioxidant molecular functions of alpha-tocopherol (vitamin E), *FEBS Lett* 519:8, 2002.

Cohn W et al: Tocopherol transport and absorption, *Proc Nutr Soc* 51:179, 1992.

Maeda H, Akaike T: Oxygen free radicals as pathogenic molecules in viral diseases, *Proc Soc Exp Biol Med* 198:721, 1991.

Vitamin K

Dowd P et al: The mechanism of action of vitamin K, *Annu Rev Nutr* 15:419, 1995.

Furie B, Furie BC: Molecular basis of vitamin K–dependent carboxylation, *Blood* 75:1753, 1990.

Shearer MJ: Vitamin K, *Lancet* 345:229, 1995.

Thiamin

Carpenter KJ: *Beriberi, white rice, and vitamin B: a disease, a cause, a cure,* Berkeley, Calif, 2000, University of California Press.

Rindi G: Thiamin. In Ziegler EE, Filer LJ Jr, eds: *Present knowledge in nutrition,* ed 7, Washington, DC, 1996, ILSI Press.

Riboflavin

McCormick D: Riboflavin. In Shils M et al, eds: *Modern nutrition in health and disease,* ed 8, Philadelphia, 1994, Lea & Febiger.

Rivlin RS: Riboflavin. In Ziegler EE, Filer LJ Jr, eds: *Present knowledge in nutrition,* ed 7, Washington, DC, 1996, ILSI Press.

Niacin

Jacob RA, Swendseid ME: Niacin. In Ziegler EE, Filer LJ Jr, eds: *Present knowledge in nutrition,* ed 7, Washington, DC, 1996, ILSI Press.

Preuss HG, Bagchi D, Bagchi M: Protective effects of a novel niacin-bound chromium complex and a grape seed proanthocyanidin extract on advancing age and various aspects of syndrome X, *Ann N Y Acad Sci* 957:250, 2002.

Vitamin B_6

Driskell J: Vitamin B_6 requirements of humans, *Nutr Res* 14(2):293, 1994.

Gospe SM: Pyridoxine-dependent seizures: findings from recent studies pose new questions, *Pediatr Neurol* 26:181, 2002.

Lecklem J: Vitamin B_6. In Ziegler EE, Filer LJ, eds: *Present knowledge in nutrition,* ed 7, Washington, DC, 1996, ILSI Press.

Folate

Antony AC: Folate receptors, *Annu Rev Nutr* 16:501, 1996.

Bailey LB: Dietary reference intakes for folate: the debut of dietary folate equivalents, *Nutr Rev* 56:294, 1998.

Moyers S, Bailey LB: Fetal malformation and folate metabolism: review of recent evidence, *Nutr Rev* 59:215, 2001.

Vitamin B_{12}

Drazkowski J, Sirven J, Blum D: Symptoms of B12 deficiency can occur in women of child bearing age supplemented with folate, *Neurol* 58:1572, 2002.

Herbert V: Vitamin B_{12}. In Ziegler EE, Filer LJ Jr, eds: *Present knowledge in nutrition,* ed 7, Washington, DC, ILSI Press.

Pantothenic Acid

Plesofsky-Vig N: Pantothenic acid. In Ziegler EE, Filer LJ Jr, eds: *Present knowledge in nutrition,* ed 7, Washington, DC, 1996, ILSI Press.

Tahiliani AG, Benlich CJ: Pantothenic acid in health and disease, *Vitam Horm* 46:165, 1991.

Biotin

A role for biotin in bone growth, *Nutr Rev* 47:157, 1989.

Dakshinamurti K: Biotin. In Shils M et al, eds: *Modern nutrition in health and disease,* ed 8, Philadelphia, 1994, Lea & Febiger.

Mock DM: Biotin. In Ziegler EE, Filer LJ Jr, eds: *Present knowledge in nutrition,* ed 7, Washington, DC, 1996, ILSI Press.

Vitamin C

Hemilä H: Vitamin C intake and susceptibility to the common cold, *Br J Nutr* 77:59, 1997.

Jacob R: Vitamin C. In Shils M et al, eds: *Modern nutrition in health and disease,* ed 8, Philadelphia, 1994, Lea & Febiger.

Machlin LJ, Bendich A: Free radical tissue damage: protective role of antioxidant nutrients, *FASEB J* 1:441, 1988.

Pauling L: *Vitamin C and the common cold,* San Francisco, 1970, Freeman.

Choline

Zeisel SH: Choline. In Shils ME et al, eds: *Modern nutrition in health and disease,* ed 8, vol 1, Philadelphia, 1994, Lea & Febiger.

Carnitine

Metabolic effects of carnitine supplementation in subjects with low plasma carnitine levels, *Nutr Rev* 48:159, 1990.

Rebouche CJ, Paulson DJ: Carnitine metabolism and function in humans, *Annu Rev Nutr* 6:41, 1986.

myo-Inositol

Aukema HM, Holub BJ: Inositol. In Shils ME et al, eds: *Modern nutrition in health and disease,* ed 8, vol 1, Philadelphia, 1994, Lea & Febiger.

Berdanier C: Is inositol an essential nutrient? *Nutrition Today* 22(2):18, 1987.

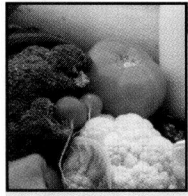

CHAPTER 5

Minerals

JOHN J.B. ANDERSON, PhD

CHAPTER OUTLINE

- Characteristics of Minerals
- Macrominerals
- Microminerals (Trace Elements)
- Ultratrace Minerals
- Other Trace Elements

KEY TERMS

bioavailability–the availability of a mineral within the small intestine for absorption and the actual absorption (efficiency) of the mineral; implies retention of the mineral in the body and its use in cellular or tissue functions

calbindins–calcium-binding proteins found in intestinal absorbing cells and other cells of the body

ceruloplasmin–a plasma protein that transports copper and acts as an oxidase (enzyme)

cretinism–a congenital condition typically caused by severe iodine deficiency during gestation; characterized by arrested physical and mental development and subnormal intelligence

ferritin–an iron-apoferritin complex that is the major storage form of iron in the liver and other tissues

glucose tolerance factor (GTF)–a biologically active chromium complex found in foods; unknown structure

glutathione peroxidase (GSH-Px)–a selenium-containing enzyme that is the major active form of selenium in cells

goiter–a chronic enlargement of the thyroid gland, visible as a swelling at the front of the neck; commonly associated with iodine deficiency

goitrogens–compounds that block the uptake and utilization of iodine by thyroid cells and contribute to iodine deficiency and goiter

heme iron–the nonprotein, insoluble, iron-containing protoporphyrin that is a constituent of hemoglobin, myoglobin, and a few other proteins

hemoglobin–a conjugated protein containing four heme groups and globin, with the property of reversible oxygenation

hemosiderin–a complex insoluble form of storage iron

hydroxyapatite–a crystalline structure in bone consisting of calcium phosphate and calcium carbonate

hypercalciuria–excessive urinary losses of calcium that may occur in individuals who have excessive intestinal absorption of calcium or high protein intakes, especially of animal protein

macrominerals (bulk elements)–minerals required by humans in amounts of 100 mg/day or more (i.e., in large quantities)

metallothionein–a nonenzymatic, zinc-binding protein found in intestinal absorbing cells and other tissues of the body, especially the liver

microminerals (trace elements)–minerals required by humans in amounts of less than 100 mg/day (i.e., in quantities of a few milligrams or even micrograms)

myoglobin–an oxygen-storing iron protoporphyrin-globin complex in striated muscle

nonheme iron–the form of iron found in plants; less well absorbed than heme iron

oxalic acid (oxalate)–an organic acid that is found in certain leafy vegetables; binds with calcium and other divalent cations, thereby inhibiting their absorption from foods

phytic acid (phytate)–a phosphorus-containing compound that is found in the outer husks of cereal grains; binds with minerals and inhibits absorption

s-containing amino acids–sulfur-containing amino acids, methionine and cysteine, which provide the bulk of the sulfur used in organic reactions.

tetany–muscle twitching, spasms, and (eventually) convulsions caused by low blood levels of calcium or magnesium

thyroxine (T_4) –an iodine-containing hormone secreted by the thyroid gland to regulate the rate of cell metabolism

transferrin–a protein that is synthesized in the liver and transports iron in the blood to the erythroblasts for use in heme synthesis and to all other tissues; also carries chromium and a few other cations in blood, especially from the small intestine to tissues

triiodothyronine (T_3) –an iodine-containing thyroid hormone with several times more biologic activity than thyroxine

ultratrace elements–minerals in the body, each of which exists in small quantities and is typically measured in micrograms

The minerals are a large class of micronutrients, most of which are considered essential. They are traditionally divided into *macrominerals (bulk elements)* and *microminerals (trace elements)*. More recently, the term ultratrace elements has been used to describe elements that are consumed in microgram (μg) quantities each day. Macrominerals such as calcium and phosphorus are required in amounts of 100 mg/day or more, whereas microminerals such as iron and selenium are required in much smaller amounts, typically less than 15 mg/day. Knowledge about the trace elements has expanded over the past few decades because of greatly improved analytic techniques. Because less information has been generated about the essentiality of a few of the ultratrace elements for human health, this group is addressed only briefly in the final section of this chapter.

Except for the few "other trace elements," fluoride, and possibly boron, all minerals covered in this chapter are recognized as essential for human function, even though specific requirements have not been established for a few of them. (Fluoride's essentiality remains in question because it has no known cellular role; see the Fluoride section.) Studies of patients receiving long-term total parenteral nutrition (TPN) have helped to determine the essentiality and the required amounts of several ultratrace elements.

CHARACTERISTICS OF MINERALS

Macrominerals exist in the body and food chiefly in the ionic state. For example, sodium, potassium, and calcium form positive ions (cations), whereas other minerals exist as negative ions (anions). The latter include chlorine (as chloride), sulfur (as sulfate), and phosphorus (as phosphates). Salts such as sodium chloride and calcium phosphate dissociate in solution, existing in body fluids and crystals as Na^+, Cl^-, Ca^{2++}, and HPO_4^{2-}. Minerals also exist as components of organic compounds such as phosphoproteins, phospholipids, metalloenzymes, and other metalloproteins such as hemoglobin. (See Chapter 6 for a discussion of the electrolytes sodium, potassium, and chloride.)

Bioavailability

Bioavailability has become a useful term in recent years to describe the chemical or physiochemical state of minerals within the lumen of the small intestine (Fairweather-Tait and Hurrell, 1996). With the exception of heme iron, other elements are absorbed in the ionic state. Therefore any elements that remain bound to organic molecules or other inorganic complexes after the digestive steps are completed are not absorbed; that is, they are not bioavailable, and these unabsorbed minerals are eliminated in the feces. (A few elements such as iron may be absorbed in a chelated form when intake from foods is inadequate.) After the ions are absorbed at the brush borders of the columnar intestinal epithelial cells or enterocytes, which are often referred to as the *mucosal surface,* they still must transfer through the cytosol of the absorbing cells before they are transported across the basolateral (serosal) membrane to the blood. This exit step of the absorptive process typically requires an active transport mechanism, at least for the mineral cations. If the cationic forms of the elements are not transported across the basolateral membrane, they remain in the absorbing cells bound to proteins. For example, calcium ions bind to calbindins, iron to intestinal ferritin, and zinc to metallothionein, only to be excreted when the intestinal cells die and slough off into the intestinal lumen. (The low intestinal absorption efficiencies of these cations may have evolved to protect the body against potential toxicities that result from excessive absorption.) For example, low bioavailability may also result from the formation of soaps, from calcium and magnesium binding to free fatty acids in the lumen, in fat malabsorption, and from precipitation when one of a pair of ions (e.g., calcium, which combines with phosphates) is present in the lumen in a very high concentration. Mineral-mineral interactions also can result in depressed absorption of elements or reduce their bioavailability.

Many molecules in foods influence bioavailability, either by enhancing absorption or interfering with or inhibiting absorption. Examples of inhibitors include the binding by phytates and oxalates of calcium and other divalent cations. Enhancers include ascorbate for nonheme iron. Vegetarians tend to consume foods with higher quantities of many of the inhibiting factors, but they typically also ingest more ascorbic acid, an enhancer. In addition, the bioavailability of elements may be influenced by many physiologic factors, such as gastric acidity, homeostatic adaptations, and stress (that affect gastrointestinal [GI] function). Bioavailability also is equated with absorption of a mineral element after its digestion from food and before its use in tissue and cells. Bioavailability cannot be quantified easily when its meaning is intended to include use in tissues or cells.

In general, certain elements typically have a low bioavailability from foods (e.g., iron, chromium, manganese), whereas others have a high bioavailability (e.g., sodium, potassium, chloride, iodide, fluoride). Other minerals, including calcium and magnesium, have a medium bioavailability. (See following discussion and Chapter 27 for additional information on calcium bioavailability.)

Mineral-Mineral Interactions

Minerals can have negative interactions with other minerals, potentially affecting intestinal absorption, transport, use, and storage. For example, the absorption of zinc is typically reduced by nonheme iron supplementation, excessive intake of zinc reduces the absorption of copper, and excessive intake of calcium may reduce the absorption of manganese, zinc, and iron (Wood and Zheng, 1997). However, interaction studies are difficult to conduct, and definitive conclusions about the cited interactions await additional investigation. Other examples of interactions are discussed in the sections on the individual elements.

Mineral Composition of the Body

Minerals represent about 4% to 5% of body weight, or 2.8 to 3.5 kg in adult women and men, respectively. Approximately 50% of this weight is calcium, and another 25% is phosphorus, existing as phosphates; almost 99% of the calcium and 70% of the phosphates are found in bones and teeth. The five other essential macrominerals (magnesium, sodium, potassium, chloride, and sulfur) and the eleven established microminerals (iron, zinc, iodide, selenium, manganese, fluoride, molybdenum, copper, chromium, cobalt, and boron) constitute the remaining 25%. The ultratrace elements without established essentiality for humans, such as arsenic, aluminum, tin, nickel, vanadium, and silicon, provide a negligible amount of weight.

Functions

Mineral elements have many essential roles, including serving as ions dissolved in body fluids and as constituents of essential molecules. The mineral ions in body fluids regulate the activities of many enzymes, maintain acid-base balance and osmotic pressure, facilitate the membrane transfer of essential nutrients and other molecules, and maintain nerve and muscular irritability. In some cases, mineral ions are structural constituents of extracellular body tissues such as bones and teeth. Several minerals such as zinc and iron are involved in different ways in the growth process as well. Selenium functions in cells only as a component of selenoproteins (Burk et al, 1998; 2001). Several minerals such as zinc and selenium have roles in immune function, but specific mechanisms have been difficult to identify (Bogden and Louria, 1999; Fortes et al, 1998; Giordon et al, 1999; Shankar and Prasad, 1998). Clearly, in very young individuals and older adults, nutrient deficits, including those of energy and protein, diminish immune responses, especially those related to cell-mediated immunity because of low mineral intakes (Lesourd, 1997).

Problem Minerals in the U.S. Diet

A few minerals such as calcium and iron continue to be consumed in less than optimal amounts by a large percentage of people in the United States. The intakes of magnesium, zinc, and possibly a couple of other trace minerals are also generally insufficient in the population. In the last decade, fortification of foods, especially of ready-to-eat cereals, has improved intakes of iron and zinc but not calcium (Berner et al, 2001), although the mean intakes still do not meet dietary reference intake (DRI) levels.

Prebiotics and Minerals

Nondigestible oligosaccharides (NDOs), which by definition are fermented by intestinal bacteria, stimulate the intestinal absorption and retention of several minerals, including calcium, magnesium, zinc, and iron (Scholz-Ahrens et al, 2001). In human investigations, NDOs have been shown to increase absorption and presumably skeletal retention of these minerals (van den Heuvel et al, 1999). Whereas NDOs have been studied primarily in animal models, they will probably become components of functional foods in the near future as they are studied more in humans.

MACROMINERALS

The macrominerals (bulk elements) that are essential for adult humans in amounts of 100 mg/day or more are calcium, phosphorus (phosphates), magnesium, sulfur (sulfate), sodium, chloride, and potassium. (Sodium, potassium, and chloride are discussed in Chapter 6.) Except for sulfur, these minerals typically exist in the ionic state as inorganic components in the body. Many organic molecules also contain phosphorus-containing groups, such as phospholipids and nucleotides that are not in a free ionic form.

Calcium

Calcium, the most abundant mineral in the body, makes up about 1.5% to 2% of the body weight and 39% of total body minerals. Approximately 99% of the calcium exists in the bones and teeth. (However, the calcium in teeth cannot be mobilized back to the blood because the minerals of erupted teeth are fixed for life.) The remaining 1% of calcium is in the blood and extracellular fluids and within the cells of all tissues, where it regulates many important metabolic functions. Figure 5-1 illustrates the pathways of calcium metabolism.

The skeleton is not simply a store of calcium and other minerals, it is also a dynamic tissue that returns calcium and other minerals to the extracellular fluids and blood on demand. Bone also takes up calcium and other minerals from the blood when they are consumed (i.e., during the postprandial period). However, late in life, bone retention of calcium derived from food and supplements is limited unless the calcium is consumed along with sufficient vitamin D or a bone-conserving drug. (The roles of calcium in bone metabolism are discussed in Chapter 27.)

Absorption, Transport, Storage, and Excretion

Calcium is absorbed by all parts of the small intestine, but the most rapid absorption after a meal occurs in the duodenum, where an acidic medium (pH <7) prevails. Absorption is slower in the remainder of the small bowel because of the alkaline pH, but the amount of calcium absorbed is actually greater in the lower segments of the small intestine, including the ileum.

Usually only 30% (or slightly less) of ingested calcium is absorbed by adults, but a few individuals may absorb as little as 10%. Although rare, some adults can absorb as much as 60% of ingested calcium.

Calcium is absorbed by two mechanisms: (1) *active transport,* which operates predominantly at low luminal concentrations of calcium ions, and (2) *passive transfer,* or paracellular movement, which operates at high luminal concentrations of calcium ions. The active transport mechanism, mainly in the duodenum and proximal jejunum, has limited capacity, and it is controlled through the action of 1,25-dihydroxyvitamin D (1,25[OH]$_2$D$_3$), or vitamin D. This hormone increases calcium uptake at the brush border of the intestinal mucosal cell by an incompletely understood

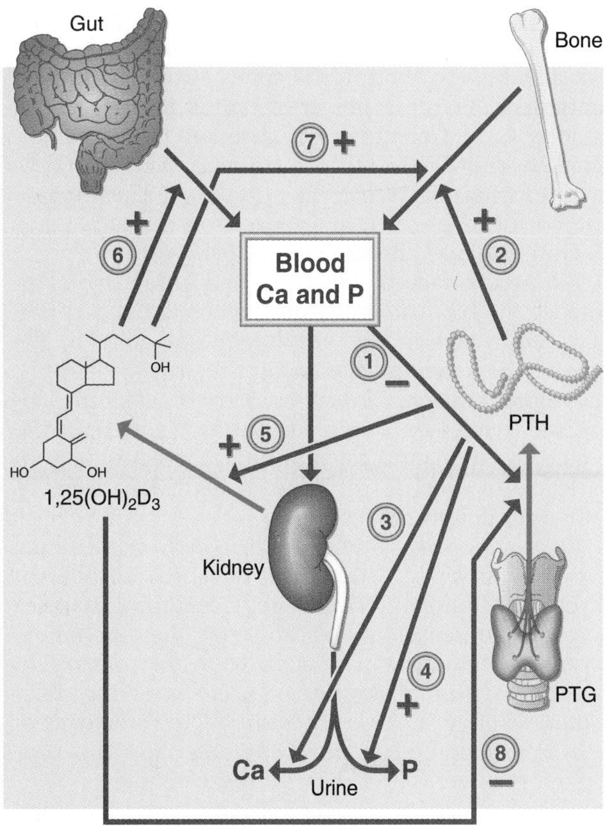

FIGURE 5-1 • Pathways of calcium metabolism. The regulation of calcium metabolism involves intestinal absorption (gut), blood calcium *(Ca)* and phosphate *(P)* concentrations, bone, the kidneys—which produce the hormonal form of vitamin D (1,25)[OH]$_2$D$_3$—and the parathyroid glands *(PTG),* which secrete parathyroid hormone *(PTH).* Steps 1 through 8 are specific regulation points. A low serum calcium or high serum phosphate level stimulates PTH secretion *(Step 1)* through negative feedback.

mechanism, and it also stimulates the production of calcium-binding proteins, or calbindins. The second transfer mechanism, which is passive, nonsaturable (with no limit), and independent of vitamin D, occurs along the entire length of the small intestine. When large amounts of calcium are consumed in a single meal (e.g., from a dairy food or a supplement), much of the calcium that is absorbed occurs by this passive route. The active transport mechanism becomes much more important when calcium intakes are low and body requirements are not being met—that is, at levels typically well below recommended intakes at any stage of the life cycle.

The role of calbindins in the actions of the intestinal absorbing cells is to store calcium ions temporarily after a meal and ferry them to the basolateral membrane for the final step of absorption. The calcium-binding proteins bind two or more calcium ions per protein molecule within the cytosol.

Most calcium is absorbed in the lower half of the small intestine, including by the ileum, as shown by the devastating effect surgical removal of the ileum has on calcium metabolism (see Chapter 30). Calcium can also be absorbed in the colon but only in small amounts. Calcium is absorbed only if it is present in an ionic form. Calcium is not absorbed if it is precipitated by another dietary constituent such as oxalate or if it forms soap with free fatty acids. These unabsorbed forms of calcium are excreted in the feces as calcium oxalates and calcium soaps.

Numerous factors, favorable and unfavorable, influence the bioavailability and hence the absorption of calcium within the gut lumen. In general, the greater the need and the smaller the dietary supply, the more efficient the absorption of calcium. Increased needs encountered during growth, pregnancy, lactation, and calcium-deficient states, as well as levels of exercise resulting in high bone density, enhance calcium absorption.

As mentioned, vitamin D in its active hormonal form, $1{,}25(OH)_2D_3$, stimulates intestinal absorption through a complex series of steps, including transfer across the mucosal brush border into the blood. Low vitamin D intake or inadequate exposure to sunlight reduces calcium absorption, especially among older adults (Gloth et al, 1995). In addition, the efficiency of skin production of vitamin D by older adults is considerably lower than that of younger people.

Calcium is best absorbed in an acidic medium; thus the hydrochloric acid secreted in the stomach, such as that secreted during a meal, increases calcium absorption by lowering the pH in the proximal duodenum. This also applies to calcium supplements; therefore taking a calcium supplement with a meal improves absorption, especially in older adults (see Chapter 27). Lactose enhances calcium absorption. Even in adults with lactose intolerance, lactose probably improves calcium absorption (see Chapter 30).

Oxalic acid (oxalate) in rhubarb, spinach, chard, and beet greens forms insoluble calcium oxalate in the digestive tract. For example, only 5% of the calcium in spinach is absorbed. Phytic acid (phytate), a phosphorus-containing compound found principally in the outer husks of cereal grains, combines with calcium to form calcium phytate, which is also insoluble and cannot be absorbed.

Dietary fiber may decrease calcium absorption, but this may only be a problem for those who consume large amounts of fiber (i.e., more than 30 g/day). Less fiber has little effect on calcium availability in the gut lumen and hence on absorption. Medications can affect bioavailability or increase calcium excretion, both of which may contribute to bone loss (see Chapter 19). Aging is characterized by decreased calcium absorption efficiency, probably because of achlorhydria (a lack of gastric acid secretion) and a blunted adaptive response of vitamin D to a decreased calcium intake (see Chapter 13).

In individuals with fat malabsorption, calcium absorption is decreased because of the formation of calcium–fatty acid soaps. Calcium absorption does not seem to be affected by the amount of phosphate in the diet unless the intake of phosphate is excessively high, or by the calcium/phosphorus ratio (see following discussion on phosphorus).

Renal Excretion

Normally, just more than 50% of the ingested calcium is excreted in the urine each day, but an almost equivalent amount is also secreted into the intestine (and joins unabsorbed calcium in the feces). Calcium resorption from the renal tubules occurs by transport mechanisms similar to those in the small intestine. Urinary calcium excretion varies throughout the life cycle, but it is typically low during periods of rapid skeletal growth. At menopause, calcium excretion increases greatly, but in postmenopausal women treated with estrogen, less calcium is excreted. After approximately 65 years of age, calcium excretion decreases, most likely because of decreased intestinal absorption of calcium. In general, urinary calcium levels correlate well with calcium intake.

A high urinary calcium excretion level, or hypercalciuria, induced experimentally by a diet high in animal protein occurs because of the generation of inorganic acids such as sulfuric acid from the sulfur-containing amino acids methionine and cysteine. However, this hypercalciuric effect has not been established in long-term studies of populations with diets high in meat, possibly because the elevated serum phosphate level partially counters the acid effect on the kidneys. A high serum concentration of phosphate induces an increase in parathyroid hormone (PTH) secretion, which leads to a decrease in renal calcium excretion. Consumption of several cups of caffeinated coffee daily increases urinary calcium loss, but results from studies have not been consistent. A high sodium intake also contributes to lower renal resorption of calcium and higher urinary calcium losses.

Skin Losses

Dermal losses of calcium occur in the form of skin exfoliation and sweat. The amount of calcium lost in sweat is about 15 mg/day. Strenuous physical activity with sweating increases the loss, even in persons with a low calcium intake.

Serum Calcium

Total serum calcium consists of three distinct fractions: (1) free, or ionized, calcium (47.6%); complexes between calcium and anions such as phosphate, citrate, or other organic anions (6.4%); and calcium that is protein bound, primarily with albumin (46%). Serum albumin binds between 70% and 90% of the calcium that is protein bound.

Ionized calcium (Ca^{2++}), the regulated form, equilibrates rapidly with protein-bound calcium in blood.

The serum ionized calcium concentration is controlled primarily by PTH, the hormone secreted by the parathyroid glands, although other hormones have minor roles in its regulation. These other hormones include calcitonin, vitamin D, estrogens, and others (see the following section). The total serum calcium level is maintained within a narrow range of 8.8 to 10.8 mg/dl, of which the ionized calcium concentrations range from 4.4 to 5.2 mg/dl. (Serum calcium level values higher than the upper limit of normal are defined as *hypercalcemic,* whereas values below the lower limit are *hypocalcemic.* Each abnormal level has a physical significant risk.) Serum levels of calcium are highest early in life, gradually decreasing throughout life and reaching the lowest levels during the older years.

Several factors affect the relative distribution of calcium in blood serum or plasma. One of these is pH; the ionized fraction is higher in acidosis and lower in alkalosis. Total calcium changes concurrently with changes in plasma protein levels; however, the ionized fraction usually remains within normal limits. The strict regulation of ionized calcium makes it a useful diagnostic tool in assessing parathyroid gland function, monitoring kidney disease, and monitoring sick neonates for whom hypocalcemia could be life-threatening.

Regulation of Serum Calcium

Calcium in bones is in equilibrium with calcium in the blood. PTH plays the major role in maintaining serum calcium at a normal concentration of about 10 mg/100 ml of blood serum (2.5 mmol/L). (The physiologic role of calcitonin in this regulation is not well established.) When the blood calcium concentration falls below this level, PTH stimulates the transfer of exchangeable calcium from the bone into the blood. At the same time, PTH promotes renal tubular resorption of calcium, and it indirectly stimulates increased intestinal absorption of calcium via the hormonal form of vitamin D ($1,25[OH]_2D_3$).

Other hormones such as glucocorticoids, thyroid hormones, and sex hormones also have important roles in calcium homeostasis. Glucocorticoids may impair calcium absorption through active and passive mechanisms. Glucocorticoid excess leads to bone loss, particularly of trabecular bone—a condition commonly found in patients receiving chronic glucocorticoid therapy at doses of 20 mg/day or higher. Thyroid hormones (T_4 and T_3) may stimulate bone resorption; chronic hyperthyroid conditions result in loss of compact and trabecular bone. In women, normal bone balance requires serum estrogen concentrations to be within normal limits. The rapid decrease of the serum estrogen concentration during menopause is a major factor contributing to bone resorption. Treating postmenopausal women with estrogen slows the rate of bone resorption (see Chapter 27). Bone resorption is also inhibited by testosterone.

Functions

Adequate dietary calcium is needed to permit optimal gains in bone mass and density in the prepubertal and adolescent years. These gains are especially critical for girls because the accumulated bone may provide additional protection against osteoporosis in the years after menopause. Peak calcium retention by girls has been shown to occur in the prepubertal and early pubertal periods (Abrams and Stuff, 1994). Other studies also support the importance of young girls obtaining sufficient calcium for bone development (Jackman et al, 1997; Matkovic et al, 1995) (see Chapter 27).

Postmenopausal women need to obtain sufficient amounts of calcium to maintain bone health and suppress PTH (McKane et al, 1996). The latter increases later in life in most individuals, perhaps as a result of inadequate calcium in the diet (see Chapters 13 and 27). Additional amounts of calcium are recommended to meet the needs of pregnancy and lactation. Calcium requirements during pregnancy, infancy, childhood, and adolescence are discussed in detail in Chapters 7 through 11. In addition to its function in building and maintaining bones and teeth, calcium also has numerous metabolic roles in cells in all other tissues. However, compared with the significant needs of the skeleton, only small amounts of calcium are required for all other cellular and extracellular functions.

The transport functions of cell membranes are influenced by calcium, which affects membrane stability in poorly understood ways. Calcium also influences the transmission of ions across membranes of cell organelles, the release of neurotransmitters at synaptic junctions, the function of hormones, and the release or activation of intracellular and extracellular enzymes.

Calcium is required for nerve transmission and regulation of heart muscle function. The proper balance of calcium, sodium, potassium, and magnesium ions maintains skeletal muscle tone and controls nerve irritability. A significant increase in the serum calcium level can cause cardiac or respiratory failure, whereas a decrease results in tetany of skeletal muscles. In addition, calcium ions play a critical role in smooth muscle contractility.

Ionized calcium initiates the formation of a blood clot by stimulating the release of thromboplastin from blood platelets. Calcium ions also serve as required cofactors for several enzymatic reactions, including the conversion of prothrombin to thrombin, which aids in the polymerization of fibrinogen to fibrin and the final step in blood clot formation.

Dietary Reference Intakes

The adequate intake (AI) for calcium recommended by the Food and Nutrition Board (1997) is based on estimates of requirements of both genders throughout the life cycle (Table 5-1) The tolerable upper intake level (UL) has also been established for this nutrient for the first time (Table 5-2). During several periods of the female life cycle, calcium intake is critical: prepuberty and adolescence, postmenopause, and during pregnancy and lactation. In a study of adolescent girls, calcium intakes of 1300 mg or more each day were necessary for maximal calcium retention by the body's skeleton (Yates et al, 1998). Men also need adequate amounts of calcium throughout the life cycle, but less is known about their requirements.

Food Sources and Intakes

Dark green leafy vegetables such as kale, collards, turnip greens, mustard greens, and broccoli; the small bones of sardines and canned salmon; and clams and oysters are good sources of calcium. Soybeans also contain ample amounts of calcium. Oxalic acid limits the availability of calcium in rhubarb, spinach, chard, and beet greens. Fortified orange juice contains as much calcium as milk. Tofu prepared by calcium precipitation is also a good source of calcium. Table 5-3 shows the calcium content of selected foods. Commercial bread and other wheat products prepared with calcium propionate are also good sources of calcium.

Calcium supplements are now commonly used to increase calcium intakes. The most common form is calcium carbonate, which is relatively insoluble, particularly at a neutral pH. Although it has less calcium than calcium carbonate by weight, calcium citrate is much more soluble. Therefore calcium citrate would be suitable for patients with achlorhydria (lack of hydrochloric acid in the stomach). In patients with achlorhydria the efficiency of calcium absorption is greatly decreased because of the higher pH of the stomach contents; however, calcium absorption is increased by the consumption of a meal, which improves the gastric solubility of calcium ions (Recker, 1985). The selection of the most appropriate calcium supplement depends on several factors, including physical and chemical properties, interactions with other medicines being taken concurrently, current medical conditions, and age (Levenson and Bockman, 1994). Beginning at the age of 11 years, median

TABLE 5-1 Dietary Reference Intakes: Calcium, Phosphorus, and Magnesium

AGE/LIFE STAGE	CALCIUM (mg/day)*	PHOSPHORUS (mg/day)*	MAGNESIUM (mg/day)*
Infants			
0-6 mo	210	100	30
7-12 mo	270	275	75
Children			
1-3 yr	500	**460**	**80**
4-8 yr	800	**500**	**130**
Males			
9-13 yr	1300	**1250**	**240**
14-18 yr	1300	**1250**	**410**
19-30 yr	1000	**700**	**400**
31-50 yr	1000	**700**	**420**
51-70 yr	1200	**700**	**420**
>70 yr	1200	**700**	**420**
Females			
9-13 yr	1300	**1250**	**240**
14-18 yr	1300	**1250**	**360**
19-30 yr	1000	**700**	**310**
31-50 yr	1000	**700**	**320**
51-70 yr	1200	**700**	**320**
>70 yr	1200	**700**	**320**
Pregnant			
≤18 yr	1300	**1250**	**400**
19-30 yr	1000	**700**	**360**
31-50 yr	1000	**700**	**320**
Lactating			
≤18 yr	1300	**1250**	**360**
19-30 yr	1000	**700**	**310**
31-50 yr	1000	**700**	**320**

From Food and Nutrition Board, National Academy of Sciences, Institute of Medicine: *Dietary reference intakes for calcium, phosphorus, magnesium, vitamin D, and fluoride,* Washington, DC, 1997, National Academy Press.

**Bold values* are recommended dietary allowances (RDAs). *Other (nonbold) values* are adequate intakes (AIs).

TABLE 5-2 Tolerable Upper Intake Levels: Calcium, Phosphorus, and Magnesium

AGE/LIFE STAGE	CALCIUM (mg/day)	PHOSPHORUS (g/day)	MAGNESIUM (mg/day)
Infants			
0-6 mo	—	—	—
7-12 mo	—	—	—
Children			
1-3 yr	2500	3	65
4-8 yr	2500	3	110
Males			
9-13 yr	2500	4	350
14-18 yr	2500	4	350
19-30 yr	2500	4	350
31-50 yr	2500	4	350
51-70 yr	2500	4	350
>70 yr	2500	3	350
Females			
9-13 yr	2500	4	350
14-18 yr	2500	4	350
19-30 yr	2500	4	350
31-50 yr	2500	4	350
51-70 yr	2500	4	350
>70 yr	2500	3	350
Pregnant			
≤18 yr	2500	3.5	350
19-30 yr	2500	3.5	350
31-50 yr	2500	3.5	350
Lactating			
≤18 yr	2500	4	350
19-30 yr	2500	4	350
31-50 yr	2500	4	350

From Food and Nutrition Board, National Academy of Sciences, Institute of Medicine: *Dietary reference intakes for calcium, phosphorus, magnesium, vitamin D, and fluoride,* Washington, DC, 1997, National Academy Press.

dietary calcium intakes in the United States are considerably less than the AIs (Figure 5-2). Therefore calcium intakes of Americans are insufficient for the critical ages of bone deposition in both genders, as well as being inadequate at other critical stages.

According to the Continuing Survey of Food Intakes of Individuals (CSFII) (U.S. Department of Agriculture, 1994), the most commonly consumed food sources of calcium in the U.S. diet are milk, cheese, bread, ice cream, sherbet, and frozen yogurt, in addition to cakes, cookies, quick breads, and doughnuts (Subar et al, 1998).

Deficiency

The development of peak bone mass requires adequate amounts of calcium and phosphorus, vitamin D, and other nutrients. Compared with adulthood, greater amounts of calcium and phosphate are required for skeletal development; therefore adequate intakes of these minerals and others have a significant impact on peak bone mass development until the time of puberty and throughout adolescence. After adolescence, bone gains may still occur, but the amounts of calcium required decrease. Vitamin D status may or may not be a problem, depending on the intakes of calcium and phosphorus. Almost any time during the life cycle when the calcium intake is well below the recommended amount, PTH concentrations in the blood increase. A persistent elevation may contribute to low bone mass (see the Phosphorus section in this chapter and Chapter 27). Calcium and vitamin D intakes of most older women are inadequate (Dawson-Hughes, 1996).

An inadequate intake of calcium, in addition to an inadequate intake of vitamin D, has also been demonstrated to contribute to osteomalacia (Marie et al, 1982) (see Chapters 4 and 27). A low calcium intake may be an important factor in several chronic diseases, such as colon cancer (see Chapter 40) and hypertension (see Chapter 36), that commonly occur in Western societies. Data from the Dietary Approaches to Stop Hypertension (DASH) study show that adequate dietary intakes of calcium, magnesium, potassium, and other micronutrients from low-fat dairy foods, fruits, and vegetables can both substantially reduce blood pressure in those with hypertension and prevent the development of hypertension (Appel et al, 1997) (see Chapter 36).

Toxicity

A very high intake of calcium (i.e., 2000 mg or more per day), especially in a person with a high level of vitamin D (e.g., from ingestion of combined supplements of calcium and vitamin D), is a potential cause of hypercalcemia. Such toxicity may lead to excessive calcification in soft tissues, especially the kidneys, which may be life-threatening. (The tolerable ULs for calcium are shown in Table 5-2.)

High intakes of calcium may also interfere with the absorption of other divalent cations such as iron, zinc, and manganese (Wood and Zheng, 1997). Therefore when a person needs to consume minerals as supplements, the iron supplement should be taken at a different time—that is, on an empty stomach if possible—whereas the calcium supplement should be taken with a meal. The same concerns have been expressed about the use of calcium supplements dur-

TABLE 5-3 Calcium Content of Selected Foods

FOOD	CONTENT (mg)
Yogurt, low fat, with fruit, 1 cup	345
Milk, skim, 1 cup	302
Ice milk, soft serve, 1 cup	274
Yogurt, frozen, 1 cup	240
Cheese, cheddar, 1 oz	204
Salmon, canned, with bones, 3½ oz	185
Ice cream, vanilla, 1 cup	176
Rhubarb, cooked, ½ cup	174
Cheese, cottage, 2% fat, 1 cup	155
Spinach, frozen, cooked, ½ cup	138
Molasses, blackstrap, 1 tbsp	137
Tofu, regular, ½ cup*	130
Milk, dry, instant, nonfat, 2 tbsp	104
Almonds, ¼ cup	92
Baked beans, white, ½ cup	64
Frankfurter, turkey, 1	58
Orange, 1 medium	52
Halibut, baked, 3 oz	51
Kale, fresh, cooked, ½ cup	47
Broccoli, cooked from fresh, ½ cup	36
Bread, whole wheat, 1 slice	32
Waffle, frozen, 4-inch diameter, 1	29
Cheese, cream, 2 tbsp	23
Oatmeal, cooked, 1 cup	19
Cream, half-and-half, 1 tbsp	16
Chicken, breast, baked, 3 oz	13
Banana, 1 medium	7
Ground beef, lean, 3 oz	4

From U.S. Department of Agriculture: *Composition of foods*, USDA Handbook No. 8 Series, Washington, DC, 1976-1986, Agricultural Research Service, The Department.
*Tofu prepared by calcium precipitation.

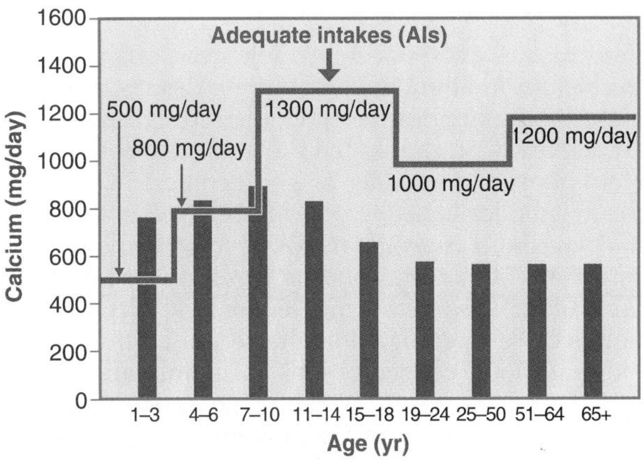

FIGURE 5-2 • Comparison of the median daily calcium intake for females in the United States and the AIs established in 1998.

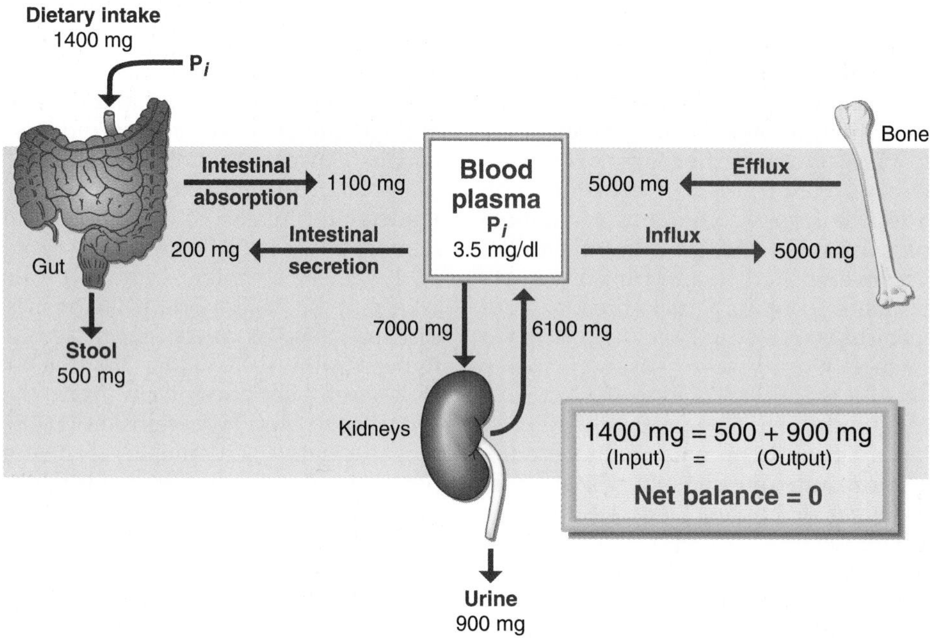

FIGURE 5-3 • Phosphorus balance is maintained primarily by the amount of phosphate absorbed versus the amount excreted by the kidneys and intestine. Bone is the major storage site for phosphate, as it is for calcium. The metabolic pathways share many similarities with the calcium pathways.

ing pregnancy. Another potential adverse, although not toxic per se, effect of excessive calcium intake is constipation. Constipation is common among older women who take calcium supplements.

Physical Immobility

Prolonged bed rest or periods of weightlessness during space travel promote significant calcium losses in response to a lack of tension or gravity on the bones. Older individuals who require a prolonged recovery with limited activity, such as those with hip fractures or other illnesses, also have increased calcium losses. Many studies have shown that physical activity promotes bone health.

Phosphorus

Phosphorus, another essential element, ranks second to calcium in abundance in human tissues; approximately 700 g of phosphorus exist in adult tissues, and about 85% is present in the skeleton and teeth as calcium phosphate crystals. The remaining 15% exists in the metabolically active pool in every cell in the body and in the extracellular fluid compartment. The serum inorganic phosphorus level is closely maintained by PTH at 3 to 4 mg/100 ml in adults, but it is not as closely regulated as the serum calcium level. Normal blood concentrations in infants are higher. In older adults, serum phosphate concentrations are typically lower; hypophosphatemia (<2.5 mg/dl) may be more common among older adults than previously thought. Phosphorus balance is illustrated in Figure 5-3 (see Chapter 27).

Almost 50% of the inorganic phosphate is present in serum as free ions (i.e., $H_2PO_4^-$ and HPO_4^{2-}. Smaller percentages are bound to protein (~10%) or complexed (~40%).

Absorption, Transport, Storage, and Excretion

The relative amounts of inorganic and organic phosphates in the diet vary with the food or supplement consumed. Regardless of the form, most phosphates are absorbed in the inorganic state. Organically bound phosphate is hydrolyzed in the lumen of the intestine and released as inorganic phosphate, primarily through the action of pancreatic or intestinal phosphatases. Bioavailability depends on the form of the phosphate and the pH. The acidic milieu of the most proximal portion of the duodenum is important in maintaining phosphorus solubility and therefore bioavailability. In vegetarian diets the major portion of the phosphorus is phytate, which is poorly digested by humans. Humans do not have the enzyme phytase to cleave the phosphorus from the phytate; however, intestinal bacteria have the enzyme needed to hydrolyze phosphates. The yeast used in making bread contains a phytase, which releases phosphate.

In general, the efficiency of phosphate absorption is 60% to 70% in adults, almost twice as high as for calcium; phosphate absorption is also much more rapid than that of calcium. For example, the peak of absorption of phosphates occurs approximately 1 hour after ingestion of a meal, whereas the peak for calcium entry into the blood occurs 3 to 4 hours after a meal (Anderson, 1996).

The primary route of phosphorus excretion is renal, which also is the primary site of phosphate regulation. Major determinants of urinary phosphorus loss are an increased intake of phosphate, an increase in phosphate absorption, and the plasma phosphorus concentration. Other factors contributing to increased urinary phosphate loss are hyperparathyroidism, acute respiratory or metabolic acidosis, the intake of diuretics, and the expansion of extracellular volume. If PTH levels are high, the urinary route excretes additional phosphate. Starvation or chronic undernutrition typically contributes to most of the alterations in metabolism that result in hypophosphatemia and renal losses of phosphate. Regulation of serum phosphate and hence urinary phosphate losses is not as precise as it is for calcium, but endogenous fecal phosphate excretion may be better regulated and provide a way to eliminate some of the excessive phosphate when PTH levels are elevated. The latter route of excretion may increase when the phosphate load in the blood and tissues is excessively high. Reduced phosphate excretion is associated with dietary phosphorus restriction; increases in plasma insulin, thyroid hormone, growth hormone, glucagon, or glucocorticoids; metabolic or respiratory alkalosis; and extracellular volume contraction.

Functions

As phosphates, phosphorus participates in numerous essential functions of the body. Deoxyribonucleic acid (DNA) and ribonucleic acid (RNA) are based on phosphate. The major cellular form of energy, adenosine triphosphate (ATP), contains high-energy phosphate bonds, as do creatinine phosphate and phosphoenolpyruvate. Cyclic adenosine monophosphate (cAMP) acts as a secondary signal within cells following peptide hormone activation of many membrane receptors. As part of phospholipids, phosphorus is present in every cell membrane in the body. Numerous phospholipid molecules also act as secondary messengers within the cytosol. Phosphorylation-dephosphorylation reactions control various steps in the activation or deactivation of cytosolic enzymes by kinases or phosphatases. Total intracellular concentrations of phosphate (but not ionic concentrations) are much higher than extracellular concentrations because phosphorylated compounds do not cross cell membranes easily and are trapped within the cell. The phosphate buffer system is important in intracellular fluid and the kidney tubules, where phosphate functions in the excretion of hydrogen ion. Filtered phosphate reacts with secreted hydrogen ions, releasing sodium in the process. In turn, the sodium can be reabsorbed under the influence of aldosterone (see Chapter 6).

Finally, phosphate ions combine with calcium ions to form hydroxyapatite, the major inorganic molecule in teeth and bones. The bone mineral, not the tooth mineral, provides phosphate ions via homeostatic regulation of serum calcium by PTH.

TABLE 5-4 Phosphorus Content of Selected Foods

FOOD	CONTENT (mg)
Macaroni and cheese, 1 cup	322
Sole, baked, 3 oz	248
Milk, 2% fat, 1 cup	232
Pizza, ⅛ of 15-inch diameter	216
Cheese, Swiss, processed, 1 oz	216
Split-pea soup, 1 cup	213
Ham, 3 oz	210
Ice milk, soft serve, 1 cup	202
Almonds, ¼ cup	184
Oatmeal, 1 cup	178
Lentils, cooked, ½ cup	178
Cheese, cottage, 2% fat, ½ cup	170
Cheese, cheddar, 1 oz	146
Yeast, brewer's, 1 tbsp	140
Shrimp, boiled, 2 large	137
Baked beans, white, ½ cup	137
Ground beef, cooked, 3 oz	135
Tofu, regular, ½ cup	120
Potato, baked, with skin, 1	115
Garbanzo beans, canned, ½ cup	108
Egg, 1	86
Bread, whole wheat, 1 slice	74
Peas, frozen, cooked, ½ cup	72
Cola beverage, 1 can, 12 oz	46
Potato chips, 14	43
Chocolate, dark, 1 oz	41
Bread, white, 1 slice	30
Lettuce, romaine, 1 cup	25
Cauliflower, fresh, ½ cup	23
Orange, 1	18

From U.S. Department of Agriculture: *Composition of foods*, USDA Handbook No. 8 Series, Washington, DC, 1976-1986, Agricultural Research Service, The Department.

Dietary Reference Intakes

In 1997, the Food and Nutrition Board recommended DRIs for phosphorus that are somewhat lower than those for calcium for all age groups (see Table 5-1). Tolerable ULs were also established (see Table 5-2) (Food and Nutrition Board, 1997).

Food Sources and Intakes

In general, good sources of protein are also good sources of phosphorus. Meat, poultry, fish, and eggs are excellent sources. Milk and milk products are good sources, as are nuts and legumes, cereals, and grains. (Phosphorus is bound to a few amino acids, especially serine, threonine, and tyrosine, in food proteins.) In the outer coating of cereal grains, particularly wheat, phosphorus exists in the form of phytic acid, which can form a complex with some minerals to create insoluble compounds. In conventional breads, phytic acid is converted to the soluble form of orthophosphate during the leavening process. However, in the unleavened breads commonly eaten in the Middle East, the availability of practically all minerals is much lower. Table 5-4 lists the phosphorus content of selected foods.

The average intakes of phosphorus by adults in the United States are approximately 1300 mg/day for men and 1000 mg/day for women. Most phosphorus (about 60%) comes from milk, meat, poultry, fish, and eggs. Cereals and legumes provide another 20%, and less than 10% is derived from fruits and their juices. Other dietary sources such as tea, coffee, vegetable oils, and spices supply only small amounts of phosphorus. The estimated amount provided by food additives is almost 10% (Calvo and Park, 1996).

Deficiency

Phosphate deficiency is rare, but it could possibly develop in individuals who are taking drugs known as *phosphate binders* (see Chapter 39). However, among older adults, phosphorus deficiencies may be more common than previously thought because of poor intakes in general. The widespread and ultimately fatal consequences of severe phosphorus depletion reflect its ubiquitous roles in body functions. Symptoms result primarily from decreased synthesis of adenosine triphosphate (ATP) and other organic phosphate molecules. Neural, muscular, skeletal, hematologic, renal, and other abnormalities occur.

Because phosphorus is so widely available from foods, including processed foods and soda types of soft drinks, little likelihood of a dietary inadequacy exists. Clinical phosphate depletion and hypophosphatemia can result from long-term administration of glucose or TPN without sufficient phosphate, excessive use of phosphate-binding antacids, hyperparathyroidism, or treatment of diabetic acidosis, and it may develop in those who have alcoholism with or without decompensated liver disease. Premature infants who are fed unfortified human milk may also develop hypophosphatemia.

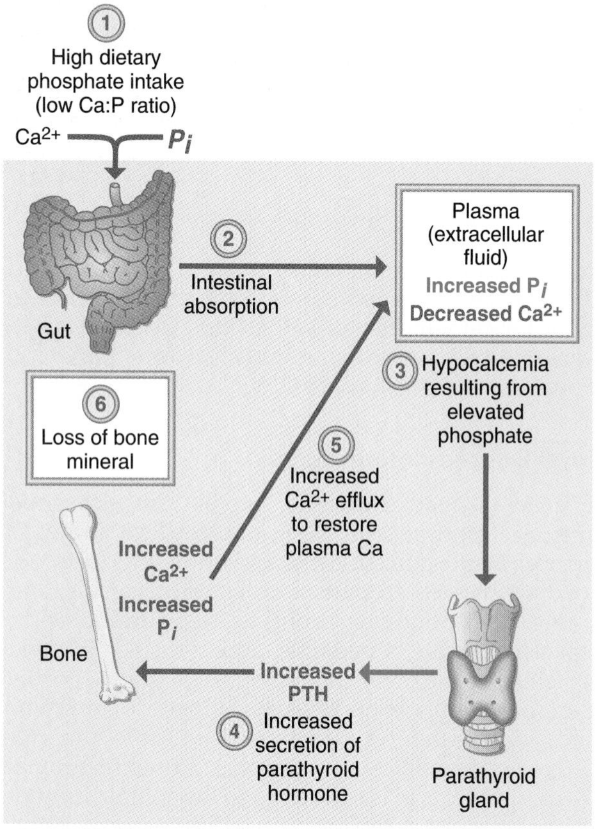

FIGURE 5-4 • Mechanism through which a low dietary calcium/phosphorus *(Ca:P)* ratio contributes to the development of a persistently high parathyroid hormone *(PTH)* concentration.

Toxicity

A persistently high concentration of PTH may result because of the chronic consumption of a low-calcium, high-phosphorus diet. This condition was often previously referred to as "nutritional secondary hyperparathyroidism." In humans the PTH levels in blood that result from a low calcium/phosphorous ratio typically remain within the normal range but usually at the high end. A persistently high PTH, even within the normal range, contributes to increased bone turnover that potentially can result in a reduction of bone mass and density (Calvo et al, 1990). If this condition is chronic, it could contribute to fragility fractures because of excessive resorption and thinning of trabecular plates at bone sites throughout the skeleton. Individuals with a low calcium/phosphorous ratio would benefit from increasing their calcium intake from foods or supplements (Anderson, 1996). Adequate calcium intakes, whether provided by food or supplements, have been shown to reduce the serum PTH concentration and presumably help inhibit bone loss (McKane et al, 1996). The effects of a low dietary calcium/phosphorous ratio on the PTH concentration is illustrated in Figure 5-4. The persistently high PTH level contributes to the limited bone mineralization during growth—that is, the inadequate peak bone mass accumulation in adolescents and young adults and the loss of bone mass in adults (Anderson, 1996).

Magnesium

Magnesium is the second-most abundant (after potassium) intracellular cation in the body. The adult human body contains approximately 20 to 28 g of magnesium, of which approximately 60% is found in bone, 26% in muscle, and the remainder in soft tissues and body fluids. Gender differences in the body content of magnesium begin before puberty. Magnesium in bone is present in exchangeable and nonexchangeable pools. Magnesium ions in the bone fluid compartment are much more exchangeable than magnesium ions that have become part of the crystal lattice. Normal serum levels are usually in the range of 1.5 to 2.1 mEq/L (0.75 to 1.1 mmol/L). About half the magnesium in plasma is free, approximately one third is bound to albumin, and the remainder is complexed with citrate, phosphate, or other anions. Magnesium homeostasis is governed by intestinal absorption and renal excretion. No hormone is known to have a major role in the control of serum magnesium, although PTH has a minor role (Rude, 1998).

Absorption, Transport, Storage, and Excretion

The efficiency of absorption of magnesium varies widely from 35% to 45%. Magnesium may be absorbed along the length of the small intestine, but most absorption occurs in the jejunum. Like other divalent cation minerals, the entry of magnesium from the gut lumen occurs by two mechanisms: a carrier-facilitated process and simple diffusion. A saturable facilitated mechanism operates at low intraluminal concentrations, whereas paracellular movement across the mucosa predominates throughout the length of the small bowel when intraluminal concentrations are high. The efficiency of absorption varies with the magnesium status of the individual, the amount of magnesium in the diet, and the composition of the diet as a whole. Vitamin D has little or no effect on magnesium absorption.

No homeostatic system for serum magnesium regulation has been identified, but the serum magnesium concentration is remarkably constant. Maintenance of these constant values depends on absorption, excretion, and transmembranous cation flux rather than on hormonal regulation. Once in the cells, magnesium is bound mainly to protein and energy-rich phosphates. The magnesium balance is illustrated in Figure 5-5.

Primarily the kidneys control magnesium balance by conserving magnesium efficiently, particularly when intake is low. Supplementing a normal intake increases urinary excretion, and the serum magnesium level remains normal. Low dietary intake of magnesium results in reduced urinary excretion of magnesium. To allow nursing mothers to meet the increased needs for magnesium, urinary excretion of the mineral tends to decrease during lactation (Dengel et al, 1994). Renal resorption varies inversely with that of calcium.

Functions

The major function of magnesium is to stabilize the structure of ATP in ATP-dependent enzyme reactions. Magnesium is a cofactor for more than 300 enzymes involved in the metabolism of food components and the synthesis of many metabolic products. Among the reactions requiring magnesium are the synthesis of fatty acids and proteins, phosphorylation of glucose and its derivatives in the glycolytic pathway, and transketolase reactions. Magnesium is important in the formation of cAMP, which was the first cytosolic *second messenger* to be identified as a mechanism for transmitting messages from outside the cells in response to hormones, local hormonelike factors, or other molecules.

Magnesium plays a role in neuromuscular transmission and activity, working in concert with and against the effects of calcium, depending on the system involved. In a normal muscle contraction, calcium acts as a stimulator and magnesium acts as a relaxant. Magnesium acts as a physiologic calcium-channel blocker and has been called "nature's blocker" (Iseri and French, 1994). High magnesium intakes are associated with greater bone density (Tucker et al, 1998).

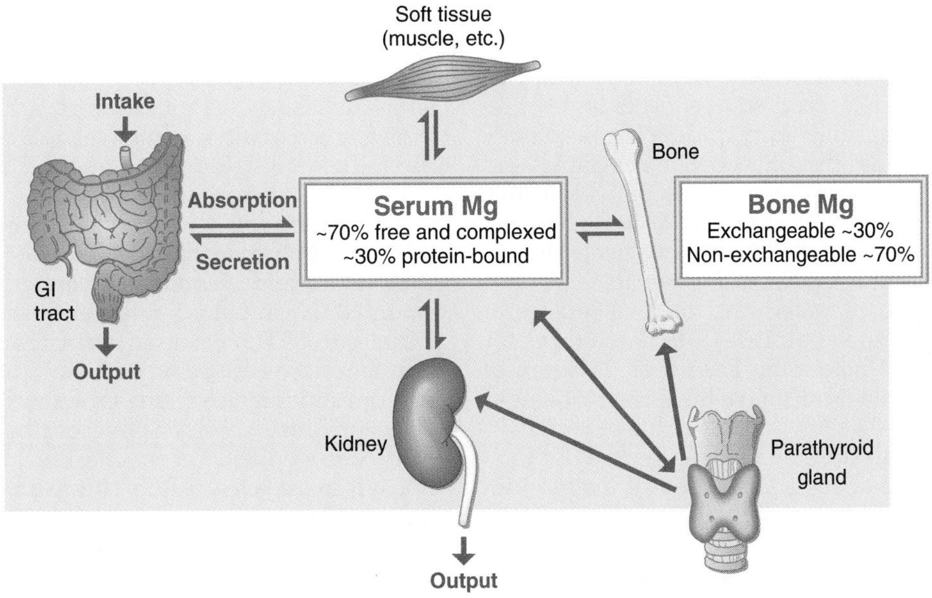

FIGURE 5-5 • Magnesium balance is maintained largely by GI absorption and renal excretion.

The reactivity of vascular and other smooth muscle cells depends on the ratio of calcium to magnesium in the blood. Large doses of magnesium can result in central nervous system depression, anesthesia, and even paralysis, especially in patients with renal insufficiency. Thus patients with renal problems should not be given magnesium supplements (see Chapter 39).

Magnesium has been implicated in clinical problems that share an underlying pathophysiologic condition involving vasospasm and increased coagulation. Experimental studies have shown that low magnesium intakes affect the ratio of prostacyclin to thromboxane in pregnancy-induced hypertension (see Chapter 7). The use of magnesium to inhibit atherogenesis or prevent ischemic heart disease remains the subject of continuing study (see Chapter 35).

Dietary Reference Intakes

The recommended dietary allowance (RDA) for magnesium was increased in 1997, and for the first time, different recommendations were made for females and males beginning at puberty (see Table 5-1). ULs were also established (see Table 5-2), as were AIs for infants (Food and Nutrition Board, 1997).

TABLE 5-5 Magnesium Content of Selected Foods

FOOD	CONTENT (mg)
Tofu, firm, ½ cup*	118
Chili with beans, 1 cup	115
Wheat germ, toasted, ¼ cup	90
Cashews, roasted, ¼ cup	89
Halibut, baked, 3 oz	78
Swiss chard, cooked, ½ cup	75
Peanuts, roasted, ¼ cup	67
Chocolate chips, semisweet, ¼ cup	58
Baked potato with skin, 1	55
Cocoa powder, 2 tbsp	52
Molasses, blackstrap, 1 tbsp	52
Cereal, raisin bran, 1 oz	48
Spinach, fresh, 1 cup	44
Cheerios, 1 oz	39
Milk, 2% fat, 1 cup	33
Bread, whole wheat, 1 slice	26
Chicken, breast, baked, 3 oz	25
Green peas, frozen, cooked, ½ cup	23
Ground beef, lean, cooked, 3 oz	16
Fruits	10-25
Coffee, brewed, ¾ cup	9
Egg, 1	5

From U.S. Department of Agriculture: *Composition of foods,* USDA Handbook No. 8 Series, Washington, DC, 1976-1986, Agricultural Research Service, The Department.
*Tofu prepared by magnesium precipitation.

Food Sources and Intakes

Magnesium is abundant in many foods, and the ordinary diet should usually provides adequate amounts. Good sources are seeds, nuts, legumes, and milled cereal grains, as well as dark green vegetables because magnesium is an essential constituent of chlorophyll. Milk is a moderately good source of magnesium, especially because milk and other dairy products are so widely consumed. Fish, meat, and the most commonly eaten fruits (i.e., oranges, apples, and bananas) are poor sources of magnesium. Tofu prepared by magnesium precipitation (e.g., when calcium is used) is a good source. Diets high in refined foods, meat, and dairy products are usually lower in magnesium than diets rich in vegetables and unrefined grains (Table 5-5). Magnesium is lost during the refining of wheat cereals and the processing of foods such as sugar, and it is not generally replaced as part of the enrichment of cereals.

Figure 5-6 shows Americans' median intakes of magnesium (Alaimo et al, 1994). Median intakes for both genders fall below the RDA after 11 years of age; however, older adults have the lowest intakes of any adult group. The low intakes of the older adults are consistent with studies of Norwegians older than 60 years of age that suggest subclinical magnesium deficiency among healthy older adults (Gullestad et al, 1994).

High intakes of calcium, protein, vitamin D, and alcohol all increase the requirements for magnesium; physical or psychologic stress may also increase magnesium needs.

The most commonly consumed food sources of magnesium in the U.S. diet according to the CSFII include milk, bread, coffee, ready-to-eat cereals, beef, potatoes, and dried beans and lentils (Subar et al, 1998).

Deficiency

Although rare, severe magnesium deficiency symptoms include tremors, muscle spasms, personality changes, anorexia, nausea, and vomiting. Tetany, myoclonic jerks, athetoid movements, convulsions, and coma have also been reported in those with a magnesium deficiency. Hypocalcemia and hypokalemia typically occur first, combined with impairment of the individual's responsiveness to PTH. Sodium retention may also occur.

The effects of severe magnesium depletion on bone metabolism include decreased PTH secretion by the parathyroid glands, very low concentrations of serum PTH, impaired responsiveness of bone and kidneys to PTH, decreased serum $1{,}25(OH)_2D_3$, vitamin D resistance, altered hydroxyapatite crystal formation, and impaired bone growth in young patients or osteoporosis in older patients (Rude, 1996). With continued depletion of magnesium, PTH concentrations decrease even further. Intravenous administration of magnesium reverses the clinical signs and symptoms within a short time.

Moderate depletion of magnesium is apparently prevalent in older populations in Western nations (Gullestad et al, 1994). Such deficiencies are typically precipitated by dietary intakes that are persistently

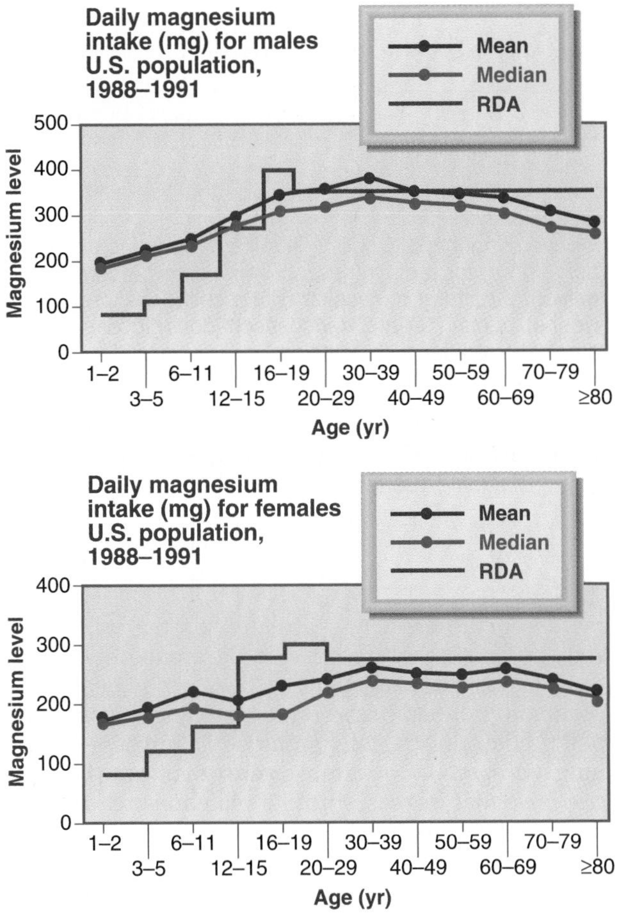

FIGURE 5-6 • Comparison of the median daily magnesium intake for Americans and the 1998 RDAs.

low in magnesium, especially in individuals who avoid consuming dark green leafy vegetables, milk, and other good sources of magnesium. Any other condition such as an increased loss of electrolytes or a shift in electrolyte balance, especially a decrease in potassium, also triggers a moderate magnesium deficiency (Rude, 1998). Conditions and situations that may cause acute deficiencies to develop include renal disease, diuretic therapy, malabsorption, hyperthyroidism, pancreatitis, kwashiorkor, diabetes, parathyroid gland disorders, postsurgical stress, and vitamin D–resistant rickets.

Magnesium status is difficult to determine from serum measurements of magnesium because the total serum magnesium level remains constant with wide range of intake levels. Leukocyte magnesium contents are much more sensitive to nutritional status, which makes them a superior marker. Urinary excretion of magnesium (and often of potassium) is less in those with a magnesium deficiency than in those with sufficient magnesium, suggesting that those with magnesium deficiencies have greater retention of magnesium and improved tissue magnesium status throughout the body. Attention has been focused on the interrelationships of magnesium and other electrolytes, particularly potassium, and the effects of these relationships on the development of various tissue abnormalities. For example, a low magnesium intake is now considered to be a potential risk factor for hypertension, as are inadequate intakes of potassium, calcium, and other micronutrients (Appel et al, 1997). Oral magnesium supplementation in middle-age and older women with mild to moderate hypertension was found to reduce systolic and diastolic blood pressure significantly (Witteman et al, 1994) (see Chapter 36). Low magnesium intakes have been associated with coronary heart disease. Studies of magnesium use by patients who had experienced acute myocardial infarction (MI) suggest that rapid post-MI magnesium treatment reduces mortality. Magnesium deficits may also be a factor in osteoporosis, although the mechanism has not been established. Researchers in Israel who administered magnesium supplements for 2 years to postmenopausal women with established osteoporosis demonstrated improved trabecular but not cortical bone mass (Stendig-Lindenberg et al, 1993). Additional research on the link between magnesium and bone in postmenopausal women is needed.

Toxicity

Although excess magnesium can inhibit bone calcification, magnesium excesses from dietary sources, including supplements, are very unlikely to result in toxicity. However, the ULs for magnesium from supplements or pharmacologic agents were established for the first time in 1998 (see Table 5-2). The only cases of toxicity that have been reported involve smelter workers who inhale or otherwise ingest toxic levels of magnesium dust.

Sulfur

Although sulfur has long been studied as a mineral, it functions almost entirely as a component of organic molecules (see *Focus On:* Sulfur: It's Not a Mineral; It's an Organic Molecule). Sulfur exists in the body as a constituent of three amino acids—cystine, cysteine, and methionine—and of many other organic molecules. As such, it exists as part of these organic molecules in all cells and extracelluar compartments such as connective tissue. The tertiary structure of proteins is attributable in part to covalent bonding between cysteine residues in which the —SH groups are oxidized to form disulfide (—S—S—) bridges. These bridges also provide the three-dimensional structural modifications necessary for the activity of some enzymes, insulin, and other proteins. Sulfhydryl groups of proteins also participate in diverse cellular reactions. For example, the poisonous effects of arsenic are caused by its ability to bind sulfhydryl groups of enzymes. The sulfur of cysteine binds to iron-sulfur clusters in electron transfer proteins involved in basic, life-sustaining processes, such as photosynthesis, nitrogen fixation, and oxidative phosphorylation.

FOCUS ON

Sulfur: It's Not a Mineral; It's an Organic Molecule

The sulfur-containing amino acids (*S*-containing amino acids), methionine and cysteine, provide almost 100% of the sulfur in the human diet. (A small percentage of the methionine molecules have selenium as a substitute for the sulfur.) The transmethylation pathway within cells, especially in the liver, converts methionine to homocysteine while transferring the methyl group to other molecules. This pathway is linked to the metabolism of other important molecules such as cysteine, adenine (a nucleoside), and polyamines. *S*-adenosylmethionine is a critical intermediate in these pathways. The sulfur atoms remain part of the organic structures until hepatic degradation (oxidation) of the cysteine and the formation of inorganic sulfate groups that are excreted by the kidneys.

Several nonhepatic cells use sulfate (bound to an organic donor) for the synthesis of iron-sulfur proteins. In addition, structural molecules within cells (i.e., proteoglycans), contain sulfated monosaccharide (glucose and galactose) residues. In addition, taurine, a sulfur-containing amino acid made by liver cells, is used to conjugate bile acids before secretion.

In summary, sulfur acts primarily as a component of organic molecules in cells rather than as an inorganic element (Stipanuk, 1986).

Glutathione, a tripeptide-containing cysteine, acts as a donor of reducing equivalents for the reduction of hydrogen peroxide and organic peroxides by glutathione peroxidase. In the broadest sense, sulfur can be considered an antioxidant. Sulfur exists as a component of *heparin*, an anticoagulant found in liver and some other tissues, and as *chondroitin sulfate* in bone and cartilage. Sulfur is also an essential component of three vitamins—thiamin, biotin, and pantothenic acid. Other important molecules such as *S*-adenosylmethionine also contain sulfur.

Excess inorganic sulfur generated as a result of hepatic or renal metabolism is excreted in the urine as sulfates. The metabolism of sulfur-containing amino acids generates inorganic acids, especially sulfate anions, in substantial amounts. The sulfates are thought to combine with calcium ions in the glomerular ultrafiltrate, thereby reducing the renal tubular resorption of calcium. This mechanism may explain as much as 50% of the calcium loss associated with protein-induced hypercalciuria, which develops after consumption of meals rich in animal proteins—proteins that are rich in sulfur. Food sources of sulfur include meat, poultry, fish, eggs, dried beans, broccoli, and cauliflower. Sulfur deficiency or toxicity is highly unlikely.

MICROMINERALS (TRACE ELEMENTS)

Numerous elements that are present in minute amounts in body tissues are essential for optimal human growth, health, and development. Microminerals (trace elements) are defined as those that have been shown through appropriately designed and corroborated experiments to be required for optimal performance of a particular function. Classically, each element exhibits a spectrum of action that depends on the element's dosage and the nutritional state of the host with respect to the element.

Deficiency of a nutrient has historically been identified and defined based on investigations using animal models. Increasing amounts of a nutrient (beginning with intake of almost zero) evokes a biologic response that increases until a plateau is reached beyond which larger intakes can produce pharmacologic effects and eventually toxicity. (Low intakes, of course, produce signs and symptoms of deficiency.)

The spectrum of effects produced by trace element deficiencies is more subtle and difficult to identify today, partly because many of these effects occur at the cellular or subcellular level. For example, iron deficiency eventually results in a type of anemia that is easy to identify. The cellular effects cannot be identified as easily but may actually be more harmful to the individual (see Chapter 34). Reports have indicated that a benign strain of a virus became virulent after infecting an individual with a selenium deficiency (Beck et al, 1994, 1995). This finding, which is discussed in greater detail in the Selenium section, illustrates the fact that current theories and knowledge about adequacy and deficiency are different than they were 10 years ago; the knowledge of the various functions of trace and ultratrace minerals must continually be improved.

DRIs and ULs have been established for nine essential trace elements—chromium, copper, iodine, iron, manganese, molybdenum, selenium, zinc, and fluoride (Tables 5-6 and 5-7). DRIs for five potentially essential trace elements—arsenic, boron, nickel, silicon, and vanadium—have not yet been published (Trumbo et al, 2001). No DRI exists for cobalt.

General Characteristics

Trace elements exist typically in two forms: (1) as charged ions or (2) bound to proteins or complexed in molecules (e.g., metalloenzymes). Each element

TABLE 5-6 Dietary Reference Intakes of Trace Elements Throughout the Life Cycle

AGE/LIFE STAGE	IRON (mg/day)*	ZINC (mg/day)*	SELENIUM (μg/day)*	COPPER (μg/day)*	CHROMIUM (μg/day)*	FLUORIDE (mg/day)*	IODINE (μg/day)*	MANGANESE (mg/day)*	MOLYBDENUM (μg/day)*
Infants									
0-6 mo	0.27	2	15	200	0.2	0.01	110	0.003	2
7-12 mo	11	3	20	220	5.5	0.5	130	0.6	3
Children									
1-3 yr	**7**	**3**	**20**	**340**	11	0.7	**90**	1.2	**17**
4-8 yr	**10**	**5**	**30**	**440**	15	1	**90**	1.5	**22**
Males									
9-13 yr	**8**	**8**	**40**	**700**	25	2	**120**	1.9	**34**
14-18 yr	**11**	**11**	**55**	**890**	35	3	**150**	2.2	**43**
19-30 yr	**8**	**11**	**55**	**900**	35	4	**150**	2.3	**45**
31-50 yr	**8**	**11**	**55**	**900**	35	4	**150**	2.3	**45**
51-70 yr	**8**	**11**	**55**	**900**	30	4	**150**	2.3	**45**
>70 yr	**8**	**11**	**55**	**900**	30	4	**150**	2.3	**45**
Females									
9-13 yr	**8**	**8**	**34**	**700**	21	2	**120**	1.6	**34**
14-18 yr	**15**	**9**	**43**	**890**	24	3	**150**	1.6	**43**
19-30 yr	**18**	**8**	**45**	**900**	25	3	**150**	1.8	**45**
31-50 yr	**18**	**8**	**45**	**900**	25	3	**150**	1.8	**45**
51-70 yr	**8**	**8**	**45**	**900**	20	3	**150**	1.8	**45**
>70 yr	**8**	**8**	**45**	**900**	20	3	**150**	1.8	**45**
Pregnant									
≤18 yr	**27**	**13**	**60**	**1000**	29	3	**220**	2.0	**50**
19-30 yr	**27**	**11**	**60**	**1000**	30	3	**220**	2.0	**50**
31-50 yr	**27**	**11**	**60**	**1000**	30	3	**220**	2.0	**50**
Lactating									
≤18 yr	**10**	**14**	**70**	**1300**	44	3	**290**	2.6	**50**
19-30 yr	**9**	**12**	**70**	**1300**	45	3	**290**	2.6	**50**
31-50 yr	**9**	**12**	**70**	**1300**	45	3	**290**	2.6	**50**

From Food and Nutrition Board, National Academy of Sciences, Institute of Medicine: *Dietary reference intakes for vitamin C, vitamin E, selenium, and carotenoids,* Washington, DC, 2000, National Academy Press; and Food and Nutrition Board, National Academy of Sciences, Institute of Medicine: *Dietary reference intakes for vitamin A, vitamin K, arsenic, boron, chromium, copper, iodine, iron, manganese, molybdenum, nickel, silicon, vanadium, and zinc,* Washington, DC, 2001, National Academy Press.

**Bold values* are recommended dietary allowances (RDAs). *Other (nonbold) values* are adequate intakes (AIs).

has different chemical properties that become critical in its functional role in cells or extracellular compartments. In blood and other tissue and cellular fluids, the trace elements do not exist in the free ionic state; they are typically bound to transporting or holding proteins. Fluoride ions become bound in the hydroxyapatite crystals of bones and teeth.

Functions

Many enzymes require small amounts of one or more trace metals for full activity. Metals function in enzyme systems by (1) participating directly in catalysis, (2) combining with substrates to form complexes on which enzymes act, (3) forming metalloenzymes that bind substrates, (4) combining with reaction end products, or (5) maintaining quaternary structures.

Minute concentrations of trace minerals affect the whole body through interactions with the enzymes or hormones that regulate masses of substrate. This ability is amplified if, in turn, the substrate has some regulatory function. Trace minerals may also interact with DNA to control the transcription of proteins important for the metabolism of that particular trace mineral.

Food Sources

Compared with other sources, foods of animal origin are generally superior sources of trace elements because concentrations of the elements tend to be higher, and the metals more available for absorption. Seafood in particular is usually rich in nearly all micronutrients except manganese, which is more readily available from plant sources. Trace elements are not distributed evenly in wheat grains, and the germ and outer layers that contain major amounts of most minerals are removed to a large extent by the milling process. However, the small quantities of minerals that remain in white flour are more biologically available than those in whole-wheat flour, which are in complexes with or bound by molecules in the inner layer, such as phytate and fiber.

Iron

Iron has been recognized as an essential nutrient for more than a century. Nutritional iron deficiency and iron deficiency anemia remain far too common in the twenty-first century given the wide availability of iron-rich foods (see Chapter 34). Indeed, iron deficiency anemia is the world's most common nutritional

TABLE 5-7 Tolerable Upper Intake Levels of Trace Elements Throughout the Life Cycle

AGE/LIFE STAGE	IRON (mg/day)	ZINC (mg/day)	SELENIUM (mg/day)	COPPER (μg/day)	CHROMIUM (mg/day)	FLUORIDE (mg/day)	IODINE (μg/day)	MANGANESE (mg/day)	MOLYBDENUM (μg/day)
Infants									
0-6 mo	40	4	45	—	—	0.7	—	—	—
7-12 mo	40	5	60	—	—	0.9	—	—	—
Children									
1-3 yr	40	7	90	1000	—	1.3	200	65	300
4-8 yr	40	12	150	3000	—	2.2	300	110	600
Males									
9-13 yr	40	23	280	5000	—	10	600	350	1100
14-18 yr	45	34	400	8000	—	10	900	350	1700
19-30 yr	45	40	400	10,000	—	10	1100	350	2000
31-50 yr	45	40	400	10,000	—	10	1100	350	2000
51-70 yr	45	40	400	10,000	—	10	1100	350	2000
>70 yr	45	40	400	10,000	—	10	1100	350	2000
Females									
9-13 yr	40	23	280	5000	—	10	600	350	1100
14-18 yr	45	34	400	8000	—	10	900	350	1700
19-30 yr	45	40	400	10,000	—	10	1100	350	2000
31-50 yr	45	40	400	10,000	—	10	1100	350	2000
51-70 yr	45	40	400	10,000	—	10	1100	350	2000
>70 yr	45	40	400	10,000	—	10	1100	350	2000
Pregnant									
≤18 yr	45	34	400	8000	—	10	900	350	1700
19-30 yr	45	40	400	10,000	—	10	1100	350	2000
31-50 yr	45	40	400	10,000	—	10	1100	350	2000
Lactating									
≤18 yr	45	34	400	8000	—	10	900	—	1700
19-30 yr	45	40	400	10,000	—	10	1100	—	2000
31-50 yr	45	40	400	10,000	—	10	1100	—	2000

From Food and Nutrition Board, National Academy of Sciences, Institute of Medicine: *Dietary reference intakes for vitamin C, vitamin E, selenium, and carotenoids,* Washington, DC, 2000, National Academy Press; Food and Nutrition Board, National Academy of Sciences, Institute of Medicine: *Dietary reference intakes for vitamin A, vitamin K, arsenic, boron, chromium, copper, iodine, iron, manganese, molybdenum, nickel, silicon, vanadium, and zinc,* Washington, DC, 2001, National Academy Press; and Food and Nutrition Board, National Academy of Sciences, Institute of Medicine: *Dietary reference intakes for calcium, phosphorus, magnesium, vitamin D, and fluoride,* Washington, DC, 1997, National Academy Press.

deficiency disease. Many advances have been made in the study of iron metabolism and iron deficiency, but questions about the mechanisms regulating the intestinal absorption of iron and iron balance persist. The adult human body contains iron in two major pools: (1) functional iron in hemoglobin, myoglobin, and enzymes and (2) storage iron in ferritin, hemosiderin, and transferrin (a transport protein in blood). Healthy adult men have about 3.6 g of total body iron, whereas women have about 2.4 g. Table 5-8 lists the relative proportions of the major categories of iron in men and women. Adult women have much lower amounts of iron in storage than do men. Iron is highly conserved by the body; approximately 90% is recovered and reused every day. The rest is excreted, primarily in the bile. Dietary iron must be available to maintain iron balance to meet this 10% gap, or else iron deficiency results.

Two concerns about iron nutritional status predominate: the incidence of iron deficiency anemia and the role of excessive iron intake in coronary heart disease and cancer. Because of food fortification and the use of iron supplements by so many individuals, high iron intakes by men and postmenopausal women may be contributing to the risk of these chronic diseases. In fact, a study of older adults replete with iron in the Framingham Heart Study cohort concluded that increased iron stores were a liability (Fleming et al, 2001).

Absorption, Transport, Storage, and Excretion

Dietary iron exists in two chemical forms: (1) heme iron, which is found in hemoglobin, myoglobin, and some enzymes and (2) nonheme iron, which is found predominantly in plant foods but also in some animal foods, as are nonheme enzymes and ferritin. Heme iron (i.e., the intact ferroporphyrin ring) is absorbed across the brush border (mucosa) of intestinal absorbing cells *(enterocytes)* after it is digested from animal sources. After heme enters the cytosol, the ferrous iron is enzymatically removed from the ferroporphyrin complex. The free iron ions combine immediately with apoferritin to form ferritin in the same way that free nonheme iron combines with apoferritin. Ferritin is an intracellular store and a ferry that carries bound iron from the brush border to the basolateral membrane of the absorbing cell. The final step of absorption by which iron ions are moved into the blood occurs at the basolateral membrane of the

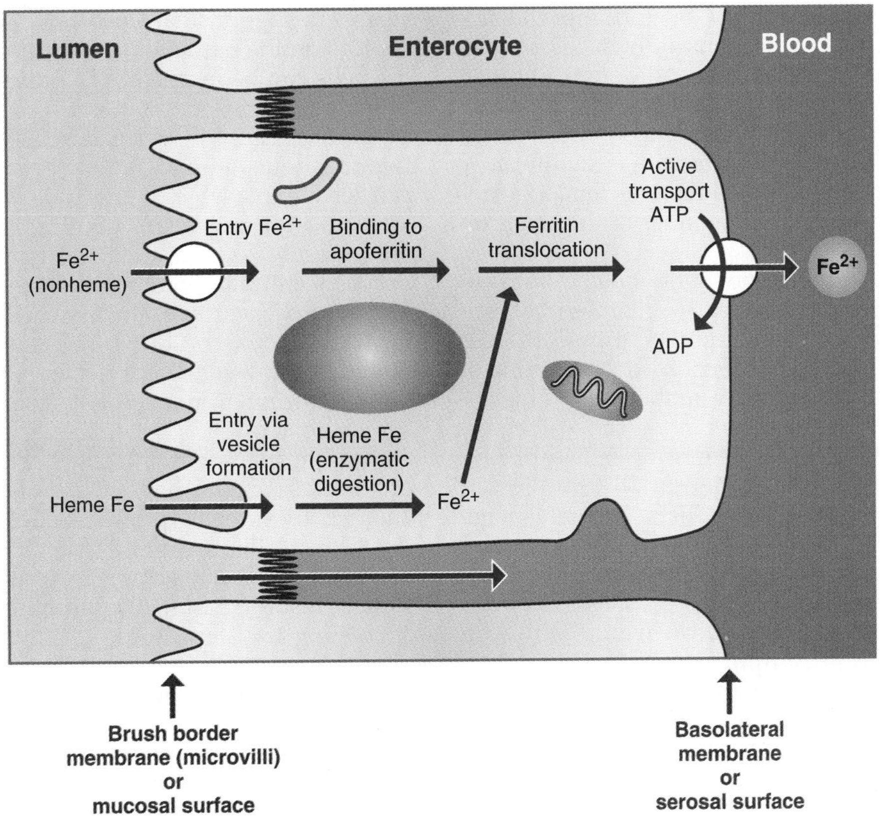

FIGURE 5-7 • Intestinal absorption of iron from heme and nonheme sources by an intestinal absorbing cell, or enterocyte. Enerocytes contain two membranes—the brush border membrane and the basolateral membrane. The entry step of nonheme iron at the brush border membrane is different from that of heme iron. Heme iron enters by vesicle formation around the heme, whereas nonheme iron (ionic iron) enters by facilitated diffusion down a concentration gradient. Absorbed ions combine with apoferritin to form ferritin complexes that move across the cell by diffusion to the basolateral membrane for the exit step of absorption by active transport. The iron of heme iron is enzymatically removed, and these ions exit at the basolateral membrane by an unknown mechanism. (*ATP,* Adenosine triphosphate; *ADP,* adenosine disphosphate.)

TABLE 5-8 Relative Proportions of Iron in Young, Healthy Adults

	MEN: IRON CONTENT		WOMEN: IRON CONTENT	
IRON TYPE	**(mg)**	**(%)**	**(mg)**	**(%)**
Functional				
Hemoglobin	2300	64	1700	73
Myoglobin	320	9	180	8
Heme enzymes	80	2	60	3
Nonheme enzymes	100	3	80	3+
Storage				
Ferritin	540	15	200	9
Hemosiderin	230	6	100	4
Transferrin	5	<1	4	<1
TOTAL	3575	100	2314	100

absorbing cell and involves an active transport mechanism. At this point, it is the same for heme and nonheme iron, and a diagram of these steps is presented in Figure 5-7. The absorption of heme iron is affected only minimally by the composition of meals and GI secretions. Heme iron represents only 5% to 10% of the dietary iron of individuals who consume a mixed diet, but absorption may be as high as 25%, compared with only 5% or so for nonheme iron. Because vegans consume only plant foods, sufficient amounts of nonheme iron must be ingested and absorbed to meet body requirements.

Three steps of absorption also precede the entry of nonheme iron into the blood circulation (see Figure 5-7). Nonheme iron must be digested free from plant sources and enter the duodenum and upper jejunum in a soluble (and ionized) form if it is to be transferred across the brush border (mucosa), the first step of absorption (Figure 5-8). The acid of gastric secretions enhances the solubility and the change of iron to the ionic state—either as ferric (+3 oxidation state) or ferrous (+2 oxidation state) iron—within the gut luminal contents. Iron in the reduced or ferrous state is preferred for the entry step of absorption, but some ferric iron is also transferred across the brush border. Iron absorption is enhanced by the coingestion of vitamin C because ascorbic acid reduces ferric to ferrous iron, and it also binds, or *chelates,* the ferrous form, which allows the two entities to be absorbed together at the brush border. Other food molecules such as sugars and sulfur-containing amino acids may also enhance iron entry by forming chelates with ionic iron. As chyme moves down the duodenum, the addition of pancreatic and duodenal secretions increases the pH of the contents to 7, at which point most ferric iron is precipitated unless it has been chelated. However, ferrous iron is significantly more soluble at a pH of 7, so these ions remain available for absorption in the remainder of the small intestine.

The efficiency of nonheme (but not heme) iron absorption seems to be controlled by the intestinal mucosa, which allows certain amounts of iron to enter the blood from the cytosolic ferritin pool according to the body's needs. The signal from the body to the absorbing cells may be *transferrin saturation,* or the percentage of iron bound to transferrin (see Figure 5-8). Normally, transferrin saturation is 30% to 35% in healthy, iron-consuming individuals. The percentage can vary greatly depending on iron intake and bioavailability.

A low percentage (e.g., 15%) of the total iron-binding capacity (TIBC) of transferrin would stimulate the absorbing cells to transport iron by the exit step at the basolateral membrane to the blood. Some researchers suggest that the amount of transferrin receptors on the basolateral membranes of the absorbing cells can be increased (i.e., up-regulated) to permit more transport of iron to awaiting transferrin molecules, each of which has the capacity to bind two iron ions (atoms). At low saturations, more vacancies are available on the transferrin molecules to take up iron and carry it to the bone marrow and other tissues to meet their needs. Conversely, if the iron concentration in the body is excessive, the TIBC may approach 40% to 50%, in which case the absorbing cells would be down-regulated, and less iron would be allowed to be absorbed. The latter situation occurs during iron overloads to protect the body against toxicity.

The life span of an intestinal absorbing cell is approximately 5 to 6 days. During this time, the cell emerges from the crypt after cell division, passes up the villus to the tip, and eventually sloughs off as a dead cell. During the early life of the individual cell, signals resulting from the saturation percentage of circulating transferrin are sent to the young cells to adjust their number of receptors for transferrin (e.g., to increase iron absorption in a state of iron defi-

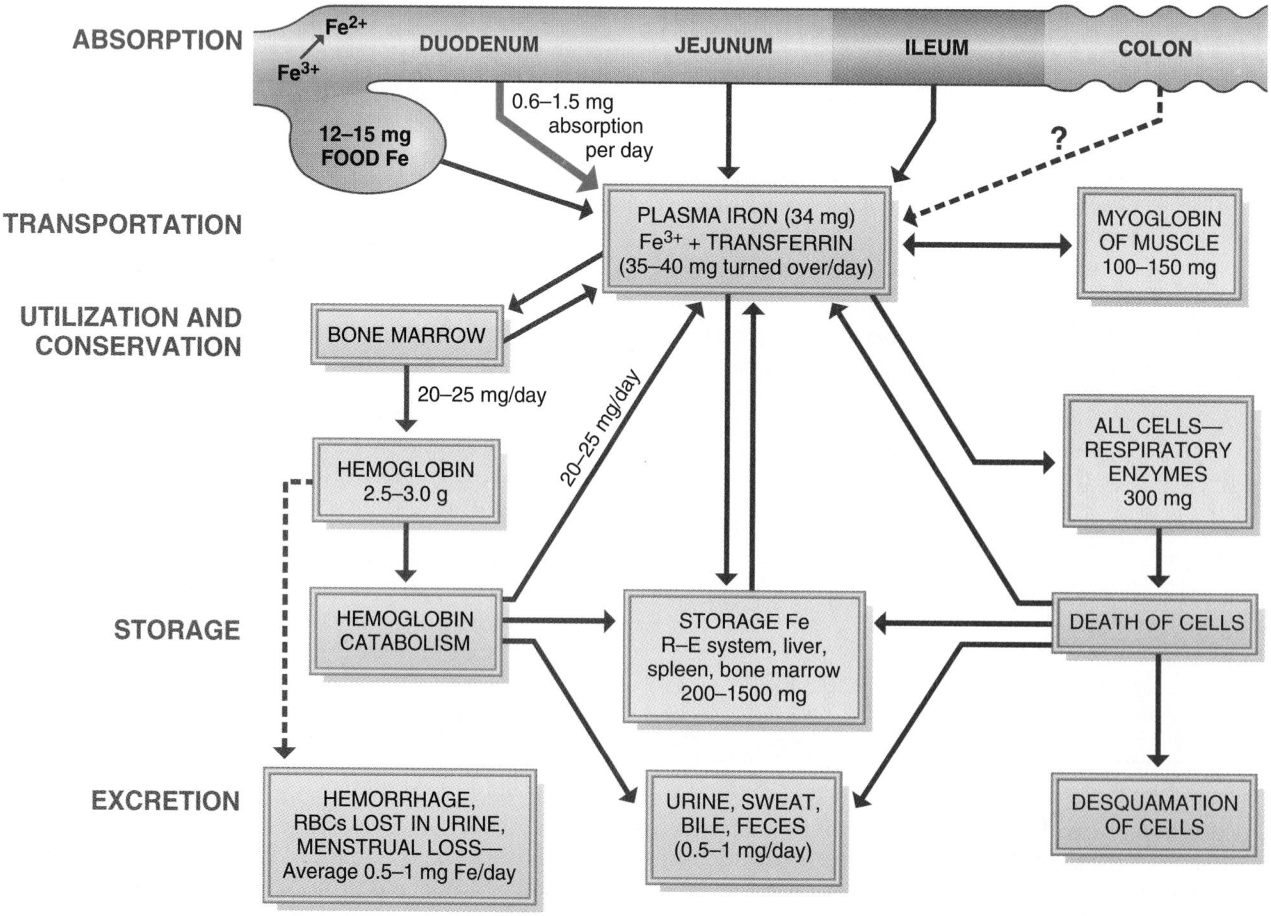

FIGURE 5-8 • Iron metabolism in adults. Most iron is absorbed from the duodenum and jejunum, after which it is transported as plasma iron or bound to transferrin. (*RBCs,* Red blood cells; *R-E system,* reticuloendothelial system.)

ciency). Other cells formed before or after may have different numbers of receptors depending on the nutritional supply of iron. In individuals who persistently consume inadequate levels of iron, especially women in their childbearing years, the number of receptors may consistently be up-regulated to maximize the efficiency of iron absorption.

The efficiency of iron absorption (from gut lumen to blood) by adults with normal hemoglobin values averages 5% to 15% of the iron (heme and nonheme combined) contained in food and supplements. Although absorption may be as high as 50% in those with iron deficiency anemia, this level of absorption is not common. Most women with an iron deficiency but no anemia probably have absorption efficiencies of 20% to 30%. From 2% to 10% of nonheme iron in vegetables is absorbed, and from 10% to 30% of iron (heme and nonheme) in animal sources is typically absorbed.

Several factors affect the intestinal absorption of iron, especially of nonheme iron. The efficiency of iron absorption is determined to some extent by the foods from which it is derived. Some foods contain absorption-enhancing substances such as ascorbic acid and the so-called "meat factor," which is explained in the next paragraph.

Both ascorbic acid and sodium ethylenediaminetetraacetic acid (EDTA) improved iron absorption from a school breakfast meal (Davidsson et al, 2001). Ascorbic acid, the most potent enhancer of iron absorption, forms a chelate with iron that remains soluble at the alkaline pH of the lower small intestine. However the effect of prolonged daily dietary increases in ascorbic acid on iron absorption from a complete diet does not seem to be strong enough to improve iron status over time (Cook and Reddy, 2001). Animal proteins from beef, pork, veal, lamb, liver, fish, and chicken enhance absorption. The substance responsible for this improved absorption—which is called the *meat factor*—remains unknown, but specific amino acids or dipeptide digestion products may enhance iron absorption.

Although the iron content of human milk is very low, it is highly bioavailable because of the presence of milk *lactoferrin,* which enhances iron absorption. Infants retain more iron from human milk than from cow's milk or infant formulas because of the presence of lactoferrin in breast milk. Whey protein (lactalbumin), which constitutes a greater percentage of the total protein in human milk than in cow's milk, may also improve iron absorption (Borch-Iohnsen et al, 1994).

The degree of *gastric acidity* enhances solubility and therefore bioavailability of iron derived from foods. Therefore achlorhydria (lack of gastric acid secretion), hypochlorhydria (inadequate acid secretion), or administration of alkaline substances such as antacids can interfere with nonheme iron absorption by not permitting the solubilization of iron in gastric and duodenal fluids. Gastric secretions also seem to increase the absorption of heme iron.

Certain physiologic states such as pregnancy and growth that involve increased blood formation stimulate iron absorption. In addition, more iron is absorbed during iron deficiencies because of adaptive mechanisms that enhance nonheme iron absorption.

Foods with a high phytate content have low iron bioavailability, but whether phytate is the cause is not clear. Oxalates can inhibit absorption. Tannins, which are polyphenols, in tea also reduce nonheme iron absorption. On the other hand, the presence of an adequate amount of calcium helps to remove phosphate, oxalate, and phytate that would otherwise combine with iron and inhibit its absorption.

The availability of iron from various compounds used for food enrichment or as supplements varies widely according to their chemical composition. Although iron in the ferrous form is most readily absorbed, not all ferrous compounds are equally available. Ferrous pyrophosphate is used frequently in products such as breakfast cereals because it does not add a gray color to the food; however, this compound and others such as ferrous citrate and ferrous tartrate, are poorly absorbed. Iron is usually added to baby foods in an elemental form, the absorbability of which depends on the iron particle size. Increased intestinal motility decreases iron absorption by decreasing contact time and rapidly removing the chyme from the area of highest intestinal acidity. Poor fat digestion leading to steatorrhea also decreases iron absorption and the absorption of other cations.

Transport

Iron (nonheme) is transported, bound to transferrin, from the intestinal absorbing cells to various tissues to meet their needs. It rarely exists in the free ionic state in serum.

Storage

Between 200 and 1500 mg of iron is stored in the body as ferritin and hemosiderin; 30% of the body's iron store is in the liver, 30% is in the bone marrow, and the rest is found in the spleen and muscles. Up to 50 mg/day can be mobilized from storage iron, 20 mg of which is used in hemoglobin synthesis. (Estimates of these amounts are listed in Table 5-8.) The amounts of circulating ferritin in blood correlate closely with total body iron stores, which make this measurement an invaluable tool for clinical evaluation of iron status (see Chapters 18 and 34).

Intestinal Excretion

Iron is only lost from the body through bleeding and in very small amounts through defecation, sweat, and the normal exfoliation of hair and skin. Most of the iron lost in the feces could not be absorbed from food. The remainder comes from bile and the cells exfoliated from the GI epithelium. Almost no iron is excreted in the urine. Daily iron loss is approximately 1 mg for men and slightly less for nonmenstruating women. The loss of iron accompanying menstruation averages about 0.5 mg/day. However, wide variations exist among individuals, and menstrual losses of more than 1.4 mg of iron daily have been reported in approximately 5% of normal women.

Functions

The functions of iron relate to its ability to participate in oxidation and reduction reactions (Beard, 2001). Chemically, iron is a highly reactive element that can interact with oxygen to form intermediates with the potential of damaging cell membranes or degrading DNA. Iron must be tightly bound to proteins to prevent these potentially destructive oxidative effects.

Iron metabolism is complex because this element is involved in so many aspects of life, including red blood cell function, myoglobin activity, and the roles of numerous heme and nonheme enzymes. Because of its oxidation-reduction *(redox)* properties, iron has a role in the blood and respiratory transport of oxygen and carbon dioxide, and it is an active component of the cytochromes (enzymes) involved in the processes of cellular respiration and energy (ATP) generation. Iron also seems to be involved in immune function and cognitive performance. Although these latter relationships have not been clearly identified, they underscore the importance of preventing iron deficiency anemia in the world population. Table 5-9 lists the major iron molecules in the body and their functions.

Hemoglobin, present in red blood cells, is synthesized in immature cells in bone marrow. Hemoglobin works in two ways: (1) the iron-containing heme combines with oxygen in the lungs, and (2) the heme releases the oxygen in tissues, where it picks up carbon dioxide and then releases it in the lungs after its return from the tissues. Myoglobin, also a heme-containing protein, serves as an oxygen reservoir within muscle.

TABLE 5-9 Iron Molecules in the Body

IRON TYPE	FUNCTION
Metabolic Proteins	
Heme proteins	
Hemoglobin	Oxygen transport from lungs to tissues
Myoglobin	Transport and storage of oxygen in muscle
Enzymes: heme	
Cytochromes	Electron transport
Cytochrome P-450	Oxidative degradation of drugs
Catalase	Conversion of hydrogen peroxide to oxygen and water
Enzymes: nonheme	
Iron-sulfur and metalloproteins	Oxidative metabolism
Enzymes: iron dependent	
Tryptophan pyrolase	Oxidation of tryptophan
Transport and Storage Proteins	
Transferrin	Transport of iron and other minerals
Ferritin	Storage
Hemosiderin	Storage

Oxidative production of ATP within the mitochondria involves many heme and nonheme *iron-containing enzymes.* The cytochromes, present in nearly all cells, function in the mitochondrial respiratory chain in the transfer of electrons and the storage of energy through the alternate oxidation and reduction (redox) of iron ($Fe^{2+++} \Longleftrightarrow Fe^{3+++}$). Numerous water-insoluble drugs and endogenous organic molecules are transformed by the iron-containing cytochrome P-450 system in the liver into more water-soluble molecules that can be secreted in the bile and eliminated. *Ribonucleotide reductase,* the rate-limiting enzyme involved in DNA synthesis, is also an iron enzyme. Although these vital enzymes represent only a small portion of the total iron in the body (see Table 5-8), a severe decrease in their concentrations can have long-term consequences. Other enzymes, including several in the brain, also require iron.

An adequate iron intake is essential for the normal function of the immune system (Beard, 2001). Iron overloads and deficiencies result in changes in the immune response. Iron is required by bacteria; therefore an iron overload (especially intravenously) may result in an increased risk of infection. Iron deficiency affects humoral and cellular immunity. Concentrations of circulating T-lymphocytes decrease in individuals with an iron deficiency, and the mitogenic response is typically impaired. Natural killer (NK) cell activity also decreases. Production of interleukin-1 has been shown to be reduced in iron-deficient animals, and depressed interleukin-2 production has been reported in humans and animals.

Two iron-binding proteins—transferrin (in blood) and lactoferrin (in breast milk)—seem to protect the body against infection by withholding iron from microorganisms that need it for proliferation. Iron is used by brain cells for normal function in people of all ages (Beard et al, 1993). Iron is involved in the function and synthesis of neurotransmitters and possibly myelin. The detrimental effects of early iron deficiency anemia in children persist for many years (Beard, 2001). For example, differences have been found between the scholastic performance, sensorimotor competence, attention, learning, and memory of children with anemia and control children (Pollitt et al, 1976). Iron supplementation in children with iron deficiency anemia has been found to improve learning, as indicated by achievement test scores (Beard, 2001). Changes occur in iron metabolism in those with certain diseases such as Alzheimer's disease. Iron distribution in the brain has also been reported to change during normal aging (Johnson et al, 1994).

Dietary Reference Intakes

DRIs have been established for iron (see Table 5-6). The old RDA for iron was 10 mg/day for men and postmenopausal women and is now 8 mg/day. The old RDA of 15 mg for women of childbearing age (to replace iron loss from menstruation and provide for iron stores sufficient to support a pregnancy) is now 18 mg/day. For teenage boys (ages 14 to 18) the iron RDA is now 11 mg/day. Full-term infants are born with a reserve supply of iron from placental transfer during gestation, but normal-term infants still require adequate iron from food sources and fortified milk products during the first year of life. Premature infants have limited iron stores because they lack most of the iron and other trace minerals that are normally transferred during the last trimester of pregnancy. The need for iron to support rapid growth in premature infants becomes apparent at approximately 2 to 3 months of age (see Chapter 9). The RDAs for ages 1 year and older are now (variably) 7, 8, or 10 mg/day until adolescence (age 14) begins. Figure 5-9 shows the physiologic requirements for iron in relation to age. Requirements are highest during infancy and adolescence. Iron needs among males decrease after the adolescent growth spurt, whereas the iron needs of their female counterparts continue to be high until the menopausal transition. Iron allowances increase during pregnancy (from 15 to 30 mg/day) but not during lactation, although many lactating women are told to continue taking supplements.

Food Sources and Intakes

By far, the best source of dietary iron is liver, followed by seafood (oysters and fish), kidney, heart, lean meat, and poultry. Dried beans and vegetables are the best plant sources. Some other foods that provide iron are egg yolks, dried fruits, dark molasses, whole-grain and enriched breads, wine, and cereal. Milk and milk products are practically devoid of iron. Corn is a notoriously poor source of iron, so it is not surprising that cultures with diets based primarily on corn have high rates of anemia. Old-fashioned iron skillets used for cooking add to the total iron intake. The median iron intakes of most women are lower than the RDA, whereas the median intakes of men generally exceed the RDA, as reported from NHANES III (Alaimo et al, 1994). An adequate diet containing meats and other animal sources typically has a high iron content, containing approximately 6 mg of iron per 1000 kcal. Therefore the average omnivorous woman of childbearing age consuming 2000 kcal takes in only 12 mg of iron, or approximately 67% of the RDA of 18 mg/day. This intake level meets the needs of almost no menstruating women. However, iron intakes totaling much less than 12 mg/day place women at more serious risk for developing deficiency anemia. Women with high daily iron losses compensate with an increased rate of absorption, but even with this adaptation, insufficient stores of iron typically exist and the risk of anemia remains high.

The availability of iron derived from food is important in the consideration of dietary sources. For example, only 50% or less of the iron in whole-grain cereals and in some green vegetables is available in a useable form. Table 5-10 presents the iron content of

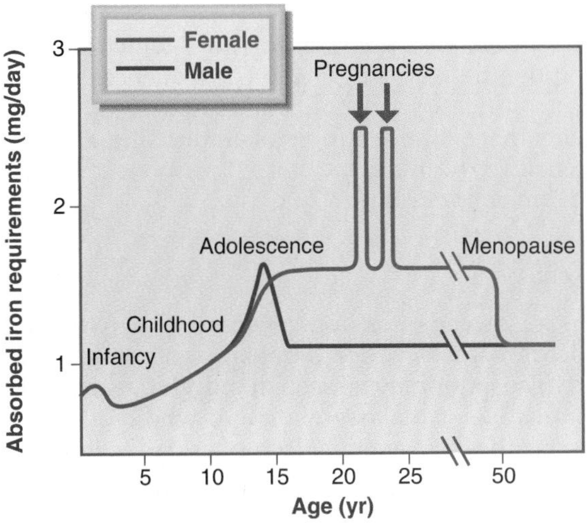

FIGURE 5-9 • The absorbed iron requirement for various ages. The greatest requirements for iron occur during infancy. During childhood, requirements are the same for boys and girls. During the adolescent growth spurt, iron needs increase and are greater for boys than girls. However, because of menstruation, the requirements after adolescence remain high for females but decrease for males.

TABLE 5-10 Iron Content of Selected Foods

FOOD	CONTENT (mg)
Cereal, ready to eat, fortified, 1 cup	1-16
Clams, canned, ¼ cup	11.2
Beef liver, fried, 3 oz	5.3
Braunschweiger, 2 oz	5.3
Baked beans, 1 cup	5.0
Molasses, blackstrap, 1 tbsp	5.0
Oysters, cooked, 1 oz	3.8
Venison, roasted, 3 oz	3.8
Baked potato, with skin, 1	2.8
Soup, lentil and ham, 1 cup	2.6
Wheat germ, toasted, ¼ cup	2.5
Burrito, bean, 1	2.5
Soup, beef noodle, 1 cup	2.4
Rice, white, enriched, 1 cup	2.3
Spaghetti with tomato sauce, 1 cup	2.3
PopTart, fortified, 1	2.2
Ground beef, lean, 3 oz	1.8
Apricots, dried halves, 10	1.7
Oatmeal, unfortified, 1 cup	1.6
Spinach, fresh, 1 cup	1.5
Cocoa powder, 2 tbsp	1.5
Peas, frozen, cooked, ½ cup	1.3
Bread, whole wheat, 1 slice	1.2
Chicken, breast, roasted, 1	0.9
Peanuts, dry roasted, ¼ cup	0.8
Pork chop, broiled, 1	0.7
Broccoli, fresh, cooked, ½ cup	0.7
Egg, 1	0.7
Blueberries, frozen, ½ cup	0.5
Wine, red, ½ cup	0.5
Raspberries, fresh, ½ cup	0.4
Cheese, cheddar, 1 oz	0.2
Milk, 2% fat, 1 cup	0.1

From U.S. Department of Agriculture: *Composition of foods*, USDA Handbook No. 8 Series, Washington, DC, 1976-1986, Agricultural Research Service, The Department.

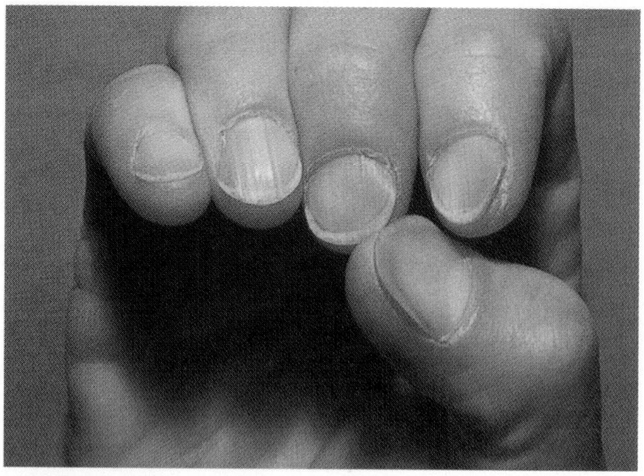

FIGURE 5-10 • Koilonychia—thin, concave nails with raised edges—may be seen on people with iron deficiency anemia. (From Callen WBS et al: *Color atlas of dermatology,* Philadelphia, 1993, WB Saunders.)

selected foods. Vegetarian or vegan women can obtain enough iron from their plant-based diet, but they must consume sufficient amounts of moderately iron-rich foods, such as legumes and dried fruits. Soy products are typically good sources of iron and zinc.

Iron fortification of cereals, flours, and bread has added significantly to the total iron intake of the U.S. population. Fortified cereals have become a substantial source of iron for infants and children, as well as for adolescents and adults. Concern about potential iron overloading from fortified breakfast foods were raised because analyzed values of iron content were considerably greater than labeled values (Whittaker et al, 2001).

The foods that supply the greatest amount of iron in the U.S. diet include ready-to-eat cereals fortified with iron; bread, cakes, cookies, doughnuts, and pasta (all fortified with iron); beef; dried beans and lentils; and poultry (Subar et al, 1998; U.S. Department of Agriculture, 1994).

Deficiency

Iron deficiency, the precursor of iron deficiency anemia, is the most common of all nutritional deficiency diseases (see Chapter 32). In the United States and worldwide, iron deficiency anemia is prevalent among children and women of childbearing age. The groups considered to be at greatest risk for iron deficiency anemia are infants younger than 2 years of age, adolescent girls, pregnant women, and older adults. Pregnant teenagers are frequently at high risk because of poor eating habits and continuing growth (see Chapters 7 and 11). Women in their childbearing years who are iron deficient benefit from either a diet rich in iron-containing foods or supplements (Patterson, 2001).

The final stages of iron deficiency include hypochromic, microcytic anemia. Anemia may be corrected by providing high-dose supplements in the form of ferrous sulfate or ferrous gluconate until blood parameters return to normal. To prevent worsening of the iron deficiency, individuals should be counseled regarding a diet that is appropriately rich in iron. Figure 5-10 shows koilonychia, a rare iron deficiency symptom of the nails.

Iron deficiency can be caused by injury, hemorrhage, or illness (e.g., blood loss from hookworms, GI diseases that interfere with iron absorption). Iron deficiency may also be aggravated by an unbalanced diet containing insufficient iron, protein, folate, and vitamins and C. Anemia typically develops because of an inadequate amount of dietary iron or faulty iron absorption. (Iron deficiency anemia is discussed in detail in Chapter 34.)

Female athletes, especially cross-country runners and others involved in endurance sports, often have an iron deficiency at some point in their training if they are not taking iron supplements or do not have diets high in iron. The source of the additional iron losses in those with athletic amenorrhea has not been determined, but it is thought that iron losses occurring through the gut may increase during the stressful conditions of training. One cross-country runner became so anemic that she developed hairline fractures in her proximal femur (hip), which illustrates the potential severity of the consequences of inadequate iron consumption (Anderson et al, 1998). It seems that without supplementation, the greater the intensity of training, the worse the iron levels become in women (see Chapter 26).

Box 5-1. Iron Overload Symptoms (Hemochromatosis)

Abnormal accumulation of iron in the liver
Excessive tissue ferritin levels
Elevated serum transferrin levels
Oxidation of LDL cholesterol
Cardiovascular complications

LDL, Low-density lipoprotein.

Toxicity

The major cause of iron overload is hereditary **hemochromatosis,** whereas transfusion iron overload is rare. The latter may be seen in individuals with sickle cell disease or thalassemia major who require transfusions for their anemia. Iron overload is linked to a distinct gene that favors excessive iron absorption if the iron is available in the diet. Genetic testing may eventually become a routine, readily available method for detecting this gene and reducing the risk of overload. The characteristic chemical parameters of iron overload are listed in Box 5-1 and described in more detail in Chapter 34.

Frequent blood transfusions or long-term ingestion of large amounts of iron can lead to abnormal accumu-

CLINICAL INSIGHT

The Role of Zinc in Children's Health

The first studies linking zinc and growth were carried out in Iran and Egypt almost 3 decades ago. "Nutritionally dwarfed" boys, characterized by short stature, iron deficiency anemia, and delayed sexual maturity, showed remarkable improvements with zinc supplementation. Some grew as much as 5 inches in 1 year and had parallel progression in gonadal development. The primary cause of zinc deficiency in these boys was identified as an impoverished diet consisting mainly of fibrous, unleavened bread. Although the whole grains used to make the bread were relatively high in zinc, they also contained phytates, which are known to form insoluble complexes with zinc and iron.

At the time, the circumstances leading to growth impairment secondary to zinc deficiency were believed to be unique to less developed countries. However, studies of preschool children from apparently well-nourished families in Denver demonstrated a correlation between short stature and low zinc levels in hair (Hambidge et al, 1976). Other studies have supported these findings.

In addition to inhibited growth, mild zinc deficiency is probably associated with reduced resistance to infection in children, but it has been difficult to establish this link (Prentice, 1993). However, children with severe zinc deficiency, as measured by plasma zinc concentrations, have been found to be at increased risk for diarrhea and respiratory diseases (Bahl et al, 1998). Therefore adequate zinc status plays a central role not only in growth and health promotion but also in disease prevention.

lation of iron in the liver. Saturation of tissue apoferritin with iron is followed by the appearance of hemosiderin, which is similar to ferritin but contains more iron and is very insoluble. *Hemosiderosis* is an iron storage condition that develops in individuals who consume abnormally large amounts of iron or in those with a genetic defect resulting in excessive iron absorption. If the hemosiderosis is associated with tissue damage, it is called *hemochromatosis* (see Chapter 34).

Iron supplements may not be beneficial for either older (postmenopausal) women or older men because of the associated increased risks for heart disease and cancer. A dietary intake of iron in excess of the RDA for adult men and postmenopausal women may contribute to an enriched oxidative environment in the body that favors oxidation of low-density lipoprotein (LDL) cholesterol, arterial vessel damage, and other adverse effects involving the cardiovascular system. In addition, excessive iron may help generate excessive amounts of free radicals that attack cellular molecules, thereby increasing the number of potentially carcinogenic molecules within cells. These potential adverse iron-disease linkages must be explored more to be confirmed.

Zinc

The most readily available form of zinc exists in animal flesh, particularly red meats and poultry. Meat intake is frequently low among preschoolers, occasionally because of personal preferences or socioeconomic reasons but usually because meats are displaced by cereal foods, milk, and milk products that children tend to prefer. For example, in Hambidge's classic study in Denver, some of the preschool children were found to eat as little as 1 oz of meat per day (Hambidge et al, 1976). This observation led to the fortification of infant and children's foods, especially cereals, with zinc. Milk is a good source of zinc, but high intakes of calcium from the milk may interfere with the absorption of iron and zinc (see Mineral Interactions section). Although the phytates from whole grains in unleavened breads may limit zinc absorption in Middle Eastern populations, this is less likely to be a problem in Western nations, where breads, breakfast foods, and other cereal-based foods are made primarily from refined grains and are typically fortified.

Nutritional assessments, including biochemical measurements, are necessary to detect the presence of a mild zinc deficiency in young children with suboptimal stature (i.e., less than the 5th percentile on the infant growth curves). However, a response of an increase in growth rate in short children to zinc supplementation would provide some confirmation of zinc deficiency.

Zinc has only been known to be essential for humans since the now classic studies of zinc deficiency in Iran and Egypt in the early 1960s (Halsted et al, 1972; Prasad et al, 1963). Severe zinc deficiency disease has been identified in undernourished populations such as those in the Middle East, but a marginal form of deficiency has also been identified among low-income preschoolers in Denver and other cities in the United States (Hambidge et al, 1976). These marginal deficits have largely been corrected by food fortification in the last 2 decades (see *Clinical Insight:* The Role of Zinc in Children's Health).

Zinc is abundantly distributed throughout the human body and is second only to iron among trace elements. The human body has about 2 to 3 g of zinc, with the highest concentrations in the liver, pancreas, kidney, bone, and muscles. Other tissues with high concentrations include various parts of the eye, prostate gland, spermatozoa, skin, hair, fingernails, and toenails. Zinc is primarily an intracellular ion, functioning in association with more than 300 different enzymes of various classes. Even though zinc is abundant in the cytosol, virtually all of it is bound to proteins, but it is in equilibrium with a small ionic fraction.

Absorption, Transport, Storage, and Excretion

Zinc absorption and excretion are controlled by poorly understood homeostatic mechanisms. The mechanism of absorption involves two pathways similar to those of calcium: (1) a saturable carrier mechanism operating most efficiently at low zinc intakes when luminal zinc concentrations are low, and (2) a passive mechanism involving paracellular movement when zinc intakes and luminal concentrations are high. Solubility of zinc in the gut lumen is critical, but zinc ions are generally bound to amino acids or short peptides in the lumen, and the ions are released at the brush border for absorption via the carrier mechanism (hZIPI family). The entry step of absorption across the brush border is followed by the binding of zinc ions to metallothionein and other proteins within the cytosol of the absorbing cell. Metallothionein carries the zinc (via transcellular movement) to the basolateral border for the exit step from the absorbing cell to the blood. The exit step occurs by active transport, because the blood concentration of zinc is significantly greater than the cytosolic ion concentration. The process of zinc absorption is illustrated in Figure 5-11.

Zinc absorption is affected not only by the level of zinc in the diet but also by the presence of interfering substances, especially phytates. After the consumption of zinc in a meal, the serum zinc level rises and then decreases in a dose-response pattern. A protein-rich diet promotes zinc absorption by forming zinc-amino acid chelates that present zinc in a more absorbable form. Zinc absorption is slightly higher during pregnancy and lactation (Fung et al, 1997). Absorbed zinc is taken up from the portal circulation initially by the liver, but most of the zinc is subsequently redistributed to other tissues. Impaired absorption is associated with a variety of intestinal diseases, such as *Crohn's disease* or pancreatic insufficiency. Several dietary factors affect zinc absorption. Phytate decreases zinc absorption, but other complexing agents (e.g., tannins) do not. Copper and cadmium compete for the same carrier protein, so they reduce zinc absorption. Concern exists that high intakes of iron may reduce the amounts of zinc absorbed. High calcium intakes reduce zinc absorption and balance (Wood and Zheng, 1997). Folic acid may also reduce zinc absorption when zinc intake is low. On the other hand, high doses of zinc can impair absorption of iron from ferrous sulfate, the form usually found in vitamin and mineral supplements (Crofton et al, 1989). Dietary fiber may also interfere with zinc absorption, but the significance of this interaction within the gut lumen is unclear.

Zinc absorption may be enhanced by glucose or lactose and by soy protein consumed alone or mixed with beef. Red table wine also increases zinc absorption, probably because of its congeners; white wine has not been studied. Like iron, zinc is better absorbed from human milk than from cow's milk.

Transport in Blood

The amount of zinc transported in the blood depends on the availability not only of zinc but also of albumin, a transport protein for many mineral cations. Albumin is the major plasma carrier, although some zinc is transported by transferrin and by α_2-macroglobulin. Most of the zinc in blood is localized in erythrocytes and leukocytes. Plasma zinc is metabolically active and fluctuates in response to dietary intake and physi-

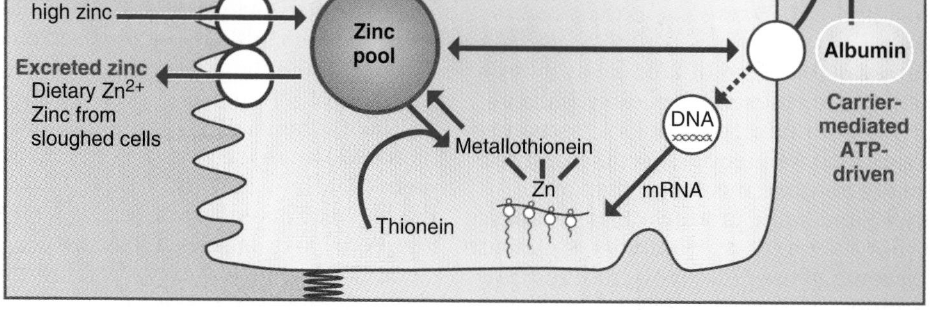

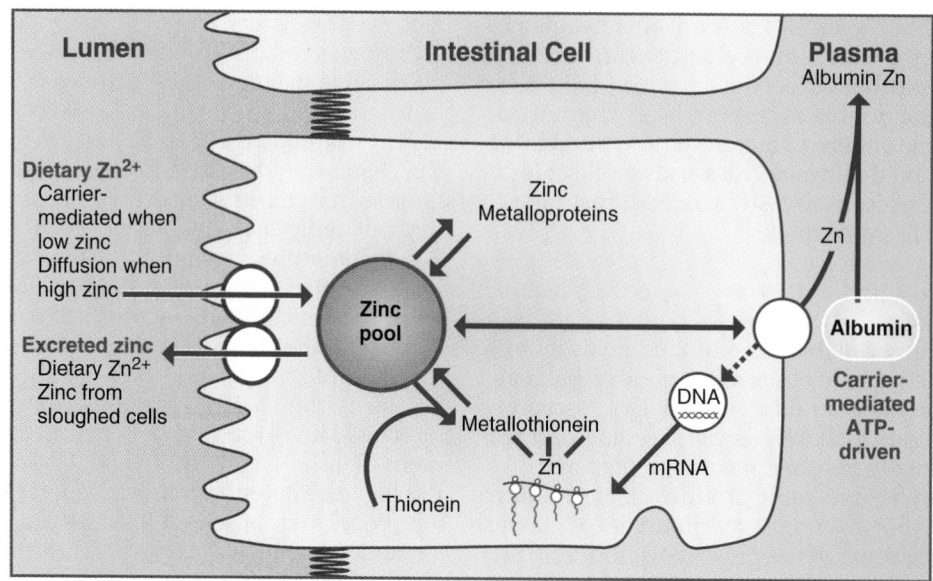

FIGURE 5-11 • Model for zinc absorption showing the relationship between metallothionein and cysteine-rich intestinal protein. (*DNA*, Deoxyribonucleic acid; *mRNA*, messenger ribonucleic acid; *ATP*, adenosine triphosphate.)

ologic factors such as injury or inflammation. Plasma zinc levels drop by 50% in the acute phase of a response to an injury, probably because of the sequestering of zinc by the liver, although transferrin may also increase its zinc content (King and Keen, 1994).

When zinc is administered intravenously, about 10% of the dose appears in the intestine within 30 minutes. Serum concentration decreases after a zinc-free meal, possibly because the pancreas removes zinc from the circulation to produce and secrete zinc metalloenzymes needed for digestion and absorption.

Intestinal Excretion

Excretion of zinc in normal individuals is almost entirely via the feces. However, increased urinary excretion has been reported in those who are starving and those with nephrosis, diabetes, alcoholism, hepatic cirrhosis, and porphyria. Plasma and urine concentrations of amino acids, specifically the zinc-binding cysteine and histidine, and other urinary metabolites, may have a role in increasing zinc losses in these patients.

Functions

Zinc, primarily an intracellular ion, functions in association with more than 300 different enzymes. It participates in reactions involving either synthesis or degradation of major metabolites—carbohydrates, lipids, proteins—and nucleic acids. This trace mineral also plays important structural roles as components of several proteins and functions as an intracellular signal in brain cells. Zinc is also involved in the stabilization of protein and nucleic acid structure and the integrity of subcellular organelles, as well as in transport processes, immune function, and expression of genetic information.

Metallothionein is the most abundant, nonenzymatic zinc-containing protein known today. This low–molecular-weight protein is rich in cysteine and exceptionally high in metals, among which are zinc and lesser amounts of copper, iron, cadmium, and mercury. The biologic role of metallothionein has not been defined conclusively, but it does have a function in zinc absorption. Metallothionein may function as an intracellular reservoir that can donate zinc ions to other proteins, or it may have a redox role that reduces oxidative stress, especially in cells with high stress. Thus metallothionein may have a role in the detoxification of metals as well as in their absorption.

Zinc is abundant in the nucleus, where it stabilizes RNA and DNA structure and is required for the activity of RNA polymerases important in cell division. Zinc also functions in chromatin proteins involved in transcription and replication.

A relationship between zinc intake and *age-related macular degenerative (AMD) disease* was suggested by previous reports, and a recent publication suggests that zinc supplementation (200 mg/day for 24 months) reduces AMD (age-related eye diseases [AREDS] Group, 2001).

Though widely touted to cure or prevent common colds, zinc gluconate lozenges were not proved to do so in a randomized, controlled trial with children and adolescents (Macknin et al, 1998) or in a study with adults (Turner and Cetnarowski, 2000). Nasal zinc sprays do not seem to be effective either (Belongia et al, 2001).

Zinc appears in the crystalline structure of bone, in bone enzymes, and at the zone of demarcation. It is thought to be needed for adequate osteoblastic activity, formation of bone enzymes such as alkaline phosphatase, and calcification. Unless bone resorption is occurring, the zinc in bone is not available (see Chapter 27).

Dietary Reference Intakes

The zinc DRIs established for adolescent and adult males are 11 mg/day. Because of the lower body weight of adolescent and adult women, their DRI is 8 mg/day. The DRIs for preadolescents are estimated to be 8 mg/day. The DRI for infants is 2 mg/day for the first 6 months and 3 mg/day for the second 6 months of life (see Table 5-6).

Food Sources and Intakes

For most Americans, almost 80% of the daily intake of zinc is provided by meat, fish, poultry, ready-to-eat breakfast cereals fortified with zinc, and milk and milk products (Subar et al, 1998). Oysters (which are especially high in zinc) and other shellfish, liver, whole-grain cereals, dry beans, and nuts are all good sources (Table 5-11). Soy products may also be fairly

TABLE 5-11 Zinc Content of Selected Foods

FOOD	CONTENT (mg)
Oysters, Eastern, ½ cup	113.0
Oysters, Pacific ½ cup	21.0
Wheat germ, toasted, ¼ cup	4.7
Ground beef, lean, 3 oz	4.6
Liver, beef, fried, 3 oz	4.6
Turkey, dark meat, baked, 3 oz	3.8
Beef enchilada, 1	2.3
Baked beans, with pork, ½ cup	1.9
Cheese, ricotta, part skim, ½ cup	1.7
Pecans, ¼ cup	1.6
Tahini (sesame butter), 1 tbsp	1.6
Peanuts, dry roasted, ¼ cup	1.4
Crab, canned, ¼ cup	1.3
Wild rice, cooked, ½ cup	1.1
Clams, canned, ¼ cup	1.1
Lobster, cooked, ½ cup	1.1
Cheese, Edam, 1 oz	1.1
Milk, 2% fat, 1 cup	1.0
Chicken, breast, baked, 1	1.0
Walnuts, English, ¼ cup	0.8
Gingerbread, 1 piece	0.6
Egg, 1	0.6
Salmon, baked, 3 oz	0.4

From U.S. Department of Agriculture: *Composition of foods*, USDA Handbook No. 8 Series, Washington, DC, 1976-1986, Agricultural Research Service, The Department.

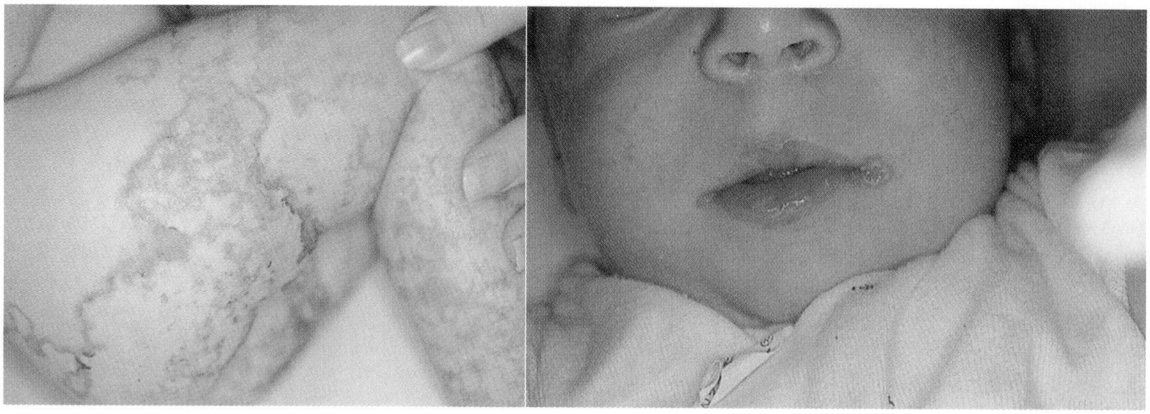

FIGURE 5-12 • Cutaneous manifestations of zinc deficiency. (From Callen WBS et al: *Color atlas of dermatology,* Philadelphia, 1993, WB Saunders.)

good sources of zinc. In general, zinc intake correlates well with protein intake.

The zinc content of typical diets of adults in Western countries ranges between 10 and 15 mg/day, but women consume less than men because of their lower caloric intakes. The zinc density of the American adult's diet is about 5.6 mg/1000 kcal (Subar et al, 1998).

Deficiency

The clinical signs of zinc deficiency in humans that were first described involved young boys in Iran and Egypt and included short stature, hypogonadism, mild anemia, and low plasma zinc level (Prasad et al, 1963) (see *Clinical Insight:* The Role of Zinc in Children's Health). This deficiency is caused by a diet high in unrefined cereals and unleavened breads, which contain high levels of fiber and phytate, both of which chelate with zinc in the intestine and prevent absorption. The anemia in the youths may have reflected a coexisting iron deficiency from the same cause. Additional symptoms of zinc deficiency include *hypogeusia* (decreased taste acuity), delayed wound healing, alopecia, and diverse forms of skin lesions. Acquired zinc deficiency may occur as the result of malabsorption, starvation, or increased losses via urinary, pancreatic, or other exocrine secretions.

Patients with alcoholism may have altered zinc metabolism. Pregnant women and older adults are also at increased risk for deficiency. In one study of older adults in institutions, low-dose zinc supplementation partially reversed measures of poor zinc status (Boukaïba et al, 1993).

Acrodermatitis enteropathica, an autosomal recessive disease characterized by zinc malabsorption, results in eczematoid skin lesions (Figure 5-12), alopecia, diarrhea, intercurrent bacterial and yeast infections, and eventually death if left untreated. Symptoms generally first develop during weaning from human milk to cow's milk. A potential adverse interaction between iron and zinc may contribute to acrodermatitis enteropathica.

Box 5-2. Zinc Deficiency Symptoms

Growth retardation
Delayed sexual maturation
Hypogonadism and hypospermia
Alopecia
Delayed wound healing
Skin lesions
Impaired appetite
Immune deficiencies
Behavioral disturbances
Eye lesions, including photophobia and night blindness
Impaired taste (hypogeusia)

Zinc deficiency results in various immunologic defects. Severe deficiency is accompanied by thymic atrophy, lymphopenia, reduced lymphocyte proliferative response to mitogens, a selective decrease in T_4-helper cells, decreased NK cell activity, anergy, and deficient thymic hormone activity. Even mild zinc deficiency can reduce immune function, producing impaired interleukin-2 production, for example. Supplementation with zinc may improve immune status, but more studies are needed to confirm this. Moderate zinc deficiency is associated with anergy and diminished NK cell activity but not with thymic atrophy or lymphopenia. Box 5-2 summarizes the clinical manifestations of human zinc deficiency. Similarities between patients with sickle cell anemia and zinc deficiency suggest the possibility of a secondary zinc deficiency in those with the anemia (see Chapter 34).

Low zinc intakes are associated with low concentrations of insulin-like growth factor 1 (IGF-l) in postmenopausal women, but the meaning of this finding is unclear (Devine et al, 1998). If calcium supplements are taken by postmenopausal women, it is possible that zinc absorption becomes suppressed, reducing IGF-l, which normally supports tissue growth. Problems caused by low zinc intakes seem to be increasing, partly because of the low bioavailability of zinc (Fairweather-Tait, 1998). Athletes may also have an increased risk for developing zinc deficiency. Physical activity may increase mobilization of zinc from bone stores for cellular needs (e.g., for the synthesis of zinc-metalloenzymes) (see Chapter 26).

Toxicity

Oral ingestion of toxic amounts of zinc (100 to 300 mg/day) is rare, but the UL for zinc in adults is 40 mg/day (Food and Nutrition Board, 2001) (see Table 5-7). Excessive zinc supplementation has long been known to interfere with copper absorption. A major form of zinc toxicity develops in patients receiving hemodialysis for renal failure. Contamination of dialysis fluids from the adhesive plastic used on the dialysis coils or from galvanized pipes has been reported. The toxic syndrome in these patients is characterized by anemia, fever, and central nervous system disturbances. Zinc sulfate in amounts of 2 g/day or more may cause GI irritation and vomiting. Inhalation of zinc fumes during welding may be toxic, but exposure to fumes can be prevented with proper precautions.

Fluoride

Fluoride is a natural element found in nearly all drinking water and soil, although the fluoride content varies greatly throughout the world (Palmer and Anderson, 2000). For example, some well water has much more fluoride than other water, so families who use well water need to monitor fluoride levels periodically to make sure that levels are not in the fluorotic range. Although fluoride is not considered an essential element, this anion is known to be important for the health of bones and teeth (see Chapters 27 and 28). The average skeleton contains 2.5 mg of fluoride.

Functions

Fluoride is considered important, if not essential, because of its benefits for tooth enamel—conferring maximal resistance to dental caries—and possibly for skeletal hydroxyapatite. Fluoride also acts as an antibacterial agent in the oral cavity, serving as an enzyme inhibitor. Fluoride has no known requirement in human metabolic pathways.

The prevalence of dental caries has decreased by 50% in recent decades because of fluoridation of drinking water and the use of topical fluorides. The prevalence of dental caries has also decreased in communities without fluoridated water. The cause of this decrease probably results from the use of fluoridated toothpaste, topical fluoride applications, and increased use of fluorides in food, especially in fluoridated water used in food processing, all of which provide fluoride for incorporation into teeth. Soft drinks typically are prepared with fluoridated waters at bottling plants in urban areas. (See Chapter 28 for fluoride supplementation recommendations.)

Fluoride substitutes for the hydroxyl group on the lattice structure of calcium phosphate salts (i.e., hydroxyapatites) of the bones and teeth to form *fluoroapatite,* which is harder and less readily resorbed than hydroxyapatite. However, after fluoridation, bone tissue formed at high flouride blood levels is not as healthy because it is subject to greater numbers of fractures from too tight binding of the flouroapatite (crystals) compared with the hydroxyapatite unfluoridated bone (see Chapter 27).

Dietary Reference Intakes

The AIs for fluoride were established for the first time in 1997. AIs for adult men and women are 4 and 3 mg/day, respectively. Depending on age, the AIs range from 2 to 3 mg/day for children and adolescents and from 0.7 to 1 mg/day for young children between the ages of 1 and 8 years (see Table 5-6) (Food and Nutrition Board, 1997). For comparison, an 8-oz glass of fluoridated water (1 ppm or 1 mg/L) provides about 0.2 mg of fluoride. ULs have also been established for fluoride (see Table 5-7).

Food Sources and Intakes

The major dietary sources of fluoride are drinking water and processed foods that have been prepared or reconstituted with fluoridated water. Seafood also is high in fluoride, but the flouride content of freshwater fish is lower than that of saltwater fish. The standard recommendation is 1 ppm in fluoridated community water supplies. Children who consume fluoridated water typically consume more fluoride than children who consume unfluoridated water. Intakes higher than 2 mg begin to raise concerns about mild fluorosis, which has been reported in a few U.S. communities.

Although fluorides exist in fruits and vegetables, the amounts in most foods other than seafood and tea are not significant. The amount in tea leaves can be quite substantial, depending on the brewing strength. One cup of tea may contain as much as 1 mg of fluoride. Soups and stews made with fish and meat bones also provide substantial fluoride. Beef liver and mechanically deboned meat and fowl are also high in fluoride. Cooking foods in Teflon pans (a fluoride-containing polymer) may increase fluoride intake, although solid scientific data are not available to support this fact.

Deficiency

Because no known metabolic function exists for fluoride, fluoride cannot have a true deficiency that results in disease. Fortuitous binding in hydroxyapatite crystals, especially from fluoridated water supplies, reduces dental caries, but it does not seem to have any effect on reducing osteoporotic fractures (Palmer and Anderson, 2000).

Toxicity

A mild fluorosis can develop from daily doses of 0.1 mg/kg—that is, greater than about 2 to 3 ppm of fluoride in the drinking water (see Chapter 28). The resulting discoloration of the teeth, or mottling, is not usually visible and has no adverse effect except cosmetically. However, higher intakes lead to tooth flaking and more serious dental effects.

Some evidence suggests that fluoride intakes are increasing among toddlers and young children because of the proliferating sources of fluoride. When drinking water contained less fluoride, the average intake was lower. Even the highest values did not exceed the recommendation of 0.08 mg/kg daily. Intakes of fluoride by young children may vary greatly because of the widespread availability of foods prepared with fluoridated water, the use of dentifrices, and other sources. Therefore some are concerned that some children may ingest total amounts of fluoride that exceed the optimal intake level (0.05 to 0.07 mg/kg daily), possibly causing dental fluorosis.

Copper

Copper, a normal constituent of blood, is another established essential micronutrient. Recent interest in copper and several other trace elements has increased because of the many tissue-related functions and the potential (though unlikely) risk of deficiency (Uauy et al, 1998). Concentrations of copper are highest in the liver, brain, heart, and kidney. Muscle contains a low level of copper, but because of its large mass, skeletal muscle contains almost 40% of all the copper in the body. Recent investigations have increased the understanding of the physiologic roles of copper, copper homeostasis, and copper needs throughout the life cycle (Lönnerdal and Uauy, 1998).

Absorption, Transport, Storage, and Excretion

Copper absorption occurs in the small intestine. Entry at the mucosal surface is by facilitated diffusion, and exit across the basolateral membrane is primarily by active transport, but facilitated transfer may also occur. Competition between copper ions and other divalent cations exists at each step. Within the intestinal absorbing cells, copper ions are bound to metallothionein with greater affinity than zinc or other ions. Some evidence suggests that the amount of copper absorbed is regulated by the amount of metallothionein in the mucosal cells. Net absorption of copper varies from 25% to 60%. Low absorption efficiencies help to regulate the retention of copper in the body; therefore the percentage of absorption decreases with increased intake. Fiber and phytate, known to affect bioavailability of several minerals, may slightly inhibit copper absorption, as shown by a study comparing a vegetarian diet with an omnivorous diet. However, because the total content of copper in the study's vegetarian diet was higher, the total amount of copper absorbed was also higher than from the nonvegetarian diet (Hunt and Vanderpool, 2001).

Approximately 90% of the copper in serum is incorporated into ceruloplasmin; the rest is bound loosely to albumin, transcuprein, and other proteins; free amino acids; and possibly histidine. Copper is transported in the blood to other tissues, primarily bound to albumin. It also exists in blood as ceruloplasmin, a functional protein that acts as an enzyme at the erythrocyte-forming cells of the bone marrow. Serum copper and immunoreactive ceruloplasmin levels tend to be higher in women than in men. The serum copper concentration is greatest in the neonate and decreases gradually during the first year of life.

Copper bound to albumin in the blood may serve as a temporary storage site for copper. In the liver, copper binds to metallothionein, which serves as a storage form, and is incorporated into ceruloplasmin and secreted into the plasma for the transport of copper to cells. Copper is also secreted from the liver as a component of bile, the major route of excretion of copper. Once in the GI tract, copper becomes part of the pool that may be reabsorbed or excreted, depending on the body's need for copper. Biliary excretion increases in response to excessive intakes of copper but may not be able to keep up with intake, allowing it to reach toxic levels.

Small amounts of copper are found in urine, sweat, and menstrual blood. Copper can be conserved by the kidney if necessary when substantial amounts are filtered through the glomeruli and reabsorbed in the tubules.

The interaction of copper with other nutrients negates the fallacy that taking excessive amounts of vitamin and mineral supplements above the recommended levels of consumption is good. In amounts of 150 mg/day, zinc has been shown to induce copper deficiency by overwhelming the capacity of metallothionein in intestinal absorbing cells to bind copper (even though metallothionein has a greater affinity for copper than for zinc). High ascorbic acid intake (1500 mg/day) also reduces blood concentrations of copper, which may decrease the role of ceruloplasmin in red cell formation.

Functions

Copper is a component of many enzymes, and symptoms of copper deficiency are attributable to enzyme failures. Copper in ceruloplasmin has a well-documented role in oxidizing iron before it is transported in the plasma. Lysyl oxidase, a copper-containing enzyme, is essential in the lysine-derived cross-linking of collagen and elastin, connective tissue proteins with great tensile strength (Rucker et al, 1998).

Through the involvement of copper-containing electron transport proteins, copper also has roles in mitochondrial energy production. As part of copper-containing enzymes such as superoxide dismutase, copper protects against oxidants and free radicals and promotes the synthesis of melanin and catecholamines. Other functions of copper-containing enzymes have not yet been completely defined.

Dietary Reference Intakes

RDAs of 900 μg/day (0.9 mg/day) for adolescents and adults of both genders have been established for copper (Food and Nutrition Board, 2001; Trumbo et al, 2001). Copper intakes should range between 200 and 220 μg/day for infants and between 340 and 440 μg for young children (see Table 5-6). Premature infants are born with low copper reserves and may require additional dietary copper during their first few months of life (see Chapter 9).

Food Sources and Intakes

Copper is distributed widely in foods, including animal products (except for milk), and most diets provide between 0.6 and 2 mg/day. Foods high in copper are shellfish (oysters), organ meats (liver, kidney), muscle meats, chocolate, nuts, cereal grains, dried legumes, and dried fruits (Table 5-12).

In general, fruits and vegetables contain little copper. Cow's milk, a poor source of copper, contains 0.015 to 0.18 mg/L, whereas the copper in human milk is well absorbed and ranges from 0.15 to 1.05 mg/L. Infants fed cow's milk may be at risk for copper deficiency because of its low copper content (Lönnerdal, 1996).

Copper intakes of individuals in several age categories in the United States have been consistently below recommended amounts, with adolescent girls consuming only about 50% of the recommended intakes, according to estimated median intakes reported in the Total Diet Study of the Food and Drug Administration (FDA) (Pennington and Schoen, 1996). Typically, the copper content of drinking water is not considered in diet surveys, but the amount of copper in water from copper pipes is considered to be very low, perhaps insignificant.

Copper intakes may be low in U.S. diets because until recently, ready-to-eat cereals typically were not fortified with copper as they were for several other trace minerals such as iron and zinc (Johnson et al, 1998). Another reason for the potential existence of low copper intakes is the inaccuracy associated with short-term assessments of dietary copper (Pang et al, 2001).

Deficiency

Copper deficiency has historically been assessed by a decrease in serum copper and ceruloplasmin levels, but more sensitive indicators of copper status—copper-containing enzymes in blood cells—have now been identified (Milne, 1998). Copper deficiency is characterized by anemia, neutropenia, and skeletal abnormalities, especially demineralization. Other changes may also develop, including subperiosteal hemorrhages, hair and skin depigmentation, and defective elastin formation. The failure of erythropoiesis, as well as cerebral and cerebellar degeneration, may lead to death. Neutropenia and leukopenia are the best early indications of copper deficiency in children. Copper deficiency anemia is discussed in Chapter 34.

Classical cases of copper deficiency were reported in the 1960s among Peruvian infants who were poorly nourished, had diarrhea, and were fed diluted cow's milk (Cordano, 1998). Other cases of deficiency have been reported since then. Premature infants are likely to have copper deficiency unless given a copper supplement, because most of the copper is normally transferred across the placenta during the last few months of a full-term pregnancy (see Chapter 9).

Copper is stored in the liver; therefore deficiency develops slowly as copper stores become depleted. Deficiencies have not been reported in otherwise healthy humans consuming a varied diet. Low serum copper, ceruloplasmin, and superoxide dismutase levels provide supportive evidence of copper deficiency, but these markers are not sensitive to marginal copper status. Bone changes, including osteoporosis, metaphyseal spur formation, and soft tissue calcification in infants receiving prolonged TPN may resolve with copper supplementation. The only signs of copper deficiency found in adults are neutropenia and microcytic anemia, but deficiency is very rare in adults, probably because copper accumulates in the liver throughout life in most individuals.

Menkes' syndrome, also known as *kinky-hair syndrome,* is a sex-linked recessive defect that results in

TABLE 5-12 Copper Content of Selected Foods

FOOD	CONTENT (mg)
Beef liver, fried, 3 oz	2.4
Cashews, dry roasted, ¼ cup	0.8
Black-eyed peas, dried, cooked, ½ cup	0.7
Molasses, blackstrap, 2 tbsp	0.6
Sunflower seeds, ¼ cup	0.6
Chocolate chips, semisweet, ¼ cup	0.5
V-8 juice, 1 cup	0.5
Tofu, firm, ½ cup	0.5
Beans, refried, ½ cup	0.5
Instant breakfast, fortified, 1 envelope	0.5
Cocoa powder, 2 tbsp	0.4
Prunes, dried, 10	0.4
Salmon, baked, 3 oz	0.3
Tahini (sesame butter), 1 tbsp	0.2
Pizza, cheese, ⅛ of 15 inch	0.2
Bread, whole wheat, 1 slice	0.1
Milk chocolate, 1 oz	0.1
Milk, 2% fat, 1 cup	0.1

From U.S. Department of Agriculture: *Composition of foods,* USDA Handbook No. 8 Series, Washington, DC, 1976-1986, Agricultural Research Service, The Department.

copper malabsorption, increased urinary copper loss, and abnormal intracellular copper transport, all of which cause an abnormal distribution of copper among organs and within cells. Affected infants have retarded growth, defective keratinization and pigmentation of the hair, hypothermia, degenerative changes in aortic elastin, abnormalities of the metaphyses of long bones, and progressive mental deterioration. These infants typically do not survive the first few months of life. Many of the features of this disorder result from interference with the cross-linking of collagen and elastin, steps that require one or more copper enzymes. Brain tissue is practically devoid of cytochrome C oxidase, and a marked accumulation of copper occurs in the intestinal mucosa, although serum copper and ceruloplasmin levels remain very low. Many defects exist in connective tissue in patients with Menkes' syndrome.

A relatively new type of copper deficiency manifests as a demyelinating neuropathy with chronic intestinal pseudoobstruction, osteoporosis, testicular failure, retinal degeneration, and cardiomyopathy. The underlying defect seems to involve hepatic incorporation of copper into ceruloplasmin (Buchman et al, 1994). Decreased plasma copper levels develop in patients with malabsorption diseases such as celiac sprue, tropical sprue, protein-losing enteropathies, and nephrotic syndrome. Like zinc, low copper intakes may also contribute to reduced immune responses in otherwise healthy individuals.

Toxicity

Copper toxicity from food consumption is considered impossible, but toxicity from excessive supplementation or copper salts used in agriculture has been reported. Liver cirrhosis typically develops from toxic intake levels, and abnormalities in red blood cell formation also occur.

Ceruloplasmin concentrations increase during pregnancy and with the use of oral contraceptives. Serum copper concentrations in pregnant women are approximately twice those in women who are not pregnant. Serum copper concentrations are also elevated in patients with acute and chronic infections, liver disease, and pellagra. The physiologic significance of these elevations is not known, but bile also contains substantial amounts of copper in these patients. Any chronic liver disease that interferes with the excretion of bile may contribute to the retention of copper. Primary biliary cirrhosis, as well as mechanical obstruction of the bile ducts, contributes to a progressive rise in liver copper content.

Wilson's disease (hepatolenticular degeneration) is characterized by excessive accumulation of copper in body tissues such as the eyes as a result of a genetic deficiency in the liver synthesis of ceruloplasmin (see Chapter 31). A strict vegetarian diet may benefit patients with Wilson's disease because of the low copper content of fruits and vegetables (Brewer et al, 1993).

ULTRATRACE MINERALS

Ultratrace minerals, such as iodine, selenium, manganese, molybdenum, chromium, and a few other nonessential minerals, are found in the body in small quantities, and their amounts are typically measured in micrograms. Each of these elements has one or more essential roles in human tissues. Because of their small quantities in human tissues, special analytic instrumentation and ultra-clean laboratories are necessary for the routine analysis or experimental work relating to the ultratrace minerals.

Of the several trace elements, only a few—copper, zinc, and iron—have been found to be consistently deficient in the diets of those living in the United States. However, American ready-to-eat cereals are now fortified with all three of these elements, so deficiencies of these trace minerals may be eliminated in the future. The full extent of the benefits of these nutritionally enhanced foods has not yet been evaluated. Other ultratrace elements such as chromium and manganese may also be consumed in inadequate amounts from the food supply today, in part because of processing; evidence supporting the prevalence of these deficiencies needs strengthening. Of all the microminerals, fluoride is most commonly associated with increased risk of toxicity (e.g., fluorosis in infants and children) (see Chapters 27 and 28), but toxicities of other trace elements (e.g., selenium) may occur, although not from food. However, toxicity is a concern because the food supply could become overfortified.

Iodine

Iodine deficiency in the United States and many Western nations has practically been eliminated with the iodinization of salt. However, people living in many mountainous areas of the world and a few low-lying delta regions still have low iodine intakes because of the low iodine content of the soil used in cultivating crops. Others living in lowlands may have high goitrogen consumption that reduces iodine use by the thyroid gland. The body normally contains 20 to 30 mg of iodine, with more than 75% in the thyroid gland and the rest distributed throughout the body, particularly in the lactating mammary gland, gastric mucosa, and blood. Dietary iodine is needed for the synthesis of thyroid hormones.

Absorption, Transport, Storage, and Excretion

Iodine is absorbed easily as iodide. In the circulation, iodine exists freely and protein bound, but the bound iodide predominates. Excretion is primarily via urine, but small amounts are found in the feces as a result of biliary secretion.

Functions

Iodine is stored in the thyroid gland, where it is used in the synthesis of triiodothyronine (T_3) and thyroxine (T_4). Uptake of iodide ions by the thyroid cells may be inhibited by goitrogens (substances that exist naturally in foods). Thyroid hormone is degraded in target cells and the liver, and the iodine is highly conserved under normal conditions. Selenium is important in iodine metabolism because of its presence in one enzyme responsible for forming active T_3 from thyroglobulin stored in the thyroid gland.

Recommended Dietary Allowances

An iodine intake of 150 μg/day has been suggested as sufficient for all adults and adolescents. The RDA for pregnant and lactating women increases to 220 μg and 290 μg, respectively. The RDA is 110 μg for infants up to 6 months of age, and 130 μg for older infants. The RDA for children is between 90 and 120 μg and increases with age (or body size) (see Table 5-6).

Food Sources and Intakes

Iodine exists in variable amounts in food and drinking water. Seafood such as clams, lobsters, oysters, sardines, and other saltwater fish is the richest source of iodine. Saltwater fish contain 300 to 3000 μg/kg of flesh; freshwater fish contain 20 to 40 μg/kg, but they are still good sources. The iodine content of cow's milk and eggs is determined by the iodides available in the diet of the animal; the iodide content of vegetables varies according to the iodine content of the soil in which they grow. Iodine also enters the food chain through *iodophors,* which are used as disinfectants in dairy processing, coloring agents, and dough conditioners. These sources add significant amounts of iodine to the food supply. Table 5-13 lists the iodine content of various foods.

TABLE 5-13 Iodine Content of Selected Foods

FOOD	CONTENT (μg)
Salt, iodized, 1 tsp	400
Bread, made with iodate dough conditioner and continuous mix process, 1 slice	142
Haddock, 3 oz	104-145
Bread, made with regular process, 1 slice	35
Cheese, cottage, 2% fat, ½ cup	26-71
Shrimp, 3 oz	21-37
Egg, 1	18-26
Cheese, cheddar, 1 oz	5-23
Ground beef, 3 oz	8

From U.S. Department of Agriculture: *Composition of foods,* USDA Handbook No. 8 Series, Washington, DC, 1976-1986, Agricultural Research Service, The Department.

The use of iodized salt should still be advocated in certain areas to prevent goiter. The best way to obtain an adequate intake of iodine is to use iodized salt (which has 60 μg of iodine per gram of salt in the United States and Canada) in food preparation (Kuhajek, 2000). More than 50% of the table salt sold in the United States is iodized; however, iodized salt is not used in processed foods. Mandatory iodinization has been adopted by many nations, including Canada, but is not legally required in the United States, where iodine deficiency is now very rare. The Total Diet Study of the FDA showed that median adult iodine intakes from 1982 to 1991 ranged from 130 to 140 μg/day for women and 182 to 204 μg/day for men. The median iodine intake for male and female teenagers was even higher, with adolescent boys consuming almost twice the RDA (Pennington and Schoen, 1996). Intakes of iodine in the United States seem adequate for most people because of iodinization of salt and the use of iodofors.

A small subset of vegans who eat only uncooked, lactobacilli-rich food were tested for thyroid function and found to be within normal limits (Rauma et al, 1994). These vegans consumed iodine in seaweed or kelp tablets. Some of the individuals in this study had iodine intakes high enough to cause potential problems, but symptoms of toxicity were not observed.

Deficiency

An estimated 2 billion people worldwide living in less developed nations remain at risk for iodine deficiency. These individuals may have a moderate iodine deficiency, even when obvious goiter, a severe condition, is not evident. In schoolchildren, iodine deficiency is associated with poor cognition. Iodine deficiency is the most common preventable cause of mental retardation in the world (Lee et al, 1999) Use of iodized salt, or the oral administration of a single dose of iodized oil would suffice to correct iodine deficiency for about 1 year. Weekly iodine supplements also are effective (Alnwick, 1998). Use of iodized salt should be encouraged during pregnancy, especially through the end of the second trimester (Xue-Yi et al, 1994). Very low iodine intakes are associated with the development of endemic or simple goiter, which is an enlargement of the thyroid gland (Figure 5-13). The deficiency may be nearly total, especially in mountainous areas and regions of high goitrogen intakes, or relative, subsequent to an increased need for thyroid hormones (e.g., by females during adolescence, pregnancy, and lactation.

Goiter may affect as many as 200 to 300 million people worldwide. In some countries, goiter is so common that it is regarded as a normal physical feature. In the United States the prevalence rate of goiter for all ages is 1.9/1000 persons.

The rate is higher in women than in men and is higher in older individuals than in younger ones.

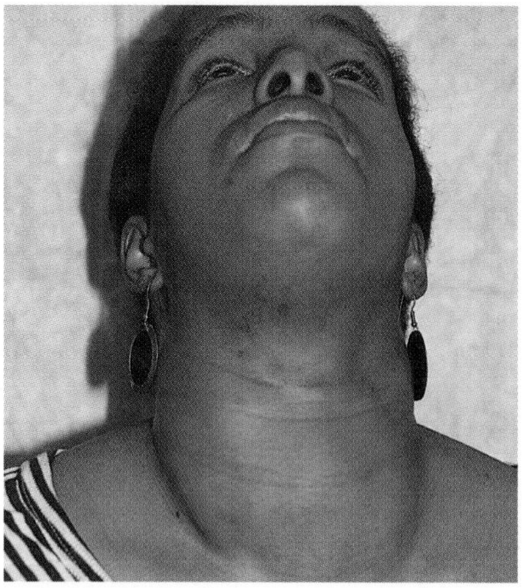

FIGURE 5-13 • Goiter caused by iodine deficiency. (From Swartz MH: *Textbook of physical diagnosis history and examination*, ed 3, Philadelphia, 1998, WB Saunders.)

Goitrogens, which exist naturally in foods, can also cause goiter by blocking uptake of iodine from the blood by thyroid cells. Foods containing goitrogens include cabbage, turnips, rapeseeds (from rape plants), peanuts, cassava, sweet potatoes, kelp, and soybeans. Goitrogens are inactivated by heating or cooking. Severe iodine deficiency during gestation and early postnatal growth results in cretinism in infants, a syndrome characterized by mental deficiency, spastic diplegia or quadriplegia, deaf mutism, dysarthria, a characteristic shuffling gait, shortened stature, and hypothyroidism. Less severe variations of this syndrome also exist, manifesting as moderate retardation in intellectual or neuromotor maturation.

Toxicity

Even though iodine intakes have a wide margin of safety, tolerable ULs have been established (Food and Nutrition Board, 2001). Adults have a UL of 1100 μg/day, and young children have a UL of 200 to 300 μg/day (see Table 5-7). In some cases, goiter develops slowly as a consequence of long-term iodine intakes that are much higher than physiologic requirements. The role of excessive iodine in thyroid disease or disorder is not clear (Lee et al, 1999). Today, the level of iodine in foods is not considered a significant public health problem in the United States or Canada. However, two different studies, one in Canada and the other in the United States, reported iodine intakes that were either greater than or approximately equal to recommended intake levels throughout the life cycle (Discher and Girous, 1987; Pennington and Schoen, 1996). The level of iodine in most American diets is appropriate for good health, but for small groups of people with underlying thyroid pathologic conditions, excessive iodine in the diet may result in hypothyroidism, goiter formation, or hyperthyroidism (Lee et al, 1999).

Selenium

A rather narrow dietary intake range exists for selenium, below which deficiency occurs and above which toxicity develops. Only in China have these extremes been shown to relate to the soil content of selenium. A dietary intake of approximately 40 μg of selenium per day seems to be necessary to maintain glutathione peroxidase (GSH-Px), an enzyme containing selenium. The diets of practically all nations other than China supply selenium in sufficient amounts to maintain adequate levels of GSH-Px, so selenium deficiency is extremely rare. GSH-Px, discovered to be a selenoenzyme in the early 1970s, is considered the major active form of selenium in tissues, although other selenium proteins have since been discovered.

Tissue levels are influenced by dietary intake and reflect the geochemical environment. Regions of North America identified as low in selenium content are the Northeast, Pacific, Southwest, and coastal plain of the southeastern region of the United States, as well as north central and eastern Canada. The lowest selenium content of soil exists in a few regions of China, especially in Keshan, where severe selenium deficiency was first reported in a human population in 1979. Other areas with low selenium content include parts of Finland and New Zealand.

Absorption, Transport, Storage, and Excretion

Absorption of selenium, which occurs in the upper segment of the small intestine, is more efficient under conditions of deficiency. Increased intake frequently results in increased excretion of selenium in the urine. Selenium status is assessed by measuring selenium or GSH-Px in serum, platelets, and erythrocytes or in whole blood. Erythrocyte selenium measurement is an indicator of long-term intake (Neve, 2000). Selenium is transported bound to albumin initially and subsequently to α_2-globulin.

Functions

Many but not all of the pathologic changes caused by selenium deficiency can be explained on the basis of inadequate levels of GSH-Px. Because GSH-Px acts together with other antioxidants and free radical scavengers, these molecules reduce cellular peroxides and free radicals in general into water and other harmless molecules.

Additional roles for selenium that are not associated with GSH-Px have been identified. Selenium, as selenomethionine or selenocysteine, exists in several proteins that are widely distributed in the body. *Cellular glutathione peroxidase (cGSH-Px)* has been found in almost all cells and extracellularly in serum and milk. This family of enzymes may help provide a reserve of selenium in proteins that can be drawn on when needed. *Phospholipid hydroperoxide glutathione peroxidase (phGSH-Px),* which has a distribution in lipid-soluble fractions of the cell, may have other roles in lipid and eicosanoid metabolism.

Type I iodothyronine 5′-deiodinase, an enzyme capable of converting thyroxine (T_4) to triiodo- thyronine (T_3), is a selenoprotein. Moderate selenium intakes (40 μg/day) seem adequate to maintain activities of these deiodinases. However, high intakes (350 μg/day) were associated with depressed T_3 levels, suggesting less activity of iodothyronine deiodinase (Neve, 2000).

Selenoprotein P, another selenium-containing molecule, may act as a free radical scavenger or a transporter of selenium. Selenium is used in the synthesis of these molecules in the anionic form, but in the molecules selenium is covalently bound, as is sulfur, which it typically replaces in some of these molecules.

The antioxidant effects of selenium and vitamin E may reinforce each other by the overlap of their protective actions against oxidative damage. These two antioxidant nutrients may participate in other cooperative activities that help maintain healthy cells. GSH-Px acts in the cytosol and the mitochondrial matrix, whereas vitamin E exerts its antioxidative actions within cell membranes.

The GSH-Px reaction step is illustrated in Figure 5-14. Other selenium-dependent enzymes exist in mammalian systems, but less is known about the requirements of these enzymes for selenium. The antioxidative roles of cellular selenium-containing enzymes may have a role in preventing cancer. For example, in the only study of its kind, modest doses of selenium supplements given to adults resulted in a great reduction in prostate cancer as well as lesser decreases in several other cancers after a period of several years (Clark et al, 1996). Many other selenoproteins have been identified, but their functions have not yet been eludicated (Burk et al, 2001).

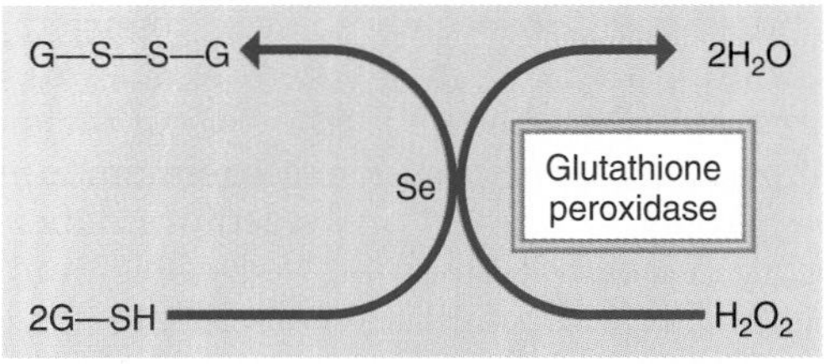

FIGURE 5-14 • Enzymatic reaction catalyzed by the selenium-containing enzyme, glutathione peroxidase (GSH-Px). Selenium is a prosthetic form of the enzyme that removes highly reactive hydrogen peroxide *(H_2O_2)* from within cells by converting it to water *(H_2O)* while simultaneously converting two molecules of reduced glutathione *(G—SH) to oxidized glutathione* (G—S—S—G).

TABLE 5-14 Selenium Content of Selected Foods

FOOD	CONTENT (μg)
Brazil nuts, ¼ cup	380
Snapper, baked, 3 oz	148
Halibut, baked, 3 oz	113
Salmon, baked, 3 oz	70
Scallops, steamed, 3 oz	70
Clams, steamed, 20	52
Oysters, raw, ¼ cup	35
Lasagna, with meat, 1 piece	34
Wheat germ, toasted, ¼ cup	28
Molasses, blackstrap, 2 tbsp	25
Sunflower seeds, ¼ cup	25
Granola, 1 cup	23
Ground beef, 3 oz	22
Chicken, breast, baked, 3 oz	17
Bread, whole wheat, 1 slice	16
Egg, 1	12
Milk, 2% fat, 1 cup	6
Cheese, cheddar, 1 oz	4

From Hands ES: *Food finder: food sources of vitamins and minerals,* ed 2, Salem, Ore, 1990, ESHA Research.

Dietary Reference Intakes

The RDAs for selenium were redefined in 2000 by the Food and Nutrition Board to be 55 μg/day for women, men, and adolescents (ages 14 to 18), whereas the RDAs for children range from 20 to 30 μg/day. The AI for infants is 15 to 20 μg/day (Trumbo et al, 2001). The RDA during pregnancy is 60 μg, and the RDA during lactation is 70 μg/day (see Table 5-6). Requirements for selenium may increase with a high consumption of saturated fatty acids because of the need for the antioxidant activity of selenium.

Food Sources and Intakes

No comprehensive table of the selenium content of foods has been published. The selenium concentration in foods depends on the selenium content of the soil and water where the food was grown. Improvements in analytic techniques have resulted in changes being made to many previously published data of the selenium content of foods during the last few decades. Table 5-14 lists the selenium contents of some foods.

Major food sources of selenium are Brazil nuts, seafood, kidney, liver, meat, and poultry; fruits and vegetables are low in selenium content. The major food source of selenium identified by the FDA's Total Diet Study was animal flesh foods. Grains vary in selenium content depending on where they are grown.

Selenium content and GSH-Px activity in human breast milk are influenced directly by maternal selenium intake and by the form of selenium consumed (McGuire et al, 1993a). Plasma selenium concentrations of infants fed unsupplemented formula are lower than those of infants fed supplemented formula or human milk (McGuire et al, 1993b).

Data summarized for the FDA's Total Diet Study (1982 to 1991) showed that the estimated median selenium intakes of adults and children were greater than the age-specific RDAs (Pennington and Schoen, 1996). Mean intakes of 19 and 13 μg/day in men and women, respectively, were reported in a low-selenium area of China where Keshan disease was prevalent (Yang et al, 1988). Typical diets consumed by Americans provide sufficient amounts of selenium daily to prevent any selenium deficiency and promote health (Levander, 1995). Selenium fortification of infant formulas with selenate has been shown to improve the selenium status of preterm infants (Tyrala et al, 1996).

Deficiency

Despite a wide range of selenium intakes from food, selenium deficiency is rare in populations throughout the world. Selenium deficiency takes years to develop when food intake is adequate. Severe selenium deficiency in a population has only been reported for regions in China, including Keshan. *Keshan disease,* a form of cardiomyopathy that mainly affects children and women, was first observed in the Keshan province of China. A viral infection combined with selenium deficiency has been suggested as the etiology of Keshan disease (Beck et al, 1994, 1995). Since its discovery, supplementation programs in Keshan have totally eradicated the disease. However, in individuals with established disease the response to supplementation is poor, probably because of other factors contributing to myopathy.

The second selenium deficiency disease, discovered in Mongolia, is known as *Kashin-Beck disease* and is common in preadolescent and adolescent children. These two human diseases occur in areas where the content of selenium in the soil is very low. This disease may also have a viral component combined with the selenium deficiency in the diet, but very little is known of its etiology. Illness initially involves symmetrical stiffness, swelling, and often pain in the interphalangeal joints of the fingers, followed by generalized osteroarthritis in which elbows, knees, and ankles are also involved (Sokoloff, 1988). Kashin-Beck disease may also have iodine deficiency as a risk factor (Moreno-Reyes et al, 1998).

Selenium deficiency has previously been reported in malnourished patients receiving long-term TPN. Supplementation resulted in improved serum selenium levels, platelet GSH-Px activity, and reduced clinical symptoms. Selenium deficiency should no longer be a problem in patients receiving long-term TPN or enteral nutrition because the preparation of these solutions now includes a trace element supplement (see Chapter 23).

Deficient selenium intakes may also contribute to carcinogenesis. Patients with some cancers have been shown to have low serum selenium levels, although the underlying mechanisms for this correlation have not been established. One possible explanation lies in the possible failure of GSH-Px to scavenge free radicals efficiently in dividing cells. In addition, patients with cirrhosis have low plasma selenium concentrations, which may predispose them to cancer (Burk et al, 1998).

Toxicity

Indicators of selenium toxicity and the level of dietary intake at which toxicity occurs have only been reported in China (Yang et al, 1983). Signs of toxicity, referred to as *selenosis,* include skin and nail changes, tooth decay, and nonspecific GI and neurologic abnormalities.

Manganese

Manganese deficiency in humans was first reported in 1972, and its essentiality in humans is well established. Symptoms of deficiency are weight loss, transient dermatitis, and occasionally nausea and vomiting, a change in hair color, and slow hair growth. Manganese deficiency in animals also affects reproductive capacity, pancreatic function, and several aspects of carbohydrate metabolism.

Absorption, Transport, Storage, and Excretion

Manganese is absorbed throughout the small intestine. Iron and cobalt compete for common binding sites for absorption. Men absorb less manganese than women, a difference that may be related to iron status according to a study by Finley et al (1994). In this study, manganese absorption was significantly associated with plasma ferritin. In another study (Greger et al, 1990), however, manganese was not found to correlate with serum iron concentrations in men. In young women, heme iron has no influence on manganese status, but diets high in nonheme iron were associated with lower serum manganese values, higher urinary manganese losses, and somewhat lower activity of a manganese-dependent enzyme called *superoxide dismutase* (Davis et al, 1992). Manganese is transported bound to a macroglobin, transferrin, and transmanganin. Excretion of manganese occurs mainly in the feces after secretion into the intestine via the bile.

Functions

The 10 to 20 mg of manganese contained in the adult human body tends to be concentrated predominantly in tissues rich in mitochondria. Manganese is a component of many enzymes, including glutamine synthetase, pyruvate carboxylase, and mitochondrial superoxide dismutase. In addition, manganese activates many other enzymes, most of which can also be activated by magnesium. Manganese is associated with the formation of connective and skeletal tissues, growth and reproduction, and carbohydrate and lipid metabolism.

Dietary Reference Intakes

The AIs for manganese are 2.3 mg/day for men and 1.8 mg/day for women. For children 9 years of age and older the AIs are 1.9 to 2.2 mg/day for boys and

1.6 mg/day for girls. For children the AIs are 1.2 to 1.5 mg/day, depending on their age (see Table 5-6).

Food Sources and Intakes

The manganese content of foods varies greatly. The richest sources are whole grains, legumes, nuts, and tea. Fruits and vegetables are moderately good sources. Animal tissues, seafood, and dairy products are poor sources. Relatively high amounts exist in instant coffee and tea. Human milk is relatively low in manganese. The Total Diet Study of the FDA (1982 to 1991) revealed that the median manganese intakes approximated the recommended intake for men and women but were too low for adolescent girls (Pennington and Schoen, 1996).

Deficiency

Even though the FDA Total Diet Study reported that manganese intakes were below recommended levels for adolescent girls (Pennington and Schoen, 1996), no physiologic evidence of insufficiency has been reported. Data on the physiologic effects resulting from manganese deficiency are confined to the results of animal studies. These studies have established the essentiality of manganese for reproduction. Sterility develops in both sexes; striking skeletal abnormalities and ataxia characterize the offspring of mothers who are manganese deficient.

Toxicity

Manganese toxicity has developed in miners as a result of absorption of manganese through the respiratory tract. The excess, which accumulates in the liver and central nervous system, produces Parkinson-like symptoms. Toxicity has also been reported in patients receiving TPN including manganese. Symptoms include headaches, dizziness, and abnormal magnetic resonance imaging (MRI) results and hepatic dysfunction (Masumoto et al, 2001). Upper limits of manganese intakes have been difficult to establish (Greger and Malecki, 1997).

Chromium

A biologic role for chromium was first proposed in 1954. Chromium was not accepted as an essential nutrient until 1977, however, when patients receiving TPN exhibited abnormalities of glucose metabolism that were reversed with chromium supplementation. The low concentrations of chromium in food, body tissues, and body fluids have required careful and appropriate analytic techniques and new standard reference materials for accurate measurements.

Absorption, Transport, Storage, and Excretion

As with other minerals, organic and inorganic forms of chromium are absorbed differently. Organic chromium is readily absorbed but quickly passes out of the body. Less than 2% of the trivalent chromium consumed is absorbed. Chromium absorption is increased by oxalate and is higher in iron-deficient animals than in animals with adequate iron, suggesting it shares some similarities with the iron absorption pathway. With dietary intakes of 40 μg or more per day, chromium absorption reaches and remains at a plateau; at such high intakes, urinary excretion increases to maintain balance. The type of dietary carbohydrate consumed modifies absorption from chromium chloride; starch, rather than sugar, increases absorption. The absorption of chromium ions from chromium picolinate is greater than that from chromium chloride, whose absorption efficiency is 2% or less.

Chromium and iron are carried by transferrin; however, albumin is also capable of assuming this role if iron transferrin saturation is high. In addition, α- and β-globulins and lipoproteins can also bind chromium.

Primarily the kidney excretes inorganic chromium, with small amounts being excreted through hair, sweat, and bile. Organic chromium is excreted through bile. Strenuous exercise, physical trauma, or an increased intake of simple sugar results in increased chromium excretion.

Functions

Chromium potentiates insulin action and as such influences carbohydrate, lipid, and protein metabolism. Although the chemical nature of the relationship between chromium and insulin activity has not been clearly identified, chromium may have a beneficial effect on serum triglyceride levels in patients with non–insulin-dependent diabetes mellitus (Lee and Reasner, 1994).

The proposed role of chromium with a so-called glucose tolerance factor (GTF) is controversial. A possible chromium-nicotinic acid (chromium polynicotinate) complex has been identified, but its structure has not been established by modem chemical techniques (Baumgartner, 1993). Chromium may regulate the synthesis of a molecule that potentiates insulin action. Another possible role for chromium, similar to that of zinc, is in the regulation of gene expression.

Twelve weeks of chromium picolinate supplementation was not shown to have any effects on plasma glucose concentrations, glucose-regulating hormones, or any other measure in moderately obese women who had completed an exercise program (Volpe et al, 2001).

Dietary Reference Intakes

The AIs recommended for chromium range from 25 to 35 μg/day for males 9 years of age and older and 21 to 25 μg/day for females of the same age. Depending on the age of the child, 11 to 15 μg/day has been established for children 1 to 8 years of age (Trumbo et al, 2001) (see Table 5-6).

TABLE 5-15 Chromium Content of Selected Foods

FOOD	CONTENT (μg)
Broccoli, 1 cup	22.0
Turkey, leg, 3 oz	10.4
Juice, grape, 1 cup	7.5
Waffle, egg, 1	6.7
Ham, 3 oz	3.6
English muffin, 1	3.6
Cookies, chocolate chip, 1 large	3.4
Potatoes, mashed, 1 cup	2.7
Bagel, egg, 1	2.5
Juice, orange, 1 cup	2.2
Green beans, 1 cup	2.2
Beef cubes, 3 oz	2.0
Lettuce, 1 wedge	1.8
Barbecue sauce, 1 tbsp	1.7
Ketchup, 1 tbsp	1.0
American cheese, 1 oz	0.56
Maple syrup, 1 tbsp	0.5

From Anderson RA, Bryden NA, Polansky MM: Dietary chromium intake, *Biol Trace Elem Res* 32:117, 1992.

Food Sources and Intakes

Precise assessment of chromium in foods is difficult; biologically available chromium and inorganic chromium cannot be distinguished from each other. Analyses done before 1980 must be considered with caution because determinations were flawed by contamination and analytic problems.

Brewer's yeast, oysters, liver, and potatoes have high chromium concentrations; seafood, whole grains, cheeses, chicken, meats, and bran have medium chromium concentrations. The refining of wheat removes chromium with the wheat germ and the bran; refining sugar fractionates the chromium into the molasses portion. Dairy products, fruits, and vegetables are low in chromium. Table 5-15 presents the chromium content of selected foods.

Usual chromium intakes range between 25 and 35 μg/day for women and men, respectively. Chromium intakes are not assessed in the USDA, NHANES, or Total Diet Study surveys because of inadequate methodology.

Human breast milk contains 3 to 8 nmol/L of chromium, which is lower than the recommended intake for infants.

Deficiency

Chromium deficiency results in insulin resistance and a few lipid abnormalities, which can be ameliorated by chromium supplementation. Insufficient chromium may be consumed by some Americans, but true deficiency is more likely to be significant in populations with very low chromium intakes, such as those in some areas of China (Anderson et al, 1997). Symptoms of chromium deficiency in animals includes impaired growth, elevated serum cholesterol and triglyceride concentrations, increased incidence of aortic plaques, corneal lesions, and decreased fertility and sperm count.

Recent claims that the ingestion of high doses of chromium (as chromium picolinate) improve strength, body composition, endurance, or other characteristics of physical fitness are controversial, with some studies supporting these claims and others not (Anderson, 1997). Lukaski et al (1996) found that chromium supplements did not improve body composition or strength in healthy men. However, both acute and chronic resistive exercise did increase urinary chromium losses in men who consumed the American Heart Association Phase I diet (with no supplements) (Rubin et al, 1998). The investigators concluded that these losses indicated increased absorption of chromium during the 16-week study.

Toxicity

Chromium toxicity from food has not been reported, but chromium picolinate taken as a supplement in high doses by athletes and power lifters has resulted in some adverse effects, primarily skin lesions.

Molybdenum

Molybdenum has been established as an essential micronutrient, particularly because of its requirement in the enzyme *xanthine oxidase.* Interrelationships among molybdenum, copper, and sulfate absorption in livestock and between molybdenum intake and copper excretion in humans and animals have been demonstrated. Individuals receiving long-term TPN have displayed symptoms of molybdenum deficiency, including mental changes and abnormalities of sulfur and purine metabolism.

Absorption, Transport, Storage, and Excretion

Molybdenum, which is found in minute amounts in the body, is readily absorbed from the stomach and small intestine, with the rate of absorption being higher in the proximal small intestine than in the distal small intestine. As with other minerals, molybdenum is absorbed by two mechanisms: carrier mediated and passive diffusion. Molybdenum is excreted primarily in the urine. Excretion, rather than absorption, is the homeostatic mechanism. Some molybdenum is also excreted in the bile.

Functions

Xanthine oxidase, aldehyde oxidase, and sulfite oxidase, all enzymes that catalyze oxidation-reduction reactions, require a prosthetic group containing molybdenum. Sulfite oxidase is important to the degradation of cysteine and methionine and catalyzes the formation of sulfate from sulfite. Genetic sulfite oxidase deficiency is a fatal disorder of cysteine metabolism. Clinical symptoms include severe brain damage with mental retardation, dislocation of the lens, and increased urinary output of sulfate (Rajagopalan, 1987). Whether molybdenum is involved in the response of some asthmatics to sulfites is not known.

Dietary Reference Intakes

The RDAs for molybdenum throughout the life cycle range from 43 to 45 μg/day for adolescent and adult males and females. Depending on age, RDAs range from 17 to 34 μg/day for children (see Table 5-6).

Food Sources and Intakes

Molybdenum is distributed widely in commonly consumed foods such as legumes, whole-grain cereals, milk and milk products, and dark green leafy vegetables. Estimated intakes, as determined by the FDA's Total Diet Study, ranged from 50 μg/day in infants to 80 and 126 μg/day for 14- to 16-year-old girls and boys, respectively. These intakes were found to decrease slowly over the lifetime of the subjects to 74 and 101 μg/day for 60- to 65-year-old women and men, respectively (Pennington and Jones, 1987).

Deficiency

Molybdenum deficiency has not been established in humans other than patients treated with TPN. Symptoms of molybdenum deficiency include mental changes and abnormalities of sulfur and purine metabolism.

Toxicity

An excessive molybdenum intake of 10 to 15 mg/day is associated with a goutlike syndrome (Nielsen, 2001). However, no good biomarkers are available to accurately assess the presence of molybdenum excess (Greger, 1997).

Boron

The essentiality of boron for humans has not yet been established, but its essentiality for plants and animals is widely accepted. Boron, an ultratrace element, is obtained from foods as sodium borate, and it is rapidly and almost completely (90%) absorbed. The highest concentrations of boron are found in bone, spleen, and thyroid, although it is present in all other tissues of the body. The roles of boron in humans have not been well studied, and symptoms of severe boron deficiency have not been established (Nielsen, 2001). Additional studies of this ultratrace element, especially its relationship to bone metabolism, are being conducted.

Functions

Boron is associated with cell membranes and in plants is involved with the functional efficiency of cell membranes. Response to boron deprivation is enhanced when other nutrients that alter membrane functions are also deficient. Boron apparently binds to the active site of some enzymes, reducing their ability to function. Boron is also thought to compete with some enzymes for the coenzyme *nicotinamide adenine dinucleotide.*

Evidence from animal studies shows that boron deprivation affects two major organs: the brain and bone. Boron deficiency alters brain composition and function and reduces bone composition, structure, and strength. Because of the role of boron in bone, studies in humans have focused on its potential role in the development of osteoporosis. Some evidence suggests that boron may have actions similar to estrogens on bone (Nielsen, 2001) (see Chapter 27). One report involving a rodent model has suggested that boron may actually improve bone strength (Chapin et al, 1997).

Dietary Reference Intakes

No DRIs have been established for boron.

Food Sources and Intakes

Foods that are good sources of boron include plant foods, especially noncitrus fruits, vegetables, nuts, and legumes. Wine, cider, and beer are other good sources of boron.

Deficiency and Toxicity

Boron deficiency has not been reported in humans, and no toxicity level has been established.

Cobalt

Most of the cobalt in the body exists with vitamin B_{12} stores in the liver, but one enzyme has an established specific requirement for cobalt. Blood plasma contains approximately 1 μg of cobalt per 100 ml.

Absorption, Transport, Storage, and Excretion

Cobalt may share at least part of the same intestinal transport mechanism as iron. Absorption is higher in patients with deficient iron intake, portal cirrhosis with iron overload, and idiopathic hemochromatosis. The major route of cobalt excretion is the urine; small amounts are excreted via feces, sweat, and hair.

Functions

The well-known essential role of cobalt is as a component of vitamin B_{12} (cobalamin). This vitamin is essential for the maturation of red blood cells and the normal function of all cells (see Chapters 4 and 34). In addition, methionine aminopeptidase, an enzyme involved in the regulation of translation (i.e., of DNA to RNA), is the only enzyme in humans known to have an established requirement of this trace element (Arfin et al, 1995).

Dietary Reference Intakes

The dietary requirement for cobalt is expressed in terms of vitamin B_{12}. Approximately 2 to 3 μg of vitamin B_{12} is needed daily (see Table 4-22 for the DRIs).

Food Sources and Intakes

Cobalt exists in foods; however, only microorganisms are able to synthesize vitamin B_{12}. Ruminant animals obtain cobalamin as the result of a symbiotic relationship with the microorganisms of their GI tract. The microorganisms of monogastric species such as humans have an extremely limited capacity for synthesis in areas where the vitamin can be absorbed; therefore, humans must obtain vitamin B_{12}—and thus cobalt—from animal foods such as organ and muscle meats. In some circumstances, ordinary bacterial contamination of foods of vegetable origin may supply the minute amounts of this vitamin required for normal function. The 1984 Total Diet Survey estimated cobalt intakes of the American population to be in the range of 6.3 to 10.8 μg/day for adults and 7.6 to 11.6 μg/day for 14- to 16-year-olds (Pennington and Jones, 1987).

Strict vegetarians who avoid all animal products may develop vitamin B_{12} deficiency. However, the deficiency may develop only after 3 to 6 years or not at all.

Deficiency

A cobalt deficiency develops only in relation to a vitamin B_{12} deficiency. Insufficient vitamin B_{12} causes a macrocytic anemia. A genetic defect limiting vitamin B_{12} absorption results in pernicious anemia, which is treated appropriately with massive doses of the vitamin. These forms of anemia are discussed in detail in Chapter 34.

Toxicity

A high intake of inorganic cobalt (existing freely from cobalamin) in animal diets produces polycythemia (an overproduction of red blood cells), hyperplasia of bone marrow, reticulocytosis, and increased blood volume.

The information on the microminerals (trace elements) known to be required by humans is summarized in Table 5-16.

OTHER TRACE ELEMENTS

Several other trace elements of uncertain essentiality exist, including aluminum, lithium, nickel, silicon, tin, and vanadium. A few other ultratrace elements, including arsenic, may be added to this list in the future. They are classified as *ultratrace elements* because of their very low quantities in human tissues. Requirements remain undefined for all of these elements because of their uncertain essentiality. The ultratrace elements continue to be enigmas because of their uncertain roles in human function. It has long been established that these elements exist in human tissues, especially in the skeleton, because of their abundance on the earth's surface, but the essentiality of any of these in humans remains questionable. These ultratrace elements have been reviewed by Nielsen (2001). The presence of several of these elements in various foods was reported in the Total Diet Study of the FDA (Pennington and Jones, 1987).

SUMMARY

The functions of macrominerals and microminerals vary significantly, but they all need to be consumed in reasonable amounts—near the recommended intake levels—each day to support certain functions. Most of these minerals have well-established deficiency diseases when intakes are insufficient and toxicities when intakes are greatly excessive. Multinutrient supplements commonly found in pharmacies and food markets typically contain recommended amounts of the nutrients, but this is not always the case (e.g., calcium); not all of the trace elements are found in these formulations. The best way to get such a variety of minerals is to consume various foods, including seafood, frequently rather than relying on a daily supplement.

Clinical Scenario

Miles is a 46-year-old Native American man with a history of high blood pressure (140/95), elevated serum cholesterol levels (240 mg/dl), and hypothyroidism. He currently takes a small dose of thyroid replacement hormone and a mild potassium-depleting diuretic. He has purchased an exercise bike for indoor use and has started a walking program. Other than increasing his activity levels, he plans to avoid all table salt and read food labels avidly when he shops for groceries.

1. What concerns do you have about his intake of iodine given his resolve to avoid table salt? Which other foods might provide sufficient iodine?
2. His usual diet, which contains few fruits and vegetables, is likely to contain an insufficient amount of which minerals? What suggestions do you have for increasing the intake of these minerals?
3. Miles drinks very little milk. What would you recommend to increase his dietary calcium intake?
4. Fluoridated water is not available to Miles. Does this concern you?

TABLE 5-16 Minerals in Human Nutrition

MINERAL	BODY LOCATION AND SELECTED BIOLOGIC FUNCTIONS	DRIs*	FOOD SOURCES	LIKELIHOOD OF DEFICIENCY
Macronutrients Essential at Daily Levels of 100 mg or More				
Calcium	99% is found in bones and teeth. Ionic calcium in body fluids is essential for ion transport across cell membranes. Calcium may also be bound to protein, citrate, or inorganic acids.	1000 mg for adults 19-50 yr; 1200 mg for adults 51+ yr (AI)	Milk and milk products, sardines, clams, oysters, kale, turnip greens, mustard greens, tofu	Dietary surveys indicate that many people do not meet AIs for calcium. Because bone serves as a homeostatic mechanism to maintain calcium levels in the blood, many essential functions are maintained, regardless of dietary intake. Long-term dietary deficiency is probably one of the factors responsible for development of osteroporosis later in life.
Phosphorus	About 80% is found in inorganic portion of bones and teeth. Phosphorus is a component of every cell, as well as of important metabolites, including DNA, RNA, ATP, and phospholipids. Phosphorus is also important for pH regulation.	700 mg for adults (RDA)	Cheese, egg yolk, milk, meat, fish, poultry, whole-grain cereals, and almost all other foods	Dietary inadequacy is not likely if protein and calcium intake are adequate.
Magnesium	About 50% is in bone; the remaining 50% is almost entirely inside body cells, with only about 1% located in extracellular fluid.	400-420 mg for men, 310-320 mg for women 14-70+ yr (RDA)	Whole-grain cereals, tofu nuts, meat, milk, green vegetables, legumes, chocolate	Dietary inadequacy is considered unlikely, but conditioned deficiency often develops and is usually associated with surgery, alcoholism, malabsorption, loss of body fluids, and certain hormonal and renal diseases.
Sulfur	Bulk of dietary sulfur is present in sulfur-containing amino acids needed for synthesis of essential metabolites. Sulfur functions in oxidation-reduction reactions, as part of thiamin and biotin.	No DRI; the need for sulfur is satisfied by essential sulfur-containing amino acids	Protein foods such as meat, fish, poultry, eggs, milk, cheese, legumes, nuts	Dietary intake is chiefly from sulfur-containing amino acids, and adequacy is related to protein intake.
Micronutrients Essential at Daily Levels of a Few Milligrams or Less				
Iron	About 70% is found in hemoglobin; about 25% is stored in liver, spleen, and bone. Iron is a component of hemoglobin and myoglobin and is important in oxygen transfer. It is also present in serum transferrin and certain enzymes. Almost none exists in ionic form.	8 mg for men, 18 mg for women (after menopause, 8 mg) (RDA)	Liver, meat, egg yolk, legumes, whole or enriched grains, dark green vegetables, dark molasses, shrimp, oysters	Iron deficiency anemia occurs in women of reproductive age and infants and preschool children. Deficiency may be associated with unusual blood loss, parasites, or malabsorption. Anemia is the last state of deficiency.
Zinc	Zinc is present in most tissues, with greatest amounts in the liver, voluntary muscle, and bone.	11 mg for men, 8 mg for women (RDA)	Oysters, shellfish, herring, liver, legumes, milk, wheat bran	The extent of dietary zinc inadequacy in the United States is not known. Conditioned deficiency may develop with systemic childhood

Date from The Food and Nutrition Board, National Academy of Sciences, Institute of Medicine: *Dietary reference intakes for vitamin A, vitamin K, arsenic, boron, chromium, copper, iodine, iron, manganese, molybdenum, nickel, silicon, vanadium, and zinc,* Washington, DC, 2001, National Academy Press; and the Food and Nutrition Board, National Academy of Sciences, Institute of Medicine: *Dietary reference intakes for vitamin C, vitamin E, selenium, and carotenoids,* Washington, DC, 2000, National Academy Press.

**DRI,* Dietary reference intake; *RDA,* recommended dietary allowance; *AI,* adequate intake.

TABLE 5-16 Minerals in Human Nutrition—cont'd

MINERAL	BODY LOCATION AND SELECTED BIOLOGIC FUNCTIONS	DRIs*	FOOD SOURCES	LIKELIHOOD OF DEFICIENCY
Micronutrients Essential at Daily Levels of a Few Milligrams or Less—cont'd				
Zinc, cont'd	A constituent of many enzymes and of insulin, zinc is important for nucleic acid metabolism.			illnesses and in patients who are nutritionally depleted or have been subjected to severe stress such as surgery.
Copper	Copper is found in all body tissues, with the bulk in the liver, brain, heart, and kidney. Copper is a constituent of enzymes and ceruloplasmin and erythrocuprein in blood. It may be an integral part of DNA or RNA.	900 μg for men and women (RDA)	Liver, shellfish, whole grains, cherries, legumes, kidney, poultry, oysters, chocolate, nuts	No evidence shows that specific deficiencies of copper occur in humans. Menkes' disease is a genetic disorder resulting in copper deficiency.
Iodine	Iodine is a constituent of T_4 and related compounds synthesized by the thyroid gland. T_4 functions in the control of reactions involving cellular energy.	150 μg for men and women (RDA)	Iodized table salt, seafood, water and vegetables in regions without goiter	Iodization of table salt is recommended, especially in areas where food is low in iodine.
Manganese	The highest concentration of manganese is in bone; relatively high concentrations also exist in pituitary, liver, pancreas, and gastrointestinal tissue. Manganese is a constituent of essential enzyme systems and is rich in mitochondria of liver cells.	2.3 mg for men, 1.8 mg for women (AI)	Beet greens, blueberries, whole grains, nuts, legumes fruit, tea	Deficiency is unlikely to occur in humans.
Fluoride	Fluoride exists in bones and teeth. In optimal amounts from water and diet, fluoride reduces dental caries and may minimize bone loss.	4 mg for men, 3 mg for women (AI)	Drinking water (1 ppm), tea, coffee, rice, soybeans, spinach, gelatin, onions, lettuce	In areas where the fluoride content of water is low, fluoridation of water (at 1 ppm) has reduced the incidence of dental caries.
Molybdenum	Molybdenum is a constituent of an essential enzyme (xanthine oxidase) and flavoproteins.	45 μg for men and women (RDA)	Legumes, cereal, grains, dark green leafy vegetbles, organ meats	No available information.
Cobalt	Cobalt is a constituent of cyanocobalamin (vitamin B_{12}), existing bound to protein in foods of animal origin. Cobalt is essential for the normal function of all cells, particularly cells of bone marrow and nervous and gastrointestinal systems.	2.4 mg vitamin B_{12}	Liver, kidney, oysters clams, poultry, milk	Primary dietary inadequacy is rare except in those who consume no animal products. Deficiency may be associated with lack of gastric intrinsic factor, gastrectomy, or malabsorption syndromes.
Selenium	Selenium is involved in fat metabolism, cooperates with vitamin E, and acts as an antioxidant.	55μg for men and women (RDA)	Grains, onions, meats, milk; varied amounts in vegetables depending on selenium content of soil	Keshan disease is a selenium-deficient state. Deficiency has occurred in patients receiving long-term TPN without selenium supplementation.
Chromium	Chromium is associated with glucose metabolism.	35 μg for men, 25 μg for women (AI)	Corn oil, clams, whole-grain cereals, brewer's yeast, meats, drinking water (amount varies)	Deficiency is found in those with severe malnutrition and may be a factor in diabetes in older adults and cardiovascular disease.

**DRI*, Dietary reference intake; *RDA*, recommended dietary allowance; *AI*, adequate intake.

Relevant Web Sites

American Society for Bone and Mineral Research
www.asbmr.org/
National Academy of Sciences Institute of Medicine
www.iom.edu/
National Dairy Council
www.nationaldairycouncil.org/

Cited References

Abrams SA, Stuff JE: Calcium metabolism in girls: current dietary intakes lead to low rates of calcium absorption and retention during puberty, *Am J Clin Nutr* 60:739, 1994.

Age-Related Eye Diseases Group: A randomized, placebo-controlled, clinical trial of high-dose supplementation with vitamins C and E, beta-carotene, and zinc for age-related macular degeneration and vision loss, *Arch Ophthalmol* 119:1417, 2001.

Alaimo K et al: *Dietary intake of vitamins, minerals, and fiber of persons aged 2 and over in the United States: third health and nutrition examination survey, phase 1, 1988-1991,* advance data from Vital and Health Statistics, No. 258, Hyattsville, Md, 1994, National Center for Health Statistics.

Alnwick D: Weekly iodine supplements work, *Am J Clin Nutr* 67:1103, 1998.

Anderson JJB: Calcium, phosphorus, and human bone development, *J Nutr* 126:1153, 1996.

Anderson JJB et al: Nutrition and bone in physical activity and sport. In Wolinsky I, ed: *Nutrition in exercise and sport,* p 219, ed 3, Boca Raton, Fla, 1998, CRC Press.

Anderson, RA: Nutritional factors influencing the glucose/insulin system: chromium, *J Am Coll Nutr* 16:404, 1997.

Anderson RA et al: Elevated intakes of supplemental chromium improve glucose and insulin variables in individuals with type 2 diabetes, *Diabetes* 46:1786, 1997.

Appel IJ et al: A clinical study of the effects of dietary patterns on blood pressure, *N Engl J Med* 336:1117, 1997.

Arfin SM et al: Eukaryotic methionyl peptidases: two classes of cobalt-dependent enzymes, *Proc Nat Acad Sci USA* 92:7714, 1995.

Bahl R et al: Plasma zinc as a predictor of diarrheal and respiratory morbidity in children in an urban slum setting, *Am J Clin Nutr* 68:414, 1998.

Baumgartner T: Trace elements in clinical nutrition, *Nutr Clin Pract* 8:251, 1993.

Beard JL: Iron biology in immune function, muscle metabolism, and neuronal functioning, *J Nutr* 131:568, 2001.

Beard JL et al: Iron in the brain, *Nutr Rev* 51:157, 1993.

Beck M et al: Increased virulence of human enterovirus (coxsackievirus B3) in selenium-deficient mice, *J Infect Dis* 170:351, 1994.

Beck M et al: Rapid genomic evolution of a non-virulent coxsackievirus B_3—in selenium-deficient mice results in selection of identical virulent isolates, *Nature Med* 1:433, 1995.

Belongia EA et al: A randomized trial of zinc spray for treatment of upper respiratory illness in adults, *Am J Med* 111:103, 2001.

Berner LA et al: Fortification contributed greatly to vitamin and mineral intakes in the United States, 1989-1991, *J Nutr* 131:2177-2183, 2001.

Bogden J, Louria D: Aging and the immune system: role of micronutrient nutrition, *Nutrition* 15:593, 1999.

Borch-Iohnsen B et al: High bioavailability to humans of supplemental iron in a whey concentrate product, *Nutr Res* 14:1643, 1994.

Boukaïba N et al: A physiological amount of zinc supplementation: effects on nutritional, lipid, and thymus V status of an elderly population, *Am J Clin Nutr* 57:566, 1993.

Brewer GJ et al: Does a vegetarian diet control Wilson's disease? *J Am Coll Nutr* 12:527, 1993.

Buchman AL et al: Copper deficiency secondary to a copper transport defect: a new copper metabolic disturbance, *Metabolism* 12:1462, 1994.

Burk RF et al: Plasma selenium in patients with cirrhosis, *Hepatology* 27:794, 1998.

Burk RF et al: Plasma selenium in specific and non-specific forms, *Biofactors* 14:107, 2001.

Calvo MS et al: Persistently elevated parathyroid hormone secretion and action in young women after four weeks of ingesting high phosphorus, low calcium diets, *J Clin Endocrinol Metab* 70:1340, 1990.

Calvo MS, Park YM: Changing phosphorus content of the U.S. diet: potential for adverse effects on bone, *J Nutr* 126:1168S, 1996.

Chapin RE et al: Effects of dietary boron on bone strength in rats, *Fund Appl Toxicol* 35:205, 1997.

Clark LC et al: Effects of selenium supplementation for cancer prevention in patients with carcinoma of the skin: a randomized controlled trial, *JAMA* 276:1957, 1996.

Cook JD, Reddy MB: Effect of ascorbic acid intake on non-heme-iron absorption from a complete diet, *Am J Clin Nutr* 73:93, 2001.

Cordano A: Clinical manifestations of nutritional copper deficiency in infants and children, *Am J Clin Nutr* 67(suppl):1012, 1998.

Crofton RW et al: Inorganic zinc and the intestinal absorption of ferrous iron, *Am J Clin Nutr* 50:141, 1989.

Davidsson L et al: Improving iron absorption from a Peruvian school breakfast meal by adding ascorbic acid or Na_2EDTA, *Am J Clin Nutr* 73:283, 2001.

Davis CD et al: Interactions among dietary manganese, heme iron, and non-heme iron in women, *Am J Clin Nutr* 56:926, 1992.

Dawson-Hughes B: Calcium and vitamin D needs of the elderly, *J Nutr* 126:1165S, 1996.

Dengel JL et al: Magnesium homeostasis: conversion mechanism in lactating women consuming a controlled-magnesium diet, *Am J Clin Nutr* 59:990, 1994.

Devine A et al: Effects of zinc and other nutritional factors on insulin-like growth factor I and insulin-like growth factor binding proteins in postmenopausal women, *Am J Clin Nutr* 68:200, 1998.

Discher PWF, Girous A: Iodine content of a representative Canadian diet, *J Can Diet Assoc* 48:24, 1987.

Fairweather-Tait SJ: Zinc in human nutrition, *Nutr Res Rev* 1:23, 1998.

Fairweather-Tait SJ, Hurrell RF: Bioavailability of minerals and trace elements, *Nutr Res Rev* 9:295, 1996.

Finley JW et al: Sex affects manganese absorption and retention by humans from a diet adequate in manganese, *Am J Clin Nutr* 60:949, 1994.

Fleming DJ et al: Iron status of the free-living, elderly Framingham Heart Study cohort: an iron-replete population with a high prevalence of elevated iron stores, *Am J Clin Nutr* 73:638, 2001.

Food and Nutrition Board, National Research Council, National Academy of Sciences: *Recommended dietary allowances,* ed 10, Washington, DC, 1989, National Academy Press.

Food and Nutrition Board, Institute of Medicine: *Dietary reference intakes for calcium, phosphorus, magnesium, vitamin D, and fluoride,* Washington, DC, 1997, National Academy Press.

Food and Nutrition Board, Institute of Medicine: *Dietary reference intakes for vitamin A, vitamin K, arsenic, boron, chromium, copper, iodine, iron, manganese, molybdenum, nickel, silicon, vanadium, and zinc,* Washington, DC, 2001, National Academy Press.

Fortes C et al: The effect of zinc and vitamin A supplementation on immune response in an older population, *J Am Geriatr Soc* 46:19, 1998.

Fung EB et al: Zinc absorption in women during pregnancy and lactation: a longitudinal study, *Am J Clin Nutr* 66:80, 1997.

Giordon F et al: Impact of trace element and vitamin supplementation on immunity and infections in institutionalized elderly patients: a randomized controlled clinical trial, *Arch Int Med* 159:748, 1999.

Gloth FM III et al: Vitamin D deficiency in homebound elderly persons, *JAMA* 274:1683, 1995.

Greger JL, Malecki EA: Manganese: how do we know our limits? *Nutr Today* 32:116, 1997.

Greger JL et al: Intake, serum concentrations, and urinary excretion of manganese by adult males, *Am J Nutr* 51:457, 1990.
Gullestad L et al: Magnesium status in healthy free-living elderly Norwegians, *J Am Coll Nutr* 13:45, 1994.
Halsted JA et al: Zinc deficiency in man—the Shiraz experiment, *Am J Med* 43:277, 1972.
Hambidge KM et al: Zinc nutrition of preschool children in the Denver Head Start program, *Am J Clin Nutr* 29:734, 1976.
Hunt JR, Vanderpool RA: Apparent copper absorption from a vegetarian diet, *Am J Clin Nutr* 74:803, 2001.
Iseri LT, French JH: Magnesium: nature's physiologic calcium blocker, *Am Heart J* 108:188, 1994.
Jackman LA et al: Calcium retention in relation to calcium intake and postmenarcheal age in adolescent females, *Am J Clin Nutr* 66:327, 1997.
Johnson MA et al: Iron nutriture in elderly individuals, *FASEB J* 8:609, 1994.
Johnson MA et al: Copper, iron, zinc, and manganese in dietary supplements, infant formulas, and ready-to-eat cereals, *Am J Clin Nutr* 67(suppl):1035, 1998.
Kelley DS et al: Effects of low-copper diets on human immune response, *Am J Clin Nutr* 62:412, 1995.
King JC, Keen C: Zinc. In Shils ME et al: *Modern nutrition in health and disease,* vol 1, ed 8, Philadelphia, 1994, Lea and Febiger.
Kuhajek EJ: Letter to the editor: iodized salt, *Nutr Rev* 58:250, 2000.
Lee K et al: Too much versus too little: the implications of current iodine intake in the United States, *Nutr Rev* 57:177, 1999.
Lee N, Reasner C: Beneficial effect of chromium supplementation on serum triglyceride levels in NIDDM, *Diabetes Care* 17:1449, 1994.
Lesourd BM: Nutrition and immunity in the elderly: modifications of immune responses with nutritional treatments, *Am J Clin Nutr* 66:478S, 1997.
Levander GA et al: Vitamin E and selenium, *Proc Nutr Soc* 54:475, 1995.
Levenson DI, Bockman RS: A review of calcium preparations, *Nutr Rev* 52:221, 1994.
Lönnerdal B: Bioavailability of copper, *Am J Clin Nutr* 63:821S, 1996.
Lönnerdal B, Uauy R, eds: Genetic and environmental determinants of copper metabolism, *Am J Clin Nutr* 67(suppl):951, 1998.
Lukaski HC et al: Chromium supplementation and resistance training: effects on body composition, strength, and trace element status of men, *Am J Clin Nutr* 63:954, 1996.
Macknin ML et al: Zinc gluconate lozenges for treating the common cold in children, *JAMA* 279:1962, 1998.
Marie PJ et al: Histological osteomalacia due to dietary calcium deficiency in children, *N Engl J Med* 307:584, 1982.
Masumoto K et al: Manganese intoxication during intermittent parenteral nutrition: report of two cases, *J Parent Ent Nutr* 25:95, 2001.
Matkovic V et al: Urinary calcium, sodium, and bone mass of young females, *Am J Clin Nutr* 62:417, 1995.
McGuire MK et al: Selenium status of infants is influenced by supplementation of formula or maternal diets, *Am J Clin Nutr* 58:643, 1993a.
McGuire MK et al: Selenium status of lactating women is affected by the form of selenium consumed, *Am J Clin Nutr* 58:649, 1993b.
McKane WR et al: Role of calcium in modulating age-related increases in parathyroid function and bone resorption, *J Clin Endocrinol Metab* 81:1699, 1996.
Milne DB: Copper intake and assessment of copper status, *Am J Clin Nutr* 67(suppl):1041, 1998.
Moreno-Reyes R et al: Kashin-Beck osteoarthropathy in rural Tibet in relation to selenium and iodine status, *N Engl J Med* 339:112, 1998.
Neve J: New approaches to assess selenium status and requirement. Nutr Rev 58:363, 2000.
Nielsen FH: Boron, manganese, molybdenum, and other trace elements. In Bowman BA, Russell RM, eds: *Present knowledge in nutrition,* ed 8, Washington, DC, 2001, ILSI Press.
Palmer C, Anderson JJB: Position of the American Dietetic Association: the impact of fluoride on health, *J Am Diet Assoc* 200:1208, 2000.
Pang Y et al: A longitudinal investigation of aggregate oral intake of copper, *J Nutr* 131:2171, 2001.
Patterson AJ et al: Dietary treatment of iron deficiency in women of child-bearing age, *Am J Clin Nutr* 74:650, 2001.
Pennington JAT, Jones JW: Molybdenum, nickel, cobalt, vanadium, and strontium in total diets, *J Am Diet Assoc* 87:1644, 1987.
Pennington JAT, Schoen SA: Total diet study: estimated dietary intakes of nutritional elements, 1982-1991, *Int J Vitam Nutr Res* 66:350, 1996.
Pollitt E et al: Behavioral effects of iron deficiency among preschool children in Cambridge, Mass, *Fed Proc* 37:487, 1976. [Classic]
Prasad AS et al: Zinc metabolism in patients with the syndrome of iron deficiency anemia, hepatosplenomegaly, dwarfism and hypogonadism, *J Lab Clin Med* 61:537, 1963.
Prentice A: Does mild zinc deficiency contribute to poor growth performance? *Nutr Rev* 51:268, 1993.
Rajagopalan KV: Molybdenum—an essential trace element, *Nutr Rev* 45:321, 1987.
Rauma AL et al: Iodine status in vegans consuming a living food diet, *Nutr Res* 14:1789, 1994.
Recker RR: Calcium absorption and achlorhydria, *New Eng J Med* 313:70, 1985.
Rubin MA et al: Acute and chronic resistive exercises increase urinary chromium excretion in men as measured with an enriched chromium stable isotope, *J Nutr* 128:73, 1998.
Rucker RB et al: Copper, lysyl oxidase, and extracellular matrix protein cross-linking, *Am J Clin Nutr* 67(suppl):996, 1998.
Rude RK: Magnesium homeostasis. In Bilezikian JP, Raisz LG, Rodan GA, eds: *Principles of bone biology,* San Diego, 1996, Academic Press.
Rude RK: Magnesium deficiency: a cause of heterogeneous disease in humans, *J Bone Miner Res* 13:749, 1998.
Scholz-Ahrens KE et al: Effects of prebiotics on mineral metabolism, *Am J Clin Nutr* 73:459S, 2001.
Shankar AH, Prasad AS: Zinc and immune function: the biological basis of altered resistance to infection, *Am J Clin Nutr* 68:447S, 1998.
Sokoloff L: Kashin-Beck disease: current status, *Nutr Rev* 46:113, 1988.
Stendig-Lindenberg G et al: Trabecular bone density in a two year controlled trial of peroral magnesium in osteoporosis, *Magnes Res* 6:155, 1993.
Stipanuk MH: Metabolism of sulfur-containing amino acids, *Annu Rev Nutr* 6:179, 1986.
Subar AF et al: Dietary sources of nutrients among US adults, 1989 to 1991, *J Am Diet Assoc* 98:537, 1998.
Trumbo P et al: Dietary reference intakes: vitamin A, vitamin K, arsenic, boron, chromium, copper, iodine, manganese, molybdenum, nickel, silicon, vanadium, and zinc, *J Am Diet Assoc* 101:294, 2001.
Tucker KL et al: Potassium, magnesium, and fruit and vegetable intakes are associated with greater bone mineral density in older men and women, *Am J Clin Nutr* 69:727, 1998.
Turner RB, Cetnarowski WE: Effect of treatment with zinc gluconate or zinc acetate on experimental and natural colds, *Clin Infect Dis* 31:1202, 2000.
Tyrala EE et al: Selenate fortification of infant formulas improves the selenium status of preterm infants, *Am J Clin Nutr* 64:860, 1996.
Uauy R et al: Essentiality of copper in humans, *Am J Clin Nutr* 67(suppl):952, 1998.
U.S. Department of Agriculture: *Continuing survey of food intakes of individuals (CSFII): diet and knowledge survey, 1991,* Springfield, Va, 1994, U.S. Department of Commerce, National Technical Information Service.
van den Heuvel EGHM et al: Oligofructose stimulates calcium absorption in adolescents, *Am J Clin Nutr* 69:544, 1999.
Volpe SL et al: Effect of chromium supplementation and exercise on body composition, resting metabolic rate and selected bio-

chemical parameters in moderately obese women following an exercise program, *J Am Coll Nutr* 20:293, 2001.

Whittaker P et al: Iron and folate in fortified cereals, *J Am Coll Nutr* 20:247, 2001.

Witteman JCM et al: Reduction of blood pressure with oral magnesium supplementation in women with mild to moderate hypertension, *Am J Clin Nutr* 60:129, 1994.

Wood RJ, Zheng JJ: High dietary calcium intakes reduce zinc absorption and balance in humans, *Am J Clin Nutr* 65:1803, 1997.

Xue-Yi C et al: Timing of vulnerability of the brain to iodine deficiency in endemic cretinism, *N Engl J Med* 331:1739, 1994.

Yang G et al: Selenium-related endemic deseases and the daily selenium requirement of humans, *World Rev Nutr Diet* 55:98, 1988.

Yang GQ et al: Endemic selenium intoxication of humans in China, *Am J Clin Nutr* 37:872, 1983.

Yates AA et al: Dietary reference intakes: the new basis for recommendations for calcium and related nutrients, B vitamins, and choline, *J Am Diet Assoc* 98:699, 1998.

Additional References

Anderson JJB, Garner SC, eds: *Calcium and phosphorus in health and disease,* Boca Raton, Fla, 1996, CRC Press.

Anderson JJB et al: Phosphorus. In Bowman BA, Russell RM, eds: *Present knowledge in nutrition,* ed 8, Washington, DC, 2001, ILSI Press.

Anderson RA: Effects of chromium on body composition and weight loss, *Nutr Rev* 56:266, 1998.

Andrews NC: Iron-transport across biologic membranes, *Nutr Rev* 57:114, 1999.

Beinert H, Kennedy MC: Aconitase: a two-faced protein: enzyme and iron regulatory factor, *FASEB J* 7:1442, 1993.

Chandra RK: Nutrition and immunity, *Am J Clin Nutr* 66:460S, 1997.

Chesters JK, Arthur JR: Early biochemical defects caused by dietary trace element deficiencies, *Nutr Res Rev* 1:39, 1998.

Clarkson PM: Effects of exercise on chromium levels. Is supplementation required? *Sports Med* 23:341, 1997.

Cousins RJ: Metal elements and gene expression, *Ann Rev Nutr* 14:449, 1994.

Dibley MJ: Zinc. In Bowman BA, Russell RM, eds: *Present knowledge in nutrition,* ed 8, Washington, DC, 2001, ILSI Press.

Failla ML et al: Copper. In Bowman BA, Russell RM, eds: *Present knowledge in nutrition,* ed 8, Washington, DC, 2001, ILSI Press.

Fleet JC, Cashman KD: Magnesium. In Bowman BA, Russell RM, eds: *Present knowledge in nutrition,* ed 8, Washington, DC, 2001, ILSI Press.

Fleming RE, Sly WS: Mechanisms of iron accumulation in hereditary hemochromatosis, *Annu Rev Physiol* 64:663, 2002.

Goyer RA: Toxic and essential metal interactions, *Ann Rev Nutr* 17:37, 1997.

Heaney RP: Calcium, dairy products, and osteoporosis, *J Am Coll Nutr* 19:835, 2000.

Hunt CD, Meacham SL: Aluminum, boron, calcium, copper, iron, magnesium, manganese, molybdenum, phosphorus: concentrations in common Western foods and estimated daily intakes by infants; toddlers; and male and female adolescents, adults, and seniors in the United States, *J Am Diet Assoc* 101:1058, 2001.

Jackson JL et al: A meta-analysis of zinc salt lozenges and the common cold, *Arch Intern Med* 157:2373, 1997.

Klimis-Tavantzis DJ: *Manganese in health and disease,* Boca Raton, Fla, 1994, CRC Press.

Nielsen FH: Boron, manganese, molybdenum, and other trace elements. In Bowman BA, Russell RM, eds: *Present knowledge in nutrition,* ed 8, Washington, DC, 2001, ILSI Press.

Salonen J et al: High stored iron levels are associated with excess risk of myocardial infarction in Eastern Finnish men, *Circulation* 86:803, 1992.

Seelig MS, Elin R: Is there a place for magnesium in the treatment of acute myocardial infarction? *Am Heart J* 132(pt 2, suppl 2):472, 496, 1996.

Sempos C et al: Body iron stores and the risk of coronary heart disease, *N Engl J Med* 330:1119, 1994.

Stanbury JB, Dunn JT: Iodine and iodine deficiency disorders. In Bowman BA, Russell RM, eds: *Present knowledge in nutrition,* ed 8, Washington, DC, 2001, ILSI Press.

Stocker BJ: Chromium. In Bowman BA, Russell RM, eds: *Present knowledge in nutrition,* ed 8, Washington, DC, 2001, ILSI Press.

Sunder R. Selenium. In Bowman BA, Russell RM, eds: *Present knowledge in nutrition,* ed 8, Washington, DC, 2001, ILSI Press.

Weaver CM: Calcium. In Bowman BA, Russell RM, eds: *Present knowledge in nutrition,* ed 8, Washington, DC, 2001, ILSI Press.

Winzerling JJ, Law JH: Comparative nutrition of iron and copper, *Annu Rev Nutr* 17:501, 1997.

Yip R: Iron. In Bowman BA, Russell RM, eds: *Present knowledge in nutrition,* ed 8, Washington, DC, 2001, ILSI Press.

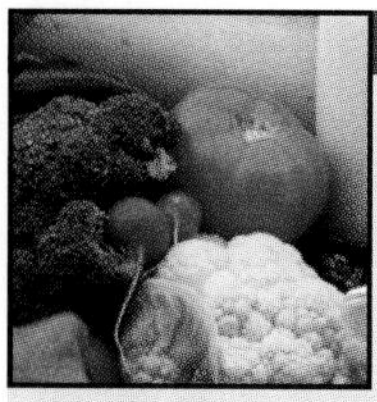

CHAPTER 6

Water, Electrolytes, and Acid-Base Balance

SUSAN J. WHITMIRE, RD, LDN, CNSD

CHAPTER OUTLINE

- Body Water
- Electrolytes
- Acid-Base Balance
- Acid-Base Disorders

KEY TERMS

acid-base balance–a dynamic equilibrium state of hydrogen ion concentration in the body

acidemia–a state in which the pH of arterial blood decreases below the normal range of 7.35 to 7.45 because of an increase in circulating acids or a reduction in bicarbonate levels

acidosis–a physiologic process or disease state that if left untreated results in acidemia

alkalemia–a state in which the pH of arterial blood exceeds the normal range of 7.35 to 7.45 because of an increase in bicarbonate levels or a reduction in circulating acids

alkalosis–a physiologic process or disease state that if left untreated results in alkalemia

anion gap–the difference between measured cations and measured anions

buffer–a proton donor and acceptor system that helps preserve homeostasis of the hydrogen ion concentration

contraction alkalosis–metabolic alkalosis resulting from hypovolemia; occurs when decreased blood flow to the kidneys stimulates reabsorption of water and sodium; bicarbonate is reabsorbed with the sodium, causing alkalosis

dehydration–excessive loss of body water

edema–an abnormal accumulation of fluid in the intercellular tissue spaces or body cavities

electrolytes–substances that dissociate into positively and negatively charged ions when dissolved in water

extracellular fluid–the water and dissolved substances in the spaces outside cells

extracellular water–water in the plasma, lymph, spinal fluid, and secretions

insensible water loss–imperceptible water loss (e.g., when water exits with air expired from the lungs or water vapor escapes the skin's surface)

intercellular (interstitial) water–water between and around the cells

intracellular fluid–the water and dissolved substances contained within cells

intracellular water (ICW)–water contained within the cell

metabolic acidosis–acidosis caused by an increase in circulating noncarbonic acids, an excessive loss of bicarbonate, or both

metabolic alkalosis–alkalosis caused by an increase in circulating bicarbonate, an excessive loss of acid, or both

metabolic water–water derived from the metabolism of carbohydrate, protein, or fat

oncotic pressure (colloidal osmotic pressure)–the pressure at the capillary membrane that is caused by dissolved proteins in the plasma and interstitial fluids

osmolality–a measure of the osmotically active particles per kilogram of solvent in which the particles are dispersed

osmolarity–a measure of the osmotically active particles per liter of solution

osmotic pressure–the pressure of a solution directly related to its solute osmolar concentration

respiratory acidosis–acidosis caused by acute or chronic retention of carbon dioxide by the lungs

respiratory alkalosis–alkalosis caused by increased ventilation and elimination of carbon dioxide

sensible water loss–water that is lost in urine, feces, and sweat

"third space" fluid–fluid that is extracellular and extravascular (e.g., in tissues and cavities), the accumulation of which results in edema.

water intoxication–a state in which excess water increases intracellular volume and dilutes body fluids.

The volume, composition, and distribution of body fluids have profound effects on cell function. A stable internal environment is requisite for optimal physiologic function. This internal environment is maintained through a sophisticated network of homeostatic mechanisms. Protein-energy malnutrition, disease, trauma, and surgery can disrupt fluid, electrolyte, and acid-base balance, causing alterations in the composition, distribution, and amount of body fluids. Even small changes in pH, electrolyte concentrations, and fluid status can have adverse effects on cell function. If these derangements are not corrected, severe consequences, including death, can ensue.

BODY WATER

Water is the largest single component of the body. Metabolically active cells of the muscle and viscera have the highest concentration of water, whereas calcified tissue cells have the lowest. Water as a percentage of body weight varies among individuals depending on the proportion of muscle to adipose tissue. Total body water is higher in athletes than in nonathletes and decreases significantly with age because of diminished muscle mass (Figure 6-1).

Functions

Water is an essential component of all body tissues. As a solvent, it makes many solutes available for cell function and is the medium needed for all reactions. It also participates as a substrate in metabolic reactions and as a structural component providing form to cells. Water is essential for the physiologic processes of digestion, absorption, and excretion. It plays a key role in the structure and function of the circulatory system and acts as a transport medium for nutrients and all body substances. Water maintains the physical and chemical constancy of intracellular and extracellular fluids and has a direct role in maintaining body temperature. Evaporation of perspiration cools the body during warm weather; 600 kcal of body heat dissipates during the evaporation of 1 L of perspired water.

Loss of 20% of body water may cause death; loss of only 10% causes severe disorders (Figure 6-2). In moderate weather, adults can live up to 10 days without water, and children can live up to 5 days. In contrast, it is possible to survive for several weeks without food.

Distribution

Intracellular water (ICU) is the water contained within cells. Extracellular water, commonly estimated to account for one third of total body water or 20% of body weight, includes the water in plasma, lymph, spinal fluid, and secretions and the intercellular (interstitial) water between and around the cells. Most interstitial water is held in a gel in the intercellular spaces and is continuous with the plasma through pores in the capillaries. Abnormal accumulation of fluid in the intercellular tissue spaces or body cavities is called edema.

The distribution of body water varies under different circumstances, but the total amount in the body remains relatively constant. The understanding of body water's role in health and disease has improved through the use of bioelectrical impedance, a measurement of electrical conduction, to estimate the amount of body water (Ellis et al, 1999).

Balance

Homeostatic regulation by the gastrointestinal (GI) tract, kidneys, and brain keeps the water content of the fat-free body weight fairly constant. The amount of water taken in daily is approximately equivalent to the amount lost (Table 6-1).

Water Intake

In healthy individuals, water intake is controlled primarily by thirst. Thirst control centers are located in the ventromedial and anterior hypothalamus, close to the centers that regulate antidiuretic hormone (ADH). Thirst is stimulated when plasma osmolality

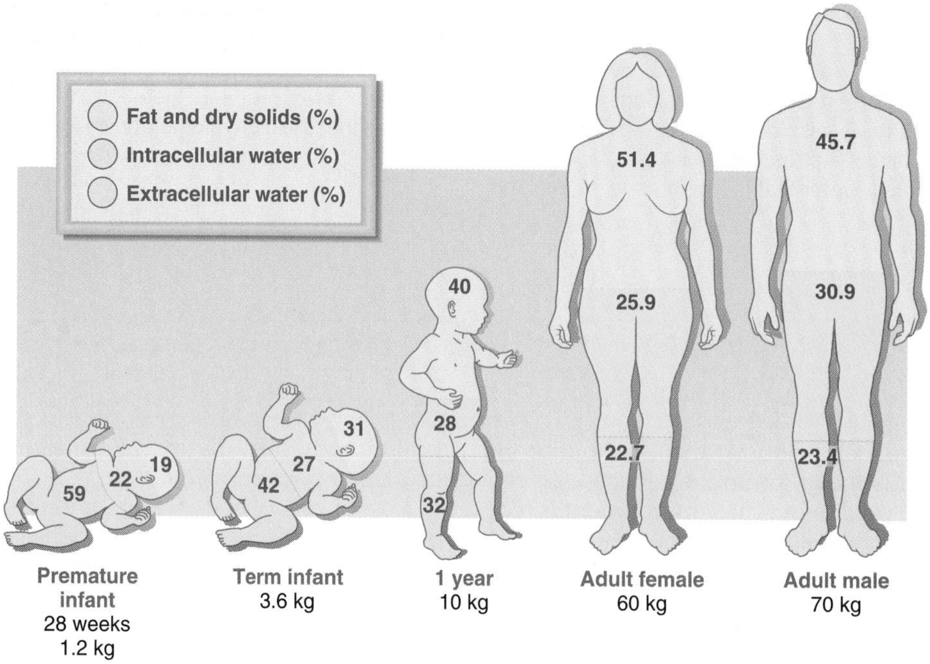

FIGURE 6-1 • Distribution of body water as a percentage of body weight.

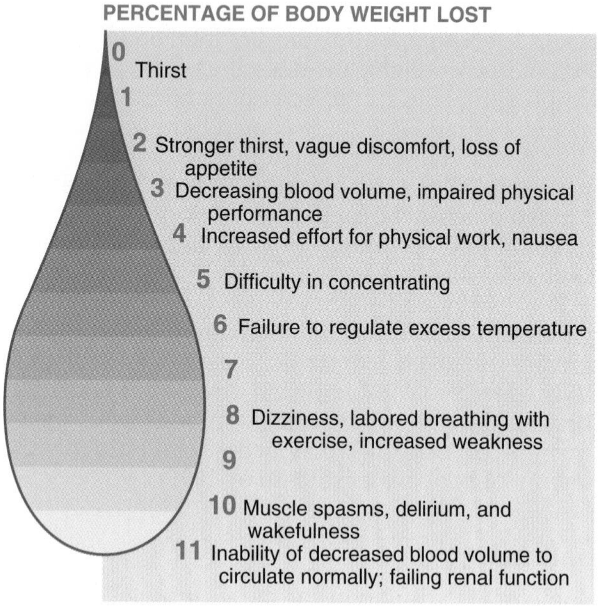

FIGURE 6-2 • Adverse effects of dehydration.

increases or intravascular volume decreases. The sensation of thirst is a signal to consume fluids.

Water is ingested as fluid and part of food (Table 6-2). The oxidation of foods in the body also produces metabolic water as an end product. The oxidation of 100 g of fat, carbohydrate, or protein yields 107, 55, or 41 g of water, respectively, for a total of approximately 200 to 300 ml/day.

Water is absorbed rapidly because it moves freely through membranes by diffusion. This movement is controlled mainly by osmotic forces generated by inorganic ions in solution in the body (see *Clinical Insight:* Osmotic Forces).

When water cannot be ingested orally or by a feeding tube, it may be administered intravenously in the form of salt (saline) solutions, which closely resemble the electrolyte content of body fluids; glucose solutions; or in blood, plasma, or protein hydrolysate mixtures. Water intoxication occurs as a result of excess water intake and increased intracellular fluid volume and is accompanied by osmolar dilution. The increased volume of intracellular fluid causes the cells, particularly the brain cells, to swell, leading to headache, nausea, vomiting, muscle twitching, convulsions with impending stupor, and possibly death. Papilledema, blurred vision, and blindness may also result.

Water Elimination

Water loss normally occurs through the kidneys in the urine and through the GI tract in the feces (which is called sensible water loss, or measurable water loss), as well as through air expired from the lungs and water vapor lost through the skin (which is called insensible water loss, or nonmeasurable water loss) (see Table 6-1). The kidney is the primary regulator of sensible water loss. Natural diuretics in the diet (i.e., substances that increase urinary excretion) include alcohol and caffeine. Insensible water loss is continuous and usually unconscious. Sweat, a de-

TABLE 6-1 Water Balance

WATER INTAKE AND OUTPUT (ml)*	WATER SOURCE
Water Intake	
1400	Fluids
700	Food
200	Cellular oxidation of food
2300	TOTAL
Water Output	
Normal temperature	
1400	Urine
100	Feces
100	Skin (perspiration)
	Insensible loss
350	Skin
350	Respiratory tract
2300	TOTAL
Hot weather	
1200	Urine
100	Feces
1400	Skin (perspiration)
	Insensible loss
350	Skin
250	Respiratory tract
3300	TOTAL
Prolonged exercise	
500	Urine
100	Feces
5000	Skin (perspiration)
	Insensible loss
350	Skin
650	Respiratory tract
6600	TOTAL

Modified from Guyton AC: *Textbook of medical physiology,* ed 9, Philadelphia, 1996, WB Saunders.
*Average values.

TABLE 6-2 Percentage of Water in Common Foods

FOOD	PERCENTAGE
Lettuce, iceberg	96
Celery	95
Cucumbers	95
Cabbage, raw	92
Watermelon	92
Broccoli, boiled	91
Milk, nonfat	91
Spinach	91
Green beans, boiled	89
Carrots, raw	88
Oranges	87
Cereals, cooked	85
Apples, raw, without skin	84
Grapes	81
Potatoes, boiled	77
Eggs	75
Bananas	74
Fish, haddock, baked	74
Chicken, roasted, white meat	70
Corn, boiled	65
Beef, sirloin	59
Cheese, Swiss	38
Bread, white	37
Cake, angel food	34
Butter	16
Almonds, blanched	5
Saltines	3
Sugar, white	1
Oils	0

From Pennington JA: *Bowes and Church's food values of portions commonly used,* ed 17, Philadelphia, 1994, JB Lippincott.

tectable source of water loss, is distinct from insensible water loss through the skin. High altitude, low humidity, and high temperatures can increase insensible fluid loss through the lungs and sensible fluid loss through sweat. Athletes can lose 3 to 4 lb from fluid loss when exercising in a temperature of 80° F and low humidity and even more at higher temperatures (see Chapter 26).

The GI tract can be a major source of water loss. Under normal conditions, the water contained in the 7 to 9 L of digestive juices and other extracellular fluids secreted daily into the GI tract is almost entirely reabsorbed in the ileum and colon, except for about 100 ml that is excreted in the feces. Because this volume of reabsorbed fluid is about twice that of the blood plasma, excessive GI fluid losses through diarrhea may have serious consequences, particularly for very young and very old individuals.

Fluid loss through diarrhea has been responsible for thousands of children's deaths in developing countries. Oral rehydration therapy with a simple mixture of water, sugar, and salt has been highly effective in reducing the number of deaths (Victora et al, 2000) (see Chapter 30). Other abnormal fluid losses may occur as a result of emesis, hemorrhage, fistula drainage, burn and wound exudates, gastric and surgical tube drainage, and the use of diuretics.

When water intake is insufficient or water loss is excessive, healthy kidneys compensate by conserving water and excreting more concentrated urine. The renal tubules increase water reabsorption in response to the hormonal action of ADH. However, the concentration of the urine made by the kidneys has a limit: approximately 1400 mOsm/L. The ability of the kidneys in older individuals to concentrate the urine may be compromised, resulting in increased risk of developing dehydration and hypernatremia, especially during illness (Beck, 1998). Signs of dehydration include headache, fatigue, decreased appetite, light-headedness, poor skin turgor (although this may be present in well-hydrated older persons), skin tenting on the forehead, concentrated urine, decreased urine output, sunken eyes, dry mucous membranes of the mouth and nose, orthostatic blood pressure changes, and tachycardia (Sanservero, 1997). In a dehydrated person, the specific gravity of urine increases above the normal levels of 1.008 to 1.030, and the urine becomes remarkably darker.

Intentional dehydration through excessive sweating or fluid restriction is a method of water loss that has frequently been used by young wrestlers trying to "make weight"—lose pounds quickly before being

CLINICAL INSIGHT

Osmotic Forces

Osmotic pressure

Osmotic pressure is directly proportional to the number of particles in solution and usually refers to the pressure at the cell membrane. It is convenient (although not entirely accurate) to consider the osmotic pressure of the intracellular fluid as a function of its potassium content because potassium is the predominant cation in the intracellular fluid. In contrast, the osmotic pressure of extracellular fluid may be considered relative to its sodium content because sodium is the major cation present in extracellular fluid. Although variations in the distribution of sodium and potassium ions are the principal causes of water shifts between the various fluid compartments, chloride and phosphate also influence water balance. Proteins, which cannot diffuse because of their size, also play a key role in maintaining osmotic equilibrium.

Oncotic pressure

Oncotic pressure, or colloidal osmotic pressure, is the pressure at the capillary membrane and is maintained by dissolved proteins in the plasma and interstitial fluids. Oncotic pressure helps to retain water within blood vessels, preventing its leakage from plasma into the interstitial spaces. In patients with an exceptionally low plasma protein content, such as those who are under physiologic stress or have certain diseases, water leaks into the interstitial spaces causing edema. This process is referred to as *third spacing,* and the fluid is called "third space" fluid.

Osmoles and milliosmoles

Concentrations of individual ionic constituents of extracellular or intracellular fluids are expressed in terms of milliosmoles per liter (mOsm/L). One mole equals the gram molecular weight of a substance; dissolved in 1 L of water, it becomes 1 osmole (osm). One milliosmole (mOsm) equals 1/1000th of an osmole. The number of milliosmoles per liter equals the number of millimoles per liter times the number of particles into which the dissolved substance dissociates. Thus 1 mmol of a nonelectrolyte (e.g., glucose) equals 1 mOsm; similarly, 1 mmol of an electrolyte containing only monovalent ions (e.g., sodium chloride [NaCl]) equals 2 mOsm. One mOsm dissolved in 1 L of water has an osmotic pressure of 17 mm Hg.

Osmolality and osmolarity

Osmolality is a measure of the osmotically active particles per kilogram of the solvent in which the particles are dispersed. It is expressed as milliosmoles of solute per kilogram of solvent (mOsm/kg). Osmolarity is the term formerly used to describe concentration—milliosmoles per liter of the entire solution; however, osmolality is now expressed in this form for most clinical work. However, in reference to certain conditions such as hyperlipidemia, it makes a difference whether osmolality is stated as *milliosmoles per kilogram of solvent or per liter of solution.*

The average sum of the concentration of all the cations in serum is about 150 mEq/L. The cation concentration is balanced by 150 mEq/L of anions, yielding a total serum osmolality of about 300 mOsm/L. Serum osmolality can be calculated as follows:

$$\text{Serum osmolality} = (\text{Serum sodium [mEq/L]} \times 2) + \text{Glucose (mg/dl)}/18 + \text{Blood urea nitrogen (mg/dl)}/2.8$$

An osmolar imbalance is caused by a gain or loss of water relative to a solute or a gain or loss of solute relative to water. An osmolality of less than 285 mOsm/L generally indicates a water excess; an osmolality of greater than 295 mOsm/L indicates a water deficit.

weighed at a competition. It is a harmful practice that can adversely affect performance (see Chapter 26).

Requirements

The body has no provision for water storage; therefore the amount of water lost every 24 hours must be replaced to maintain health and body efficiency. Under ordinary circumstances a reasonable allowance based on recommended caloric intake is 1 ml/kcal for adults and 1.5 ml/kcal for infants. This translates into approximately 35 ml/kg of usual body weight in adults, 50 to 60 ml/kg in children, and 150 ml/kg in infants. In most cases a suitable daily allowance for adults is 2.0 to 2.5 L, depending on body size (see *Focus On:* Drink Up! Why Eight Glasses per Day?). Infants need more water because of the limited capacity of their kidneys to handle the renal solute load, their higher percentage of body water, and their large surface area per unit of body weight. A lactating woman's need for water also increases—theoretically by an additional 600 to 700 ml/day—because of the large amount required for milk production (see Chapter 7).

Thirst is usually an adequate signal for the need consume water, except in infants, heavily exercising athletes, those who are ill, and sometimes older adults, who may have a diminished thirst sensation (see Chapter 13). Anyone sick enough to be hospitalized, regardless of the diagnosis, is at risk for water and electrolyte imbalance. Older adults are particularly susceptible because of other factors such as impaired renal concentrating ability, polypharmacy, fever, diarrhea, vomiting, and a decreased ability to care for themselves. In situations involving extreme heat or excessive sweating, thirst may not keep pace with the actual water requirements of the body.

FOCUS ON

Drink Up! Why Eight Glasses per Day?

The primary determinants of maintenance water requirements are metabolic. Ultimately, the body's water intake must be sufficient to meet metabolic demands, balance sensible and insensible water losses, and maintain a tolerable renal solute load. Sound easy? Metabolic demand is influenced by body size, composition, physical activity, and fever. Sensible nonrenal water loss such as perspiration varies greatly according to activity, altitude, humidity, and temperature, as does insensible water loss via the lungs. The renal solute load depends on a person's dietary intake and composition. Considering these and other variables that affect water requirements, it is obvious that estimating water requirements for individuals is anything but easy, and individual requirements are highly variable. Nonetheless, most people are familiar with the recommendation that adults consume at least 8 glasses (8 cups) of water per day. How did that recommendation come to be, and does it apply to everyone?

The recommendation for 8 glasses of water per day likely arose from the need to have a guideline that stresses the importance of adequate water intake but at the same time is easily understood by the public. For practical purposes, the National Research Council recommends 1 ml/kcal energy expenditure for adults under "average conditions of energy expenditure and environmental conditions." Clinical models are typically based on an "average" 70-kg (154-lb) male. The energy allowance for men ages 19 to 50 years is 38 to 41 kcal/kg/day for light to moderate activity (Food and Nutrition Board, National Research Council, 1989). This translates to 2660 to 2870 ml, or about 11 to 12 cups of water, each day. Solid food typically contributes about 750 ml (approximately 3 cups) of water, and oxidative metabolism contributes another 250 ml (approximately 1 cup), leaving a *minimum* of 7 to 8 cups of *noncaffeinated, nonalcoholic fluids* to be consumed daily. Caffeine and alcohol are diuretics, so drinking 8 cups of coffee does not result in the same net water gain as drinking 8 cups of water!

Because this guideline is based on the average 70-kg man model, is its usage limited? Large deviations from this average, whether deviations in weight, body composition, activity, or environmental condition, make the recommendation less applicable. For individuals who are markedly less than or more than this average weight, the daily water requirement is calculated as follows (Grant and DeHoog, 1999): 100 ml/kg for the first 10 kg and 50 ml/kg for the next 10 kg and either 20 ml/kg thereafter (for those younger than 50 years) or 15 ml/kg thereafter (for those older than 50 years). For example, the water requirement for a 40-year-old, 170-kg man is calculated as follows:

$$\text{(First 10 kg} = \text{1000 ml)} + \text{(Second 10 kg} = \text{500 ml)} + \text{(Remaining 150 kg} = \text{3000 ml)} = \text{4500 ml}$$

An individual of this size may receive more water from solid food and oxidative metabolism because of his overall increased dietary intake. Even so, his fluid intake requirement could be as high as 14 cups per day. The daily water requirement using this method for a 70-kg man is 2500 ml. *Roughly* translated, every 25 pounds that a person (who is less than 50 years old) is above the ideal 70-kg weight increases the water requirement by about another 1 cup ($\approx$240 ml):

$$\text{(25 lb)} \times \text{(1 kg/2.2 lb)} \times \text{(20 ml/kg)} = \text{227 ml (about 1 cup)}$$

Healthy individuals are seldom at risk for water intoxication when their intake exceeds their water requirements. In terms of health and performance, people are more at risk for chronic underhydration. Dehydration causing as little as a 2% loss of body weight results in impaired physiologic and performance responses (Kleiner, 1999). Chronic mild dehydration is also associated with diminished salivary gland function (see Figure 6-2) (Ship and Fischer, 1997), an increased risk of kidney stones in susceptible individuals (Borghi et al, 1996), an increased risk of colon cancer (Shannon et al, 1996), an increased risk of breast cancer (Stookey, 1997), an increased risk of childhood obesity (Levine, 1996), and an increased risk of mitral valve prolapse in susceptible individuals (Lax et al, 1992). Therefore drink . . . noncaffeinated, nonalcoholic beverages . . . to your health!

ELECTROLYTES

Electrolytes are substances that dissociate into positively and negatively charged ions (*cations* and *anions*) when dissolved in water. Electrolytes can be simple inorganic salts of sodium, potassium, or magnesium or complex organic molecules, and they play a key role in a host of normal metabolic functions (Table 6-3). One milliequivalent (mEq) of any substance has the capacity to combine chemically with 1 mEq of a substance with an opposite charge. For univalent ions, 1 millimole (mmol) equals 1 mEq; for divalent ions, 1 mmol equals 2 mEq, and so on. (See Appendix 4 for milligram-to-milliequivalent conversion guidelines.)

Three indispensable dietary constituents—sodium, potassium, and chloride—commonly known as the *electrolytes,* are related in the body. Sodium constitutes 2%, potassium 5%, and chloride 3% of the total mineral content of the body. These elements, which exist as ions in body fluids, are distributed throughout all body fluids and involved in maintaining at least four important physiologic body functions: (1) water

TABLE 6-3 Normal Electrolyte Concentration of Serum

ELECTROLYTE	NORMAL RANGE
Cations	
Sodium	136-145 mEq/L
Potassium	3.5-5 mEq/L
Calcium	4.5-5.5 mEq/L (9-11 mg/dl)
Magnesium	1.5-2.5 mEq/L (1.8-3 mg/dl)
Anions	
Chloride	96-106 mEq/L
CO_2 (content) TCO_2*	24-28.8 mEq/L
Phosphorus (inorganic)	3-4.5 mg/dl (1.9-2.85 mEq/L as HPO_4^{2-})
Sulfate (as S)	0.8-1.2 mg/dl (0.5-0.75 mEq/L as SO_2^{2-})
Lactate	0.7-1.8 mEq/L (6-16 mg/dl)
Protein	6-7.6 g/dl (14-18 mEq/L); depends on albumin level

*TCO_2, Total CO_2.

balance and distribution, (2) osmotic equilibrium, (3) acid-base balance, and (4) intracellular and extracellular concentration differentials.

Sodium

Sodium (Na^+) is the major cation of extracellular fluid, the water and dissolved substances in the spaces outside cells. The normal serum sodium concentration is 136 to 145 mEq/L. Various intestinal secretions such as bile and pancreatic juice, contain substantial amounts of sodium. Approximately 35% to 40% of the total body's sodium is in the skeleton; however, most of it is unexchangeable or slowly exchangeable with that in body fluids. Contrary to common belief, sweat is hypotonic and contains a relatively small amount of sodium.

Functions

As the predominant ion of extracellular fluid, sodium regulates its volume and the plasma volume. Sodium also aids in nerve impulse conduction and muscle contraction control.

Absorption and Excretion

Sodium is readily absorbed from the intestine and carried to the kidneys, where it is filtered and returned to the blood to maintain appropriate levels. The amount absorbed is proportional to the intake.

About 90% to 95% of normal body sodium loss is through the urine; the rest is lost in feces and sweat. Normally the quantity of sodium excreted daily is equal to the amount ingested. Sodium excretion is maintained by a mechanism involving the glomerular filtration rate, the cells of the juxtaglomerular apparatus of the kidneys, the renin-angiotensin-aldosterone system, the sympathetic nervous system, circulating catecholamines, and blood pressure (see Chapter 39).

Sodium balance is regulated by *aldosterone,* a mineralocorticoid secreted by the adrenal cortex (see Chapter 36). When blood sodium levels rise, the thirst receptors in the hypothalamus stimulate the thirst sensation. Ingestion of fluids returns sodium levels to normal. When blood sodium levels are low, sodium excretion through the urine decreases. Under certain circumstances, sodium and fluid regulation can be disrupted, resulting in abnormal blood sodium levels. The *syndrome of inappropriate antidiuretic hormone secretion (SIADH)* is characterized by concentrated, low-volume urine and dilutional hyponatremia as water is retained. ADH secretion is inappropriate when it occurs in the absence of dehydration. SIADH can result from central nervous system disorders, pulmonary disorders, tumors, and certain medications.

Estrogen, which is slightly similar to aldosterone, also causes sodium and water retention. Changes in water and sodium balance during the menstrual cycle, during pregnancy, and while taking oral contraceptives are partially attributable to changes in progesterone and estrogen levels.

Recommended Intakes

Actual minimum requirements for sodium are not known but have been estimated to be as low as 200 mg/day. Because the Food and Nutrition Board did not release any new guidelines for sodium in its 1998 to 2002 publications, the *estimated minimum requirements* for healthy persons of all ages, as cited in the *1989 Recommended Dietary Allowances,* are shown in Table 6-4. The mean daily salt intake in Western societies is about 10 to 12 g (4 to 5 g of sodium) per capita, far in excess of the estimated minimum requirements. Approximately 3 g of the daily salt exists naturally in foods, 3 g is added during processing, and 4 g is added by the individual. Increased reliance on restaurants, fast food, and commercially prepared convenience foods has contributed to this high per capita salt intake (Clemens et al, 1999).

An isolated excessive intake of sodium leads to edema and hypertension; however, the kidneys are usually able to excrete the excess sodium. Of greater concern is persistent excessive sodium intake. In addition to its role in hypertension, excessive salt intake is associated with increased urinary calcium excretion (Dawson-Hughes et al, 1996). Currently, studies linking salt intake to bone mineral density are suggesting that high salt intake may be a risk factor for osteoporosis (Burger et al, 2000). An upper limit of 2400 mg of sodium per day (or 6.4 g sodium chloride per day) has been recommended, given the potential role of sodium in hypertension (see Chapter 36) (Food and Nutrition Board, 1989; The Sixth Report of the Joint National Committee on Prevention, Detection, Evaluation, and Treatment of High Blood Pressure, 1997). Results of the Dietary Approaches to Stop

Hypertension (DASH) clinical study support that people need to go beyond restricting sodium chloride intake (to approximately 3 g/day) and take additional dietary measures to prevent and control hypertension. The DASH diet is rich in fruits, vegetables, and low-fat dairy products, making it not only low in sodium but also low in saturated fat, total fat, and cholesterol; high in dietary fiber, potassium, calcium, and magnesium; and moderately high in protein (Appel et al, 1997) (see Chapter 36).

Sources

The major source of sodium is sodium chloride, or common table salt, of which sodium constitutes 40% by weight. Protein foods generally contain more naturally existing sodium than do vegetables and grains, whereas fruits contain little or none. The addition of table salt, flavored salts, flavor enhancers, and preservatives during food processing accounts for the high sodium content of most convenience and fast-food products. For instance ½ cup of frozen vegetables prepared without salt contains 10 mg of sodium, whereas ½ cup of canned vegetables contains approximately 260 mg of sodium. Similarly, 1 ounce of plain meat contains 30 mg of sodium, whereas 1 ounce of luncheon meat contains approximately 400 mg of sodium. The larger portion sizes that are being offered by dining establishments to consumers are increasing the sodium intake even more. (See Tables 36-5 to 36-8 for additional information on the sodium content of foods and food additives.)

Chloride

Chloride (Cl^-) is widely distributed throughout the body as the principal anion of extracellular fluids. The normal serum chloride concentration is 96 to 106 mEq/L. The highest concentrations of chloride are found in cerebrospinal fluid, bile, and gastric and pancreatic juices. In the stomach, chloride is secreted by the gastric mucosa as hydrochloric acid, providing an acid medium for digestion and enzyme activation.

Functions

In addition to sodium, chloride helps to maintain water balance and osmotic pressure. Chloride is crucial in maintaining the acid-base balance and has been implicated in regulating the renin-angiotensin-aldosterone system (William and Dluhy, 1994). (See Chapter 36 for a discussion of the possible role of chloride in hypertension.)

Absorption and Excretion

Chloride is almost completely absorbed in the intestine and excreted in urine and sweat. Chloride loss parallels sodium loss. Excessive loss through sweat is minimized by aldosterone, which acts directly on the sweat glands. Extra chloride may be necessary to correct the metabolic alkalosis resulting from disease, the use of diuretics, or gastric losses from gastric suctioning or vomiting.

Sources

Most dietary chloride comes from sodium chloride (table salt), which is 60% chloride by weight. The amount in food and added table salt provides approximately 3 to 9 g/day. Chloride in water contributes only a very small fraction of the chloride consumed in the diet.

Recommended Intakes

The safe range of chloride intake for all ages, as determined by the Food and Nutrition Board, is shown in Table 6-4. As with sodium, the Food and Nutrition

TABLE 6-4 Estimated Minimum Requirements for Sodium, Chloride, and Potassium in Healthy Persons

AGE	WEIGHT (kg)	SODIUM (mg)*	CHLORIDE (mg)*	POTASSIUM (mg)†
Months				
0-5	4.5	120	180	500
6-11	8.9	200	300	700
Years				
1	11.0	225	350	1000
2-5	16.0	300	500	1400
6-9	25.0	400	600	1600
10-18	50.0	500	750	2000
>18‡	70.0	500	750	2000

From National Academy of Sciences: *Recommended dietary allowances,* ed 10, Washington, DC, 1989, National Academy Press.

*No allowance has been included for large, prolonged losses from the skin through sweat. No evidence shows that higher intakes of sodium or chloride confer any health benefit.

†Desirable intakes of potassium may considerably exceed these values (e.g., 3500 mg for adults).

‡No allowance is included for growth. Values for those younger than 18 years assume a growth rate at the 50th percentile reported by the National Center for Health Statistics and averaged for males and females. (See Chapter 7 for information on pregnancy and lactation.)

Board did not release any new guidelines for chloride in their 1998 to 2002 publications. A chloride deficiency syndrome has been described in infants receiving chloride-deficient formula. The syndrome is characterized by loss of appetite, failure to thrive, muscle weakness, lethargy, and severe metabolic alkalosis with resultant hypokalemia (Grossman et al, 1980).

Potassium

Potassium (K^+), the major cation of intracellular fluid, is present in small amounts in extracellular fluid. The normal serum potassium concentration is 3.5 to 5 mEq/L.

Functions

With sodium, potassium is involved in maintaining a normal water balance, osmotic equilibrium, and the acid-base balance. In addition to calcium, it is important in the regulation of neuromuscular activity. Potassium also promotes cellular growth. The potassium content of muscle is related to muscle mass and glycogen storage; therefore if muscle is being formed, an adequate supply of potassium is essential.

Absorption and Excretion

Potassium is readily absorbed from the small intestine. Approximately 80% to 90% of ingested potassium is excreted in the urine; the remainder is lost in the feces. The kidneys maintain normal serum levels through their ability to filter, reabsorb, and excrete potassium under the influence of aldosterone. Ionized potassium is excreted in place of ionized sodium through the renal tubule exchange mechanism.

Sources

As a rule, fruits, vegetables, fresh meat, and dairy products are good sources of potassium. Box 6-1 categorizes select foods according to their potassium content.

Recommended Intakes

The minimum potassium requirement for adults is 1600 to 2000 mg (40 to 50 mEq) per day, but higher levels are recommended because of the possibility that potassium can prevent hypertension (see Chapter 36). The safe range of recommended intakes for all ages is given in Table 6-4; no new guidelines were provided for this element in the 1998 to 2002 Food and Nutrition Board publications. Potassium intake is inadequate in a large number of Americans, perhaps as many as 50% of adults. The reason for the poor potassium intakes is simply inadequate consumption of fruits and vegetables. Insufficient potassium intakes have been linked to hypertension (Cohn et al, 2000) and osteoporosis (Tucker et al, 1999) (see Chapters 27 and 36).

ACID-BASE BALANCE

An *acid* is any substance that tends to release hydrogen ions in solution, whereas a *base* is any substance that tends to accept hydrogen ions in solution. The hydrogen ion concentration, or $[H^+]$, determines acidity. Because the magnitude of hydrogen ion concentration is small compared with that of other serum electrolytes, acidity is more readily expressed in terms of pH units, determined by $^1/[H^+]$. A low blood pH indicates a higher hydrogen ion concentration, whereas a high pH value indicates a lower hydrogen ion concentration.

Acid-base balance is the dynamic equilibrium state of hydrogen ion concentration. Maintaining the arterial blood pH level within the normal range of 7.35 to 7.45 is crucial for many physiologic functions and biochemical reactions. Regulatory mechanisms of the kidneys, lungs, and buffering systems enable the body to maintain the blood pH level despite the enormous acid load from food consumption and tissue metabolism. A disruption of the acid-base balance occurs when acid or base losses or gains exceed the body's regulatory capabilities or when normal regulatory mechanisms become ineffective. These regulatory disturbances may develop in association with certain diseases, toxin ingestion, shifts in fluid status, and certain medical and surgical treatments (Table 6-5). If a disrupted acid-base balance is left untreated, multiple detrimental effects ranging from electrolyte abnormalities to death can ensue.

Acid Generation

Acids are introduced exogenously through the ingestion of food, acid precursors, and toxins. They are also generated endogenously through normal tissue metabolism. Fixed acids such as phosphoric and sulfuric acids are produced from the metabolism of phosphate-containing substrates and sulfur-containing amino acids, respectively. Organic acids such as lactic and keto acids typically accumulate only during acute illness. Carbon dioxide (CO_2), a volatile acid, is generated from the oxidation of carbohydrates, amino acids, and fat.

Regulation

Various regulatory mechanisms maintain the pH level within very narrow physiologic limits. At the cellular level, buffer systems composed of weak acids or bases and their corresponding salts minimize the effect on pH of the addition of a strong acid or base.

Box 6-1. Classification of Select Foods by Potassium Content

Low (0 to 100 mg/serving)*

Fruits
- Applesauce
- Blueberries
- Cranberries
- Lemon, ½ medium
- Lime, ½ medium
- Pears, canned
- Pear nectar
- Peach nectar

Vegetables
- Cabbage, raw
- Cucumber slices
- Green beans, frozen
- Leeks
- Lettuce, iceberg, 1 cup
- Water chestnuts, canned
- Bamboo shoots, canned

Medium (100 to 200 mg/serving)*

Fruits
- Apple, 1 small
- Apple juice
- Apricot nectar
- Blackberries
- Cherries, 12 small
- Fruit cocktail
- Grape juice
- Grapefruit, ½ small
- Grapes, 12 small
- Mandarin oranges
- Peaches, canned
- Pineapple, canned
- Plum, 1 small
- Raspberries
- Rhubarb
- Strawberries
- Tangerine, 1 small
- Watermelon, 1 cup

Vegetables
- Asparagus, frozen
- Beets, canned
- Broccoli, frozen
- Cabbage, cooked
- Carrots
- Cauliflower, frozen
- Celery, 1 stalk
- Corn, frozen
- Eggplant
- Green beans, fresh raw
- Mushrooms, fresh raw
- Onions
- Peas
- Radishes
- Turnips
- Zucchini, summer squash

Miscellaneous
- Chocolate, 1½-oz bar

High (200 to 300 mg/serving)*

Fruits
- Apricots, canned
- Grapefruit juice
- Kiwi, ½ medium
- Nectarine, 1 small
- Orange, 1 small
- Orange juice
- Peach, fresh, 1 medium
- Pear, fresh, 1 medium

Vegetables
- Asparagus, fresh, cooked, 4 spears
- Beets, fresh, cooked
- Brussels sprouts
- Kohlrabi
- Mushrooms, cooked
- Okra
- Parsnips
- Potatoes, boiled or mashed
- Pumpkin
- Rutabagas

Miscellaneous
- Granola
- Nuts and seeds, 1 oz
- Peanut butter, 2 tbsp

Very High (>300 mg/serving)*

Fruits
- Avocados, ¼ small
- Banana, 1 small
- Cantaloupe, ¼ small
- Dried fruit, ¼ cup
- Honeydew melon, ⅛ small
- Mango, 1 medium
- Papaya, ½ medium
- Prune juice

Vegetables
- Artichoke, 1 medium
- Bamboo shoots, fresh
- Beet greens, ¼ cup
- Corn on the cob, 1 ear
- Chinese cabbage, cooked
- Dried beans
- Potatoes, baked, ½ medium; French fried, 1 oz
- Spinach
- Sweet potatoes, yams
- Swiss chard, ¼ cup
- Tomato, fresh, sauce, or juice; tomato paste, 2 tbsp
- Winter squash

Miscellaneous
- Bouillon, low sodium, 1 cup
- Cappuccino, 1 cup
- Chili, 4 oz
- Coconut, 1 cup
- Lasagna, 8 oz
- Milk, chocolate milk, 1 cup
- Milkshakes, 1 cup
- Molasses, 1 tbsp
- Pizza, 2 slices
- Salt substitutes, ¼ tsp
- Soy milk, 1 cup
- Spaghetti, 1 cup
- Yogurt, 6 oz

*One serving equals ½ cup unless otherwise specified.

The buffering effect involves formation of a weaker acid or base in an amount equivalent to the strong acid or base that has been added to the system (Figure 6-3). Proteins and phosphates are the primary intracellular buffers, whereas the bicarbonate and carbonic acid system is the primary extracellular buffer. The acid-base balance is also maintained by the kidneys and lungs. The kidneys regulate hydrogen ion (H^+) secretion and bicarbonate reabsorption. The lungs control alveolar ventilation by altering either the depth or rate of breathing. In turn, changes in breathing alter the amount of carbon dioxide expired.

TABLE 6-5 Four Major Acid-Base Imbalances and Selected Etiologies

CHARACTERISTICS OF FAILURE	ASSOCIATED DISEASES AND CONDITIONS
Respiratory Imbalance	
Respiratory acidosis	
↑ H_2CO_3 level from retention of CO_2	Conditions involving decreased lung surface area, such as emphysema Restrictive or obstructive lung diseases Certain neuromuscular disease in which respiratory function is impaired
Respiratory alkalosis	
↓ H_2CO_3 level from excessive expiration of CO_2 and H_2O	Aftermath of intense exercise Anxiety reaction Early sepsis
Metabolic Imbalance	
Metabolic acidosis	
↑ H^+ (↓pH) concentration from increased production, increased ingestion, or increased retention *or* ↓ HCO_3^- from excretion of large amounts of base from extracellular fluid	Diarrhea Uremia Ketoacidosis from uncontrolled diabetes mellitus Starvation High-fat, low-carbohydrate diet Drugs
Metabolic alkalosis	
↓ H^+ (↑pH) concentration from increased losses *or* ↑ HCO_3^- from abnormal retention of base in extracellular fluid	Diuretics use Increased ingestion of alkali Loss of chloride Vomiting

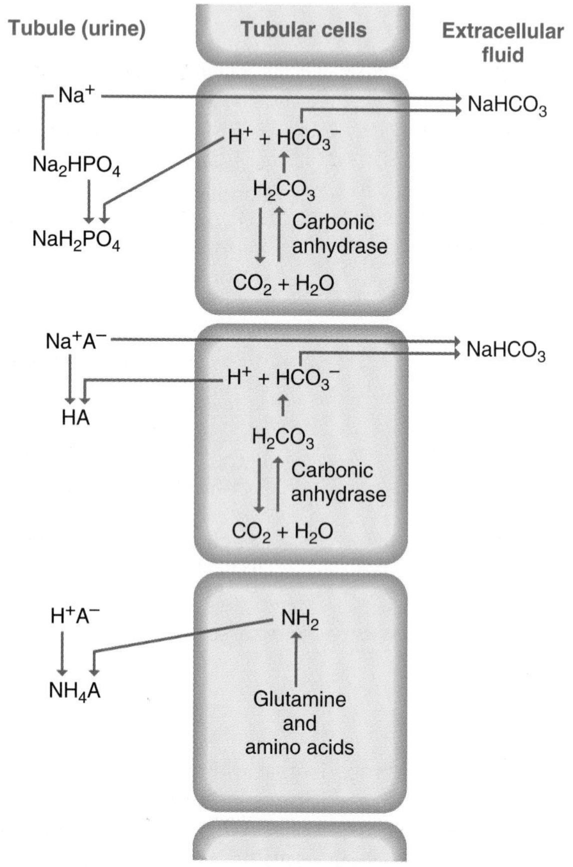

FIGURE 6-3 • Generation of $NaHCO_3$ and clearance of H^+ by the three buffer systems that function in the kidney. (*HA*, Any acid in the body.)

TABLE 6-6 Normal Arterial Blood Gas Values

CLINICAL TEST	ABG* VALUE
pH	7.35-7.45
P_{CO_2}	35-45 mm Hg
P_{O_2}	80-100 mm Hg
HCO_3^-	22-26 mEq/L
O_2 saturation	>95%

**ABG*, Arterial blood gas.

ACID-BASE DISORDERS

Acid-base disorders can be differentiated based on whether they have metabolic or respiratory etiologies. The evaluation of acid-base status requires analysis of serum electrolytes (see Table 6-3) and arterial blood gas (ABG) values (Table 6-6). Metabolic acid-base imbalances result in changes in bicarbonate (i.e., base) levels, which are reflected in the *total carbon dioxide* (TCO_2) portion of the electrolyte profile. TCO_2 includes bicarbonate (HCO_3^-), carbonic acid (H_2CO_3), and dissolved carbon dioxide; however, all but 1 to 3 mEq/L is in the form of bicarbonate. Thus for ease of interpretation, TCO_2 should be equated with bicarbonate. Respiratory acid-base imbalances result in changes in the *partial pressure of dissolved carbon dioxide* (PCO_2). This is reported in the ABG values in addition to the pH, which reflects the overall acid-base status.

CLINICAL INSIGHT

Anion Gap

The number of positively charged ions (cations) in the body equals the number of negatively charged ions (anions). However, not all cations and anions are measured routinely. Sodium is the principal measured cation, whereas chloride and bicarbonate are the principal measured anions. The term anion gap refers to the difference between measured cations and measured anions (and is normally 12 to 14 mEq/L):

Anion gap (AG) = Serum sodium − (Serum chloride + bicarbonate)

Nongap metabolic acidosis

Nongap metabolic acidosis occurs when a decrease in bicarbonate concentration is balanced by an increase in chloride concentration, resulting in a normal anion gap. This type of acidosis, which is also referred to as *hyperchloremic metabolic acidosis,* may develop in association with the following (which are represented by the acronym *USED CARP*) (Wilson, 1992):

Ureterosigmoidostomy	Carbonic anhydrase inhibitor
Small bowel fistula	Adrenal insufficiency
Extra chloride ingestion	Renal tubular acidosis
Diarrhea	Pancreatic fistula

Anion gap metabolic acidosis

Anion gap metabolic acidosis occurs when a decrease in bicarbonate concentration is balanced by increased acid anions other than chloride. This causes the calculated anion gap to exceed the normal range of 12 to 14 mEq/L. This type of acidosis, which is also referred to as *normochloremic metabolic acidosis,* may develop in association with the following conditions (which are represented by the acronym *MUD PILES*) (Wilson, 1992):

Methanol ingestion	Paraldehyde ingestion
Uremia	Iatrogenic
Diabetic ketoacidosis	Lactic acidosis
	Ethylene glycol or ethanol ingestion
	Salicylate ingestion

Metabolic Acidosis

Metabolic acidosis results from increased generation or accumulation of acids or loss of base (i.e., bicarbonate). Simple, acute metabolic acidosis results in a low blood pH, or acidemia. Possible etiologies include diabetic ketoacidosis, lactic acidosis, toxin ingestion, uremia, and excessive bicarbonate loss via the kidneys or intestinal tract. Multiple deaths have been attributed to lactic acidosis caused by administration of parenteral nutrition devoid of thiamin (Centers for Disease Control and Prevention [CDC], 1997; Romanski and McMahon, 1999). In patients with metabolic acidosis the anion gap is calculated to help determine etiology and appropriate treatment (see *Clinical Insight:* Anion Gap and Table 6-5).

Metabolic Alkalosis

Metabolic alkalosis results from the administration or accumulation of bicarbonate (i.e., base) or its precursors, excessive loss of acid (e.g., during gastric suctioning), or loss of extracellular fluid containing more chloride than bicarbonate (e.g., from villous adenoma or diuretic use). Simple, acute metabolic alkalosis results in a high blood pH, or alkalemia. Metabolic alkalosis may also result from volume depletion; decreased blood flow to the kidneys stimulates reabsorption of sodium and water, increasing bicarbonate reabsorption. This condition is known as contraction alkalosis. Alkalosis can also result from severe hypokalemia (serum potassium concentration <2 mEq/L). As potassium moves from the intracellular to the extracellular fluid, hydrogen ions move from the extracellular to the intracellular fluid to maintain electroneutrality. This process produces intracellular acidosis, which increases hydrogen ion excretion and bicarbonate reabsorption by the kidneys.

Respiratory Acidosis

Respiratory acidosis is caused by decreased ventilation and consequent carbon dioxide retention. Simple, acute respiratory acidosis results in a low pH, or acidemia. Acute respiratory acidosis can occur as a result of sleep apnea, asthma, aspiration of a foreign object, or acute respiratory distress syndrome (ARDS), also known as *adult respiratory distress syndrome* (see Chapter 38). Chronic respiratory acidosis is associated with obesity hypoventilation syndrome, chronic obstructive pulmonary disease (COPD) or emphysema, certain neuromuscular diseases, and starvation cachexia.

Respiratory Alkalosis

Respiratory alkalosis results from increased ventilation and elimination of carbon dioxide. The condition may be mediated centrally (e.g., from head injury, pain, anxiety, cerebrovascular accident, or tumors) or by peripheral stimulation (e.g., from pneumonia, hypoxemia, high altitudes, pulmonary embolism,

TABLE 6-7 Primary and Compensatory Laboratory Value Changes in Acid-Base Disorders*

ACID-BASE DISORDER	PH	HCO_3^-	Pco_2
Metabolic acidosis	↓↓/↑ (net pH remains less than normal)	↓↓	↓ (compensatory respiratory alkalosis)
Metabolic alkalosis	↑↑/↓ (net pH remains greater than normal)	↑↑	↑ (compensatory respiratory acidosis)
Respiratory acidosis	↓↓/↑ (net pH remains less than normal)	↑ (compensatory metabolic alkalosis)	↑↑
Respiratory alkalosis	↑↑/↓ (net pH remains greater than normal)	↓ (compensatory metabolic acidosis)	↓↓

*↑↑/↓↓, Primary change; ↑/↓, compensatory change.

congestive heart failure, or interstitial lung disease). Simple, acute respiratory alkalosis results in a high pH, or alkalemia.

Compensation

When an acid-base imbalance occurs, the body attempts to restore the normal pH by developing an opposite acid-base imbalance to offset the effects of the primary disorder (Table 6-7), a response known as *compensation.* For example, the kidneys of a patient with a primary respiratory acidosis (decreased pH) compensate by increasing bicarbonate reabsorption, thereby creating a metabolic alkalosis. This response helps to increase the pH. Similarly, in response to a primary metabolic acidosis (decreased pH), the lungs compensate by increasing ventilation and carbon dioxide elimination, thereby creating a respiratory alkalosis. This compensatory respiratory alkalosis helps increase pH. Respiratory compensation for metabolic acid-base disturbances occurs quickly—within minutes. In contrast, renal compensation for respiratory acid-base imbalances may take 3 to 5 days to be maximally effective. Compensation does not always occur and when it does, it is not completely successful (i.e., does not result in a pH of 7.40). The pH level still reflects the underlying primary disorder. It is imperative to distinguish between primary disturbances and compensatory responses because treatment is always directed toward the primary acid-base disturbance and its underlying cause. As the primary disturbance is treated, the compensatory response corrects itself. Predictive values for compensatory responses are available and may aid the clinician in differentiating between primary acid-base imbalances and compensatory responses (Whitmire, 2002). Alternatively, clinicians can also use acid-base maps and nomograms (DuBose et al, 1996; Goldberg et al, 1973).

SUMMARY

Despite wide daily variations in intake of water and minerals that function as electrolytes, the body strives to maintain a stable internal environment to maintain physiologic functioning. When normal homeostatic mechanisms are rendered ineffective by disease or injury or intakes exceed the body's normal regulatory capacities, the internal environment and ultimately cell function are disrupted. A basic knowledge of fluid, electrolyte, and acid-base balance is important for understanding many aspects of nutrition in health and disease. Information in this and other chapters, as well as additional references, can help complete the case studies that follow.

Clinical Scenario I

Cynthia is a 62-year-old, 60-kg woman status post stroke CVA. She received a percutaneous endoscopic gastrostomy (PEG) in anticipation of long-term home enteral nutrition therapy. Following a brief rehabilitative stay, Cynthia is discharged and moves in with her family. She is fed solely by the tube feedings (and receives nothing by mouth); her gravity tube feedings consist of 300 ml of fiber-enriched 1 kcal/ml formula given five times each day with 120-ml water flushes after each feeding.

Her outpatient follow-up appointments in January, March, and May are favorable; her weight is stable, and her bowel habits and serum electrolytes are normal. Several days before Cynthia's scheduled July appointment, her daughter calls and is concerned because Cynthia seems lethargic and is light-headed when she stands. She does not have a fever or diarrhea and has not been vomiting. In fact, Cynthia is somewhat constipated. Cynthia's urine is darker and smells stronger. Her tube-feeding regimen has not changed.

Cynthia is brought to the clinic for evaluation and treatment. She has sunken eyes, dry mucous membranes, tenting, and mild orthostatic hypotension. Her weight is 126.7 lb (5.7 lb less than she weighed in May). Her lab results are as follows: sodium, 154 mEq/L; chloride, 111 mEq/L; blood urea nitrogen, 29 mg/dl; glucose, 108 mg/dl; potassium, 4.3 mEq/L; bicarbonate, 29 mEq/L; creatinine, 0.9, mg/dl; urine specific gravity, 1.04.

1. What is Cynthia's fluid-electrolyte disorder?
2. What information supports your diagnosis?
3. What may have caused Cynthia's fluid-electrolyte disorder?
4. Outline treatment for Cynthia.

Clinical Scenario 2

Richard is a 54-year-old man who has been admitted to the hospital; he has been vomiting for 2 days. He is receiving intravenous fluids of 5% dextrose in 0.45% sodium chloride (NaCl) with 20 mEq of potassium chloride per liter at 75 ml/hr. He has a nasogastric tube (NGT) inserted (KCl). Richard has been diagnosed with gastric outlet obstruction. On his third day in the hospital, he begins receiving total parenteral nutrition (TPN) therapy, with 2 L of a standard total nutrient admixture. The maintenance intravenous fluids are discontinued. His nasogastric output remains fairly consistent at 1.5 to 2 L/day. On his fifth day in the hospital, Richard's laboratory results are as follows: sodium, 135 mEq/L; chloride, 93 mEq/L; blood urea nitrogen, 29 mg/dl; glucose, 108 mg/dl; potassium, 3.3 mEq/L; bicarbonate, 33 mEq/L; creatinine, 0.9 mg/dl; pH, 7.51.

1. What are Richard's fluid-electrolyte and acid-base disorders?
2. What information supports this diagnosis?
3. List the probable causes of his fluid-electrolyte and acid-base disorders?
4. Outline treatment for Richard, including but not limited to, TPN adjustments.

■ Relevant Web Sites

Harrison's Online
www.harrisons.accessmedicine.com/
Chapter 49: Fluid and Electrolyte Disturbances
Chapter 50: Acidosis and Alkalosis
The Merck Manual of Diagnosis and Therapy
www.merck.com/pubs/mmanual/section2/chapter12/12a.htm
Chapter 1: Nutrition: General Considerations
Chapter 12: Water, Electrolyte, Mineral, and Acid-Base Metabolism

■ Cited References

Appel IJ et al: A clinical study of the effects of dietary patterns on blood pressure, *N Engl J Med* 336:1117, 1997.

Beck LH: Changes in renal function with aging, *Clin Geriatr Med* 14:199, 1998.

Borghi L et al: Urinary volume, water, and recurrences in idiopathic calcium nephrolithiasis: a 5-year randomized prospective study, *Urology* 155:839, 1996.

Burger H et al: Osteoporosis and salt intake, *Nutri Metab Cardiovasc Dis* 10(1):46-53, 2000.

Centers for Disease Control and Prevention: Lactic acidosis traced to thiamine deficiency related to nationwide shortage of multivitamins for total parenteral nutrition—United States, 1997, *MMWR Morb Wkly Rep* 46:523, 1997.

Clemens LH et al: The effect of eating out on the quality of diet in premenopausal women, *J Am Dietetic Assoc* 99:442, 1999.

Cohn JN et al: New guidelines for potassium replacement in clinical practice: a contemporary review by the National Council on Potassium in Clinical Practice, *Arch Int Med* 160:2429, 2000.

Dawson-Hughes B et al: Sodium excretion influences calcium homeostasis in elderly men and women, *J Nutr* 126(9):2107, 1996.

DuBose TD et al: Acid-base disorders. In Brenner BM, Rector FC, eds: *The kidney,* pp 929-998, ed 5, Philadelphia, 1996, WB Saunders.

Ellis KJ et al: Bioelectrical impedance methods in clinical research: a follow-up to the NIH Technology Assessment Conference, *Nutrition* 15:874, 1999.

Food and Nutrition Board, National Research Council: *Recommended dietary allowances,* ed 10, Washington, DC, 1989, National Academy Press.

Goldberg M et al: Computer-based instruction and diagnosis of acid-base disorders, *JAMA* 223:269, 1973.

Grant A, DeHoog S: *Nutrition assessment support and management,* pp 287-288, ed 5, Seattle, 1999, Grant/DeHoog.

Grossman H et al: The dietary chloride deficiency syndrome, *Pediatrics* 66:366, 1980.

Kleiner SM: Water: an essential but overlooked nutrient, *J Am Diet Assoc* 99:200, 1999.

Lax D et al: Mild dehydration induces echocardiographic signs of mitral valve prolapse in healthy females with prior normal cardiac findings, *Am Heart J* 124:1533, 1992.

Levine B: Role of liquid intake in childhood obesity and related diseases, *Curr Concepts Persp Nutr* 8:2, 1996.

New SA et al: Nutritional influences on bone density: a cross-sectional study in premenopausal women, *Am J Clin Nutr* 123:1615, 1993.

Pennington JA: *Bowes and Church's food values of portions commonly used,* ed 17, Philadelphia, 1998, JB Lippincott.

Romanski SA, McMahon MM: Metabolic acidosis and thiamine deficiency, *Mayo Clinic Proceedings* 74:259, 1999.

Sanservero AC: Dehydration in the elderly: strategies for prevention and management, *Nurse Pract* 22:41, 1997.

Shannon J et al: Relationship of food groups and water intake to colon cancer risk, *Cancer Epidemiol Biomarkers Prev* 5:495, 1996.

Ship JA, Fischer DJ: The relationship between dehydration and parotid salivary gland function in young and older healthy adults, *J Gerontol* 52A:310, 1997.

The Sixth Report of the Joint National Committee on Prevention, Detection, Evaluation, and Treatment of High Blood Pressure: NIH Pub No 98-4080, *Arch Intern Med* 157:2413, 1997.

Stookey JD et al: Correspondence: relationship of food groups and water intake to colon cancer risk, *Cancer Epidemiol Biomarkers Prev* 6:657, 1997.

Tucker KL et al: Potassium, magnesium, and fruit and vegetable intakes are associated with greater bone mineral density in elderly men and women, *Am J Clin Nutr* 69:727, 1999.

Victora CG et al: Reducing deaths from diarrhea through oral rehydration therapy, *Bull WHO* 78:1246, 2000.

Whitmire SJ: Fluids, electrolytes, and acid-base balance. In Matarese LE, Gottschlich MM, eds: *Contemporary nutrition support practice: a clinical guide,* ed 2, Philadelphia, 2002, WB Saunders.

William GH, Dluhy RG: Hypertensive states: associated fluid and electrolyte disturbances. In Narins RG, ed: *Maxwell and Kleeman's clinical disorders of fluid and electrolyte metabolism,* pp 1621-1622, ed 5, New York, 1994, McGraw-Hill.

Wilson RF: Acid-base problems. In Tintinalli JE, Krome RL, Ruiz E, eds: *Emergency medicine: a comprehensive study guide,* ed 3, New York, 1992, McGraw-Hill.

■ Additional References

Adrogué HJ, Madias NE: Management of life-threatening acid-base disorders, Parts I and II, *N Engl J Med* 338:26, 107, 1998.

Adrogué HJ, Madias NE: Hypernatremia, *N Engl J Med* 342(20): 1493, 2000.

Adrogué HJ, Madias NE: Hyponatremia, *N Engl J Med* 342(21): 1581, 2000.

Cohn JN et al: New guidelines for potassium replacement in clinical practice: a contemporary review by the National Council on Potassium in Clinical Practice, *Arch Intern Med* 160:2429, 2000.

Gennari FJ: Hypokalemia, *N Engl J Med* 339:451, 1998.

Gluck SL: Acid-base [Electrolyte Quintet], *Lancet* 352:474, 1998.

Halperin ML, Goldstein MB: *Fluid, electrolyte, and acid-base physiology: a problem-based approach,* ed 3, Philadelphia, 1999, WB Saunders.
Hood VL, Tannen RL: Protection of acid base balance by pH regulation of acid production, *N Engl J Med* 12:819, 1998.
Kumar S, Berl T: Sodium, *Lancet* 352:220, 1998.
Kumar S, Berl T: Approach to the hyponatremia patient. In Berl T, ed: *Atlas of diseases of the kidney. Part 1: Disorders of water, electrolytes, and acid-base,* vol 1, Philadelphia, 1999, Blackwell Science.
Mange K et al: Language guiding therapy: the case of dehydration versus volume depletion, *Ann Intern Med* 127:848, 1997.
Miller M: Hyponatremia: age-related risk factors and therapy decisions, *Geriatrics* 53:32, 1998.
Oh MS, Uribarri J: Electrolytes, water, and acid-base balance. In Shils ME et al, eds: *Modern nutrition in health and disease,* ed 9, Baltimore, 1999, Williams & Wilkins.
Oster JR, Singer I: Hyponatremia, hyposmolality, and hypotonicity: tables and fables, *Arch Intern Med* 159:333, 1999.
Palevsky PM: Hypernatremia, *Semin Nephrol* 18:20, 1998.

Piazza-Barnett R, Matarese LE: Electrolyte management in total parenteral nutrition, *Support Line* 21:8, 1999.

Shires GT et al: Fluid, electrolyte, and nutritional management of the surgical patient. In Schwartz SI, ed: *Principles of surgery,* ed 7, New York, 1999, McGraw-Hill.

Singer GG, Brenner BM: Fluid and electrolyte disturbances. In Fauci SA et al, eds: *Harrison's principles of internal medicine,* vol 1, ed 14, New York, 1998, McGraw-Hill.

Verbalis J: Adaptation to acute and chronic hyponatremia: implications for symptomatology, diagnosis, and therapy, *Sem Nephrol* 18:3, 1998.

Vogelzang JL: Overview of fluid maintenance/prevention of dehydration, *J Am Diet Assoc* 99:605, 1999.

Whitmire SJ: Fluid and electrolytes. In Gottschlich MM et al, eds: *The science and practice of nutrition support: a case-based core curriculum,* American Society for Parenteral and Enteral Nutrition, Dubuque, Iowa, 2001, Kendall/Hunt.

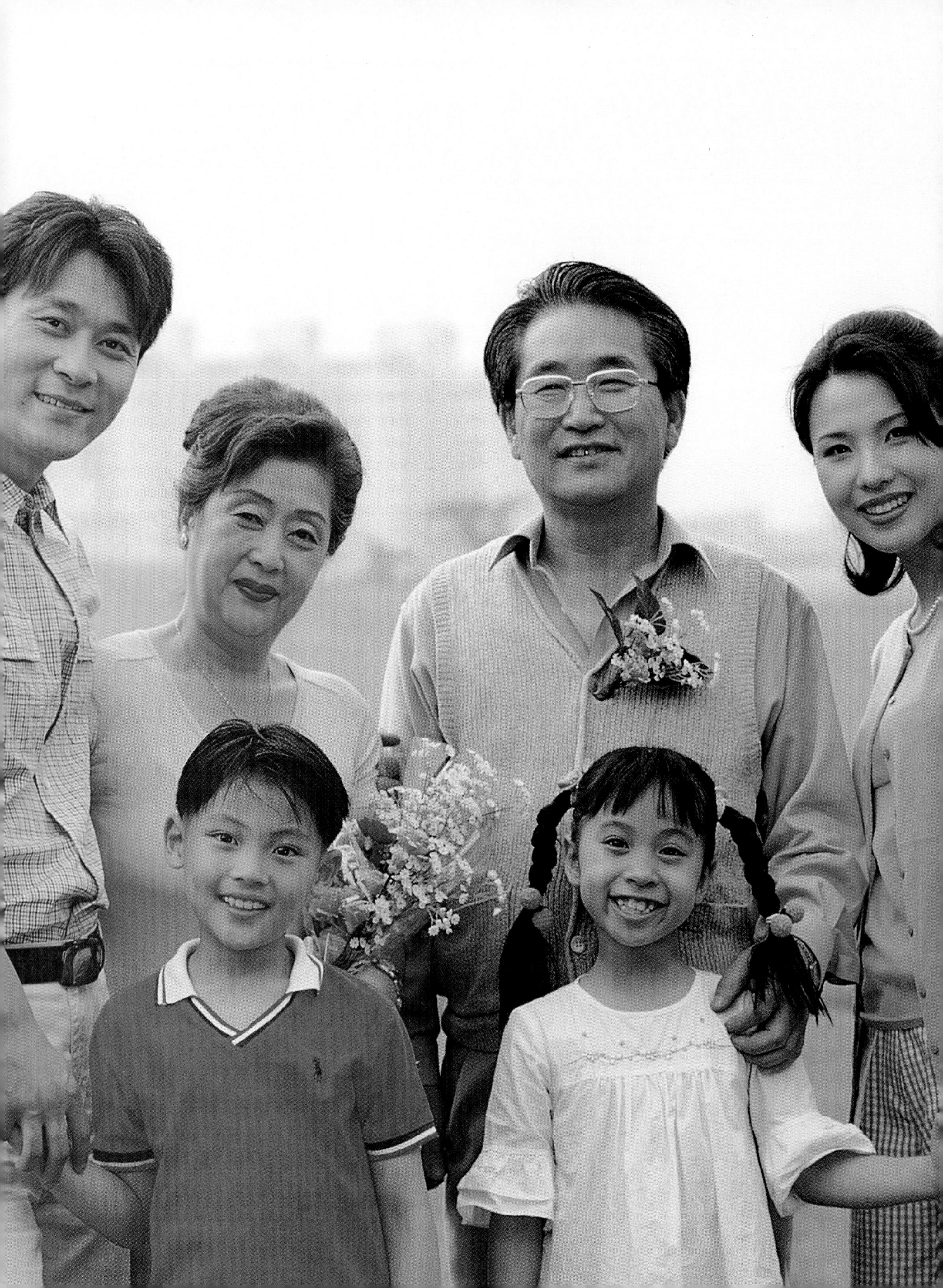

PART 2

NUTRITION IN THE LIFE CYCLE

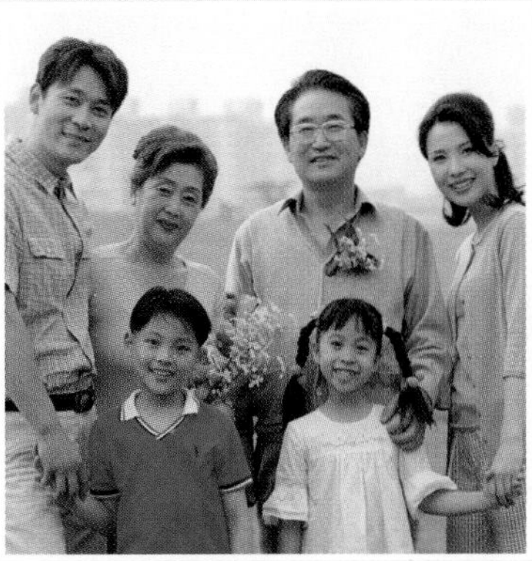

The importance of nutrition throughout the life cycle cannot be refuted—after all, people must eat to live. However, the significance of nutrition during specific times of growth, development, and aging is becoming increasingly appreciated.

Health professionals have recognized for quite some time the effects of proper nutrition during pregnancy on the health of the infant and mother after her childbearing years. Maternal nutrition and possibly even paternal nutrition before conception affect the health of the newborn. It is now recognized that "fetal origin" has far more lifelong effects than originally thought.

Establishing good dietary habits during childhood lessens the possibility of inappropriate eating behavior (a phenomenon that occurs with disturbing frequency during adolescence) later in life. Although the influence of proper nutrition on a person's own morbidity and mortality usually remains unacknowledged until adulthood, recent studies suggest that dietary practices aimed at preventing the degenerative diseases that develop later in life should be instituted in childhood.

Clearly, during early adulthood, many changes begin that lead to the development of diseases of aging several years later. What is only beginning to become clear is that many of these changes can be accelerated or slowed over the years depending on the quality of the individual's nutritional intake, the health of the gut, and the function of the immune system.

With the rapid growth of the older adult population has evolved a need to expand the limited nutrition data currently available for these individuals. Although it is known that energy needs decrease with aging, little is known about whether requirements for specific nutrients increase or decrease. Identifying the unique nutritional differences among the various stages of aging is becoming even more important as the life span of the population increases.

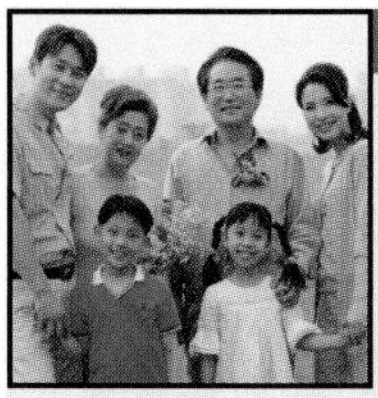

CHAPTER 7

Nutrition During Pregnancy and Lactation

JUDITH K. SHABERT, MD, RD, MPH

CHAPTER OUTLINE

- Pregnancy
- Lactation
- Nutrition, Fertility, and Conception

KEY TERMS

amenorrhea–cessation of menses in a female who has previously menstruated

amylophagia–a form of pica characterized by the consumption of nonnutritive starch (such as laundry starch)

colostrum–an antibody-rich, thin, yellow, milky fluid secreted by the mammary gland a few days before and after birth and before the secretion of mature milk

eclampsia–the late stage of pregnancy-induced hypertension characterized by proteinuria and grand mal seizures; occurs after the twentieth week of gestation

fetal alcohol syndrome–a specific set of abnormal features resulting from exposure of the fetus to alcohol during gestation

geophagia–a form of pica characterized by the consumption of substances such as dirt and clay

gestational diabetes–diabetes that exists only during pregnancy

gestational hypertension–hypertension without proteinuria developing after the twentieth week of gestation; one of two types of pregnancy-induced hypertension

hyperemesis gravidarum–prolonged and persistent vomiting during pregnancy

intrauterine fetal demise (IUFD)–intrauterine death after the twentieth week of gestation

intrauterine growth restriction (IUGR)–a fetal growth condition resulting in a birth weight at or below the tenth percentile for age and gender and a fetus that does not reach its full potential

lactation–the period of milk secretion

let-down–a distinct, tingling sensation in the breast accompanying the movement of milk from the alveoli through the duct system and lactiferous sinuses to the nipple

macrosomia–an infant birth weight greater than 4000 g

neural crest defect–a birth defect resulting in cleft lip, facial anomalies, and heart valve abnormalities; associated with the ingestion of a vitamin A analogue used to treat acne

neural tube defect (NTD)–a developmental anomaly resulting in anencephaly or spina bifida; related to folic acid deficiency

oxytocin–a posterior pituitary hormone that stimulates the movement of milk down to the nipple and uterine contractions during labor and after birth

perinatal mortality–the number of infant deaths occurring from 28 weeks gestation to 4 weeks after birth per 1000 live births per year

pica–compulsive ingestion of unsuitable substances having little or no nutritional value, such as cornstarch *(amylophagia)* and soil or clay *(geophagia)*

preeclampsia–pregnancy-induced hypertension with proteinuria developing after the twentieth week of gestation; one of two types of pregnancy-induced hypertension

pregnancy-induced hypertension–gestational hypertension (hypertension without proteinuria) or preeclampsia (hypertension with proteinuria) developing after the twentieth week of gestation

prolactin–an anterior pituitary gland hormone that stimulates milk production by alveolar breast cells

spina bifida–cleft spine, or a failure of the spinal column to close

teratogen–any agent (e.g., infectious, environmental, nutritional) that causes a malformation in the fetus

PREGNANCY

Various factors determine the outcome of a pregnancy, including the nutritional status of the mother before she became pregnant. Some nutritional factors can affect the newborn's birth weight, the risk of neural tube defects, and fetal alcohol syndrome. Birth weight is highly correlated with infant mortality and morbidity. Newborns who are small for gestational age (SGA) are at increased risk for long-term adverse health outcomes such as hypertension, obesity, glucose intolerance, and cardiovascular disease (Barker, 1995).

Effect of Nutritional Status on Pregnancy Outcome

Historical Perspective

In the early 1900s, it was documented that women with a poor nutritional status had adverse pregnancy outcomes and infants with compromised birth weights (Smith, 1916). During World War II the effects of inadequate nutrition on previously well-nourished populations were explored because severe food deprivation occurred in many parts of Europe. Retrospective studies in Germany, the Netherlands, and Russia indicate that the incidence of amenorrhea, the cessation of menses in females, increased significantly and was accompanied by a subsequent decrease in fertility. These nutritionally and energy-deprived females were physiologically unable to conceive. In the Netherlands, 50% of the female population stopped menstruating. Those less affected by amenorrhea and therefore infertility lived in rural areas or had much better access to food rations. The incidence of spontaneous abortion, stillbirths, neonatal deaths, and congenital malformations increased in females who conceived during the famine. Surviving infants had significantly lower mean birth weights and lengths (Susser and Smith, 1994). As living conditions improved, mean birth weights rose steadily, returning to normal by 1948.

Attitudes regarding weight gain in pregnancy have changed dramatically. In the early 1900s, when cesarean sections were rarely performed because surgery carried such high risk, the accepted practice was to discourage maternal weight gain during pregnancy. Health professionals reasoned that a smaller infant could fit more easily through the birth canal. This philosophy prevailed in the United States through the 1960s.

Perinatal Mortality and Birth Weight

Low birth weight (LBW; <2500 g), and especially very-low-birth weight (VLBW; <1500g), play a major role in perinatal mortality (the number of infant deaths occurring from 28 weeks gestation to 4 weeks after birth per 1000 live births per year), necrotizing enterocolitis, and respiratory distress syndrome, particularly if the fetus has intrauterine growth restriction (IUGR) or a birthweight at or below the 10th percentile for age and gender (Bernstein et al, 2000). Other risks include long-term morbidity such as developmental disabilities and learning disorders. Although many congenital defects or perinatal defects cannot be prevented, poor nutrition and low maternal weight gain—factors implicated in LBW—can be modified. In addition, it seems that poor nutritional status and being underweight before conception can decrease infant birth weight; being underweight can also increase the risk of *gastroschisis* (protrusion of intestines through the abdominal wall) (Lam et al, 1999).

Two indicators of maternal nutritional status have consistently been shown to correlate with infant birth weight: maternal size (height and prepregnancy weight) and the amount of weight gained during pregnancy.

Maternal Size

Females of large stature tend to have large babies, and it has been proposed that maternal size plays a role in the ultimate size of the placenta. The size of the placenta is an indicator of placental health, which determines the amount of nutrition available to the fetus and ultimately the birth weight of the neonate. Females with less-than-ideal prepregnancy weights have lighter weight placentas and an increased risk for LBW and delivering premature infants than do females who conceive with normal body weight. An adequate prepregnancy weight and satisfactory weight gain are particularly important for the offspring of mothers with short stature (Luke et al, 1984). Attaining a normal prepregnancy weight may improve pregnancy outcome. Recommended weight gain goals are based on prepregnancy body mass index (BMI). (The BMI calculation is explained in Chapter 17 and Appendix 17.)

Maternal Weight Gain During Pregnancy

The normal distribution of weight gain during pregnancy is illustrated in Figure 7-1. Less than half of the

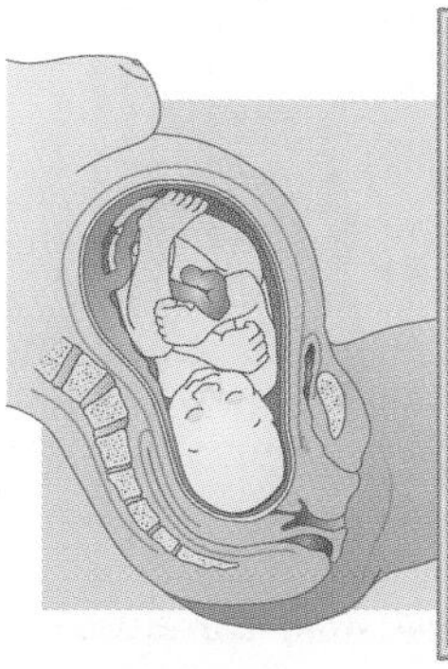

WEIGHT IN POUNDS	
7.5–8.5	Fetus
7.5	Stores of fat and protein
4.0	Blood
2.7	Tissue fluids
2.0	Uterus
1.8	Amniotic fluid
1.5	Placenta and umbilical cord
1.0	Breasts
28–29 pounds	

FIGURE 7-1 • Distribution of weight gain during pregnancy.

TABLE 7-1 Recommended Weight Gains During Pregnancy Based on Body Mass Index

WEIGHT CATEGORY*	TOTAL WEIGHT GAIN†		FIRST TRIMESTER GAIN		SECOND AND THIRD TRIMESTERS WEEKLY GAIN	
	lb	kg	lb	kg	lb	kg
Underweight (BMI <19.8)	28-40	12.5-18.0	5.0	2.3	1.07	0.49
Normal weight (BMI = 19.8-26)	25-35	11.5-16.0	3.5	1.6	0.97	0.44
Overweight (BMI >26-29)	15-25	7.0-11.5	2.0	0.9	0.67	0.3
Obese (BMI >29)	At least 15	6.0				

Data from Subcommittee on Nutritional Status and Weight Gain During Pregnancy and Subcommittee on Dietary Intake and Nutrient Supplements During Pregnancy, Food and Nutrition Board, National Academy of Sciences: *Nutrition during pregnancy, Parts I and II,* Washington, DC, 1990, National Academy Press.
*Body mass index (BMI) = weight (kg)/height (m)^2 (see Appendix 17)
†Young adolescents and black women should strive for gains at the upper end of the recommended range. Short women (<62 inches or <157 cm) should strive for gains at the lower end of the range.

total weight gain is in the fetus, placenta, and amniotic fluid; the remainder comprises maternal reproductive tissues, fluid, blood, and *maternal stores,* a component composed largely of body fat. Gradually increasing amounts of subcutaneous fat in the abdomen, back, and upper thigh serve as an energy reserve for pregnancy and lactation.

In normal-weight females, a weight gain of 26 to 35 lb during gestation is associated with an optimal outcome. The Institute of Medicine (IOM) recommends a weight gain of 25 to 35 lb for women of normal weight, 28 to 40 lb for underweight women, and 15 to 25 lb for overweight women (IOM, 1990) (Table 7-1).

Accepted ranges for BMI that define *underweight, normal weight, overweight,* and *obesity* may vary. A normal BMI ranges from 20 to 25. A BMI of less than 20 indicates underweight, a BMI of 25 to 29 indicates overweight, and a BMI exceeding 29 indicates obesity. For example, a female with a BMI of 22 is considered normal weight and should gain 25 to 35 lb during her pregnancy.

The pregnancy weight gain curves currently in use reflect the prepregnancy weight, height, and age of the mother. Figure 7-2 presents curves of desirable weight gain during pregnancy as recommended by the Subcommittee on Nutritional Status and Weight Gain During Pregnancy (IOM, 1990). A weight gain during pregnancy that is more than the upper limits recommended in the 1990 IOM report is associated with postpartum weight retention (Caulfield et al, 1996).

Obesity

Trends among American women reveal an increasing prevalence of obesity. For example, the prevalence of individuals, with *overweight* being defined in one study as a BMI of greater than 27.8, among women 20 to 29 years increased from 12.6% in 1971 through 1974 to 20.2% in 1988 through 1991 (Kuczmarski et al, 1994).

The risk of gestational diabetes, pregnancy-induced hypertension, and cesarean section increases in females who are obese (Brost et al, 1997). Overweight and obese females are also at increased risk for late-pregnancy (>28 weeks gestation) and term intrauterine fetal demise (IUFD) (Cnattingius et al, 1998; Stephansson et al, 2001). The risk for delivery of a *very preterm* (≤32 weeks) infant, an infant with a cardiac defect, an infant with neural tube defects, and an infant with macrosomia (a birth weight of greater than 4000 g) increases for females who are obese (Watkins and Botto, 2001; Werler et al, 1996).

Obese pregnant females have an increased risk of delivering an infant with a neural tube defect (NTD), and the risk of having a infant with spina bifida increases twofold compared with normal-weight females; the risk for anencephaly is not higher (Shaw et al, 1996). The etiology of the association of maternal obesity and an increased incidence of NTDs is unknown but is not related to lower dietary folic acid intake, vitamin supplementation containing folic acid, diabetes, or a history of NTDs in a previous pregnancy. An adequate folate intake did not help prevent NTDs in a study of obese females, although it does in normal-weight pregnant females (Werler et al, 1996).

Weight gains of 15 to 25 lb have been recommended by the IOM for overweight females. These recommendations allow for adequate fetal growth without increasing maternal adipose tissue. However, recent investigators report that in females with a BMI of greater than 26, weight gains of 0.5 lb/wk (for a 20-lb weight gain during the entire pregnancy) were associated with a higher risk of preterm delivery than for females with a BMI greater than 26 who had weight gains of greater than 20 lb (Schieve et al, 2000). Weight gains of less than 15 lb are associated with an increased risk of IUFD (Edwards et al, 1996). Even though obese females may be hesitant to gain weight during pregnancy, they should be told that pregnancy is not a time for weight loss. An appropriate nutritional goal would be to choose nutritional foods and avoid unnecessary, calorie-rich foods. Because obese females have an increased incidence of

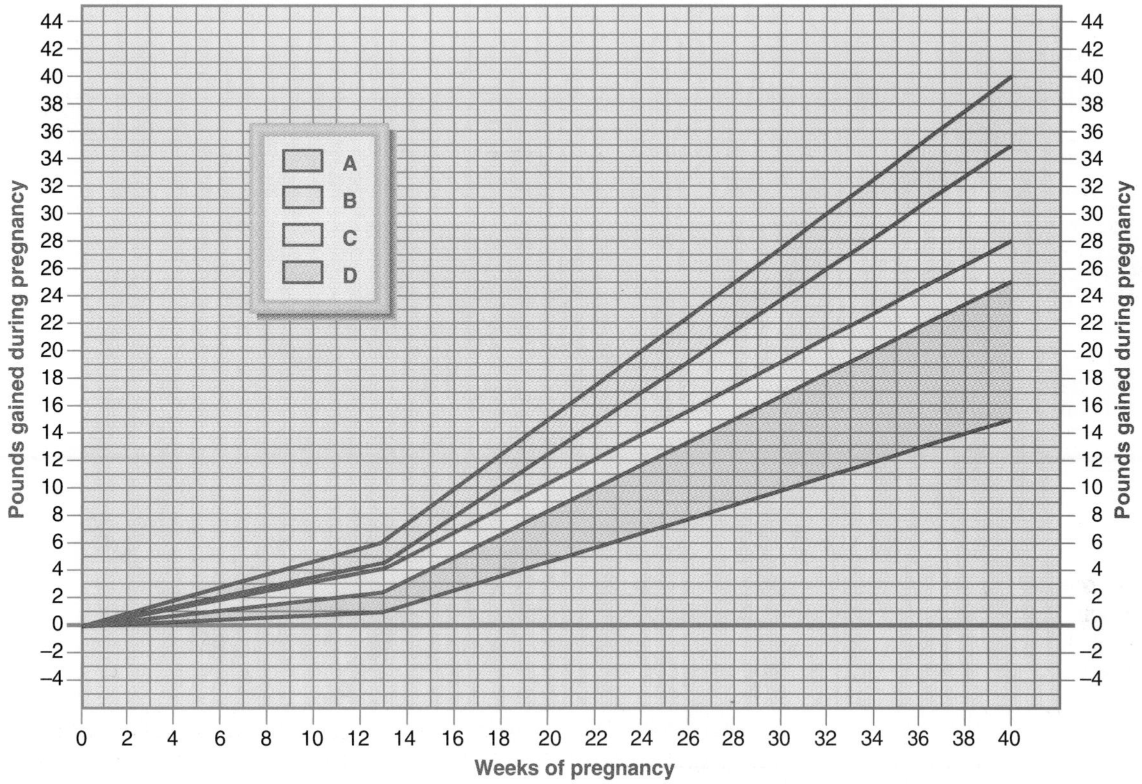

FIGURE 7-2 • Desirable weight gain during pregnancy. Females who are of normal weight before their pregnancy should aim for a weight gain in the *B* to *C* range (25 to 35 lb) during the pregnancy. Underweight females should gain in the *A* to *B* range (28 to 40 lb). Females who are overweight before pregnancy should gain in the *D* range (15 to 25 lb).

obstetric complications, the weight gain pattern during pregnancy should be monitored carefully by a nutrition professional who prescribes appropriate dietary interventions as necessary.

Adolescence

About 1 million adolescents in the United States become pregnant every year. Teenagers have a higher incidence of delivering LBW infants; low birth weight carries the highest risk for infant death and disability. Risk factors for poor pregnancy outcome in pregnant adolescents are listed in Box 7-1 (Story, 1990). Even though the teenage birth rate is decreasing (Martin, Park, and Sutton, 2002), teenage pregnancy continues to be considered one of the major public health problems in the United States and is associated with significant medical and nutritional risks (Figure 7-3). Many teenagers who become pregnant already have iron deficiency anemia and consume a poor diet that is low in calcium and folic acid. Improved dietary practices is one of the most important and controllable factors for a pregnant teenager and her infant. When counseling pregnant teenagers, nutrition professionals must be aware of the social, economic, and educational frameworks

✓ Box 7-1. Risk Factors for Poor Pregnancy Outcome in Teenagers

- Maternal age, especially 15 years or younger
- Pregnancy less than 2 years after onset of menarche
- Poor nutrition and low prepregnancy weight
- Poor weight gain
- Infection
- Sexually transmitted disease infection
- Preexisting anemia
- Substance abuse: smoking, drinking, drugs
- Poverty
- Lack of social support
- Lack of education
- Rapid repeat pregnancies
- Lack of access to age-appropriate prenatal care
- Late entry into the health care system
- Unmarried status

Data from Story M, ed: *Nutrition management of the pregnant adolescent*, Washington, DC, 1990, U.S. Departments of Agriculture and Health and Human Services, March of Dimes Birth Defects Foundation, National Clearing House.

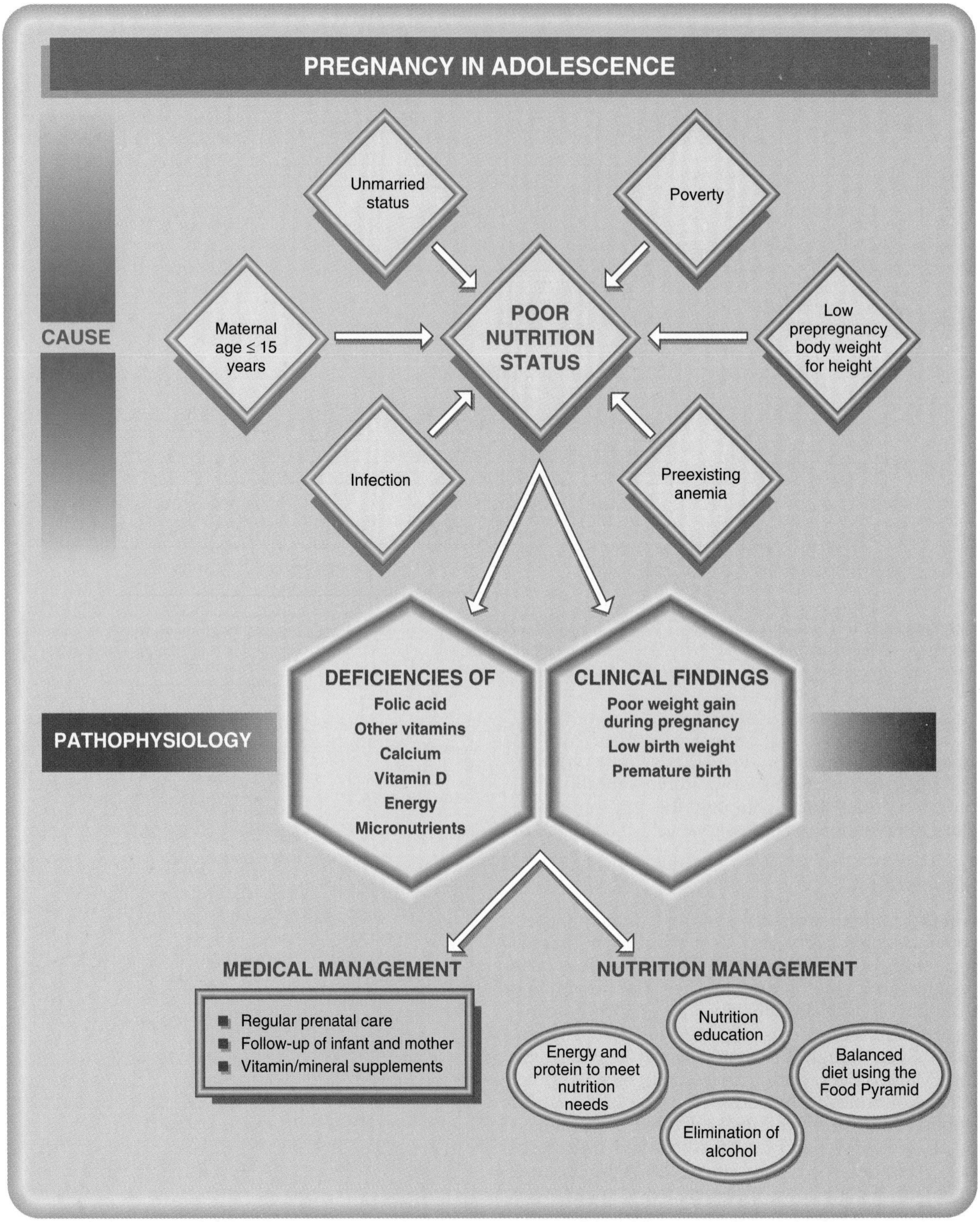

FIGURE 7-3 • Pathophysiology algorithm: management of pregnancy in adolescence. (Algorithm content developed by John Anderson, PhD, and Sanford C. Garner, PhD, 2000.)

that influence food choices. It is recommended that adolescents gain 28 to 40 lb during pregnancy; the recommended weight gain is modified according to the prepregnant weight and gynecologic age (i.e., years since menarche) (see Chapter 11). The benefits of prenatal counseling for teenagers are noted in Figure 7-4.

Multiple Births

The incidence of multiple births in the United States is rising in part because of the increased use of fertility drugs and increased incidence of pregnancy in older women (both of which increase the chance of multiple births). Infants of multiple-birth pregnancies have a much greater risk of being born premature with IUGR or LBW than do infants of single births. An adequate maternal weight gain has been shown to be particularly important in these high-risk pregnancies. Optimal weight gains and infant gestational ages for multiple-fetus pregnancies are presented in Table 7-2 (Luke, 1994).

Nutritional Supplementation During Pregnancy

Supplementation of a mother's diet during pregnancy may take the form of energy, protein, vitamins, or minerals that exceed her routine daily intake. The more compromised the nutritional status of the mother, the more beneficial improved diet and nutritional supplementation are for pregnancy outcome. Table 7-3 gives the most current dietary reference intakes (DRIs).

Under the auspices of the U.S. Department of Agriculture (USDA), pregnant females at risk for nutritional inadequacies are encouraged to enroll in the Special Supplemental Nutrition Program for Women, Infants, and Children (WIC). The WIC program, which was originally authorized in 1972, serves pregnant females, non–breast-feeding mothers until 6 months after birth, breast-feeding mothers until 1 year after birth, and infants and children up to age 5 years. To qualify for WIC services, participants must live in an area served by WIC, be at nutritional risk, and have an income that does not exceed 185% of the federal poverty guidelines. Criteria for "nutritional risk" vary by state but may include anemia, poor gestational weight gain, a diet record showing an inadequate diet, or failure to thrive of an infant or a child. WIC provides vouchers for foods high in vitamin A, vitamin C, iron, protein, and calcium, such as iron-fortified breakfast cereals, milk, eggs, peanut butter, and juice. WIC participants receive individual or group nutrition education and referrals to other health care resources. Many WIC clinics also offer prenatal and well-child health services. In addition, the WIC program is actively involved in breast-feeding promotion. Outcome studies have found than infants born to WIC participants have a higher mean birth weight and mean gestational age than infants born to women who were eligible for WIC but did not participate in the program. WIC participants also have a decreased prevalence of LBW and VLBW infants, and their toddlers and preschool-age children have a lower prevalence of iron deficiency anemia (Owen and Owen, 1997).

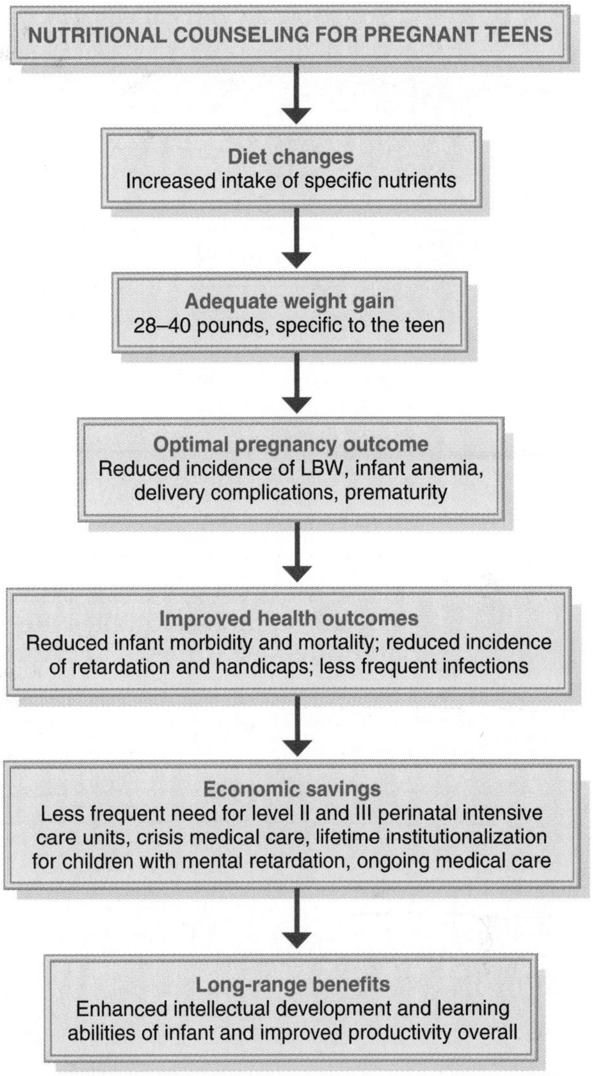

FIGURE 7-4 • Benefits of nutritional counseling for pregnant adolescents.

A balanced diet that results in appropriate weight gain during pregnancy generally supplies the required vitamins and minerals needed for pregnancy. The IOM did not find sufficient evidence to recommend routine use of most vitamins except for those with high-risk pregnancies (e.g., undernourished females, females with substance abuse problems, teenagers, females with a short interval between pregnancies, females with a history of delivering an LBW infant, females with multiple gestation) (IOM,

1990). However, supplementation with folate and iron is recommended for all pregnant females, and most physicians prescribe a prenatal vitamin and mineral supplement because of the uncertainty of the mother's nutritional status and intake (see Nutritional Requirements section).

Physiologic Changes During Pregnancy

Blood Volume and Composition

Physiologic and biochemical changes that occur during a normal pregnancy include a blood volume expansion of 50%, resulting in a decreased hemoglobin,

TABLE 7-2 Weight Gains of Mothers and Multiple-Birth Babies*

PLURALITY	LIVE-BORN INFANTS†	LBW (%)* (<2500 g)	VLBW (%)* (<1500 g)	MATERNAL WEIGHT BY 24 WK	WEIGHT GAIN TOTAL (lb)	WEEKS GESTATION	MEAN BIRTH WEIGHT (g)
Singletons	3,899,627	6	1	12	25-35	38-41	3700-4000
Twins	96,445	50	10	24	40-45	36-37	2500-2800
Triplets‡	4168	90	32	36	50-60	34-35	1900-2200

From Luke B: Managing maternal nutrition: prenatal and postpartum, *Perinat Nutr Rep* 3:2, 1997.
**LBW*, Low birth weight; *VLBW*, very low birth weight.
†Based on 1994 U.S. vital statistics.
‡Those pregnant with quadruplets should have gained at least 50 lb by 24 weeks.

TABLE 7-3 Dietary Reference Intakes: Recommended Dietary Allowances and Adequate Intakes for Women

	14-18 YR OF AGE	19-50 YR OF AGE	PREGNANT	LACTATING
Energy (kcal)	2368	2403	+0 1st trimester +340 2nd trimester +452 3rd trimester	+330 1st 6 mo +400 2nd 6 mo
Protein (g)	46	46	71	71
Vitamin A (μg RE)	700	700	770 (>18 yr) 750 (≤18 yr)	1300 (>18 yr) 1200 (≤18 yr)
Vitamin D (μg)* AI	5	5	5	5
Vitamin E (mg α-TE)	8	15	15	19
Vitamin K (μg)	55	90	90 (>18 yr) 75 (≤18 yr)	90 (>18 yr) 75 (≤18 yr)
Vitamin C (mg)	60	75	85 (>18 yr) 80 (≤18 yr)	120 (>18 yr) 115 (≤18 yr)
Thiamin (mg)	1	1.1	1.4	1.4
Riboflavin (mg)	1	1.1	1.4	1.6
Niacin (mg NE)	14	14	18	17
Vitamin B_6 (μg)	1.2	1.3	1.9	2
Folate (μg)†	400	400	600	500
Vitamin B_{12} (μg)	2.4	2.4	2.6	2.8
Biotin (μg)* AI	25	30	30	35
Pantothenic acid (mg)* AI	5	5	6	7
Choline (mg)* AI	400	425	450	550
Calcium (mg)* AI	1300	1000	1000 (>18 yr) 1300 (≤18 yr)	1000 (>18 yr) 1300 (≤18 yr)
Phosphorus (mg)	1250	700	700 (>18 yr) 1250 (≤18 yr)	700 (>18 yr) 1250 (≤18 yr)
Magnesium (mg)	360	310	350 (>18 yr) 400 (≤18 yr)	310 (>18 yr) 360 (≤18 yr)
Fluoride (mg)* AI	3	3	3	3
Iron (mg)	15	18	27	9 (>18 yr) 10 (≤18 yr)
Zinc (mg)	9	8	11 (>18 yr) 12 (≤18 yr)	12 (>18 yr) 13 (≤18 yr)
Iodine (μg)	150	150	220	290
Selenium (μg)	55	55	60	70

Modified from Institute of Medicine, Food and Nutrition Board, National Academy of Sciences: *Dietary reference intakes for energy, carbohydrate, fiber, fat, fatty acids, cholesterol, protein, and amino acids*, Washington, DC, 2002, National Academy Press; *Dietary reference intakes for calcium, phosphorus, magnesium, vitamin D, and fluoride*, Washington, DC, 1997, National Academy Press; *Dietary reference intakes for thiamin, riboflavin, niacin, vitamin B_6, folate, vitamin B_{12}, pantothenic acid, biotin and choline*, Washington, DC, 1998, National Academy Press; *Dietary reference intakes for vitamin C, vitamin E, selenium, and carotenoids*, Washington, DC, 2000, National Academy Press; *Dietary reference intakes for vitamin A, vitamin K, boron, chromium, copper, iodine, iron, manganese, molybdenum, nickel, silicon, vanadium, and zinc*, Washington, DC, 2001, National Academy Press.
tri., trimester; *RE*, retinol equivalents; *α-TE*, alpha-tocopherol; *NE*, niacin equivalents.
*Adequate Intake (AI).
†This is synthetic folic acid from fortified foods or supplements.

serum albumin, and other serum protein concentrations, and water-soluble vitamin concentration. The decline in serum albumin concentration may contribute to extracellular water accumulation, or *edema*. The decrease in water-soluble vitamin concentrations makes determination of an inadequate nutrient intake or a deficient nutritional status difficult. In contrast, serum concentrations of fat-soluble vitamins and other lipid fractions, such as triglycerides, cholesterol, and free fatty acids, increase.

Cardiovascular and Pulmonary Function

Cardiac output increases during pregnancy, and the cardiac size increases by 12%. Diastolic blood pressure decreases during the first two trimesters because of peripheral vasodilation but returns to prepregnancy levels in the third trimester.

Mild lower extremity edema is a normal condition of pregnancy resulting from the pressure of the expanding uterus on the inferior vena cava. The blood return to the heart decreases, leading to decreased cardiac output, a decrease in blood pressure, and lower extremity edema. Mild physiologic lower extremity edema is associated with slightly larger babies and a lower rate of prematurity (Worthington-Roberts and Williams, 1993).

Maternal oxygen requirements increase as the threshold for carbon dioxide decreases, making the mother feel dyspneic—a feeling that increases as the growing uterus pushes the diaphragm upward. The body compensates through more efficient pulmonary gas exchange.

Gastrointestinal Function

During pregnancy the gastrointestinal system changes in several ways that affect nutritional status. In the first trimester the mother may experience nausea and vomiting, which may be followed by a return of a possibly ravenous appetite (see Nausea and Vomiting section). Cravings for and aversions to foods may be accompanied by a decreased ability to taste saltiness. Increased progesterone concentrations relax the uterine muscle to allow for fetal growth, but they also decrease gastrointestinal motility and increase reabsorption of water, often resulting in constipation. In addition, relaxation of the lower esophageal sphincter and pressure on the stomach from the growing uterus can cause regurgitation and gastric reflux (see Heartburn section).

Renal Function

The glomerular filtration rate (GFR) increases by 50% during pregnancy, although the volume of urine excreted each day does not increase. The blood volume increases because of the increased glomerular filtration rate with lower serum creatinine and blood urea nitrogen (BUN) concentrations. Renal tubular reabsorption is less efficient than it was before pregnancy, and glucosuria may develop in addition to increased excretion of water-soluble vitamins.

Placenta

Not only is the placenta the principal site for production of several hormones responsible for regulating fetal growth and development of maternal support tissues, it is also the conduit for the exchange of nutrients, oxygen, and waste products. Placental insult compromises the ability to nourish the fetus, regardless of how well nourished the mother is or how optimal her dietary intake. Placental size and cell number can be 15% to 20% below normal in infants with IUGR. A small placenta has a smaller surface area of placental villi, which are responsible for the transfer of nutrients to the fetus.

Nutritional Requirements

Fetal growth and pregnancy demand additional nutrients, and these requirements are defined in the new DRIs, which include adequate intakes (AIs) and recommended dietary allowances (RDAs) (see Table 7-3).

Energy

Additional energy is required during pregnancy to support the metabolic demands of pregnancy and fetal growth. Metabolism increases by 15% during pregnancy. The 2002 DRIs for energy for pregnant females in the first trimester are the same as for females who are not pregnant, but they increase about an additional 340 to 360 kcal/day during the second trimester and another 112 kcal/day in the third trimester (IOM, 2002). However, if the maternal weight gain is within the desirable limits, the range of acceptable energy intakes is wide because of individual differences in energy output and basal metabolic rate.

Exercise

Energy expended in voluntary physical activity is the largest variable in overall energy expenditure. Physical activity increases energy expenditure in proportion to a person's body weight. However most pregnant females compensate for their increased weight gain by slowing their activity pace, so their total daily energy expenditure may not be substantially greater than it was before the pregnancy (see *Focus On:* Exercise During Pregnancy).

Excessive exercise combined with inadequate energy intake may lead to a suboptimal maternal weight gain and poor fetal growth. Therefore a pregnant female should always discuss exercise with her primary health practitioner. Nutrition counseling may also be necessary to create an adequate meal plan that promotes weight gain.

FOCUS ON

Exercise During Pregnancy

Exercise programs have become increasingly popular with heightened concerns about weight control, particularly during the reproductive years, when some females have a tendency to gain weight. Health care providers need sound scientific information on the benefits and risks of exercise during pregnancy to provide appropriate advice to such mothers.

Research shows that continuing a regular exercise regimen throughout pregnancy reduces subcutaneous fat deposition during midpregnancy and subcutaneous fat retention during late pregnancy. The rate of weight gain decreases after the fifteenth week, and the overall weight gain is lower but remains well within the normal range (Clapp and Little, 1995). Additional outcome data confirm that the incidence of obstetric complications in females who continue a regular exercise regimen throughout pregnancy is either the same as or lower than those who do not (Clapp, 1993; Dewey and McCrory, 1994).

The potential benefits of prenatal exercise include improved fitness, prevention of gestational diabetes, facilitation of labor, and reduced stress. A healthy fetus is generally able to compensate for periods of transitory stress that occur during maternal exercise. However, pregnant females should follow particular guidelines to avoid extreme stress for either themselves or their fetuses. Guidelines for exercise during pregnancy have been developed by the American College of Obstetricians and Gynecologists (ACOG, 2002).

A woman who is just beginning an exercise program during pregnancy should exercise at a level that keeps her heart rate below 140 bpm. A good fitness program would be 1 hour of physical activity 3 days per week, with an intensity that keeps the maternal heart rate between 120 and 130 bpm (Revelli et al, 1992). The types of exercise that provide the best cardiovascular and psychological benefits with the least pregnancy risks are walking, jogging, stationary cycling, and swimming.

Consequences of Energy Restriction

A once popular concept was that the fetus develops at the expense of the mother during periods of nutritional deprivation. However, evidence from famines in Holland and Germany during World War II clearly contradicts this assumption. It is now accepted that an inadequately nourished mother is proportionately less affected than her fetus.

One consequence of severe energy restriction is increased ketone production. Although the fetus has a limited ability to metabolize ketone bodies, the short- and long-term effects of maternal ketonemia are unclear. Animal and human data indicate that ketone bodies are normally transferred to the fetal brain at various times during pregnancy. After an overnight fast, maternal blood ketone body concentrations are greater in pregnant females than in those who are not pregnant, and ketonuria may even develop. However, extreme ketonemia may be an indicator of maternal energy deficiency, with the mother and the fetus competing for nutrients and with an increased metabolic risk for the fetus.

Protein

Pregnant females have additional protein requirements to support the synthesis of maternal and fetal tissues, but the magnitude of this requirement is uncertain. Protein use in pregnant females is about 70%, the same as those of the fetus. Protein requirements increase throughout gestation and peak during the third trimester. The current RDA of 71 g of protein for pregnant females is 25 g more than the RDA for females who are not pregnant. It is based on 1.1 g/kg/day using the prepregnant weight. (IOM, 2002).

Protein deficiency during pregnancy has adverse consequences, but because limited intakes of protein and energy are usually simultaneous, it is difficult to distinguish between the effects of energy deficiency and those of protein deficiency. Providing extra energy to a pregnant female influences pregnancy outcome in the same way that providing energy *and* protein influences outcome (Zlatnick and Burmeister, 1983). Thus it seems that an energy deficit rather than a protein deficit is the factor that can result in an unfavorable pregnancy outcome.

Carbohydrates

For the first time, the Institute of Medicine has established DRIs for carbohydrate intake during pregnancy. The estimated average requirement (EAR) is 135 g/day, and the adequate intake (AI) is 175 g/day (IOM, 2002). (EAR and AI are defined in Chapter 15.) The recommended amount of 135 to 175 g/day is the quantity needed to provide enough calories in the diet, prevent ketosis, and maintain appropriate blood glucose levels during pregnancy.

Fiber

Daily consumption of whole-grain breads and cereals, leafy green and yellow vegetables, and fresh and dried fruits should be encouraged to provide additional minerals, vitamins, and fiber. The DRI for fiber during pregnancy is 28 g/day (IOM, 2002). Pregnant females should select foods that are good sources of iron and folic acid (see Chapters 4, 5, and 34).

Lipids

No DRIs for total lipids during pregnancy have been established. The amount of fat in the diet should depend on energy requirements for proper weight gain. However, for the first time the IOM recommends an AI of 13 g/day for the amount of *n*-6 polyunsaturated fatty acids (linoleic acid) and an AI of 1.4 g/day for the amount of *n*-3 polyunsaturated fatty acids (α-linolenic acid) in the diet (IOM, 2002).

Vitamins

Certain vitamins have particular significance in an optimal pregnancy outcome. In some instances the need for these specific vitamins may be met through diet, and some are met through supplements. Periconceptional multivitamin supplementation has been documented to reduce the risk of heart defects in infants by 43%; this decreased risk did not result when multivitamin supplementation began in the second month of pregnancy or later (Bolto et al, 1996).

Folic Acid

Folic acid requirements increase during pregnancy in response to the demands for maternal erythropoiesis, for fetal and placental growth, and most important for the prevention of NTDs. The RDA for folic acid during pregnancy (established in 1998) is 600 μg, 200 μg higher than the RDA for females who are not pregnant. The IOM recommends that 400 μg of the 600 μg/day be provided by folate-fortified foods or supplements and 200 μg be from food and beverages (IOM, 1998). The tolerable upper intake level (UL) is 800 to 1000 μg/day from fortified foods or supplements (IOM, 1998).

Folic acid deficiency is marked by a reduced rate of deoxyribonucleic acid (DNA) synthesis and mitotic activity in individual cells. Megaloblastic anemia is the most advanced stage of folate deficiency, and its symptoms may not develop until the third trimester; however, white cell morphologic and biochemical changes signaling deficiency may precede overt anemia (see Chapter 34).

In experimental animals, maternal folate deficiency is associated with an increased incidence of congenital malformations. Malformations can also develop in fetuses of mothers using folate-antagonist drugs, such as the anticonvulsant medications dilantin, phenatoin, carbamazepine, and diphenylhydantoin. Oral contraceptives and some antibiotics (e.g., trimethoprim, triamterene, and carbamazepine) may also cause folate insufficiency (see Chapter 19).

Limited evidence from humans also suggests that folate deficiency may be associated with spontaneous abortion and obstetric complications such as preterm labor and LBW. In one study, pregnant females with folate intakes of 240 μg/day or less were found to have twice the risk of having an LBW or a premature infant compared with females with intakes greater than 240 μg/day (Scholl et al, 1996).

Folic acid's greatest significance during pregnancy is its role in preventing NTDs, which are among the most common birth defects (Fleming, 2001). Approximately 2500 infants with NTDs are born in the United States each year. Moreover, mothers who give birth to infants with an NTD have a 2% to 10% chance of having another infant with an NTD.

Two randomized trials in Europe have strengthened the association between periconceptional folic acid supplementation and the prevention of NTDs. In the Medical Research Council (MRC) Vitamin Study, 1817 mothers who had previously given birth to an infant with an NTD were either given a folic acid supplement, a multivitamin supplement, folic acid and multivitamin supplements, or a placebo. The group who received the folic acid supplement had a 72% lower risk of having another infant with an NTD. So striking were the results that the trial was halted early (MRC, 1991). The second study of 5520 European women demonstrated that periconceptional supplementation with a multivitamin containing 800 μg of folic acid reduced the incidence of NTDs (Czeizel et al, 1994). In these studies, folic acid supplementation was associated not only with a significant reduction in birth defects but also with an increased incidence of recognized spontaneous abortions or *terathanasia,* the selective promotion of spontaneous abortion of a defective fetus (Hook and Czeizel, 1997). However, another study involving approximately 24,000 females reported no association between folic acid supplementation and spontaneous abortion (Gindler et al, 2001).

Red blood cell (RBC) folate concentrations exceeding 906 mmol/L (400 ng/ml) are associated with the fewest NTDs. In a study of 189 healthy females attempting to become pregnant, only one in four had RBC folate levels greater than 906 mmol/L. Females who only consumed food sources of folate had the lowest folate intake and the lowest RBC folate concentrations. Only those who consumed folic acid supplements in addition to dietary folate had RBC folate concentrations considered optimal for protection against NTDs (Brown et al, 1997).

The Centers for Disease Control and Prevention (CDC) have recommended that all females of childbearing age increase their intake of folic acid (CDC, 1992) because 50% of all pregnancies in the United States are unplanned, and the neural tube closes by 28 days of gestation (before most mothers realize they are pregnant). Therefore supplementation with folic acid should begin before conception, hence the CDC's recommendation. The Food and Drug Administration (FDA) has mandated that grain products such as bread, rice, and pasta be enriched with folic acid (see Chapter 13). All females of childbearing age should be encouraged to take a folic acid supplement and include generous amounts of folic acid food sources in their diets (see Chapters 4 and 34).

Females who smoke, have moderate to heavy alcohol consumption (more than one serving of alcohol per day), or use recreational drugs are at risk for marginal folate levels. In addition, females taking oral contraceptives or antiseizure medications, and those with malabsorption syndromes, may have low serum or RBC folate concentrations. Females taking antiseizure medications must be closely monitored when they begin taking folic acid because folic acid supplementation can reduce the seizure threshold.

Despite a CDC-supported nationwide folate and pregnancy educational program, a 1997 Gallup survey sponsored by the March of Dimes demonstrated that only 6% of the respondents—women 18 to 45 years of age—knew that folic acid should be taken before pregnancy (Johnston and Staples, 1997).

Vitamin B_6

The 1998 RDA for vitamin B_6 during pregnancy is 1.9 mg/day—0.6 mg more than the amount recommended for women who are not pregnant. The extra vitamin helps the pregnant female synthesize the nonessential amino acids needed for growth and synthesize vitamin B_6–dependent niacin from tryptophan. The UL for vitamin B_6 is 80 to 100 mg/day (IOM, 1998).

Vitamin B_6 has also been used to manage severe nausea and vomiting during pregnancy. Although it catalyzes numerous reactions involving neurotransmitter production, it is not known whether these reactions are involved in the relief of symptoms. Megadoses of vitamin B_6 (i.e., 25 mg three times per day) are necessary to achieve antiemetic effects; therefore its administration for nausea and vomiting should be closely monitored (Jewel and Young, 2002; Sahakian et al, 1991).

Ascorbic Acid

An additional 10 mg/day of vitamin C is recommended for pregnant females. The total recommendation of 80 to 85 mg/day is easily met by the typical American diet (IOM, 2000).

Although ascorbic acid deficiency has not been associated with adverse pregnancy outcome in large population studies, a few studies have suggested an association between low plasma levels of vitamin C and preeclampsia, as well as premature rupture of the membranes (Casanueva et al, 1995; Woods, 2001).

Vitamin A

The RDA for vitamin A is 750 μg retinol equivalents (RE), or 2800 IU, for pregnant females 18 and under and 770 μg retinol equivalents [RE] (3000 IU) for women over the age of 18. Maternal stores of vitamin A easily meet the fetal accretion rate. Vitamin A deficiency is teratogenic in experimental animals, but confirmatory evidence of its teratogenicity in humans is lacking.

In contrast to earlier reports that 10,000 IU or more of vitamin A increased the risk for neural crest defects, a National Institutes of Health (NIH) alert announced that moderate doses of vitamin A (i.e., 8,000 to 10,000 IU) do not increase the risk of birth defects (Mills et al, 1997; National Institute for Child Health and Human Development [NICHD], 1997). However, the alert continues to discourage large doses of vitamin A. A review of retinoids in embryonal development presents a summary of the studies where supplementation with vitamin A during pregnancy had both positive and detrimental effects (Ross et al, 2000). Females who are taking the vitamin A analogue Accutane for acne and become pregnant are at extremely high risk for fetal anomalies.

Vitamin D

The AI for vitamin D is 5 μg (200 IU) per day for pregnant and non-pregnant women. The DRIs also suggest a UL of 5 μg/day during pregnancy (IOM, 1997).

Vitamin D has long been appreciated for its positive effects on calcium balance during pregnancy. This vitamin and its metabolites cross the placenta and have fetal blood concentrations that are the same as those in the maternal circulation.

Maternal vitamin D deficiency is associated with neonatal hypocalcemia and hypoplasia of tooth enamel. Fetal bone mineralization may be affected by maternal vitamin D deficiency (Namgung et al, 1998). Vitamin D blood concentrations are often low in infants born to mothers with vitamin D deficiency, and vitamin D deficiency is increasingly being recognized in dark-skinned women and in those who wear veils and cover their bodies with clothing for religious reasons (Pugliese et al, 1998). However, excessive amounts of vitamin D may also be harmful during gestation. Severe infantile hypercalcemia was reported in a newborn born to a mother who ingested excessive amounts of vitamin D (Forbes, 1979).

Vitamin E

Vitamin E requirements increase during pregnancy, but vitamin E deficiency in humans is rare and has not been linked to reduced fertility or fetal malformations as it has in animals. However, the 2000 RDA of 15 mg of α-tocopherol for women who are not pregnant is the same as the RDA for those who are pregnant (IOM, 2000). The UL is 800 mg/day for pregnant females 18 years of age or younger and 1000 mg/day for pregnant women 19 to 50 years old (IOM, 2000).

Vitamin K

The RDA for vitamin K during pregnancy is 90 mg/day for women over age 18 and 75 mg/day for females 18 years of age and younger (IOM, 2001). The typical diet provides an adequate amount of vitamin

K; no ULs for vitamin K during pregnancy have been defined. Given the recent association of vitamin K and bone health, adequate intakes of vitamin K during pregnancy are further supported (Zittermann, 2001).

Minerals

Calcium

Hormonal factors strongly influence calcium metabolism in pregnant females. Human chorionic somatomammotropin from the placenta increases the rate of maternal bone turnover. Estrogen is also largely derived from the placenta and inhibits bone resorption, provoking a compensatory release of parathyroid hormone, which maintains the maternal serum calcium concentration while enhancing maternal absorption of calcium across the gut. The net effect of these changes, which occur before fetal skeletal mineralization, is the promotion of progressive calcium retention to meet progressively increasing fetal skeletal demands for mineralization. Fetal hypercalcemia and subsequent endocrine adjustments ultimately stimulate the mineralization process.

Approximately 30 g of calcium accumulates during pregnancy, most of which (25 g) is in the fetal skeleton. The remainder is stored in the maternal skeleton, presumably as a reserve for the calcium needed during lactation. Most fetal accretion occurs during the last trimester of pregnancy at an average of 300 mg/day.

The latest AI for calcium during pregnancy is 1300 mg/day for females 18 years of age or younger and 1000 mg/day for women 19 years of age and older. This recommendation is the same as that for females who are not pregnant because the hormonal changes of pregnancy increase the absorption and use of calcium. Daily intakes of less than the AI may increase calcium loss from the maternal skeleton. Multiparous women with an inadequate calcium intake can develop osteomalacia. The UL for calcium during pregnancy is 2500 mg/day.

Phosphorus

The RDA for phosphorus is the same for females who are pregnant and those who are not: 1250 mg/day for females younger than 19 years of age and 700 mg/day for those 19 years of age and older. Phosphorus is found in such a wide variety of foods that deficiency is rare. The UL during pregnancy is 3500 mg/day.

Iron

The marked increase in the maternal blood supply during pregnancy greatly increases the demand for iron. The normal erythrocyte volume increases by 20% to 30% during pregnancy. A pregnant female must consume an additional 700 to 800 mg of iron throughout her pregnancy—500 mg for hematopoiesis and 250 to 300 mg for fetal and placental tissues. Most accretion occurs after the twentieth week of gestation, when maternal and fetal demands are greatest. Iron requirements increase; therefore the 2001 RDA for iron during pregnancy is 27 mg/day, 9 mg/day more than the RDA for women who are not pregnant and 12 mg/day more than the RDA for adolescents who are not pregnant. The UL is 45 mg/day (IOM, 2001).

Rarely do females become pregnant with sufficient iron stores to meet the physiologic needs of pregnancy. Therefore iron supplementation, usually in the form of ferrous salts, is often necessary to prevent iron deficiency anemia.

Maternal anemia, defined by a hematocrit of less than 32% and a hemoglobin level of less than 11 g/dl, develops in some pregnant females who do not use iron supplements or are anemic when they become pregnant. A female with anemia poorly tolerates hemorrhage during childbirth and is more prone to develop puerperal infection. The fetal effects of maternal anemia are poorly understood. Some data suggest that fetal effects are relatively mild, but several reports suggest that pregnancy outcome may be compromised. It could be hypothesized that inadequate iron consumption leads to poor hemoglobin production and resulting compromised oxygen delivery to the uterus, placenta, and developing fetus. The added workload of the heart, with its increased cardiac output, could compromise the pregnancy.

It is recommended that all pregnant females who are consuming a well-balanced diet should take 30 mg in divided doses of ferrous iron supplements daily during the second and third trimesters (IOM, 1990). In addition, for optimal absorption, the iron supplement should ideally be taken between meals and not with milk, tea, or coffee because they interfere with absorption. Beverages containing ascorbic acid enhance absorption. For females with iron deficiency anemia, therapy consists of 60 to 120 mg of ferrous iron in divided doses throughout the day. Iron supplements greater than 56 mg per dose interfere with zinc absorption and should be avoided (Fairweather-Tait, 1995). When the hemoglobin returns to a level appropriate for the mother's stage of pregnancy, 30 mg/day in divided doses may be resumed (IOM, 1990) (see Chapter 34).

Zinc

The 2001 RDA for zinc is 11 mg (for those age 19 and older) and 12 mg (for those age 18 and younger) during pregnancy (IOM, 2001). The average zinc intake of pregnant females is 11.1 mg/day (Murtaugh and Weingart, 1995). Pregnant women with a zinc-deficient diet cannot effectively mobilize the zinc stored in the skeleton; therefore a compromised zinc status rapidly develops.

Animal studies of zinc status during gestation have shown that zinc deficiency is highly teratogenic in rats and leads to the development of various congenital malformations. Nonhuman primates are also affected by zinc deficiency, which results in abnormal fetal brain development and abnormal newborn behavior.

Zinc supplementation for females with low prepregnancy weights and low plasma zinc concentrations resulted in an increase in infant birth weight (Goldenberg et al, 1995). However, in another study infants at 13 months of age whose mothers received 30 mg of zinc during pregnancy scored lower on measures of development than the group of infants whose mothers received a placebo (Hamadani et al, 2002). Until further research resolves the concern of zinc and delayed development, zinc supplementation should bring the mother's intake only up to the level of the RDA.

Maternal zinc status may be inversely related to the degree of prenatal iron supplementation because excess iron ingestion inhibits zinc absorption (IOM, 1990). The UL for zinc intake during pregnancy is 34 mg/day for pregnant teenagers and 40 mg/day for pregnant women 19 to 50 years of age.

Copper

Diets of pregnant females often have marginal copper contents; however, it has not been determined whether moderate dietary copper intake deficiency affects the developing human fetus. Copper deficiency is teratogenic in animals. The RDA for copper during pregnancy is 1000 μg/day, 100 μg/day more than for females who are not pregnant (IOM, 2001). Excessive iron supplementation inhibits copper absorption. The UL for copper is 8000 μg/day for females 18 years of age and younger and 10,000 μg/day for 19- to 50-year-old pregnant women, the same as for those who are not pregnant.

Sodium

The hormonal milieu of pregnancy affects sodium metabolism. The increased maternal blood volume leads to an increased glomerular sodium filtration rate of 5,000 to 10,000 mEq/day. Compensatory mechanisms maintain fluid and electrolyte balance.

Restricting the dietary sodium of or prescribing diuretics for pregnant females with edema is not recommended. Rigorous sodium restriction in pregnant animals stresses the renin-angiotensin-aldosterone system and results in water intoxication and renal and adrenal tissue necrosis. Neonatal hyponatremia (a low blood sodium concentration) can result when pregnant females severely restrict their sodium intake before delivery.

Although moderation in the consumption of salt and sodium-rich foods is appropriate for everyone, aggressive restriction is usually unwarranted during pregnancy, and consumption of sodium should remain higher than 2 to 3 g/day.

Magnesium

The RDA of 360 to 400 mg of magnesium during pregnancy is 40 to 90 mg more than the RDA for females who are not pregnant. A term fetus accumulates 1 g of magnesium during gestation. The IOM reports that magnesium supplementation during pregnancy reduces the incidence of preeclampsia and IUGR. However, the IOM has also set a UL for magnesium from supplements or pharmacologic agents (i.e., from substances other than food and beverages) during pregnancy of 350 mg/day (IOM, 1997) (see also Edema and Leg Cramps section).

Fluoride

The role of fluoride in prenatal development is controversial. Development of primary dentition begins at 10 to 12 weeks of gestation; from the sixth to the ninth month, the first four permanent molars and eight of the permanent incisors form. Thus 32 teeth develop during gestation. Controversy involves the extent to which fluoride is transported across the placenta and its value in utero in the development of caries-resistant permanent teeth (see Chapter 28). The AI for fluoride during pregnancy is 3 mg/day, and the UL is 10 mg/day (IOM, 1997).

Iodine

An additional 70 μg of iodine for pregnant females has been added to the RDA of 150 μg for females who are not pregnant—making the RDA for iodine during pregnancy 220 μg/day. This amount should be adequate to provide for fetal iodine demands. The UL in pregnancy is 900 to 1100 μg/day (IOM, 2001).

Maternal iodine deficiency has long been recognized as a cause of neonatal cretinism. A suboptimal iodine intake by pregnant females without an overt deficiency may compromise fetal development, even in the absence of cretinism, leading to developmental delays in the infant (Glinoer, 2003). Previous studies established that preconception iodine supplementation prevents endemic cretinism, but recent findings indicate that supplementation before the end of the second trimester for pregnant females who may not have taken preconception iodine supplements can also protect the fetal brain from the effects of iodine deficiency (Xue-Yi et al, 1994) (see Chapter 5).

Guide for Eating During Pregnancy

Recommended Food Intake

The increased food requirements during pregnancy can be met by following the Daily Food Guide presented in Table 7-4.

Calcium

Three 1-cup servings of milk or the equivalent per day provide 24 g protein, close to the additional requirement for protein in pregnancy of 25 g/day; it also provides 900 mg of calcium. An additional 270 kcal (from skim milk) or 480 kcal (from whole milk) are also provided. Numerous milk choices are avail-

TABLE 7-4 Daily Food Guide for Females

FOOD GROUP	MINIMUM NUMBER OF SERVINGS: NONPREGNANT 11- TO 24-YEAR-OLDS	NONPREGNANT 25- TO 50-YEAR-OLDS	PREGNANT OR LACTATING 11- TO 50-YEAR-OLDS
Protein, foods	5*	5*	7†
Milk products	3	2	3
Breads, grains	7	6	7
Whole-grain	4	4	4
Enriched	3	2	3
Fruits, vegetables	5	5	5
Vitamin C rich	1	1	1
β carotene rich	1	1	1
Folate rich	1	1	1
Other	2	2	2
Unsaturated fats	3	3	3

Modified from *Nutrition during pregnancy and the postpartum period: a manual for health care professionals,* 1990, California Department of Health Services, Maternal Child Health Branch.
*Equivalent in protein to 5 oz of animal protein; at least three servings per week should be from the vegetable proteins.
†Equivalent in protein to 7 oz of animal protein; at least one of these servings should be a vegetable protein.

able, such as whole milk, low-fat milk, skim milk, nonfat powdered milk, buttermilk, acidophilus milk, Lactaid-treated milk, evaporated milk, enriched soy milk, and yogurt. Milk products can be consumed plain or in soups, custards, puddings, ice cream, or flavored beverages. Nonfat milk powder can be added to meat loaf, soups, scrambled eggs, mashed and scalloped potatoes, sandwich spreads, cooked cereals, homemade breads, cookies, or pastries. Approximately ⅓ cup of dried skim milk equals 1 cup of fluid milk. Fluid milk can be made richer in calcium, protein, and calories by the addition of 2 tbsp of dried nonfat milk per glass of fluid milk. Three cups of cow or soy milk fortified with vitamin D provide 7.5 μg of cholecalciferol (300 IU). If fluid milk is used in limited amounts, a vitamin D supplement may be desirable, especially if exposure to sunlight is limited.

Many females, primarily those who are not white, are unable to digest the lactose in milk (see Chapter 30) unless it is consumed in small amounts. Commercial enzyme preparations such as Lactaid can be added to fluid milk to improve lactose digestion. Cheese or yogurt, which contain only small amounts of lactose, or calcium-enriched soy milk (which is lactose free) can be substituted. If necessary, clinicians can prescribe preparations such as calcium lactate or calcium carbonate (see Chapter 30).

Fluids

Drinking six to eight glasses of fluid daily is encouraged. Intestinal stasis often occurs as a result of limited activity and the pressure of the enlarging uterus. However, the high fiber suggested diet in addition to the suggested fluid intake tends to counteract constipation in most females. Regardless, a fiber supplement may be needed by some.

Pregnant females are usually very receptive to well-presented nutritional advice. A full discussion of individual needs and involvement of the mother (and perhaps her partner or other siblings) in planning dietary changes is usually an effective strategy (Figure 7-5). See Box 7-2 for a suggested menu and Box 7-3 for a summary of nutritional care for pregnant females.

Alcohol

Abundant evidence from animal studies and human experience associates heavy (more than 1 drink per day) alcohol consumption by a pregnant female with teratogenicity and a specific pattern of abnormalities in the neonate. The resulting condition is known as the fetal alcohol syndrome (Streissguth et al, 1980). Features of this syndrome include prenatal and postnatal growth failure, developmental delays, microcephaly, eye changes (including involvement of the epicanthal fold), facial abnormalities, and skeletal joint abnormalities (Figure 7-6). When a limited number of these features is present, the infant is said to have *fetal alcohol effects.* Use of alcohol during pregnancy has been associated with an increased rate of spontaneous abortion, abruptio placentae, and LBW infants.

The mechanisms by which alcohol affects the fetus are not completely understood. Alcohol may be toxic during blastogenesis and cell differentiation (Figure 7-7), or fetal damage could be the result of dietary deficiencies or altered metabolism of key nutrients, such as vitamin A, vitamin C, or folate (Cogswell et al, 2003).

The data on the impact of binge drinking on pregnancy outcome are limited, so the question of what amount of alcohol is safe during pregnancy remains unanswered. A 1995 survey of American pregnant or childbearing-age females indicated that they consume more alcohol than females in past generations (Zuger, 1997). Because current data are insufficient to recommend any safe level of alcohol consumption during

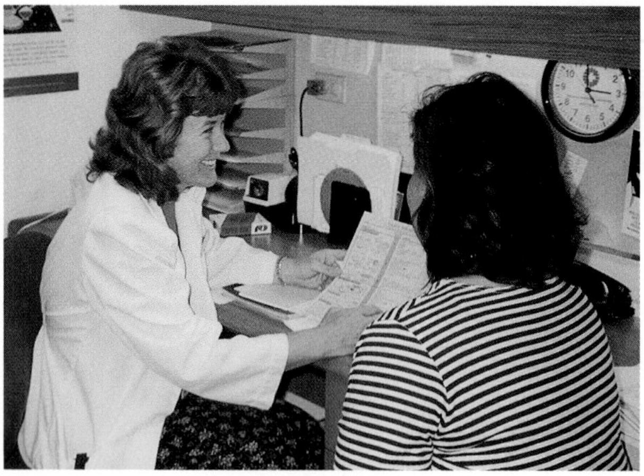

FIGURE 7-5 • Nutritionist with client. A prospective mother learns about nutrition during pregnancy.

Box 7-2. Suggested Menu During Pregnancy*

Breakfast

Orange juice, ½ cup
Oatmeal, ½ cup
Whole-grain or enriched toast, 1 slice
Peanut butter, 2 tsp
Decaffeinated coffee or tea

Midmorning Snack

Apple
High-bran cereal, ¼ cup
Nonfat or reduced-fat milk, ½ cup

Lunch

Turkey (2 oz) sandwich on rye or whole-grain bread with lettuce and tomato and 1 tsp mayonnaise
Green salad
Salad dressing, 2 tsp
Fresh peach
Nonfat or low-fat milk, 1 cup

Midafternoon Snack

Nonfat or low-fat milk, 1 cup
Graham crackers, 4 squares

Dinner

Baked chicken breast, 3 oz
Baked potato with 2 tbsp sour cream
Peas and carrots, ½ cup
Green salad
Salad dressing, 2 tsp

Evening Snack

Nonfat, yogurt, ½ cup
Fresh strawberries

*Quantities of food should be adjusted to meet individual energy needs to promote appropriate weight gain. Pregnant adolescents and very active or underweight pregnant women require greater quantities.

pregnancy, health care providers should promote abstinence from alcohol among females who are pregnant or planning a pregnancy (Eustace et al, 2003).

Some evidence shows that the course and outcome of pregnancy can be significantly improved if females with a drinking problem abstain from alcohol or decrease their consumption even after conception or the first few weeks of pregnancy (Rosett et al, 1983). However, those who do reduce or eliminate alcohol consumption are usually those who drink moderately, not heavily (Streissguth et al, 1983).

Nonnutritive Substances in Foods

Caffeine

The effect of caffeine on pregnancy has been extensively researched. Caffeine intake seems to increase the risk of first trimester spontaneous abortions, and the risk increases as consumption increases from 100 mg/day to more than 500 mg/day (Cnattingius et al, 2000). Caffeine may not contribute to IUGR or other major complications after the first trimester; however, it seems sensible to limit caffeine intake during pregnancy, although insufficient data exist to make a specific recommendation (Grosso et al, 2001; Nehlig and Debry, 1994).

Artificial Sweeteners

Four types of artificial sweeteners are sold in the United States; their chemical names are *saccharin* (Sweet 'n' Low), *acesulfame-K* (Sunette and Sweet One), *sucralose* (Splenda), and *aspartame* (Equal or Nutrasweet).

Saccharin is not classified as a teratogen; however, in very high doses, it is weakly carcinogenic in rats.

Box 7-3. Summary of Nutritional Care During Pregnancy

1. Energy intake to meet nutritional needs and allow for about a 0.4-kg (14-oz) weight gain per week during the last 30 weeks of pregnancy
2. Protein intake to meet nutritional needs (about an additional 25 g/day)
3. Sodium intake that is not be excessive but is no less than 2 g/day
4. Mineral and vitamin intakes to meet the RDA (For folic acid, this requires supplementation, and for iron, it is also likely that it is required.)
5. Alcohol omitted
6. Caffeine in moderation: less than 200 mg/day—equivalent of 2 cups of coffee

Its consumption in pregnancy has not been restricted. Acesulfame-K consumption by pregnant females is classified as safe; however, few or no long-term studies have been done on its consumption during human pregnancy. Saccharin and acesulfame-K cross the placenta and appear in breast milk but have no known adverse effect on the fetus or infant.

Sucralose was approved for general use in all foods by the FDA in 1998. It is a carbohydrate derived from sucrose but is 600 times sweeter. Approximately 93% to 97% of radiolabeled sucralose is eliminated unchanged through the urine and feces within 5 days of ingestion. Approximately 3% is eliminated as glucuronide conjugates of sucralose (Roberts et al, 2000). Sucralose has not been found to be mutagenic or teratogenic in high doses in animals. No studies of sucralose in breast milk or during lactation have been reported.

The use of aspartame is unsafe for females with phenylketonuria (PKU), regardless of whether they are pregnant. Aspartame is metabolized to phenylalanine and aspartic acid. In people without PKU, phenylalanine is rapidly broken down into a relatively harmless substance; those with PKU lack the enzyme necessary for its conversion. Individuals with PKU can develop brain damage from high blood phenylalanine concentrations. High circulating concentrations of phenylalanine are known to damage the fetal brain (see Chapter 45).

Because pregnant females may drink artificially sweetened soft drinks as substitutes for water or more nutritional beverages such as milk or juice, artificially sweetened beverage use during pregnancy should be discouraged.

Contaminants

Contaminants found in food may adversely affect pregnancy outcomes. Most heavy metals are embryotoxic; mercury, lead, cadmium, and potentially nickel and selenium are possibilities. Pregnant females

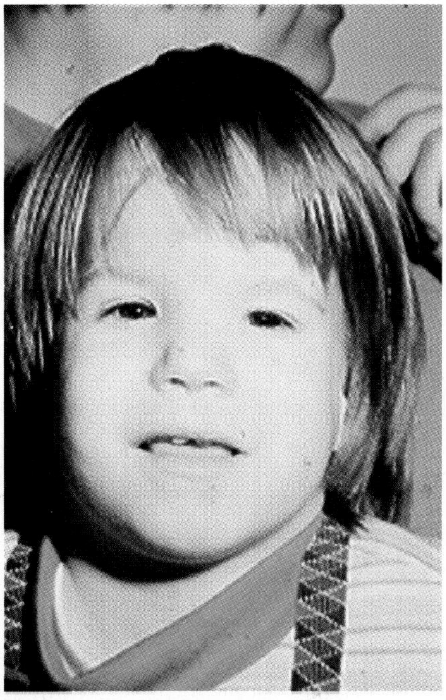

FIGURE 7-6 • One-year-old child with fetal alcohol syndrome. (From Streissguth AP et al: Teratogenic effects of alcohol in humans and laboratory animals, *Science* 209:353, 1980.)

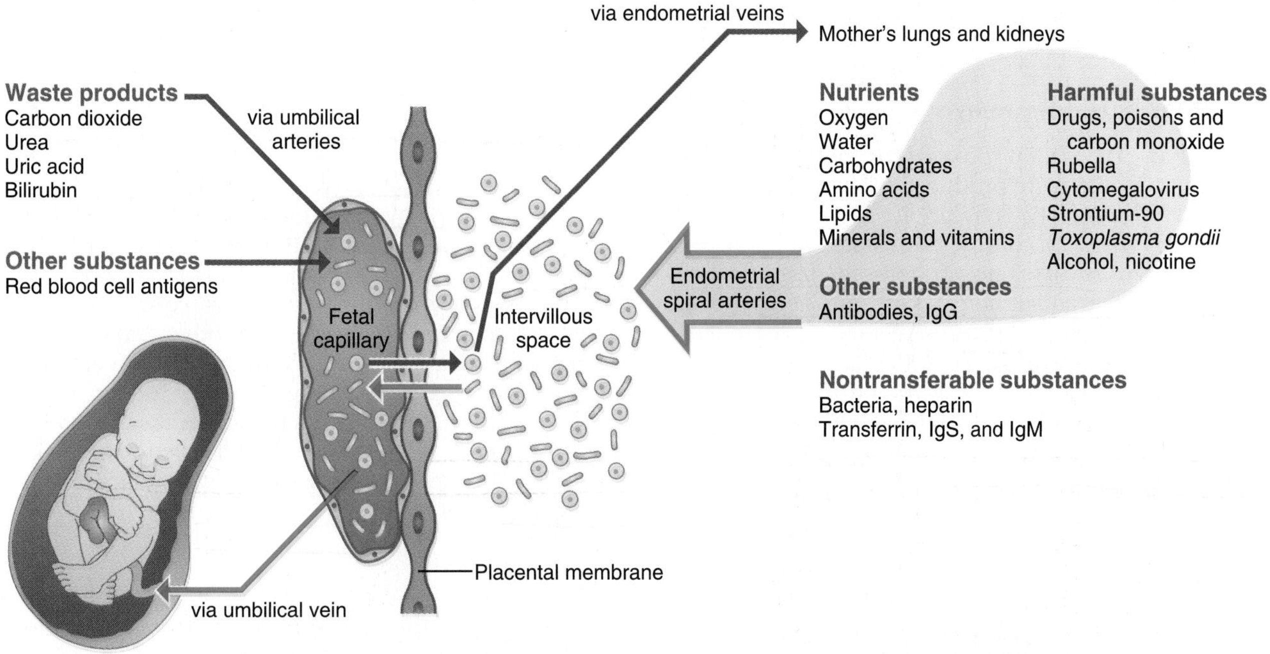

FIGURE 7-7 • Transfer of substances across the placental membrane. (*Ig*, Immunoglobulin.)

should be advised not to use dolomite as a calcium supplement because it often contains lead.

Methyl Mercury

In January 2001 the USDA and FDA issued a warning that pregnant and lactating females and females of childbearing age should limit their consumption of shark, mackerel, tilefish, and swordfish to no more than once a month. Traces of methyl mercury are found in most fish, but concentrations may be higher in areas with industrial mercury pollution. The usual concentration of methyl mercury in most fish ranges from less than 0.01 ppm to 0.5 ppm. Few species of fish reach the FDA limit for human consumption of 1 ppm except shark, swordfish, large tuna (the type used to make sushi or fresh steaks), tilefish, and king mackerel. Freshwater predatory species such as pike and walleye occasionally have methyl mercury levels in the 1 ppm range (FDA, 2001).

The types of seafood that comprise 80% of the market—canned tuna, shrimp, pollock, salmon, cod, catfish, clams, flatfish, crabs, and scallops—all have methyl mercury levels of less than 0.2 ppm. Their consumption is not restricted unless a person eats more than 2.2 pounds of these types of seafood per week. Farm-raised fish are an exception and are acceptable for consumption without restriction.

The Canadian government has established more stringent methyl mercury guidelines than those in the United States. Their designated acceptable level of methyl mercury in fish is 0.5 ppm (Health Canada, 2001). In addition to the fish that the United States restricts, they advise that fresh and frozen tuna consumption also be restricted in the diets of pregnant and lactating females and females of childbearing age.

Polychlorinated Biphenyls

More than 1.2 billion pounds of polychlorinated biphenyls (PCBs) were produced in the United States before 1976; half still remain in the environment, where they have primarily been taken up through water systems. PCBs concentrate in the fatty flesh of larger fish such as salmon, lake trout, and carp as they move up the food chain (Agency for Toxic Substances and Disease Registry, 2001).

Although PCBs can be absorbed through the skin and lungs, they primarily enter the body through ingestion of contaminated fatty fish. They readily pass through the placenta and breast milk, so pregnant and nursing females and females of childbearing age should avoid eating fish from water known to be contaminated with PCBs. State land and natural resources departments usually regulate freshwater fish, so they can answer questions regarding methyl mercury, PCBs, and other contaminants.

Listeria monocytogenes

Listeria monocytogenes infects 2500 Americans each year, and 500 of those infected die. Pregnant females are 20 times more likely than other healthy adults to become infected with *Listeria* bacteria. Infection is a known cause of spontaneous abortion and fetal and newborn meningitis (CDC, 2001). *Listeria* bacteria are soil-borne organisms, and infection results from eating contaminated foods of animal origin and raw vegetables. Raw milk, smoked seafood, frankfurters, pâté, soft cheeses, cold cuts from the deli counter, and uncooked meats are likely *Listeria* bacteria sources, so nutritionists should inform their clients of these risks.

Food Beliefs, Avoidances, and Preferences

Beliefs

Most females change their diets during their pregnancies. These changes may be a result of medical advice, folk medicine beliefs, or a varying food preferences and appetite. The changes may be idiosyncratic or culturally patterned and because they affect a female's willingness to follow prescribed dietary regimens, the health care provider should be aware of their existence.

Two harmful practices are the elimination of animal proteins from the diet, and the attempt to limit weight gain to produce a smaller fetus for an easier delivery. It is mistakenly assumed that the infant's growth catches up to normal rates after birth.

Avoidances

Food avoidances are a mother's conscious choice not to consume certain foods during her pregnancy, usually for a reason she can articulate and that seems reasonable to her. The four most commonly avoided foods are sources of animal protein: milk, lean meats, pork, and liver.

Cravings and Aversions

Cravings and *aversions* are powerful urges to consume or not consume particular foods, including foods that were neither craved nor considered aversive before pregnancy. The most commonly craved foods are sweets and dairy products. The most common aversions are to alcohol, coffee and other caffeinated drinks, and meat. However, cravings and aversions are not limited to any particular food or food groups.

The nutritional implications of cravings and aversions should be assessed with reference to the individual's entire diet. Cravings and aversions are not necessarily deleterious.

Pica

Pica—the consumption of substances with little or no nutritional value—of pregnancy most often involves geophagia (the consumption of dirt or clay) or amylophagia (the consumption of nonnutritive starchy substances such as laundry starch). Additional nonfood substances associated with pica of pregnancy include ice, paper, burnt matches, stones or gravel, charcoal, soot, cigarette ashes, antacid tablets, milk of magnesia, baking soda, and coffee grounds. The incidence of pica is not limited to any geographic area, race, sex, culture, or social status, nor is it limited to those who are pregnant.

Malnutrition can be a consequence of pica because the nonfood substances do not provide essential nutrients needed in the diet. Excessive amounts of starch consumption can contribute to obesity, and it is especially deleterious in women with diabetes mellitus. Some substances contain toxic compounds such as heavy metals, and others can interfere with the absorption of minerals such as iron. Excessive intake of nonfood substances such as starch and clay can lead to intestinal obstruction.

The etiology of pica is poorly understood. One theory suggests that the ingestion of nonfood substances relieves nausea and vomiting. It has also been hypothesized that a deficiency of an essential nutrient such as calcium or iron causes a person to eat nonfood substances that contain these nutrients (Rainville, 1998). Much pica behavior seems to be based on superstition, customs, and traditions that are often passed from mother to daughter.

Complications of Pregnancy and Their Dietary Implications

Nausea and Vomiting

Morning sickness, or nausea, is common during the first trimester of pregnancy and usually resolves around the thirteenth to fourteenth week of gestation, often as spontaneously as it developed. However, when a female vomits excessively during early pregnancy, a deficit in protein, energy, vitamins, and minerals may result. Females with fluid and electrolyte imbalances may need to be hospitalized for rehydration and the prevention of ketosis.

The common form of morning sickness may be ameliorated by simple dietary measures. Small, frequent, dry meals of easily digested carbohydrate-containing foods are usually tolerated best. Liquids are best consumed between meals. Fats are often not tolerated, and they are relatively hard to digest. Unfortunately, no cure-all exists for morning sickness. It has been suggested that females with morning sickness should eat whatever makes them feel good and avoid odors that trigger nausea (Erick, 1994).

Pregnant females should be advised of the importance of eating and be encouraged to eat as much as possible when they are not nauseated. As stated previously, vitamin B_6 has been demonstrated to relieve symptoms (Jewel and Young, 2002; Sahakian et al, 1991).

Hyperemesis gravidarum, prolonged and persistent vomiting, develops in about 2% of pregnant females (Erick, 1995) and is associated with an increase in maternal free thyroid hormone (Panesar et al, 2001). Hospitalization is usually needed when dehydration occurs. Parenteral nutritional support may be required in unusually persistent cases. Tube feeding may be successful and should be attempted before parenteral nutrition because of the relatively few associated complications (see Chapter 23).

Heartburn

Gastric reflux is common during the latter part of pregnancy and often occurs at night. In most cases, it is an effect of pressure from the enlarged uterus on the intestines and stomach, which, combined with the relaxation of the esophageal sphincter, may result in regurgitation of stomach contents into the esophagus. Limiting food intake before bedtime, limiting the amount of food consumed at one time, and drinking fluids between meals rather than with meals may help relieve the condition. Wearing clothing that is loose around the waist, eating slowly, sitting upright after meals for at least 3 hours, and elevating the head of the bed may also help (see Chapter 29).

Constipation and Hemorrhoids

Pregnant females may develop constipation, and it usually occurs in the third trimester. Causes include reduced gut motility, physical inactivity, and pressure exerted on the bowel by the enlarged uterus. The weight of the fetus and downward pressure on the veins also may lead to the development of hemorrhoids during this period. Increased consumption of fluids, fiber-rich foods, and dried fruits (especially prunes and figs) usually controls these problems, but some women may also require a bulking type of stool softener (see Chapter 30).

Edema and Leg Cramps

Mild, physiologic edema usually develops in the extremities in the third trimester and should not be confused with the pathologic, generalized edema associated with pregnancy-induced hypertension. Normal, lower-extremity edema during pregnancy is caused by the pressure of the enlarging uterus on the vena cava, obstructing the return of blood flow to the heart. Extravascular fluid is often mobilized in the evening when the woman is lying on her side. No dietary intervention is required.

Although calcium supplementation for leg cramps during pregnancy is used extensively, only three studies met the criteria for analysis by the Cochrane Review, and the use of calcium for leg cramps in pregnancy is not supported (Young and Jewell, 2000). The authors suggest that the best evidence exists for the use of magnesium lactate or citrate to relieve leg cramps (Young and Jewell, 2000).

Magnesium supplementation may relieve leg cramps because pregnancy and lactation can lead to a magnesium deficiency, which is indicated by low serum magnesium levels (Dahle et al, 1995). Signs of magnesium deficiency include muscle tremor, ataxia, tetany, constipation, and cramps, thus supplemental magnesium may relieve the leg cramps associated with pregnancy or lactation. A placebo-controlled study demonstrated that females with pregnancy-related leg cramps had low serum magnesium levels. The magnesium-treated group, who received 122 mg of magnesium (as lactate and citrate) in the morning and 244 mg in the evening, reported a significantly greater reduction of distress than the control group. However, the low serum magnesium level initially detected in the magnesium-treated group did not return to normal levels, even though their leg cramps improved. This suggests that the participants had a significant magnesium deficit because only a severe total body magnesium deficiency is reflected in serum magnesium concentrations (Dahle et al, 1995).

Diabetes Mellitus

Individualized, expert care is needed for the nutritional management of a pregnant female with diabetes. Based on a nutritional history and assessment early in pregnancy or preferably before conception, a meal plan should be adapted for each patient by a skilled nutritionist as part of the health care team (see Chapter 33).

The risk of pregnancy-induced hypertension, macrosomia, chorioamnionitis, prematurity, IUFD, and fetal morbidity is significantly greater in pregnant females with diabetes than in pregnant females without diabetes. Recent evidence suggests that females who do not meet the criteria to be classified as having diabetes but who have elevated blood glucose levels during pregnancy have a significant risk for pregnancy complications, including macrosomia, prematurity, and chorioamnionitis (Scholl et al, 2001). Adverse outcomes can be reduced significantly with specialized care, including ongoing involvement with the nutritionist. The risk of complications can be reduced to the same level typical of pregnant females who do not have diabetes (Cousins, 1991).

Infants born to females with diabetes are usually larger than those of females who do not have diabetes. Fetal macrosomia is caused by in utero hyperglycemia from maternal blood. The fetus responds to maternal hyperglycemia by increasing its own insulin production, leading to excessive growth and adiposity. After birth, the infant's pancreas continues to secrete elevated amounts of insulin. Because the maternal supply of glucose is no longer available, many infants of mothers with diabetes rapidly develop hypoglycemia and require a glucose infusion.

A successful pregnancy requires a dietary intake that is adequate to meet the growth needs of the fetus, prevent ketosis, and prevent depletion of maternal nutritional stores. Maintaining optimal blood glucose levels and avoiding ketosis are important goals of therapy for pregnant females with diabetes. Frequent glucose monitoring and appropriate insulin adjustments are crucial. Insulin requirements decrease in the first half of pregnancy because the fetus uses some of the mother's glucose, and she may need only two thirds of her usual amount. During the second half of pregnancy, hormone changes induce an increase in insulin requirements that is 70% to 100% higher than prepregnancy requirements. This increase occurs rather abruptly during the fifth month and may last until birth. During this time, pregnant females whose diabetes was adequately controlled by diet when they were not pregnant may need insulin. Frequent changes in diet and insulin dosage may be necessary.

Gestational diabetes, which usually develops after 20 weeks of gestation, may affect as many as 5% to 10% of all pregnant females. Although symptoms are similar to those of diabetes mellitus, including glycosuria and elevated blood glucose levels, the degree of hyperglycemia does not usually reach the markedly high levels of classic diabetes mellitus, nor does diabetic-induced ketosis develop. However, infants whose mothers have gestational diabetes have an increased risk of perinatal mortality and prematurity, with its associated complications. If the mother's blood glucose is not well controlled, the infant is at risk for macrosomia. In addition, females who develop gestational diabetes are at risk for developing type 2 diabetes mellitus in the future.

Currently, most obstetric health care providers perform a routine 50-g oral glucose challenge between 24 and 28 weeks of gestation to screen for gestational diabetes. If values are not in the normal range, an oral glucose tolerance test is scheduled to confirm the diagnosis (see Chapter 33). Gestational diabetes is treated largely through dietary changes (with possible calorie restrictions) and moderate exercise to maintain appropriate weight gain. Insulin is rarely administered, but blood glucose levels are monitored daily. Through these venues, gestational diabetes can be controlled and result in a favorable pregnancy outcome.

Pregnancy-Induced Hypertension

Pregnancy-induced hypertension includes gestational hypertension and preeclampsia or eclampsia. Gestational hypertension, which develops after midpregnancy, is a maternal blood pressure of 140/90 mm Hg or higher with no proteinuria. Females with gestational hypertension may develop preeclampsia, which is defined as a systolic blood pressure of 140 mm Hg or higher or a diastolic blood pressure of 90 mm Hg and/or a urinary protein level of 300 mg or more in a 24-hr urine sample. Severe preeclampsia is defined as a systolic blood pressure of 160 mm Hg or higher or a diastolic blood pressure of 110 mm Hg or higher and 5 g of protein in a 24-hr urine sample. Preeclampsia is associated with decreased uterine blood flow, leading to a reduced placental size, compromised fetal nourishment, and a fetus with IUGR. Vasospasm, intravascular volume depletion, and subsequent hemoconcentration also develop in females with severe **pregnancy-induced hypertension.** The condition usually develops in the third trimester and affects about 5% to 8% of pregnant females, particularly those who are nulliparous, older than 40 years, black, and have a family history of pregnancy-induced hypertension. Other risk factors include chronic hypertension, chronic renal disease, antiphospholipid syndrome, diabetes mellitus, being pregnant with twins, and homozygosity or heterozygosity for the angiotensinogen gene T235 (American College of Obstetricians and Gynecologists [ACOG], 1996). Dietary related risk factors include a high intake of energy, sucrose, and polyunsaturated fatty acids (Clausen et al, 2001). Insulin resistance syndrome has also been suggested as a cause for pregnancy-induced hypertension (Solomon and Sealy, 2001) (see Chapters 12, 33, and 35).

Eclampsia

Eclampsia is pregnancy-induced hypertension resulting in grand mal seizures. Symptoms of pregnancy-induced hypertension that may indicate imminent seizures are dizziness, headache, visual disturbances, facial edema, anorexia, and nausea and vomiting. Fetal death often occurs in women who develop eclampsia.

Calcium and Magnesium Supplementation

A double-blind, placebo-controlled trial of more than 4500 healthy, nulliparous women who were provided with calcium supplements revealed that calcium supplementation during pregnancy does not prevent pregnancy-induced hypertension (Levine et al, 1997). These results are in contrast to a previous study that also involved a large cohort of patients and demonstrated the effectiveness of calcium supplementation (Bucher et al, 1996).

Magnesium supplementation has also been recommended to prevent and treat preeclampsia and eclampsia (Roberts, 1995). Magnesium sulfate is better than phenytoin for preventing seizures in females with preeclampsia and managing convulsions in females with eclampsia (Lucas et al, 1995; Magpie Trial Collaborative Group, 2002).

Previous attempts to treat preeclampsia have included severe sodium restriction and use of diuretics. Sodium restriction and diuretics do not reduce blood pressure, limit weight gain, or reduce the amount of proteinuria in those with preeclampsia, and they have no place in the treatment or prevention of the condition. Females with pregnancy-induced hypertension who take diuretics experience fluid loss and a decrease in intravascular volume, thus further compromising the fetus. Restricted energy intake also has no role in the prevention of pregnancy-induced hypertension.

A growing body of evidence shows that antioxidants help prevent preeclampsia; serum and placental concentrations of vitamins C and E and carotenoids were significantly reduced in females with preeclampsia and eclampsia (Kharb, 2000; Palan et al, 2001). Females at risk for preeclampsia who were provided with vitamins C and E had a significant reduction in preeclampsia compared with females at risk who received placebos (Chappell et al, 1999).

LACTATION

Exclusive breast-feeding is unequivocally the preferred method of infant feeding for the first 4 to 6 months of life. The American Dietetic Association (ADA) and the American Academy of Pediatrics (AAP) have issued position statements in support of breast-feeding (AAP, 1995; ADA, 1997). Some of the distinct advantages of breast-feeding are listed in Box 7-4. Females infected with the human immunodeficiency virus (HIV) should be counseled not to breast-feed, and females who are at risk for being infected with the virus (e.g., those who use injection drugs, those with sexual partners who are infected with HIV or are active drug users) should be educated about the risk of infecting their infant with HIV through breast milk (AAP, 1995).

Box 7-4. Advantages of Breast-Feeding

1. Breast milk is nutritionally superior to any alternative.
2. Breast milk is bacteriologically safe and always fresh.
3. Breast milk contains various antiinfectious factors and immune cells.
4. Breast milk is the least allergenic of any infant food.
5. Breast-fed babies are less likely to be overfed.
6. Breast-feeding promotes good jaw and tooth development.
7. Breast-feeding generally costs less than the commercial infant formulas currently available.
8. Breast-feeding automatically promotes close mother-child contact.
9. Breast-feeding is generally more convenient once the process is established.

CLINICAL INSIGHT

The Baby Friendly Hospital Initiative

Ten steps to successful breast-feeding

1. Have a written breast-feeding policy that is routinely communicated to all health care staff.
2. Train all health care staff in the skills necessary to implement this policy.
3. Inform all pregnant females about the benefits and management of breast-feeding.
4. Help the mother initiate breast-feeding within a half hour of birth.
5. Show mothers how to breast-feed and how to maintain lactation, even if they are separated from their infants.
6. Give newborn infants no food or drink other than breast milk unless medically indicated.
7. Practice rooming-in; allow mothers and infants to remain together 24 hours a day.
8. Encourage breast-feeding on demand.
9. Give no artificial teats or pacifiers (also called *dummies* or *soothers*) to breast-feeding infants.
10. Foster the establishment of breast-feeding support groups, and refer mothers to them on discharge from the hospital or clinic.

From Ebrahim GJ: The baby friendly hospital initiative, *J Trop Pediatr* 39:2, 1993.

Numerous national health promotion strategies support breast-feeding. In the early 1980s, up to 62% of infants in the United States were discharged from the hospital with mothers who were breast-feeding. However, this declined in the 1990s to approximately 50%. Efforts to promote the practice and duration of breast-feeding need to be strengthened in hospitals, health maintenance organizations, private physician's offices, and public health clinics.

The World Health Organization (WHO) and the United Nations Children's Fund (UNICEF) have adopted the Baby Friendly Hospital Initiative (BFHI), a global effort to increase the incidence and duration of breast-feeding. To become "baby friendly," a hospital must agree to implement the "Ten Steps to Successful Breast-Feeding," which suggest guidelines for mother and infant management in the hospital. These guidelines include training hospital staff in breast-feeding education and prohibiting supplementary bottles of formula for breast-feeding infants unless medically indicated (Ebrahim, 1993) (see *Clinical Insight:* The Baby Friendly Hospital Initiative).

Physiology

Mammary gland growth during menarche and pregnancy prepares the body for lactation. (The human mammary gland is illustrated in Figure 7-8.) Hormonal changes markedly increase breast, areola, and nipple size and growth of mammary ducts and alveoli. In the later stages of pregnancy, the lobules of the alveolar system are maximally developed, and small amounts of colostrum may be released for several weeks before term. After birth the mother experiences a rapid drop in circulating levels of estrogen and progesterone accompanied by a rapid increase in prolactin secretion, setting the stage for the onset of lactation.

The usual stimulus for milk production and secretion is suckling. Subcutaneous nerves of the areola send a message via the spinal cord to the hypothalamus, which in turn transmits a message to the pituitary gland, where the anterior and posterior areas are stimulated. Prolactin from the anterior pituitary stimulates alveolar cell milk production (Figure 7-9). Oxytocin from the posterior pituitary stimulates the myoepithelial cells of the mammary gland to contract, causing movement of milk through the ducts and lactiferous sinuses, a process referred to as let-down. Oxytocin also stimulates uterine muscle contractions; therefore lactation is useful in preventing hemorrhage in the postpartum period.

The process of let-down is highly sensitive to small changes in circulating oxytocin, which is influenced by stress; thus the stress from labor and delivery can delay lactogenesis (Chen et al, 1998). The attitude of the mother toward the process of breast-feeding is a powerful factor in determining her success. The support of the mother's partner, physician, nurse, extended family, and friends is also an important determinant of the degree of satisfaction and success derived from the breast-feeding experience (Figure 7-10).

Nutritional Requirements

Lactation is nutritionally demanding, especially for the mother who nurses her infant exclusively for several months. Increased intake of most nutrients is advised (see Table 7-3).

Milk production is most affected by the frequency of suckling, and volume can be affected by maternal hydration. However, milk composition varies according to the mother's diet.

For example, the fatty acid composition of a mother's milk reflects her dietary intake. In addition, milk concentrations of selenium, iodine, and some of the water-soluble B vitamins vary according to the

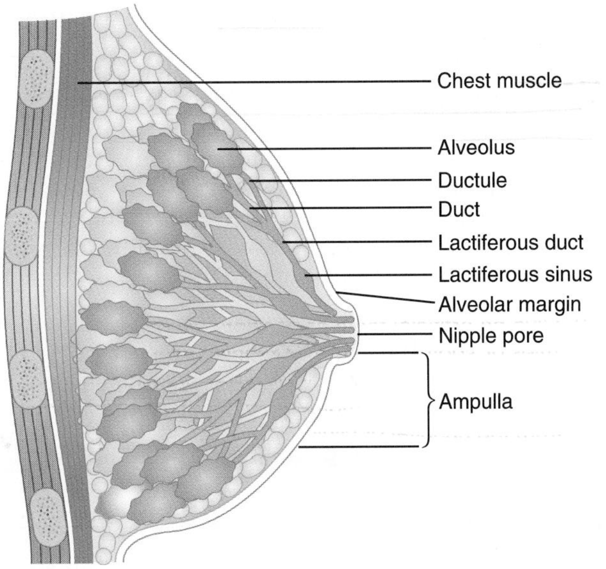

FIGURE 7-8 • Structural features of the human mammary gland. The terminal glandular (alveolar) tissue of each lobule leads into the duct system, which enlarges eventually into the *lactiferous duct* and *lactiferous sinus.* The lactiferous sinuses rest beneath the *areola* and converge at the *nipple pore.*

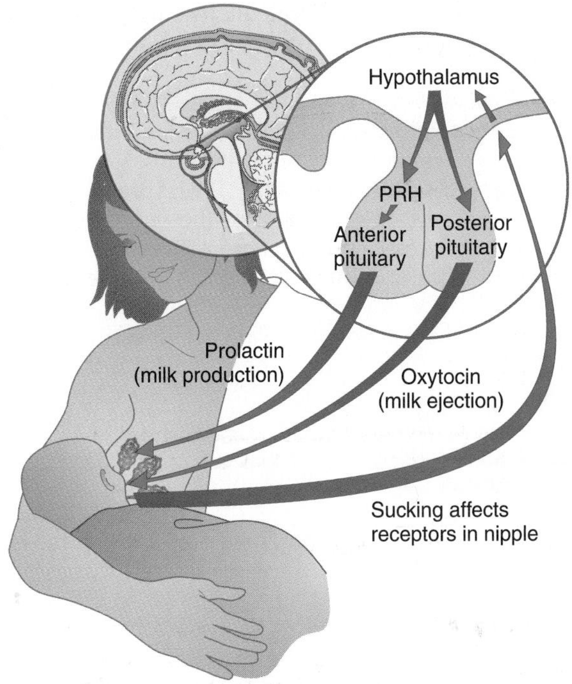

FIGURE 7-9 • Physiology of milk production and the let-down reflex. (*PRH,* Pituitary-releasing hormone.)

maternal diet. Most other nutrients are present at remarkably constant levels, regardless of diet. However, one study suggests that antimicrobial proteins provided by human milk may be secreted in reduced amounts if the mother is malnourished (Chang, 1990).

Energy

Milk production is 80% efficient; production of 100 ml of milk (about 67 kcal) requires an 85-kcal expenditure. During the first 6 months of lactation, the average milk production is 750 ml/day, with a range of 550 to more than 1200 ml/day (IOM, 1990). Recall that milk production is a function of the frequency of infant feeding; therefore infants who feed often are likely to stimulate the production of larger volumes of milk.

The RDA for energy during lactation is 330 kcal greater during the first 6 months of lactation and 400 kcal greater during the second 6 months of lactation than the RDA for a female who is not pregnant. It is about the same as the RDA during the second trimester of pregnancy (IOM, 2002). Obese and overweight females may not need to add the entire 330 to 400 kcal/day. Maternal fat stores accumulated during pregnancy provide about 100 to 150 kcal/day during the early months of lactation. When the reserve fat pad has been depleted, dietary energy must be increased if the mother intends to provide all or most of her infant's nutrition through breast milk alone. During the second 6 months of lactation, production generally drops to an average of 600 ml/day. Most infants are also consuming solid foods by this age, so

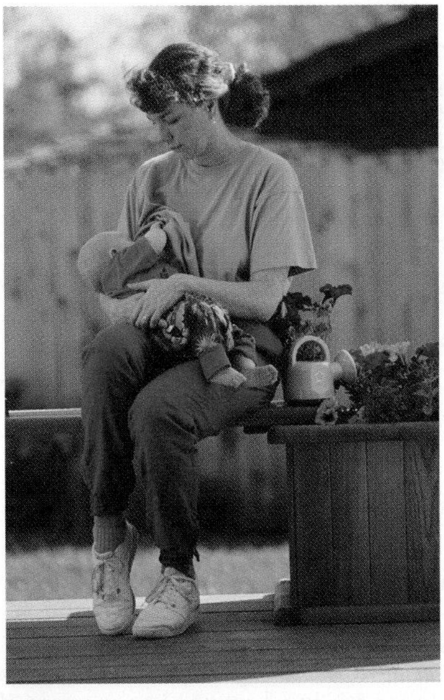

FIGURE 7-10 • A nursing mother and her infant enjoy the close physical contact that accompanies breast-feeding. (Courtesy Kathryn Abbe, New York.)

the frequency of breast-feeding usually declines, as do the energy requirements for the nursing mother.

Milk production decreases if the mother is undernourished; for example, nursing women who follow rigorously calorie-restricted diets may not receive the proper nutrients. However, a mother can reduce her energy intake modestly while increasing fat use without adversely affecting milk production after lactation is well established.

One study demonstrated that healthy breast-feeding mothers could lose as much as 1 lb/wk and still supply an adequate amount of milk to maintain infant growth (Dusdieker et al, 1994). Breast-feeding mothers should be reminded of the energy drain of lactation and that exclusive breast-feeding with no reduction in caloric intake can still promote the loss of body fat (Dewey et al, 1993). However, mothers who are already lean may be at risk for reduced milk production if they restrict their energy intake. It is generally advisable for lactating mothers to maintain an energy intake of at least 1800 kcal/day (Dewey and McCrory, 1994).

Inadequate maternal fluid intake affects milk volume. Approximately 2 to 3 quarts of fluid daily, perhaps more in very hot weather, should be encouraged. Oral contraceptives may also suppress lactation, especially during the first 6 to 10 weeks after birth.

Protein

The RDA for lactating mothers suggests an additional 25 g of protein. The average protein requirement for lactation is estimated from milk composition data and the mean daily volume of 750 ml, assuming an efficiency of 70% in conversion of dietary protein to milk protein.

Carbohydrates

The DRIs for carbohydrates during lactation are presented in Table 7-3. The EAR is 160 g/day, and the AI is 210 g/day (IOM, 2002). (EAR and AI are defined in Chapter 15.) The EAR and AI provide enough calories in the diet for an adequate volume of milk, to prevent ketonemia, and to maintain appropriate blood glucose levels during lactation.

Lipids

The amount and type of fat in breast milk directly reflects the maternal diet, so adjustments in the diet can increase or decrease the amounts of specific fatty acids in the milk (Francois et al, 1998). Severe energy restriction results in body fat mobilization, and the milk produced has a fatty acid composition resembling that of the mother's depot fat. No DRI for lipids during lactation exists because it depends on the amount of energy required by the mother to maintain milk production, but it is recommended that fat provide 20% to 35% of total calories (IOM, 2002).

The presence of long-chain polyunsaturated fatty acids in the maternal diet is crucial for fetal and infant retina and brain development (Birch et al, 2002). In fact, the new DRIs provide recommended amounts of fatty acids for the first time. The AI for *n*-6 polyunsaturated fatty acids is 13 g/day, and the AI for *n*-3 polyunsaturated fatty acids (a-linolenic acid) is 1.3 g/day (IOM, 2002) (see *Focus On:* Omega-3 Fatty Acids During Pregnancy and Lactation).

Human milk contains 10 to 20 mg/dl of cholesterol, so a breast-feeding infant consumes approximately 100 mg/day. The amount of cholesterol in milk does not vary according to the mother's diet; however, the cholesterol content of the milk decreases over time as lactation progresses.

Vitamins and Minerals

The requirements for zinc during lactation are greater than those during pregnancy (Krebs, 1998). In the process of normal lactation, the zinc content of breast milk drops dramatically during the first few months from 2 to 3 mg/day to 1 mg/day by the third month after birth. In lactating mothers with deficient zinc levels, normal zinc concentrations are maintained in breast milk for at least the first 2 months of lactation through increased fractional absorption of zinc and intestinal conversion of endogenous fecal zinc (Sian et al, 2002). The DRIs for zinc during lactation are 12 to 14 mg/day (IOM, 2001). The UL is 34 to 40 mg/day, depending on the age of the lactating mother. (See Table 7-3 for the DRIs for minerals and vitamins for lactating women.)

The vitamin D content of milk is related to the mother's vitamin D intake and degree of sun exposure. Numerous case reports document marginal or significant vitamin D deficiencies in pregnant females and in infants of lactating mothers who are veiled or dark skinned or living in northern latitudes with little sun exposure (Daaboul et al, 1997; Pugliese et al, 1998; Waiters et al, 1999). Mothers with lactose intolerance who do not drink vitamin D–fortified milk or take a vitamin supplement may be at higher risk for vitamin D deficiency. The AI for vitamin D during lactation is 5 μg/day (IOM, 1997).

The calcium content of breast milk is not related to the mother's diet, and no convincing evidence shows that maternal changes in bone mineral density are influenced by calcium consumption in a broad range of calcium intakes—up to 1600 mg/day (Kalkwarf et al, 1997). Maternal bone loss during lactation is approximately 3% to 7%, which is rapidly regained after weaning (Kalkwarf and Specker, 2002). The AI for calcium during pregnancy and lactation and in females who are not pregnant or lactating is 1300 mg/day for 9- to 18-year-olds and 1000 mg/day for 19- to 50-year-old women; the UL is the same, 2500 mg/day (IOM, 1997). (The DRIs for lactating mothers are presented in Table 7-3.)

Breast-Feeding an Infant

Preparation

The advantages of breast-feeding should be presented to females throughout their childbearing years. The process of lactation and the benefits of breast-feeding should be a part of high school family and health curricula. Females should be encouraged to express and discuss their opinions and feelings so that any misinformation can be corrected. During the last months of pregnancy, counseling on the process of lactation should be made available to mothers who have decided to breast-feed. Fathers should be encouraged to participate in counseling sessions because the emotional support they provide contributes to the success of breast-feeding. Many mothers have never seen another mother nursing an infant, so they may find it especially helpful to talk with a mother who is successfully nursing an infant and who can answer questions and provide positive reinforcement.

Technique

The infant should be put to the breast as soon after birth as the mother feels ready. It is not essential that suckling occur immediately after delivery, but the wishes of mothers who want this experience should be accommodated if possible. Milk typically begins to flow between 48 and 96 hours after delivery. Before this time, the thin yellow fluid called colostrum should appear. Higher in protein and lower in fat and carbohydrate than mature milk, colostrum provides approximately 15 kcal/oz and is a rich source of antibodies. As colostrum is replaced by transitional and mature milk, the breasts become enlarged and firm as they fill.

For breast-feeding to be successful, it is important that the mother and infant get into a comfortable position either sitting or lying down. If she is sitting up, the mother should hold the infant close, cradling the infant in her arm to support the head. If the infant's cheek is touched, the infant will turn toward that side (a reaction called the *rooting reflex*). The mother should hold her breast so that as much of the areola and nipple are in the infant's mouth as possible. If the breast is very full, the mother can press it gently away from the infant's nose so that the infant can breathe more easily. Alternatively, it may be helpful for the mother to express a little milk before letting the infant nurse. The infant should be allowed to nurse for at least 10 minutes on each side initially, and then longer if the mother and infant wish. The length of time spent nursing should not be unduly limited because this could prevent establishment of successful lactation.

Lactating mothers experience a tingling sensation in the breast that is being suckled, signaling the let-down reflex. This is often accompanied by milk dripping from the other breast and occasionally by uterine cramps. It may take some time for the let-down reflex to become fully functional and conditioned. Some mothers never feel the milk let-down, but swallowing by the infant is a definite sign that it has occurred. Rest or a hot shower before nursing may facilitate the let-down reflex. If the mother has too much breast milk, the infant may need to nurse on only one side at each feeding for a while. This method reduces the overall stimulation and eventually the milk supply. Having too much milk is also an ideal opportunity for the mother to express milk from the other breast so that it can be stored for a

FOCUS ON

Omega-3 Fatty Acids During Pregnancy and Lactation

Our ancestors consumed a diet with equal amounts of omega-3 and omega-6 fatty acids. American diets are currently estimated to contain a 1 : 10 ratio of omega-3 to omega-6 fatty acids. The dramatic decrease in the consumption of the omega-3 fatty acids over many centuries is thought to affect overall disease prevalence and pregnancy outcome (Leaf and Weber, 1987; McGregor et al, 2001).

Fatty acids are found in all cell membranes. They compose 60% of the dry weight of fetal brain, half of which is omega-6 and half of which is omega-3 (arachidonic acid [AA] and docosahexaenoic acid [DHA], respectively]. Because DHA is important for the growth and development of the fetal central nervous system and the retina, it has been suggested that the prenatal diet should include adequate amounts of preformed DHA (Crawford, 1993; Monique et al, 1996). In fact, the new DRIs specify 1.4 g/day during pregnancy and 1.3 g/day during lactation (IOM, 2002).

The main food source of DHA is fatty, cold-water fish, and two to three meals with fish per week during pregnancy seem to provide adequate amounts of DHA and have been recommended (Olsen et al, 1993). However, given the recent advice that childbearing-age, pregnant, and lactating females should limit their consumption of certain fish during pregnancy because of mercury and PCB exposure, dietary strategies must be highly specific. Fish with elevated concentrations of DHA that are not on the FDA advisory are sardines. Other options for increasing the DHA content in the diet of pregnant and lactating females include consuming omega-3–enriched eggs and using DHA supplements (Cherian and Sim, 1996). Vegetable sources of omega-3 fats include flax seeds and nuts, especially walnuts and walnut oil.

The breast-fed infant obtains DHA through breast milk, and some infant formulas sold in the United States just recently have had AA and DHA added. Japan has included these fatty acids it in their infant formulas for years (see Chapter 8).

future feeding when she needs to be away from the infant.

To remove the infant from the breast, the mother places a finger in the corner of the infant's mouth until the suction is broken. The breast can then be removed from the infant's mouth comfortably. Most infants need to be burped before they are fed from the second breast; however, burping needs are highly individual.

Because breast milk is more easily digested than infant-feeding formula, breast-fed infants may want to feed more often than formula-fed babies. If the infant wants to nurse, the mother should allow the infant to nurse; breast-fed babies consume what they need when they need it. Breast-feeding whenever an infant is hungry is easy because the milk is always ready. Some infants may be hungry as frequently as every hour or two on some days, whereas others may not become hungry until 4 hours after the previous feeding. The more often the infant nurses, the more milk the breasts produce. Therefore whenever a mother's supply is low (e.g., during or after an illness, provided there is no risk of the infant contracting the disease through breast-feeding), she should nurse more often.

Feeding time is perfectly suited for establishing and maintaining close mother-child interactions (see Figure 7-10). However, the mother need not be with her infant all of the time. On occasions when she wants or needs to be away at the usual feeding time, a bottle of breast milk that has been expressed earlier or a commercial infant formula can be given. It is best to avoid supplemental bottles until the mother is satisfied that her milk supply is well established and regulated, which is usually around 6 weeks after birth.

Infants who are introduced to artificial nipples in the first few weeks of life may experience *nipple confusion.* Because the muscle action required by the infant to empty a bottle is quite different from that needed to nurse at the breast, a very young infant may be easily confused if both feeding methods are offered. Because it is more work to suck at the breast, infants in such situations may refuse the breast, leading to lactation failure. In the early weeks it is important to minimize mother and infant separations. It is unnecessary to offer breast-fed babies additional water from a bottle; human milk usually provides all the fluid the infant needs.

Duration

The length of time a mother breast-feeds her infant depends on her own feelings and situation. If she is working, she can continue to breast-feed by expressing milk and instructing a caregiver to provide it in a bottle. Milk continues to be produced as long as a demand for it exists and it is taken from the breast, even though a breast may not be emptied at any given feeding.

Some mothers prefer to breast-feed until the infant is weaned to a cup (thus avoiding bottles altogether); this can be accomplished when the infant is about 9 to 10 months of age. Some mothers choose to breast-feed much longer—some for several years—and let

TABLE 7-5 Drugs for Which the Effect on Nursing Infants Is Unknown but May Be of Concern*

DRUG	REPORTED OR POSSIBLE EFFECT
Antianxiety	
Alprazolam	None
Diazepam	None
Lorazepam	None
Midazolam	—‡
Perphenazine	None
Prazepam†	None
Quazepam	None
Temazepam	—‡
Antidepressant	
Amitriptyline	None
Amoxapine	None
Bupropion	None
Clomipramine	None
Desipramine	None
Dothiepin	None
Doxepin	None
Fluoxetine	Colic, irritability, feeding and sleep disorders, slow weight gain
Fluvoxamine	—‡
Imipramine	None
Nortriptyline	None
Paroxetine	None
Sertraline†	None
Trazodone	None
Antipsychotic	
Chlorpromazine	Galactorrhea in mother, drowsiness and lethargy in infant, decline in developmental scores
Chlorprothixene	None
Clozapine†	None
Haloperidol	Decline in developmental scores
Mesoridazine	None
Trifluoperazine	None
Other	
Amiodarone	Possible hypothyroidism
Chloramphenicol	Possible idiosyncratic bone marrow suppression
Clofazimine	Possible transfer of high percentage of maternal dose, possible increase in skin pigmentation
Lamotrigine	Potential therapeutic serum concentrations in infant
Metoclopramide†	None described, dopaminergic blocking agent
Metronidazole	In vitro mutagen, may discontinue breast-feeding for 12-24 hr to allow excretion of dose when single-dose therapy is given to mother
Tinidazole	See *metronidazole*

Modified from American Academy of Pediatrics, Committee on Drugs: The transfer of drugs and other chemicals into human milk, *Pediatrics* 108(3):776, 2001.

*Psychotropic drugs—the compounds listed as *anti-anxiety, antidepressant,* and *antipsychotic*—are of special concern when given to nursing mothers for long periods. Although very few case reports of adverse effects in breast-feeding infants are known, these drugs do appear in human milk and thus could conceivably alter short-term and long-term central nervous system function.

†Drug is concentrated in human milk relative to simultaneous maternal plasma concentrations.

‡—Data not sufficient to confidently assess risk.

TABLE 7-6 Drugs That Have Been Associated With Significant Effects on Some Nursing Infants and Should Be Given to Nursing Mothers With Caution

DRUG	REPORTED EFFECT*
Acebutolol	Hypotension, bradycardia, tachypnea
5-Aminosalicylic acid	Diarrhea (one case)
Aspirin (salicylates)	Metabolic acidosis (one case)
Atenolol	Cyanosis, bradycardia
Bromocriptine	Suppresses lactation; may be hazardous to the mother
Clemastine	Drowsiness, irritability, refusal to feed, high-pitched crying, neck stiffness (one case)
Ergotamine	Vomiting, diarrhea, convulsions (in doses used in migraine medications)
Lithium	One third to one half therapeutic blood concentration in infants
Phenindione	Anticoagulant: increased prothrombin and partial thromboplastin time in one infant; not used in United States
Phenobarbital	Sedation, infantile spasms after weaning from milk containing phenobarbital, methemoglobinemia (one case)
Primidone	Sedation, feeding problems
Sulfasalazine (salicylazosulfapyridine)	Bloody diarrhea (one case)

Modified from American Academy of Pediatrics, Committee on Drugs: The transfer of drugs and other chemicals into human milk, *Pediatrics* 108(3):776, 2001.
*Blood concentration in infant may be of clinical importance.

TABLE 7-7 Food and Environmental Agents: Effects on Breast-Feeding

AGENT	REPORTED SIGN OR SYMPTOM IN INFANT OR EFFECT ON LACTATION
Aflatoxin	None
Aspartame	Caution if mother or infant has phenylketonuria
Bromide (photographic laboratory)	Potential absorption and bromide transfer into milk
Cadmium	None reported
Chlordane	None reported
Chocolate (theobromine)	Irritability or increased bowel activity if excess amounts (≥16 oz/day) consumed by mother
Dichloro-diphyenyl-trichloroethane (DDT), benzene hexachlorides, dieldrin, aldrin, hepatachlorepoxide	None
Fava beans	Hemolysis in patient with glucose-6-phosphate dehydrogenase (G6PD) deficiency
Fluorides	None
Hexachlorobenzene	Skin rash, diarrhea, vomiting, dark urine, neurotoxicity, death
Hexachlorophene	None, possible contamination of milk from nipple washing
Lead	Possible neurotoxicity
Mercury, methyl mercury	Possible neurodevelopmental effects
Methylmethacrylate	None
Monosodium glutamate	None
Polychlorinated biphenyls and polybrominated biphenyls	Lack of endurance, hypotonia, sullen, expressionless facies
Silicon	Esophageal dysmotility
Tetrachlormethylene cleaning fluid (Perchloroethylene)	Obstructive jaundice, dark urine
Vegetarian diet	Signs of B_{12} deficiency

Modified from American Academy of Pediatrics, Committee on Drugs: The transfer of drugs and other chemicals into human milk, *Pediatrics* 108(3):776, 2001.

the infant decide when to be weaned. Ease of weaning varies widely, depending on the infant's overall interest in nursing, the relationship between mother and child, and the use of bottles. Infants who have had frequent supplemental bottles from birth are likely to wean themselves at an early age.

When a mother decides to wean her infant, it should be done gradually over a period of several weeks. At first, one feeding can be omitted for several days; two feedings may then be skipped and so on until the infant has one feeding a day (usually the night or early morning feeding). Eventually, this last feeding can be discontinued. Weaning gradually is easier on the mother because it prevents engorgement of her breasts and eases the infant's transition to the new routine.

Exercise

The breast-feeding mother should be encouraged to get back to exercising a few weeks after birth and after lactation is well established. Aerobic exercise at 60% to 70% of the maximal heart rate has no adverse effect on lactation; infants gain weight at the same rate, and the mother's cardiovascular fitness improves (Dewey et al, 1994). However, strenuous exercise resulting in lactic acid production is not recommended. In some mothers, lactic acid levels rise in their breast milk and remain high for 90 minutes after strenuous exercise, giving the milk a sour taste that infants may not like (Wallace et al, 1992). Mothers who want to do anaerobic exercise should nurse before they exercise and wait until at least 90 minutes after exercise to nurse again.

Transfer of Drugs Into Human Milk

The AAP has issued a statement on the transfer of drugs and other chemicals into human milk (AAP, 2001). Many drugs are known to have detrimental effects (e.g., cytotoxic drugs), and some drugs have unknown effects but may be of concern (e.g., antidepressant, antianxiety, and neuroleptic drugs) (Tables 7-5 to 7-7).

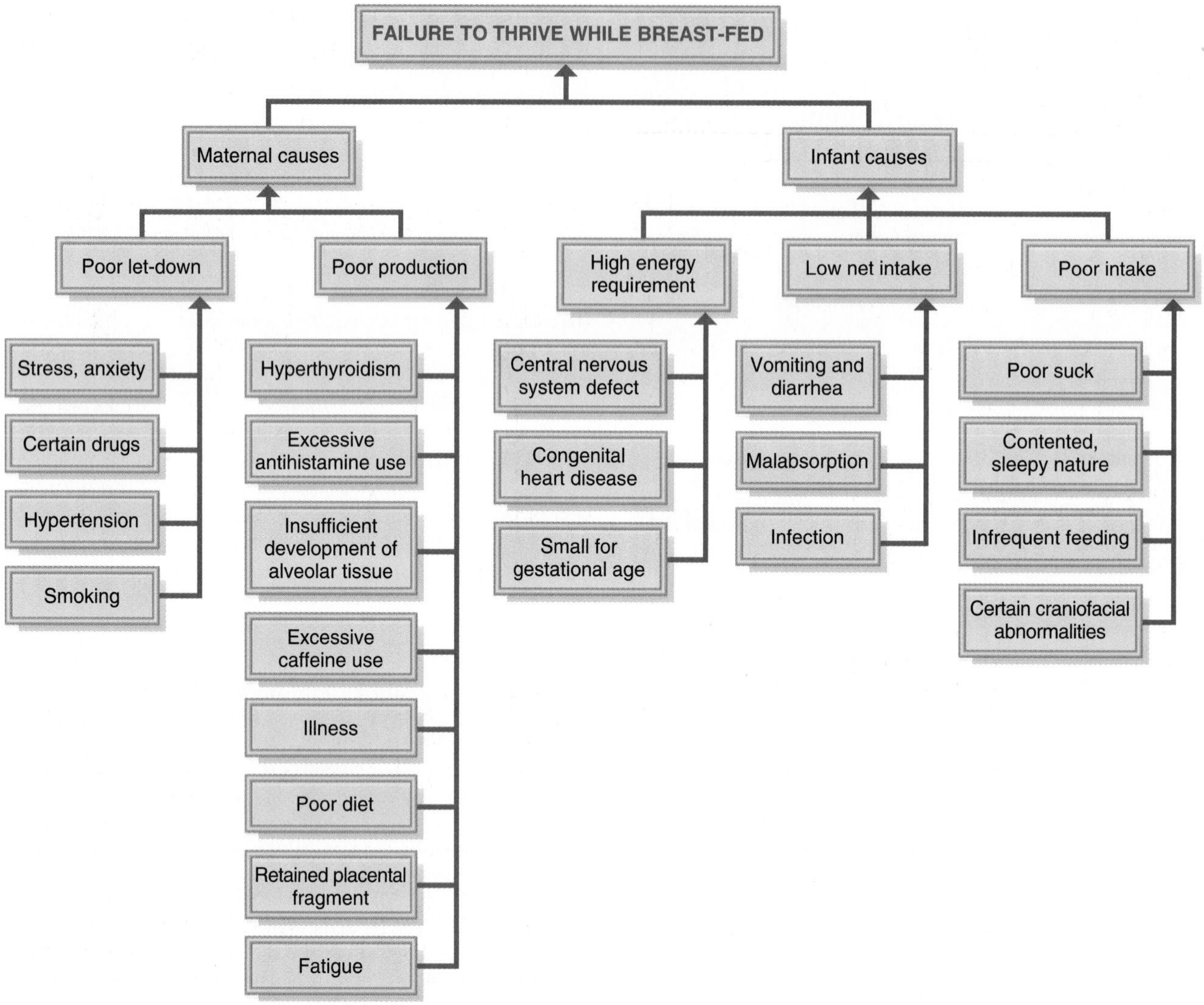

FIGURE 7-11 • Diagnostic flow chart for failure to thrive while breast-feeding.

TABLE 7-8 Management of Breast-Feeding Problems

PROBLEM	APPROACHES TO MANAGEMENT
Retracted nipple(s)	Before feeding the infant, roll the nipple gently between the fingers until erect.
Baby's mouth not open wide enough	Before feeding, depress the infant's lower jaw with one finger as the nipple is guided into the mouth.
Baby sucks poorly	Stimulate sucking motions by pressing upward under the baby's chin. Expression of colostrum often occurs, and the taste may stimulate sucking.
Baby demonstrates rooting but does not grasp the nipple; eventually cries in frustration	Interrupt the feeding, comfort the infant; the mother should take time to relax before trying again.
Baby falls asleep while nursing	If the infant falls asleep early in the feeding, the mother should awaken the infant by holding him or her upright, rubbing his or her back, talking to him or her, or providing similar quiet stimuli; another effort at feeding can then be made. If the baby falls asleep again, the feeding should be postponed.

Breast-Fed Infants and Failure to Thrive

Insufficient milk supply is rarely a problem for the well-fed mother. Because sucking stimulates the flow of milk, feeding on demand for an adequate duration should supply ample amounts of milk to the infant. If the infant continues steadily to gain weight and length, has at least six to eight wet diapers daily, and has frequent stools, the milk supply is probably adequate.

Occasionally, an infant fails to thrive while seeming to nurse properly. Various circumstances can be explored as likely causes of an unsatisfactory breast-feeding experience. The diagram in Figure 7-11 illustrates potential problems of the mother or infant that should be investigated during the course of evaluation. If the cause of the problem cannot be identified or the defined problem cannot be corrected, it may be necessary to encourage the mother to use commercial infant formula for at least partial nutritional support of the infant.

Common Breast-Feeding Problems

A mother may have to overcome numerous hurdles to successfully breast-feed her infant. These problems and their solutions are discussed in Table 7-8.

NUTRITION, FERTILITY, AND CONCEPTION

Although most American females have access to sufficient food sources of energy, protein, and micronutrients, individual circumstances sometimes prevent a female from achieving nutritional well-being. The problem may involve limited resources, but it is just as likely that self-selected behaviors have led to nutritional imbalances over time. Poor dietary habits during childhood or adolescence can temporarily or permanently limit growth and development. Stunted linear growth or incomplete development of the pelvic girdle in a female infant may interfere later with *her* fetus's development because of restricted space.

Chronic dieting may lead to amenorrhea, which would obviously reduce fertility (see Chapter 25). Deficiencies of specific nutrients may lead to eventual depletion of nutrient stores, adversely affecting the function of many physiologic and biochemical processes and resulting in recurrent pregnancy losses. One example involves selenium deficiency as assessed by maternal blood concentrations (Al-Kunani et al, 2001).

Overeating combined with lack of exercise may lead to excessive deposition of body fat, anovulation, and infertility. Obese females (BMI ≥29) who smoke are more likely to take longer to conceive, although females who are obese but do not smoke do not take longer to conceive than normal-weight females (Bolumar et al, 1997).

Elevated plasma homocysteine concentrations and vitamin B_{12} deficiencies are associated with infertility and recurrent fetal loss (Bennett, 2001; Nelen et al, 2000). Elevated lipid peroxidation with decreased concentrations of vitamin A, E, and β-carotene have also been demonstrated in females with habitual spontaneous abortions (Simsek et al, 1998).

Caffeine has been associated with infertility in healthy females. Daily consumption by females of caffeine greater than the amount in one cup of coffee (or three cans of caffeinated soda) was associated with a 50% lower conception rate in a given menstrual cycle than for females who consumed less caffeine (Christianson et al, 1989). More recent evidence supports the association between caffeinated coffee consumption and delayed conception but raises issues about whether caffeine intake is related to other job- and life-related stress variables (Bolumar et al, 1997).

SUMMARY

The Dietary Guidelines for Americans provide an appropriate base for counseling females of reproductive age (see Chapter 15), but a continued focus on individualized counseling is still needed. Whether defined problems are attributable to lack of resources, lack of nutrition knowledge, self-imposed dietary manipulations, genetic individuality, or a combination of these factors, solutions to defined problems can often be found. Although the value of nutritional counseling may not be immediately measurable, the ultimate result may be improved preparation for reproduction.

Clinical Scenario 1

Melissa is a 15-year-old who is in the twelfth week of her first pregnancy. She is 5 ft, 5 inches tall and weighs 120 lb. Her prepregnancy weight was 118 lb. Her diet history reveals that she does not have a regular eating pattern, and her meals usually consist of convenience foods and carbonated beverages. She is not married and still living with her parents. The physician has prescribed a prenatal vitamin, mineral supplement, and nutrition counseling. Her hemoglobin and hematocrit values are within normal limits.

1. What weight gain goals would you give this pregnant adolescent?
2. What nutritional advice would you give Melissa for a healthy pregnancy?
3. How would you design an eating plan that Melissa can follow?
4. Which complications might occur during Melissa's pregnancy?

Clinical Scenario 2

Tina is a 40-year old who abuses intravenous drugs and alcohol. While in rehabilitation last year, she became pregnant and is now at 26 weeks gestation. She is thrilled about her pregnancy, knowing that she is carrying twins. She is currently using drugs and alcohol again but wants to stop. The perinatologist referred her to you because she wants to discuss breast-feeding.

1. What are Tina's risks during this pregnancy?
2. What are the risks for Tina's two fetuses?
3. What advice would you give her about breast-feeding?

Clinical Scenario 3

Claire is a 23-year-old woman who has a 2-year-old child and a 10-day-old infant. She has come to the WIC clinic for certification as a breast-feeding mother. She is breast-feeding her infant every 3 hours but is concerned that he may not be getting enough milk. While with the nutritionist in the clinic, she begins to cry and talk about her sore nipples, profound fatigue, and worry. A 24-hour recall of foods eaten the day before reveal that Claire skipped breakfast and ate some microwaved meals for lunch and dinner.

The nutritionist asks permission to watch Claire nurse her infant. Because she is not supporting the infant's back and buttocks firmly, the infant tugs at the nipple and causes the soreness.

The nutritionist then weighs the infant and finds that he has already regained his birth weight.

1. What would you say to Claire regarding her concern that her son may not be getting enough milk?
2. What would you recommend to improve the infant's position during nursing? How would this improve the nursing experience?
3. What advice would you give Claire about her fatigue?
4. How would you design an eating plan that Claire could follow?

■ Relevant Web Sites

Agency for Toxic Substances and Disease Registry
www.atsdr.cdc.gov/tfacts17.html
Centers for Disease Control and Prevention
www.cdc.gov/ncidod/dbmd/diseaseinfo/listeriosis
Food and Drug Administration, Center for Food Safety and Applied Nutrition
www.cfsan.fda.gov/~dms/admehg.html

■ Cited References

Agency for Toxic Substances and Disease Registry: *Polychlorinated biphenyls (PCBs)*, 2001, http://www.atsdr.cdc.gov/tfacts17.html

Al-Kunani AS et al: The selenium status of women with a history of recurrent miscarriage, *Br J Obstet Gynecol* 108:1094, 2001.

American Academy of Pediatrics, Committee on Drugs: The transfer of drugs and other chemicals into human milk, *Pediatrics* 108:776, 2001.

American Academy of Pediatrics, Committee on Pediatric AIDS: Human milk, breast-feeding, and transmission of human immunodeficiency virus in the United States (RE9542), *Pediatrics* 96:977, 1995.

American College of Obstetrics and Gynecology: Exercise during pregnancy and the postpartum period, ACOG Tech Bull No 267, *Obstet Gynecol* 99:171, 2002.

American College of Obstetrics and Gynecology: *Hypertension in pregnancy*, ACOG Tech Bull No 219, January 1996, ACOG.

American Dietetic Association: Position of the American Dietetic Association: promotion and support of breast-feeding, *J Am Diet Assoc* 97:662, 1997.

Barker DJP: Fetal origins of coronary heart disease, *BMJ* 311:171, 1995.

Bennett M: Vitamin B_{12} deficiency, infertility, and recurrent fetal loss, *J Reprod Med* 46:209, 2001.

Bernstein IM et al: Morbidity and mortality among very-low-birth-weight neonates with intrauterine growth restriction, *Am J Obstet Gynecol* 182:198, 2000.

Birch EE et al: A randomized controlled trial of long-chain polyunsaturated fatty acid supplementation of formula in term infants after weaning at 6 weeks of age, *Am J Clin Nutr* 75:570, 2002.

Bolto LD et al: Periconceptual multivitamin use and the occurrence of conotruncal heart defects: results from a population-based case control study, *Pediatrics* 98:911, 1996.

Bolumar F et al: Caffeine intake and delayed conception: a European multicenter study on infertility and subfecundity, *Am J Epidemiol* 145:324, 1997.

Brost BC et al: The Preterm Prediction Study: association of cesarean delivery with increases in maternal weight and body mass index, *Am J Obstet Gynecol* 179:333, 1997.

Brown JE, Toma RB: Taste changes during pregnancy, *Am J Clin Nutr* 43:414, 1986.

Brown JE et al: Predictors of red cell folate level in women attempting pregnancy, *JAMA* 277:548, 1997.

Bucher HC et al: Effect of calcium supplementation on pregnancy-induced hypertension and preeclampsia, *JAMA* 275:1113, 1996.

Casanueva E et al: Vitamin C status, cervico-vaginal infections and premature rupture of amniotic membranes, *Arch Med Res* 26:S149, 1995.

Canlfield LE et al: Determinants of gestational weight gain outside the recommended ranges among black and white women, *Obstet Gynecol* 87:760, 1996.

Centers for Disease Control and Prevention: *Listerosis*, 2001, http://www.cdc.gov/ncidod/dbmd/diseaseinfo/listeriosis

Centers for Disease Control and Prevention: Recommendations for use of folic acid to reduce the number of cases of spina bifida and other neural tube defects, *MMWR* 41:1, 1992.

Chang SJ: Antimicrobial proteins of maternal and cord sera and human milk in relation to maternal nutritional status, *Am J Clin Nutr* 51:183, 1990.

Chappell LC et al: Effect of antioxidants on the occurrence of preeclampsia in women at increased risk: a randomized trial, *Lancet* 354:810, 1999.

Chen DC et al: Stress during labor and delivery and early lactation performance, *Am J Clin Nutr* 68:335, 1998.

Cherian G, Sim JS: Changes in the breast milk fatty acids and plasma lipids of nursing mothers following consumption of *n*-3 polyunsaturated fatty acid-enriched eggs, *Nutrition* 12:8, 1996.

Christianson RE et al: Caffeinated beverages and decreased fertility, *Lancet* 1:378, 1989.

Clapp JF: Exercise in pregnancy—good, bad, or indifferent? In Lee RV et al, eds: *Current obstetric medicine, vol 3*, p 4, Chicago, 1993, CV Mosby.

Clapp JF, Little KD: Effect of recreational exercise on pregnancy weight gain and subcutaneous fat deposition, *Med Sci Sports Exerc* 27:170, 1995.

Clausen T et al: High intake of energy, sucrose, and polyunsaturated fatty acids is associated with increased risk of preeclampsia, *Am J Obstet Gynecol* 185:451, 2001.

Cnattingius S et al: Prepregnancy weight and the risk of adverse pregnancy outcomes, *N Engl J Med* 337:147, 1998.

Cnattingius S et al: Caffeine intake and the risk of first-trimester spontaneous abortion, *N Engl J Med* 343:1839, 2000.

Cogswell ME et al: Cigarette smoking, alcohol use, and adverse pregnancy outcomes: implications for micronutrient supplementation, *J Nutr* 133:1722S, 2003.

Cousins L: The California Diabetes and Pregnancy Program: a statewide collaborative program for the preconception and prenatal care of diabetic women, *Clin Obstet Gynecol* 5:443, 1991.

Crawford MA: The role of essential fatty acids in neural development: implications for perinatal nutrition, *Am J Clin Nutr* 57:703, 1993.

Czeizel AE et al: Pregnancy outcomes in a randomized controlled trial of periconceptional multivitamin supplementation, *Arch Gynecol Obstet* 255:131, 1994.

Daaboul J et al: Vitamin D deficiency in pregnant and breastfeeding women and their infants, *J Perinatol* 17:10, 1997.

Dahle LO et al: The effect of oral magnesium substitution on pregnancy-induced leg cramps, *Am J Obstet Gynecol* 173:175, 1995.

Dewey KG, McCrory MA: Effects of dieting and physical activity on pregnancy and lactation, *Am J Clin Nutr* 59(suppl):446, 1994.

Dewey KG et al: Maternal weight-loss patterns during prolonged lactation, *Am J Clin Nutr* 58:162, 1993.

Dewey KG et al: A randomized study of the effects of aerobic exercise by lactating women on breast-milk volume and composition, *N Engl J Med* 330:449, 1994.

Dusdieker LB et al: Is milk production impaired by dieting during lactation? *Am J Clin Nutr* 59:833, 1994.

Ebrahim GJ: The baby friendly hospital initiative (editorial), *J Trop Pediatr* 39:2, 1993.

Edwards LE et al: Pregnancy complications and birth outcomes in obese and normal-weight women: effects of gestational weight change, *Obstet Gynecol* 87:389, 1996.

Erick M: Battling morning (noon and night) sickness: new approaches for an age-old problem, *J Am Diet Assoc* 94:147, 1994.

Erick M: Hyperolfaction and hyperemesis gravidarum: what is the relationship? *Nutr Rev* 53:289, 1995.

Eustace LW et al: Fetal alcohol syndrome: a growing concern for health professionals, *J Obstet Gynecol Neonatal Nurs* 32:215, 2003.

Fairweather-Tait SJ: Iron-zinc and calcium-iron interactions in relation to zinc and iron absorption, *Proc Nutri Soc* 54:465, 1995.

Fleming A: The role of folate in the prevention of neural tube defects: human and animal studies, *Nutri Rev* 59(supp):13, 2001.

Food and Drug Administration, Center for Food Safety and Applied Nutrition: *Consumer advisory,* 2001, http://www.cfsan.fda.gov/~dms/admehg.html

Forbes, GB. Vitamin D in pregnancy and the infantile hypercalcemic syndrome, *Pediatric Res* 13:1382, 1979.

Francois CA et al: Acute effects of dietary fatty acids on the fatty acids of human milk, *Am J Clin Nutr* 67:301, 1998.

Gindler J et al: Folic acid supplements during pregnancy and risk of miscarriage, *Lancet* 35:796, 2001.

Glinoer D: Feto-maternal repercussions of iodine deficiency in pregnancy. *Ann Endocrinol* (Paris) 64:37, 2003.

Goldenberg RL et al: The effect of zinc supplementation on pregnancy outcome, *JAMA* 274:463, 1995.

Grosso LM et al: Maternal caffeine intake and intrauterine growth retardation, *Epidemiology* 12:447, 2001.

Hamadani JD et al: Zinc supplementation during pregnancy and effects on mental development and behavior of infants: a follow-up study, *Lancet* 360:290, 2002.

Health Canada: *Advisory: information on mercury levels in fish,* 2001, http://www.hcsc/ca/english/archives/warnings/2001/2001.

Hook EB, Czeizel AE: Can terathanasia explain the protective effect of folic acid supplementation on birth defects? *Lancet* 350:513, 1997.

Institute of Medicine, Food and Nutrition Board: *Nutrition during pregnancy, Parts I and II,* Washington, DC, 1990, National Academy Press.

Institute of Medicine, Food and Nutrition Board: *Dietary reference intakes for calcium, phosphorus, magnesium, vitamin D, and fluoride,* Washington, DC, 1997, National Academy Press.

Institute of Medicine, Food and Nutrition Board: *Dietary reference intakes for dietary antioxidants and related compounds,* Washington, DC, 2000, National Academy Press.

Institute of Medicine, Food and Nutrition Board: *Dietary reference intakes for energy and the macronutrients, carbohydrate, fiber, fat, and fatty acids,* Washington, DC, 2002, National Academy Press.

Institute of Medicine, Food and Nutrition Board: *Dietary reference intakes for thiamin, riboflavin, niacin, vitamin B_6, folate, vitamin B_{12}, pantothenic acid, biotin, and choline,* Washington, DC, 1998, National Academy Press.

Institute of Medicine, Food and Nutrition Board: *Dietary reference intakes for vitamin A, vitamin K, arsenic, boron, chromium, copper, iodine, iron, manganese, molybdenum, nickel, silicon, vanadium, and zinc,* Washington, DC, 2001, National Academy Press.

Jewell D, Young G: Interventions for nausea and vomiting in early pregnancy, *Cochrane Database Syst Rev* 1:CD000145, 2002.

Johnston RB, Staples DA: Knowledge and use of folic acid by women of childbearing age—United States, 1997, *MMWR* 46:721, 1997.

Kalkwarf HJ, Specker BL: Bone mineral changes during pregnancy and lactation, *Endocrine* 1:49, 2002.

Kalkwarf HJ et al: The effect of calcium supplementation on bone density during lactation and after weaning, *N Engl J Med* 337:523, 1997.

Kharb S: Vitamin E and C in preeclampsia, *Eur J Obstet Gynecol Reprod Bio* 93:37, 2000.

Krebs NF: Zinc supplementation during lactation, *Am J Clin Nutr* 68(suppl 2):509, 1998.

Kuczmarski RJ et al: Increasing prevalence of overweight among U.S. adults: the National Health and Nutrition Examination Surveys 1960 to 1991, *JAMA* 272:205, 1994.

Lam PK et al: A low pregnancy body mass index is a risk factor for an offspring with gastroschisis, *Epidemiology* 10:717, 1999.

Leaf A, Weber PC: A new era for science in nutrition, *Am J Clin Nutr* 45:1048, 1987.

Levine R et al: Trial of calcium to prevent preeclampsia, *N Engl J Med* 337:69, 1997.

Life Sciences Research Office: Executive summary: assessment of nutrient requirements for infant formulas, *Am Soc Nutr Sci,* 1998.

Lucas M et al: A comparison of magnesium sulfate with phenytoin for the prevention of eclampsia, *N Engl J Med* 333:201, 1995.

Luke B et al: A consideration of height as a function of prepregnancy nutritional background and its potential influence on birth weight, *J Am Diet Assoc* 84:176, 1984.

Luke B: The changing pattern of multiple births in the United States: maternal and infant characteristics, 1973 and 1990, *Obstet Gynecol* 84:101, 1994.

McGregor JA et al: The omega-3 story: nutritional prevention of preterm birth and other adverse pregnancy outcomes, *Obstet Gynecol Surv* 56(5 suppl 1):1, 2001.

Magpie Trial Collaborative Group: Do women with pre-eclampsia and their babies benefit from magnesium sulphate? The Magpie Trial: a randomized placebo-controlled trial, *Lancet* 359: 1877, 2002.

Martin JA, Park MM, Sutton PD: Births: preliminary data for 2001, *Natl Vital Stat Rep* 6, 50:1, 2002.

Medical Research Council Vitamin Study Research Group: Prevention of neural tube defects: results of the Medical Research Council vitamin study, *Lancet* 338:131, 1991.

Mills JL et al: Vitamin A and birth defects, *Am J Obstet Gynecol* 177:31, 1997

Monique A et al: Fat intake of women during normal pregnancy—relationships with maternal and neonatal essential fatty acid status, *J Am Coll Nutr* 15:49, 1996.

Murtaugh MA, Weingart J: Individual nutrient effects on length of gestation and pregnancy outcome, *Semin Perinatol* 19:197, 1995.

Namgung R et al: Low total body bone mineral content and high bone resorption in Korean winter-born versus summer-born newborn infants, *J Pediatr* 132:421, 1998.

National Institute for Child Health and Human Development, National Institutes of Health: *Moderate doses of vitamin A do not pose risk of birth defects,* 2001, http://www.nichd.nih.gov//new/releases/vitama.cfm.

Nehlig A, Debry G: Potential teratogenic and neurodevelopmental consequences of coffee and caffeine exposure: a review of human and animal data, *Neurotox Teratol* 16:531, 1994.

Nelen WL et al: Hyperhomocysteinemia and recurrent early pregnancy loss: a meta-analysis, *Fertil Steril* 74:1196; 2000.

Olsen SF et al: Frequency of seafood intake in pregnancy as a determinant of birth weight: evidence for a dose-dependant relationship, *J Epidemiol Comm Hlth* 47:436, 1993.

Owen AL, Owen GM: Twenty years of WIC: a review of some effects of the program, *J Am Diet Assoc* 97:777, 1997.

Palan PR et al: Placental and serum levels of carotenoids in preeclampsia, *Obstet Gynecol* 98:459, 2001.

Panesar NS et al: Are thyroid hormones or hCG responsible for hyperemesis gravidarum? A matched paired study in pregnant Chinese women, *Acta Obstet Gynecol Scan* 80:519, 2001.
Pugliese MT et al: Nutritional rickets in suburbia, *J Am Coll Nutr* 17:637, 1998.
Rainville A: Pica practices of pregnant women are associated with lower maternal hemoglobin level at delivery, *J Am Diet Assoc* 98:293, 1998.
Revelli A et al: Exercise and pregnancy: a review of maternal and fetal effects, *Obstet Gynecol Surv* 47(6):355, 1992.
Roberts A et al: Sucralose metabolism and pharmacokinetics in man, *Food Chem Toxicol* 30(suppl 2):31, 2000.
Roberts J: Magnesium for preeclampsia and eclampsia, *N Engl J Med* 333:250, 1995.
Rosett HL et al: Treatment experience with pregnant problem drinkers, *JAMA* 249:2029, 1983.
Ross SA et al: Retinoids in embryonal development, *Physiol Rev* 80:1021, 2000.
Sahakian V et al: Vitamin B_6 is effective therapy for nausea and vomiting of pregnancy: a randomized, double-blind, placebo controlled study, *Obstet Gynecol* 78:33, 1991.
Schieve LA et al: Prepregnancy body mass index and pregnancy weight gain: associations with preterm delivery, the NMIHS Collaborative Study Group, *Obstet Gynecol* 96:194, 2000.
Scholl TO et al: Dietary and serum folate: their influence on the outcome of pregnancy, *Am J Clin Nutr* 63:520, 1996.
Scholl TO et al: Maternal glucose concentration influences fetal growth, gestation, and pregnancy complications, *Am J Epidemiol* 154:514, 2001.
Shaw GM et al: Risk of neural tube defect–affected pregnancies among obese women, *JAMA* 275:1093, 1996.
Sian L et al: Zinc homeostasis during lactation in a population with a low zinc intake, *Am J Clin Nutr* 75:99, 2002.
Simsek M et al: Blood plasma levels of lipoperoxides, glutathione peroxidase, β-carotene, vitamin A and E in women with habitual abortion, *Cell Biochem Funct* 16:227, 1998.
Smith GFD: Effects of the state of nutrition of the mother during pregnancy and labour on the condition of the child at birth and for the first few days of life, *Lancet* 2:54, 1916.
Solomon CG, Seely EW: Brief review: hypertension in pregnancy: a manifestation of the insulin resistance syndrome? *Hypertension* 37:232, 2001.
Story M, ed: *Nutrition management of the pregnant adolescent,* Washington, DC, 1990, March of Dimes Birth Defects Foundation, National Clearing House, U.S. Department of Agriculture and Health and Human Services.
Streissguth AP et al: Comparison of drinking and smoking patterns during pregnancy over a six-year interval, *Am J Obstet Gynecol* 145:716, 1983.
Streissguth AP et al: Teratogenic effects of alcohol in humans and laboratory animals, *Science* 209:353, 1980.
Stephansson O et al: Maternal weight, pregnancy weight gain, and the risk of antepartum stillbirth, *Am J Obstet Gynecol* 184:463, 2001.
Susser M, Smith Z: Timing in prenatal nutrition: a reprise of the Dutch Famine Study, *Nutr Rev* 52:84, 1994.
Waiters B et al: Perinatal vitamin D and calcium status of northern Canadian mothers and their newborn infants, *J Am Coll Nutr* 18:122, 1999.
Wallace JP et al: Infant acceptance of postexercise breast milk, *Pediatrics* 89:1245, 1992.
Watkins ML, Botto LD: Maternal prepregnancy weight and congenital heart defects in the offspring, *Epidemiology* 11:439, 2001.
Werler MM et al: Prepregnant weight in relation to risk of neural tube defects, *JAMA* 275:1089, 1996.
Woods JR: Reactive oxygen species and premature rupture of membranes: a review, *Placenta Tropht Res* 15 (suppl A): 38, 2001.
Worthington-Roberts BS, Williams SR: Nutrition in pregnancy and lactation, 5th ed, St. Louis, 1993, Mosby.
Xue-Yi C et al: Timing of vulnerability of the brain to iodine deficiency in endemic cretinism, *N Engl J Med* 331:1739, 1994.
Young GL, Jewell D: Interventions for leg cramps in pregnancy, *Cochrane Database Syst Rev* CD000121, 2000.
Zittermann A: Effects of vitamin K on calcium and bone metabolism, *Curr Opin Clin Nutr Metab Care* 4:483, 2001.
Zlatnick FJ, Burmeister LF: Dietary protein in pregnancy: effect on anthropometric indices of the newborn infant, *Am J Obstet Gynecol* 146:199, 1983.
Zuger A: Alcohol consumption among pregnant and childbearing-aged women: United States, 1991 and 1995, *MMWR* 46:346, 1997.

Additional References

Allen LH, ed: Recent developments in maternal nutrition and their implication for practitioners, *Am J Clin Nutr* 59(suppl 2), 1994.
American Dietetic Association: Position of The American Dietetic Association: nutrition care for pregnant adolescents, *J Am Diet Assoc* 94:450, 1994.
Bagwell J et al: Knowledge and attitudes toward breast-feeding: differences among dietitians, nurses, and physicians working with WIC clients, *J Am Diet Assoc* 93:801, 1993.
Barclay B: Experience with enteral nutrition in the treatment of hyperemesis gravidarum, *Nutr Clin Pract* 4:153, 1990.
Barrett J et al: Absorption of non-heme iron from food during normal pregnancy, *Br Med J* 309:79, 1994.
Benke PJ: The isotretinoin teratogen syndrome, *JAMA* 251:3267, 1984.
Bunin G et al: Relation between maternal diet and subsequent primitive neuroectodermal brain tumors in young children, *N Engl J Med* 329:536, 1993.
Dewey KG, McCrory MA: Effects of dieting and physical activity on pregnancy and lactation, *Am J Clin Nutr* 59(suppl):446, 1994.
Duque AG: The role of lipids in fetal brain development, *Perinatol Nutr Rep* Spring:4, 1997.
Durnin JVGA: *Energy requirements of pregnancy: an integration of the longitudinal data from the 5-country study,* Nestle Foundation Annual Report, Lausanne, Switzerland, 1986, Nestle Foundation.
Erick M: *No more morning sickness,* New York, NY, 1993, Penguin Books.
Eskes TKAB: Open or closed? A world of difference: a history of homocysteine research, *Nutr Rev* 56:236, 1998.
Fly AD et al: Major mineral concentrations in human milk do not change after maximal exercise testing, *Am J Clin Nutr* 68:345, 1998.
Fraser A et al: Association of young maternal age with adverse reproductive outcomes, *J Am Diet Assoc* 332:1113, 1995.
Freed G et al: National assessment of physicians' breast-feeding knowledge, attitudes, training, and experience, *JAMA* 273:472, 1995.
Frequent alcohol consumption among women of childbearing age: Behavioral Risk Factor Surveillance System, *MMWR* 48:328, 1994.
Glenn FB et al: Fluoride tablet supplementation during pregnancy for caries immunity: a study of the offspring produced, *Am J Obstet Gynecol* 143:560, 1982.
Grummer-Strawn L: Does prolonged breast-feeding impair child growth? *Pediatrics* 91:766, 1993.
Harsham J et al: Growth patterns of infants exposed to cocaine and other drugs in utero, *J Am Diet Assoc* 94:999, 1994.
Hatch et al: Maternal exercise during pregnancy, physical fitness, and fetal growth, *Am J Epidemiol* 137:1105, 1993.
Hilson J et al: Maternal obesity and breast-feeding success in a rural population of white women, *Am J Clin Nutr* 66:1371, 1997.
Huggins K, Ziedrich L: *The nursing mother's guide to weaning,* Boston, 1994, The Harvard Common Press, 1994.
Institute of Medicine, Food and Nutrition Board: *Nutrition during lactation,* Washington, DC, 1991, National Academy Press.
Krebs N et al: Bone mineral density changes during lactation: maternal, dietary, and biochemical correlates, *Am J Clin Nutr* 65:1738, 1997.
Kritz-Silverstein D et al: Relation of pregnancy history to insulin levels in older, nondiabetic women, *Am J Epidemiol* 140:375, 1994.

Lenders C et al: Gestational age and infant size at birth are associated with dietary sugar intake among pregnant adolescents, *J Nutr* 127:1113, 1997.

Mackey A et al: Self-selected diets of lactating women often fail to meet dietary recommendations, *J Am Diet Assoc* 98:297, 1998.

Mannan S, Picciano MF: Influence of maternal selenium status on human milk selenium concentration and glutathione peroxidase activity, *Am J Clin Nutr* 46:95, 1987.

Mills J et al: Moderate caffeine use and the risk of spontaneous abortion and intrauterine growth retardation, *JAMA* 269:593, 1993.

Oakley GP, Erickson JO: Vitamin A and birth defects (editorial), *N Engl J Med* 333:1414, 1995.

Pettit D et al: Comparison of World Health Organization and National Diabetes Group procedure to detect abnormalities of glucose tolerance during pregnancy, *Diabetes Care* 17:1264, 1994.

Sharma M, Petosa R: Impact of expectant fathers in breast-feeding decisions, *J Am Diet Assoc* 97:1311, 1997.

Smithells RW et al: Further experience of vitamin supplementation for prevention of neural tube defect recurrences, *Lancet* 1:1027, 1983.

Stacy L, Mizumoto D: *Breast-feeding: nature's best for you and your baby*, Chicago, 1993, American Dietetic Association.

Strode MA et al: Effects of short-term caloric restriction on lactational performance of well-nourished women, *Acta Paediatr Scand* 75:222, 1986.

Wolfe H: High prepregnancy body-mass index—a maternal-fetal risk factor (Editorial), *N Engl J Med* 338:191, 1998.

Wolfe L, Mottola M: Aerobic exercise in pregnancy: an update, *Can J Appl Physiol* 18:119, 1993.

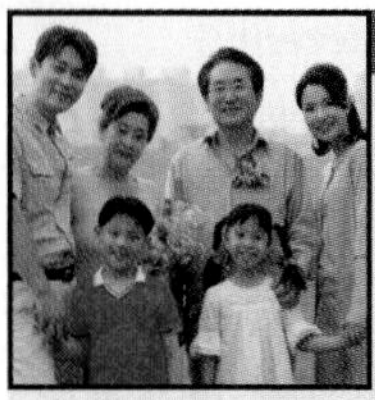

CHAPTER 8

Nutrition During Infancy

CRISTINE M. TRAHMS, MS, RD, CD, FADA

CHAPTER OUTLINE

- Physiologic Development
- Nutrient Requirements
- Milk
- Food
- Feeding

KEY TERMS

arachidonic acid (AA)–a very-long-chain fatty acid (C20:4*n*-6), known to be a derivative of linoleic acid, that is found in breast milk

casein–the principal protein in cow's milk

casein hydrolysate–casein that has been split into smaller components by acid, alkali, or enzymes

catch-up–the growth phenomenon in the first year of life that occurs when the rate of growth increases to the genetic potential

colic–severe abdominal pain in infants

docosahexaenoic acid (DHA)–a very-long-chain fatty acid (C22:6*n*-3), known to be a derivative of linolenic acids, that is found in breast milk

electrolytically reduced iron–iron that has been fractionated into small particles for improved absorption; used in the fortification of foods

hemorrhagic disease of the newborn–a self-limiting hemorrhagic disorder that develops during the first few days of life and is caused by a vitamin K deficiency; develops more frequently in breast-fed infants than in formula-fed infants

lactalbumin–an easy-to-digest protein found in human milk

lag-down–the growth phenomenon in the first year of life that occurs when the rate of growth decreases to the genetic potential

palmar grasp–an immature way of holding an object with the palm

pincer grasp–a more refined and mature way (than the palmar grasp) of holding an object with the fingers

renal solute load–the amount of nitrogenous waste and minerals that must be excreted by the kidney

whey proteins–the proteins remaining in the watery fraction of milk after the curd and cream have been removed, contains lactalbumin

During the first 2 years of life, which are characterized by rapid physical and social growth and development, many changes occur that affect feeding and nutrient intake. The adequacy of infants' nutrient intakes affects their interaction with their environment. Healthy, well-nourished infants have the energy to respond to and learn from the stimuli in their environment and to interact with their parents and caregivers in a manner that encourages bonding and attachment.

PHYSIOLOGIC DEVELOPMENT

The length of gestation, the mother's prepregnancy weight, and the mother's weight gain during gestation determine an infant's birth weight. After birth, the growth of an infant is influenced by genetics and nourishment (Figure 8-1). Most infants who are genetically determined to be larger reach their growth channel between 3 and 6 months of age. However, many infants born at or below the 10th percentile for height may not reach their appropriate growth channel until 1 year of age. Larger infants at birth who are genetically determined to be smaller grow at their fetal rate for several months and often do not reach their growth channel until 13 months of age (Smith et al, 1976).

Infants lose weight during the first few days of life, but their birth weight is usually regained by the seventh to tenth day. Growth thereafter proceeds at a rapid but decelerating rate. Infants usually double their birth weight by 4 to 6 months of age and triple it by the age of 1 year. The amount of weight gained by the infant during the second year approximates the birth weight. Infants increase their length by 50% during the first year of life and double it by 4 years. Total body fat increases rapidly during the first 9 months, after which the rate of fat gain tapers off throughout the rest of childhood. Total body water decreases throughout infancy from 70% at birth to 60% at 1 year. The decrease is almost all in extracellular water, which declines from 42% at birth to 32% at 1 year of age (see Figure 6-1).

The stomach capacity of infants increases from a range of 10 to 20 ml at birth to 200 ml by 1 year, enabling infants to consume more food at a given time and at less frequent intervals as they grow older. During the first weeks of life, gastric acidity decreases and for the first few months remains lower than that of older infants and adults. The rate of emptying is relatively slow, depending on the size and composition of the meal.

Although gastric secretion of pepsin remains low during the first 3 months of life, it is not a limiting factor for protein digestion. Trypsin activity in duodenal fluids is lower in infants than in older children, as is the activity of *enterokinase* (the enzyme responsible for the activation of trypsin) (see Chapter 1). However, the enzymatic activity is sufficient to digest the milk protein that infants normally consume.

Fat absorption varies in the neonate. Human milk fat is well absorbed, but butterfat is poorly absorbed, with fecal excretions of 20% to 48%. The fat combinations in commercially prepared infant formula are well absorbed. Human milk contains two lipases; one of them, which is found in the lipid fraction of milk, is essential for the milk lipid formation in the mammary gland but is of no known nutritional importance to the infant. The other lipase—*bile-stimulated lipase*—hydrolyzes triglycerides into three fatty acids and glycerol. The infant's lingual and gastric lipases hydrolyze short- and medium-chain fatty acids in the stomach. Gastric lipase also hydrolyzes long-chain fatty acids.

Most long-chain triglycerides pass unhydrolyzed into the small intestine, where they are broken down by pancreatic lipase; the bile salt–stimulated lipase in human milk, which is stimulated by the infant's bile salts, hydrolyzes the triglycerides in the small intestine. Bile salts, which are effective emulsifiers when combined with monoglycerides, fatty acids, and lecithin, aid in the intestinal digestion of fat.

The activities of the enzymes responsible for the digestion of disaccharides—maltase, isomaltase, and sucrase—reach adult levels by 28 to 32 weeks of gestation. Lactase activity (responsible for digesting the disaccharide in milk) increases near birth and reaches adult levels by birth, whereas pancreatic amylase, which digests starch, continues to remain low during the first 6 months after birth. If the infant consumes starch before this time, increased activity of salivary amylase and digestion in the colon usually compensate.

The neonate has functional but physiologically immature kidneys that increase in size and concentrating capacity in the early weeks of life. The kidneys double in weight by 6 months and triple in weight by 1 year of age. The last renal tubule is estimated to form between the eighth fetal month and the end of the first postnatal month. The glomerular tuft is covered by a much thicker layer of cells throughout neonatal life than at any later time, which may explain why the glomerular filtration rate is lower during the first 9 months of life than it is in later childhood and adulthood. In the neonatal period the ability to form acid urine and concentrate solutes is often limited. The renal concentrating capacity at birth may be limited to as little as 700 mOsm/L in some infants. Others have the concentrating capacity of adults (1200 to 1400 mOsm/L). By 6 weeks, most infants can concentrate urine at adult levels. Renal function in a normal newborn infant is rarely a concern; however, difficulties may arise in infants with diarrhea or those who are fed formula that is too concentrated.

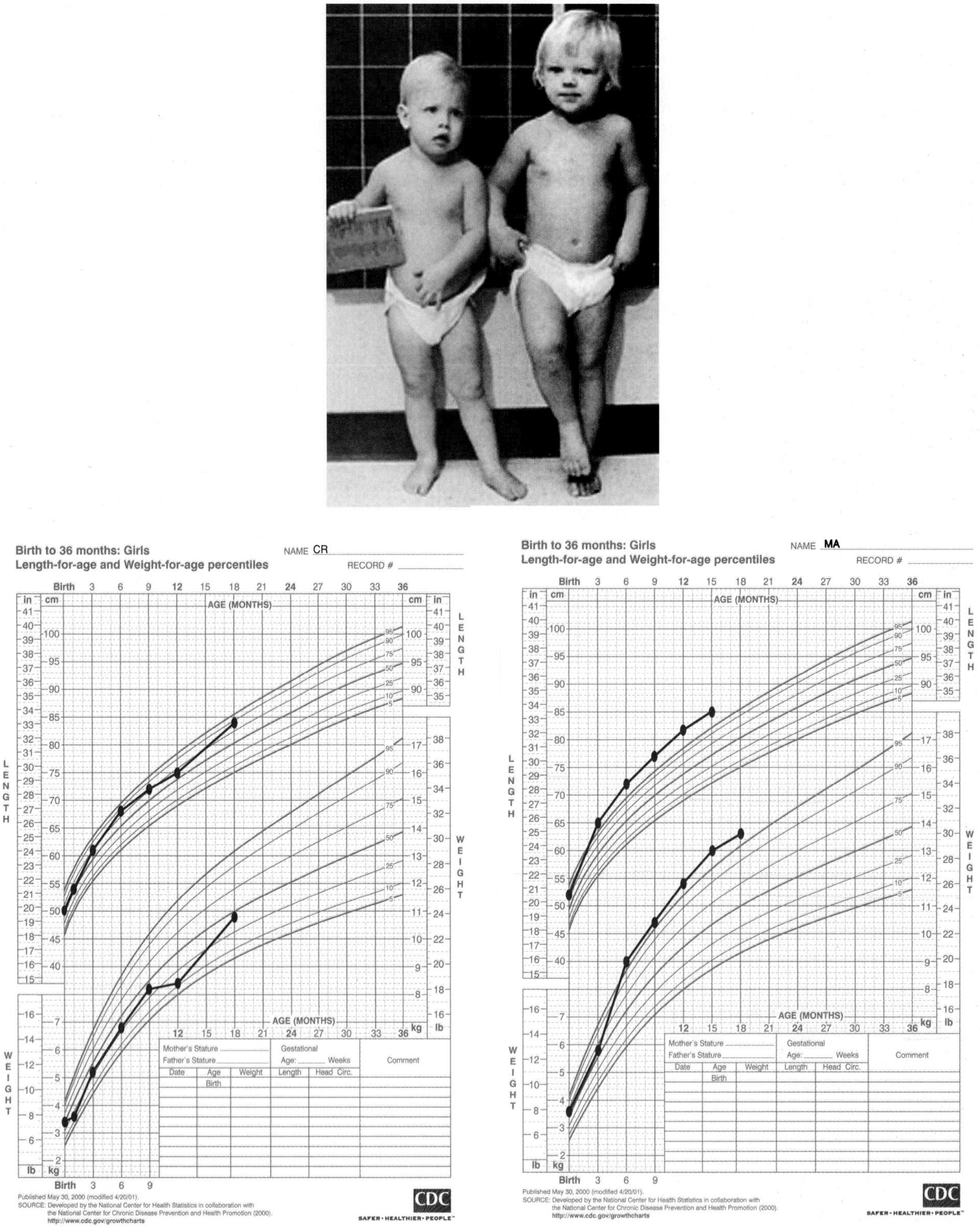

FIGURE 8-1 • Two girls born just 1 month apart with only a 1-lb difference in birth weight; note the marked difference in growth. (The girls are approximately 20 months of age.) In the growth chart, note M.A.'s early catch-up growth to above the 95th percentile for height and weight by 6 months of age. In addition, note the effect of an illness on C.R.'s weight gain and linear growth at the age of 12 months, as well as the subsequent catch-up growth. (Data from The National Center for Health Statistics, in collaboration with the National Center for Chronic Disease Prevention and Health Promotion, 2000, http://www.cdc.gov/growthcharts.)

NUTRIENT REQUIREMENTS

Nutrient needs of infants reflect rates of growth, energy expended in activity, basal metabolic needs, and the interaction of the nutrients consumed. Balance studies have defined minimal acceptable levels of intakes for a few nutrients, but for most nutrients the suggested intakes have been extrapolated from the intakes of normal, thriving infants. The dietary reference intakes (DRIs) for infants are shown in Table 8-1.

Energy

Full-term infants who are breast-fed to satiety and infants who are fed a standard 20-kcal/oz formula generally adjust their intake to meet their energy needs when caregivers are sensitive to the infants' hunger and satiety cues. An effective method for determining the adequacy of an infant's energy intake is to carefully monitor gains in weight, length, and weight-for-length for age and to plot these data on the growth charts shown in Appendix Tables 6, 7, 9, and 10. It is important to recognize that during the first year, a catch-up or lag-down period in growth may occur.

If infants begin to experience a decrease in their rate of weight gain, do not gain weight, or lose weight, their energy and nutrient intake should be monitored carefully. If the rate of growth in length decreases or ceases, potential malnutrition, an undetected disease, or both should be investigated thoroughly. If the

TABLE 8-1 Dietary Reference Intakes: Adequate Intakes and Recommended Dietary Allowances for Infants and Children from Birth to 3 Years

NUTRIENT (AMOUNT/DAY)	AGE		
	BIRTH-6 MO	6 MO-1 YR	1-3 YR
Protein (g)	9.1	13.5	13
Energy (kcal)	M:570 F:520	M:743 F:676	M:1046 F:992
Carbohydrate (g)	60	95	M:130* F:130*
Fiber (g)	ND	ND	19
Total fat (g)	31	30	ND
n-6 Polyunsaturated fatty acids [omega-6, linoleic] (g)	4.4	4.6	7
n-3 Polyunsaturated fatty acids [omega-3, linolenic] (g)	0.5	0.5	0.7
Vitamin A (μg)†	400	500	300*
Vitamin D (μg)‡	5	5	5
Vitamin E (mg)	4	5	6*
Vitamin K (μg)	2	2.5	30
Vitamin C (mg)	40	50	15*
Thiamin (mg)	0.2	0.3	0.5*
Riboflavin (mg)	0.3	0.4	0.5*
Niacin (mg)§	2	4	6*
Vitamin B6 (mg)	0.1	0.3	0.5*
Folate (μg)¶	65	80	150*
Vitamin B_{12} (μg)	0.4	0.5	0.9*
Pantothenic acid (mg)	1.7	1.8	2
Biotin (μg)	5	6	8
Choline (mg)	125	150	200
Calcium (mg)	210	270	500*
Phosphorus (mg)	100	275	460*
Magnesium (mg)	30	75	80*
Iron (mg)	0.27	11*	7*
Zinc (mg)	2	3*	3*
Iodine (μg)	110	130	90*
Selenium (μg)	15	20	20*
Fluoride (mg)	0.01	0.5	0.7
Manganese (mg)	0.003	0.6	1.2
Molybdenum (μg)	2	3	17*
Chromium (μg)	0.2	5.5	11
Copper (μg)	200	220	340*

Data from Institute of Medicine, Food and Nutrition Board: *Dietary reference intakes: vitamins,* January 2002, Washington, DC, http://www4.nationalacademies.org/iom/iomhome.nsf/WFiles/webtablevitamins/$file/webtablevitamins.pdf; Institute of Medicine, Food and Nutrition Board: *Dietary reference intakes: elements,* Washington, DC, January 2002, http://www4.nationalacademies.org/iom/iomhome.nsf/WFiles/webtableminerals/$file/webtableminerals.pdf; and Institute of Medicine, Food and Nutrition Board: *Dietary reference intakes: energy, carbohydrates, fiber, protein, and amino acids (macronutrients),* Washington, DC, September 2002, http://books.nap.edu/books

*RDA. RDAs and AIs may both be used as goals for individual intakes. RDAs are set to meet the needs of almost all (98%) individuals in a group. For healthy breast-fed infants, the AI is the mean intake. An AI is set instead of an RDA if there is insufficient data to set an RDA.

†Retinol activity equivalents (REA): 1 REA = 1 μg retinol = 12 μg β-carotene = 24 μg α-carotene.

‡1 μg calciferol = 40 IU vitamin D.

§Niacin equivalents (NE): 1 mg niacin = 60 mg tryptophan; for 0-6 months value is preformed niacin (not NE).

¶Dietary folate equivalents (DFE): 1 DFE = 1 μg food folate = 0.6 μg folate from fortified food.

weight gain proceeds at a much more rapid rate than growth in length, the energy concentration of the formula, the quantity of formula consumed, and the amount and type of semisolid and table foods offered should be evaluated. The activity level of the infant should also be assessed.

Formula-fed infants consume more kilocalories of energy per unit of body size than breast-fed infants during the first year. Gains in weight are greater in formula-fed infants, as are increases in body mass per gram of protein intake. However, no functional advantage has been ascribed to the more rapid growth rate (Dewey et al, 1993; Heinig et al, 1993).

Protein

Protein is needed for tissue replacement and growth. Protein requirements during the rapid growth of infancy are higher per kilogram of weight than those for adults or older children. Recommendations for protein intake are based on the composition of human milk, and it is assumed that the efficiency of human milk use is 100%. Table 8-1 lists the protein DRIs for children from birth to 3 years of age.

Infants require a larger percentage of total amino acids as essential amino acids than do adults. Histidine seems to be an essential amino acid for infants but not for adults. Tyrosine, cystine, and taurine may be essential for premature infants.

Human milk or formula provides the major portion of protein during the first year of life. The amount of protein in human milk is adequate for the first 6 months of the infant's life, even though the amount of protein in human milk is considerably less than in infant formula. In the last 6 months of the first year, diets of infants should be supplemented with additional sources of high-quality protein such as yogurt, strained meats, or cereal mixed with formula or milk.

Infants whose formula is excessively diluted because of a prolonged regimen designed to treat diarrhea after an enteric illness or who have multiple food allergies may receive inadequate amounts of protein.

Lipids

The current recommendation for infants younger than 1 year of age is to consume a minimum of 30 g of fat per day. This quantity is present in human milk and all infant formulas. Significantly lower fat intakes (e.g., with skim-milk feedings) may result in an inadequate total energy intake. An infant may try to correct the energy deficit by increasing the volume of milk ingested but usually cannot make up the entire deficit this way.

Human milk contains a generous amount of the essential fatty acids linoleic acid and linolenic acid, as well as the longer-chain derivatives arachidonic acid (AA) and docosahexaenoic acid (DHA), which are found in large amounts in the retina of the eye and the brain. Many infant formulas are supplemented with linoleic acid and linolenic acid, from which AA and DHA are derived.

TABLE 8-2 Linoleic Acid Content of Selected Infant Formulas

FORMULA	LINOLEIC ACID (mg per 100 kcal energy)
Alimentum (Ross)	1900
Pregestimil (Mead Johnson)	1040
Isomil (Ross)	1000
Isomil 2 (Ross)	1000
Similac (Ross)	1000
Similac 2 (Ross)	1000
Alsoy (Carnation)	920
Enfamil (Mead Johnson)	860
Follow-Up Soy (Carnation)	860
LactoFree (Mead Johnson)	860
Prosobee (Mead Johnson)	860
Good Start (Carnation)	850
Nutramigen (Mead Johnson)	820
Next Step (Mead Johnson)	810
Next Step Soy (Mead Johnson)	720
Follow-Up (Carnation)	680

Linoleic acid, which is essential for growth and dermal integrity, should provide 3% of the infant's total kilocalories or 4.4 g/day for infants younger than 6 months of age and 4.6 g/day for infants 9 months to 1 year of age. Smaller amounts of *α-linolenic* acid, a precursor of the *n*-3 fatty acids DHA and eicosapentaenoic acid (EPA), should be included. The current recommendation is 0.5 g/day during the first year of life. Five percent of the kilocalories in human milk and 10% in most infant formulas are derived from linoleic acid. Table 8-2 indicates the linoleic acid content of infant formulas. Because DHA can be formed by desaturation of α-linolenic acid, the importance of dietary DHA intake is uncertain. In addition, the concentration of DHA in human milk varies depending on the amount of DHA in the mother's diet.

Recently the importance of *n*-3 fatty acids in infant visual and neurologic development has been studied. Although findings suggest that DHA facilitates early development of visual acuity in premature infants, studies with full-term infants are less clear. For example, randomized trials reveal that DHA supplementation increases visual acuity in infants who are fed formula (Birch et al, 1998; Carlson et al, 1996), but other studies have not found any effects (Auestad et al, 1997; Makrides et al, 2000; Scott et al, 2000). One study, in which DHA concentration was related to visual acuity at 2 months and 12 months of age, seems to suggest that factors other than breast-milk sources of DHA may be important (Innis, Gilley, and Werker, 2001.)

Carbohydrates

Carbohydrates should supply 30% to 60% of the energy intake during infancy. Thirty-seven percent of the energy in human milk and 40% to 50% of the energy in infant formulas is derived from lactose or

TABLE 8-3 Water Requirements of Infants and Children

AGE	WATER REQUIREMENT (ml/kg/day)
10 days	125-150
3 mo	140-160
6 mo	130-155
1 yr	120-135
2 yr	115-125
6 yr	90-100
10 yr	70-85
14 yr	50-60

From Barness LA: Nutrition and nutritional disorders. In Behrman RE, Kliegman RM: *Nelson textbook of pediatrics,* ed 17, Philadelphia, 2003, WB Saunders.

other carbohydrates. Although rare, some infants cannot tolerate lactose and require a special diet (see Chapters 30 and 45).

Botulism in infancy is caused by the ingestion of *Clostridium botulinum* spores, which germinate and produce toxin in the bowel lumen. Honey and corn syrup, occasionally used in home-prepared foods, have been identified as the only food sources of these spores in infants' diets. The spores are extremely resistant to heat treatment and are not destroyed by current methods of processing. Thus honey and corn syrup should not be fed to infants younger than 1 year of age because they have not yet developed the immunity required to resist botulism spore development.

Water

The water requirement for infants is determined by the amount lost from the skin and lungs and in the feces and urine, in addition to a small amount needed for growth. The National Research Council recommends an intake of 1.5 ml/kcal/day. Water requirements per kilogram of body weight are shown in Table 8-3.

Because the renal concentrating capacity of young infants may be less than that of older children and adults, they may be vulnerable to developing a water imbalance. Under ordinary conditions, human milk and formula that is properly prepared supply adequate amounts of water. However, when a formula is boiled, the water evaporates and the solutes become concentrated; therefore boiled milk or formulas are inappropriate for infants. In very hot, humid environments, infants may require additional water. When other than renal losses of water are high (e.g., in infants with vomiting and diarrhea), infants should be monitored carefully for any fluid electrolyte imbalance.

Water deficits result in *hypernatremic dehydration* and its associated neurologic consequences (e.g., seizures, vascular damage). Hypernatremic dehydration has been reported in breast-fed infants who had a weight loss of greater than 10% of their birth weight in the first few days of life. (Manganaro et al, 2001; Oddie, Richmond, and Coulthard, 2001). Because of the potential for hypernatremic dehydration, careful monitoring of volume of intake, weight gain, and hydration status (e.g., number of wet diapers) in all newborns is warranted.

Water intoxication results in hyponatremia, restlessness, nausea, vomiting, diarrhea, and polyuria or oliguria; seizures can also result. This condition may occur when water is provided as a replacement for milk, the formula is excessively diluted, or bottled water instead of an electrolyte solution is provided as treatment for diarrhea.

Minerals

Calcium

The previous RDA of 400 to 800 mg/day of calcium was set to meet the needs of infants fed cow's milk-based formula, who retain approximately 25% to 30% of the intake. This is not applicable to breast-fed infants, who retain approximately two thirds of their calcium intake. The recommended adequate intake (AI) of 210 mg/day is for infants ages 0 to 6 months and for infants ages 7 to 12 months the mean intake of healthy breast-fed infants.

Iron

Full-term infants are considered to have adequate stores of iron for enough growth to double their birth weight. This weight doubling occurs at approximately 4 months of age in full-term infants and much earlier in prematurely born infants. Recommended intakes of iron increase depending on age, growth rate, and iron stores. At 4 to 6 months of age, infants who are fed only breast milk are at risk for developing a negative iron balance and may deplete their reserves by 6 to 9 months (Kim et al, 1996). Iron in human milk is highly bioavailable; however, breast-fed and formula-fed infants should receive an additional source of iron by 4 to 6 months of age. Iron-fortified cereals and infant formula are common food sources.

Iron deficiency and iron deficiency anemia are common health concerns for the older infant. Recent data suggest that the prevalence of iron deficiency in children 1 to 2 years of age who are living in the United States is 9% and the prevalence of iron deficiency anemia is 3% (Looker et al, 1997) (see Chapter 34).

The iron status of infants fed whole milk during the first year of life is less satisfactory than that of breast-fed infants or those fed formula with iron. Not only is milk a poor source of iron, it also contains factors that inhibit iron absorption (Fuchs et al, 1993).

Monitoring iron status is important because of the fully acknowledged, long-term cognitive effects of iron deficiency in infancy. Low hemoglobin concentrations at 8 months of age correlated with impaired motor development at 18 months of age (Sherriff et al, 2001). In addition, children with chronic iron deficiency in infancy demonstrated long-term developmental deficits and behavioral issues in early adolescence (Lozoff et al, 2000)

Zinc

Newborn infants are immediately dependent on a dietary source of zinc. Zinc is better absorbed from human milk than from infant formula. Human milk and infant formulas provide adequate zinc (0.3 to 0.5 mg per kilogram of body weight) for the first year of life; other foods (e.g., meats, cereals) should provide most of the zinc required during the second year. See Table 8-1 for the RDAs and AIs for zinc.

Fluoride

The importance of fluoride in preventing dental caries has been well documented. However, fluoride can also cause dental fluorosis (ranging from fine white lines to entirely chalky teeth) at intake levels of 4 to 1000 mg/day (see Chapter 28).

Human milk has a very low fluoride content. Commercially prepared infant cereals, wet pack cereals, and fruit juice produced with fluoridated water are significant sources of fluoride in infancy. Currently, fluoride supplementation is not recommended for infants younger than 6 months of age. After tooth eruption, it is recommended that fluoridated water be offered several times per day to breast-fed infants, those who receive cow's milk, and those fed formulas made with water that contains less than 0.3 mg of fluoride/L (American Academy of Pediatrics [AAP], 1998a).

Vitamins

Commercially prepared infant formulas are fortified with all necessary vitamins. Homogenized cow's milk, which is often offered to older infants, is fortified with vitamin D but contains little vitamin C.

Vitamin D

Human milk derived from an adequately fed, lactating mother supplies all the vitamins that the term infant needs except for vitamin D; human milk contains only 40 to 50 IU/L (1 to 1.25 μg calciferol) of vitamin D. Breast-fed infants should receive a vitamin D supplement or be exposed regularly to sunlight. Exposure for 30 minutes per week with the infant wearing only a diaper, or 2 hours per week if fully clothed without a hat, is sufficient to meet vitamin D needs (Specker et al, 1985). Cases of rickets have been diagnosed in breast-fed infants with dark skin and little exposure to sunlight (Kreiter et al, 2000; Tomashek et al, 2001).

Vitamin B_{12}

Milk from lactating mothers who follow a strict vegan diet may be vitamin B_{12} deficient, especially if the mother followed the regimen for a long time before and during the pregnancy. Vitamin B_{12} deficiency has also been diagnosed in infants breast-fed by mothers with pernicious anemia (Higgenbottom, 1978; Johnson and Roloff, 1982).

Vitamin K

The vitamin K requirements of the neonate need special attention. Deficiency may result in bleeding or hemorrhagic disease of the newborn. This condition is more common in breast-fed infants than in other infants because breast milk contains only 15 μg/L of vitamin K, whereas cow's milk and cow's milk-based formulas contain approximately four times this amount. Breast-fed infants consume less milk during the first few days of life than do formula-fed infants, which also accounts for their low vitamin K intake. All infant formulas contain a minimum of 4 μg of vitamin K per 100 kcal of formula. The suggested intake of 5 to 15 μg/day can be supplied by mature breast milk (15 μg/L), although perhaps not during the first few days to 1 week of life. Vitamin K supplementation may be necessary during that time (Greer, 2001). Many states require that infants receive an injection of vitamin K as a prophylactic measure while they are in the nursery. Previous reports that vitamin K injections may increase the risk of leukemia or cause cancer have not been supported by studies (Greer, 1995) (see Chapter 4).

Vitamin and mineral supplements should be prescribed only after careful evaluation of the infant's intake and exposure to sunlight. Infants who are fed commercially prepared formula rarely need supplements. Breast-fed infants need additional vitamin D supplementation by 2 months of age and iron by 4 to 6 months of age (see *Focus On:* Vitamin and Mineral Supplementation). Older infants who are fed homogenized milk need a food source or supplement of vitamin C. (Chapter 9 discusses the feeding of premature or high-risk infants and their special needs.)

MILK

Human milk is unquestionably the food of choice for the infant. Its composition is designed to provide the necessary energy and nutrients in appropriate amounts. It contains specific and nonspecific immune factors that support and strengthen the immature immune system of the newborn and thus protect the body against infections (Oddy, 2001). Breast milk also helps prevent diarrhea and otitis media (AAP, 1997; Scariati et al, 1997). Allergic reactions to human milk protein are rare. Moreover, the closeness of the mother and infant during breast-feeding facilitates attachment and bonding (see Figure 7-10), and breast milk provides nutritional benefits (i.e., optimal nourishment in an easily digestible and bioavailable form), decreases infant morbidity, provides maternal health benefits (e.g., lactation amenorrhea, maternal weight loss, some cancer protection), and has economic and environmental benefits (American Dietetic Association [ADA], 2001).

Population-based and metaanalysis studies indicate that breast-feeding benefits cognitive development (Angelsen et al, 2001), helps prevent childhood asthma (Dell and To, 2001; Gdalevich, Mimouni, Mimouni, 2001), and may help prevent children from becoming overweight as a dose-dependent effect (Hediger et al, 2001; von Kries et al, 1999) or because it mediates maternal control over feeding (Fisher et al, 2000). For these reasons the *Healthy Children 2010* Objectives propose to support breast-feeding among mothers of newborn infants (see *Focus On:* Healthy Children 2010 Objectives: Nourishment of Infants).

The American Dietetic Association (ADA) and the American Academy of Pediatrics (AAP) support exclusive breast-feeding for the first 4 to 6 months of life and breast-feeding supplemented by weaning foods for at least 12 months (AAP, 1997; American Dietetic Association, 1997). The ages are important because adding other foods at too young of an age decreases breast milk intake and increases early weaning (Hill et al, 1997).

Breast-feeding may not be appropriate for mothers with certain infections or who are taking medications that may have untoward effects on the infant; for example, a mother who is infected with HIV can transmit the infection to the infant (Humphrey and Iliff, 2001), and a mother using psychotropic drugs or other pharmacologic drugs may pass the medication to the infant through her breast milk (AAP, 2001)

Unmodified cow's milk is inappropriate for infants. The tough, hard curd is difficult for young infants to digest, and less fat is absorbed from cow's milk than from human milk. The much higher protein and ash content of cow's milk results in a higher renal solute load, which is the amount of nitrogenous waste and minerals that must be excreted by the kidneys.

Commercial formulas made from heat-treated nonfat milk and supplemented with adequate carbohydrates, fats, vitamins, and minerals are designed to provide necessary nutrients in an easily absorbed form. The manufacture of infant formulas is regulated by the Food and Drug Administration (FDA) through the Infant Formula Act (Nutrient Requirements for Infant Formulas, 1985). By law, infant formulas are required to have a nutrient level that is consistent with these guidelines (Table 8-4).

Composition of Human and Cow's Milk

The composition of human milk is different from that of cow's milk; for this reason, cow's milk is not recommended for infants until at least 1 year of age. Both provide 20 kcal/oz; however, the nutrient sources of the energy are different. For example, protein provides 6% to 7% of the energy in human milk and 20% of the energy in cow's milk. Human milk is 60% whey proteins (mainly lactalbumins) and 40% casein; by contrast, cow's milk is 20% whey and 80% casein. Casein forms a tough, hard-to-digest curd in the infant's stomach, whereas lactalbumin in human milk forms soft, flocculent, easy-to-digest curds. The amino acids taurine and cystine are present in higher concentrations in human milk than in cow's milk. These amino acids may be essential for premature infants. Lactose provides 42% of the energy in human milk and only 30% of the energy in cow's milk.

Lipids provide 50% of the energy in human and cow's milk. Monounsaturated oleic acid is the predominant fatty acid in both milks. Linoleic acid, an essential fatty acid, provides 4% of the energy in human milk and only 1% of that in cow's milk. The cholesterol content of human milk is 7 to 47 mg/dl, compared with 10 to 35 mg/dl in cow's milk. An additional lipase in the nonfat fraction of human milk is stimulated by bile salts and contributes significantly to the hydrolysis of milk triglycerides.

FOCUS ON

Healthy Children 2010 Objectives: Nourishment of Infants

Healthy People 2010 is a comprehensive set of health objectives for the United States to achieve during the first decade of 2000. Healthy People 2010 identifies a wide range of public health priorities and specific, measurable objectives. The objectives have 28 focus areas, one of which is Maternal, Infant, and Child Health. The objectives related to nourishment of infants are as follows:

GOAL: Improve the health and well-being of women, infants, and families

Objective 16-19. Increase the proportion of mothers who breast-feed their infants to 75% in the early postpartum period, to 50% until their infants are 6 months old, and to 25% until their infants are 12 months old

GOAL: Promote health and reduce chronic disease associated with diet and weight

Objective 19-4. Reduce growth retardation among low-income children ages 5 years and younger to less than 5%

Objective 19-12. Reduce iron deficiency among children ages 1 to 2 years to less than 5%

GOAL: Prevent and control oral and craniofacial diseases, conditions, and injuries and improve access to related services

Objective 21-1a. Reduce the proportion of young children with dental caries in their primary teeth

The complete text of the *Healthy People 2010 Objectives* can be found at www.healthypeople.gov/documents/.

TABLE 8-4 Nutrient Levels in Infant Formulas as Specified by the Infant Formula Act

SPECIFIED NUTRIENT COMPONENT	MINIMUM LEVEL REQUIRED (per 100 kcal of energy)
Protein (g)	1.8
Fat (g)	3.3
Percentage of calories	30.0
Linoleic acid (mg)	300.0
Percentage of calories	2.7
Vitamin A (IU)	250.0
Vitamin E (IU)	0.7
Vitamin D (IU)	40.0
Vitamin K (μg)	4.0
Thiamin (μg)	40.0
Riboflavin (μg)	60.0
Niacin (μg)	250.0
Ascorbic acid (mg)	8.0
Pyridoxine (μg)	35.0
Vitamin B_{12} (μg)	0.15
Folic acid (μg)	4.0
Biotin (μg) (non–milk-based formulas only)	1.5
Pantothenic acid (μg)	300.0
Choline (mg) (non–milk-based formulas only)	7.0
Inositol (mg) (non–milk-based formulas only)	4.0
Calcium (mg)	60.0
Phosphorus (mg)	30.0
Iron (mg)	0.15
Zinc (mg)	0.5
Magnesium (mg)	6.0
Manganese (μg)	5.0
Sodium (mg)	20.0
Potassium (mg)	80.0
Iodine (μg)	5.0
Chloride (mg)	55.0
Copper (μg)	60.0

From Nutrient requirements for infant formulas, Final Rule (21 CFR 107), *Federal Register* 50:45106, 1985.

All of the water-soluble vitamins in human milk reflect maternal intake. Cow's milk contains adequate quantities of the B-complex vitamins but little vitamin C. Both milks provide sufficient vitamin A. Human milk, which provides 2 IU/L (2 mg of α-tocopherol), is a richer source of vitamin E than cow's milk. Human milk contains five metabolites of vitamin D, providing 40 to 50 IU/L (1 to 1.25 μg cholecalciferol) of vitamin D activity; however, the need for additional vitamin D becomes progressively important with increasing age. Cow's milk is usually fortified with 400 IU/L (10 μg of cholecalciferol) of vitamin D.

The quantity of iron in human and cow's milk is small (0.3 mg/L). Approximately 49% of the iron in human milk, but less than 1% of the iron in cow's milk, is absorbed. The bioavailability of zinc in human milk is higher than in cow's milk. Cow's milk contains three times as much calcium and six times as much phosphorus as human milk, and its fluoride concentration is twice that of human milk.

The sodium and potassium concentrations in human milk are about one third those in cow's milk, thus reducing the renal solute load. The osmolality of human milk averages 286 mOsm/kg, whereas that of cow's milk is 400 mOsm/kg.

Antiinfective Factors

Human milk and colostrum contain antibodies and antiinfective factors that are not present in infant formulas. Secretory immunoglobulin A (sIgA) is the predominant immunoglobulin in human milk, and it plays a role in protecting the infant's immature gut from infection. However, research indicates that breast-feeding must be maintained until the infant is at least 3 months of age to obtain this benefit.

The iron-binding protein lactoferrin in human milk deprives bacteria of iron and thus slows their growth. *Lysozymes,* which are bacteriolytic enzymes found in human milk, destroy the cell membranes of bacteria after the peroxides and ascorbic acid that are also present in human milk have inactivated them. Breast milk enhances the growth of the bacterium *Lactobacillus bifidus,* which produces an acidic gastrointestinal environment that interferes with the growth of certain pathogenic organisms. Because of these antiinfective factors, the incidence of infections is lower in breast-fed infants than in formula-fed infants.

Formulas

Infants whose mothers are unwilling or unable to breast-feed are usually fed a formula based on cow's milk or a soy product. Those who have special requirements receive specially designed products.

Formulas based on nonfat milk with added vegetable fats and vitamins and minerals are available for healthy infants and are formulated to approximate as closely as possible the composition of human milk. For example, Enfamil formula has been modified to provide a whey/casein protein ratio similar to that of human milk. Similac formulas are heat treated to reduce the curd tension. Good Start formula contains reduced-mineral whey and is higher in protein and lower in fat than other commercially available formulas. Vegetable oils are added to ensure fat absorption levels similar to those from human milk, and vitamins and minerals are added to meet the recommended intake for infants.

Formulas are also available for older infants (e.g., Follow-Up and Follow-Up Soy formulas) and toddlers (e.g., Next Step and Next Step Soy formulas). However, most pediatricians believe "older infant" formulas are unnecessary unless toddlers are not receiving adequate amounts of infant or table foods.

The declining prevalence of anemia in infants is credited to the use of iron-fortified formula; for this reason, the AAP recommends iron-fortified formulas for all formula-fed infants. The widespread theory that iron-fortified formula may cause constipation, loose stools, colic (severe abdominal pain), and spitting up has not been confirmed by clinical studies (AAP, 1999). Formulas are available with and without additional iron. Table 8-5 shows the

TABLE 8-5 Composition of Milk and Selected Infant Formulas per Liter

MILK OR FORMULA	ENERGY (KCAL)	PROTEIN (g)	FAT (g)	CARBOHYDRATE (g)	CALCIUM (mg)	PHOSPHORUS (mg)	SODIUM (mg)	SODIUM (mEq)	POTASSIUM (mg)	POTASSIUM (mEq)	IRON (mg)	PROTEIN SOURCE	FAT SOURCE	CARBOHYDRATE SOURCE	COMMENTS
Human Milk	750	11.0	45.0	70.0	340	140	161	7.0	570	15.0	0.2	Lactalbumin, casein	Human breast milk	Lactose	Protein readily digested; adequate in all nutrients except vitamin D and fluoride
Cow's Milk–Based Infant Formulas															
Similac (Ross)	680	14.0	36.5	73.0	530	280	162	7.0	710	18.0	12.0/1.5*	Nonfat milk, whey	High oleic safflower, soy, coconut oils	Lactose	Vitamins and minerals added
Enfamil (Mead Johnson)	666	13.9	35.3	72.6	525	357	182	7.8	725	18.4	12.1/4.7*	Reduced-mineral whey, nonfat milk	Palm olein, soy, coconut, high oleic safflower oils	Lactose	Vitamins and minerals added
LactoFree (Mead Johnson)	666	14.0	35.3	72.6	546	366	200	8.6	733	18.6	12.0	Milk protein isolate	Palm olein, soy, coconut, high oleic sunflower oils	Corn syrup solids	Vitamins and minerals added
Good Start (Carnation)	666	16.0	34.0	73.3	426	240	160	6.9	653	16.5	10.0	Enzymatically hydrolyzed reduced-mineral whey	Palm olein, soy, coconut, high oleic safflower oils	Lactose, maltodextrin	Whey-predominant formula for normal infants; vitamins and minerals added
Cow's Milk															
Skim	357	35.0	2.0	50.0	1256	1028	524	23.0	1689	43.0	Trace	Casein	None	Lactose	Inappropriate for infants
2%	503	34.0	20.0	49.0	1236	965	508	22.0	1568	40.0	Trace	Casein	Butterfat	Lactose	Inappropriate for infants
Whole	624	33.0	34.0	47.0	1211	948	499	22.0	1539	39.0	Trace	Casein	Butterfat	Lactose	Inappropriate for infants younger than 12 months of age
Soy-Based Infant Formulas															
Prosobee (Mead Johnson)	666	16.6	35.3	70.6	699	553	240	10.4	799	20.3	11.9	Soy protein isolate with L-methionine	Palm olein, soy, coconut, high oleic sunflower oils	Corn syrup solids	Vitamins and minerals added
Isomil (Ross)	680	16.6	36.9	69.6	710	510	300	13.0	730	19.0	12.0	Soy protein isolate with L-methionine	High oleic safflower, coconut, soy oils	Corn syrup sucrose	Vitamins and minerals added

Data from Mead Johnson Nutritionals: *The very best professional handbook,* PHB0500, Nestle', 2000; *Ross Laboratories Product Handbook,* January 2002, http://www.ross.com/productHandbook/pedNut.asp; and *Mead Johnson nutritionals handbook,* January 2002, http://www.meadjohnson.com/products/index.html.
MCT, medium-chain triglycerides.
*Without added iron

Continued

TABLE 8-5 Composition of Milk and Selected Infant Formulas per Liter—cont'd

MILK OR FORMULA	ENERGY (KCAL)	PROTEIN (g)	FAT (g)	CARBOHYDRATE (g)	CALCIUM (mg)	PHOSPHORUS (mg)	SODIUM (mg)	SODIUM (mEq)	POTASSIUM (mg)	POTASSIUM (mEq)	IRON (mg)	PROTEIN SOURCE	FAT SOURCE	CARBOHYDRATE SOURCE	COMMENTS
Soy-Based Infant Formulas—cont'd															
Alsoy (Carnation)	666	18.6	33.0	73.9	699	406	220	9.5	773	19.6	12.0	Soy protein isolate with L-methionine	Palm olein, soy, coconut, high oleic safflower oils	Corn maltodextrin, sucrose	Vitamins and minerals added
Casein Hydrolysate Formulas															
Nutramigen (Mead Johnson)	666	18.6	33.3	73.3	626	420	313	13.5	733	18.6	12.0	Casein hydrolysate with added amino acids	Palm olein, soy, coconut, high oleic sunflower oils	Corn syrup solids, modified cornstarch	Vitamins and minerals added
Pregestimil (Mead Johnson)	666	18.6	37.3	67.9	766	500	313	13.5	733	18.6	12.0	Casein hydrolysate with added amino acids	Medium-chain triglyceride (55%), corn, soy, high oleic safflower oils	Corn syrup solids, dextrose, modified cornstarch	Vitamins and minerals added
Alimentum (Ross)	680	18.6	37.5	69.0	710	510	300	13.0	800	20.0	12.2	Casein hydrolysate with added amino acids	Safflower, medium-chain triglyceride (33%), soy oils	Sucrose, modified tapioca starch	Vitamins and minerals added
Formulas for Feeding Beyond 4 to 6 Months of Age															
Follow-Up (Carnation)	666	17.3	27.3	87.9	799	533	260	11.2	899	22.8	12.0	Nonfat milk	Palm olein, soy, coconut, high oleic safflower oils	Corn syrup solids, lactose, maltodextrin	Vitamins and minerals added
Follow-Up Soy (Carnation)	666	20.8	29.5	80.4	905	603	281	12.1	791	20.1	12.1	Soy protein isolate with L-methionine	Palm olein, soy, coconut, high oleic safflower oils	Corn syrup solids, maltodextrin, sucrose	Vitamins and minerals added
Formulas for Feeding Beyond 1 Year of Age															
Next Step (Mead Johnson)	666	17.3	33.8	73.9	799	559	273	11.8	866	21.9	12.0	Nonfat milk	Palm olein, soy, coconut, high oleic sunflower oils	Corn syrup solids, lactose	Vitamins and minerals added
Next Step Soy (Mead Johnson)	666	21.9	29.3	78.5	766	599	320	13.8	999	25.4	12.0	Soy protein isolate with L-methionine	Palm olein, soy, coconut, high oleic sunflower oils	Corn syrup solids, sucrose	Vitamins and minerals added
Similac 2 (Ross)	675	13.9	37.1	71.6	797	432	162	7.0	708	17.9	12.1	Nonfat milk, whey	High oleic safflower, coconut, soy oils	Lactose	Vitamins and minerals added
Isomil 2 (Ross)	675	16.5	36.8	69.5	911	608	297	12.8	729	18.5	12.1	Soy protein isolate with L-methionine	High oleic safflower, coconut, soy oils	Corn syrup sucrose	Vitamins and minerals added

Data from Mead Johnson Nutritionals: *The very best professional handbook,* PHB0500, Nestle', 2000; *Ross Laboratories Product Handbook,* January 2002, http://www.ross.com/productHandbook/pedNut.asp; and *Mead Johnson nutritionals handbook,* January 2002, http://www.meadjohnson.com/products/index.html.
MCT, medium-chain triglycerides.

composition of various formulas, human milk, and cow's milk.

Recently, soy-based formulas have come under scrutiny. Infants ingesting soy formulas grow as well as and absorb minerals as well as infants fed cow's milk–based formulas, but they are exposed to several thousand times higher levels of phytoestrogens (see Chapter 12) or isoflavones than infants fed breast milk or cow's milk–based formulas (Setchell et al, 1997). The concern is whether this exposure poses a developmental hazard. The amount of soy protein isolate used in the manufacture of soy-based infant formulas determines the isoflavone content. One study estimates that a typical 4-month-old infant ingesting soy formula is exposed to 28 to 47 mg of isoflavones each day. Plasma isoflavone concentrations in infants receiving soy-based formula were significantly greater than in infants fed breast milk or cow's milk–based formulas (Irvine et al, 1998). However, the biologic impact of these elevated isoflavone levels on long-term infant development is not yet understood.

In an ongoing effort to manufacture infant formulas that closely approximate breast milk, the long-chain polyunsaturated fatty acid intake of formula-fed infants has been evaluated (Auestad et al, 1997; Jensen et al, 1997; Koletzko et al, 1996). AA and DHA are found in breast milk but not in cow's milk. Current research indicates that these very-long-chain fatty acids may be associated with accelerated cognition and vision development (Angelsen et al, 2001). However, no current documentation shows that the growth or development of formula-fed infants is compromised when they consume formulas without AA or DHA supplementation. However, many infant formulas now have these very-long-chain fatty acids added (Innis, Gilley, and Werker, 2001). The new DRIs for infants recommend 0.5 g/day of omega-3 fatty acids.

Various products are available for infants who cannot tolerate the protein in cow's milk–based formulas. Soy products designed to meet all nutrient needs are recommended for (1) children in vegetarian families, (2) children with galactosemia or primary lactase deficiency and those recovering from secondary lactose intolerance, and (3) infants who may be allergic to cow's milk protein but who have not shown clinical manifestations of the allergy. These products are not recommended for children known to have protein allergies because many infants who are allergic to cow's milk protein also develop allergies to soy milk protein (AAP, 1998b) (see Chapter 32).

Infants who cannot tolerate soy products can be fed formulas made from a casein hydrolysate which is casein that has been split into smaller components by treatment with acid, alkali, or enzymes. These formulas are Nutramigen, Pregestimil, and Alimentum (AAP, 2000). In addition, these formulas do not contain lactose. Other formulas are available for children with problems such as malabsorption or metabolic disorders (e.g., phenylketonuria) (see Chapters 9 and 45).

Infants who receive adequate breast milk, infant formula, or both require few supplemental nutrients (see *Focus On:* Vitamin and Mineral Supplementation Recommendations for Full-Term Infants).

Whole Cow's Milk

Although it is generally recommended that infants receive human milk or iron-fortified formula for the first year of life, many parents make the transition from formula to fresh cow's milk when the infant is between 5 and 9 months of age. However, the AAP

FOCUS ON

Vitamin and Mineral Supplementation Recommendations for Full-Term Infants

Iron

Breast-Fed Infants

About 1 mg/kg/day by 4 to 6 months of age, preferably from supplemental foods, and only iron-fortified formulas for weaning or supplementing breast milk

Formula-Fed Infants

Only iron-fortified formula during the first year of life

Vitamin D

Recommended intake of 400 IU/day (10 μg cholecalciferol/day), and most formulas contain 62 IU/100 kcal (6.45 μg of cholecalciferol per 100 kcal) to meet this recommendation; adequate sun exposure—for white infants, is 30 min/wk if wearing diaper only or 2 hours/wk if fully clothed (but with no hat).

Vitamin K

Supplementation soon after birth to prevent hemorrhagic disease of the newborn

Fluoride

Intake of 0.25 mg/day after 6 months of age if water contains less than 0.3 ppm.

Modified from American Academy of Pediatrics, Committee on Nutrition: *Handbook of pediatric nutrition,* ed 4, Elk Grove Village, Ill, 1998.

Committee on Nutrition has concluded that infants should not be fed whole cow's milk during the first year of life (AAP, 1998). Infants who are fed whole cow's milk have been found to have lower intakes of iron, linoleic acid, and vitamin E and excessive intakes of sodium, potassium, and protein. Cow's milk may cause a small amount of gastrointestinal blood loss.

Low-fat (2%) and nonfat milk are also inappropriate for infants during the first 2 years of life. In addition, substitute or imitation milks, such as rice, oat, or nut milks, are inappropriate and should not be fed to infants unless they are properly supplemented.

Formula Preparation

Commercial infant formulas are available in ready-to-feed forms that require no preparation, as concentrates prepared by mixing with equal parts of water, and in powder form that is designed to be mixed with 2 oz of water per level tablespoon or scoop of powder.

In most households that maintain a reasonable level of sanitation, formulas are seldom sterilized. However, formulas should be made in a very clean environment. All equipment, including bottles, nipples, mixers, and the top of the can of formula, should be washed thoroughly. The infant should be fed immediately after the formula is prepared, and any formula not consumed at that feeding should be discarded. Any opened cans of formula should be covered and refrigerated.

Box 8-1. Directions for Home Preparation of Infant Foods

1. Select fresh, high-quality fruits, vegetables, or meats.
2. Be sure that all utensils, including cutting boards, grinder, knives, and other items, are thoroughly cleaned.
3. Wash hands before preparing the food.
4. Clean, wash, and trim the food in as little water as possible.
5. Cook the foods until tender in as little water as possible. Avoid overcooking, which may destroy heat-sensitive nutrients.
6. Do not add salt or sugar. Do not add honey to food intended for infants younger than 1 year of age.*
7. Add enough water for the food to be easily puréed.
8. Strain or purée the food using an electric blender, a food mill, a baby food grinder, or a kitchen strainer.
9. Pour purée into an ice cube tray and freeze.
10. When the food is frozen hard, remove the cubes and store in freezer bags.
11. When ready to serve, defrost and heat in a serving container the amount of food that will be consumed at a single feeding.

**Clostridium botulinum* spores, which cause botulism, have been reported in honey, and young infants do not have the immune capacity to resist this infection.

FOOD

Various commercially prepared foods and organically grown products are available for infants. These products vary widely in their nutrient value. Foods for infants should be thoughtfully selected to meet their nutritional and developmental needs.

Ready-to-serve dry infant cereals are fortified with electrolytically reduced iron. Three level tablespoons of cereal provide about 5 mg of iron, or from one half to one third the amount the infant requires. Therefore cereal is usually the first food added to the infant's diet. Jarred cereal and fruit mixtures are fortified with ferrous sulfate and provide 7 to 9 mg of iron per 4.5-oz jar.

Strained and "junior" vegetables and fruits provide carbohydrates and various amounts of vitamins A and C. Vitamin C is added to numerous jarred fruits and all fruit juices. In addition, tapioca is added to several of the jarred fruits. Milk is added to the creamed vegetables, and wheat is incorporated into the mixed vegetables.

Most strained and junior meats are prepared with water. Strained meats, which have the highest energy density of any of the commercial baby foods, are an excellent source of high-quality protein and heme iron.

Numerous dessert items are also available such as puddings and fruit desserts. The nutrient composition of these products varies, but all contain excess energy in the form of sugar and modified cornstarch or tapioca starch. Most infants do not need this excess energy.

Mothers who would like to make their own infant food can easily do so by following the directions in Box 8-1. Home-prepared foods are generally more concentrated in nutrients than commercially prepared foods because less water is used. Salt and sugar should not be added to foods prepared for infants.

FEEDING

Initial Feeding Patterns

Because milk from a mother with an adequate diet is uniquely designed to meet the needs of the human infant, breast-feeding for the first 6 months of life is strongly recommended. Most chronic medical conditions do not contraindicate breast-feeding.

A mother should be encouraged to nurse her infant immediately after birth. Those who care for and counsel parents during the first postpartum days should acquaint themselves with ways in which they can be supportive. Ideally, counseling and preparation for breast-feeding start in the last few months or weeks of pregnancy (see Chapter 7).

During the first few days of life, a breast-feeding infant receives colostrum, a yellow, transparent fluid that meets the infant's needs during the first week. It contains less fat and carbohydrate but more protein and greater concentrations of sodium, potassium, and chloride than mature milk.

Infants who are formula fed are likely to receive ready-to-feed formula in the hospital. At home, products that have been refrigerated such as concentrated formulas should be mixed with warm water or heated to body temperature in a water bath. Refrigerated, read-to-feed formula also needs to be warmed. Microwave heating is not recommended because of the risk of burns from formula that is too hot or unevenly heated.

Regardless of whether infants are breast-fed or formula fed, they should be held and cuddled during feedings. Once a feeding rhythm has been established, infants become fussy or cry to indicate they are hungry, whereas they often smile and fall asleep when they are satisfied (Table 8-6). Infants, not adults, should establish the feeding schedules. Initially, most infants feed every 2 to 3 hours; by 4 weeks of age, most feed every 4 hours. By 2 to 4 months of age, infants have usually matured enough to allow the mother to omit night feedings.

TABLE 8-6 Satiety Behaviors in Infants

AGE (WEEKS)	BEHAVIOR
4-12	Draws head away from the nipple Falls asleep When nipple is reinserted, closes lips tightly Bites nipple, purses lips, or smiles and lets go
16-24	Releases nipple and withdraws head Fusses or cries Obstructs mouth with hands Pays more attention to surroundings Bites nipple
28-36	Changes posture Keeps mouth tightly closed Shakes head as if to say "no" Plays with utensils Uses hands more actively Throws utensils
40-52	See behaviors listed for previous age range Sputters with tongue and lips Hands bottle or cup to mother

From Pipes PL: Health care professionals. In Garwood G, Fewell R, eds: *Educating handicapped infants*, Rockville, Md, 1982, Aspen Systems.

Development of Feeding Skills

At birth, infants coordinate sucking, breathing, and swallowing and are prepared to suckle liquids but not foods with texture. During the first year, typical infants develop head control, the ability to move into and sustain a sitting posture, and the ability to grasp, first with a palmar grasp and then with a refined pincer grasp (Figure 8-2, *B*). They develop mature sucking and rotary chewing abilities and progress from being fed to feeding themselves using their fingers. In the second year, they learn to feed themselves independently with a spoon (Figure 8-3).

Addition of Semisolid Foods

Developmental readiness and nutrient needs are the criteria that determine appropriate times for the addition of various foods. Table 8-7 lists developmental landmarks and their indications for semisolid and table food introduction. During the first 4 months of life, the infant attains head and neck control, and oral motor patterns progress from a suck to a suckling to the beginnings of a mature sucking pattern. Puréed foods introduced during this phase are consumed in the same manner as are liquids, with each suckle being followed by a tongue-thrust swallow.

Between 4 and 6 months of age, when the mature sucking movement is refined and munching movements (up-and-down chopping motions) begin, the introduction of strained foods is appropriate. Infant cereal is usually introduced first. To support developmental progress, cereal is offered to the infant from a spoon, not combined with formula in a bottle. Thereafter, various commercially or home-prepared foods may be offered. The sequence in which these foods are introduced is not important; however, it is important that only one food (e.g., peaches, not peach cobbler, which has many ingredients) be introduced at a time. This helps parents to identify any allergic responses or food intolerances. Introducing vegetables before fruits may increase vegetable acceptance.

Infants demonstrate their acceptance of new foods by slowly increasing the quantity of solids they accept. Breast-fed infants seem to accept greater quantities than do formula-fed infants (Sullivan and Birch, 1994).

As oral-motor maturation proceeds, an infant's rotary chewing ability develops, indicating a readiness for more textured foods such as well-cooked mashed vegetables, casseroles, and pasta from the family menu. Learning to grasp—with the palmar grasp, then with an inferior pincer grasp, and finally with the refined pincer grasp—indicates a readiness for finger foods such as oven-dried toast, arrowroot biscuits, or cheese sticks (see Figure 8-2). Table 8-8 presents recommendations for adding foods to an infant's diet. Foods with skins or rinds and foods that stick to the roof of the mouth (e.g., hot dogs, grapes, bread with peanut butter) may cause choking and should not be offered to young infants.

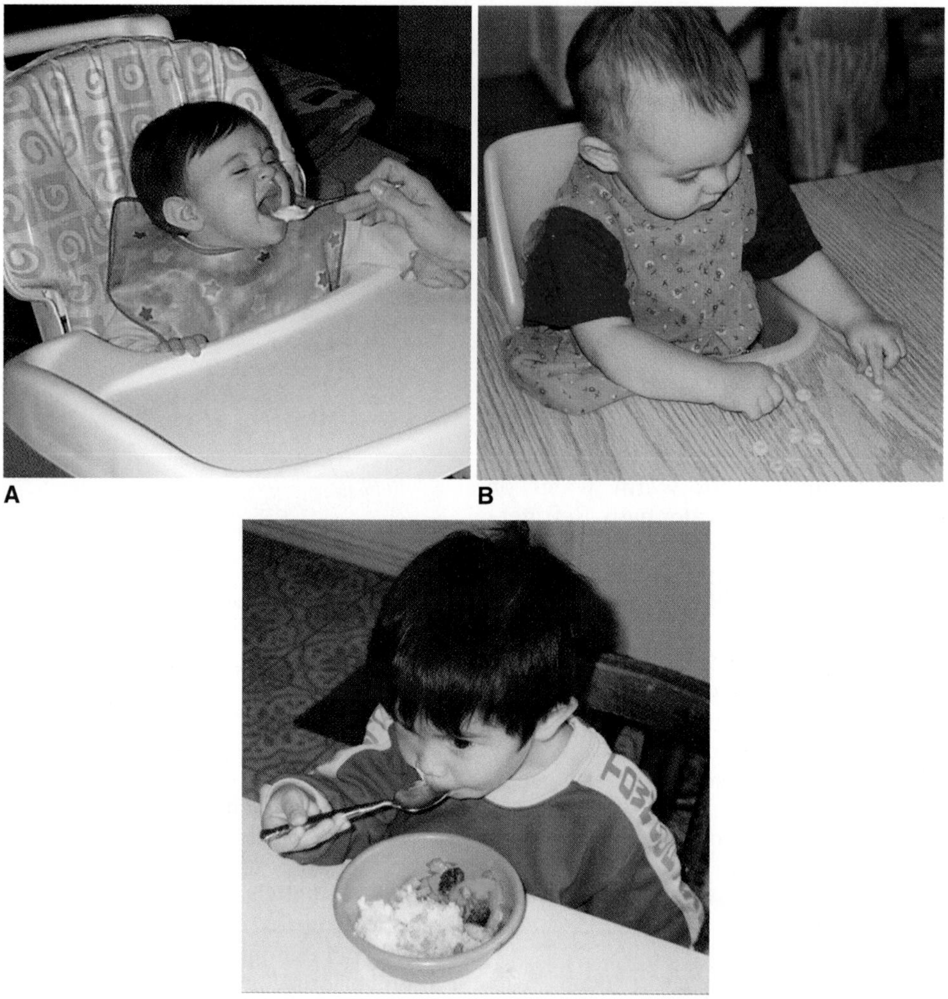

A B

C

FIGURE 8-2 • Development of feeding skills in infants and toddlers. **A,** This 7-month-old child shows the beginnings of involvement with feeding by anticipating the spoon. **B,** This 9-month-old girl is using a refined pincer grasp to pick up her food. **C,** This 19-month-old boy is beginning to use his spoon independently, although he is not yet able to rotate his wrist to keep food on it.

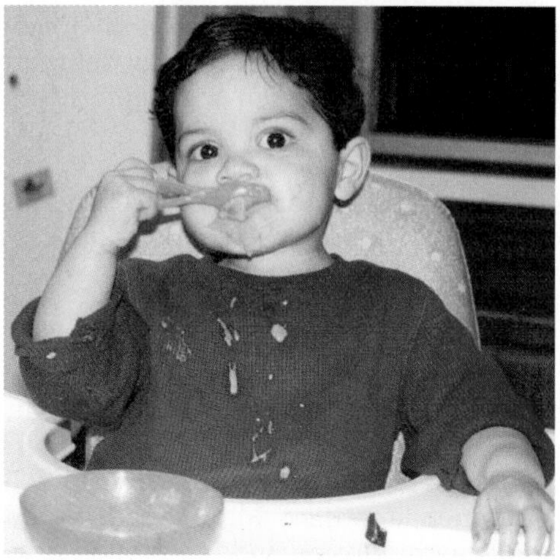

FIGURE 8-3 • This 2-year-old is skilled at self-feeding because he has the ability to rotate his wrist and elevate his elbow to keep food on the spoon.

During the last quarter of the first year, infants can approximate their lips to the rim of the cup and can drink if the cup is held for them. During the second year, they gain the ability to rotate their wrists and elevate their elbows, thus allowing them to hold the cup themselves and manage a spoon. They are very messy eaters at first, but by 2 years of age, most typical children skillfully feed themselves (see Figure 8-3).

Weaning From Breast or Bottle to Cup

The introduction of solids into an infant's diet begins the weaning process in which the infant transitions from a diet of only breast milk or formula to a more varied one. Weaning should proceed gradually and be based on the infant's rate of growth and developmental skills. Weaning foods should be carefully chosen to complement the nutrient needs of the infant, promote appropriate nutrient intake, and maintain

TABLE 8-7 Feeding Behaviors: Developmental Landmarks During the First 2 Years of Life

DEVELOPMENTAL LANDMARKS	CHANGE INDICATED	EXAMPLES OF APPROPRIATE FOODS
Tongue laterally transfers food in the mouth Shows voluntary and independent movements of the tongue and lips Sitting posture that can be sustained Shows beginning of chewing movements (up and down movements of the jaw)	Introduction of soft, mashed table food	Tuna fish; mashed potatoes; well-cooked, mashed vegetables; ground meats in gravy and sauces; soft, diced fruit, such as bananas, peaches, and pears; flavored yogurt
Reaches for and grasps objects with scissors (palmar) grasp Brings hand to mouth	Finger feeding (large pieces of food)	Oven-dried toast, teething biscuits; cheese sticks (Should be soluble in the mouth to prevent choking)
Voluntarily releases food (refined digital [pincer] grasp)	Finger feeding (small pieces of food)	Bits of cottage cheese, dry cereal, peas and other bite-size vegetables; small pieces of meat
Shows rotary chewing pattern	Introduction of food of varied textures from family menu	Well-cooked, chopped meats and casseroles; cooked vegetables and canned fruit (not mashed); toast; potatoes; macaroni; spaghetti; peeled ripe fruit
Approximates lips to rim of the cup	Introduction of cup for sipping liquids	
Understands relationship of container and its contents	Beginning of self-feeding (though messiness should be expected)	Food that when scooped adheres to the spoon, such as applesauce, cooked cereal, mashed potatoes, cottage cheese, yogurt
Shows increased movements of the jaw Shows development of ulnar deviation of the wrist	More skilled at cup and spoon feeding	Chopped, fibrous meats, such as roast and steak Raw vegetables and fruit (introduced gradually)
Walks alone	May seek food and obtain food independently	Foods of high nutritional value
Names food, expresses preferences; prefers unmixed foods Goes on food jags Appetite appears to decrease		Balanced food choices, with child permitted to develop food preferences (Parents should not be concerned that these preferences will last forever.)

Modified from Trahms CM, Pipes P: *Nutrition in infancy and childhood,* ed 6, New York, 1997, McGraw-Hill.

TABLE 8-8 Suggested Ages for the Introduction of Juice, Semisolid Foods, and Table Foods

FOOD	AGE (MONTHS) 4-6	6-8	9-12
Iron-fortified cereals for infants	Add.		
Vegetables		Add strained.	Gradually eliminate strained foods and introduce table foods.
Fruits		Add strained.	Gradually eliminate strained foods; introduce chopped, well-cooked, or canned foods.
Meats		Add strained or finely chopped table meats.	Decrease the use of strained meats; increase the varieties of table meats offered.
Finger foods, such as arrowroot biscuits, oven-dried toast		Add foods that can be secured with a palmar grasp.	Increase the use of small finger foods as the pincer grasp develops.
Well-cooked mashed or chopped table foods prepared without added salt or sugar			Add.
Juice or formula by cup			Add.

From Trahms CM, Pipes P: *Nutrition in infancy and childhood,* ed 6, New York, 1997, McGraw-Hill.

growth. Many infants begin the process of weaning with the introduction of the cup at about 6 to 9 months of age and complete the process when they are able to ingest an adequate amount of milk from a cup at 18 to 24 months of age. Parents of infants who are breast-fed may choose to transition the infant directly to a cup or have an intermittent transition to a bottle before the cup is introduced.

Early Childhood Caries

Early childhood caries (ECC), or *baby bottle tooth decay,* is the most common chronic disease of childhood (Mouradian, Wehr, and Crall, 2000). ECC is a pattern of tooth decay that involves the upper anterior and sometimes lower posterior teeth. ECC is common among infants and children who are allowed to bathe their teeth in sugar (sucrose or lactose) throughout the day and night. If infants are given sugar-sweetened beverages or fruit juice in a bottle during the day or at bedtime after teeth have erupted, the risk of dental caries increases (see Chapter 28 and Figure 28-5). Infants should be fed and burped and then put to bed without milk, juice, or food. Juice should be limited to 4 to 6 oz/day for infants and young children and offered to children from a cup (AAP, 2001).

Feeding Older Infants

As maturation proceeds and the rate of growth slows down, infants' interest in and approach to food change. Between 9 and 18 months of age, most reduce their breast-milk or formula intake. They become finicky about what and how much they eat (see *Clinical Insight:* Self-Selected Diets of Infants and Young Children).

In the weaning stage, infants have to learn many manipulative skills, including the ability to chew and swallow solid food and use utensils. They learn to tolerate various textures and flavors of food, eat with their fingers, and then feed themselves with a utensil. Very young children should be encouraged to feed themselves.

At the beginning of a meal, children are hungry and should be allowed to feed themselves; when they become tired, they can be helped quietly. Emphasis on table manners and the fine points of eating should be delayed until they have the necessary maturity and developmental readiness for such training.

The food should be in a form that is easy to handle and eat. Meat should be cut into bite-size pieces. Potatoes and vegetables should be mashed so that they can be easily eaten with a spoon. Raw fruits and vegetables should be in sizes that can be picked up easily. In addition, the utensils should be small and manageable. Cups should be easy to hold, and dishes should be designed so that they do not tip over easily.

Type of Food

In general, children prefer simple, uncomplicated foods. Food from the family meal can be adapted for the child and served in child-size portions. Children younger than 6 years of age usually prefer mild-flavored foods. Because a young child's stomach is small, a snack may be required between meals. Fruit, cheese, crackers, dry cereal, fruit juices, and milk contribute nutrients and energy. Children ages 2 to 6 years often prefer raw instead of cooked vegetables and fruits.

Infants should be offered foods that vary in texture and flavor. Infants who are accustomed to many kinds of foods are less likely to limit their variety of food choices later. To add variety to an infant's diet, add vegetables and fruits to cereal feedings. It is important to offer various foods and not allow the in-

CLINICAL INSIGHT

Self-Selected Diets of Infants and Young Children

If left to their own devices with a wide variety of wholesome foods at their disposal, young children instinctively choose an adequate diet. This was documented by research conducted in the late 1920s by Davis, who was attempting to demonstrate that the prevailing practice of withholding solid foods until 1 year of age was not in the best interest of the child (Davis, 1928). At the onset of the study, Davis studied three children, ages 7 to 9 months, for 6 months to 1 year. Later, she studied 12 additional children for 6 months to 4½ years, during which time their diets were entirely self-selected. They were offered various fresh, unprocessed, and unseasoned foods and were allowed to eat as little or as much as they pleased of any or all items (Davis, 1939). A modern evaluation of their intakes indicates that the nutrients in the foods consumed equaled or exceeded the recommendations for all nutrients except iron.

Though some of the foods offered are unfamiliar to today's families, it seems difficult for a child with a typical appetite to fail to obtain an adequate diet when his or her choices are limited to the following: beef, lamb, chicken, liver, kidney, brains, sweetbreads, haddock, whole wheat bread, oatmeal, barley, cornmeal, Ry-Krisp, bone marrow, bone jelly, eggs, raw milk, apples, oranges, bananas, peaches, pineapples, lettuce, cabbage, spinach, cauliflower, peas, beets, carrots, turnips, potatoes, tomatoes, and sea salt.

No desserts or snacks commonly eaten during those times were included, and certainly none of the highly refined, energy-rich, and nutrient-dilute foods available today were offered.

A preference for sweetness that is present at birth and persists throughout childhood suggests that infants who are offered dietary selections that include desserts and sweetened snack foods are unable to make the choices appropriate for a nutritious diet (Story and Brown, 1987).

However, a similar study of children ages 1½ to 4 years who were presented with wholesome foods that are common today also demonstrated the ability to select foods to meet their energy requirements. Unfortunately, the nutrient adequacy of their selected diets was not determined (Birch, 1991).

fant to continue consuming a diet consisting of one or two favorite foods. Older infants generally reject unfamiliar foods the first time they are offered. When parents continue to offer small portions of these foods without comment, infants become familiar with them and often accept them. It is important that fruit juice does not replace more nutrient-dense foods. If excessive amounts of juice are consumed, children may *fail to thrive* (Smith and Lifshitz, 1994) (see Chapter 10).

Serving Size

The size of a serving of food offered to a child is very important. At 1 year, infants eat one third to one half the amount an adult normally consumes. This proportion increases to one half an adult portion by the time the child reaches 3 years of age and increases—to about two thirds—by 6 years of age. Young children should not be served a large plateful of food; the size of the plate and the amount should be in proportion to their age. A tablespoon (not a *heaping* tablespoon) of each food for each year of age is a good guide to follow. Serving less food than parents think or hope will be eaten helps children eat successfully and happily. They will ask for more food if their appetite is not satisfied.

Forced Feeding

Children should not be forced to eat; instead, the cause for the unwillingness to eat should be determined. A typical, healthy child eats without coaxing. Children may refuse food because they are too inactive to be hungry or too active and overtired. Fatigue can be avoided by planning a short rest period for the child or providing a picture book for the child's quiet enjoyment before meals. A child who is fed snacks or given a bottle too close to mealtime is not hungry for the meal and may refuse it. Omitting all eating or drinking for 1 to 1½ hours before a meal helps solve the problem.

An overanxious parent can affect the appetite of an infant or child because strong emotions can retard the flow of gastric juice and inhibit digestion. Refusal to eat may also be the result of too much attention. Children enjoy the attention of their parents and soon learn that refusing to eat is one way to obtain it.

If a child refuses to eat, the family meal should be completed without comment, and the plate should be removed. This procedure is usually harder on the parent than on the child. At the next mealtime, the child will be hungry enough to enjoy the food presented.

Eating Environment

Young children should eat their meals at the family table because it gives them an opportunity to learn table manners while enjoying meals with a family group. Sharing the family fare strengthens ties and makes mealtime pleasant. However, if the family meal is delayed, the children should receive their meal at the usual time. When children eat with the family, everyone must be careful not to make unfavorable comments about any food. Children are great imitators of the people they admire; thus if the father or older siblings make disparaging remarks about squash, for example, young children are likely to do the same.

Clinical Scenario 1

Lela is a 12-week-old female infant who was born by cesarean section at 42 weeks of gestation to an 18-year-old unmarried mother. Her mother gained 70 lb during the pregnancy. Lela's weight-for-length is plotted at the 95th percentile, and her length and weight continue in the same channels as at birth.

Lela's mother chose to feed Lela infant formula rather than breast feed. Lela is offered Similac with iron that is prepared with 1 scoop of powder mixed in 2 oz of water. Lela consumes about six 8-oz bottles per day and is fed on demand. She usually sleeps during the night, but if she is fussy, her mother gives her small amounts of commercially prepared infant cereal, vegetables, and fruit.

1. What additional information is needed to get an accurate assessment of this infant's intake?
2. Is Lela growing appropriately? Explain your answer.
3. What is Lela's estimated energy intake? Is this appropriate?
4. Would you guess that Lela is ready for semisolid foods? Which infant skills would you assess in a feeding evaluation?

Clinical Scenario 2

Shana is 12 months old and has been growing at the 50th percentile for weight and the 25th percentile for length since early infancy. She consumes formula from a bottle (24 oz per day of Enfamil with iron), table and finger foods (e.g., crackers, toast fingers, cooked carrot sticks, cooked green beans, cheese cubes, mashed potatoes, applesauce, and canned pears), and 12 to 14 oz of apple juice each day. Shana's mother wonders if Shana is drinking enough formula each day.

1. Do you need additional information to accurately assess Shana's nutrient intake?
2. Do you think Shana is drinking enough formula each day? What if any changes would you suggest to her mother?
3. How would you evaluate the foods offered to Shana in terms of her motor development? Her oral health? Her growth? The adequacy of her nutrient intake?
4. What suggestions might you make to Shana's mother so that she can use food to support Shana's developmental progress?

SUMMARY

Basic concepts of infant growth and development and nourishment are related. Infants grow rapidly in the first year of life; thus the types of infant feedings (human milk or formula), the composition of feedings, and the addition of solids to infants' diets are important considerations. The use of solid foods (with thought given to the types of foods and portion sizes served) to support nourishment and developmental progress sets the stage for lifelong food habits that promote appropriate growth and healthy food choices.

Relevant Web Sites

American Academy of Pediatrics
www.aap.org/
University of Washington
Assuring pediatric nutrition in the community
http://depts.washington.edu/nutrpeds
National Center for Education in Maternal and Child Health
Bright Futures: *Nutrition in practice*
www.brightfutures.org/nutrition/about.html
National Center for Health Statistics
Healthy People 2010: Objectives for Improving Health
www.health.gov/healthy people/

Cited References

American Academy of Pediatrics, Committee on Drugs: Transfer of drugs and other chemicals into human milk, *Pediatrics* 108: 776, 2001.

American Academy of Pediatrics, Committee on Nutrition: The use of whole cow's milk in infancy, *Pediatrics* 91:515, 1992 (reaffirmed April 1998).

American Academy of Pediatrics, Committee on Nutrition: *Handbook of pediatric nutrition*, ed 4, Elk Grove Village, Ill, 1998a, The Academy.

American Academy of Pediatrics, Committee on Nutrition: Soy protein-based formulas: recommendations for use in infant feeding (RE9806), *Pediatrics* 101:148, 1998b.

American Academy of Pediatrics, Committee on Nutrition: Iron fortification of infant formulas (RE9865), *Pediatrics* 104:119, 1999.

American Academy of Pediatrics, Committee on Nutrition: Hypoallergenic infant formulas (RE0005), *Pediatrics* 106:346, 2000.

American Academy of Pediatrics, Committee on Nutrition: The use and misuse of fruit juice in pediatrics (RE0047), *Pediatrics* 107:1210, 2001.

American Academy of Pediatrics, Work Group on Breast-Feeding: Breastfeeding and the use of human milk, *Pediatrics* 100:1035, 1997.

American Dietetic Association: Position of the American Dietetic Association: promotion of breastfeeding, *J Am Diet Assoc* 97: 662, 1997.

American Dietetic Association: Position of the American Dietetic Association: breaking the barriers to breastfeeding, *J Am Diet Assoc* 101:1213, 2001.

Angelsen NK et al: Breast feeding and cognitive development at age 1 and 5 years, *Arch Dis Child* 85:183, 2001.

Auestad N et al: Visual acuity, erythrocyte fatty acid composition, and growth in term infants fed formula with long chain polyunsaturated fatty acids for one year, *Pediatr Res* 41:1, 1997.

Birch EE et al: Visual acuity and essentiality of docosahexaenoic acid in the diet of term infants, *Pediatr Res* 44:201, 1998.

Birch L et al: The variability of young children's energy intake, *N Engl J Med* 324:232, 1991.

Carlson SE et al: Visual acuity and fatty acid status of term infants fed human milk and formula with and without docosahexaenoate and arachidonate from egg yolk lecithin, *Pediatr Res* 39:882, 1996.

Davis CM: Self-selection of diet by newly weaned infants: an experimental study, *Am J Dis Child* 36:651, 1928.

Davis CM: Results of the self-selection of diets by young children, *Can Med Assoc J* 41:257, 1939.

Dell S, To T: Breastfeeding and asthma in young children: findings from a population based study, *Arch Pediatr Adolesc Med* 155:1261, 2001.

Dewey KG et al: Breast-fed infants are leaner than formula-fed infants at 1 year of age: the DARLING study, *Am J Clin Nutr* 57:140, 1993.

Fisher JO et al: Breast-feeding through the first year predicts maternal control in feeding and subsequent toddler energy intakes, *J Am Diet Assoc* 100:641, 2000.

Fuchs GJ et al: Iron status and intake of older infants fed formula vs cow's milk with cereal, *Am J Clin Nutr* 58:343, 1993.

Gdalevich M, Mimouni D, Mimouni M: Breast-feeding and the risk of bronchial asthma in childhood: a systematic review with meta-analysis of prospective studies, *J Pediatr* 139:261, 2001.

Greer FR: Vitamin K deficiency and hemorrhage in infancy, *Clin Perinatol* 22:759, 1995.

Greer FR: Are breast-fed infants vitamin K deficient? *Adv Exp Med Biol* 501:391, 2001.

Hediger ML et al: Association between infant breastfeeding and overweight in young children, *JAMA* 285:2453, 2001.

Heinig MJ et al: Energy and protein intakes of breast-fed and formula-fed infants during the first year of life and their association with growth velocity: the DARLING STUDY, *Am J Clin Nutr* 58:152, 1993.

Higgenbottom L: A syndrome of megaloblastic anemia and neurological abnormalities of a vitamin B_{12} deficient breast fed infant of a strict vegetarian, *N Engl J Med* 299:317, 1978.

Hill PD et al: Does early supplementation affect long-term breastfeeding? *Clin Pediatr* 56:345, 1997.

Humphrey J, Iliff P: Is breast not best? Feeding babies born to HIV-positive mothers: bringing balance to a complex issue, *Nutr Rev* 59:119, 2001.

Innis SM, Gilley J, Werker J: Are human milk long-chain polyunsaturated fatty acids related to visual and neural development in breast-fed term infants? *J Pediatr* 139:532, 2001.

Irvine CH et al: Phyto-estrogens in soy-based infant foods: Concentrations, daily intake, and possible biological effects, *Proc Soc Exp Biol Med* 217:247, 1998.

Jensen CL et al: Effect of dietary linoleic/alpha–linolenic acid ratio on growth and visual function in term infants, *J Pediatr* 131:200, 1997.

Johnson PR, Roloff JS: Vitamin B_{12} deficiency in an infant strictly breast-fed by a mother with latent pernicious anemia, *J Pediatr* 100:917, 1982.

Kim SK et al: Red blood cell indices and iron status according to feeding practices in infants and young children, *Acta Paediatr* 85:139, 1996.

Koletzko B et al: Arachidonic acid supply and metabolism in human infants born at full term, *Lipids* 31:79, 1996.

Kreiter SR et al: Nutritional rickets in African-American breast-fed infants, *J Pediatr* 137:153, 2000.

Looker AC et al: Prevalence of iron deficiency in the United States, *JAMA* 277:973, 1997.

Lozoff B et al: Poorer behavioral and developmental outcome more than 10 years after treatment for iron deficiency anemia in infancy, *Pediatrics*, vol 105, 2000.

Makrides M et al: A critical appraisal of the role of dietary long-chain polyunsaturated fatty acids on neural indices of term infants: a randomized controlled trial, *Pediatrics* 105:32, 2000.

Manganaro R et al: Incidence of dehydration and hypernatremia in exclusively breast-fed infants, *J Pediatr* 139:673, 2001.

Mehta KC et al: Trial on timing of introduction to solids and food type on infant growth, *Pediatr* 102:569, 1998.
Mouradian W, Wehr E, Crall JJ: Disparities in children's oral health and access to dental care, *JAMA* 284:2625, 2000.
Nutrient Requirements for Infant Formulas, Final Rule (21 CFR 107), *Federal Register* 50:45106, 1985.
Oddie S, Richmond S, Coulthard M: Hypernatremic dehydration and breast feeding: a population study, *Arch Dis Child* 85:318, 2001.
Oddy WH: Breastfeeding protects against illness and infection in infants and children: a review of the evidence, *Breastfeed Rev* 9:11, 2001.
Scariati PD et al: Longitudinal analysis of infant morbidity and the extent of breastfeeding in the United States, *Pediatrics* 99:E51, 1997.
Scott DT et al: Formula supplementation with long-chain polyunsaturated fatty acids: are there developmental benefits? *Pediatrics* 102:E59, 1998.
Setchell KD et al: Exposure of infants to phtyoestrogens from soy based formula, *Lancet* 350:23, 1997.
Sherriff A et al: Should infants be screened for anemia? A prospective study investigating the ratio between hemoglobin at 8, 12, and 18 months and development at 18 months, *Arch Dis Child* 84:480, 2001.
Smith D et al: Shifting linear growth during infancy: illustration of genetic factors in growth from fetal life through infancy, *J Pediatr* 89:225, 1976.
Smith MM, Lifshitz F: Excess fruit juice consumption as a contributing factor in nonorganic failure to thrive, *Pediatrics* 93:438, 1994.
Specker B et al: Sunshine exposure and serum-25-hydroxyvitamin D concentrations in exclusively breast-fed infants, *J Pediatr* 107:372, 1985.
Story M, Brown JE: Do young children instinctively know what to eat? *N Engl J Med* 316:103, 1987.
Sullivan SA, Birch LL: Infant dietary experience and acceptance of solid foods, *Pediatrics* 93:271, 1994.
Tomashek KM et al: Nutritional rickets in Georgia, *Pediatrics* 107:46, 2001.
Von Kries R et al: Breastfeeding and obesity: a cross sectional study, *Br Med J* 319:147, 1999.

Additional References

American Academy of Pediatrics, Work Group on Cow's-Milk Protein and Diabetes Mellitus: Infant feeding practices and their possible relationship to the etiology of diabetes mellitus, *Pediatrics* 94:752, 1994.
Calvo EB et al: Iron status in exclusively breast fed infants, *Pediatrics* 90:375, 1992.
Churella H et al: Growth and protein status of term infants fed soy protein formulas differing in protein content, *J Am Coll Nutr* 13:262, 1994.
Campbell CM: Preventing obesity: prevention starts in infancy, *Br Med J* 326(7380):102, 2003.
Forsyth JS et al: Long chain polyunsaturated fatty acid supplementation in infant formula and blood pressure in later childhood: follow up of a randomized control trial, *Br Med J* 326(7396):953, 2003.
Garza C, Frongillo EA: Infant feeding recommendations (Editorial), *Am J Clin Nutr* 67:815, 1998.
Holman SR: Infant feeding in Roman antiquity, *Nutr Today* 33:113, 1998.
Neuringer MD, Connor WE: *n*-3 fatty acids in the brain and retina: evidence for their essentiality, *Nutr Rev* 44:285, 1986.
Trahms C, Pipes P: *Nutrition in infancy and childhood,* ed 6, New York, 1997, McGraw-Hill.

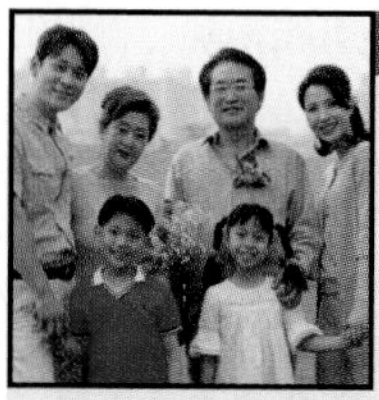

CHAPTER 9

Nutrition for Low-Birth-Weight Infants

DIANE M. ANDERSON, PhD, RD, CSP, FADA

CHAPTER OUTLINE

- Physiologic Development
- Nutritional Requirements: Parenteral Feeding
- Transition From Parenteral to Enteral Feeding
- Nutritional Requirements: Enteral Feeding
- Feeding Methods
- Selection of Enteral Feeding
- Growth and Nutritional Assessments
- Discharge Care
- Neurodevelopmental Outcome

KEY TERMS

Apgar score–a score given to newborn infants at 1 and 5 minutes of age to describe their clinical condition; neonatal resuscitation and neurologic signs such as respirations, heart rate, skin color, reflex irritability, and tone are evaluated

appropriate for gestational age (AGA)–describes the size of an infant whose birth weight is between the 10th and 90th percentiles for gestational age on an intrauterine growth grid

extremely low birth weight (ELBW)–a birth weight of less than 1000 g (2¼ lb)

gastric gavage–a feeding method that involves inserting a soft feeding tube through the mouth or nose into the stomach

gestational age–the age of an infant at birth as determined by the length of the pregnancy (the number of weeks since the last menstrual period) or a clinical assessment

glucose load–the amount of glucose received intravenously

hemolytic anemia–anemia caused by oxidative destruction of mature red blood cells; sometimes caused by vitamin E deficiency

human milk fortifiers–supplements of protein, carbohydrate, fat, minerals, and vitamins added to human milk to meet the increased nutrient needs of premature infants

infancy–birth to 1 year of age

infant mortality rate–the number of infant deaths in the first year of life per 1000 live births

large for gestational age (LGA)–refers to the size of an infant whose birth weight is above the 90th percentile of the standard weight for gestational age according to the intrauterine growth chart

low birth weight (LBW)–a birth weight of less than 2500 g (5½ lb)

necrotizing enterocolitis–inflammation or death of the gastrointestinal tract

neonatal period–the first 28 days of life

neutral thermal environment–the environmental temperature at which an infant expends the least amount of energy to maintain body temperature

osteopenia of prematurity–reduced bone mass in a premature infant resulting from a decreased bone synthesis rate; often attributable to inadequate calcium and phosphorus intake

perinatal period–from 28 weeks of gestation to 4 weeks after birth

premature (preterm) infant–an infant born before 37 weeks of gestation

respiratory distress syndrome–lung disease caused by a surfactant deficiency; develops shortly after birth and is common in preterm infants

small for gestational age (SGA)–referring to the size of an infant whose birth weight is lower than the 10th percentile of the standard weight for gestational age

surfactant–a mixture of lipoproteins secreted by alveolar cells into the alveoli and respiratory air passages that contributes to the elastic properties of pulmonary tissue

term infant–an infant born between 37 and 42 weeks of gestation

very low birth weight (VLBW)–a birth weight of less than 1500 g (3⅓ lb)

The management of *low-birth-weight (LBW)* infants requiring intensive care continues to improve dramatically. With new technologies, improved understanding of perinatal (from 28 weeks of gestation to 4 weeks after birth) pathophysiology, current nutrition management principles, and regionalization of perinatal care, the mortality rates during infancy, that period from birth to 1 year of age, continue to decrease in the United States. In particular, the development and use of surfactant—a mixture of lipoproteins secreted by alveolar cells into the alveoli and respiratory air passages that contributes to the elastic properties of pulmonary tissue—have increased the survival of preterm infants, as has the use of antepartum corticosteroids. Most LBW infants have the potential for long and productive lives (Wilson-Costello and Hack, 2002).

Nutrition can be provided to LBW infants in many ways, each of which has certain benefits and limitations. The infant's size, age, and clinical condition dictate the nutritional requirements and the way they can be provided. Because of the complexities involved in the neonatal intensive care setting, a team that includes a registered dietitian trained in neonatal nutrition should make the decisions necessary to facilitate optimal nutrition. In regionalized perinatal care systems, the neonatal nutritionist may also consult with health care providers in community hospitals and public health settings.

PHYSIOLOGIC DEVELOPMENT

Gestational Age and Size

At birth, an infant who weighs less than 2500 g (5½ lb) is classified as having a low birth weight (LBW); an infant weighing less than 1500 g (3⅓ lb) has a very low birth weight (VLBW); and an infant weighing less than 1000 g (2¼ lb) has an extremely low birth weight (ELBW). LBW may be attributable to a shortened period of gestation, or prematurity, or a retarded intrauterine growth rate, which makes the infant small for gestational age.

The term infant is born between the thirty-seventh and forty-second weeks of gestation. A premature (preterm) infant is born before 37 weeks of gestation, whereas a postterm infant is born after 42 weeks of gestation.

Antenatally, an estimate of the infant's gestational age is based on the date of the mother's last menstrual period, clinical parameters of uterine fundal height, the presence of quickening (the first movements of the fetus that can be felt by the mother), fetal heart tones, or ultrasound evaluations. After birth, gestational age is determined by clinical assessment. Clinical parameters fall into two groups: (1) a series of neurologic signs, which depend primarily on postures and tone, and (2) a series of external characteristics that reflect the physical maturity of the infant. The New Ballard Score (Ballard et al, 1991) examination is a frequently used clinical assessment tool. An accurate assessment of gestational age is important for establishing nutritional goals for individual infants and differentiating the premature infant from the term SGA infant.

An infant who is small for gestational age (SGA) has a birth weight that is lower than the 10th percentile of the standard weight for that gestational age. An SGA infant whose intrauterine weight gain is poor but whose linear and head growth are between the 10th and 90th percentiles on the intrauterine growth grid has experienced *asymmetrical intrauterine growth retardation (IUGR)*. An SGA infant whose length and occipital frontal circumference are also below the 10th percentile of the standards has *symmetrical IUGR*. Symmetrical IUGR, which usually reflects early and prolonged intrauterine deficit, is apparently more detrimental to later growth and development. An infant whose size is appropriate for gestational age (AGA) has a birth weight between the 10th and 90th percentiles on the intrauterine growth chart. An infant whose birth weight is above the 90th percentile on the intrauterine growth chart is large for gestational age (LGA). Figure 9-1 shows the classification of neonates based on maturity and intrauterine growth.

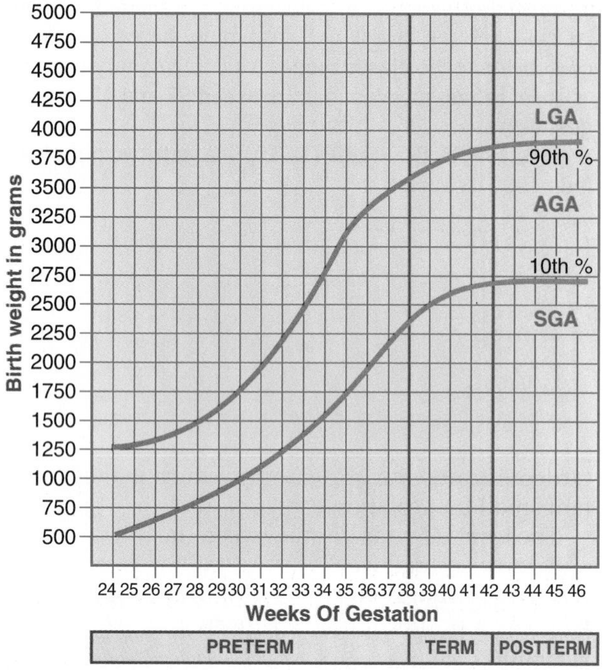

FIGURE 9-1 • Classification of neonates based on maturity and intrauterine growth (small for gestational age [SGA], appropriate for gestational age [AGA], or large for gestational age [LGA].) (From Battaglia FC, Lubchenco LO: A practical classification of newborn infants by weight and gestational age, *J Pediatr* 71:159, 1967).

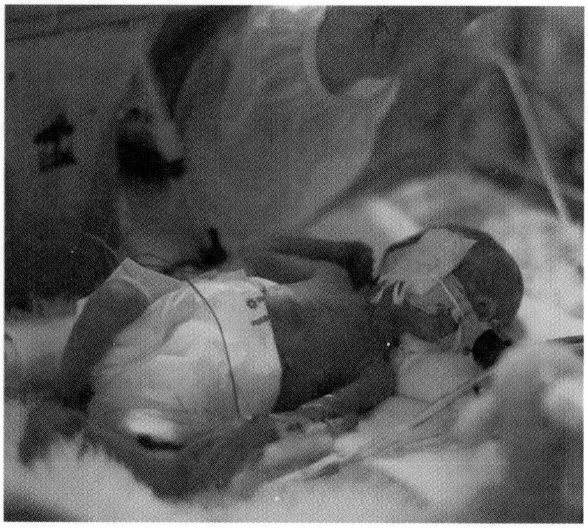

FIGURE 9-2 • A.R., born at 27 weeks of gestation, had a birth weight of 870 g (1 lb, 14 oz).

Infant Mortality and Statistics

Although the infant mortality rate in the United States continues to decrease, it is still higher than in many Western countries. This discrepancy may be attributable to the inconsistent collection of mortality data among nations, which may falsely lower mortality rates in other countries. However, the high incidence of LBW infants born in the United States contributes to this high infant mortality rate. Greater than 64% of the infant mortality rate is linked to LBW infants (Hoyert et al, 2001). An inverse relationship exists between birth weight and infant mortality rate. The risk for infant death for those who weigh 1500 to 2499 g is six times higher than for infants who weigh more than 2500 g; for infants who weigh less than 1500 g, the risk is 96 times higher (Hoyert et al, 2001). Even though the United States has a high incidence of LBW and VLBW infants, it still has one of the best birth weight–specific survival rates (American Academy of Pediatrics and American College of Obstetrics and Gynecology, 1997). The high incidence of teenage pregnancy also contributes to the high infant mortality rate; teenagers have a 2.3% to 6% higher incidence of giving birth to LBW infants (MacKay et al, 2000).

The incidence of multiple births has increased, which is also associated with a higher infant mortality rate. Multiple births are nine times more likely to result in LBW infants than singleton births. In 1999 the number of twin births was 67% higher than it was in 1980 (Hoyert et al, 2001). The number of triplet or greater births soared 470% from 1980 to 1998 but decreased by 4% from 1998 to 1999 (Hoyert et al, 2001). This growth in the number of multiple births is related to women delaying childbirth, because multiple gestations are associated with mothers of older ages. In addition, fertility-enhancing therapies are frequently used.

Characteristics of Immaturity

The premature or LBW infant has not had the chance to develop fully in utero and is physiologically different from the term infant (Figure 9-2). Because of this, LBW infants have various clinical problems in the early neonatal period, depending on their intrauterine environment, degree of prematurity, birth-related trauma, and function of immature or stressed organ systems. Certain problems occur with such frequency that they are considered typical of prematurity (Table 9-1). Premature infants are at high risk for poor nutritional status because of poor nutrient stores, physiologic immaturity, illness (which may interfere with nutritional management and needs), and the nutrient demands required for growth.

Most fetal nutrient stores are deposited during the last 3 months of pregnancy; therefore the premature infant begins life in a compromised nutritional state. Because metabolic (i.e., energy) stores are limited, nutritional support in the form of parenteral nutrition (PN), enteral nutrition, or both should be initiated as soon as possible. In the preterm infant weighing 1000 g, fat constitutes only 1% of total body weight; by contrast the term infant (3500 g)

TABLE 9-1 Common Problems Among Premature Infants

SYSTEM	PROBLEM
Respiratory	Respiratory distress syndrome, chronic lung disease (bronchopulmonary dysplasia)
Cardiovascular	Patent ductus arteriosus (PDA)
Renal	Fluid and electrolyte imbalance
Neurologic	Intraventricular hemorrhage, periventricular leukomalacia (cerebral necrosis)
Metabolic	Hypoglycemia, hyperglycemia, hypocalcemia, metabolic acidosis
Gastrointestinal	Hyperbilirubinemia, feeding intolerance, necrotizing enterocolitis
Hematologic	Anemia
Immunologic	Sepsis, pneumonia, meningitis
Other	Apnea, bradycardia, cyanosis, osteopenia

Modified from Zerzan J, O'Leary MJ: Nutrition for preterm and low-birth-weight infants. In Trahms CM, Pipes PL, eds: *Nutrition in infancy and childhood,* ed 6, New York, 1997, WBC/McGraw-Hill.

has a fat percentage of about 16%. For example, a 1000-g AGA premature infant has a glycogen and fat reserve equivalent to about 110 kcal per kilogram of body weight. With basal metabolic needs of approximately 50 kcal/kg/day, it is obvious that this infant will rapidly run out of fat and carbohydrate fuel unless adequate nutritional support is established. The depletion time is even shorter for preterm infants weighing less than 1000 g at birth. Nutrient reserves are depleted most quickly by tiny infants who have IUGR as a result of their increased basal metabolic rate.

However, it is often difficult to provide adequate nutrition during the first several days of life because of immature organ systems and severe medical problems. When an adequate dietary intake cannot be established and fat and glycogen reserves have been exhausted, the infant begins to catabolize vital body protein tissue for energy. Theoretical estimates of survival time of starved and semistarved infants are shown in Table 9-2. These estimates assume depletion of all glycogen and fat and about one third of body protein tissue at a rate of 50 kcal/kg/day. The effects of fluids such as intravenously provided water (which has no exogenous calories) and 10% dextrose solution ($D_{10}W$) are shown. Even with protein tissue catabolism, the projected survival times are alarmingly short.

The small premature infant is particularly vulnerable to undernutrition. Malnutrition in premature infants may increase the risk of infection, prolong chronic illness and adversely affect brain growth and function. In fact, Lucas et al (1998) reported that the type of milk used for the neonatal diet may be directly linked to neurodevelopment at 18 months of age. Human milk or premature infant formula fed the first month of life resulted in improved development.

TABLE 9-2 Expected Survival Time of Starved (H_2O Only) and Semistarved ($D_{10}W$) Infants

BIRTH WEIGHT (g)	ESTIMATED SURVIVAL TIME (DAYS) H_2O	ESTIMATED SURVIVAL TIME (DAYS) $D_{10}W$
1000	4	11
2000	12	30
3500	32	80

Data from Heird WC et al: Intravenous alimentation in pediatric patients, *J Pediatr* 80:351, 1972.

NUTRITIONAL REQUIREMENTS: PARENTERAL FEEDING

Many critically ill preterm infants have difficulty progressing to full enteral feedings in the first several days or even weeks of life. The infant's small stomach capacity, immature gastrointestinal tract, and illness make the progression of enteral feedings difficult (Figure 9-3). PN becomes essential for nutrition support, either as a supplement to enteral feedings or as the total source of nutrition. Chapter 23 offers a complete discussion of PN; only those aspects related to feeding of the preterm infant are presented here.

Fluid

Because fluid needs vary widely for preterm infants, fluid balance must be monitored. Inadequate intake can lead to dehydration, electrolyte imbalances, and hypotension; excessive intake can lead to edema, congestive heart failure, and possible opening of the ductus arteriosus. Additional neonatal clinical complications reported with high fluid intakes include necrotizing enterocolitis, bronchopulmonary dysplasia (BPD) (see Chapter 38), and intraventricular hemorrhage. The premature infant has a greater percentage of body water (especially extracellular water) than the term infant (see Figure 6-1). The amount of extracellular water should decrease in all infants during the first few days of life. This reduction is accompanied by a normal loss of 10% to 15% of body weight and improved renal function. ELBW infants often lose up to 20% of their birth weight without complications. Failure of this transition in fluid dynamics and lack of diuresis may complicate the course of preterm infants with respiratory disease.

Water requirements are estimated by the sum of the predicted losses from the lungs and skin, urine, and stool and the water needed for growth. A major route of water loss in preterm infants is evaporation through the skin and respiratory tract. This insensible water loss is highest in the smallest and least mature infants because of their larger body surface area relative to body weight, increased permeability of the skin epidermis to water, and greater skin blood flow relative to metabolic rate. Insensible water loss is increased by radiant warmers and phototherapy lights and decreased by heat shields, thermal blankets, and humidified incubators. Insensible water loss can vary from 50 to 100 ml/kg/day on the first day of life and increase up to 120 to 200 ml/kg/day, depending on the infant's size, gestational age, day of life and environment. The use of humidified incubators can decrease insensible water losses and thereby reduce fluid requirements.

Excretion of urine, the other major route of water loss, varies from 40 to 85 ml/kg/day. This loss depends on the fluid volume and solute load presented to the kidneys. The infant's ability to concentrate urine increases with maturity. Stool water loss is generally 5 to 10 ml/kg/day, and 10 ml/kg/day is suggested as optimal for growth (Bell and Oh, 1999).

Because of the many variables affecting neonatal fluid losses, fluid needs must be determined on an individual basis. Usually, fluid is administered at a rate of 80 to 105 ml/kg/day the first day of life to meet insensible losses and urine output. Fluid needs are then evaluated by assessing fluid intake and comparing it with the clinical parameters of urine volume output, specific gravity or osmolality, and serum electrolyte, creatinine, and urea nitrogen levels. Assessments of weight, blood pressure, peripheral perfusion, skin turgor, and mucous membrane moisture are performed daily. Daily fluid administration generally increases by 10 to 20 ml/kg/day. By the end of the second week of life, preterm infants may receive fluids

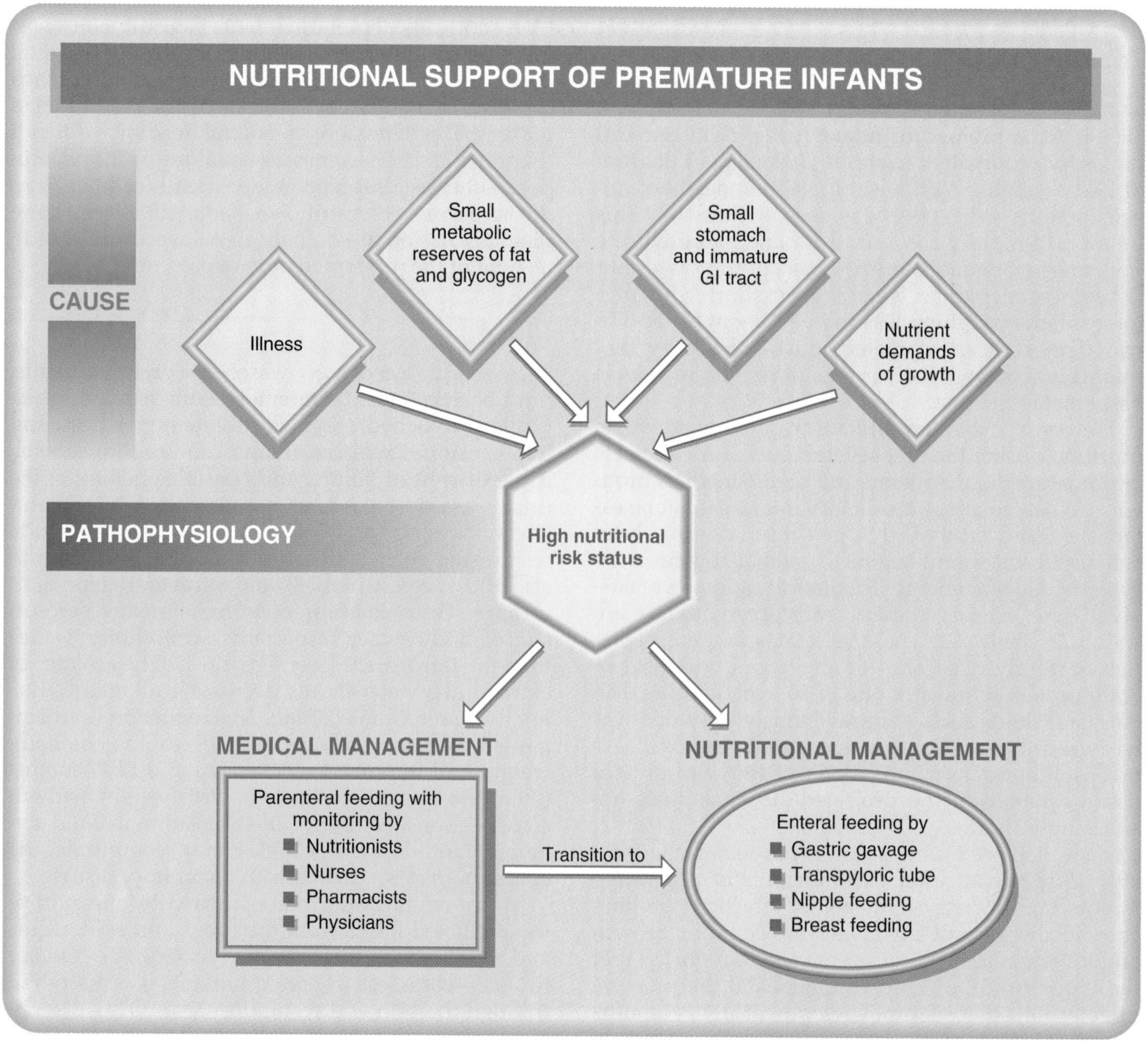

FIGURE 9-3 • Pathophysiology algorithm: nutritional support of premature infants. (Developed by John Anderson, Ph.D., and Stanford C. Garner, Ph.D., 2000. Updated by Diane M. Anderson, 2002.)

at a rate of 140 to 160 ml/kg/day. Fluid restriction may be necessary in preterm infants with patent ductus arteriosus (PDA), congestive heart failure, renal failure, or cerebral edema. More fluids are needed by preterm infants who are placed under phototherapy lights or a radiant warmer or when the environmental or body temperature is elevated.

Energy

The energy needs of preterm infants fed parenterally are less than those of enterally fed infants because absorption loss does not occur when nutritional intake bypasses the intestinal tract. Enterally fed preterm infants usually require 105 to 130 kcal/kg/day to grow, whereas parenterally fed premature neonates can grow well receiving 80 to 90 kcal/kg/day (AAP, 1998). Minimal maintenance energy needs and adequate protein should be provided as soon as possible to prevent tissue catabolism. Providing VLBW infants with 1 to 2 g of protein and 30 to 50 kcal/kg/day promotes nitrogen balance during the first 3 days of life (Heird, 1999). Energy and protein intake should be increased as the infant's condition stabilizes and growth becomes the goal (Table 9-3).

Glucose

Glucose or dextrose is the principal energy source (3.4 kcal/g). However, glucose tolerance is limited in premature infants, especially in VLBW infants, because of inadequate insulin production, insulin resistance, and continued hepatic glucose release while intravenous glucose is infusing. Hyperglycemia is less likely when glucose is administered with amino acids than when it is infused alone. Amino acids exert a stimulatory effect on insulin release. Prevention of hyperglycemia is important because it can lead to diuresis and dehydration.

To prevent hyperglycemia in VLBW infants, glucose should be administered in small amounts. The glucose load is a function of the concentration of the dextrose infusion and the rate at which it is administered (Table 9-4). The administration of exogenous insulin may be necessary for infants with persistent or very high glycemia, but changes in the infant's blood glucose level are common problems associated with its use. In addition, protein synthesis may be inhibited by insulin administration in premature infants (Poindexter et al, 1998).

In general, preterm infants should receive an initial glucose load of less than 6 mg/kg/min, with a gradual increase to 11 to 12 mg/kg/min. ELBW infants tolerate a lower initial glucose load of 4 to 6 mg/kg/min. The glucose load can be advanced by 1 to 2 mg/kg/min per day. Hypoglycemia is not as common a problem as hyperglycemia, but it may occur if the glucose infusion is abruptly decreased or interrupted.

Amino Acids

Protein guidelines range from 2.5 to 3.8 g/kg/day. However, an intrauterine growth rate of protein accretion can be achieved at 3 g/kg/day (Hanning and Zlotkin, 1997). ELBW infants may need as much as 3 to 4 g/kg/day (Hanning and Zlotkin, 1997). Protein in excess of these parenteral requirements should not be administered because additional protein offers no apparent advantage and increases the risk of metabolic problems. In practice, preterm infants are usually given 1 to 2 g of protein per kilogram for the first few days of life, and then protein is provided as tolerated.

In the United States, two pediatric solutions are in use: Trophamine (McGaw Laboratories) and Aminosyn PF (Abbott Laboratories). The use of pediatric solutions results in plasma amino acid profiles similar to those of healthy infants fed breast milk, and appropriate acid-base status has been noted (Heird and Gomez, 1996). These solutions promote adequate weight gain and nitrogen retention. Standard amino acid solutions such as Aminosyn (Abbott Laboratories), FreAmine (McGaw Laboratories), and Travasol (Clintec) were not designed to meet the particular needs of immature infants and may provoke imbalances in plasma amino acid levels. For example, cysteine, tyrosine, and taurine levels in these solutions are low relative to the needs of the preterm infant,

TABLE 9-3 Comparison of Parenteral and Enteral Energy Needs of Premature Infants

	PARENTERAL	ENTERAL
Maintenance		
Gradually increase intake to meet energy needs by the end of the first week	40-50 cal/kg/day	50 kcal/kg/day
Growth		
Meet energy needs as soon as the infant's condition is stable	80-90 cal/kg/day	105-130 kcal/kg/day

TABLE 9-4 Guidelines for Glucose Load in Premature Infants

BIRTH WEIGHT (g)	INITIAL LOAD (mg/kg/min)*	DAILY INCREMENTS (mg/kg/min)	MAXIMUM LOAD (mg/kg/min)
<1000	4-6	1-2	11-12
1001-2000	≤6	1-2	11-12

*Use the following formula to calculate glucose load: (% Glucose × ml/kg/day) × (1000 mg/g glucose) ÷ (1440 min/day). *For example:* (0.10 × 150 ml/kg/day) × (1000 mg/g glucose) ÷ (1440 min/day) = 10.4 mg/kg/min.

TABLE 9-5 Guidelines for Administration of Parenteral Amino Acids for Premature Infants

INITIAL RATE (g/kg/day)*	INCREMENTS (g/kg/day)	MAXIMUM RATE (g/kg/day)
1.5	0.5-1	3.5-3.8†

*Use the following formula to calculate protein load: % Protein × ml/kg/day = Protein g/kg/day.
For example: 0.02 × 150 ml/kg/day = 3 g/kg/day.
†3.8 g/kg/day is recommended for infants weighing less than 1000 g. (From Hansen JW: Appendix Table A.1. Consensus recommendations. In Tsang RC et al, eds: *Nutritional needs of the preterm infant,* Baltimore, 1993, Williams & Wilkins.)

but the methionine and glycine levels are relatively high. Because premature infants do not effectively synthesize cysteine from methionine because of decreased concentrations of the hepatic enzyme cystathionase, a cysteine supplement has been suggested. Cysteine is insoluble and unstable in solution, so it is added as cysteine hydrochloride when the PN solution is prepared. In one study, nitrogen retention was increased with cysteine supplementation, although this finding has not consistently been reported (Heird and Gomez, 1996; Rivera et al, 1993). Metabolic acidosis can also occur with the use of cysteine hydrochloride, but it can be corrected by decreasing the dose of the supplement or by adding additional acetate to the solution.

In addition to plasma amino acid imbalances, other metabolic problems associated with amino acid infusions in preterm infants include metabolic acidosis, hyperammonemia, and azotemia. These problems can be minimized by using the crystalline amino acid products that are available today and by keeping the protein load within the recommended guidelines (Table 9-5).

Lipids

Intravenous fat emulsions are used for two reasons: (1) to meet essential fatty acid (EFA) requirements and (2) to provide a concentrated source of energy. EFA needs can be met by providing 0.5 to 1 g/kg/day of lipids. Biochemical evidence of EFA deficiency has been noted during the first week of life in VLBW infants fed parenterally without fat. The clinical consequences of EFA deficiency may include coagulation abnormalities, abnormal pulmonary surfactant, and adverse effects on lung metabolism.

Lipids should be introduced slowly in preterm infants, with periodic monitoring of plasma triglyceride levels, which should remain less than 150 mg/dl. Elevated plasma triglyceride levels may develop in infants with a decreased ability to hydrolyze triglycerides. This problem is most commonly associated with decreasing gestational age, SGA status infection, surgical stress, and malnutrition. Under these conditions, close monitoring of serum triglyceride levels is indicated, and less than 3 g/kg/day of fat may need to be provided. Further, hyperbilirubinemia can increase the risk of lipid toxicity. Kernicterus can occur in infants with hyperbilirubinemia if free fatty acids displace bilirubin from albumin-binding sites, raising the level of free bilirubin in the blood. In preterm infants with severe hyperbilirubinemia, lipid loads may be limited to avoid possible complications. Once the infant is medically stable and additional energy is needed for growth, lipid loads can slowly be increased.

TABLE 9-6 Guidelines for Administration of Parenteral Lipids for Premature Infants

INITIAL RATE (g/kg/day)*	INCREMENTS (g/kg/day)	MAXIMUM RATE (g/kg/day)
0.5	0.5-1	3

*Use the following formula to calculate lipid load:
% Lipid × ml/kg/day = Lipid g/kg/day. *For example:* 0.20 × 15 ml/kg = 3 g/kg/day.

Lipids should be administered over 24 hours at a maximum rate of 0.15 g/kg/hr to prevent a rise in triglycerides and free fatty acids. A daily increment of 0.5 to 1 g/kg/day is provided until a rate of 3 g/kg/day is being provided (Table 9-6). The total lipid load is usually less than 30% to 40% of nonprotein calories, but it should not exceed 60% of nonprotein calories. (The lipid emulsions currently in use are described in Chapter 23.) In preterm infants, 20% solutions providing 2 kcal/ml are recommended because plasma triglyceride, cholesterol, and phospholipid levels are generally lower with these than with the 10% emulsions. The lower plasma fat levels may be attributable to a decreased phospholipid load per gram of fat in the 20% emulsion.

It has been suggested that continuous administration of heparin to infants receiving parenteral lipids may improve lipid clearance by stimulating the release of the enzymes lipoprotein lipase and hepatic lipase into the circulation, thus promoting the intravascular lipolysis of fat. Heparin is commonly administered at 1 U/ml. Higher heparin concentrations may lead to increased serum free fatty acid levels. Heparin also prevents thrombosis formation and, with the administration of lipids, prolongs the life of peripheral veins.

Carnitine is frequently added to PN solutions provided to premature infants. Carnitine facilitates the mechanism by which fatty acids are transported across the mitochondrial membrane, allowing their oxidation to provide energy. Enhanced lipid utilization has been documented with carnitine supplementation in LBW infants receiving PN for longer than 1 month (Christensen et al, 1989). Other short-term investigations have failed to show an improvement in

TABLE 9-7 Guidelines for Administration of Parenteral Electrolytes for Premature Infants

ELECTROLYTE	AMOUNT (mEq/kg/day)
Sodium	2-3
Chloride	2-3
Potassium	2-3

fatty acid oxidation. One study reported increased protein oxidation and decreased weight gain (Sulkers et al, 1990). Carnitine supplementation may be helpful for preterm infants who are receiving only PN at 2 to 4 weeks of age.

Electrolytes

After the first few days of life, sodium, potassium, and chloride are added to parenteral solutions to compensate for the loss of extracellular fluid. To prevent hyperkalemia and cardiac arrhythmia, potassium should be withheld until renal flow is demonstrated. In general, the preterm infant has the same electrolyte requirements as the term infant, but actual requirements vary depending on factors such as renal function, state of hydration, and the use of diuretics (Table 9-7). Very immature infants may have a limited ability to conserve sodium and so may require increased amounts of sodium to maintain a normal serum sodium concentration. Serum electrolyte levels should be monitored periodically. Urine electrolytes should be quantified when serum levels are abnormal to detect inappropriate electrolyte excretion.

Minerals

Calcium and phosphorus are important components of the PN solution. Premature infants who receive PN with low calcium and phosphorus concentrations are at risk for developing osteopenia of prematurity. This poor bone mineralization is most likely to develop in VLBW infants who receive PN for prolonged periods. Calcium and phosphorus status should be monitored using serum calcium, phosphorus, and alkaline phosphatase levels and radiographic bone studies.

Preterm infants have higher calcium and phosphorus needs than term infants. However, it is difficult to add enough calcium and phosphorus to parenteral solutions to meet these higher requirements without causing precipitation of the minerals. Calcium and phosphorus should be provided simultaneously in PN solutions. Alternate-day infusions are not recommended because abnormal serum mineral levels and decreased mineral retention develop.

TABLE 9-8 Guidelines for Administration of Parenteral Minerals for Premature Infants

MINERALS	AMOUNT (mg/L)*
Calcium	500-600
Phosphorus	400-500
Magnesium	50-70

Modified from Greene HL et al: Guidelines for the use of vitamins, trace elements, calcium, magnesium and phosphorus in infants and children receiving total parenteral nutrition: report of the Subcommittee on Pediatric Parenteral Nutrient Requirements from the Committee on Clinical Practice Issues of the American Society for Clinical Nutrition, *Am J Clin Nutr* 48: 1324, 1988.
*Guidelines are given per liter to prevent administration of excessively high concentrations of calcium and phosphorus with intakes expressed per kilogram of body weight or with fluid restriction.
These recommendations assume an average fluid intake of 120 to 150 ml/kg/day with 2.5 g of amino acids per 100 ml. These doses should be administered only by central venous infusion.

Current recommendations for parenteral administration of additional calcium, phosphorus, and magnesium are presented in Table 9-8. The intakes are expressed per liter of solution, at a rate of 120 to 150 ml/kg/day, with 2.5 g of amino acids or protein. Lower fluid volumes or lower protein concentrations may cause the minerals to precipitate out of solution. The addition of cysteine hydrochloride further increases the acidity of the fluid, which inhibits precipitation of calcium and phosphorus.

Trace Elements

Zinc should be given to all preterm infants receiving PN. If enteral feedings cannot be started by 2 weeks of age, then additional trace elements should be added. However, the amounts of copper and manganese should be reduced for infants with obstructive jaundice, and the amounts of selenium, chromium, and molybdenum should be reduced in infants with renal dysfunction. Parenteral iron is not routinely provided because treated infants often receive blood transfusions soon after birth, and enteral feedings, which provide a source of iron, can often be initiated. The dosage for parenteral iron is approximately 10% of the enteral dosage; guidelines range from 0.1 to 0.2 mg/kg/day (Greene et al, 1988). Recommended guidelines have not yet been established for parenteral administration of fluoride to preterm infants (Table 9-9).

Vitamins

Shortly after birth, all newborn infants receive an intramuscular injection of 0.5 to 1 mg of vitamin K to prevent hemorrhagic disease of the newborn from vitamin K deficiency. Stores of vitamin K are low in newborn infants, and little intestinal bacterial production of vitamin K occurs until bacterial colonization takes place. Because initial dietary intake of vitamin K may be limited, neonates would be at nutritional risk if they did not receive this intramuscular supplement.

Only intravenous multivitamin preparations currently approved and designed for use in infants should be given to provide the appropriate vitamin intake and prevent toxicity from additives used in adult multivitamin injections. The AAP (1998) recommends using the American Society of Clinical Nutrition's guideline of 40% of the MVI-Pediatric 5-ml vial per kilogram of weight. The maximum dose of 5 ml would be given to an infant with a weight of 2.5 kg (Greene et al, 1988). (Table 9-10)

Large supplemental doses of vitamin A have been suggested for the prevention of BPD because of the vitamin's role in facilitating tissue repair and because of reports of preterm infants having low vitamin A stores. Several reports suggest that providing premature infants with intramuscular injections of vitamin A at 5000 IU per day three times per week during the first month of life decreases the incidence of BPD (Tyson et al, 1999). However, this practice remains controversial because more research is needed regarding dose toxicity and effects from additional medical management practices that may decrease the development of BPD (Greer, 2000).

The sugar *inositol* is present in human milk and infant formula but is only present in low concentrations in PN solutions. It is a component of membrane phospholipids and may be involved in signal transduction. Hallman et al (1992) reported that the addition of inositol to PN solutions was associated with increased survival and a decreased incidence of BPD and retinopathy of prematurity in preterm infants with respiratory distress syndrome (a lung disease that is caused by a surfactant deficiency, develops shortly after birth, and is common in preterm infants). However, inositol supplementation is not used clinically because its effectiveness has not been definitively established. Inositol was studied before the many other therapies, including surfactant therapy, that are used today to effectively treat respiratory distress syndrome (Barrington and Finer, 1998).

TRANSITION FROM PARENTERAL TO ENTERAL FEEDING

It is beneficial to begin enteral feedings for preterm infants as early as possible because the feedings stimulate gastrointestinal enzymatic development and activity, promote bile flow, increase villous growth in the small intestine, and promote mature gastrointestinal motility. These initial enteral feedings can also decrease the incidence of cholestatic jaundice and the duration of physiologic jaundice and can improve subsequent feeding tolerance in preterm infants. At times, small, initial feedings are used only to prime the gut and are not intended to optimize enteral nutrient intake until the infant demonstrates feeding tolerance or is clinically stable.

When making the transition from parenteral to enteral feeding, it is important to maintain parenteral feeding until enteral feeding is well established to maintain adequate net intake of fluid and nutrients. In VLBW infants, it may take 7 to 14 days to provide a full enteral feeding, and it may take longer for infants with feeding intolerances or illness. The smallest, sickest infants usually receive increments of only 10 ml/kg/day. Larger, more stable preterm infants may tolerate increments of 20 to 30 ml/kg/day. (See Chapter 23 for a more detailed discussion of transitional feeding.)

TABLE 9-9 Guidelines for Administration of Parenteral Trace Elements for Premature Infants

TRACE ELEMENTS	AMOUNT (μg/kg/day)
Zinc	400
Copper	20*
Manganese	1*
Selenium	2†
Chromium	0.2†
Molybdenum	0.25†
Iodine	1

Modified from Greene HL et al: Guidelines for the use of vitamins, trace elements, calcium, magnesium, and phosphorus in infants and children receiving total parenteral nutrition: report of the Subcommittee on Pediatric Parenteral Nutrient Requirements from the Committee on Clinical Practice Issues of the American Society for Clinical Nutrition, *Am J Clin Nutr* 48:1324, 1988.
*Reduced or not provided for infants with obstructive jaundice.
†Reduced or not provided for infants with renal dysfunction.

TABLE 9-10 Guidelines for Administration of Parenteral Vitamins for Premature Infants

	PRETERM*	<1000 g†	1001-3000 g†	>3000 g†
Percentage of one 5-ml vial of MVI-Pediatric‡	40%/kg	30%/day	65%/day	100%/day

*Data from Greene HL et al: Guidelines for the use of vitamins, trace elements, calcium, magnesium, and phosphorus in infants and children receiving total parenteral nutrition: report of the Subcommittee on Pediatric Parenteral Nutrient Requirements from the Committee on Clinical Practice Issues of the American Society for Clinical Nutrition, *Am J Clin Nutr* 48:1324, 1988. Maximum volume intake is 5 ml/day, which is achieved at 2.5 kg body weight.
†Data from MVI-Pediatric Insert, Amour Pharmaceuticals, 1996.
‡MVI-Pediatric (5 ml) contains the following vitamins: 80 mg of ascorbic acid, 0.7 mg of vitamin A, 10 μg of vitamin D, 1.2 mg of thiamin, 1.4 mg of riboflavin, 1 mg of vitamin B_6, 17 mg of niacin, 5 mg of pantothenic acid, 7 mg of vitamin E, 20 μg of biotin, 140 μg of folic acid, 1 μg of vitamin B_{12}, and 200 μg of vitamin K.

NUTRITIONAL REQUIREMENTS: ENTERAL FEEDING

Enteral alimentation is preferred for preterm infants because it is more physiologic than parenteral alimentation and is nutritionally superior. Initiating a tiny amount of an appropriate milk feeding whenever possible is beneficial. However, determining when and how to provide enteral feedings is often difficult and involves consideration of the degree of prematurity, history of perinatal insults, current medical condition, function of the gastrointestinal tract, respiratory status, and several other individual concerns (Table 9-11).

Preterm infants should be fed enough to promote growth similar to that of a fetus at the same gestational age but not so much that nutrient toxicity develops. Although the exact nutrient requirements are unknown for preterm infants, several useful guidelines exist. In general, the requirements of premature infants are higher than those of term infants because the preterm infant has smaller nutrient stores, decreased digestion and absorption capabilities, and a rapid growth rate. Stress, illness, and certain therapies for illness may further influence nutrient requirements. It is also important to remember that in general, enteral nutrient requirements are different from parenteral requirements.

Energy

The energy requirements of premature infants vary with individual biologic and environmental factors. It has been estimated that an intake of 50 kcal/kg/day is required to meet maintenance energy needs, compared with 105 to 130 kcal/kg/day for growth (Table 9-12). However, energy needs may be increased by stress, illness, and rapid growth. Likewise, energy needs may be decreased if the infant is placed in a neutral thermal environment (the environmental temperature at which an infant expends the least amount of energy to maintain body temperature). It is important to consider the infant's rate of growth in relation to average energy intakes. Some premature infants may need at least 130 to 150 kcal/kg/day to sustain an appropriate rate of growth; SGA infants or those with BPD often require such increased amounts. To provide such a large number of calories to infants with a limited ability to tolerate large fluid volumes, it may be necessary to concentrate the feedings to a level of more than 24 kcal/oz.

Protein

The amount and quality of protein must be considered when establishing protein requirements for the preterm infant. Amino acids must be provided at a level that meets demands without inducing amino acid or protein toxicity.

Amount

A reference fetus model has been used to determine the amount of protein that needs to be ingested to match the quantity of protein deposited into newly formed fetal tissue (Ziegler et al, 1976). To achieve these fetal accretion rates, additional protein must be supplied to compensate for intestinal losses and obligatory losses in the urine and skin.

Based on this method for determining protein needs, the advisable protein intake is 3.5 to 4 g/kg/day. This amount of protein is apparently well tolerated by stable infants who are growing rapidly. However, this amount of protein may increase stress for sick infants who are not growing.

TABLE 9-11 Factors to Consider Before Initiating or Increasing the Volume of Enteral Feedings

CATEGORY	FACTORS
Perinatal	Birth asphyxia
Respiratory	Stability of ventilation, blood gases, apnea, bradycardia, cyanosis
Medical	Vital signs (heart rate, respiratory rate, blood pressure, temperature)
Gastrointestinal	Anomalies (gastroschisis, omphalocele), patency, GI tract function (bowel sounds present, passage of stool), risk of necrotizing enterocolitis
Procedure	Pending intubation or extubation

Modified from Zerzan J, O'Leary MJ: Nutrition for preterm and low-birth-weight infants. In Trahms CM, Pipes PL, eds: *Nutrition in infancy and childhood,* ed 6, New York, 1997, WCB/McGraw-Hill.

TABLE 9-12 Estimation of the Energy Requirement of the Low-Birth-Weight Infant

ACTIVITY	AVERAGE ESTIMATION (kcal/kg/day)
Energy expended	40-60
Resting metabolic rate	40-50*
Activity	0-5*
Thermoregulation	0-5*
Synthesis	15†
Energy stored	20-30†
Energy excreted	15
Energy intake	90-120

Modified from American Academy of Pediatrics, Committee on Nutrition: Nutritional needs of preterm infants. In Kleinman RE, ed: *Pediatric nutrition handbook,* ed 4, Elk Grove, Ill, 1998, AAP; Committee on Nutrition of the Preterm Infant, European Society of Paediatric Gastroenterology and Nutrition (ESPGAN): Nutrition and feeding of preterm infants, Oxford, 1987, Blackwell Scientific.

*Energy for maintenance.

†Energy cost of growth.

Type

The quality or type of protein is an important consideration because premature infants have different amino acid needs than term infants because of immature hepatic enzyme pathways. The amino acid composition of *whey protein,* which differs from that of *casein* (see Chapter 8), is more appropriate for premature infants. The essential amino acid cysteine is more highly concentrated in whey protein, and premature infants do not synthesize cysteine well. In addition, the amino acids phenylalanine and tyrosine are lower, and the preterm infant has difficulty oxidizing them. Furthermore, metabolic acidosis decreases with consumption of whey-predominant formulas. Because of the advantages of whey protein for premature infants, breast milk or formulas containing predominantly whey proteins should be chosen whenever possible.

Taurine is a sulfonic amino acid that may be important for preterm infants. Human milk is a rich source of taurine, and taurine is added to most infant formulas. Term and preterm infants develop low plasma and urine concentrations of taurine without a dietary supply, but the clinical significance of this requires additional study.

Energy must be provided at sufficient levels to allow protein to be used for growth and not merely for energy expenditure. A range of 10.2% to 12.4% of calories from protein has been suggested. Inadequate protein intake is growth limiting, whereas excessive intake causes elevated plasma amino acid levels, azotemia, and acidosis.

Lipids

Amount

The growing preterm infant needs an adequate intake of well-absorbed dietary fat to help meet the high energy needs of growth, provide essential fatty acids, and facilitate absorption of other important nutrients such as the fat-soluble vitamins and calcium. However, neonates in general, and premature and SGA infants in particular, digest and absorb lipids inefficiently.

The percentage of total calories as fat relative to carbohydrate and protein is another important consideration. Fat should constitute 40% to 50% of total calories. Furthermore, a diet that is high in fat and low in protein may yield more fat deposition than is desirable for the growing preterm infant. To meet essential fatty acid needs, *linoleic acid* should comprise 3.1% of the total calories, and 0.7% of the total calories should be *linolenic acid* (Raiten et al, 1998). Additional longer-chain fatty acids—*arachidonic acid* and *docosahexaenoic acid*—are present in human milk and have recently been added to standard infant formulas for term infants meeting the Food and Drug Administration's (FDA's) guidelines for amounts and sources. The addition of these fatty acids to premature infant formulas has also been approved by the FDA. Both of these fatty acids play a role in visual and neurologic development and physical growth (Heird, 2001).

Type

Preterm infants have low levels of pancreatic lipase and bile salts, and this decreases their ability to digest and absorb fat. Lipases are needed for triglyceride breakdown, and bile salts solubilize fat for ease of digestion and absorption. Because medium-chain triglycerides (MCTs) do not require pancreatic lipase and bile acids for digestion and absorption, they have been added to the fat mixture in premature infant formulas.

Human milk and vegetable oils contain the EFA linoleic acid, but MCT oil does not. Premature infant formulas must contain vegetable oil and MCT oil to provide the essential long-chain fatty acids.

The composition of dietary fat also plays a role in the digestion and absorption of lipid. In general, infants absorb vegetable oils more efficiently than saturated animal fats, although one exception is the saturated fat in human milk. Infants digest and absorb human milk fat better than the saturated fat in cow's milk or the vegetable oil in standard infant formulas. Human milk contains two lipases that facilitate fat digestion and has a special fatty acid composition that aids absorption.

Carbohydrates

Carbohydrates are an important source of energy, and the enzymes for endogenous production of glucose from carbohydrate and protein are present in preterm infants.

Amount

Approximately 40% of the total calories in human milk and standard infant formulas is derived from carbohydrates. Too little carbohydrate may lead to hypoglycemia, whereas too much may provoke osmotic diuresis or loose stools. The recommended range for carbohydrate intake is 40% to 50% of total calories.

Type

Lactose, a disaccharide composed of glucose and galactose, is the predominant carbohydrate in almost all mammalian milks and may be important to the neonate for glucose homeostasis, perhaps because galactose can be used for either glucose production or glycogen storage (Narkewicz and Girard, 1998). Galactose generally is used for glycogen formation first, and then it becomes available for glucose production as blood glucose levels decrease. Because infants born before 28 to 34 weeks of gestation have low lactase activity, the premature infant's ability to digest lactose may be marginal. In practice, malabsorption is not a clinical problem because lactose is hydrolyzed in the intestine or fermented in the colon and absorbed. *Sucrose* is another disaccharide that is commonly found in commercial infant formula products. Because sucrase activity early in the third trimester is at 70% of newborn levels, sucrose is well tolerated by most premature infants. Sucrase and lactase are sensitive to changes in the intestinal milieu. Infants who have diarrhea, are undergoing antibiotic therapy, or are undernourished may develop temporary intolerances to lactose and sucrose.

Glucose polymers are common carbohydrates in the preterm infant's diet. These polymers, consisting mainly of chains of five to nine glucose units linked together, are used to achieve the isoosmolality of certain specialized formulas. Glucosidase enzymes for digesting glucose polymers are active in small preterm infants.

TABLE 9-13 Recommendations for Enteral Administration of Vitamins in the Premature Infant

VITAMIN	AMOUNT (kg/day)
Vitamin A	700-1500 IU
Vitamin D	150-400 IU
Vitamin E	6-12 IU
Vitamin K	8-10 μg
Ascorbic acid	18-24 mg
Thiamin	180-240 μg
Riboflavin	250-360 μg
Pyridoxine	150-210 μg
Niacin	3.6-4.8 mg
Pantothenate	1.2-1.7 μg
Biotin	3.6-6 μg
Folate	25-50 μg
Vitamin B_{12}	0.3 μg

Modified from Hansen JW: Appendix Table A.1. Consensus recommendations. In Tsang RC et al, eds: *Nutritional needs of the preterm infant,* Baltimore, 1993, Williams & Wilkins.

Minerals and Vitamins

Premature infants require the same vitamins and minerals as term infants, but poor body stores, physiologic immaturity, illness, and rapid growth increase their needs (Table 9-13). Formulas and human milk fortifiers, which are developed especially for preterm infants, contain higher vitamin and mineral concentrations to meet the needs of the infant, obviating the need for additional supplementation in most cases. The major exception is infants receiving human milk with a fortifier that does not contain iron. An iron supplement of 2 to 4 mg/kg/day should be sufficient to meet their needs (AAP, 1998).

Calcium and Phosphorus

Calcium and phosphorus are just two of many nutrients that growing premature infants require for optimal bone mineralization. Intake guidelines have been established at levels that promote the bone mineralization rate that would occur with the fetus. An intake of 175 mg/100 kcal/day of calcium and 91.5 mg/100 kcal/day of phosphorus is recommended. Two thirds of the calcium and phosphorus body content of the term neonate is accumulated through active transport mechanisms during the last trimester of pregnancy. Infants who are born prematurely are deprived of this important intrauterine mineral deposition. With poor mineral stores and low dietary intake, preterm infants can develop osteopenia of prematurity, a disease characterized by demineralization of growing bones and documented by radiologic evidence of "washed-out" or thin bones. Very immature babies are particularly susceptible to osteopenia and may develop bone fractures or florid rickets with a prolonged dietary deficiency. Osteopenia of prematurity is most likely to develop in preterm infants who are (1) fed infant formula that is not specifically formulated for preterm infants, (2) fed human milk that is not supplemented with calcium and phosphorus, or (3) receiving long-term PN without enteral feedings.

Vitamin D

Human milk with human milk fortifier or infant formula for preterm infants provides adequate vitamin D when infants consume the entire calorie intake suggested. It was once common practice to provide 400 to 1000 IU/day of vitamin D as a supplement to prevent osteopenia of prematurity, but this was later shown to be ineffective. In fact, the current recommendations for intake range from 150 to 400 IU/day for preterm infants.

Vitamin E

Preterm infants require more vitamin E than term infants because of their limited tissue stores, decreased absorption of fat-soluble vitamins, and rapid growth. Vitamin E protects biologic membranes against oxidative lipid breakdown. Because iron is a biologic oxidant, a diet high in either iron or polyunsaturated fatty acids (PUFAs) increases the risk of vitamin E deficiency. The PUFAs are incorporated into the red blood cell membranes and are more susceptible to oxidative damage than when saturated fatty acids comprise the membranes.

A premature infant with vitamin E deficiency may experience hemolytic anemia (oxidative destruction of red blood cells). However, this anemia is uncommon today because of changes that have been made in infant formula composition. The fat blends in human milk and premature infant formulas now contain appropriate vitamin E/PUFA ratios for preventing hemolytic anemia. Preterm infants do not generally receive additional iron unless they are receiving recombinant erythropoietin therapy; these infants receive vitamin E supplementation of 15 to 25 IU/day (Ohls et al, 2001).

Because the dietary requirement for vitamin E depends on the PUFA content of the diet, the recommended intake of vitamin E is commonly expressed as a ratio of vitamin E to PUFA. The recommendation for vitamin E is 0.7 IU (0.5 mg of d-α-tocopherol) per 100 kcal, and at least 1 IU of vitamin E per gram of linoleic acid.

Pharmacologic dosing of vitamin E (50 to 100 mg/kg/day) has not proven to be helpful in preventing BPD or retinopathy of prematurity by reducing the toxic effects of oxygen. Furthermore, high doses of vitamin E have been associated with intraventricular hemorrhage, sepsis, necrotizing enterocolitis, liver and renal failure, and death.

Iron

Preterm infants are at risk for iron deficiency anemia because of the reduced iron stores associated with early birth. At birth, most of the available iron is in the circulating hemoglobin. Thus frequent blood sampling further depletes the amount of iron available for erythropoiesis. Transfusions of red blood cells are often needed to treat the early physiologic anemia of prematurity. Recombinant erythropoietin therapy has been used to prevent anemia. Iron supplementation is indicated to facilitate red blood cell production, and a dosage of 6 mg/kg/day of enteral iron has been used (AAP, 1998). This therapy has not consistently prevented anemia and the need for blood transfusions (Ohls et al, 2001).

In general, the recommendation for iron intake is 2 to 4 mg/kg/day. Infants fed human milk should be given ferrous sulfate drops. Formulas fortified with iron usually contain sufficient iron for preterm infants. The optimal time to introduce iron into the preterm infant's diet is unclear; suggestions range from 2 weeks to 2 months of age (AAP, 1998).

Folic Acid

Premature infants seem to have higher folic acid needs than infants born at term. Although serum folate levels are high at birth, they decrease dramatically, probably as a result of high folic acid use by the premature infant for deoxyribonucleic acid and tissue synthesis needed for rapid growth.

A mild form of folic acid deficiency causing low serum folate concentrations and hypersegmentation of neutrophils is not unusual in premature infants. Megaloblastic anemia is much less common. A daily folic acid intake of 25 to 50 μg effectively maintains normal serum folate concentrations. Fortified human milk and formulas for premature infants meet these guidelines when full enteral feedings are established.

Sodium

Preterm infants, especially those with VLBW, are susceptible to hyponatremia during the neonatal period. These infants may have excessive urinary sodium losses because of renal immaturity and an inability to conserve adequate sodium. Furthermore, their sodium needs are high because of their rapid growth rate.

Daily sodium intakes of 4 to 8 mEq/kg or more may be required by some infants to prevent hyponatremia. Routine sodium supplementation of fortified human milk and infant formulas is not necessary. However, it is important to consider the possibility of hyponatremia and monitor infants by assessing serum or urinary sodium concentrations. Milk can be supplemented with sodium if repletion is necessary.

FEEDING METHODS

Decisions about breast-feeding, bottle-feeding, or tube-feeding depend on the gestational age and the clinical condition of the preterm infant. The goal is to feed the infant via the most physiologic method possible and supply nutrients for growth without creating clinical complications.

Gastric Gavage

Gastric gavage by the *oral route* is often chosen for infants who are unable to suck because of immaturity or problems with the central nervous system. Infants less than 32 to 34 weeks' gestational age, regardless of birth weight, may be expected to have poorly coordinated sucking and swallowing abilities because of their developmental immaturity. Consequently, they have difficulty with nipple-feeding. With the oral gastric gavage method, a soft feeding tube is inserted through the infant's mouth and into the stomach. The major risks of this technique include aspiration and gastric distention. Because of weak or absent cough reflexes and poorly developed respiratory muscles, the tiny infant may not be able to dislodge milk from the upper airway, which can cause reflex bradycardia or airway obstruction. However, electronic monitoring of vital functions and proper positioning of the infant during feeding minimize the risk of aspiration from regurgitation of stomach contents. Gastric distention and vagal nerve stimulation, with resultant bradycardia, are potential problems when oral gastric gavage feedings are delivered on an intermittent bolus schedule. Occasionally, elimination of the distention and vagal bradycardia requires the use of an indwelling tube for continuous gastric gavage feedings rather than intermittent administration of boluses. Continuous drip feedings are sometimes preferred for tiny, immature infants whose small gastric capacity and slow intestinal motility may impede the tolerance of large-volume bolus feeds. However, a randomized, control trial was conducted with premature infants of 26 to 30 weeks gestation to compare continuous and bolus feedings (Schanler et al, 1999b). Bolus feedings resulted in better weight gain and feeding tolerance than continuous infusion of feedings.

Nasal gastric gavage is sometimes better tolerated than oral tube-feeding. However, because neonates must breathe through the nose, this technique may compromise the nasal airway in preterm infants and cause an associated deterioration in respiratory function. However, this method is helpful for infants who are learning to nipple-feed. An infant with a nasal gastric tube can still form a tight seal on the bottle nipple, but it can be difficult if an oral feeding tube is in place during feedings.

Transpyloric Feeding

Transpyloric tube-feeding is indicated for infants who are at risk for aspirating formula into the lungs or who have slow gastric emptying. The goal of this method is to circumvent the often slow gastric emptying of the immature infant by passing the feeding tube through the stomach and pylorus and placing its tip within the duodenum or jejunum. Infants with severe gastrointestinal reflux do well with this method, which prevents aspiration of feedings into the lungs. This method is also used for infants whose respiratory function is compromised and who are at risk for formula aspiration. The possible disadvantages of transpyloric feedings include decreased fat absorption, diarrhea, dumping syndrome, alterations of the intestinal microflora, intestinal perforation, and bilious fluid in the stomach. In addition, the placement of transpyloric tubes also requires considerable expertise and radiographic confirmation of the catheter tip location. Although associated with many possible complications, transpyloric feedings are used when gastric feeding is not successful.

Nipple-Feeding

Nipple-feeding may be attempted with infants whose gestational age is greater than 32 weeks. Before this time, they are unable to coordinate sucking, swallowing, and breathing. The ability to feed from a nipple is usually indicated by evidence of an established sucking reflex and sucking motion. Because sucking requires effort by the infant, any stress from other causes such as hypothermia or hypoxemia diminishes the sucking ability. Therefore nipple-feeding should be initiated only when the infant is under minimal stress and is sufficiently mature and strong to sustain the sucking effort. Initial oral feedings may be limited to one to three times per day to prevent undue fatigue or too much energy expenditure, either of which can slow the infant's weight gain.

Before oral feedings begin, a standardized oral stimulation program can help infants successfully nipple-feed more quickly (Fucile, Gisel, and Lau, 2002). Healthy premature infants who are younger than 32 weeks of gestation may tolerate the introduction of one nipple-feeding per day (Simpson, Schanler, and Lau, 2002). This daily feeding can help infants learn and improve their oral feeding skills.

Breast-Feeding

When the mother of a premature infant chooses to breast-feed, nursing at the breast should begin as soon as the infant is ready. Before this time, the mother must express her milk so that it can be tube-fed to her infant. These mothers need emotional and educational support for successful lactation. One study reports that premature breast-fed infants have better sucking, swallowing, and breathing coordination and less breathing disruptions than bottle-fed infants (Meier, 2001). *Kangaroo baby care*—allowing the mother to maintain skin-to-skin contact while holding her infant—facilitates her lactation. In addition, this type of contact promotes continuation of breast-feeding and enhances the mother's confidence in caring for her high-risk infant. The latter benefit may also apply to fathers who engage in kangaroo care with their infants (Meier, 2000).

Feeding infants with cups instead of bottles to supplement breast-feeding has recently been suggested for preterm infants based on the rationale that it may prevent infant "nipple confusion" (i.e., confusion between nursing at the breast and from a bottle). However, additional research is needed to document the benefits and complications of this practice. Milk aspiration, refusal to breast-feed, and low volume intakes are possible problems (Meier, 2001).

Tolerance of Feedings

All preterm babies receiving enteral nutrition should be monitored for signs of feeding intolerance. *Vomiting* of feedings usually signals the infant's inability to retain the provided amount of milk. When not associated with other signs of a systemic illness, vomiting may indicate that feeding volumes were increased too quickly or are excessive for the infant's size and maturity. Simply reducing the feeding volume may resolve the problem. If it does not or if the infant has signs of a systemic illness, feedings may need to be interrupted until the infant's condition has stabilized. Bile-stained emesis may indicate the infant has an intestinal blockage and needs additional evaluation or that the feeding tube has slipped into the intestine.

Abdominal distention may be caused by excessive feeding, organic obstruction, excessive swallowing of air, resuscitation, or sepsis (i.e., systemic infection).

Observing infants for abdominal distention should be a routine practice for nurses. Intermittent measurements of abdominal circumference aid in the early detection of distention. Abdominal distention often indicates the need to interrupt feeding until its cause is determined and the abdomen becomes soft and is not distended.

Gastric residuals, measured by aspiration of the stomach contents, should be determined routinely before each bolus gavage feeding, and intermittently in all continuous drip feedings. Whether a residual amount is significant depends partly on its volume in relation to the total volume of the feeding. For example, a residual volume of more than 50% of a bolus feeding or equal to the continuous infusion rate might be a sign of feeding intolerance. However, when interpreting the significance of a gastric residual measurement, it is important to consider other concurrent signs of feeding intolerance and the previous pattern of residual volumes established for a particular infant. Bloody or bilious gastric residuals are more alarming than those that seem to be undigested milk.

The *frequency and consistency of bowel movements* should be constantly monitored when feeding preterm infants. Simple inspections can detect the presence of gross blood. However, occult blood is not always visible; a specific assay to detect small amounts of blood in the stool can be performed.

All feeding methods for preterm infants have associated complications. Unless close attention is paid to symptoms that indicate poor feeding tolerance, serious complications may ensue. Certain diseases can be recognized by recognizing signs of feeding intolerance. For example, necrotizing enterocolitis is a serious and potentially fatal disease associated with specific symptoms such as abdominal distention and tenderness, abnormal gastric residuals, and grossly bloody stools.

SELECTION OF ENTERAL FEEDING

During the initial feeding period, premature infants may often require additional time to adjust to enteral nutrition feedings and may experience concurrent stress, weight loss, and diuresis. The primary goal of enteral feeding during this initial period is to establish tolerance to the milk being provided. When aggressive nutritional support is provided and expected to be tolerated from the onset of enteral feeding, the effort often fails. Infants seem to need a period of adjustment to be able to assimilate a large volume and concentration of nutrients. Thus enteral feedings often require supplementation with parenteral fluids until infants can tolerate adequate amounts of feedings by mouth.

After the initial period of adjustment, the goal of enteral feeding changes from establishing milk tolerance to providing complete nutritional support for growth and rapid organ development. All essential nutrients should be provided in quantities that support sustained growth. The following feeding choices are appropriate: (1) human milk supplemented with human milk fortifier and iron, (2) iron-fortified premature infant formula for infants who weigh less than 2 kg, or (3) iron-fortified standard infant formula for infants who weigh more than 2 kg.

Premature infants who are discharged from the hospital and going home can be given a transitional formula unless they have osteopenia. Infants with osteopenia need calcium- and phosphorus-enriched premature infant formula until the condition improves. Breast-fed infants with osteopenia should also receive supplementation with bottles of fortified human milk or premature infant formula. Breast-fed infants without osteopenia should receive a multivitamin and mineral supplement that contains vitamin D and iron.

Human Milk

Human milk is the ideal food for healthy term infants and premature infants. Although human milk requires nutrient supplementation to meet the needs of premature infants, its benefits for the infant are numerous. During the first month of lactation, the composition of milk from mothers who have given birth to premature infants differs from that of mothers who have given birth to term infants; the protein and sodium concentrations of breast milk are higher in mothers with preterm infants (Klein, 2002). When premature infants are fed their own mother's milk, they grow more rapidly than infants fed banked, or mature, breast milk (Gross, 1983).

In addition to its nutrient concentration, human milk offers nutritional benefits because of its unique mix of amino acids and long-chain fatty acids. The zinc and iron in human milk are more readily absorbed, and fat is more easily digested because of the presence of lipases. Moreover, human milk contains factors that are not present in formulas. These components include (1) live cells, macrophages, and T and B lymphocytes; (2) antimicrobial factors, secretory immunoglobulin A (SIgA), lactoferrin, and others; (3) hormones; (4) enzymes; and (5) growth factors. The significance of many of these factors is currently being investigated. It has also been suggested that human milk fed to preterm infants reduces the incidence of necrotizing enterocolitis and sepsis and improves neurodevelopment (Lucas et al, 1998; Schanler et al, 1999a).

However, one well-documented problem is associated with feeding human milk to preterm infants. Whether preterm, term, or mature, human milk does not meet the calcium and phosphorus needs for normal bone mineralization in premature infants. Therefore calcium and phosphorus supplements are recommended for rapidly growing preterm infants who are fed predominantly human milk. Currently, three human milk fortifiers are available: Similac Natural

TABLE 9-14 Comparison of the Nutritional Content of Human Milk and Formulas

	HUMAN MILK	FORTIFIED HUMAN MILK*	STANDARD FORMULA†	TRANSITIONAL FORMULA‡	PREMATURE FORMULA§
Caloric density (kcal/oz)	20	24	20	22	20, 24
Protein whey/casein ratio	70:30	Whey predominant	60:40, 48:52, 100:0	60:40, 50:50	60:40
Protein: (g/L)	9-14	19-20	14-16	19-21	18-24
Carbohydrate	Lactose	Lactose, glucose polymers	Lactose or lactose and glucose polymers	Lactose, glucose polymers	Lactose, glucose polymers
Carbohydrate (g/L)	66-73	77-88	73-74	77-79	72-90
Fat	Human fat	Human fat, MCTs	Vegetable	Vegetable, MCT oil	Vegetable, MCT oil
Fat (g/L)	39-42	44-52	34.1-36.5	39-41	34.5-43.8
Calcium (mg/L)	248-280	1180-1411	429-530	784-890	1115-1452
Phosphorus (mg/L)	128-147	650-790	241-360	463-490	561-806
Vitamin D (IU/L)	20-21	1190-1520	402-410	522-590	1014-2200
Vitamin E (IU/L)	2.8-10.7	34-49	10.1-13.5	26.9-30	27-51
Folic acid (μg/L)	33-85	306-335	60-108	187-192	237-298
Sodium (mEq/L)	7.9-10.8	14-15	7-8	10.7-11.3	11.5-15.1

Data compiled from *Carnation—the very best professional handbook*, PHB0500, Nestlé, 2000; *Ross Laboratories Product Handbook* [Internet] http://www.ross.com/productHandbook/pedNut.asp [cited Jan. 28, 2002]; and *Mead Johnson Nutritionals Handbook* [Internet] http://www.meadjohnson.com/products/index.html [cited Jan. 28, 2002].

*Based on the composition of term human milk fortified with either Similac or Enfamil Human Milk fortifiers at four packets per 100 ml.

†Based on the composition of Enfamil, Similac, and Good Start formulas.

‡Based on the composition of EnfaCare and Similac NeoSure formulas.

§Based on the composition of Enfamil Premature Formula and Similac Special Care formulas.

Care (Ross Laboratories), which is available in liquid form, and Similac and Enfamil Human Milk Fortifiers (Ross Laboratories, Mead Johnson Nutritionals), which are available in powdered form. These contain calcium and phosphorus, as well as protein, carbohydrates, fat, vitamins, and minerals, and are designed to be added to expressed breast milk fed to premature infants (Table 9-14).

Providing human milk to a premature infant can be a very positive experience for the mother, one that promotes involvement and interaction. Because many preterm infants are neither strong enough nor mature enough to nurse at their mother's breast in the early neonatal period, their mothers usually express their milk for several days (and occasionally for several weeks) before nursing can be established. The proper technique of expression, storage, and transport of milk should be reviewed with the mother (see Chapter 7). Many summaries of the special considerations for nursing a preterm infant have been published (Lawrence and Lawrence, 1999; Meier, 2001).

Premature Infant Formulas

Formula preparations have been developed to meet the unique nutritional and physiologic needs of growing preterm infants. The quantity and quality of nutrients in these products promote growth at intrauterine rates. These formulas, which have caloric densities of 20 and 24 kcal/oz, are available only in a ready-to-feed form. These premature formulas differ in many respects from standard cow's milk–based formulas (see Table 9-14). The types of carbohydrate, protein, and fat differ to facilitate digestion and absorption of nutrients. These formulas also have higher concentrations of protein, minerals, and vitamins.

Transitional Infant Formulas

Formulas containing 22 kcal/oz have been designed as transition formulas for the premature infant. Their nutrient content is less than that of the nutrient-dense premature infant formulas and more than that of the standard infant formula (see Table 9-14). These formulas can be introduced when the infant reaches a weight of 1800 g or more, and they can be used throughout the first year of life. Not all premature infants need these formulas to grow appropriately. Infants who weigh less than 1250 g (2 lb, 11 oz) at birth and do not consume enough nutrients while hospitalized or cannot consume adequate amounts of standard formula to grow when discharged may benefit from these formulas (Carver et al, 2000; Worrell et al, 2002). Transitional formulas are available in powder form for home use and in ready-to-feed form for use in hospitals.

Formula Adjustments

Occasionally, it may be necessary to increase the energy content of the formulas fed to small infants. This may be appropriate when the infant is not growing quickly enough and is already consuming as much as possible during feedings.

Concentration

One approach to providing hypercaloric formula is to prepare the formula with less water, thus concentrating all its nutrients, including energy. Concentrated infant formulas with energy contents of 24 kcal/oz are available to hospitals as ready-to-feed nursettes. However, when using these concentrated formulas, it is important to consider the infant's fluid intake and fluid losses in relation to the renal solute load of the concentrated feeding, to ensure that a positive water balance is maintained. This method of increasing formula density is often preferred because the nutrient balance remains the same; infants who need more energy also need additional nutrients. As mentioned, the transitional formulas are available in ready-to-feed and powder form and can be concentrated from 24 to 30 kcal/oz. However, this formula is still inadequate for infants who need additional calcium (e.g., infants with osteopenia).

Because premature infant formulas are available only as ready-to-feed preparations, altering the concentration by preparing them with less water is impossible. Instead, these premature formulas should be provided in amounts tolerated by the infant, and caloric supplements can be added as needed. When infants consume less because of an illness, infant formula powder is often added to provide more calories and nutrients. These formulas provide enough calcium, phosphorus, magnesium, and vitamin D to treat osteopenia.

Caloric Supplements

Another approach to increasing the energy content of a formula involves the use of caloric supplements such as corn oil, MCT oil (Mead Johnson Nutritionals), and glucose polymers such as Polycose (Ross Laboratories). These supplements increase the formula's caloric density without markedly altering solute load or osmolality. However, they do alter the relative distribution of total calories derived from protein, carbohydrate, and fat. Because even small amounts of oil or carbohydrate dilute the percentage of calories derived from protein, adding these supplements to human milk or standard (20 kcal/oz) formulas is not advised. Caloric supplements should be used only when a formula already meets all nutrient requirements other than energy or when the renal solute load is a concern.

When a high-energy formula is needed, MCT oil and Polycose can be added to a base that has a concentration of 24 kcal/oz or greater (either full-strength premature formula or a concentrated standard formula), with a maximum of 50% of total calories from fat and a minimum of 9% of total calories from protein. For the infant who can tolerate long-chain fatty acids, an emulsified fatty acid product (Microlipid, Sherwood Medical) may be appropriate because it stays in solution better than the MCT oil, or the corn oil, both of which cling to the sides of the container. Adding fat at each feeding rather than mixing it with the daily supply of formula may prevent the oil from adhering to the storage container and thus not being taken in by the infant.

GROWTH AND NUTRITIONAL ASSESSMENTS

Growth Rates and Growth Charts

All neonates typically lose some weight after birth. Preterm infants are born with more extracellular water than term infants and thus tend to lose more weight than term infants. However, the postnatal weight loss should not be excessive. Preterm infants who lose more than 15% to 20% of their birth weight may become dehydrated from the inadequate fluid intake or experience tissue wasting from poor energy intake. An infant's birth weight should be regained by the second or third week of life. The smallest and sickest infants take the longest time to regain their birth weights.

During the first 98 days of life, the Ehrenkranz growth chart is commonly used to assess weight progress (Ehrenkranz et al, 1999). This chart (Figure 9-4) longitudinally depicts daily weight changes and actual growth curves for 1660 infants who were born with a weight of 501 to 1500 g (1¹⁄₁₆ to 3⅓ lb). These infants received care in 12 different neonatal intensive care units (NICUs) for various neonatal medical problems. Charts are also available for length, head circumference, and midarm circumference (Ehrenkranz et al, 1999). (See Relevant Web sites for a source to create a growth curve for an individual infant.)

Intrauterine growth curves have also been developed using birth weight data of infants born at several successive weeks of gestation. However, these curves do not depict the initial period of postnatal weight loss and probably set unrealistic goals for preterm infants in the neonatal period. After an infant's condition stabilizes and the infant begins consuming all needed nutrients, the infant may be able to grow at a rate that parallels these curves. An intrauterine weight gain of 15 g/kg/day can be achieved before 38 weeks of gestation.

Although weight is an important anthropometric parameter, measurements of length and head circumference can also be helpful. A growth curve can be used to evaluate the adequacy of growth in all three areas (Figure 9-5). This chart has a built-in correction factor for prematurity, and the infant's growth can be followed on one chart through the first year of corrected age. This chart represents cross-sectional data constructed from the anthropometric measurements taken at birth of infants with different gestational ages and infants in a health maintenance program (Babson and Benda, 1976).

The Centers for Disease Control and Prevention (CDC) 2000 Growth Charts from birth to 3 years of

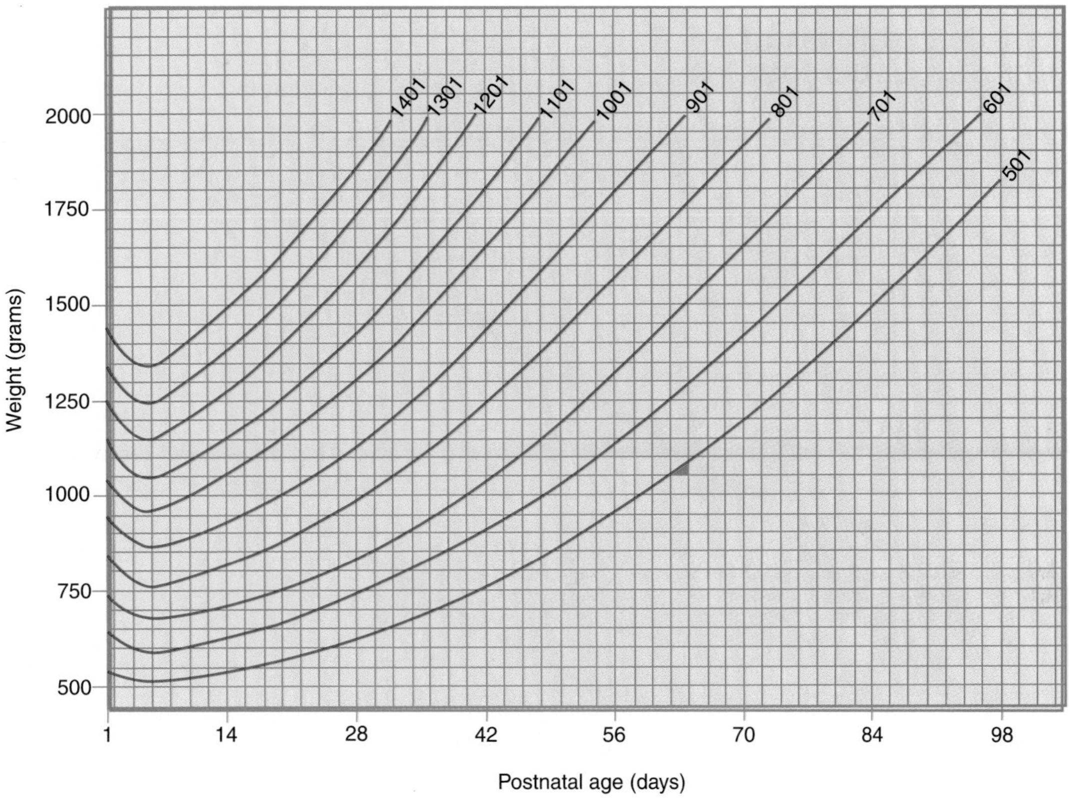

FIGURE 9-4 • Weight chart for premature infants based on actual growth data. From Ehrenkranz RA et al: Longitudinal growth of hospitalized very–low-birth-weight infants. Reproduced with permission from *Pediatrics* 104:283, Figure 1, Copyright, 1999.

age can also be used for preterm infants after 40 weeks of gestation, as long as the age is adjusted. For example, an infant born at 28 weeks of gestation is 12 weeks premature (40 weeks of term gestation − 28 weeks of birth gestational age). Four months after birth, the growth parameters of a premature infant born at 28 weeks of gestation can be compared with those of a 1-month-old infant born at term (Box 9-1). When using growth grids, age should be adjusted for prematurity until at least 2½ to 3 years of corrected age. In Figure 9-6, A.R.'s pattern of growth is shown through 18 years of age. These charts are based on infants born with a birth weight greater than 1500 g (3⅓ lb).

Anthropometric measurements of premature infants can also be plotted on the Casey charts (Casey et al, 1991; Ogden et al, 2002). These charts contain weight, length, and head circumference references for the first 3 years of corrected age (Casey et al, 1991) (see *Focus On*: Long-Term Outcome for Premature Infants).

Laboratory Indices

Laboratory assessments usually involve measuring the following parameters: (1) fluid and electrolyte balance, (2) PN tolerance, (3) bone mineralization status, and (4) hematologic status. In addition, serum protein, prealbumin, and retinol-binding protein levels may reflect recent changes in nutritional intake. However, these levels are also influenced by the infant's gestational age, illness, level of stress, and vitamin A and zinc status.

DISCHARGE CARE

Establishment of successful feeding is the pivotal factor determining whether a preterm infant can be discharged from the hospital nursery and go home. Preterm infants must be able to (1) tolerate their feedings and usually obtain all of their feedings from the breast or bottle; (2) grow adequately on a modified-demand feeding schedule (usually every 3 to 4 hours during the day for bottle-fed infants or every 2 to 3 hours for breast-fed infants); and (3) maintain their body temperature without the help of an incubator. In addition, it is important that any ongoing chronic illnesses, including nutritional problems, be manageable at home. Most important, the parents must be ready to care for their infant. In hospitals that allow parents to visit their infants in the nursery 24 hours a

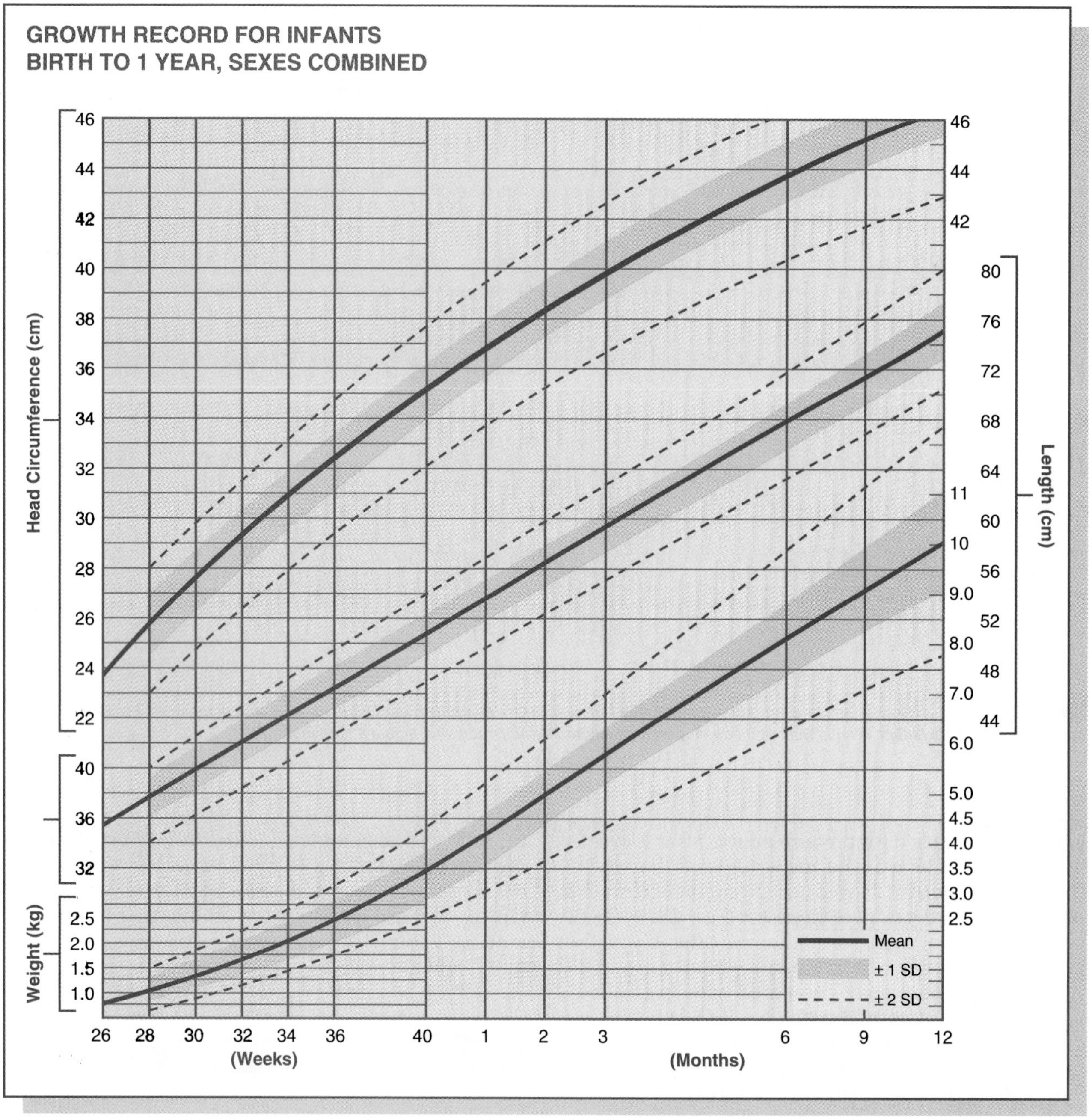

FIGURE 9-5 • Example of a growth record of weight, length, and head circumference for infants from 26 weeks of gestation to 1 year of age. This chart has a built-in correction factor for prematurity. (Modified from Babson SG, Benda GI: Growth graphs for the clinical assessment of infants of varying gestational age, *J Pediatr* 89:814, 1976.)

day, staff can help parents develop their caregiving skills and learn care for their infant at home. Often, parents are permitted to "room in" with their infant (i.e., stay with the infant all day and night) before discharge, which helps build confidence in their ability to care for a high-risk infant (Figure 9-7).

Box 9-1. Steps for Adjusting Age for Prematurity in Growth Charts

Calculate the number of weeks the infant was premature:

- 40 weeks (term) − birth gestational age = number of weeks premature.
- The resulting number of weeks is the *correction factor.*

Calculate the adjusted age for prematurity:

- Chronologic age − correction factor = adjusted age for prematurity.

  For example:

  40 weeks − 28 weeks of gestation = 12 weeks, therefore 12 weeks (3 months) is the correction factor.

  4 months (chronologic age) − 3 months (correction factor) = 1 month adjusted age.

Many preterm infants who are discharged from the hospital weigh less than 5½ lb. Although these infants must meet certain discharge criteria before they can go home, the stress of a new environment may lead to setbacks. Small preterm infants should be followed very closely during the first month after discharge, and parents should be given as much information and support as possible. Within the first week of discharge, a home visit by a nurse, nutritionist, or both, and an office visit to the pediatrician can be extremely helpful educationally and because they can provide early intervention for developing problems.

Factors that affect the feeding skills and behavior of preterm infants are particularly important after the infants have been discharged. Physical factors such as a variable heart rate, a rapid respiratory rate, and tremulousness are examples of physiologic events that interfere with feeding. In addition, infants weighing less than 5½ lb have poor muscle tone. Although muscle tone gradually improves as an infant becomes larger and more mature, it can deteriorate quickly in infants who are tired or weak. Feeding is often difficult for infants who have limited muscle flexion and strength and poor head and neck control, which are needed to maintain a good feeding posture. Positioning these infants in a manner that supports normal body flexion and ensures proper alignment of the head and neck during feedings may be helpful. Premature infants may also need their chin and cheeks supported while bottle-feeding.

FOCUS ON

Long-Term Outcome for Premature Infants

As the survival of premature infants continues to improve, their physical growth, mental development, health, and quality of life are being investigated. Previously, it was believed that if premature infants experienced catch-up growth, it would only occur during the first few years of life. However, catch-up growth for weight, length, and head circumference can continue throughout the first 18 years of life (Doyle, 2000). In fact, even ELBW infants may reach their predicted genetic height.

Only recently have tools been developed and validated that assess how children report their health status and quality of life. Saigal and group (2000) compared two groups of adolescents, who ranged in age from 12 to 16 years. The first group included 150 children who were born premature with ELBW. The second group consisted of 124 children who were born at term and were not LBW infants. All children were interviewed in the same way except for nine ELBW children who were severely neurologically impaired. Their parents completed the interviews on their behalf. Neurosensory impairments were present in 27% of the children who were born prematurely and in 1.6% of the children born at term. The impairments included cerebral palsy, hydrocephalus, cognitive impairments, autism, blindness, and deafness. Of the children who were preterm infants, 34% rated their health as "perfect," compared with 58% of the children who were born at term. Quality of life was also rated lower by the children who had been born prematurely. However, when the parents' scores for the nine adolescents with neurologic impairments were not included in the calculations, no difference was found between the two groups' assessments of their quality of life. Although children who were born prematurely may be more likely to have neurosensory impairments, they are optimistic about their quality of life. In addition, no difference was found between assessments of self-esteem by children who were born prematurely and children who were born at term (Saigal et al, 2002).

Therefore not only are more premature infants surviving, but they also are growing into children who are enjoying their lives. The medical and nutritional care in the hospital nursery continues to progress, which improves outcome in the nursery and sets the stage for later development.

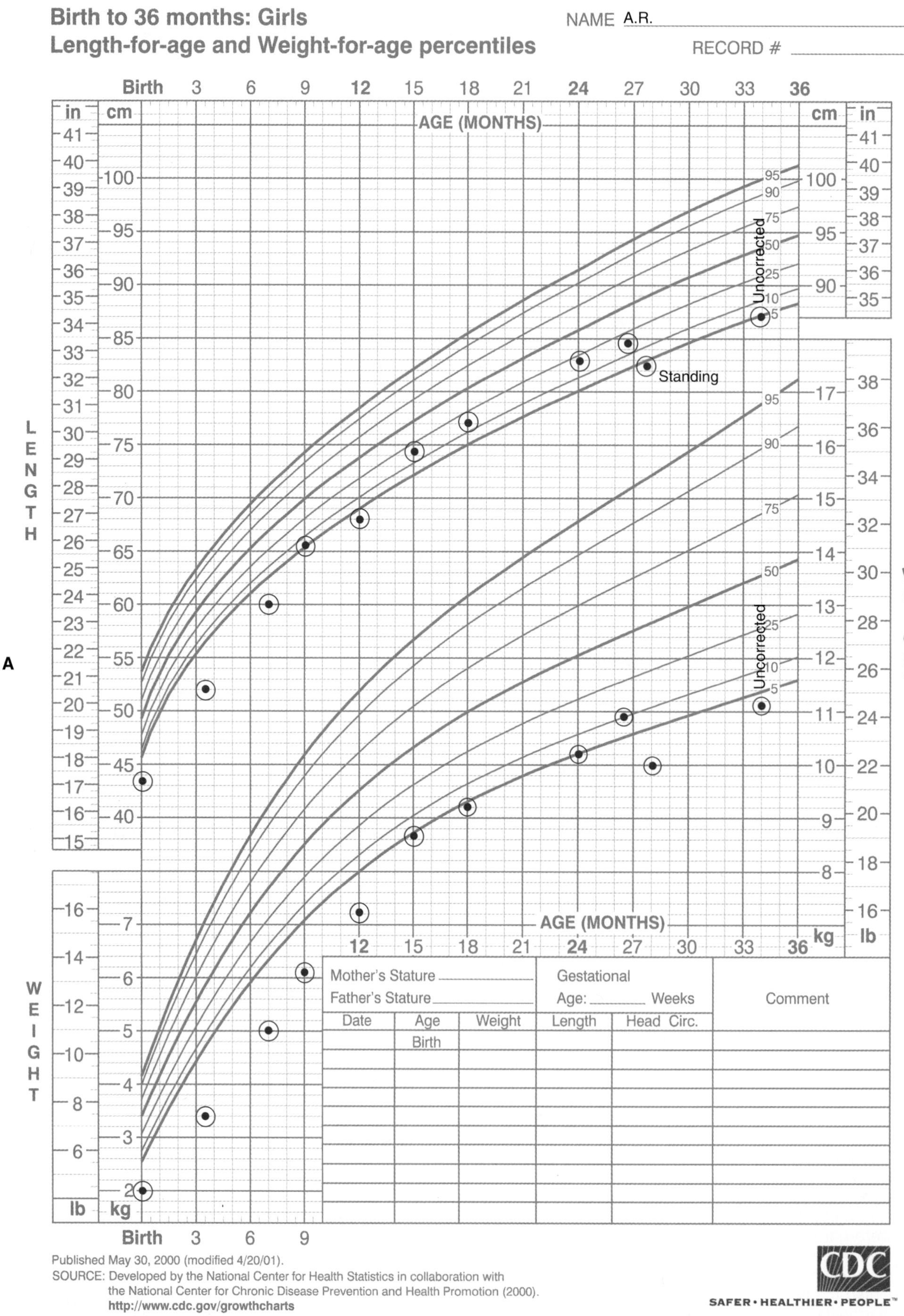

FIGURE 9-6 • **A,** Graphs showing how A.R. (from Figure 9-2), who was born at 27 weeks of gestation, grew after leaving the neonatal unit 1 day before her due date at a weight of 4½ lb. Heights and weights until age of 28 months are plotted on the grid at "corrected age" points and thereafter at "uncorrected age" points. A.R. experienced catch-up growth during the first 15 months. (Data from the National Center for Health Statistics in collaboration with the National Center for Chronic Disease Prevention and Health Promotion, 2000, http://www.cdc.gov/growthcharts.)

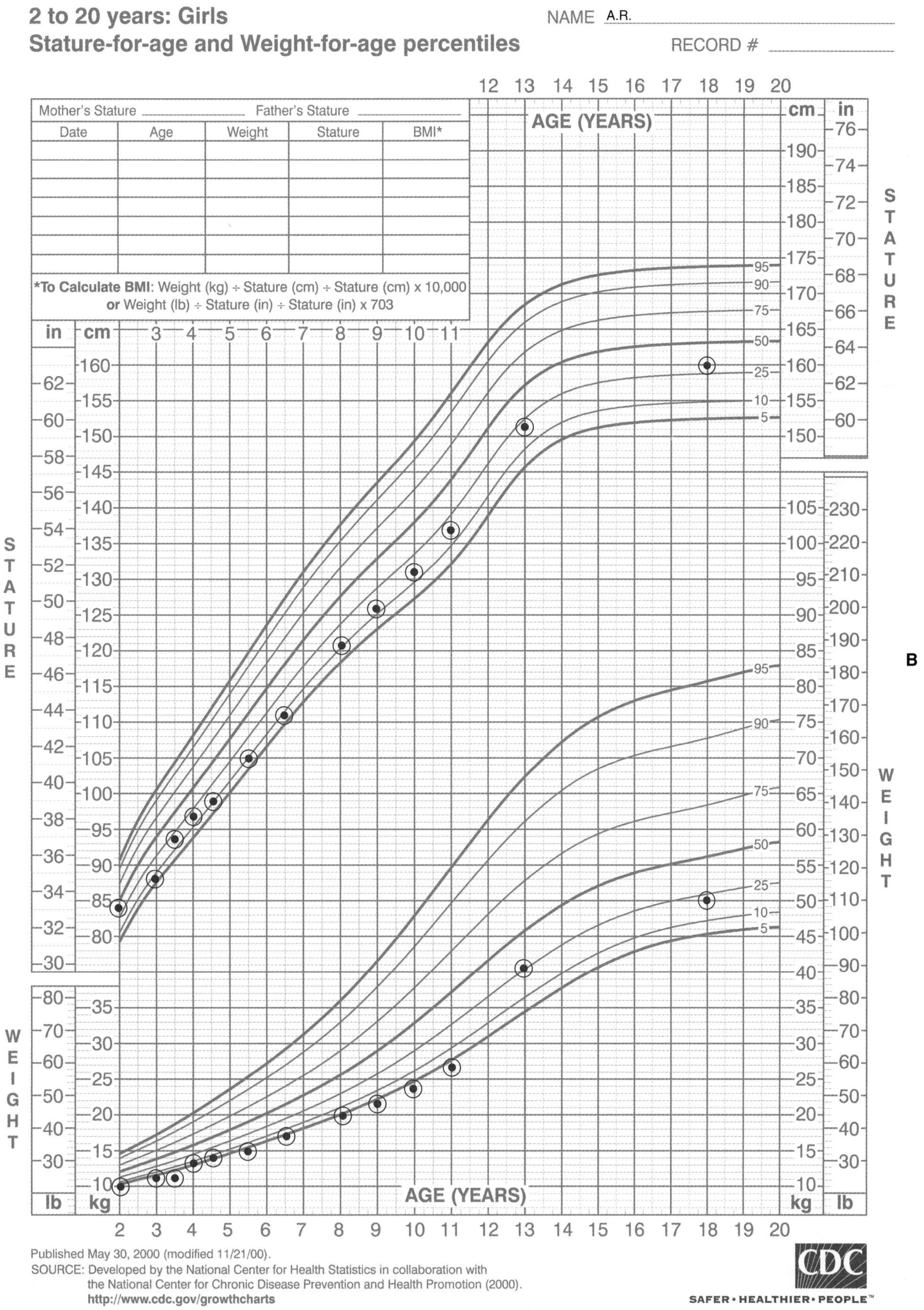

FIGURE 9-6, cont'd • **B,** A.R.'s growth pattern from the age of 2 to 18 years. During the first 10 years, she grew at the 5th percentile for weight and the 10th percentile for height. She followed her channel of growth but did not experience catch-up growth. However, between the ages of 10 and 13, she began to change growth channels and moved to the 25th percentile for weight and the 25th percentile for height (catch-up growth). At 18 years, she crossed the 25th percentile for height and fell slightly below the 25th percentile for weight.

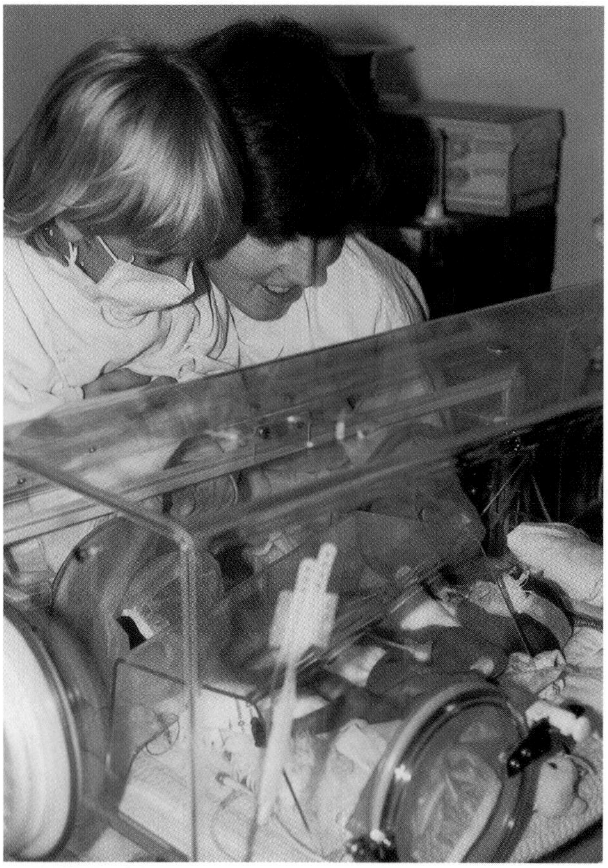

FIGURE 9-7 • Family in the nursery with their premature infant before discharge.

Clinical Scenario

Sara, an infant born at 26 weeks of gestation, was admitted to the NICU. Her birth weight was 850 g, which meant her size was AGA. Sara had respiratory distress syndrome and had to receive a tube for mechanical ventilation. During the first few hours of her life, she was given surfactant and her ventilator settings were lowered. She was also placed in a humidified incubator and given 100 ml/kg/day of $D_{10}W$ intravenously. On the second day after her birth, she had gained 20 g, and her serum sodium concentration and urine volume output were low. She was diagnosed with a PDA and was given indomethacin to close the ductus arteriosus. On the fourth day after birth, her body weight had decreased 50 g—6% of her birth weight—and her serum electrolyte levels were normal. The protein concentration of her parenteral fluids was increased, as was the volume of intravenous fat being provided. By the sixth day, Sara was clinically stable. She began receiving feedings of milk from her mother—0.7 ml every 2 hours (10 ml/kg of her birth weight)—via bolus oral gastric tube. The feedings were tolerated well. She then began receiving 10 ml/kg/day of her mother's breast milk and less parenteral fluids. The ventilation tube was removed after full enteral feedings were established, and Sara was successfully breathing on her own.

1. On the second day after birth, should Sara's intravenous fluid volume have been (1) increased because she needed more calories, (2) decreased because she was overhydrated, or (3) changed to enteral feedings because she was clinically stable?
2. How should the intravenous fat that was given to Sara have been administered?
3. The breast milk from Sara's mother may have inadequate amounts of which nutrients? What do you recommend to resolve this?

Small infants tend to sleep more than larger and term infants. It is much easier for preterm infants to feed effectively if they are fully awake. To awaken a preterm infant, the caregiver should provide one type of gentle stimulation for a few minutes and then change to a different type, repeating this pattern until the infant is fully awake. Lightly swaddling infants and then placing them in a semiupright position may also help.

The feeding environment should be as quiet as possible. Preterm infants are easily distracted and have difficulty focusing on feeding when noises or movements interrupt their attention. They also tire quickly and are easily overstimulated. When they are overstimulated, they may show only subtle signs of distress. It is important to teach parents of premature infants to recognize the subtle cues that indicate the need for rest or comfort and to respond to them appropriately.

After discharge, most preterm infants need approximately 180 ml/kg/day (2¾ oz/lb/day) of breast milk or standard infant formula containing 20 kcal/oz. This amount of milk provides 120 kcal/kg/day (55 kcal/lb/day). Alternatively, transitional formula with a concentration of 22 kcal/oz can be provided at a rate of 160 ml/kg/day (or 2½ oz/lb/day). The best way to determine whether these amounts are adequate for individual infants is to compare their intake with their growth progress over time. Some infants may need a formula that provides 24 kcal/oz. As mentioned previously, powdered transitional formula can be readily altered to a concentration of 24 kcal/oz because ready-to-feed premature formulas providing 24 kcal/oz are highter in calcium and phosphorus than the concentrated formulas. Premature infants with osteopenia should continue to receive the ready-to-feed premature formula.

It is important to evaluate needs based on the three growth parameters: weight, length, and head circumference. Patterns of growth should be assessed to determine whether (1) individual curves at least parallel reference curves, (2) growth curves are shifting inappropriately across growth percentiles, (3) weight is appropriate for length, and (4) growth is proportionate in all three areas.

NEURODEVELOPMENTAL OUTCOME

It is possible to meet the metabolic and nutritional needs of premature infants sufficiently to sustain life

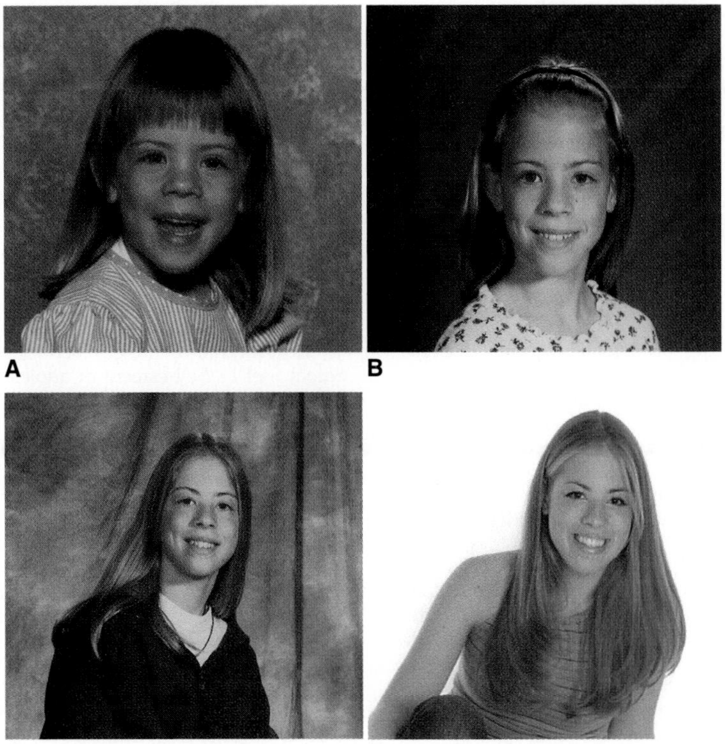

A B C D

FIGURE 9-8 • The premature infant A.R. (from Figures 9-2 and 9-6) as she grows up. **A,** $3\frac{1}{2}$ years. **B,** 10 years. **C,** 14 years. **D,** 18 years. (*D,* Courtesy Yuen Lui Studio, Seattle, Wash.)

and promote growth and development. In fact, more tiny premature infants are surviving than ever before because of adequate nutritional support and the recent advances in neonatal intensive care technology. However, the incidence of infants born with neurosensory and developmental handicaps has remained constant, despite the increase in the total number of surviving children (Wilson-Costello and Hack, 2002).

The increased survival rate of VLBW infants has increased concerns about their short- and long-term neurodevelopmental outcomes. Many questions have been raised about the quality of life awaiting infants who receive neonatal intensive care. As a rule, VLBW infants should be referred to a follow-up clinic to evaluate their development and growth and begin early interventions. Surviving ELBW infants, particularly those with birth weights of less than 750 g, have an increased risk of developing handicapping central nervous system conditions, which vary in severity and type of functional impairment (Wilson-Costello and Hack, 2002). However, many of these premature infants reach childhood with no evidence of any disability (Figure 9-8).

SUMMARY

Nutritional management of the premature infant is a dynamic process because the nutritional needs change based on the rapid growth of the infant. Parenteral, enteral, and transitional nutrition guidelines are used to feed them; nutrition fortifiers for human milk and infant formulas, which are specially designed for the premature infant, help tremendously. Assessments and concerns for the neurodevelopmental outcome of premature infants reveal that the nutritional efforts provided help them reach adulthood in good health.

Relevant Web Sites

American Academy of Pediatrics
www.pediatrics.org
National Center for Education in Maternal and Child Health
www.ncemch
National Institute of Child Health and Human Development (NICHD), Neonatal Research Network
http://neonatal.rti.org/dsp_birthcurves.cfm

Cited References

American Academy of Pediatrics and American College of Obstetricians and Gynecologists: Introduction. In *guidelines for perinatal care,* ed 4, Evanston, Ill, 1997, AAP.

American Academy of Pediatrics, Committee on Nutrition: Nutritional needs of preterm infants. In Kleinman RE, ed: *Pediatric nutrition handbook,* ed 4, Elk Grove, Ill, 1998, AAP.

Babson SG, Benda GI: Growth graphs for the clinical assessment of infants of varying gestational age, *J Pediatr* 89(5):814, 1976.

Ballard JL et al: New Ballard score, expanded to include extremely premature infants, *J Pediatr* 119:417, 1991.

Barrington KJ, Finer NN: Treatment of bronchopulmonary dysplasia: a review. *Clin Peri Natol* 25:177, 1998.

Bell EF, Oh W: Fluid and electrolyte management. In Avery GB, Fletcher MA, MacDonald MG, eds: *Neonatology: pathophysiology and management of the newborn*, ed 5, Philadelphia, 1999, JB Lippincott.

Carver JD et al: Growth of preterm infants fed nutrient-enriched or term formula after hospital discharge, *Pediatrics* 107:683, 2001.

Casey PH et al: Growth status and growth rates of a varied sample of low birth weight, preterm infants: a longitudinal cohort from birth to three years of age, *J Pediatr* 119:599, 1991.

Christensen ML et al: Plasma carnitine concentration and lipid metabolism in infants receiving parenteral nutrition, *J Pediatr* 115:794, 1989.

Doyle LW: Growth and respiratory health in adolescence of the extremely low-birth-weight survivor, *Clin Peri Natol* 27:421, 2000.

Ehrenkranz RA et al: Longitudinal growth of hospitalized very low birth weight infants, *Pediatrics* 104:280, 1999.

Fucile S, Gisel E, Lau C: Oral stimulation accelerates the transition from tube to oral feeding in preterm infants, *J Pediatr* 141:230, 2002.

Greene HL et al: Guidelines for the use of vitamins, trace elements, calcium, magnesium, and phosphorus in infants and children receiving total parenteral nutrition: report of the Subcommittee on Pediatric Parenteral Nutrient Requirements from the Committee on Clinical Practice Issues of the American Society for Clinical Nutrition, *Am J Clin Nutr* 48(5):1324, 1988.

Greer FR: Vitamin metabolism and requirements in the micropremie, *Clin Peri Natol* 27:95, 2000.

Gross SJ: Growth and biochemical response of preterm infants fed human milk or modified infant formula, *N Engl J Med* 308:237, 1983.

Hallman M et al: Inositol supplementation in premature infants with respiratory distress syndrome, *N Engl J Med* 326:1233, 1992.

Hanning RM, Zlotkin SA: Parenteral proteins. In Baker RD, Baker SS, Davis A: *Pediatric parenteral nutrition,* New York, 1997, Chapman & Hall.

Hansen JW: Appendix Table A.1. Consensus recommendations. In Tsang RC et al, eds: *Nutritional needs of the preterm infant,* Baltimore, 1993, Williams & Wilkins.

Heird WC: Early use of parenteral amino acids. In Ziegler EE, Lucas A, Moro GE, eds: *Nutrition of the very low birthweight infant,* Philadelphia, 1999, Nestec and Lippincott Williams & Wilkins.

Heird WC: The role of polyunsaturated fatty acids in term and preterm infants and breastfeeding mothers, *Pediatr Clin North Am* 48:173, 2001.

Heird WC, Gomez MR: Parenteral nutrition in low-birth-weight infants, *Ann Rev Nutr* 16:471, 1996.

Hoyert DL et al: Annual summary of vital statistics, 2000, *Pediatrics* 108:1241, 2001.

Klein CJ, ed: Nutrient requirements for preterm infant formula, *J Nutr* 132:1395S, 2002.

Lawrence RA, Lawrence RM: *Breastfeeding: a guide for the medical profession,* ed 5, St Louis, 1999, Mosby.

Lucas A et al: Randomised trial of early diet in preterm babies and later intelligence quotients, *BMJ* 317:1481, 1998.

MacKay AP et al: *Adolescent health chartbook. Health, United States, 2000,* Hyattsville, Md, 2000, National Center for Health Statistics.

Meier PP: Breastfeeding in the special care nursery: prematures and infants with medical problems, *Pediatr Clin North Am* 48:425, 2001.

Narkewicz MR , Girard J: Role of glucoregulatory hormones in hepatic glucose metabolism during the perinatal period. In Poland RA, Fox WW, ed: *Fetal and neonatal physiology,* ed 2, Philadelphia, 1998, WB Saunders.

Ogden CL et al: Centers for Disease Control and Prevention 2000 growth charts for the United States, *Pediatrics* 109:45, 2002.

Ohls RK et al: Effects of early erythropoietin therapy on the transfusion requirements of preterm infants below 1250 grams birth weight: a multicenter, randomized, controlled trial, *Pediatrics* 108:934, 2001.

Poindexter BB et al: Exogenous insulin reduces proteolysis and protein synthesis in extremely low birth weight infants, *J Pediatr* 132:948, 1998.

Raiten DJ et al, eds: Assessment of nutrient requirements for infant formulas, *J Nutr* 128:2059S, 1998.

Rivera A et al: Effects of intravenous amino acids on protein metabolism of preterm infants during the first three days of life, *Pediatr Res* 33:106, 1993.

Saigal S: Perception of healthy status and quality of life of extremely low-birth weight survivors: the consumer, the provider, and the child, *Clin Perinatol* 27:403, 2000.

Saigal S et al: Self-esteem of adolescents who were born prematurely, *Pediatrics* 109:429, 2002.

Schanler RJ et al: Feeding strategies for premature infants: randomized trial of gastrointestinal priming and tube-feeding method, *Pediatrics* 103:434, 1999a.

Schanler RJ et al: Feeding strategies for premature infants: beneficial outcomes of feeding fortified human milk versus preterm formula, *Pediatrics* 103:1150, 1999b.

Simpson C, Schanler RJ, Lau C: Early introduction of oral feeding in preterm infants, *Pediatrics* 110:517, 2002.

Sulkers EJ et al: Effects of high carnitine supplementation on substrate utilization in low-birth-weight infants receiving total parenteral nutrition, *Am J Clin Nutr* 52:889, 1990.

Tyson JE et al: Vitamin A supplementation for extremely-low-birth-weight infants, *N Eng J Med* 340:1962, 1999.

Wilson-Costello DE, Hack M: Follow-up for high risk neonates. In Fanaroff AA, Martin RJ, eds: *Neonatal-perinatal medicine diseases of the fetus and infant, vol 2,* ed 7, St Louis, 2002, Mosby.

Worrell LA et al: The effects of the introduction of a high-nutrient transitional formula on growth and development of very-low-birth-weight infant, *J Perinatol* 22:112, 2002.

Ziegler EE et al: Body composition of the reference fetus, *Growth* 40:329, 1976.

Additional References

American Academy of Pediatrics, Work Group on Breastfeeding: Breastfeeding and the use of human milk, *Pediatrics* 100:1035, 1997.

American Dietetic Association: Position of the American Dietetic Association: promotion of breast-feeding, *J Am Diet Assoc* 97:662, 1997.

Anderson DM: Nutritional assessment and therapeutic interventions for the preterm infant, *Clin Perinatol* 29:313, 2002.

Balistreri WF, Farrell MK, Bove KE: Lessons from the E-Ferol tragedy, *Pediatrics* 78:503, 1986.

Berseth CL: Feeding and maturation of gut motility. In Ziegler EE, Lucas A, Moro GE, eds: *Nutrition of the very low birthweight infant,* Philadelphia, 1999, Nestec and Lippincott Williams & Wilkins.

Groh-Wargo S, Thompson M, Cox JH, eds: *Nutritional care for high-risk newborns,* rev ed 3, Chicago, 2000, Precept Press.

Hack M et al: Outcomes in young adulthood for very-low-birth-weight infants, *N Engl J Med* 346:149, 2002.

Lucas A, Cole TJ: Breast milk and neonatal necrotizing enterocolitis, *Lancet* 336:1519, 1990.

Schanler RJ: The use of human milk for premature infants, *Pediatr Clin North Am* 48:207, 2001.

Thureen PJ, Hay WW: Intravenous nutrition and postnatal growth of the micropremie, *Clin Peri* 27:197, 2000.

Wilson DC et al: Randomised controlled trial of an aggressive nutritional regimen in sick very low birthweight infants, *Arch Dis Child* 77:F4, 1997.

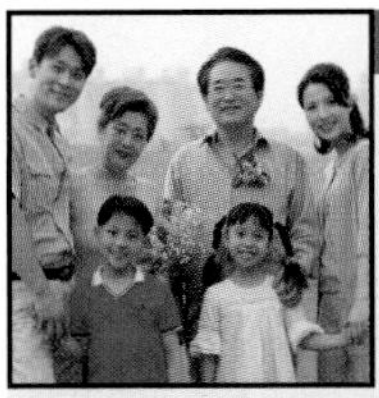

CHAPTER 10

Nutrition in Childhood

BETTY L. LUCAS, MPH, RD, CD

CHAPTER OUTLINE

- Growth and Development
- Nutrient Requirements
- Providing an Adequate Diet
- Nutritional Concerns
- Preventing Chronic Disease

KEY TERMS

adiposity rebound–a phenomenon of normal growth, occurring at approximately 6 years of age, which is when a child's body fat increases

appetite–a natural desire to eat, especially when food is present

catch-up growth–a higher-than-normal growth rate after a period of growth suppression as a result of extended illness or deprivation

failure to thrive (FTT)–weight loss or lack of weight gain in a child because of an acute or a chronic illness, a restricted diet, poor appetite, lack of food, lack of social interaction, or a harsh or disruptive environment

food insecurity–having limited or uncertain availability of nutritionally adequate and safe foods or a limited ability to acquire appropriate foods in socially acceptable ways

food jags–periods during which foods that were previously liked are refused or a particular food is requested at every meal; common in children ages 2 to 6 years

growth channel–a curve of weight and height gain throughout the period of growth; stated as a percentile based on a standard growth chart

The period that begins after infancy and lasts until puberty is often referred to as the *latent* or *quiescent* period of growth—a contrast to the dramatic changes that occur during infancy and adolescence. Although physical growth may be less remarkable and proceed at a steadier pace than it did during the first year, these preschool and middle-school years are a time of significant growth in the social, cognitive, and emotional areas.

GROWTH AND DEVELOPMENT

Growth Patterns

The rate of growth slows considerably after the first year of life. In contrast to the usual tripling of birth weight that occurs in the first 12 months, another year passes before the birth weight quadruples. Likewise, birth length increases by 50% in the first year but does not double until approximately the age of 4 years. Increments of change are small compared with those of infancy and adolescence; weight typically increases an average of 2 to 3 kg (4½ to 6½ lb) per year until the child is 9 or 10 years old. Then the rate increases, signaling the approach of puberty. Height increase increments average 6 to 8 cm (2½ to 3½ inches) per year from 2 years of age until puberty.

Growth is generally steady and slow during the preschool and school-age years, but it can be erratic in individual children, with periods of no growth followed by growth spurts. These patterns usually parallel similar changes in appetite and food intake. For parents, periods of slow growth and poor appetite can cause anxiety, leading to mealtime struggles.

Body proportions of young children change significantly after the first year. Head growth is minimal, trunk growth slows substantially, and limbs lengthen considerably, all of which create more mature body proportions. Because of walking and increased physical activity, the legs straighten, and the abdominal and back muscles strengthen to support the now erect child. These changes are gradual and subtle, occurring over years.

The body composition of preschool and school-age children remains relatively constant. Fat gradually decreases during the early childhood years, reaching a minimum between 4 and 6 years of age. Children then experience the adiposity rebound, or increase in body weight in preparation for the pubertal growth spurt. Earlier adiposity rebound has been associated with increased adult body mass index (BMI) (Whitaker et al, 1998). Sex differences in body composition become increasingly apparent—boys have more lean body mass per centimeter of height than girls. Females have a higher percentage of weight as fat than males, even in the preschool years, but these differences in lean body mass and fat do not become significant until adolescence.

Catch-Up Growth

A child who is recovering from an illness or undernutrition and whose growth has slowed or ceased experiences a greater-than-expected rate of recovery. This recovery is referred to as catch-up growth, a period during which the body strives to get back into the child's normal growth channel. The degree of growth suppression is influenced by the timing, severity, and duration of the precipitating cause; that is, a severe illness or prolonged nutritional deprivation during a period of rapid growth has the most dramatic impact (Berhane and Dietz, 1999).

Initial studies supported the thesis that malnourished infants who did not experience immediate catch-up growth would have permanent growth retardation. However, studies of malnourished children from developing countries who subsequently received adequate nourishment, as well as reports of children who were malnourished because of chronic diseases, such as celiac disease (see Chapter 30) or cystic fibrosis (see Chapter 38), have reported that these children caught up to their normal growth channels after the first year or two of life.

Rates of catch-up weight gain can be 20 times faster than normal in children who are both stunted (have low height for their age) and wasted (have low weight for their height); that is, their weight deficit is greater than their length deficit. Once catch-up growth has resulted in an appropriate weight for their height, the rate of subsequent weight gain is approximately three times the usual rate expected for age. The catch-up in linear growth reaches its peak about 1 to 3 months after treatment starts, whereas weight gain begins immediately (Ashworth and Millward, 1986).

Nutrient requirements, especially for energy and protein, vary depending on the rate and stage of catch-up growth. For instance, more protein and energy are needed during the very rapid weight gain period and for those in whom lean tissue is the major component of the weight gain. Guidelines for determining nutrient requirements are discussed in *Clinical Insight:* Obtaining Optimal Catch-Up Growth.

Assessing Growth

Because children are constantly growing and changing, periodic assessments allow any problems to be detected and treated early. Unfortunately, many children are seen by health care professionals only when they are ill, so growth and development may not be the focus of care.

A complete assessment of nutritional status includes the collection of anthropometric data. This includes length or height, weight, weight for length, and body mass index (BMI), all of which are plotted as percentiles on the Centers for Disease Control (CDC) growth charts (see Appendixes 6 through 11 and 18 and 19). Other measurements that are less

CLINICAL INSIGHT

Obtaining Optimal Catch-Up Growth

Clinical management of a child who has retarded growth as a result of malnourishment, a chronic disorder, or malabsorptive disease begins with a thorough assessment. The assessment includes determining the nature, severity, and duration of the nutritional problem, as well as the usual components of a nutritional assessment (e.g., anthropometric, dietary, biochemical, clinical, and social and environmental assessments). Growth data (height, weight, weight-for-length or BMI, head circumference of infants) are important criteria to monitor over time, and arm circumference and triceps skin-fold measurements can provide estimates of body composition.

The nutritional feeding goals depend on whether the child has stunted growth and is *chronically malnourished* or *primarily wasted* (i.e., has a weight deficit that exceeds the height deficit). A chronically malnourished child may not be expected to gain more than 2 to 3 g/kg/day, whereas a child who is primarily wasted may gain as much as 20 g/kg/day (Ashworth and Millward, 1986). Formulas are available to estimate the energy required to support the increased growth in an individual child. Current growth parameters are used to determine the child's *weight age* (the age corresponding to the child's weight at the 50th percentile), *ideal* (median) *weight for age,* and *ideal* (median) *weight for actual stature.* Formulas are then used to calculate the minimum and maximum energy needed for catch-up growth (Cunningham and McLaughlin, 1999). After a child who is wasted catches up in weight, dietary management changes to slow down the weight and height growth catch-up rate.

In addition to energy, other nutrients are important. Vitamin A supplementation improves linear growth and weight gain in infants who are infected with HIV and malaria, respectively, and decreases stunting that is associated with persistent diarrhea. Supplementation is a low-cost, effective intervention to decrease growth retardation in those with infectious diseases (Villamor et al, 2002.) The possibility of an iron deficiency also must be evaluated and corrected (Dewey, 1998.)

The following table illustrates the varying requirements for energy and protein at different rates of weight gain. Generally, the protein requirement increases proportionately more than the energy requirement when the weight gain is greater.

Dietary Requirements for Energy and Protein According to Weight Gain Rate

RATE OF WEIGHT* GAIN (g/kg/day)	ENERGY* (kcal/kg/day)	PROTEIN† (g/kg/day)	PROTEIN† (g/100 kcal)	NUMBER OF WEEKS NEEDED TO RENOURISH WASTED CHILD‡
—	85	0.62	0.73	—
1	90	0.83	0.92	50.0
2	94	1.04	1.11	25.0
5	108	1.67	1.55	10.0
10	130	2.72	2.09	5.0
20	174	4.82	2.77	2.5

From Ashworth A, Millward DJ: Catch-up growth in children, *Nutr Rev* 44:157, 1986.

*Assuming that the intake for zero energy balance is 85.5 kcal/kg/day and the cost of weight gain is 4.4 kcal/kg, which indicates that the composition of the tissue deposited is 73.5% lean and 26.5% fat.

†Assuming that the intake for zero nitrogen (N) balance is 100 mg of N/kg/day, the protein content of weight gain is 14.7%, and the efficiency of dietary protein utilization for tissue deposition is 70%.

‡Assuming that the child has an initial weight deficit of 3 kg and an average body weight, during rehabilitation, of 8.5 kg.

The child's health and medical condition, developmental readiness, meal and snack patterns, and family resources and lifestyle should be considered when providing nutrition services. Milk or a milk-based formula often provides the basis of the diet for young children during catch-up growth, in addition to developmentally appropriate foods. Frequent, small meals are usually better tolerated than infrequent, large ones. Because the total volume of food and the child's stomach capacity can be limiting factors, energy and nutrients can be concentrated or adjusted with commercial liquid or powder supplements, formula concentration, increased use of fats and oils, or the addition of glucose polymers and medium-chain triglyceride (MCT) oil.

Growth and nutritional status should be monitored frequently and nutrition interventions modified as needed. The medical, social, and environmental concerns related to the growth retardation must be addressed and resolved.

commonly used but that provide estimates of body composition include upper arm circumference and triceps or subscapular fat folds. Care should be taken to use standardized equipment and techniques for obtaining and plotting growth measurements. For instance, charts designed for birth to 36 months of age are based on length measurements and nude weights, whereas charts used for 2- to 20-year-olds are based on standing height and weight with light clothing and without shoes (see Chapter 17).

Growth measurements obtained at regular intervals provide a growth pattern. One-time height and weight measurements do not allow for an interpretation of growth status. Children generally maintain their heights and weights in the same growth channels during the preschool and childhood years, although the channels are not well established until after 2 years of age. Individual children sometimes grow at faster or slower rates; nonetheless, they should follow along the same channels.

The proportion of weight to length or height is a critical element of growth assessment. This parameter is determined by plotting the weight-for-length measurement on the CDC birth to 36 months growth charts or calculating BMI and plotting it on the 2 to 20 year old CDC growth charts (see Appendixes 7, 10, 18, 19). Midarm circumference and skin-fold measurements can yield additional information regarding the composition of the child's weight but require standardized equipment and techniques.

Regular monitoring of growth enables problematic trends to be identified early and intervention or education initiated so that long-term growth is not compromised. Weight that increases rapidly and crosses growth channels suggests the development of obesity. Lack of weight gain or loss of weight over a period of months may be a result of undernutrition, an acute illness, an undiagnosed chronic disease, or significant emotional or family problems. Figure 10-1 demonstrates these changes in growth parameters.

NUTRIENT REQUIREMENTS

Because children are growing and developing bones, teeth, muscles, and blood, they need more nutritious food in proportion to their size than do adults. They may be at risk for malnutrition when they have a poor appetite for a long period, eat a limited number of foods, or dilute their diets significantly with nutrient-poor foods.

The dietary reference intakes (DRIs) are based on current knowledge of nutrient intakes needed for optimal health (Institute of Medicine [IOM], 1997, 1998, 2000, 2002; Trumbo et al, 2001). They include estimated average requirements (EARs), recommended dietary allowances (RDAs), adequate intakes (AIs), and tolerable upper intake levels (ULs). Most data for preschool and school-age children are values interpolated from data on infants and adults (see Tables 8-1 and 15-1). These reference intakes are meant to improve the long-term health of the population by reducing the risk of chronic disease and preventing nutritional deficiencies. Thus when intakes are less than the recommended level, it cannot be assumed that a particular child is inadequately nourished.

Energy

The energy needs of healthy children are determined on the basis of basal metabolism, rate of growth, and energy expenditure. Dietary energy must be sufficient to ensure growth and spare protein from being used for energy but not so excessive that obesity results. Suggested intake proportions of energy are 50% to 60% as carbohydrate, 25% to 35% as fat, and 10% to 15% as protein.

Newer techniques for assessing energy expenditure suggest that the RDAs for energy may be too high for today's children. Using a doubly labeled water determination, the energy RDAs for infants may be overestimated by about 15% and by up to 25% for children 4 to 6 years of age (Cryan and Johnson, 1997; Goran, 2001). The new DRIs for energy do in fact change the energy requirements for children, and these new findings will be applied to child nutrition programs and other guidelines (IOM, 2002) (Table 10-1; see also Chapter 2).

Energy intakes of healthy, growing children of the same age and sex vary depending on their activity level. A 9-year-old boy and a 12½-year-old girl approaching puberty have significantly different factors determining their energy needs even though they are in the same DRI age category. It is useful to determine energy requirements on an individual basis using energy per kilogram of weight or per centimeter of height. Results of energy intake were 13 to 15 kcal/cm for children ages 2 to 5 years and 13 to 14 kcal/cm for girls and 16 to 17 kcal/cm for boys ages 6 to 11 years (Beal, 1970).

Protein

The need for protein per kilogram of body weight decreases from approximately 1.1 g in early childhood to 0.95 g in late childhood (see Box 10-1). Although this amount of protein is approximately 5% to 6% of the energy DRI, reported intakes from national surveys have shown that protein intakes are considerably higher—in the range of 10% to 16% of kilocalories (U.S. Department of Agriculture [USDA], 1997).

Protein deficiency is uncommon in American children, partly because of the cultural emphasis on protein foods. Children who are most likely to be at risk for inadequate protein intake are those on strict vegan diets, with multiple food allergies, or who have limited food selections because of fad diets, behavioral problems, or inadequate access to food.

Minerals and Vitamins

Minerals and vitamins are necessary for normal growth and development. Insufficient intake can cause impaired growth and result in deficiency dis-

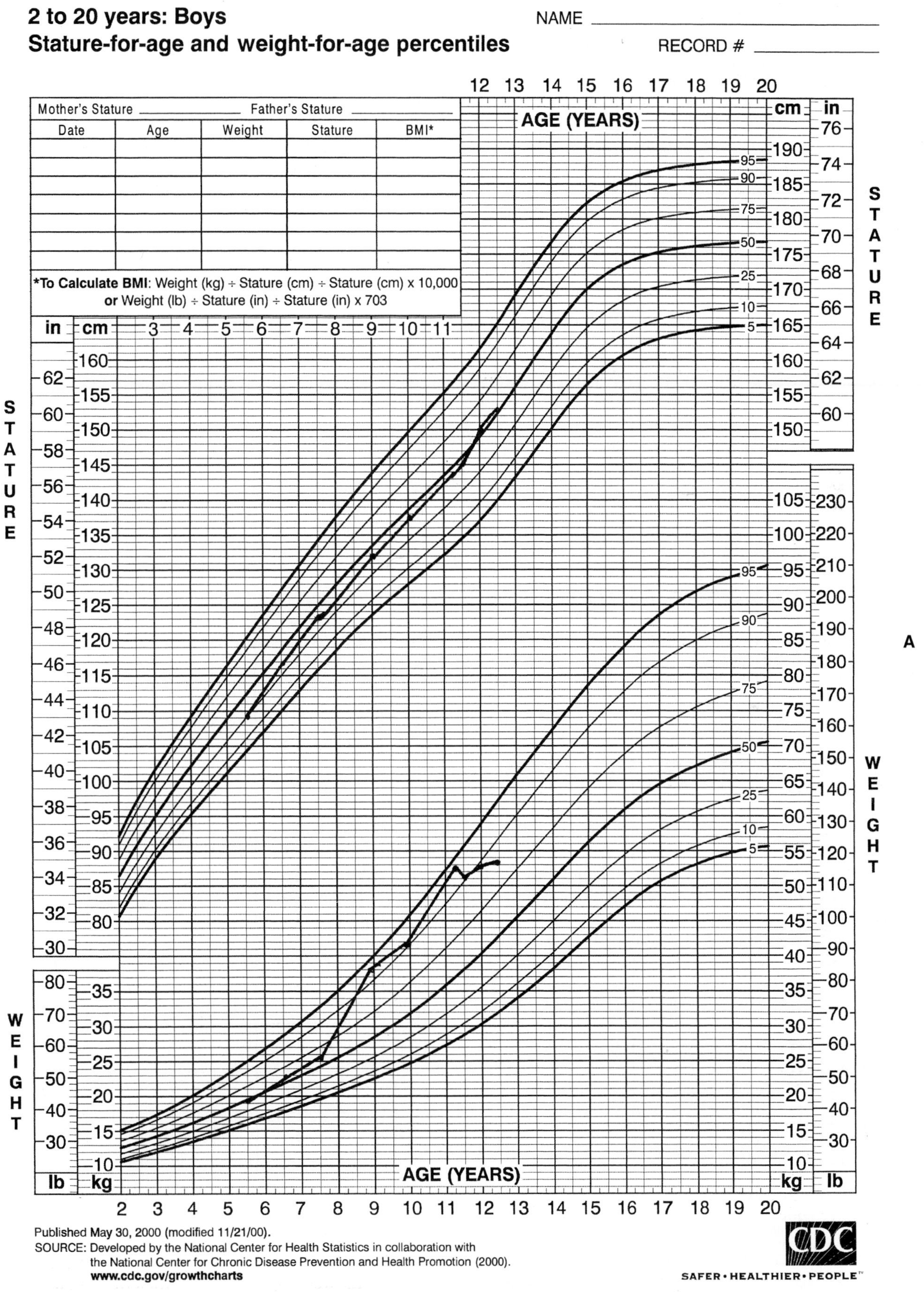

FIGURE 10-1 • **A,** Growth chart for an 8-year-old boy who gained excessive weight after having leg surgery and being immobilized in a body cast for 2 months. The surgery and immobilization were followed by a long period of stress from family problems. At the age of 11 years, he became involved in a weight management program. (Source of growth charts only: The National Center for Health Statistics in collaboration with the National Center for Chronic Disease Prevention and Health Promotion, 2000.)

Continued

2 to 20 years: Boys
Body mass index-for-age percentiles

NAME ____________________

RECORD # ____________

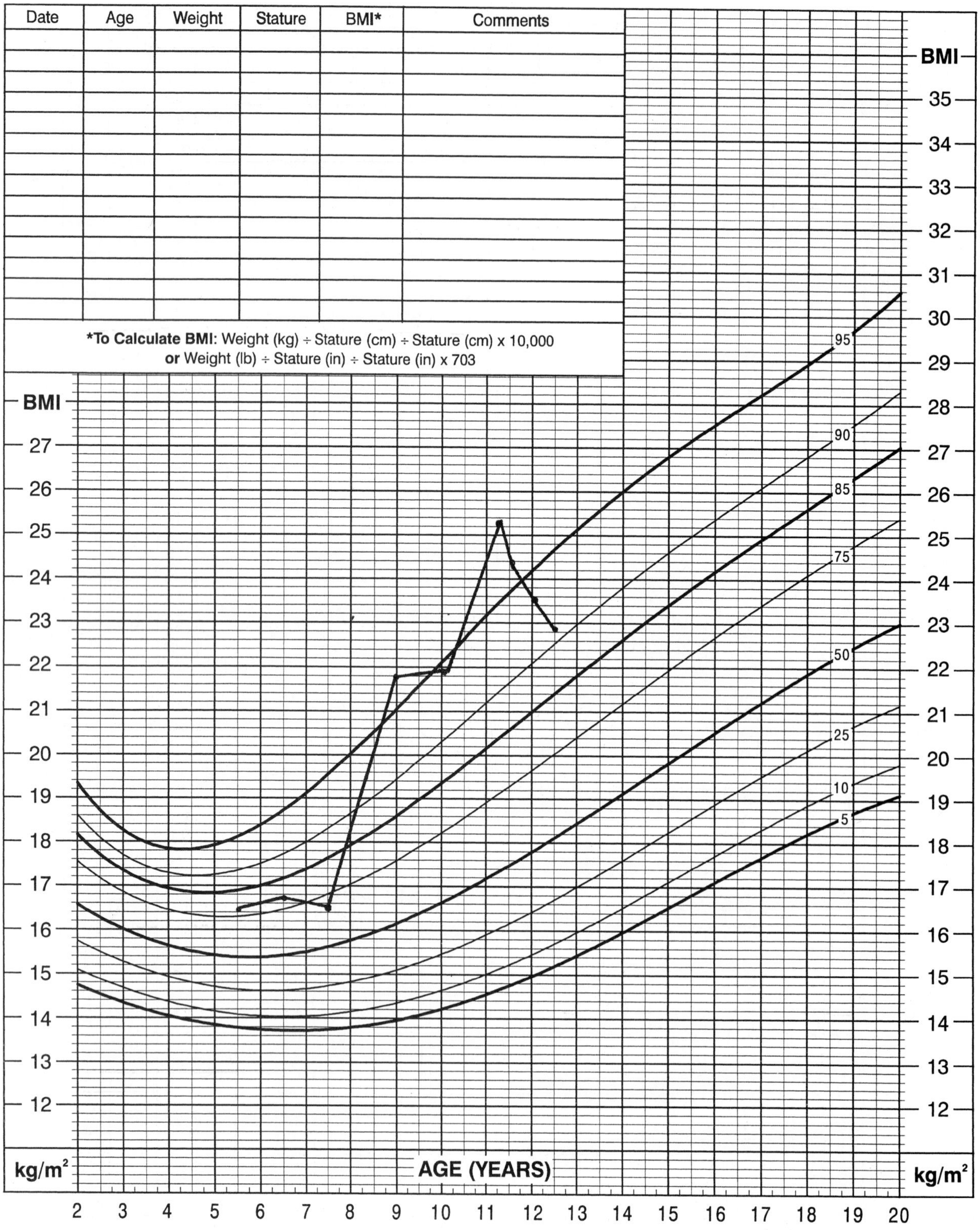

Published May 30, 2000 (modified 11/21/00).
SOURCE: Developed by the National Center for Health Statistics in collaboration with the National Center for Chronic Disease Prevention and Health Promotion (2000).
www.cdc.gov/growthcharts

CDC
SAFER • HEALTHIER • PEOPLE™

FIGURE 10-1, A cont'd • **A**, Growth chart for an 8-year-old boy who gained excessive weight after having leg surgery and being immobilized in a body cast for 2 months. The surgery and immobilization were followed by a long period of stress from family problems. At the age of 11 years, he became involved in a weight management program. (Source of growth charts only: The National Center for Health Statistics in collaboration with the National Center for Chronic Disease Prevention and Health Promotion, 2000.)

Birth to 36 months: Girls
Length-for-age and weight-for-age percentiles

NAME ____________________
RECORD # ____________

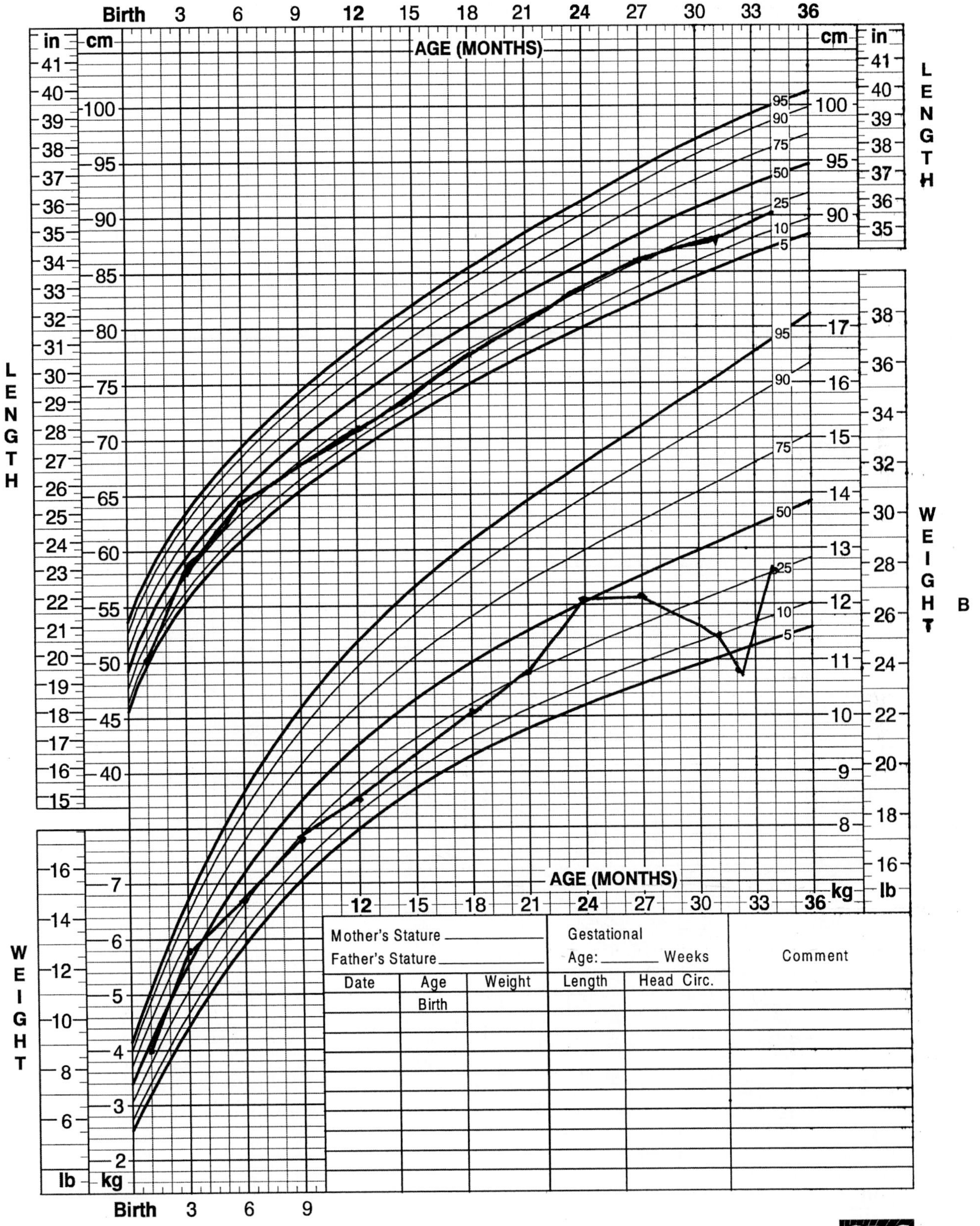

Published May 30, 2000 (modified 4/20/01).
SOURCE: Developed by the National Center for Health Statistics in collaboration with the National Center for Chronic Disease Prevention and Health Promotion (2000).
www.cdc.gov/growthcharts

CDC
SAFER • HEALTHIER • PEOPLE™

FIGURE 10-1, cont'd • **B,** Growth chart for a 2-year-old girl who experienced significant weight loss during a prolonged period of diarrhea and feeding problems. After being diagnosed with celiac disease, she began following a gluten-free diet and entered a period of catch-up growth. (Source of growth charts only: The National Center for Health Statistics in collaboration with the National Center for Chronic Disease Prevention and Health Promotion, 2000.)

Continued

Birth to 36 months: Girls
Head circumference-for-age and weight-for-length percentiles

NAME ______________________

RECORD # ______________

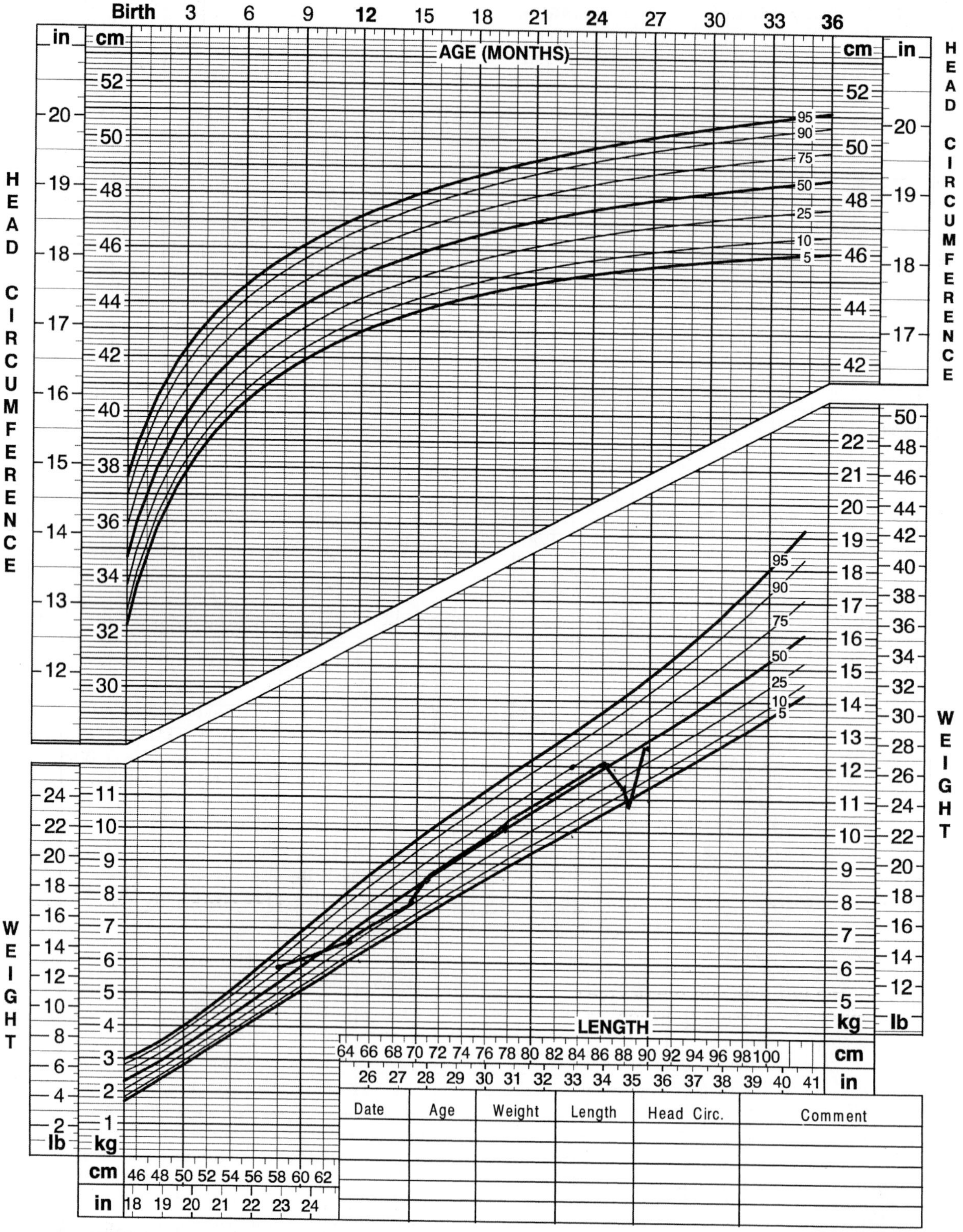

Published May 30, 2000 (modified 10/16/00).
SOURCE: Developed by the National Center for Health Statistics in collaboration with the National Center for Chronic Disease Prevention and Health Promotion (2000).
www.cdc.gov/growthcharts

CDC
SAFER • HEALTHIER • PEOPLE™

FIGURE 10-1, B cont'd • **B,** Growth chart for a 2-year-old girl who experienced significant weight loss during a prolonged period of diarrhea and feeding problems. After being diagnosed with celiac disease, she began following a gluten-free diet and entered a period of catch-up growth. (Source of growth charts only: The National Center for Health Statistics in collaboration with the National Center for Chronic Disease Prevention and Health Promotion, 2000.)

TABLE 10-1 Daily Dietary Reference Intakes for Energy and Protein for Children

Energy AGE (yr)	MALES (kcal)	FEMALES (kcal)
1-2	1046	992
3-8	1742	1642
9-13	2279	2071
Protein AGE (yr)	**GRAMS**	**GRAMS (per kg)**
1-3	13	1.1
4-8	19	0.95
9-13	34	0.95

Data from Institute of Medicine, Food and Nutrition Board: *Dietary reference intakes for energy and the macronutrients, carbohydrate, fiber, fat, fatty acids, cholesterol, protein, and amino acids,* Washington, DC, 2002, National Academy Press.

eases (see Chapters 4 and 5). (The DRIs for different age groups are listed in Tables 8-1 and 15-1.)

Iron

Children between 1 and 3 years of age are at high risk for iron deficiency anemia. The rapid growth period of infancy is marked by an increase in hemoglobin and total iron mass. In addition, the diet may not be rich in iron-containing foods. Recommended intakes must factor in the absorption rate and quantity of iron in foods, especially those of plant origin (see Chapters 5 and 34).

Calcium

Calcium is needed for adequate mineralization and maintenance of growing bone in children. The DRI for calcium is higher for children 9 to 18 years of age (1300 mg of calcium per day) than it was in the past (Trumbo, 2001). For 1- to 3-year-olds, it is 500 mg/day; for children 4 to 8 years, it is 800 mg/day. Actual need depends on individual absorption rates and dietary factors such as quantities of protein, vitamin D, and phosphorus. Because calcium intake has very little influence on the degree of urinary calcium excretion during periods of rapid growth, children need two to four times more calcium per kilogram than adults. Because milk and other dairy products are the primary sources of calcium, children who consume no or limited amounts of these foods are at risk for poor bone mineralization (Figure 10-2). Other calcium-fortified foods such as soy and rice milks and fruit juices are now available.

Zinc

Zinc is essential for growth; a deficiency results in growth failure, poor appetite, decreased taste acuity, and poor wound healing. An allowance of 3 mg/day of zinc is recommended for 1- to 3-year-olds, 5 mg/day for children 4 to 8 years of age, and 8 mg/day for those 9 to 13 years of age (Trumbo, 2001). Because the best sources of zinc are meats and seafood, some children may regularly have a low intake. Marginal zinc deficiency has been reported in preschool and school-age children from middle- and low-income families (Roberts and Heyman, 2000). Diagnosis may be difficult because laboratory parameters including plasma, serum, erythrocyte, hair, and urine levels are of limited value in determining zinc deficiency. In some cases, a carefully controlled, short-term trial of zinc supplementation may be the only conclusive way to diagnose a problem (Krebs and Hambidge, 1996) (see Chapter 5).

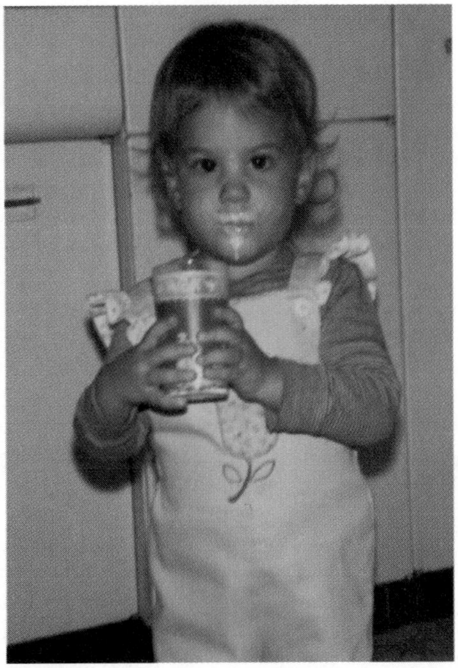

FIGURE 10-2 • Milk and other dairy products supply preschool children with the calcium and vitamin D needed for growing bones.

Vitamin D

Vitamin D is needed for calcium absorption and deposition of calcium in the bones. Because this nutrient is also formed from sunlight exposure on the skin, the amount required from dietary sources depends on nondietary factors such as geographic location and time spent outside. Children living in tropical areas may need no dietary vitamin D or only 2.5 μg (100 IU) or less for optimal calcium (see Chapter 4, *Focus On:* Sunshine, Vitamin D, and Fortification). However, in the temperate zones, some dietary source is needed; the DRI is 5 μg (200 IU) for children. Vitamin D–fortified milk is the primary source of this nutrient; however, dairy products such as cheese and yogurt are not usually made from fortified milk. Regardless, many breakfast cereals and nondairy milks are fortified with vitamin D.

Vitamin-Mineral Supplements

More than 50% of preschool children use supplements (commonly a multivitamin-mineral with iron), but use usually decreases in older children. Families with more education, insurance coverage, and higher incomes have higher rates of supplement use, although these may not be the families that are at greatest risk for having inadequate diets (Yu et al, 1997). Supplements do not necessarily fulfill specific nutrient needs. For instance, although many consume less than the recommended amount of calcium, children's vitamin-mineral supplements do not contain significant amounts of calcium.

Evidence shows that fluoride can help prevent caries. If a community's water supply is not fluoridated (i.e., has <0.6 ppm), fluoride supplements are recommended from 6 months until 16 years of age (see Chapter 28). However, individual family practices should be assessed, because some children in communities with adequately fluoridated water primarily drink bottled water, juice, or other beverages, and thus drink little fluoridated tap water.

The American Academy of Pediatrics (AAP) does not support giving healthy children routine supplements of any vitamins or minerals other than fluoride. However, children at risk for inadequate nutrition who may benefit from supplementation include those (1) from deprived families; (2) with anorexia, poor appetites, and poor eating habits; (3) with chronic diseases such as cystic fibrosis or liver disease; (4) enrolled in dietary programs for weight management; and (5) who have vegetarian diets with an inadequate intake of dairy products or calcium-containing foods (AAP, 1998a).

Children who routinely take a multiple vitamin or vitamin-mineral supplement do not have any negative effects if the supplement contains nutrients in amounts that do not exceed the RDA. However, they should not take megadoses, particularly of the fat-soluble vitamins because large amounts can result in toxicity (see Chapter 4).

Complementary nutrition therapies and herbal products are becoming more common for children (Sawni-Sikand et al, 2002), especially those with special needs such as children with Down syndrome, autism spectrum disorder, or cystic fibrosis. Practitioners should include the use of these products and therapies in nutrition assessments, be knowledgeable about their efficacy and safety, and help families to determine whether they are beneficial and how to use them (see Chapter 20).

PROVIDING AN ADEQUATE DIET

Food and eating are more than the simple provision of nutrients for body growth and maintenance. The development of feeding skills, food habits, and nutrition knowledge parallels the cognitive development that takes place in a series of stages, each laying the groundwork for the next. Table 10-2 outlines the development of feeding skills in terms of Piaget's theory of child psychology and development.

Intake Patterns

Children are most likely to consume inadequate amounts of calcium, iron, zinc, vitamin B_6, and vitamin A (Roberts and Heyman, 2000; USDA, 1997). However, clinical signs of malnutrition in American children are rare.

Studies of children have shown that food patterns have changed over the years. They drink more low-fat and nonfat milk, consume less whole milk and eggs, eat more snacks, and are more likely to consume food in environments other than the home. Data from national food intake studies of children and adolescents indicates that most of their diets do not meet the national recommendations for food groups as presented in the U.S. Dietary Guidelines and Food Guide Pyramid. Except for the dairy group, the mean numbers of servings reported for each group were less than the minimum recommendations for children ages 2 to 11 years. Only about 30% of children of this age consumed the recommendations for fruit, grains, and meat; 36% consumed the vegetable recommendations. The total fat intake averaged 35% of the energy intake (Munoz et al, 1997). Some children receive almost 50% of their energy from the pyramid's "tip," additional fat and sugar food groups (Brady et al, 2000).

Population studies of nutritional status have reported an increased frequency of low nutrient intake and higher cholesterol in children from low-income families (Casey et al, 2001; Cook and Martin, 1997). In addition, inner-city, low-income children and homeless children are at more risk for poor dietary intake and lead exposure and toxicity (see *Focus On:* Childhood Lead Exposure and Toxicity: The Role of Nutrition).

Like physical growth patterns, food intake patterns are not smooth and consistent. Although subjective, appetites usually follow the rate of growth and nutrient needs. A good appetite in infants often becomes a fair or poor appetite in young, preschool-age children, which frequently causes parents to become anxious.

By a child's first birthday, milk consumption begins to decline. In the next year, vegetable intake decreases, whereas intakes of cereals, grain products, and sweets increase. Children prefer ground beef and hot dogs to meats that are harder to chew.

Changes in food consumption are reflected in nutrient intakes. Compared with nutrient intake in infancy, that in the early preschool years shows a decrease in calcium, phosphorus, riboflavin, iron, and vitamin A. Intakes of most other key nutrients remain relatively stable. During the early school years,

TABLE 10-2 Feeding, Nutrition, and Piaget's Theory of Cognitive Development

DEVELOPMENTAL PERIOD	COGNITIVE CHARACTERISTICS	RELATIONSHIPS TO FEEDING AND NUTRITION
Sensorimotor (birth-2 yr)	Neonate progresses from automatic reflexes to a child with intentional interaction with the environment and the beginning use of symbols.	Progression involves advancing from sucking and rooting reflexes to the acquisition of self-feeding skills. Food is used primarily to satisfy hunger, as a medium to explore the environment, and as an opportunity to practice fine motor skills.
Preoperational (2-7 yr)	Thought processes become internalized; they are unsystematic and intuitive. Use of symbols increases.	Eating becomes less the center of attention and is secondary to social, language, and cognitive growth. Food is described by color, shape, and quantity, but the child has only a limited ability to classify food into "groups."
	Reasoning is based on appearances and happenstance.	
	The child's approach to classification is functional and unsystematic.	Foods tend to be categorized into "like" and "don't like."
	The child's world is viewed egocentrically.	Foods can be identified as "good for you," but reasons they are healthy are unknown or mistaken.
Concrete operations (7-11 yr)	The child can focus on several aspects of a situation simultaneously.	The child begins to realize that nutritious food has a positive effect on growth and health but has a limited understanding of how or why.
	Cause-and-effect reasoning becomes more rational and systematic. The ability to classify, reclassify, and generalize emerges.	
	A decrease in egocentrism permits the child to take another's view.	Mealtimes take on a social significance.
		The expanding environment increases the opportunities for and the influences on food selection; for example, peer influence increases.
Formal operations (11 yr and beyond)	Hypothetical and abstract thought expand.	The concept of nutrients from food functioning at physiologic and biochemical levels can be understood.
	The child's understanding of scientific and theoretical processes deepens.	Conflicts in making food choices may be realized; that is, knowledge of the nutritious value of foods may conflict with preferences and non-nutritive influences.

a pattern of consistent and steady increased intakes of most nutrients is seen until adolescence. For any age and sex group, a wide variability of nutrient intake is seen in healthy children.

Factors Influencing Food Intake

Numerous influences, some obvious and others subtle, determine the food intake and habits of children. Habits, likes, and dislikes are established in the early years and are carried through to adulthood, when change is often met with resistance. The major influences on food intake in the developing years include family environment, societal trends, the media, peer pressure, and illness or diseases.

Family Environment

For toddlers and preschool children, the family is the primary influence in the development of food habits. In young children's immediate environment, parents and older siblings are significant models . Food attitudes of parents can be strong predictors of food likes and dislikes and diet complexity in children of primary-school age. Similarities between children's and their parents' food preferences are likely to reflect genetic and environmental influences.

Contrary to common belief, young children do not have the innate ability to choose a balanced, nutritious diet; they can choose one only when presented with nutritious foods (see Chapter 8, *Clinical Insight: Self-Selected Diets of Infants and Young Children*). Parents and other adults are responsible for offering various nutritious and developmentally appropriate foods. A positive feeding relationship includes a division of responsibility between parents and children. The parents provide safe, nutritious food as regular meals and snacks, and the children decide how much, if any, they eat.

National trends indicate that eating together at family meals is becoming less common, partly because of family schedules, more time eating in front of the television, and the decreasing amount of time devoted to planning and preparing family meals. In a recent report, school-age children and adolescents who ate more dinners with their families consumed more fruits and vegetables, less soda, and fewer fried foods than those who rarely ate dinner with their families (Gillman et al, 2000).

The atmosphere around food and mealtime also influences attitudes toward food and eating. Unrealistic expectations for a child's mealtime manners, arguments, and other emotional stress can have a negative effect. Meals that are rushed create a hectic atmosphere and reinforce the tendency to eat too fast. A positive environment is one in which sufficient time is set aside to eat, occasional spills are tolerated, and conversation that includes all family members is encouraged (Figure 10-3).

Societal Trends

Because almost three fourths of women with school-age children are employed outside the home, children eat one or more meals at child-care homes, day-care centers, or schools. Because of time constraints, food shopping and meal preparation may be modified to include more convenience or fast foods. However, having a mother who is employed outside the home does not seem to affect children's dietary intakes negatively.

Approximately one in five American children live in families with incomes below the poverty line; these children constitute 40% of all the poor in the United States. The increasing numbers of single-parent households predominantly headed by women have a lower income and less money for all expenses, including food, than households headed by men. The poverty rate for children younger than 6 years old who live in families headed by a single female is almost 60%. This phenomenon, referred to as the *feminization of poverty,* makes these families increasingly vulnerable to multiple stressors, such as marginal health and nutritional status, partly because of lack of jobs, child care, adequate housing, and health insurance. Moreover, recent studies suggest that intermittent hunger in American children is associated with poor psychosocial function (Kleinman RE et al, 1998; Murphy JM et al, 1998) (see *Focus On:* Childhood Hunger and Its Effect on Behaviors and Emotions).

Media Messages

By the time average American children have graduated from high school, they have watched 15,000 hours of television and spent 11,000 hours in the classroom. School-age children watch an average of 23 hours or more per week, whereas preschool children average about 27 hours per week. One half of all commercials in children's programs advertise food—

FOCUS ON

Childhood Lead Exposure and Toxicity: The Role of Nutrition

Elevated blood lead levels in toddlers and children can result in developmental regression, irritability, anorexia, gastrointestinal symptoms (e.g., abdominal pain, constipation, vomiting), and ataxia. High levels can cause growth impairment and mental retardation. Children living in poverty are at greatest risk, partly because they are more likely to be exposed to lead-based paint and contaminated soil, dust, and air emissions in industrial areas. Lead exposure can also result from consuming contaminated drinking water (from lead pipes or solder) and contaminated food (from lead glazing or lead crystal). Toddlers who typically put everything in their mouths and children with mental retardation who exhibit pica are exposed to lead from many environmental sources.

When correlations were found between middle-class toddler blood lead levels and the toddlers' subsequent IQ scores at ages 5 and 10, the CDC lowered the blood lead threshold to 10 μg/dl and established screening guidelines (CDC, 1997). Although the effect of lead exposure varies with its intensity and timing (with younger children being the most susceptible to its effects), it is now accepted that moderate blood lead levels of 10 to 25 μg/dl can have a negative impact a child's attention, adaptive behaviors, and emotional reactivity, all of which affect learning, school achievement, and life functioning.

Because more lead is absorbed from an empty stomach, nutrition guidelines include regular meals and snacks. Increased calcium and iron intakes are also recommended to minimize the lead absorption in children with mineral deficiencies. However, the associations that have been found between high blood lead levels and calcium and iron deficiencies could also be a result of poverty and other environmental factors. Because studies of lead uptake and calcium and iron intake have not had consistent results, practitioners can promote a mineral-rich diet but should not assume that it can ameliorate the negative effects of lead ingestion (Ballew and Bowman, 2001). In addition to ensuring that children at risk for lead exposure follow a nutrient-rich diet, regular screening and education should be provided and public health policies should be developed to decrease environmental lead levels.

primarily foods low in fiber and high in sugar, fat, or sodium.

Preschool children are generally unable to distinguish commercial messages from regular programs. In fact, they often pay more attention to the commercials, so they remember and request the advertised items (Borzekowski and Robinson, 2001). Many schools include a short television "news" segment as part of the school day; however, the content is accompanied by advertisements aimed at children. As children get older, they gain knowledge about the purpose of commercial advertising and become more critical of its validity but are still susceptible to the commercial message. Media literacy education programs teach children and adolescents about the intent of advertising and media messages and how to evaluate and interpret their obvious and subtle influences.

Television can also be detrimental to growth and development because it encourages inactivity and passive use of leisure time. Indeed, television viewing and its multiple media cues to eat have been suggested as a factor contributing to excessive weight gain in school-age children and adolescents (Dietz and Gortmaker, 2001).

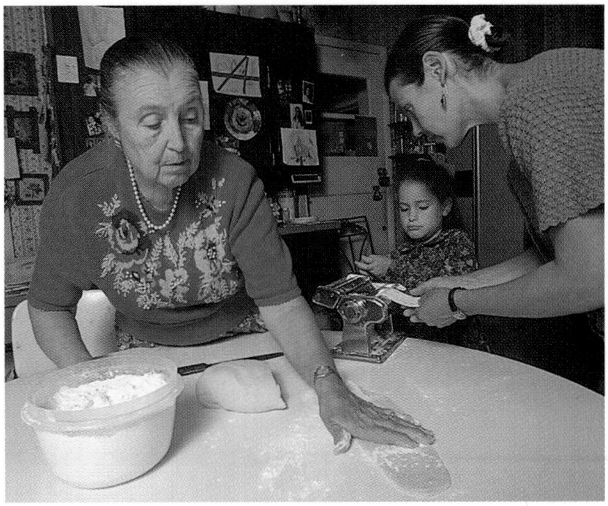

FIGURE 10-3 • Three generations of Italian Americans make a pasta dinner. The custom of eating authentically prepared foods gives meals a place of prominence in this home—meals that will not be replaced with fast foods eaten on the run. (From Leahy J, Kisilay P: *Foundations of nursing practice: a nursing process approach,* Philadelphia, 1998, WB Saunders.)

FOCUS ON

Childhood Hunger and Its Effect on Behaviors and Emotions

It is well accepted that malnourished children are less responsive, less inquisitive, and participate in less exploratory behavior than well-nourished infants. Specific nutrient deficiencies such as iron-deficiency anemia can also result in a decreased ability to pay attention and poorer problem-solving skills. Less clear is the impact of periodic hunger or food insecurity on a child's behavior and functioning. With recent federal welfare reform legislation and economic downturns, an increasing number of children from low-income families are at risk for limited food resources.

The Community Childhood Hunger Identification Project (CCHIP) conducts surveys using standardized questions and large, rigorously selected samples to categorize families as "hungry," "at-risk for hunger," or "not hungry" (Kleinman et al, 1998). Results estimate that 8% of the children younger than 12 years of age living in the United States experience prolonged periods in which they have insufficient food each year. Children make up about 40% of all individuals with food insecurity, with an overall increase in total numbers during the late 1990s. In one study a group of 328 parents from a larger CCHIP study were asked to complete the Pediatric Symptom Checklist, which was related to their child's emotional and behavioral symptoms. "Hungry" children were three times more likely than "at-risk for hunger" children and seven times more likely than "not hungry" children to have scores indicative of characteristics such as aggression, irritability, oppositional behavior, and anxiety (Kleinman et al, 1998).

In a similar CCHIP study, 204 school-age children and their parents and teachers provided information on psychosocial function using the parent Child Behavior Checklist (CBCL), the Connors Teacher Rating Scale, and a global assessment scale (Murphy et al, 1998). Results showed that "hungry" and "at-risk for hunger" children were twice as likely as "not hungry" children to be considered functionally impaired, and a significant association was found between hunger and CBCL scores. Teachers reported an increased incidence of hyperactivity, absenteeism, and tardiness in the "hungry" and "at-risk for hunger" children. Although these studies have limitations because of other factors (e.g., stress, family dysfunction, or substance abuse) that may affect a child's functioning, a correlation exists between children's lack of sufficient food and their behavioral and academic functioning. If future studies provide more evidence of this relationship, it will be clear that social policies need to ensure the provision of children's basic needs for optimal growth and development.

Peer Influence

As children grow, their world expands and their social contacts become more important. Peer influence increases with age and affects food attitudes and choices. This may result in a sudden refusal of a food or a request for a currently popular food. Decisions about whether to participate in school meals may be made more on the basis of friends' choices than on the menu. Such behaviors are developmentally typical. Positive behaviors, such as a willingness to try new foods, can be reinforced. Parents need to set limits for undesirable influences but also need to be realistic; struggles over food are self-defeating.

Illness or Disease

Children who are ill usually have a decreased appetite and limited food intake. Acute viral or bacterial illnesses are often short-lived but may require an increase in fluids, protein, or other nutrients. Chronic conditions such as asthma (see Chapter 38), chronic renal disease (see Chapter 39), and cystic fibrosis (see Chapter 38) may make it difficult to obtain sufficient nutrients for optimal growth. Children with these types of conditions are more likely to have behavior problems relating to food. Children requiring special diets (e.g., those who have diabetes or phenylketonuria) not only have to adjust to the limits of foods allowed but also have to deal with issues of independence and peer acceptance as they grow older. Some rebellion against the prescribed diet is typical, especially as children approach puberty.

Feeding Preschool Children

The period from 1 to 6 years of age is marked by vast development and the acquisition of skills. Children learn to talk, run, and become social beings. One-year-old children primarily use fingers to eat and may need assistance with a cup. By 2 years of age, they can hold a cup in one hand and use a spoon well (see Figure 8-3) but may still prefer to use their hands at times. Six-year-old children have refined skills and are beginning to use a knife for cutting and spreading.

Because growth is slower during these years, the appetite decreases, which often concerns the parents. Children have a decreased interest in food and an increased interest in the world around them. They develop food jags during this time, refusing previously accepted food or asking for the same food at each meal. This behavior may be attributable to boredom with the usual foods or may be a means of asserting newly discovered independence.

This can be a difficult time for parents, who may have concerns about the adequacy of their child's diet and be frustrated with their child's seemingly irrational food behavior. Struggles over control of the eating situation are fruitless; no child can be forced to eat. Parents need to understand that this period is developmental and temporary. They still retain control over what foods are offered, and they have the opportunity to set limits on inappropriate behaviors. Neither rigid control nor a laissez-faire approach is likely to succeed. Parents and other caregivers should continue to offer a variety of foods, including the child's favorite ones, and not make substitutions a routine. Preschool children tend to vary considerably in their meal intakes during the day, but their total daily energy intake remains fairly constant.

Because of their smaller stomach capacity and variable appetites, preschool children eat best with small servings of food offered several times a day. A general rule of thumb is to offer 1 tablespoon of each food for every year of age and to serve more food according to the child's appetite. Table 10-3 is a guide for food and portion sizes and is designed to provide an adequate diet for preschoolers. Most children eat four to six times a day, making snacks as important as meals in contributing to the total daily nutrient intake. Snacks should be chosen carefully so that they are dense in nutrients and least likely to promote dental caries. Wholesome snacks enjoyed by many young children include fresh fruit, cheese, raw vegetable sticks, milk, fruit juices, whole-grain crackers, dry cereal, and peanut butter sandwiches.

Senses other than taste play an important part in food acceptance by young children. They tend to avoid food with extreme temperatures, and some foods are rejected because of odor rather than taste. A sense of order in the food presentation is often required; many children will not accept foods that touch each other on the plate, and mixed dishes or casseroles with unidentifiable foods are not popular. Broken crackers may go uneaten or a sandwich may be refused because it is "cut the wrong way."

The physical setting of children's meals is as important as the emotional atmosphere. Children should not be made to eat with feet dangling and arms reaching up to a table at chest height. Sturdy, child-sized tables and chairs are ideal, or a high chair or booster seat should be used. Bowls, plates, and cups should be unbreakable and heavy enough to resist tipping. For very young children, a shallow bowl is often better than a plate for scooping. Thick, short-handled spoons and forks allow for an easier, less tiring grasp.

Young children do not eat well if they are tired, so this should be considered when meal and play times are scheduled. A quiet activity or rest immediately before eating is conducive to a relaxed, enjoyable meal. However, children need active, large-motor activities and time in the fresh air to stimulate a good appetite.

Children should not be given any food or drink within 1½ hours of a meal. It takes little to satisfy a young child's appetite, so even small snacks may result in poor eating at mealtime.

TABLE 10-3 Feeding Guide for Preschool Children*

FOOD	2- TO 3-YEAR-OLDS PORTION SIZE	2- TO 3-YEAR-OLDS NUMBER OF SERVINGS	4- TO 6-YEAR-OLDS PORTION SIZE	4- TO 6-YEAR-OLDS NUMBER OF SERVINGS	COMMENTS
Milk and Dairy Products	½ cup (4 oz)	4-5	½-¾ cup	3-4 (4-6 oz)	The following may be substituted for ½ cup of liquid milk: ½-¾ oz cheese, ½ cup yogurt, 2½ tbsp nonfat dry milk powder.
Meat, Fish, Poultry, or Equivalent	1-2 oz	2	1-2 oz	2	The following may be substituted for 1 oz of meat, fish, or poultry: 1 egg, 2 tbsp peanut butter, 4-5 tbsp cooked legumes.
Fruits and Vegetables		4-5		4-5	Include one green leafy or yellow vegetable for vitamin A, such as spinach, carrots, broccoli, or winter squash.
Vegetables					
Cooked	2-3 tbsp		3-4 tbsp		
Raw†	Few pieces		Few pieces		
Fruit					Include one vitamin C–rich fruit, vegetable, or juice, such as citrus juices, an orange, grapefruit sections, strawberries, melon in season, a tomato, or broccoli.
Raw	½-1 small		½-1 small		
Canned	2-4 tbsp		4-6 tbsp		
Juice	3-4 oz		4 oz		
Bread and Grain Products		3		3	The following may be substituted for 1 slice of bread: ½ cup spaghetti, macaroni, noodles, or rice; 5 saltines; 1 tortilla; or ½ bagel.
Whole-grain or enriched bread	½-1 slice		1 slice		
Cooked cereal	¼-½ cup		½ cup		
Dry cereal	½-1 cup		1 cup		

Modified from Lowenberg ME: Development of food patterns in young children. In Trahms CM, Pipes P: *Nutrition in infancy and childhood,* ed 6, St Louis, 1997, WCB/McGraw-Hill.

*This is a guide to a basic diet. Fats, oils, sauces, desserts, and snack foods provide additional kilocalories to meet the needs of a growing child. Foods can be selected from this pattern for meals and snacks.

†Do not give to children until they can chew well.

Fruit juices, especially apple juice and juice drinks, are an increasingly common beverage for young children, at home and in group settings; they frequently replace water and milk in children's diets. In addition to altering the diet's nutrient content, excessive intake of fruit juice can result in carbohydrate malabsorption and chronic, nonspecific diarrhea (AAP, 2001). This suggests that juices, especially apple and pear, should be avoided when using clear liquids to treat acute diarrhea. For children with chronic diarrhea, a trial of restricting fruit juices may be warranted before more costly diagnostic tests are done.

Excessive fruit juice consumption (12 to 30 oz/day) has been identified as a contributing factor in some cases of failure to thrive in toddlers. A reduction in juice intake, in addition to nutritional education designed to increase total energy intake, resulted in improved growth (AAP, 2001). Although some have suggested that excess fruit juice intake (>12 oz/day) is linked with short stature and obesity, a longitudinal study of children 24 to 72 months of age showed no association (Skinner and Carruth, 2001). Excess juice intake by young preschool children may replace the consumption of higher-energy foods and decrease a child's appetite, resulting in decreased food intake and poor growth. It is also possible that large volumes of juice, combined with other dietary and activity factors, may contribute to or sustain an overweight condition in a child. The AAP recommends that fruit juice be limited to 4 to 6 oz daily for infants older than 6 months of age and toddlers and to 6 to 12 oz per day for older children and adolescents (AAP, 2001).

A generation ago, the food experiences of most preschool children centered on home and family. Today, many children spend part or most of their days in day-care homes or centers, preschools, or Head Start programs. Depending on the time the children are in these settings, they may consume only a snack, or they may eat as many as two meals and two snacks per day. Therefore many children consume more than half of their nutrients outside the home.

Food service in group settings such as day-care centers, Head Start programs, and preschool programs in elementary schools is regulated by federal or state guidelines. Many facilities and some day-care homes may participate in the USDA Child and Adult Care Food Program. However, the quality of meals and snacks can vary greatly; parents should investigate food service when considering child-care options. In addition to providing children with optimal nutrients, a program should offer food that is appealing, safely prepared, and appropriate, incorporating cultural and developmental patterns (see Chapter 14).

Because of peer influence, children usually eat well in group settings; group settings are also ideal environments for nutrition education programs during mealtimes and as the focus for various learning activities (Figure 10-4). Experiencing new foods, participating in simple food preparation, and planting a garden are activities that develop and enhance positive food habits and attitudes.

Feeding School-Age Children

Growth from ages 6 to 12 years is slow but steady, paralleled by a constant increase in food intake. Children are in school a greater part of the day, and they begin to participate in clubs, organized sports, and recreational programs. The influence of peers and significant adults such as teachers, coaches, or sports idols increases. Except for severe issues, most behavioral problems connected with food have been resolved by this age, and children enjoy eating to alleviate hunger and obtain social satisfaction.

School-age children may participate in the school lunch program or bring a lunch from home. The National School Lunch Program, established in 1946 and administered by the USDA, provides approximately one third of the DRI for students. Children from low-income families are eligible for free or reduced-price meals. In addition, the School Breakfast Program that began in 1966 has expanded, and more than three fourths of the schools participate in the lunch program. The USDA also offers the Summer Food Service Program, which offers meals and snacks to children in programs during school vacations (see Chapter 14).

Over the years, efforts have been made to decrease food waste by altering menus to accommodate student preferences, allowing students to decline one or two menu items, and offering salad bars. Ongoing concerns over excessive amounts of fat, salt, and sugar in school meals resulted in changes to school meals that incorporated the Dietary Guidelines for Americans. Specific changes in the school and child nutrition programs included reducing the fat content of recipes and offering a greater variety of fresh fruits and vegetables, whole-grain products, and fewer baked items (see Chapter 14). By 1999, significantly more elementary and secondary schools were meeting the lower fat and sodium standards for school lunches (USDA, 2001).

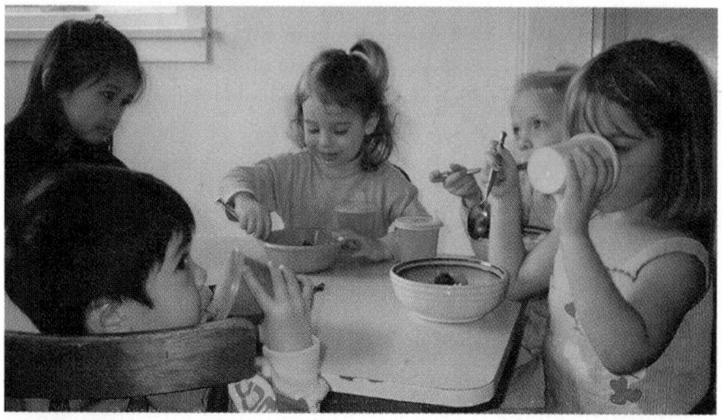

FIGURE 10-4 • Children who eat with each other in an appropriate environment often eat more nutritiously and try a wider variety of foods than they do when alone.

Consumption of school meals is also affected by the daily school schedule and the amount of time allotted for children to eat. A study of elementary school students found that food waste significantly decreased when recess was scheduled before, rather than after, the lunch period (Getlinger et al, 1996).

Children who require a special diet because of certain medical conditions such as diabetes, hyperlipidemia, or documented food allergy are eligible for modified school meals. Children with special health care needs are eligible to attend public school from ages 3 to 21 years, and some of them need modified school meals (e.g., meals that are texture modified, high in calories, or low in calories). To receive modified meals, students must submit written documentation by a medical professional of the diagnosis, meal modification, and rationale. For children receiving special education services, the documentation for meals and feeding (e.g., modified meals, snacks and supplement needs, feeding therapy programs) can be incorporated as objectives in the child's individual education plan (IEP), the school education plan developed collaboratively between school personnel and the family (Horsley et al, 1996).

Studies of lunches packed at home indicate that they usually provide fewer nutrients but less fat than school lunch meals. Favorite foods tend to be packed, so children have less variety. Food choices are limited to those that travel well and require no heating or refrigeration. A typical well-balanced lunch brought from home could include a sandwich with whole-grain bread and a protein-rich filling (lean meat, egg, cheese, peanut butter); fresh fruit, vegetables, or both; low-fat milk; and possibly a cookie, a graham cracker, or another simple dessert. Food safety measures (e.g., keeping perishable foods well chilled) must be observed when packing lunches for school.

Because of changes in family lifestyles, many school-age children are responsible for preparing their own breakfasts. It is not uncommon for children to skip this meal altogether, even children in the primary grades. Children who skip breakfast tend to consume less energy and fewer nutrients than those who eat breakfast. Reviews of the effects of breakfast on cognition and school performance suggest that children who go to school without breakfast are more likely to experience performance deficits than those who eat breakfast (Kleinman et al, 1998) (see *Focus On:* Breakfast: Does It Affect Learning?).

Snacks are commonly eaten by school-age children, primarily after school and in the evening. As children grow older and have money to spend, they tend to consume more snacks from vending machines, fast-food restaurants, and neighborhood groceries. Families can continue to offer wholesome snacks at home and support nutrition education efforts in the school. In most cases, good eating habits established in the first few years help children through this period of decision-making and responsibility.

Nutrition Education

As children grow, they acquire knowledge and assimilate concepts by leaps and bounds. The early years are ideal for providing nutrition information and promoting positive attitudes about all foods. This education can be informal and natural and take place in the home, with parents as models and a diet with a wide variety of foods. Food can be used in daily experiences for the toddler and preschooler and to promote the development of language, cognition, and self-help behaviors (i.e., labeling; describing size, shape, and color; sorting; assisting in preparation; and tasting).

More formal nutrition education is provided in preschools, Head Start programs, and public schools. Some programs such as Head Start have federal guidance and standards that incorporate healthy eating and nutrition education for the families involved. Nutrition education in schools is less standard and frequently has minimal or no requirements for inclusion in the curriculum or the training of teachers. Teachers attempting to teach children nutrition concepts and information should take into account the children's developmental level. The play approach, based on Piaget's theory of learning, is one method for teaching nutrition and fitness to school-age children (Rickard et al, 1995). Many written and electronic resources on nutrition education for children exist, such as the National Center for Education in Maternal and Child Health.

The concept of nutrition is abstract and so may not be understood by preschoolers and most primary school children. Some nutrition curricula are too sophisticated for the children's conceptual abilities, and modifications may be necessary to make the educational experiences meaningful. Activities and information that focus on children's real-world relationships with food are most likely to yield positive results. Meals, snacks, and food-preparation activities provide children an opportunity to practice and reinforce their nutrition knowledge and demonstrate their cognitive understanding. Parental involvement in nutrition education projects can produce positive outcomes that are also beneficial in the home.

NUTRITIONAL CONCERNS

Obesity

The increasing prevalence of obesity in children is a significant and alarming public health problem. The most recent National Health and Nutrition Examination Survey (NHANES) documented an overweight (i.e., BMI > 95th percentile) prevalence of 11% in children ages 6 to 11 years (NHANES, 1999). This prevalence is 2% more than the prevalence in the 1988 to 1994 NHANES survey and does not show a leveling-off trend. During the 1990s, the percentage of overweight children (BMI > 95th percentile) continued to

FOCUS ON

Breakfast: Does It Affect Learning?

The educational benefits of school meal programs, and especially the role of breakfast in better school performance, have been debated and discussed for decades. Experimental studies of healthy 9- to 11-year-old children have shown that those who skipped breakfast and were then given a variety of tests made more errors, had slower stimulus discrimination, and had slower memory recall (Pollitt et al, 1998). Similar studies in other countries with children who were at nutritional risk (i.e., had wasted and stunted growth) and skipped breakfast demonstrated even poorer performance on the learning tasks (Pollitt et al, 1998). These studies suggest that brain functioning is sensitive to short-term variations in nutrient availability. A short fast may impose greater stress on young children than on adults, resulting in metabolic alterations as various homeostatic mechanisms work to maintain circulating glucose concentrations.

One report on breakfast and cognitive function in elementary-school children suggests that the timing of the meal may play a role (Vaisman et al, 1996). Those receiving breakfast 30 minutes before testing scored higher than those who had breakfast 2 hours before testing. Although the results may be related to glucose concentration, additional controlled studies on meal timing are needed.

A field study in a predominantly low-income school district compared academic achievement before and after introducing the School Breakfast Program. The children who received the school breakfast had significantly improved basic skills test scores and less tardiness than those who did not receive the breakfast (Meyers et al, 1989). Similar school-based studies in Jamaica and other developing countries have also shown that the introduction of breakfast programs results in better school performance and attendance (Powell et al, 1998).

These studies underscore the potential benefits—not only for low-income and at-risk children but also for all school children—of school meal programs that include breakfast. Pollitt and Mathews have reviewed the breakfast and cognition studies and challenged research design, appropriate cognitive and biochemical measures, and relevance to nutrition public policy (Pollitt and Mathews, 1998).

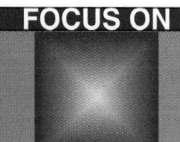

increase, particularly for African-American and Hispanic children (Strauss and Pollack, 2001).

Even more alarming is the degree to which the children are overweight—overweight children are heavier than they were in the previous decade. When factoring in children who are at risk for becoming overweight (those in the 85th to 95th BMI percentiles), the rates are even higher. A similar increasing prevalence of obesity among preschool children from low-income families has been reported from the national Pediatric Nutrition Surveillance System. Using weight-for-height criteria, 10.2% of children younger than 5 years of age are overweight with a BMI greater than the 95th percentile, and 21.6% are overweight with a BMI greater than the 85th percentile (Mei et al, 1998). Although more people are recognizing the role of inheritability in obesity development because of studies of molecular genetics and animal obesity phenotypes, the recent increases in the prevalence of overweight children cannot be explained by genetics alone (Rosenbaum and Leibel, 1998).

Obesity in childhood is not a benign condition, despite the popular belief that overweight children will outgrow their condition. The longer a child has been overweight, the more likely the child is to be overweight during adolescence and adulthood (Goran, 2001). Consequences of obesity in childhood include psychosocial difficulties such as discrimination from others, a negative self-image, depression, and decreased socialization. In the past the health consequences of childhood overweight were thought to be manifested in adulthood, but current evidence shows that many overweight children have one or more cardiovascular risk factors such as hyperlipidemia, hypertension, or hyperinsulinemia (Freedman et al, 1999). An even more dramatic health consequence of overweight is the rapid increase in the incidence of type 2 diabetes in children and adolescents, which has a serious impact on adult health, development of other chronic diseases, and health care costs (Fagot-Campagna et al, 2000; Rocchini, 2002) (see Chapters 24 and 33).

The BMI growth charts show the *adiposity rebound*, which normally occurs in children between 5 and 7 years of age. Children whose normal growth adiposity rebound occurs before 5½ years of age are more likely to weigh more as adults than those whose adiposity rebound occurs after 7 years of age. The timing of the adiposity rebound and excess fatness in adolescence are two critical factors in the development of obesity in childhood, with the latter being the most predictive of adult obesity and related morbidity (Whitaker et al, 1998).

Factors contributing to excess energy intake for the pediatric population include the proliferation of eating and food establishments, eating tied to leisure activities (many of which are sedentary), children making more food and eating decisions, larger portion sizes, and inactivity (French et al, 2001). Inactivity plays a major role in obesity development, whether it results from television and computer use, limited opportunities for physical activity, or safety concerns that prevent children from enjoying free play outdoors. In the past 2 decades, time spent watching television has been related to obesity (Crespo et al, 2001). Obesity prevalence is highest among those who watch 4 or more hours of television per day, particularly among females. A recent report of 6- to 12-year-old children found an association between increased television viewing and more meals eaten while watching television (Saelens et al, 2002). Using automobiles for short trips limits children's opportunities to walk to local destinations, a phenomenon particularly relevant to children in the suburbs.

Determining whether growing children are obese is difficult. Some excess weight may be gained at either end of the childhood spectrum; the 1-year-old toddler and the prepubescent child may weigh more for developmental and physiologic reasons, but this extra weight is often not permanent. Only considering height and weight when determining whether a child's weight is appropriate does not take into account children with significant muscle mass. BMI, a useful clinical tool for assessing weight in comparison to height, has limitations in determining obesity because of variability related to sex, race, and maturation stage (Daniels et al, 1997). However, the CDC Growth Charts allow tracking of BMI from age 2 into adulthood, so children can be monitored frequently and prevention or intervention provided at a young age. The AAP has developed guidelines for overweight screening and assessment for children from age 2 through adolescence (Barlow and Dietz, 1998). Screening parameters include overweight defined as a BMI that is greater than the 95th percentile, and at risk for overweight defined as a BMI in the 85th to 95th percentile.

Management of obesity in children should include considerations of nutrient needs for growth. Success is most likely to result from a program that includes family involvement, dietary modifications, nutrition information, physical activity, and behavioral components. A follow-up study of 158 obese children who participated in regular, long-term group meetings revealed that 10 years after treatment, 30% were not obese, and 34% had decreased their percentage of overweight by 20% or more (Epstein et al, 1994).

Health care providers generally promote healthy eating and activity with minimal use of highly restrictive diets or medication to control weight (Barlow et al, 2002.) The best outcomes are experienced by children who participate in programs that are family based and include a physical activity component. The children's long-term outcomes are better than those in similar programs for adults.

Incorporating behavioral intervention in obesity treatment improves outcomes and is most effective with a team approach (Epstein et al, 2001). Depending on the child, goals for weight change may include a decrease in the rate of weight gain, maintenance of weight, or in severe cases, gradual weight loss (see Chapter 24).

Practitioners should avoid treating overweight children too aggressively. The hazards of treating children who are overweight or obese include the following: alternate periods of undereating and overeating, feelings of failure in meeting external expectations, ignoring of internal cues for appetite and satiation, feelings of deprivation and isolation, an increased risk for eating disorders, and a poor or an increasingly poor self-image.

Some children with special health care needs, such as those with Down syndrome, Prader-Willi syndrome, short stature, and limited mobility, are at increased risk for being overweight. Their size, level of activity, and developmental status need to be considered when estimating energy intake and providing dietary guidance to their families. Prader-Willi syndrome is a genetic disorder characterized by hypotonia in early life, short stature, cognitive delays, low energy needs, and a preoccupation with food. To avoid gaining excessive weight, children with this syndrome usually need a lower energy intake than typical for children their height; they also need their food access controlled in all situations.

Prevention of childhood obesity is beginning to be addressed as an important public health policy in the United States. Families are the logical target for education and anticipatory education regarding food choices and healthy eating, physical and sedentary activities, and healthy parent-child interactions and behaviors. Epstein reported that a target of decreasing sedentary behaviors was just as effective in reducing the percentage of overweight children ages 8 to 12 years as was a target of increasing activity (Epstein et al, 2000). Schools are a natural but challenging environment for obesity prevention, which can include nutrition and health curricula, opportunities for physical education and activity, and appropriate school meals. Although most schools do not have coordinated programs, several school-based obesity prevention programs have been successful (Dietz and Gortmaker, 2001). More federal support of obesity prevention and community collaboration is underway to develop policies and programs that will support healthy lifestyles for children and families.

Underweight and Failure to Thrive

Weight loss, lack of weight gain, or failure to thrive (FTT) can be caused by an acute or chronic illness, a restricted diet, a poor appetite, feeding problems, a poor appetite because of constipation or medication, deprivation, or a simple lack of food. Some experts prefer the terms *pediatric undernutrition* or *growth deficiency* to FTT. Infants and toddlers are most at risk for FTT and poor growth, often as a result of being born premature, medical conditions, developmental delays, inadequate parenting, or all of these. A careful assessment of FTT is critical and must include the social and emotional environment of the child and any physical findings. Because of the complexity of FTT, an interdisciplinary team would be ideal for assessments and interventions.

Studies have documented growth failure (poor weight gain, short stature, and delayed puberty) in pubescent children who are restricting their diets because of a fear of becoming obese. Many preadolescent children have the same body image concerns, dieting patterns, and eating patterns (e.g., consumption of diet soft drinks) as adolescents. Some FTT in preschool children has been associated with food restrictions stemming from (1) parents' concerns about obesity, atherosclerosis, or other potential health problems and (2) excess fruit juice intake (AAP, 2001; Pugliese et al, 1987).

Lack of fiber in the diet or poor bowel habits that lead to chronic constipation can result in poor appetite, diminished intake, and failure to thrive. Adding legumes and fruits (especially dried fruits), vegetables, high-fiber breakfast cereals, bran muffins, or all of these to the diet can help relieve constipation, improve appetite, and eventually promote weight gain. Because the fiber intake of children is often low, especially in children who are picky eaters, fiber intake should always be addressed in the evaluation. If the child is also of short stature, the possibility of a zinc deficiency should be investigated (see Chapter 5).

The provision of adequate energy and nutrients and nutrition education should be among the goals of the management plan. Nutrition is often one part of an overall interdisciplinary plan to assist children and their families. Attempts should be made to increase children's appetites and modify the environment to ensure optimal intake (Cunningham and McLaughlin, 1999). Energy requirements for catch-up growth are discussed in *Clinical Insight:* Obtaining Optimal Catch-Up Growth.

Iron Deficiency

Iron deficiency is one of the most common nutrient disorders of childhood, affecting approximately 9% of toddlers (Looker et al, 1997). Iron deficiency is less of a problem among older preschool and school-age children. Certain low-income populations and other groups such as Native Alaskans have an increased incidence of iron deficiency, even in older children (Looker et al, 1997). Possible factors associated with iron deficiency, with or without anemia, include parents' educational level and access to medical care, as well as dietary intake.

In addition to growth and the increased physiologic need for iron, dietary factors also play a role. For example, a 1-year-old child who continues to consume a large quantity of milk and excludes other foods may develop *milk anemia.* Many young preschool children do not like meat, so most of their iron is consumed in the nonheme form, which is absorbed less efficiently.

Infants with iron deficiency, with or without anemia, tend to score lower on standardized tests of mental development and pay less attention to relevant information needed for problem-solving. Lozoff reevaluated 11- to 14-year-old children who had been treated for iron deficiency anemia in infancy . In addition to poor performance on developmental tests when they were 5 years old, the children continued to score lower on measures of mental and motor functioning when they were older (Lozoff et al, 2000). A recent report assessed the academic performance of children 6 to 16 years of age who had iron deficiency (some with and some without anemia), and the children had lower scores on standardized academic tests (Halterman et al, 2001). These data should be considered during assessments of the nutrient quality of individual diets and in policy-making decisions intended to address the nutritional needs of low-income, high-risk children.

Consuming good dietary sources of iron can help prevent iron deficiency anemia. To enhance absorbability of nonheme iron sources, parents should be taught to increase the amount of ascorbic acid and meat, fish, and poultry in their children's diets. (See Chapter 34 for a more detailed discussion of anemia.)

Dental Caries

Nutrition and eating habits are important factors affecting dental health. An optimal nutrient intake is needed to produce strong teeth and healthy gums. The composition of the diet and an individual's eating habits (e.g., dietary carbohydrate intake, retentiveness of foods, eating frequency) are significant factors in the development of dental caries. Infants and young children who drink sweetened liquids from a bottle at bedtime or frequently throughout the day are susceptible to early childhood caries (ECC) or *baby bottle tooth decay (BBTD)* (see Chapter 28).

Because children tend to consume snacks regularly, those that are least cariogenic (i.e., least likely to cause caries) should be emphasized. When protein foods such as cheese, nuts, and meats are eaten with more fermentable, sticky foods, they prevent the decrease in the plaque pH that usually accompanies ingestion of these foods and may help protect the teeth against caries. For older school-age children, chewing sugarless gum after cariogenic snacks may be beneficial because it raises the salivary pH. Desserts and sweet foods should be consumed infrequently and incorporated into meals to reduce their cariogenicity. Parents are strong role models for their children and should have positive food habits and practice good dental hygiene. A toothbrush should be introduced to toddlers and a daily oral hygiene routine developed. Because fluoride is highly effective in caries prevention, it should be supplied to children via a fluoridated water supply or a fluoride supplement (see Chapter 28).

Allergies

Food allergies usually develop during infancy and childhood and are more likely when a child has a family history of allergies. Allergic responses most often include respiratory or gastrointestinal symptoms and skin reactions, but they may be more vague, such as fatigue, lethargy, and behavior changes. Controversy exists over the true definition of *food allergy*, and tests for food allergies are unspecific and unequivocal (see Chapter 32).

Attention Deficit Hyperactivity Disorder

Attention deficit hyperactivity disorder (ADHD) is a clinical diagnosis based on specific criteria—excessive motor activity, impulsiveness, a short attention span, a low tolerance for frustration, and an onset before 7 years of age. Because dietary factors have been suggested as a cause of this disorder, various dietary treatments have been promoted, such as the Feingold diet, the omission of sugar, allergy elimination diets, and megavitamin therapy.

In the 1970s, Feingold proposed that many children were hyperactive because they were sensitive to salicylates and artificial colorings and flavorings in food. The Feingold plan removed these substances and the preservatives BHA and BHT from the child's diet. Despite initial positive anecdotal reports, controlled double-blind dietary challenge studies using objective behavior rating scales did not support the Feingold hypothesis. Of the children with ADHD who seemed to respond most favorably to the diet (about 5% to 10%), most were preschoolers. Other reports have shown some behavior improvements when the Feingold diet was paired with removal of specific foods believed to bother the children.

Conflicting study results may be explained in part by a placebo effect or by altered interactions between the family and the child with ADHD. However, a child with ADHD who tries the Feingold diet is at little risk for an insufficient nutrient intake as long as the child is offered and accepts a wide variety of foods from the family menu. Periodic nutritional counseling should be provided, and the family should be urged to consider proven interventions for the child's disorder, such as behavioral management, special education, and medication.

Although sugar has often been implicated as a cause of hyperactive behavior in children, controlled challenge studies have not demonstrated that it has any negative behavioral effects (Wolraich et al, 1995). Although little evidence supports that sugar has behavioral effects, the benefits of decreasing sugar consumption (e.g., improved dental health, a more nutrient-dense diet) should be emphasized.

Another theory suggests that altered fatty acid metabolism may play a role in ADHD, either through inefficient conversion of essential fatty acids to long-chain polyunsaturated fatty acids or enhanced cellular metabolism of these fatty acids. One study found significantly lower concentrations of key fatty acids, including docosahexaenoic acid (DHA) and arachidonic acid (AA), in boys with ADHD compared with controls (Burgess et al, 2000). Some of the boys also showed general symptoms of essential fatty acid deficiency, but their dietary intake of fatty acids was not low. No cause-and-effect relationship between fatty acid metabolism and ADHD has been documented, but future supplementation studies may provide answers.

Children who have allergies may exhibit some of the behaviors (e.g., irritability, poor ability to pay attention) of children with ADHD, but it remains questionable whether elimination diets can alleviate these symptoms or alter negative behaviors. Likewise, the value of megavitamin therapy for ADHD has not been supported in controlled studies.

Autism Spectrum Disorders

Autism spectrum disorders (ASDs) affect 1 in 500 children and are diagnosed by impairments in three behavioral categories: social interactions, verbal and nonverbal communication, and restricted or repetitive behaviors. The impairments affect the children's nutrient intake and eating behaviors. They typically eat only specific foods, have hypersensitivities (e.g., to texture, temperature, color, and smell), and have difficulty in making transitions. Although most children have normal growth parameters, their restricted diet makes them at risk for marginal or inadequate nutrient intake. They usually refuse fruits and vegetables and may only eat a few foods from the other food groups. They are also commonly very resistant to taking a vitamin-mineral supplement.

A popular dietary intervention is the gluten-free, casein-free diet, which was developed based on a theory that the children have a "leaky gut," allowing peptides to act as brain opiates. (See Chapter 30 for a gluten-free diet and Chapter 32 for a casein-free diet.) Despite positive anecdotal reports, no controlled studies have been done to test the effectiveness of the diet. The diet can increase the risk for inadequate nutrient consumption. For children with ASD, the nutrition assessment should include the possibility of medication (e.g., anticonvulsants, selective serotonin reuptake inhibitors, antipsychotics) and nutrient interactions, the use of any alternative therapies, herbals and supplement use, and possible lead exposure. A nutrition intervention may include a behavioral program to increase the types of food accepted at home and school (Lucas et al, 2002).

PREVENTING CHRONIC DISEASE

The roots of chronic adult diseases, such as heart disease, cancer, diabetes, and obesity, are often based in childhood—a phenomenon that is particularly relevant to the increasing rates of obesity-related diseases, such as type II diabetes, resulting from pediatric and adult obesity. To help decrease the prevalence of chronic conditions in Americans, governmental and nonprofit agencies have been promoting healthy eating habits. Their recommendations include the Dietary Guidelines for Americans, the USDA Food Guide Pyramid, the National Cholesterol Education Program (NCEP), and the National Cancer Institute Dietary Guidelines (see Chapter 15).

Dietary Fat and Cardiovascular Health

Compared with their counterparts in many other countries, American children and adolescents have higher blood cholesterol levels and higher intakes of saturated fatty acids and cholesterol. Autopsy studies demonstrate that early coronary atherosclerosis begins in childhood and adolescence and is related to high serum total cholesterol levels, low-density lipoprotein (LDL) cholesterol and very–low-density lipoprotein (VLDL) cholesterol levels, and low high-density lipoprotein (HDL) levels (AAP, 1998b).

The NCEP recommendations for prevention of cardiovascular disease in children older than 2 years of age are the same as those for adults: (1) no more than 30% of calories from fat (10% or less from saturated fat, up to 10% from unsaturated fat, and 10% to 15% from monosaturated fat) and (2) no more than 300 mg of cholesterol per day. Cholesterol screening is also recommended for children with family risk factors—parents or grandparents who have had a cardiac event (heart attack, angina, or cardiac surgery) before the age of 55 years or at least one parent with a cholesterol level of 250 mg/dl or more (National Heart, Lung, and Blood Institute, 1991) (see Chapter 35).

The AAP (1998b) advises that children older than 2 years of age gradually adopt a lower fat diet so that by age 5 their diet contains no more than 30% of calories from fat. Dietary trends have demonstrated a decrease in total fat, saturated fat, and percentage of calories from fat (36% in 1987-1988 to 32%-33% in 1994-1996) in children's diets, but these levels have not yet met the NCEP guidelines (USDA, 1997). Reports have shown that from the age of 4 years to adolescence, children can consume diets that comply with the NCEP guidelines without compromising energy or nutrient intake (Ballew et al, 2000; Obarzanek et al, 2001). Field intervention studies of children on low-fat diets have shown little effect on blood cholesterol levels, blood pressure measurements, or body weight (Luepker et al, 1996). However, a long-term dietary intervention study demonstrated improved lipid levels in children with elevated LDL cholesterol levels (Obarzanek et al, 2001). Some critics warn of the risks from broad implementation of low-fat diets for children (Olson, 2000).

Because no apparent risks to appropriate growth or nutrient intake are associated with a diet meeting the NCEP guidelines, a gradual transition to a lower-fat diet after the age of 2 years is appropriate (Obarzanek et al, 2001). However, health practitioners should assess the dietary fat intake of children with poor growth, inquire about excessive consumption of low-fat and nonfat foods (especially by preschool children), and provide appropriate nutrition guidance.

Calcium and Bone Health and Obesity

Osteoporosis prevention begins in childhood by maximizing calcium retention and bone density in the growing years. Osteoporosis prevention is most efficient during childhood and adolescence, when bones are growing rapidly and are most sensitive to environmental influences such as diet and physical activity (Leonard and Zemel, 2002) (see Chapter 27). Regardless, many pediatricians are not sharing information about the prevention of osteoporosis with their patients (Fleming and Patrick, 2002.)

Balance studies of adolescent girls suggest that to reach the maximum calcium balance, young teenage girls may need to consume more than the recommended amount (Matkovic and Heany, 1992). However, only about 10% of girls and 25% of boys meet the current DRI for calcium—1300 mg/day—the AI for children and adolescents 9 to 18 years of age. Although calcium supplementation coupled with an average calcium dietary intake in prepubescent children was found to increase bone mineral density significantly, it is less certain whether this benefit is permanent (Slemenda et al, 1997).

Data from trials in which calcium intake was the independent variable reveal the consistent effects of higher calcium intakes on lower body fat, body weight, or both, and less weight gain during midlife (Heaney et al, 2002). Each 300-mg increase in regular calcium intake has been associated with approximately 1 kg less body fat in children and 2.5 to 3 kg lower body weight in adults. Increasing calcium intake by the equivalent of two dairy servings per day could reduce the risk of overweight substantially, perhaps by as much as 70% (Heaney et al, 2002).

Because recent food consumption surveys show children are drinking more soft drinks and noncitrus juices and less milk, education is needed to encourage young people to consume an appropriate amount of calcium from food sources. Different types of reinforcement for better calcium intake are needed according to cultural and male/female differences (Lytle et al, 2002).

Fiber

Education about dietary fiber and disease prevention has mainly been focused on the adult population, and only limited information is available on the dietary fiber intake of children. National survey data indicate that 3- to 5-year-olds consume a mean of 10.7 g of dietary fiber per day, up slightly from the late 1980s; school-age children consume approximately 13 g/day (USDA, 1997). Dietary fiber is needed for health and normal laxation in children. The DRI for children ages 1 to 3 years is an AI of 19 g/day and the DRI for children 4 to 8 years is an AI of 25 g/day. For children 9 to 13 years, the AI for boys is 31 g/day, and the AI for girls is 26 g/day (IOM, 2002). However, education is needed to help increase fiber intake by children.

Physical Activity

A decreased level of physical activity in children has been noted for several decades, and it is thought to be a substantial contributor to obesity in children. Participation in school physical education programs generally decreases with increasing age, with high school girls having the lowest participation rates (Kohl and Hobbs, 1998). Regular physical activity not only helps control excess weight gain but also improves strength and endurance, enhances self-esteem, and reduces anxiety and stress. Activity, combined with an optimal calcium intake, is associated with increased bone mineral density in children and adolescents. The Council on Physical Education for Children has recommended that elementary-school children be active for at least a total of 60 minutes a day, with activity including moderate to vigorous activities (Corbin and Pangrazi, 1998). The CDC has developed guidelines for school and community programs to promote lifelong physical activity among young people (CDC, 1997).

In an effort to promote dietary habits that can reduce the incidence of chronic diseases later in life, the Dietary Guidelines for Americans and the Food Guide Pyramid have been applied to children and their parents. The USDA has also developed a Food Guide Pyramid for Young Children (ages 2 to 6), which also incorporates physical activity. Some experts and professional groups support the development of separate dietary guidelines for children to ensure that their primary nutritional needs for growth and development are met and to prevent disease (American Dietetic Association, 1999; Picciano et al, 2000).

SUMMARY

Overall, children's diets should provide enough energy to support optimal growth and development without causing them to gain excess weight. Emphasis should be placed on their intake of fruits and vegetables, whole-grain products, low-fat dairy products, legumes, and lean meat, fish, and poultry. Fermentable carbohydrate intake should be controlled for good dental health. Adherence to these general dietary guidelines is beneficial for children because their total fat intake decreases and their dietary fiber and β-carotene and other phytochemical intake increases, resulting in a more nutrient-dense diet.

Although changes in the years between infancy and adolescence are slower and steadier than those taking place before and after, these growing years add significant cognitive, physical, and socioemotional growth. Nutrition education and resources for families and children can help establish healthy, positive eating and activity patterns that can help children during adolescence and adulthood.

Clinical Scenario

Brian is a 7-year, 4-month-old boy who gained 15 lb during the last school year. His height is 50½ inches and his weight is 70 pounds. An evaluation revealed that Brian moved to a new home and began a new school a year ago after his parents' divorce. After-school care has been provided by an older neighbor, who loves to bake for Brian. Because he has no friends in the neighborhood, his main leisure activities have been watching television and playing video games. His mother reports that they have been relying more on take-out and fast-food meals because of the time constraints of her full-time job, and she has gained weight herself. However, she has recently started an aerobics class with a friend and is interested in developing healthier eating habits.

After joint sessions with Brian and his mother, the following goals were identified by the family: (1) explore after-school care at the local community center, which has sports activities; (2) alter shopping and food preparation to emphasize the Food Guide Pyramid and low-fat choices; (3) begin weekend swimming or bicycling for the family; and (4) limit television and video games to no more than 2 hours daily.

It is 4 months later, and most of the changes have been made except for participating in the weekend family activity and watching less television on the weekends. However, Brian is now playing soccer, has lost 4 pounds, and has grown taller. He is 51 inches tall and weighs 66 pounds.

1. What recommendations should be made to prevent Brian and his mother from resuming their old habits?
2. Calculate and plot Brian's BMI over time. Discuss the changes.
3. What other activities can Brian try to help him avoid or reduce the tendency to overeat?
4. How can Brian's mother alter some of his favorite recipes to lower the fat content? For example, his favorite meal is fried chicken with gravy, mashed potatoes, and ice cream.

Relevant Web Sites

Assuring Pediatric Nutrition in the Community
http://depts.washington.edu/nutrpeds/
Bright Futures
www.brightfutures.org/
Centers for Disease Control and Prevention
BAM!
www.bam.gov/
Growth Charts
www.cdc.gov/growthcharts/
Guidelines for Physical Activity
www.cdc.gov/nccdphp/dash/guidelines/physact.htm
Nutrition and Physical Activity
www.cdc.gov/nccdphp/dnpa/
Eat well, Play Hard
www.eatwellplayhard.org/
National Center for Education in Maternal and Child Health
www.ncemch.org
Pediatric Nutrition Practice Group
www.pediatricnutrition.org/

Cited References

American Academy of Pediatrics: *Pediatric nutrition handbook,* ed 4, Elk Grove Village, Ill, 1998a, AAP.

American Academy of Pediatrics, Committee on Nutrition: Cholesterol in childhood, *Pediatrics* 101:141, 1998b.

American Academy of Pediatrics, Committee on Nutrition: The use and misuse of fruit juice in pediatrics, *Pediatrics* 107:1210, 2001.

American Dietetic Association: Position of the American Dietetic Association: Dietary guidance for healthy children aged 2 to 11 years, *J Am Diet Assoc* 99:93, 1999.

Ashworth A, Millward DJ: Catch-up growth in children, *Nutr Rev* 44:157, 1986.

Ballew C, Bowman B: Recommending calcium to reduce lead toxicity in children: a critical review, *Nutr Rev* 59:71, 2001.

Ballew C et al: Nutrient intakes and dietary patterns of young children by dietary fat intakes, *J Pediatr* 136:181, 2000.

Barlow SE, Dietz WH: Obesity evaluation and treatment: expert committee recommendations, *Pediatrics* 102(3):e29, 1998.

Barlow SE et al: Treatment of child and adolescent obesity: reports from pediatricians, pediatric nurse practitioners, and registered dietitians, *Pediatrics* 110:229 (1, part 2), 2002.

Beal VA: Nutritional intake. In McCammon RW, ed: *Human growth and development,* Springfield, Ill, 1970, Charles C Thomas.

Berhane R, Dietz WH: Clinical assessment of growth. In Kessler DB, Dawson P, eds: *Failure to thrive and pediatric undernutrition,* Baltimore, 1999, Brookes Publishing.

Borzekowski DLG, Robinson TN: The 30-second effect: an experiment revealing the impact of television commercials on food preferences of preschoolers, *J Am Diet Assoc* 101:42, 2001.

Brady LM et al: Comparison of children's dietary intake patterns with US dietary guidelines. *Br J Nutr* 84:361, 2000.

Burgess JR et al: Long-chain polyunsaturated fatty acids in children with attention-deficit hyperactivity disorder, *Am J Clin Nutr* 71:327, 2000.

Casey PH et al: Children in food-insufficient, low-income families: prevalence, health, and nutrition status, *Arch Ped Adol* 155:508, 2001.

Centers for Disease Control and Prevention, National Center for Chronic Disease Prevention and Health Promotion: *Guidelines for school and community programs to promote lifelong physical activity among young people,* 1997, http://www.cdc.gov/nccdphp/dash/guidelines/physact.htm.

Centers for Disease Control and Prevention: *Screening young children for lead poisoning: guidance for state and local public health officials,* 1997, US Department of Health and Human Services, Public Health Service.

Cook JT, Martin LS: *Differences in nutrient adequacy among poor and non-poor children,* Medford, Mass, May 1995, Tufts University School of Nutrition, Center on Hunger, Poverty and Nutrition Policy, 1997.

Corbin CB, Pangrazi RP: *Physical activity for children: a statement of guidelines.* Reston, Va, 1998, National Association for Sport and Physical Education, Council on Physical Education for Children.

Crespo CJ et al: Television watching, energy intake, and obesity in U.S. children: results from the third National Health and Nutrition Examination Survey, 1988-1994, *Arch Pediatr Adolesc Med* 155:360, 2001.

Cryan J, Johnson RK: Should the current recommendations for energy intake in infants and young children be lowered? *Nutr Today* 32:69, 1997.

Cunningham KF, McLaughlin M: Nutrition. In Kessler DB, Dawson P, eds: *Failure to thrive and pediatric undernutrition,* Baltimore, 1999, Brookes Publishing.

Daniels SR et al: The utility of body mass index as a measure of body fatness in children and adolescents: differences by race and gender, *Pediatrics* 99:804, 1997.

Dewey KG: Cross-cultural patterns of growth and nutritional status of breast-fed infants, *Am J Clin Nutr* 67:10, 1998.

Dietz WH, Gortmaker SL: Preventing obesity in children and adolescents, *Annu Rev Public Health* 22:337, 2001.

Epstein LH et al: Ten-year outcomes of behavioral family-based treatment for childhood obesity, *Health Psychol* 13:373, 1994.

Epstein LH et al: Decreasing sedentary behaviors in treating pediatric obesity, *Arch Pediatr Adolesc Med* 154:220, 2000.

Epstein LH et al: Behavioral therapy in the treatment of pediatric obesity, *Pediatr Clin North Am* 48:981, 2001.

Fagot-Campagna A et al: Type 2 diabetes among North American children and adolescents: an epidemiologic review and a public health perspective, *J Pediatr* 136:664, 2000.

Fleming R, Patrick K: Osteoporosis prevention: pediatricians' knowledge, attitudes, and counseling practices, *Prev Med* 34:411, 2002.

Freedman DS et al: Relationship of childhood obesity to coronary heart disease risk factors in adulthood: the Bogalusa Heart Study, *Pediatrics* 108:712, 2001.

French SA et al: Environmental influences on eating and physical activity, *Annu Rev Public Health* 22:309, 2001.

Getlinger MJ et al: Food waste is reduced when elementary-school children have recess before lunch, *J Am Diet Assoc* 96:906, 1996.

Gillman MW et al: Family dinner and diet quality among older children and adolescents, *Arch Fam Med* 9:235, 2000.

Goran MI: Metabolic precursors and effects of obesity in children: a decade of progress, 1990-1999, *Am J Clin Nutr* 73:158, 2001.

Halterman JS et al: Iron deficiency and cognitive achievement among school-aged children and adolescents in the United States, *Pediatrics* 107:1381, 2001.

Heaney RP et al: Calcium and weight: clinical studies, *J Am Coll Nutr* 21(2):152S, 2002.

Horsley JW et al: *Nutrition management of school age children with special needs: a resource manual for school personnel, families and health professionals,* ed 2, Richmond, Va, 1996, Virginia Department of Health and Virginia Department of Education.

Institute of Medicine, Food and Nutrition Board: *Dietary reference intakes for calcium, phosphorus, magnesium, vitamin D, and fluoride,* Washington, DC, 1997, National Academy Press.

Institute of Medicine, Food and Nutrition Board: *Dietary reference intakes for thiamin, riboflavin, niacin, vitamin* B_6*, folate, vitamin* B_{12}*, pantothenic acid, biotin, and choline,* Washington, DC, 1998, National Academy Press.

Institute of Medicine, Food and Nutrition Board: *Dietary reference intakes for dietary antioxidants and related compounds,* Washington, DC, 2000, National Academy Press.

Institute of Medicine, Food and Nutrition Board: *Dietary reference intakes for energy and the macronutrients, carbohydrate, fiber, fat, fatty acids, cholesterol, protein, and amino acids,* Washington, DC, 2002, National Academy Press.

Kleinman RE et al: Hunger in children in the United States: potential behavioral and emotional correlates, *Pediatrics* 101(1):e3, 1998.

Kohl HW, Hobbs KE: Development of physical activity behaviors among children and adolescents, *Pediatrics* 101:549, 1998.

Krebs NF, Hambidge KM: Trace elements in human nutrition. In Walker WA, Watkins JB: *Nutrition in pediatrics,* ed 2, Hamilton, Ontario, 1996, BC Decker.

Leonard MB, Zemel BS: Current concepts in pediatric bone disease, *Pediatr Clin North Am* 49:143, 2002.

Looker AC et al: Prevalence of iron deficiency in the United States, *JAMA* 277:973, 1997.

Lozoff B et al: Poorer behavioral and developmental outcome more than 10 years after treatment for iron deficiency in infancy, *Pediatrics* 105(4):e51, 2000.

Lucas B et al: Nutrition concerns of children with autism spectrum disorders, *Nutrition Focus* 17(1):1, 2002.

Luepker RV et al: Outcomes of a field trial to improve children's dietary patterns and physical activity: the Child and Adolescent Trial for Cardiovascular Health (CATCH), *JAMA* 275:768, 1996.

Lytle LA et al: Nutrient intake over time in a multi-ethnic sample of youth, *Public Health Nutr* 5:319, 2002.

Matkovic V, Heany RP: Calcium balance during human growth: evidence for threshold behavior, *Am J Clin Nutr* 55:992, 1992.

Mei Z et al: Increasing prevalence of overweight among U.S. low-income preschool children: The Centers for Disease Control and Prevention Pediatric Nutrition Surveillance, 1983-1995, *Pediatrics* 101:e12, 1998.

Meyers AF et al: School breakfast program and school performance, *Am J Dis Child* 143:1234, 1989.

Munoz KA et al: Food intakes of U.S. children and adolescents compared with recommendations, *Pediatrics* 100:323, 1997.

Murphy JM et al: Relationship between hunger and psychosocial functioning in low-income American children, *J Am Acad Child Adolesc Psychiatry* 37:163, 1998.

National Health and Nutrition Examination Survey (1988-1994): Summary of findings, Hyattsville, Md, 1999, Centers for Disease Control and Prevention, National Center for Health Statistics.

National Heart, Lung, and Blood Institute, National Cholesterol Education Program: *Report of the expert panel on blood cholesterol levels in children and adolescents,* Bethesda, Md, 1991, National Heart, Lung, and Blood Institute.

Obarzanek E et al: Long-term safety and efficacy of a cholesterol-lowering diet in children with elevated low-density lipoprotein cholesterol: seven-year results of the Dietary Intervention Study in Children (DISC), *Pediatrics* 107:256, 2001.

Olson RE: Is it wise to restrict fat in the diets of children? *J Am Diet Assoc* 100:28, 2000.

Picciano MF et al: Nutritional guidance is needed during dietary transition in early childhood, *Pediatrics* 106:109, 2000.

Pollitt E, Mathews R: Breakfast and cognition: an integrative summary, *Am J Clin Nutr* 67(suppl):804, 1998.

Pollitt E et al: Fasting and cognition in well- and undernourished school children: a review of three experimental studies, *Am J Clin Nutr* 67(suppl):779, 1998.

Powell CA et al: Nutrition and education: a randomized trial of the effects of breakfast in rural primary school children, *Am J Clin Nutr* 68:873, 1998.

Pugliese MT et al: Parental health beliefs as a cause of nonorganic failure to thrive, *Pediatrics* 80:175, 1987.

Rickard KA et al: The play approach to learning in the context of families and schools: an alternative paradigm for nutrition and fitness education in the 21st century, *J Am Diet Assoc* 95:1121, 1995.

Roberts SB, Heyman, MB: Micronutrient shortfalls in young children's diets: common, and owing to inadequate intakes both at home and at child care centers, *Nutr Rev* 58:27, 2000.

Rocchini AP: Childhood obesity and a diabetes epidemic, *N Eng J Med* 346:854, 2002.

Rosenbaum MD, Leibel RL: The physiology of body weight regulation: relevance to the etiology of obesity in children, *Pediatrics* 101:525, 1998.

Saelens BE et al: Home environmental influences on children's television watching from early to middle childhood, *J Dev Behav Pediatr* 23:127, 2002.

Sawni-Sikand A et al: Use of complementary/alternative therapies among children in primary care pediatrics, *Ambul Pediatr* 2:99, 2002.

Skinner JD, Carruth, BR: A longitudinal study of children's juice intake and growth: the juice controversy revisited, *J Am Diet Assoc* 101:432, 2001.

Slemenda CW et al: Reduced rates of skeletal remodeling are associated with increased bone mineral density during the development of peak skeletal mass, *J Bone Min Res* 12:676, 1997.

Strauss RS, Pollack HA: Epidemic increase in childhood overweight, 1986-1998, *JAMA* 286:2845, 2001.

Trumbo P et al: Dietary reference intakes: vitamin A, vitamin K, arsenic, boron, chromium, copper, iodine, iron, manganese, molybdenum, nickel, silicon, vanadium, and zinc, *J Am Diet Assoc* 101:294, 2001.

U.S. Department of Agriculture, Agricultural Research Service Food Surveys Research Group: *1997 data tables: results from USDA's 1994-96 Continuing Survey of Food Intakes by Individuals and 1994-96 Diet and Health Knowledge Survey,* http://www.barc.usda. gov/bhnrc/foodsurvey/home.html.

U.S. Department of Agriculture: *School Nutrition Dietary Assessment Study—II: summary of findings,* Washington, DC, 2001, USDA.

Vaisman N et al: Effect of breakfast timing on the cognitive functions of elementary school students, *Arch Pediatr Adolesc Med* 150:1089, 1996.

Villamor E et al: Vitamin A supplements ameliorate the adverse effect of HIV-1, malaria, and diarrhea/infections on child growth, *Pediatrics* 109:E6, 2002.

Whitaker RC et al: Early adiposity rebound and the risk of adult obesity, *Pediatrics* 101(3):e5, 1998.

Wolraich ML et al: The effect of sugar on behavior or cognition in children: a meta-analysis, *JAMA* 274:1617, 1995.

Yu SM et al: Vitamin-mineral supplement use among preschool children in the United States, Pediatrics 100(5):e4, 1997.

Additional References

American Dietetic Association: Position of the American Dietetic Association: local support for nutrition integrity in schools, *J Am Diet Assoc* 100:108, 2000.

American Dietetic Association: Position of the American Dietetic Association: nutrition standards for child-care programs, *J Am Diet Assoc* 99:981, 1999.

Baxter SD et al: Low accuracy and low consistency of fourth-graders' school breakfast and school lunch recalls, *J Am Diet Assoc* 102:386, 2002.

Is fruit juice a "no-no" in children's diets? *Nutrition Rev* 58:180, 2000.

Kleinman RE et al: Diet, breakfast and academic performance in children, *Ann Nutr Metab* 46(suppl 1):24, 2002.

Nicklas TA et al: Efficiency of breakfast consumption patterns of ninth graders: nutrient-to-cost comparisons, *J Am Diet Assoc* 102:226, 2002.

Samour PQ, Helm KK, Lang CE, eds: *Handbook of pediatric nutrition,* ed 2, Gaithersburg, Md, 1999, Aspen Publishers.

Satter EM: *Child of mine: feeding with love and good sense,* Palo Alto, Calif, 2000, Bull.

Story M, Holt K, Sofka D, eds: *Bright futures in practice: nutrition,* Arlington, Va, 2000, National Center for Education in Maternal and Child Health.

Trahms CT, Pipes PL: *Nutrition in infancy and childhood,* ed 6, St Louis, 1997, WCB/McGraw-Hill.

Wosje KS, Specker BL: Role of calcium in bone health during childhood, *Nutr Rev* 58(9):253, 2000.

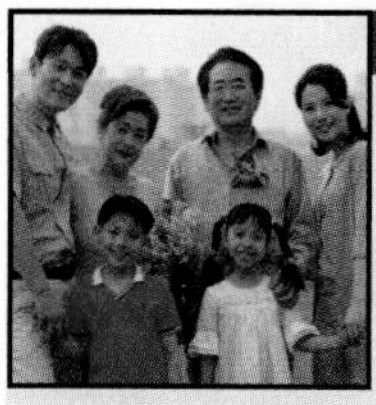

CHAPTER 11

Nutrition in Adolescence

BONNIE A. SPEAR, PhD, RD

CHAPTER OUTLINE

- Growth and Development
- Nutrient Requirements
- Food Habits
- Special Situations
- Strategies for Improving Nutritional Well-Being

KEY TERMS

adolescence–the period of life beginning with the appearance of secondary sex characteristics and ending with the cessation of somatic growth

body image–a mental self-concept related to growth rate and changes in body proportions

eating disorder–abnormal behaviors related to food and eating; may include starving, bingeing, vomiting, laxative abuse, or excessive exercise accompanied by unrealistic ideas about food, a distorted body image, and psychologic and developmental abnormalities

growth spurt–the 18- to 24-month period of adolescence when the growth rate is the fastest

gynecologic (postmenarchal) age–the number of years between the onset of menses and the current chronologic age

menarche–onset of menses

peak height gain velocity–the fastest rate of growth during the growth spurt

physiologic anemia of growth–a low serum hematocrit or hemoglobin level that is not accompanied by decreased iron stores; caused by rapid growth and a significant increase in lean body mass; often develops in adolescents

puberty–the period during which the secondary sex characteristics begin to develop and a person becomes capable of sexual reproduction

sexual maturity ratings (SMRs)–used to assess a person's stage of sexual development; usually expressed as *sexual maturation stages* or *Tanner stages*

tasks of adolescence–the accomplishments expected in adolescence that lead to maturity in emotional and intellectual development

Adolescence is one of the most challenging periods in human development. The relatively uniform growth of childhood is suddenly altered by a rapid increase in the growth rate. These sudden changes create special nutritional needs. Adolescents are considered especially vulnerable nutritionally for several reasons. First, they have an increased demand for nutrients because of the dramatic increase in physical growth and development. Second, the changes in lifestyle and food habits of adolescents affect nutrient intake and needs. Third, adolescents have special nutrient needs associated with participation in sports, pregnancy, development of an eating disorder, excessive dieting, use of alcohol and drugs, or other situations common to adolescents (Spear, 1996).

GROWTH AND DEVELOPMENT

Physiologic Changes

Puberty, the process of physically developing from a child into an adult, is initiated by physiologic factors and includes maturation of the entire body. Adolescence is the only time after birth when the velocity of growth actually increases. Figure 11-1 shows the rate of linear growth during the teenage years compared with the rate during the childhood years. Adolescents gain about 20% of their adult height and 50% of their adult weight during this period.

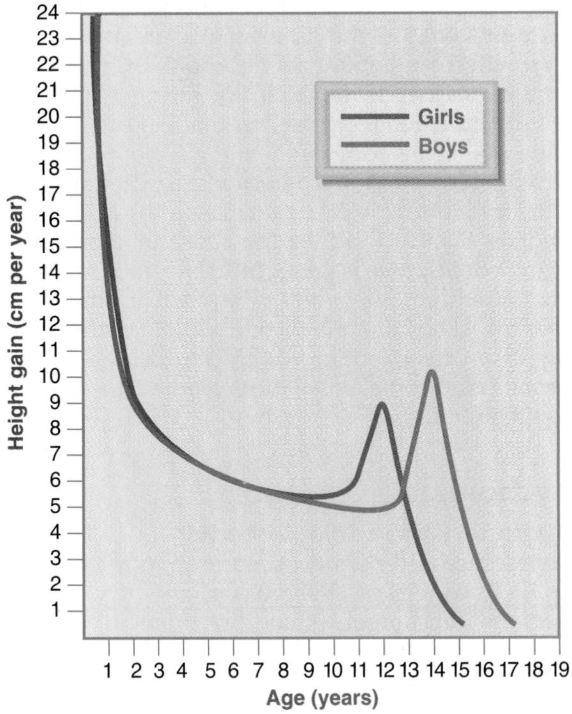

FIGURE 11-1 • Typical individual velocity curves for supine length or height in boys and girls. Curves represent the growth velocity of the typical boy and girl at any given age.

This growth continues throughout the approximately 5 to 7 years of pubertal development. A great percentage of this height is gained during the 18- to 24-month period of the growth spurt. The peak height gain velocity is the fastest rate of growth during the growth spurt and occurs at different ages for different individuals, as does the initiation of puberty. For example, Figure 11-2 shows a group of adolescent boys, all of whom are 13 years of age. All are at different levels of maturation and therefore have different nutritional needs.

In general, girls begin the pubertal process approximately 2 years before boys. Factors known about the timing and milestones of pubertal development are summarized in Figure 11-3 and Appendixes 12 and 13. Although growth slows after the achievement of sexual maturity, linear growth and weight acquisition continue into the late teens for females and early 20s for males. Most girls gain no more than 2 to 3 inches after menarche, although girls who have early menarche tend to grow more after its onset than do those having later menarche.

During the process of total body maturation, the composition of the body changes. Prepubertal boys and girls tend to be similar, with their body fat averaging about 15% and 19%, respectively. Girls gain more fat than boys during puberty, and in adulthood, they have about 22% to 26% body fat, compared with around 15% to 18% in men. During puberty, men gain twice as much lean tissue as women.

Growth Assessments

Weight and height can be plotted on growth grids to determine whether individuals are maintaining their growth pattern or growth channel. The relationship between weight and height can be evaluated by using the Centers for Disease Control (CDC) NCHS body mass index (BMI) tables (www.cdc.gov/growthcharts). Appropriate weights-for-height ac-

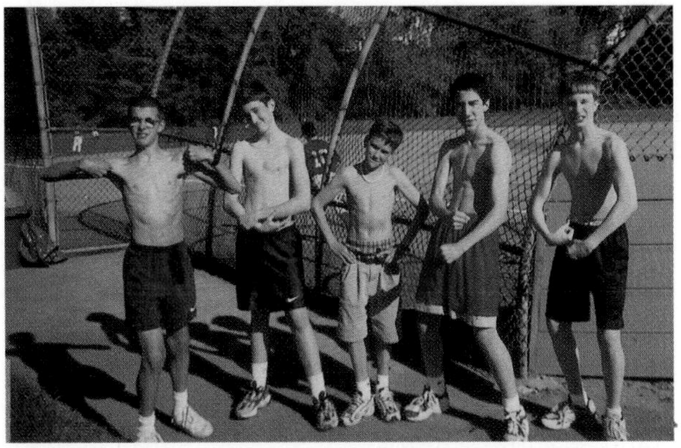

FIGURE 11-2 • These boys are all 13 years old, but their energy needs vary according to their individual growth rates.

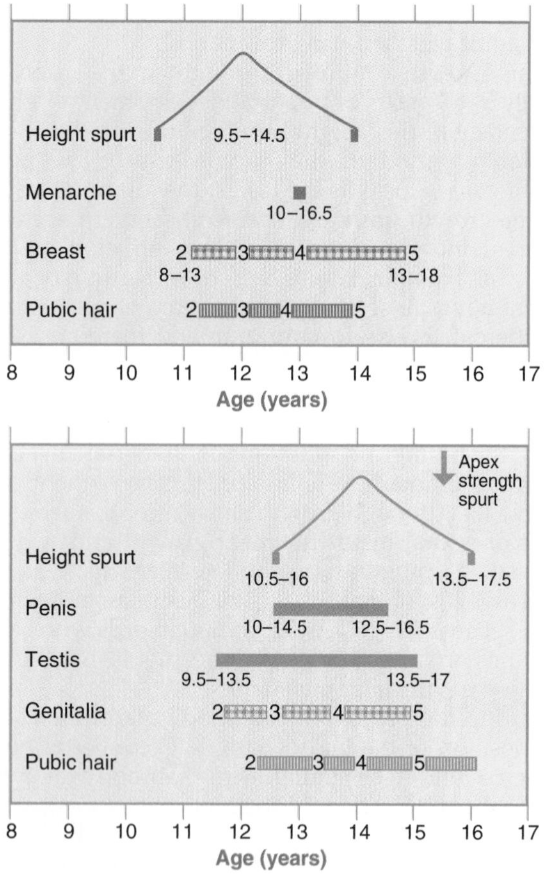

FIGURE 11-3 • Sequence of events during puberty in girls *(upper chart)* and boys *(lower chart).* Breast, genitalia, and pubic hair development are numbered 2 to 5 based on the Tanner developmental stages. (From Marshall WA, Tanner JM: Variations in the pattern of pubertal changes in boys, *Arch Dis Child* 45:13, 1970.)

cording to age and sex lie between the 10th and 85th percentiles, a range that allows for individual differences in body build (Story, Holt, and Sofka, 2000) (see Appendixes 8, 11, 18, and 19).

Use of BMI, which is highly correlated with body fat, can also indicate weight status. An adolescent's BMI is calculated by dividing body weight (in kilograms) by the square of the adolescent's height (in meters); that is, BMI = kg/m^2. Adolescents with BMIs below the 5th percentile should be assessed for organic diseases or eating disorders. Adolescents with BMIs between the 85th and 95th percentiles are at risk for overweight, and a nutritional screening or assessment should be performed to determine their health risk. Adolescents with BMIs at the 95th percentile or greater for age and gender are overweight and should have an in-depth medical assessment (Barlow and Dietz, 1998) (see Chapter 24).

A skin-fold evaluation is even more precise. For example, a low skin-fold measurement in an individual who is above the 85th percentile BMI indicates the person is overweight but not that the person has too much fat. An assessment of muscle and arm circumference can confirm a person's muscular composition. However, a skin-fold in the 90th percentile or greater with a BMI greater than the 95th percentile suggests that a person has too much fat, or is truly overweight (WHO, 1995). (Measurement of skin folds is discussed in more detail in Chapter 17.)

Sexual Maturity Ratings (Tanner Stages)

Because adolescents of the same age often differ markedly in size (see Figure 11-2), it is impossible to use age alone in evaluating pubertal growth. An assessment of the degree of maturation of secondary sexual characteristics is useful not only in evaluating physical growth but also in detecting certain diseases and disorders associated with adolescence. Sexual maturity ratings (SMRs), often called *Tanner stages,* are widely used to evaluate growth and developmental age during adolescence. These ratings are based on the development of secondary sex characteristics and are assigned on a scale of 1 (prepubertal) to 5 (adult). For boys, this scale is based on the progression of genital and pubic hair development (see Appendix 13); for girls, the rating is based on the stage of breast and pubic hair development (see Appendix 12). These stages of growth correlate highly with other pubertal events.

Table 11-1 explains the changes in the secondary sex characteristics. Because nutrition professionals are often unable to evaluate breast and genital development, Table 11-1 also gives other characteristics that correspond with each SMR level. Knowledge of the relationship between these milestones and physical growth enables the clinician to assess the progress of growth in an adolescent at a particular time, give some indication of the extent of future growth, and provide nutritional counseling that is geared toward individual needs for growth and development.

Excessive or less-than-normal growth can be detected by plotting height changes on the grids in Appendixes 8 and 11. The major cause of short stature during adolescence is genetically late initiation of puberty, although other conditions such as chronic diseases or skeletal and chromosomal abnormalities may also cause certain children to be shorter than normal. Hormonal imbalances leading to abnormal growth are rare.

Psychological Changes

Characteristics of Adolescents

Adolescence is a period of maturation for the mind and body. Along with the physical growth of puberty, emotional and intellectual development is rapid. Adolescents' capacity for abstract thinking, as opposed to the concrete thought patterns of childhood, enables them to accomplish the tasks of adolescence. These tasks are the expected accomplishments that lead to maturity in emotional and intellectual development, many of which have implications for their nutritional well-being.

TABLE 11-1 Ratings of Sexual Maturation*

	PUBIC HAIR	GENITALIA	CORRESPONDING CHANGES
Boys			
Stage 1	None	Prepubertal	
Stage 2	Small amount at outer edges of pubis, slight darkening	Beginning penile enlargement Testes enlarged to 5-ml volume Scrotum reddened and changed in texture	Increased sweat gland activity
Stage 3	Covers pubis	Penis longer Testes enlarged to 8-10 ml Scrotum enlarged	Voice changes Faint mustache/facial hair Axillary hair Beginning of peak height gain velocity (growth spurt of 6-8 inches)
Stage 4	Adult type, does not extend to thighs	Penis wider and longer Testes enlarged to 12 ml Scrotal skin darker	End of peak height gain velocity Voice deeper Possibly severe acne More facial hair Darker hair on legs
Stage 5	Adult type, spreads to thighs	Adult penis Testes enlarged to 15 ml	Significantly increased muscle mass
Girls			
Stage 1	None	No change from childhood	
Stage 2	Small amount, downy, on medial labia	Breast buds	Increased sweat gland activity Beginning of peak height gain velocity (growth spurt of 3-5 inches)
Stage 3	Increased, darker, curly	Larger, but no separation of the nipple and the areola	End of peak height gain velocity Beginning of acne Axillary hair
Stage 4	More abundant, coarse texture	Larger Areola and nipple form secondary mound	Possibly severe acne Menarche begins
Stage 5	Adult, spreads to medial thighs	Adult distribution of breast tissue, continuous outline	Increased fat and muscle mass

Modified from Tanner JM: *Growth at adolescence,* ed 2, Oxford, 1962, Blackwell Scientific Publications.
*See Appendix Tables 12 and 13.

Cognitive and emotional development can be divided into *early, middle,* and *late* adolescence. Determining the adolescent's stage can be very helpful when providing nutritional counseling and designing educational programs.

In *early adolescence* the adolescent has the following characteristics:

- Is preoccupied with body and body image
- Trusts and respects adults
- Is anxious about peer relationships
- Is ambivalent about autonomy

The nutritional implications are that adolescents in this stage are willing to do or try anything that makes them look better or improves their body image. However, adolescents at this stage want immediate results, so nutrition counseling should be geared toward short-term goals and addressing nutritional concerns that affect the teenager's appearance, performance (e.g., dance, sports), or both.

Teenagers in *middle adolescence* have the following characteristics:

- Are greatly influenced by their peer group
- Are mistrustful of adults
- Consider independence to be very important
- Experience significant cognitive development

During this stage the teenager listens to peers more than to parents or other adults. Teenagers are becoming more in charge of the food they eat. The drive toward independence often results in temporary rejection of the family dietary patterns. It is during middle adolescence that adolescents often experiment with vegetarianism. Nutritional counseling should include making wise decisions when eating away from home.

Teenagers in *late adolescence* have the following characteristics:

- Have established a body image
- Are oriented toward the future and are making plans
- Are increasingly independent
- Are more consistent in their values and beliefs
- Are developing intimacy and permanent relationships

By late adolescence, teenagers are thinking about the future and are interested in improving their overall health. Nutritional counseling during this stage can address long-term goals. Adolescents in this stage still want to make their own decisions but are open to information provided by health care providers. Nutritional counselors not only should present current recommendations, but they also should explain the rationale behind them.

As adolescents strive for independence, they often take risks. Many of these risks are important for becoming independent (e.g., trying out for a sports

CLINICAL INSIGHT

Body Image and Dieting Practices of Adolescents

Regardless of how they look to others, adolescents are seldom satisfied with their appearance. Girls are often unhappy with their weight and body shape, and boys envision having masculine physiques that often do not coincide with their own. This disparity between the perceived and the desired often leads to inappropriate eating behaviors. The Youth Risk Behavior Survey (YRBS) of 1999 obtained information from 10,904 students about their body image and their behaviors to change it. The survey included a self-administered, 75-item questionnaire given to a random sample of high school students from public and private schools in grades 9 through 12 who were representative of the U.S. high school population (CDC, 2002). The survey revealed large differences in the way female and male adolescents viewed themselves.

Female adolescents (34%) were twice as likely as their male counterparts (15%) to view themselves as "too fat." The boys were twice as likely to view themselves as "too thin" (16% versus 7%). Male and female black students were less likely to view themselves as "too fat." Overall, white and Hispanic students (29% and 32%, respectively) were significantly more likely than black students (21%) to identify themselves as being overweight (CDC, 2002).

Among the female students, 60% were attempting to lose weight at the time of the survey, whereas only 24% of the male students were participating in weight loss behaviors. Even more disturbing is the fact that 25% of the girls who considered themselves to be the "right weight" were still trying to lose weight. Of the boys, 24% were trying to lose weight, but 26% were trying to gain weight. Overall, white and Hispanic students (43% and 45%, respectively) were significantly more likely than black students (33%) to be attempting to lose weight (CDC, 2002).

The most popular method for losing weight was exercising, which was followed closely by skipping meals, particularly among the female students. White students were more likely to report exercise as a method of weight control than black students. Eight percent of the female students and 2% of the male students reported using vomiting or laxatives to control their weight during the 7 days preceding the survey, but the numbers jumped to 14% and 4%, respectively, when they were asked whether they had ever used vomiting to manage their weight. In addition, 9% of the female students and 2% of the male students had taken diet pills to lose weight.

As these studies show, adolescents with a normal-appearing physique may have a very different body image, leading to dissatisfaction and inappropriate behaviors to change their shape. Clinicians need to be aware of this disparity in some teenagers and may need to probe further to determine the extent of inappropriate eating and exercise behaviors. Adolescents may be dieting even when they are not overweight, and they need help to accept having more realistic body weights (Emmons, 1994).

team, applying to college, dating), but many risky behaviors can be dangerous. Resnick et al (1993) found that certain serious behaviors called *acting-out behaviors* can be categorized and include the following: using drugs, skipping school, and taking unintended injury risks, such as drinking and driving, not wearing a seatbelt, and not using a bicycle helmet. Another group of serious behaviors, called *quietly disturbed behaviors,* are of concern to nutritionists because they include behaviors related to poor body image; disordered eating, including bingeing, bulimia, and chronic dieting; fear of loss of control over eating; emotional stress; and suicidal ideation.

Body Image

Developing a body image—an image of the physical self that includes an adult body—is an intellectual and emotional task that is intertwined with nutritional issues. Adolescents often feel uncomfortable with their rapidly changing bodies, yet at the same time, they want to be like their most perfect peers and cultural idols (see *Clinical Insight:* Body Image and Dieting Practices of Adolescents). Their sense of worth may be derived from feelings about their own physical attributes, a trait that causes them to be vulnerable to severe distortions if an eating disorder develops.

The desire to change their rate of growth or body proportions can lead adolescents to be exploited by commercial interests and be subject to dietary manipulations that may have negative consequences. The rapid weight gain accompanying the development of secondary sexual characteristics causes many girls to unnecessarily restrict the amount of food they eat. Boys are tempted to use nutritional supplements, hoping to achieve the muscular appearance of adults. The importance to teenagers of fitting in and having body images they think will help them fit in cannot be overlooked in nutritional counseling (Moore, 1988; Moore, 1990; Story, Holt, and Sofka 2002).

NUTRIENT REQUIREMENTS

Recommendations for fulfilling the nutritional needs of adolescents arise from a small research base. Often

TABLE 11-2 Estimated Energy Requirements for Male Adolescents

AGE	REFERENCE WEIGHT (kg [lb])	REFERENCE HEIGHT (m [in])	ESTIMATED ENERGY REQUIREMENTS (kcal/day) SEDENTARY PAL*	LOW ACTIVE PAL*	ACTIVE PAL*	VERY ACTIVE PAL*
10	31.9 (70.3)	1.39 (54.7)	1601	1875	2149	2486
11	35.9 (79.1)	1.44 (56.7)	1691	1985	2279	2640
12	40.5 (89.2)	1.49 (58.7)	1798	2113	2428	2817
13	45.6 (100.4)	1.56 (61.4)	1935	2276	2618	3038
14	51.0 (112.3)	1.64 (64.6)	2090	2459	2829	3283
15	56.3 (124)	1.70 (66.9)	2223	2618	3013	3499
16	60.9 (134.1)	1.74 (68.5)	2320	2736	3152	3663
17	64.6 (142.3)	1.75 (68.9)	2366	2796	3226	3754
18	67.2 (148)	1.76 (69.3)	2383	2823	3263	3804

Data from Institute of Medicine, Food and Nutrition Board: *Dietary reference intakes for energy, carbohydrate, fiber, fat, fatty acids, cholesterol, protein, and amino acids,* Washington, DC, 2002, National Academies Press.
*PAL, Physical activity level. PAL categories, which are based on walking per day at 2-4 mph, are as follows: *sedentary,* no additional activity; *low active,* 1.5-2.2 miles/day; *active,* 3-4.4 miles/day; and *very active,* 7.5-10.3 miles/day.

TABLE 11-3 Estimated Energy Requirements for Female Adolescents

AGE	REFERENCE WEIGHT (kg [lb])	REFERENCE HEIGHT (m [in])	ESTIMATED ENERGY REQUIREMENTS (kcal/day) SEDENTARY PAL*	LOW ACTIVE PAL*	ACTIVE PAL*	VERY ACTIVE PAL*
10	32.9 (72.5)	1.38 (54.3)	1470	1729	1972	2376
11	37.2 (81.9)	1.44 (56.7)	1538	1813	2071	2500
12	40.5 (89.2)	1.49 (58.7)	1798	2113	2428	2817
13	44.6 (91.6)	1.51 (59.4)	1617	1909	2183	3640
14	49.4 (108.8)	1.60 (63)	1718	2036	2334	3831
15	52.0 (114.5)	1.62 (63.8)	1731	2057	2362	2870
16	53.9 (118.7)	1.63 (64.2)	1729	2059	2368	2883
17	55.1 (121.4)	1.63 (64.2)	1710	2042	2353	2871
18	56.2 (123.8)	1.63 (64.2)	1690	2024	2336	2858

Data from Institute of Medicine, Food and Nutrition Board: *Dietary reference intakes for energy, carbohydrate, fiber, fat, fatty acids, cholesterol, protein, and amino acids,* Washington, DC, 2002, National Academies Press.
*PAL, Physical activity level. PAL categories, which are based on walking per day at 2-4 mph, are as follows: *sedentary,* no additional activity; *low active,* 1.5-2.2 miles/day; *active,* 3-4.4 miles/day; and *very active,* 7.5-10.3 miles/day (see Table 2-3).

the amounts recommended are extrapolated from studies in adults or children. Part of the difficulty lies in the fact that studies of requirements must consider not only age but also the stage of physical maturity or SMR. The dietary reference intakes (DRIs), which include the recommended dietary allowances (RDAs), adequate intakes (AIs), and tolerable upper intake levels (ULs) for adolescents, have been established for three age groups (see Table 15-1).

Energy

Marked variability exists for the estimated energy requirements (EERs) among males and females because of variations in growth rate and physical activity. Energy requirements of adolescents are designed to maintain health, promote optimal growth and maturation, and support a desirable level of physical activity. It is important to ensure adequate energy for growth. Adolescents who limit their energy intake or have food security issues that limit their energy intake may limit their ultimate adult growth. In 2002, the Food and Nutrition Board released new guidelines for energy requirements (Institute of Medicine [IOM], 2002). The EERs of adolescents are based on energy expenditure, requirements for growth, and level of physical activity. To derive the EERs, the adolescent's gender, age, height, weight, and physical activity level (PAL) were used in calculations with an additional 25 kcal/day added for energy deposition or growth. To determine adequate energy intake (in kilocalories), physical activity assessment is required. The energy requirements allow for four levels of activity (*sedentary, low active, active,* and *very active*). This physical activity reflects the energy expended in activities other than the activities of daily living. Tables 11-2 and 11-3 show the EER (kcal/day) for each activity level based on PALs (see Chapter 2 and Table 2-3).

Protein

During adolescence, protein needs, like those for energy, correlate more closely with the growth pattern than with chronologic age. The 2002 DRIs for protein are based on the amount of protein needed for growth and positive nitrogen balance (IOM, 2002).

The DRIs provide for the estimated average requirements (EAR) and the recommended dietary allowances (RDAs). The DRIs recommend using the EAR when assessing nutrient intakes of groups. The EAR provides for adequate intake for 50% of the population. The RDA is recommended to be used when assessing the intake of an individual. Table 11-4 shows the protein EARs and RDAs for adolescents. Average intakes of protein are well above the RDA for all age groups. In fact, when comparing protein intakes of adolescents from the United States with teenagers from other countries, studies show that U.S. adolescents have a much higher intake of protein. Insufficient protein intake is uncommon in the adolescent population. However, if energy intake is inadequate for any reason (e.g., food security issues, chronic illness, attempts to lose weight), dietary protein may be used to meet energy needs and therefore be unavailable for synthesis of new tissue or for tissue repair. This may result in a state of insufficient protein, which leads to a reduction in growth rate and a decrease in lean body mass. Current dieting patterns in some adolescent girls can result in restricted calorie intakes that are potentially harmful, especially when protein sources are used to meet energy needs.

Excessive intakes of protein can also have an impact on nutritional status. For example, a high protein intake can interfere with calcium metabolism (see Chapters 4 and 27) and increase fluid needs. These increased fluid needs may put adolescent athletes at high risk for dehydration (see Chapter 26).

Minerals and Vitamins

Micronutrients (i.e., vitamins and minerals) play an important role in the growth and health of adolescents. Inadequate fruit and vegetable consumption has been linked to certain types of cancer and other diseases (see Chapters 12 and 40). National recommendations support increased consumption of fruits and vegetables because of their contributions of vitamins, minerals, and phytonutrients. The recommendation is to eat five servings of fruits and vegetables per day. Unfortunately, surveys show that adolescents consume significantly less than the recommended amount. The 1999 Youth Risk Behavior Surveillance (YRBS) revealed that only 22.5% of whites, 27.8% of blacks and 24.0% of Hispanics ate more than five servings of fruits and vegetables per day. Although this is low, it is higher than the 1995 YRBS results indicating that only 9% ate five servings of fruit and vegetables (CDC, 2002). This increase in consumption is encouraging and shows that educating adolescents about the "five-a-day" recommendation may have had an impact on their food consumption patterns. Although the consumption of vitamins and minerals has increased, 75% of adolescents still do not eat adequate amounts of fruits and vegetables. This inadequate intake has a tremendous impact on the amount of vitamins and minerals adolescents need for growth. Adolescents incorporate two times more calcium, iron, zinc, and magnesium into their bodies during the years of their growth spurt than they do at other times.

TABLE 11-4 Protein: Estimated Average Requirements and Recommended Dietary Allowances for Adolescents

AGE (yr)	EAR* (g/kg/day)	RDA† (g/kg/day)
9-13	0.76	0.95 or 34 g/day*
14-18		
Boys	0.73	0.85 or 52 g/day*
Girls	0.71	0.85 or 46 g/day*

Data from Institute of Medicine; Food and Nutrition Board: *Dietary reference intakes for energy, carbohydrate, fiber, fat, fatty acids, cholesterol, protein, and amino acids,* Washington, DC, 2002, National Academies Press.
*EAR, Estimated average requirement.
†RDA, Recommended dietary allowance. Based on average weight for age.

Calcium

Because of accelerated muscular, skeletal, and endocrine development, calcium needs are greater during puberty and adolescence than during childhood or adult years. At the peak of the growth spurt the daily deposition of calcium can be twice that of the average deposition during the rest of the adolescent period. In fact, 45% of the skeletal mass is added during adolescence (Lytle, 2002).

The DRI for calcium is 1300 mg for all adolescents (Yates et al, 1998); calcium requirements are expressed as adequate intakes (AIs). The AI recommendation is believed to supply the needs of all individuals in a group, but lack of data or uncertainty in the data preclude confidently specifying the percentage of those adequately addressed by this intake (IOM, 1997). This is especially true for adolescents. The National Institutes of Health (NIH) Consensus Development Conference Statement on Optimal Calcium Intake (NIH, 1994) recommended 1200 to 1500 mg of calcium per day for adolescents 11 to 24 years of age. In their statement, the committee acknowledged that a certain threshold level of dietary calcium is necessary to allow growing adolescents to achieve their genetically predetermined peak bone mass. Dietary survey data indicate that adolescents, particularly girls, are at greatest risk for inadequate calcium intake (American Academy of Pediatrics [AAP], 1999; Alaimo et al, 1994; Harnack, Stang, and Story, 1999; Johnson, Panely, and Wang 1998). Calcium intake tends to decline among girls 10 to 17 years of age. Consumption surveys show an average intake for females to be 780 to 820 mg/day. Among boys, the average intake is 800 to 920 mg/day. The National Health and Nutrition Examination Survey III (NHANES III, 1988-1991) results also revealed a decrease in young adolescents' dietary calcium intakes compared with NHANES II (1976-1980) (Albertson, 1997), as shown in the following chart:

Age	NHANES II (1976-1980)	NHANES III (1988-1991)
6-11	1209	867
12-15	854	796
16-19	725	822

In addition, evidence suggests that high soft drink consumption in the adolescent population contributes to low calcium intake because of the likelihood that soda is being substituted for milk. It is estimated that 9% of the total caloric intake of male adolescents and 8% of total caloric intake of female adolescents can be attributed to soft drink consumption (Golden, 2000; Jacobson, 1998). Male adolescents average 2½ 12-oz servings of soft drinks per day but only 1 cup of milk per day. Female adolescents average 2 12-oz servings of soft drinks per day and less than 1 cup of milk per day. As teenagers have begun doubling and tripling their consumption of soft drinks, they have begun decreasing their consumption of milk by more than 40%.

The risk of developing osteoporosis depends partially on how much bone mass is built early in life. Girls build 92% of their bone mass by the age of 18 (IOM, 1997; Golden, 2000), but an inadequate intake of calcium may limit their ultimate bone growth. This is the reason why the IOM committee recommends higher levels of calcium for youths ages 9 to 18 than for adults ages 19 to 50. Although osteoporosis takes decades to develop, preliminary research suggests that drinking soft drinks can increase the risk of broken bones in children. Wyshak found that active teenagers who drink sodas are more likely to break a bone than active teenagers who do not drink sodas (Wyshak, 2000). Wyshak states that the amount of bone people have when they are older is related to the peak bone mass they reached in adolescence. The less bone laid down during adolescence, the greater the risk for osteoporosis in later life.

Iron

All adolescents have high requirements for iron. The build-up of muscle mass in boys is accompanied by greater blood volume; girls lose iron monthly with the onset of menses. During periods of rapid growth, adolescents often have low serum hematocrit or hemoglobin concentrations. The majority of these teenagers have adequate iron stores but because of the rapid growth and significant increase in lean body mass, their circulating iron may be low (see Chapters 18 and 34). This condition is referred to as physiologic anemia of growth. During adolescence, anemia secondary to iron deficiency may impair the immune response and decrease resistance to infection. Iron deficiency anemia can also affect learning, as shown by studies revealing that children and adolescents with anemia have problems with short-term memory (Halterman et al, 2001) (see Chapter 34). In their recommendations to prevent and control iron deficiency in the United States (CDC, 1998), the CDC presents guidelines for prevention, screening, and treatment of iron deficiency anemia.

Zinc

Zinc is known to be essential for growth and sexual maturation. Although plasma zinc levels decline during pubertal development, retention of zinc increases significantly during the growth spurt. This increased use may lead to more efficient use of dietary sources. However, limited intake of zinc-containing foods may affect physical growth and the development of secondary sex characteristics (see Chapter 5).

Other Minerals

Although the role of other minerals in the nutrition of adolescents has not been studied extensively, the importance of magnesium, iodine, phosphorus, copper, chromium, cobalt, and fluoride is well known. The possibility of interactions among these nutrients cannot be overlooked. Recommendations for estimated safe and adequate dietary intakes are made on the basis of the best data currently available (see Table 15-1).

Vitamins

The need for vitamins increases during adolescence. Because of increased energy demands during this period, increased quantities of thiamin, riboflavin, and niacin are required for the release of energy from carbohydrates. Because of tissue synthesis, the body has an increased demand for vitamin B_6, folic acid, and vitamin B_{12}. It also needs more vitamin D for rapid skeletal growth and vitamins A, C, and E for new cell growth. Although few reports have been made about low serum vitamin C levels in teenagers, those who habitually avoid eating fruits and vegetables and those who smoke cigarettes may be at increased risk for deficiency (see Chapter 4).

Folic Acid

In 1998, new DRIs for folic acid were released, and the DRI for folic acid increased to 400 μg/day (IOM, 1998). This increase was designed to reduce the risk of fetal neural tube defects in females capable of becoming pregnant. It is recommended that the 400 μg/day come from a varied diet with foods containing folic acid, as well as from fortified foods, supplements, or both. Before the fortification of food with folic acid, the median intake of folate was approximately 250 μg/day. Because of the Food Fortification Act (January 1,

1998), the average intake of folic acid is expected to increase 100 μg/day (Suitor and Bailey, 2000).

Like other nutrients, vitamin needs are primarily determined by an individual's degree of physical maturity rather than chronologic age because of varying growth demands. Adolescents who diet, have an eating disorder or a chronic disease, or consistently make poor food choices are the exceptions to this rule.

Supplement Use by Adolescents

The American Dietetic Association's position statement on vitamin and mineral supplementation states that consuming a wide variety of foods is preferred to nutrient supplementation as a method for obtaining adequate vitamins and minerals (American Dietetic Association, 2001). Despite this recommendation, studies show that adolescents do not consume nutrient-dense foods and usually have inadequate intakes of many vitamins and minerals.

Results from the 1994 Continuing Survey of Food Intake of Individuals (CSFII) showed that only 15.6% of adolescents reported daily use of supplements, and 8.2% reported less frequent use. Adolescents who used supplements had higher mean dietary intakes of most micronutrients and carbohydrates and lower intakes of total and saturated fat than those who did not take supplements. More that one third of all adolescents had dietary intakes of vitamin A and E, calcium, and zinc that were less than 75% of the U.S. RDA. In addition, 35% of the females who did not use supplements consumed inadequate amounts of every micronutrient in the study (Stang et al, 2000). It is evident that prevention and education programs are needed to improve the dietary intakes of America's adolescents—programs that promote appropriate food intakes and use of fortified foods and supplements as needed.

Physical Activity

Physical Activity and Health: A Report of the Surgeon General is a comprehensive overview of research related to physical activity and health (CDC, 1996). The report (1) summarizes the benefits of physical activity, (2) reinforces the importance of promoting physical activity, (3) states that many children and adolescents are at risk for health problems because of inactive lifestyles, and (4) states that everyone should participate in a moderate amount of physical activity (e.g., 15 minutes of running, 30 minutes of brisk walking, 45 minutes of playing volleyball) on most if not all days of the week. The report revealed the following findings on adolescents' physical activity behavior:

- About 14% of children and adolescents did not participate in light to moderate or vigorous physical activity.
- Nearly half of adolescents ages 12 to 21 did not participate regularly in vigorous physical activity.
- Female adolescents were less active than male adolescents, and black females were less active than white females.
- Adolescents' participation in physical activity declined considerably as they got older.
- Daily attendance of high school students in physical education classes declined from 42% in 1991 to 25% in 1995.
- Only 19% of high school students were physically active for 20 minutes or more in daily physical education classes.

These findings are disturbing in view of the numerous health benefits that children and adolescents derive by being physically active on a regular basis. Physical activity can lead to improved body composition (i.e., increased lean muscle mass, reduced total body fat) and can help reduce other coronary heart disease (CHD) risk factors among adolescents. For example, increased physical activity levels can improve blood lipid profiles in adolescents at high risk for CHD (e.g., children and adolescents who are obese or who have type 1 or 2 diabetes mellitus) and can reduce blood pressure in adolescents whose blood pressure is high. Physical activity plays a substantial role in the development of bone mass during adolescence and can help maintain the structure and functional strength of bone throughout life (Patrick and Spear, 2002; Sallis and Patrick, 1994).

Efforts to increase physical activity levels among children and adolescents have been most successful in school settings. However, little attention has been focused on promoting physical activity among children and adolescents in settings other than schools such as health care settings. For example, during health supervision visits, health professionals could counsel children and adolescents about physical activity (Corbin and Pangrazi, 1998).

Health professionals, families, peers, and communities can influence children's and adolescents' physical activity levels. Parents who participate in physical activity and support and encourage physical activity in their children have a positive influence on physical activity levels. In addition, older children and adolescents whose friends are physically active tend to be more physically active themselves.

Little is known about which factors motivate children and adolescents to become physically active, remain physically active, and increase their physical activity levels as they become older. In addition, the reason these factors differ between females and males and among different racial and ethnic groups is unclear. However, it is clear that females are less likely than males to participate in vigorous physical activity, participate in strengthening or toning activities, or participate on sports teams. Strategies different from those used to promote physical activity in male children and adolescents should be needed to promote physical activity in female children and adolescents (Patrick et al, 2002). Strategies that take into account children's and adolescents' race or cultural background could also be beneficial. The Surgeon General's report recommends the following intervention strategies to promote physical activity in children and adolescents:

- Make physical activity enjoyable.
- Help adolescents succeed and increase their confidence in their ability to be physically active.
- Support adolescents' efforts to be physically active.
- Help adolescents learn about the benefits of physical activity, and help them develop positive attitudes toward it.
- Help adolescents overcome barriers that keep them from being physically active.

FOOD HABITS

Adolescents are maturing not only physically but also cognitively and psychosocially. They search for their identity, strive for independence and acceptance, and are concerned about appearance. Irregular meals, snacking, eating away from home, and following alternative dietary patterns characterize the food habits of adolescents. These habits are further influenced by family, peers, and the media.

Irregular Meals and Snacking

Meal patterns of adolescents are often chaotic. Teenagers miss an increasing number of meals at home as they get older. Breakfast and lunch are often the meals most frequently missed, but social and school activities may cause a teenager to miss an evening meal as well. Female adolescents tend to miss more meals than their male counterparts (Story et al, 2002).

Although concern has been expressed about the habit of snacking, teenagers may obtain substantial nourishment from snacks. Thus the choice of foods being eaten is more important than the time or place in which the food is eaten.

As a result of health and science education at school, most adolescents know what they should and should not eat (Story, Neumark-Sztainer, and French, 2002; Story and Resnick, 1986). However, overcoming barriers to act on this knowledge is the concern. Teenagers identify time as the biggest barrier to eating properly. They perceive themselves as too busy to worry about food, nutrition, meal planning, or eating well. In addition, adolescents tend to form different associations with healthy foods and junk foods. As shown in Box 11-1, adolescents form mainly negative associations with healthy foods and positive associations with "junk" foods (Chapman and Maclean, 1993). For adolescents to improve their eating habits, counseling must center on fitting proper nutrition into allowable time, making selection of healthy foods easier, and making healthy foods appealing to teens and their peers (see Chapter 22).

During the peak growth velocity, adolescents usually need to eat large amounts of food often. They are able to use foods with a high concentration of energy; however, they need to be careful to adjust the amounts and frequency they are eating when their growth slows. Habits of overeating adopted during adolescence may ultimately contribute to numerous debilitating diseases.

Fast Foods and the Media

Eating fast foods for meals or snacks is especially popular with busy adolescents (Figure 11-4). Fast foods include foods from vending machines, self-

Box 11-1. Situations and Feelings Associated With Eating Junk Foods and Healthy Foods

JUNK FOODS	HEALTHY FOODS
Being with friends	Being with parents
Being away from home or parents	Staying home
Being at the mall or store	Eating meals
Snacking	Being concerned with weight and appearance
Enjoyment and pleasure	Self-control
Not being in control, over-eating, guilt, disgust	

Modified from Chapman G, Maclean H: "Junk food" and "healthy food": meanings of food in adolescent women's culture, *J Nutr Educ* 25:108, 1993.

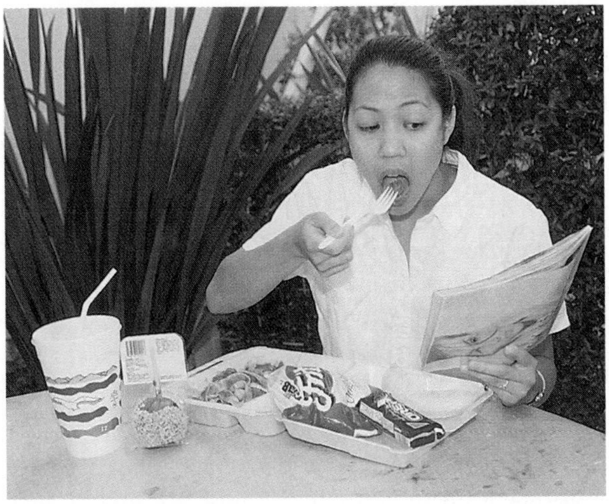

FIGURE 11-4 • For teenagers who eat meals or snacks in addition to traditional meals, the choice of food is more important than the time it is eaten or place in which it is eaten. (From Bowden VR, Dickey SB, Greenberg CS: *Children and their families: the continuum of care*, Philadelphia, 1998, WB Saunders.)

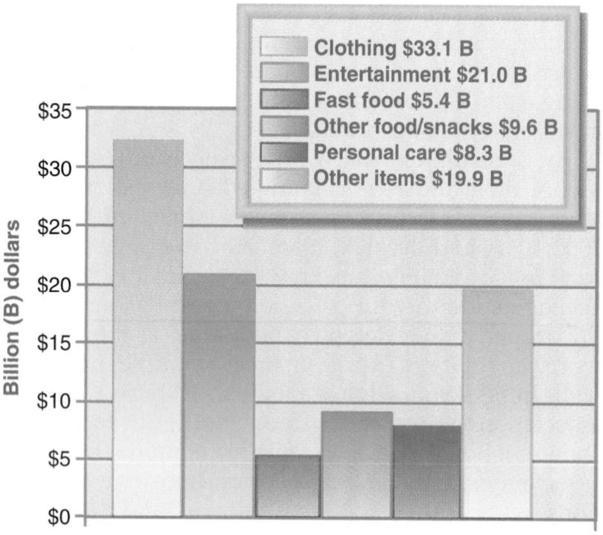

FIGURE 11-5 • The buying power of teenagers. (Data from Channel One Network, New York, 2000.)

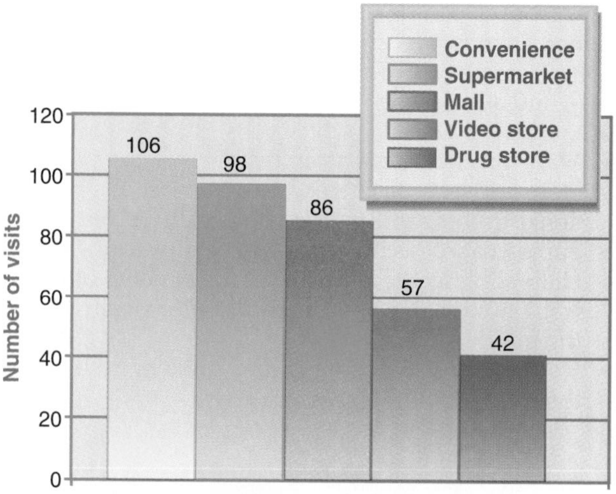

FIGURE 11-6 • Store visits by teenagers in a 30-day period. (Data from Channel One Network, New York, 2000.)

service restaurants, convenience groceries, and franchised food restaurants. Fast foods tend to be low in iron, calcium, riboflavin, and vitamin A, and few of them are good sources of folic acid. The vitamin C content of fast foods is also low unless fruit or fruit juice is consumed. Although most places offer a selection of healthy foods, most of the food items provide more than 50% of their calories from fat. Adolescents should be counseled on how to make wise and healthy choices when eating in one of these establishments.

Television and magazines probably have a greater influence on adolescents' eating habits than any other form of mass media. It is estimated that by the time average children reach the teenage years, they have viewed 100,000 food commercials, most of them for products with high concentrations of fat and simple carbohydrates. More than 65% of food advertisements promote beverages (primarily alcoholic) and sweets (Brown and Witherspoon, 1998; Story, Neumark-Sztainer, and French, 2002).

Potential Nutritional Inadequacies

Surveys of nutrient intakes have shown that adolescents are likely to obtain less vitamin A, vitamin B_6, folate, riboflavin, iron, calcium, and zinc than recommended. Young women are also likely to obtain less magnesium, copper, and manganese than recommended (Alaimo et al, 1994).

Studies also show that teenagers' intakes of fat, saturated fat, protein, and sodium are higher than needed. The School Nutrition Dietary Assessment Study revealed that dietary fat represented 33% to 35% of the participants' energy intake, and that the intake of saturated fat was 12% to 13%—higher than the recommended level of 10% (Devaney et al, 1995). Although the intake of fat as a percentage of calories has decreased from 37% to approximately 33% to 34%, the levels still remain higher than the recommended 30%. Even though the fat intakes of adolescents seem to be decreasing, the incidence of obesity in this population continues to increase.

Adolescents as Food Purchasers

For marketers, being a teenager involves a certain lifestyle and typical spending habits that are attractive. Marketing to teenagers has become a multibillion-dollar business. It is estimated that the nation's approximately 23 million teenagers spend nearly $100 billion annually (Channel One Network, 2000) (Figure 11-5). About one third of their spending is for clothing, another 22% is for entertainment, and another $15 billion annually is for fast food and other food and snacks. Teenagers not only spend money themselves, they also wield a tremendous influence over purchases made by their parents (Channel One Network, 2000).

Teenagers are frequent visitors to different stores. In a 30-day period the most common two types of stores teenagers visit are food stores, with more than 200 million visits to convenience stores and supermarkets (Figure 11-6). Teenagers also frequent fast-food restaurants; the highest number of visits occur immediately after school (Figure 11-7), and the next highest number occur during weekday dinnertime. Teenagers watch the least amount of television, but it still averages to be more than 3 hours per day (Figure 11-8). It is critical to incorporate information about consumer habits of teenagers into nutrition assessment and counseling of teenagers. It is important to determine where they eat, how much they spend, and what they buy. This information is vital in helping provide nutrition care plans for adolescents.

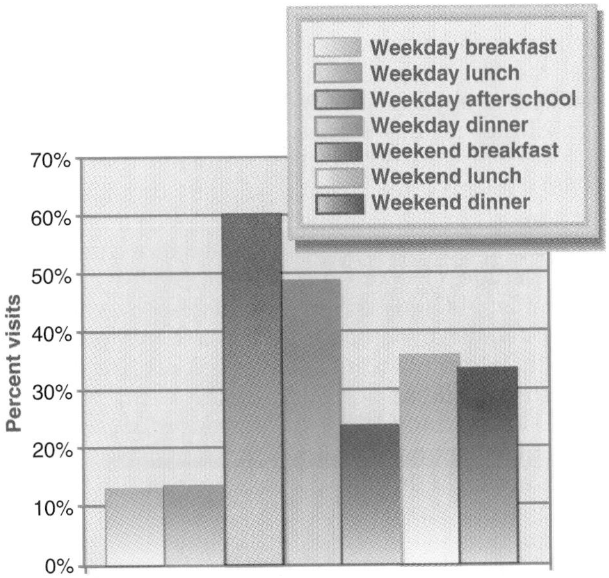

FIGURE 11-7 • Fast-food restaurant visits by teenagers in a 2-week period. (Data from Channel One Network, New York, 2000.)

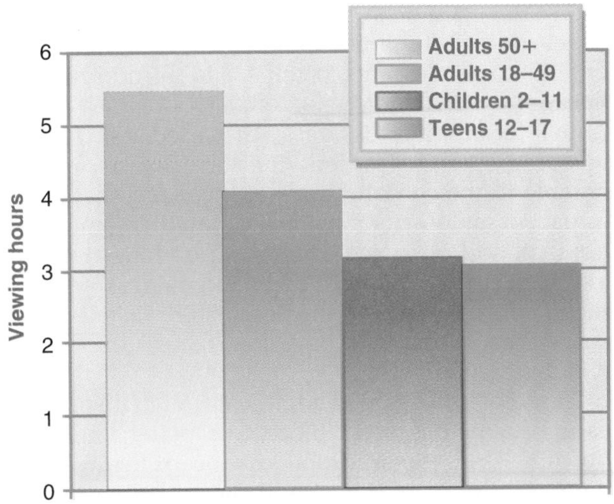

FIGURE 11-8 • Average number of hours of television viewing per day. (Data from Channel One Network, New York, 2000.)

SPECIAL SITUATIONS

Vegetarians

Adolescence is a time of experimentation, so as adolescents experience cognitive changes and broaden their perspectives, they often become concerned about social and environmental issues. Especially during middle or late adolescence, adolescents tend to be attracted to vegetarian eating practices because of their concerns about animal welfare, ecology, the environment, or personal health. In addition, concerns about body weight also motivate some adolescents to adopt a vegetarian diet because it is a socially acceptable way to reduce dietary fat. Vegetarian diets are often followed by adolescents with anorexia nervosa, who adopt the diet in an attempt to hide their restriction of food intake (Story et al, 2002).

Vegetarian diets are consistent with the *Dietary Guidelines for Americans* and can meet the DRIs and RDAs for nutrients. With planning, vegetarian diets can provide various nutrient-dense foods that promote health, growth, and development (Table 11-5). Diets need to be planned to provide adequate energy, protein, calcium, iron, zinc, and vitamins B_{12} and D. The bioavailablity of calcium, iron, and zinc should also be ensured. When adolescents become vegetarians, parents are often concerned about the diet's nutritional adequacy and especially about their children meeting their protein requirements. Parents need reassurance that a vegetarian diet can meet their children's nutrition needs, and they should receive information on the principles of healthy vegetarian eating for adolescents. In addition, parents and adolescents should be informed that overly restricted or inappropriately selected vegetarian diets can result in significant malnutrition. A delayed growth spurt, iron deficiency anemia, and vitamin B_{12} deficiency have developed in vegetarian adolescents who have inadequate intakes (Sanders, 1995; Story, Holt, and Sofka, 2000).

Eating Disorders

Eating disorders are the third most common chronic illness in adolescent females, with an incidence of up to 5%. The prevalence has increased dramatically over the past 3 decades (Kreipe and Birndorf, 2000; Spear and Stellefson-Myers, 2001). Although vastly more prevalent in teenage girls, boys can have eating disorders, especially boys participating in sports that require a low body weight. Girls and boys who compete in sports such as wrestling, dancing, track, or rowing and sports that require low body fat, such as body building or gymnastics, are at risk for developing eating disorders (Herbold and Frates, 2000). Numerous adolescents who have eating disorders do not meet the strict DSM-IV (Diagnostic and Statistical Manual-IV) criteria for either anorexia nervosa or bulimia nervosa but can be classified as having *eating disorders not otherwise specified (EDNOS)* (see Chapter 25). In one study, more than half of the adolescents evaluated for eating disorders had experienced a degree of psychologic distress similar to those who met strict diagnostic criteria (Bunnell, 1990). Diagnostic criteria for eating disorders such as those provided by the DSM-IV may not be entirely applicable to adolescents. The wide variability in the rate, timing, and magnitude of height and weight gain during normal puberty; the absence of menstrual periods in early puberty combined with the unpredictability of menses soon after menarche; and the cognitive lack of abstract concepts limit the application of the diagnostic criteria to adolescents (Kreipe and Birndorf, 2000; Spear and Sellefson-Myers, 2001).

Just as adolescents are at increased risk for developing eating disorders, they are also more vulnerable to the complications of these disorders. The impact of malnutrition on linear growth, brain development, and bone acquisition can be long-standing and irreversible. Yet with early and aggressive treatment, adolescents have the potential for a better outcome than adults who have had the disease longer (Golden, 2000).

Early identification of adolescents with disordered eating habits has been linked to a better long-term outcome, but identification can be difficult. Often parents bring a teenager with an unknown eating disorder to a doctor for another reason, such as gastrointestinal complaints, amenorrhea, or unexplained weight loss. A screening for disordered eating can easily be done and should include questions about fear of becoming fat, amount of dieting, use of laxatives, fasting or frequently skipping meals to lose weight, fear of certain foods (e.g., foods containing fat or sugar), vomiting, bingeing, and excessive exercise (see Chapter 25).

Because adolescents have the greatest risk for developing an eating disorder, efforts must be made to reduce the incidence of malnutrition or at least provide early intervention to prevent its serious complications (Striegel-Moore, 1997) (see Chapter 25).

Obesity

The incidence of obesity in teenagers is increasing. Among 12- to 19-year-olds in the United States, the prevalence of overweight is 21%, which is 6% higher than it was in the previous decade. Although the underlying causes of obesity are not fully understood, obesity seems to be a complex, multifactorial, chronic disease. Contributing factors include genetics, metabolic physiology, and environmental and psychosocial factors (Greger and Edwin, 2001). The eating habits and physical inactivity patterns of adolescents contribute to the increase in adolescent obesity (Christoffel and Ariza, 1998; Troiano and Flegal, 1998). However, teenagers are merely duplicating recent trends in the adult population, which has had a similar increase in overweight incidence during the past decade (Troiano and Flegal, 1998). Work by Gilman et al (2001) shows that adolescent who were breast-fed for more than 7 months or had more breast milk than formula were at lower risk for obesity during later childhood and adolescence.

This disturbing trend of increasing obesity warrants the attention of health professionals because being overweight during adolescence seems to be associated with a range of adverse physical health effects that are independent of adult weight. This fact was demonstrated in a 55-year follow-up of the Harvard Growth Study. An increased risk of morbidity from coronary heart disease and arteriosclerosis was found in men and women who were overweight as teenagers. In men who were overweight teenagers, the risk of colorectal cancer and gout increased, whereas in women who were overweight teenagers, the risk of arthritis was higher that of their leaner counterparts (Must et al, 1992).

The social and economic consequences of being overweight in adolescence are perhaps even greater than the long-term physical health effects. In fact, social consequences such as rejection seem to be greater for teenagers who are overweight than for those with chronic diseases such as asthma, musculoskeletal abnormalities, diabetes, and epilepsy, and the consequences are more severe for women than for men. Remaining unmarried, earning a low income, and obtaining fewer years of education have been found to be related to a higher incidence of obesity and the persistence of societal discrimination against the obese (Gortmaker, 1993) (see Chapter 24).

An obese teenager may gain weight as a result of a combination of psychologic, physiologic, and cultural factors (see Chapter 24). It seems that the longer teenagers have been obese, the greater the chance that they will remain obese. By adolescence, they often have adopted a restricted lifestyle and do not want to be seen in settings requiring vigorous exercise.

Accurate identification of the overweight adolescent is important because early, family-centered, behavior-based treatment can be successful (Williams et al, 1998). The adolescent can be evaluated based on BMI (weight/height^2 [kg/m^2]) as shown in Appendixes 17, 18, and 19. Adolescents with a BMI above the 95th percentile for age and sex should be considered overweight for screening purposes. These adolescents should be referred for additional in-depth medical assessments and treatment. Adolescents with BMIs at or above the 85th percentile for age and sex, but less than the 95th percentile, are

TABLE 11-5 Suggested Daily Food Intake Guide for Vegetarian Adolescents

FOOD GROUP	SERVINGS/DAY*
Bread, grains, cereal	9-11
Legumes	2-3
Vegetables	4-5
Fruits	4
Nuts, seeds	1
Milk, yogurt, cheese	3
Eggs (limit 3/week)	½
Fats, oils (added)	4-6
Sugar (added teaspoons)	6-9

Data from Story M, Holt K, Sofka D, eds: *Bright futures in practice: nutrition*, ed 2, Arlington, National Center for Education in Maternal and Child Health, 2002.
*Age ≥11 years; 2200-2800 kcal.

considered to be at risk for becoming overweight. These teenagers should be referred for second-level screening, which includes data on family history, blood pressure, total cholesterol level, any major change in BMI, and concerns about weight (Dietz, 1998; Story, 2002).

Teenagers are vulnerable to unrealistic attitudes about the amount of time and effort necessary for effective weight management. Many think that diet fads, drugs, and equipment provide the quick remedy they seek. Meanwhile, realistic educational and comprehensive therapeutic programs are scarce; thus the obese teenager is very likely to be obese throughout life.

Education about weight control can be designed effectively for a wide range of audiences in various settings, including youth programs and organizations. To be successful, therapeutic programs must include an individualized nutrition plan, a physical activity plan, and psychologically supportive components involving families and the individual adolescent (Flodmark et al, 1993; Greger and Edwin, 2001; Williams et al, 1998). Family therapy is an important factor in preventing progression from obesity in childhood to severe obesity in adolescence (see Chapter 24).

Hyperlipidemia

The major adult cardiovascular diseases—coronary artery disease and essential hypertension—begin in childhood and adolescence. Cardiovascular risk factors change during periods of growth and development, and distinct differences between blacks and whites and between males and females relate to adult heart disease (Freedman et al, 2001). These risk factors have been shown to "track" with age and predict adult risk levels (Berenson et al, 1998). Cardiovascular risk factors also tend to cluster; for example, obesity correlates with high blood pressure and adverse serum lipoprotein changes. Adolescents with high blood cholesterol levels are also likely to have elevated cholesterol levels as adults. Children and adolescents in families with a history of premature cardiovascular disease or parental hypercholesterolemia should have screening of blood cholesterol (National Cholesterol Education Program [NCEP], 1991). Other individuals who should be screened are (1) children and adolescents whose parents or grandparents, at age 55 years or younger, were found through diagnostic coronary arteriography to have coronary arteriosclerosis or who suffered a documented cardiovascular or cerebrovascular event or sudden cardiac death; (2) children and adolescents with a parent who has an elevated blood cholesterol level; and (3) adolescents who are at high risk for heart disease because they smoke or because they are obese.

The nutritional recommendations of the NCEP (see Chapter 35) are appropriate for all children older than 2 years of age. Helping adolescents understand the importance of current lifestyle factors on later disease is challenging, but not impossible. The challenge is to make the information practical for the adolescent's hectic lifestyle, much of which revolves around consuming food that is high in fat, low in fiber and nutrients, and of a limited variety. Promoting healthy lifestyle behaviors should include a discussion not only of food choices but also of the risks of smoking and alcohol use and the benefits of regular physical activity.

The Child and Adolescent Trial of Cardiovascular Health (CATCH), initiated in 1987, is a study of 12,000 elementary school children and adolescents and is designed to evaluate the effectiveness of school-based interventions in reducing subsequent cardiovascular risk (Nicklas et al, 1998). The results of this program demonstrate that a school-based program involving school food service, physical education, classroom curricula, and the family can help children and adolescents make healthy changes in behavior. If these changes can be continued for several years, they have a great potential for producing cardiovascular health benefits.

Sports Nutrition

Adolescent athletes are particularly vulnerable to nutritional misinformation and unsafe practices that promise enhanced performance. Pressures to achieve optimal performance encourage athletes to experiment with supplements and ergogenic aids to obtain a competitive edge. Inappropriate use of supplements, unsafe weight loss practices, and inadequate nutrient intakes can adversely affect their health and limit their growth (see Chapter 26).

Adequate fluid intake and prevention of dehydration are critical for young athletes, especially for younger adolescents. In fact, heat illness is second to head injury as a cause of reported noncardiac causes of death in secondary school athletes (Patrick et al, 2002). Compared with adults, children and young adolescents are at higher risk for becoming dehydrated and developing hypothermia because of the following factors (Steen, 1996):

- They sweat less (overall and per sweat gland), which potentially decreases their capacity to dissipate heat through the evaporation of the sweat.
- They produce more heat production during exercise but have less ability to transfer heat from the muscles to the skin.
- They have a greater body surface area, which can result in excessive heat gain in extreme heat and excessive heat loss in the cold.
- They have a lower cardiac output, which reduces their capacity for heat transport from the core to the skin during strenuous exercise.
- They acclimatize to exercising in heat more gradually than adults. A young adolescent may require five to six sessions to achieve the same degree of

acclimatization acquired by an adult in two to three sessions in the same environment.

It is not only the actual temperature but also the degree of humidity that affects an individual's ability to dissipate heat. The higher the humidity, the less sweat evaporates from the skin, decreasing the body's ability to cool itself and increasing the risk of heat-related illness (see Chapter 26).

Adolescents with certain diseases or medical conditions are at increased risk for developing heat-related illness. Children or adolescents with bulimia, congenital heart disease, diabetes mellitus, gastroenteritis, fever, or obesity may experience excessive fluid loss. In addition, those with anorexia nervosa, cystic fibrosis, mental retardation, or kidney disease may have insufficient fluid intake. Children who are obese develop heat-related illnesses more frequently than children of normal weight because (1) only a small amount of heat is needed to increase the temperature of a large amount of fat mass, (2) fat mass has a lower water content than lean body mass (so those with a high fat mass lose a greater amount of fluid), and (3) obese children expend greater effort than lean children, to perform at the same level which increases their overall body temperature more quickly.

Teenagers with these diseases or medical conditions should be considered to be at high risk for heat-related illnesses and should be monitored more closely when they are physically active, although they should not be prevented from participating in activities. If kept properly hydrated, their medical conditions can often be improved with a consistent physical activity program.

Although the benefits of participating in physical activity greatly outweigh the risks, physically active female adolescents and their parents, physical education teachers, coaches, and health professionals should be aware of certain issues and concerns. A major concern is the relationship among unhealthy eating behaviors, amenorrhea, and osteoporosis—a relationship known as the *female athlete triad* (see Chapter 26.) Physically active female adolescents whose caloric intake does not provide the energy needed to participate in physical activity are at risk for weight loss and an energy drain. This can lead to menstrual irregularities—usually amenorrhea—and negative consequences for bone health (e.g., premature bone loss, decreased bone density, increased risk of stress fractures) (Patrick et al, 2001).

Substance Use

Use of tobacco, alcohol, marijuana, and other drugs is a major public health problem. The effect of these chemicals on nutritional status depends on the amount and length of use and the individual's general state of health. Studies have indicated that although adolescents who abuse alcohol and drugs generally consume adequate quantities of principal nutrients and do not develop nutrient deficiencies, they obtain these nutrients from a narrower range of foods than those who do not abuse alcohol and drugs. However, current data indicate that most smokers become nicotine dependent as adolescents, which places them at risk for chronic disease associated with continuous oxidative damage (Hampi and Betts, 1999). Any initial nutrition assessment should screen for substance use. For example, a simple question such as "How often do you smoke cigarettes?" would be a good screening question for cigarette use. The adolescents will either answer that they never smoke or tell you how often they smoke. More questions can be asked about amounts and length of time smoking. Adolescent smokers need more antioxidants than nonsmokers, especially vitamin C. In addition, adolescents who drink alcohol are at higher risk for many nutrient deficiencies (see Chapter 31).

Pregnancy

Recommended weight gains during pregnancy may be slightly higher for the teenager than for the adult. The current recommendation is that pregnant adolescents should gain weight within the upper range currently recommended for adults (i.e., 30 to 35 lb) (IOM, 1990). For adolescents with a low prepregnancy weight, a 35- to 40-lb weight gain may be desirable (IOM, 1990; Story and Stang, 2000) (see Chapter 7).

Pregnant adolescents with a young gynecologic (postmenarchal) age (the number of years between the onset of menses and the date of conception), or who are undernourished at the time of conception, have the greatest nutritional needs. A young woman who conceives soon after her first menstrual period is at greatest physiologic risk for complications. It was once thought that adolescents with more physiologic maturity had no more physical complications during pregnancy than adult women, but the Camden study (Scholl et al, 1998) has shown that these adolescents and their infants are at increased risk. This longitudinal study sought to explain why the infant birth weights remained low even as maternal weight gain increased. This increased risk of fetal growth restriction may be attributed to disruption in the fetal-placental blood flow and the transmission of nutrients to the fetus as a result of the physiologic changes associated with maternal growth. Perhaps the increased concentrations of insulin, human growth hormone, and insulin-like growth factors that are characteristic of adolescent growth (even in late adolescence) combined with the normal milieu of pregnancy enhance accrual of fat stores and maternal weight gain but diminish circulating nutrients, ultimately impairing fetal growth.

Adolescents who begin having children at a young age (i.e., while still growing themselves) may be at particular risk for being overweight and obese. The Camden Study (Hediger et al, 1998) has documented that the excessive accrual of subcutaneous fat stores at central body sites often leads to the development of cardiovascular disease, type 2 diabetes, and hypertension in later life.

A clinically practical method of ensuring nutritional adequacy is to encourage the pregnant adolescent to gain the recommended amount of weight by consuming nutrient-rich foods. Most important, contact with health professionals during prenatal care is an opportunity to teach adolescents about feeding themselves and their families (American Dietetic Association, 1994). Because of the economic instability of pregnant adolescents, it is impossible to assume that they have an adequate food supply. Health professionals can help provide access to and information about resources such as food stamps, food banks, and the Women, Infants, and Children (WIC) program. (Table 7-4 lists recommended amounts of nutrients for pregnant women.)

STRATEGIES FOR IMPROVING NUTRITIONAL WELL-BEING

Nutritional Status Assessments

Nutritional status assessments of adolescents are typical of most nutritional assessments but have some specific differences (see Chapters 17 and 18). It is important to use an age-specific database for each aspect of the assessment. Standards based on stage of maturity are even more exact and should be used if available.

Nutritional assessments also should include an evaluation of the nutritional environment, including parental, peer, school, cultural, and personal lifestyle factors. The attitude of the adolescent toward food and nutrition is also a primary component of a comprehensive evaluation (Stang, 2002). A prime component of nutritional counseling for adolescents is helping them overcome their perceived barriers to eating well.

Prerequisites for Change

Because of their increasing independence, any attempt to help adolescents improve their nutritional status requires careful planning. For a plan to succeed, the adolescent must be willing to change; therefore, an assessment of a teenager's desire to change is essential. Encouraging the desire to change usually requires most of the nutrition counselor's attention. A recommended eating plan for adolescents is shown in Box 11-2.

Knowledge, attitude, and behavior must be addressed when guiding adolescents toward acquiring healthful food habits. Information can be provided in various settings ranging from the classroom to the hospital. The clinician must understand the change process and how to meaningfully communicate this process (see Chapter 22). Parents may be included in the process and encouraged to be supportive but not intrusive (Sigman-Grant, 2002).

SUMMARY

Adolescence is a period of tremendous physical and cognitive changes. It is considered a nutritionally vulnerable period because of the increased needs for all nutrients and the changes in lifestyle and food

Box 11-2. Recommended Daily Eating Guide for Adolescents

- 3-4 cups of nonfat or low-fat milk or yogurt to provide calcium, vitamin D, riboflavin, and for some vegetarian teens, adequate protein
- 5 or more servings of fresh, frozen, dried, raw, or cooked fruits and/or vegetables; mostly yellow, orange, dark green, or red
- 2 servings (2-3 oz each) of lean protein foods, such as chicken, turkey, fish, lean beef, or lean pork
- 6-11 servings of grains, breads, and cereals (preferably whole grain), rolls, pasta, rice, potatoes, and other starches to meet energy needs
- Small amounts, perhaps one serving per day, of high-fat, high-sugar items, such as desserts, soda, candy, cookies, and pastries that have little nutritional value

Clinical Scenario 1

Joe is a 17-year-old who lives at home with his parents and younger sister. He has no prior medical problems but recently complained about lack of energy during sports and athletic activities at school. He has been scheduled to meet with you, a nutrition counselor, because his pediatrician recommended it. When he arrives, he shares his food diary with you, which indicates that he skips lunch on the days that he wrestles after school. Otherwise, he eats the same meals each day—black coffee and sugar-sweetened cereals with whole milk for breakfast, a luncheon-meat sandwich and two candy bars on days when he eats lunch, and a typical family meal for dinner.

1. What suggestions would you make about his breakfast and lunch meals?
2. How much calcium does he need at the age of 17 years? If he drinks only one glass of milk each day, what percentage of his daily requirement is he missing?
3. Which other nutrients might be inadequate in Joe's diet? How can he change his diet to include the proper types of foods that he needs at his age?

Clinical Scenario 2

Carly is a 14-year-old girl who has been referred to you by her mother and family doctor. Her mother is concerned that Carly is not eating the proper foods, and her doctor wants you to give her some nutritional advice, especially because she has expressed a desire to be a vegetarian. She has heard that red meat contains a lot of fat, and she "does not want to get fat." A physical examination by her doctor shows that she is between Tanner (SMR) stages 1 and 2 for development, she weighs 89 lb, and she is 5 ft tall. She is extremely active, spending every afternoon after school involved in some kind of sport—basketball, swimming, track, or soccer.

1. List at least four questions you would include in your assessment session with Carly. Why would you include these questions?
2. What are the particular nutritional requirements for a teenage girl in Tanner stage 1?
3. How would you address Carly's concern about meat and her desire to be a vegetarian?
4. How would you address her concerns about getting fat?
5. What advice would you give to Carly's parents regarding their food-related interactions with her?

habits that affect nutrient intake. Adolescents with special needs, such as those who participate in sports, have a chronic illness, are pregnant, diet excessively, or use alcohol and drugs, need to pay even more attention to their nutrition. Understanding the nutrition and physical activity needs of adolescents is important in helping them to develop a healthy body and lifestyle.

Relevant Web Sites

American College of Sports Medicine
www.acsm.org
American Diabetic Association
www.eatright.org
American School Health Association
www.ashaweb.org
Bright Futures
www.brightfutures.org
www.cdc.gov/growthcharts
National Eating Disorder Association
www.edap.org

Cited References

Alaimo K et al: *Dietary intake of vitamins, minerals, and fiber of persons ages 2 months and over in the United States: third National Health and Nutrition Examination Survey, Phase 1, 1988-91. Advance data from vital and health statistics,* No. 258, Hyattsville, Md, 1994, National Center for Health Statistics.

Albertson AM et al: Estimated dietary calcium intake and food sources for adolescent females: 1980-92, *J Adolesc Health Care* 20:20, 1997.

American Academy of Pediatrics: Position committee. Calcium requirements of infants, children and adolescents, *Pediatrics,* 104(5):1152, 1999.

American Dietetic Association: Position on nutrition care for pregnant adolescents, *J Am Diet Assoc* 94:449, 1994.

American Dietetic Association: Position of the American Dietetic Association: food fortification and dietary supplements, *J Am Diet Assoc* 101:115, 2001.

Barlow SE, Dietz WH: Obesity evaluation and treatment: expert committee recommendations, *Pediatrics* 102(3):1, 1998.

Berenson GS et al: Precursors of cardiovascular risk in young adults from a biracial (black-white) population: the Bogalusa Heart Study. In Jacobson MS et al, eds: *Adolescent nutritional disorders: prevention and treatment,* New York, 1998, The New York Academy of Science.

Brown JD, Witherspoon EM: *The mass media and American adolescents' health.* Proceedings of the Health Futures of Youth! Pathways to Adolescent Health Conference, Annapolis, Md, September 14, 1998.

Bunnell DW et al: Subclinical versus formal eating disorders: differentiating psychological features, *Int J Eating Disorder* 9:357, 1990.

Centers for Disease Control and Prevention, National Center for Chronic Disease Prevention and Health Promotion, President's Council on Physical Fitness and Sports: *Physical activity and health: a report of the Surgeon General,* Washington, DC, 1996, CDC.

Centers for Disease Control and Prevention: Recommendations and reports: recommendations to prevent and control iron deficiency in the United States, *MMWR Morb Mortal Wkly Rep* 47:(RR-3), 1998.

Centers for Disease Control and Prevention: Surveillence summaries: youth risk behavior surveillance, United States, *MMWR Morb Mortal Wkly Rep* 51:(SS-4), 2002.

Channel One Network: *Teen fact book,* New York, 2000, Channel One Network.

Chapman G, Maclean H: "Junk food" and "healthy food": meanings of food in adolescent women's culture, *J Nutr Educ* 25:108, 1993.

Christoffel KK, Ariza A: The epidemiology of overweight in children: relevance for clinical care, *Pediatrics* 101:103, 1998.

Corbin CB, Pangrazi RP: *Physical activity for children: a statement of guidelines,* Reston, Va, 1998, National Association for Sport and Physical Education.

Devaney BL et al: Dietary intakes of students, *Am J Clin Nutr* 61(suppl):205, 1995.

Dietz WH: Use of the body mass index (BMI) as a measure of overweight in children and adolescents, *J Pediatr* 132:191, 1998.

Emmons L: Predisposing factors differentiating adolescent dieters and nondieters, *J Am Diet Assoc* 94:725, 1994.

Flodmark C-E et al: Prevention of progression to severe obesity in a group of obese schoolchildren treated with family therapy, *Pediatrics* 91:880, 1993.

Food and Nutrition Board, National Academy of Sciences: *Recommended dietary allowances,* ed 10, Washington, DC, 1989, National Academy of Sciences, National Academy Press.

Freedman DS et al: Relationship of childhood obesity to coronary heart disease risk factors in adulthood: the Bogalusa heart study, *Pediatrics* 108:712, 2001.

Gilman MW et al: Risk of overweight among adolescents who were breastfed as infants, *JAMA* 285(19):2461, 2001

Golden NH: Osteoporosis prevention: a pediatric challenge, *Arch Pediatr Adolesc Med* 154:542, 2000.

Gortmaker SL et al: Social and economic consequences of overweight in adolescence and young adulthood, *N Engl J Med* 329:1008, 1993.

Greger N, Edwin CM: Obesity: a pediatric epidemic, *Pediatr Ann* 30(1):694-700, 2001.

Halterman, JS et al: Iron deficiency and cognitive achievement among school-aged children and adolescents in the United States, *Pediatrics* 107:1381, 2001.

Hampi JS, Betts NM: Cigarette use during adolescence: effects on nutritional status, *Nutr Rev* 57:215, 1999.

Harnack L, Stang J, Story M: Soft drink consumption among U.S. children and adolescents: nutritional consequences, *J Am Diet Assoc* 99:436, 1999.

Hediger ML et al: Implications of the Camden Study of adolescent pregnancy: interactions among maternal growth, nutrition status, and body composition. In Jacobson MS et al, eds: *Adolescent nutritional disorders: prevention and treatment,* New York, 1998, New York Academy of Science.

Herbold NH, Frates SE: Update of nutrition guidelines for the teen: trends and concerns, *Curr Opin Pediatr* 12(4):303-309, 2000.

Institute of Medicine, Committee on Nutrition Status During Pregnancy and Lactation: *Nutrition during pregnancy, part 1. Weight gain,* Washington, DC, 1990, National Academy Press.

Institute of Medicine, Food and Nutrition Board: *Dietary reference intakes for calcium, phosphorus, magnesium, vitamin D, and fluoride,* Washington, DC, 1997, National Academy Press.

Institute of Medicine, Food and Nutrition Board: *Dietary reference intakes for energy, and the macronutrients, carbohydrate, fiber, fat, fatty acids, cholesterol, protein and amino acids,* Washington, DC, 2002, National Academy Press.

Institue of Medicine, Food, and Nutrition Board: *Dietary reference intakes for thiamin, riboflavin, niacin, vitamin B-6, folate, vitamin B-12, pantothenic acid, biotin and choline,* Washington, DC, 1998, National Academy Press.

Jacobson MF: *Liquid candy: how soft drinks are harming Americans' health,* Washington, DC, 1998, Center for Science in the Public Interest.

Johnson RK, Panely C, Wang MQ: The association between noontime beverage consumption and the diet quality of school-aged children, *J Child Nutr Mgt* 2:95-100, 1998.

Kreipe RE, Birndorf DO: Eating disorders in adolescents and young adults, *Med Clin North Am* 84(4):1027-1049, 2000.

Lytle L: Nutritional issues for adolescents, *JADA* 102:S8, 2002.

Marshall WA, Tanner JM: Variations in the pattern of pubertal changes in boys, *Arch Dis Child* 45:13, 1970.

Moore DC: Body image and eating behavior in adolescent girls, *Am J Dis Child* 142:144, 1988.

Moore DC: Body image and eating behavior in adolescent boys, *Am J Dis Child* 144:475, 1990.

Must A et al: Long-term morbidity and mortality of overweight adolescents, *N Engl J Med* 327:1350, 1992.

National Cholesterol Education Program: *Report of the Expert Panel on Blood Cholesterol Levels in Children and Adolescents,* National Institutes of Health Pub No 91-2732, September, 1991, National Heart, Lung and Blood Institute, Public Health Service.

National Institutes of Health: *Consensus Development Conference statement: optimal calcium intake, JAMA* 272:1942, 1994.

Nicklas TA et al: School-based programs for health-risk reduction. In Jacobson MS et al, eds: *Adolescent nutritional disorders: prevention and treatment,* New York, 1998, The New York Academy of Science.

Patrick K et al, eds: *Bright futures in practice: physical activit*y, Arlington, Va, 2002, National Center for Education in Maternal and Child Health.

Resnick MD et al: Health and risk behaviors of urban adolescent males involved in pregnancy, *Fam Soc* 74:366, 1993.

Sallis JF, Patrick K: Physical activity guidelines for adolescents: consensus statement, *Pediatr Exer Sci* 6(4):302-314, 1994.

Sanders T: Vegetarian diets and children, *Pediatr Clin North Am* 42(4):955-965, 1995.

Scholl TO et al: Maternal growth and fetal growth: pregnancy course and outcome in the Camden Study. In Jacobson MS et al, eds: *Adolescent nutritional disorders: prevention and treatment,* New York, 1998, The New York Academy of Science.

Sigman-Grant M: Strategies for counseling adolescents, *JADA* 102:S32, 2002.

Spear BA: Adolescent growth and development. In Rickert VI, ed: *Adolescent nutrition: assessment and management, pp 3-24,* New York, 1996, Chapman and Hall.

Spear BA, Stellefson-Myers E: Position of the American Dietetic Association: nutrition intervention in the treatment of anorexia nervosa, bulimia nervosa, and eating disorders not otherwise specified (EDNOS), *JADA* 101:810, 2001.

Stang J: Assessment of nutritional status and motivation to make behavior changes among adolescents, *JADA* 102:S13, 2002.

Stang J et al: Relationship between vitamin and mineral supplement use, dietary intake and dietary adequacy among adolescents, *JADA* 100:905, 2000.

Steen SN: Timely statement of the American Dietetic Association: nutrition guidance for adolescent athletes in organized sports, *J Am Diet Assoc* 96:610, 1996.

Story M, Holt K, Sofka D, eds: *Bright futures in practice: nutrition,* ed 2, Arlington, Va, 2002, National Center for Education in Maternal and Child Health.

Story M, Neumark-Sztainer D, French S: Individual and environmental influences on adolescent eating behaviors, *JADA* 102:S40-S51; 2002.

Story M, Resnick MD: Adolescents' views on food and nutrition, *J Nutr Educ* 18:188, 1986.

Story M, Stang J: *Nutrition and the pregnant adolescent,* 2000, University of Minnesota, Center for Leadership Education and Training in Maternal and Child Health.

Striegel-Moore R: Risk factors for eating disorders. In Jacobson MS et al, eds: *Adolescent nutritional disorders: prevention and treatment,* pp 98-109, New York, 1997, The New York Academy of Science.

Suitor CW, Bailey LB: Dietary folate equivalents: interpretation and application, *JADA* 100:88-94, 2000.

Troiano RP, Flegal KM: Overweight children and adolescents: description, epidemiology and demographics, *Pediatrics* 101(suppl): 497, 1998.

Williams CL et al: Management of childhood obesity in pediatric practice. In Jacobson MS et al: *Adolescent nutritional disorders: prevention and treatment,* New York, 1998, The New York Academy of Science.

World Health Organization: Physical status: the use and interpretation of anthropometry: report of a WHO Expert Committee, *WHO Tech Rep Ser* 854:1-452, 1995.

Wyshak G: Teenage girls, carbohydrate beverage consumption and bone fractures, *Arch Pediatr Adolesc Med* 154:610-613, 2000.

Yates AM et al: Dietary reference intakes: the new basis for recommendations for calcium and related nutrients, B vitamins and choline, *J Am Diet Assoc* 98:699, 1998.

■ Additional References

Frisancho AR et al: Developmental and nutritional determinants of pregnancy outcome among teenagers, *Am J Phys Anthropol* 66:247, 1985.

Frisch RE: Fatness of girls from menarche to age 18 years, with a nomogram, *Hum Biol* 48:353, 1976.

Gong EJ, Spear BA: Adolescent growth and development: Implications for nutritional needs, *J Nutr Educ* 20:273, 1988.

Hammer LD et al: Standardized percentile curves of body-mass index for children and adolescents, *Am J Dis Child* 145:259, 1991.

Himes JH, Dietz WH: Guidelines for overweight in adolescent preventive services: recommendations from an expert committee, *Am J Clin Nutr* 59:307, 1994.

Johnson RK et al: Characterizing nutrient intakes of adolescents by sociodemographic factors, *J Adolesc Health* 15:149, 1994.

Merzenich H et al: Dietary fat and sports activity as determinants for age at menarche, *Am J Epidemiol* 138:217, 1993.

Meserole LP et al: Prenatal weight gain and postpartum weight loss pattern in adolescents, *J Adolesc Health Care* 5:21, 1984.

Must A et al: Reference data for obesity: 85th and 95th percentiles of body mass index (wt/ht^2) and triceps skinfold thickness, *Am J Clin Nutr* 53:839, 1991.

Must A et al: Reference data for obesity: 85th and 95th percentiles of body mass index (wt/ht^2)—a correction, *Am J Clin Nutr* 54:773, 1991.

Results from the National Adolescent Student Health Survey, *JAMA* 261:2025, 1989.

Schlicker SA et al: The weight and fitness status of United States children, *Nutr Rev* 52:11, 1994.

Spear BA, ed: Adolescent nutrition: a springboard for health, *J Am Diet Assoc* 102:7-111(suppl), 2002.

Stettler N: Environmental factors in the etiology of obesity in adolescents, *Ethn Dis* 12(1):S1-41, 2002.

Tanner JM: *Fetus into man: physical growth from conception to maturity,* Cambridge, Mass, 1978, Harvard University Press.

Wright LS: Physiological development in adolescence. In Mahan LK, Rees JM: *Nutrition in adolescence,* St Louis, 1984, Mosby.

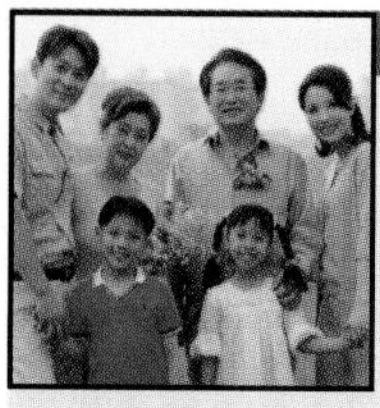

CHAPTER 12

Nutrition in the Adult Years

KIMBERLY MATHAI, MS, RD, CN

CHAPTER OUTLINE

- Eating and the Food Environment
- Defensive Nutrition Paradigm
- Gastrointestinal Integrity
- Detoxification Systems
- Guidelines for a Defensive Nutrition Paradigm

KEY TERMS

allyl sulfides–organosulfur phytochemicals found in allium vegetables; may act as cancer-blocking or cancer-suppressing agents

butyric acid (butyrate)–a short-chain fatty acid that is the preferred fuel of intestinal cells; produced by bacterial fermentation of dietary fiber

carotenoids–a subclass of terpene phytochemicals found in some vegetables, including tomatoes, parsley, oranges, pink grapefruit, and spinach

cytochrome P-450 (mixed-function oxidase system [MFOS])–a family of enzymes involved in phase I of the liver detoxification system

defensive nutrition paradigm–a nutrition plan that includes plant-based foods and balancing the intake of healthy fats to prevent disease and promote wellness

detoxification–a process that decreases the negative impact of xenobiotics or toxins on the body.

dithiolthiones, indoles, isothiocyanates–organosulfur phytochemicals; a subclass of thiols found in cruciferous vegetables

flavonoids–a subclass of phenol phytochemicals; pigments that act as free radical scavengers in plants

glycemic index–a ranking of the effect on blood glucose of the consumption of a single food relative to a reference carbohydrate (e.g., white bread, glucose)

glycemic load–the glycemic index of a food multiplied by the carbohydrate present in the food; measures both the quantity and the quality (i.e., nature and source) of a carbohydrate's effect on blood glucose and insulin release

gut-associated lymphoid tissue (GALT)–lymphoid tissue surrounding the digestive tract; generates almost 70% of the body's antibodies and contains the greatest number of lymphocytes in the body

insulin resistance–a defect in glucose metabolism at the cellular level

isoflavones–a subclass of phenol phytochemicals; found in beans and other legumes (especially soybeans) and may have cancer-preventing properties, especially against hormone-linked cancers

***Lactobacillus* organisms**–beneficial intestinal organisms that produce organic acids to retard the growth of pathogenic bacteria

lignans–phytoestrogens found in flax seed, wheat bran, and other whole grains; affect sex hormone metabolism and may reduce the risk of hormone-linked cancer

limonoids–a subclass of terpenes found in citrus fruits; identified as chemopreventive agents that induce enzymes in phases I and II of the liver's enzyme detoxification system

lycopene–one of the carotenoid phytochemicals found in tomatoes; acts as a free radical scavenger

metabolic syndrome–a cluster of metabolic disorders, including non–insulin-dependent diabetes mellitus, hypertension, and dyslipidemia, that are characterized by insulin resistance

phase I and phase II detoxification system–the sequential two-stage enzyme detoxification process of the liver during which toxic molecules are biotransformed from lipid-soluble substances into water-soluble molecules that can then be excreted from the body

phenols–a class of phytochemicals that function in plants as blue, blue-red, and violet pigments and provide protection against oxidative damage

phytochemicals–biologically active, naturally existing substances in plants that act as natural defense systems in plants and show potential for reducing risk for cancer and cardiovascular disease

phytoestrogens–phytochemicals that are nonsteroidal estrogens of dietary origin; structurally similar to estrogens and act as weak estrogens and antiestrogens

plant-based diet–an eating plan in which plant foods (e.g., vegetables, fruit, legumes, grains) provide a significant portion of the nutrients and calories

prebiotics–nondigestible food products that stimulate the growth of symbiotic bacterial species already present in the colon

probiotics–microbial foods or supplements that can be used to change or reestablish the intestinal flora and improve the health of the host

terpenes–the largest class of phytochemicals; found in a wide variety of plants

thiols–sulfur-containing phytonutrients found in cruciferous vegetables

xenobiotics–substances foreign to the body

Nutrition in the adult years emphasizes the importance of diet in maintaining wellness and preventing disease. The role of nutrition has expanded significantly, and it is now viewed as a tool that can be used not just to prevent disease but to promote health. *Healthy People 2010,* a U.S. Department of Health and Human Services (DHHS) report, recognizes the importance of nutrition and other lifestyle factors in achieving health goals and increasing the years and quality of healthy life of Americans. This report states that "the leading causes of death—heart disease, cancer, stroke, chronic obstructive pulmonary disease, and unintentional injuries—can be attributed, at least in part, to behaviors and environmental factors." (USDHHS, 2000).

EATING AND THE FOOD ENVIRONMENT

What Americans Eat

Information about prevalent adult food patterns in the United States can be culled from government reports. Researchers examined data from the U.S. Department of Agriculture (USDA) Economic Research Service to describe U.S. dietary patterns (Putnam, Kantor, and Allshouse, 2000). They contrasted per capita food supply trends with government recommendations as stated in the Food Guide Pyramid and found the following:

- Five foods—iceberg lettuce, frozen potatoes (primarily French fries), fresh potatoes, potato chips, and canned tomatoes—accounted for 52% of the total vegetable consumption in 1999. Potatoes are the dominant vegetable, and the consumption of dark-green leafy vegetables and deep yellow vegetables was extremely low.
- Cheese accounts for more than two fifths of total daily dairy servings. Whole milk consumption decreased by 21% between 1970-1979 and 1999, but consumption of high-fat cheeses increased 76% in the same period.
- American adults eat less than half of the recommended three fruit servings per day. Six foods—orange juice (19%), bananas (11%), fresh apples (7%), apple juice (6%), watermelon (6%), and fresh grapes (6%)—represent more than half (55%) of all fruit servings consumed in 1999.
- The per capita grain consumption has increased almost 50% since the early 1970s, but cakes, cookies, pastries, and pies accounted for 13% of the grain consumption in 1994-1996. Less than 2% of total wheat flour consumed was whole-wheat flour (in 1992, the last year for which data are available).
- Consumption of added fats increased dramatically during the survey period, with the per capita daily intake increasing to 64 g of added fat in 1999, a 32% increase from the early 1970s. Shortening and margarine (major sources of *trans* fats) added to processed foods such as baked goods, French fries, and snack foods, accounted for more than one third of added fats. Other sources of added fat included cooking and salad oils and animal fat (e.g., lard, butter, and other dairy fats).
- The consumption of added sugars is almost triple the recommended amounts. In 1999, Americans were eating 34 teaspoons of added sugars daily—three times the suggested 12 teaspoons per 2200 calories suggested in the Food Guide Pyramid.

These food patterns are a distorted version of the Food Guide Pyramid (Figure 12-1). The grain group, at the base of the pyramid, is heavily weighted with highly refined grain foods. Vegetable and fruit consumption is below the recommended amounts and includes little variety. Dairy and calcium-rich food consumption is half of the recommended amount, and far too many unhealthy fats and sugars are consumed (Putnam, Kantor, and Allshouse, 2000).

The result of these dietary patterns is escalating rates of obesity among Americans of all ages. Almost 64% of American adults are either overweight or obese, and 31% of American adults are at least 30 lb overweight (i.e., obese) according to the Centers for Disease Control and Prevention (CDC). Larger portion sizes, increased consumption of fast foods, and sedentary lifestyles are linked to increasing obesity (CDC, 2000). Overweight adults are at increased risk for many acute and chronic diseases, including hypertension, dyslipidemia, coronary heart disease, gallbladder disease, some types of cancer, and arthritis (Flegal et al, 2002).

How Americans Eat

Adult social models influence food shopping, food preparation, and the frequency of sit-down meals in a home environment. Social models include single adulthood, partnered adulthood without children, single-parent adulthood, adulthood in a two-parent working family, and adulthood in a two-parent family with one parent at home as caretaker. Responsibilities of working or single parents and stresses related to long working or commuting hours affect eating habits. Too little time for food planning may lead to meal patterns that rely heavily on processed foods, take-out foods, or restaurant-prepared meals, with only sporadic meals prepared and eaten at home. According to government researchers, Americans spend 47% of their food dollars away from home. From 1998 to 1999, food expenditures for eating out grew faster than retail food expenditures (Clauson, 1999).

Many adults, especially young adults, have food intake patterns that rely on restaurant or take-out convenience foods. Indeed, one survey found that of more than 18,000 persons who frequented restaurants three or more times per week, more than 20% were in their 20s (Leach, 1998).

The discussed psychosocial factors contribute to food choices and patterns that may lead to steady weight gain in adulthood. Unhealthy food choices not only lead to weight gain but also contribute to the probability that an individual can develop a chronic disease.

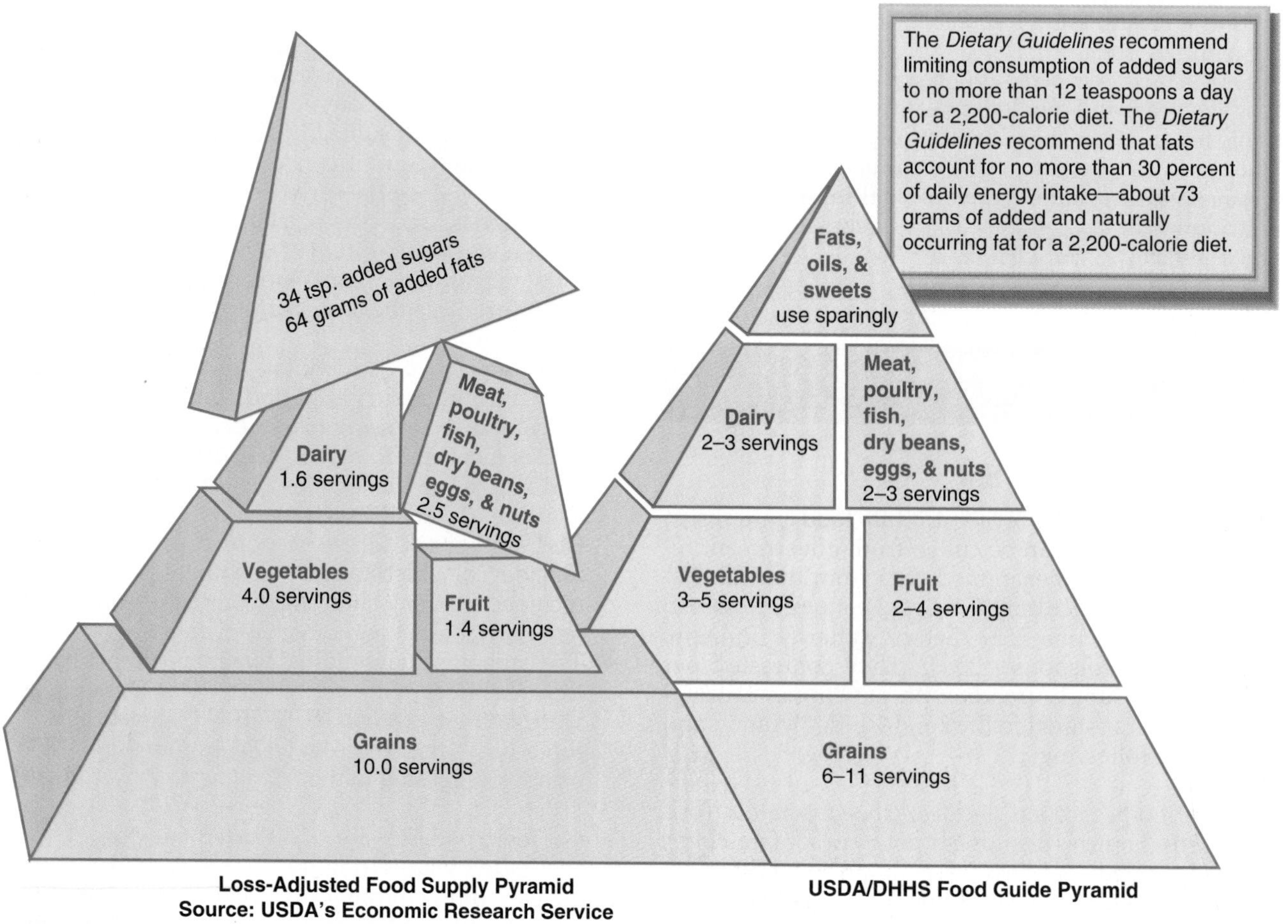

FIGURE 12-1 • The unbalanced American diet. (From Economic Research Service of the U.S. Department of Agriculture: *Food review* 23(3):13, 2001.)

DEFENSIVE NUTRITION PARADIGM

A defensive nutrition paradigm for adults in the twenty-first century emphasizes making food choices to promote wellness and support organ systems for optimal functioning during aging. This nutrition paradigm organizes the new American diet using more plant-based foods: fruits, vegetables, whole grains, and nuts and legumes. Other foods in a defensive nutrition paradigm include fish and eggs and lean animal proteins such as poultry or wild game. Consumption of red meats such as beef, pork, and lamb is limited. Healthy fats, including monounsaturated and omega-3 essential fatty acids, low-fat dairy products, and fermented food products, should also be added.

Combined with a regular exercise program, a plant-based diet can help adults maintain a healthy weight. Plant-based food programs can have a significant and positive impact on aging by reducing the risk of cardiovascular disease, cancer, diabetes, and other chronic diseases (Lampe, 1999). Increased fruit and vegetable intake reduces incidence of diseases like cardiovascular disease and cancer. Researchers who monitored almost 10,000 American adults for 19 years found that fruit and vegetable intake is inversely related to cardiovascular disease and all causes of mortality in general (Bazzano et al, 2002). In a landmark study an international panel of experts reviewed more than 4500 research studies to determine the relationships among food, nutrition, and cancer, the second leading cause of death among Americans. These experts estimated that cancer rates would decrease by as much as 20% if people would eat five or more servings of fruits and vegetables per day (American Institute for Cancer Research, 1997).

To understand the value of plant-based diets, it is important to (1) understand the components in plant-based foods that specifically protect cellular mechanisms in humans and (2) learn how these plant-based foods support organ systems in the body that protect against chronic disease.

Phytochemicals

Plant foods contain not only major nutrient components (e.g., protein, fat, carbohydrates, fiber, and micronutrients such as vitamins and minerals) but also large numbers of nonnutrient compounds called *phytochemicals.* Phytochemicals (from the Greek word *phyto,* meaning "plant") are biologically active, naturally occurring chemical components in plant foods. In plants, phytochemicals act as natural defense systems for their host plants, protecting the plants from infections and microbial invasions and providing color, aroma, and flavor. More than 2000 plant pigments are considered phytochemicals—pigments such as flavonoids, carotenoids, and anthocyanins. Dietary sources of phytochemicals (Table 12-1) include fruits, vegetables, legumes, whole grains, nuts, seeds, fungi, herbs, and spices (Craig, 1997; King and Young, 1999).

Phytochemicals are the subject of intense scientific research focusing on the prevention or treatment of chronic diseases such as cancer and heart disease. As protection against cancer, plant-based chemicals detoxify drugs, toxins, carcinogens, and mutagens. These detoxification actions have overlapping and complementary mechanisms such as neutralizing free radicals, inhibiting enzymes that activate carcinogens, and inducing enzymes that detoxify carcinogens (Lampe, 1999; Steinmetz and Potter, 1996).

Because they act as blocking, or suppressing, agents, phytochemicals may reduce the risk of cancer. Blocking agents prevent the active carcinogen or tumor promoter from reaching the target tissue by several mechanisms or a combination of mechanisms: (1) by inducing activities of enzyme systems that detoxify carcinogens, (2) by trapping and se-

TABLE 12-1 Phytochemicals and Their Sources

PHYTOCHEMICAL	SOURCE
Butyrate	Fruits, vegetables, legumes
Carotenoids	Dark yellow, dark orange, and deep green vegetables and fruit
Diallyl sulfide	Onions, garlic, scallions, leeks, chives
Flavonoids and phenols	Parsley, carrots, citrus fruits, broccoli, cabbage, cucumbers, squash, yams, tomatoes, eggplant, peppers, soy products, berries, potatoes, broad beans, pea pods, colored onions, radishes, horseradish, tea, onions, apples
Indoles	Cabbage, Brussels sprouts, cauliflower, spinach, broccoli
Isoflavones	Soybeans, soybean products
Isothiocyanates	Cabbage, cauliflower, broccoli, Brussels sprouts, mustard, horseradish, radishes
Flavonoids	Fruits, vegetables, wine, green tea, onions, kale, beans
Lignans	Flax seed, whole-grain products
Limonene	Citrus oil
Lycopenes	Tomatoes, red grapefruit, guava, dried apricots
Organosulfuric compounds	Garlic, onions, chives, citrus fruits, broccoli, cabbage, cauliflower, Brussels sprouts
Terpenes and monoterpenes	Citrus fruits, parsley, carrots, celery, broccoli, cabbage, cauliflower, cucumbers, squash, yams, tomatoes, eggplant, peppers, mint, basil, caraway seeds

questering reactive carcinogens, or (3) by blocking cellular events required for tumor promotion. Suppressing agents, the actions of which are less well defined, may arrest carcinogenesis by acting on the cellular level and preventing malignant expression of cells that have been exposed to cancer-causing agents (Wattenberg, 1997) (see Chapter 40). Phytochemicals seem to reduce the risk of coronary heart disease by protecting low-density lipoprotein (LDL) cholesterol from oxidation, reducing the synthesis or absorption of cholesterol, and affecting blood pressure and clotting (Craig and Beck, 1999) (see Chapters 35 and 36).

Phytochemicals are grouped into classes on the basis of their similar protective functions and individual physical and chemical characteristics. The major classes of phytochemicals include the terpenes, phenols, and thiols.

Terpenes

The terpenes, one of the largest classes of phytonutrients, are found in a wide variety of plant foods and act as powerful antioxidants. Carotenoids comprise one subclass of terpenes that has been studied extensively. More than 600 naturally occurring carotenoids exist; they are yellow, orange, and red plant pigments. The most prevalent carotenoids include α-carotene, β-carotene, β-cryptoxanthin, lycopene, lutein, and zeaxanthin. Fruits and vegetables that contain carotenoids include apricots, papayas, sweet potatoes, mangoes, corn, pumpkins, carrots, tomatoes, parsley, oranges, pink grapefruit, and spinach. Processed tomato products such as spaghetti sauce have carotenoids with the highest availability. (Holden et al, 1999) (see Appendix 47).

Lycopene, a carotenoid in tomatoes, has been called one of the most effective biologic singlet oxygen quenchers; it is two times as powerful as β-carotene in the destruction of free radicals. Researchers who reviewed 57 of 72 studies found that consumption of tomatoes and tomato-containing foods was correlated with reduced risks of prostate, lung, and stomach cancer (Giovannucci et al, 1999).

Limonoids are another subclass of terpenes *(monoterpenes)* found in citrus fruits such as grapefruit and orange juice. The limonoids have been identified as chemopreventive agents that induce enzymes in the liver's *phase I and II enzyme detoxification* system. This system detoxifies carcinogens by making them more water soluble for excretion from the body (Craig, 1997).

Phenols

Phenols are phytochemicals that protect plants from oxidative damage; they include the subclass flavonoids. More than 800 flavonoids, which are the blue, blue-red, and violet plant pigments, have been identified. Flavonoids scavenge free radical compounds, such as superoxide anion and singlet oxygen, and sequester metal ions. Anthocyanins are phytochemicals in the flavonoid family that give the bluish-red pigments to blueberries, cherries, grapes, cranberries, currants, red cabbage, and raspberries. Blueberries, whether wild or cultivated, may be one of the richest sources of plant-derived antioxidants (Halvorsen et al, 2002).

Phenolic flavonoids are antioxidants that may help prevent some chronic diseases. Flavonoids have free radical scavenging properties and are chelators of metal ions; thus they may protect tissues against free oxygen radicals and lipid peroxidation (Knekt et al, 2002). Researchers studied the eating habits and examined the disease history of more than 10,000 Finnish men and women to determine the link between phytochemicals and disease. They found that people who ate foods high in *quercetin,* a flavonoid antioxidant found in foods such as apples and onions, had 21% lower risk of mortality from ischemic heart disease and were 19% less likely to have type 2 diabetes (Knekt et al, 2002) (see Chapter 35).

Isoflavones are a phenol subclass found in beans and other legumes, especially soybeans and soy foods. Isoflavones have a wide range of health effects, including reduction of the risk of heart disease. An elevated serum cholesterol level, one risk factor associated with heart disease, can be significantly lowered by consuming soy protein. A meta-analysis of 38 research studies on the effect of soy on blood lipids revealed that 25 to 50 g of soy protein daily decreases LDL cholesterol levels by approximately 10% in those with hypercholesterolemia (Anderson et al, 1995) (Table 12-2). Soy's amino acid profile and isoflavones seem to be the bioactive components that improve arterial elasticity and protect LDL cholesterol from oxidation (Potter, 1998).

Some isoflavones are phytoestrogens (also known as *phytosterols*), which are weak, nonsteroidal versions of estrogens. Phytoestrogens have 1/100,000 to 1/1000 the strength of steroidal estrogens, and they exert biologic effects as they fit estrogen receptor sites. They act as weak estrogens (agonists) and as antiestrogens (antagonists). Phytoestrogens in soy foods act as antioxidants, carcinogen blockers, or tumor

TABLE 12-2 Soy Protein Content of Soy Foods

SOY FOOD	SERVING SIZE	SOY PROTEIN (grams)
Soy "sausage" link	One link	6.0
Soy "burger"	One burger	10.0-12.0
Tofu (firm)	4 oz	13.0
Roasted soy nuts	¼ cup	19.0
Tempeh	½ cup	19.5
Plain soy milk	8 oz	10.0

From Henkel J: Soy: health claims for soy protein: questions about other components, U.S. Food and Drug Administration, *FDA Consumer,* May-June 2000, www.cfsan.fda.gov/~dms/fdsoypr.html.

suppressors and may help prevent hormone-related tumors (e.g., breast cancer) by reducing estrogen binding at receptor sites, down-regulating estrogen receptors, or favorably altering estrogen metabolism (Xu et al, 2000). Phytoestrogens may be useful in preventing or helping people survive prostate cancer because they act as estrogen-like agonists and seem to inhibit prostate cancer cell growth. Isoflavones, particularly, *genistein,* may modulate prostate-specific antigen (PSA) expression in prostate cancer cells and decrease secreted and intracellular levels of PSA (Davis, Kucuk, and Sarkar, 2002) (see *Focus On:* Soy).

Thiols

Thiol is a sulfur-containing phytonutrient found in cruciferous vegetables such as broccoli, cauliflower, brussels sprouts, kale, and cabbage. Cruciferous vegetables contain subclasses of thiols called dithiolthiones, indoles, and isothiocyanates. These organosulfuric compounds up-regulate enzymes involved in the detoxification of carcinogens and other foreign compounds (Talalay and Fahey, 2001).

In cohort and case control studies, researchers have found an inverse relationship between the consumption of broccoli, cabbage, and cauliflower and the risk of cancer. The association between increased vegetable consumption and decreased cancer risk is most consistent for cancers of the lung, stomach, colon, and rectum (van Poppel et al, 1999).

Organosulfur compounds are also found in the allium, or onion, family, which includes garlic, shallots, and leeks. The phytochemicals in garlic, the allyl sulfides, and other organosulfur compounds seem to prevent carcinogen activation. Allyl sulfides have several actions, including (1) increasing the production of glutathione-*S*-transferase, a phase II enzyme of the liver's detoxification system; (2) inhibiting mutagenesis; and (3) increasing the activity of macrophages and T lymphocytes (Milner, 2001).

Lignans

Lignans, phytochemicals found in flax seed, wheat bran, rye meal, buckwheat, oatmeal, and barley, are a focus of research because of their anticancer and phytoestrogen properties. The richest source of lignans is flax seed, which contains 75 to 800 times more lignans than any other plant food (Serraino and Thompson, 1992). The plant lignans are converted to mammalian lignans by gut bacteria and have biologic properties that include antimitotic and antioxidant activity.

Lignans are phytoestrogens that may help prevent hormone-sensitive cancers because of their interference with endogenous sex hormone production. Studies of premenopausal and postmenopausal women suggest that the plant lignans in flax stimulate sex-hormone-binding globulin and modulate the ratio of estrogen metabolites used as biomarkers for breast cancer risk (Dai et al, 2002; Hutchins et al, 2001).

In summary, phytochemicals in plants and plant-based foods are powerful antioxidants and metabolism regulators that may help prevent the development of chronic disease.

FOCUS ON

Soy

Soy foods are the richest source of isoflavones (soy phytochemicals); genistein, daidzein, and glycitein are the major isoflavones in soy. Consumption of this class of phytoestrogens has documented health benefits, including reduction of hypercholesterolemia, maintenance of prostate health, and possibly increased bone density and reduction of the risk of hormone-dependent cancers (Messina and Erdman, 1998).

The ancient Chinese considered soy, which is native to eastern Asia, to be one of the five sacred grains vital for life. The United States is now the world's largest producer of soybeans. Soybeans are 13% to 25% oil, 30% to 50% protein, and 14% to 24% carbohydrate—2% to 5% is fiber. Soy protein is nutritionally equivalent to proteins derived from animal sources such as eggs, milk, and meat (Young et al, 1984).

Asian populations are known to have a lower incidence of breast, prostate, and other cancers, which epidemiologists hypothesize may be attributable to their average daily intake of one serving of soy (equal to approximately 40 mg of isoflavones). Japanese women consume large amounts of soy foods, which may account for their lower incidence of menopausal symptoms (Adlercreutz et al, 1991). Studies investigating the health benefits of soy foods have involved participants with intakes of 45 to 90 mg of isoflavones per day (approximately two to three servings of soy foods).

In October 1999 the FDA approved food label claims of reduced risk of heart disease on food that contains 6.25 g of soy protein per serving. To qualify for the claim, the food must also be low in fat (less than 3 g) and saturated fat (less than 1 g), low in cholesterol (less than 20 mg), and have a sodium value of less than 480 mg if it is an individual food, less than 720 mg if it is considered a main dish, and less than 960 mg if it is considered an entire meal (Henkel, 2000).

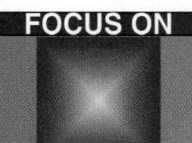

Organ Support

A defensive nutrition paradigm also provides nutritional support for organ systems that defend the body against chronic disease. These major body systems include (1) the gastrointestinal (GI) system, which absorbs nutrients for the body, protects the body from toxins, and acts as part of the body's immune system; and (2) the liver, with its two-phase enzyme detoxification system that acts as a disposal system for procarcinogens and other toxins. These two organ systems have a profound effect on immune, nervous, and endocrine systems that help maintain health.

GASTROINTESTINAL INTEGRITY

The GI system has a vital and unique function in each person. The gut is a conduit for nutrients into systemic circulation and a barrier against toxins from various sources (see Chapter 1). These toxins include exotoxins, such as drugs and chemicals, and endotoxins, such as bacterial waste, food antigens (foreign proteins), and the breakdown products of metabolism. Optimal functioning of the GI system is based on intestinal integrity; the mucous membrane absorbs and assimilates foods and serves as a barrier against pathogens or other antigens. When intestinal integrity is compromised, the permeability of the gut may be altered and gut function erodes. Two factors that influence intestinal integrity are the health of the gut mucosa and a balanced bacterial population in the gut. The gut's mucosa and bacteria are affected by nutrients.

Intestinal Mucosa

One of the major functions of the intestinal mucosa is to block antigenic or pathogenic molecules or microorganisms from entering the systemic circulation. The GI mucosa is composed of close-fitting, thin, and semipermeable epithelial cells that are separated by tight junctures. When the mucosa is disrupted, the intestine's permeability may increase and allow bacteria from the gut, undigested food, or toxins to cross the barrier (see Chapters 32 and 42).

The exact etiology of altered intestinal permeability is unclear, but dietary intake and bacterial imbalances in the gut have been suggested as factors. Conditions that have been linked to excessive gut permeability include (1) delayed transit of food through the intestine and (2) delayed peristalsis (Levin, 1994). Both of these conditions are linked to a lack of dietary fiber, the addition of which not only improves bowel transit time and intestinal muscle activity but also protects gut integrity by nourishing intestinal cells (see Chapters 1, 3, and 30).

Gut integrity is related to a balance of intestinal bacteria and the healthy nourishment of enterocytes and colonocytes, the intestinal mucosal cells. More than 50% of the energy needs of the small intestine and more than 80% of the large intestine's energy needs must come from food components in the organ. The preferred fuels of the intestinal cells are the short-chain fatty acids (SCFAs) *butyrate, acetate,* and *propionate.* Dietary fibers, particularly soluble fiber, are the sources of these fuels. In the colon, beneficial gut bacteria, primarily the bifidobacteria, metabolize SCFAs from indigestible carbohydrates in dietary fiber. Butyric acid, or butyrate, is the preferred cellular food of the large intestine (i.e., the colonocytes) and is produced only by fermentation action of gut bacteria on dietary fiber. The SCFAs *proprionate* and *acetate* are used primarily by the liver for energy production, but the by-products of their metabolism, including glutamine, glutamate, and acetoacetate, are preferred to glucose as fuels for enterocytes, the cells of the small intestine (Windmueller and Spaeth, 1990) (see Chapter 1).

Intestinal Microflora

General Properties

The intestinal microflora, estimated to include 100 trillion bacteria, comprises hundreds of different species of microbiota that have a significant impact on human health (Gibson and Roberfroid, 1995). The large intestine hosts the largest population of microorganisms, with an estimated 400 different bacterial species (Kopp-Hoolihan, 2001). Approximately 35% to 50% of the contents of the human colon is composed of bacteria. In the optimally functioning gut, bacteria that are pathogenic (e.g., hemolytic *Escherichia coli, Clostridium perfringens, Campylobacter* organisms, and *Listeria* organisms) coexist with beneficial bacteria (e.g., bifidobacteria, *Lactobacillus* organisms, and *E. coli* [a nonpathogenic strain]), and the two populations are balanced.

Healthy GI microflora (1) form a barrier against invading organisms by enhancing the host's defense mechanisms against pathogens, (2) improve gut immunity by adhering to the intestinal mucosa and stimulating local immune responses, and (3) help digest foods and produce certain vitamins (Salminen et al, 1995). Table 12-3 outlines some properties, functions, and effects on the host of intestinal microflora. Molecular tools are illuminating the species of this interior ecosystem and improving understanding of bacteria-bacteria and host-bacteria interactions. Modifications of this intestinal environment may either promote or retard certain disease processes such as inflammatory bowel disease and arthritis (Hart et al, 2002). The use of broad-spectrum antibiotics has a negative impact on intestinal integrity. Although antibiotics are used to prevent serious bacterial infections from becoming life-threatening, they also kill beneficial bacteria. Antibiotics cause changes in intestinal microflora and may alter the balance between beneficial and pathogenic microflora. Disruption of the normal flora of the GI tract makes the host sus-

TABLE 12-3 Intestinal Microflora and Their Functions*

SOME FUNCTIONS OF INTESTINAL MICROFLORA	EFFECTS ON HOST	PRIMARY BACTERIA INVOLVED AND THEIR PROPERTIES†
Health-Promoting Properties		
Produce vitamins, short-chain fatty acids, and protein, which are partly absorbed and used by the host	Maintain good health	**Predominantly Health-Promoting Properties** Bifidobacteria (1,2,3,4) *Lactobacillus* orgainisms (3) *Eubacterium* organisms (3)
Supplement the digestive and absorptive process	Maintain good health	
Protect the host from overgrowth and infection by exogenous organisms such as pathogenic bacteria and yeasts	Maintain good health	
Stimulate the immune system	Maintain good health	
		Combination of Health-Promoting and Virulent Properties Bacteroidaceae (1,2,3,4,5,7,8) Peptococcaecea (3,8) *Escherichia coli* (4,5,6,7,8) Streptococci (3,8)
Virulent Properties		**Predominantly Virulent Properties**
Produce certain putrefactive substances (e.g., ammonia, hydrogen sulfide, amines, phenols, indoles) and secondary bile acids	May cause diarrhea, constipation, and growth inhibition; may also injure the intestine directly and be partially absorbed, potentially contributing throughout the host's life to aging and geriatric diseases such as arteriosclerosis, hypertension, liver disorders, autoimmune diseases, and immunosuppression	*Veillonella* organisms (8) *Clostridium perfringens* (7,8) Staphylococci (7,8) *Proteus* organisms (7,8)
Produce other toxins		
Produce carcinogens	May cause cancer	
Stimulate pathogenicity	May contribute to the establishment of a pathologic condition (e.g., spontaneous infections such as diarrhea, gastroenteritis, or superinfection [cerebromeningitis, endocarditis, septicemia, urinary tract infection, brain abscess, liver abscess, pulmonary abscess])	

Modified from Percival M: Intestinal health, *Clin Nutr Insights* 5:1, 1997.
*It is important to maintain a balance in the intestinal flora. If an imbalance results in more bacteria with virulent properties, illness can result.
†The numbers that follow the name of the bacteria identify their functions as defined in the first column.

ceptible to disease such as antibiotic-induced diarrhea (Rolfe, 2000). Repopulation of gut bacteria with bacteria-containing supplements (probiotics) may be used to reestablish healthy microflora populations when the populations have been devastated by the use of antibiotics.

Nourishing Microflora

Healthy microflora can be supported by prebiotics and probiotics. Prebiotics are nondigestible food products that stimulate the growth of symbiotic bacterial species, already in the colon, that improve the health of the host. Probiotics are microbial foods or supplements that can be used to change or improve intestinal bacterial balance to improve the health of the host (Teitelbaum and Walker, 2002) (see Chapters 1 and 30).

Prebiotics include foods containing substrates that nourish beneficial gut microbiota. These substrates include dietary fiber and fructooligosaccharides (FOSs) (see Chapter 3). The sugars of FOSs are linked together by indigestible bonds that cannot be hydrolyzed by enzymes in the small intestine, so carbohydrates from FOSs pass undigested into the large intestine. Food sources of these FOSs include honey, beer, onions, burdock root, asparagus, rye, Jerusalem artichokes, bananas, maple sugar, oats, and Chinese chives (Bournet and Brouns, 2002).

FOSs have been shown to selectively stimulate the growth of beneficial bacteria, including bifidobacteria and *Lactobacillus* organisms, which reduces the levels of pathogenic bacteria such as *Salmonella* organisms and clostridia in the GI tract. One study revealed that increasing these neosugars causes an increase in numbers of bifidobacteria and a decrease in the activity of β-glucuronidase, an enzyme that converts procarcinogens to carcinogens in the bowel (Buddington, Donahoo, and Buddington, 2002). Components of dietary fiber, including pectin, hemicellulose, and inulin, a storage carbohydrate in chicory, onions, asparagus, and Jerusalem artichokes, also function as prebiotics and stimulate the production of SCFAs.

A second avenue for supporting intestinal integrity is direct repopulation of the intestine with probiotics, which are organisms and substances that contribute to the intestinal microbial balance. The most common forms of probiotics include *Lactobacillus* organisms and bifidobacteria. These organisms maintain intestinal health by inhibiting the overgrowth of pathogenic bacteria through competition for attachment sites and nutrients.

Intestinal bacteria, such as *Lactobacillus* organisms and other strains of beneficial bacteria, also produce organic acids that reduce intestinal pH and retard the growth of pathogenic acid-sensitive bacteria. At the optimal pH, the organic acids produced by beneficial bacteria solubilize cell membranes of pathogenic bacteria, block transport of their necessary growth substances, acidify the cell interiors, and exert other inhibitory influences on their growth.

Fermented dairy products, including live-culture yogurts, kefir, and commercial probiotic preparations, contain forms of beneficial bacteria. Other fermented foods, such as sauerkraut, miso, and tempeh, may also be cultured with beneficial bacteria, especially *Lactobacillus* strains. However, the concentration of bacteria contained in food products varies significantly. For example, yogurt food products labeled with "contains live active cultures" are more likely to contain viable beneficial bacteria than products without this designation. Specific bacterial strains have been developed and researched, such as *Lactobacillus GG.* Clinical studies of *Lactobacillus GG* show that this patented bacteria restores and helps maintain healthy intestinal flora in general and helps maintain healthy intestinal flora during and after oral antibiotic therapy (Madsen, 2001).

DETOXIFICATION SYSTEMS

Optimal health for a lifetime involves the body's ability not only to assimilate nutrients but also to limit the accumulation of potentially harmful endogenous and exogenous toxins. The body is somewhat protected from xenobiotics (compounds foreign to the body) by its natural barriers, which include the GI system, the lungs, and the skin. However, foreign compounds that cross these barriers are shuttled to the body's detoxification systems, which decrease the negative impact of xenobiotics or toxins on the biochemistry and cellular integrity of the body. The two major detoxification pathways in the body are (1) the immune tissue in the gut and (2) the detoxification enzyme systems in the liver. Food and nutrients have significant effects on both of these pathways.

Gastrointestinal System: Gut-Associated Lymphoid Tissue

Because the gut mucosa is a barrier, the GI tract plays a major role in keeping endogenous and exogenous toxins from entering the systemic circulation. When toxins breach this barrier, further migration of these compounds is arrested by the gut-associated lymphoid tissue (GALT).

The gut is the largest organ in the body's immune system, and more than 50% to 60% of the body's lymphoid tissue surrounds the digestive tract. GALT generates almost 70% of the body's antibodies and contains the greatest number of lymphocytes in the body (Mayer, 2000). This major immune system in the gut is composed of secretory immunoglobulin A (sIgA), which often operates separately from the systemic immune system (Walker, 1994). GALT immunoglobulins attach to bacteria, viruses, and other foreign particles to prevent absorption of these compounds into the body. In addition, bacterial enzymes and toxins such as those from pathogenic *E. coli* are directly inactivated by sIgA (Lei and Walker, 2001).

Increased production of sIgA is promoted by certain strains of beneficial bacteria, such as bifidobacteria (Yasui et al, 1992). *Saccharomyces boulardii* is a beneficial yeast that also seems to stimulate humoral immunity (i.e., immunity mediated by body fluids such as lymph). This patented yeast is used to prevent and treat GI disorders caused by use of antimicrobial agents (Rolfe, 2000) (see Chapter 30).

Liver: Two-Phase Detoxification System

Antigens or toxins that are not processed by the intestinal lumen or gut bacteria and get into the bloodstream are delivered via the hepatic portal vein to the liver for detoxification. The liver's actions on these toxins, actions called *biotransformations,* involve a two-phase sequential system—the phase I and phase II detoxification system. Toxic molecules are transformed from lipid-soluble substances into water-soluble molecules that can be excreted from the body.

In phase I a family of enzymes—the cytochrome P-450, or mixed-function oxidase system (MFOS)—is activated. In this phase, endogenous compounds (e.g., hormones and prostaglandins produced in the body) and xenobiotics are transformed by biochemical reactions, primarily by glutathione conjugation, into more water-soluble compounds. In phase II, the metabolites produced in phase I are conjugated in a series of reactions controlled by a different series of enzymes called *conjugases.* The conjugases attach a substance to the phase I biotransfomed compounds to make them less toxic and more easily eliminated. Conjugators involved in phase II reactions include glucuronic acid, glutathione, and glycine. Enzymes that catalyze phase II reactions include glutathione-*S*-transferase and nicotinamide adenine dinucleotide phosphate (NADP) quinone reductase. The conjugated water-soluble metabolites produced by phase II are excreted in the urine or feces. Achieving a balance between these two phases of detoxification is critical because phase I metabolites that are not biotransformed by phase II agents can be more toxic than the original molecule. For example, a component of cigarette smoke that is relatively harmless is transformed during phase I into a metabolically activated carcinogen; in phase II the metabolite is biotransformed, detoxified, and eliminated.

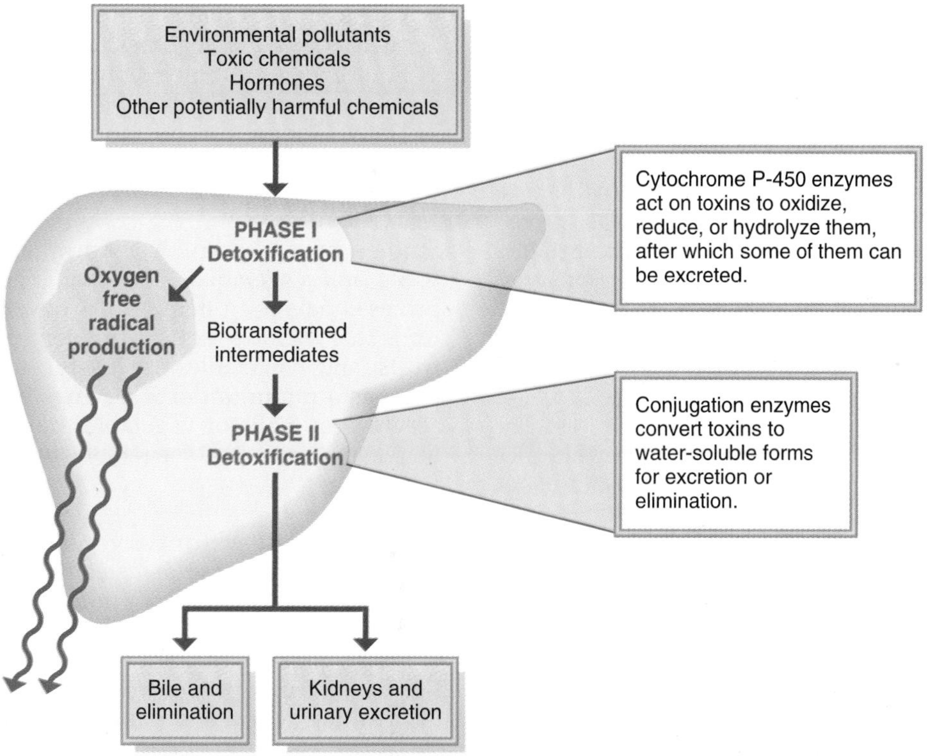

FIGURE 12-2 • Detoxification in the liver. (Modified from Percival M: Phytonutrients and detoxification, *Clin Insights* 5:1, 1997.)

Phase I and phase II balance is also important in minimizing the free radical damage produced by cytochrome P-450 activity. The more efficiently these metabolites are processed by the two-phase system, the less likely it is that cells or tissues will be damaged by free radicals (Lampe, 1999) (Figure 12-2).

Supporting Detoxification Pathways

An individual's nutritional status and the presence of nutrients drive phase I and phase II detoxification; nutrient deficiencies affect the functioning of these systems. Foods, especially those high in specific phytochemicals, provide key nutrients that support these detoxification pathways. Indoles, phytochemicals found in broccoli, cauliflower, and other cruciferous vegetables, markedly enhance phase I pathways (Waladkhani and Clemens, 1998). The dithiolthiones and isothiocyanates, other phytochemicals in the cruciferous family, and liminoids, the phytochemicals in citrus, increase phase II enzymes, including glutathione-*S*-transferase, which blocks carcinogens from damaging cellular DNA (Craig, 1997). The organosulfuric compounds found in vegetables of the allium family—garlic, onions, shallots, and leeks—have also been shown to induce phase II enzymes (Wattenberg, 1997).

Phytochemicals in certain foods can also function as agents to retard the detoxification process. Grapefruit juice contains the flavonoids and other compounds such as furanocoumarins that act as blocking agents in the cytochrome P-450 system. This downregulation of the P-450 system slows the clearance rate of certain drugs, increasing their therapeutic activity (Ho and Saville, 2001). For example, cholesterol-lowering *statin* drugs become 12 times more concentrated in the blood when taken with grapefruit juice. Calcium-channel blockers, tranquilizers (the benzodiazepines), and some antihistamines are also affected by grapefruit juice (Fuhr, 1998) (see Chapter 19).

GUIDELINES FOR A DEFENSIVE NUTRITION PARADIGM

A defensive nutrition paradigm for adults should (1) maximize support for organ systems, (2) optimize GI integrity and immunologic function, (3) ensure maintenance of a healthy body weight and adiposity level, and (4) help prevent metabolic syndrome and related chronic diseases (see *Clinical Insight:* Insulin Resistance and the Metabolic Syndrome). A widely used educational tool for guiding people to make food choices is the USDA Food Guide Pyramid (see Figure 15-1). Introduced in 1992, the USDA Food Guide Pyramid gives adults guidelines for constructing an optimal diet. More than a decade old, the USDA pyramid is being revised to reflect current research in nutrition and health such as the beneficial role of healthy fats in the diet. Other health organizations and researchers have proposed versions of the pyramid that address these nutrition issues. For example, the Mayo Clinic has introduced a version of the Food Guide Pyramid entitled the *Healthy Weight Pyramid* (Mayo Clinic, 2002). This pyramid places fruits and vegetables at the base of the pyramid, places whole grains in the second tier of the pyramid, and highlights exercise as an important component. The *Mediterranean Diet Food Pyramid* emphasizes beans, legumes, and nuts as protein sources; daily intake of olive oil, fruits and vegetables, and cheese and yogurt; and only monthly consumption of red meat (Oldways, 2000) (see Figure 15-6). The *Healthy Eating Food Pyramid,* developed at Harvard School of Public Health, emphasizes plant oils, whole grains, vegetables, fruits, legumes, and nuts, as well as fish, poultry and eggs, as daily food choices. This pyramid suggests eating red meat, butter, white rice, white bread, pasta, sweets, and potatoes only sparingly (Willett, 2001) (Figure 12-3).

Food pyramids provide a general overview of healthy eating objectives; nutrition professionals should tailor food and meal plans based on specific calorie needs and unique physical, psychologic, and genetic characteristics of individuals. Therefore general guidelines for a defensive nutrition eating plan should include the following:

- Nine to 10 servings daily of fruits and vegetables
- Three to five servings daily of fats from monounsaturated and polyunsaturated sources such as olive oil, canola oil, avocados, nuts, and seeds
- Two to three servings daily of protein from beans, fish (especially those rich in omega-3 fatty acids), lean meat, and low-fat dairy products
- One to three servings daily of nonanimal proteins such as nuts and legumes
- Four to eight servings daily of whole grains
- A 1-hour/day activity program
- Daily vitamin-mineral supplementation

Increasing Fruit and Vegetable Intake

Studies have shown that Americans eat too few fruits and vegetables. The challenge for nutrition professionals is to help adults develop eating patterns that include regular, frequent consumption of fruits and vegetables. A useful target for meal plans is a minimum of 5 servings but optimally 10 servings of fruits or vegetables daily. Strategies for increasing fruit and vegetable intake include the following:

1. Trying one new fruit or vegetable each week
2. Doubling the normal vegetable serving size
3. Eating fruit on cereal or muesli
4. Regularly consuming all-vegetable–based meals (e.g., vegetable chili or stew)
5. Eating fruit or vegetables as snacks
6. Adding vegetables to favorite entrees (e.g., tacos, pizza, lasagna)
7. Having salad or soup that has vegetables
8. Adding lettuce, spinach, onions, peppers, cucumbers, and tomatoes to sandwiches
9. Keeping favorite frozen vegetables in the freezer for a quick addition to meals
10. Making fruit smoothies using frozen fruit and dairy or nondairy milk or yogurt

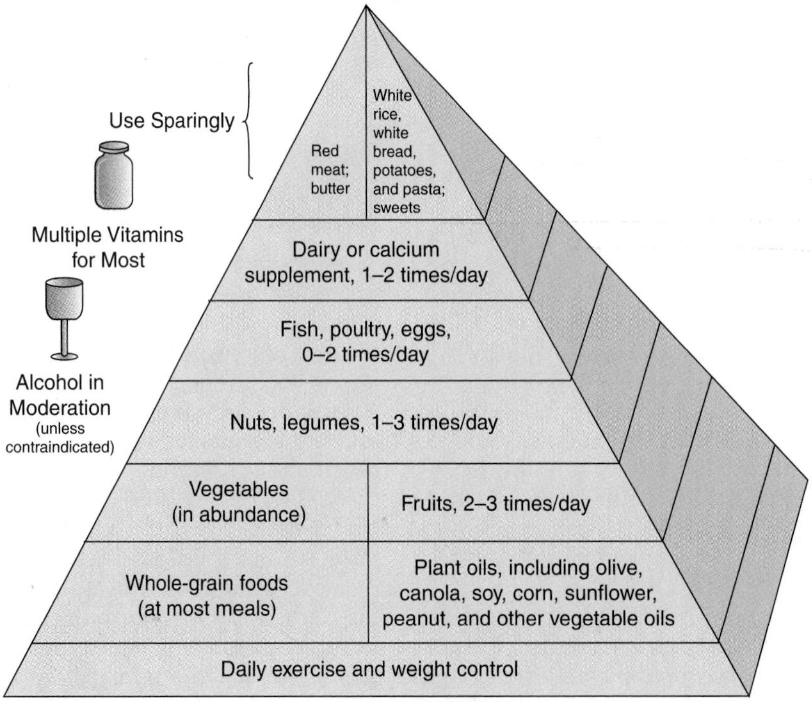

FIGURE 12-3 • Healthy Eating Food Pyramid. (From Willet WC: Eat, drink and be healthy, New York, 2001, Simon & Schuster.)

CLINICAL INSIGHT

Insulin Resistance and Metabolic Syndrome

Metabolic syndrome refers to cluster of metabolic disorders, including high fasting blood glucose levels, hypertension, dyslipidemia, and abdominal obesity (although metabolic syndrome can also develop in those who are not obese). Approximately 47 million people in the United States have metabolic syndrome (Ford, Giles, and Dietz, 2002). A major factor in metabolic syndrome is a defect in glucose metabolism, insulin resistance—cellular resistance to insulin that results in *hyperinsulinemia,* or excess insulin secretion by the body in an attempt to regulate blood sugar (Figure 12-4).

Hyperinsulinemia and impaired glucose tolerance are characteristic of type 2 diabetes mellitus but also develop in other people. (See Chapter 34 for a more detailed discussion of diabetes mellitus.) Resistance to insulin-mediated glucose uptake may be more common than currently thought; approximately 60 to 70 million Americans are insulin resistant. Diet plays an important role in improving insulin resistance and moderating hyperinsulinemia. Factors that have a positive impact on insulin include exercising, reducing caloric intake, and reducing body weight.

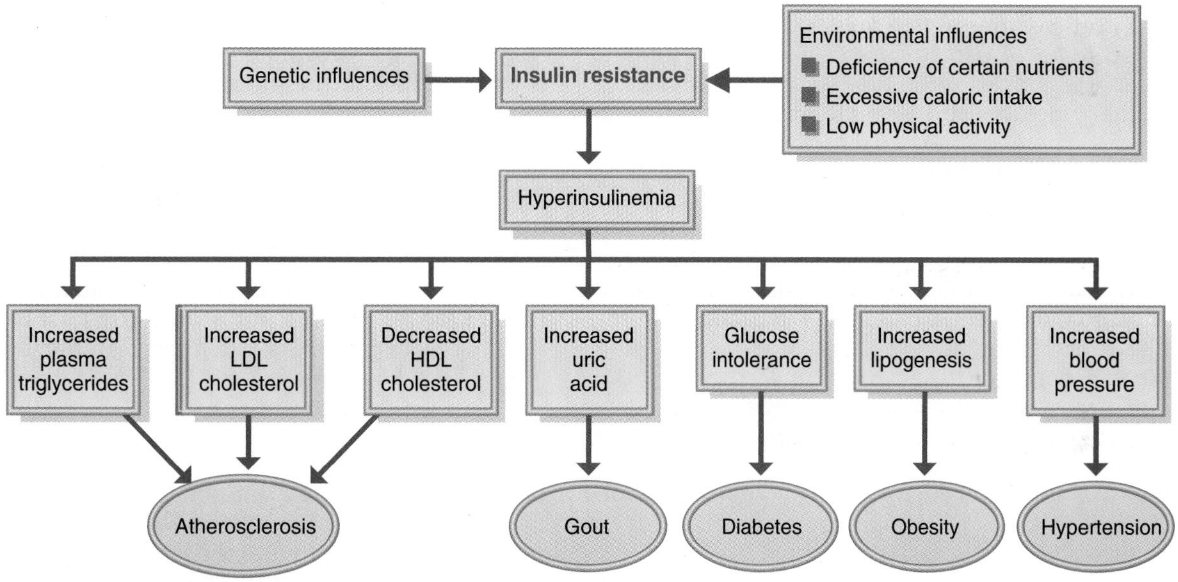

FIGURE 12-4 • Pathophysiologic etiology of insulin resistance and the metabolic syndrome.

Choosing foods that supply glucose to the cells at a steady rate and result in moderate insulin demands may help prevent insulin resistance. One useful tool for measuring the rate at which foods provide glucose to the blood and thus stimulate insulin release is the glycemic index (Ludwig and Eckel, 2002). The glycemic index measures the effect on blood glucose of equivalent amounts of carbohydrate contained in different foods (Wolever, 1990). The glycemic load (the glycemic index multiplied by the dietary carbohydrate content) is a more sensitive measure of glycemic response. The glycemic load measures the quantity and quality (i.e., nature or source) of carbohydrate's effect on blood glucose and insulin release (Foster-Powell, Holt, and Brand-Miller, 2002; Pi-Sunyer, 2002).

Factors that influence the glycemic index include (1) the physical form of a food (e.g., apple juice versus apples, with apple juice having a higher index); (2) the botanical variety of a food (e.g., various species of rice, all of which have different glycemic indexes); (3) the presence of fat; (4) ripeness (i.e., of fruit); (5) whether protein and fat are eaten with carbohydrates; and (6) the starch structure of the carbohydrate in the food (e.g., foods with greater amylose content, which have lower glycemic indexes, versus foods with less amylose) (Foster-Powell, Holt, and Brand-Miller, 2002; Pi-Sunyer, 2002).

In general, foods high in soluble (i.e., gel-forming) fiber with low glycemic indexes (e.g., beans, vegetables, whole fruit, and whole grains such as oatmeal, basmati rice, and barley) are the preferred forms of carbohydrates. Planning the types of food eaten during meals is also an important factor in managing blood glucose levels. Combining protein, fat, and carbohydrate during meals and snacks (e.g., eating fruit with nuts or celery sticks with peanut butter) can lead to better control of blood glucose levels and less insulin release than consuming meals or snacks that consist primarily of carbohydrate (e.g., a white-flour bagel). A food plan to manage metabolic syndrome includes 15% of total calories as protein, 5% to 10% as saturated fat, 30% to 35% as monounsaturated and unsaturated fat, and 45% as carbohydrate (Reaven, Stom, and Fox, 2000).

When plant-based foods form the core of meal plans in adults, the benefits can be maintenance of healthy weight and a decreased incidence of heart disease, cancer, diabetes, and other chronic diseases. For example, targeted fruit and vegetable intake combined with physical activity, maintenance of a healthy weight, and abstinence from smoking may reduce cancer risk by 60% to 70%, especially if started in early adulthood (American Institute for Cancer Research, 1997).

Increasing Omega-3 Fatty Acid Intake

A balanced intake of the essential fatty acids—omega-6 (linoleic acid [LA] and γ-linolenic acid [GLA]) and omega-3 fatty acids (α-linolenic acid [ALA], eicosapentaenoic acid [EPA], and docosahexaenoic acid DHA])—is an important component of an optimal wellness nutrition plan. The current dietary ratio of omega-6 to omega-3 fatty acids is estimated to be 14:1 to 20:1 (see Chapter 3). Humans cannot interconvert *n*-6 and *n*-3 essential fatty acids, and their metabolism uses the same desaturation enzymes. Therefore the two essential fatty acid families are in competition, and *n*-6/*n*-3 imbalances may develop.

Scientific studies have shown that *n*-3 fats help prevent coronary artery disease (see Chapter 35), hypertension (see Chapter 36), and other diseases such as inflammatory (see Chapter 44) and autoimmune diseases (Krauss et al, 2000). Recently the Food and Nutrition Board of the Institute of Medicine (IOM) defined dietary reference intakes (DRIs) as adequate intakes (AIs) for omega-3 and omega-6 fatty acids for men and women (see Chapter 15). The AI for ALA is 1.6 g/day for adult men and 1.1 g/day for adult women. The AI for LA is 17 g/day for men and 12 g/day for women (IOM, 2002).

Flax seed is the richest source of ALA, an omega-3 fatty acid that can be converted in the body to other omega-3 fatty acids, EPA, and DHA. Other sources include canola and soybean oils, walnuts, butternuts, and red and black currant seeds. However, in humans, conversion of omega-3-rich plant sources to EPA and DHA may not be optimal (see Chapter 3).

Recognizing that the current intakes of *n*-3 fats are low, nutrition professionals should encourage increased consumption of omega–3 fatty acid food sources such as fish, especially fatty fish such as salmon and sardines, and plant sources of ALA such as flax seed meal and oil, canola oil, soybean oil, and nuts, especially walnuts. The American Heart Association recommends consuming at least two servings of fish weekly.

Vitamin and Mineral Supplementation

Studies have shown that few Americans are able to meet recommended nutritional guidelines promoted by programs such as "Five a Day," which encourage people to eat five or more servings of fruits and vegetables daily. A telephone survey of 24,000 adults in 16 states found that only 20% of the respondents had eaten the recommended five or more daily servings of fruits and vegetables (Li et al, 2000). A study of the nutrient intake levels of the offspring of participants involved in the Framingham Heart Study revealed that only 50% of the study's 2520 participants met the recommended dietary allowances (RDAs) for vitamins A, E, and B_6; only 25% of the women in the study had daily intakes of 800 mg of calcium or more; and 75% of the population consumed less than the suggested amount of β-carotene. The researchers concluded that ". . . large proportions of adults fall short of the guidelines for some key nutrients" (Millen and Quatromoni, 2001).

Medical researchers now recognize ". . . that most people do not consume an optimal amount of all vitamins by diet alone" and ". . . suboptimal intake of some vitamins, above levels causing classic vitamin deficiency, is a risk factor for chronic diseases and common in the general population." The researchers concluded that all American adults should take vitamin supplements (Fletcher and Fairfield, 2002).

Dietetic professionals should be prepared to (1) assess and recommend appropriate nutrient supplements when necessary and (2) educate supplement users that supplements may meet certain nutrient needs but should be combined with a healthy diet, not replace it. Tufts University has created an excellent guide to reliable nutrition (Tufts University, 2003) (see Chapter 4, *Clinical Insight:* Vitamin Supplements: To Take or Not to Take).

Women's Health

Women have monthly hormonal shifts that trigger the female reproductive cycle. These hormones, such as estrogen and progesterone, signal physiologic changes in the ovaries and uterus that prepare these organs for possible egg fertilization. While women are fertile, they can experience menses-related mood fluctuations and general discomfort. Approximately 10% to 20% of women who experience this discomfort have symptoms that are sufficiently severe to create personal hardships. The most common symptoms include anxiety, depression, mood swings, fatigue, weight gain, swelling, breast pain, cramps, and backache. This complex of physical and psychologic symptoms, known as premenstrual syndrome (PMS), generally begins 7 to 10 days before the onset of menses and increases in severity as menses approaches. Because peak severity usually occurs during menses, the term *perimenstrual symptoms* has been proposed to describe more accurately what most women experience.

No one consistent imbalance or deficiency has been identified in the etiology of PMS, although some promising theories have been developed that are related to hormone imbalance (estrogen and progesterone), neurotransmitter synthesis defects, disorders of essential fatty acid metabolism, and deficiencies of certain nutrients such as vitamin B_6 and calcium.

In a meta-analysis of published research on the efficacy of vitamin B supplementation to relieve PMS symptoms, researchers concluded that limited evidence suggested that 100 mg (and possibly 50 mg) of vitamin B_6 supplementation was significantly better than placebo in managing PMS symptoms such as depression, breast tenderness, and bloating. However, the authors of this study cautioned that the trials examined had small sample sizes; they suggested that a large-scale clinical study was needed to establish definitive recommendations for treating PMS symptoms with vitamin B_6. None of the studies examined found that doses of B_6 higher than 50 to 100 mg were warranted (Wyatt et al, 1999).

In a study that examined the relationship between PMS symptoms and calcium regulation, women who took 1200 mg of calcium daily in the form of calcium carbonate throughout the course of three menstrual cycles reported a significantly lower incidence of PMS symptoms than the placebo group (Thys-Jacobs et al, 1998).

Improved nutrition and stress reduction may also help decrease premenstrual symptoms. Women who experience PMS symptoms report higher intakes of refined carbohydrates, sugar, sodium, and dairy products than women without PMS (Abraham, 1987). When combined with regular exercise and stress reduction or relaxation techniques, a healthy diet that includes fruits and vegetables (especially dark green vegetables), whole grains, legumes, and quality fats and proteins can help women cope with PMS.

Women have special health and nutrition concerns in their later adult years because of perimenopause and menopause. Perimenopause and menopause typically begin when a woman enters her late 40s. During menopause, which the average woman experiences at about age 50, estrogen production decreases (with endogenous estrogen circulation decreasing approximately 60%), signaling the end of the reproductive years. However, women are not completely without estrogen, even after the ovaries cease production, because the adrenal glands continue to produce weaker forms of estrogen. Women in developed countries live more than one half of their lives in the postmenopausal stage (Barrett-Connor et al, 2002).

With diminished production of estrogen, women may experience symptoms associated with menopause, including vasomotor symptoms such as hot flashes. Bone health is also affected as a result of the decrease in circulating estrogen as the body's ability to keep up with the natural process of bone turnover slows in response. Bone mass decreases, and osteoporosis may develop (see Chapter 28). Lower levels of circulating estrogen also affect blood lipid levels, resulting in an increase in total cholesterol and LDL cholesterol levels and a decrease in high-density lipoprotein (HDL) cholesterol levels (see Chapter 35).

Plant-based foods can be used for nutritional management of menopause symptoms. For example, protein from soy foods can help prevent osteoporosis. Researchers compared the effects of soy protein with those of casein-whey protein on bone mineral density. Results of this study showed markedly decreased calcium excretion in participants consuming the soy protein, which suggests that soy protein may possess nonestrogenic properties that retard osteoporosis. (Spence, 2001). Research results on the relationship between soy isoflavones and bone health are mixed. In one study, postmenopausal women who consumed soy milk with a high isoflavone content and 100 mg of isoflavone daily for 2 years had a higher bone mineral density (Lydeking-Olsen, 2001). In another study, those who followed a diet with a moderate, yet significant, isoflavone content (58 mg) did not have any increase in bone mineral density (Vitolins, 2001) (see Chapter 27).

Men's Health

Leading causes of death among American men include heart disease, prostate cancer, and lung cancer. Plant-based foods, especially foods rich in the phytochemical lycopene, are strongly associated with reduced risk of developing these diseases (Rao and Agarwal, 2000). Cardiovascular disease is the leading cause of death among men of all races and ethnic groups in the United States. Men develop cardiovascular disease at younger ages and more frequently than women (see Chapter 35). Several studies have established an association between reduced risk of heart disease and lycopene. In one study, men with the lowest serum lycopene levels had a three times higher risk of having an acute coronary event or a stroke (Rissanen et al, 2001). Researchers found an inverse relationship between low plasma lycopene levels and carotid intima-media thickness, an index of atherosclerotic severity suggesting that lycopene is a dietary antioxidant. They concluded that lycopene helped prevent atherosclerosis (Gianetti et al, 2002) (see Chapter 35).

Prostate cancer is the second leading cause of death and the most common cancer among American men. Tomatoes, which contain lycopene are associated with reduced risk of prostate cancer (Millen and Quatromoni, 2001). In a study of almost 48,000 health care professionals, researchers found that the highest level of lycopene intake (from dietary sources) was associated with a 16% reduction in prostate cancer (Giovannucci et al, 2002).

SUMMARY

Nutrition in the adult years focuses on maintaining health by using foods, particularly plant-based foods and their constituents (phytonutrients), to optimize the functions of the digestive and liver detoxification systems and other organ systems of the body, including the immune system. With a nutrition program based on a nutrition paradigm that promotes defensive eating, adults of all ages can maintain and promote health and productivity while preventing disease.

Clinical Scenario

JoAnn is a 48-year-old woman who works full-time and is the single parent of two teenagers. She is 5 ft, 9 inches tall and currently weighs 175 lb. In the past 2 years, she has gained 10 lb. Her recent blood glucose test results were borderline high, and her family has a history of diabetes and cancer. She recently completed a course of antibiotics for an ear infection and has been experiencing mood swings and night sweats, which she thinks may be related to perimenopause.

JoAnn has called to make an appointment for dietary counseling and has expressed interest in getting more information about how diet can help her maintain her health, manage her risk for diabetes and cancer, and prevent any further weight gain. Her typical meals are as follows: a bagel, coffee, and orange juice for breakfast; a sandwich with ham, cheese, lettuce, tomato, and mayonnaise and fat-free cookies for lunch; and pasta with chicken and carrots, a green salad with blue cheese dressing, and a small slice of cake or a dish of ice cream for dinner. Her beverages include diet colas, and her snacks are usually rice cakes or popcorn. She has no regular exercise program.

1. Which kinds of foods are lacking in JoAnn's diet that could help (1) manage her blood glucose levels, (2) relieve her perimenopausal symptoms, and (3) help reduce her risk of cancer?
2. Explain to JoAnn the way that adding or increasing the amounts of certain foods in her diet may help address her concerns. What type of background information can you give her so that she can understand the rationale for your recommendations?
3. With JoAnn's input, design a 3-day meal plan that reflects your recommendations. Plan the menus for all breakfasts eaten at home, lunches prepared at home and taken to work, and two dinners—one prepared at home and one eaten at a restaurant.
4. Would you recommend any dietary supplements for JoAnn? What type of information or assessment tools can you use to determine whether supplementation is necessary?
5. How would you help JoAnn formulate goals for an exercise program?

Relevant Web Sites

Agricultural Research Service, U.S. Department of Agriculture
www.ars.usda.gov/is/np/fnrb/fnrb0403.htm#flavonoid
Centers for Disease Control and Prevention, National Center for Health Statistics
www.cdc.gov/nchs/products/pubs/pubd/hestats/obese/obese99.hym
Mayo Clinic:
Healthy Weight Pyramid:
www.mayo.edu/news/pyramid1.jpg). -
Mediterranean Diet Food Pyramid
www.oldwayspt.org/
National Agricultural Library, USDA Food Composition data
www.nal.usda.gov/fnic/foodcomp/Data
National Center for Biotechnology Information
www.ncbi.nlm.nih.gov
Tufts University Guide to Reliable Nutrition Information
www.foodnavigator.com
U.S. Department of Agriculture
www.ers.usda.gov/publications/FoodReview/septdec00/)
U.S. Department of Health and Human Services
www.health.gov/healthypeople/document/).
U.S. Food and Drug Administration
www.cfsan.fda.gov/~dms/fdsoypr.html) - health claims for soy protein

Cited References

Abraham GE: Role of nutrition in managing the premenstrual tension syndromes, *J Reprod Med* 32:405,1987.

Adlercreutz H et al: Urinary excretion of lignans and isoflavonoid phytoestrogens in Japanese men and women consuming a traditional Japanese diet, *Am J Clin Nutr* 54:1093, 1991.

American Institute for Cancer Research: *Food, nutrition and the prevention of cancer: a global perspective,* Washington, DC, 1997, American Institute for Cancer Research.

Anderson J et al: Meta-analysis of the effects of soy protein on serum lipids. *N Engl J Med* 333:276, 1995.

Barrett-Connor E et al: *Women's health and menopause: a comprehensive approach,* Best clinical practices, Chapter 13, International Position Paper, National Institutes of Health Office of Research on Women's Health, March 2002, www.nhlbi.nih.gov/health/prof/heart/other/wm_menop.htm.

Bazzano LA et al: Fruit and vegetable intake and risk of cardiovascular disease in U.S. adults: the first National Health and Nutrition Examination Survey epidemiologic follow-up study, *Am J Clin Nutr* 76:93, 2002.

Bournet FRJ, Brouns F: Immune stimulating and gut health–promoting properties of short chain fructo-oligosaccharides, *Nutr Rev* 60:326, 2002.

Buddington KK, Donahoo JB, Buddington RK: Dietary oligofructose and inulin protect mice from enteric and systemic pathogens and tumor inducers, *J Nutr* 132:472 2002.

Centers for Disease Control and Prevention, National Center for Health Statistics: Prevalence of overweight and obesity among adults in the United States, 2000, www.cdc.gov/nchs/products/pubs/pubd/hestats/obese/obse99.htm.

Clauson A: Share of food spending for eating out reaches 47%, *Food Rev* 22(3), September-October, 1999, www.ers.usda.gov/publications/foodreviews/sep.1999/contents.htm.

Craig W: Phytochemicals: guardians of our health, *J Am Diet Assoc* 97(suppl 2):199, 1997.

Craig W, Beck L: Phytochemicals: health protective effects, *Can J Diet Pract Res* 60(2):78, 1999.

Dai Q et al: Urinary excretion of phytoestrogens and risk of breast cancer among Chinese women in Shanghai, *Cancer Epidemiol Biomarkers Prev* 11(9):815, 2002.

Davis JN, Kucuk O, Sarkar FH: Expression of prostate-specific antigen is transcriptionally regulated by genistein in prostate cancer cells, *Mol Carcinog* 34(2):91, 2002.

Flegal K et al: Prevalence and trends in obesity among US adults, 1999-2000, *JAMA* 288:1723, 2002.

Fletcher RH, Fairfield KM: Vitamins for chronic disease prevention in adults: clinical applications, *JAMA* 287:3127, 2002.

Ford ES, Giles WH, Dietz WH: Prevalence of the metabolic syndrome among U.S. adults: findings from the third National Health and Nutrition Examination Survey, *JAMA* 287:356, 2002.

Foster-Powell K, Holt SHA, Brand-Miller JC: International table of glycemic index and glycemic load values, *Am J Clin Nutr* 76:5, 2002.

Fuhr U: Drug interactions with grapefruit juice. Extent, probable mechanism and clinical relevance, *Drug Safety* 18:251, 1998.

Gianetti J et al: Inverse association between carotid intima-media thickness and the antioxidant lycopene in atherosclerosis, *Am Heart J* 143:467, 2002.

Gibson GR, Roberfroid MB: Dietary modulation of the human colonic microbiota: introducing the concept of prebiotics, *J Nutr* 125:1401, 1995.

Giovannucci E: Tomatoes, tomato-based products, lycopene and cancer: review of the epidemiologic literature, *J Natl Cancer Inst* 91:317, 1999.

Giovannucci E et al: A prospective study of tomato products, lycopene and prostate cancer risk, *J Natl Cancer Inst* 94:391, 2002.

Halvorsen BL et al: A systematic screening of total antioxidants in dietary plants, *J Nutr* 132:461, 2002.

Hart Al et al: The role of the gut flora in health and disease, and its modification as therapy, *Aliment Pharmacol Ther* 16:1383, 2002.

Henkel J: Soy: health claims for soy protein. Questions about other components, U.S. Food and Drug Administration, *FDA Consumer,* May-June 2000, (http://www.cfsan.fda.gov/~dms/fdsoypr.html).

Ho PC, Saville DJ, Wanwimolruk S: Inhibition of human CYP3A4 activity by grapefruit flavonoids, furanocoumarins and related compounds, *J Pharm Pharm Sci* 4(3):217, 2001.

Holden JM et al:. Carotenoid content of U.S. foods: an update of the database, *J Food Comp Anal* 12:169, 1999.

Hutchins AM et al: Flaxseed consumption influences endogenous hormone concentrations in postmenopausal women, *Nutr Cancer* 39(1):58, 2001.

Institute of Medicine, Food and Nutrition Board: *Dietary reference intakes (DRIs) for energy and the macronutrients, carbohydrate, fiber, fat, fatty acids, cholesterol, protein and amino acids,* Washington, DC, 2002, National Academy of Sciences.

King A, Young G: Characteristics and occurrence of phenolic phytochemicals, *J Am Diet Assoc* 99:213, 1999.

Knekt P et al: Flavonoid intake and risk of chronic diseases, *Am J Clin Nutr* 76:560, 2002.

Kopp-Hoolihan L: Prophylactic and therapeutic uses of probiotics: a review, *J Am Diet Assoc* 101:229,241, 2001.

Krauss RM et al: AHA Dietary Guidelines: revision 2000. A statement for healthcare professionals from the Nutrition Committee of the American Heart Association, *Circulation* 102:2284, 2000.

Lampe J: Health effects of vegetables and fruit: assessing mechanisms of action in human experimental studies, *Am J Clin Nutr* 70(suppl 3):475, 1999.

Leach P: New survey targets eating trends, *Wall Street J,* April 17, 1998.

Lei L and Walker WA: Pathologic and physiological interactions of bacteria with the gastrointestinal epithelium, *Am J Clin Nutr* 73:11245-11305, 2001.

Levin B: Intestinal permeability and nutritional support of intestinal integrity, *Q Rev Nat Med* Summer, p 141, 1994.

Li R et al: Trends in fruit and vegetable consumption among adults in 16 U.S. states: Behavioral Risk Factor Surveillance System, 1990-1996, *Am J Public Health* 90:777, 2000.

Ludwig DS, Eckel RH: The glycemic index at 20 y, *Am J Clin Nutr* 76:264S, 2002.

Lydeking-Olsen E et al: *Isoflavone-rich soymilk prevents bone loss in the lumbar spine of postmenopausal women: a 2-yr study,* Abstract from the Fourth International Symposium on the role of Soy, 2001, http://talksoy.com/Media/ChronDiseaseSym.htm.

Madsen KL: The use of probiotics in gastrointestinal disease, *Can J Gastroenterol* 15:817, 2001.

Mayer L: Mucosal immunity and gastrointestinal antigen processing, *J Pediatr Gastroenterol Nutr* 30(suppl):4, 2000.

Mayo Clinic: www.mayo.edu/news/pyramid.jpg, 2002.

Messina M, Erdman JW, eds: The role of soy in preventing and treating chronic disease, *Am J Clin Nutr* 68(suppl 6):1329S, 1998.

Millen BE, Quatromoni PA: Nutritional research within the Framingham Heart Study, *J Nutr Health Aging* 5(3):139, 2001.

Milner JA: Mechanisms by which garlic and allyl sulfur compounds suppress carcinogen bioactivation: garlic and carcinogenesis, *Adv Exp Med Biol* 492:69, 2001.

Oldways Preservation and Exchange Trust and Harvard School of Public Health, www.oldwayspt.org, 2000.

Pi-Sunyer FX: Glycemic index and disease, *Am J Clin Nutr* 76(suppl):290, 2002.

Potter SM: Soy protein and cardiovascular disease: the impact of bioactive components, *Nutr Rev* 56:231, 1998.

Putnam J, Kantor LS, Allshouse J: Per capita food supply trends: progress toward dietary guidelines, 2000, *Food Rev* 23(3):2, 2000, http://www.ers.usda.gov/publications/FoodReview/septdec00/).

Rao AV, Agarwal S: Role of antioxidant lycopene in cancer and heart disease, *J Am Coll Nutr* 19:563, 2000.

Reaven G, Stom R, Fox B: *Syndrome X,* New York, 2000, Simon & Schuster.

Rissanen TH et al: Low serum lycopene concentration is associated with an excess incidence of acute coronary events and stroke: the Kuopio Ischaemic Heart Disease Risk Factor Study, *Br J Nutr* 85:749 2001.

Rolfe RD: The role of probiotic cultures in the control of gastrointestinal health, *J Nutr* 130(suppl):396, 2000.

Salminen S et al: Gut flora in normal and disordered states, *Chemotherapy* 41(suppl 1):5, 1995.

Serraino M, Thompson LU: Flaxseed supplementation and early markers of colon carcinogenesis, *Cancer Lett* 63:159, 1992.

Spence L et al: Effect of soy isoflavones on calcium metabolism in postmenopausal women, Abstract from the Fourth International Symposium on the role of Soy, 2001, www.talksoy.com/Media/ChronDiseaseSym.htm.

Steinmetz K, Potter J: Vegetables, fruit, and cancer prevention: a review, *J Am Diet Assoc* 96:1037, 1996.

Talalay P, Fahey JW: Phytochemicals from cruciferous plants protect against cancer by modulating carcinogen metabolism, *J Nutr* 131(suppl 11):3027, 2001.

Teitelbaum JE, Walker WA: Nutritional impact of pre- and probiotics as protective gastrointestinal organisms, *Ann Rev Nutr* 22:255, 2002.

Thys-Jacobs S et al: Calcium carbonate and the premenstrual syndrome: effects on premenstrual and menstrual symptoms. Premenstrual Syndrome Study Group, *Am J Obstet Gynecol* 179: 444, 1998.

Tufts University Center on Nutrition Communication, Nutrition Navigator, www.navigator.tufts.edu, 2003.

U.S. Department of Health and Human Services: *Healthy People 2010,* ed 2, With Understanding and improving health and objectives for improving health, 2 vols, Washington, DC, 2000, U.S. Goverment Printing Office.

van Poppel G et al: Brassica vegetables and cancer prevention: epidemiology and mechanisms, *Adv Exp Med Biol* 472:159, 1999.

Vitolins M: Does soy protein and its isoflavones prevent bone loss in peri- and postmenopausal women? Results of a 2-yr randomized clinical trial, Abstract from the Fourth International Symposium on Soy 2001. http://talksoy.com/Media/ChronDiseaseSym.htm.

Waladkhani AR, Clemens MR: Effect of dietary phytochemicals on cancer development, *Int J Mol Med* 1:747, 1998 (review).

Walker W: Uptake of antigens: role in gastrointestinal disease, *Acta Paediatr Jpn* 36:597, 1994.

Wattenberg LW: An overview of chemoprevention: current status and future prospects, *Proc Soc Exp Biol Med* 216:133, 1997.

Willett W: *Eat, drink and be healthy,* New York, 2001, Simon & Schuster.

Windmueller H, Spaeth A: Uptake and metabolism of plasma glutamine by the small intestine, *Nutr Rev* 48:310, 1990.

Wolever T: The glycemic index. In Bourne GH, ed: Aspects of Some vitamin, minerals, and enzymes in health and disease, *World Rev Nutr Diet.* 62:120, 1990.

Wyatt KM et al: Efficacy of vitamin B-6 in the treatment of premenstrual syndrome: systematic review, *BMJ* 318(7195):1375, 1999.

Xu X et al: Soy consumption alters endogenous estrogen metabolism in postmenopausal women, *Cancer Epidemiol Biomarkers Prev* 9:781, 2000.

Yasui I et al: Detection of bifidobacterium that induces large quantities of IgA, *Microbial Ecol Health Dis* 5:155, 1992.

Young VR et al: Evaluation of the protein quality of an isolated soyprotein in young men: relative nitrogen requirements and effect of methionine supplementation, *Am J Clin Nutr* 39:16, 1984.

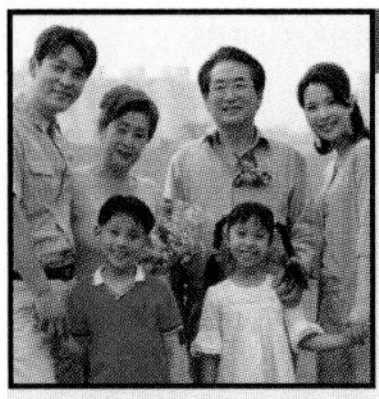

CHAPTER 13

Nutrition in Aging

NANCY G. HARRIS MS, RD, LDN, FADA

CHAPTER OUTLINE

- The Older Population
- Theories of Aging
- Physiologic Changes
- Multidisciplinary Assessment
- Nutrition Screening
- Nutrition Needs
- Dietary Planning
- Nutrition Issues
- Supportive Services

KEY TERMS

activities of daily living–everyday tasks requiring individual skills; include ambulation and locomotion, eating, toileting, grooming, personal hygiene, and bathing

assisted living–a care setting that combines housing, personalized supportive services, and health care designed to meet the needs of those who need help with activities of daily living.

Centers for Medicare and Medicaid Services (CMS)–a federal agency responsible for administering the federal Medicare and Medicaid programs

cross-link theory–a theory of aging stating that the chemical conversion of soluble forms of collagen into insoluble collagen via cross-linkages causes a decrease in elasticity and cell permeability

free radical theory–a theory of aging stating that normal metabolic processes—or exposure to free radicals—damages cells and eventually causes aging

genetic theory–a theory of aging stating that aging is determined by inherited genes

instrumental (independent) activities of daily living–daily tasks such as meal preparation, housework, managing finances or medications, telephone use, shopping, and transportation

long-term care–a general term used to describe the care provided in nursing homes; also describes a broader continuum of care for those with chronic diseases and disabilities, including nursing homes, assisted living facilities, board-and-care facilities, and community care providers such as home health agencies

pacemaker theory–a theory of aging stating that aging is determined by a biologic clock paced by the neuroendocrine and immune systems, which regulates the rate of aging

pressure ulcers–skin injuries that can result from an inadequate dissipation of pressure, fragile vessels and connective tissue, a reduction in dermal blood vessels, impaired healing, and malnutrition

rate of living theory–a theory suggesting that all people have a finite amount of a vital substance that when depleted results in aging and death

sarcopenia–age-related loss of skeletal muscle

senescence–the period of life beginning after age 30 years when changes occur that reflect normal decreases in all organ systems

skilled nursing facility–a nursing home that meets the requirements for Medicare certification as defined in 1919(a) of the Federal Social Security Act; a term previously used to define a nursing home type that was licensed to provide the highest level of care

somatic mutations theory–a theory stating that spontaneous changes in the structure of genes that cannot be corrected or eliminated will accumulate and cause cells to malfunction and die

wear-and-tear theory–a theory of aging suggesting that several years of damage to cells, tissues, and organs eventually destroy them

THE OLDER POPULATION

Demographic trends in the older adult population are changing dramatically. In fact, the chronologic age at which a person is considered to be an "older adult" varies among groups and increases over time. The U.S. Census Bureau defines those 55 years and older as the "older population" and those 65 and older as the "elderly population," whereas those 50 years and older are eligible for membership in the American Association of Retired Persons. The decrease in infant mortality in the twentieth century and the increase in life expectancy have had an impact on vital statistics related to aging. The increase in aging is not distributed proportionately around the world; developing regions lag behind. In 2000 the median age in the developing countries was 24.3 years, compared with 37.4 years in more advanced countries. The United Nations projects that by 2050, the median age will be 35 years in the developing countries and 46.4 years in the more developed countries (United Nations, 2001).

In the United States in 2000, the average life expectancy—the average length of life projected for a population of a given age—was 76.9 years, with a male newborn having a life expectancy of 74.1 years and a female newborn having a life expectancy of 79.5 years (Centers for Disease Control and Prevention [CDC], 2002). The increase in life expectancy for Americans is affected by the decrease in number of deaths from cancer and certain heart diseases. However, with longer life comes an increase in diseases such as Alzheimer's disease, influenza, pneumonia, kidney disease, hypertension, and other conditions that affect older adults. These changes have resulted in a growing demand for information on the health status of older Americans, including measures of activity limitations, sensory impairments, quality of life, and the availability and use of preventive health services.

In 2000 the United States had approximately 35 million people—almost 13% of the total population, age 65 or older. This number is expected to reach 70 million by 2030, with the population group comprising those 85 and older experiencing the largest growth. In 2000, approximately 2% of the U.S. population was 85 years or older, and this number is predicted to reach 5% by 2050. Demographic trends indicate that women constitute 58% of the population age 65 and older and 70% of the population age 85 and older (Figure 13-1). Racial and ethnic diversity will also continue to change (Figure 13-2).

Life span, the maximum number of years of life that humans have lived, continues to increase. The size of the population of *centenarians*—those living to 100 years of age or longer—is expected to increase from about 65,000 in 2000 to 381,000 by 2030 (Figures 13-3 and 13-4).

In addition to chronologic age, many factors—such as gender, race and ethnic composition, marital status, educational level, living arrangements, economic status, presence of disease, and health behaviors—can provide valuable insight for identifying opportunities for research, legislation, and preventive and service delivery. The National Center for Health Statistics, with support from the National Institute on Aging, maintains databases that improve the quality of data, identify trends in the aging population, and promote collaboration among governmental and other agencies.

THEORIES OF AGING

Gerontology is the study of late adulthood and aging; *gerontologists,* scientists who study aging, have developed various theories to explain aging. Today, two broad types of theories on the causes of aging exist. One group of theories describes aging as a result of random events, and the other group views aging as a result of programmed events.

The major theories of aging as a consequence of random events are the *cross-link, wear-and-tear, free radical, rate of living,* and *somatic mutations* theories. The cross-link theory states that it is the chemical conversion of the soluble forms of collagen into insoluble collagen via cross-linkages that causes a decrease in elasticity and cell permeability. The protein *elastin* also experiences cross-link damage and becomes more soluble. The wear-and-tear theory suggests that years of damage to cells, tissues, and organs eventually destroy them, whereas the free radical theory states that normal metabolic processes, or exposure to free radicals, will damage cells and eventually cause aging. The rate of living theory suggests that we have a finite amount of a vital substance that when depleted results in aging and death. The somatic mutations theory suggests that spontaneous

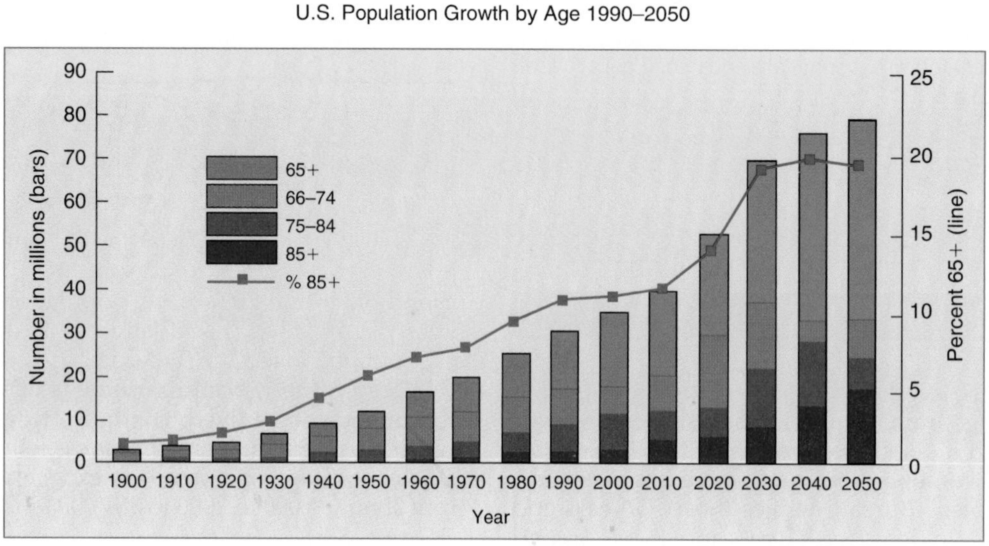

FIGURE 13-1 • U.S. population growth by age, 1990-2050. (From U.S. Census Bureau Publications: *65+ in America,* Washington, DC, 2002, NAIC website: www.aoa.dhhs.gov/naic/.)

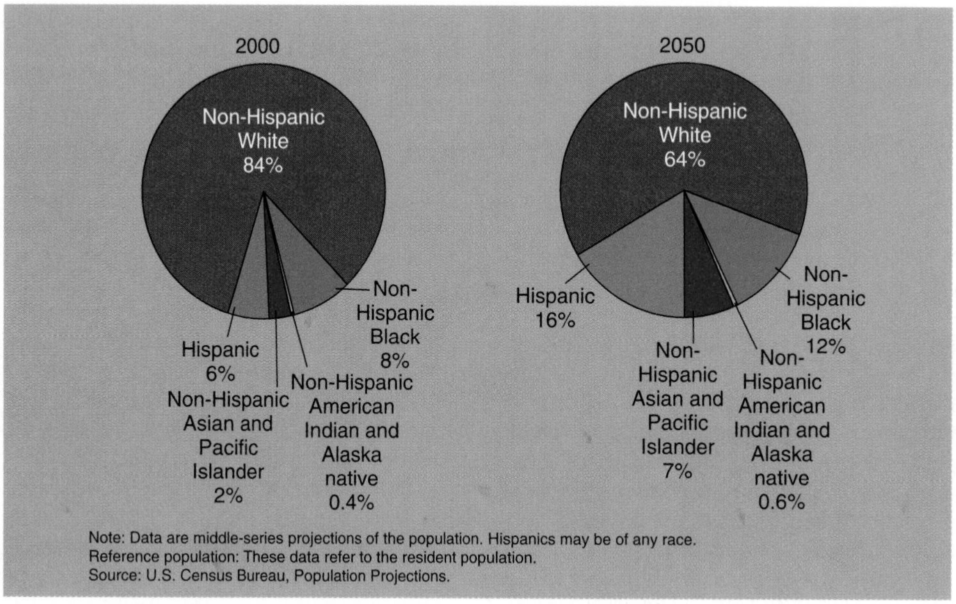

FIGURE 13-2 • Projected distribution of the population age 65 and older by race and Hispanic origin, 2000 and 2050. (From U.S. Census Bureau: *Population projections,* Washington, DC, 2002.)

changes in the structure of our genes—changes that cannot be corrected or eliminated—will accumulate and cause cells to malfunction and die.

Theories of aging based on predetermined or programmed events include the genetic theory and the pacemaker theory. The genetic theory describes aging as being determined by inherited genes. Genes can be either helpful by promoting longevity or harmful by shortening the life span (see Chapter 16). Proponents of the theory recognize that genes can be affected by external conditions such as free radicals, toxins, ultraviolet light, and radiation. The pace-

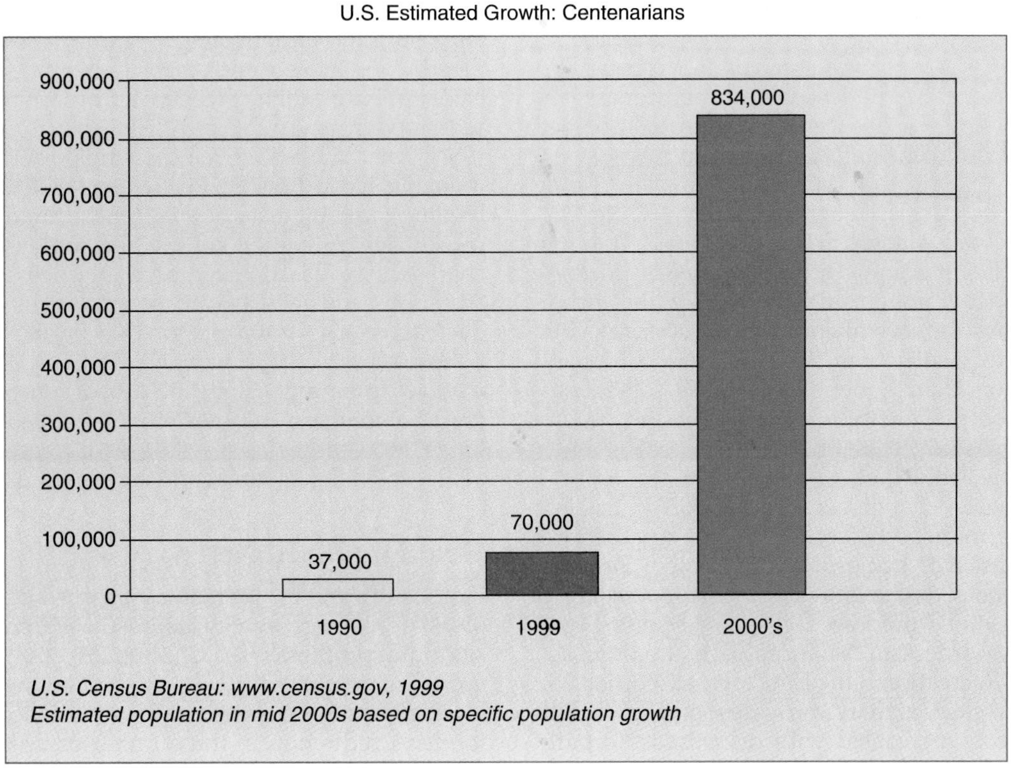

FIGURE 13-3 • U.S. estimated centenarian population in mid 2000s. (From U.S. Census Bureau: www.census.gov, 1999.) (Courtesy Ihab Hajjar, MD.)

maker theory describes aging as a biologic clock paced by the neuroendocrine and immune systems, which regulate the rate of aging.

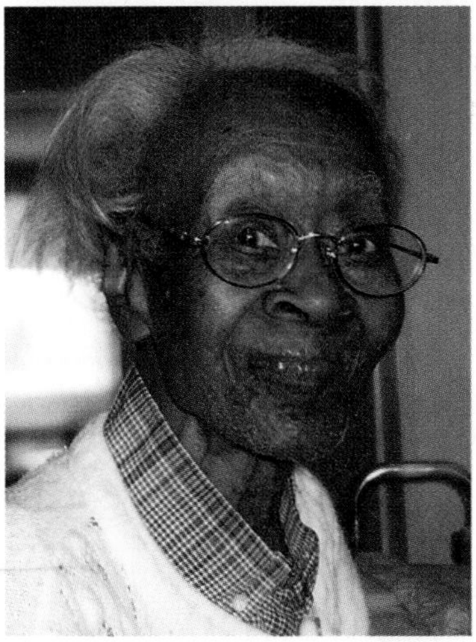

FIGURE 13-4 • Healthy centenarian.

PHYSIOLOGIC CHANGES

Aging is a normal process that begins at conception and ends at death. Senescence, the period of life after age 30, is a process that involves the whole body. During periods of growth, anabolic processes outnumber catabolic changes. Once the body reaches physiologic maturity, the rate of catabolic or degenerative change may become greater than the anabolic regeneration. The resultant loss of cells can lead to varying degrees of decreased efficiency and impaired function. Gerontologists view aging in terms of chronologic, biologic, psychological, and social processes. These changes can be influenced by life events, illness, genetics, and socioeconomic and lifestyle factors. Therefore a person's physiologic age reflects health status but may or may not reflect chronologic age. Lifestyle factors that seem to influence physiologic age are adequacy and regularity of sleep, frequency of consumption of well-balanced meals, sufficiency of physical activity, smoking status, extent of alcohol consumption, and body weight. Disease and disability are not always inevitable consequences of aging. The use of preventive services, elimination of risk factors, and adoption of healthy lifestyle behaviors are some of the major determinants of how well a person ages.

Body Composition Changes

Aging is marked by an approximate 2% to 3% loss of lean body mass per decade. Sarcopenia—age-related loss of skeletal muscle—contributes to decreases in muscle strength, changes in gait and balance, loss of physical function, and increased risk for chronic diseases (Dutta, 1997). The loss of lean body mass, the most metabolically active tissue, is often accompanied by an increase in body fat and a proportionate decrease in metabolic rate (Hurley, 1997). The resting metabolic rate decreases approximately 15% to 20% during life. These changes in lean body mass, body fat, and metabolic rate can reduce energy needs, decrease ability to function independently in daily life, and increase the risk for several chronic diseases associated with obesity. Results from the 1999 National Health and Nutrition Examination Survey (NHANES) indicates that the prevalence of overweight and obesity measured by body mass index (BMI) among older adults is increasing (Table 13-1).

Energy needs change because the person has less lean muscle, more body fat, and a sedentary lifestyle. The importance of being physically active throughout life has been documented by the American Heart Association, the American College of Sports Medicine, and the American Alliance for Health, Physical Education, Recreation, and Dance (see Chapter 25). Regular physical activity provides myriad health benefits and is associated with decreased mortality and age-related morbidity in older people. Currently, more than 60% of adult Americans do not exercise with any regularity, and 25% are sedentary. Physical activity levels often decrease with age and become quite low after age 75 (Pollock et al, 1998) (see *Clinical Insight:* Active Living for Healthy Aging).

Sensory Losses

The senses of taste, smell, sight, hearing, and touch often diminish at individual rates in the older adult. Less acute senses of taste *(dysgeusia)* and smell *(hyposmia)* are common and may result from various factors, including degenerative aging processes such as decreased numbers of papilla on the tongue and olfactory nerve endings, use of dentures, certain diseases such as Alzheimer's disease, medications, medical or surgical interventions, and environmental exposure. A reduction in taste and smell acuity may not only reduce appetite and the pleasure and comfort associated with food but may also be a risk factor for contracting foodborne illnesses or being overexposed to environmentally hazardous chemicals that would otherwise be detectable by taste or smell (Schiffman, 1997). Because taste and smell stimulation induces metabolic changes such as salivary, gastric acid, and pancreatic secretions and increases in plasma levels of insulin, decreased sensory stimulation may impair these metabolic processes (Schiffman and Warwick, 1992). Hearing loss, impaired vision, and loss of functional status are also common in older adults and may lead to a lower food intake as a result of decreased appetite, ability to recognize food, and self-feeding ability.

TABLE 13-1 Age-Adjusted* Prevalence of Overweight and Obese U.S. Adults (Ages 20-74 Yr)

	NHANES II (1976-1980) (*N* = 11,207)	NHANES III (1988-1994) (*N* = 14,468)	NHANES IV (1999) (*N* = 14,446)
Overweight or obese (BMI ≥25)	47	56	61
Overweight (BMI 25-29.9)	32	33	34
Obese (BMI ≥30)	15	23	27

From National Center for Health Statistics, Division of Data Services, 1999, www.cdc.gov/nchs/products/pubs/pubd/hestats/obese/obse99t2.htm.
*Age adjusted by the direct method to 2000 U.S. Bureau of the Census estimates using the age groups 20-34, 35-44, 45-54, 55-64, and 65-74 years.

Oral Health Status

Oral health can be affected by factors such as inadequate dental care, which can result in dental and periodontal problems (see Chapter 29). *Xerostomia* (dry mouth) can cause difficulty with chewing and swallowing, which can result in the avoidance of certain foods. A reduction in the number of taste buds can alter taste perception and the palatability of certain foods. Untreated dental caries and periodontitis are major causes of tooth and bone loss in older adults and can lead to edentulousness and dentures. People who are missing teeth or who wear dentures often chew less efficiently, which can cause them to eat less hard-to-chew foods such as meats, fresh fruits, and raw vegetables. Using moist food preparation techniques (e.g., stewing); adding sauces and gravies; grinding, chopping, or pureeing foods; or adding thickeners or thinners to foods can make chewing and swallowing easier. Modifications of food texture or consistency may make some foods easier to eat and therefore improve a person's overall nutrient intake. Food fortification may also help improve nutrient density when food consumption is inadequate.

Gastrointestinal Function

Numerous changes that can affect nutrient intake, digestion, absorption, and metabolism occur in the gastrointestinal (GI) system during the aging process (MacIntosh et al, 2001). Age-related changes in GI-associated mucosal immune responses also occur but have not been well studied (Beharka et al, 2001).

Dysphagia, a weakening of the gag reflex that causes swallowing difficulties, can affect a person's ability to safely consume foods. A person with dysphagia may need modifications in the texture or consistency of food, method of eating, or both (see Chapter 43). Gastric atrophy, alterations in gastric acidity, delayed gastric emptying, changes in bowel motility rates, decreased lactase activity, and medication usage can affect intake and availability of nutrients. These conditions can affect the bioavailability of nutrients, overall nutritional status, and the risk for developing chronic diseases such as osteoporosis.

Achlorhydria, loss of hydrochloric acid in the stomach, also develops in those who are aging. *Atrophic gastritis,* which results when a person has insufficient amounts of stomach acid to break protein-bound bonds necessary for the absorption of vitamin B_{12}, can cause a vitamin B_{12} deficiency (Ziesel, 2000).

Constipation, which makes it difficult to pass stools or causes incomplete or infrequent passage of stools, is one of the most common digestive complaints in older adults. It can be caused by a prolonged rectosigmoid transit time, an insufficient fluid intake, an inadequate dietary fiber intake, limitations in mobility or activity, psychologic factors, and medications (Evans et al, 1998). Constipation can often be resolved by increasing intake of dietary fiber, fluid, and kilocalories and increasing physical activity (see Chapters 29 and 30).

Cardiovascular Function

During the aging process, blood vessels become less elastic and total peripheral resistance increases, leading to an increased risk for and prevalence of hypertension. Increased vascular resistance can also cause inadequate blood flow to the heart, resulting in cardiovascular disease, which continues to be one of the leading causes of death in the United States. The risk factors that influence the development of cardiovascular disease in older adults are similar to those for middle-age adults (see Chapter 35). Treatment interventions such as the correction of hypertension and hyperlipidemia have been shown to be cost-effective ways to reduce cardiovascular morbidity and mortality in the older adult.

Renal Function

Renal function and the glomerular filtration rate can diminish as much as 60% between the ages of 30 and 80 years, primarily from a reduction in the number of *nephrons,* the functional unit of urine formation in the kidney, resulting in reduced blood flow (see Chapter 39). These anatomic changes produce a general decrease in the ability of the kidneys to concentrate urine. Consequently, older adults are often less able to respond to changes in fluid status and challenges to the acid-base balance. Excessive amounts of protein waste products and electrolytes may become increasingly difficult to metabolize, so dietary modifications may be needed. Additional complications involving kidney function can result from dehydration, hemorrhage, cardiac failure, systemic infection, improper use of diuretics, or toxic antibiotics. Compromised renal function may also result in alterations in the normal metabolism of medications, which can pose physical risks (see Chapter 39).

CLINICAL INSIGHT

Active Living for Healthy Aging

Physically active lifestyles benefit individuals throughout life. Age 50 marks an age wherein the benefits of regular physical activity can strategically prevent, minimize, or reverse many of the physical, psychological, and social declines that often accompany aging. These benefits help most individuals, regardless of their health or disease status. Reaping many of these benefits requires regular, continuous participation in activity, and the benefits are lost with inactivity.

Although scientific evidence clearly shows that regular physical activity has powerful positive effects on psychological and physical well-being, functional improvement, and quality of life, older adults are often sedentary. Sedentary lifestyles contribute to a loss of independence; to increases in health care expenditures related to chronic diseases such as hypertension, diabetes, heart disease, and some cancers; and to premature death.

Few contraindications to exercising exist. People can benefit from even moderate levels of physical activity, which can improve endurance, strength, balance, and flexibility. Individuals who have been extremely sedentary should start with short physical activity sessions with light intensity and then gradually increase the duration and intensity. Physical activity is important for individuals with medical and physical limitations, and programs can be individualized to prevent injury and help them overcome barriers and meet personal goals. Physicians can play key roles in developing activity programs by identifying physical limitations and comorbidities.

Advantages of physical activity include improvement in joint movement and degenerative joint disease symptoms; maintenance of strong bone and muscle, which reduces the risk for falls and fractures; improved flexibility, agility, coordination, balance, and range of motion; improved cardiovascular endurance from involvement of large muscle groups; preservation of independence; enhanced general well-being; changes in stereotypic perceptions of older adults; control of specific conditions such as overweight, obesity, and stress; management of diseases such as type 2 diabetes mellitus and hypercholesterolemia; and reduced risk for developing diseases such as hypertension and coronary heart disease.

Neurologic Function

Neurologic function in the older adult may be compromised for various reasons, including alterations in cerebral functioning, decreased synthesis of neurotransmitters, and less efficient nerve conduction. Smaller amounts of neurotransmitters may predispose an individual to depression and sleep disturbances. Changes in the central nervous system can cause diminished coordination and balance, changes in mental acuity and sensory interpretation, less dexterity, mood alterations, and difficulties with information retrieval. It is important for an assessment to establish a baseline for independence in activities of daily living to detect changes over time and identify those at risk for depression, dementia, Alzheimer's disease, and Parkinson's disease. Depression in the older adult may be associated with failing health, loss of independence, an inability to perform daily tasks, grief over deaths of relatives and friends, feelings of being unproductive, social isolation, financial concerns, fear of victimization, or a decrease in cognitive function. Depression can affect appetite, dietary intake, digestion, weight status, fatigue, and overall sense of well-being.

Immunocompetence

Immune function decreases with age. Although humoral and cell-mediated immunities are affected, the primary defects seem to be in the T-cell component. These changes result in a diminished ability to fight infections, leading to an increased prevalence of infections in older adults. Development of biomarkers of immune senescence may eventually help identify groups of older adults who are at risk for infections, malignancies, and possibly autoimmune diseases (Yung, 2000).

Medications

Approximately one third of the medications prescribed in the United States are considered unnecessary (Morrison and Hark, 1999). *Polypharmacy,* the unnecessary and excessive use of prescribed and over-the counter medications, increases the risk of adverse drug reactions and drug-nutrient interactions (see Chapter 19). Use of multiple medications is common among older adults. The nutritional implications of medications, which are affected by their dose, frequency, and duration, should be carefully considered, as should age-related changes in drug metabolism involving absorption, distribution, metabolism, and excretion. Pathologic factors such as cardiovascular disease, liver disease, renal disease, and GI malabsorption should also be considered. In addition, side effects of medications can affect nutrient needs, appetite, cognition, the ability to eat independently, metabolic function, and laboratory values. A complete drug history can reduce risks and lead to safer medication usage. Appropriate nutrition assessment, intervention, and counseling should be implemented to prevent or correct drug-nutrient interactions and improve nutritional status (Nelms and Anderson, 2002).

MULTIDISCIPLINARY ASSESSMENT

Based on the multidimensional changes in the older adult, it is understandable that an optimal assessment would include a multidisciplinary approach with a team of health professionals. This team would include a physician, a physician assistant, a nurse, a registered dietitian, a certified dietary manager, a social worker, a physical therapist, an occupational therapist, a speech therapist, a psychologist, an activities director, and a physical trainer. An evaluation of social functioning, economic status, and values related to advanced directive issues such as living wills and durable power of attorney for health care are also important in the overall plan of care.

A multidisciplinary assessment format significantly improves the overall care provided. Measures of mobility include an assessment of whether an individual is fully ambulatory, ambulatory with assistance, or confined to a wheelchair, room, or bed. Measures of functional status evaluate the ability of individuals to perform the survival tasks necessary to negotiate everyday life in their own environment. Measures of functional status include an assessment of level of independence related to activities of daily living and instrumental activities of daily living (Box 13-1).

Box 13-1. Activities of Daily Living and Instrumental Activities of Daily Living

Activities of Daily Living

- Eating
- Moving into and out of beds and chairs
- Being mobile indoors and outdoors
- Dressing
- Bathing
- Toileting
- Maintaining continence

Instrumental Activities of Daily Living

- Using the telephone
- Traveling
- Shopping
- Preparing meals
- Doing light housework
- Taking medication
- Managing money

NUTRITION SCREENING

Data from the third NHANES (NHANES III) suggest that the older adult is at risk for malnutrition because of the presence of disease, physical disabilities, poor dental and oral health, polypharmacy, social isolation, financial limitations, or impaired mental health (www.cdc.gov/nchs/nhanes.htm). In the national *Healthy People* objectives, nutrition screening is emphasized as a necessary component of primary care. Nutrition screening and interventions have been shown to be cost effective, improve the quality of life, promote health, reduce complications and hospital length of stay, reduce health care costs, and delay admissions into nursing homes (see Chapter 17).

Several tools are available to screen older adults to identify risks for malnutrition. The Mini Nutritional Assessment (MNA) is an efficient, innovative, noninvasive method for detecting the risk for malnutrition. The MNA consists of questions and anthropometric measures to determine a malnutrition indicator score (Vellas et al, 1999; www.nestleclinicalnutrition.com).

The Nutrition Screening Initiative (NSI) is a broad, multidisciplinary effort led by the American Academy of Family Physicians (AAP), the American Dietetic Association, the National Council on Aging, and a diverse coalition of organizations related to health, aging, and medicine. The initiative was established as a multifaceted campaign to improve the incorporation of nutrition screening and intervention in the nation's health care delivery system for older adults (NSI, 1991). The initiative developed and validated the *Determine Your Nutritional Health Checklist* to serve as a public awareness tool (Figures 13-5 and 13-6).

The NSI also developed more comprehensive assessment tools to be used for those identified through the screening process to be at risk for poor nutrition. More comprehensive assessment tools include data on medical history, current diagnoses, medications, anthropometric values, biochemical indexes, and physical or clinical evaluations. A new tool is available at www.aafp.org/nsi/palm.html.

Health professionals consider inadequate third-party reimbursements to be a primary obstacle to routine screening and treatment. Because the broad consensus is that nutritional screening and treatment should be included as part of a reimbursable basic benefits package, the initiative team is working on several approaches to expand reimbursement for nutrition screening and services. The NSI promoted alliances to ensure that nutritional status is considered

The Nutrition Checklist is based on the Warning Signs described below.
Use the word DETERMINE to remind you of the Warning signs.

Disease Any disease, illness or chronic condition which causes you to change the way you eat, or makes it hard for you to eat, puts your nutritional health at risk. Four out of five adults have chronic diseases that are affected by diet. Confusion or memory loss that keeps getting worse is estimated to affect one out of five or more of older adults. This can make it hard to remember what, when or if you've eaten. Feeling sad or depressed, which happens to about one in eight older adults, can cause big changes in appetite, digestion, energy level, weight and well-being.

Eating Poorly Eating too little and eating too much both lead to poor health. Eating the same foods day after day or not eating fruit, vegetables, and milk products daily will also cause poor nutritional health. One in five adults skip meals daily. Only 13% of adults eat the minimum amount of fruit and vegetables needed. One in four older adults drink too much alcohol. Many health problems become worse if you drink more than one or two alcoholic beverages per day.

Tooth Loss/Mouth Pain A healthy mouth, teeth, and gums are needed to eat. Missing, loose, or rotten teeth, or dentures which don't fit well or cause mouth sores, make it hard to eat.

Economic Hardship As many as 40% of older Americans have incomes of less than $6,000 per year. Having less—or choosing to spend less— than $25–30 per week for food makes it very hard to get the foods you need to stay healthy.

Reduced Social Contact One-third of all older people live alone. Being with people daily has a positive effect on morale, well-being and eating.

Multiple Medicines Many older Americans must take medicines for health problems. Almost half of older Americans take multiple medicines daily. Growing old may change the way we respond to drugs. The more medicines you take, the greater the chance for side effects, such as increased or decreased appetite, change in taste, constipation, weakness, drowsiness, diarrhea, nausea, and others. Vitamins or minerals, when taken in large doses, act like drugs and can cause harm. Alert your doctor to everything you take.

Involuntary Weight Loss/Gain Losing or gaining a lot of weight when you are not trying to do so is an important warning sign that must not be ignored. Being overweight or underweight also increases your chance of poor health.

Needs Assistance in Self-Care Although most older people are able to eat, one out of every five has trouble walking, shopping, or buying and cooking food, especially as they get older.

Elder Years Above Age 80 Most older people lead full and productive lives. But as age increases, the risk of frailty and health problems increases. Checking your nutritional health regularly makes good sense.

FIGURE 13-5 • *Determine Your Nutritional Health* checklist. (Courtesy Nutrition Screening Initiative, a project of the American Academy of Family Physicians, the American Dietetic Association, and the National Council of the Aging and funded in part by a grant from Ross Products Division, Abbott Laboratories, 1991.)

DETERMINE YOUR NUTRITIONAL HEALTH

The Warning Signs of poor nutritional health are often overlooked. Use this checklist to find out if you or someone you know is at nutritional risk.

Read the statements below. Circle the number in the yes column for those that apply to you or someone you know. For each yes answer, score the number in the box. Total your nutrition score.

	YES
I have an illness or condition that made me change the kind and/or amount of food I eat.	2
I eat fewer than 2 meals per day.	3
I eat few fruits or vegetables, or milk products.	2
I have 3 or more drinks of beer, liquor or wine almost every day.	2
I have tooth or mouth problems that make it hard for me to eat.	2
I don't always have enough money to buy the food I need.	4
I eat alone most of the time.	1
I take 3 or more different prescribed or over-the-counter drugs a day.	1
Without wanting to, I have lost or gained 10 pounds in the last 6 months.	2
I am not physically able to shop, cook and/or feed myself.	2
TOTAL	

Total Your Nutritional Score. If it's —

0–2 **Good!** Recheck your nutritional score in 6 months.

3–5 **You are at moderate nutritional risk.** See what can be done to improve your eating habits and lifestyle. Your office on aging, senior nutrition program, senior citizens center or health department can help. Recheck your nutritional score in 3 months.

6 or more **You are at high nutritional risk.** Bring this checklist the next time you see your doctor, dietitian or other qualified health or social service professional. Talk with them about any problems you may have. Ask for help to improve your nutritional health.

Remember that warning signs suggest risk but do not represent diagnosis of any condition.

FIGURE 13-6 • *Determine Your Nutritional Health* checklist. (Courtesy Nutrition Screening Initiative, a project of the American Academy of Family Physicians, the American Dietetic Association, and the National Council of the Aging and funded in part by a grant from Ross Products Division, Abbott Laboratories, 1991.)

a fundamental component of health care (Wellman, 1994). The first Medicare coverage, which was effective January 2002, provided coverage for nutrition services by a registered dietitian for those with diabetes and pre–end-stage renal disease.

NUTRITION NEEDS

Each older adult has unique needs, so dietary recommendations should be individualized. The current dietary reference intakes (DRIs), established to optimize health for individuals and groups, provide a guideline for assessing intake and estimating needs and reflect the latest understanding about nutrient requirements (Table 13-2) (Bryant, Cadogan, and Weaver, 1999).

Energy

Energy requirements generally decrease with age because of changes in body composition, a decrease in the basal metabolic rate, and a reduction in physical activity. An estimation of energy needs can be determined based on an actual or a desired body weight, basal energy expenditure, resting energy expenditure, or total energy expenditure (see Chapter 2). Meeting the nutritional needs of the older adult can be challenging because although energy requirements decrease, most requirements for protein, vitamins, and minerals remain the same or increase. Although obesity in humans is associated with a shorter life expectancy, the extent of the effect is somewhat controversial. Some data have indicated that the mortality rate associated with being underweight is the same as the rate associated with moderate obesity, particularly in those older than 60 years of age. A desirable BMI can be estimated in relation to a person's age to determine a more appropriate estimate of energy needs (Table 13-3).

An average caloric intake is 2000 kcal/day for older men and 1600 kcal/day for women. Health problems arise when intakes are less than 1500 kcal/day; supplementation is often needed for those who have a severely restricted caloric intake.

Protein

As people age and experience a loss of skeletal tissue mass, stores of protein in skeletal muscle may be inadequate to meet the needs for protein synthesis, making dietary protein intake more important. Decreased food intake, a sedentary lifestyle, and reduced energy expenditure in older adults become critical risk factors for malnutrition and especially for insufficient intake of protein and micronutrients (Meydani, 2001). Although the recommended intake for protein has not changed, some studies have demonstrated that an intake of 1 g/kg is needed to maintain a positive nitrogen balance in an older adult (Campbell, 1996). A protein intake of 1 to 1.25 g/kg is generally safe for older adults (*Merck Manual of Geriatrics,* 2001).

Protein needs increase in relation to acute and chronic diseases. Stressful physical and psychological stimuli can induce a negative nitrogen balance. Infection, altered GI function, and metabolic changes caused by chronic disease can reduce the efficiency of dietary nitrogen use and increase nitrogen excretion.

The serum albumin level is the most reliable indicator of protein status in older adults, whereas other short-lived proteins such as prealbumin and retinal binding protein may be used in more serious situations to evaluate a person's response to therapy (*Merck Manual of Geriatrics,* 2001). Healthy, ambulatory older adults can have serum albumin levels greater than 4 g/dl or 3.5 g/dl because of fluid shifts when lying down for long periods (*Merck Manual of Geriatrics,* 2001). Other serum protein values such as transferrin, urea nitrogen, and total protein, are less reliable but may help evaluate an individual's response to therapy. Serum albumin levels can be used to estimate protein needs (Table 13-4).

Carbohydrates

Abundant carbohydrates are needed to protect protein from being used as an energy source. Current dietary guidelines recommend that approximately 45% to 65% of the total daily calories come from carbohydrates. Emphasis should be placed on increasing the intake of complex carbohydrate sources such as legumes, vegetables, whole grains, and fruits to provide fiber, phylochemicals, and essential vitamins and minerals.

Lipids

Current adult dietary guidelines recommend that no more than 25% to 35% of the total daily caloric intake come from lipids. Emphasis should be placed on reducing the intake of saturated fat and choosing monounsaturated or polyunsaturated fat sources. Although only limited available evidence shows that dietary changes can reduce the risk of cardiovascular events in older adults, people have no reason to doubt that the same environmental factors leading to a decreased risk in the younger population will continue to be effective in later years. The recommended modified use of dietary fat also supports principles of weight control and cancer prevention. Conversely, restricting dietary fat to less than 20% of the caloric intake may affect the overall quality of the diet and negatively affect taste, satiety, and intake.

Minerals

Aging produces physiologic changes that affect the need for several essential nutrients. Whereas overt mineral deficiencies are less common in the healthy adult, subclinical nutrient deficiencies that affect metabolic function can develop. Poor mineral status in the older adult can be attributed to inadequate dietary intake, physiologic changes that affect the need for a nutrient, and medications. Some older adults may have to increase the variety of their diet and take a nonfood dietary nutrient supplement to consume adequate levels of nutrients (Marshal et al, 2001).

Diminished lactase secretion can cause lactose intolerance and GI complaints, which can result in decreased consumption of dairy products. Dietary modifications, including controlled intake of lactose-containing products, substitution of less problematic dairy products, and use of lactase-treated products, can help alleviate the discomfort from cramping, flatulence, and diarrhea. As people age, they experience an intrinsic decrease in calcium absorption, primarily because of a change in calcium transport (Nordin et al, 1998). As the calcium decreases below its necessary level, calcium is mobilized from the bones to maintain the calcium concentration of extracellular fluid, destroying whole bone. Bone loss resulting in osteoporosis, the presence of **hypochlorhydria** (a deficiency of hydrochloric acid in the gastric juice), and failure to efficiently absorb calcium can affect calcium status. Because approximately 10 million people in the United States have osteoporosis and 18 million have low bone mass, calcium-rich products should be included in the diet (see Chapter 27).

Iron deficiency anemia is uncommon in older adults than in younger people, especially in women after menopause. In older adults, anemia is most likely to be related to blood loss from disease and medications or decreased absorption caused by medications or hypochlorhydria.

Intakes of zinc in older adults decrease in relation to the decrease in energy intake and are much lower than the recommended level of 15 mg/day for men and 12 mg/day for women. Definite indicators of zinc status are not available, which impedes its assessment in older adults. Older people who avoid eating meat and fish may be at increased risk of poor zinc status because of the reduced bioavailabilty of zinc from other food sources. Zinc deficiency is associated with impaired immune function, anorexia, *dysgeusia* (the loss of the sense of taste), delayed wound healing, and pressure ulcers.

Sodium intake is often associated with hypertension, but it is difficult to identify individuals who are sensitive to dietary sodium. Therefore it is prudent to limit the dietary sodium intake to approximately 2 to 4 g/day and increase intakes of other minerals such as potassium, magnesium, and calcium (see Chapter 36).

TABLE 13-2 Dietary Reference Intakes for Older Adults

VITAMINS AND ELEMENTS

	VITAMIN A (μg)[d,e]	VITAMIN C (mg)	VITAMIN D (μg)[f,g]	VITAMIN E (mg)[h,i,j]	VITAMIN K (μg)	THIAMIN (mg)	RIBOFLAVIN (mg)	NIACIN (mg)[j,k]	VITAMIN B_6 (mg)	FOLATE (μg)[j,l]
RDA or AI[b]										
Age 51-70										
Men	900	90	*10*	15	*120*	1.2	1.3	16	1.7	400
Women	700	75	*10*	15	*90*	1.1	1.1	14	1.5	400
Age 70+										
Men	900	90	*15*	15	*120*	1.2	1.3	16	1.7	400
Women	700	75	*15*	15	*90*	1.1	1.1	14	1.5	400
UL[c]										
Age 51-70										
Men	3000	2000	50	1000	ND[a]	ND	ND	35	100	1000
Women	3000	2000	50	1000	ND	ND	ND	35	100	1000
Age 70+										
Men	3000	2000	50	1000	ND	ND	ND	35	100	1000
Women	3000	2000	50	1000	ND	ND	ND	35	100	1000

	VITAMIN B_{12} (μg)[m]	PANTOTHENIC ACID (mg)	BIOTIN (μg)	CHOLINE (mg)[n]	BORON (mg)	CALCIUM (mg)	CHROMIUM (μg)	COPPER (μg)	FLUORIDE (mg)	IODINE (μg)
RDA or AI[b]										
Age 51-70										
Men	2.4	*5*	*30*	*550*	ND	*1200*	*30*	900	*4*	150
Women	2.4	*5*	*30*	*425*	ND	*1200*	*20*	900	*3*	150
Age 70+										
Men	2.4	*5*	*30*	*550*	ND	*1200*	*30*	900	*4*	150
Women	2.4	*5*	*30*	*425*	ND	*1200*	*20*	900	*3*	150
UL[c]										
Age 51-70										
Men	ND	ND	ND	3500	20	2500	ND	10,000	10	1100
Women	ND	ND	ND	3500	20	2500	ND	10,000	10	1100
Age 70+										
Men	ND	ND	ND	3500	20	2500	ND	10,000	10	1100
Women	ND	ND	ND	3500	20	2500	ND	10,000	10	1100

ELEMENTS AND MACRONUTRIENTS

	IRON (mg)	MAGNESIUM (mg)[o]	MANGANESE (mg)	MOLYBDENUM (mg)	NICKEL (mg)	PHOSPHORUS (mg)	SELENIUM (μg)	VANADIUM (mg)[p]	ZINC (mg)
RDA or AI[b]									
Age 51-70									
Men	8	420	*2.3*	45	ND[a]	700	55	ND	11
Women	8	320	*1.8*	45	ND	700	55	ND	8
Age 70+									
Men	8	420	*2.3*	45	ND	700	55	ND	11
Women	8	320	*1.8*	45	ND	700	55	ND	8

UL[c]									
Age 51-70									
Men	45	350	11	2000	1	4000	400	1.8	40
Women	45	350	11	2000	1	4000	400	1.8	40
Age 70+									
Men	45	350	11	2000	1	3000	400	1.8	40
Women	45	350	11	2000	1	3000	400	1.8	40

	ENERGY (kcal)	PROTEIN (g)	CARBOHYDRATES[r]	TOTAL FAT[r]	SATURATED FAT[r]	CHOLESTEROL (mg)	SODIUM (mg)	FIBER (mg)[s]
1989 RDAs								
Age 51+[q]								
Men	2204	56	**130**	20-35%	<10%	<300	<2400	30
Women	1978	46	**130**	20-35%	<10%	<300	<2400	21

Data from Institute of Medicine, Food and Nutrition Board: *Dietary reference intakes: applications in dietary assessment,* Washington, D.C., 2000, National Academy Press. *Health implications of dietary fiber.* Position of the American Dietetic Association, *J Am Diet Assoc* 97:1157-1159, 1997, compiled by the National Policy and Resource Center on Nutrition and Aging, Miami, Fla, Florida International University, Spring 2003.

[a]*ND,* Values not determined.

[b]Recommended dietary allowances (RDAs) are in **bold,** and adequate intakes (AIs) are in *italics.* RDAs and AIs may both be used as goals for individual intake. RDAs are set to meet the needs of almost all (97% to 98%) of the individuals in a group. The AI for life-stage and gender groups (other than healthy, breast-fed infants) is believed to address needs of all individuals in the group, but lack of or uncertainty in data prevent specification of the percentage of individuals addressed by this intake.

[c]*UL,* Tolerable upper intake level. The maximum level of daily nutrient intake that is likely to pose no risk of adverse effects. Unless otherwise specified, the UL represents total intake from food, water, and supplements. Because of a lack of suitable data, ULs could not be established for vitamin K, thiamin, riboflavin, vitamin B_{12}, pantothenic acid, biotin, or carotenoids. In the absence of ULs, use caution when consuming levels above recommended intakes.

[d]As retinal activity equivalents (RAEs). 1 RAE = 1 μg retinal, 12 μg β-carotene, or 24 μg β-cryptoxanthin. To calculate RAEs from the REs of provitamin A carotenoids in foods, divide the REs by 2. For preformed vitamin A in foods or supplements and for provitamin A carotenoids in supplements, 1 RE = 1 RAE.

[e]ULs: As preformed vitamin A only.

[f]Cholecalciferol. 1 μg cholecalciferol = 40 IU vitamin D.

[g]In the absence of adequate exposure to sunlight.

[h]As α-tocopherol. α-Tocopherol includes RRR-α-tocopherol, the only form of α-tocopherol that exists naturally in foods, and the 2R-steroisomeric forms of tocopherol (RRR-, RSR-, RRS-, and RSS-α-tocopherol) that exist in fortified foods and supplements. It does not include the 2S-stereoisomeric forms of α-tocopherol (SRR-, SSR-, SRS-, SSS-α-tocopherol), also found in fortified foods and supplements.

[i]ULs: As α-tocopherol; applies to any form of supplemental α-tocopherol.

[j]The ULs for vitamin E, niacin, and folate apply to synthetic forms obtained from supplements, fortified foods, or a combination of the two.

[k]As niacin equivalents (NE). 1 mg of niacin = 60 mg of tryptophan: 0-6 months = preformed niacin (not NE).

[l]As dietary folate equivalents (DFE). 1 DFE = 1 μg food folate = 0.6 μg of folic acid from fortified food or as a supplement consumed with food = 0.5 ?g of a supplement taken on an empty stomach.

[m]Because 10%-30% of older people may malabsorb food-bound B_{12}, it is advisable for those older than 50 years of age to meet their RDA mainly by consuming foods fortified with B_{12} or a supplement containing B_{12}.

[n]Although AIs have been set for choline, few data assess whether a dietary supply of choline is needed at all stages of the life cycle, and the choline requirement may be able to be met by endogenous synthesis at some of these stages.

[o]The ULs for magnesium represent intake from a pharmacologic agent only and do not include intake from food and water.

[p]Although vanadium in food has not been shown to have adverse effects in humans, adding vanadium to food cannot be justified and vanadium supplements should be used with caution. The UL is based on adverse effects in laboratory animals; these data could be used to set a UL for adults but not children and adolescents.

[q]The 1989 RDAs are used because no new DRIs have been established for energy, protein, and other macronutrients.

[r]The Food and Nutrition Board's Committee on Diet and Health recommendations base intake on the percentage of total calories in the diet (NCR, 1989).

[s]The National Cancer Institute and American Dietetic Association recommend 20-35 g dietary fiber daily (ADA, 1997).

TABLE 13-3 Desirable Body Mass Index by Age

AGE (YEARS)	BMI (WEIGHT/HEIGHT [kg/m^2])
19-24	19-24
25-34	20-25
35-44	21-26
45-54	22-27
55-65	23-28
>65	24-29

From Food and Nutrition Board, Committee on Diet and Health, National Research Council: *Implications for reducing chronic disease risk,* Washington, DC, 1989, National Academies Press.

TABLE 13-4 Protein Requirements for Repletion of Low Serum Albumin Levels

CONDITION	ALBUMIN (g/dl)	PROTEIN REQUIREMENT (g/kg/day)
Normal nutritional status	>3.5	0.8
Mild depletion	2.8-3.5	1.0-1.2
Moderate depletion	2.1-2.7	1.2-1.5
Severe depletion	<2.1	1.5-2.0

Modified from *North Carolina Dietetic Association diet manual* and *Nutritional aspects of sound healing,* 1993, Nestle/Clintec Nutrition Co.

Vitamins

Much remains to be learned about vitamin requirements and the efficiency of vitamin absorption, use, and excretion in the older adult. Oxidative mechanisms may play an important role in the aging process. It is important to emphasize the relationship between health and nutrition, particularly in relation to requirements for antioxidant vitamins such as tocopherols, carotenoids, and vitamin C (Richard and Roussel, 1999). Antioxidants act as a buffer against cell damage that can occur during normal cell function. If this cell damage is allowed to accumulate, the risk of certain diseases such as cataracts, heart disease, and cancer increases (Ausman and Mayer, 1999). Suboptimal intakes of key vitamins may place a person at risk for chronic illness, especially in the elderly (Fletcher and Fairfield, 2002).

Assessments of vitamin A intake are important because it is often deficient in diets of older adults. However, consumption of too much vitamin A is not beneficial. A recent study (Feskanich et al, 2002) suggests that high doses may contribute to the incidence of hip fractures. Dietary sources of vitamin A such as dark green, leafy, and yellow-orange fruits and vegetables should be carefully included in the diet to provide adequate but not excessive β-carotene, the precursor to vitamin A.

Older adults often have lower serum levels of vitamin C than younger adults. However, no age-related alterations seem to be associated with the absorption or use of vitamin C. Stress, smoking, and some medications can increase vitamin C requirements, so an assessment of dietary intake is especially important for individuals who may be at risk. Encouraging the consumption of vitamin C–rich foods may be the most effective way of improving vitamin C status in the older adult.

The requirement for vitamin D depends on the concentration of calcium and phosphorus in the diet and the person's age, sex, degree of exposure to sunlight, and amount of skin pigmentation. The ability to synthesize vitamin D from the sun is approximately 60% lower in the older adult (Miesler, 1999). The influence of age on vitamin D absorption from the GI tract is unclear. The lower levels of vitamin D in older adults who are institutionalized or homebound may result from decreased exposure to sunlight, less efficient synthesis of vitamin D in the skin, or a decrease in renal mass that causes insufficient production of vitamin D (Nordin et al, 1998; Ryan, Eleazer, and Egbert, 1995). A decrease in skin thickness is partially related to the lower levels of 25-hydroxyvitamin D levels that are associated with aging (Need et al, 1993). Vitamin D may help heal skin lesions, especially those caused by psoriasis (Cather and Menter, 2002); hyperproliferative disorders of cancer; and actinic keratoses. Moderate dietary supplementation with calcium and vitamin D improves bone density and may prevent fractures in healthy older adults (Dawson-Hughes et al, 1997).

It may be beneficial to enhance the vitamin E content in diets for older adults. From epidemiologic studies, the antioxidant properties of vitamin E may help reduce the risk of cardiovascular disease, in part by reducing the susceptibility of low-density lipoproteins to oxidation, thus decreasing the vascular endothelial cell expression of proinflammatory cytokines (Meydani, 2001). However, clinical trials have not demonstrated clear evidence of prevention. Vitamin E may have also a role in cancer prevention, but more clinical trials are needed to establish its activities (see Chapter 40).

Many studies have demonstrated that older adults do not consume enough vitamin B_6. Because of atrophic gastritis (which interferes with absorption), alcoholism, and liver dysfunction, requirements for the vitamin are increased in some older adults.

No specific age-related impact on folate requirements are known; however, alcoholism could result in a folate deficiency. Severe deficiencies in an older adult may result in anemia and elevated serum homocysteine levels, increasing the risk for cardiac disease (see Chapter 26). Diets are often lacking in folate, so consumption of folate-fortified foods (e.g., cereals, flour products) or folate-rich foods (e.g., liver, dried beans, broccoli, avocados, asparagus, spinach) should be encouraged (see Chapter 4).

Screening for vitamin B_{12} levels in older adults is needed because of the prevalence of deficiency related to GI and metabolic changes. Vitamin B_{12} deficiency affects 10% to 15% of those older than age 60 (Baik and Russell, 1999). The usual causes of vitamin B_{12} deficiency are atrophic gastritis, bacterial overgrowth, pernicious anemia, and decreased absorption related to conditions such as Crohn's disease, ileal resection, or malabsorption syndromes (Hoffbrand and Provan, 1997). People with these conditions may require a higher dietary vitamin B_{12} intake and need oral or injectable vitamin supplementation. Vitamin B_{12} is important for all older adults, not just those with deficiencies (Dharmarajan and Norhus, 2001).

Water

Hydration status is a critical component of the initial and ongoing assessment of a person at any age. Fluid needs are affected by variations in activity, insensible water losses, medications, and urinary solute load. Daily fluid replacement is essential, particularly in those who exercise regularly, consume large amounts of protein, use laxatives or diuretics, or live in areas with high temperatures. In general, daily fluid needs are approximately 30 to 35 ml per kilogram of actual body weight, with a minimum of 1500 ml/day or 1 to 1.5 ml per kilocalorie consumed. With age, total body water decreases. Water accounts for approximately 50% of an older person's weight, which is 10% less than in a young adult's; the decrease is associated with a corresponding decrease in lean body mass. Reduced thirst sensation, reduced fluid intake, limited access to fluid, diminished renal function, and urinary incontinence all increase the risk for dehydration.

Dehydration is more common in older adults than recognized. Symptoms of dehydration include electrolyte disturbances, altered drug effects, headache, constipation, thirst, loss of skin elasticity, weight loss, cognitive status deterioration, dizziness, dry mouth and nose mucous membranes, a swollen or dry tongue, blood pressure changes, recessed or sunken eyes, changes in urine color or output, and speech difficulties. An insufficient fluid intake in a person with frequent diarrhea or vomiting, fever, illness, infection, organ failure, or some chronic disease can lead to clinical dehydration requiring hospitalization. Careful monitoring of fluid intake and output is important.

DIETARY PLANNING

People of all ages need various nutrients to stay healthy. They can obtain them by having a balanced diet with regular consumption of foods from all food groups. With age, nutrient density becomes even more important; a person's diet must provide enough fluid, calcium, fiber, iron, protein, folic acid, and vitamins A, D, B_{12}, and C without extra calories. Often, older adults do not include adequate fruits, vegetables, and dairy products, which can affect their nutritional status. The USDA Food Consumption Survey and the NHANES I, II, and III correlate with studies that demonstrate that the older adult may be at nutritional risk because of an inadequate intake of vitamin D, vitamin E, folate, and calcium and excessive intake of protein and fat (Foote, Guiliano, and Harris, 2000).

Food is the best source of nutrients, and supplements are often unnecessary for the healthy older adult. However, use of vitamin and mineral supplements is common in the older population (Kaufman et al, 2002), so older adults should be advised about potentially toxic doses (Chandra et al, 1991). Vitamins, minerals, and herbal supplements are frequently used for nonspecific reasons such as "to stay healthy" (Kaufman et al, 2002.) Questions about over-the-counter supplements and herbal products should always be included in a comprehensive nutritional assessment.

Basic diet planning principles that include moderation, balance, and variety apply to the older adult and comply with the Dietary Guidelines for the United States and the USDA Food Guide Pyramid. An important guideline is to consume meals and snacks that are nutrient dense, visually appealing, tasty, and of the appropriate consistency. Four or five smaller meals are often better tolerated than three substantial ones. The American Dietetic Association modified the USDA Food Guide Pyramid to reflect dietary intake recommendations for those 50 years and older (Figure 13-7).

A different Food Guide Pyramid for those 70 years of age and older has been developed at the USDA Human Nutrition Research Center on Aging at Tufts University and recognizes the nutrient needs of this age group (Figure 13-8). This pyramid has water as its foundation to reinforce the need for adequate hydration and highlights foods that are good sources of calcium and vitamins D and B_{12} and the need for supplements.

NUTRITION ISSUES

Certain groups within the aging population are at risk of malnutrition for various reasons, including lack of nutrition education, financial constraints, decreasing physical and psychological abilities, social isolation, and treatments for multiple, concomitant disorders or diseases. Secondary causes of malnutrition include feeding impairments, anorexia, malabsorption from GI dysfunction, increased nutrient needs as a result of injury or disease, drug-nutrient interactions resulting from polypharmacy, and substance abuse such as alcoholism. Some common at-risk issues in the older population include dysphagia, pressure ulcers, Alzheimer's disease, Parkinson's

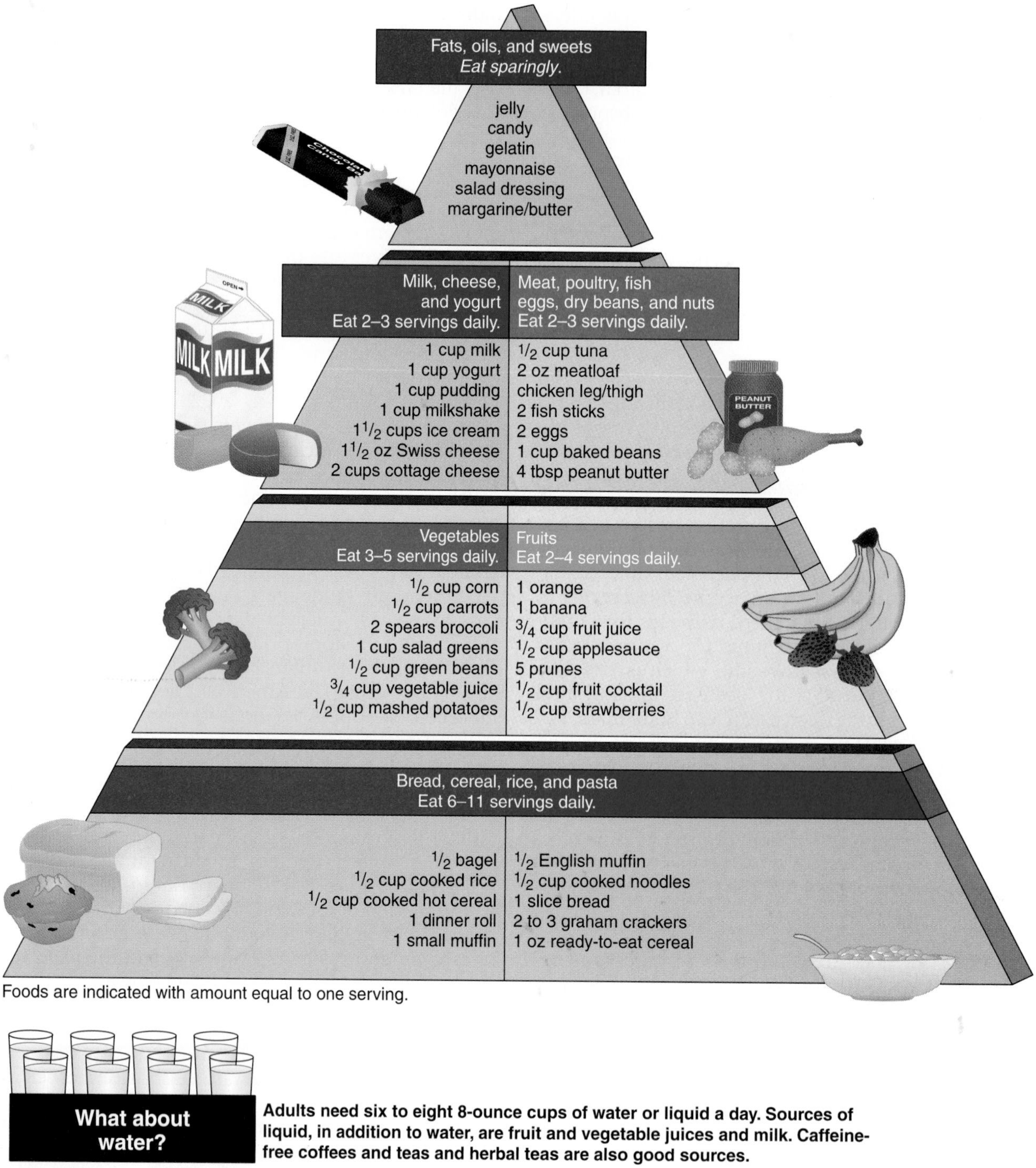

FIGURE 13-7 • Food Guide Pyramid for adults 50 years of age and older. (From American Dietetic Association: *Nutrition management and restorative dining,* 2001 Chicago, The Association.)

disease, geriatric failure to thrive, osteoporosis, type 2 diabetes, hypertension, and constipation.

Dysphagia

Speech therapists, physicians, nurses, and dietitians work together to assess an individual's swallowing ability and design an individualized diet. The evaluation and monitoring of dysphagia can include an assessment of the cause of drooling of liquids or solids, coughing during or after swallowing, facial or tongue weakness, difficulty managing secretions, pocketing food or beverages, poor head or posture control, a prolonged eating time, and a change in

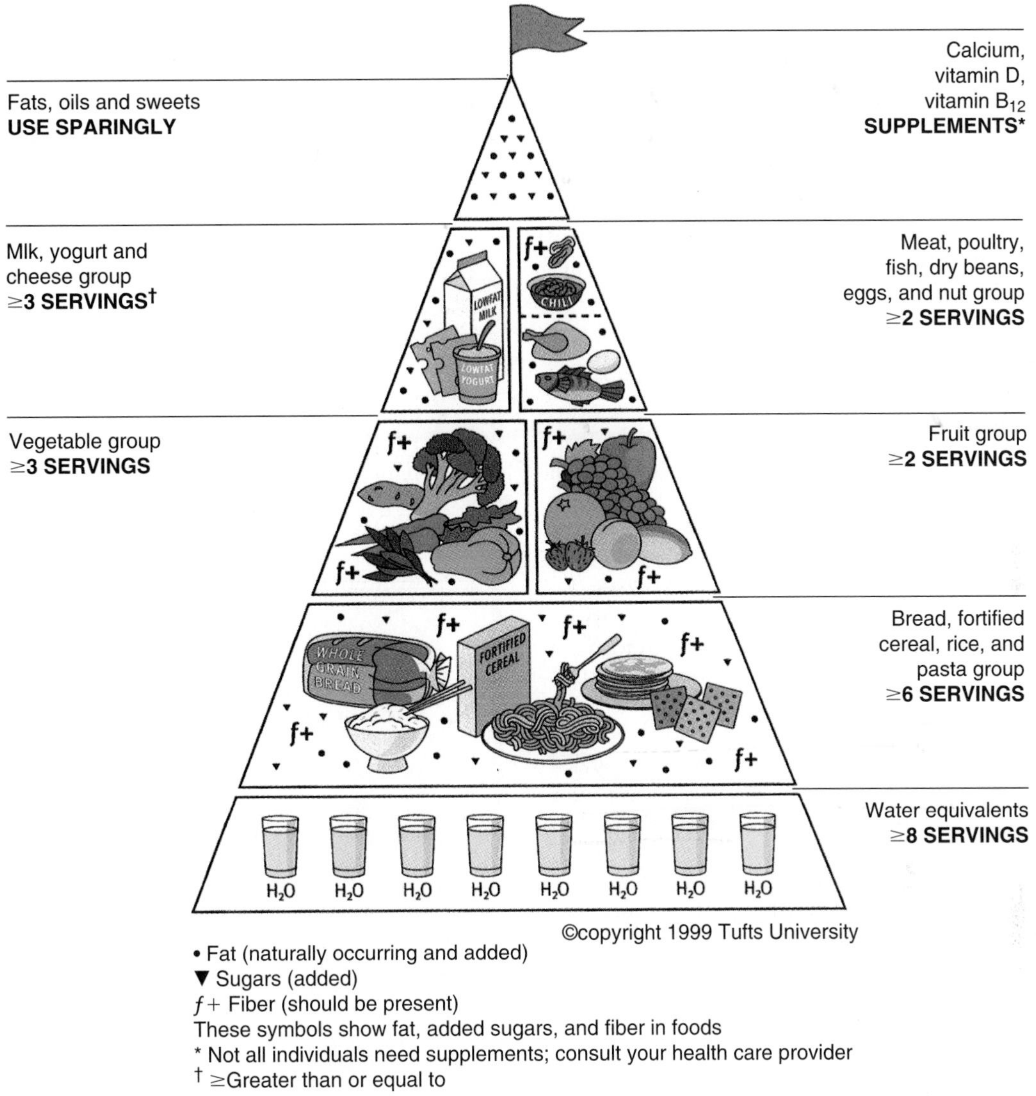

FIGURE 13-8 • Tufts University Modified Food Pyramid for adults 70 years of age and older. (Copyright 1999, Tufts University, Boston, Mass.)

voice quality from normal to hoarse or wet sounds. Careful selection and seasoning of foods are important. Food can chopped, ground, or pureed until the individual is able to begin eating food with regular consistencies. The consistency of liquids can be modified to thin, nectar, honey, or pudding consistency using a thickening agent. Appropriate body positioning also helps reduce the risk of choking. (See Chapter 43 for a detailed dysphagia discussion.)

Pressure Ulcers

Pressure ulcers are most common in older adults who are confined to a bed or wheelchair or are unable to position themselves. They usually develop below the waist but can develop anywhere on the body. People at risk for developing pressure ulcers include those who have medical conditions such as diabetes mellitus or peripheral vascular disease, a chronic illness, cognitive impairments, mobility problems, incontinence, or neurologic impairments. In addition, those who are unable to feed themselves sufficiently may be at risk for pressure ulcers because of their inadequate intake of nutrients such as kilocalories, protein, zinc, and vitamin C. Frequent monitoring of body weight, skin integrity, and relevant laboratory values for nutritional status are important in the prevention and treatment of pressure ulcers.

Pressure ulcers are categorized into four stages according to the depth of damage. Clinical practice guidelines developed by the U.S. Department of Health and Human Services (DHHS) for the treatment of pressure ulcers are based on these stages and include pressure reduction by frequent repositioning, use of support surfaces, moisture reduction, debridement, and nutritional support (DHHS, 1994). Risk factors for pressure ulcer formation include a weight decrease of more than 15%, a serum albumin level of <3.5 mg/dl, and a low total lymphocyte count <1800/L. High-protein, high-energy diets with vitamin C and zinc supplementation and adequate fluid intake are usually used to spare protein for wound healing and tissue epithelialization. Commercial oral supplements or tube feedings can help meet higher nutrient needs.

Alzheimer's and Parkinson's Diseases

Alzheimer's disease is a degenerative brain disorder that results in irreversible memory loss and intellectual and personality deterioration; it affects at least 2.5 million people in the United States. As the disease progresses, the risk for malnutrition increases. Appetite and food intake fluctuate with emotional state, agitation level, and confusion level. Feeding skills decrease with cognitive and physical deterioration. Strategies to improve care can involve providing a simple, predictable environment and frequent cues relating to daily activities (see Chapter 43).

Parkinson's disease is a neurodegenerative disease that affects voluntary movement. It is characterized by the loss of brain cells that produce dopamine, a chemical that helps direct muscle activity. Constipation, difficulty chewing and swallowing, dribbling, and mental confusion contribute to an increased risk for malnutrition. Intervention often includes medication, exercise, and nutrition management, particularly in the coordination of dietary protein adequacy and timing of intake with medication regimens (see Chapter 43).

Failure to Thrive

Malnutrition compromises the immune system and can contribute to the development of infection or sepsis, pressure ulcers, delayed wound healing, multisystem organ failure, disability, longer hospital stays, increased health care costs, and death. Malnutrition is associated with higher morbidity and mortality, as well as a poor quality of life (Huffman, 2002). Because it is more difficult to correct nutritional status once it has deteriorated, early detection of malnutrition is very important. When malnutrition is detected with proper screening techniques, nutritional intervention can be started early, and further deterioration can be prevented (Box 13-2). Involuntary weight loss is the best single factor for predicting who is at risk for malnutrition. Unexplained, involuntary weight loss, especially if it is significant and progressive, is cause for concern. *Significant weight loss* is defined as a documented continued weight loss of greater than 5% or more than 10 lb in 6 to 12 months. Inadequate food consumption because of psychosocial and other factors is one of the most common causes of unplanned weight loss (Roberts, 2000).

Box 13-2. Key Factors for Assessing Those at Risk for Malnutrition

- Weight Loss
- BMI <21
- Serum albumin level <3.5 g/dl
- Cholesterol level <160 mg/dl
- Decreased food, fluid, and nutrient intake
- Loss of interest in food or decreased desire to eat
- Anorexia
- Early satiety
- Oral health
- Dysphagia
- Functional status
- Cognitive and emotional status (depression)
- Medications
- Alcohol intake
- Institutionalization
- Poverty
- Presence of infectious disease
- Early Alzheimer's disease
- Increased loss of ingested nutrients through stools or urine
- Increased metabolic rate from congestive heart failure

The release of cytokines in a person with a chronic disease may be an important predictor of malnutrition (Bales and Ritchie, 2002). Cytokines contribute to lipolysis, muscle protein breakdown, and nitrogen loss. Clinical interventions for weight loss, *sarcopenia* (age-related loss of skeletal muscle), and cytokine alterations have been used with modest success (Bales and Ritchie, 2002).

Nutrition intervention guidelines include weight restoration through increased intake of protein, energy, and fluids. Restorative interventions may involve nutrient fortification of foods or beverages, frequent oral feeding, or use of enteral or parenteral nutrition support (see Chapter 23). Referrals for medical, psychological, dental, and support services may also be indicated.

SUPPORTIVE SERVICES

Various food and nutrition programs have been implemented at the federal, state, and local levels to provide food assistance to the older population. The

Older Americans Act (OAA) of 1965 established the Administration on Aging (AOA) under the U.S. DHHS, and the most recent reauthorization was in 2000. This legislation provides support for research, training, needs identification, program development, and service delivery. Target populations include caregivers and homebound, Native American, low-income, minority, and frail older individuals. The OAA Amendments of 2000 supported the new National Family Caregiver Support Program, which helps provide care for older adults who are ill or have disabilities.

Community Nutrition Programs

Community-based nutrition programs to assist older adults with obtaining adequate food and maintaining their nutritional status are administered by governmental, private, nonprofit, and volunteer agencies throughout the United States. Nutrition services of the *Elderly Nutrition Programs (ENP)* under the OAA are valuable for helping older individuals remain independent at home and in the community. This program authorizes funds for congregate and home-delivered nutrition programs. These meals and other nutrition services are provided in various community settings. Through this program, one meal that provides one third of the recommended dietary allowance (RDA) for persons older than 50 years of age is served weekdays to senior citizens in congregate meal settings or in the home if the citizens are unable to come to the sites. To be eligible to receive services at the congregate meal sites, participants must be 60 years of age or older or be the spouse or primary caretaker of an eligible participant. Because American Indians, Alaskan natives, and native Hawaiians tend to have lower life expectancies and higher rates of illness at earlier ages, the tribal organizations have the authority to adjust the age of eligibility.

Other services, including outreach, transportation, recreational activities, nutrition screening, and assessment, are provided. A donation or contribution for the meals is often requested but is not required. Food stamps are accepted as donations. Many of the advantages of this program are related to the social interaction that occurs at the meal sites.

Additional sources for food include the Food Stamp Program, the Commodity Supplemental Food Program (CSFP), The Emergency Food Assistance Program (TEFAP), the Nutrition Services Incentive Plan (NSIP), the Child and Adult Care Food Program (CACFP), and the Seniors Farmers' Market Nutrition Pilot Program (SFMNPP). Other community support resources include home health care agencies, hospice organizations, commodity food sources, food banks, food co-ops, and home-delivered grocery services. Support services can assist in shopping and meal preparation for senior citizens who are unable to shop or prepare their own meals (see Chapter 14).

Assisted Living and Skilled Care Facilities

As the size of the older population increases and the needs of the population change, new housing and health care alternatives have been created that combine independence with personal care in a supportive, dignified, community setting. Assisted living is a combination of safe housing, personalized supportive services, and health care designed to meet the needs of those who need assistance with activities of daily living. Assisted living residences offer cost-effective, quality care that fosters independence in each resident. Residents are treated with dignity and respect, and individuality is promoted. Assisted living residents maintain active social lives with planned activities, exercise classes, religious and social functions, and field trips directed by the facilities. Others who require skilled care may reside in a skilled nursing facility or skilled care units in retirement communities. These facilities must undergo certification by Centers for Medicare and Medicaid Services (CMS). Long-term care services are for those who have lost the capacity to function independently as a result of chronic illness or conditions that require intervention for an extended period.

The nutritional care of those in institutions must be directed toward long-term identification and responses to changing physiologic and psychological needs. Serving attractive and palatable food in an atmosphere that encourages independent eating or provides assistance when necessary helps promote the nutritional well-being of the residents. Overall health goals for older adults may not warrant the implementation of strict therapeutic diets, which are often unpalatable and can have a negative impact on quality of life (American Dietetic Association, 2002).

It is important to use resident assessment and intervention protocols and evaluate outcomes. Periodic reassessments of nutritional status are critical for preventing the use of unnecessary dietary restrictions or missing important nutrient needs. In certain situations, such as hospice care, intervention strategies may be limited to providing comfort foods and emotional support for family and friends.

In 1987, Congress approved the initial nursing home reform legislation as a part of the Omnibus Reconciliation Act (OBRA) to improve the quality of services furnished to residents of nursing homes by strengthening the standards that must be met to obtain reimbursement under the federal and state Medicaid program. Nursing homes are required to conduct periodic assessments to determine the residents' needs; provide services to ensure that residents maintain the highest possible physical, mental, and psychological well-being; and ensure that residents are not being harmed. Surveyors from regulatory agencies use criteria established by the CMS to regulate the care given in nursing homes, and they have the authority to close down a facility immediately if many violations or substandard care, neglect, or abuse is noted. It may be difficult for consultant dietitians to provide all the necessary services if their onsite time is limited. Facilities are now often encouraged to hire full-time registered dietitians to provide more comprehensive medical nutrition therapy.

Clinical Scenario

Mary L. is an 85-year old female who lives alone. She has no children and generally receives a meal from her local Meals on Wheels program at lunch on weekdays. Mary has limited resources and skips breakfast daily. Lately Mary has felt lightheaded and has been sleeping more than usual during the day. Neighbors who provide shopping assistance for Mary have been away for a week. When they return home and notice a difference in Mary's cognitive functioning, they call the doctor's office. He refers Mary to you after a complete medical examination, during which nothing unusual is noted.

1. What types of nutrition screening and assessment questions will you ask Mary?
2. What suggestions do you have for Mary and her neighbors about shopping and preparing regular meals?
3. With no medical conditions that warrant long-term care placement, what other options are available that might assist Mary's capability to stay at home and continue "aging in place?"

Relevant Web Sites

Administration on Aging
www.aoa.dhhs.gov
American Association of Homes and Services for the Aging
www.aahs.org
American Association of Retired Persons
www.aarp.org
American Geriatrics Society
www.americangeriatrics.org
Centers for Disease Control and Prevention
www.cdc.gov/nchs/fastats/lifexpec.htm.
Centers for Medicare and Medicaid Services (CMS)
www.hhs.gov/siteinfo/
Food and Nutrition Service, U.S. Department of Agriculture
Seniors and food safety—preventing foodborne illness
www.cfsan.fda.gov/~dms/seniors.html
Geriatric Net
www.e-geriatric.net/index.html.
Meals on Wheels Association of America
www.projectmeal.org/
The Merck Manual of Geriatrics
www.merck.com
National Institute on Aging
www.nih.gov/nia
National Policy and Resource Center on Aging and Nutrition
www.fiu.edu/~ntreldr/Aging_Network/aging_network.htm
Nutrition Management and Restorative Dining for Older Adults (U.S. Health Care Financing Administration)
www.hcfa.gov/medicaid/siq/siqnhpg.htm

Cited References

American Dietetic Association: Liberalized diets for older adults in long term care—position paper, *J Am Diet Assoc* 98:201, 1998.

Ausman LM, Mayer J: Brief critical reviews: criteria and recommendations for vitamin C intake, *Nutr Rev* 57:222, 1999.

Baik HW, Russell RM: Vitamin B_{12} deficiency in the elderly, *Annu Rev Nutr* 19:357, 1999.

Bales CW, Ritchie CS: Sarcopenia, weight loss, and nutritional frailty in the elderly, *Annu Rev Nutr* 22:309, 2002.

Beharka AA et al: Effect of age on the gastrointestinal-associated mucosal immune response of humans, *J Gerontol A Biol Sci Med Sci* 56:218, 2001.

Bryant RD, Cadogan J, Weaver CM: The new dietary reference intakes for calcium: implications for osteoporosis, *J Am Coll Nutr* 18:406S, 1999.

Campbell W: Dietary protein requirements of older people: is the RDA adequate? *Nutr Today* 31:192, 1996.

Cather J, Menter A: Novel therapies for psoriasis, *Am J Clin Dermatol* 3:159, 2002.

Chandra RK: Graying of the immune system, *JAMA* 277:1398, 1997.

Chandra RK et al: Nutrition of the elderly, *Can Med Assoc J* 145:1475, 1991.

Dawson-Hughes B et al: Effect of calcium and vitamin D supplementation on bone density in men and women 65 years of age or older, *N Engl J Med* 337:670, 1997.

Department of Health and Human Services: Clinical practice guideline number 15, *Treatment of pressure sores,* AHCPR Pub No 95-0652, December 1994.

Dharmarajan TS, Norhus EP: Approaches to vitamin B_{12} deficiency, *Postgrad Med* 11:99, 2001.

Dutta C: Significance of sarcopenia in the elderly, *J Nutr* 127(suppl):992, 1997.

Evans J et al: Relation of colonic transit to functional bowel disease in older people: a population-based study, *J Am Geriatr Soc* 46:83, 1998.

Feskanich D et al: Vitamin A intake and hip fractures among postmenopausal women, *JAMA* 287:47, 2002.

Fletcher RH, Fairfield KM: Vitamins for chronic disease prevention in adults: clinical applications, *JAMA* 287:3127, 2002.

Foote A, Guiliano A, Harris R: Older adults need guidance to meet nutritional recommendations, *J Am Coll Nutr* 19:628, 2000.

Harrell R et al: How geriatricians identify elder abuse and neglect, *Am J Med Sci* 323:34, 2002.

Hoffbrand V, Provan D: ABC of clinical haematology: macrocytic anaemias, *BMJ* 314(7078):430, 1997.

Huffman G: Evaluating and treating unintentional weight loss in the elderly, *Am Fam Physician* 65:640, 2002.

Hurley R et al: Comparative evaluation of body composition in medically stable elderly, *J Am Diet Assoc* 97:1105, 1997.

Kaufman DW et al: Recent patterns of medication use in the ambulatory adult population of the United States: the Slone survey *JAMA* 287:337, 2002.

MacIntosh CG et al: Effect of small intestinal nutrient infusion on appetite, gastrointestinal hormone release, and gastric myoelectrical activity in young and older men, *Am J Gastroenterol* 96:997, 2001.

Marshal TA et al: Inadequate nutrient intakes are common and are associated with low diet variety in rural, community-dwelling elderly, *J Nutr* 131:2192, 2001.

Meydani M: Nutrition interventions in aging and age-associated disease, *Ann NY Acad Sci* 928:226, 2001.

Miesler JG: Toward optimal health: the experts respond to dietary supplement use, *J Womens Health Gend Based Med* 8:297, 1999.

Morrison G, Hark L: *Medical nutrition and disease,* ed 2, Malden, MA, 1999, Blackwell Science.

Need A et al: Effects of skin thickness, age, body fat and sunlight on serum 25-hydroxyvitamin D, *Am J Clin Nutr* 58:882, 1993.

Nelms M, Anderson S: Medical nutritional therapy: a case study approach, Belmont, Calif, 2002, Wadsworth.

Nordin BE et al: Nutrition, osteoporosis and aging, *Ann NY Acad Sci* 854:336, 1998.

Nutrition Screening Initiative: *Nutrition screening manual for professionals caring for older Americans,* Washington, D.C., 1991, NSI.

Pollock M et al: Physical activity and exercise training in the elderly: a position paper from the Society of Geriatric Cardiology, *Am J Geriatr Cardiol* 7:45, 1998.

Protein-energy undernutrition. In *Merck manual,* ch. 293, Geratric medicine, Whitehouse Station, NJ, 2001, Merck.

Richard MJ, Roussel AM: Micronutrients and aging: intakes and requirements, *Proc Nutr Soc* 58:573, 1999.

Roberts SB: Regulation of energy intake in older adults: recent findings and implications, *J Nutr Health Aging* 4:170: 2000.

Ryan C, Eleazer P, Egbert J: Vitamin D in the elderly, *Nutr Today* 30:228, 1995.

Schiffman SS: Changes in taste and smell: drug interactions and food preferences, *Nutr Rev* 52:11, 1994.

Schiffman SS: Taste and smell losses in normal aging and disease, *JAMA* 278:1357, 1997.

Schiffman SS, Warwick ZS: Effect of flavor enhancement of foods for the elderly on nutritional status: food intake, biochemical indices, and anthropometric measures, *Physiol Behav* 53:395, 1992.

United Nations: *World population prospects: the 2000 revision highlights,* pp 14-15, February 2001.

Vellas B et al: *Mini nutritional assessment (MNA): research and practice in the elderly,* Nestle Nutrition Workshop Series—Clinical and Performance Programme, vol 1, 1999.

Wellman N: The Nutrition Screening Initiative, *Nutr Rev* 52:544, 1994.

Yung RL: Changes in immune function with age, *Rheum Dis Clin North Am* 26(3):455, 2003.

Ziesel SH: Is there a metabolic basis for dietary supplementation? *J Clin Nutr* 72:5075(2S); 2000.

■ Additional References

American Dietetic Association: Position of The American Dietetic Association: Nutrition, aging and the continuum of care, *J Am Diet Assoc* 100:580, 2000.

Ames BN: The metabolic tune-up: metabolic harmony and disease prevention, *J Nutr* 133(5 Suppl 1):1544S; 2003.

Covinsky KE et al: The relationship between clincial assessments of nutritional status and adverse outcomes in older hospitalized medical patients, *J Am Geriatr Soc* 47:532, 1999.

Diet manual for long term care residents—2000 revision, Catonsville, Md, Office of Health Care Quality, Maryland Department of Health and Mental Hygiene.

Morley JE: Pathophysiology of anorexia, *Clin Geriatr Med* 18(4):661, 2002.

Saltzman E: Nutrition in disease prevention & treatment, *Caring* 21(8):22, 2002.

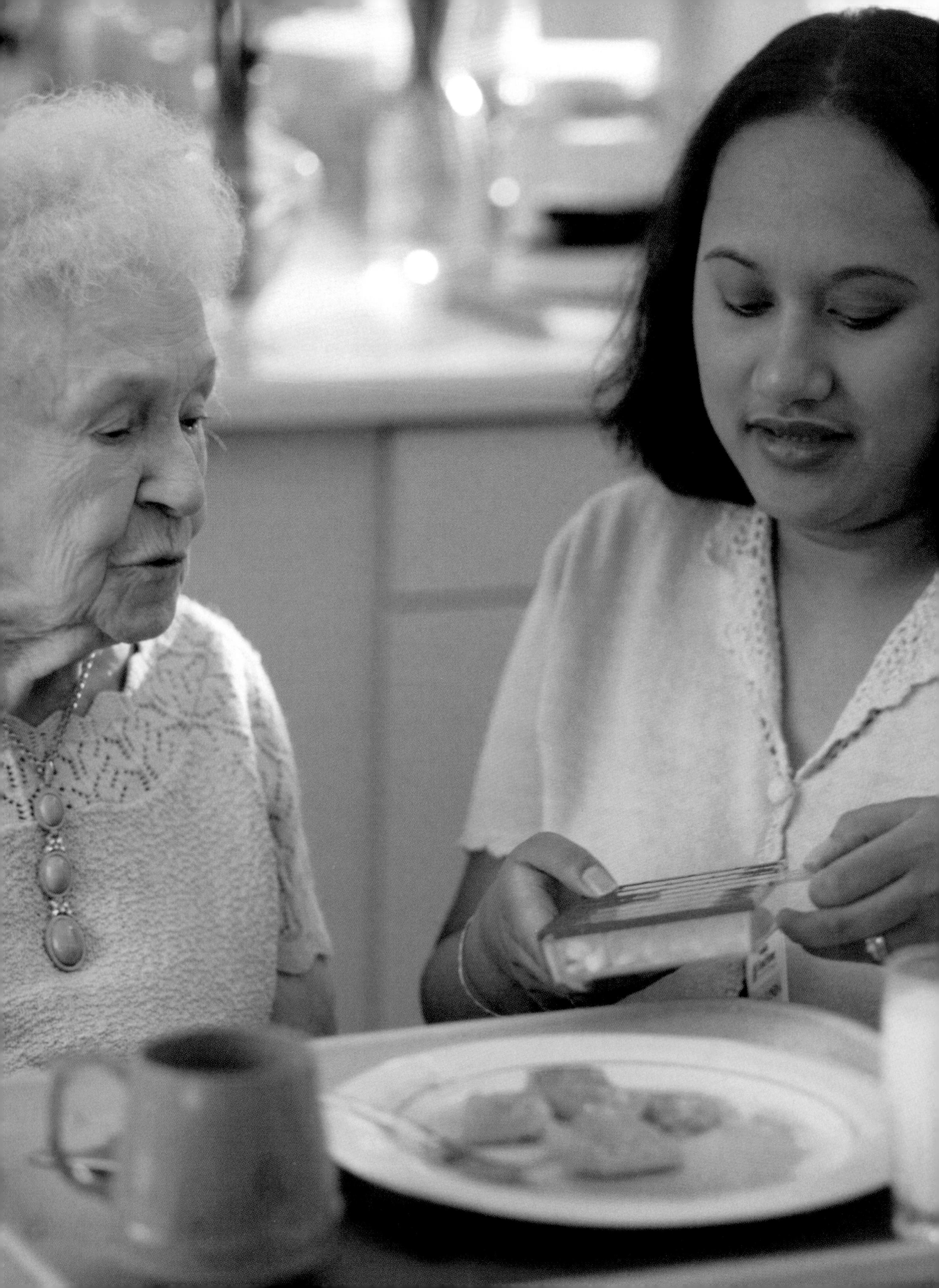

PART 3

NUTRITION CARE

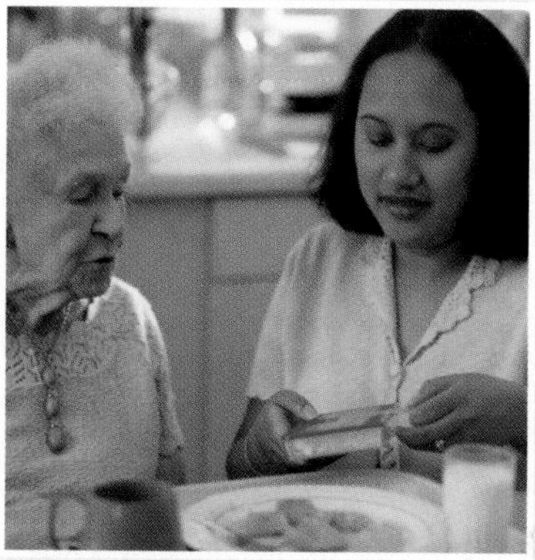

Part 3 includes background chapters related to the nutrition care process, starting with the population in general (i.e., community nutrition) and methods for dietary planning. The nutritive assessment of the individual is addressed in chapters on dietary and clinical evaluation and biochemical assessment, the human genome, and the use of herbs, other plants, and phytochemicals. Nutrition care is discussed in the chapters on the nutrition care process, methods of nutrition support, counseling, guidelines for dietary planning, and drug-nutrient interaction. The chapter on complementary therapy and the use of herbs and phytonutrients is important because of the rapidly growing interest in and knowledge of this field.

The reader is encouraged to refer to these chapters when providing nutrition services for population groups or individuals. Although it is essential to assess each person individually, practitioners must also be aware that certain parameters are meaningful for groups of people with specific diagnoses. Knowledge of common problems or symptoms related to diseases provides practitioners with the basic skills needed to prepare an effective nutrition care plan and evaluate or alter it throughout the intervention.

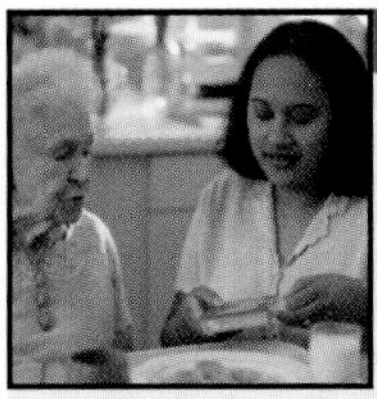

CHAPTER 14

Nutrition in the Community

JUDITH L. DODD, MS, RD, FADA, LD
CYNTHIA TAFT BAYERL, MS, RD, LDN

CHAPTER OUTLINE

- Nutrition Practice in the Community
- Needs Assessment for Community-Based Nutrition Services
- National Food and Nutrition Data Sources
- National Nutrition Guidelines and Goals
- Food Assistance and Nutrition Programs
- Food Safety: Laws, Regulations, and Issues
- Food Technology
- Agricultural Products and Concerns
- Other Concerns About Food and Water Safety

KEY TERMS

acceptable daily intake (ADI)–the amount of a chemical or nutrient that if ingested daily throughout a lifetime seems to be without appreciable risk

child nutrition programs–Programs funded by the U.S. Department of Agriculture aimed at improving the nutritional status of children in the United States; include school lunches and breakfasts, summer feeding programs, after-school snacks, provision of the Special Milk Program, Child and Adult Care Food Program, and WIC program

Commodity Supplemental Food Program (CSFP)–a program that is administered by the states and offers donated foods from the U.S. Department of Agriculture to eligible schools, institutions, summer feeding programs, and food assistance programs

community assessment–one of the three public health core functions that involves all of the activities related to the concept of community diagnosis (e.g., surveillance, identifying needs, analyzing the causes of problems, collecting and interpreting data, case finding, monitoring and forecasting trends, research, and evaluation of outcomes)

congregate meals, home-delivered meals–established in 1965 by the Older Americans Act, Title VII section, under the Department of Health and Human Services Elderly Nutrition Program (ENP) for senior adults; combined with the Title III program in 1978 in concert with the U.S. Department of Agriculture Nutrition Program for the Elderly (NPE), which provides cash and commodity foods for use in these programs

Continuing Survey of Food Intake of Individuals (CSFII)–part of the U.S. Department of Agriculture National Nutrition Monitoring System, a nationwide dietary intake survey originally designed to be conducted every 2 years; merged in 2002 with the National Health and Nutrition Examination Survey (NHANES)

Delaney Clause–a component of the Food Additive Amendment of 1959 that prohibits the use in food of any substance shown to cause cancer in animals or humans; repealed for pesticides in 1996 with passage of the Food Quality Protection Act

Department of Health and Human Services (DHHS; USDHHS)–a federal agency; formerly the "U.S. Depart-

Elizabeth A. Yakes, Public Health Nutrition Program, Case Western Reserve University, assisted in the updates to the references for this chapter.

ment of Health, Education, and Welfare"; houses the Food and Drug Administration and Centers for Disease Control and Prevention

food additive–any natural or synthetic material other than the basic raw ingredients used in the production of a food item to enhance the final product

food irradiation–the exposure of food to sufficient radiant energy to destroy insects and microorganisms; used in food protection or preservation; also called *cold pasteurization*

foodborne illness–formerly called "food poisoning"; usually accompanied by gastrointestinal symptoms and initiated by organisms or their toxins in food or water

food security–having a readily available supply of nutritionally adequate and safe foods and an ensured ability to acquire acceptable foods

Food Stamp Program–an entitlement program established in 1964 and administered by the U.S. Department of Agriculture to provide more food-buying power to low-income persons or families through monthly allotments of food purchasing credits

generally recognized as safe (GRAS)–describes 675 commonly used food ingredients considered safe and in use when the 1959 Food Additives Amendment was enacted

Hazard Analysis Critical Control Points (HACCP)–a food safety system developed to identify key danger points in food handling and service

Head Start–a comprehensive child development program with a food component; targets low-income preschool children and their families; administered by the Department of Health and Human Services with meals under the U.S. Department of Agriculture

National Food and Nutrition Survey (NFNS)–created from the January 2002 merge of the NHANES and the CSFII

National Health and Nutrition Examination Survey (NHANES)–a series of surveys that include information from medical histories, physical measurements, biochemical evaluations, physical examinations, and dietary intakes of a representative sample of U.S. population groups; a responsibility of the National Center for Health Statistics of the Department of Health and Human Services; merged with the U.S. Department of Agriculture Continuing Survey of Food Intake of Individuals study in January 2002 to become the National Food and Nutrition Survey (NFNS)

National Nutrient Data Bank–the United States' primary resource for information on the nutrient content of foods

National School Lunch Program, School Breakfast Program (NSLP)–child nutrition programs administered by the U.S. Department of Agriculture; offer cash reimbursement, commodities, and technical assistance for schools to provide a free or reduced-price meal that meets specified nutritional requirements and the *Dietary Guidelines for Americans*

nutrition epidemiology–the study of nutrition and diet as they relate to the etiology, pathogenesis, and prevention of disease

Nutrition Program for the Elderly (NPE)–a U.S. Department of Agriculture program that provides cash and commodity foods for home-delivered meals or congregate feeding sites; meals must follow a specified nutritionally adequate pattern

Nutrition Screening Initiative (NSI)–an effort to improve the nutrition and well-being of senior adults who are not in institutions; offers screening tools to evaluate nutritional risks and identify targets for early preventive efforts

nutrition surveillance–the ongoing monitoring of the nutritional status of population groups; monitors dietary intake, anthropometric, biochemical, clinical, and environmental data

policy development–one of the three public health core functions; the process by which society makes decisions about problems, chooses goals, and prepares the means to reach them; handles conflicting views about what should be done; and allocates resources

primary prevention–a disease prevention strategy targeting generally healthy individuals to decrease the probability that they will develop a disease or disability

public health assurance–one of the three core public health functions; addresses the implementation of legislative mandates, maintenance of statutory responsibilities, support of crucial services, regulation of services and products provided in the public and private sectors, and maintenance of accountability

secondary prevention–a disease prevention strategy that focuses on detection, diagnosis, and intervention early in the disease process to minimize detrimental and disabling effects

Special Supplemental Nutrition Program for Women, Infants, and Children (WIC)–established in 1972 to provide nutritious, supplemental food and nutrition education and to improve the nutritional status of medically high-risk, low-income pregnant and lactating females and children up to 5 years of age; administered by the U.S. Department of Agriculture

tertiary prevention–rehabilitation of an individual to optimal function by correcting or ameliorating a health defect or disability; may involve medical treatment

Total Diet Study (Market Basket Sample)–analysis of a sampling of food items purchased throughout the United States that are representative of the diets of consumers; used for comparison with acceptable daily intakes of pesticides and food contaminants; administered by the Food and Drug Administration of the Department of Health and Human Services

U.S. Department of Agriculture (USDA)–a federal agency with responsibility for ensuring a safe, affordable, nutritious, and accessible food supply and supporting the production of agriculture

Community nutrition is an evolving area of practice with the broad focus of serving the population at large. Although this practice area encompasses the goals of public health, the current model has been shaped and expanded as emphasis in the U.S. population moves toward prevention and wellness.

Historically, public health was defined as "the science and art of preventing disease, prolonging life, and promoting health and efficiency through organized community effort, so organizing these benefits as to enable every citizen to realize his birthright of health and longevity" (Winslow, 1920). The *public health approach,* also known as a *population-based* or an *epidemiologic approach* (nutrition epidemiology), differs from the clinical or patient care model generally seen in hospitals and other clinical settings. In the public health model, the client is the community, a geopolitical entity. The focus of the traditional public health approach was primary prevention (health promotion) rather than secondary prevention (risk reduction) or tertiary prevention (treatment and rehabilitation) (Egan, 1994). Changes in the health care system, technology, and attitudes of the nutrition consumer have influenced the expansion of the responsibilities of community nutrition (American Dietetic Association [ADA], 1998b).

A 1998 report of the Institute of Medicine (IOM) reinforces the concept that the scope of community nutrition is a work in progress. The IOM report defines a mission and delineates roles and responsibilities. The scope of community-based nutrition encompasses efforts to prevent disease and promote positive health and nutritional messages for individuals and groups in settings where they live and work. The focus is on well-being and building potential for the best possible quality of life; "well-being" encompasses more than physical and mental health.

Community nutrition includes numerous factors that affect the quality of life within a community. Community members need a safe environment and adequate housing, food, income, employment, and education. This echoes the IOM intent that the mission of community nutrition is to fulfill society's interest in ensuring that individuals live in conditions in which they can be healthy (IOM, 1998).

The potential audience for programming and services is any segment of the population; the segment should reflect the diversity of the designated community. A community can be defined by politics, geography, culture and ethnicity, age, gender, socioeconomic issues, and overall health status. In addition to primary prevention, community nutrition has links to programs and services with goals of risk reduction and rehabilitation. Heart-healthy cooking classes and demonstrations are an example of multifaceted programming and services offered under the community nutrition umbrella. Depending on the audience, the program is primary prevention (e.g., through the general public) or secondary or tertiary prevention (e.g., through cardiovascular support groups).

In the traditional model, funding for public health efforts was money allocated from official sources (i.e., the government) at the local, state, or federal level. The community is now beginning to share the responsibility for meeting the mission (IOM, 1998). Currently, nutrition programs and services are funded alone or in partnership by a broad range of sources, including public (government), private, and voluntary health sectors. For example, heart-healthy cooking classes might receive funding from the American Heart Association (a voluntary, nonprofit agency), a health care insurer (nonprofit or for profit), a supermarket or business (for profit), or a demonstration grant from a government source. The potential size and diversity of a designated community makes collaboration critical. A single agency may be unable to fund or deliver the full range of services.

NUTRITION PRACTICE IN THE COMMUNITY

Nutrition professionals have recognized that successful delivery of food and nutrition services involves people in their own community. The pool of nutrition professionals delivering medical nutrition therapy and nutrition education in community-based or public health facilities continues to expand. Community practice has core functions in public health. The objectives of *Healthy People 2010* offer a common framework of outcomes.

The three roles of the public, or government, agencies involved in community practice are the core functions of public health—community assessment, policy development, and public health assurance (IOM, 1998). These areas are components of practice for the community nutrition professional. This chapter includes information on community assessment, which is also known as *needs assessment.* The assessment shapes policy development and the components of ensuring that the health of the public is protected.

Although the responsibility for core functions is shared, the IOM report designates that personnel of the official state health agencies have primary responsibility. Under this model, state public health agencies in conjunction with community organizations and leaders are responsible for assessing the capacity of their state to perform the essential functions of public health nutrition and supporting attainment and monitoring of the goals and objectives of *Healthy People 2010.*

Local health agencies are responsible for protecting the health of their population groups by ensuring that effective service delivery systems are in place. The role of the federal government is to support the development and dissemination of public health knowledge and provide funds to strengthen the capacity to carry out the core functions (IOM, 1998). Table 14-1 lists federal surveys that are relevant to food and nutrition concerns of the community.

TABLE 14-1 Food, Nutrition, and Health Surveys

NAME OF SURVEY	TIMING	AGENCY*	PURPOSE/COMMENTS
Ten State Nutrition Survey	1968-1970	DHEW	To evaluate dietary intake, nutritional status, and economic status
Preschool Nutrition	1968-1970	DHEW	To evaluate dietary intake, nutritional status, and economic status in children 1-6 yr in 36 states
National Health and Nutrition Examination Survey (NHANES)	1971-1974	DHEW	First nationwide health survey to include nutrition; includes ages 1-74 yr
NHANES II	1976-1980	DHEW	Includes ages 6 mo to 74 yr
Hispanic Hanes (HHANES)	1982-1984	DHHS	To remedy underreporting of Hispanics
National Food Consumption Survey	1987-1988; discontinued	USDA	To assess the nutritional adequacy of American diets and track changes in dietary intake over time; includes low-income sample
NHANES III	1988-1994	DHHS	Ages 2 mo and older; to monitor health and nutrition over time, especially of older adults
Continuing Survey of Food Intakes by Individuals (CSFII)	1985-1986	USDA	To determine the types and amounts of foods eaten by Americans; includes women 19-50 yr and their children and men 19-50 yr; includes low-income sample
CSFII	1989-1991	USDA	Data collected through 24-hr dietary recall (in-person interview) and 2-day diet record (self-administered); includes men, women, and children of all ages and low-income sample
CSFII	1994-1996	USDA	Data collected through two nonconsecutive 24-hr dietary recalls (in-person interviews); includes oversampled low-income population, larger samples of children and older adults
Diet and Health Knowledge Survey (DHKS)	1989-1991; 1994-1996	USDA	To assess the impact that knowledge and attitudes about healthy eating have on food choice and nutrient intake; telephone follow-up to CSFII
Cholesterol Awareness Study	1986	DHHS/NIH	To assess cholesterol knowledge of consumers
Pregnancy and Infant Feeding Survey	1988-1989	DHHS/FDA	To assess feeding practices of pregnant females and of infants
NHANES	1999-2001	DHHS/USDA	Changed to a continuous, annual format with detailed data released every 3 years; piloted integration of CSFII
National Food and Nutrition Survey (NFNS)	2002+	DHHS/USDA	To allow diet and health data to be linked; NHANES and CSFII fully integrated under new name
Total Diet Study	Ongoing	DHHS/FDA	Specific age-sex groups; market basket sample
Food Disappearance Data	Annual	USDA	To monitor total available food used; waste not accounted for
Coordinated State Surveillance System	Ongoing	DHHS/CDC	Includes pregnant women, children

**CDC,* Centers for Disease Control and Prevention; *DHEW,* Department of Health, Education, and Welfare until 1980, then renamed *DHHS,* Department of Health and Human Services; *FDA,* Food and Drug Administration; *HNIS,* Human Nutrition Information Service; *NIH,* National Institutes of Health; *USDA,* U.S. Department of Agriculture.

The expansion of community-based practice beyond the scope of traditional public health has opened new employment opportunities for nutrition professionals. Such professionals are found in agencies or organizations that provide primary care, promote health, and prevent chronic diseases in the community or community groups. Nutrition professionals also serve as consultants or maintain community-based private practices. Some examples of community settings that employ nutritionists include public health agencies (state and local), the WIC program, services for senior adults, community health centers, early intervention programs such as Head Start, health maintenance organizations and health insurers, food pantries and shelters, physicians' offices, and schools (Bayerl and Ries, 1995).

In a study of 7550 public health nutrition personnel, the participants described the responsibilities and positions of nutritionists within public health and community nutrition as being on a continuum (Probert,

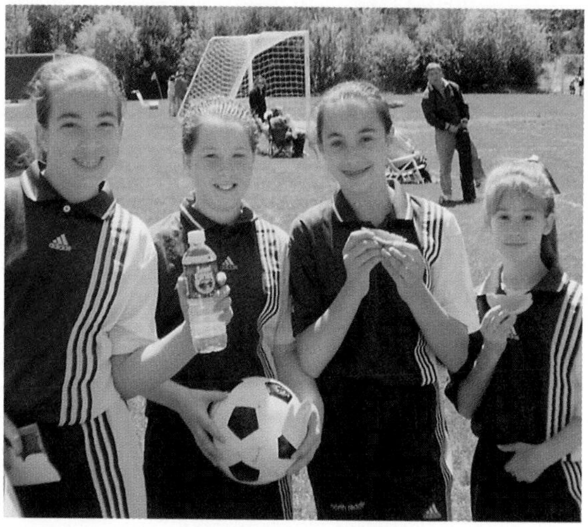

FIGURE 14-1 • Community nutritionists are involved in advising athletes on nutrition.

FOCUS ON

Legislation and Advocacy

Nutrition and health professionals can be valuable advocates for legislation (local, state, or federal) that supports the nutritional well-being of the population, especially of those who are underserved or underrepresented. They can advocate in the following ways:

- Visiting, writing, or calling legislators and their aides to provide important information and establish communication links
- Encouraging community members to provide testimony on their successes or the consequences of having unavailable or insufficiently funded medical nutrition therapy or nutrition services—a step that is especially important when legislation is pending
- Inviting legislators to visit local agencies, schools, or hospitals to showcase the benefits of nutrition services provided by qualified professionals
- Serving on campaign committees, donating time and money, or running for office

1996). This continuum extends from direct or client-based service to population and system–focused services. Client-based services are likely to be education, counseling, or care management, whereas population-based services include program planning, policy making, evaluation, or management (Figure 14-1).

Effective practice in the community requires a nutrition professional who understands the impact of economic, social, and political issues on health. Because many community-based efforts are funded or guided by legislation and the resulting regulations and public policies, community practice requires an understanding of the legislative process and an ability to translate policies into action (see *Focus On:* Legislation and Advocacy). In addition, community practice requires a working knowledge of funding sources and resources at the federal, state, and local level.

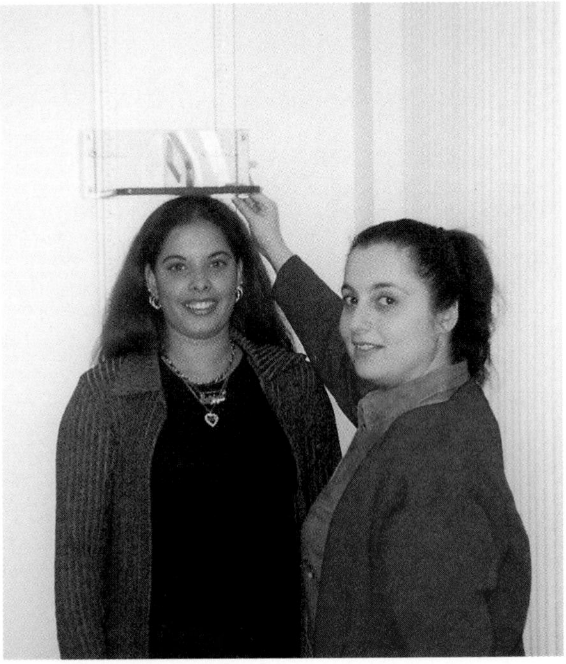

FIGURE 14-2 • Anthropometric measurement training in progress.

NEEDS ASSESSMENT FOR COMMUNITY-BASED NUTRITION SERVICES

Community based services should be organized to meet the needs of a defined community. Once a community has been defined, a needs assessment can be used to shape the planning, implementation, and evaluation phases. An assessment provides a current glimpse of the community and is useful in identifying the health risks or areas of greatest concern to community well-being. A needs assessment should be viewed as a dynamic document that continues to change. A plan is only as good as the research used to shape the decisions, meaning that the plan should have a built-in mechanism for ongoing review and revision.

Needs Assessment: General Information

A needs assessment is based on objective data, including demographic information and health statistics (Figure 14-2). When possible, information should be segmented by such factors as age, gender, socioeconomics, disability factors, and ethnicity, and should represent the community's diversity. Examples of information to be gathered include current morbidity and mortality statistics, number of low-birth-weight infants, deaths attributed to chronic diseases that are associated with poor nutrition, and health risk indicators such as incidence of smoking or obesity. Subjective information such as input from community members, leaders, and health and nutrition professionals may be useful. The process mirrors what the business world knows as market research.

In addition to studying the health indicators of the community and conducting interviews with community leaders, community resources and services should be assessed. During nutrition planning, the goal is to determine who and what are available for community members when they need food or nutrition-related products or services. What is available in the areas of medical nutrition therapy (screening, assessment, monitoring), nutrition and food education, and child care or homemaker skills training? Do people have safe areas for exercise or recreation? Does the community have access to transportation, and does it comply with disability legislation? Are programs such as those involving food stamps, food pantries, congregate and home-delivered meals, and child nutrition programs available? Are supermarkets and other food sources available?

At first glance, some of the data gathered in this process may not seem to relate directly to nutrition. An experienced community nutritionist or a community-based advisory group with public health professionals can help associate this information with nutrition- and diet-related issues. Often the nutritional problems identified as a result of a review of nutrition indicators are associated with dietary inadequacies, excesses, or imbalances that can be triggers for disease risk. Some trigger areas include the presence of risk factors for cardiovascular disease, diabetes, and stroke, including elevated blood cholesterol and lipid levels, inactivity, smoking, elevated blood glucose levels, a high body mass index (BMI), and an elevated blood pressure; risk factors for osteoporosis; evidence of eating disorders; teenage pregnancy; and evidence of hunger and food insecurity. Careful attention should be paid to the special needs of adults and children with disabilities or other lifestyle-limiting conditions. Once evaluated, the information is used to propose needed services, including medical nutrition therapy, as part of the strategy for improving the overall health of the community. Other chapters discuss the protocols for meeting these needs.

Sources for Needs Assessment Information

Census information can be a starting point. Morbidity and mortality and other health data collected by state and local public health agencies, the Centers for Disease Control and Prevention (CDC), and the National Center for Health Statistics (NCHS) are useful. Federal agencies and their state counterparts that administer programs are sources, including the U.S. Department of Agriculture (USDA), the Department of Health and Human Services (DHHS), and the Office on Aging. Local providers such as community hospitals, the Special Supplemental Nutrition Program for Women, Infants, and Children (WIC), child-care agencies, health centers, and universities with a public health or nutrition department are additional sources of information. Volunteer organizations such as the March of Dimes, the American Heart Association, and the American Diabetes Association also maintain population statistics. Inclusion of community leaders and other professionals in the needs assessment process can help ease access to these resources and information. The face of the community and its resources are constantly in flux.

Technology has made it simpler to stay abreast of current resources because much of the information is now available through web sites. However, it is critical that community practitioners know how to locate relevant and valid resources. Knowing the background and intended use of any data sources and the dates when the information was collected are critical when selecting and using such sources.

NATIONAL FOOD AND NUTRITION DATA SOURCES

Nutrition and health surveys at the federal and state level are basic data sources. Such surveys are useful in providing information on the dietary status of a population, assessing the nutritional adequacy of the food supply, determining the economics of food consumption, and evaluating the effects of food assistance and regulatory programs. Public guidelines for food selection such as the *Dietary Guidelines for Americans* are based on surveys. The data are also used in policy setting, program development, and funding at the national, state, and local levels. Until the late 1960s, the USDA was the primary source of food and nutrient consumption data. Although much of the data collection is still at the federal level, other agencies and states are now generating information that provides comprehensive information on the health and nutrition of the public.

National Health and Nutrition Examination Surveys

The National Health and Nutrition Examination Surveys (NHANES) provide a framework for describing the health status of the nation. Sampling the noninstitutionalized population, the current NHANES is the eighth in a series conducted in the United States since 1960. In January 2002, the USDA Continuing Survey of Food Intake of Individuals (CSFII) study merged with NHANES to provide a more comprehensive study design. The integrated survey—the National Food and Nutrition Survey (NFNS)—is a joint effort of NCHS and USDA and expands on the components of NHANES and CSFII. Since 1999, information on representative population groups from newborns to senior adults has been collected continuously. The process of continuous nutrition surveillance should provide quicker access to the NFNS data (NCHS, 2000). Each survey has included changes or additions that made NHANES more responsive as a measurement of the health status of the population. NHANES I, II, and III include (1) medical history, (2) physical measurements, (3) biochemical evaluation, (4) physical signs and symptoms, and (5) diet information using food frequency questionnaires and a 24-hour recall. Some previous design changes added special population studies to increase information on underrepresented groups such as the 1982 to 1984 Hispanic HANES (Kuczmarski et al, 1994; Woteki et al, 1988).

NHANES III (1988 to 1994) included a large proportion of persons age 65 years and older and broadened the available information on the growing and changing population of senior adults. After the information was gathered, reports were generated on the health profile of the community in relation to 30 topics, including blood pressures and the prevalence of hypertension, cholesterol levels and cardiovascular risk, measurements of height and weight and prevalence of overweight and obesity, and levels of energy and nutrient intakes and iron status and other hematologic data. The current NHANES began in 1999 and will be continuous, involving 15 U.S. locations each year, with a goal of studying 5000 people annually (NCHS, 2000). Information on past and current NHANES is available through the NCHS of the CDC (see Table 14-1).

Nationwide Food Consumption Survey

The Nationwide Food Consumption Survey (NFCS) of the USDA monitored the nutrient intake of a representative sampling of the U.S. public. The NFCS compiled information on food consumption of households and individuals using a food use and food cost questionnaire on food eaten at home and away from home during a 3-day period. The first survey was conducted in 1935, and the data were updated approximately every 10 years until 1988. The information collected is still quoted (Nutrition Monitoring Division, 1989).

Continuing Survey of Food Intake of Individuals: Diet and Health Knowledge Survey

The CSFII is a nationwide dietary survey instituted in 1985 by the USDA. In 1990, the CSFII became part of the USDA National Nutrition Monitoring System. The Diet and Health Knowledge Survey (DHKS), a telephone follow-up to the CFSII, began in 1989. The combined DHKS and CFSII surveys are known as *What We Eat in America.* Information from these surveys is available from 1985 to 1986, 1989 to 1991, and 1994 to 1996. As discussed, by January 2002, both surveys merged with NHANES to become part of the NFNS.

The DHKS was designed as a personal interview questionnaire that allowed individual attitudes and knowledge about healthy eating to be linked with reported food choices and nutrient intakes. Initial studies focused on dietary history and 24-hour recalls of food choices (through personal interviews) of adult men and women ages 19 to 50. The 1989 and 1994 surveys questioned men, women, and children of all ages and included the 24-hour recall and a 2-day food diary. Household data for these studies were determined by calculating the nutrient content of foods reported to be used in the home during the survey. These results were compared with nutrition recommendations for those of relevant age and gender. The information derived from the CSFII and DHKS are useful for decision-makers and researchers who monitor the nutritional adequacy of American diets, measure the impact of food fortification on nutrient intakes, track trends, and develop dietary guidance and related programs. In 1998 the CFSII released information on intakes from 1994 through 1996 (USDA CSFI, 1998).

National Nutrition Monitoring and Related Research Act

In 1990, Congress passed Public Law 101-445, the National Nutrition Monitoring and Related Research (NNMRR) Act. This law was created as an umbrella to provide organization, consistency, and unification to the survey methods that monitor the food habits and nutrition of the U.S. population (Sims, 1993). The intent was to coordinate efforts of the 22 federal agencies that implemented or reviewed nutrition services or surveys at that time.

Data obtained through NNMRR are used to direct research activities, develop programs and services, and make policy decisions. Food labeling, food and nutrition assistance programs, food safety, and education activities are areas shaped by the information gathered through the NNMRR. Reports of the various activities are issued approximately every 5 years and summarize the dietary, nutrition, and related health status of Americans and the nutritional quality of the food they consume. NNMRR provides information on trends in nutrition and health, knowledge, attitude and behavior assessments, food composition, and food supply determinants (Federation of American Societies for Experimental Biology, 1995; Kuczmarski et al, 1994). Nutrition monitoring reports can be obtained through the National Agricultural Library database.

Nutrition Screening Initiative

The Nutrition Screening Initiative (NSI) was created in 1990 by a partnership of the ADA, the American Academy of Family Physicians (AAFP), and the National Council on the Aging (NCA), with the goal of improving nutrition and nutrition care for the older population. NSI was a response to studies indicating that early detection and interventions addressing nutrition-related problems could improve the quality of life and reduce the number of hospitalizations. A result of the NSI is a series of validated screening tools that can be used to assess senior adults who are living independently. The initial screen is an assessment that can be self-administered by an older adult or used by persons without medical or nutrition training. The Level 1 Screen is more in-depth and is designed to be used by nonprofessionals with some guidance from professionals. Level 1 can help identify warning signs of nutritional risk, such as altered body weight, eating habits, living environment, and functional status. The Level 2 and 3 Screens provide progressively more comprehensive nutritional assessment to be used by nutrition and health care professionals. By 2000, the screening tools had been used with more than 300,000 individuals nationwide. The information collected using these screens is used to build a valuable database about senior adults and to provide guidance for community-based caregivers (NSI, 1997). (See Chapter 13 for a more detailed discussion of the NSI.)

National Nutrient Data Bank

The National Nutrient Data Bank, maintained by USDA, is the United States' primary resource of information on the nutrient content of foods. The information is obtained from private industry, academic institutions, and government laboratories. Historically, the information was published as a series called the *Agriculture Handbook 8.* Currently the databases are available through public access on tapes and on the Internet. The database is updated frequently and includes supplemental sources, the databases of other countries, and links to other sites. This database is a standard source of nutrient information for commercial references and data systems. When using sources other than the USDA site, check their reliability and when they have last been updated to ensure that accurate and current information is being provided.

Centers for Disease Control and Prevention

The Centers for Disease Control and Prevention (CDC) is a component of the DHHS, monitoring the nation's health, detecting and investigating health problems, and conducting research to enhance prevention. CDC is also the source of health information for those traveling outside of the United States. Housed at CDC is the National Center for Health Statistics, which is the lead agency for NHANES and information on mortality, morbidity, BMI, and other health-related measures. Hard copies of reports and publications are available to professionals through a publications list or the Web site.

NATIONAL NUTRITION GUIDELINES AND GOALS

Frequently, established health priorities include dietary guidance. Table 14-2 lists some landmark reports that have influenced the development of dietary guidance or affected the content and scope of health priorities.

Healthy People and *The Surgeon General's Report on Nutrition and Health*

Healthy People, a 1979 report of the Surgeon General, and *Promoting Health/Preventing Disease: Objectives for the Nation* outlined the prevention agenda for the nation with a series of health objectives to be accomplished by 1990 (*Healthy People,* 1979; *Promoting Health/Preventing Disease,* 1980). In 1988, *The Surgeon General's Report on Nutrition and Health* further stimulated the health promotion and disease prevention movement (*The Surgeon General's Report on Nutrition and Health,* 1988), providing information on dietary practices and health status. In addition to specific health recommendations, the report provided documentation of the scientific basis for the recommendations (Box 14-1). Because its focus includes implications for individuals as well as for future public health policy decisions, this report is still considered a useful tool.

Healthy People 2000: National Health Promotion and Disease Prevention Objectives and *Healthy People 2010* are the next generations of these landmark public health efforts. The reports outline the progress made on previous objectives and set new objectives for the next decade (*Healthy People 2000,* 1990; *Healthy People 2010,* 2000).

During the evaluation phase for setting the 2010 objectives, it was found that the United States has made progress in reducing the number of deaths from cardiovascular disease, stroke, and certain cancers. Dietary evaluations reveal a slight decrease in total dietary fat intake; however, in the last decade the number of people who are overweight or obese has increased. Reducing the incidence of overweight and obesity (and increasing physical activity) are targeted priorities in 2010 for all segments of the population (Box 14-2). Other areas continuing to be targeted are improving the health of minorities, increasing the numbers of breast-feeding mothers, and reducing the incidence of iron deficiency anemia (*Healthy People 2010,* 2000) (Figure 14-3).

Dietary Guidelines for Americans

Senator George McGovern and the Senate Select Committee on Nutrition and Human Needs presented the first *Dietary Goals for the United States* in 1977 (Senate Select Committee on Nutrition and Human Needs, 1977). In 1980 the goals were modified and issued jointly by the DHHS and the USDA as the *Dietary Guidelines for Americans (DGAs).* Updated every 5 years, the current revision is the fifth edition, *Nutrition and Your Health: Dietary Guidelines for Americans.* The original guidelines were a response to an increasing national concern about the increase in inci-

TABLE 14-2 History of Dietary Recommendations for the U.S. Public

PUBLICATION	YEAR	ORGANIZATION OR AGENCY*	RECOMMENDATION
Food for Young Children	1916	USDA	First U.S. government dietary guidance pamphlet
Food Guide	1917	USDA	Five food groups: flesh, starches, fats, watery fruits and vegetables, sweets
Food Guide	1933	USDA	Twelve food groups
Recommended Dietary Allowances	1941	FNB/NAS	Recommended intakes for known nutrients
Food Guide	1946	USDA	"Basic 7" food groups
Food for Fitness (daily food guide)	1958	USDA	"Basic 4" food groups based on RDA†
Dietary Goals for the United States, ed 1	1977	Senate Select Committee on Nutrition and Human Needs	First government publication to address macronutrient intake and excess
Dietary Goals for the United States, ed 2	1978	Senate Select Committee on Nutrition and Human Needs	Refined recommendations of first edition
Nutrition and Your Health: Dietary Guidelines for Americans	1980	USDA/DHHS	Generic recommendations similar in content to the *Dietary Goals* without specified amounts
Toward Healthful Diets	1980	FNB/NAS	Similar to *Dietary Guidelines* and goals except for fat recommendations
Various guidelines on nutrition	1980	AMA, AHA, NCI, American Society for Clinical Nutrition, NAS	Several organizations published similar recommendations
Diet, Nutrition, and Cancer	1982	Committee on Diet, Nutrition, and Cancer; NRC; NAS	Dietary guidelines to reduce risk of cancer
Nutrition and Your Health: Dietary Guidelines for Americans, ed 2	1985	USDA/DHHS	
National Cholesterol Education Program (NCEP): Adult Treatment Panel I	1987	DHHS/NHLBI	Guidelines for the clinical treatment of patients with hyperlipoproteinemia
NCI Dietary Guidelines: Rationale	1988	DHHS/NCI	Recommendations to reduce risk of cancer
Nutrition and Your Health: Dietary Guidelines for Americans, ed 3	1990	USDA/DHHS	
Food Guide Pyramid	1992	USDA/HNIS	New eating guide based on RDA that also considers salt, fat, and sugar
NCEP: Adult Treatment Panel II	1994	DHHS/NHLBI	Established categories of risk; more aggressive clinical measures for patients at a higher risk for coronary heart disease
Dietary Guidelines for Americans, ed 4	1995	USDA/DHHS	
Dietary Reference Intakes	1996	FNB/NAS	Reference values for nutrient intake; contain three components: estimated average requirement (EAR), recommended dietary allowance (RDA), and tolerable upper intake level (UL)
Dietary Guidelines for Americans, ed 5	2000	USDA/DHHS	Guidelines grouped into three categories: (1) aim for fitness, (2) build a healthy base, (3) choose sensibly (the ABC approach)
American Heart Association Eating Plan for Healthy Americans	2000	AHA	Dietary guidelines to reduce the risk of hypertension, hyperlipoproteinemia, and overweight and obesity
NCEP: Adult Treatment Panel III	2001	DHHS/NHLBI	Adds recommendations for primary prevention of hyperlipoproteinemia in people with multiple risk factors

**AHA,* American Heart Association; *AMA,* American Medical Association; *DHHS,* Department of Health and Human Services; *FNB,* Food and Nutrition Board; *HNIS,* Human Nutrition and Information Services; *NAS,* National Academy of Sciences; *NCI,* National Cancer Institute; *NHLBI,* National Heart, Lung, and Blood Institute; *NRC,* National Research Council; *USDA,* U.S. Department of Agriculture.
†Recommended dietary allowances (RDAs) revised approximately every 5 years since 1943.

dence of overweight, obesity, and chronic diseases that had a nutrition cause (e.g., diabetes, coronary artery disease, hypertension, certain cancers). The guidelines are still being produced with the goals of promoting health and preventing disease (*Nutrition and Your Health,* 2000) and have become a central component of community nutrition assessments, program planning, and evaluation. The guidelines are incorporated into programs such as school lunch and congregate meal programs (see Chapter 15).

Other Dietary Guidance

Until the release of the DGAs, dietary guidelines often had a specific disease approach. The American Heart Association (AHA) guidelines were updated in 2000

Box 14-1. Recommendations of *The Surgeon General's Report on Nutrition and Health*

Issues for Most People

- *Fats and cholesterol:* Reduce consumption of fat (especially saturated fat) and cholesterol. Choose foods relatively low in fat and cholesterol, such as vegetables, fruits, whole-grain foods, fish, poultry, lean meats, and low-fat dairy products. Use food preparation methods that add little or no fat.
- *Energy and weight control:* Achieve and maintain a desirable body weight by choosing a dietary pattern in which energy (caloric) intake is consistent with energy expenditure. To reduce energy intake, limit consumption of foods relatively high in calories, fats, and sugars, and minimize alcohol consumption. Increase energy expenditure through regular and sustained physical activity.
- *Complex carbohydrates and fiber:* Increase consumption of whole-grain foods and cereal products, vegetables (including dried beans and peas), and fruits.
- *Sodium:* Reduce intake of sodium by choosing foods relatively low in sodium and limiting the amount of salt added in food preparation and at the table.
- *Alcohol:* To reduce the risk for chronic disease, consume alcohol only in moderation (no more than two drinks a day), if at all. Avoid drinking any alcohol before or while driving, operating machinery, taking medications, or engaging in any other activity requiring judgment. Avoid drinking alcohol while pregnant to lessen the risk of birth defects.
- *Overweight and obesity:* Focus on health rather than appearance. Incorporate principles of portion control into the diet, and increase intake of fruits and vegetables. Make physical activity a part of everyday life, and reduce time spent engaged in sedentary activities (e.g., television watching). As a society, encourage breast-feeding and physical activity in schools, workplaces, and the community.

Other Issues for Certain People

- *Fluoride:* Community water systems should contain fluoride at optimal levels for prevention of tooth decay. If fluoridated water is not available, use other appropriate sources of fluoride.
- *Sugars:* Those who are particularly vulnerable to dental caries (i.e., cavities), especially children, should limit their consumption of foods high in sugars.
- *Calcium:* Adolescent girls and adult women should increase consumption of foods high in calcium, including low-fat dairy products.
- *Iron:* Children, adolescents, and women of childbearing age should be sure to consume foods that are good sources of iron, such as lean meats, fish, certain beans, and iron-enriched cereals and whole-grain products. This issue is of special concern for low-income families.

Updated from *The Surgeon General's report on nutrition and health—summary and recommendations,* U.S. Department of Health and Human Services (Public Health Service), Pub No 88-50211, Washington, DC, 1988, U.S. Government Printing Office.

and provide guidance for those at risk for hypertension and coronary artery disease. The National Heart, Lung, and Blood Institute provided landmark guidelines for identifying and treating hyperlipoproteinemia in 1987 and updated them in 2001 (see Chapter 35) (ADA, 1998). The National Cancer Institute landmark report, *Diet, Nutrition, and Cancer,* led to the *Dietary Guidelines for Cancer Prevention* (National Research Council, 1982). In 2001, they were updated and broadened and became the Recommendations for Nutrition and Physical Activity for Cancer Prevention.

A consumer-friendly, single guideline—sponsored by the National Cancer Institute with the National Institutes of Health (NIH) and the Produce for Better Health Foundation—was released in 1991 as a part of the 5-A-Day for Better Health program. The 5-A-Day message is simple: try to eat at least five servings of fruits and vegetables daily (two servings of fruit and three servings of vegetables).Fruits and vegetables are naturally low in fat and good sources of fiber, several vitamins and minerals, and phytochemicals (US DHHS, 1991).

Recommended Dietary Allowances and Dietary Reference Intakes

The recommended dietary allowances (RDAs) were developed in 1943 by the Food and Nutrition Board of the National Research Council of the National Academy of Sciences. Revised approximately every 10 years, the RDAs have kept pace with current research and population needs. The first tables were developed at a time when the U.S. population was recovering from a major economic depression and World War II, so nutrient deficiencies were a concern (Food and Nutrition Board, 1989). The guidelines were intended to promote optimal health by establishing nutrient intakes that would lower the risk of nutrient deficiencies. As the food supply and the nutrition needs of the population changed, the intent of the RDAs was modified and the goal became preventing nutrition-related diseases.

The RDAs have always reflected gender, age, and life cycle differences. Nutrients have been added and age groupings have been revised. Beginning in 1998, a new form of nutrient guidelines known as the *dietary reference intakes (DRIs)* was introduced. DRIs include the RDAs, adequate intakes (AIs), and guidance on safe upper limits of certain nutrients (IOM, 2000). (See Chapter 15 for a more detailed discussion of DRIs.)

Box 14-2. *Healthy People 2010* Nutrition Objectives

Goal

To promote health and reduce chronic diseases associated with diet and weight

Objectives

Eighteen measurable nutrition objectives addressing a wide range of issues

1. Healthy weight in adults
2. Obesity in adults
3. Overweight or obesity in children and adolescents
4. Growth retardation in children
5. Fruit intake
6. Vegetable intake
7. Grain product intake
8. Saturated fat intake
9. Total fat intake
10. Sodium intake
11. Calcium intake
12. Iron deficiency in young children and females of childbearing age
13. Anemia in low-income pregnant females
14. Iron deficiency in pregnant females
15. Meals and snacks at school
16. Worksite promotion of nutrition education and weight management
17. Nutrition counseling for medical conditions
18. Food security

Modified from http://healthy.gov/healthypeople, Healthy People 2010, accessed 2002.

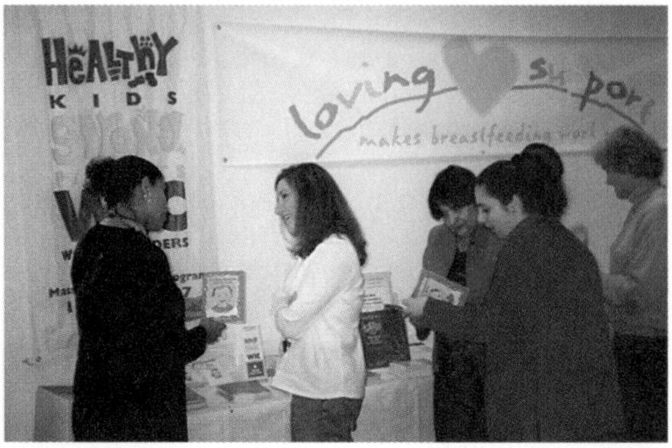

FIGURE 14-3 • Strategies for reaching 2010 objectives: Breast-Feeding Works.

Food Guides

In 1916 the USDA initiated the idea of food grouping in a pamphlet called *Food for Young Children.* Food grouping systems have changed in shape (e.g., wheels, boxes, pyramids) and numbers of groupings (four, five, seven), but the intent has remained the same—to present a simple guide for healthy eating. The current guide is the USDA Food Guide Pyramid, which was introduced in 1992. Like other current public health tools, the Food Guide Pyramid focuses on health promotion and disease prevention (Davis et al, 2001; Human Nutrition Information Service, 1992). Ongoing discussion revolves around the relevancy of specific food guides for various members of the population, but the Food Guide Pyramid remains useful as a basic assessment and education tool that can be adapted to various food styles and diverse needs. (See Chapter 15 for more information on this and other food guides.)

FOOD ASSISTANCE AND NUTRITION PROGRAMS

Having food security is having access to an adequate amount of healthy and safe foods. Although an increase in the incidence of obesity and overweight in the U.S. population has been documented, a segment of the population is also at risk for hunger and poor nutrition. The ADA addressed the issues related to domestic food and nutrition security in a position paper (ADA, 2002) that describes the impact of hunger and undernutrition on vulnerable groups such as infants, children, pregnant females, and older adults. Having adequate access to food means that the food is readily available and that resources are available for obtaining the food. Historically, public health nutritionists have advocated for food and nutrition programs that help provide consumers with adequate and safe food.

The USDA and the DHHS support many of the community-based health-related programs (Table 14-3), including child nutrition programs. Such programs can affect the nutritional status of the population throughout the life span, from before birth through old age.

National School Lunch Program and After-School Snack Program

Providing food for children in school began in the early 1900s when universal, free compulsory education was established. Early efforts were often initiated by philanthropic organizations, local school districts, and private individuals. Momentum grew as states and municipalities received federal assistance, primarily in the form of donations of surplus food.

TABLE 14-3 Food Programs Administered by the USDA

PROGRAM AND YEAR STARTED	ELIGIBLE INDIVIDUALS OR GROUPS	OBJECTIVES OF PROGRAM	COMPONENTS OF PROGRAM
Food Distribution Program (Donatable Foods), 1930s	Supplemental food program for mothers and infants; older adult food program; schools and institutions	To distribute food to individuals and institutions to support agriculture and add value	Distribution of food; previously, to low income families but currently to eligible schools, institutions, and food programs
National School Lunch Program (NSLP), 1946	All children enrolled at participating schools, residential child-care institutions—including homes for those with developmental disabilities up to 21 yr—juvenile detention centers, and orphanages	To provide a nutritious lunch (one that has as its objective to provide one third of the RDA for a child) at a reasonable cost to school children; to provide reduced-price or free lunches to needy eligible children	Donated food to participating schools; federal monetary support
Food Stamp Program, 1964	Needy families and individuals in participating counties (almost all counties); entitlement program based on income for all Americans	To supplement an individual's or a family's food-buying power	Limited monthly allotment of food vouchers at a reduced price, depending on income; coupons are used to pay for food
Child and Adult Care Food Program, 1968 ("Adult" added in 1989)	Preschool children enrolled in day-care, Head Start, and Even Start programs; children up to 18 yr enrolled in after-school care programs; children up to 12 yr living in homeless centers (children with disabilities up to 18 yr); migrant children up to 15 yr; functionally impaired adults in day-care programs	To provide nutritious meals and snacks to children enrolled in day-care, after-school, Head Start, and Even Start programs, children without a permanent residence, and adults with functional impairments	Federal monetary support; cash in lieu of commodities available
Special Milk Program,* 1968	Schools, child-care centers, summer camps, and institutions	To reduce the cost of milk for children or provide it free to children who are also eligible for free meals	Federal reimbursement to schools or centers for all or part of the cost of the milk served
Summer Food Service Program for Children, 1968	Public agency–sponsored programs for preschool and school-age children in schools, recreation centers, and summer camps and during vacations in areas with a continuous school calendar	To provide free lunches to children in summer	Federal monetary support
School Breakfast Program, 1973	All children enrolled in participating schools	To provide children a low-cost nutritious breakfast	Donated food to participating schools; federal monetary support
Supplemental Nutrition Program for Women, Infants, and Children (WIC), 1974 (renamed "Nutrition" versus "Food" in 1993-1994)	Pregnant and lactating females, infants and children up to 5 yr who are judged to be at nutritional risk because of inadequate nutrition and family income	To improve the nutritional status of pregnant and lactating females and of children up to 5 yr in low-income areas	Cash grants to state health departments and comparable agencies who make available supplemental foods through participating health clinics; health clinics providing specified nutritious food supplements or vouchers for these foods; requires regular health examination of the mother and the children and nutrition education
Farmer's Market Nutrition Program (FMNP)	Women, infants (older than 4 mo), and children eligible for the WIC program† Low income older adults‡	To encourage WIC participants to include fresh fruits and vegetables in their diets while promoting the use of local farmers' markets	Federal and state monetary support; nutrition education from local WIC agency

*If a school is on the School Lunch Program, it cannot receive the Special Milk Program and vice versa.
†Farmer's Market Nutrition Program, 1992.
‡Farmer's Market Nutrition Program, 2003.

Legislation in 1946 established the National School Lunch Program (NSLP). Administered by the USDA, this program offered nutritious school meals at a low cost or free. The strategy was to provide nutritious food to children and maintain food prices for the nation's farmers through distribution of surplus foods. The program provided federal cash reimbursement and donated foods to schools serving a lunch that met specified nutritional requirements. This pattern, known as the *Type A Lunch,* was set to provide about one third of the RDA for an 11-year-old child.

Although the NSLP has undergone several revisions, many of the basic guidelines are still in place. Since 1998 the nutrition pattern has incorporated the DGAs. The government still provides a cash reimbursement for meals at three levels—the regular-price meal, the reduced-price meal, and the free meal. Children from households above income guidelines of 185% of poverty pay the cost of the meal minus the small reimbursement. Reduced-price meals are offered to children from households with incomes between 130% and 185% of poverty guidelines. Children of families with an income below 130% of the poverty level are offered free meals.

The participating school receives the predetermined cash reimbursement for each meal offered; some states offer additional reimbursement. Although surplus foods no longer exist, commodity foods in lieu of cash are offered through the Commodity Supplemental Food Program (CSFP). These are foods purchased by the government and offered to qualifying food assistance programs.

The passage of the Rehabilitation Act of 1973 and the Americans with Disabilities Act in 1991 brought changes that have relevance to community nutrition. Under these provisions, children who need special choices or textures of food or certain feeding modalities have access to meals at schools.

The newest program under the NSLP umbrella offers nutritious snacks to children in after-school education or recreation programs. The after-school snack program began in 1998 and is provided to children in eligible sites who are younger than age 18. The NSLP operates in more than 98,000 public and nonprofit private schools and residential child-care institutions. Each day more than 27 million children receive meals supported by the NSLP (USDA, 2002). Studies have shown that children who participate in the NSLP are more likely to reach the RDA for key nutrients.

School Breakfast Program

The School Breakfast Program began as a pilot project in 1966 and became permanent in 1975. Eligibility criteria are the same as those in the NSLP. The meal should offer about one fourth of the RDA. Participating schools receive a set reimbursement and are eligible for benefits under the CSFP. Approximately 7.4 million children in more than 72,000 schools and institutions participate in school breakfast programs. Research indicates that children who participate in the School Breakfast Program have higher standardized achievement test scores than eligible nonparticipants (USDA, 2002). (See Chapter 10 for a more detailed discussion on the impact of eating breakfast on the nutrition of children.)

Special Milk Program

The Special Milk Program was established in 1955 by the USDA to reimburse institutions for half-pints of milk served to children. It is available to schools and child-care institutions that are ineligible for other federal child nutrition service programs. Children who are eligible for free school lunches or breakfasts are eligible for milk through this program. Expansion of the breakfast and lunch programs has led to a decrease in the Special Milk Program since the 1960s. In 2000, 120 million half-pints of milk were offered through this program (USDA, 2002).

Child and Adult Care Food Program

USDA's Child and Adult Care Food Program (CACFP) provides meals and snacks to 2.6 million children and 74,000 adults who receive day care outside of their home. Authorized under the National School Lunch Act, this program follows nutrition and eligibility guidelines similar to those in the NSLP. Qualifying nonprofit day-care centers, institutions, and Head Start programs are reimbursed for meals and snacks that meet nutrition requirements. Participants are provided the meals and snacks for free or at a reduced rate based on income (USDA, 2002).

Summer Food Service Program

The Summer Food Service Program is a USDA program that was established in 1975 after a 1968 pilot program proved it would be beneficial for the nutritional status of children. The program provides nutritious meals to children from low-income families during the summer school break. Sponsors include day camps and recreation programs in which at least half of the children are from households with incomes below 185% of the poverty level. The program provides one or two meals per day, although in special situations three daily meals are provided. All meals are free to eligible participants, and set fees are reimbursed to the sites for meal costs (USDA, 2002).

WIC Program

The Special Supplemental Nutrition Program for Women, Infants, and Children (WIC) is funded as part of child nutrition legislation. Administered by the USDA, this program was established in 1974 to improve the nutritional status of pregnant and lactating females and children up to 5 years of age from low-income families (Figure 14-4). Participants must meet income and medical risk guidelines. As an example of the reach of the WIC program, in May 2002, approximately 7 million people were receiving WIC benefits each month. Programs are active in all states and the District of Columbia, 32 Indian tribal organizations, Puerto Rico, the Virgin Islands, American Samoa, and Guam (USDA, 2002).

WIC provides cash grants to state health departments and comparable agencies, which make available specific supplemental foods and nutrition education. It is not an entitlement program, so the state caseload is limited by the funding available. Eligible participants are provided vouchers for a specific food package tailored to meet their health needs. Most clients are seen by WIC staff, including nutrition professionals, at least every 2 months during their 6-month period of eligibility. At the end of the 6 months, clients must be reevaluated and recertified for eligibility.

The foods are selected based on their nutritional value to women, infants, and children. The food package is reviewed and revised routinely. The vouchers are used like checks at WIC-certified vendors in the community. Ongoing monitoring of vendors ensures that program regulations are followed. Nutrition education is mandated and funded, and nutrition professionals are key personnel. Studies have shown that participants have lower medical costs for themselves and their infants, longer gestation periods, and higher birth weights, all resulting in lower infant mortality (USDA, 2002).

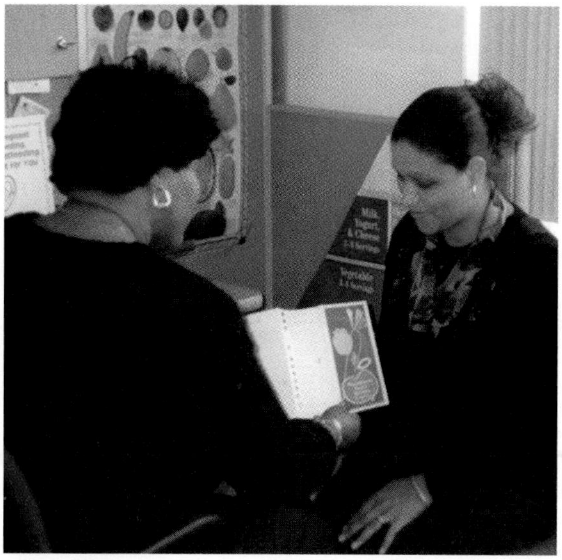

FIGURE 14-4 • WIC Works: a community-based nutrition service for pregnant women.

Head Start Program

Started in 1965, Head Start is a comprehensive child health and development program for children between the ages of 3 and 5 who are from low-income families. Head Start, administered by DHHS, funds community centers so that they can offer half-day and full-day programs providing education, nutritious meals and snacks, and access to social services and health guidance. Parents and caregivers are encouraged to be involved, and special services are available for home-based children with disabilities. Meals and snacks are offered under the guidance of the Child Care Food Program of the USDA.

Food Stamp Program

The Food Stamp Program is an entitlement program administered by USDA. Established in 1964, the program's goal is to supplement the food-buying power of low-income individuals and families. Monthly allotments are based on household size and gross monthly income. The allotments must be used for purchasing food from a business eligible to accept food stamps. Most foods, including some take-out establishment and restaurant foods, are allowed under this program. Cleaning items, medicine, paper goods, and pet food are examples of ineligible items. Electronic benefit transfer (EBT) cards are now being used in most areas of the country. A major effort is currently underway to provide support for food and nutrition education and thus increase the buying power and nutrition status of those who use food stamps.

Senior Adult Meals

Senior adults comprise a large and growing segment of the population. In 1965 a federal program was established to provide meals and support services for senior adults. The Title III Elderly Nutrition Program (ENP) of the Older Americans Act authorizes funding for nutritious meals (that provide at least one third of the RDA) and other services at a community site or for home-delivered meals for qualified senior adults. A later reauthorization added the consultation of nutrition professionals to the program regulations. Partially funded through federal legislation, the Administration on Aging (AoA) of DHHS administers these programs with assistance from state and local agencies. No income stipulation for eligibility in these programs has been made. In addition to the ENP, the USDA Nutrition Program for the Elderly (NPE) provides cash and commodity foods for meals. Participants are expected to pay a small fee, or contribution, for the meals.

Most congregate sites offer lunch three to five times a week. The meals (which are also known as *Meals-on-Wheels*) are delivered Monday through Friday, and occasionally snacks are included. Volunteers often play a significant role in the congregate and home-delivered services. Transportation to the sites, counseling, nutrition education, and recreation may also be offered and funded. Congregate meals and visits with those receiving home-delivered meals increase socialization, which is important for many otherwise isolated senior adults. Studies indicate that participation in congregate or home-delivered meals improves the nutrient intake of older adults and contributes to their mental well-being. Because these programs must be reauthorized under the Older Americans Act, advocacy is important (AoA, 2002).

Cooperative Extension and the Expanded Food and Nutrition Education Program

The Cooperative Extension program is a USDA initiative administered by land grant or state universities. The program provides hands-on training in homes and community settings for community residents. Originally intended for rural settings, Cooperative Extension is still active in such programs as 4H and homemaker training. Since 1969, one component of the program has been the Expanded Food and Nutrition Education Program (EFNEP), which serves low-income families, many in urban settings. Childcare, nutrition education, food preservation, food safety, and budgeting are some of the major topics addressed by these programs. EFNEP is also involved in food stamp recipient education.

FOOD SAFETY: LAWS, REGULATIONS, AND ISSUES

One of the major responsibilities of the public health system is to ensure the safety of the food supply. A multitiered approach to enhance safety, monitor systems, and prevent epidemics of foodborne illness is in place. The tiers include federal regulatory agencies, state and local public health agencies, and the private sector (e.g., food producers and manufacturers). Recently, professional organizations such as the ADA, the American Medical Association, and the School Food Service Association have emphasized the need to enhance public education about food safety (Cody and Kunkel, 2002).

The goal is disease prevention, but the etiologies of foodborne illnesses are constantly changing. In the past, foodborne illness was most likely to be associated with a large event such as a picnic or a wedding reception. Outbreaks were linked to improper food handling that resulted in bacterial contamination of a single food item (e.g., potato salad, sliced meat). Foodborne illness occurred when people ate the contaminated food. Another previous focus was prevention of the contamination of human food with sewage or animal manure—sources of pathogens.

Although these types of threats to food safety still exist, the issues of today and the future are more complicated. New pathogens have emerged, some of which have spread worldwide. Examples of pathogens in healthy animals and foods that can be spread to other foods are *Salmonella* organisms, *Staphylococcus aureus, Escherichia coli (157:H7), Campylobacter* organisms, and *Yersinia enterocolitica.* These pathogens have caused millions of cases of sporadic illness and chronic complications throughout the world. Future prevention issues include controlling the accidental contamination of food and water consumed by animals and passed on to humans and the purposeful contamination of food and water supplies. Research into ways that pathogens can persist in animal reservoirs is important for the long-term prevention of outbreaks (Tauxe, 1997). Another key to prevention is an enhanced surveillance system to rapidly identify the offending organisms and halt outbreaks.

Surveillance Systems

The public health surveillance and response systems involve local, state, and national agencies. The local county or city health department provides basic surveillance, investigation, and prevention. At the state level, public health epidemiologists, inspectors, and educators conduct statewide surveillance and prevention activities in conjunction with local authorities. Federal agencies are involved when the geographic boundaries are crossed or the public health threat has national ramifications.

When a foodborne illness develops, agencies work as a team. The local health agency is the first defense in identifying and controlling an immediate or potential source of contamination. Emergency action (e.g., restaurant closing, product recall) can be localized and rapid. The next step is to identify ways to prevent similar outbreaks in the future.

Regulatory Agencies

At the federal level, several agencies have responsibility for food safety; laws and rules regulating food safety and quality are found in Table 14-4. CDC is responsible for the risk assessment of public health hazards. CDC also conducts the primary national surveillance and supports state health departments in managing their response to outbreaks. The Food and Drug Administration (FDA) and USDA's Food Safety Inspection Service (FSIS) regulate food safety. Each agency has specific responsibilities for the nation's food and water, although they do overlap.

The FDA has responsibilities and programs that keep it in the public spotlight. In addition to food concerns, the FDA oversees the safety of cosmetics, medicines and medical devices, and the radiation-emitting products used daily such as microwave ovens. Other responsibilities include the regulation of low-acid canned foods, imported foods, pasteurized milk, certain types of seafood, rabbits raised for meat, and the food and water provided on aircraft

TABLE 14-4 Legislation Milestones in Health Claim Regulation

NAME OF LEGISLATION	YEAR*	TYPE	PRIMARY PROVISIONS
Pure Food and Drug Act	1906 (F) 1906 (E)	Law	Prohibited false and misleading statements on labels of foods and drugs.
Federal Food, Drug, and Cosmetics Act	1933 (I) 1938 (E)	Law	Regulated and defined misbranding ". . . labeling represents, suggests, or implies that the food because of the presence or absence of certain dietary properties is adequate or effective in the prevention, cure, mitigation, or treatment of any disease or symptom." Continued prohibition of false and misleading claims in food labeling. Required "common and usual name" of food, net quantity of contents, ingredient statements, name and address of manufacturer and distributor. Required labeling of imitation and special dietary foods.
Label Statements Concerning Dietary Properties of Food Purporting to be or Represented for Special Dietary Uses	1941 (F)	Regulation	Created regulations for vitamin and mineral supplements, fortified food products, and special dietary foods.
Fair Packaging and Labeling Act	1966 (F) 1966 (E)	Law	Gave the US FDA jurisdiction over regulation of package size, provision of label information, and measurement of content.
Public Health Messages on Food Labels	1987 (I); reproposed 1990	Regulation	Proposed procedures for allowing reliable and valid consumer information on food labels. Proposed criteria for appropriate health messages. Proposed interagency health committee on health messages. Withdrawn with the passage of the National Labeling and Education Act.
Food Labeling, Advance Notice of Proposed Rule-Making	1989 (I)	Regulation	Asked for comments on the need for revision of food labels, including health messages, nutrition label format, requirements for nutrition labeling, food descriptors, and ingredient labeling. Four national public hearings across the nation to gather comments on ways to improve the rules.
Nutrition Labeling and Education Act	1990 (I) 1990 (F) 1990 (E)	Law	Provided for mandatory nutrition labeling of most foods under the FDA's jurisdiction. Allowed health claims for the first time but only if consistent with the FDA final regulations. Mandated that standardized serving sizes represent amounts customarily consumed and be expressed in appropriate common household measures. Expanded list of required nutrients. Provided for consistent, defined nutrient content claims based on standardized serving sizes (reference amounts). Federal preemption for nutrient labeling. Provided for consumer education.
Food Labeling: General Requirements for Health Claims for Foods	1991 (I)	Regulation	Proposed general health claim requirements: definitions to clarify the meaning of specific terms used in the regulation; preliminary requirements a food must meet to be eligible for a health claim; a scientific standard for assessing the validity of claims for dietary supplements and conventional foods and general labeling requirements for health claims permitted by regulation and prohibitions on certain types of health claims; and the required content of petitions for health claims.
Food Labeling: General Requirements for Health Claims for Foods	1993 (F)	Regulation	Discussed general health claim requirements—contained (1) definitions: health claim, substance, nutritive value, and disqualifying level to clarify the meaning of specific terms used in the regulation; (2) requirements a component of food must meet to be eligible for a health claim; (3) general labeling requirements for health claims permitted by regulation and prohibitions on certain types of health claims; and (4) the required content of petitions for health claims.
Nutrition Labeling: Health Claims on Meat and Poultry Products	1994 (I)	Regulation	Proposed to permit the use of health claims and an application process for such health claims. Would permit health claims that are designed to parallel those issued by the FDA.
Dietary Supplement Health and Education Act	1994	Law	Outlined marketing regulations for dietary supplements. Allowed supplements to carry "structure/function" claims describing the structural or functional role of a nutrient in the human body (e.g., "Calcium builds strong bones."). Required that FDA be notified within 30 days after a dietary supplement is marketed with a structure/function claim, and that supplements carrying structure/function claims must have the following words on their label: "This statement has not been evaluated by the Food and Drug Administration. This product is not intended to diagnose, treat, cure, or prevent any disease." Prohibited supplements from claiming to be able to "diagnose, prevent, mitigate, treat, or cure" a specific disease, with the exception of classic nutrient deficiency

Data from Geiger C: Health claims: history, current regulatory status, and consumer research, *J Am Diet Assoc* 98:1313, 1998, http://vm.cfsan.fda.gov/~dms/dietsupp.html; www.cfsan.fda.gov/label.html, 2002. Copyright American Dietetic Association.

*I, Year initialized; F, year finalized; E, year enacted.

Continued

TABLE 14-4 Legislation Milestones in Health Claim Regulation—cont'd

NAME OF LEGISLATION	YEAR*	TYPE	PRIMARY PROVISIONS
Dietary Supplement Health and Education Act—cont'd	1994	Law	diseases such as scurvy; if claims are made about deficiency disease, the disease's prevalence in the United States must be included on the label. Supplements can use FDA-authorized health claims if they meet the criteria. The 1999 court decision in the case of *Pearson v. Shalala* authorized dietary supplements to use "qualified" health claims—qualified claims have the bulk of scientific evidence in their favor, but they have not yet met the standards required to become FDA authorized.
Food Labeling: Nutrient Content Claims, General Principles; Health Claims, General Requirements and Other Specific Requirements for Individual Health Claims	1995 (I)	Regulation	Proposal that would permit the use of shortened versions of authorized health claims under certain circumstances, eliminate some of the required elements for health claims, permit health claims on certain foods that do not currently qualify because they do not contain 10% of certain required nutrients, and provide additional guidance for petitioners seeking exemption from the disqualification of some foods from bearing a health claim because they contain high levels of certain nutrients. Would also provide refinements to those regulations to allow additional synonyms for nutrient content claims without specific preclearance by the agency.
Food and Drug Administration Modernization Act	1997	Law	Stipulated that health claims could be made based on authoritative statements made by scientific entities of the U.S. government or the National Academy of Sciences as long as the FDA is notified. Specified the wording for these claims and required they be used. Did not authorize dietary supplements to carry these claims.

Data from Geiger C: Health claims: history, current regulatory status, and consumer research, *J Am Diet Assoc* 98:1313, 1998, http://vm.cfsan.fda.gov/~dms/dietsupp.html; www.cfsan.fda.gov/label.html, 2002.
**I*, Year initialized; *F*, year finalized; *E*, year enacted.

and trains. In addition, the FDA monitors foods and drugs for pets and farm animals and is responsible for food labeling.

The USDA regulates pasteurized eggs, meat, poultry—including their slaughter and packaging—and pasteurized eggs. Animal and plant health, including investigations of any diseases, is another responsibility of the USDA under the Cooperative Extension outreach program. The USDA regulates the grading of shell eggs for quality, but the FDA has responsibility for their microbiologic safety (FDA, 2002)—an example of the previously mentioned agency overlap.

Approaches to Foodborne Illness Prevention

Although the U.S. food supply is considered one of the safest in the world, the CDC estimates that 76 million people become sick each year from a food-related illness. About 300,000 are hospitalized and 5000 Americans die as a result of foodborne illness (CDC, 2002). Food handling has gained more attention as Americans have begun to eat out more and use more food prepared away from home. More foods are imported from other countries or brought to market from long distances (Food Marketing Institute, 2001). In addition, unskilled laborers—from those in the fields to those in the dining rooms—are likely to need training in safe food handling. Emphasis is on continuing research into new ways to prevent foodborne illness outbreaks and contamination of the food supply, development of multilingual educational tools, and an enhanced, quick-response surveillance system (ADA, 1997).

One national resource available to educators, trainers, producers, and the public is the USDA and FDA Foodborne Illness Education Information located at the National Agricultural Library (www.nalusda.gov/fnic/foodborne/). This center is part of an interagency agreement between the FSIS (of the USDA) and the FDA (of the DHHS). The mission of the center is to reduce the risk of foodborne illness and increase knowledge of food-related risks from production through consumption. The center maintains two databases. One database includes sources of educational materials, including software, audiovisual information, and printed information for a wide range of audiences from children through adults, including food handlers. The other database addresses the Hazard Analysis Critical Control Points (HACCP) training programs and resources. Another important resource is FIGHT BAC, a national partnership of industry and government for food safety education (FIGHT BAC, 1998).

Hazard Analysis Critical Control Points

Hazard Analysis Critical Control Points (HACCP) is an approach to food safety focusing on identifying and controlling critical points in the food production chain that may lead to food hazards. HAACP incorporates a set of food safety strategies specific to the tasks and the settings of the food chain; these strategies apply to farmers working in the field and those responsible for food handling and production before it reaches a consumer's table. Food handlers at all levels are trained to implement key strategies to eliminate or control foodborne illness triggers at critical points in the operation. The FDA and USDA have adopted the HACCP system to replace older strategies. For example, an HACCP strategy to prevent bacterial growth on fresh fruits would be to (1) refrigerate or chill the fruit, and (2) use bottled or distilled water for the ice cubes used to chill the fruit rather than using potentially polluted water. Multilevel HACCP strategies for reducing the risk of *E. coli* contamination in ground beef could include sanitation inspections of the slaughterhouses, sanitization of plant equipment, use of proper hand-washing techniques by meat handlers, irradiation of the meat after slaughter, safe handling and storage of the raw meat, and thorough cooking of the beef to a safe internal temperature (FDA, 2001; National Advisory Committee, 1997).

Health Claims

Health claims are yet another way to ensure the safety of food and supplements. The FDA is the oversight agency for labeling and health claims. The 1990 Nutrition Labeling and Education Act (NLEA) supports a process through which all health claims on food must be thoroughly researched and approved before the claim can be added to a label. Dietary supplements do not follow the same regulations.

In foods, health claims are permitted for specific nutrients and diseases and limited to those that have been determined to have sufficient supporting research. An application must be submitted, evidence provided, and permission granted before a claim can appear on a label. The roles of calcium in osteoporosis, fat in cancer, sodium in hypertension, folate in birth defects, and soy protein in heart disease are examples of current health claims on food labels (Food and Nutrition Science Alliance [FANSA], 1997; Geiger, 1998). When such claims appear on a label, consumers can be assured that they are supported by scientific evidence. Even the word "healthy" can only be used as an implied claim under the NLEA if the food meets a defined set of criteria. The reference amount of the food must contain 3 g or less of fat, 1 g or less of saturated fat, 15% or less of the total kilocalories as saturated fat, and 60 mg or less of cholesterol, and it must provide at least 10% of the recommended daily allowance (RDA) or daily recommended value (DRV) of one micronutrient such as vitamin A or C, protein, calcium, iron, and fiber or 480 mg or less of sodium (Geiger, 1998).

Dietary supplements are addressed by the 1994 Dietary Supplement Health and Education Act (DSHEA) and include traditional nutrient supplements (vitamins and minerals) and botanicals (herbs), functional foods and beverages, and amino acids. Currently, supplements addressed by the DSHEA are not required to meet the same rigid standards as food. Although responsible for ensuring that a supplement is safe before it is marketed, a manufacturer does not have to have prior approval before producing or selling it. Dietary supplements may advertise "true" claims stating the effect of the product on the body but not suggesting that the product treats, prevents, or mitigates a certain disease (Storlie, 1999). If adverse effects are reported after a product appears in the market, the FDA has the responsibility of taking action. The Federal Trade Commission (FTC) regulates the advertising of supplements (FDA, 2002). This disparity between label claims on foods and for dietary supplements can be confusing to the public and professionals (see Chapter 15). Table 14-4 delineates the history of health claims and their current regulatory status.

FOOD TECHNOLOGY

Technology can enhance food properties, resulting in such benefits as higher crop yields, better freshness, and improved nutrition. Food processing, food safety, pharmacology, and waste management are likely to be affected by new trends in technology. *Biotechnology* is a term used to describe gene splicing, cell fusion, and protein purification. The advances and the issues connected to food technology are changing rapidly, as are the associated emotions (Hodgson, 2001).

Additives

Additives are used in food processing to maintain or improve the quality and palatability of foods. The Federal Food, Drug and Cosmetic (FFD&C) Act of 1938 gives the FDA authority over food ingredients. The 1958 Food Additives Amendment to the FFD&C Act specifies that the manufacturer is responsible for proving an additive's safety before it can be approved. The Delaney Clause, which is currently under review, prohibits approval of any food additive that has been found to cause cancer in animals and humans. The generally recognized as safe (GRAS) list includes more than 600 ingredients such as salt, sugar, and spices that do not have to be tested by the prescribed procedures required for every new food item. The GRAS list is reviewed and changed as technology advances.

Food Fortification and Enrichment

Assuring and improving the nutritional adequacy of an ever-changing food supply includes both enrichment and fortification of foods that are widely consumed. Enrichment is the addition of nutrients to restore the nutritional value lost in processing. An example is enriched flour with additions of iron and certain B vitamins lost in the milling process. Iron enrichment is considered a major public health measure to improve the iron status of the U.S. population. Fortification is the addition of nutrients to enhance a food's nutritional value. Adding folate to flour and grain products, iodine to salt, and calcium to orange juice are examples of fortification being used as a public health measure.

Irradiation

Despite food safety efforts, microbiologic hazards exist. Food irradiation is one way to reduce potential pathogens and enhance the safety and quality of the food supply. By using low levels of radiant energy, pathogens and other biologic contaminants can be rendered harmless. Studies have shown that the irradiated food is structurally and nutritionally of high quality and does not emit radioactivity. Newer methods of irradiation use electronic beams. Spices, certain fresh fruits, and meat are examples of foods currently being irradiated. Some states require labeling of irradiated foods with a symbol or statement (ADA, 2000).

AGRICULTURAL PRODUCTS AND CONCERNS

A survey conducted for the International Food Information Council (IFIC) in 2001 found that most Americans (61%) believe and can state the ways biotechnology will benefit them or their families in the next 5 years. Approximately 39% of consumers anticipate benefits such as improved health and nutrition; 33% expect improved food quality, taste, and variety; 21% anticipate reduced chemical and pesticide use on plants; 9% expect reduced food costs and improved crops and crop yields (IFIC, 2002).

Pesticides

The Environmental Protection Agency (EPA) approves the use of and establishes tolerance levels for pesticides at the field, or commodity, level and the processed food level. The FDA monitors and enforces the tolerance levels. To obtain approval for a particular pesticide, a manufacturer must supply the EPA with data from toxicologic studies and residue data. The pesticide's use must be justified in relation to maintaining or improving the economics and adequacy of the food supply. A risk/benefit analysis of the information leads to rejection or acceptance and establishment of a legal tolerance. Approval is granted for the specific commodity requested on the application. For example, using a chemical approved for use on lettuce is a violation if it is used on cabbage or any other food. Consumers often misunderstand the levels of residue they should expect in the marketplace. The Total Diet Study (Market Basket) monitors the food supply and provides information that allows authorities to take action as needed.

Interest in *natural* or *organically grown* products has been growing—that is, foods grown without the use of pesticides and herbicides. Although organically grown foods may provide the consumer with psychological benefits, they often do not have any nutrition or safety advantages. Safety of organically grown food is still a concern, especially if manure is used as a fertilizer or safe food handling procedures are not implemented. In addition, regulation of the organic food supply is limited and inconsistent. The public depends on the integrity of the producer when a food is labeled *organic.* Beginning in 2002, a national voluntary label system was established to make it easier for the public to identify authentic organically grown food (see *Focus On:* Is it Really Organic?).

Total Diet Study (Market Basket Sample)

In an effort to monitor the level of residues in food being served, the FDA routinely analyzes table-ready foods. Four times each year, 234 food items representing the diets of American consumers are purchased in different cities in the United States. Sampled foods are prepared as they would be in the home and analyzed for actual levels of pesticides, industrial chemicals, heavy metals, radionucleotides, and essential minerals. The intakes for eight age-sex groups are compared with the acceptable daily intakes (ADIs) established by the Food and Agriculture Organization and World Health Organization of the United Nations. The ADI is the acceptable daily intake of a chemical that if ingested throughout a lifetime seems to be associated with no appreciable risk. Twenty-five years of data have revealed that levels of pesticide residue are consistently lower than the ADI. Actual pesticide intakes as determined by the Total Diet Study (Market Basket Sample) are usually considerably lower than the ADI.

Genetically Modified Foods and Biotechnology

Genetically modified (GM) foods (or *genetically modified organisms [GMOs]*) are being debated by consumers and professionals. Also known as *bioengineered foods,* GM foods are produced by a form of biotechnology that uses deoxyribonucleic acid (DNA) recombinant technology to design protein molecules and other compounds. In existence for more 8000 years, various forms of biotechnology have been used throughout history in the natural production of vinegar, alcoholic beverages, cheese, and sourdough bread. Much of the current debate focuses on processes that genetically modify plants or use gene splitting. Consumers

FOCUS ON

Is It Really Organic?

Environmental, social, and political issues are as important as nutrition in organic farming. The popularity of organic or natural foods continues to increase. Although the word *natural* is not regulated, some have taken actions to establish voluntary standards for the use of *organic* as a description for food. As of October 2002, a food designated as *Aorganic@* has met production and handling standards identified and regulated by USDA; in the marketplace, the food is labeled with the word *Aorganic@* or a small sticker with the *USDA Organic* seal. For a food to earn the designation Aorganic@, 95% of the ingredients must have been produced in fields that use renewable resources and conserve soil and water to enhance environmental quality. Aorganic@ meat, poultry, eggs, and dairy are produced from animals grown without antibiotics or growth hormones. Fruits and vegetables are grown without conventional pesticides, petroleum-based fertilizers, or sewage sludge-based fertilizers. The land on which organic crops are grown is required to be pesticide and herbicide free for 3 years before a crop is harvested. In addition, bioengineering or ionizing radiation cannot be used in the food's production. For a product or farm to use the designation *Aorganic@*, a government-approved certifier must inspect the farm or processor; obtaining this designation is voluntary (Data from *Organic foods get national standards,* 2001).

are often concerned about the safety of the resulting food, especially for people who have or may develop allergies or food intolerances (see Chapter 32). Some states are considering obtaining voluntary statements from food processors ensuring that their foods have not been genetically modified. Because no easy way exists to identify foods that have been modified and no official regulations have been established, the public has to depend on the integrity of the producer or processor. All areas of biotechnology are being pursued cautiously. The goals are to use biotechnology techniques to add or enhance qualities such as disease resistance, a higher yield, or better keeping qualities. Public confidence continues to be an issue, so this topic should be monitored by community nutrition professionals (Hodgson, 2001).

Antibiotics and Hormones

Use of antibiotics at subtherapeutic levels to improve growth of food animals is a concern or issue to some consumers. Some are concerned that the antibiotics may result in the development of resistant strains of bacteria. To date, data do not support the concern that subtherapeutic amounts of antibiotics in animals are implicated in human illness (National Research Council, 1997). Other than penicillin and tetracycline, antibiotics currently being added to animal feed are not prescribed for human use.

Another consumer concern is the use of hormones in cattle feed. The use of such additives is permitted as long as the residues are not found in meat and milk when they arrive at the marketplace. The use of the estrogen *diethylstilbesterol* was discontinued when more precise analytic techniques enabled the identification of extremely small amounts of the hormone in some meat products.

Use of bovine growth hormone (bovine somatotropin [BST], or gonadotropin) has resulted in significant increases in milk production (20% to 40%) and meat production (10% to 20%). Growth hormones from other species are postulated to be inactive in humans. Because it is a protein, growth hormone is inactivated and digested by enzymes in the stomach before it enters the circulation.

OTHER CONCERNS ABOUT FOOD AND WATER SAFETY

Mad cow disease (bovine spongiform encephalopathy) and foot-and-mouth disease were problems in Great Britain and Europe in 2001 and made headlines around the world. The two diseases are not related, and the supply of beef in the United States remains the safest in the world.

Bioterrorism is a concern in today's political environment. Government agencies remain alert to potential foodborne pathogens being introduced to the food or water supply (Box 14-3). Suggestions for decreasing the risk of being affected by bioterrorism include only accepting foods from reputable vendors, checking carefully to ensure that packaging is intact, washing cans before opening them to keep debris from falling into foods, keeping 3 or more days' worth of food and water available in the home, washing all produce before use, and removing the outer layers of salad greens before preparation (Cody and Kunkel, 2002).

USDA has a question hotline: 1 (800) 601-9327. For information about animal diseases when traveling outside the United States, the number is 1 (866) 723-4827.

Box 14-3. Government Agencies Related to Food and Nutrition

Central Web Site for Access to All U.S. Government Information on Nutrition: http://www.nutrition.gov

Centers for Disease Control and Prevention
1600 Clifton Road, NE
Atlanta, GA 30333
Phone: (404) 639-3311
Internet: http://www.cdc.gov

Environmental Protection Agency
Ariel Rios Building
1200 Pennsylvania Avenue, NW
Washington, DC 20460
Phone: (202) 260-2090
Internet: http://www.epa.gov

Federal Trade Commission
Public Reference Branch
600 Pennsylvania Avenue, NW
Room 130
Washington, DC 20580
Phone: (202) 326-2222
Internet: http://www.ftc.gov

Food and Agriculture Organization of the United Nations
Viale delle Terme di Caracalla
00100 Rome, Italy
Internet: http://www.fao.org

Food and Drug Administration
Office of Public Affairs
5600 Fishers Lane
Rockville, MD 20857-0001
Phone: (888) 463-6332
Internet: http://www.fda.gov

Food and Drug Administration Advisory Committees
Phone: (800) 741-8138
Food Advisory Committee, ext. 10564
National Center for Toxicological Research Science Advisory Committee, ext. 12559
Internet: http://www.fda.gov/nctr/

Food and Drug Administration Center for Food Safety and Applied Nutrition
Phone: (800) FDA-4010
Internet: http://www.vm.cfsan.fda.gov

National Cancer Institute
NCI Public Inquiries Office
6116 Executive Boulevard, MSC8322
Suite 3036A
Bethesda, MD 20892-8322
Phone: (301) 496-6641
Internet: http://www.nci.nih.gov

National Health Information Center
P.O. Box 1133
Washington, DC 20013-1133
Phone: (800) 336-4797
Internet: http://www.health.gov/nhic

National Institutes of Health
Office of Communications and Public Liaison
1 Center Drive, MSC0188
Building 1, Room 344
Bethesda, MD 20892
Phone: (301) 496-4461
Internet: http://www.nih.gov

National Institutes of Health
Office of Dietary Supplements
31 Center Drive, MSC2086
Building 31, Room 1B29
Bethesda, MD 20892-2086
Phone: (301) 435-2920
E-mail: ods@nih.gov
Internet: http://dietary-supplements.info.nih.gov

National Marine Fisheries Service
National Oceanic Atmospheric Administration Office of Public and Constituent Affairs
1305 East-West Highway, #1W514
Silver Spring, MD 20910
Phone: (301) 713-1208
Internet: http://www.nmfs.noaa.gov

USDA Center for Nutrition Policy and Promotion
3101 Park Center Drive
Room 1034
Alexandria, VA 22302-1594
Phone: (703) 305-7600
Internet: http://www.usda.gov/cnpp

USDA Food and Nutrition Service
Public Information Staff
3101 Park Center Drive
Room 819
Alexandria, VA 22302-1594
Phone: (703) 305-2286
Internet: http://www.fns.usda.gov/fns

USDA Food Safety and Inspection Service
1400 Independence Avenue, SW
Room 2932—South
Washington, DC 20250-3700
Meat and Poultry Hotline: (800) 535-4555
Internet: http://www.fsis.usda.gov
Gateway to Government Food Safety Information
Internet: http://www.foodsafety.gov

USDA National Agriculture Library
Food and Nutrition Information Center
10301 Baltimore Avenue
Beltsville, MD 20705-2351
Phone: (301) 504-5719
Internet: http://www.nal.usda.gov/fnic

World Health Organization
Headquarters Office in Geneva (HQ)
Avenue Appia 20
1211 Geneva 27
Switzerland
Telephone: (+ 00 41 22) 791 21 11
Fax: (+00 41 22) 791 31 11
Telex: 415 416
Telegraph: UNISANTE GENEVA
Internet: http://www.who.org

SUMMARY

Promoting a positive health profile in the community includes addressing all aspects of food and nutrition throughout the life cycle. The broad issues in today's community continue to be the same as they have been in the past; however, the complexity of today's environment, the speed of technology and communication, and the interactions among health promotion, disease prevention, and community-level interventions have broadened the focus of community-based practice. The community should be a safe venue for education, health promotion, and disease prevention and qualified professionals should be active members. Nutrition services and medical nutrition therapy in community and public health agencies offer exciting opportunities. The scope of practice may involve direct care services such as individual counseling or broader administrative roles such as managing a health promotion program or developing public policies. Being qualified to practice in the community means having enough knowledge of the tools, resources, and processes to provide relevant food and nutrition services.

Clinical Scenario

You are employed as a health professional in a community center. Marie has been referred to you to discuss the results of her pregnancy test, which reveals that she is 6 weeks pregnant. She wants to receive prenatal care because she has many concerns about her health and the health of her baby. During the intake interview, you learn that Marie is 17 years old and has a toddler. She lives at home with her mother, who is a widow. Her mother speaks limited English and has recently been diagnosed with type 2 diabetes and hypertension. You refer Marie to case management services to discuss enrolling the family into primary care services at your facility and possibly refer her to other community-based services.

1. For which health and nutrition programs is Marie (herself) eligible?
2. Which programs could help her toddler?
3. Which health and nutrition programs are available in your community to promote optimal health and education of infants and children? What are the eligibility guidelines?
4. Describe Marie's age-related nutrition care issues.
5. In addition to nutrition programs, which other health and safety programs and resources are available in your community for this family? (Consider issues related to food and water safety, budgeting assistance, and food assistance.)
6. Which programs might help Marie's mother manage her current health problems?
7. Which resources are available to address the varied cultural and linguistic needs of Marie's family and other families?

Relevant Web Sites

Agency on Aging
www.aoa.dhhs.gov
Agricultural Research Service (ARS)
USDA Nutrient Database for Standard Reference, Release 15:
www.nai.usda.gov/fnic/foodcomp/
American Academy of Family Physicians, Nutrition Screening Initiative
www.aafp.org/nsi/
American Cancer Society
www.cancer.org
American Dietetic Association
www.eatright.org/gov
American Heart Association
www.americanheart.org
American Medical Association
www.ama-assn.org
Center for Food Safety and Applied Nutrition (CFSAN)
www.cfsan.fda.gov
Centers for Disease Control and Prevention
www.cdc.gov
Fight Bac! Food safety
www.fightbac.org
Food and Drug Administration
www.fda.gov
Healthy People 2010
www.healthypeople.gov/
Institute of Food Technologists
www.ift.org
International Food Information Center
ificinfo.health.org
National Center for Health Statistics of the CDC
www.cdc.gov/nchs
U.S. Dairy Association, Agricultural Research Service, Food Surveys Research Group
www.barc.usda.gov/bhnrc/foodsurvey/home.htm
U.S. Dairy Association, National Agricultural Library, food composition
www.nal.usda.gov/fnic/foodcomp.html
U.S. Department of Agriculture Food, Nutrition and Consumer Services
www.fns.usda.gov/fncs
U.S. Department of Health and Human Services
www.hhs.gov
U.S. Government Access to All Nutrition and Food Information
www.nutrition.gov
U.S. Government Food Safety
www.foodsafety.gov

Cited References

Administration on Aging: *The elderly nutrition program fact sheet: administration on aging fact sheet,* Washington, DC, 2002, The Administration.

American Dietetic Association: Position of the American Dietetic Association: food and water safety, *J Am Diet Assoc* 97:184, 1997.

American Dietetic Association: Position of the American Dietetic Association: domestic food and nutrition security, *J Am Diet Assoc* 102:184, 2002.

American Dietetic Association: Position of the American Dietetic Association: the role of nutrition in health promotion and disease prevention programs, *J Am Diet Assoc* 98:205, 1998b.

American Dietetic Association: Position of the American Dietetic Association: food irradiation, *J Am Diet Assoc* 100:246, 2000.

Bailar JC III, Travers K: Review of assessments of the human health risk associated with the use of antimicrobial agents in agriculture, *Clin Infect Dis* 34:135S, 2002.

Bayerl C, Ries J: *EARLY START: nutrition services in early intervention,* Boston, 1995, Department of Public Health.

Centers for Disease Control and Prevention: *Food safety initiative activity,* 2002, http://www.cdc.gov/foodsafety.

Cody MC, Kunkel ME: *Food safety for professionals,* ed 2, Chicago, 2002, American Dietetic Association.

Davis CA et al: Past, present, and future of the Food Guide Pyramid, *J Am Diet Assoc* 101:881-885, 2001.

Egan M: Public health nutrition: a historical perspective, *J Am Diet Assoc* 94:298, 1994.

Federation of American Societies for Experimental Biology, Interagency Board for Nutrition Monitoring and Related Research: *Third report on nutrition monitoring in the United States: executive summary,* Washington, DC, 1995, U.S. Government Printing Office.

FIGHT BAC Partnership for Food Safety Education: *FIGHT BAC: A national public education campaign to reduce the risk of foodborne illness,* Washington, DC, 1998, USDA.

Food and Drug Administration: FDA Backgrounder, 2001; HACCP Principles and Application Guidelines, Washington, DC, 1997.

Food and Drug Administration: *Overview and history of FDA and the Center for Food Safety and Applied Nutrition (CFSAN),* Washington, DC, 2002, FDA.

Food Marketing Institute: *Trends in the United States,* Washington, DC, 2001, FMI.

Food and Nutrition Board, National Research Council, National Academy of Sciences: *Recommended dietary allowances,* ed 10, Washington, DC, 1989, National Academy Press.

Food and Nutrition Science Alliance (FANSA): What does the public need to know about dietary supplements? *J Am Diet Assoc* 97:728, 1997.

Geiger C: Health claims: history, current regulatory status, and consumer research, *J Am Diet Assoc* 98:1312, 1998.

HACCP Principles and Application Guidelines: *National Advisory Committee on Microbiological Criteria for Foods,* Washington, DC, 1997, Food and Drug Administration and U.S. Department of Agriculture.

Haughton B et al: Profile of public health nutrition personnel: challenges for population/systems–focused roles and state-level monitoring, *J Am Diet Assoc* 98:664, 1998.

Healthy People: Surgeon General's report on health promotion and disease prevention, Washington, DC, 1979, U.S. Department of Health and Human Services.

Healthy People 2000: National health promotion and disease prevention objectives, Washington, DC, 1990, U.S. Department of Health and Human Services.

Healthy People 2010: National health promotion and disease prevention objectives, Washington, DC, 2000, U.S. Department of Health and Human Services.

Hodgson E: Genetically modified plants and human health risks: can additional research reduce uncertainties and increase public confidence? *Toxicol Sci* 63:153-156, 2001.

Human Nutrition Information Service, U.S. Department of Agriculture: *The Food Guide Pyramid,* Home Garden Bulletin 249, Washington, DC, 1992, U.S. Government Printing Office.

Institute of Medicine, Committee for the Study of Public Health: *The future of public health: a vision of public health in America: an attainable level,* Washington, DC, 1998, National Academy Press.

Institute of Medicine, National Academy of Sciences: *Dietary reference intakes: applications in dietary assessment,* Washington, DC, 2000, National Academy Press.

International Food Information Council Foundation: *Medical guide on food safety and nutrition,* Washington, DC, 2002, The Foundation.

Kuczmarski M et al: Update on nutrition monitoring activities in the United States, *J Am Diet Assoc* 94:753, 1994.

National Center for Health Statistics: *National health and nutrition examination survey, Background history, 2000,* http://www.cdc.gov/nchs/about/major/nhanes/bhistory.htm.

National Research Council, Committee on Diet, Nutrition and Cancer: *Diet, nutrition and cancer,* Washington, DC, 1982, National Academy Press.

National Research Council, Committee on Drug Use in Food Animals: *The use of drugs in food animals: benefits and risks,* Washington, DC, 1997, National Academy Press.

Nutrition Monitoring Division, Human Nutrition Information Service: USDA nationwide food consumption survey: continuing survey of food intakes by individuals—1986, *Nutr Today* 24(5):35, 1989.

Nutrition Screening Initiative: *The role of nutrition in chronic disease care,* Washington, DC, 1997, Greer, Margolis, Mitchell, Burns and Associates.

Organic foods get national standards, *Tufts Univ Health Nutr Lett* 18(12):2, 2001.

Probert KL, ed: *Moving to the future: developing community-based nutrition services,* Washington, DC, 1996, Association of State and Territorial Public Health Nutrition Directors.

Promoting health/preventing disease: objectives for the nation, Washington, DC, 1980, U.S. Government Printing Office.

Senate Select Committee on Nutrition and Human Needs: *Dietary goals for the United States,* Pub No 052-070-03913-2, Washington, DC, 1977, U.S. Government Printing Office.

Senate Select Committee on Nutrition and Human Needs: *Dietary goals for the United States,* ed 2, Pub No 052-070-04376-8, Washington, DC, 1978, U.S. Government Printing Office.

Sims L: *Research aspects of public policy in nutrition generating research questions to determine the impact of nutritional, agricultural, and health care policy and regulation on the health and nutrition status of the public,* The Research Agenda for Dietetics Conference Proceedings, Chicago, 1993, American Dietetic Association.

Storlie J: *DSHEA revisited: understanding and using the supplement facts label,* Chicago, Winter 1999, SCAN's Pulse.

The Surgeon General's report on nutrition and health—Summary and recommendations, U.S. Department of Health and Human Services Public Health Service Pub No 88-50211, Washington, DC, 1988, U.S. Government Printing Office.

Tauxe R: Emerging foodborne diseases: an evolving public health challenge, *Emerg Infect Dis* 3(4):1, 1997.

U.S. Department of Agriculture: *Continuing survey of food intakes by individuals (CSFI) 1994-96,* Beltsville, Md, 1998, The Department.

U.S. Department of Agriculture: *FNS OnLine: child nutrition fact sheets,* Washington, DC, 2002, http:www.fns.usda.gov/cnd.

U.S. Department of Agriculture and U.S. Department of Health and Human Services. *Nutrition and your health:* dietary guidelines for Americans, Home and Garden Bulletin No 232, Washington DC, 2000.

U.S. Department of Health and Human Services: *Eat more fruits and vegetables: 5-a-day for better health,* NIH Pub No 92-3248, Washington, DC, 1991, Public Health Service and National Institutes of Health.

Winslow CEA: The untilled field of public health, *Mod Med* 2:183, 1920.

Woteki CE et al: National Health and Nutrition Examination Survey—NHANES: plans for NHANES III, *Nutr Today* 23(1):25, 1988.

Additional References

Horrigan L et al: How sustainable agriculture can address the environmental and human health harms of industrial agriculture, *Environ Health Perspect* 110:445, 2002.

Lathers CM: Clinical pharmacology of antimicrobial use in humans and animals, *J Clin Pharmacol* 42:587, 2002.

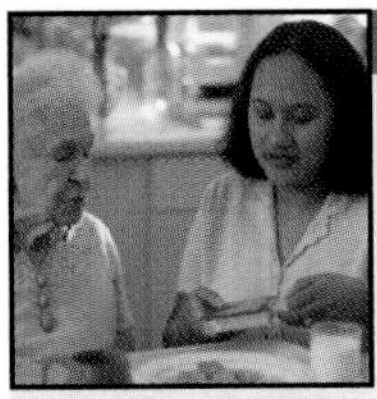

CHAPTER 15

Guidelines for Dietary Planning

ROBERT EARL, MPH, RD

CHAPTER OUTLINE

- Determining Nutrient Needs
- Nutritional Status of Americans
- National Guidelines for Diet Planning
- Food Labeling
- Cultural Aspects of Dietary Planning

KEY TERMS

adequate intake (AI)–the recommended daily intake level based on observed or experimentally determined approximations of nutrient intake by a group (or groups) of healthy people; used when a recommended dietary allowance (RDA) cannot be determined

daily reference values (DRVs)–a set of food labeling reference values for which no nutrient recommendation previously existed; established for fat, saturated fatty acids, cholesterol, total carbohydrate, protein, dietary fiber, sodium, and potassium

daily value (DV)–reference term on food labels to aid consumers in selecting a healthy diet; consists of two sets of references—the reference daily intakes (RDIs) and daily reference values (DRVs)—expressed as percentages

***Dietary Guidelines for Americans* (DGAs)**–dietary recommendations that promote health and reduce risk of chronic disease for people ages 2 years and older

dietary reference intake (DRI)–an overall term designed to encompass the four specific types of nutrient recommendations (adequate intake [AI], estimated average requirement [EAR], recommended dietary allowance [RDA], and tolerable upper intake level [UL]); used for nutrient recommendations for the United States and Canada

estimated average requirement (EAR)–nutrient intake value that is estimated to meet the requirements of half the healthy individuals in a group

estimated safe and adequate daily dietary intakes (ESADDIs)–recommended intake ranges of nutrients for which not enough information is available to establish a recommended dietary allowance

Food Guide Pyramid–translates the *Dietary Guidelines for Americans* and nutrient recommendations into a visual form of the kinds and amounts of food to eat each day

food insecurity–having inadequate and insufficient access to food on a daily basis

health claims–any claims on a food package label or other label (such as an advertisement) of a food, including fish and game meat, that characterize the relationship of any nutrient or other substance in the food to a disease or health-related condition

Healthy Eating Index (HEI)–summary measure of overall diet quality; designed to assess and monitor the dietary status of Americans

nutrition facts label–nutrient content information on food products designed to help consumers (4 years of age and older) select foods to incorporate into a healthy diet using the Food Guide Pyramid and *Dietary Guidelines for Americans*

recommended dietary allowances (RDAs)–the amount of a nutrient needed to meet the requirements of almost all (97% to 98%) of the healthy population

Former contributions by Susan T. Borra, RD, ed 10, and Paul R. Thomas, EdD, RD, ed 9.

KEY TERMS—Continued

recommended nutrient intakes (RNIs)–the Canadian recommended dietary allowance; replaced by the joint American and Canadian dietary reference intake grouping of nutrient recommendations

reference daily intakes (RDIs)–set of dietary references for food labels based on the 1968 recommended dietary allowances for vitamins and minerals; replaces the U.S. recommended daily allowances that were previously used with nutrition labeling on food products

tolerable upper intake level (UL)–the highest daily intake amount of a nutrient that is likely to pose no risk of adverse health effects for almost all individuals in the general population

An appropriate diet is adequate and balanced and incorporates the individual's variations such as age and stage of development, taste preferences, and food habits. It also reflects the availability of foods, socioeconomic conditions, storage and preparation facilities, and cooking skills. An adequate and balanced diet meets all the nutritional needs of an individual for maintenance, repair, living processes, growth, and development. It includes energy and all nutrients in proper amounts and proportion to each other. The presence or absence of one essential nutrient may affect the availability, absorption, metabolism, or dietary need for others. The recognition of nutrient interrelationships provides further support for the principle of maintaining variety in foods to provide the most complete diet.

With increasing knowledge of diet and disease links that lead to premature disability and mortality among Americans, an appropriate diet is now considered one that helps reduce the risk of developing chronic degenerative diseases and conditions. In this era of vastly expanding scientific knowledge and information about food components, the way the public thinks about food intake for health promotion and disease prevention is changing rapidly. In addition to traditional nutrient requirements, the public often hears references to *functional foods,* which are foods or food components that provide more benefits than basic nutritional benefits (see Chapter 12). Dietitians and other health professionals are essential translators of food, nutrition, and health information into dietary choices and patterns for groups and individuals.

DETERMINING NUTRIENT NEEDS

Worldwide Guidelines

Numerous standards serve as guides for planning and evaluating diets and food supplies for individuals and population groups. Many countries have issued guidelines appropriate for the circumstances and needs of their populations. The Food and Agriculture Organization and the World Health Organization (WHO) of the United Nations have established international standards in many areas of food quality and safety, as well as dietary and nutrient recommendations. In the United States, the Food and Nutrition Board (FNB) of the Institute of Medicine (IOM) has led the development of nutrient recommendations since the 1940s. Since the mid-1990s, nutrient recommendations developed by the FNB have been used by the United States and Canada. The U.S. Department of Agriculture (USDA) and Department Health and Human Services (DHHS) have a shared responsibility for issuing dietary recommendations, collecting and analyzing food composition data, and formulating regulations for nutrition information on food products. In Canada, Health Canada is the agency responsible for Canadian dietary recommendations and food labeling regulations.

Dietary Reference Intakes (Formerly "Recommended Dietary Allowances")

American standards for nutrient requirements have been the recommended dietary allowances (RDAs) established by the FNB of the IOM. They were first published in 1941 and most recently revised between 1997 and 2002. Each revision incorporated the most recent research findings.

In 1993 the FNB developed a framework for the development of future nutrient recommendations to be called dietary reference intakes (DRIs) (IOM, 1994) (Figure 15-1). DRIs encompass four types of nutrient recommendations for healthy individuals—adequate intake (AI), estimated average intake (EAR), recommended dietary allowance (RDA), and tolerable upper intake level (UL). From 1997 to the present the FNB's DRI panels have been completing reports on groupings of related nutrients and a report on applications of DRIs for dietary assessment (IOM, 1997, 1998, 2000, 2001, 2002a, 2002b) (Tables 15-1 to 15-3).

DRI reports for nutrients are now complete, except for the panel on water and electrolytes (i.e., sodium, potassium, chloride). Thus DRIs are now available for all nutrients for which RDAs had been established through the 1989 edition, in addition to new DRIs for macronutrients and several micronutrients. Because measurements have changed for several nu-

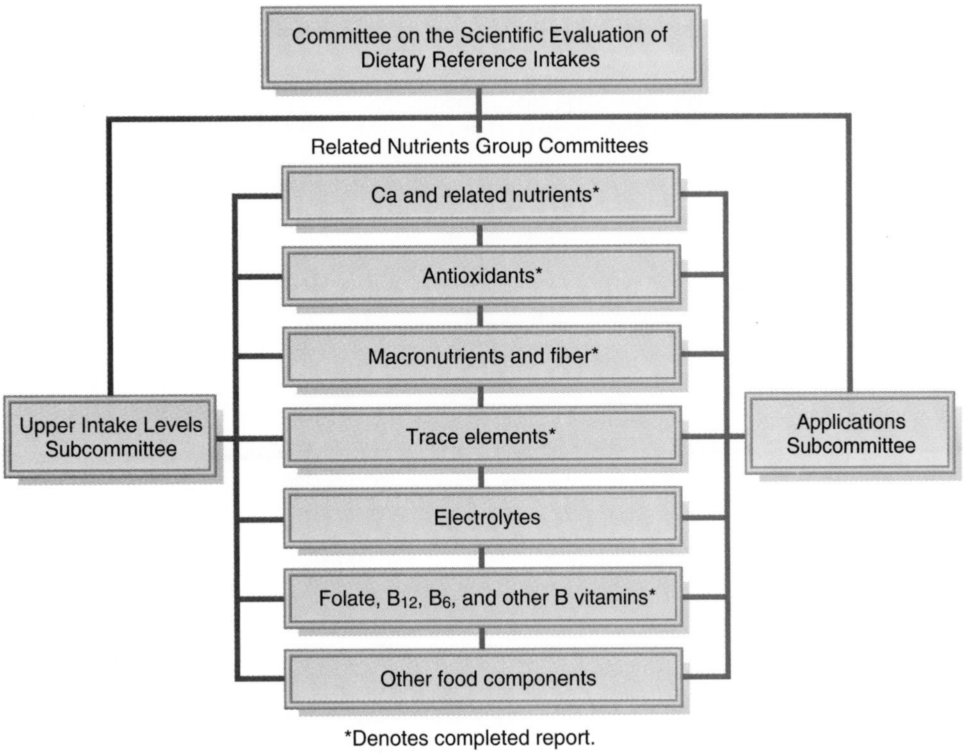

FIGURE 15-1 • The organizational structure of the subcommittee on scientific evaluation of dietary reference intakes.

trients (e.g., vitamin A changing from retinol equivalents [RE] to retinol activity equivalents [RAE]), food composition databases are being updated to reflect the new values. Nutrition and health professionals should use the most updated food composition databases and tables and inquire whether data used in computerized nutrient analysis programs have been revised.

Components

The DRI model expands the previous RDA, which focused on establishing AIs of nutrients for healthy populations to prevent deficiency diseases. To respond to scientific advances in diet and health throughout the life cycle, the DRI model now includes four reference points.

The adequate intake (AI) is a nutrient recommendation based on observed or experimentally determined approximation of nutrient intake by a group (or groups) of healthy people when sufficient scientific evidence is not available to calculate an RDA or an EAR.

The estimated average requirement (EAR) is the average requirement of a nutrient for healthy individuals; a functional or clinical assessment has been conducted, and measures of adequacy have been made at a specified level of dietary intake. An EAR is the amount of a nutrient with which about one half of individuals would have their needs met and one half would not. The EAR should be used for assessing the nutrient adequacy of populations, not individuals.

The new RDA is the amount of a nutrient needed to meet the requirements of almost all (97% to 98%) of the healthy population of individuals for whom it is developed. An RDA for a nutrient should serve as a goal for intake for individuals, not as a benchmark of adequacy of diets of populations.

Tolerable upper intake levels (ULs) have been established (for nutrients for which adequate data are available) to reduce the risk of adverse or toxic effects from increased consumption of nutrients in concentrated form—either alone or combined with others (not in food)—or from enrichment and fortification. A UL is the highest level of daily nutrient intake that is unlikely to have any adverse health effects on almost all individuals in the general population.

Target Population

Each of the nutrient recommendation categories in the emerging DRI system is used for specific purposes among individuals or populations. The EAR is used for evaluating the nutrient intake of populations. The new RDA can be used for individuals. Nutrient intakes between the RDA and the UL may further define intakes that may promote health or prevent disease.

TABLE 15-1 Dietary Reference Intakes for Vitamins and Minerals: RDAs or AIs*

LIFE-STAGE GROUP	BIOTIN (μg/day)	CALCIUM (mg/day)	CHOLINE (mg/day)	CHROMIUM (μg/day)	COPPER (μg/day)	FLUORIDE (mg/day)	FOLATE (μg/day)	IODINE (μg/day)	IRON (mg/day)	MAGNESIUM (mg/day)	MANGANESE (mg/day)	MOLYBDENUM (μg/day)	NIACIN (mg/day)
Infants													
0-6 mo	5	210	125	0.2	200	0.01	65	110	0.27	30	0.003	2	2
7-12 mo	6	270	150	5.5	220	0.5	80	130	**11**	75	0.6	3	4
Children													
1-3 yr	8	500	200	11	**340**	0.7	**150**	**90**	**7**	**80**	1.2	**17**	**6**
4-8 yr	12	800	250	15	**440**	1	**200**	**90**	**10**	**130**	1.5	**22**	**8**
Males													
9-13 yr	20	1300	375	25	**700**	2	**300**	**120**	**8**	**240**	1.9	**34**	**12**
14-18 yr	25	1300	550	35	**890**	3	**400**	**150**	**11**	**410**	2.2	**43**	**16**
19-30 yr	30	1000	550	35	**900**	4	**400**	**150**	**8**	**400**	2.3	**45**	**16**
31-50 yr	30	1000	550	35	**900**	4	**400**	**150**	**8**	**420**	2.3	**45**	**16**
51-70 yr	30	1200	550	30	**900**	4	**400**	**150**	**8**	**420**	2.3	**45**	**16**
>70 yr	30	1200	550	30	**900**	4	**400**	**150**	**8**	**420**	2.3	**45**	**16**
Females													
9-13 yr	20	1300	375	21	**700**	2	**300**	**120**	**8**	**240**	1.6	**34**	**12**
14-18 yr	25	1300	400	24	**890**	3	**400**	**150**	**15**	**360**	1.6	**43**	**14**
19-30 yr	30	1000	425	25	**900**	3	**400**	**150**	**18**	**310**	1.8	**45**	**14**
31-50 yr	30	1000	425	25	**900**	3	**400**	**150**	**18**	**320**	1.8	**45**	**14**
51-70 yr	30	1200	425	20	**900**	3	**400**	**150**	**8**	**320**	1.8	**45**	**14**
>70 yr	30	1200	425	20	**900**	3	**400**	**150**	**8**	**320**	1.8	**45**	**14**
Pregnant													
≤18 yr	30	1300	450	29	**1000**	3	**600**	**220**	**27**	**400**	2	**50**	**18**
19-30 yr	30	1000	450	30	**1000**	3	**600**	**220**	**27**	**350**	2	**50**	**18**
31-50 yr	30	1000	450	30	**1000**	3	**600**	**220**	**27**	**360**	2	**50**	**18**
Lactating													
≤18 yr	35	1300	550	44	**1300**	3	**500**	**290**	**10**	**360**	2.6	**50**	**17**
19-30 yr	35	1000	550	45	**1300**	3	**500**	**290**	**9**	**310**	2.6	**50**	**17**
31-50 yr	35	1000	550	45	**1300**	3	**500**	**290**	**9**	**320**	2.6	**50**	**17**

Data from Food and Nutrition Board, Institute of Medicine: *Dietary reference intakes,* Washington, DC, 1997, 1998, 2000, and 2002, National Academy Press.
*Values represent recommended dietary allowances (RDA) in bold type and average intakes (AIs) in plain type. Table does not include estimated average requirements (EARs) or tolerable upper intake levels (ULs), if established.
RDAs and AIs may both be used as goals for individual intake. RDAs are set to meet the needs of almost all (97%-98%) individuals in a group. For healthy breastfed infants, the AI is the mean intake. The AI for other life stage and gender groups is believed to cover the needs of all individuals in the group, but lack of data prevent being able to specify with confidence the percentage of individuals covered by this intake.

Age and Sex Groups

Because nutrient needs are highly individualized depending on age, sexual development, and the reproductive status of females, the RDAs were listed for 10 groups based on age. Those older than 10 years of age were divided according to gender. Recommendations for pregnancy and lactation were also included. The new DRI framework retains 10 age groupings, including age group categories for children, men and women 51 to 70 years of age and 70 years of age and older. It also establishes three age group categories each for pregnancy and lactation—less than 18 years, 19 to 30 years, and 31 to 50 years of age.

Reference Men and Women

The requirement for many nutrients is based on body weight. The RDAs are listed according to *reference men and women* of designated height and weight. These values for age-sex groups of individuals older than 19 years of age are based on actual medians obtained for the American population by the third National Health and Nutrition Examination Survey (NHANES III [1988 to 1994]). Although this does not necessarily imply that these weight-for-height values are ideal, at least they make it possible to define recommended allowances appropriate for the largest number of people. Recommended energy intakes for median heights and weights are shown in Table 15-4.

Estimated Safe and Adequate Daily Dietary Intakes

Numerous nutrients are known to be essential for life and health, but data for some have been insufficient to establish a recommended intake. Intakes for these nutrients are estimated safe and adequate daily dietary intakes (ESADDIs) (Table 15-5). Most intakes

PANTOTHENIC ACID (mg/day)	PHOSPHORUS (mg/day)	RIBOFLAVIN (mg/day)	SELENIUM (μg/day)	THIAMIN (mg/day)	VITAMIN A (μg/day)	VITAMIN B_6 (mg/day)	VITAMIN B_{12} (μg/day)	VITAMIN C (mg/day)	VITAMIN D (μg/day)	VITAMIN E (mg/day)	VITAMIN K (μg/day)	ZINC (mg/day)
1.7	100	0.3	15	0.2	400	0.1	0.4	40	5	4	2	2
1.8	275	0.4	20	0.3	500	0.3	0.5	50	5	5	2.5	3
2	460	0.5	20	0.5	300	0.5	0.9	15	5	6	30	3
3	500	0.6	30	0.6	400	0.6	1.2	25	5	7	50	5
4	1250	0.9	40	0.9	600	1	1.8	45	5	11	60	8
5	1250	1.3	55	1.2	900	1.3	2.4	75	5	15	75	11
5	700	1.3	55	1.2	900	1.3	2.4	90	5	15	120	11
5	700	1.3	55	1.2	900	1.3	2.4	90	5	15	120	11
5	700	1.3	55	1.2	900	1.7	2.4	90	10	15	120	11
5	700	1.3	55	1.2	900	1.7	2.4	90	15	15	120	11
4	1250	0.9	40	0.9	600	1	1.8	45	5	11	60	8
5	1250	1	55	1	700	1.2	2.4	65	5	15	75	9
5	700	1.1	55	1.1	700	1.3	2.4	75	5	15	90	8
5	700	1.1	55	1.1	700	1.3	2.4	75	5	15	90	8
5	700	1.1	55	1.1	700	1.5	2.4	75	10	15	90	8
5	700	1.1	55	1.1	700	1.5	2.4	75	15	15	90	8
6	1250	1.4	60	1.4	750	1.9	2.6	80	5	15	75	12
6	700	1.4	60	1.4	770	1.9	2.6	85	5	15	90	11
6	700	1.4	60	1.4	770	1.9	2.6	85	5	15	90	11
7	1250	1.6	70	1.4	1200	2	2.8	115	5	19	75	13
7	700	1.6	70	1.4	1300	2	2.8	120	5	19	90	12
7	700	1.6	70	1.4	1300	2	2.8	120	5	19	90	12

are shown as ranges to indicate that not only are specific recommendations not known but also at least the upper and lower limits of safety should be observed. If applicable, DRIs will replace ESADDIs for electrolytes. The DRI report on water and electrolytes was delayed but is expected in 2003.

Interpretation and Use of Dietary Reference Intakes

A separate DRI subcommittee expanded interpretation of the new terms and concepts integral to the overall project and provided guidance for their use in dietary assessments (IOM, 2001). A second report from this subcommittee is being completed and will focus on use of DRIs in planning food and nutrition assistance programs, nutrition education programs, food guides, and public health programs. A separate FNB panel is preparing a framework for use of DRIs in nutrition labeling and food fortification.

NUTRITIONAL STATUS OF AMERICANS

Food and Nutrient Intake Data

Twenty-two federal agencies collect information about the dietary and nutritional status of Americans and the relationship between diet and health. This effort is coordinated by the USDA and DHHS through the National Nutrition Monitoring and Related Research Program (NNMRRP). The NHANES and the Continuing Survey of Food Intakes by Individuals (CSFII) are the cornerstone surveys of the NNMRRP (see Chapter 14).

Status Report From the NNMRRP

The third report on nutrition monitoring in the United States from the NNMRRP (1995) addressed

TABLE 15-2 Dietary Reference Intakes for Macronutrients: EERs, RDAs, and AIs*†

LIFE-STAGE GROUP	ENERGY‡	PROTEIN	FAT								CARBOHYDRATE§				
			TOTAL	SATURATED	*TRANS-*	MONOUNSATURATED	POLYUNSATURATED	α-LINOLENIC ACID (*n*-3)	LINOLEIC ACID (*n*-6)	CHOLESTEROL	TOTAL	COMPLEX	SIMPLE	ADDED SUGAR	TOTAL FIBER¶
Infants															
0-6 mo	570/520	9.1	31	ND	ND	ND	ND	0.5	4.4	ND	60	ND	ND	ND	ND
7-12 mo	743/676	**13.5**	30	ND	ND	ND	ND	0.5	4.6	ND	95	ND	ND	ND	ND
Children															
1-3 yr	**1046/992**	**13**	ND†	ND	ND	ND	ND	0.7	7	ND	**130**	ND	ND	ND	19
4-8 yr	**1742/1642**	**19**	ND	ND	ND	ND	ND	0.9	10	ND	**130**	ND	ND	ND	25
Males															
9-13 yr	**2279**	**34**	ND	ND	ND	ND	ND	1.2	12	ND	**130**	ND	ND	ND	31
14-18 yr	**3152**	**52**	ND	ND	ND	ND	ND	1.6	16	ND	**130**	ND	ND	ND	38
19-30 yr	**3067-2957**	**56**	ND	ND	ND	ND	ND	1.6	17	ND	**130**	ND	ND	ND	38
31-50 yr	**2947-2757**	**56**	ND	ND	ND	ND	ND	1.6	17	ND	**130**	ND	ND	ND	38
51-70 yr	**2747-2557**	**56**	ND	ND	ND	ND	ND	1.6	14	ND	**130**	ND	ND	ND	30
>70 yr	**≤2547**	**56**	ND	ND	ND	ND	ND	1.6	14	ND	**130**	ND	ND	ND	30
Females															
9-13 yr	**2071**	**34**	ND	ND	ND	ND	ND	1	10	ND	**130**	ND	ND	ND	26
14-18 yr	**2368**	**46**	ND	ND	ND	ND	ND	1.1	11	ND	**130**	ND	ND	ND	26
19-30 yr	**2403-2326**	**46**	ND	ND	ND	ND	ND	1.1	12	ND	**130**	ND	ND	ND	26
31-50 yr	**2319-2186**	**46**	ND	ND	ND	ND	ND	1.1	12	ND	**130**	ND	ND	ND	26
51-70 yr	**2179-2046**	**46**	ND	ND	ND	ND	ND	1.1	11	ND	**130**	ND	ND	ND	21
>70 yr	**≤2039**	**46**	ND	ND	ND	ND	ND	1.1	11	ND	**130**	ND	ND	ND	21
Pregnant															
≤18 yr	**2368-2820**	**+25**	ND	ND	ND	ND	ND	1.4	13	ND	**175**	ND	ND	ND	28
19-30 yr	**2403-2855**	**+25**	ND	ND	ND	ND	ND	1.4	13	ND	**175**	ND	ND	ND	28
31-50 yr	**2403-2855**	**+25**	ND	ND	ND	ND	ND	1.4	13	ND	**175**	ND	ND	ND	28
Lactating															
≤18 yr	**2689-2768**	**+25**	ND	ND	ND	ND	ND	1.3	13	ND	**210**	ND	ND	ND	29
19-30 yr	**2733-2803**	**+25**	ND	ND	ND	ND	ND	1.3	13	ND	**210**	ND	ND	ND	29
31-50 yr	**2733-2803**	**+25**	ND	ND	ND	ND	ND	1.3	13	ND	**210**	ND	ND	ND	29

Modified from Food and Nutrition Board, Institute of Medicine: *Dietary reference intakes for energy, carbohydrate, fiber, fat, fatty acids, cholesterol, protein, and amino acids,* Washington, DC, 2002, National Academy Press.

*Values represent energy expenditure requirement (EER; kcal/day) for energy and recommended dietary allowances (RDAs; g/day) in bold type and average intakes (AIs; g/day) in plain type. Tolerable upper intake levels (ULs) were not established for energy or macronutrients. Table does not include estimated average requirements (EARs), if established by the Food and Nutrition Board.

†*ND,* Not determined.

‡Energy values for infants and children separated by a (/) denote males, then females; energy values for adults separated by a (-) denote the range within life-stage group (decreasing each year 10 kcal/day for men, 7 kcal/day for women); energy ranges for pregnancy are from first trimester through third trimester; energy ranges for lactation range from birth through 6 mo, then 7 mo onward.

§Carbohydrate RDA is based on the average minimum amount needed by the brain without using protein or fat as an energy source. Dietary patterns should include 45%-65% kcal/day from carbohydrate.

¶Total fiber = Dietary fiber + Functional fiber.

TABLE 15-3 Acceptable Macronutrient Distribution Ranges

NUTRIENT	AMDR (PERCENTAGE OF ENERGY AS kcal/day) 1-3 YEARS	4-18 YEARS	>19 YEARS	AMDR SAMPLE DIET (ADULT, 2000-kcal/day DIET) % REFERENCE§	g/DAY
Protein*	5-20	10-30	10-35	10	50
Carbohydrate	45-65	45-65	45-65	60	300
Fat	30-40	25-35	20-35	30	67
α-Linolenic acid (*n*-3)†	0.6-1.2	0.6-1.2	0.6-1.2	0.8	1.8
Linoleic acid (*n*-6)	5-10	5-10	5-10	7	16
Added sugars‡	≤25% of total calories			500	125

Modified from Food and Nutrition Board, Institute of Medicine: *Dietary reference intakes for energy, carbohydrate, fiber, fat, fatty acids, cholesterol, protein, and amino acids,* Washington, DC, 2002, National Academy Press.
*Higher number in protein AMDR is set to complement AMDRs for carbohydrate and fat, not because it is a recommended upper limit in the range of calories from protein.
†Up to 10% of the AMDR for α-linoenic acid can be consumed as EPA, DHA, or both (0.06%-0.12% of calories).
‡Suggested maximum.
§Reference percentages chosen based on average dietary reference intake (DRI) for protein for adult men and women, then calculated back to percentage of calories. Carbohydrate and fat percentages chosen based on difference from protein and balanced with other federal dietary recommendations.

TABLE 15-4 Reference Heights and Weights for Children and Adults in the United States

SEX	AGE	MEDIAN BODY MASS INDEX (kg/m^2)	REFERENCE HEIGHT (cm [in])	REFERENCE WEIGHT* (kg [lb])
Male, female	2-6 mo	—	64 (25)	7 (16)
	7-11 mo	—	72 (28)	9 (20)
	1-3 yr	—	91 (36)	13 (29)
	4-8 yr	15.8	118 (46)	22 (48)
Male	9-13 yr	18.5	147 (58)	40 (88)
	14-18 yr	21.3	174 (68)	64 (142)
	19-30 yr	24.4	176 (69)	76 (166)
Female	9-13 yr	18.3	148 (58)	40 (88)
	14-18 yr	21.3	163 (64)	57 (125)
	19-30 yr	22.8	163 (64)	61 (133)

Data from Third National Health and Nutrition Examination Survey, 1988-1994; Briefel R: U.S. Department of Health and Human Services, 1997, personal communication; and Institute of Medicine, 1998.
*Calculated from median body mass index and median heights for ages 4-8 yr and older.

TABLE 15-5 Estimated Sodium, Chloride, and Potassium Minimum Requirements of Healthy Persons*

AGE	WEIGHT (kg)	SODIUM (mg)†	CHLORIDE (mg)†	POTASSIUM (mg)‡
Months				
0-5	4.5	120	180	500
6-11	8.9	200	300	700
Years				
1	11	225	350	1000
2-5	16	300	500	1400
6-9	25	400	600	1600
10-18	50	500	750	2000
>18§	70	500	750	2000

From National Academy of Sciences: *Recommended dietary allowances,* ed 10, Washington, DC, 1989, National Academy Press.
*No allowance has been included for large, prolonged losses from the skin through sweat.
†No evidence shows that higher intakes confer any health benefits.
‡Desirable intakes of potassium may considerably exceed these values (~3500 mg for adults).
§No allowance included for growth. Values for those younger than 18 yr assume a growth rate at the 50th percentile reported by the National Center for Health Statistics and averaged for males and females.

two questions: "What is the nutrition-related health status of Americans?" and "What is the nutritional quality of the American diet?" The nutritional quality of the American diet shows that the population is slowly changing eating patterns and adopting more healthy diets, although gaps exist between consumption and government recommendations among population subgroups. Intake of total fat, saturated fatty acids, and cholesterol has decreased among some portions of the population. The average consumption of servings of fruits and vegetables has risen to four per day, approaching the recommendation of five servings per day. However, many Americans experience food insecurity, or hunger from not getting enough to eat.

Nutrition-related health measurements indicate that overweight and obesity are increasing from lack of physical activity. The number of people with acceptable serum cholesterol levels is increasing, although some individuals still have high levels, a major risk factor for coronary heart disease. Hypertension remains a major public health problem in middle-age and older adults; among non-Hispanic blacks, it increases the risk of stroke and coronary heart disease. Osteoporosis, which increases the risk for broken bones and impaired mobility among women 50 years of age and older, develops more often among non-Hispanic whites than non-Hispanic blacks or Mexican Americans.

Nutrition Monitoring Report

At the request of the DHHS and USDA, the Expert Panel on Nutrition Monitoring was established by the Life Sciences Research Office of the Federation of American Societies for Experimental Biology (FASEB) to review the dietary and nutritional status of the American population. The report of the committee summarized the results of data from NHANES II, Hispanic HANES, and the Nationwide Food Consumption Survey (NFCS) and CSFII surveys. In general, the committee concluded that the food supply in the United States is abundant, although some people may not receive enough nutrients for various reasons. Nutrient intakes are most likely to be low in persons living below the poverty level. Intakes of nutrients reported to be low in the general population are even lower in the poverty group.

Among the evaluations carried out by the committee were categorizations of various food components by the degree to which their intakes constituted public health issues (FASEB, 1995).

Current Public Health Issues

Nutrients

According to the NNMRRP report, the following food components were identified as current or potential public health issues (Box 15-1):

- **Energy:** Median reported energy intakes in the 1988 to 1991 CSFII were below recommended levels, yet approximately one fifth of adolescents and one half of adults were overweight. The high prevalence of overweight indicates that an energy imbalance exists among Americans because of physical inactivity and underreporting of energy intake or food consumption in national surveys.
- **Total fat, saturated fat, and cholesterol:** Intakes of fat, saturated fatty acids, and cholesterol among

Box 15-1. Classification of Food Components as Public Health Issues in the TRONM

Current Public Health Issues	Potential Public Health Issues That Need Additional Study	Not Current Public Health Issues
Food energy	Total carbohydrate*	Thiamin
Total fat	Dietary fiber	Riboflavin
Saturated fatty acids	Sugars†	Niacin
Cholesterol	Polyunsaturated and monounsaturated fatty acids†	Iodine†
Alcohol	*Trans*-fatty acids†	
Iron	Fat substitutes†	
Calcium	Protein*	
Sodium	Vitamin A	
	Antioxidant vitamins	
	Vitamin C	
	Vitamin E*	
	Carotenes	
	Folate	
	Vitamin B_6	
	Vitamin B_{12}*	
	Magnesium*	
	Potassium	
	Zinc	
	Copper*	
	Selenium†	
	Phosphorus*	
	Fluoride	

From *Third report on nutrition monitoring in the United States (TRONM), Executive summary,* Life Sciences Research Office, Federation of American Societies for Experimental Biology, Interagency Board for Nutrition Monitoring and Related Research, 1995.
*Monitoring status has changed since the second report on nutrition monitoring was published (LSRO, 1989).
†Components that are being evaluated for the first time for the NNMRRP.

all age groups older than 2 years of age were higher than recommended levels (<30% of calories for total fat and 8% to 10% of calories for saturated fatty acids). Cholesterol intakes were generally within the recommended range of 300 mg/dl or less.

- **Alcohol:** Intake of alcohol is a public health concern because it displaces food energy from food sources of nutrients and has potential health consequences.
- **Iron and calcium:** Low intakes of iron and calcium continue to be a public health concern, particularly among infants and females of childbearing age. Prevalence of iron deficiency anemia was higher among these groups than among other age-sex groups. Low calcium intake is a particular concern among adolescent girls and adult women in most racial and ethnic groups.
- **Sodium:** Sodium intake continues to exceed government recommendations of 2400 mg/day in most age-sex groups.

Food Components

Some nutrient intakes are considered potential problems, but additional study of their requirements or associations with risk is needed to establish this. The nutrients include total carbohydrate and carbohydrate constituents; dietary fiber; polyunsaturated and monounsaturated fatty acids, *trans*-fatty acids, and fat substitutes; protein; vitamin A; antioxidant vitamins (vitamins C and E and carotenes); and in certain groups, folate, vitamins B_6 and B_{12}, magnesium, potassium, zinc, copper, selenium, phosphorus, and fluoride.

TABLE 15-6 Healthy Eating Index: Overall and Component Mean Scores, 1989 Versus 1996*

	1989	1996
Overall	*61.5*	*63.8*
Components		
Grains	6.1	6.7
Vegetables	5.9	6.3
Fruits	3.7	3.8
Milk	6.2	5.4
Meat	7.1	6.4
Total fat	6.3	6.9
Saturated fat	5.4	6.4
Cholesterol	7.5	7.9
Sodium	6.7	6.3
Variety	6.6	7.6

*The overall healthy eating index (HEI) score ranges from 0 to 100. An HEI score higher than 80 implies a "good" diet, an HEI score between 51 and 80 implies a diet that "needs improvement," and an HEI score less than 51 implies a "poor" diet. HEI component scores range from 0 to 10. High component scores indicate intakes close to recommended ranges or amounts; low component scores indicate less compliance with recommended ranges or amounts. The 1989 scores are based on 1-day intake data.

Healthy Eating Index

The Center for Nutrition Policy and Promotion of the USDA released newly updated Healthy Eating Index (HEI) data for 1994 to 1996 (Bowman et al, 1998). The HEI measures how well people's diets conform to recommended healthy eating patterns. The index provides a picture of foods people are eating, the amount of variety in their diets, and compliance with specific recommendations in the *Dietary Guidelines for Americans.* The HEI is designed to assess and monitor the dietary status of Americans by using data from USDA's CSFII and evaluating 10 components, each representing different aspects of a healthy diet. The dietary components used in the evaluation include grains, vegetables, fruits, milk, meat, total fat, saturated fat, cholesterol sodium, and variety (Table 15-6).

Overall, the HEI score for 1994 to 1996 is 63.8, which is a slight but significant improvement from 61.5 in 1989. An HEI score higher than 80 implies a person has a "good" diet, an HEI score between 51 and 80 implies a person has a diet that "needs improvement," and an HEI score less that 51 implies a person has a "poor" diet. Scores from 1989 to 1996 increased for all HEI components except milk, meat, and sodium. Scores improved the most for saturated fat and variety.

Data from the HEI over time show that Americans are reducing total fat and saturated fat in their diets and eating a wider variety of foods but still need to eat more fruit, drink more milk, and reduce their sodium intake. Women generally have scores 1 point higher than men, and children ages 2 to 3 have the highest HEI scores.

NATIONAL GUIDELINES FOR DIET PLANNING

Current Health Issues

Within the past 30 years, attention has been focused increasingly on the relationship of nutrition to chronic diseases and conditions. Although this interest derives somewhat from the rapid increase in number of older adults and incremental longevity, it is also prompted by the desire to prevent premature deaths from diseases such as coronary heart disease, diabetes mellitus, and cancer.

Approximately two thirds of deaths in the United States are caused by chronic disease. Of the 10 leading causes of death, almost half are associated with diet (heart disease, some types of cancer, stroke [as a subset of cerebrovascular diseases], diabetes mellitus, and kidney disease), and many accidental deaths result from excessive alcohol consumption (Anderson, 2001) (Table 15-7).

TABLE 15-7 Ten Leading Causes of Death (United States, 1999)

CAUSE OF DEATH*	NUMBER	PERCENTAGE†
Heart disease	725,192	30.3
Cancers	549,838	23.0
Cerebrovascular diseases	167,366	7.0
Chronic lower respiratory diseases	124,181	5.2
Accidents	97,860	4.1
Diabetes mellitus	68,399	2.9
Influenza and pneumonia	63,730	2.7
Alzheimer's disease	44,536	1.9
Kidney diseases	35,525	1.5
Septicemia	30,680	1.3

Modified from Anderson RN: Deaths: leading causes for 1999, *Nat Vital Stat Rep* 49(11):8, 2001.
*Causes of death in 1999 are based on the tenth revision of the *International Classification of Diseases*, 1992.
†Numbers do not add up to 100% because of other causes of death.

Current Dietary Guidance in the United States and Canada

Eating can be one of life's greatest pleasures. People eat for enjoyment and to obtain energy and nutrients. Although many genetic, environmental, behavioral, and cultural factors affect health, diet is equally important for promoting health and preventing disease.

In 1969, President Nixon convened the White House Conference on Nutrition and Health (White House, 1970). Increased attention was being given to prevention of hunger and disease. The development of dietary guidelines in the United States began with the 1977 report of the U.S. Senate Select Committee on Nutrition and Human Needs called *Dietary Goals for the United States* (U.S. Senate Select Committee on Nutrition and Human Needs, 1977).

Dietary recommendations have evolved during the past 30 years. Although numerous federal agencies are involved in the issuance of dietary guidance, USDA and DHHS lead the effort. Following the Senate's *Dietary Goals* report, the *Dietary Guidelines for Americans* was first published in 1980. The guidelines were revised in 1985 (second edition), 1990 (third edition), and 1995 (fourth edition) (Dietary Guidelines Alliance, 1996). The most recent guidelines were released in 2000 (USDA, DHHS, 2000). With the passage of the Nutrition Monitoring Act in 1990, the dietary guidelines are now required to be reviewed every 5 years (Table 15-8).

In addition to these dietary guidelines, several other important government or expert reports have addressed dietary recommendations for healthy Americans. The Surgeon General's Report on Nutrition and Health (Public Health Service, 1988) and the National Academy of Sciences (NAS) Diet and Health Report (Food and Nutrition Board, 1989) provide similar and different qualitative or quantitative dietary recommendations. In Canada, dietary recommendations appear in Nutrition Recommendations for Canadians, which were prepared by Health Canada (Minister of National Health and Welfare, 1992; National Institute of Nutrition, 1990) (see *Clinical Insight:* Nutrition Recommendations for Canadians).

The specific dietary recommendations of the Senate Select Committee on Nutrition and Human Needs and the previously mentioned documents are compared in Table 15-8. Except for minor differences, they are surprisingly similar to those established by the Senate Select Committee in 1977. Some, such as the dietary guidelines, the Surgeon General's recommendations, and the *Nutrition Recommendations for Canadians*, are deliberately general, whereas others, such as the NAS Committee's *Diet and Health* recommendations, are more specific. Other differences reflect differences in specific amounts of or even the need to include items such as cholesterol, sodium, sugar, or alcohol. Because of heightened awareness of food safety, the dietary guidelines (2000) added a new guideline: "Keep food safe to eat."

Guidelines directed toward prevention of a particular disease, such as the National Cancer Institute's *Cancer Guidelines* (Public Health Service, 1987) and the National Heart, Lung, and Blood Institute's cholesterol education guidelines, contain recommendations unique to the particular condition (see Chapter 35). In addition, dietary recommendations have been published by private health organizations such as the American Heart Association and the American Cancer Society.

In addition, the American Dietetic Association (2002) published a position statement citing the following:

> . . . all foods can fit in a healthful eating style. The ADA strives to communicate healthful eating messages to the public that emphasize the total diet, or overall pattern of food eaten, rather than any one food or meal. If consumed in moderation with appropriate portion size and combined with regular physical activity, all foods can fit into a healthful diet.

The various counseling guidelines to be used by dietitians can be summarized as follows:

A basic universal prescription for health and fitness includes the following:

- Adjust energy intake and exercise level to achieve and maintain appropriate body weight.
- Eat a wide variety of foods to ensure nutrient adequacy.
- Increase total carbohydrate intake; increase complex carbohydrate intake.
- Eat less total fat and less saturated fat.

To this can be added the following (from most, but not all, guidelines):

- Eat more fiber.
- Eat more fruits and vegetables.

TABLE 15-8 Comparison of Selected Dietary Recommendations in the United States and Canada, 1977-2000

TOPIC	U.S. DIETARY GOALS, 1997	DIETARY GUIDELINES FOR AMERICANS, ED 1, 1980	THE SURGEON GENERAL'S REPORT ON NUTRITION AND HEALTH, UNITED STATES, 1988	DIET AND HEALTH, UNITED STATES 1989	NUTRITION RECOMMENDATIONS FOR CANADIANS, 1990	DIETARY GUIDELINES FOR AMERICANS, ED 5, 2000
Weight	To avoid overweight, consume only as much energy (calories) as is expected; if overweight, decrease energy intake and increase energy expenditure.	Maintain ideal weight.	Achieve and maintain a desirable body weight.	Balance food intake and physical activity to maintain appropriate body weight.	Provide energy needed to maintain body weight within the recommended range.	Aim for a healthy weight.
Physical activity				See Weight entry.	Include essential nutrients in amounts specified in the recommended nutrient intakes on food labels.	Be physically active each day.
Food choices		Eat a variety of foods.				Use the Food Guide Pyramid as a model for food choices.
Carbohydrates and whole grains	Increase the consumption of complex carbohydrates (naturally occurring sugars) from about 28% of energy intake to about 48% of energy intake.	Eat foods with adequate starch and fiber.	Increase consumption of whole-grain foods and cereal products, vegetables, and fruits.		Provide 55% of energy as carbohydrates (138 g/100 kcal or 185 g/5000 kJ) from a variety of sources.	Choose a variety of grains daily, especially whole grains.
Fruits and vegetables			See Carbohydrates and Whole Grains entry.			Choose a variety of fruits and vegetables daily.
Food safety						Keep food safe to eat.
Fats and cholesterol	Reduce overall fat consumption from approximately 40% to about 30% of energy intake. Reduce saturated fat consumption to account for about 10% of total energy intake; balance that with polyunsaturated and monounsaturated fats, which should each account for about 10% of energy intake. Reduce cholesterol consumption to about 300 mg/day.	Avoid consuming too much fat, saturated fat, and cholesterol.	Reduce consumption of fat (especially saturated fat) and cholesterol.		Include no more than 30% of energy as fat (33 g/1000 kcal or 39 g/5000 kJ) and no more than 10% as saturated fat (11g/1000 kcal or 13 g/5000 kJ).	Choose a diet that is low in saturated fat and cholesterol and moderate in total fat.
Sugars	Reduce the consumption of refined and processed sugars by 45% to account for about 10% of total energy intake.	Avoid consuming too much sugar.				Choose beverages and foods to moderate intake of sugars.

Continued

TABLE 15-8 Comparison of Selected Dietary Recommendations in the United States and Canada, 1977-2000—cont'd

TOPIC	U.S. DIETARY GOALS, 1997	DIETARY GUIDELINES FOR AMERICANS, ED 1, 1980	THE SURGEON GENERAL'S REPORT ON NUTRITION AND HEALTH, UNITED STATES, 1988	DIET AND HEALTH, UNITED STATES 1989	NUTRITION RECOMMENDATIONS FOR CANADIANS, 1990	DIETARY GUIDELINES FOR AMERICANS, ED 5, 2000
Salt or sodium	Limit the intake of sodium by reducing the intake of salt to about 5 g/day.	Avoid consuming too much sodium.	Reduce intake of sodium by choosing foods relatively low in sodium and limiting the amount of salt added during food preparation and at the table.	Limit total daily intake of salt (sodium chloride) that you eat to 6 g/day or less.	The sodium content should be reduced.	Choose and prepare foods with less salt.
Alcohol		If drinking alcohol, do so in moderation.	Take alcohol only in moderation (no more than two drinks a day).	Alcohol intake is not recommended.	Include no more than 50% of total energy intake as alcohol, or two drinks daily, whichever is less.	If drinking alcoholic beverages, do so in moderation.
Food safety						Keep food safe to eat.
Other				Maintain adequate calcium intake. Maintain optimal intake of fluoride, particularly during the years of primary and secondary tooth formation and growth.	Should contain no more caffeine than the equivalent of 4 cups of regular coffee per day. Community water supplies containing less than 1 mg/L of fluoride should be fluoridated to that level.	

CLINICAL INSIGHT

Nutrition Recommendations for Canadians

Canada's Food Guide to Healthy Eating was released in 1992. Suggestions include 5 to 12 servings of grain products, 5 to 10 servings of vegetables and fruits, 2 to 4 servings of milk (specified for age or for pregnancy or lactation), and 2 to 3 servings of meat or meat alternatives. Unlike the Food Guide Pyramid in the United States, *Canada's Food Guide to Healthy Eating* contains four food groupings presented in a rainbow shape, with grains representing the largest component (Health Canada, 1992). Tips include:

- The Canadian diet should provide energy consistent with the maintenance of body weight within the recommended range.
- The Canadian diet should include essential nutrients in amounts specified in the recommended nutrient intakes (RNIs), which will be replaced with DRIs in the future.
- The Canadian diet should include no more than 30% of energy as fat (33 g/1000 kcal) and no more than 10% of energy from saturated fat (11 g/1000 kcal).
- The Canadian diet should provide 55% of energy from carbohydrates (138 g/1000 kcal) from various sources.
- The sodium content of the Canadian diet should be reduced.
- The Canadian diet should include no more than 5% of total energy from alcohol or no more than two drinks daily, whichever is less.

The Canadian food guide also provides recommendations for caffeine intake and fluoridation of the water supply:

- Canadians should consume no more caffeine than the equivalent of four cups of regular coffee per day.
- Community water supplies containing less than 1 mg/L of fluoride should be fluoridated to that level.

Modified from Health Canada: *Action towards healthy eating,* Catalogue No H39-166/199, Ottawa, Canada, 1990, Branch Publications Unit.

- Eat less cholesterol.
- Eat less sodium.
- Reduce intake of sugars.
- Drink alcohol in moderation or not at all.

Included in a few recommendations are the following recommendations:

- Meet the RDA for calcium, a recommendation especially important for adolescents and women.
- Meet the RDA for iron, a recommendation especially for children, adolescents, and women of childbearing age.
- Limit protein to no more than twice the RDA.
- If using a daily multivitamin, choose dietary supplements that do not exceed the DRI.
- Drink fluoridated water.

Implementing the Guidelines

The task of planning nutritious meals centers on including the essential nutrients in sufficient amounts as outlined in the new DRIs, in addition to appropriate amounts of energy, protein, carbohydrates (including fiber and sugars), fat (especially saturated fat), cholesterol, and salt. Suggestions are included to help people meet the specifics of the recommendations. When specific numerical recommendations differ, they are presented as ranges.

The Food Guide Pyramid shown in Figure 15-2 offers a pattern for daily food choices based on servings from the five major food groups (USDA, 1992). For comparison, *Canada's Food Guide to Healthy Eating* is shown in Figure 15-3. When planned to include a wide variety of foods within each food group, this eating pattern creates a diet that is adequate in nutrients (see *Focus On:* What Is a Varied Diet?). The Food Guide Pyramid also was designed to help consumers put the dietary guidelines into action. To help people select an eating pattern that achieves specific health promotion or disease prevention objectives, nutritionists should assist individuals in making food choices (e.g., to reduce fat, to increase fiber).

In 1999, the USDA Center for Nutrition Policy and Promotion (CNPP) published the *Food Guide Pyramid for Young Children, 2 to 6 Years Old* (CNPP, 1999). The children's Food Guide Pyramid includes dimensions of physical activity and play in addition to modification of recommended serving sizes from food groupings (Figure 15-4). The serving sizes are described for children 4 to 6 years of age, with guidance for reduced amounts (except for milk) for children 2 to 3 years of age.

By combining the dietary guidelines, the Food Guide Pyramid, and the nutrition facts information from food labels, consumers design healthy diets. Because the dietary guidelines form the basis of federal policy related to nutrition and diet and address the needs of individual consumers, the committee recommended a two-step process to address dietary policy needs and those related to communicating the guidelines to the pubic. Accordingly, a group of health and food professional associations in liaison

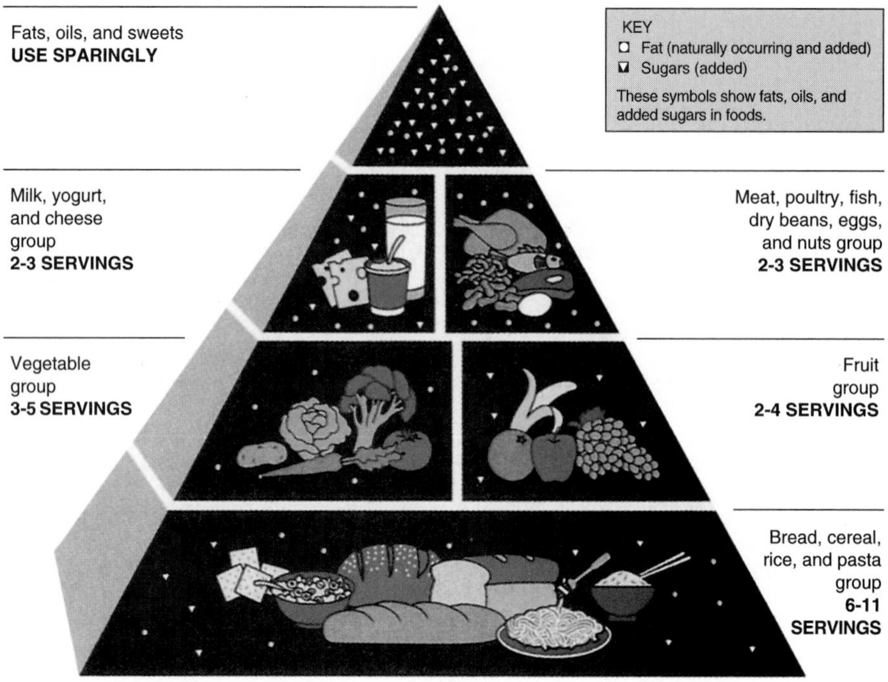

FIGURE 15-2 • The Food Guide Pyramid (From U.S. Department of Agriculture and U.S. Department of Health and Human Services.)

FOCUS ON

What Is a Varied Diet?

Many food guides and other recommendations for Americans emphasize eating a "wide variety of foods" to achieve dietary adequacy. Lack of complete information makes it impossible to establish dietary recommendations for all the known nutrients; a possibility always exists, albeit remote, that other essential nutrients will be discovered (Food and Nutrition Board, 1989; IOM, 1994).

According to the Food and Nutrition Board, choosing various foods to meet dietary recommendations (DRIs) should provide adequate amounts of the nutrients that do not have well-defined recommended levels. A varied diet also ensures that a person is consuming sufficient amounts of food constituents that although not defined as nutrients have biologic effects and may influence health and susceptibility to disease. Examples include dietary fiber and carotenoids, as well as lesser known phytochemicals (substances found in plant products) such as isothiocyanates in broccoli or other cruciferous vegetables and lycopene in tomato products. Diets rich in phytochemicals may help reduce the risk of developing certain types of cancer, but their exact mechanisms are not currently understood (see Chapter 12).

Although it is impossible to measure the effect of a varied diet on these intangibles, it does seem that increasing the number of foods eaten over a period of time improves food choices in general. Some studies have shown that the nutritional adequacy of the diet increases as people eat a greater number of different foods. Such diets tend to include less protein, meat, and meat alternatives and more carbohydrates, fruits, and vegetables. Diets that limit food intakes, such as energy-restricted weight-reduction diets, have better nutritional adequacy when they include a larger number of different foods.

with USDA and DHHS developed the Dietary Guidelines Alliance (DGA).

The mission of the DGA was to motivate consumers to change their eating and activity patterns by providing them with positive, simple messages based on the principles of the dietary guidelines. Using consumer research, the DGA developed messages that would expand the influence of the dietary guidelines to encourage consumers to adopt them and ultimately change their behaviors. The DGA message, "It's All About You," reaches out to consumers' motivations, individual needs, and life goals

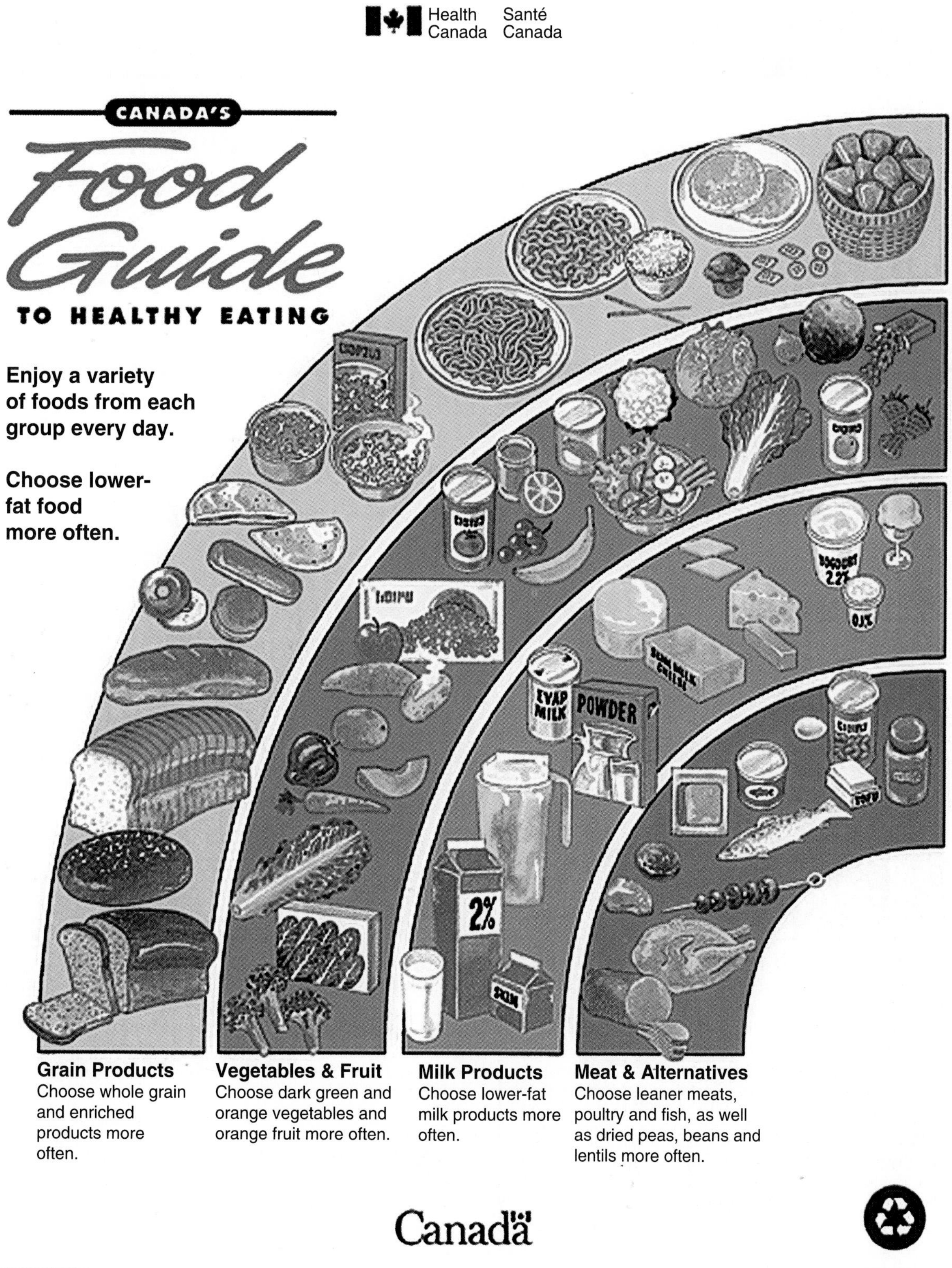
Health Canada
Santé Canada
CANADA'S
Food Guide
TO HEALTHY EATING
Enjoy a variety of foods from each group every day.
Choose lower-fat food more often.
EVAP MILK
POWDER
2%
SKIM
Grain Products
Choose whole grain and enriched products more often.
Vegetables & Fruit
Choose dark green and orange vegetables and orange fruit more often.
Milk Products
Choose lower-fat milk products more often.
Meat & Alternatives
Choose leaner meats, poultry and fish, as well as dried peas, beans and lentils more often.
Canada

FIGURE 15-3 • *Canada's Food Guide to Healthy Eating.* (From the Office of Nutrition Policy and Promotion, Health Canada, 2002. Courtesy the Minister of Public Works and Government Services, 2003. For the complete *Canada's Food Guide to Healthy Eating,* please visit the Health Canada website at www.hc-sc.gc.ca/hpfb-dgpsa/onpp-bppn/food_guide_rainbow_e.html.)

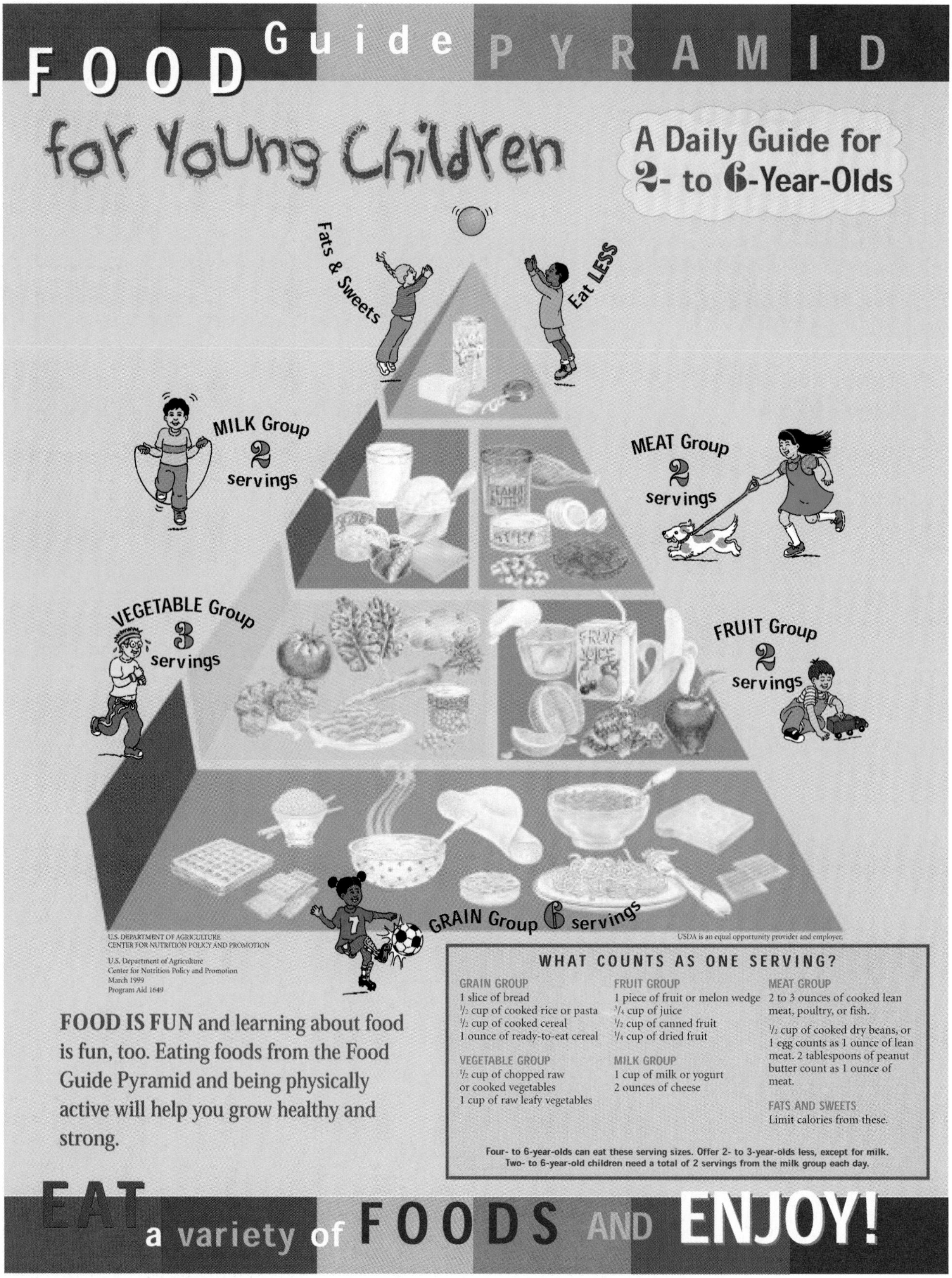

FOOD Guide PYRAMID
for Young Children
A Daily Guide for 2- to 6-Year-Olds
Fats & Sweets
Eat LESS
MILK Group 2 servings
MEAT Group 2 servings
VEGETABLE Group 3 servings
FRUIT Group 2 servings
GRAIN Group 6 servings
U.S. DEPARTMENT OF AGRICULTURE
CENTER FOR NUTRITION POLICY AND PROMOTION
USDA is an equal opportunity provider and employer.
U.S. Department of Agriculture
Center for Nutrition Policy and Promotion
March 1999
Program Aid 1649
FOOD IS FUN and learning about food is fun, too. Eating foods from the Food Guide Pyramid and being physically active will help you grow healthy and strong.
WHAT COUNTS AS ONE SERVING?
GRAIN GROUP
1 slice of bread
1/2 cup of cooked rice or pasta
1/2 cup of cooked cereal
1 ounce of ready-to-eat cereal
VEGETABLE GROUP
1/2 cup of chopped raw or cooked vegetables
1 cup of raw leafy vegetables
FRUIT GROUP
1 piece of fruit or melon wedge
3/4 cup of juice
1/2 cup of canned fruit
1/4 cup of dried fruit
MILK GROUP
1 cup of milk or yogurt
2 ounces of cheese
MEAT GROUP
2 to 3 ounces of cooked lean meat, poultry, or fish.
1/2 cup of cooked dry beans, or 1 egg counts as 1 ounce of lean meat. 2 tablespoons of peanut butter count as 1 ounce of meat.
FATS AND SWEETS
Limit calories from these.
Four- to 6-year-olds can eat these serving sizes. Offer 2- to 3-year-olds less, except for milk. Two- to 6-year-old children need a total of 2 servings from the milk group each day.
EAT a variety of FOODS AND ENJOY!

FIGURE 15-4 • Children's Food Guide Pyramid. (From U.S. Department of Agriculture.)

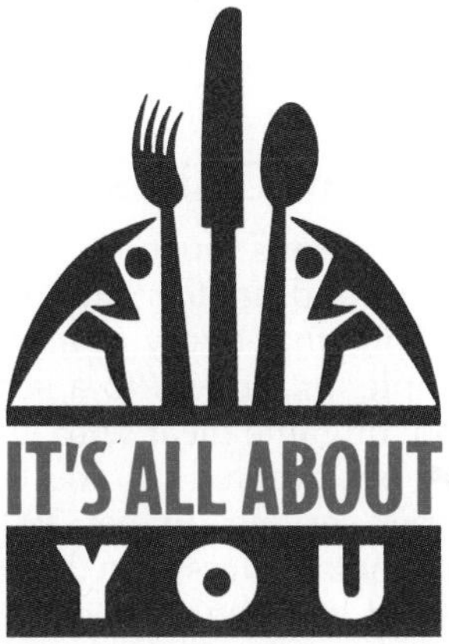

Make healthy choices that fit your lifestyle so you can do the things you want to do

BE REALISTIC

Make small changes over time in what you eat and the level of activity you do. After all, small steps work better than giant leaps.

BE ADVENTUROUS

Expand your tastes to enjoy a variety of foods.

BE FLEXIBLE

Go ahead and balance what you eat and the physical activity you do over several days. No need to worry about just one meal or one day.

BE SENSIBLE

Enjoy all foods, just don't overdo it.

BE ACTIVE

Walk the dog, don't just watch the dog walk.

FIGURE 15-5 • "It's All About You" guidelines. (From the Dietary Guidelines Alliance, 1996.)

and can be used in education, counseling, and communications initiatives (Figure 15-5).

The USDA created the publication, *Putting the Guidelines Into Practice: How Much Are You Eating?* to assist consumers with choosing sensible portions to control energy intake and promote weight loss or maintenance (USDA, 2002). Over time, USDA plans to create a series of consumer education brochures to supplement the *Dietary Guidelines for Americans* and the Food Guide Pyramid.

FOOD LABELING

To help consumers make choices between similar types of food products that can be incorporated into a healthy diet, the Food and Drug Administration (FDA) established a voluntary system of providing selected nutrient information on food labels (Figure 15-6 and Box 15-2). The regulatory framework for nutrition information on food labels was revised and updated by the USDA (which regulates meat and poultry products and eggs) and the FDA (which regulates all other foods) with enactment of the Nutrition Labeling and Education Act (NLEA) in late 1990. The new labels became mandatory in 1994.

Mandatory Nutrition Labeling

As a result of the NLEA, nutrition labels must appear on most foods except products that provide few nutrients (such as coffee and spices), restaurant foods, and ready-to-eat foods prepared on site, such as supermarket bakery and deli items (FDA, 1993).

Providing nutrition information on many raw foods is voluntary. However, the FDA and USDA have called for a voluntary point-of-purchase program in which nutrition information is available in most supermarkets. Nutrition information is provided through brochures or point-of-purchase posters for the 20 most popular fruits, vegetables, and fresh fish and the 45 major cuts of fresh meat and poultry.

Nutrition information for foods purchased in restaurants is widely available at the point of purchase or from Internet sites or toll-free numbers. Ready-to-eat, unpackaged foods in delicatessens or supermarkets may provide nutrition information voluntarily. However, if nutrition claims are made, nutrition labeling is required at the point of purchase.

Standardized Serving Sizes

Serving sizes of products are set by the government based on reference amounts commonly consumed (RACC). For example, a serving of milk is 8 oz, and a serving of salad dressing is 2 tbsp. Standardized serving sizes make it easier for consumers to compare the nutrient contents of similar products.

Nutrition Facts Label

The nutrition facts label on a food product (see Figure 15-6) provides information on its per-serving calories and calories from fat. The label then lists the amount (in grams) of total fat, saturated fat, cholesterol, sodium, total carbohydrate, dietary fiber, sugar, and protein. For most of these nutrients, the label also shows the percentage of the daily value (DV) supplied by a serving. A product's content of vitamins A and C, calcium, and iron is listed in terms of DV percentage only. DVs show how a product fits into an overall diet by comparing its nutrient content with recommended intakes of those nutrients.

It is important to remember that DVs are not recommended intakes for individuals; no one nutrient standard applies to everyone. They are simply reference points to provide some perspective on daily nutrient needs. DVs are based on a 2000-kcal diet; however, the bottom of the nutrition label also provides the DVs for a 2500-kcal diet. For example, individuals who consume diets supplying more or fewer calories can still use the DVs as a rough guide to ensure that they are getting adequate amounts of vitamin C but not too much saturated fat.

The DVs exist for nutrients for which RDAs already exist (in which case they are known as reference daily intakes [RDIs]) and for which no RDAs exist (in which case they are known as daily reference values [DRVs]) (Table 15-9). However, food labels use only the term "daily value." RDIs provide a large margin of safety; in general, the RDI for a nutrient is greater than the RDA for a specific age group. The term "RDI" replaces the term "U.S. RDAs," used on previous food labels (Table 15-10).

The previously mentioned nutrients must be listed on the food label. Nutrients that a manufacturer or processor may voluntarily disclose include those for which a DV has been established, such as monounsaturated and saturated fat, potassium, vitamins such as thiamin and riboflavin, and minerals such as iodine and magnesium. As new DRIs are developed in various categories (see Figure 15-6), labeling laws will most likely be updated. This issue is currently being explored by a Food and Nutrition Board committee sponsored by the FDA, the USDA, and Health Canada. Implementation of updated DVs is unlikely until 2008 or 2010.

Nutrient Content Claims

Nutrient content terms such as *reduced sodium, fat-free, low-calorie,* and *healthy* must now meet government definitions that apply to all foods (see Box 15-2). For example, *lean* refers to a serving of meat, poultry, seafood, or game meat with less than 10 g of fat, less than 4 g of saturated fat, and less than 95 mg of cholesterol per serving, or per 100 g. *Extra lean* meat or poultry contains less than 5 g of fat, less than 2 g of saturated fat, and the same cholesterol content as *lean* per serving, or per 100 g of product.

Health Claims

Health claims are allowed only on appropriate food products that meet specified standards. The government requires that health claims be worded in ways that are not misleading; for example, the claim cannot imply that the food product itself helps prevent disease. Health claims cannot appear on foods that supply more than 20% of the DV for fat, saturated fat, cholesterol, and sodium.

Manufacturers can use health claims for the following diet-disease relationships on food labels: calcium and a reduced risk of osteoporosis; dietary fat

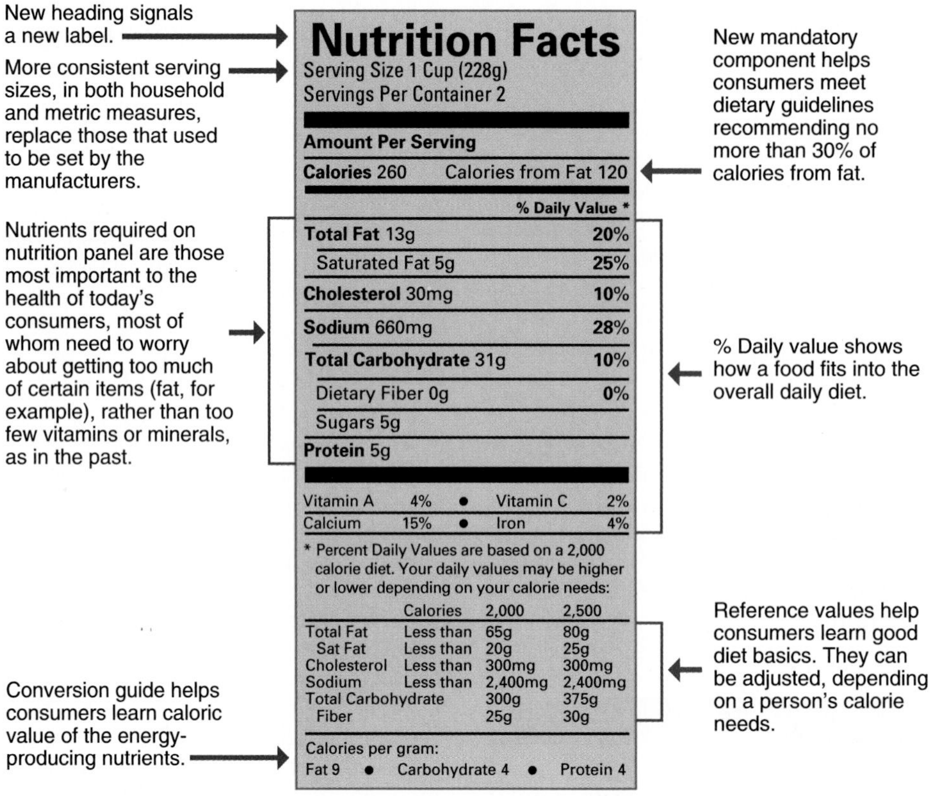

FIGURE 15-6 • Nutrition facts label information. (From Food and Drug Administration, www.fda.gov/ora/inspect_ref/igs/nleatxt.html.)

and an increased risk of cancer; dietary saturated fat and cholesterol and an increased risk of coronary heart disease; fiber-containing grain products, fruits, and vegetables and a reduced risk of cancer; fruits, vegetables, and grain products that contain fiber, particularly soluble fiber (with specific claims allowed for whole oats or psyllium seed husks), and a reduced risk of coronary heart disease; sodium and an increased risk of hypertension; potassium and a decreased risk of hypertension; fruits and vegetables and a reduced risk of cancer; folic acid during pregnancy and a reduced risk of neural tube defects; sugar alcohols and a reduced risk of dental caries; soy protein and a reduced risk of coronary heart disease; and stanol and sterol esters (in vegetable oil spreads and salad dressings) and a reduced risk of coronary heart disease. The following is an example of a health claim for dietary fiber and cancer: "Low-fat diets rich in fiber-containing grain products, fruits, and vegetables may reduce the risk of some types of cancer, a disease associated with many factors."

Box 15-2. Food Label Terminology

Calories

Calorie free: Fewer than 5 calories per serving

Low calorie: 40 calories or less per serving, or per 50 g of the food

Reduced or *fewer calories:* At least 25% fewer calories per serving than reference food

Fat

Fat free: Less than 0.5 g of fat per serving

Saturated fat free: Less than 0.5 g per serving and the level of *trans*-fatty acids does not exceed 1% of total fat

Low fat: 3 g or less per serving, or per 50 g of the food

Low saturated fat: 1 g or less per serving and not more than 15% of calories from saturated fatty acids

Reduced or *less fat:* At least 25% less per serving than reference food

Reduced or *less saturated fat:* At least 25% less per serving than reference food

Cholesterol

Cholesterol free: Less than 2 mg of cholesterol and 2 g or less of saturated fat per serving

Low cholesterol: 20 mg or less and 2 g or less of saturated fat per serving, or per 50 g of the food

Reduced or *less cholesterol:* At least 25% less and 2 g or less of saturated fat per serving than reference food

Sodium

Sodium free: Less than 5 mg per serving

Low sodium: 140 mg or less per serving, or per 50 g of the food

Very low sodium: 35 mg or less per serving, or per 50 g of the food

Reduced or *less sodium:* At least 25% less per serving than reference food

Fiber

High fiber: 5 g or more per serving. (Foods with high-fiber claims must meet the definition for low fat, or the level of total fat must appear next to the high-fiber claim.)

Good source of fiber: 2.5 g to 4.9 g per serving

More or *added fiber:* At least 2.5 g more per serving than reference food

Sugar

Sugar free: Less than 0.5 g per serving

No added sugar, without added sugar, or *no sugar added:*

- No sugars are added during processing or packing, including ingredients that contain sugars (e.g., fruit juices, applesauce, or dried fruit).
- Processing does not increase the sugar content to an amount higher than is naturally present in the ingredients. (A functionally insignificant increase in sugars is acceptable from processes used for purposes other than increasing sugar content.)
- The food that resembles it and for which it substitutes normally contains added sugars.
- If the food doesn't meet the requirements for a low- or reduced-calorie food, the product bears a statement that the food is not low calorie or reduced calorie and directs consumers' attention to the nutrition panel for additional information on sugars and calorie content.

Reduced sugar: At least 25% less sugar per serving than reference food

Healthy

Products using the term "healthy" in the product name or as a claim on the label must contain, per serving, no more than 3 g of fat, 1 g of saturated fat, 480 mg of sodium (350 mg by the end of 1997), or 60 mg of cholesterol. They must also supply at least 10% of the daily value for at least one of six nutrients: vitamins A and C, calcium, iron, protein, and fiber. Raw meat, poultry, and fish can be labeled "healthy" if they contain, per serving, no more than 5 g of fat, 2 g of saturated fat, and 95 mg of cholesterol.

Modified from Stehlin D: A little "lite" reading. In Food and Drug Administration: *Focus on food labeling,* Washington, DC, 1993, Department of Health and Human Services; and Federal Register 59(24219), May 10, 1994; 59(27143), May 25, 1994.

TABLE 15-9 Daily Reference Values

FOOD COMPONENT	DRV*
Fat	65 g
Saturated fatty acids	20 g
Cholesterol	300 mg
Total carbohydrate	300 g
Fiber	25 g
Sodium	2400 mg
Potassium	3500 mg
Protein†	50 g

From Kurtzweil P: "Daily values" encourage healthy diet. In Food and Drug Administration: *Focus on food labeling,* Washington, DC, 1993, Department of Health and Human Services.

*Daily reference value (DRV) based on 2000 cal/day for adults and children older than 4 only.

†DRV for protein does not apply to certain populations; reference daily intake (RDI) for protein has been established for these groups: children 1-4 yr, 16 g; infants younger than 1 yr, 14 g; pregnant females, 60 g; nursing mothers, 65 g.

TABLE 15-10 Reference Daily Intakes

NUTRIENT	AMOUNT	NUTRIENT	AMOUNT
Vitamin A	5000 IU	Folic acid	0.4
Vitamin C	60 mg	Vitamin B_{12}	6 μg
Thiamin	1.5 mg	Phosphorus	1 g
Riboflavin	1.7 mg	Iodine	150 μg
Niacin	20 mg	Magnesium	400 mg
Calcium	1 g	Zinc	15 mg
Iron	18 mg	Copper	2 mg
Vitamin D	400 IU	Biotin	0.3 mg
Vitamin E	30 IU	Pantothenic acid	10 mg
Vitamin B_6	2 mg		

Data from *National Academy of Sciences' 1968 Recommended Dietary Allowances.* In Kurtzweil P: "Daily values" encourage healthy diet. In Food and Drug Administration: *Focus on food labeling,* Washington, DC, 1993, Department of Health and Human Services.

CULTURAL ASPECTS OF DIETARY PLANNING

To plan diets for individuals or groups that are appropriate from a health and nutrition perspective, it is important that the nutritionists and health professionals develop a cultural awareness (i.e., become culturally competent) and use resources that are targeted to the specific group. Numerous population subgroups in the United States have specific cultural, ethnic, or religious beliefs and practices that must be considered. These groups have their own set of dietary practices or beliefs, which are important when considering dietary planning. Their cultural, ethnic, or religious rules can have an effect on access to food, food choices, preparation, and storage methods. For example, the Mediterranean Diet Pyramid has been developed to represent the eating pattern of the Mediterranean culture and to demonstrate a reasonable diet for reducing chronic disease (Figure 15-7) (see *Focus On:* The Mediterranean Diet: Pros and Cons).

Cultural aspects of dietary planning may include vegetarianism, ethnic heritage practices, and religious customs or rules. The following questions may help nutritionists accommodate food habits while meeting dietary recommendations:

- Which individual foods are the major components of the food or mixed dish to be classified?
- To which Food Guide Pyramid groups do the foods seem most related?
- What are the important nutrient sources and their contribution to overall nutrient adequacy?
- How is the food used, and in what quantity is the food consumed?
- Do any food handling, preparation, or storage considerations compromise food safety or limit food choices?

Dietary Patterns of Southeast Asians

During the past few decades, the number of Southeast Asian refugees has increased dramatically worldwide. In the United States, immigrants from Southeast Asia have become the third-largest ethnic group after blacks and Hispanics. Among these immigrants are numerous groups, each with a distinct language, culture, and food habits. From Laos, Cambodia, and Vietnam come the native ethnic groups, as well as Muslims and ethnic Chinese. From Laos, Thailand, and Southern China come the nomadic hill people, the Hmong (Tripp, 1982). Urban and rural immigrants may have lifestyles that differ considerably even when the people come from the same country.

The traditional Hmong (Southeast Asian) diet is high in complex carbohydrates and low in refined carbohydrates, predominantly from rice that is eaten at every meal (American Dietetic Association and American Diabetes Association [ADA/ADA], 1999). The Southeast Asian Hmong diet includes large amounts of fruits, vegetables, and soy products (mostly tofu), and smaller amounts of meat, poultry, and fish.

The Hmong value freshness in their diet. Pork is the preferred meat, and chicken is popular as well. Numerous fruits and vegetables are included in the diet, with substitutions for domestically available products. Foods are boiled, grilled, steamed, and stir fried, and lard is commonly used for frying. The most common spices used in Southeast Asian cuisine are lemon grass, coriander, chili peppers, green onion, basil, cilantro, ginger, and garlic. Lemon and lime juice often are used in place of salad dressings and salt; soy and fish sauces and monosodium glutamate (MSG) are common seasonings.

Lactose intolerance has been reported to be a problem in many Southeast Asians (Anh et al, 1977). However, most children accept milk readily, and many adults are able to drink it in small amounts without any discomfort.

If the immigrants are refugees, they may be at nutritional risk for various reasons. They come from countries with limited food supplies caused by long histories of war and political strife. They may have

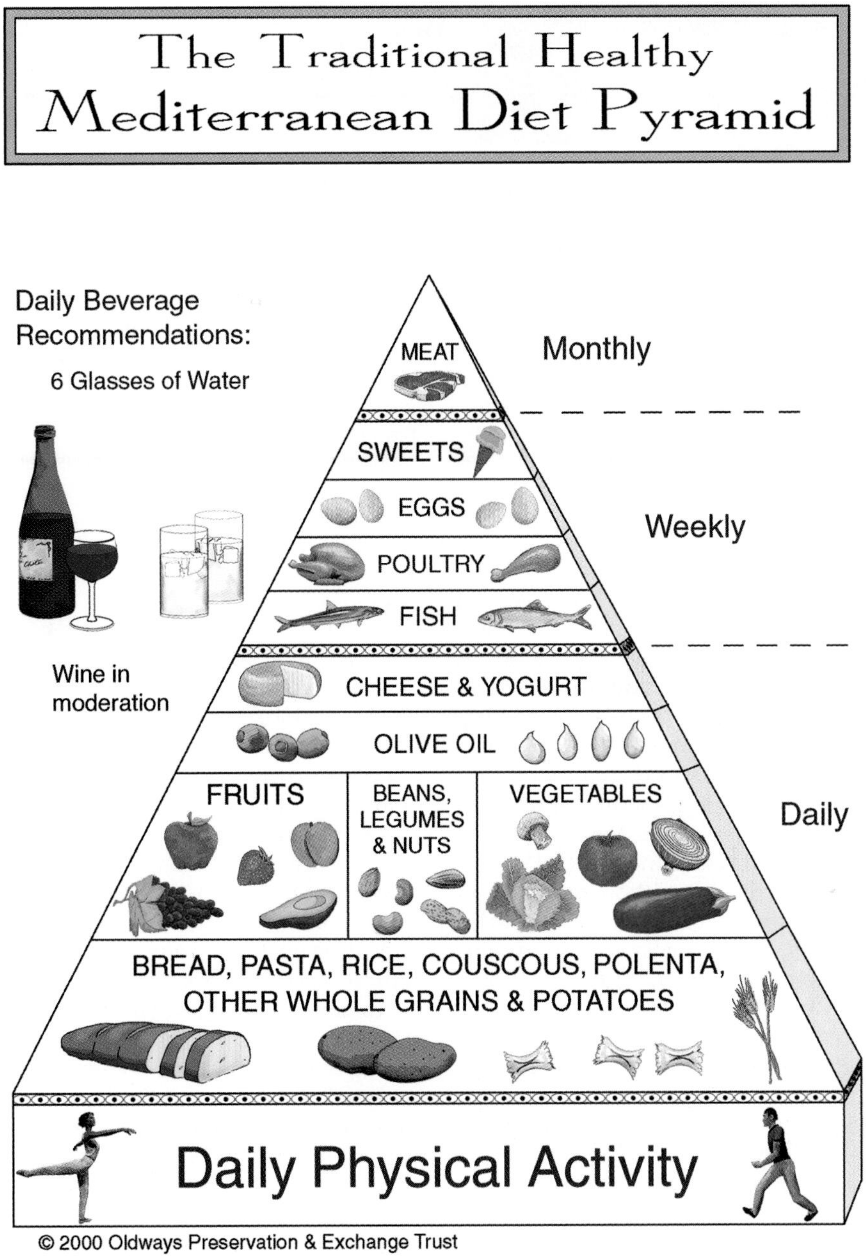

FIGURE 15-7 • The traditional healthy Mediterranean Food Guide Pyramid. (Courtesy Oldways Preservation and Exchange Trust, http://oldwayspt.org.)

spent as many as 5 years in refugee camps with limited food supplies. Poor sanitation has led to a proliferation of parasites and therefore an increase in anemia. General malnutrition, hypertension, dental caries, and iron deficiency anemia have been identified as problems among incoming refugees.

Dietary Patterns of Chinese Americans

In Chinese culture, food is much more than something to eat. What, how often, in what season, and in what order food is eaten are all carefully planned (ADA/ADA, 1998a). Food is thought to play a vital role in preventing and treating diseases and addressing certain health conditions. For example, foods and herbs are frequently boiled in soup or tea to create treatments for various diseases and conditions. A Chinese pagoda food guide was developed and published in 2000.

Most Chinese food in the United States is created for the American palate. The traditional Chinese diet is much richer in carbohydrates (i.e., rice) and has various meats, poultry, and seafood but in smaller quantities than in the American version. The Chinese diet obtains more than 80% of its calories from grains, legumes, and vegetables. The remaining 20% comes

FOCUS ON

The Mediterranean Diet: Pros and Cons

The Mediterranean diet has received attention because of its potential for protecting the body against cardiovascular disease and cancers. The diet is rich in fruits, vegetables, grains, and sources of monounsaturated and polyunsaturated fatty acids (such as omega-3 fatty acids).

A trial involving this diet was conducted as part of the Lyon Diet Heart Study; 605 patients with coronary heart disease were randomly selected to follow either a Mediterranean-type diet or a control diet (Hakim, 1998). Those following the Mediterranean pattern ate less delicatessen food, beef, pork, butter, and cream and more vegetable oils, vegetable oil margarine-type spreads, and olive oil. The control diet was similar to the Step 1 American Heart Association (AHA) Prudent Diet (30% energy from fat). Participants were monitored for 4 years.

Compared with the control diet, the Mediterranean diet provided more fiber, vitamin C, and omega-3 fatty acids and less cholesterol and saturated fatty acids. Risk ratios were lower for cancers, cardiac death, and overall mortality rates. More use of these strategies in dietary planning may be beneficial in the U.S. populations when combined with adequate daily physical activity.

from animal protein, fruits, and fats. Most typical Chinese meals include 2- to 3-cup bowls of rice. Northern Chinese cuisine may include more noodles, dumplings, and steamed buns made from wheat flour. Stir frying, deep-fat frying, braising, roasting, smoking, and steaming are common food preparation techniques. When foods are fried, peanut or corn oil is used rather than lard, which is more common in Southeast Asian cuisine.

Pork is the staple meat in the Chinese diet. Poultry and eggs are also favored, in addition to fish and shellfish. When animal products are included in traditional Chinese dishes, almost every part of an animal may be consumed—the liver, kidneys, lungs, stomach, intestines, marrow, brains, feet, and tail. Other protein sources include soybeans, which may be sprouted, dried, or fermented as tofu. Dairy products are rarely consumed.

Fruits and vegetable are abundant in Chinese cuisine. Vegetables are rarely eaten raw and are most often stir-fried, steamed, or added to soups just before serving, allowing for maximum retention of nutrients.

The beverage of choice for most Chinese is clear, hot green tea. Older Chinese rarely drink cold beverages. Chinese children and adults also drink a wide range of fermented beverages and juices.

Although Chinese meals are eaten communally, each region has its own set of foods, ingredients, and cooking methods. Northern cuisine is characterized by garlic, leeks, and scallions, with noodles rather than rice. In the Western region, Hunan cuisine includes liberal use of chili peppers and hot pepper sauces. Hunan dishes are spicier and oilier than dishes in other regions. Southern Chinese cuisine, or Cantonese, includes primarily steamed and stir-fried dishes with a lot of fish and shellfish. As Chinese adopt traditional American foods, their diet begins to include more sweets such as cookies, chocolate, soft drinks, and snacks.

Dietary Patterns of Hispanics

Hispanics are the second-largest and most rapidly growing ethnic group in the United States (ADA/ADA, 1998b). Forecasts indicate that Hispanics will outnumber blacks early in the twenty-first century. Mexican Americans are the largest subgroup of Hispanics, and older Mexican Americans are the fastest growing group of older Americans.

Hispanic cuisine and Mexican and Latin American foods are based on the concept of foods having "hot" and "cold" properties and on beliefs about food's contribution to health and well-being. "Cold" foods include most vegetables, tropical fruits, dairy products, and inexpensive cuts of meat. "Hot" foods include chili peppers, garlic, onions, most grains, expensive cuts of meat, oils, and alcohol. For example, pregnancy is considered a "hot" condition, so "hot" foods upset the stomach. Thus some Hispanics may not eat chili peppers while pregnant for cultural reasons, not because of safety issues for the mother or developing fetus.

Depending on the part of the world, the main dishes of Hispanic diets may include meat (pork, veal, sausage), poultry, or fish. Rice and tortillas are mainstays of the diet, as are fruits and vegetables. Milk and cheese are consumed when available but are uncommon in some parts of the world. Fried foods are often eaten and may need to be limited for those with diabetes or who are obese.

Hispanic cuisine often incorporates chili peppers, which are a rich source of vitamin C. Chili peppers can range from mild to very hot and from small to very large. As with Chinese cuisine, Hispanic and Latin American foods are often modified for the American palate.

Dietary Patterns of Native Americans

Native Americans (American Indians and Alaska Natives) comprise more than 500 federally recognized groups who live on federal Indian reservations and in small rural communities (ADA/ADA, 1991, 1993). In Native American culture, food has great religious and social significance. It is an integral part of many celebrations, including powwows and other ceremonies. Food is more of a social or religious obligation than it is simple nourishment. Likewise, communication about food is linked closely to cultural practices.

Common foods may be prepared and used in different ways in various regions and tribal organizations. Fry bread (fried dough) is a central part of American Indian cuisine and is eaten with foods such as stews, soups, and bean dishes. Fried foods are generally prepared with lard.

Corn is the carbohydrate staple of the American Indian diet, in addition to protein-rich dried beans. Fruits and vegetables were traditionally gathered from the wild but are also cultivated on small farms. Sheep, or mutton, and goat are more common than pork or beef. Other animal food sources include game and some poultry.

The Alaska Native diet is changing and consists of a mixture of traditional foods and American prepared and processed foods. The diet is high in protein and fat and is based on meat and fish more than plant foods. Meat, fish, sea mammals, and game are staple foods. Seaweed, willow leaves, and sour dock are some of the few edible plants consumed.

Nutrition professionals who work with Native Americans will find that they have a higher incidence of obesity and diabetes mellitus than the general American population. Nutrition professionals should merge cultural sensitivity with options to balance diet and health issues.

Dietary Restrictions and Patterns of Religious Groups

Jewish Food Customs, Dietary Laws, and Holidays

The Jewish dietary laws are biblical ordinances that are interpreted as rules regarding food (ADA/ADA, 1989; Kaufman, 1957). The rules pertain chiefly to the selection, slaughter, and preparation of meat. Animals allowed to be eaten are quadrupeds that have cloven hooves and chew cud, specifically cattle, sheep, goats, and deer; they are considered "clean." Permissible fowl are chicken, turkey, goose, pheasant, and duck. All animals and fowl must be inspected for disease and killed by a ritual slaughterer according to specific rules. Only the forequarter of the quadruped may be used, except when the hip sinew of the thigh vein can be removed, in which case the hindquarter is also allowed.

Blood is forbidden as food because blood is synonymous with life. The traditional process of *koshering* meat and poultry removes all blood before cooking. Koshering involves soaking meat in water, salting it thoroughly, allowing it to drain, and then washing it three times to remove the salt.

Meat and milk cannot be combined in the same meal. Milk or milk-related foods can be eaten immediately before a meal but not with a meal. After eating meat, Jewish people must wait 6 hours before consuming milk products. Because of the rules related to separating meat and milk products, those in traditional orthodox Jewish homes must keep two completely separate sets of dishes, silver, and cooking equipment—one for meat meals and one for dairy meals. Only fish with fins and scales can be eaten, so no shellfish or eel is permissible. Fish can be eaten with dairy or meats. Eggs can also be combined with meat or milk. However, an egg yolk containing a drop of blood cannot be eaten because the blood is considered a chick embryo, or a sign of a new life.

Fruits, vegetables, cereal products, and all of the other foods that generally comprise a diet can be consumed with no restrictions. Bakery products and prepared food mixtures must be produced under acceptable kosher standards.

The most important of the Jewish holy days is the Sabbath, or day of rest, which is observed on Saturdays. The Friday night meal is the best of the week and usually includes fish and chicken. No food is allowed to be cooked or heated on Saturday; thus all food eaten on the Sabbath is cooked on Friday and either kept warm in the oven or eaten cold.

The festival holidays are Rosh Hashanah—the New Year—in September; Succoth, the fall harvest holiday; Chanukah—the Feast of Lights—in midwinter; and Purim, a joyous holiday in spring. Each holiday has certain associated food delicacies.

Yom Kippur, or the Day of Atonement, occurs 10 days after Rosh Hashanah and is a day of fasting. Jewish people abstain from all food and drink, including water, from sundown on the eve of the holiday to sundown on the holiday. Pregnant females and those who are ill do not fast.

Passover, a spring commemorative festival lasting 8 days, includes special dietary requirements. During the Passover holiday, leavened bread or cake is prohibited. Matzo, an unleavened bread, is eaten, and all cake and baked products are made of flour from ground-up matzo or potato starch and leavened only with beaten egg whites. No salt is allowed in traditional Passover matzo. Variations of fried matzo or matzo-meal pancakes are prepared with generous amounts of fat.

Muslim Food Customs, Dietary Laws, and Holidays

Islam promotes the concept of eating to live rather than living to eat (ADA/ADA, 1996). Prayers are offered before food is eaten. Muslims are advised not to eat until they are full and always to share food. Although many foods are allowed, certain codes must be observed and some dietary restrictions exist.

The flesh of animals slaughtered in a humane way as outlined by Islamic law is considered *halal* (according to Islamic law). All meat to be consumed as food must be slaughtered with a ritual letting of blood while speaking the name of God. The slaughter can be done by anyone—no special person is designated for this function. Muslims eat kosher meat products because they know that they have been slaughtered properly. Although all foods not specifically prohibited are allowed to be eaten, certain foods are recommended such as milk, dates, meat, seafood, sweets, honey, and vegetable oil, especially olive oil.

If an animal is slaughtered improperly, the meat becomes *haram,* or forbidden. Pork and pork products such as gelatin are prohibited, as are alcoholic beverages and alcohol products (e.g., vanilla extract or other alcohol-based food or flavoring extracts).

Muslims fast every year during the month of Ramadan, which occurs during the ninth month of the Islamic lunar calendar. Muslims fast completely from dawn to sunset and eat only twice a day—before dawn and after sunset. The end of Ramadan is marked by the Feast of Breaking the Fast *(Eid-ul-Fitr).*

Muslims are also encouraged to fast 3 days of every month. Menstruating, pregnant, or lactating females are not required to fast but must make up the fasting days at some other time.

Vegetarianism

Vegetarian diets of various descriptions have enjoyed increased popularity in recent years. Those who choose them may be motivated by philosophical, religious, or ecologic concerns or a desire to have a healthier lifestyle.

Considerable evidence attests to the health benefits of a vegetarian diet. Epidemiologic data, particularly from studies of Seventh-Day Adventists, indicate that the diet results in lower rates of type 2 diabetes, breast and colon cancer, and cardiovascular and gallbladder disease. However, data are not sufficient to prove that an omnivorous diet based on the recommended guidelines and combined with a healthy lifestyle is not equally beneficial (National Institute of Nutrition, 1990).

Of the 8 to 10 million people in the United States who profess to be vegetarians, most eliminate "red" meats but eat fish, poultry, and dairy products (Tufts University, 1988). A *lactovegetarian* does not eat meat, fish, poultry, or eggs but does consume milk, cheese, and other dairy products; a *lactoovovegetarian* also consumes eggs. A true vegetarian, or *vegan,* does not eat any food of animal origin. The vegan diet is the only vegetarian diet that incorporates any real risk of obtaining inadequate nutrition, but this risk can be avoided by careful planning.

Vegetarian diets tend to be lower in iron than omnivorous diets, although the non-heme iron in fruits, vegetables, and unrefined cereals is usually accompanied either in the food or in the meal by large amounts of ascorbic acid that aids in iron assimilation. Vegetarians do not have a greater risk of iron deficiency than those who are not vegetarians (American Dietetic Association, 1997).

Vegetarians who consume no dairy products may have low calcium intakes, and vitamin D intakes may be inadequate among those in northern latitudes. The calcium in some vegetables is inactivated by the presence of oxalates. Phytates in unrefined cereals also can inactivate calcium; however, this is not a problem for Western vegetarians, whose diets tend to be based more on fruits and vegetables than on the unrefined cereals of Middle Eastern cultures.

Long-term vegans may develop megaloblastic anemia because of a deficiency of vitamin B_{12}, a vitamin found only in foods of animal origin. This deficiency is less of a problem in areas where sanitation is poor because contaminating bacteria can serve as a source of this vitamin. The high levels of folate in vegan diets may mask the neurologic damage of a vitamin B_{12} deficiency. Vegans should have a reliable source of vitamin B_{12}, such as fortified breakfast cereals or soy beverages, or take a supplement (American Dietetic Association, 1997).

Although most vegetarians meet or exceed the RDA for protein, their diets tend to be lower in protein than those of omnivores. This lower intake may help vegetarians retain more calcium from their diets. Furthermore, lower protein intake usually results in lower dietary fat because many high-protein animal products are also rich in fat (American Dietetic Association, 1997).

Well-planned vegetarian diets are safe for infants, children, and adolescents and can meet all of their nutritional requirements for growth. They are also adequate for pregnant and lactating females. The key is that the diets be well planned. Vegetarians should pay special attention to ensure they get adequate calcium, iron, zinc, and vitamins B_{12} and D. Calculated combinations of complementary protein sources do not seem to be necessary (American Dietetic Association, 1997). Although vegetarians tend to eat less protein than those who are not vegetarians, the total intake still exceeds the RDA in the United States (Auld, 1994). Protein sources should be reasonably varied.

SUMMARY

Dietetics and health professionals are essential translators of food, nutrition, and health information into dietary choices and patterns for groups or individuals. An understanding of nutrient needs and requirements, dietary guidelines, food guides, and ethnic and religious practices is an important basis for counseling patients or providing group education. Also important are the educational level, lifestyle patterns, and socioeconomic status of individuals or groups. With a knowledge of dietary planning, nutrient needs, and food and nutrient information, as well as developed skills in counseling for change (see Chapter 22), clients and counselors can work together to develop diets that promote health.

Clinical Scenario 1

Marty is a 45-year-old Jewish man who emigrated from Israel to the United States 3 years ago. He follows a strict kosher diet. In addition, he does not drink milk but does consume other dairy products. He has a body mass index (BMI) of 32 and a family history of heart disease.

1. What type of dietary guidance would you offer Marty?
2. What type of dietary plan following strict kosher protocols would meet his daily dietary needs and promote weight loss?
3. What suggestions would you offer him about dietary choices for a healthy heart?
4. Which special steps should Marty to take meet calcium requirements without using supplements?
5. How can food labeling information be used to help Marty meet his weight loss and nutrient goals and incorporate his religious dietary concerns?

Clinical Scenario 2

Nan is a 20-year-old college student who has decided to become a vegetarian for nonreligious reasons. She does not eat red meat, chicken, or fish and also avoids dairy products. She is 5 ft, 2 inches and weighs 95 lb. Her health is stable, but she does have iron deficiency anemia and her blood pressure is 100/75 mm Hg.

1. What type of dietary guidance would you offer Nan?
2. Nan is at risk for developing deficiencies of which nutrients?
3. Plan a 3-day menu for Nan that excludes the foods she does not eat but provides adequate amounts of the key nutrients she needs.
4. What other dietary health-related advice would you give Nan?

Relevant Web Sites

American Dietetic Association
www.eatright.org
Center for Nutrition Policy and Promotion, USDA
www.usda.gov/cnpp/
Centers for Disease Control, NHANES Survey
www.cdc.gov/nchs/nhanes.htm
Ethnic and Cultural Food Guides
www.nal.usda.gov/fnic/etext/000023.html#xtocid2381818
Food and Drug Administration, Center for Food Safety and Applied Nutrition
www.cfsan.fda.gov
Food and Nutrition Board, Institute of Medicine, National Academy of Sciences
www.iom.edu/IOM/IOMHome.nsf/Pages/Food+and+Nutrition+Board
Food and Nutrition Information Center, National Agricultural Library, USDA
www.nal.usda.gov/fnic/
Food Guide Pyramid
www.usda.gov/cnpp/pyramid.htm
Food Guides for Ethnic and Cultural Groups, and Special Audiences
www.nal.usda.gov/fnic/etext/000023.html#xtocid2381818
Health Canada
www.hc-sc.gc.ca/english/
Healthy Eating Index
www.usda.gov/cnpp/usda_healthy_eating_index.htm
International Food Information Council
http://ific.org
Kids' Food Guide Pyramid
www.usda.gov/cnpp/KidsPyra/index.htm
National Center for Health Statistics
www.cdc.gov/nchs/nhanes.htm
Nutrition.gov (U.S. government nutrition site)
www.nutrition.gov
U.S. Department of Agriculture
www.usda.gov

Cited References

American Dietetic Association: Position of the American Dietetic Association: vegetarian diets, *J Am Diet Assoc* 97:1317, 1997.

American Dietetic Association: Position of the American Dietetic Association: total diet approach to communicating food and nutrition information, *J Am Diet Assoc* 102:100, 2002.

American Dietetic Association and American Diabetes Association: *Jewish food practices, customs, and holidays,* Ethnic and Regional Food Practices Series, Chicago, 1989, American Dietetic Association.

American Dietetic Association and American Diabetes Association: *Navajo food practices, customs, and holidays,* Ethnic and Regional Food Practices Series, Chicago, 1991, American Dietetic Association.

American Dietetic Association and American Diabetes Association: *Alaska Native food practices, customs, and holidays,* Ethnic and Regional Food Practices Series, Chicago, 1993, American Dietetic Association.

American Dietetic Association and American Diabetes Association: *Indian and Pakistani food practices, customs, and holidays,* Ethnic and Regional Food Practices Series, Chicago, 1996, American Dietetic Association.

American Dietetic Association and American Diabetes Association: *Chinese American food practices, customs, and holidays,* Ethnic and Regional Food Practices Series, Chicago, 1998a, American Dietetic Association.

American Dietetic Association and American Diabetes Association: *Mexican American food practices, customs, and holidays,* Ethnic and Regional Food Practices Series, Chicago, 1998b, American Dietetic Association.

American Dietetic Association and the American Diabetes Association: *Hmong American food practices, customs, and holidays,* Ethnic and Regional Food Practices Series, Chicago, 1999, American Dietetic Association.

Anderson RN: Deaths: leading causes for 1999, *Natl Vital Stat Rep* 49(11):8, 2001.

Anh NT et al: Lactose malabsorption in adult Vietnamese, *Am J Clin Nutr* 5:676, 1977.

Auld E: *Getting to the roots of a vegetarian diet: food insight,* Washington, DC, 1994, International Food Information Council Foundation.

Bowman SA et al: *The Healthy Eating Index: 1994-1996,* Publication CNPP-5, Center for Nutrition Policy and Promotion, U.S. Department of Agriculture, Washington, DC, 1998, U.S. Government Printing Office.

Center for Nutrition Policy and Promotion: *Food Guide Pyramid for young children 2 to 6 years old,* U.S. Department of Agriculture, Washington, DC, 1999, Center for Nutrition Policy and Promotion.

Dietary Guidelines Alliance: *Reaching consumers with meaningful health messages: a handbook for nutrition and food communicators,* Washington, DC, 1996, International Food Information Council.

Federation of American Societies for Experimental Biology, Life Sciences Research Office: *Third report on nutrition monitoring in the United States,* Prepared for the Interagency Board for Nutrition Monitoring and Related Research, Washington, DC, 1995, U.S. Government Printing Office.

Food and Drug Administration: *Focus on food labeling,* Special Issue of *FDA Consumer Magazine,* Department of Health and Human Services Pub No (FDA) 93-2262, Washington, DC, May 1993, U.S. Government Printing Office.

Food and Nutrition Board, Committee on Diet and Health, National Research Council: *Diet and health: implications for reducing chronic disease risk,* Washington, DC, 1989 National Academy Press.

Hakim I: Mediterranean diets and cancer prevention, *Arch Intern Med* 158(11):1169, 1998.

Institute of Medicine: *How should the recommended dietary allowances be revised?* Report of the Food and Nutrition Board, 1994, National Academy Press.

Institute of Medicine, Food and Nutrition Board: *Dietary reference intakes for calcium, phosphorus, magnesium, vitamin D, and fluoride,* Washington, DC, 1997, National Academy Press.

Institute of Medicine, Food and Nutrition Board: *Dietary reference intakes for thiamin, riboflavin, niacin, vitamin B_6, folate, vitamin B_{12}, pantothenic acid, biotin, and choline,* Washington, DC, 1998, National Academy Press.

Institute of Medicine, Food and Nutrition Board: *Dietary Reference intakes for vitamin C, vitamin E, selenium, and carotenoids,* Washington, DC, 2000, National Academy Press.

Institute of Medicine, Food and Nutrition Board: *Dietary reference intakes: applications in dietary assessment,* Washington, DC, 2001, National Academy Press.

Institute of Medicine, Food and Nutrition Board: *Dietary reference intakes for energy, carbohydrate, fiber, fat, fatty acids, cholesterol, protein, and amino acids,* Washington, DC, 2002a, National Academy Press.

Institute of Medicine, Food and Nutrition Board: *Dietary reference intakes for vitamin A, vitamin K, arsenic, boron, chromium, copper, iodine, iron, manganese, molybdenum, nickel, silicon, vanadium, and zinc,* Washington, DC, 2002b, National Academy Press.

Kaufman M: Adapting therapeutic diets to Jewish food customs, *Am J Clin Nutr* 5:676, 1957.

Minister of National Health and Welfare: *Canada's food guide to healthy eating,* Catalogue No H39-253/1992E, Ottawa, Canada, 1992, Health Canada.

National Institute of Nutrition (Canada): Risks and benefits of vegetarian diets, *Nutr Today* 25(2):27, 1990.

National Nutrition Monitoring and Related Research Program: *Third report on nutrition monitoring in the United States: executive summary,* Life Sciences Research Office, Federation of American Societies for Experimental Biology, Washington, DC, 1995, U.S. Government Printing Office.

Public Health Service: *The Surgeon General's report on nutrition and health: summary and recommendations,* Department of Health and Human Services, Public Health Service, Pub No 88-50211, Washington, DC, 1988, U.S. Government Printing Office.

Public Health Service; Department of Health and Human Services; National Heart, Lung, and Blood Institute: *National Cholesterol Education Program (NCEP),* Second Report of the Expert Panel on Detection, Evaluation, and Treatment of High Blood Cholesterol in Adults, National Institutes of Health Pub No 93-3095, Washington, DC, 1993, U.S. Government Printing Office.

Public Health Service, Department of Health and Human Services, National Institutes of Health: *Diet, nutrition, and cancer prevention: a guide to food choices,* rev ed, Pub No 87-2878, Washington, DC, 1987, U.S. Government Printing Office.

Tripp RR: *World refugee survey, 1982,* New York, 1982, U.S. Committee for Refugees.

Tufts University: Lessons we can learn from vegetarians, *Tufts Univ Nutr Lett* 6(5):3, 1988.

U.S. Department of Agriculture: *The Food Guide Pyramid,* Home and Garden Bulletin No 252, Washington, DC, 1992, U.S. Government Printing Office.

U.S. Department of Agriculture: *Putting the guidelines into practice: How much are you eating?* Home and Garden Bull No 267-1, Washington, DC, 2002, U.S. Government Printing Office.

U.S. Department of Agriculture and U.S. Department of Health and Human Services: *Nutrition and your health: dietary guidelines for Americans,* ed 5, USDA Home and Garden Bulletin No 232. Washington, DC, 2000, U.S. Government Printing Office.

U.S. Senate Select Committee on Nutrition and Human Needs: *Dietary goals for the United States,* ed 2, Washington, DC, U.S. Senate, 95th Congress—1st session, December 1977.

White House: *White House conference on food, nutrition, and health,* Final report, Washington, DC, 1970, U.S. Government Printing Office.

Additional References

Anderson SL: A look at the Japanese dietary guidelines, *J Am Diet Assoc* 90:1527, 1990.

Barr SI et al: Interpreting and using the dietary references intakes in dietary assessment of individuals and groups, *J Am Diet Assoc* 102:780, 2002.

Chang KC, ed: *Food in Chinese culture,* New Haven, Conn, 1977, Yale University Press.

Communications/Implementation Committee, Minister of National Health and Welfare: *Action toward healthy eating: Canada's guidelines for healthy eating and recommended strategies for implementation,* Catalogue No H39-166/1990E, Ottawa, Canada, 1990, Minister of Supply and Services.

Duyff R et al: Food behavior and related factors of Puerto Rican American teenagers, *J Nutr Educ* 7:99, 1975.

Fanelli-Kuczmarski M, Woteki CE: Monitoring the nutritional status of the Hispanic population: selected findings for Mexican Americans, Cubans, and Puerto Ricans, *Nutr Today* 25(3):6, 1990.

Food and Drug Administration: *The new food label summaries,* Washington, DC, January 6, 1993, Department of Health and Human Services.

Food Safety Information Service: *Nutrition labeling of meat and poultry products, FSIS Backgrounder,* Washington, DC, 1993, U.S. Department of Agriculture.

Lenfant C, Ernst N: Daily dietary fat and total food energy intakes—Third National Health and Nutrition Examination Survey, Phase 1, 1988-91, *MMWR* 43:116, 1994.

Monsen ER: New dietary reference intakes proposed to replace the recommended dietary allowances, *J Am Diet Assoc* 96:754, 1996.

Pennington JAT: *Bowes and Church's food values of portions commonly used,* ed 17, Philadelphia, 1998, Lippincott Williams & Wilkins.

Scientific Review Committee and Communications/Implementation Committee, Minister of National Health and Welfare: *Nutrition recommendations: a call for action,* Catalogue No. H39-162, 1990E, Ottawa, Canada, 1990, Minister of Supply and Services.

U.S. Department of Agriculture: *Report of the Dietary Guidelines Advisory Committee on the dietary guidelines for Americans,* 2000, Agricultural Research Service, http://www.usda.gov/cnpp/Pubs/DG2000/FullReport.pdf.

Welsh S et al: Development of the Food Guide Pyramid, *Nutr Today* 27(6):12, 1992.

Wiecha JM et al: Differences in dietary patterns of Vietnamese, white, African-American, and Hispanic adolescents in Worcester, Mass, *J Am Diet Assoc* 101:248, 2001.

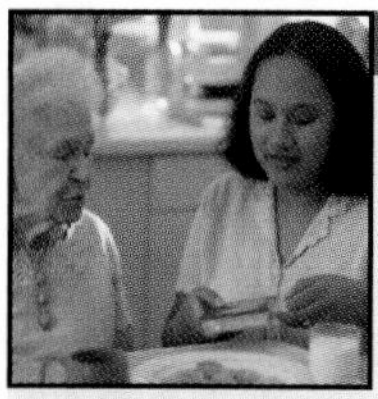

CHAPTER 16

Introduction to Nutritional Genomics

RUTH M. DEBUSK, PhD, RD

CHAPTER OUTLINE

- The Human Genome Project
- Genetic Fundamentals
- Genetics and Nutrition Therapy

KEY TERMS

alleles–variants of a gene; refers to the different variations in deoxyribonucleic acid (DNA) sequence that a gene may have within a population

autosomal dominant–refers to inheritance resulting when an allele on an autosome gives rise to a phenotype that is essentially the same whether a single copy of the allele is present *(heterozygous)* or two copies are present *(homozygous)*

autosomal recessive–refers to inheritance resulting when a mutant allele carried on an autosome gives rise to a phenotype only when two copies of that allele are present; when only a single copy is present, the phenotype of the dominant normal allele masks that of the recessive mutant allele

autosome–one of the 22 pairs of non-sex (X or Y) chromosomes

carriers–heterozygous individuals; in humans, usually refers to those who have a single copy of a disease-causing gene but may not overtly express the disease

chromosomes–subunits of deoxyribonucleic acid (DNA) that are composed of DNA and protein; a means of packaging the large amount of DNA into the nucleus of a cell; humans have 23 pairs of chromosomes, and each gene has an address at a discrete location on a specific chromosome

codon–a set of three nucleotides in deoxyribonucleic acid (DNA) arranged side-by-side; specifies an amino acid in the gene's protein product or a signal to start or stop transcription

deletion–loss of genetic material; may be loss of a portion of a chromosome or a single nucleotide

deoxyribonucleic acid (DNA)–the genetic material for humans and most organisms; consists of two strands of nucleotide building blocks arranged side by side on each strand; a linear arrangement of nucleotides that encodes the information needed to create and operate a living organism

ELSI–ethical, legal, and social implications of genetic research; initiative of the Human Genome Project to ensure that genetic information is used positively and fairly

exons–the parts of a gene that code for the amino acids in the gene's protein product

genes–segments of DNA that code for a protein

genetic code–the combination of codons that specify the amino acids used to synthesize proteins

genetic engineering–the alteration of genetic material, typically by recombinant deoxyribonucleic acid (DNA) technology

genetics–the science of inheritance

genome–the total of an organism's genetic information

genomics–a broader concept of genetics that includes not only genes, their proteins, and associations with diseases, but also the interaction among susceptibility factors and environmental factors and the potential for multiple genes, proteins, and environmental factors to influence health and well-being

genotype–an individual's unique genetic makeup

heterozygous–two different alleles at a single genetic locus; a carrier of these two different alleles is a *heterozygote*

homology–refers to deoxyribonucleic acid (DNA) or amino acid sequences that are highly similar to each other

homozygous–two identical alleles at a single genetic locus; a carrier of these two identical alleles is called a *homozygote*

Human Genome Project–a multinational collaborative effort to completely identify the sequence of nucleotides in the deoxyribonucleic acid (DNA) of human beings and several other organisms, associate this sequence with genes and their protein products, and identify the function of these proteins

intervening sequences–the deoxyribonucleic acid (DNA) sequences between two genes

introns–deoxyribonucleic acid (DNA) sequences between two exons; transcribed into messenger ribonucleic acid (mRNA) and then removed before translation

karyotype–a visual display of chromosomes arranged in pairs from largest to smallest, with the X and Y chromosomes at the end

ligands–molecules or cofactors that bind to another chemical entity to form a larger complex; often refers to molecules binding to their specific receptor or transcription factors binding to their activator

linked genes–genes physically close enough to each other on a chromosome that the frequency of recombination between them is less than 50%; such genes tend to be inherited together most of the time

Mendelian inheritance–the predictable inheritance pattern of a single gene trait; named after Gregor Mendel, who first described the rules of inheritance for single gene traits

messenger RNA (mRNA)–a class of ribonucleic acid (RNA) in which the formation in double-stranded DNA is converted into a single-stranded RNA molecule composed of nucleotides containing the sugar ribose, the mineral phosphorus, and one of four nitrogen-containing bases (adenine, cytosine, guanine or uracil); serves as an intermediary between deoxyribonucleic acid (DNA) and the amino acid sequence of the protein being synthesized

mitochondrial inheritance–the inheritance pattern of a trait carried on mitochondrial deoxyribonucleic acid, which is typically passed from mother to child

model system–an experimental system in which phenomena can be studied, often in great detail, and the results extrapolated to other organisms; for example, the transgenic mouse model system that is often used to study gene-disease associations

mutation–a change in the deoxyribonucleic acid (DNA) sequence, which may change the protein whose synthesis is directed by the information in the DNA sequence; if the change alters the function of the protein significantly, a disease can result

nucleotide–the building block of deoxyribonucleic acid (DNA) and ribonucleic acid (RNA); consists of the sugar ribose, the mineral phosphorus, and a nitrogen-containing purine or pyrimidine base; in DNA the base is *adenine, cytosine, guanine,* or *thymine,* and in RNA it is *adenine, cytosine, guanine,* or *uracil*

nutritional genomics–the study of the consequences of the interaction of nutrients and food components with the genetic material; also called *nutrigenomics*

pedigree–a visual method of tracing the inheritance of traits through multiple generations of a family

penetrance–the proportion of a population that has a disease-causing genotype and expresses the associated phenotype; when that proportion is less than 100%, the gene is said to have *reduced penetrance*

pharmacogenomics–the study of the way genetic variations in key drug-metabolizing enzymes affect drug efficacy and safety; the genetic uniqueness of each individual confers different drug-metabolizing abilities, so the same dosage of a drug can be toxic for one person, effective for another, and ineffective for another

phenotype–the measurable expression of a gene; observed through the physical characteristics of an individual

polymorphism–results from a variant of a gene that occurs in greater than 1% of a population

promoter–the deoxyribonucleic acid (DNA) sequence on the 5′ end ("upstream") of the gene to which ribonucleic acid (RNA) polymerase binds to transcribe the DNA into messenger RNA (mRNA)

proteins–molecules composed of amino acids; carry out the work of the living cell by serving as enzymes, receptors, transporters, hormones, antibodies, or communicators

proteomics–the study of the structure and function of proteins

recombinant DNA–hybrid deoxyribonucleic acid (DNA) made from two different sources by cutting out a segment of DNA from one organism and inserting it into the DNA of another; recombinant DNA technology is also called *genetic engineering*

response elements–deoxyribonucleic acid (DNA) sequences in the regulatory region of a gene to which transcription factors bind and control the expression of the gene

restriction endonucleases (restriction enzymes)–bacterial enzymes that recognize a specific deoxyribonucleic acid (DNA) sequence and cut the DNA at that location; bacteria contain thousands of these enzymes, and each has a particular DNA recognition site; useful as "molecular scissors" for precisely excising a sequence of DNA that can then be transferred into the DNA of another organism

sex chromosomes–the X and Y chromosomes in humans

sex-linked disorders–diseases caused by a mutation on the X or Y chromosome in humans

single nucleotide polymorphism (SNP)–results from single-base-change variants of a gene that occur in greater than 1% of the population

spectral karyotyping–the use of fluorescent probes and computer software to "paint" each pair of chromosomes with a unique color; helps scientists pair the chromosomes to form a *karyotype*

transcription–the process of transferring information encoded in deoxyribonucleic acid (DNA) to ribonucleic acid (RNA); messenger RNA (mRNA) serves as an intermediary between DNA and the amino acid sequence of the protein to be synthesized

transcription factors–proteins that bind to deoxyribonucleic acid (DNA) to increase or decrease transcription of DNA into messenger ribonucleic acid (mRNA); many nutrients bind to transcription factors and thus influence gene expression

KEY TERMS—Continued

translation–the process of transferring information encoded in the messenger ribonucleic acid (mRNA) intermediate into the amino acid sequence of a protein

xenobiotics–chemicals that are foreign to the body

X-linked dominant–refers to an inheritance pattern resulting from an allele carried on the X chromosome; gives rise to the phenotype when only a single copy of that allele is present

X-linked recessive–refers to an inheritance pattern resulting from an allele carried on the X chromosome; only gives rise to the phenotype in males who have a single copy or females who have two copies of the allele

Y-linked inheritance–refers to an inheritance pattern resulting from an allele carried on the Y chromosome; expressed only in males

Nutrition professionals have long been intrigued and more than a little puzzled by the fact that one person can be lean and have an identical twin who is overweight, that the Pima Indians living in northern Mexico are lean even though their genetic counterparts in Arizona are obese and have a high incidence of type 2 diabetes, and that a low-fat diet can reduce blood lipid levels in many people, but not in everyone. What has become obvious but is still not well understood is that although people's genetic makeup sets the stage for their susceptibilities to various diseases, environmental factors such as nutrition and other lifestyle choices determine who among the susceptible actually develop diseases. The role of nutrients and other biologically active food components on gene expression is the focus of an exciting emerging field in nutrition called nutritional genomics.

Genetic research is rapidly clarifying the association between genes and physiologic function. Mistakes in the genes are being correlated with dysfunction and disease. This evolving appreciation for the central role of genetics in health and disease is having a significant impact on the way medicine is practiced. As the details of the connections among genes, protein products, and disease unfold, the focus of the health care system is shifting. During the past 50 years, the focus has been on treating manifest disease, and physicians have had increasingly sophisticated drugs and technology available with which to meet this challenge. However, with the understanding that disease is genetically based but environmentally influenced, the focus is on targeted intervention and prevention based on an understanding of the involved genes and environmental factors and the metabolic consequences of their interaction.

The immediate applications of this changed focus involve the medical and pharmaceutical aspects of health care, but ultimately nutrition therapy is expected to figure prominently as a cornerstone of preventive health care. Genetic research will help clarify the pathogenesis of disease, which includes the influence of nutrient and nonnutrient food components. From these advances will come diagnostic tests and susceptibility profiles that, coupled with genetic testing and family history analysis, will allow health care professionals to predict those at risk for particular disorders. Nutrition can mitigate the harmful effects of many genetic errors that result in disease, from supplying missing metabolites to altering gene expression. Therefore nutrition therapy will become an increasingly important therapeutic tool for maximizing health and minimizing the risk of disease in susceptible individuals.

Nutrition professionals need to be familiar with the genetic basis for the medical and pharmaceutical therapies that physicians order and need to be able to play a prominent role in recommending preventive therapy using nutrition and lifestyle approaches. Therapies will increasingly be customized to the genetic uniqueness of individuals and their particular susceptibilities. Nutrition professionals need to have a firm foundation in genetics; the associations among genes, disease, and environmental influences; and the role of nutrients and other food components in the modulation of gene expression. This chapter is a brief overview of the anticipated emergence of the new field of nutritional genomics.

THE HUMAN GENOME PROJECT

The basis for the fundamental shift in health care focus is the Human Genome Project. This project began in 1990 as a 15-year multinational cooperative effort, with the goal of identifying each of the nucleotides in the deoxyribonucleic acid (DNA), which comprises the genetic material of human beings (the human genome). The project has consistently exceeded its benchmarks, so the vision for the project has been expanding and new goals have been set regularly. The current goals include (1) completely sequencing the genome of human beings and those of numerous organisms (or model systems) that have played a significant role in genetic research, (2) identifying each gene, (3) identifying the protein products of each of these genes (functional units within the genome that contain information for making proteins) and understanding their function (a new science called proteomics), (4) associating genes and their products with specific diseases, and (5) understanding the way genes, proteins, and environmental factors interact to cause the physiologic dysfunction that results in disease. The expectation is that this type of detailed knowledge will lead to an understanding of ways to prevent disease and help people stay healthy.

The Human Genome Project has several other goals, one of which is to address the ethical, legal, and social implications (ELSI) of genetic research. This focus has been a commitment of the project from the beginning (see *Focus On:* ELSI: Ethical, Legal, and Social Implications of Genetics Research).

In addition, those involved with the Human Genome Project are concerned with developing genetic technology that is accurate, fast, and inexpensive; developing sophisticated computer technology that can handle the vast amount of data generated by the project and enable scientists to rapidly compare a sequence in multiple species; developing the field of *bioinformatics,* in which scientists specialize in the interface between computer technology and molecular biology; educating genetic scientists and clinicians; and applying results of genetic research in clinics.

Significant progress has been made. A rough draft of the human genome sequence was published in June 2001 (International Human Genome Sequencing Consortium, 2001; Venter, 2001), and scientists continue to work on converting the rough draft to an error-free final draft. The genomes of numerous model systems have been sequenced and compared with the human sequence, revealing considerable similarity (homology) among species. One of the more widely used model systems in human genetic research is the mouse, and its genome has been found to be quite similar to that of the human (Mural et al, 2002). This similarity means that experiments with the mouse provide useful data that are relevant to humans.

Among the other aspects of progress are significant strides in the improvement of existing genetic technologies and the development of new technologies that make available sufficient quantities of DNA for experimental use and allow DNA sequencing to be a routine process. In addition, the ability to manipulate

FOCUS ON

ELSI: Ethical, Legal, and Social Implications of Genetics Research

Genetic technology gives humans the power to read the information in each of their genes and tell them who is likely to remain healthy or become ill—and with which type of illness. Genetic technology also gives humans the power to change their genetic information through gene therapy. Not surprisingly, such power raises many concerns. From its inception, the Human Genome Project has addressed such implications of genetic research. Professionals from diverse disciplines are working together to identify and address the *ethical, legal, and social implications (ELSI)* that are emerging.

Among the issues being addressed are (1) ways to ensure that genetic information about an individual will be used fairly and that the individual's privacy will be protected, (2) the best ways to implement genetic technologies into the practice of health care to ensure more targeted therapy with increased benefits and decreased side effects, (3) ways to handle the many developing ethical issues, and (4) the best ways to educate health care professionals so that they can meet the growing demand for genetics-savvy practitioners.

Protecting the privacy of the individual is of paramount concern. People are extremely concerned that genetic information can be misused; for example, they might be discriminated against based on their genotypic profile. Federal legislation helps to ensure that such discrimination does not occur, but it is likely to take some time before people are comfortable with the way genetic information is used. Ready and open access to such information is critical if the benefits of presymptomatic testing are to be realized. Ideally, a person's genotypic profile should be just another important piece of information in analyzing health risk—like height, weight, and blood pressure. Reaching this point will take a concerted effort on many fronts.

In considering how best to implement genetic technologies into the practice of health care, the issue becomes "*who* should be tested?" Ethical issues abound. For example, should individuals be tested for a disease for which there is no cure? Do parents have the right to have their children, if they are minors, tested for a genetic disease—without the children's consent? Do they have the right to withhold the results from the children? Should gene therapy be allowed on reproductive cells so that any corrected genes can be inherited by subsequent generations? Should human cloning be allowed? The basis of health care is becoming more intertwined with genetics and genetic technology, so what is the best way to educate those who are already in practice as health care professionals? What changes are needed so that future health care practitioners can be properly educated?

the genetic makeup of various organisms has enabled scientists to develop model systems in which a gene can be eliminated, overproduced, or subjected to the influence of various environmental factors, and the effect of these manipulations on the health of the organism can be observed.

The Human Genome Project is a stellar accomplishment in terms of the basic science and application outcomes and the worldwide collaboration that has been achieved. The project is administered by the United States through two governmental agencies: the National Human Genome Research Institute of the National Institutes of Health and Oak Ridge National Laboratory of the U.S. Department of Energy. In addition, numerous private and university laboratories in this and several countries worldwide are also contributing to the program's success.

Much of the knowledge and technologic advances gained from the Human Genome Project have clinical applications. Knowing the gene associated with a particular disease and its DNA sequence, its protein product, and the function of its protein product in maintaining health or leading to illness provides the basis for diagnostic assays. For example, tumors that appear identical physically can now be distinguished by their genetic profiles. This distinction is important for effective therapy because different types of tumors respond to different therapeutic approaches. Not only can such assays be used to definitively reach a diagnosis, they also can be used for detection in those without symptoms, which allows interventions to be initiated before a disease's symptoms become apparent.

Another initial application of the information gained from the Human Genome Project is in the field of pharmacogenomics, which is involved in screening people for their ability to metabolize drugs. Each human being has the same basic set of drug-metabolizing enzymes, but the genes responsible for these enzymes can have numerous variations, which means that the resulting enzyme function varies also. One drug may have the intended effects on one person, be ineffective for another person, and actually be harmful to a third person. The ability to assess an individual's genetic makeup as it relates to the major drug-metabolizing genes helps the physician select the drug and dosage that will have the desired effect on that individual. Like drugs, food requires numerous enzymatic processes to be digested, absorbed, and used by the body's cells. The ability to tailor food to the genetic makeup of individuals is expected to be an important application of genetic research, similar to the way it has been applied in pharmacogenomics.

Another aspect of genetic research relevant to nutrition professionals is the applicability of the research to food production and safety. The field of food biotechnology is based on genetic manipulation and diagnostics for detecting contaminating organisms. Although modern biotechnology began long before the Human Genome Project, many of the same basic genetic techniques are used, and the progress in streamlining genetic technology has had a positive effect on food biotechnology applications.

The application that is likely to have the most impact on the way nutrition professionals approach their work is the ability to associate a genotype with a person's susceptibility to developing a particular disease. Genetic science and nutritional science are identifying the influence of specific food components and other environmental factors on gene expression. As this knowledge unfolds, protocols will be developed to guide the nutrition professional in the most efficacious therapy for ameliorating or, ideally, preventing the development of various nutrition-related diseases. Clients will arrive for nutrition counseling sessions with their genetic profiles in hand. Nutrition professionals will need to be able to read the genotypes and know to which diseases clients are susceptible and which therapeutic approaches will be most effective in reducing their susceptibility. If nutrition professionals are going to be prepared for the era of genomic medicine, they must build a foundation in genetics, biochemistry, metabolism, and other aspects of nutrition science.

GENETIC FUNDAMENTALS

It is assumed that the readers have a basic understanding of DNA as the genetic material for humans and of chromosomal and molecular genetics. Among the key concepts at the chromosomal level are the packaging of DNA into chromosomes within the nucleus, the processes of meiosis and mitosis, autosomal and sex-linked inheritance, linkage and the mapping of genes, and chromosomal mutation and its consequences. At the molecular level, key basic concepts include the replication of DNA, the nature of a gene, regulatory sequences and their control of gene expression, exons, introns, the processes of transcription, translation, and posttranslational processing, mutation at the molecular level, and the connection between molecular mutations and disease. An overview is provided to discuss the connection between genetics and nutrition. Those who would like additional information about these genetic fundamentals and their application to health care can refer to the Additional References list.

Genetics and Genomics

Genetics is the science of inheritance—the inheritance of an organism's genetic material and the consequences of that inheritance. Its focus and scope have changed over the years as the details of inheritance and the underlying chromosomal and molecular processes have unfolded. Study of the inheritance of traits in humans initially focused on readily observable characteristics such as eye color and the mechanism by which these characteristics were passed from parent to child. Certain rare diseases were found to be inherited from generation to generation, so genetic disease came to be thought of as a separate disease category. Today scientists realize that, directly or indirectly, all disease is connected to the information in the genes. Genetic research is actively involved in identifying the associations between genes and disease and the influence of environmental factors on gene expression. By understanding the details of these associations, genetics has progressed from being a descriptive science to a science that can predict mechanisms of disease and suggest logical interventions.

As a result, the science of genetics has significantly expanded in scope and includes the whole set of genetic information in an organism—its *genome*—and the interactions of the various genes and their protein products with each other and the environment. The term *genomics* is often used now instead of *genetics* because the term genomics suggests a more global role for genes—a more important role in the functioning of living organisms. Whereas genetics was initially concerned with diseases that arose from a mistake in a single gene, genomics is more concerned with today's chronic diseases that result from the influence of multiple genes and multiple influencing factors. More emphasis is being placed on determining the way various environmental factors influence whether individuals develop diseases to which they are susceptible.

Exact terminology is not as important as the changing view of genes' central role in health and disease and the realization that environmental influences (especially lifestyle choices) have a profound effect on whether genes predispose people to health or illness. Among the more important lifestyle influences are food choices and how those choices influence gene expression and ultimately health. The field of nutritional genomics involves the processes by which food and food components influence genetic outcomes (DeBusk, 2003).

Genetic Basics

The genetic material of human beings is deoxyribonucleic acid (DNA), which comprises nucleotide subunits consisting of a sugar molecule, the mineral phosphorus, and one of four nitrogen-containing bases: *adenine (A)*, *thymine (T)*, *guanine (G)*, or *cytosine (C)*. These bases are arranged side by side in long strands. Sets of three nucleotides make up a codon that specifies an amino acid in the gene's protein product. In humans, approximately 3 billion nucleotides make up the genome, which is housed in the nucleus of cells. The genome is distributed among 23 chromosomes, each one containing thousands of genes and each gene containing within its nucleotide sequence the information needed to form the proteins that carry out the work of the cells (Figure 16-1). The human genome contains approximately 30,000 to 40,000 genes (Baltimore, 2001; International Human Genome Sequencing Consortium, 2001; Venter, 2001).

The information within the genes is in a code. To be useful to the cells, the information must be decoded and translated into proteins. The genetic code sequence of nucleotides or codons in the DNA determines the sequence of the amino acids in the protein. Long stretches of nucleotides are often found between one gene and the next along the chromosome. Such sequences are called intervening sequences and comprise the majority of the DNA in humans. These sequences do not code for proteins, and their function is currently unknown.

Information decoding from the gene occurs in two steps: (1) the process of transcription, during which the enzyme *ribonucleic acid polymerase (RNA polymerase)* converts DNA into an intermediate messenger RNA (mRNA) molecule, and (2) a subsequent translation step in which mRNA directs the assembly of amino acids into the protein molecule. The average gene is approximately 1000 nucleotides long. Genes have a common structure, with a promoter region where the RNA polymerase binds and a coding (informational) region where the RNA polymerase transcribes the DNA into mRNA. Within the coding region is the sequence of nucleotides (exons) that directs the assembly of amino acids into the gene's protein product. Exons are interspersed with DNA sequences called introns that do not code for amino acids. RNA polymerase transcribes the exons and introns into mRNA, which then must be processed so that the introns are removed before protein synthesis.

Upstream from the 5′ end of the promoter region is the regulatory region, where control of the transcriptional process takes place. Within this region certain sequences, called response elements, serve as binding sites for transcription factors and the ligands that bind to them. Depending on the particular ligand bound, gene expression may increase or decrease. Binding of the transcription factor and its attached ligand to the response element changes the conformation of the promoter region and increases or decreases the ability of RNA polymerase to attach and begin transcription. The array of response elements within the promoter region can be quite complex, allowing for the binding of multiple transcription factors and fine tuning of the control of gene expression. It is through the binding of transcription factors to response elements that environmental factors such as nutrients and other nonnutrient components of food communicate to a gene that more or less of its protein product is needed.

The proteins coded for by the genes provide the metabolic machinery for the cells. They have various roles, such as enzymes, receptors, transporters, antibodies, hormones, and communicators. An error, or mutation, within a gene can alter the amino acid sequence of the protein, which in turn can severely

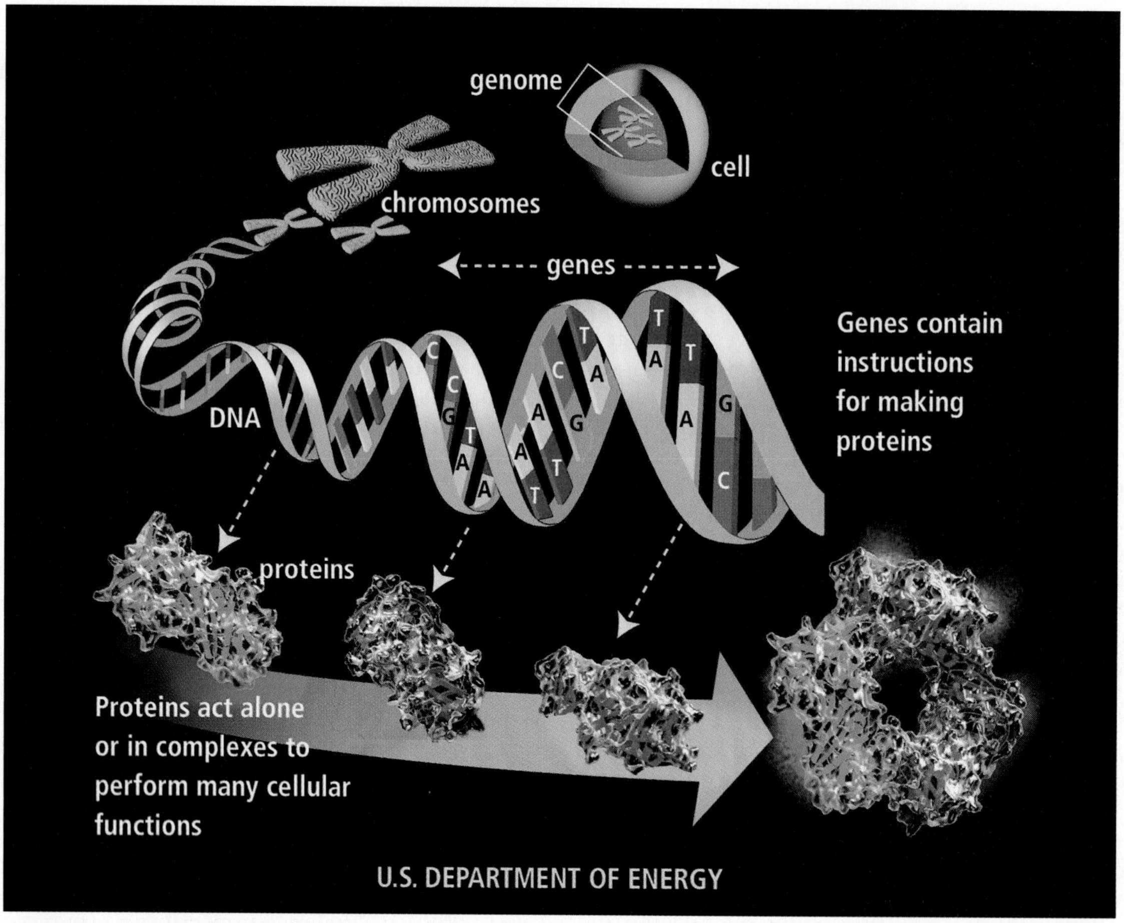

FIGURE 16-1 • Overview of cells, chromosomes, DNA, genes, amino acids, and proteins. (From U.S. Department of Energy, Human Genome Program: www.ornl.gov/hgmis.)

impair the function of that protein and harm the functioning of the organism. It only takes one change in a single nucleotide to cause a devastating disease. For example, in those with *sickle cell disease* a single nucleotide change causes a single amino acid change in the hemoglobin molecule, resulting in severe anemia and considerable pain because the defective hemoglobin molecules cannot adequately carry oxygen to the cells (see Chapter 34).

Not all mutations are harmful; some actually improve certain functions, and many, referred to as *silent mutations,* have no effects. Mutation frequency is not equal throughout the genome. Some genes accumulate mutations far more quickly than others and exist in slightly various forms, called alleles. As a result, they have protein products with differing amino acid sequences *(isoforms)* and often different functions. When a particular allele exists in greater than 1% of the population, it is called a genetic polymorphism, and the gene is said to be *polymorphic.* Polymorphism is an important concept because it explains why human beings are basically alike yet distinctively different. Polymorphism is the basis for the obvious physical differences among humans. It is also the basis for more subtle differences that may not be readily observable, such as in the functional ability of a key metabolic enzyme. Such differences may explain many of the inconsistencies in therapeutic outcomes and nutritional intervention research despite the relationships suggested by large epidemiologic studies.

Each person has slightly different DNA sequences and therefore slightly different enzymes and other proteins, a finding that is changing the focus in health care from diagnostics to therapeutics. Each person is susceptible to a different set of diseases, handles environmental toxins differently, metabolizes drugs differently, and has slightly different nutritional requirements. These exciting discoveries are revolutionizing the way people think about health and disease and the clinical aspects of medicine, pharmacology, and nutrition. They have laid the foundation for personalized therapy in many aspects of health care.

Modes of Inheritance and Penetrance

Each cell nucleus contains a complete set of nuclear DNA divided among 23 pairs of chromosomes. Each person has one pair of sex chromosomes—with females having two X chromosomes and males having one X and one Y chromosome—and 22 pairs of nonsex chromosomes, or autosomes. During *mitosis* (cell division), all 23 pairs are duplicated and distributed to each new cell. During *meiosis,* which is the specialized cell division that forms the haploid egg and sperm cells, one member of each of the 23 pairs is distributed to each egg or sperm. During fertilization, the zygote formed has the full set of 23 pairs of chromosomes.

Because genes are carried on chromosomes, the rules governing the distribution of chromosomes during mitosis and meiosis also govern the distribution of genes. These rules describe the Mendelian inheritance of a gene, a process named after Gregor Mendel, who first deduced that the inheritance of traits was governed by a predictable set of rules. It is possible to track a gene through multiple generations by knowing the rules of inheritance. This transmission can be depicted as a pedigree, which shows the journey of a gene through multiple generations of a family and can be used to predict the probability of a gene being inherited by a particular family member. When a gene is associated with a disease, pedigrees are used to predict the probability that an individual will inherit that disease.

The Mendelian modes of inheritance are logical and can be traced to the movement of chromosomes during meiosis and gamete formation. The genes carried on each of the chromosomes are inherited in the same way as the chromosomes on which they reside. Females receive 22 autosomes and one X chromosome from their mothers and 22 autosomes and one X chromosome from their fathers. Males receive 22 autosomes from each parent, their X chromosome from their mothers, and their Y chromosome from their fathers.

Although a gene may be inherited appropriately and exist on a chromosome, whether it is expressed depends on whether it is dominant or recessive and its degree of *penetrance.* (The *genotype* refers to the genetic basis for a trait; the phenotype refers to the measurable expression of that trait.) Genes with characteristics that are expressed when only a single copy of the gene is present are called *dominant*—they have a dominant phenotype. Genes that are not expressed when only a single copy is present and only express their phenotype when two copies are present are called *recessive*—they have a recessive phenotype; the gene exists, but is not expressed. In general, mutations that affect the structural makeup of an organism are dominant; those involved with metabolic processes tend to be recessive and require two mutated genes to be expressed.

Even when a pedigree suggests that a gene should cause a particular individual to display a certain phenotype, the disease may not be evident. Such a gene is said to have reduced penetrance, meaning that not everyone who has the gene expresses it in a measurable form. Penetrance is a fascinating concept and of particular interest to nutrition professionals because it is likely the result of environmental factors modulating the expression of the gene, which suggests that modifying such factors may improve outcomes for those with some disorders.

The classic modes of Mendelian inheritance are autosomal dominant, autosomal recessive, X-linked dominant, X-linked recessive, and Y linked. Remember that each gene is present in two copies (alleles), one on each chromosome. When the alleles are the same (either both normal or both mutated), the individual is said to be homozygous for that gene. If the alleles are different (one normal, one mutant), the individual is heterozygous.

Autosomal dominant disorders are inherited equally by males and females and typically evident in each generation of a pedigree. Autosomal recessive disorders are also inherited equally by males and females but require two mutant copies of a gene to be expressed; therefore autosomal recessive diseases typically skip a generation. Numerous metabolic disorders are inherited in an autosomal recessive pattern because they are caused by a mutation resulting in a faulty enzyme that can no longer meet the metabolic needs of the cell. These types of mutations are usually not harmful in those who are heterozygous (carriers) because the normal gene's output of the critical protein is sufficient to meet the needs of the cells.

Sex-linked disorders include X-linked and Y-linked disorders. Males carrying a mutation on their X chromosome express the disorder. Females with a mutation on one X chromosome express the disorder if the mutation is dominant but must have the mutated gene on both of their X chromosomes to express the disorder if the mutation is recessive.

In a pedigree of an X-linked recessive disorder, all male offspring of females with the disease also have the disease-causing gene. In a pedigree of an X-linked dominant trait, half the sons of a female with the disease inherit the disease gene. The other half inherit the normal X chromosome and do not have the disease. For Y-linked inheritance disorders, all males in the family are expected to have the disease because the Y chromosome determines maleness, and they inherit their Y chromosome from their fathers. Obviously, the concept of dominance and recessiveness in reference to the sex chromosomes applies only to the female because the male has a single X chromosome and a single Y chromosome.

In addition to the genetic material in the nucleus, the mitochondria in each cell also contain DNA that gives rise to a limited number of proteins. The majority of these genes are involved in housekeeping needs related to maintenance of the mitochondrion and its activities but, like nuclear DNA, mutation in mitochondrial genes can lead to disease.

Traits resulting from mitochondrial genes have a characteristic inheritance pattern, but it is non-Mendelian because mitochondria and their genetic material typically pass from mother to child.

Disease at the Chromosomal Level

Disease can be caused by a change in a single gene or changes in multiple genes through chromosomal abnormalities. Because chromosomes contain thousands of genes, changes in the number of chromosomes or the arrangement of the DNA within a chromosome can affect numerous genes. Such changes are typically harmful to the individual and often fatal. Examples of nonfatal chromosomal abnormalities include trisomy 21 (Down syndrome), trisomy 18 (cri du chat syndrome), and Klinefelter syndrome, in which an extra chromosome 21, 18, or X is present, respectively. In addition, females with Turner syndrome have a single X chromosome. These disorders result from the gain or loss of all or a significant portion of a chromosome. Nutrition professionals play an important role in the therapy of such individuals because they typically have oral-motor problems that affect their nutritional status and cause growth problems in early life. Later in development, obesity is common in those with trisomy 21, Klinefelter syndrome, and Turner syndrome, and nutrition therapy is helpful in controlling weight and preventing the diabetes and cardiovascular complications that typically accompany obesity.

In contrast to syndromes caused by extra chromosomes, some syndromes are caused by the loss of a portion of a chromosome (or a partial deletion); examples include Williams syndrome (chromosome 7 deletion), Beckwith-Wiedemann syndrome (chromosome 11 deletion), Prader-Willi syndrome (chromosome 15 deletion), and Angelman syndrome (chromosome 15 deletion). People with these syndromes often have feeding difficulties and require the assistance of a knowledgeable nutrition professional. Williams syndrome in particular is characterized by cardiac defects that have nutritional effects. The other deletion syndromes are quite interesting because the expression of the syndromes is distinctively influenced by sex. When the Beckwith-Wiedemann syndrome is inherited from the mother, it is caused by a partial deletion of chromosome 11; when inherited from the father, the person has only a single copy of chromosome 11. The characteristics are similar whether inherited from the mother or father (e.g., an enlarged tongue, an enlarged body size, ear creases). The oversized tongue leads to feeding difficulties and, for many infants, hypoglycemia.

Prader-Willi and Angelman syndromes affect food intake in similar ways. Typically individuals with these syndromes have abnormal feeding behaviors. They often do not register the bodily signal that they are full, so they continue to eat. Obesity is a common problem. Prader-Willi syndrome results from inheriting a partial deletion of chromosome 15 from the mother; Angelman syndrome results from inheriting two copies of a deletion in chromosome 15 from the father, a mutation that was originally inherited from the father's mother.

In people with any of these chromosomal abnormalities, therapy is often complicated by mental retardation, ranging from mild to severe. Clearly, many unanswered questions exist regarding these syndromes, but the important issue is that nutrition professionals play a significant role in the treatment of each of them.

Chromosomal disorders of the type just described are detected by developing a karyotype. Nucleated cells are collected from drawn blood or a swab from the oral cavity, grown in culture, and arrested in metaphase, and the chromosomes are then counted and arranged in matched pairs. Until recently, this analysis was performed manually and was quite time-consuming. Advances in genetic technology have led to computer-assisted karyotyping. Each chromosome can be "painted" a different color so that the chromosomal pairs can be readily identified, a process called spectral karyotyping (Figure 16-2).

Many more chromosomal disorders that have nutritional consequences are known, and additional disorders are being discovered regularly as a result of the Human Genome Project and advances in genetic research. The expertise of a knowledgeable nutrition professional is invaluable in mitigating the detrimental effects of these disorders.

Disease at the Molecular Level

Insight into disease at the molecular level has been among the major advances of genetic research and its applications to medicine. Whereas mutations at the chromosomal level involve numerous genes, mutation at the molecular level can involve a single nucleotide change. Mutation typically results in the substitution of one nucleic acid base for another or the deletion or addition of one or more bases. Such changes in the genetic material may occur within the protein coding region or the regulatory region. Alterations in the regulatory region may increase or decrease the quantity of protein produced or alter the ability of the regulatory region to respond to environmental signals. Alterations in the coding region may affect the amino acid sequence of the protein, which

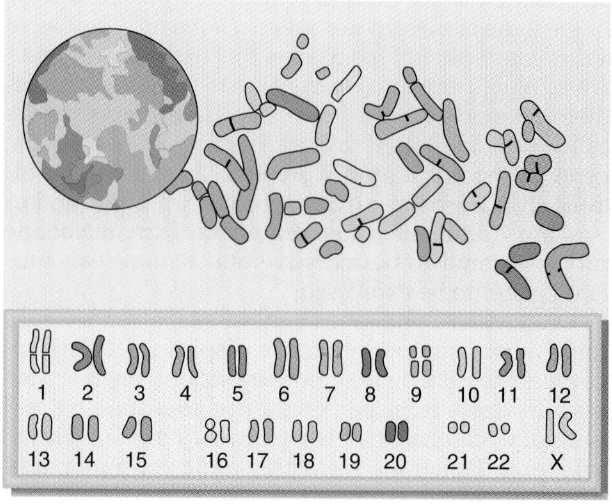

FIGURE 16-2 • Spectral karyotype. (Redrawn from photo courtesy National Human Genome Research Institute, Division of Intramural Research, 2003, National Institutes of Health.)

may in turn affect the conformation and therefore function of the protein. Altered proteins may be less functional than the *wild type* (normal), be unaffected by the mutation, or have enhanced activity and provide a selective advantage to the organism.

The vast majority of the genes in a human being reside on the nuclear chromosomes and are passed on through generations by Mendelian inheritance. The autosomal dominant disorders that have nutritional implications include several that result in oral-motor problems, growth problems, increased weight gain, and occasionally difficulties with constipation. Examples include Albright hereditary osteodystrophy, which commonly results in dental problems, obesity, hypocalcemia, and hyperphosphatemia; chondrodysplasias, which often result in oral-motor problems and obesity; and Marfan's syndrome, which promotes cardiac disease susceptibility and excessive growth and its concomitant nutritional needs. Familial hypercholesterolemia results in a defective low-density lipoprotein receptor and elevated levels of cholesterol, which leads to atherosclerosis.

Autosomal recessive disorders are by far the most common of the Mendelian inherited disorders and include numerous metabolic disorders of amino acid, carbohydrate, and lipid metabolism—disorders called *inborn errors of metabolism* (see Chapter 45). These disorders are chronic, and diet modifications are a primary treatment modality. The classic example of this type of disorder is *phenylketonuria (PKU).* A defect in the gene coding for the enzyme phenylalanine hydroxylase leads to an inability to convert the amino acid phenylalanine to tyrosine. Tyrosine levels become inadequate, and phenylalanine is converted to phenylpyruvate, which is harmful to the developing brain. Lifelong dietary restriction of phenylalanine, although challenging, enables individuals with PKU to live into adulthood and to enjoy a quality life.

Similarly, *tyrosinemia* is an inborn error of amino acid metabolism and is caused by a mutation in the gene that codes for the enzyme fumarylacetoacetate hydrolase. Tyrosine and phenylalanine accumulate and can lead to liver disease and the aforementioned characteristics of phenylketonuria. Dietary restriction of tyrosine and phenylalanine is essential. In *maple syrup urine disease,* the metabolic defect involves a step in the catabolism of the branched-chain amino acids valine, leucine, and isoleucine. To serve as energy sources, these amino acids are converted to their α-keto acid forms and then decarboxylated. The mutant enzyme that causes maple syrup urine disease is branched-chain α-keto acid decarboxylase, a multimeric enzyme complex encoded by six genes. A mutation in any one of these genes can result in accumulation of α-keto acids in the urine, which gives the urine an odor similar to maple syrup. Failure to limit branched-chain amino acid intake leads to mental retardation, seizures, and deaths (see Chapter 45).

Galactosemia and hereditary fructose intolerance are examples of autosomal recessive inborn errors of carbohydrate metabolism. A mutation in the gene encoding galactose-1-phosphate uridyl transferase is the most common cause of galactosemia, a condition in which the sugar galactose cannot be converted to glucose. Accumulation of galactose leads to failure to thrive, developmental delay, and hepatic insufficiency. Dietary restriction of galactose is the treatment of choice. Hereditary fructose intolerance is caused by a deficiency in the enzyme fructose 1,6-biphosphate aldolase, so fructose cannot be converted to glucose. Breast-fed infants are typically asymptomatic until fruit is added to the diet. Nutrition therapy involves the elimination of fructose and sucrose, because sucrose is composed of glucose and fructose. Autosomal recessive disorders of lipid metabolism also exist. The most common is a deficiency of medium-chain acyl-coenzyme A (acyl-CoA) dehydrogenase. Toxic fatty acid intermediates accumulate and can lead to death unless fatty acid intake is controlled (see Chapter 45).

Another inborn error of metabolism, classic *homocystinuria,* is of particular interest because it led to the realization that elevated levels of homocysteine are an independent risk factor for cardiovascular disease, an idea originally proposed by McCully in 1969. A defect in the vitamin B_6–requiring enzyme cystathionine β-synthase leads to an inability to convert homocysteine to cystathionine. Homocysteine accumulates and can promote atheroscleosis and form homocystine, which leads to abnormal collagen cross-linking and osteoporosis. Nutrition therapy for homocystinuria is multipronged. Some individuals have an enzyme defect that requires a high concentration of the vitamin B_6 cofactor for activity. Others are not responsive to B_6 and need a combination of folate, vitamin B_{12}, choline, and betaine to convert homocysteine to methionine, and others must limit their methionine intake. At least three forms of homocystinuria exist, and they all require different nutritional therapies. The ability to distinguish the disorders using genetic analysis will be helpful (see Chapter 18).

Examples of X-linked disorders with nutritional implications include the X-linked dominant *fragile X syndrome* and the X-linked recessive *nephrogenic diabetes insipidus, adrenoleukodystrophy,* and *Duchenne muscular dystrophy* disorders. Fragile X syndrome is characterized by developmental delays and mental retardation. The name "fragile X" comes from the discovery that cells grown in a culture medium deficient in the B vitamin folic acid break near the tip of the long arm of the X chromosome. Whether folate nutriture influences the in vivo expression of this syndrome is unclear. Individuals with X-linked recessive nephrogenic diabetes insipidus are unable to concentrate urine and exhibit polyuria and polydipsia. This disorder is usually detected in infancy and can manifest as dehydration, poor feeding, vomiting, and failure to thrive. Management with thiazide diuretics is common, usually with a low-salt diet to decrease water retention and supplemental dietary

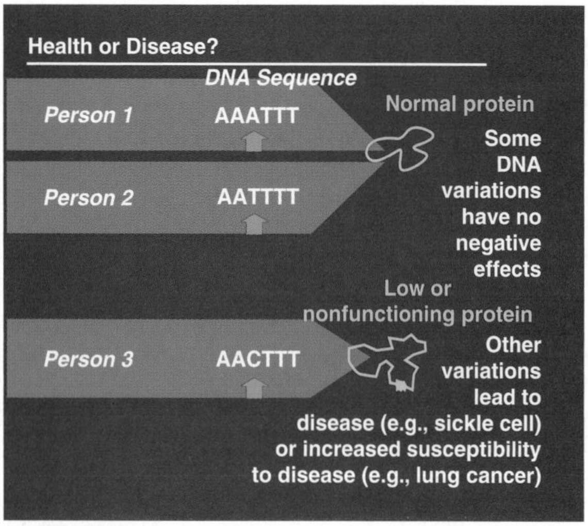

FIGURE 16-3 • Health or disease? (Courtesy U.S. Department of Energy.)

potassium to counter the potassium wasting induced by this class of diuretics. X-linked recessive *adrenoleukodystrophy* results from a defect in the enzyme that breaks down very-long-chain fatty acids. These fats accumulate and lead to brain and adrenal dysfunction and, ultimately, motor dysfunction. X-linked recessive Duchenne muscular dystrophy is characterized by fatty infiltration of muscles and extreme muscle wasting. Children are typically confined to a wheelchair by age 11 and need assistance with feeding.

Y-linked disorders involve male sex determination and physiological "housekeeping functions." No nutrition-related disorders have been conclusively assigned to the Y chromosome.

Progressing beyond knowing the chromosomal position of a disease trait to associating the disease with a particular gene and understanding its functional consequences has required the development of sophisticated genetic technologies for analyzing the molecular basis of mutation. One of the key technologic advances is recombinant DNA. Using bacteria-derived restriction endonucleases (also called *restriction enzymes*), researchers are able to cut DNA in precise places along the nucleotide chain. The DNA fragments from one organism can then be inserted into the genetic material of another organism. The development of recombinant DNA technology has provided a major technologic advance in terms of studying genes, their functions, and the regulation of their expression.

Recombinant DNA technology has been the cornerstone of many molecular techniques that are now routinely used. It is the foundation for genetic engineering and the production of human therapeutic proteins such as insulin and growth hormone. It paved the way for DNA sequencing, which is used to identify the sequence of nucleotides within a gene and pinpoint the exact location of any change (mutation) that has occurred. Recombinant DNA is also the basis for diagnostic tests that detect mutated DNA sequences in an individual and thereby predict susceptibility to disease. Still another important application is its role in gene therapy, by which a corrected gene sequence can be introduced into the cells of an individual with a disease-causing mutation (Figure 16-3).

Additional genetic technologies that have been critical in the development of molecular medicine and the ability to associate genes with diseases include *transgenic technology* and single nucleotide polymorphisms (SNPs, pronounced "snips") technology. Transgenic mice are an example of a model system, which is an experimental approach used in research laboratories to explore questions in a system that is relatively simpler than a human being. Because the mouse and human share many of the same genes, the ability to manipulate the genetic material of the mouse and examine the impact on metabolism and physiologic function has been invaluable for understanding health and disease in the human.

In a transgenic mouse, a gene can be mutated so that the normal protein is no longer made; the resulting mouse is called a *knockout mouse.* In addition, a gene can be altered so that it expresses too much or too little of its product, and regulatory sequences can be altered so that a gene no longer responds appropriately to environmental signals. In this way, the normal function of a gene can be determined, the effects of overexpressing or underexpressing a gene can be studied, and the details of the communication process between signals outside the organism and the genetic material inside the organism can be determined. Transgenic mice are particularly valuable for studying gene-nutrient interactions.

SNPs are those variations of a gene that are found in greater than 1% of the population. It is the total of these subtle variations that is thought to distinguish one member of a species from another. When the subtle variations include genes associated with disease, the potential exists to create an individual profile of a person's number of disease susceptibilities. Once risk for a disease has been identified, early detection coupled with appropriate therapeutic intervention can potentially minimize the disease's impact. Because an increasing number of SNPs are being associated with the susceptibility of developing specific diseases, therapy is focusing on medical surveillance for early detection and educating individuals about their genetic risks and the lifestyle choices that minimize those risks.

Food and dietary supplement choices, exercise habits, alcohol and tobacco usage, and handling of chronic stressors are all important lifestyle choices that individuals need to consider when attempting to minimize their risk. A genetics-savvy nutrition professional is invaluable in helping people understand their disease susceptibilities and their options for enjoying lifelong health.

Disease at the Mitochondrial Level

Human mitochondrial DNA codes for 13 proteins and the 2 ribosomal RNAs and 22 transfer RNAs needed to synthesize these proteins (Report of the Committee of the Human Mitochondrial Genome, 2002). A major function of mitochondria is to produce cellular energy through the respiratory system. Not surprisingly, mutations in mitochondrial DNA are typically degenerative, affect tissues with a high demand for oxidative phosphorylation, and have considerably varied clinical manifestations, including neurologic disease, cardiomyopathy, and skeletal myopathy (MITOMAP, 2002; Shoffner and Wallace, 1992). Maternally inherited diabetes and deafness have also been traced to changes in mitochondrial DNA (MITOMAP, 2002).

Mitochondrial inheritance is non-Mendelian and normally passes from mother to child. This biologic principle has become the basis for anthropologic studies that trace lineage and population migration patterns through the centuries. It also has provided a way to trace familial diseases caused by gene defects in mitochondrial DNA. However, as with other biologic processes, occasional mistakes occur; reports exist of mitochondrial DNA being passed from father to child. This phenomenon was first noted in mice but was more recently found in an unusual case study involving humans (Gyllensten et al, 1991; Schwartz and Vissing, 2002).

GENETICS AND NUTRITION THERAPY

Of particular relevance to nutrition professionals are mutations that affect nutritional status or whose effects can be influenced by nutrients or other food components. The impact of numerous chromosomal and single-gene mutations on nutritional status is an area in which nutrition professionals have long made valuable contributions and will continue to do so. An expanding role for the nutrition professional is emerging in the current era of *nutritional genomics.* Genetic research is suggesting ways in which food and food components can be used to specifically target the consequences of mutations, thereby mitigating the effects of genetic limitations.

Examples of gene-nutrient interactions include interactions in which the nutrient effect is direct and reasonably well defined, such as when a missing metabolite is supplied or a nutrient is involved with regulating gene expression. The vast majority of gene-nutrient interactions have yet to be clearly defined, particularly in reference to the chronic diseases, but continued research is expected to clarify these relationships as well.

Influences of Gene-Nutrient Interactions on Metabolic Processes

The interplay between nutrition and genetics varies from being straightforward to being intriguingly complex. The most straightforward is the direct correlation between a faulty gene, a defective protein, a deficient level of a metabolite, and a resultant disease state that is passed on through Mendelian inheritance and is responsive to nutrition therapy. Inborn errors of metabolism, such as those already discussed, were among the initial examples of this type of relationship. Another example concerns the essential nutrients such as amino acids, fatty acids, vitamins, and minerals that cannot be synthesized by the body and must be provided through the diet to prevent dysfunction and disease. For example, human beings lack the enzyme gulonolactone oxidase and cannot synthesize vitamin C. If dietary vitamin C intake is below needed levels, individuals develop disease.

The situation is similar with the amino acids and fatty acids and is one that is well understood by nutrition professionals—the diet must supply certain essential nutrients—but a new understanding has developed. The reason the diet must supply these nutrients is because humans have mutations in key metabolic pathways. Nutrition therapy is actually circumventing the genetic limitation by supplying the missing nutrient. This provides a hint of what is to come in nutritional genomics—nutrition therapy as a tool for treating a disease-causing mutation.

In addition to mutations in biosynthetic pathways, disease-causing changes can develop in any gene coding for a cellular protein, such as transport proteins, receptors, and hormones. Mutations that increase the transport of iron *(hereditary hemochromatosis)* or copper *(Wilson's disease)* to higher than normal levels have nutritional implications. Medical therapy is the primary treatment for these particular disorders, but nutrition is an important adjunctive therapy because it can help limit the intake of potentially harmful nutrients. Mutations in vitamin D receptors are associated with vitamin D–dependent rickets and likely with several other consequences because the active form of vitamin D is a hormone that is involved in several different metabolic and regulatory processes. Errors in the gene coding for insulin can result in structural changes in the insulin hormone and lead to dysglycemia, as can mutations in insulin receptors. Many proteins such as cytokines and transcription factors that are involved in critical signaling cascades are subject to mutational changes and altered activities.

In addition, a mutation may affect the conformational ability of a protein and prevent it from binding with cofactors or prevent membrane proteins from being able to insert themselves into a membrane and carry out their activities. Approximately fifty metabolic reactions have been described that are caused by gene defects, result in enzymes with a decreased affinity for their vitamin cofactors, and require high levels of vitamin supplementation to restore function (Ames et al, 2002). Most of the supplementation levels are well in excess of the normally recommended levels, which highlights the importance of remembering that each individual is genetically unique and has distinct metabolic needs. Although generalized guidelines for recommended nutrient levels are helpful, individuals may have mutations that require them to consume significantly more or less nutrients than recommended.

An interesting example of gene-nutrient interactions and their effects on metabolic processes is the B vitamin folate and its role in maintaining normal homocysteine levels. Homocysteine is a precursor to *S*-adenosylmethionine, a critical methyl donor to numerous metabolic reactions, including those involved in synthesizing nucleic acids. An elevated blood level of homocysteine is an independent risk factor for vascular disease. It also increases the risk of neural tube defects in fetuses, which led to the fortification of cereal grains with folate to help ensure adequate levels in women of childbearing age. Elevated homocysteine levels have been linked to inadequate levels of the B vitamins folate, B_{12}, and B_6 and to mutations in genes coding for enzymes involved in homocysteine metabolism (see Chapter 35).

A common mutation is the base substitution of thymine for cytosine at position 677 in the gene for the enzyme 5,10-methylenetetrahydrofolate reductase (MTHFR), which produces the biologically active form of folate (5-methyltetrahydrofolate). This form is needed to convert homocysteine to methionine. The mutation results in an enzyme that is thermolabile and has reduced activity, causing homocysteine to accumulate (Kang et al, 1988). This polymorphism has implications for people of all ages; the extent to which homocysteine accumulates and responds to supplementation with folate or B_{12} and the forms of folate that are most effective are related to the genotype of the individual (Bailey et al, 2002; Fohr et al, 2002; Kauwell et al, 2000a, 2000b). Such findings suggest that supplementation recommendations tailored to genotype are needed.

Influences of Gene-Nutrient Interactions on Gene Expression

Clearly, nutrients and other food components can change the outcomes of individuals who have mutations that affect metabolic processes. A more complex interplay between nutrition and genetics involves the ability of nutrients to modulate gene expression. One of the known examples of gene-nutrient interactions is the ability of nutrients to bind to transcription factors. Binding either enhances or interferes with the ability of transcription factors to bind to response elements in the gene's promoter region, which in turn controls RNA polymerase binding. In this way, nutrients help control gene expression in positive and negative ways.

Such a system provides an elegant sensing pathway that amplifies an environmental trigger through a signaling cascade of biochemical reactions. It links this trigger with the binding of a transcriptional factor and nutrient ligand complex to a response element in the promoter region of a gene. Multiple transcription factors and response element interactions may be required to control a single gene's expression, which provides a mechanism for fine-tuning control of gene expression by multiple environmental and endogenous factors.

Nutrient involvement in the control of gene expression is an active area of genetic research. Investigators are focusing on which nutrients affect transcription, the mechanism of control, and the nature of the signaling cascades that ultimately translate the environmental stimuli into nutrient-associated changes in gene expression that are mediated by specific transcription factors. Among the key players in this sensing system are nuclear receptors, such as the retinoid X receptors (RXRs), the peroxisome proliferator-activated receptors (PPARs), the liver X receptors (LXRs), the farnesoid X receptor, the constitutive androstane receptor (CAR), the steroid X receptor (SXR)/pregnane X receptor (PXR), the sterol regulatory element binding proteins (SREBPs), and the nuclear vitamin D receptor (VDR_{nuc}). These nuclear receptors serve as transcription factors and are either activated by fat-soluble ligands provided by the diet or made endogenously, as are cholesterol, steroid hormones, bile acids, xenobiotics (foreign chemicals), and the active form of vitamin D (Chawla et al, 2001; Jacobs and Lewis, 2002).

Through their ability to interact directly with DNA and regulate expression of a diverse set of genes, transcription factors coordinate an intricate metabolic signaling cascade that senses the environment and regulates the cells' responses. The RXRs do not function alone; they form heterodimers with other lipid-sensing receptors (Wei, 2002). The vitamin A derivative 9-*cis*-retinoic acid and the omega-3 polyunsaturated fatty acid docosahexaenoic acid (DHA) are ligands for these receptors. The LXRs act as cholesterol sensors that regulate genes involved with cholesterol homeostasis (Lu et al, 2001), whereas the farnesoid X receptor is a bile acid receptor that also affects lipoprotein metabolism (Edwards et al, 2002). The CAR and SRX/PXR receptors are involved in protecting the body against xenobiotics, so they respond to potentially toxic molecules such as drugs and environmental contaminants (Willson and Kliewer, 2002). The SREBPs are another example of nuclear receptors that are responsive to nutrients and food components (Horton et al, 2002; Jump, 2002; Müller-Wieland and Kotzka, 2002; Müller-Wieland et al, 2001; Shimano, 2001; Zannis et al, 2001).

The vitamin D receptor seems increasingly complex as it becomes apparent that it has nuclear and membrane receptors and is involved in maintenance of extracellular calcium levels, bone mineralization, muscle function, immune function, and cell growth and differentiation, including of breast and prostate cancer cells (DeLuca and Cantorna, 2001; Norman et al, 2001).

Each of these transcription factors is an example of gene-nutrient interactions and control of gene expression. PPARs, RXRs, and SREBPs are of particular interest because of their impact on glycemic and lipid control. The PPARs exist in various isoforms that are encoded by different genes and are active in different tissues. They are important in insulin resistance and obesity caused by a high-fat diet (Clarke et al, 1999; Hihi et al, 2002; Kadowaki et al, 2002). They function as lipid sensors and regulate lipid and lipoprotein metabolism, glucose homeostasis, and cell proliferation and differentiation, especially of adipocytes and in the formation of foam cells from monocytes (Tontonoz et al, 1998). Their natural ligands include the omega-3 and omega-6 fatty acids and certain eicosanoids. Synthetic ligands such as the fibrates and thiazolidinediones can also bind and are useful for treating dyslipidemia and dysglycemia (Berger and Wagner, 2002). However, before the PPARs can bind to their DNA response element, they must first bind to an RXR to form a heterodimer of PPAR-RXR. RXRs are also ligand-activated transcription factors and bind retinoids, which are derived from retinol (vitamin A), another example of gene-nutrient interactions (Wei, 2002). Once the heterodimer is formed with the RXR and PPAR ligands attached, it can bind to DNA. Binding increases gene expression related to fatty acid oxidation and decreases expression related to fatty acid synthesis.

The PPARs also have a negative effect on the expression of proinflammatory genes (Delerive et al, 2001). The implications for nutrition therapy include the potential use of omega-3 fatty acids to enhance PPAR transcriptional control of such processes as glucose homeostasis, adipocyte proliferation, and atherogenesis. Increasing the amount of omega-3 fatty acids may be helpful in enhancing the negative control of the expression of the proinflammatory cytokine genes by PPARs.

The SREBPs regulate several genes involved in cholesterol homeostasis and fatty acid and triglyceride synthesis (Brown and Goldstein, 1997; Magaña et al, 2000; Stoeckman and Towle, 2002). The omega-3 fatty acids are again important activators, but in this case they affect the transcription of the actual SREBPs (Stoeckman and Towle, 2002; Xu et al, 1999). By decreasing SREBP transcription, the omega-3 fatty acids decrease lipogenesis. The SREBPs promise to be an interesting set of regulatory proteins—one of the isoforms, SREBP-1c, seems to be a major factor in increasing the expression of lipogenic genes in response to carbohydrate feeding (Stoeckman and Towle, 2002). Practical applications may include using omega-3 fatty acids to suppress the lipogenesis that results from high-carbohydrate diets by decreasing the synthesis of the SREBP-1c transcription factor, thereby reducing expression of the lipogenic genes.

Complex Genetic-Nutrition Connections

The majority of gene-nutrient interactions are not yet defined, although the expectation is that they will be found to affect virtually every key physiologic process. Observations have detected considerably varied responses among individuals, from food selection to digestion and absorption to therapeutic intervention responses. For example, genetic variations affecting the sense of taste are a critical factor in determining the foods a person likes and dislikes (Duffy and Bartoshuk, 2000). The extent to which a person responds to bitter, sweet, sour, salty, and fatty tastes influences his or her choice of foods and affects his or her nutritional status. The details of this genetic variability are not yet known, but the applications to nutrition counseling are obvious. For example, recommending a diet high in cruciferous vegetables to an individual with a heightened sense of the taste for bitterness would be unlikely to yield the needed therapeutic results. A genetic profile of taste sensations is helpful for working with clients to develop diets that address their nutritional needs as well as their food preferences.

Practitioners are familiar with the variability in response to therapeutic interventions for nutrition-related disorders such as cardiovascular disease, cancer, diabetes, obesity, and osteoporosis. Each of these diseases is likely a heterogeneous category of related disorders, some of which are caused by single-gene mutations and others that are far more complex in their etiology. Coupled with the fact that each individual has a unique set of genetic variants that affect the numerous processes that contribute to these conditions, it is not surprising that a high degree of variability in response to nutrition therapy is the norm.

For example, a challenging situation for physicians and nutrition professionals has been the variability in blood levels of low-density lipoprotein cholesterol (LDL-C) in response to dietary changes, whether short-term or long-term. Some individuals are responsive to lowering the fat in the diet; others are not. Normally LDL-C levels rise right after a fat-rich meal and subside with time. In some individuals the levels rise quite high for an extended period. Others respond in this way to some high-fat foods but not to others. Not surprisingly, genetic makeup has been correlated with the lipemic response, and it is on this topic that considerable research effort is being concentrated. The expectation is that by identifying the genes involved and the effects of particular mutations on specific proteins, researchers will gain a clearer understanding of the interactions between nutrients and genes—an understanding that will form the basis for effective therapeutic interventions. However, the situation is complex, and it may take some time before a clear picture emerges.

Numerous single-gene effects are already known. For example, familial hypercholesterolemia (FH) is passed on through an autosomal dominant inheritance pattern with strong penetrance and causes extremely high cholesterol levels. The mutation affects the LDL receptor, which prevents cholesterol from being cleared from the bloodstream and causes it to accumulate in the arteries as plaque, ultimately resulting in occlusion of the blood vessels. Individuals homozygous for the FH gene have an early onset of heart disease and death. Heterozygotes have LDL-C levels that are considerably higher than normal but lower than those of homozygotes; the condition can be managed with medication and a supportive diet and exercise. Obviously, individuals with either one or two copies of the FH gene must be very careful of food components that can increase blood cholesterol levels.

Although the previous example is straightforward, some suspect that environmental factors influence an individual's response. A study of multiple generations—spanning 150 years—of a family who had FH found that several of the carrier individuals who lived in the nineteenth century and early part of the twentieth century did not develop the disease (Sijbrands et al, 2001). Numerous other genes have been implicated in the response of LDL-C levels to dietary lipids: the *APOE, APOA-IV, APOB*, and *APOA-I* genes and their various polymorphisms have all been implicated (López-Miranda et al, 1997; Marín et al, 2002; Mata et al, 1998; Nikkilä M et al, 1994; Ostos et al, 1998; Weintraub et al, 1987; Ye and Kwiterovich, 2000). People with certain genotypes respond positively to food's ability to blunt this response, whereas others do not. The complexity revealed by the number of genes identified thus far, as well as diet responses that vary based on which alleles of these genes are present, suggests that genotype is an important determinant of dietary response.

Clearly, genetic variations influence the response to dietary fat. Some individuals, because of their genetic makeup, do not need to pay serious attention to the kinds and quantity of fat they eat. If their genotypes were known, it would not be necessary to recommend changing their eating habits with respect to fat. It is tempting to think that the easiest approach is to recommend a low-fat diet for everyone because most people will benefit from it, and conventional wisdom holds that this approach is beneficial. Aside from the quality-of-life issue, can it be assumed that a low-fat diet is beneficial for all? Perhaps it depends on an individual's genotype. In fact, this seems to be the case. However, in a subset of the population a low-fat diet actually seems to increase the risk of atherogenesis (Dreon et al, 1994).

Today is a time of many discoveries involving the genes that affect development or prevention of chronic diseases and involving particular nutrients and other bioactive components from food that seem to affect genetic outcomes. For example, among the components being studied in reference to cancer are the vitamins A, C, D, and E and the B vitamin folate; the minerals calcium, selenium, iron, and zinc; the carotenoids lycopene, lutein, and α- and β-carotene; fiber and butyrate; the flavonoids genistein, resveratrol, quercetin, rutin, catechins, and (-)-epigallocatechin-3-gallate; sulphoraphane and other isothiocyanates; indole-3-carbinol and its metabolite diindolylmethane; monoterpenes such as D-limonene; and phenolic acids such as curcumin, caffeic acid, and ferulic acid. Fruits and vegetables are major sources of these potentially beneficial compounds, in addition to dairy products, soybeans, and green and black teas.

Milner and colleagues at the National Cancer Institute have provided an overview of the many ongoing investigations that relate to gene-nutrient interactions and carcinogenesis (Milner et al, 2001) (see Chapters 12 and 40).

SUMMARY

The genetic revolution is providing many new opportunities for the genetics-savvy nutrition professional, and it is an exciting time. The rapid advances in genetic science are opening up new applications for nutrition and related health care disciplines. The emerging focus is on the molecular basis of disease, which is providing the means for personalizing therapy. As genetics is integrated into health care, medical, pharmacologic, and nutritional therapies will become more oriented toward the genotype of each person. Nutrition will be the key to preventing or mitigating the expression of diseases for which an individual is susceptible. Nutrition will also be the key

Clinical Scenario

Jared and Matthew are identical twins who grew up together but have lived apart since college. Jared stayed in the northeast and majored in accounting. He is now a CPA in a high-profile accounting firm, working long hours in a stressful environment. Matthew went to school on the West Coast, where he studied nutrition and exercise physiology and now manages the wellness program at a large fitness center. At age 30, the two brothers are noticeably different in weight and body shape. Jared has developed central obesity, hypertension, and problems with blood sugar regulation, all signs of a tendency toward developing type 2 diabetes. Matthew is lean and has a normal blood pressure and normal blood sugar regulation.

1. Because they are identical twins, would you have expected the two brothers to have similar health profiles?
2. What is going on? Does Matthew not have the same genetic susceptibilities that Jared has? If not, why not? If so, why doesn't Matthew exhibit the same symptoms as Jared?
3. What would you advise Jared to do to decrease his genetic susceptibility to diabetes?

to improving the quality of life for those individuals who have already developed a disease because specific nutrients will be used to alter biochemical outcomes.

In addition to working with therapies designed to improve existing disease conditions, nutrition professionals will have a deeper understanding of the underlying genetic and biochemical basis for disorders and a new set of tools that will focus on preventing disease through early detection and intervention. Nutrition professionals who have a strong base in genetics will be in higher demand.

Relevant Web Sites

Basic Genetics and Genomics
www.nhgri.nih.gov/DIR/VIP
www.ornl.gov/hgmis/project/info.html
www.genetics.com.au/
www.dnaftb.org/dnaftb
Core Competencies in Genetics Essential for All Health Care Professionals
www.nchpeg.org/core/core.asp
Ethical, Legal, and Social Issues
www.ornl.gov/hgmis/elsi/elsi.html
www.nhgri.nih.gov/ELSI
www.ornl.gov/hgmis/publicat/genechoice/index.html
Genetic Counseling
www.nsgc.org/
www.ornl.gov/hgmis/medicine/genecounseling.html
www.gradschools.com/biomed_health.html
Genetic Diseases and Testing
www.genetests.org
Genetics and Health
www.cdc.gov/genetics
www.ornl.gov/hgmis/medicine/medicine.html
Genetics Glossaries
www.genome.gov/
www.ornl.gov/TechResources/Human_Genome/glossary
Human Genome Project
www.nhgri.nih.gov
www.ornl.gov/hgmis/toc_expand.html
Genomics and Medicine
www.genetests.org
National Center for Biotechnology Information
www.ncbi.nlm.nih.gov/omim
www.ornl.gov/hgmis/publicat/primer2001
Public Health and Genetics
www.cdc.gov/genomics/training/competencies/default.html

Cited References

Ames BN et al: High-dose vitamin therapy stimulates variant enzymes with decreased coenzyme binding affinity (increased Km): relevance to genetic disease and polymorphisms, *Am J Clin Nutr* 75:616, 2002.

Bailey LB et al: Vitamin B-12 status is inversely associated with plasma homocysteine in young women with C677T and/or A1298C methylenetetrahydrofolate reductase polymorphisms, *J Nutr* 132:1872, 2002.

Baltimore D: Initial sequencing and analysis of the human genome, *Nature* 409:814, 2001.

Berger J, Wagner JA: Physiological and therapeutic roles of peroxisome proliferator-activated receptors, *Diabetes Technol Ther* 4:163, 2002.

Brown MS, Goldstein JL: The SREBP pathway: regulation of cholesterol metabolism by proteolysis of a membrane-bound transcription factor, *Cell* 89:331, 1997.

Chawla A et al: Nuclear receptors and lipid physiology: opening the X-files, *Science* 294:1866, 2001.

Clarke SD et al: Peroxisome proliferator-activated receptors: a family of lipid-activated transcription factors, *Am J Clin Nutr* 70:566, 1999.

DeBusk RM: *Genetics: the nutrition connection,* Chicago, 2002, American Dietetic Association.

Delerive P et al: Peroxisome proliferator-activated receptors in inflammation control, *J Endocrinol* 169:453, 2001.

DeLuca HF, Cantorna MT: Vitamin D: its role and uses in immunology, *FASEB J* 15:2579, 2001.

Dreon DM et al: Low-density lipoprotein subclass patterns and lipoprotein response to a reduced-fat diet in men, *FASEB J* 8:121-126, 1994.

Duffy VB, Bartoshuk LM: Food acceptance and genetic variation in taste, *J Am Diet Assoc* 100:647, 2000.

Edwards PA et al: BAREing it all: the adoption of LXR and FXR and their roles in lipid homeostasis, *J Lipid Res* 43:2, 2002.

Fohr IP et al: 5,10-Methylenetetrahydrofolate reductase genotype determines the plasma homocysteine-lowering effect of supplementation with 5-methyltetrahydrofolate or folic acid in healthy young women, *Am J Clin Nutr* 75:275, 2002.

Gyllensten U et al: Paternal inheritance of mitochondrial DNA in mice, *Nature* 352:255, 1991.

Hihi AK et al: PPARs: transcriptional effectors of fatty acids and their derivatives, *Cell Mol Life Sci* 59:790, 2002.

Horton JD et al: SREBPs: activators of the complete program of cholesterol and fatty acid synthesis in the liver, *J Clin Invest* 109:1125, 2002.

Human Genome Project Web sites: U.S. Department of Energy: www.ornl.gov/hgmis/project/info.html; and U.S. National Institutes of Health: www.nhgri.nih.gov., accessed 2003.

International Human Genome Sequencing Consortium: Initial sequencing and analysis of the human genome, *Nature* 409:860, 2001.

Jacobs MN, Lewis DF: Steroid hormone receptors and dietary ligands: a selected review, *Proc Nutr Soc* 61:105, 2002.

Jump DB: Dietary polyunsaturated fatty acids and regulation of gene transcription, *Curr Opin Lipidol* 13:155, 2002.

Kadowaki T et al: The role of PPARgamma in high-fat diet–induced obesity and insulin resistance, *J Diabetes Complications* 16:41, 2002.

Kang et al: Intermediate homocysteinemia: a thermolabile variant of methylenetetrahydrofolate reductase, *Am J Hum Genet* 43:414, 1988.

Kauwell GP et al: Methylenetetrahydrofolate reductase mutation (677C—>T) negatively influences plasma homocysteine response to marginal folate intake in elderly women, *Metabolism* 49:1440, 2000a.

Kauwell GP et al: Folate status of elderly women following moderate folate depletion responds only to a higher folate intake, *J Nutr* 130:1584, 2000b.

López-Miranda J et al: Dietary fat clearance in normal subjects is regulated by genetic variation in apolipoprotein B, *Arterioscler Thromb Vasc Biol* 17:1765, 1997.

Lu TT et al: Orphan nuclear receptors as eLiXiRs and FiXeRs of sterol metabolism, *J Biol Chem* 276:37735, 2001.

Magaña MM et al: Different sterol regulatory element-binding protein-1 isoforms utilize distinct co-regulatory factors to activate the promoter for fatty acid synthase, *J Biol Chem* 275:4726, 2000.

Marín C et al: Effects of the human apolipoprotein A-I promoter G-A mutation on postprandial lipoprotein metabolism, *Am J Clin Nutr* 76:319, 2002.
Mata P et al: Human apolipoprotein A-I gene promoter mutation influences plasma low density lipoprotein cholesterol response to dietary fat saturation, *Atherosclerosis* 137:367, 1998.
McCully KS: Vascular pathology of homocysteinemia: implications for the pathogenesis of arteriosclerosis, *Am J Pathol* 56:111, 1969.
Milner JA et al: Molecular targets for nutrients involved with cancer prevention, *Nutr Cancer* 41:1, 2001.
Müller-Wieland D, Kotzka J: SREBP-1: gene regulatory key to syndrome X? *Ann N Y Acad Sci* 967:19, 2002.
Müller-Wieland D et al: Insulin-regulated transcription factors: molecular link between insulin resistance and cardiovascular risk factors, *Int J Obes Relat Metab Disord* 25:S35, 2001.
Mural RJ et al: A comparison of whole-genome shotgun-derived mouse chromosome 16 and the human genome, *Science* 296:1661, 2002.
Nikkilä M et al: Postprandial plasma lipoprotein changes in relation to apolipoprotein E phenotypes and low density lipoprotein size in men with and without coronary artery disease, *Atherosclerosis* 106:149, 1994.
Norman AW et al: Ligands for the vitamin D endocrine system: different shapes function as agonists and antagonists for genomic and rapid response receptors or as a ligand for the plasma vitamin D binding protein, *J Steroid Biochem Mol Biol* 76:49, 2001.
Ostos MA et al: Dietary fat clearance is modulated by genetic variation in apolipoprotein A-IV gene locus, *J Lipid Res* 39:2493, 1998.
Report of the Committee of the Human Mitochondrial Genome, 2002, www.mitomap.org/mitomap/report.html.
Schwartz M, Vissing J: Paternal inheritance of mitochondrial DNA, *N Engl J Med* 347:576, 2002.
Shimano H: Sterol regulatory element-binding proteins (SREBPs): transcriptional regulators of lipid synthetic genes, *Prog Lipid Res* 40:439, 2001.
Shoffner JM, Wallace DC: Mitochondrial genetics: principles and practice, *Am J Hum Genet* 51:1179, 1992.
Sijbrands EJG et al: Mortality over two centuries in large pedigree with familial hypercholesterolaemia: family tree mortality study, *BMJ* 322:1019, 2001.
Stoeckman AK, Towle HC: The role of SREBP-1c in nutritional regulation of lipogenic enzyme gene expression, *J Biol Chem* 277:27029, 2002.
Tontonoz P et al: PPARgamma promotes monocyte/macrophage differentiation and uptake of oxidized LDL, *Cell* 93:241, 1998.
Venter JC et al: The sequence of the human genome, *Science* 291:1304, 2001.
Wallace DC, Lott MT: *MITOMAP: a human mitochondrial genome database,* University of Calif, Irvine, www.mitomap.org, 2003.
Wei LN: Retinoid receptors and their coregulators, *Annu Rev Pharmacol Toxicol* 10, 2002.
Weintraub MS et al: Dietary fat clearance in normal subjects is regulated by genetic variation in apolipoprotein E, *J Clin Invest* 80:1571, 1987.
Willson TM, Kliewer SA: PXR, CAR and drug metabolism, *Nat Rev Drug Discov* 1:259, 2002.
Xu J et al: Sterol regulatory element binding protein-1 expression is suppressed by dietary polyunsaturated fatty acids, *J Biol Chem* 274:23577, 1999.
Ye SQ, Kwiterovich Jr PO Jr: Influence of genetic polymorphisms on responsiveness to dietary fat and cholesterol, *Am J Clin Nutr* 72:S1275, 2000.
Zannis VI et al: Transcriptional regulation of the human apolipoprotein genes, *Front Biosci* 6:D456, 2001.

■ Additional References

Baker C: *Your genes, your choices,* 2002, ehrweb.aaas.org/ehr/books/index.html.
Bowers DF, Allred JB: Advances in molecular biology: implications for the future of clinical nutrition practice, *J Am Diet Assoc* 95:53, 1995.
Boyden LM et al: High bone density due to a mutation in LDL receptor-related protein 5, *N Engl J Med* 346:1513, 2002.
Clark DP et al: *Molecular biology made simple and fun,* ed 2, Vienna, Ill, 2000, Cache River Press.
Collins FS, Jegalian KG: Deciphering the code of life, *Sci Am* 281:86, 1999.
Collins FS, McKusick V: Implications of the Human Genome Project for medical science, *JAMA* 285:540, 2001.
Collins FS et al: New goals for the U.S. Human Genome Project: 1998-2003, *Science* 282:682, 1998.
Daniel H: Genomics and proteomics: importance for the future of nutrition research, *Br J Nutr* 87:S305, 2002.
Fafournoux P et al: Amino acid regulation of gene expression, *Biochem J* 351:1, 2000.
Ferraris RP: Dietary and developmental regulation of intestinal sugar transport, *Biochem J* 360:265, 2001.
Foufelle F, Ferre P: New perspectives in the regulation of hepatic glycolytic and lipogenic genes by insulin and glucose: a role for the transcription factor SREBP-1c, *Biochem J* 366(2):377, 2002.
Gennari L et al: Genetics of osteoporosis: role of steroid hormone receptor gene polymorphisms, *J Steroid Biochem Mol Biol* 81:1-24, 2002.
Guengerich FP: Functional genomics and proteomics applied to the study of nutritional metabolism, *Nutr Rev* 59:259, 2001.
Jorde LB et al: *Medical genetics,* ed 3, St Louis, 2002, Mosby.
Klug WS, Cummings MR: *Concepts of genetics,* ed 7, Upper Saddle River, NJ, 2003, Prentice Hall.
Klug WS, Cummings MR: *Genetics: a molecular perspective,* Upper Saddle River, NJ, 2003, Prentice Hall.
Konety BR, Getzenberg RH: Vitamin D and prostate cancer, *Urol Clin North Am* 29:95, 2002.
Moustaïd-Moussa N, Berdanier CD: *Nutrient-gene interactions in health and disease,* Boca Raton, Fla, 2001, CRC Press.
Ntambi JM, Bene H: Polyunsaturated fatty acid regulation of gene expression, *J Mol Neurosci* 16:273, 2001.
Nussbaum RL et al: *Thompson and Thompson genetics in medicine,* ed 6, Philadelphia, 2001, WB Saunders.
Nussbaum RL et al: Electronic image collection for *Thompson and Thompson genetics in medicine,* Philadelphia, 2002, WB Saunders.
Orphanides G, Reinberg D: A unified theory of gene expression, *Cell* 108:439, 2002.
Osborne TF: Sterol regulatory element-binding proteins (SREBPs): key regulators of nutritional homeostasis and insulin action, *J Biol Chem* 275:32379, 2000.
Patterson RE, Eaton DL, Potter JD: The genetic revolution: change and challenge for the dietetics profession, *J Am Diet Assoc* 99:1412, 1999.
Ren MQ et al: Isoflavones, substances with multi-biological and clinical properties, *Eur J Nutr* 40:135, 2001.
Schnyder G et al: Effect of homocysteine-lowering therapy with folic acid, vitamin B12, and vitamin B6 on clinical outcome after percutaneous coronary intervention. The Swiss Heart Study: a randomized controlled trial, *JAMA* 288:973, 2002.
Sigmund CD: Regulation of renin expression and blood pressure by vitamin D(3), *J Clin Invest* 110:155, 2002.
Understanding Gene Testing, The National Health Museum, www.accessexcellence.org/AE/AEPC/NIH/index.html.
Vaulont S et al: Glucose regulation of gene transcription, *J Biol Chem* 275:31555, 2000.

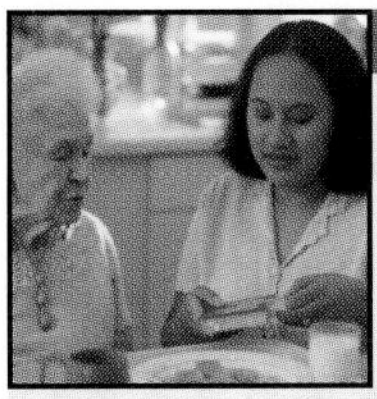

CHAPTER 17

Dietary and Clinical Assessment

KATHLEEN A. HAMMOND, MS, RD, LD, CNSD, RN, BSN, CNSN

CHAPTER OUTLINE

- Nutritional Imbalance
- Nutritional Screening
- Nutritional Assessment
- Nutrition-Focused Physical Examination
- Classifying Malnutrition

KEY TERMS

anthropometry–the science of measuring the size, weight, and proportions of the human body

bioelectrical impedance analysis (BIA)–a precise body composition analysis technique that uses a small electrical current to estimate total body water, fat-free mass, fat mass, and body cell mass

body mass index (BMI)–weight (kg)/height $(m)^2$; a definition of the degree of adiposity

dietary history–a detailed dietary record; may include a 24-hour recall, food frequency questionnaire, and other information such as weight history, previous diet changes, use of supplements, and food intolerances

dietary intake data–data about food consumption, including information on appetite, eating patterns, and estimations of typical nutrient intake

food diary–a written record of the amounts of all foods and liquids consumed during a set time, usually 3 to 7 days; often includes information on eating time, place, and situation

food frequency questionnaire–a method of dietary assessment in which the data collected relate to how often and in what amount foods are consumed (e.g., servings per week, month, or year)

height-for-age curve–assessment of stature for a child at a specific age, compared with a norm

kwashiorkor–a state of malnutrition characterized by preservation of somatic (body) fat stores and wasting of visceral proteins

marasmus–a state of malnutrition characterized by gradual wasting of somatic (body) fat and muscle stores and preservation of visceral proteins

nutrient intake analysis (NIA)–a process by which food, beverage, and supplement intake is evaluated for nutrient content over a specified time period

nutritional assessment–the science of determining nutritional status by analyzing an individual's medical, dietary, and social history; anthropometric data; biochemical data; clinical data; and drug-nutrient interactions

nutritional screening–a process used to identify nutritional problems and risk factors

nutritional status–a measurement of the extent to which an individual's physiologic need for nutrients is being met

24-hour recall–a method of dietary assessment in which an individual is asked to remember everything eaten during the previous 24 hours

waist circumference–the distance around the smallest area below the rib cage and above the umbilicus (belly button); provides a risk prediction for obesity-related disease; used in patients with a body mass index (BMI) of up to 35

weight-for-length curve–a standard for evaluating the growth of children that gives the percentile rankings for weight according to specific heights, but disregarding age

An individual's nutritional status reflects the degree to which physiologic needs for nutrients are being met. The balance between nutrient intake and nutrient requirements for optimal health is shown in Figure 17-1. Nutrient intake depends on actual food consumption, which is influenced by factors such as economic situation, eating behavior, emotional climate, cultural influences, effects of various disease states on appetite, and the ability to consume and absorb adequate nutrients. Nutrient requirements, are also influenced by many factors, including physiologic stressors such as infection, chronic or acute disease processes, fever, or trauma; normal anabolic states of growth, pregnancy, or rehabilitation; body maintenance and well-being; and psychological stress.

When adequate nutrients are consumed to support the body's daily needs and any increased metabolic demands, the person develops an optimal nutritional status. This status promotes growth and development, maintains general health, supports activities of daily living, and helps protect the body from disease and illness. Appropriate assessment techniques can detect a nutritional deficiency in the early stages of development, allowing dietary intake to be improved through nutritional support and counseling before a more severe condition develops.

A nutritional status assessment should be performed routinely for all individuals. However, the type of assessment for those who are basically healthy differs from assessments for those who are critically ill. Persons at nutritional risk can be identified on the basis of screening information that is routinely obtained at the time of admission to a hospital or nursing home or after returning to home-based care. Information obtained in the nutritional assessment is used to design an individual nutritional care plan (see Chapter 21). A thorough nutritional assessment increases the effectiveness of nutritional support and nutritional education/counseling (see Chapter 22).

NUTRITIONAL IMBALANCE

Nutrition is an important factor in the etiology and management of several major causes of death and disability in contemporary society. Atherosclerotic heart disease, obesity, hypertension, anemia, osteoporosis, diabetes, and cancer are common diseases in which nutrition is significantly involved. Table 17-1 shows the top ten causes of death in 1999 according to the *National Vital Statistics Reports* (2001).

Several of the leading causes of death, including coronary heart disease, stroke, diabetes, and some types of cancer, have a strong link with the type and amount of food consumed (*Healthy People 2010*, 2000). In addition, cirrhosis of the liver and some accidents

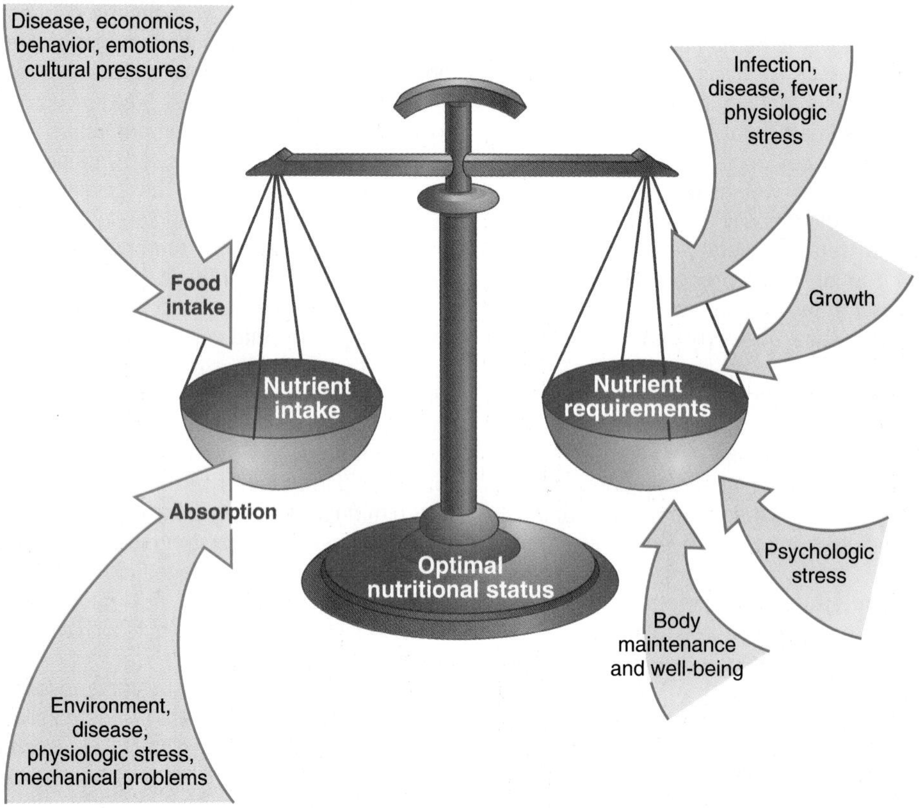

FIGURE 17-1 • Optimal nutritional status: a balance between nutrient intake and nutrient requirements.

may be associated with excessive alcohol intake. Modifications in dietary intake may assist in the prevention of some diseases and events, particularly overweight and obesity, which are included in the 10 major health issues for our nation (*Healthy People 2010,* 2000) (see Chapter 14).

States of nutritional deficiency or excess occur when the nutrient intake is not balanced with specific requirements for optimal health. Within the safe range of intake, homeostatic mechanisms of the body seem to use nutrients equally effectively, with no detectable advantage being gained by a given level of intake. As nutritional deficiencies or excesses develop, adaptations are made to achieve a new steady state without any significant loss in physiologic function. As the intake departs further from the accepted range, the organism accommodates to the changing supply of nutrients by reducing its function or changing the size or status of the affected body compartments. The nutritional status of an individual is determined by identifying the presence or absence of these adaptations (see figure in Appendix 33).

For example, before iron deficiency anemia develops (and is diagnosed by measures of hematocrit, hemoglobin, and appropriate clinical signs), a gradual diminution in iron stores can be diagnosed on the basis of increased iron absorption, decreased serum ferritin levels, or bone marrow evaluation (see Chapter 34).

When nutritional reserves are depleted or nutrient intake is inadequate to meet the body's daily metabolic needs, a state of *undernutrition* develops. Nutrient deficiency may stem from inadequate ingestion, impaired digestion or absorption, dysfunctional metabolic processing, or increased excretion of essential nutrients. Infants, children, pregnant females, individuals with low incomes, hospitalized persons, and older adults are at the greatest risk for becoming undernourished. Undernourishment may result in impaired growth and development, lowered resistance to infection, poor wound healing, and poor clinical outcome with increased morbidity and mortality.

It is estimated that in academic hospitals in the United States, 25% of patients show some type of malnutrition, marasmus (generalized wasting), or protein depletion (kwashiorkor). Other studies show that approximately 50% of hospitalized patients exhibit signs of moderate malnutrition (Pfau and Rombeau, 2000).

Overnutrition also presents major nutritional problems, manifesting as obesity and related disease states such as diabetes, atherosclerotic heart disease, hypertension, and the metabolic syndrome. These conditions may also result in poor clinical outcomes with increased morbidity and mortality. Overweight and obesity have reached epidemic proportions in the United States. In 1999, approximately 61% of adults were overweight or obese, and 13% of children and adolescents were overweight. Today, almost two times more children and about three times more adolescents are overweight than were overweight in 1980. These staggering statistics are associated with approximately 300,000 deaths per year related to overweight and obesity (*The Surgeon General's Call to Action to Prevent and Decrease Overweight and Obesity,* 2001) (see Chapter 24).

The evaluation of nutrient deficiencies consists of a review of dietary and medical histories, weight, physical examination, laboratory evaluation (see Chapter 18), and review of the use of medications and herbal products (see Chapters 19 and 20). Figure 17-2 illustrates the general sequence of steps leading to the development of a nutritional deficiency, as well as areas in which an assessment can identify problems and clinical intervention can prevent poor nutrition before it develops.

Many different factors help measure whether a person is at *nutritional risk* (Table 17-2). Factors to consider include food and nutrient intake patterns, psychosocial factors, physical conditions associated with particular disease states and disorders, biochemical abnormalities, and medication regimens (Council on Practice, 1994).

Nutritional screening and assessment are integral parts of *medical nutrition therapy (MNT),* which is the use of specific nutritional interventions to treat an illness, injury, or condition (Council on Practice, 1994). MNT has two phases: (1) assessment of nutritional status and (2) treatment, which may include diet therapy, counseling, or specialized nutritional supplementation. To provide cost-effective MNT in today's health care environment, it is important to first identify patients who are at nutritional risk. Nutritional screening and nutritional assessment are the first steps in this identification process.

TABLE 17-1 Leading Causes of Death in the United States, 1999

CAUSE OF DEATH	RANK	PERCENTAGE OF TOTAL DEATHS*
Diseases of the heart	1	30.3
Malignant neoplasms, including lymphatic and hematopoietic tissues	2	23.0
Cerebrovascular diseases	3	7.0
Chronic obstructive pulmonary diseases and allied conditions	4	5.2
Accidents and adverse effects	5	4.1
Diabetes mellitus	6	2.9
Pneumonia and influenza	7	2.7
Alzheimer's disease	8	1.9
Nephritis, nephrotic syndrome, and nephrosis	9	1.5
Septicemia	10	1.3

Modified from Anderson RN: Deaths: leading causes for 1999, *Natl Vital Stat Rep* 49(11):8, 2001 and Centers for Disease Control and Prevention, National Center for Health Statistics, Vital Statistics, Hyattsville, Md.

*Percentages do not add up to 100 because of other causes of death in addition to the top 10.

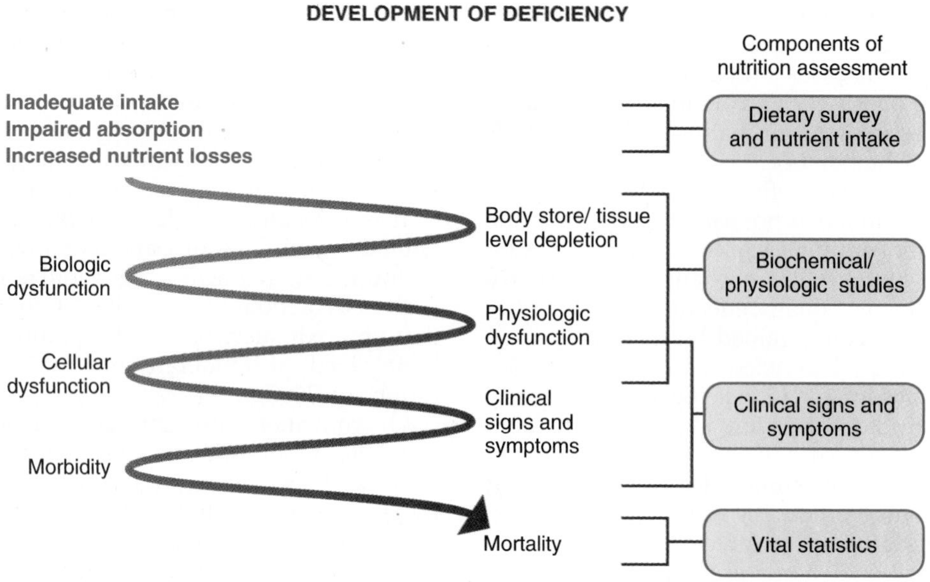

FIGURE 17-2 • Development of clinical nutritional deficiency with corresponding dietary, biochemical, and clinical evaluations.

NUTRITIONAL SCREENING

Ideally, everyone should undergo periodic nutritional status screening and assessment throughout their lives, not just when they are ill. Different approaches are used for those who are critically ill. Although the assessment process involves two phases—screening and assessment—the components of nutritional screening and assessment may vary slightly from one setting to another.

Nutritional screening begins the nutrition assessment process. A nutritional screening is the process of identifying characteristics known to be associated with nutritional problems. The purpose of a nutritional screen is to quickly identify individuals who are malnourished or at nutritional risk and determine whether a more detailed assessment is warranted (ASPEN, 2002; Council on Practice, 1994). The nutritional screen can usually be completed by a dietitian, dietetic technician, nurse, physician, or other qualified health-care professional. In many settings the nutritional screen is completed by a health professional other than the dietitian; once completed though, patients who are at nutritional risk are usually referred to a registered dietitian. Box 17-1 outlines the characteristics of a nutritional screening tool.

The information collected during a nutritional screen depends on (1) the setting in which the information is obtained (e.g., home, clinic, hospital), (2) the population group (e.g., older adults, pregnant females, patients with cancer), (3) the type of data that can easily be obtained, (4) a definition of risk, and (5) the goals of the screen. Examples of information that may be obtained using a screening tool include height, usual body weight, recent or significant loss or increase in weight; diagnosis; whether the person is receiving a modified diet for a particular disease, intravenous (parenteral) or tube feeding (enteral nutrition), or nothing by mouth (NPO); laboratory values, such as serum albumin, hemoglobin and hematocrit, and total lymphocyte levels; a history of gastrointestinal (GI) disturbances, such as distention, diarrhea, or nausea and vomiting; functional status (as determined by hand-grip dynamometry); and current medication and herbal product profile.

Regardless of the information gathered, the goal of screening is to identify individuals who are at nutritional risk or are likely to become at nutritional risk, as well as to identify those who need further assessment and the best source for that assessment. Several screening tools exist. Box 17-2 is a short screening tool used for patients who are not suspected to be at risk. Box 17-3 is a nutritional questionnaire that can be used in a clinic setting, where a patient can complete it while waiting for an appointment. Figure 17-3 is an example of a nutritional screen used in an acute care setting, whereas the questionnaire in Figure 17-4 is used in a perinatal service and Figure 17-5 is an example of a screen that could be used in a pediatric practice.

The Nutrition Screening Initiative, a joint project of the American Academy of Physicians, the American Dietetic Association, and the National Council on the Aging, was developed to focus specifically on and improve the nutritional care available to older adults (*Nutrition Interventions Manual,* 1991). These tools are simple, brief, and generic and are designed to be flexible, allowing adaptation for particular

TABLE 17-2 Nutritional Risk Factors

RISK CATEGORY	RISK FACTORS
Food and nutrient intake patterns	• Calorie and protein intake greater or less than that required for age and activity level • Vitamin and mineral intake greater or less than that required for age • Swallowing difficulties • Gastrointestinal disturbances • Unusual food habits (e.g., pica) • Impaired cognitive function or depression • Nothing by mouth for more than 3 days • Inability or unwillingness to consume food • Increase or decrease in activities of daily living • Misuse of supplements • Inadequate transitional feeding, tube feeding or parenteral nutrition, or both • Bowel irregularity (e.g., constipation, diarrhea) • Restricted diet • Feeding limitations
Psychological and social factors	• Low literacy • Language barriers • Cultural or religious factors • Emotional disturbances associated with feeding difficulties (e.g., depression) • Limited resources for food preparation or obtaining food and supplies • Alcohol or drug addiction • Limited or low income • Lack of or inability to communicate needs • Limited use or understanding of community resources
Physical conditions	• Extreme age: adults older than 80 years, premature infants, very young children • Pregnancy: adolescent, closely spaced, or three or more pregnancies • Alterations in anthropometric measurements: marked overweight or underweight for height, age, or both; head circumference less than normal; depressed somatic fat and muscle stores; amputation • Fat or muscle wasting • Obesity or overweight • Chronic renal or cardiac disease and related complications • Diabetes and related complications • Pressure ulcers or altered skin integrity • Cancer and related treatments • Acquired immune deficiency syndrome • Gastrointestinal complications (e.g., malabsorption, diarrhea, digestive or bowel changes) • Catabolic or hypermetabolic stress (e.g., trauma, sepsis, burns, stress) • Immobility • Osteoporosis, osteomalacia • Neurologic impairments, including impairment in sensory function • Visual impairments
Abnormal laboratory values	• Visceral proteins (e.g., albumin, transferrin, prealbumin) • Lipid profile (cholesterol, high-density lipoproteins, low-density lipoproteins, triglycerides) • Hemoglobin, hematocrit, and other hematologic tests • Blood urea nitrogen, creatinine, electrolyte levels • Fasting serum blood glucose level • Other laboratory indexes as indicated
Medications	• Chronic use • Multiple and concurrent administration (polypharmacy) • Drug-nutrient interactions and side effects

Data from Council on Practice, Quality Management Committee: ADA's definitions for nutrition screening and nutrition assessment, *J Am Diet Assoc* 94:838, 1994.

patient populations (Nutrition Screening Initiative, 1991). Three tools are available that focus attention on nutrition in older adults:

1. The DETERMINE Your Nutritional Health checklist is a public awareness tool designed to highlight the warning signs of poor nutritional status (see Figures 13-5 and 13-6).
2. The Level I Screen (Figure 17-6) is a tool to identify individuals who should be referred for a more comprehensive nutritional or medical follow-up, in addition to other health and community services (Barrocas et al, 1995; Nutrition Screening Initiative, 1991).
3. The Level II Screen (Figure 17-7) is used when the checklist or Level I Screen identifies potentially serious nutrition or medical problems. This screen incorporates nutritional screening and assessment measures (Barrocas et al, 1995; Nutrition Screening Initiative, 1991).

NUTRITIONAL ASSESSMENT

Nutritional assessment, according to the American Dietetic Association (Council on Practice, 1994), is a comprehensive approach—carried out by a registered dietitian—for defining nutritional status using medical, social, nutritional, and medication histories; physical examination; anthropometric measurements; and laboratory data. Nutritional assessment involves interpretation of data from the nutritional screen and incorporates additional information. The nutrition assessment organizes and evaluates the information gathered to make a professional judgment about nutritional status (ASPEN, 2002). Once the nutritional assessment process is complete, the nutritional plan of care can be developed, implemented, and tailored for the appropriate setting (e.g., hospital, clinic, home).

The goals of nutritional assessment are to (1) identify individuals who require aggressive nutritional support, (2) restore or maintain an individual's nutritional status, (3) identify appropriate medical nutrition therapies, and (4) monitor the efficacy of these

Box 17-1. Characteristics of a Nutritional Screen

- Is simple and can be completed quickly
- Relies on data that are routinely gathered in a particular setting
- Facilitates completion of early intervention goals
- Includes collection of relevant data on risk factors and data interpretation for intervention or treatment
- Determines the need for a nutrition assessment
- Is cost-effective

Data from Council on Practice Quality Management Committee: ADA's definitions for nutrition screening and nutrition assessment, *J Am Diet Assoc* 94:838, 1994.

Box 17-2. Example of a Short Nutritional Screen

O: Diagnosis
Diet order
A: Per review of medical record; patient is not nutritionally compromised at this time.
P: Will reevaluate in 5 to 7 days or per consult

Signature: ______________

O, Objective; *A*, assessment; *P*, plan.

Box 17-3. Nutritional Questionnaire

1. Height: __________ Usual weight: __________ Actual weight: __________
2. Have you had a recent weight loss of greater than 10 lb within 30 days?
3. Have you been on a weight reduction diet? ____ yes ____ no
4. Have you had a recent change in appetite? ____ yes ____ no
5. Do you have any problems with: swallowing? ____ yes ____ no
   chewing? ____ yes ____ no
   nausea? ____ yes ____ no
   diarrhea? ____ yes ____ no
   vomiting? ____ yes ____ no
   constipation? ____ yes ____ no
6. Do you follow any special diet? ____ yes ____ no
   If yes, what type of diet? ______________
7. What foods are you allergic to?
8. Do you take any vitamin/mineral supplements? ____ yes ____ no
   If yes, please list: ______________
9. Do you take any medications?
   If yes, please list:

	Prescription	*Over-the-counter*

interventions. Studies indicate that when admitted to acute care facilities, between 33% and 65% of all patients have some degree of malnutrition. Furthermore, the nutritional status of patients who are hospitalized for longer than 2 weeks deteriorates (see *Focus On:* Malnutrition in Hospitals). All patients with acute or chronic illnesses have the potential for malnutrition and should be evaluated. Malnutrition is not uncommon in those who are obese, cachexic, older, or traumatized.

Histories

The information collected about individuals or populations is used as part of the nutritional status assessment. Frequently the information is in the form of histories—medical, social, dietary, and medication.

Medical and Social Histories

The medical history usually includes the following information: chief complaint, present and past illness, current health, allergies, past or recent surgeries, family history of disease, psychosocial aspects, and a review of problems—by body system—from the patient's perspective (Hammond, 1998). These histories usually provide much insight into nutrition-related problems. Alcohol and drug use, increased metabolic needs, increased nutritional losses, chronic disease, recent major surgery or illness, disease or

NUTRITION SERVICES SCREENING ASSESSMENT FORM

ADDRESSOGRAPH

Admission Date: ____________

Medical Record Review

Diagnosis ____________ Age ____________

Ht. ______ Wt. ______ IBW ______ % IBW ______ UBW ______ % UBW ______

Albumin ______ Other Labs ____________

Appetite: >50% ≤50% Poor

Medication ____________

Other ____________

Diet Order______Date______Diet Order______Date______Diet Order______Date______

Evaluation Criteria *(Check all that apply)*

☐ Loss of appetite >48 hr.
☐ Difficulty chewing/swallowing
☐ Significant food allergies/intolerances
☐ Malnourished appearance
☐ Length of stay ≥7 days
☐ >65 years of age with a surgery this admission
☐ <50% meals consumed
☐ Modified diet ____________

Pt. identified to be at nutritional risk based on meeting >2 criteria above.

Plan

Pt. not at high nutritional risk at this time. Basic nutritional care services and follow-up will be provided per policy.
☐ Pt. seen for snacks/food preferences.
☐ Pt. to receive comfort measures only. No intervention planned unless requested/ordered by staff or pt.
☐ Pt./care provider familiar with dietary modifications. No education planned.
☐ Other ____________

X ____________
Signature Date

Nutrition Services Screening Assessment Form

3/97
Piedmont Graphics

Original - Chart
Yellow - Department

FIGURE 17-3 • Nutrition screen. (*IBW,* Ideal body weight; *UBW,* usual body weight.) (Courtesy Northside Hospital, Atlanta, Ga.)

Perinatal Nutrition Screening/Assessment Form

ADDRESSOGRAPH

SCREENING CRITERIA FOR POTENTIAL NUTRITIONAL RISK *(full assessment if one checked)*

SCREENING CRITERIA FOR POTENTIAL NUTRITIONAL RISK

ANTEPARTUM

- ☐ Obstetrical Condition (Multiple Gestation, PIH, IUGR, Diabetes, Hyperemesis, Anemia)
- ☐ Chronic/Systemic Condition Affecting Nutritional Status or Intake
- ☐ Adolescence (≤17 years)
- ☐ Inappropriate Weight Change
- ☐ Albumin ≤2.5 mg/dl
- ☐ Therapeutic or Limited Diet
- ☐ Lack of Knowledge re Pregnancy Diet
- ☐ Length of Stay ≥5 days

POSTPARTUM

☐ Gestational Diabetes this Pregnancy ☐ Albumin ≤2.5 mg/dl ☐ Hg <8.0 g/dl

Breastfeeding mother meeting the following criteria:

- ☐ ≤17 Years Old
- ☐ Therapeutic or Limited Diet
- ☐ Lack of Knowledge re Lactation Diet
- ☐ Multiple Birth with Infants in Special Care Nursery

COMPREHENSIVE ASSESSMENT

SUBJECTIVE

Weight Gain/Expected Weight Gain ______

Cultural/Social Concerns ______

Activity Level ______

Plans to Breastfeed? ☐ Yes ☐ No

Other ______

OBJECTIVE

Diagnosis ______ Parity ______ EGA/EDC ______

Medical/Obstetrical History ______

Age ______ Ht ______ Pregravid Wt ______ BMI ______ Current Wt ______

Medications ______ Vitamin/Mineral Supplements ______

Physical Exam ______ GI Function ______

Food Allergies/Intolerance ______ Diet Order ______

Labs ______

ASSESSMENT

Estimated Energy Needs ______ Protein ______ Other ______

Adequacy of Intake/Evaluation of Nutritional Status ______

FIGURE 17-4 • Perinatal nutrition assessment form. (*PIH,* Pregnancy-induced hypertension; *IUGR,* intrauterine growth retardation; *EGA,* estimated gestational age; *EDC,* estimated date of confinement; *BMI,* body mass index.) (Courtesy Northside Hospital, Atlanta, Ga.)

Shriners Burns Hospital
Rehabilitation Nutrition Screening Form

Date: ______________________ Level ______________________

Name: ______________________ Unit# ______________________

Age ____ __M __F

Birthdate ______________________

Reason for admission ______________________

Weight ____ ____ %NCHS
Height ____ ____ %NCHS

Recent weight loss/gain ____Y ____N
If yes, intended ____Y ____N
How much ______
Time frame ______

Recent: ____Nausea ____Vomiting TX:____
____Diarrhea ____Constipation
____HX of anemia ____Change in appetite
____Dentition concerns ____Difficulty swallowing

Food allergies ____N ____Y ______________________

Diet restrictions ____N ____Y ______________________

Cooking facilities ____Stove ____Refrigerator

Drinks ____Bottle ____Straw ____Sippee cup ____Cup

Vitamin supplementation ____N ____Y Type ____
Reason ____

Medications ____N ____Y Type(s) ____
Reason ____

Caretaker/relationship ______________________

Nutritional concerns stated by patient/caretaker:

Nutritional intervention proposed:

FIGURE 17-5 • Pediatric screening form. (Courtesy Shriners Burn Hospital, Cincinnati, Ohio.)

surgery of the GI tract, and recent significant weight loss all may contribute to malnutrition. In older patients, an additional review is recommended to detect mental deterioration, constipation or incontinence, poor eyesight or hearing, slowed reactions, major organ diseases, effects of prescription and over-the-counter drugs, and physical disabilities (Box 17-4).

Social aspects of the medical history may also relate to nutritional status, aspects such as information pertaining to socioeconomic status, the individual's ability to purchase food independently, whether the person is living or eating alone, physical or mental handicaps, smoking, or drug or alcohol addiction. In older adults, confusion caused by environmental changes, unsuitable housing conditions, lack of socialization at meals, psychological problems, or poverty may add to the risks.

Knowledge of various cultures is important during the interviewing process to meet the needs of diverse groups of clients (Curry, 2000; Spruhan, 1996). Components or factors that affect a person's cultural values include religious beliefs; rituals; symbols; language; dietary practices; education; communication style; views on health, wellness, and illness; and racial identity. Establishing a bond with clients of different cultures is important for positive outcomes (Heineken and McCoy, 2000) (see *Clinical Insight:* Cultural Awareness) (see Chapter 15).

Medication History

Food and drugs interact in many ways that affect nutritional status and drug therapy effectiveness, so a medication history is an important part of any nutritional assessment. Those who are older, are chronically ill, have a history of marginal or inadequate nutritional intake, or are receiving multiple drugs for a period are susceptible to drug-induced nutritional deficiencies. The effects of drug therapy can be altered by specific foods and the timing of food and meal consumption (see Chapter 19 and Appendix 34). Use of herbal products may also alter the effects of medications (see Appendix 35).

Nutrition or Diet History

Anorexia, ageusia, dysgeusia, loss of smell, excessive alcohol intake, poor-fitting dentures, fad dieting, chewing or swallowing problems, frequent meals away from home, adverse food and drug interactions, cultural or religious restrictions of diet, an inability to eat for more than 7 to 10 days, intravenous fluid therapy for more than 5 days, taste changes, or feeding dependence can lead to inadequate nutrient intake and nutritional inadequacy. For many older adults, the inability to eat independently, denture problems, changes in taste and smell, long-established poor

LEVEL I SCREEN

LEVEL I SCREEN

Name:

Date:

Body Weight

Measure height to the nearest inch, and weigh to the nearest pound. Record the values below and mark them on the Body Mass Index (BMI) scale to the right. Then use a straightedge (ruler) to connect the two points and circle the spot where this straight line crosses the center line (body mass index). Record the number below.

Healthy older adults should have a BMI between 24 and 27.

Height (in): ____________________

Weight (lb): ____________________

Body Mass Index: ____________________
(number from center column)

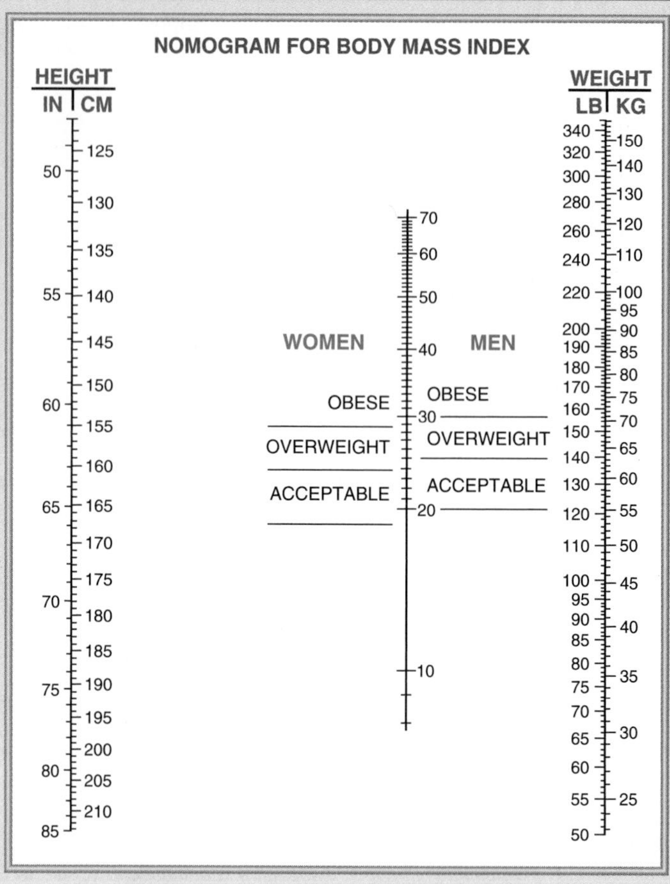

Check any boxes that are true for the individual:

- ☐ Has lost or gained 10 pounds (or more) in the past 6 months.
- ☐ Body mass index <24
- ☐ Body mass index >27

A physician should be contacted if the individual has gained or lost 10 pounds unexpectedly or without intending to during the past 6 months. A physician should also be notified if the individual's body mass index is above 27 or below 20.

For the remaining sections, please ask the individual which of the statements (if any) is true for him or her and place a check by each that applies.

Eating Habits

- ☐ Does not have enough to eat each day
- ☐ Usually eats alone
- ☐ Does not eat anything on one or more days each month
- ☐ Has poor appetite
- ☐ Is on a special diet
- ☐ Eats vegetables two or fewer times daily
- ☐ Eats milk or milk products once or not at all daily
- ☐ Eats fruit or drinks fruit juice once or not at all daily
- ☐ Eats breads, cereals, pasta, rice, or other grains five or fewer times daily
- ☐ Has difficulty chewing or swallowing
- ☐ Has more than one alcoholic drink per day (if woman); more than two drinks per day (if man)
- ☐ Has pain in mouth, teeth, or gums

Living Environment

- ☐ Lives on an income of less than $6000 per year (per individual in the household)
- ☐ Lives alone
- ☐ Is housebound
- ☐ Is concerned about home security
- ☐ Lives in a home with inadequate heating or cooling
- ☐ Does not have a stove and/or refrigerator
- ☐ Is unable or prefers not to spend money on food (<$25–$35 per person spent on food each week)

Functional Status

Usually or always needs assistance with (check all that apply):

- ☐ Bathing
- ☐ Dressing
- ☐ Grooming
- ☐ Toileting
- ☐ Eating
- ☐ Walking or moving about
- ☐ Traveling (outside the home)
- ☐ Preparing food
- ☐ Shopping for food or other necessities

If you have checked one or more statements on this screen, the individual you have interviewed may be at risk for poor nutritional status. Please refer this individual to the appropriate health care or social service professional in your area. For example, a dietitian should be contacted for problems with selecting, preparing, or eating a healthy diet, or a dentist if the individual experiences pain or difficulty when chewing or swallowing. Those individuals whose income, life-style, or functional status may endanger their nutritional and overall health should be referred to available community services: home-delivered meals, congregate meal programs, transportation systems, counseling services, day-care programs, etc.

Please repeat this screen at least once each year — sooner if the individual has a major change in his or her health, income, immediate family (e.g., spouse dies), or functional status.

FIGURE 17-6 • Level I screen. (Courtesy Nutrition Screening Initiative, Washington, DC, and Ross Products Division, Abbott Laboratories, Columbus, Ohio.)

LEVEL II SCREEN

Complete the following screen by interviewing the patient directly and/or by referring to the patient chart. If you do not routinely perform all of the described tests or ask all of the listed questions, please consider including them, but do not be concerned if the entire screen is not completed. Try to conduct a minimal screen on as many older patients as possible; and try to collect serial measurements, which are extremely valuable in monitoring nutritional status. Please refer to the manual for additional information.

Anthropometrics

Measure height to the nearest inch and weigh to the nearest pound. Record the values below and mark them on the Body Mass Index (BMI) scale to the right. Then use a straightedge (paper, ruler) to connect the two points and circle the spot where this straight line crosses the center line (body mass index). Record the number below. Healthy older adults should have a BMI between 24 and 27; check the appropriate box to flag an abnormally high or low value.

Height (in): ______________________

Weight (lb): ______________________

Body Mass Index: ______________________
(number from center column)

Please place a check by any statement regarding BMI and recent weight loss that is true for the patient:

- ☐ Body mass index <20
- ☐ Body mass index >27
- ☐ Has lost or gained 10 pounds (or more) in the past 6 months.

Record the measurement of mid-arm circumference to the nearest 0.1 centimeter and of triceps skinfold to the nearest millimeter (m).

Mid-arm circumference (cm): ______________________

Triceps skinfold (mm): ______________________

Mid-arm muscle circumference (cm): ______________________

Refer to the table and check any abnormal values:

- ☐ Mid-arm muscle circumference <10th percentile
- ☐ Triceps skinfold <10th percentile
- ☐ Triceps skinfold >95th percentile

Note: mid-arm circumference (cm) – {0.314 × triceps skinfold (mm)} = mid-arm *muscle* circumference (cm)

Percentile	Men		Women	
	55–65 y	65–75 y	55–65 y	65–75 y
Arm circumference (cm)				
10th	27.3	26.3	25.7	25.2
50th	31.7	30.7	30.3	29.9
95th	36.9	35.5	38.5	37.3
Arm muscle circumference (cm)				
10th	24.5	23.5	19.6	19.5
50th	27.8	26.8	22.5	22.5
95th	32.0	30.6	28.0	27.9
Triceps skinfold (mm)				
10th	6	6	16	14
50th	11	11	25	24
95th	22	22	22	36

For the remaining sections, please place a check by any statements that are true for the patient.

Laboratory Data

- ☐ Serum albumin below 3.5 g/dl
- ☐ Serum cholesterol below 160 mg/dl
- ☐ Serum cholesterol above 240 mg/dl

Drug Use

- ☐ Three or more prescription drugs, OTC medications, and/or vitamin/mineral supplements daily

Clinical Features

Presence of (check all that apply)

- ☐ Problems with mouth, teeth, or gums
- ☐ Difficulty chewing
- ☐ Angular stomatitis
- ☐ Glossitis
- ☐ History of bone pain
- ☐ History of bone fractures
- ☐ Skin changes (dry, loose, nonspecific lesions, edema)

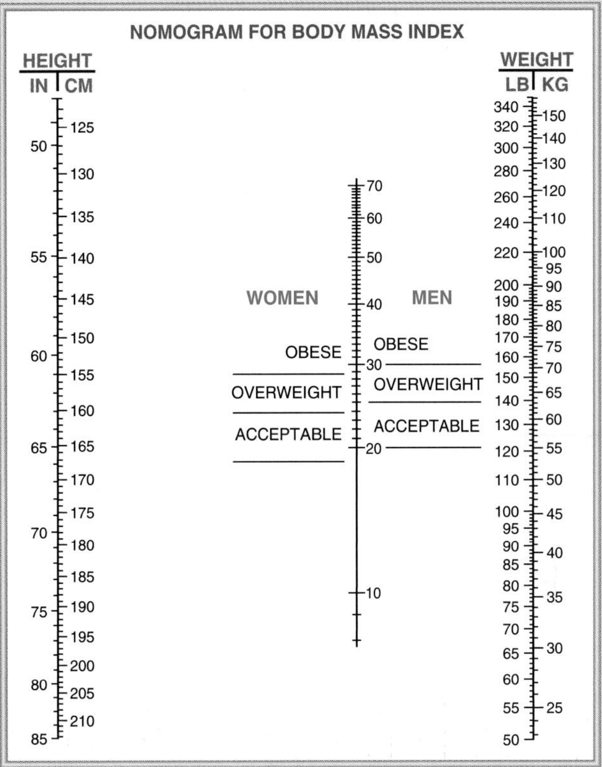

Eating Habits

- ☐ Does not have enough to eat each day
- ☐ Usually eats alone
- ☐ Does not eat anything on one or more days each month
- ☐ Has poor appetite
- ☐ Is on a special diet
- ☐ Eats vegetables two or fewer times daily
- ☐ Eats milk or milk products once or not at all daily
- ☐ Eats fruit or drinks fruit juice once or not at all daily
- ☐ Eats breads, cereals, pasta, rice, or other grains five or fewer times daily
- ☐ Has more than one alcoholic drink per day (if woman); more than two drinks per day (if man)

Living Environment

- ☐ Lives on an income of less than $6000 per year (per individual in the household)
- ☐ Lives alone
- ☐ Is housebound
- ☐ Is concerned about home security
- ☐ Lives in a home with inadequate heating or cooling
- ☐ Does not have a stove and/or refrigerator
- ☐ Is unable or prefers not to spend money on food (<$25–$35 per person spent on food each week)

Functional Status

Usually or always needs assistance with (check all that apply)

- ☐ Bathing
- ☐ Dressing
- ☐ Grooming
- ☐ Toileting
- ☐ Eating
- ☐ Walking or moving about
- ☐ Traveling (outside the home)
- ☐ Preparing food
- ☐ Shopping for food or other necessities

Mental/Cognitive Status

- ☐ Clinical evidence of impairment (e.g., Folstein <26)
- ☐ Clinical evidence of depressive illness (e.g., Beck Depression Inventory >15, Geriatric Depression Scale >5)

LEVEL II SCREEN

Name:

Date:

FIGURE 17-7 • Level II screen. (Courtesy Nutrition Screening Initiative, Washington, DC, and Ross Products Division, Abbott Laboratories, Columbus, Ohio.)

FOCUS ON

Malnutrition in Hospitals

In a landmark article, Butterworth (1974) showed that malnutrition could indeed be found in the United States—in hospitals, where it was frequently not recognized. Over the course of the next few years, malnutrition was noted in many hospitalized patients, and attempts were made to evaluate its severity and reverse its course. The past 30 years have had periods of heightened awareness and periods of minimal awareness. With only minimal training in nutrition (e.g., nutrition courses spread throughout the curriculum or having very few hours in nutrition studies) offered in many medical schools, physicians graduate with little practical knowledge about nutrition and therefore little awareness of malnutrition. To maintain a high level of awareness, physician education programs in nutrition should be conducted regularly. The American Dietetic Association has provided a Physician Nutrition Education program for many years. In this program, physicians, dietitians, and office staff team up to help patients screen their own eating habits using the Food Guide Pyramid (see Chapter 15). If problems are identified, the practitioner then refers the patient to a dietitian or qualified nutrition educator for follow-up services.

food habits, food fads, and inadequate knowledge of nutrition are common problems. Alternative nutrition therapies, including use of megadoses of vitamins and minerals, various herbs, macrobiotic diets, probiotics, and amino acid supplements, must be addressed because they have an effect on the person's health care.

A dietary history is perhaps the best means of obtaining dietary intake information (Box 17-5). The term *dietary history* refers to a review of an individual's usual patterns of food intake and the food selection variables that dictate the food intake. Dietary intake data are assessed either by collecting retrospective intake data or summarizing prospective intake data. Each method has specific purposes, strengths, and weaknesses. The choice depends on the purpose and setting in which the assessment is completed. The goal is to determine the nutrient content of the food and the appropriateness of the intake for a particular individual. The prospective method involves recording data at the time the food is consumed or shortly thereafter.

Nutrient Intake Analysis

A nutrient intake analysis (NIA) is also referred to as *nutrient intake record* or *calorie count,* depending on the setting and information collected. The NIA is a tool used in various settings to identify nutritional inadequacies by monitoring intakes before deficiencies develop. Information about actual intake is collected through direct observation or an inventory of foods eaten based on observation of what remains on the individual's tray or plate.

NIAs should be recorded for 72 hours. Complete records for this period usually accurately reflect an average intake for most individuals. If the record is incomplete, it may be necessary to extend the duration of the intake until a full 72-hour record can be completed. It should be kept in mind that eating habits or meals consumed during the weekend and during the week may differ.

The results of the NIA can be charted daily or at the end of the 3 days. The patient or a family member can participate by recording on a menu or a special form what was eaten. A graph, which can be kept in the patient's room or outside the door, can be used to record all types of dietary intake, including enteral or parental nutrition. The record of intake can then be analyzed for its nutrient content using one of several available computerized methods.

Daily Food Record or Diary

A daily food record, or food diary, involves documenting dietary intake as it occurs and is often used in outpatient clinic settings (Figure 17-8). A food record is usually most accurate if the food eaten is recorded on the same day. The individual's nutrient intake is calculated and averaged at the end of the desired period (usually 3 to 7 days) and then compared with dietary reference intakes (DRIs) or guidelines in the Food Pyramid Guide.

Retrospective Data

Retrospective data are obtained from recollection. Two examples of this form of data collection are the *food frequency questionnaire* and the *24-hour recall.*

Food Frequency

The food frequency questionnaire is a retrospective review of intake frequency—that is, food consumed per day, per week, or per month. For ease of evaluation the food frequency chart organizes foods into groups that have common nutrients (Box 17-6). Because the focus of the food frequency questionnaire is the frequency of consumption of food groups rather than of specific nutrients, the information obtained is general—not specific for certain nutrients. During illness, food consumption patterns can change depending on the stage of illness. Therefore it is helpful to

Box 17-4. Factors Associated With Risk of Poor Nutritional Status in Older Americans

Inappropriate Food Intake

Meal and Snack Frequency
- Inadequate intake
- Skipping of one or more meals daily
- Replacement of meals by snacks that are not nutritious

Inadequate Quantity and Quality
- Milk and milk products
- Meat and meat substitutes
- Fruits and vegetables
- Breads and cereals

Excess Fats or Sweets
- Use of desserts, sweetened beverages more than twice daily
- Exclusion of nutrient-dense foods

Dietary Modifications
- Self-imposed
- Prescribed
- Poor compliance
- Impact on intake, appetite

Alcohol Use or Abuse
- Chronicity
- Frequency

Dependency/Disability

Functional Status
- Problems with daily activities
- Inactivity, immobility

Disabling Conditions
- Lack of manual dexterity
- Need for assistive devices

Acute and Chronic Diseases or Conditions

Abnormalities of Body Weight
Cognitive or Emotional Impairments
- Depression
- Dementias

Oral Health Problems
Pressure Ulcers
Sensory Impairments
Other Medical Conditions

Chronic Medication Use

Prescribed or Self-Administered
Polypharmacy
Nutritional Supplements
Use of Unusual Remedies

Advanced Age
- Older than 80 years
- Older than 90 years
- 100+ years

Poverty

Income
- Source
- Adequacy

Food Expenditures and Resources
- Food
- Housing
- Medical
- Other
- Adequacy

Social Isolation

Support Systems
- Availability
- Use

Living Arrangements
- Cooking and food storage
- Transportation
- Other

Modified from Nutrition Screening Initiative: *Incorporating nutrition screening and interventions into medical practice: a monograph for physicians,* Washington, DC, June 1994, The Initiative.

complete food frequency questionnaires for the period immediately before hospitalization and before illness to obtain a complete and accurate history.

24-Hour Recall

The 24-hour recall method of data collection requires individuals to remember the specific foods and amounts of foods they consumed in the past 24 hours. The information is then analyzed by the person or professional gathering the information. Problems commonly associated with this method of data collection include (1) an inability to recall accurately the kinds and amounts of food eaten, (2) difficulty in determining whether the day being recalled represents an individual's typical intake, and (3) the tendency for persons to overreport low intakes and underreport high intakes of foods. Concurrent use of food frequency and 24-hour recall questionnaires—which is called doing a *cross-check*—improves the accuracy of intake estimates.

Reliability and validity of dietary recall methods are important concerns (Kant, 2002). *Validity* is the degree to which the method actually reflects the usual intake. When attention is directed toward the diet, people may consciously or unconsciously alter their intake either to simplify recording or impress the interviewer, thus decreasing the information's validity. The validity of dietary recall methods with obese indi-

CLINICAL INSIGHT

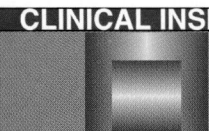

Cultural Awareness

A cross-cultural assessment tool that includes the following questions can be used in the acute care setting, home, or other care sites and may be useful in addressing sensitive issues during the initial assessment.

If the patient is an immigrant, ask the following:

- How is this kind of illness treated in your country?
- How would you describe this problem you have? *Or,* Is there someone else I should talk to?
- What does this sickness do to you?
- How long have you had the problem? Why has the problem happened to you?
- Why do you think the problem began when it did?
- What do you think is wrong, out of balance, or causing the problem?
- What has been done so far?
- What do you think will help your problem clear up? What should be done?
- What does your family think should be done?
- Apart from me, who else do you think can help get you better?
- How serious do you think this situation or problem is?

Data from Heineken J, McCoy N: Establishing a bond with clients of different cultures, *Home Healthcare Nurs* 18(1):45, 2000.

Box 17-5. Dietary History Information

Economics

Income: frequency and steadiness of employment
Amount of money for food each week or month and individual's perception of its adequacy for meeting food needs
Eligibility for food stamps and cost of stamps
Public aid assistance status

Physical Activity

Occupation: type, hours/week, shift, energy expenditure
Exercise: type, amount, frequency (seasonal?)
Sleep: hours/day (uninterrupted?)
Handicaps

Ethnic or Cultural Background

Influence on eating habits
Religion
Education

Home Life and Meal Patterns

Number in household (eat together?)
Person who does shopping
Person who does cooking
Food storage and cooking facilities (e.g., stove, refrigerator)
Type of housing (e.g., home, apartment, room)
Ability to shop and prepare foods

Appetite

Good, poor, any changes
Factors that affect appetite
Taste and smell perception (any changes?)

Attitude Toward Food and Eating

Disinterest in food
Irrational ideas about food, eating, or body weight
Parental interest in child's eating

Allergies, Intolerances, or Food Avoidances

Foods avoided and reason for avoidance
Length of time of avoidance
Description of problems caused by foods

Dental and Oral Health

Problems with chewing
Foods that cannot be eaten
Problems with swallowing, salivation, food sticking

Gastrointestinal Factors

Problems with heartburn, bloating, gas, diarrhea, vomiting, constipation, distention
Frequency of problems
Home remedies
Antacid, laxative, or other drug use

Chronic Disease

Treatment
Length of treatment time
Dietary modification: self-imposed or physician prescribed, date of modification, education, compliance with diet

Medication

Vitamin and/or mineral supplements: frequency of administration, type, amount
Medications: type, amount, frequency of administration, length of time on medication

Recent Weight Change

Loss or gain: how many pounds and over what length of time?
Intentional or nonvolitional

Dietary or Nutritional Problems (as Perceived by Patient)

viduals is often questionable because they tend to underreport their intake. The same can be true for children, patients with eating disorders, those who are critically ill, those who abuse drugs or alcohol, individuals who are confused, and those whose intake may be unpredictable.

Another problem with such retrospective methods of data collection is that people tend to forget what they have actually consumed. *Reliability* refers to the consistency of the data obtained. To have significance, dietary intake data should reflect typical food patterns of an individual. Memory lapses, inaccurate knowledge of portion sizes, and overestimation or underestimation of the amounts consumed may jeopardize the reliability of any food intake method. Table 17-3 describes the advantages and disadvantages of the various methods used to obtain accurate dietary intake data.

Anthropometry

Anthropometry involves obtaining physical measurements of an individual and relating them to standards that reflect the growth and development of the individual. These physical measurements are another component of the nutritional assessment and are useful for evaluating overnutrition or undernutrition. They can be used to monitor the effects of nutritional intervention.

Anthropometric data are most valuable when they reflect accurate measurements and are recorded over a period of time. Common, valuable measurements are height, head circumference, weight, skin-fold thicknesses, and other girth measurements. Birth weight and ethnic, familial, and environmental factors affect these parameters, and so should be taken into consideration when anthropometric measures are evaluated. Individuals conducting these measurements should be trained in the proper technique; if more than one professional is conducting these measurements, then measures of accuracy between them should be established. Measurements of accuracy can be established by several clinicians taking the same measurement and comparing results. It may take more than 20 practice sessions to become proficient (Lee and Nieman, 1996).

Interpretation of Height and Weight

Reference standards in current use are based on a statistical sample of the U.S. population. Therefore an individual measurement shows how a person's measurement compares with that of the total population, not with an absolute standard.

Height and weight measurements of children are evaluated against various norms. They are recorded as percentiles, which reflect the percentage of the total population of children of the same sex who are at

Food Diary: DAY ____________________

MEAL Foods (list)	AMOUNT EATEN	HOW PREPARED	WHERE EATEN (home, work, etc.)
Breakfast:			
Snack:			
Lunch:			
Dinner:			
Snack:			

Food Supplements Name: ________________ Cans/Day: __________
Vitamins/Mineral Supplement: ________________

FIGURE 17-8 • Food diary.

Box 17-6. General Food Frequency Questionnaire*

1. Do you drink milk? If so, how much? What kind? Whole Skim Low-fat
2. Do you use fat? If so, what kind? How much?
3. How often do you eat meat? Eggs? Cheese? Beans?
4. Do you eat snack foods? If so, which ones? How often? How much?
5. Which vegetables (in each group) do you eat? How often?
   a. Broccoli Green peppers Cooked greens Carrots Sweet potatoes
   b. Tomatoes Raw cabbage
   c. Asparagus Beets Cauliflower Corn Cooked cabbage Celery Peas Lettuce
6. Which fruits do you eat? How often?
   a. Apples or applesauce Apricots Bananas Berries Cherries Grapes or grape juice Peaches Pears Pineapple Plums Prunes Raisins
   b. Oranges Orange juice Grapefruit Grapefruit juice
7. Bread and cereal products
   a. How much bread do you usually eat with each meal? How much between meals?
   b. Do you eat cereal? (daily? weekly?) What type? Cooked Dry
   c. How often do you eat foods such as macaroni, spaghetti, and noodles?
   d. Do you eat whole-grain breads and cereals? How often?
8. Do you use salt? Do you salt your food before tasting it? Do you cook with salt? Do you crave salt or salty foods?
9. How many teaspoons of sugar do you use daily? (Be sure to remind the patient to include sugar on cereal, fruit, toast, and in beverages such as coffee and tea.)
10. Do you eat desserts? How often?
11. Do you drink sugar-containing beverages such as soda pop or sweetened juice drinks? How often? How much?
12. How often do you eat candy or cookies?
13. Do you drink water? How often during the day? How much each time? How much water do you drink each day?
14. Do you use sugar substitutes in packet form or in drinks? What type do you use? How often?
15. Do you drink alcohol? How often? How much? Which type? Beer, wine, liquor?
16. Do you drink caffeinated beverages? How often? How much per day?

*To determine the frequency of food consumption, the following pattern of questions may be useful. However, questions may need to be modified based on information from the 24-hour recall. For instance, if a woman states that she drank a glass of milk the day before, do not ask, "Do you drink milk?" rather, "How much milk do you drink?" Record answers with the appropriate time frame designated (e.g., 1/day, 1/wk, 3/mo) or as accurately as possible. The frequency may need to be recorded as "occasionally" or "rarely" if the patient cannot be more specific.

TABLE 17-3 Methods of Obtaining Dietary Intake Data

METHOD	ADVANTAGES	DISADVANTAGES
Nutrient intake analysis	Allows actual observation of food intake	May yield inconsistent and subjective estimates of food consumption Possible variation in portion size
Daily food record or diary	Provides daily record of food consumption Can provide information on quantity of food, how food is prepared, and timing of meals and snacks	Variable literacy skills of participants Requires ability to measure or judge portion sizes Actual food intake possibly influenced by the recording process Questionable reliability of records
Food frequency	Easily standardized Can be beneficial when considered in combination with usual intake Provides overall picture of intake	Requires literacy skills Does not provide meal pattern data Requires knowledge of portion sizes
24-hour recall	Quick Easy	Relies on memory Requires knowledge of portion sizes May not represent usual intake Requires interviewing skills

Data from Hopkins B: Assessment of nutritional status. In Gottschlich MM, Matarese LE, Shronts EP, eds: *Nutrition support dietetics*, ed 2, Silver Spring, Md, 1993, American Society for Parenteral and Enteral Nutrition.

or below the same height or weight at a certain age. Children's growth at every age can be monitored by mapping data on growth curves, known as height-for-age, length-for-age, and weight-for-length curves. Appendixes 6 through 11 describe percentiles and growth charts for infants, children, and adolescents up to the age of 20 years. Height and weight are useful in determining nutritional status in adults. Both should be measured because the tendency is to overestimate height and underestimate weight, resulting in an underestimation of the relative weight or body mass index (BMI).

Length and Height

Various methods may be used to measure height and weight. Measurements of height can be obtained using a direct or an indirect approach. The direct method involves a measuring rod, or *statiometer,* and the person must be able to stand or recline flat. Indirect methods, including arm span, recumbent length (using a tape measure), and knee height measurements, may be options for those who cannot stand or stand straight, such as individuals with scoliosis, cerebral palsy, muscular dystrophy, contractures, or paralysis or those who are bedridden (see Appendix 15). Recumbent bed height measurements made with a tape measure may be appropriate for individuals in institutions who are comatose, critically ill, or unable to be moved. However, this method can only be used with patients who do not have musculoskeletal deformities or contractures.

Sitting heights are used for children who cannot stand, and recumbent length measurements are used for infants and children younger than 2 or 3 years of age (Figure 17-9). Heights of children should be recorded on a growth grid (see Appendixes 6 to 11). The chart provides a record of a child's gain in height over time and compares the child's height with that of other children of the same age. The rate of length or height gain reflects long-term nutritional adequacy.

Weight

Weight is another measure that is easy to obtain but is very telling. In children, it is a more sensitive measure of nutritional adequacy than height, and it reflects recent nutritional intake (Box 17-7). Weight also provides a crude evaluation of overall fat and muscle stores (Hopkins, 1993). Body weight may be measured by several methods, including (1) BMI, (2) usual weight, and (3) actual weight.

Ideal weight for height (UBW) is no longer used from reference standards such as the Metropolitan Life Insurance Tables from 1959 and 1983 and the National Health and Nutrition Examination Survey (NHANES) percentiles. Estimation for an ideal weight can be determined using the Hamwi method (see *Clinical Insight:* Calculating Ideal Body Weight).

Usual body weight (UBW) is a more useful parameter than ideal body weight for those who are ill. Comparing their present weight to their usual body weight allows weight status changes to be assessed. One problem with using a usual body weight measurement is that it depends on the patient's memory.

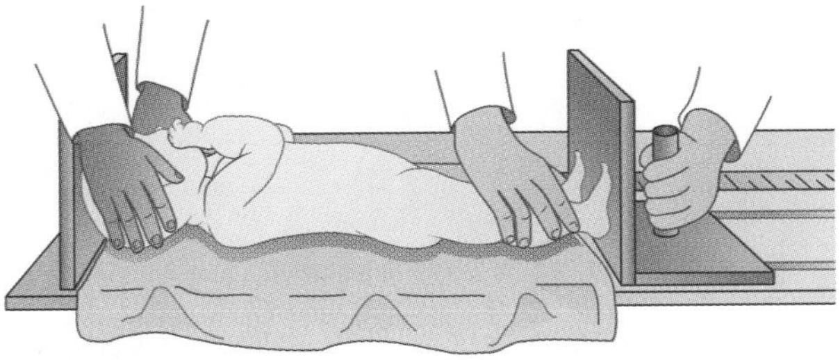

FIGURE 17-9 • Measurement of the length of an infant. Crown-to-heel length of children 3 years and younger should be measured as follows: (1) Lay the child on a ruled board that has an attached piece of wood at one end and a movable piece at the other. (2) Stretch the child out on the board for the most accurate measurement. (3) Place the movable end flat against the bottom of the child's foot, and read the length from the side of the board.

Box 17-7. Using Height and Weight to Assess a Hospitalized Patient's Nutritional Status

- Measure height.
- Measure weight (at admission, current, and usual).
- Determine percentage of weight change over time (weight pattern).
- Determine percentage above or below usual or ideal body weight.

Actual body weight is the weight measurement obtained at the time of examination. This measurement may be influenced by changes in the individual's fluid status. Weight loss (in pounds or kilograms) reflects an immediate inability to meet nutritional requirements and thus may indicate nutritional risk. The percentage of weight loss is highly indicative of the extent and severity of an individual's illness. The following formula (Blackburn, 1977) is useful in determining *the percentage of recent weight change:*

Significant weight loss: 5% loss in 1 month, 7.5% loss in 3 months, 10% loss in 6 months

Severe weight loss: >5% weight loss in 1 month, >7.5% weight loss in 3 months, >10% weight loss in 6 months

Another method for determining the percentage of weight loss is to determine an individual's current weight as a percentage of the usual weight. Minimum weight for survival is 48% to 55% of usual body weight (Buchman, 1997). The percentage of usual or

CLINICAL INSIGHT

Calculating Ideal Body Weight

Ideal body weight for an individual can be calculated using the Hamwi method, which follows:

Females: 100 lb for the first 5 feet of height and 5 lb for every inch over 5 feet

Males: 106 lb for the first 5 feet of height and 6 lb for every inch over 5 feet

An adjustment is then made for a large frame (+10%) or a small frame (−10%). Frame size is determined by measuring wrist circumference or elbow breadth (see Appendix 16).

For example, the ideal body weight for a medium-frame woman with a height of 63 inches is calculated as follows:

Step 1: *100 lb* for the first 5 feet (60 inches) + *15 lb* (5 feet + 3 inches): 100 lb + 15 lb = *115 lb*

Step 2: 10% of 115 lb = 11.5 lb

Step 3: 115 lb − 11.5 lb = 103.5 lb; 115 + 11.5 lb = 126.5 lb

Step 4: 103.5 to 126.5 lb = Ideal body weight range

---

ideal body weight can be used to assess the degree of malnutrition as follows:

- Patients with weight within 85% to 90% of usual body weight: Mild malnutrition
- Patients with weight within 75% to 84% of usual body weight: Moderate malnutrition
- Patients with weight <74% of usual body weight: Severe malnutrition

To determine whether an adult's weight is appropriate for height, the individual is usually compared with a reference standard (see Appendixes 17 and 20).

Body Mass Index

The Quetelet's index (W/H^2), the most widely used height-weight index (Lee and Nieman, 1996), is commonly referred to as body mass index (BMI) and is a validated measure of nutritional status. BMI measurement requires weight and height measurements; based on the result, it can indicate overnutrition or undernutrition. BMI accounts for differences in body composition by defining the level of adiposity according to the relationship of weight to height, thus eliminating dependence on frame size (Stensland and Margolis, 1990). BMI can be calculated using any of the following formulas:

- *Metric formula:* BMI = Weight (kg) ÷ Height $(m)^2$
- *English formula:* BMI = (Weight [lb] ÷ Height [in] ÷ Height [in]) – 703 (Centers for Disease Control and Prevention, 2002)

  Nomograms: Also available to calculate BMI, as are various *charts* (see Appendix 17 for adults and Appendixes 18 and 19 for children)

The BMI index has the least correlation with body height and the highest correlation with independent measures of body fat for adults, including older adults (Balcombe et al, 2001; Keys et al, 1972). BMI ranges are based on the relationships among body weight, disease processes, and mortality (Centers for Disease Control and Prevention, 2002).

Obesity is categorized into three BMI grades: *grade I* (25 to 29.9), *grade II* (30 to 40), and *grade III* (40+). In general, a BMI of 27 or more indicates obesity and an increased risk of developing health problems (Bray et al, 1976; Gilmore, 1999). New standards for BMI published in 1998 classify a BMI less than 18.5 as underweight, a BMI between 25 and 29 as overweight, and a BMI greater than 30 as obese. A healthy BMI for adults is considered between 18.5 and 24.9 (Centers for Disease Control and Prevention, 2002).

Although a strong correlation exists between total body fat and BMI, individual variations need to be recognized before the final assessment (Shopbell et al, 2001). Differences in race, sex, and age must be considered when evaluating the BMI (Sanchez, Reed, and Price, 2000; Tam, et al, 1999). The National Health Examination Survey I (NHES) and the NHANES I, II, and III show the mean BMI for Americans according to race, sex, and age (see Chapter 24).

BMI values tend to increase with age (Nutrition Screening Initiative, 1991; Vaccarino and Krumholz, 2001). Recent studies report an association between BMI and mortality for nonhospitalized patients 65 years of age and older, but the data do not support the BMI range of 25 to 27 as a risk factor for all-cause and cardiovascular mortality. The conclusion is that federal guideline standards for ideal weight (BMI of 18.7 to less than 25) may be too restrictive for older adults. Careful interpretation of risk factors must be part of the total assessment. Recent tables for BMI for children have been published (see Appendixes 18A and 19A).

Body Composition

Differences in skeletal size and the proportion of lean body mass can contribute to body weight variations among individuals of similar height. For example, muscular athletes may be classified as overweight because their excess muscle mass, not their adipose mass, increases their weight. Older adults tend to have lower bone density and may therefore weigh less than younger adults of the same height. Indirect

Box 17-8. Skin-Fold Measurement Techniques

1. Take measurement on the right side of the body.
2. Mark the site to be measured, and use a flexible, nonstretchable tape.
3. The tape measure can be used to locate the midpoints on the body.
4. Firmly grasp the skin fold with the thumb and index finger of the left hand about 1 cm or ½ inch proximal to the skin-fold site, pulling it away from the body.
5. Hold the caliper in the right hand, perpendicular to the long axis of the skin fold and with the caliper's dial face up. Place the caliper tip on the site and about 1 cm or ½ inch distal to the fingers holding the skin fold. (Pressure from the fingers does not affect the measurement.)
6. Do not place the caliper too deeply into the skin fold or too close to the tip of the skin-fold.
7. Read the caliper approximately 4 seconds after pressure from the measurer's hand has been released from the lever. Exerting force longer than 4 seconds results in smaller readings because fluids are forced from the compressed tissue. Measurements should be recorded to the nearest 1 mm.
8. Take a minimum of two measurements at each site to verify results. Wait 15 seconds between measurements to allow the skin-fold site to return to normal. Maintain pressure with thumb and index finger during measurements.
9. Do not take measurements immediately after the person has exercised or if the person is overheated because the shift in body fluid makes the result larger.
10. When measuring obese clients, it may be necessary to use both hands to pull the skin away while a second person makes the measurement. If the calipers do not fit, another technique may be required.

Data from Lee RD, Nieman DC: *Nutritional assessment*, ed 2, St. Louis, 1996, Mosby.

methods for measuring body composition include triceps skin fold (TSF), midarm muscle circumference (MAMC), and midarm circumference (MAC) (Shopbell et al, 2001). However, keep in mind that these measures are useful in the assessment of individuals over time but not in critical and acute care settings because changes in body fluid and composition may influence the results. When conducting body composition measurements, strict adherence to established protocols must be followed to yield accurate results. For example, most North American investigators use the right side of the body to take skin-fold measurements, and the standards are based on this. The methods used to gather meaningful data should be considered carefully (Lee and Nieman, 1996).

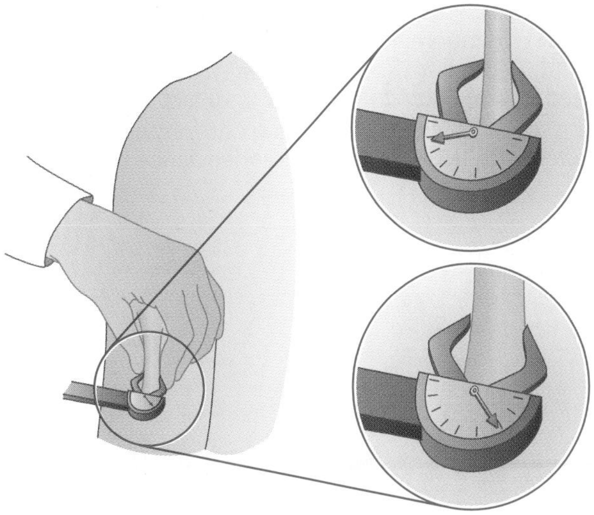

FIGURE 17-10 • Skin-fold calipers measuring the thickness of subcutaneous fat (in millimeters), giving a rough measurement of adiposity. Measurements are read counterclockwise. (Courtesy Dorice Czajka-Narins, Ph.D.)

Subcutaneous Fat (Skin-Fold Thickness)

The fat-fold or skin-fold thickness measurement is a means of assessing the amount of body fat in an individual. It is practical in clinical settings, although its validity depends on the accuracy of the measuring technique (Figure 17-10 and Box 17-8) and repetition of measurements over time. Changes, if they are going to occur, take 3 to 4 weeks. This measurement bases total body fat estimates on the assumption that 50% of body fat is subcutaneous. Accuracy decreases with increasing obesity. The skin-fold sites identified as most reflective of body fatness are over the triceps and the biceps, below the scapula, above the iliac crest (suprailiac), and on the upper thigh. The triceps skin-fold and subscapular measurements are the most useful because the most complete standards and methods of evaluation are available for these sites (Figures 17-11 and 17-12). (See Appendixes 20 to 22 for various tables related to arm and skin-fold measurements.)

Circumference Measurements

If more complete information on actual body composition is needed, additional anthropometric data can be obtained. These data include additional skin-fold and circumference measurements (Figure 17-13).

Because of the recognition that fat distribution is an indicator of risk, circumferential or girth measurements are used more frequently today. The presence of excess body fat around the abdomen out of proportion to total body fat is considered a risk factor for ailments associated with obesity and the metabolic syndrome. Waist circumference measurements are often used. An older method, *waist-to-hip circumference ratio (WHR),* is used less often; WHR is used to detect possible signs of excess fat deposition (lipodystrophy) in those infected with the human immunodeficiency virus (HIV).

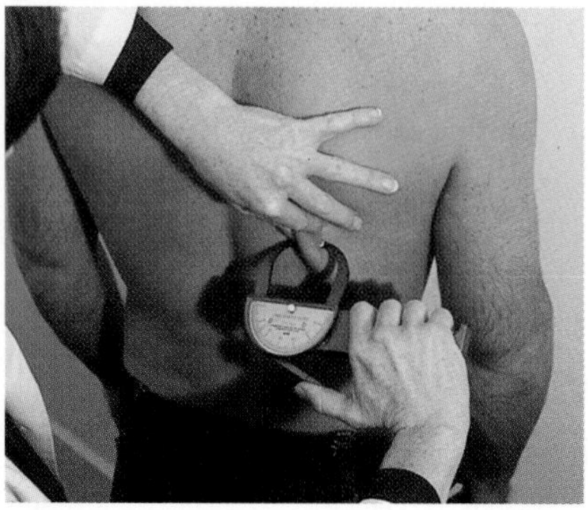

FIGURE 17-11 • Measurement of the subscapular skin-fold thickness.

Waist Circumference

Waist circumference is obtained by measuring the distance around the smallest area below the rib cage and above the umbilicus (belly button) with the use of a nonstretchable tape measure. Waist circumference measurements assess abdominal fat content. A measurement of greater than 40 inches (102 cm) for men and greater than 35 inches (88 cm) for women are independent risk factors for disease when out of proportion to total body fat (Centers for Disease Control and Prevention, 2002). These measurements may not be as useful for those less than 60 inches tall or with a BMI of 35 or above (Centers for Disease Control and Prevention, 2002). Figure 17-14 shows the proper way to measure waist (abdominal) circumference.

Mid Arm Circumference

Mid arm circumference (MAC) is measured halfway between the acromion process of the scapula and the tip of the elbow. Combining MAC with TSF measurements allows indirect determination of the arm muscle area (AMA) and arm fat area (AFA). Bone-free

A

B

C

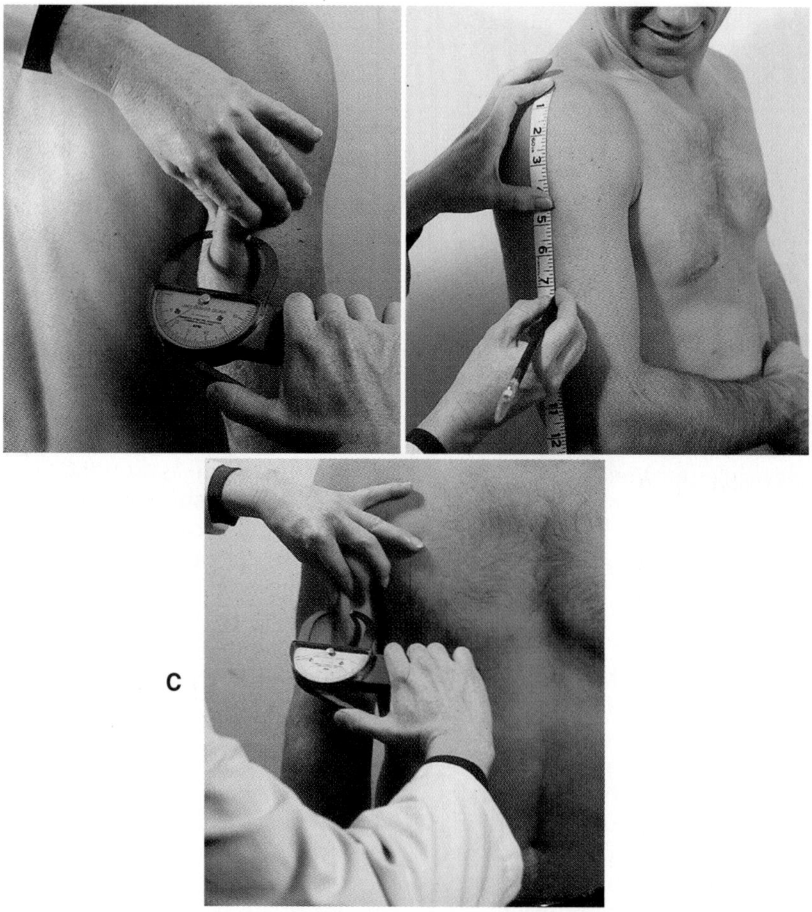

FIGURE 17-12 • **A,** Measurement of the midpoint between the acromion process at the shoulder and the olecranon process at the elbow. **B,** Marking of the midpoint. **C,** Measurement of the arm circumference (in centimeters) at the midpoint.

AMA is calculated by using the formula shown in Figure 17-15; for men, a factor of 10 is subtracted from the AMA, whereas for women, a factor of 6.5 is subtracted (Frisancho, 1984).

The AMA, or bone-free muscle area, is a good indication of lean body mass and thus an individual's skeletal protein reserves. The AMA is important in growing children and is especially valuable in evaluating possible protein-energy malnutrition as a result of chronic illness, stress, an eating disorder, multiple surgeries, or an inadequate diet (see Appendixes 21, 22, and 28 to 31).

Head Circumference

Head circumference measurements are useful in children younger than 3 years of age, primarily as an indicator of nonnutritional abnormalities. Undernutrition must be very severe to affect head circumference (see *Clinical Insight:* Head Circumference).

Calf Circumference

Measurements of calf circumference, combined with other anthropometric measures, can be used to estimate body weight in older adults (Lohman et al, 1988).

Other Methods of Measuring Body Composition

Underwater Weighing

A more direct measure of determining whole-body density is *densitometry,* which includes *underwater (hydrostatic) weighing.* Underwater weighing is based on Archimedes' principle: the volume of an object submerged in water equals the volume of water the object displaces. Once the volume and mass are known, the density can be calculated. Although this method is considered the gold standard (Indorato, 2001), it is not always practical, involves significant training to perform, and requires considerable cooperation on the part of those being measured because they must be submerged under water and remain motionless long enough for the measurements to be made (Lee and Nieman, 1996).

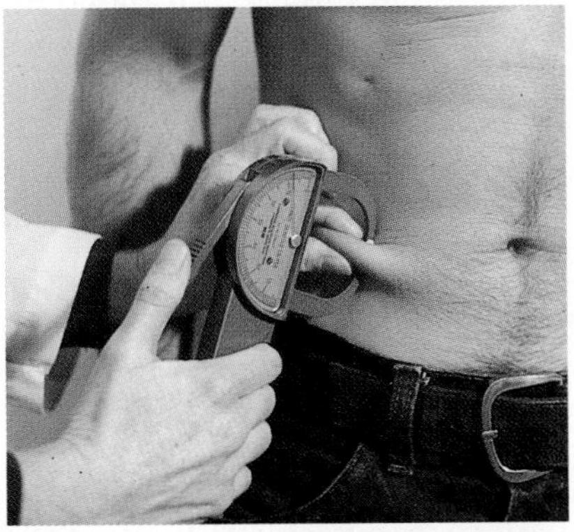

FIGURE 17-13 • Waist skin-fold measurement using calipers.

Total Body Potassium

Total body potassium can be used to study body composition because more than 90% of the body's potassium is found in fat-free tissues. Measurements are made with a special counter that is fitted with

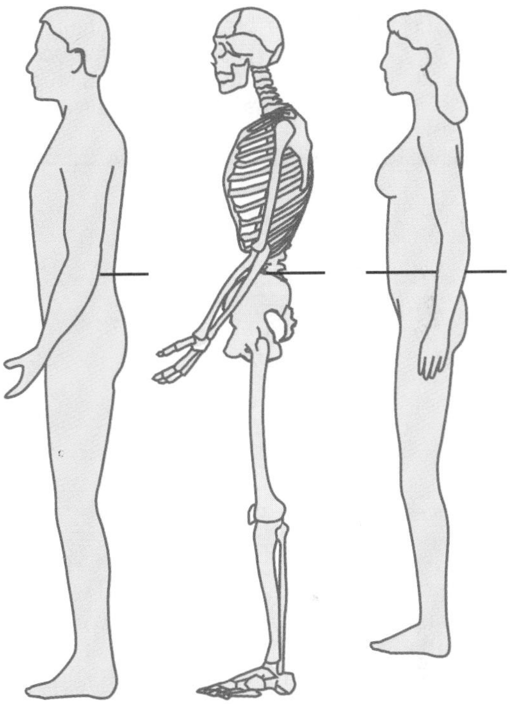

FIGURE 17-14 • Measuring tape position for waist (abdominal) circumference measurement. (From www.nhlbi.nih.gov/guidelines/obesity/e_txtbk/txgd/4142.htm.)

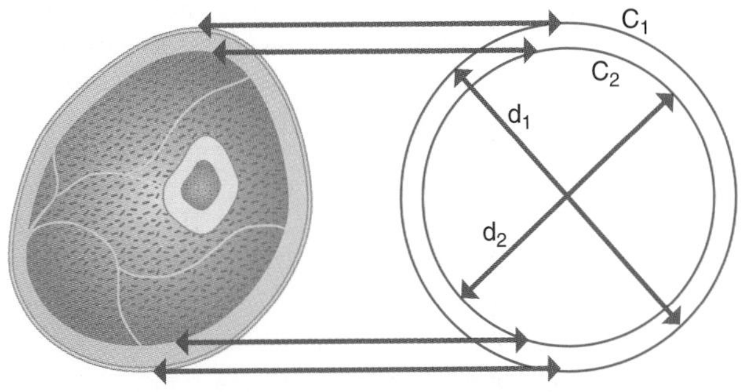

$$AA\ (mm^2) = \pi/4 \times d_1^2 \text{ where } d_1 = C_1/\pi$$

$$AMA\ (mm^2) = (C_1 - \pi T)^2/4\pi = (C_1 = \pi T)^2/12.56$$

$$AFA\ (mm2) = AA - AMA$$

$$\text{bone-free AMA} - AMA - 10 \text{ for males}$$

$$= AMA - 6.5 \text{ for females}$$

FIGURE 17-15 • Upper arm area (AA), upper arm muscle area (AMA), and upper arm fat area (AFA) are derived from measurements of upper arm circumference *(C_1)* and triceps skin-fold (T) in millimeters.

CLINICAL INSIGHT

Head Circumference

Head circumference is a standard measurement for serial assessment of growth in patients from birth to 36 months.

1. With the aid of an assistant, hold the child's head completely still.
2. Use a cloth tape measure, and place the tape measure over the most prominent part of the occiput and around the forehead, just above the supraorbital ridge. All measurements should be taken around fixed landmarks.
3. Tighten the tape measure and hold it securely; note the measurement over the forehead.
4. The circumference should be read to the nearest 0.1 cm or 1/8 inch and then recorded.
5. Compare the measurement with the National Center for Health Statistics (NCHS) standard curves for head circumference (see Appendixes 7 and 10).

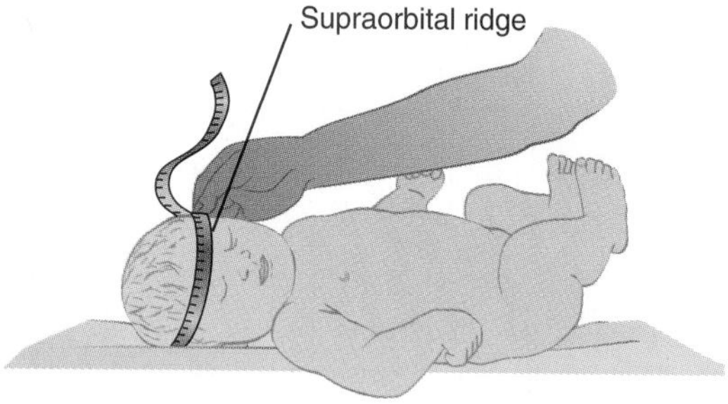

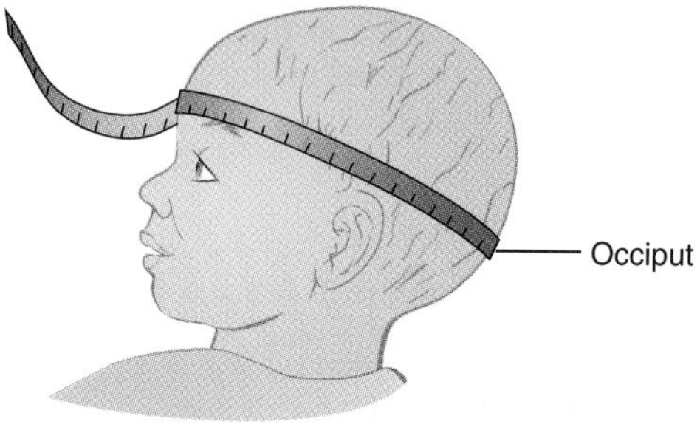

multiple gamma-ray detectors interfaced with a computer that is expensive and not always readily available. Not all researchers agree on the exact concentration of potassium in fat-free tissue and the differences between sexes, during the aging process, and in obese individuals.

Neutron Activation Analysis

The *neutron activation analysis* allows measurements of the body's calcium, iodine, hydrogen, sodium, chloride, phosphorus, carbon, and nitrogen contents (Lee and Nieman, 1996). Neutron activation measures lean body mass. The analysis is based on the assumption that fat-free tissue conducts electricity better than fat (Shopbell et al, 2001). This type of measurement is expensive and impractical in a daily clinical setting.

Bioelectrical Impedance Analysis

Bioelectrical impedance analysis (BIA) is a body composition analysis technique based on the principle that relative to water, lean tissue has a higher electrical conductivity and lower impedance than fatty tissue because of its electrolyte content. BIA has been found to be a reliable measurement of body composition (fat-free mass and fat mass) when compared with BMI or skin-fold measurements or even height and weight measurements (Kyle et al, 2001). BIA involves attaching electrodes to the right hand, wrist, ankle, and foot of a patient and passing a small electrical current through the body (Figure 17-16).

The BIA method is becoming very popular as a means of assessment because it is safe, noninvasive, portable, and rapid. For accurate results, the patient should be well hydrated, have not exercised in the previous 4 to 6 hours, and have not consumed alcohol in the previous 24 hours. If the person is dehydrated, a higher percentage of body fat than really exists is measured. Fever, electrolyte imbalance, and extreme obesity also affect the reliability of measurements (Shronts et at, 1998). Depending on the type of system used, additional recommendations for the person being measured include avoiding caffeine and over-the-counter diuretics, drinking two to four glasses of water approximately 2 hours before the test, and emptying the bladder just before the test is given (Indorato, 2001).

Several companies manufacture BIA systems, and the different systems have different advantages. For example, the Bodystat and the Tanitaone systems require sensors to be attached, whereas another sensor is a hand-held unit that is easy to pack for travel. Professional systems range in price from $1200 to $5000, and software packages add an additional cost; personal models range from $49 to $250. Professionals who would like to use BIA equipment need to speak with the various manufacturers to decide which system is best for their particular practice; factors to consider include details such as cost, ages and types of clients seen, ease of transport, and convenience (Indorato, 2001).

Computed Tomography

Computed tomography, or *CT scan,* has been useful for studying nutritional status. It has been particularly helpful for assessing the deposition of subcutaneous and intraabdominal fat, which aids in determining nutritional risk associated with morbidity and mortality.

Ultrasound and Magnetic Resonance Imaging

Magnetic resonance imaging (MRI) can be used to measure the size of visceral organs, the size of the skeleton, and the amount and distribution of intraabdominal fat. MRI has several advantages, two of which are that it is noninvasive and involves no ionizing radiation, which makes it safe for children, females of childbearing age, and multiple studies on the same individual. The disadvantages of MRI include the expense and limited availability (Lee and Nieman, 1996; Shopbell et at, 2001).

Dual-Energy X-Ray Absorptiometry

Dual-energy x-ray absorptiometry, or *DEXA,* is a means of assessing bone mineral density and can be used for measuring fat and boneless lean tissue. The energy source in DEXA is an x-ray tube that contains an energy beam (Lee and Nieman, 1996). The amount of energy loss depends on the type of tissue the beam passes through, and the result can be used to measure mineral, fat, and lean tissue compartments (Shopbell et al, 2001). DEXA is easy to use, emits low levels of radiation, is relatively available in the hospital setting, and requires little cooperation from the patient, thus making it a useful tool. Differences in hydration status and the presence of bone or calcified soft tissue can result in inaccurate measurements (Lee and Nieman, 1996).

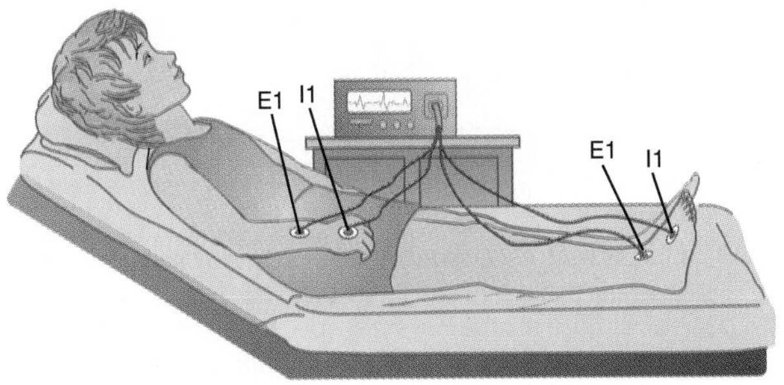

FIGURE 17-16 • Bioelectrical impedance analysis.

TABLE 17-4 Physical Examination Techniques

TECHNIQUE	DESCRIPTION
Inspection	General observation that progresses to a more focused observation using the senses of sight, smell, and hearing; most frequently used technique
Palpation	Tactile examination to feel pulsations and vibrations; assessment of body structures, including texture, size, temperature, tenderness, and mobility
Percussion	Assessment of sounds to determine body organ borders, shape, and position; not always used in a nutrition-focused physical examination
Auscultation	Use of the naked ear or a stethoscope to listen to body sounds (e.g., heart and lung sounds, bowel sounds, blood vessels)

From Hammond K: Nutrition focused physical assessment, *Support Line* 18(4):4, 1996.

NUTRITION-FOCUSED PHYSICAL EXAMINATION

A nutrition-focused physical examination is an important component of overall nutritional assessment because some nutritional deficiencies may not be identified by other assessment approaches. Keep in mind that some signs of nutritional deficiency are not specific and must be distinguished from those with a nonnutritional etiology.

Physical Signs

A systems approach is used when performing the examination, which should be conducted in an organized, logical way that progresses from head to toe to ensure efficiency and thoroughness. The examination moves from a global to a more defined or focused examination based on the results of the medical and nutrition histories. The nutrition-focused physical examination is tailored for each patient. In other words, every body system may not have to be assessed in all people; clinical judgment guides this decision (Hammond, 1996, 1997, 1998).

Equipment

The extent of the nutrition-focused physical examination dictates the necessary equipment. Any or all of the following may be used: a stethoscope, a penlight or flashlight, a tongue depressor, scales, a reflex hammer, calipers, a tape measure, a blood pressure cuff, and an ophthalmoscope.

Examination Techniques

Four basic physical examination techniques are used during the nutrition-focused physical examination. These techniques include inspection, palpation, percussion, and auscultation (Table 17-4).

CLINICAL INSIGHT

Hydration Status

It is important to recognize the fluid volume status of an individual during the nutrition-focused physical examination. Fluid disturbances can be associated with other imbalances such as electrolyte imbalance.

Fluid Volume Deficit

From the history: Note any loss of water and electrolytes from vomiting, diarrhea, excessive laxative abuse, fistulas, GI suction, polyuria, fever, excessive sweating, and edema (third-space fluid shifts). Fluid volume deficit can also be caused by decreased intake, which may be prominent in those with anorexia, nausea, depression, and inability to gain access to fluids.

Associated characteristics: Characteristics of a fluid volume deficit include weight loss that occurs over a short period, decreased skin and tongue turgor, dry mucous membranes, postural hypotension, a weak and rapid pulse, slow-filling peripheral veins, a decrease in body temperature (95° to 98° F), decreased urine output, cold extremities, disorientation, changes in laboratory test results (e.g., a blood urea nitrogen [BUN] level elevated out of proportion to serum creatinine, elevated hematocrit).

Fluid Volume Excess

From the history: Note any history of renal failure, congestive heart failure, cirrhosis of the liver, or Cushing's syndrome; excess use of sodium-containing intravenous fluids; and excessive intake of sodium-containing food or medication products.

Associated characteristics: Characteristics of fluid volume excess include weight gain that occurs over a short period, peripheral edema, distended neck veins, slow emptying of peripheral veins, rales in lungs, polyuria, ascites, pleural effusion, a bounding and full pulse, changes in laboratory test results (e.g., decreased BUN, decreased hematocrit), and in severe cases, pulmonary edema.

Data from Methany N: *Fluid and electrolyte balance: nursing considerations*, Philadelphia, 1992, JB Lippincott.

Findings

Some significant nutritional findings from the physical examination that should alert the clinician to the need for further assessment and intervention may include temporal wasting, proximal muscle weakness, depleted muscle bulk, dehydration, overhydration, poor wound healing, and chewing or swallowing difficulties. The appearance of the skin should be evaluated for any pallor, scaly dermatitis, wounds, quality of wound healing, bruising, and hydration status. Membranes (conjunctiva or pharynx) should be examined for integrity, hydration, pallor, and bleeding (see *Clinical Insight:* Hydration Status).

Special attention should be given to the areas where signs of nutritional deficiencies appear (e.g., skin, hair, teeth, gums, lips, tongue, eyes, genitalia [in men]). The hair, skin, and mouth are susceptible because of the rapid cell turnover of epithelial tissue. Mucosal changes in the GI tract are indicated by problems such as diarrhea and anorexia. Symptoms of nutrient deficiencies may or may not be apparent during the physical examination. Many signs result from a lack of several nutrients, as well as from nonnutritional causes. (Appendix 32 discusses the physical examination and findings in more detail; potential International Classification of Diseases [ICD-9] codes for classifying diagnoses with a nutritional implication can be found in Appendix 3.)

Immune Function

Skin testing, or *delayed hypersensitivity reactivity (DHR),* and *total lymphocyte count (TLC)* are two measures of immune function that can be used as screening and assessment parameters. DHR measures cell-mediated immunity and involves the intradermal injection of small amounts of antigen, most commonly tuberculin, *Candida* organisms, mumps, or trichophyton, just under the skin to determine the person's reaction. A healthy person reacts with induration, indicating that exposure has probably taken place and immunocompetence is intact; no reaction may be associated with malnutrition. Of course, DHR is not useful for individuals with an electrolyte imbalance, an infection, cancer, liver disease, renal failure, trauma, or immunosuppression (Shopbell et al, 2001). DHR is not always a useful component of the nutrition assessment for hospitalized patients (Shronts et al, 1998). TLC is also an indicator of immune function reflective of B and T cells (see Chapter 18).

Handgrip Dynamometry

Handgrip dynamometry can provide a baseline nutritional assessment of muscle function by measuring grip strength and endurance and is useful in serial measurements. Measurements are expressed as a percentage of a standard for men and women (Guenter et al, 1989):

Men: 48.8 +/− 7.0 kg; Women: 34.4 +/− 4.7 kg.

Biochemical Analysis

Biochemical tests are the most objective and sensitive measures of nutritional status, but not all are appropriate. Caution must be used when interpreting re-

TABLE 17-5 Classification of Protein-Energy Malnutrition

ICD-9-CM*	DIAGNOSIS AND DESCRIPTION	CRITERIA AND CHARACTERISTICS
260.0	Kwashiorkor: nutritional edema with dyspigmentation of skin and hair	1. Normal anthropometrics: weight >90% of standard weight for height 2. Depressed visceral protein concentrations: serum albumin <3 g/dl, transferrin <180 mg/dl 3. Caused by acute energy and protein deficiency or a metabolic response to injury 4. Characterized by edema, catabolism of muscle tissue, weakness, neurologic changes, loss of vigor, secondary infections, stunted growth in children, and changes in hair
261.0	Marasmus: nutritional atrophy; severe, chronic calorie deficiency; severe malnutrition	1. Depressed anthropometrics: weight <80% of standard weight for height, weight loss >10% of usual weight in last 6 months with muscle wasting, or both 2. Relative preservation of visceral proteins: serum albumin >3 g/dl 3. Caused by chronically deficient energy intake 4. Characterized by catabolism of fat and muscle tissue, lethargy, generalized weakness, and weight loss
262.0	Other severe PEM: nutritional edema without dyspigmentation of skin and hair	1. Depressed anthropometrics: weight <60% of standard weight for height 2. Depressed visceral protein concentration: serum albumin <3 g/dl 3. Occurs when a patient with marasmus is exposed to stress (e.g., trauma, surgery, acute illness) 4. Characterized by combined symptoms of marasmus and kwashiorkor, a high risk of infection, and poor wound healing
263.0	Malnutrition of moderate degree	1. Depressed anthropometrics: weight 60% to 75% of standard weight for height 2. Relative preservation of visceral proteins: serum albumin 3 to 3.5 g/dl
263.1	Malnutrition of mild degree	1. Depressed anthropometrics: weight 75% to 90% of standard weight for height 2. Preservation of visceral proteins: serum albumin 3.5 to 5 g/dl

From *Manual of clinical dietetics,* ed 5, Chicago, 1996, The American Dietetic Association.
**International classification of diseases,* ed 9, Clinical Modification.

sults because they can be affected by disease state and therapy. Chapter 18 provides a complete discussion of the role of laboratory data in nutritional assessment.

CLASSIFYING MALNUTRITION

Once a nutritional assessment is completed, the extent of nutritional adequacy, deficiency, or excess is apparent. Malnutrition can then be classified based on several indexes, including body weight, body fat, somatic and visceral protein stores, and laboratory values. Table 17-5 characterizes protein-energy malnutrition using the ICD-9 codes (see Appendix 3).

Once the nutritional assessment is completed and the nutritional status determined, a nutritional care plan can be formulated (see Chapter 21). Implementing a nutritional care plan involves defining the nutritional problem to be addressed (based on assessment), identifying the appropriate nutritional "diagnoses, establishing therapeutic goals or desired outcomes, determining appropriate interventions to be implemented as they relate to the nutritional therapy goals, identifying the educational needs of the patient, and formulating a plan for evaluation. In many cases the plan of care is included on the nutritional assessment form (Figure 17-17) (see Appendix 56).

SUMMARY

Careful and meticulous nutritional screening and assessment are important tools in patient management. Adaptations of the exact content of the screen or assessment vary according to the patient's diagnosis and clinical setting. A skilled dietitian uses the screening and assessment process to make the best possible decisions about the plan of care and its implementation.

Clinical Scenario I

Carl is a 32-year-old man who is 5 ft, 9 inches tall. He was diagnosed as having acquired immunodeficiency syndrome (AIDS) 1 year ago. In the past year, his weight has gradually decreased from a usual weight of 175 lb to the current low of 130 lb. His visceral proteins are depleted, and a TSF measurement reveals a body fat value that is 55% of standard. Carl's oral intake ability has gradually decreased; he can only take sips of an enteral supplement and occasional bites of food.

1. Is Carl exhibiting a degree of undernutrition? If so, classify the type of malnutrition he has.
2. Carl's current weight is what percentage of his usual body weight?
3. What is Carl's BMI?
4. Develop a nutritional assessment questionnaire for Carl.

Name: ______________________________

Number: ______________________________

Date/Time: ______________________________

Dx: ______________________________

☐ Routine Assessment
☐ Comprehensive Assessment
☐ Nutrition Care Note: Follow-up
☐ Education/Instruction
☐ Calorie Counts

CLINICAL NUTRITION SERVICES
Medical Nutrition Therapy

Subjective:

Appetite : ☐ Excellent ☐ Good ☐ Fair ☐ Poor % of meals consumed: ☐ 25% ☐ 50% ☐ 75% ☐ 100%	Food Allergies/Intolerance:
Diet Prior to Admission:	Previous Diet Counseling: ☐ Yes ☐ No
Other:	
Ethnic/Cultural:	

☐ **Write in/Type in Field:** ______________

Objective: Antropometric/Biological Indices/Nutritional Parameters

Diet Order/Feeding:					Supplements: (List all supplements – jump screen)
Ht (in/cm)	Wt (lbs/kg)	Usual Wt	Desired Wt	Frame Size: sm. med. lg.	Body Mass Index: Obese 30–40 Morbidly >40 obese
Wt change (lbs/kg) Time Period ______ wks Date: __________ Intentional Unintentional				Assessed Needs: BEE: __________ kcal	
Total Kcal: __________		Protein: __________ gms/day			Fluid: __________ cc/day

Lab/Biochemical Test		Results	Lab/Biochemical Test	Results
☐ Alb	Albumin	______ g/dl	☐ Prealbumin	______ mg/dl
☐ BG	Blood Glucose	______ mg/dl	☐ HgbAlc	______ %
☐ K	Potassium	______ mmol/l	☐ SGOT	______ U/L
☐ NA	Sodium	______ mmol/l	☐ SGPT	______ U/L
☐ BUN	BUN	______ mg/dl	☐ Alk. Phos.	______ U/L
☐ HDL	HDL	______ mg/dl	☐ Lipase	______ Units
☐ LDL	LDL	______ mg/dl	☐ Amylase	______ SomU/dl
☐ CR	Creatine	______ mg/dl		
☐ TG	Triglyceride	______ mg/dl		
☐ CHO	Cholesterol	______ mg/dl		
☐ MG	Magnesium	______ mg/dl		
☐ PO4	Phosphorus	______ mg/dl		
☐ CA	Calcium	______ mg/dl		

Values may be:
☐ falsely elevated ☐ falsely decreased ☐ secondary to hydration status
☐ Question Accuracy

Conditions That Currently Exist:
☐ Nausea
☐ Vomiting
☐ Diarrhea
☐ Chewing/Swallowing Difficulties

Other Factors:
☐ Dentures/Dentition
☐ Skin Score ≤16
☐ Age: ______
☐ Activity Level: ______________

FIGURE 17-17 • Assessment form. (Courtesy Saint Joseph's Hospital, Atlanta, Ga.)

Pertinent Medications:	
Oral Intake:	Other:
Allergies:	

❑ **Write in/Type in Field:** ____________

Assessment:

MALNUTRITION INDICATORS	DATE	VALUE	MILD	MODERATE	SEVERE
❑ Prealbumin			10–15 mg/dl	10–5 mg/dl	<5 mg/dl
❑ Albumin			2.8–3.5 gm/dl	2.1–2.7 gm/dl	<2.1 gm/dl
❑ Total Lymphocyte Count			1500–1800/mm^3	900–1500/mm^3	<800/mm^3
❑ Hematocrit (%)					
❑ % Desirable Weight/Height			75%–90%	60%–75%	<60%
❑ % Weight Loss				5% in 1 month	>5% in 1 month
				10% in 6 months	>10% in 6 months

Malnutrition indicators: ❑ Mild: ________ ❑ Moderate: ________ ❑ Severe: ________

PLANS/RECOMMENDATIONS:

MD please ❑ order ❑ ordered:

Pt. at nutritional risk secondary to: ❑ age ❑ Dx
❑ wt change albumin recent surgery
❑ poor p.o. swallowing compromise
❑ Sending diet as ordered
❑ Please change consistency of diet to:
____
❑ Honor food preferences ❑ No preferences stated
❑ Diet counseling to be provided before discharge
❑ Recommend enteral/parenteral support, refer for further evaluation and follow-up (F/U)
❑ Current nutritional parameters limited, MD please order: REQUESTED
❑ Prealbumin ❑ Albumin ❑ Weight
❑ Wt 3×/wk ❑ Wt 3×/wk ❑ Ht/Wt
❑ Cholesterol ❑ Nitrogen Balance Study
❑ Swallow evaluation per SLP ❑ Check HgbAlc
❑ Accuchecks ❑ Nutrition Support Team consult from Pharmacy Dept.
❑ Assistance with feeding during meals
❑ Snacks ❑ 1000 ❑ 1500 ❑ QHS
❑ Supplements/Changes (jump screen)
❑ Calorie Count ❑ 2d ❑ 3d
❑ RD ordered:

❑ Write-in list/Substitutions/Cafe options
❑ "Special" Meal
❑ Chef visit
❑ H.A. assist with menu
❑ If diet cannot be advanced within 72 hours recommend nutrition support or alternative mode of intake
❑ Will change diet to
❑ Suggest diet change to
❑ Continue with present diet management
❑ Referred to out-patient (OP) heart school
❑ Referred to OP diabetes school
❑ Referred to OP-RD for medical nutrition therapy and F/U
❑ Will F/U with diet instruction
❑ Diet education materials provided along with phone number for F/U
❑ Referred to social service, pastoral care, rehab
❑ Will monitor progress for any status changes
❑ Changes for intolerance of supplements
❑ Poor progress noted
❑ Comfort measures only
❑ Care plan forwarded for external care facility
❑ Patient left before instructions completed
❑ Information given to setup OP visit and follow-up

RD PRIORITY LISTING
Automatic Screen Flags to RD

1. NPO/CL >3d
2. TF/TPN/PPN → NSS + FS alb.
3. Calorie Count Orders (code)
4. 80 yrs. or >
5. Albumin ≤2.8
6. Nutrition Score ≥3
7. Wt. ≤80% ideal body weight or >140%
8. All orders for consult/assessment/instruction
9. Applicable drug-nutrient interaction (DNI) medications as coded
10. Supplements specified (including nourishment and pharmacy supplements)

FIGURE 17-17—cont'd

Clinical Scenario 2

Laverne, a 66-year-old black woman, has contacted you to set up an outpatient nutritional screening appointment. She has a 20-year history of diabetes mellitus, a 10-year history of colon cancer, and hypertension. She is 5 ft, 8 inches tall and weighs 202 lb. Her current medications are gluconase and a diuretic. (She does not know its name.)

1. What would you include in a nutrition screen for Laverne?
2. How would you identify her medications?
3. Should any laboratory tests be ordered?
4. If you need more details, what questions would you ask her physician?
5. What other information do you need to develop a nutritional care plan?

Relevant Web Sites

Bioelectrical impedance
www.odp.od.nih.gov/consensus/ta/015/015_statement.htm
Centers for Disease Control and Prevention
www.cdc.gov/nchs/about/major/nhanes/growthcharts/charts.htm
www.cdc.gov/nchs/nhanes.htm
www.cdc.gov/nccdphp/dnpa/obesity/basics.htm
MCHB Training Modules
www.depts.washington.edu/growth/
National Heart, Lung, and Blood Institute
www.nhlbi.nih.gov/index.htm
National Institutes of Health
www.cc.nih.gov/nutr.care.htm
U.S. Department of Agriculture
www.nal.usda.gov/fnic/etext/000108.html

Cited References

American Dietetic Association: Nutrition assessment of adults. In *Manual of clinical dietetics,* Chicago, 1996, The American Dietetic Association.

ASPEN Board of Directors: Guidelines for the use of parenteral and enteral nutrition in adults and pediatric patients, *J Parent Ent Nutr* 2002.

Balcombe NR et al: Nutritional status and well being: is there a relationship between body mass index and the well-being of older people? *Curr Med Res Opin* 17(1):1-7, 2001.

Barrocas A et al: Nutrition assessment practical approaches, *Clin Geriatr Med* 11(4):675, 1995.

Blackburn GL et al: Nutritional and metabolic assessment of the hospitalized patient, *J Parent Ent Nutr* 1:11, 1977.

Bray GA et al: Evaluation of the obese patient. I. An algorithm, *JAMA* 235:1487, 1976.

Buchman AL: *Handbook of nutritional support,* Baltimore, 1997, Williams & Wilkins.

Butterworth CE: The skeleton in the hospital closet, *Nutr Today* March/April, p 4, 1974.

Centers for Disease Control and Prevention: Basics about overweight and obesity, 2002, www.cdc.gov/nccdphp/dnpa/obesity/basics.htm.

Council on Practice, Quality Management Committee: ADA's definitions for nutrition screening and nutrition assessment, *J Am Diet Assoc* 94:838, 1994.

Curry KR: Mutlicultural competence in dietetics and nutrition, *J Am Diet Assoc* 100:1142, 2000.

Detsky AS et al: What is subjective global assessment? *J Parent Ent Nutr* 11:8, 1987.

Duerksen DR et al: The validity and reproducibility of clinical assessment of nutritional status in the elderly, *Nutrition* 16:740, 2000.

Frisancho AR: New standards of weight and body composition by frame size and height for assessment of nutritional status of adults and the elderly, *Am J Clin Nutr* 40:808, 1984.

Gilmore J: Body mass index and health, *Health Rep* 11:31, 1999.

Guenter PA et al: Anthropometric measurements. In Rombeau JL et al, eds: *Atlas of nutritional support techniques,* Boston, 1989, Little, Brown.

Hammond KA: Nutrition-focused physical assessment, *Support Line* 18(4):4, 1996.

Hammond KA: Physical assessment: a nutritional perspective, *Nurs Clin North Am* 32(4):779, 1997.

Hammond KA: The history and physical exam. In Matarese LE, Gottschlich M, eds: *Contemporary nutrition support practice,* Philadelphia, 1998, WB Saunders.

Healthy People 2010, Washington, DC, 2000, U.S. Department of Health and Human Services.

Heineken J, McCoy N: Establishing a bond with clients of different cultures, *Home Healthcare Nurs* 18(1):45, 2000.

Hopkins B: Assessment of nutritional status. In Gottschlich MM, Matarese LE, Shronts EP, eds: *Nutrition support dietetics,* ed 2, Silver Spring, Md, 1993, American Society for Parenteral and Enteral Nutrition.

Indorato D: Body composition analysis, *Today's Dietitian* 3:9, 2001.

Kant AK: Nature of dietary reporting by adults in the third National Health and Nutrition Examination Survey, 1988-1994, *J Am Coll Nutr* 21:315, 2002.

Keys A et al: Indices of relative weight and obesity, *J Chronic Dis* 25:329, 1972.

Kyle UG et al: Fat-free mass percentiles in 5225 healthy subjects aged 15 to 98 years, *Nutrition* 17:7/8, 2001.

Lee RD, Nieman DC: *Nutritional assessment,* ed 2, St Louis, 1996, Mosby.

Lohmann TG et al, eds: *Anthropometric standardization reference manual,* Champaign, Ill, 1988, Human Kinetics Publishers.

Methany N: *Fluid and electrolyte balance: nursing considerations,* Philadelphia, 1992, JB Lippincott.

National Center for Health Statistics: Leading causes of death, *Natl Vital Stat Rep* 47(19), 1999.

Nutrition interventions manual for professionals caring for older Americans: Executive summary: AAFP, ADA, and National Council on Aging, Washington, DC, 1991, Nutrition Screening Initiative.

Nutrition Screening Initiative: Washington, DC, 1991, AAFP, ADA, and National Council on Aging.

Nutritional assessment present and future, *Nutr Support Serv* 8:7, 1988.

Pfau PR, Rombeau JL: Nutrition, *Adv Gastroenterol* 84(5), 2000.

Sanchez AM, Reed DR, Price RA: Reduced mortality associated with body mass index (BMI) in African Americans relative to Caucasians, *Ethn Dis* 10(1):24, 2000.

Shopbell et al: Nutrition screening and assessment. In *The science and practice of nutrition support: American Society for Parenteral and Enteral Nutrition,* Dubuque, Iowa, 2001, Kendall/Hunt.

Shronts EP et al: Nutrition assessment. In *Nutrition support practice manual,* Silver Spring, Md, 1998, American Society for Parenteral and Enteral Nutrition.

Spruhan JB: Beyond traditional nursing care: cultural awareness and successful home healthcare nursing, *Home Healthcare Nurs* 14(6):445-449, 1996.

Stensland SH, Margolis S: Simplifying the calculation of body mass index for quick reference, *J Am Diet Assoc* 90:856, 1990.

The Surgeon General's call to action to prevent and decrease overweight and obesity, Rockville, Md, 2001, Office of the Surgeon General.

Tam SY et al: Body mass index is different in normal Chinese and Caucasian infants, *J Pediatr Endocrinol Metab* 12:507, 1999.

Vaccarino HA, Krumholz HM: An evidence-based assessment of federal guidelines for overweight and obesity as they apply to elderly persons, *Arch Int Med* 161:1194, 2001.

■ Additional References

Chumlea WC et al: Estimating stature from knee height for persons 60 to 90 years of age, *J Am Geriatr Soc* 33:116, 1985.

Duerksen DR: Teaching medical students the subjective global assessment, *Nutrition* 18:313, 2002.

Escott-Stump S: *Nutrition and diagnosis-related care,* ed 5, Baltimore, 2002, Lippincott Williams & Wilkins.

Evans-Stoner N: Nutrition assessment: a practical approach, *Nurs Clin North Am* 32(4):637, 1997.

Falciglia G et al: Upper arm anthropometric norms in elderly white subjects, *J Am Diet Assoc* 88:563, 451988.

Freedman DS et al: Relation of body fat patterning to lipid and lipoprotein concentrations in children and adolescents: the Bogalusa Heart Study, *Am J Clin Nutr* 50:930, 1989.

Harris TB et al: Waist circumference and sagittal diameter reflect total body fat better than visceral fat in older men and women: the health, aging and body composition study, *Ann N Y Acad Sci* 904:462, 2002.

Heiat A et al: An evidence-based assessment of federal guidelines for overweight and obesity as they apply to elderly persons, *Arch Intern Med* 161:1194, 2001.

Lissner L et al: Body composition and energy intake: do overweight women overeat and underreport? *Am J Clin Nutr* 49:320, 1989.

Trujillo EB, Robinson MK, Jacobs DO: Nutrition assessment in the critically ill, *Crit Care Nurse* 19:1, 1999.

Winkler M, Lysen L, eds: *Dietitians in Nutrition Support Dietetic Practice Group: suggested guidelines for nutrition and metabolic management of adult patients receiving nutrition support,* Chicago, 1993, American Dietetic Association.

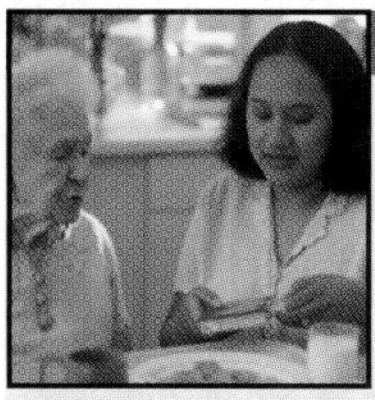

CHAPTER 18

Laboratory Data in Nutrition Assessment

TIMOTHY H. CARLSON, PhD, RD, NRCC

CHAPTER OUTLINE

- Definition and Usefulness of Nutrition Laboratory Data
- Assessment of Protein-Energy Status
- Laboratory Data for Nutritional Anemias
- Markers of Malabsorption
- Wellness Assessment
- Nutritional Interpretation of Routine Medical Laboratory Data

KEY TERMS

albumin–the most abundant (55% to 65% of total) and most often measured plasma protein; a negative acute-phase respondent with a long half-life ($t_{1/2}$ = 21 days); maintains plasma oncotic pressure and acts as a transport protein

anemia of chronic disease (ACD)–a condition associated with chronic inflammation in which hemoglobin or hematocrit values fall below reference values because iron transport from storage to the bone marrow is blocked

C-reactive protein (CRP)–a very sensitive plasma protein marker of inflammatory status

creatinine–a chemical breakdown product of creatine phosphate; used as a marker of renal function and muscle mass

ferritin–a protein that sequesters iron in a form readily activated for transport; found primarily inside the liver and other iron storage sites; plasma ferritin is proportional to intracellular ferritin and useful in assessing iron status

functional assay–the appraisal of nutrient pool size by measurement of the activity of a biochemical or physiologic function dependent on a specific nutrient

high sensitivity C-reactive protein (hsCRP)–a special CRP test to detect slight elevations of CRP, which are associated with increased risk for occlusive cardiovascular diseases

homocysteine–an amino acid that is an intermediate in the synthesis of methionine and the methyl group donor, *S*-adenosylmethionine; because the *S*-adenosylmethionine cycle requires vitamin B_{12} and folate, deficiencies in these vitamins are associated with hyperhomocysteinemia, an independent risk factor for occlusive cardiovascular disease

macrocytic anemia–a condition marked by a mean red cell volume of greater than 100 femtoliters (fl); most often caused by vitamin B_{12} or folate deficiencies

microcytic anemia–a condition marked by a mean red cell volume of greater than 80 femtoliters (fl); commonly associated with iron deficiency

negative acute-phase respondents–a group of plasma proteins, including albumin and transthyretin, whose concentrations decrease during inflammatory conditions (the acute-phase reaction)

nutrition-specific laboratory data–tests on body fluids (e.g., plasma, serum, saliva), tissues (e.g., whole blood, cells, hair, nails), and waste (e.g., urine, feces, sweat) that are performed by controlled physical, chemical, biochemical, molecular diagnostic, or microscopic examination, primarily to provide information about nutrient pool status

oxidative stress–the balance between the formation of toxic, free radical oxidation products and the reactions that convert these compounds to benign end products

positive acute-phase respondents–a group of plasma proteins, including C-reactive protein and alpha$_1$-acid glycoprotein (orosomucoid), whose concentrations increase during inflammatory states (the acute-phase reaction)

reactive oxidation species (ROS)–free radical species, including hydrogen peroxide (H_2O_2), superoxide radicals (O_2^-), and hydroxyl radicals (OH), that are formed during metabolic processes or metabolism of xenobiotic compounds

retinol-binding protein (RBP)–a negative acute-phase respondent plasma protein with a half-life ($t_{1/2}$ = 12 hours) whose concentration correlates with protein-energy status; binds and transports retinol

static assay–appraisal of nutrient pool size by direct measurement of the nutrient in a biologic fluid, tissue, or waste

total iron-binding capacity (TIBC)–a measurement of the potential for plasma to bind ferric ion (Fe^{3+})

transferrin–the plasma protein that transports iron from one organ to another; a negative acute-phase respondent that has a medium half-life ($t_{1/2}$ = 8 days) and is responsive to protein-energy status

transthyretin (TTHY)–a negative acute-phase respondent plasma protein that is frequently called *prealbumin;* binds thyroxine and retinol-binding protein and is commonly used to monitor protein-energy status; because of its short half-life ($t_{1/2}$ = 2 days), it rapidly responds to improving protein-energy status

zinc protoporphyrin/heme ratio (ZPPH)–a measurement of the proportion of zinc protoporphyrin (a hemelike compound with a substitution of zinc for iron) to heme in red blood cells; ZPPH increases in proportion to depletion of iron stores

Changes in nutritional status may occur slowly compared with changes in medical status. Deteriorating nutritional status, at least initially, may not affect medical status. When a disease develops, it is not always clear whether nutrition issues are contributing to the condition. However, disease or injury very frequently lead to rapid deterioration in nutritional status. To assess nutritional status, the data that indicate changes in clinical status must be integrated with changes in anthropometric indexes, dietary history, and laboratory markers.

DEFINITION AND USEFULNESS OF NUTRITION LABORATORY DATA

Nutrition-specific laboratory data can be defined as information about nutrition status obtained from controlled physical, chemical (biochemical), molecular diagnostic, or microscopic examination of specimens of body tissues, fluids, and wastes. Because laboratory data can be obtained from several disciplines, including clinical biochemistry and hematology, it is incorrect to use the terms biochemical assessment and laboratory assessment synonymously. In this text, laboratory data include, but are not limited to, biochemical data. Laboratory assessment of nutrients, not discussed in this chapter, is presented in Appendix 33.

Because nutrition status usually changes relatively slowly, the laboratory data used to assess it should be interpreted differently than that used to diagnose disease. Often, laboratory results are available from only a single point in time. Although a single laboratory result may be adequate for medical diagnosis, such data are less useful than serial data for performing nutrition assessment. However, one laboratory value can be helpful in screening or to confirm an assessment based on changing clinical, anthropometric, and dietary status.

The great advantage of laboratory data is that quality control can be stringently maintained inside the laboratory environment. This is primarily accomplished by analyzing control samples, which have predetermined analyte concentrations, with every batch of patient specimens. The results obtained from the control samples analyzed with a particular batch of patient samples must compare favorably with the predetermined acceptable values before the patient data are considered valid. Characterization of body dimensions, density, permeability to radiation, radiation from the body, and other biophysical properties cannot be accomplished in the same controlled environment of a clinical laboratory.

When data are obtained from a laboratory with a well-designed and faithfully practiced quality control program, the clinician can be confident that the resulting data are not compromised by inadequate analytical methods or operator error or bias (Figure 18-1). Conversely, data from laboratories that do not

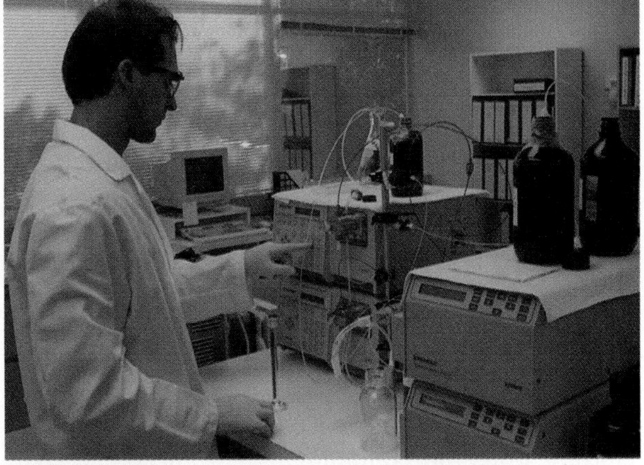

FIGURE 18-1 • A technician sets up a high-performance liquid chromatography (HPLC) assay to measure various levels such as plasma, homocysteine, vitamins, and carotenoids.

CLINICAL INSIGHT

Hair Analysis

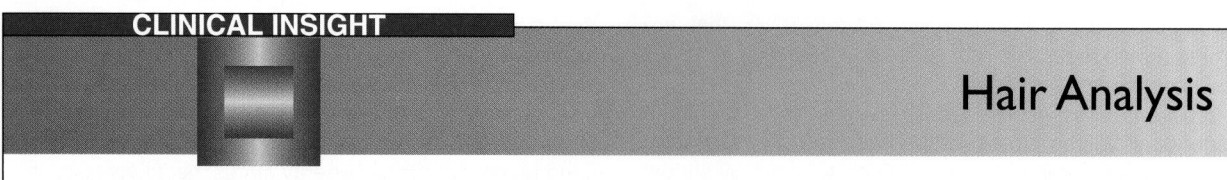

Hair analysis is not particularly useful for assessing levels of minerals such as sodium, magnesium, phosphorus, potassium, calcium, iron, and iodine because good tests already exist for evaluating body functions related to these minerals. However, hair analysis may be helpful in assessing levels of trace elements such as zinc, copper, chromium, and manganese—for which measurements of functional status are not well developed—and levels of cadmium and lead, which have negative biologic effects.

However, to be clinically useful, hair analysis procedures must be refined and standardized, and "normal" values for hair mineral content defined and accepted. Currently, hair analysis is more useful in experimental efforts than in clinical medicine. The technique is most useful when used to analyze levels of a single element rather than several elements at one time because the probability of an abnormal test result increases as the specificity of the test decreases.

Even if hair analysis results are judged to be "abnormal," it is not known whether these results reflect abnormal exposure to an element and thus a cause of the disease or whether the abnormal result is an effect of the disease. Use of hair dyes and other chemical processes may also affect results. No evidence shows that nutritional therapy based on hair analysis is of any benefit.

maintain rigorous quality control lose much of their potential to be primary indicators of nutritional imbalance. The accuracy of laboratory assessment depends not only on interpretation of the data but also on confidence that the laboratory carefully maintains quality.

Specimen Types

Several specimen types are used to test for nutrients and nutrient-related substances, including the following:

- Serum (the fluid obtained from blood after the blood has been clotted and then centrifuged to remove the clot and blood cells)
- Plasma (the fluid obtained after centrifugation of blood collected with anticoagulants, such as ethylenediaminetetraacetic acid [EDTA], heparin, trisodium citrate, or potassium oxalate)
- Erythrocytes (red blood cells)
- Leukocytes (white blood cells) and leukocyte fractions
- Other tissues (obtained from scrapings or biopsy samples)
- Urine (from random samples or timed collections)
- Feces (from random samples or timed collections)

Less commonly used specimens include the following:

- Saliva
- Nails
- Hair
- Sweat
- Blood spots

The latter specimens have significant drawbacks, including potential contamination from contact with the environment; lack of standardized procedures for processing, assay, and quality control; and nutrient levels or indexes that are less than the amounts that can be measured accurately and precisely (see *Clinical Insight:* Hair Analysis). However, because these specimens can be collected at the point of care, considerable research is being done to improve their usefulness. Point-of-care testing may include analysis of the specimen at the site of collection. Because point-of-care testing is often more convenient for the patient and caregiver and saves time and money, it is favored by medical economists and reimbursement administrators.

Types of Assays

The two fundamental types of laboratory assays are *static assays* and *functional assays.* Static assays measure the actual level of nutrient in the specimen. Examples of this kind of assay include serum iron, white blood cell ascorbic acid, and hair zinc. Although this kind of assay has the advantage of being absolutely specific for the nutrient of interest, specimen nutrient concentrations do not reflect the amount of that substance stored in body pools that are not sampled. The other major limitation of static assays is that recent dietary intake can influence the amount of a nutrient found in serum, plasma, or any other fluid or tissue. This problem can be overcome, at least partially, by collecting the specimen when the person is fasting. An overnight (8- to 12-hour) fast is usually adequate.

Functional assays quantitatively measure a biochemical or physiologic activity that depends on the nutrient of interest. This type of assay can be very sensitive for a nutrient at its functional site. A good example of a functional assay is serum ferritin. The concentration of ferritin released into the blood is a function of the iron present in the cellular storage pool. Unfortunately, functional assays are not always specific for the nutrient of interest because many physiologic and biochemical functions depend on various biologic factors in addition to the specific nutrient.

ASSESSMENT OF PROTEIN-ENERGY STATUS

Hormonal and Cell-Mediated Response to Stress

Acute illness or trauma causes inflammatory stress (Chang and Bistrian, 1998), and protein-energy malnutrition (PEM) often develops simultaneously (Moldawer and Copeland, 1997) (see Chapter 42); these result from the release of cytokines such as interleukin-1, interleukin-6, and tumor necrosis factor. The cytokines reorient hepatic synthesis of plasma proteins and increase the breakdown of muscle protein to meet the demand for protein and energy during the inflammatory response. Proteins that are designated negative acute-phase respondents, such as albumin, transferrin, transthyretin (or *prealbumin*), and retinol-binding protein, decrease during the acute-phase response. Others, designated positive acute-phase respondents (and often called *acute-phase proteins,* although the term is less accurate), increase to varying degrees. Positive acute-phase respondents include C-reactive protein, orosomucoid, and fibrinogen (Box 18-1). The change in the levels of these proteins is generally proportional to the severity of the tissue injury associated with the trauma, infection, or other physiologic insult.

The decrease in the plasma levels of albumin and in the levels of the other negative acute-phase proteins that occurs during the acute phase is caused by (1) down-regulation of gene expression and translation, (2) increases in catabolism, (3) transport to extravascular pools, and (4) a probable reduction in synthesis caused by decreased levels of dietary essential amino acids.

The shift of albumin (and similarly sized negative acute-phase proteins) to the extravascular space during the acute inflammatory response is different from the process that occurs during uncomplicated starvation *(marasmus)* without inflammatory stress. In the latter, even though albumin synthesis decreases somewhat, plasma albumin is maintained by a shift of albumin from the extravascular space into the plasma.

Box 18-1. Classification of Certain Plasma Proteins by Function*

Immunoglobulins

IgG, IgA, IgM, IgD, IgE

Complement Components

C1q, C1r, C1s, C2, **C3, C4,** C5, C6, C7, C8, and C9; properdin; factors D, H, I, and P; C4bp; S-protein; C8bp

Coagulation and Fibrinolytic Factors

Fibrinogen; prothrombin; factors V, VII, VIII, IX, XI, XII, and XIII; protein C and protein S; prekallikrein; HMW-kininogen; von Willebrand's factor; plasminogen

Enzyme Inhibitors

α_1-antitrypsin, α_2-macroglobulin, inter-α-trypsin inhibitor antithrombin III, C1-inhibitor, **α_1-chymotrypsin,** α_2-antiplasmin, heparin cofactor II, cystatin C, pregnancy-associated α_2-glycoprotein, tissue factor pathway inhibitor (lipoprotein-associated coagulation inhibitor [LACI])

Lipid Transport–Associated Proteins

Apoproteins A-I, A-II, B, C-I, C-II, C-III, D, and E; β_2-glycoprotein I; **serum amyloid A**

Transport Proteins

Albumin, TTHY (prealbumin), transferrin, RBP, thyroxin-binding protein, vitamin D–binding protein, sex hormone–binding protein, transcobalamin I, transcobalamin II, corticosteroid-binding globulin, transcortin, **hemopexin, haptoglobin, ceruloplasmin**

Proteins of Uncertain or Other Functions

α_1-Acid glycoprotein (orosomucoid), α_1B-glycoprotein, serum amyloid P component, α_1-microglobulin, Zn-α_2-glycoprotein, fibronectin, α-HS-glycoprotein, histidine-rich glycoprotein, **CRP**

Positive acute-phase proteins* are shown in **bold type; *negative acute-phase proteins* are in ***bold italics;*** proteins that are used in protein-energy assessment are underlined. Note that the positive acute-phase proteins are distributed among almost all functional classes, whereas the main negative acute-phase proteins are transport proteins.

Nitrogen Balance

Nitrogen balance is the oldest biochemical technique for assessing protein status. Currently, it is the only biochemical measurement that truly reflects changes in the somatic and visceral protein pools. Nitrogen balance calculations are based on the knowledge that approximately 16% of the mass of proteins is nitrogen. Therefore if daily protein intake can be determined accurately, measurements of nitrogen excretion, combined with corrections for insensible losses (e.g., from skin and gastrointestinal [GI] sloughing, hair loss, and sweat), allow nitrogen balance to be determined. In healthy adults the nitrogen balance is zero. The nitrogen balance is negative during starvation and several forms of PEM (in which nitrogen loss exceeds intake); it is positive in growing children, pregnant females, and adults who are adding mass (weight) or recovering from injury or illness. The nitrogen balance is calculated as follows:

$$\text{Nitrogen balance} = \text{Nitrogen intake (g/24 hr)} - (\text{Urinary nitrogen [g/24 hr]} + 2\ \text{g/24 hr})$$

If urinary nitrogen is replaced by a urinary urea measurement, the correction factor becomes *+4 g/24 hr* to account for nitrogenous compounds such as uric acid, ammonia, creatinine, and amino acids in the urine. The use of urea nitrogen in nitrogen balance determinations is not recommended because of the considerable variation among patients in the secretion of the non–urea nitrogen–containing compounds (see Konstantinides et al, 1991).

The total urinary nitrogen level can be measured by *Kjeldahl analysis,* which is laborious and generally not suitable for most clinical laboratories, or by *pyrochemiluminescence,* a rapid and simple technique for quantifying urinary nitrogen. Pyrochemiluminescence takes advantage of the heat and light produced by the product of the reaction of nitric oxide (produced by heating the various forms of nitrogen in urine to 1100° C) and ozone (Nussbaum, Baertschi, and Jansen, 2002).

Pyrochemiluminescence is easier and cheaper than the older Kjeldahl analysis. Furthermore, the results are superior to urinary urea values for determining nitrogen levels; although urinary non–urea nitrogen averages about 4 g/day, it ranges from 0 to about 6 g/day in normal persons and may exceed 10 g/day in those who are critically ill.

The chief difficulty with nitrogen balance measurements is that it may be impossible to estimate the protein intake of those who are consuming food by mouth. However, these measurements are extremely valuable for monitoring the appropriateness of a completely defined intake (e.g., in those receiving parenteral nutrition or enteral tube feeding therapy). Nitrogen balance should be measured at least weekly in those receiving short-term nutrition support—perhaps more often during the initial stages (see Chapter 23). These measurements allow the dietitian, pharmacist, and physician to assess not only whether the patient is in nitrogen balance but also whether the patient is able to use the amount of protein that total parenteral nutrition or enteral nutrition is providing. Thus even if the nitrogen balance is positive, it may be appropriate to decrease the protein being provided to prevent large-scale deamination of amino acids that cannot be used in de novo protein synthesis. The appropriate amount of protein decreases the energy expenditure for amino acid deamination and urea formation.

Visceral (Plasma) Protein Indicators

Proteins in plasma and extravascular fluids represent approximately 3% of the total body protein, whereas visceral organ protein constitutes about 10%. Because albumin and many other plasma proteins are synthesized in the liver—a surrogate for all visceral organs—plasma proteins can be thought of as functional indices of visceral protein balance. Of course, the metabolic balance of hepatic protein and somatic tissue protein is related, so the total body protein status is reflected by measurements of certain plasma proteins to some extent. Unlike nitrogen balance measurements, which assess only short-term changes in whole body protein status, plasma protein levels (and measurements of muscle mass) integrate protein synthesis and degradation over longer periods. As compared with other methods of assessing changing protein-energy status, plasma protein measurements are quicker, more precise, and less expensive. Furthermore, proper interpretation of plasma protein data can make these data very valuable to nutrition professionals, especially in institutional environments.

More than 300 proteins have been identified in human plasma. Box 18-1 shows how acute-phase respondent proteins and proteins that have been studied as indicators of protein nutrition status fit into a functional classification of plasma proteins.

Albumin

Because albumin is abundant in serum, stable, highly soluble in water, and easily purified, it has been one of the most intensively studied of all proteins. However, some of the diagnostic uses of serum albumin values are now outdated, especially in the area of nutrition assessment and monitoring. In truth, albumin likely reflects protein intake only in specialized experimental conditions, such as when animals who are housed in stressful facilities are fed diets deficient only in protein. Studies in which the albumin levels during total starvation have been compared with the levels during consumption of protein-limited diets have shown that albumin decreases dramatically in those consuming protein-free diets but is more preserved in those with total starvation. These effects are similar to the effects of marasmus and kwashiorkor on albumin levels. Inflammation is an almost universal finding in those with kwashiorkor (protein deficiency); it is likely that many hospitalized patients with low albumin levels also have inflammation (e.g., infection, trauma, another physiologic stress).

In addition to the mentioned limitation, albumin is a negative acute-phase reactant and has a long half-life (~20 days), meaning that the plasma albumin concentration increases slowly in patients recovering from stress and those receiving nutrition intervention. Another shortcoming of albumin for monitoring changes in those with PEM is related to the large extravascular albumin pool. Albumin that is not in the bloodstream (extravascular albumin) is 1.5 to 2 times higher than albumin in the blood. Some of this large albumin pool returns to the circulation when blood concentrations decrease, which tends to blunt changes in plasma albumin concentration. Therefore when synthesis decreases, large amounts of albumin can return to the circulation; when synthesis increases, albumin leaves to replenish the extravascular pool. In conclusion, albumin is at best a mediocre index of PEM.

Transferrin

Transferrin is one of several proteins functioning exclusively in the transport of other essential compounds and that are used in the assessment of PEM. Like albumin, it is a negative acute-phase respondent, but it has a shorter half-life (8 days) (Table 18-1).

In addition to being responsive to dietary protein and energy, the plasma transferrin level is controlled by the size of the iron storage pool. When iron stores are depleted, transferrin synthesis increases. Therefore its level may reflect iron status, as well as protein-energy status.

Although the half-life of transferrin is shorter than that of albumin, it still does not respond rapidly enough to protein-energy status to be useful in acute care settings. This, in addition to its nonspecificity, makes transferrin only slightly more useful than albumin as a marker of protein-energy status.

Transthyretin

For more than two decades, there has been interest in the use of transthyretin (TTHY), or *prealbumin*, for the assessment of protein-energy status (Beck and Rosenthal, 2002; Mears, 1996). TTHY is a transport protein that binds retinol-binding protein. As indicated by its alternate name, *thyroxin-binding prealbumin*, TTHY also binds thyroxin.

TTHY levels have been shown to correlate with short-term changes in PEM status. However, the use of TTHY in the assessment of PEM is associated with some of the same problems that plague the use of albumin and transferrin. Most important, it is a negative acute-phase protein. Hence, its use in screening for PEM is limited because a low level could result from either inadequate nutrition or inflammatory stress. On the other hand, because TTHY has a half-life of just 2 days, it is useful in monitoring improvements in protein-energy status (see Table 18-1). If a baseline value is obtained at or near its *nadir*—when the hypermetabolic period of the inflammatory response wanes—subsequent increases in TTHY values correlate with a positive nitrogen balance. Thus the short half-life of TTHY allows a short-term and sensitive assessment of improving status.

One other drawback to the use of TTHY is that a zinc deficiency affects hepatic TTHY synthesis and secretion. Therefore zinc status, in addition to inflammation, should be taken into account when interpreting low plasma TTHY levels.

TABLE 18-1 Properties of Proteins Commonly Used in Protein-Energy Assessments

PROTEIN	APPROXIMATE HALF-LIFE	MOLECULAR WEIGHT	REFERENCE RANGE
Albumin	3 wk	65,000	3.5-5.2 g/dl
Transferrin	1 wk	80,000	200-400 mg/dl
TTHY	2 days	55,000	19-43 mg/dl
RBP	12 hr	21,000	2.1-6.4 mg/dl

Retinol-Binding Protein

Another protein with a short half-life that has been used to assess PEM is retinol-binding protein (RBP). RBP has a half-life of about 12 hours. It is small for a plasma protein but does not pass through the renal glomerulus because it circulates in a complex with TTHY. As implied by its name, RBP binds retinol, and transport of this vitamin A metabolite seems to be its exclusive function (see Chapter 4). RBP is synthesized in the liver and released with retinol. After RBP releases retinol in peripheral tissue, its affinity for TTHY decreases, leading to dissociation of the TTHY-RBP complex and filtration of apo-RBP by the glomerulus. The protein is then catabolized in the renal tubule.

The plasma RBP concentration has been shown to correlate with protein-energy status in uncomplicated PEM. However, confounding the interpretation of RBP levels is RBP's actions in those with inflammatory stress. Like albumin, transferrin, and TTHY, RBP is a negative acute-phase protein, meaning that RBP does not reflect protein-energy status in acutely stressed patients.

The simultaneous secretion of RBP and retinol from the liver means that retinol status also complicates the interpretation of reduced RBP values. RBP cannot reliably be used to assess protein-energy status when the vitamin A status is compromised.

The use of RBP in assessing PEM is complicated by the normal catabolism of apo-RBP by the kidney. Patients with renal failure are likely to have elevated RBP levels, regardless of their protein-energy status, because the RBP is not being catabolized by the renal tubule.

C-Reactive Protein

When used as indicators of protein-energy status, the major difficulty associated with each of the four plasma proteins discussed thus far is their behavior during inflammatory stress. Indeed, most patients in acute-care settings experience some type of inflammatory response, making it difficult to interpret accurately decreases in levels of albumin, transferrin, TTHY, or RBP. Perhaps the best way to circumvent this shortcoming is not to use these plasma proteins for protein-energy assessment during various phases of the inflammatory response. Determining the optimal time for initiating aggressive nutrition intervention during the resolution of inflammation is difficult.

Standardization of nutrition therapy during the inflammatory response can be aided by the use of an objective serum marker of the acute phase. One approach that is being used more frequently is using one of the positive acute-phase respondent proteins to monitor the progress of the stress reaction and to begin more aggressive nutritional intervention when this indicator shows that the inflammatory reactions are subsiding. The best protein for this purpose is likely C-reactive protein (CRP). Although the exact function of CRP is unclear, it increases in the initial stages of acute stress—usually within 4 to 6 hours of surgery or other trauma. Furthermore, its level can increase as much as 1000-fold depending on the intensity of the stress response (Thompson et al, 1992). Experience indicates that when the CRP level begins to decrease, the patient has entered the anabolic period of the inflammatory response, and more intensive nutrition therapy is beneficial. Because TTHY levels begin to increase at about the same time that CRP starts to decrease and because increasing levels of TTHY correlate well with improving protein-energy status, starting nutrition intervention can be tied to changes in the levels of both of these plasma proteins.

Recent interest in CRP has been generated by the observation that slightly increased levels of the protein are associated with increased risk for the development of disease associated with atherosclerosis (Blake and Ridker, 2001), and evidence shows that nutrition affects this response (Liu et al, 2002). This chronic subclinical inflammation of atherosclerosis is marked by a moderate increase in serum CRP. A different test, highly sensitive CRP (hsCRP), is used to measure these slightly elevated CRP levels.

Somatic Indicators of Protein-Energy Malnutrition

Urinary Creatinine and Creatinine/Height Ratio

Creatinine is formed from *creatine,* a compound found almost exclusively in muscle tissue. Creatine is synthesized from the amino acids glycine and arginine with addition of a methyl group from the folate- and cobalamin-dependent methionine-*S*-adenosylmethionine-homocysteine cycle. It is a high-energy phosphate buffer, maintaining a constant supply of adenosine triphosphate (ATP) for muscle contraction. When creatine is dephosphorylated, some of it is spontaneously converted to creatinine by an irreversible, nonenzymatic reaction. Creatinine has no specific biologic function; it is continuously released from the muscle cells and excreted by the kidneys with little reabsorption. When a patient follows a meat-restricted diet, the size of the patient's somatic (muscle) protein pool is directly proportional to the amount of creatinine excreted. This means men generally excrete larger amounts of creatinine than women and that individuals with greater muscular development excrete larger amounts than those who are less muscular. Total body weight is not proportional to creatinine excretion, but muscle mass is. Creatinine excretion rate is related to muscle mass, as shown by the following equation:

$$\text{Muscle mass} = k + k' \times \text{Urinary creatinine}$$

where:

$$k \text{ and } k' = \text{Empirical constants}$$

Using computed tomography as the gold standard, the following equation was developed:

$$\text{Skeletal muscle mass (kg)} = 4.1 + 18.9 \times \text{24-hr creatinine excretion (g/day)}$$

This equation works well for most individuals but not for body builders, and it has not been tested with sick or injured patients.

An approach formerly used to assess somatic protein status involved the creatinine/height index (CHI):

$$\text{CHI} = \frac{\text{24-hr urine volume (dl)} \times \text{Urine creatinine concentration (mg/dl)}}{\text{Expected 24-hr urine creatinine excretion (mg)}}$$

The expected 24-hour creatinine excretion is related to the patient's height, and tables have been constructed that contain the expected values. Clearly, muscle mass does not depend entirely on height, so the CHI must be used with caution to assess tall, thin, or muscular individuals.

The use of creatinine and CHI to assess somatic protein status is also confounded by omnivorous diets. As already mentioned, creatine is stored in muscle, so muscle meats, which are rich in creatine, and the creatinine that is formed from dietary creatine cannot be distinguished from endogenously produced creatinine. Another factor confounding interpretation of urinary creatinine data is that daily creatinine excretion varies significantly within individuals, probably because of sweat losses. In addition, the test is based on 24-hour urine collections, and it is often difficult to obtain quantitative urine collections. Because of these limitations, the use of urinary creatinine concentration as a marker of muscle mass is primarily semiquantitative.

3-Methylhistidine Excretion

Muscle mass is also related to the excretion of the amino acid *3-methylhistidine.* This amino acid is found only in the actin and myosin of muscle tissue and is produced by biosynthetic modification of the histidine residues of these proteins after synthesis is complete. During the normal turnover of muscle proteins, 3-methylhistidine is released and cannot be recycled. Therefore its level in urine is related to somatic protein mass. 3-Methylhistidine is not often used in protein-energy assessments because it requires labor-intensive assay procedures. In addition, like creatinine, the amount supplied by the diet (i.e., through consumption of muscle meats) is difficult to estimate accurately, and 24-hour urine collections are required.

LABORATORY DATA FOR NUTRITIONAL ANEMIAS

Anemia is a condition characterized by a reduction in the number of erythrocytes per unit of blood volume, or a decrease in the blood's hemoglobin to below the level of usual physiologic need. By convention, *anemia* is defined as a hemoglobin concentration below the 95th percentile for healthy reference populations of men, women, or age-grouped children. Anemia is not a disease but is a symptom of various conditions, including extensive blood loss, excessive blood cell destruction, or decreased blood cell formation. Clinical nutritionists are primarily concerned with distinguishing between nutritional anemia caused by nutritional inadequacies and anemia caused by other factors (see Chapter 34).

Classification of Anemia

Nutritional deficits are a major cause of decreased hemoglobin and erythrocyte production. The initial, descriptive classification of anemia is derived from the hematocrit value or complete blood count (CBC) and associated calculations. Anemias associated with a mean red blood cell volume of less than 80 fl (femtoliters) are called *microcytic,* whereas those with values of 80 to 99 fl are termed normocytic, and those associated with values of 100 fl or more are macrocytic (Massey, 1992) (see Chapter 34).

Data from the complete blood count are helpful in differentiating nutritional causes for anemia. Microcytic anemia is most often associated with iron deficiency, whereas macrocytic anemia is generally caused by either folate- or vitamin B_{12}–deficient erythropoiesis. However, because of the low specificity of these indexes, additional data are needed to distinguish between the various nutritional causes of microcytic and macrocytic anemias and their nonnutritional causes, such as thalassemia trait and chronic renal insufficiency. Microcytosis can also be associated with inadequate iron use, most commonly in the anemia of chronic disease. The latter type of anemia is associated with rheumatic diseases, chronic infection, cancer, severe tissue injury, multiple fractures, and Hodgkin's disease. Hence, anemia with microcytosis is not a sufficient cause for recommending iron supplementation.

Other information from the CBC that helps to differentiate the nonnutritional causes of anemia includes leukocyte and platelet counts. When these are low, marrow failure is indicated; high counts are associated with anemia caused by leukemia or infection. If anemia is associated with normal-size red cells, it is most likely caused by acute blood loss. However, in those with hemolytic anemias and early iron deficiency anemia, the red blood cell size may also be normal (see Figure 34-1).

An additional way to rule out nonnutritional causes of anemia is to evaluate the reticulocyte count. Reticulocytes are large, nucleated, immature red blood cells that are released in small numbers with mature cells. When red blood cell production rates increase, reticulocyte counts also increase. Any time anemia is accompanied by a high reticulocyte count, elevated erythropoietic activity in response to bleeding should be considered. In such cases, stool specimens can be tested for occult blood to rule out chronic GI blood loss. Other causes of a high reticulocyte count include intravascular hemolysis syndromes and an erythropoietic response to therapy for iron, vitamin B_{12}, or folic acid deficiencies.

Laboratory Tests for Iron Deficiency Anemias

Serum Iron

Of the various tests used to establish iron deficiency in those with microcytic anemia, serum iron and total iron-binding capacity are often the first to be determined (Worwood, 1997).

Although it is widely available and a relatively easy test to perform, the serum iron level is a relatively poor index of iron status because of large day-to-day changes, even in healthy individuals. Diurnal variations also occur, with the highest concentrations occurring midmorning (from 6 AM to 10 AM), and a nadir, averaging 30% less than the morning level, occurs at midafternoon. Hence, other tests are needed to definitively assess iron status.

Total Iron-Binding Capacity and Transferrin Saturation

Total iron-binding capacity (TIBC) depends on the number of free binding sites on the plasma iron-transport protein, transferrin. Each transferrin molecule binds ferric ions (Fe[III]) at each of two binding sites and two bicarbonate ions at separate sites.

Intracellular iron availability regulates the synthesis and secretion of transferrin. Therefore the plasma transferrin concentration increases in those with iron deficiency. In addition, when the amount of stored iron available for release to transferrin decreases and dietary iron intake is low, saturation of transferrin decreases.

In people with sufficient iron levels, the normal plasma transferrin concentration is 200 to 400 mg/dl (25 to 50 μmol/L). Therefore because transferrin has two iron binding sites and iron has an atomic weight of 56 daltons, the expected TIBC is 2800 to 5600 mg/L (280 to 560 mg/dl). However, the range of normal TIBC values is 270 to 400 mg/dl, indicating that full occupation of all transferrin binding sites does not occur. Because bicarbonate binding by transferrin is required to activate iron binding fully, loss of this ion from the serum after standing in a tube or intrinsically inadequate amounts of the ion could explain the incomplete saturation of transferrin, even in the presence of excess iron. Because of this discrepancy, direct correlation of TIBC with transferrin level is not a 1:1 relationship.

There are exceptions to the general rule that transferrin saturation decreases and TIBC increases in patients with iron deficiency. For example, TIBC increases in those with hepatitis. It also increases in people with hypoxia, who are pregnant, or who are taking oral contraceptives or receiving estrogen replacement therapy. On the other hand, TIBC decreases in those with malignant disease, nephritis, acute and chronic inflammatory diseases, megaloblastic anemias, and hemolytic anemias. Furthermore, the plasma level of transferrin may be decreased in those with PEM, fluid overload, and liver disease. Thus, although TIBC and transferrin saturation are more specific then hematocrit or hemoglobin values, they are not perfect indicators of iron status.

An additional concern about the use of serum iron, TIBC, and transferrin saturation values is that normal values persist until frank deficiency actually develops. Thus, these tests cannot detect decreasing iron stores and preanemic iron deficiencies.

Zinc Protoporphyrin/Heme Ratio and Free-Erythrocyte Protoporphyrin

A simple, cost-effective test for iron status is the zinc protoporphyrin/heme ratio (ZPPH) (Wong et al, 1996). This test, which can be performed using a single drop of blood, is based on the finding that protoporphyrin IX, the molecule that binds iron to form the heme portion of the hemoglobin molecule, may also bind zinc. Because of a nonenzymatic process, 1 out of approximately 20,000 hemoglobin molecules in people with sufficient iron levels contains protoporphyrin IX bound to Zn(II) rather than Fe(II). As the iron available for erythropoiesis decreases, the fraction of zinc protoporphyrin increases. Iron stores are considered to be depleted when the ratio of zinc protoporphyrin in red blood cells to heme molecules increases to more than 1:12,000. The conventional way of reporting these data is as a ratio of the micromoles of zinc protoporphyrin per mole of heme in red blood cells. Abnormal ZPPH ratios are 80 μmol/mol and higher. Because the ZPPH measurement is a ratio of intracellular porphyrin species, it is better than concentration-based measurements because it is unaffected by hydration status or recent blood loss.

Unlike TIBC and transferrin saturation, the ZPPH ratio is very stable in people with sufficient iron levels, and it is minimally affected by the physiologic and pathophysiologic factors that influence many other iron tests. In addition, depletion of the storage pool can be monitored by the ZPPH ratio. Factors other than iron deficiency that increase the ZPPH ratio are limited to lead poisoning, protoporphyria (rare), and chronic inflammation (common).

A test that is analogous to the ZPPH ratio is free-erythrocyte protoporphyrin (FEP). This test does not actually measure iron-free protoporphyrin, as the name suggests. Rather, it measures a chemically derived product of zinc protoporphyrin. Therefore even though measuring this compound is much more laborious, it measures essentially the same phenomenon gauged by direct measurement of ZPPH. In addition to being a less costly procedure, the ZPPH ratio is a preferred screening test because it is independent of hematocrit, not affected by hydration status, and not altered by recent blood loss or causes of anemia not related to iron deficiency.

Ferritin

To obtain laboratory confirmation of iron deficiency anemia after screening for ZPPH ratio, FEP, or red-cell distribution width (RDW), the serum ferritin level is often measured as an indicator of iron stores (Ponka et al, 1998). The only other test currently available for this purpose is staining a bone marrow aspirate for iron. Because collection of a marrow aspirate is a very involved procedure and unpleasant for the patient, it is impractical for routine assessment of iron status. However, serum ferritin levels are used routinely for this purpose.

Ferritin is the storage protein that sequesters the iron normally gathered in the liver (reticuloendothelial system), spleen, and marrow. As the iron supply increases, the intracellular level of ferritin increases to accommodate iron storage. A small amount of this ferritin leaks into the circulation. This ferritin can be measured by assays that are available in most clinical laboratories. The serum ferritin concentration is directly proportional to the amount of ferritin inside storage cells and indirectly proportional to the amount of iron in those cells. Therefore measurement of ferritin that has leaked into the serum is an excellent indicator of the size of the body's iron storage pool.

Effect of Inflammation on Anemia

Unfortunately, under some circumstances, ferritin levels may give a skewed representation of iron status because the ferritin level increases during inflammation. Cytokines and other inflammatory mediators can increase ferritin synthesis, ferritin leakage from cells, or both. This means that patients with iron deficiency could have a normal or elevated serum ferritin level if they have a chronic or an acute inflammatory condition.

Anemia of chronic disease (ACD) is the primary condition in which ferritin fails to correlate with iron stores (Haurani, 2002; Ozatli et al, 2000). ACD, probably the most common form of anemia in hospitalized patients, occurs in those with inflammatory, infectious, and neoplastic disorders (Bron et al, 2001). It occurs during inflammation because red cell production decreases as the result of inadequate mobilization of iron from its storage sites. This is apparently caused by the release of cytokines such as interleukin-1 and tumor necrosis factor (TNF), which also inhibit division of erythroid progenitors and may inhibit erythropoietin production. In those with arthritis, a classic chronic inflammatory condition, depletion of stored iron develops partly because of reduced absorption of iron from the gut. In contrast, the regular use of nonsteroidal antiinflammatory drugs can cause occult GI blood loss. This form of anemia is usually mild and normocytic (i.e., not microcytic or macrocytic).

However, in 30% to 50% of patients, hypochromic (i.e., having inadequate amounts of hemoglobin), microcytic red cells are made, serum iron levels and TIBC are low, and iron stores are normal or elevated. Because iron stores do not decrease, normal amounts of ferritin should be present in the plasma. However, in some cases, iron stores may be depleted, but inflammatory mediators may cause ferritin levels to remain normal. Certain patients with complicated clinical conditions, such as those with rheumatoid arthritis, may have reduced or deficient stores. Thus ACD has many forms and must be distinguished from iron deficiency anemia so that inappropriate iron supplementation is not initiated.

Serum Transferrin Receptor Test

Several tests for iron deficiency are currently being developed, some of which are not affected by inflammatory status. One of the most promising tests—the *serum transferrin receptor (sTfR)* test—is now being used in clinical laboratories. This receptor protein binds holotransferrin (transferrin-Fe[III]) during cellular iron uptake. When cellular iron levels decrease, synthesis of sTfR increases. sTfR reflects the amount of this protein on the surface of cells, and an increase in serum levels correlates with iron deficiency. It seems that sTfR effectively monitors iron status in normal conditions, inflammatory conditions, and conditions of iron overload. It is possible that sTfR will soon be used with ferritin to confirm iron deficiency in those with ACD (Suominen et al, 2000).

Laboratory Assessment of Macrocytic Anemias Associated With B Vitamin Deficiencies

The nutritional causes of macrocytic anemia (also referred to as *megaloblastic anemia* because of the presence of giant red cell precursors in the blood) are related to the availability of folate and vitamin B_{12} (cobalamin) in the bone marrow. It remains to be determined which vitamin is associated with this condition and, if vitamin B_{12} deficiency is the cause, the etiology of this deficit.

Static Tests for Folate and Vitamin B_{12} Status

Usually, patients with macrocytic anemia are tested for folate and vitamin B_{12} deficiency by static measurement of the vitamins in blood. They can be assayed by testing the ability of the patient's blood specimen to support the growth of microbes that require either folate or vitamin B_{12}. However, today, radiobinding assays and various kinds of immunoassays are more commonly used.

Folate is most often simultaneously measured in whole blood (i.e., combined plasma and blood cells) and in the serum alone. The difference between whole blood folate and serum folate levels is then used to calculate the red blood cell folate concentration. It is generally thought that the level of folate in red blood cells better reflects the size of the total folate pool than does the folate level in serum. However, considerable evidence shows that a serum sample obtained after scrupulous fasting is as good for assessing folate status as red blood cell folate levels. The advantage of the serum measurement is that it is considerably less laborious and thus less expensive. Vitamin B_{12} is usually measured in the serum, and all indications are that the serum level gives as much information about vitamin B_{12} status as does the red blood cell level.

Functional Tests to Determine Causes of Macrocytic Anemias

Homocysteine

Folate and vitamin B_{12} are required for the synthesis of *S*-adenosylmethionine, the biochemical precursor involved in the transfer of one-carbon (methyl) groups during many biochemical syntheses. *S*-adenosylmethionine is synthesized from the amino acid methionine by a reaction that includes the addition of a methyl group and the purine base adenine (from ATP). For example, when *S*-adenosylmethionine donates a methyl group for the synthesis of thymine, choline, creatine, epinephrine, and protein (e.g., 3-methylhistidine formation) and DNA methylation, it is converted to *S*-adenosyl homocysteine. After losing the adenosyl group, the remaining homocysteine can either be converted to cysteine by the vitamin B_6–dependent transsulfuration pathway or converted back to methionine in a reaction that depends on folate and vitamin B_{12} (see Figure 34-7 and Chapters 4 and 35).

When either folate or vitamin B_{12} is lacking, the homocysteine-to-methionine reaction is virtually blocked, causing homocysteine to build up in the affected tissue and spill into the circulation. The vitamin B_6–dependent transsulfuration pathway can metabolize excess homocysteine. Therefore an elevated homocysteine level is expected to indicate either genetic defects involved in the enzymes that catalyze these reactions or a deficiency in folate, vitamin B_{12}, or vitamin B_6. Indeed, homocysteine has been shown to be very sensitive to folate and vitamin B_{12} deficiency (Savage et al, 1994; 2000).

Methylmalonic Acid

Once a genetic cause is ruled out, the most straightforward biochemical method for differentiating folate and vitamin B_{12} deficiencies is to monitor the hyperhomocysteinemia by measuring the serum or urinary methylmalonic acid level. The latter metabolite is formed during the degradation of the amino acid valine and odd-chain fatty acids. Methylmalonic

TABLE 18-2 Screening Tests for Malabsorption Syndromes

TEST	REFERENCE RANGE	COMMENTS
Serum carotene	60-200 μg/dl	Good test if fruit and vegetable intake are normal; is a mixture of several fat-soluble substances, of which β-carotene is only a fraction
Prothrombin time	11-15 sec	Quite sensitive but not specific
Serum calcium	8.5-10.5 mg/dl	Not very sensitive or specific
Serum magnesium	1.6-2.6 mg/dl	Not very sensitive or specific
Serum albumin	3.5-5 mg/dl	Not sensitive or specific
Serum cholesterol	>150 mg/dl	Not sensitive or specific
Qualitative stool fat	No fat globules in microscopic field	Reveals numerous stained globules in individuals with syndromes; inexpensive follow-up to nonspecific indicators, but not completely specific

acid is the side product in this metabolic pathway that increases when the conversion of methylmalonyl CoA to succinyl CoA is blocked by lack of vitamin B_{12}, a coenzyme for this reaction. Therefore deficiency leads to an increase in the methylmalonic acid pool, which is reflected by the serum or urinary methylmalonic acid level.

The advantage that homocysteine and methylmalonic acid testing has over assaying serum vitamin B_{12} levels or serum and red cell folate levels is that homocysteine and methylmalonic acid tend to detect impending vitamin deficiencies better than the static assays. This is especially important when assessing the status of certain patients, such as vegans or older adults, who could have vitamin B_{12} deficiency associated with central nervous system (CNS) impairment.

Although plasma homocysteine measurements are routinely available in many clinical laboratories because elevated plasma homocysteine is a risk factor for cardiovascular disease (see Chapter 35), methylmalonic acid measurements to determine B_{12} deficiency are done in only a few specialized laboratories. Hence, it is recommended that individuals with a risk of folate or vitamin B_{12} deficiency be screened by plasma homocysteine measurements; those individuals with positive test results should be given additional tests assessing folate and vitamin B_{12} levels or just the latter.

Vitamin B_{12} Malabsorption

If vitamin B_{12} status is compromised, the *Schilling test* may be used to detect defects in vitamin B_{12} absorption. The patient is given an oral dose of radiolabeled cobalamin and an injection of unlabeled vitamin. The vitamin saturates vitamin B_{12} storage sites so that all of the radiolabeled vitamin absorbed is excreted in the urine within approximately 24 hours. If less than the expected amount of radioactivity appears in the urine, vitamin B_{12} malabsorption is confirmed. The test can then be repeated with administration of a combination of radiolabeled cobalamin and intrinsic factor. If urinary radioactivity reaches the expected levels, intrinsic factor deficiency is the cause of the malabsorption. The term *pernicious anemia* is commonly applied to vitamin B_{12} deficiency resulting from lack of intrinsic factor (see Chapter 34).

Folate malabsorption may also develop. Folate is absorbed by the jejunum, and its malabsorption has several causes; but a specific test for folate absorption has not been developed. However, the presence and extent of deficiency should be assessed in patients with celiac disease or those with a history of long-term use of certain drugs, including anticonvulsants and sulfasalazine. Alcohol consumption interferes with folate utilization.

MARKERS OF MALABSORPTION

The *malabsorption syndrome* is a condition in which several nutrients are abnormally absorbed (see Chapter 30). In almost all such disorders, fat is not absorbed normally. These disorders are also associated with decreased absorption of fat-soluble substances, including vitamins A, E, D, and K and β-carotene. Malabsorption results from such diverse causes as pancreatic exocrine insufficiency, gastric surgery, reduced bile salt secretion, a wide variety of conditions associated with abnormal intestinal mucosa, short-gut syndrome, infection, lymphatic obstruction, some cardiovascular diseases, certain drugs, and unexplained causes associated with diseases not commonly considered to affect the GI tract. Table 18-2 provides a list of common tests that can be useful in screening for malabsorption. Several of these tests are not sensitive and are nonspecific, but if clinical symptoms are consistent with a diagnosis of malabsorption and several of these tests are positive, a microscopic stool fat test is warranted. If this test is positive, more sophisticated and disease-specific tests should be performed.

WELLNESS ASSESSMENT

Lipid Indices of Cardiovascular Risk

Serum lipoprotein and cholesterol levels are directly implicated in the development of atherosclerosis and are affected by modifiable factors, including the diet. The National Cholesterol Education Program

Box 18-2. New Lipid and Lipoprotein Cardiovascular Disease Risk Factors

Small (more dense) LDL particles
Increased apoprotein B concentration
Decreased apoprotein A-I concentration
Increased remnant lipoprotein cholesterol and triglyceride concentrations

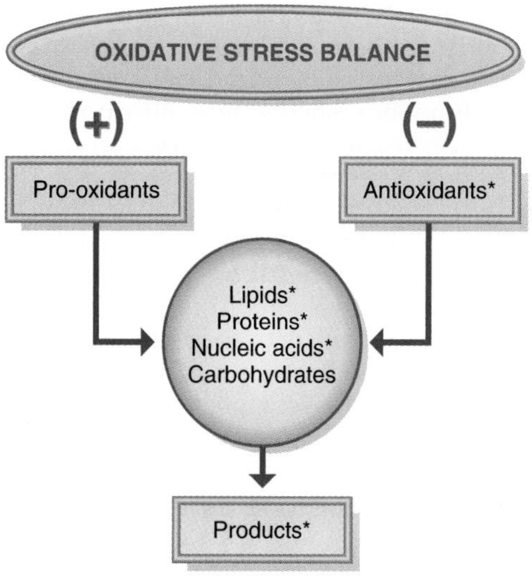

FIGURE 18-2 • Steps in maintaining the balance between pro-oxidants (reactive oxygen species) and antioxidants. The compounds marked with an asterisk *(*)* have been used as markers of oxidative stress balance.

(NCEP) Adult Treatment Panel (ATP III) has established guidelines for serum levels of total cholesterol, low-density lipoprotein (LDL) cholesterol, and high-density lipoprotein (HDL) cholesterol that are associated with risk of coronary heart disease (CHD) or cardiovascular disease (CVD). The ATP III recommendations are based on the assumption that the laboratory responsible for the lipid measurements produces precise (coefficients of variation, 3%) and unbiased (bias, 3%) results (Meyers et al, 1997). To be confident in the validity of their recommendations, health professionals must be confident that laboratories performing these analyses meet these requirements.

Patients undergoing lipid assessments should be fasting (for a recommended 12 hours) at the time of blood sampling. Fasting is necessary primarily because triglyceride levels rise and fall dramatically in the postprandial state, and LDL cholesterol values are calculated from measured total serum cholesterol and HDL cholesterol concentrations. This calculation, based on a formula called *the Friedewald equation,* is most accurate for triglyceride concentrations of less than 400 mg/dl. The Friedewald equation gives an estimate of fasting LDL cholesterol levels that is generally within 4 mg/dl of the true value when triglyceride concentrations are less than 400 mg/dl.

New methods for directly measuring serum LDL cholesterol levels have been developed. When the accuracy, precision, and cost of these assays become acceptable, laboratories may no longer use the Friedewald equation for LDL cholesterol measurement. However, triglyceride concentrations will still need to be assayed when a lipid profile is determined, so fasting will still be necessary.

In addition to the standard serum lipid risk factors, recent research has linked other lipid and lipoprotein indices to CHD. All of these are measured in the laboratory, but most have either not been studied enough to demonstrate a clear link to CHD risk or are too costly to measure except in rare cases. Several examples of these new lipid-related risk factors are listed in Box 18-2. It is not yet known how nutrition and the other modifiable risk factors for CHD will affect these indexes.

Indices of Oxidative Stress

Current research indicates that many chronic diseases, including CVD and at least some forms of cancer, are initiated by free radical oxidation of lipids, nucleic acids, or proteins (Figure 18-2). For example, the underlying mechanism for the development of atherosclerosis is now thought to be at least partially mediated by free-radical compounds called reactive oxidation species (ROS). These products include the superoxide radial (O_2^-), hydroxyl radical (OH), and hydrogen peroxide (H_2O_2). The formation of ROS is sometimes but not always mediated by certain essential trace elements (e.g., iron, copper, chromium, and nickel). Once formed, ROS react with unsaturated fatty acids in LDL, creating lipid peroxides, another free radical species. Like all free radicals, lipid peroxides initiate the oxidation of other compounds, including the proteins, *apolipoproteins,* present in lipoproteins. The oxidation leads to the formation of free radical products throughout the large, heterogeneous lipoprotein particle. Cells associated with the arterial wall ingest the resulting oxidized lipoproteins. Once present in these cells, additional metabolism of this modified complex does not seem to occur. Over time, other pathophysiologic responses stabilize the deposited oxidized lipoprotein as atherosclerotic plaque (Anderson, 1997; Hulthe and Fagerberg, 2002).

In addition to the oxidized compounds in lipoproteins, oxidized products of other lipids, proteins, and carbohydrates are also present in body fluids. These compounds can be measured in the laboratory, and some of these tests are now being used in clinical practice. Evidence shows that nutritional supplements can decrease the level of some of these markers, and a few research studies have shown that diet alone affects these markers.

Until additional research becomes available, these tests may not help nutrition professionals advise their clients definitively about how and to what degree these markers relate to their risk for chronic diseases or about the effects of nutritional intervention on their risk. On the other hand, if these potential markers of oxidative stress are ignored completely, clients may not receive information that could help them decrease their risk of developing certain chronic diseases.

Antioxidant Status

An indirect way of assessing the level of oxidative stress is to measure the levels of antioxidant compounds present in body fluids (Reaven and Witztum, 1996). Oxidative stress is related to levels of the following:

- Antioxidant vitamins (tocopherols and ascorbic acid)
- Minerals with antioxidant roles (e.g., selenium)
- Dietary phytochemicals with antioxidant properties (e.g., carotenoids, lycopene) (see *New Directions:* Biophotonic Measurement of Antioxidant Capacity)
- Endogenous antioxidant compounds and enzymes (e.g., superoxide dismutase, glutathione)

More precisely, the concentration of these compounds correlates with the balance between their intake and production and their use during the inhibition of free radical compounds (Halliwell, 1999).

Markers of Oxidative Stress

The most commonly used chemical markers of oxidative stress are presented in Table 18-3. Some tests measure the presence of one class of free radical products, and others measure the global antioxidant capacity of plasma or a plasma fraction (Halliwell, 1999). These tests have been promoted on the assumption that knowledge of the individual concentrations of free radical markers or antioxidants might be less useful than knowledge of the total antioxidant capacity of the plasma or plasma fraction. This total antioxidant activity is determined by a test that assesses the combined antioxidant capacities of the constituents. Unfortunately, the results of these tests include the antioxidant capacities of compounds such as uric acid and albumin, which are not compounds of interest. In other words, no one type of assay is likely to provide a global picture of the oxidative stress to which an individual is exposed.

Despite this lack of correlation or specificity of assays of oxidative stress, two assays seem promising. One is the *immunoassay of oxidatively modified LDL particles* (see Table 18-3). Because it measures a product that may directly participate in atherogenesis, this assay (which may be available in clinical laboratories in the next few years) may allow a specific correlation of CVD risk with dietary and supplemental antioxidant consumption. The second assay is the measurement of the compound *isoprostane* $F_{2\alpha}$ (Patrono and Fitzgerald, 1997). This test measures the presence of a continuously formed free radical compound that is produced by free radical oxidation of specific polyunsaturated fatty acids (Basu, 1998; Basu

NEW DIRECTIONS

Biophotonic Measurement of Antioxidant Capacity

Noninvasive measurements of clinical parameters are always preferable to those requiring blood, urine, or tissue. Raman spectroscopy is just such a measurement technique and may become widely used in the future. Using a laser light that is pointed toward the fat pad of the palm, the amount of carotenoids is measured at the cellular level as they "light up." Because carotenoids are powerful antioxidants, their levels can give a good assessment of the antioxidant capacity of the cell.

Serum carotenoids, which are significantly covalated with skin carotenoids, are a good measure of the absorptive capacity of the individual. Thus an individual with a diet high in fruits and vegetables, and therefore large amounts of carotenoids, has a high, optimal carotenoid antioxidant score. The antioxidant score, or the numerical result from this scan, can be used to determine how well a person is processing antioxidants and whether the antioxidants are reaching the cell, where they exert their protective functions. The number, which seems to be in the range of 25,000 and higher in those with optimal health, increases with greater consumption of carotenoid-containing fruits and vegetables, consumption of carotenoid-containing nutritional supplements, smoking cessation, and loss of excess body fat. The measurement is quick, easy, and inexpensive, making it a likely assessment tool for nutrition professionals in the future.

et al, 2001). Isoprostane $F_{2\alpha}$ has a structure similar to that of the prostaglandins and has already been shown to reflect the oxidative stress status of infants receiving therapeutic levels of oxygen (Goil et al, 1998).

Homocysteine

Many individuals who die of atherosclerotic disease do not have lipoprotein cholesterol and triglyceride concentrations that categorize them as at risk for the disease. One possible explanation for this is that many factors may be involved in the development of atherosclerosis. Recent research strongly supports the hypothesis that an elevated plasma concentration of the sulfur-containing amino acid homocysteine is an independent risk factor for developing CVD (see Chapter 35).

Although homocysteine plays an important role in the synthesis of methionine, the bulk of the current research suggests that when cellular homocysteine leaks into the circulation, even in slightly elevated amounts, the risk of CHD, stroke, peripheral vascular disease, and venous thrombosis and pulmonary embolism increases significantly (Stein and McBride, 1998). Just as the mechanism for the effect of plasma lipoproteins on the development of atherosclerosis was initially unclear, the mechanism of the effects of homocysteine on atherogenesis is not yet known.

Table 18-4 presents data on the association of CVD risk and plasma homocysteine concentrations. Because the study of homocysteine is new, values must be considered to be rough guidelines. Even individuals with a plasma homocysteine concentration within the population reference (normal) range may be at increased risk for developing CVD. In addition, almost all individuals can reduce their homocysteine levels by adding vitamin B supplements to their diet, and evidence now suggests that replacing fat intake with fruits and vegetables can also produce a significant decrease in serum homocysteine levels. Box 18-3 contains a summary of tests of oxidative stress.

TABLE 18-3 Markers of Oxidative Stress

CLASS	FUNCTIONS	COMMENT
Class I: Antioxidant Markers		
Vitamin C (plasma or leukocyte)	Specific inhibitor of water-soluble radicals	Measured by chromatography, capillary electrophoresis, or an automated enzymatic assay
α-Tocopherol	Inhibitor of lipid peroxidation	Measured by chromatography or capillary electrophoresis
γ-Tocopherol	An inhibitor of the nitrous oxide radical	Measured by chromatography or capillary electrophoresis
Carotenoids	Primarily inhibitors of lipid peroxidation	Measured by chromatography; includes α- and β-carotenes, lycopene, cryptoxanthin, zeaxanthin, and lutein
Class II: Endogenous Systems		
Glutathione assay	Detoxifies the ROS hydrogen peroxide (H_2O_2)	Measured by plasma or erythrocyte glutathione or ratio of reduced to oxidized glutathione
Class III: Global Tests of Antioxidant Capacity		
LDL oxidative susceptibility	Reflects the concentration of antioxidants in LDLs	In vitro determination of the rate of formation of LDL oxidation products called *conjugated dienes*
Oxygen radical absorbance capacity (ORAC)	NA	Measures decrease in fluorescence over time; reflects the total antioxidant capacity of the specimen
Total peroxyl radical trapping parameter (TRAP)	NA	Measures total antioxidant capacity; reflects the levels of uric acid and albumin
2,2′-Azino-bis (3-ethyl benzythiazoline-sulfonic acid (ABTS)	NA	ABTS assay in commercial by available kit; also called *total antioxidant status (TAS)*
Class IV: Products of Free Radical Reactions		
Modified LDL	NA	Immunoassay of oxidized LDL proteins; may directly reflect risk of atherosclerosis; may become commercially available, allowing assay to be performed by clinical laboratories
Isoprostane	No known function	Primary form, isoprostane $F_{2\alpha}$, measured by chromatography or an immunoassay that is available commercially and can be rapidly performed
Thiobarbituric acid reactive substances (TBARS)	NA	A colorimetric assay that is easy to perform but not specific for oxidation products; measures products of lipid peroxidation called *aldehydes* (e.g., malondialdehyde)

NA, Not applicable.

TABLE 18-4 Cardiovascular Disease Risk and Plasma Homocysteine Concentration

RANGE TYPE	CONCENTRATION (μmol/L)	COMMENTS
Usual reference ("normal") range	5-15	The range that is consistently quoted in the literature, although it is higher than the ranges cited in recent studies
Updated reference range	6-12	Reference range for healthy, well-nourished adults; increased homocysteine concentration with age and after menopause
Moderate-risk range	12-30	Has upper and lower limits that are not well established
High-risk range	>30	Usually associated with extreme nutrient deficiency or genetic defects in homocysteine metabolism
Target levels	<9	Risk minimal below this level
Optimal levels	<7	Range of lowest risk of CVD

Box 18-3. Homocysteine and Cardiovascular Disease

Known Facts

- Homocysteine is an independent risk factor for the development of CVD.
- Most studies suggest that individuals with a plasma homocysteine level of 15 μmol/L or higher have an increased risk for the development of CVD.
- A normal but high homocysteine level may still be associated with increased CVD risk.
- Supplementation with folate, vitamin B_{12}, and vitamin B_6 reduces the level of homocysteine in almost all individuals.

Persisting Questions

- What mechanism is responsible for homocysteine's effects on atherosclerosis or CVD-related events?
- What level of serum homocysteine results in the lowest risk of CVD?
- Does lowering serum homocysteine levels by vitamin supplementation decrease the risk of CVD?
- Can reasonable dietary changes decrease homocysteine concentration?
- Is homocysteine associated with risk for developing chronic diseases other than CVD (e.g., Alzheimer's disease)?

NUTRITIONAL INTERPRETATION OF ROUTINE MEDICAL LABORATORY DATA

From routine laboratory screening of patients with medical complaints or routine laboratory monitoring of patients during medical treatment, various data are generated that can be helpful in screening for nutritional deficiencies. Although the abundance of this kind of nonspecific data has decreased as the result of attempts to decrease the cost of medical diagnosis and treatment, much information is still available.

Clinical Chemistry Panels

Until recently, large panels of medical tests were extremely common. In part, this is because the autoanalyzers that were initially developed for the determination of routine blood chemistry and hematology analytes could perform many tests on the same blood or serum sample for only a slightly higher cost than the cost for one or two tests. One of these panels—called the *chem 7*, or *mini-panel*—still exists. The components of this panel, which are now designated the *basic metabolic panel* by the Centers for Medicare and Medicaid Services Common Procedure Coding System, are discussed in Table 18-5.

A panel that is often performed during routine screening, now called the *comprehensive metabolic panel*, includes all the tests in the basic metabolic panel except CO_2, in addition to all the remaining tests profiled in Table 18-5 except phosphorus, cholesterol, and triglyceride. Because the last three tests are often ordered with the comprehensive metabolic panel, they are included in the table. Well-informed nutritionists can use their understanding of the nutritional and basic medical significance of these tests to support their nutrition assessments. The information provided in Table 18-5 is not exhaustive; see the various textbooks on the topic and Appendix 33 to obtain more detailed information.

The Complete Blood Count

Another panel of tests that is commonly available for review by nutritionists is the complete blood count (CBC). The CBC is often accompanied by a differential count (often called a *differential*, or *diff*), which enumerates each of the specific classes of leukocytes. Table 18-6 provides a list of the basic elements of the CBC and differential (which are collectively called a

TABLE 18-5 Constituents of the Common Serum Chemistry Panels

ANALYTES	REFERENCE RANGE*	SIGNIFICANCE
Serum Electrolytes		
Na^+ K^+ Cl^- HCO_3^- (or total CO_2)	135-145 mEq/L† 3.6-5 mEq/L† 101-111 mEq/L† 21-31 mEq/L†	Of general interest in monitoring various patients, such as those receiving total parenteral nutrition or who have renal conditions, chronic obstructive pulmonary disease, uncontrolled diabetes mellitus (DM), various endocrine disorders, ascitic and edematous symptoms, or acidotic or alkalotic conditions; decreased K^+ associated with diarrhea, vomiting or nasogastric aspiration, some drugs, licorice ingestion, and diuretics; increased K^+ associated with renal diseases, crush injuries, infection, and hemolyzed blood specimens
Glucose	70-110 mg/dl (fasting)	Fasting glucose >125 mg/dl indicates DM (oral glucose tolerance tests are not needed for diagnosis); fasting glucose >110 mg/dl is indicator of insulin resistance Monitor levels along with triglycerides in those receiving total parenteral nutrition for glucose intolerance
Creatinine	0.8-1.4 mg/dl (males) 0.6-1.2 mg/dl (females)	Increased in those with renal disease and decreased in those with PEM (i.e., blood urea nitrogen [BUN]/creatinine ratio >15:1)
Blood Urea Nitrogen (BUN) or Urea	5-20 mg urea nitrogen/dl 1.8-7 mmol/L	Increased in those with renal disease and excessive protein catabolism; decreased in those with liver failure and negative nitrogen balance and in females who are pregnant
Albumin	3.5-5 mg/dl	Decreased in those with liver disease or acute inflammatory disease; prognostic index
Serum Enzymes		
Alkaline phosphatase AST (SGOT) ALT (SGPT)	25-140 units/L 1-40 units/L 0-45 units/L	Increased in those with any of a variety of malignant, muscle, bone, intestinal, and liver diseases or injuries AST and ALT useful in monitoring liver function in those receiving total parenteral nutrition
Bilirubin, Total	0.1-1 mg/dl	Increased in association with drugs, gallstones and other biliary duct diseases, intravascular hemolysis, and hepatic immaturity; decreased with some anemias
Total Calcium	8.5-10.5 mg/dl	Hypercalcemia associated with endocrine disorders, malignancy, and hypervitaminosis D Hypocalcemia associated with vitamin D deficiency and inadequate hepatic or renal activation of vitamin D, hypoparathyroidism, magnesium deficiency, renal failure, and nephritic syndrome
Phosphorus (Phosphate)	2.5-4.5 mg/dl	Hypophosphatemia associated with hypoparathyroidism and decreased intake; hyperphosphatemia associated with hyperparathyroidism, chronic antacid ingestion, and renal failure
Total Cholesterol	>150 mg/dl	Decreased in those with protein-calorie malnutrition, liver diseases, and hyperthyroidism
Triglycerides	40-300 mg/dl (age and sex dependent)	Increased in those with glucose intolerance (e.g., in those receiving total parenteral nutrition, who have combined hyperlipidemia) or in those who are not fasting

*Reference ranges may vary slightly among laboratories.
†1 mEq/L = 1 mmol/L.
AST, Aspartate transaminase; *ALT*, alanine transaminase; *SGOT*, serum glutamic oxalecetic transaminase; *SGPT*, serum glutamic pyruvic transaminase.

hemogram), with reference ranges and explanatory comments.

Urinalysis

A panel of tests that is routinely performed on urine is the urinalysis. The urinalysis test can be done in medical facilities that are not licensed to do more complex laboratory testing, so it is often part of a patient's medical record. Because it is so commonly available, it is advisable that the nutritionist become familiar with the components of a urinalysis and be able to interpret them. Urinalysis data are qualitative or semiquantitative, and much of the data reflects the urinary tract status. However, some urinalysis data have broader medical and nutritional significance. The full urinalysis includes a record of (1) the urine's appearance, (2) the results of basic tests done with chemically impregnated reagent strips (often called *dipsticks*) that can be read visually or by an automated reader, and (3) the microscopic examination of urine sediment. Table 18-7 provides a list of the chemical tests performed in a urinalysis and their significance.

TABLE 18-6 Constituents of the Hemogram: Complete Blood Count and Differential

ANALYTES	REFERENCE RANGE*	SIGNIFICANCE
Red blood cells	$4.3\text{-}5.9 \times 10^6/mm^3$ (men) $3.5\text{-}5.9 \times 10^6/mm^3$ (women)	In addition to nutrition deficits, may be decreased in those with hemorrhage, hemolysis, genetic aberrations, marrow failure, or renal disease or who are taking certain drugs; not sensitive for iron, vitamin B_{12}, or folate deficiencies
Hemoglobin concentration	14-17 g/dl (men) 12-15 g/dl (women) <11g/dl (pregnant females) 14-24 g/dl (newborns)	In addition to nutrition deficits, may be decreased in those with hemorrhage, hemolysis, genetic aberrations, marrow failure, or renal disease or who are taking certain drugs; not sensitive for iron, vitamin B_{12}, or folate deficiencies
Hematocrit	39%-49% (men) 33%-43% (women) <33% (pregnant females) 44%-64% (newborns)	In addition to nutrition deficits, may be decreased in those with hemorrhage, hemolysis, genetic aberrations, marrow failure, or renal disease or who are taking certain drugs; not sensitive for iron, vitamin B_{12}, or folate deficiencies
Mean cell volume (MCV)	80-95 fl 96-108 fl (newborns)	Decreased (microcytic) in presence of iron deficiency, thalassemia trait, and chronic renal failure, anemia of chronic disease; increased (macrocytic) in presence of vitamin B_{12} or folate deficiency and genetic defects in DNA synthesis; neither microcytosis nor macrocytosis sensitive to marginal nutrient deficiencies
Mean cell hemoglobin (MCH)	27-31 pg 23-34 pg (newborns)	Causes of abnormal values similar to those for MCV
Mean cell hemoglobin concentration (MCHC)	32-36 g/dl 32-33 g/dl (newborns)	Decreased in those with iron deficiency and thalassemia trait; not sensitive to marginal nutrient deficiencies
White blood cell count (WBC)	$5\text{-}10 \times 10^3/mm^3$ (>2 yr) $6\text{-}17 \times 10^3/mm^3$ (< 2 yr) $9\text{-}30 \times 10^3/mm^3$ (newborns)	Increased (leukocytosis) in those with infection, neoplasia, and stress; decreased (leukopenia) in those with PEM, autoimmune diseases, or overwhelming infections or who are receiving chemotherapy or radiation therapy
Differential	55%-70% neutrophils 40%-60% lymphocytes 4%-8% monocytes 1%-4% eosinophils 0.5%-1% basophils	*Neutrophilia:* Ketoacidosis, trauma, stress, pus-forming infections, leukemia *Neutropenia:* PEM, aplastic anemia, chemotherapy, overwhelming infection *Lymphocytosis:* Infection, leukemia, myeloma, mononucleosis *Lymphocytopenia:* leukemia, chemotherapy, sepsis, AIDS *Eosinophilia:* Parasitic infestation, allergy, eczema, leukemia, autoimmune disease *Eosinopenia:* Increased steroid production No disease noted for altered basophils

*Reference ranges may vary slightly among laboratories.

TABLE 18-7 Chemical Tests in a Urinalysis

ANALYTE	EXPECTED VALUE	SIGNIFICANCE
Specific gravity	1.010-1.025 mg/ml	Can be used to test and monitor the concentrating and diluting abilities of the kidney; low in those with diabetes insipidus, glomerulonephritis, or pyelonephritis; high in those with vomiting, diarrhea, sweating, fever, adrenal insufficiency, hepatic diseases, or heart failure
pH	6-8 (normal diet)	Acidic in those with a high-protein diet or acidosis (e.g., uncontrolled diabetes mellitus [DM] or starvation), during administration of some drugs, and in association with uric acid, cystine, and calcium oxalate kidney stones; alkaline in individuals consuming diets rich in vegetables or dairy products and in those with a urinary tract infection, immediately after meals, with some drugs, and in those with phosphate and calcium carbonate kidney stones
Protein	2-8 mg/dl	Marked proteinuria in those with nephrotic syndrome, severe glomerulonephritis, or congestive heart failure; moderate in those with most renal diseases, preeclampsia, or urinary tract inflammation; minimal in those with certain renal diseases or lower urinary tract disorders
Glucose	Not detected (2-10 g/dl in DM)	Positive in those with DM; rarely in benign conditions
Ketones	Negative	Positive in those with uncontrolled DM (usually type 1); also positive in those with a fever, anorexia, certain GI disturbances, persistent vomiting, or cachexia or who are fasting or starving
Blood	Negative	Indicates urinary tract infection, neoplasm, or trauma; also positive in those with traumatic muscle injuries or hemolytic anemia.
Bilirubin	Not detected	Index of unconjugated bilirubin; increased in those with certain liver diseases (e.g., gallstones)
Urobilinogen	0.1-1 units/dl	Index of conjugated bilirubin; increased in those with hemolytic conditions; used to distinguish among hepatic diseases
Nitrite	Negative	Index of bacteriuria
Leukocyte esterase	Negative	Indirect test of bacteriuria; detects leukocytes

SUMMARY

In summary, laboratory data can be used to assess specific nutrient deficiencies (e.g., determine the causes of nutritional anemia), or they can be useful for screening and monitoring (e.g., assessing the risk of CVD). Tests are available that can be used to screen, assess, and monitor protein-calorie status. Because laboratory data are currently increasing our knowledge of the mechanisms involved in the development of chronic disease, new laboratory tests are consistently being developed. Although the efficacy of these tests has not been proven, it is expected that eventually many (but not all) will be. Determining when to start using these tests in nutrition and dietary practice is a subjective and often philosophical decision. Finally, a wealth of routinely available laboratory data may give suggestive although not specific evidence of nutritional deficiency. These data, which are ubiquitous in patients' medical records, can be used by informed practitioners to confirm and strengthen nutrition assessments.

Clinical Scenario

Leanne is the 18-month-old daughter of immigrant parents. She has two older siblings (brothers) and has been enrolled in the Women, Infants, and Children (WIC) program since the age of 6 months. During a recent visit to the WIC clinic, Leanne appeared pallid and listless and was found to have a hematocrit value of 34%. The clinic staff was evaluating the use of the hematofluorometer (zinc protoporphyrin/heme [ZPPH] ratio) in their clinic and found that Leanne's ZPPH ratio was 135 μmol/mol. Her head circumference was 45 cm (compared with 44.5 cm at 12 months); she was 30 inches tall (compared with 28.5 inches at 12 months); and she weighed 21 lb (compared with 19 lb at the age of 12 months).

Her mother reported that Leanne had been increasingly less active in the past 3 months. She began to walk at 13 months but now prefers to play in her bed or sit on the floor or sofa. During the past 2 months, Leanne has had at least three colds and now has a nasal discharge but no fever or other symptoms. Leanne's mother reported that her daughter usually consumes five or six 6-oz bottles of cow's milk (whole milk) each day and eats a small amount of solid food (primarily polished rice).

A complete blood count (CBC) was ordered, and the following values were obtained: hematocrit, 33.5%; hemoglobin, 11 g/dl; red blood cell count, 3.8 million/mm^3; mean cell volume, 80 fl; platelet count, 195 × 10^3/mm^3; white blood cell count, 16,000/mm^3; mean cell hemoglobin, 27 pg; mean cell hemoglobin concentration; 33 g/dl; reticulocytes, 0.8%.

1. Comment on Leanne's growth and development. Does she have a problem?
2. How would you interpret her CBC?
3. What does the ZPPH ratio indicate? Why was it fortunate that a ZPPH ratio happened to be available to the clinic on the day that Leanne was evaluated?
4. Why was a serum ferritin level done?
5. Considering Leanne's diet, which nutritional inadequacies might she have?

Relevant Web Sites

National Center for Health Statistics, National Health and Nutrition Examination Survey–NHANES
www.cdc.gov/nchs/nhanes

National Cholesterol Education Program–NCEP, ATPIII Guidelines
www.nhlbi.nih.gov/guidelines/cholesterol/index.htm

The Merck Manual of Diagnosis and Therapy Section I–Nutritional Disorders
www.merck.com/pubs/mmanual/section1/sec1.htm

Cited References

Anderson TJ: Oxidative stress, endothelial function and coronary atherosclerosis, *Cardiologia* 42:701, 1997.

Basu S: Metabolism of 8-isoprostaglandin F2α, *Fed Exp Biol Soc Lett* 428:32, 1998.

Basu S et al: Biomarkers of free radical injury during spinal cord ischemia, *FEBS Lett* 508(1):36, 2001.

Beck FK, Rosenthal TC: Prealbumin: a marker for nutritional evaluation, *Am Fam Physician* 65:1575, 2002.

Blake GJ, Ridker PM: Novel clinical markers of vascular wall inflammation, *Circ Res* 89:763, 2001.

Bron D et al: Biological basis of anemia, *Semin Oncol* 28(2; suppl 8):1, 2001.

Chang HR, Bistrian B: The role of cytokines in the catabolic consequences of infection and injury, *J Parent Ent Nutr* 22:156, 1998.

Goil S et al: Eight-epi-PGF2alpha: a possible marker of lipid peroxidation in term infants with severe pulmonary disease, *J Pediatr* 132:349, 1998.

Halliwell B: Establishing the significance and optimal intake of dietary antioxidants: the biomarker concept, *Nutr Rev* 57:104, 1999.

Haurani FI: Interpretation of serum ferritin in anemia of chronic disease, *Am J Hematol* 69:296, 2002.

Hulthe J, Fagerberg B: Circulating oxidized LDL is associated with subclinical atherosclerosis development and inflammatory cytokines (AIR Study), *Arterioscler Thromb Vasc Biol* 122(7):1162, 2002.

Konstantinides FN et al: Urinary urea nitrogen: too insensitive for calculating nitrogen balance studies in surgical clinical nutrition, *JPEN* 15:189, 1991.

Liu S et al: Relation between a diet with a high glycemic load and plasma concentrations of high-sensitivity C-reactive protein in middle-aged women, *Am J Clin Nutr* 75:492-498, 2002.

Massey AC: Microcytic anemia, differential diagnosis and management of iron deficiency anemia, *Med Clin North Am* 76:549, 1992.

Mears E: Outcomes of continuous process involvement of a nutritional care program incorporating serum prealbumin measurements, *Nutrition* 12:479, 1996.

Meyers GL et al: Standardization of lipid and lipoprotein measurements. In Rifai N, Warnick GR, Sominiczak MH, eds: *Handbook of lipoprotein testing*, Washington, DC, 1997, AACC Press.

Moldawer LL, Copeland EM III: Proinflammatory cytokines, nutritional support, and the cachexia syndrome: interactions and therapeutic options, *Cancer* 79:1828, 1997.

Nussbaum MA, Baertschi SW, Jansen PJ: Determination of relative UV response factors for HPLC by use of a chemiluminescent nitrogen-specific detector, *J Pharm Biomed Anal* 27:983, 2002.
Ozatli D et al: Erythrocytes: anemias in chronic liver diseases, *Hematol* 5:69, 2000.
Patrono C, Fitzgerald GA: Isoprostanes: potential markers of oxidant stress in atherothrombotic disease, *Arterioscler Thromb Vasc Biol* 17:2309, 1997.
Ponka P et al: Function and regulation of transferrin and ferritin, *Semin Hematol* 35:35, 1998.
Reaven PD, Witztum JL: Oxidized low density lipoproteins in atherogenesis: role of dietary modification, *Ann Rev Nutr* 16:51, 1996.
Savage DG et al: Sensitivity of serum methylmalonic acid and total homocysteine determinations for diagnosing cobalamin and folate deficiencies, *Am J Med* 96:239, 1994.
Savage DG et al: Etiology and diagnostic evaluation of macrocytosis, *Am J Med Sci* 319:343, 2000.
Suominen P et al: Single values of serum transferrin receptor and transferrin receptor ferritin index can be used to detect true and functional iron deficiency in rheumatoid arthritis patients with anemia, *Arthritis Rheum* 43:1016, 2000.
Stein JH, McBride PE: Hyperhomocysteinemia and atherosclerotic vascular disease: pathology, screening and treatment, *Arch Intern Med* 158:1301, 1998.
Thompson D et al: The value of acute phase protein measurements in clinical practice, *Ann Clin Biochem* 29:123, 1992.
Wong SS et al: Detection of iron-deficiency anemia in hospitalized patients by zinc protoporphyrin, *Clin Chim Acta* 244:91, 1996.
Worwood M: The laboratory assessment of iron status—an update, *Clin Chim Acta* 259:3, 1997.

Additional References

Bernstein LH: Relationship of nutritional markers to length of hospital stay, *Nutrition* 11(suppl 2):205, 1995.
Halliwell B, Gutteridge JMC: *Free radicals in biology and medicine,* ed 3, Oxford, England, 1999, Oxford University Press.
Hoffbrand V, Procan D: ABC of clinical haematolog: macrocytic anemias, *Br Med J* 314:430, 1997.
Jacobsen DW: Homocysteine and vitamins in cardiovascular disease, *Clin Chem* 44: 1833, 1998.
Lee RD, Nieman DC: *Nutritional assessment,* ed 3, St Louis, 2002, Mosby.
Siegel RM, LaGrone DH: The use of zinc protoporphyrin in screening young children for iron deficiency, *Clin Pediatr* 33:473, 1994.
Veldee MS: Nutritional assessment, therapy, and monitoring. In Burtis CA, Ashwood ER, eds: *Tietz textbook of clinical chemistry,* ed 3, Philadelphia, 1999, WB Saunders.

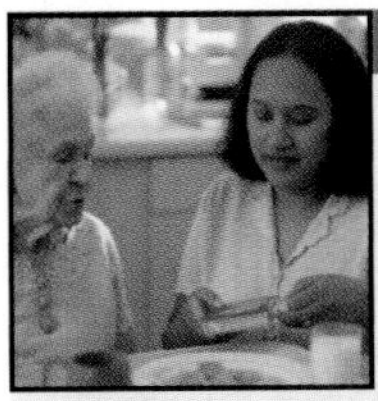

CHAPTER 19

Food-Drug Interactions

ZANETA M. PRONSKY, MS, RD, LDN, FADA
SR. JEANNE P. CROWE, PharmD, RPH

CHAPTER OUTLINE

- Pharmacologic Aspects of Food-Drug Interactions
- Risk Factors for Food-Drug Interactions
- Effects of Food on Drug Therapy
- Effects of Drugs on Food and Nutrition
- Modification of Drug Action by Food and Nutrients
- Effects of Drugs on Nutritional Status
- Excipients and Food-Drug Interactions
- Medical Nutrition Therapy

KEY TERMS

absorption–the process of movement of a drug from the site of administration into the systemic circulation

acetylation–a conjugation reaction involving the hepatic enzyme acetyl transferase, which metabolizes and inactivates amines, hydrazines, and sulfonamides

adsorption–the adhesion of drug molecules to the surface of another substance by physical or chemical attraction

bioavailability–the degree to which a drug or other substance reaches the general circulation and becomes available to the target organ or tissue

biotransformation–the metabolism of drugs by reactions such as oxidation, reduction, hydrolysis, or conjugation

cytochrome P-450 enzyme system–a multienzyme system in the smooth endoplasmic reticulum of numerous tissues that is involved in phase I of liver detoxification and is the major catalyst of drug biotransformation reactions

drug-nutrient interaction–the result of the action between a drug and a nutrient that would not happen with the nutrient or the drug alone

excipient–substance added to a drug, such as a buffer, binder, filler, diluent, disintegrant, glidant, flavoring, dye, preservative, suspending agent, or coating; also called *inactive ingredient*

food-drug interaction–a broad term that includes drug-nutrient interactions and the effect of a medication on nutritional status

half-life–the amount of time it takes for the blood concentration of a drug to decrease by one-half its steady-state level

pharmacodynamics–the study of the physiologic and biochemical effects of a drug or combination of drugs

pharmacogenomics–the study of genetically determined variations that are revealed solely by the effects of drugs in the body

pharmacokinetics–the movement of a drug through the body by absorption, distribution, metabolism, and excretion

physical incompatibility–a food-drug interaction involving granulation, gel formation, or separation of the enteral nutritional product when food and drug are combined

polypharmacy–the use of multiple drugs to treat one or more health conditions

pressor agents–organic compounds, including tyramine, dopamine, phenylethylamine, and histamine,

Sections of this chapter were written by Victoria Haken, RD, for the previous edition of this text.

KEY TERMS—Continued

that cause vasoconstriction and an increase in blood pressure

side effect–adverse effect, reaction, or any undesirable outcome of a drug

unbound fraction–the amount of a drug that is not bound to serum proteins, is able to leave the vasculature, and produces a pharmacologic effect at a target organ

The management of many diseases requires drug therapy, frequently involving the use of multiple drugs. Food-drug interactions can change the effects of drugs, and the therapeutic effects or side effects of medications can affect the nutritional status. Alternatively, the diet and the use of supplements or the nutritional status of the patient can decrease a drug's efficacy or increase its toxicity.

The terms *drug-nutrient interaction* and *food-drug interaction* are often used interchangeably. In actuality, drug-nutrient interactions are some of the many possible food-drug interactions. Drug-nutrient interactions include specific changes to the pharmacokinetics of a drug caused by a nutrient(s) or changes to the kinetics of a nutrient(s) caused by a drug. Food-drug interactions is a broader term that also includes the effects of a medication on nutritional status. Nutritional status may be impacted by the side effects of a medication, which could include an effect on appetite or the ability to eat.

For clinical, economic, and legal reasons, it is important to recognize food-drug interactions. Food-drug interactions that reduce the efficacy of a drug can result in longer or repeated stays in health care facilities, the use of multiple drugs, and deterioration of the patient because of the effects of the disease. Additional health problems can occur because of long-term drug-nutrient interactions. An example of this type of interaction would be the long-term effects of corticosteroids on calcium metabolism and resulting osteoporosis. Medical team members should be aware that *therapeutically important* food-drug interactions can do the following:

- Alter the intended response to the medication
- Cause drug toxicity
- Alter normal nutritional status

Awareness of these interactions enables the health care professional and patient to work together to avoid or minimize problems (Box 19-1).

The Joint Commission on Accreditation of Healthcare Organizations (JCAHO) requires education about potential drug-nutrient interactions. In the publication, *2002 Comprehensive Accreditation Manual for Hospitals*, education section, is Standard PF.3.1: "Patients are educated how to safely use medication. . . ." Twelve parameters necessary to meet this standard are listed; one of these parameters specifies that the patient and family must be educated about food-drug interactions.

Box 19-1. Benefits of Minimizing Drug Interactions

Medications achieve their intended effects.
Patients do not discontinue their drug.
The need for additional medication is minimized.
Fewer caloric or nutrient supplements are required.
Adverse side effects are avoided.
Optimal nutritional status is preserved.
Accidents and injuries are avoided.
Disease complications are minimized.
The cost of health care services is reduced.
There is less professional liability.
Licensing agency requirements are met.

Courtesy *Food medication interactions*, ed 13, Birchrunville, Pa, 2004, Food Medication Interactions.

PHARMACOLOGIC ASPECTS OF FOOD-DRUG INTERACTIONS

Medication is administered to produce a pharmacologic effect in the body or, more specifically, in a target organ or tissue. To achieve this goal, the drug must move from the site of administration to the bloodstream and eventually to the site of drug action. In due course, the drug may be changed to active or inactive metabolites and ultimately eliminated from the body. An interaction between the drug and food, a food component, or a nutrient can alter this process at any point. Food-drug interactions may be divided into two broad types: (1) *pharmacodynamic interactions,* which affect the pharmacologic action of the drug; and (2) *pharmacokinetic interactions,* which affect the movement of the drug into, around, or out of the body.

Pharmacodynamics

Pharmacodynamics is the study of the biochemical and physiologic effects of a drug. The mechanism of action of a drug might include the binding of the drug molecule to a receptor, enzyme, or ion channel, resulting in the observable physiologic response. Ultimately, this response may be enhanced or attenuated by the addition of other substances with similar or opposing actions.

Pharmacokinetics

Pharmacokinetics is the study of the time course of a drug in the body involving the *absorption, distribution, metabolism* (biotransformation), and *excretion* of the drug. Absorption is the process of the movement of the drug from the site of administration to the bloodstream. This process is dependent on the (1) route of administration, (2) the chemistry of the drug and its ability to cross biologic membranes, (3) the rate of gastric emptying (for orally administered drugs) and gastrointestinal movement, and (4) the quality of the product formulation. Food, food components, and nutritional supplements can interfere with the absorption process, especially when the drug is administered orally.

Distribution occurs when the drug leaves the systemic circulation and travels to various regions of the body. Body areas of distribution vary with different drugs, depending on the drug's chemistry and ability to cross biologic membranes. The rate and extent of blood flow to an organ or tissue strongly affect the amount of drug that reaches the area. Many drugs are highly bound to plasma proteins such as albumin. The bound fraction of drug does not leave the vasculature and therefore does not produce a pharmacologic effect. Only the unbound fraction is able to produce an effect at a target organ.

A drug is eliminated from the body as either unchanged drug or as a metabolite of the original compound. The major organ of metabolism, or biotransformation, in the body is the liver, although other sites contribute to a lesser degree. One of the more important enzyme systems that facilitate drug metabolism is the cytochrome P-450 enzyme system (see Figure 12-2). Substances such as food or dietary supplements, which either increase or inhibit the activity of this enzyme system, can significantly change the rate or extent of drug metabolism. The general tendency of the process of metabolism is to transform a drug from a lipid-soluble to a more water-soluble compound that can be handled more easily by the kidneys and excreted in the urine.

Renal excretion is the major route of elimination for drugs and drug metabolites either by glomerular filtration or tubular secretion. To a lesser extent, drugs may be eliminated in bile and other body fluids. Under certain circumstances, such as a change in urinary pH, drugs that have reached the renal tubule may pass back into the bloodstream. This process is known as *tubular reabsorption.* The recommended dose of a drug generally assumes normal liver and kidney function. The dose or dosing interval of a renally excreted drug or active metabolite must be altered to meet the degree of renal dysfunction in patients with kidney disease (see Chapter 39).

RISK FACTORS FOR FOOD-DRUG INTERACTIONS

Patients must be assessed individually for the effect of food on drug action and the effect of drugs on nutritional status. Interactions can be caused or complicated by polypharmacy, nutritional status, genetics, underlying illness, special diets, nutritional supplements, tube feeding, herbal or phytonutrient products, alcohol intake, drugs of abuse, nonnutrients in food, excipients in drugs or food, allergies, or intolerances. Poor patient compliance and physicians' prescribing patterns further complicate the risk. Drug-induced malnutrition occurs most commonly during long-term treatment for chronic disease, and older patients are at a particularly high risk for many reasons (see *Focus On:* Food-Drug Interactions in Older Adults).

Existing malnutrition also places patients at greater risk for drug-nutrient interactions. Protein alterations—specifically, low albumin levels—and changes in body composition secondary to malnutrition can affect drug disposition by altering protein binding and drug distribution. Patients with active neoplastic disease or active acquired immunodeficiency syndrome (AIDS) with significant anorexia and wasting are at special risk because of the high prevalence of malnutrition in these groups. The presence of the tumor and resulting illness may lead to reduced intake. Treatment modalities, such as chemotherapy and radiation, may exacerbate nutritional disturbances. Cisplatin (Platinol-AQ) and other cytotoxic agents commonly cause nausea, vomiting, diarrhea, anorexia, and reduced food intake.

Drug disposition can be affected by alterations in the gastrointestinal tract, such as vomiting, diarrhea, hypochlorhydria, mucosal atrophy, and motility changes. Malabsorption caused by intestinal damage from disease such as cancer, celiac disease, or inflammatory bowel disease creates greater potential for food-drug interactions.

Body composition is an important consideration in determining drug response. In obese or older patients, the proportion of adipose tissue to lean body mass is increased. In theory, accumulation of fat-soluble drugs such as the long-acting benzodiazepines (e.g., diazepam [Valium]) is more likely to occur. Accumulation of a drug and its metabolites in adipose tissue may result in prolonged clearance and increased toxicity. In older patients, this interaction may be complicated by decreased hepatic clearance of the drug (Ritschel and Kearns, 1999).

The developing fetus, infant, and pregnant woman are also at high risk for drug-nutrient interactions. Many drugs have not been tested on these populations,

FOCUS ON

Food-Drug Interactions in Older Adults

Older patients are more likely to be taking multiple drugs, both prescription and over the counter, than are younger patients. They have a higher risk of food-drug interactions because of physical changes related to aging, such as the increase in the ratio of fat tissue to lean body mass, a decrease in liver mass and blood flow, and impairment of kidney function. Illness, cognitive or endocrine dysfunction, and ingestion of restricted diets also increase this risk. Malnutrition and dehydration affect drug kinetics. The use of herbal or phytonutrient products has increased significantly in all developed countries, including use by older adults. Drugs of abuse or excessive alcohol intake are often missed in the older patient (see Chapter 13).

Central nervous system side effects of drugs can interfere with the ability or desire to eat. Drugs that cause drowsiness, dizziness, ataxia, confusion, headache, weakness, tremor, or peripheral neuropathy can lead to nutritional compromise, particularly in older patients. Recognition of these problems as a drug side effect, rather than a consequence of disease or aging, is often overlooked.

Care must be taken to evaluate intake of interacting nutrients (in the oral diet, supplements, or tube feedings) when specific drugs are used. Examples are vitamin K with warfarin (Coumadin); calcium and vitamin D with alendronate (Fosamax); and potassium, sodium, and magnesium with loop diuretics such as furosemide (Lasix). Parkinson's patients may be concerned with the amount and timing of protein intake because of interaction with levodopa (Sinemet, Dopar) (Duarte et al, 1993) (see Chapter 43, MNT for neurologic disorders). Special diets often need to be liberalized in older patients to improve caloric or protein intake. For instance, a malnourished older patient should not be prescribed a low-fat, low-cholesterol diet even if blood cholesterol levels are elevated. High-fat, calorie-dense foods, particularly if they are favorites, may be essential to provide adequate calories and protein.

The interdisciplinary team, which includes physician, pharmacist, nurse, and dietitian, must work together to plan and coordinate the medication regimen and diet and nutritional supplements to preserve optimal nutritional status and minimize food-drug interactions (Figure 19-1).

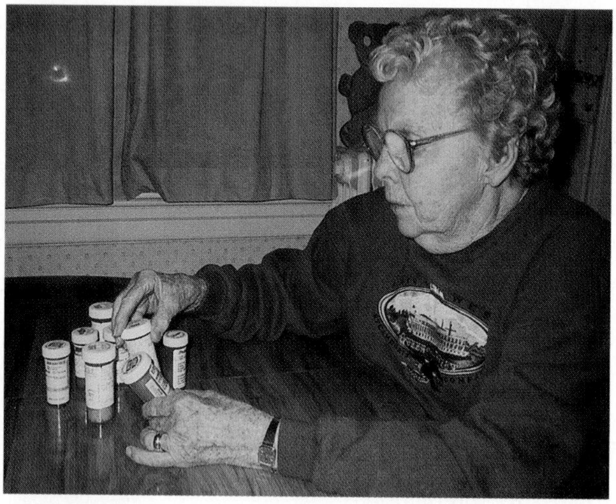

FIGURE 19-1 • As a result of the increased potential for illness with aging, older adults often take multiple drugs, both prescription and over-the-counter preparations. This places them at increased risk for drug-drug and drug-nutrient interactions.

making it difficult to assess the risks of negative drug effects, including food-drug interactions.

Pharmacogenomics

Genetic variations in an enzyme or enzyme system affect individual response to specific drug(s) (see Chapter 16). Pharmacogenomics is defined as "genetically determined variations that are revealed solely by the effects of drugs" (Tischio, 1995). Examples that have food-drug interaction ramifications are G6PD (glucose-6-phosphate dehydrogenase) enzyme deficiency, warfarin (Coumadin) resistance, and slow inactivation of isoniazid (INH) or phenelzine (Nardil). Warfarin resistance can affect individual requirements for and response to warfarin.

Slow inactivation of isoniazid or phenelzine are examples of the effect of slow acetylation. Acetylation is a conjugation reaction that metabolizes and inactivates amines, hydrazines, and sulfonamides. "Slow acetylators" are persons who metabolize these drugs more slowly than average because of inherited lower levels of the hepatic enzyme acetyl transferase. Therefore, unacetylated drug levels remain higher for longer periods in these persons than in those who are "rapid acetylators." For example, the half-life of isoniazid for fast acetylators is about 70 minutes, whereas the half-life is more than 3 hours for slow acetylators (Roth, 1995). A dose of drug prescribed normally for fast acetylators can be toxic for slow acetylators. Elevated blood levels of affected drugs in slow acetylators increase the potential for food-drug interactions. Slow inactivation of isoniazid increases the risk of pyridoxine deficiency and peripheral neuropathy. Slow inactivation of phenelzine, a monoamine oxidase (MAO) inhibitor, increases the risk for hypertensive crisis if foods high in tyramine are consumed (Box 19-2). Dapsone (DDS) and hydralazine (Apresoline) are also metabolized by acetylation and affected by inherited differences in acetylase enzymes.

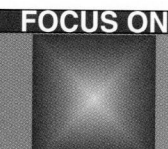

Box 19-2. Pressor Agents in Foods and Beverages (Tyramine, Dopamine, Histamine, Phenylethylamine)

Foods That Must Be Avoided

Aged cheeses: e.g., cheddar, blue, Gorgonzola, Stilton	Fermented soya beans, soya bean paste	Sauerkraut, kim chee
Aged meats: e.g., dry sausage such as salami, mortadella, Chinese dried duck	Tofu/fermented bean curd	Tap beer, Korean beer
Soy sauce	Miso soup	Concentrated yeast extracts (Marmite)
	Fava (broad) beans or pods, snowpea pods (contain dopamine)	Banana peel
		All casseroles made with aged cheese

Foods That May Be Used With Caution

Red or white wine 2-4 oz per day	Bottled beer, two 12-oz bottles, maximum
Coffee, cola*	Alcohol-free beer, two 12-oz bottles, maximum
Pizza (homemade or gourmet pizzas may have higher content)	

Foods Not Limited (based on current analyses)

Unfermented cheeses (cream, cottage, ricotta, processed)	Canned figs, raisins	Baked raised products, English cookies
Smoked white fish, salmon, carp, or anchovies	Fresh pineapple	Boiled egg, yogurt, junket, ice cream
Pickled herring	Beetroot, cucumber	Avocado, figs, banana, raspberries
Fresh meat poultry or fish	Sweet corn, mushrooms	Brewer's yeast (vitamin supplements)
	Salad dressings, tomato sauce	Curry powder
	Worcestershire sauce	Peanuts, chocolate

All packaged or processed meats: e.g., hot dogs, bologna, liverwurst, although they should be stored in refrigerator immediately and eaten as soon as possible. Histamine content is highest in improperly stored or spoiled fish, tuna.

From Pronsky ZM: *Food medication interactions*, ed 13, Birchrunville, Pa, 2004, Food Medication Interactions.
*Contains caffeine, a weak pressor agent, in quantities >500 mg per day may exacerbate reactions.

Deficiency of G6PD is an X-chromosome-linked deficiency of G6PD enzyme in red blood cells. It can lead to neonatal jaundice, hemolytic anemia, or acute hemolysis. Most common in African, Middle Eastern, and South East Asian populations, it is also called *favism*. Fava *(Vicia faba)* beans or pollen can cause acute hemolysis in some G6PD-deficient persons, particularly those of Mediterranean origin. Some drugs, such as aspirin, sulfonamides, and antimalarial drugs, can cause hemolysis and acute anemia. Several reports have been made of acute hemolysis induced in G6PD deficiency because of high-dose vitamin K or ascorbic acid (Rees, Kelsey, and Richards et al, 1993). Therefore, the potential exists for food-drug interactions in G6PD deficiency resulting from the ingestion of fava beans (also called *broad beans*), vitamin C, or vitamin K.

EFFECTS OF FOOD ON DRUG THERAPY

Drug Absorption

The presence of food and nutrients in the stomach or lumen of the intestinal tract has the potential to reduce the absorption of a drug. Examples of a critically significant reduction in drug absorption are the antiosteoporosis drugs alendronate (Fosamax) or risedronate (Actonel). Absorption is negligible if these drugs are given with food and reduced by 60% if taken with coffee or orange juice. The manufacturer's instructions are to take the drug on an empty stomach at least 30 minutes before breakfast. In one study, however, bioavailability was reduced by 40% when 10 mg of alendronate was taken 30 to 60 minutes before breakfast, compared with 2 hours before breakfast (Fosamax, 2001).

The absorption of the iron from supplements may be decreased by 50% when taken with food. Iron is best absorbed when taken with 8 oz of water or juice on an empty stomach. If iron must be taken with food to avoid gastrointestinal distress, it should not be taken with bran, eggs, high-phytate foods, fiber supplements, tea, coffee, dairy products, or calcium supplements, because each of these can decrease iron absorption.

Various mechanisms may contribute to the reduction in the rate or extent of drug absorption in the presence of food or nutrients. The presence and type of meal or food ingested influence the rate of gastric emptying. Gastric emptying may be delayed by the consumption of high-fiber meals and meals with high fat content. In general, a delay in drug absorption is not clinically significant as long as the extent of absorption is not affected. Absorption of antibiotics or analgesics may be examples of clinically significant problems with delayed absorption. Chelation reactions occur between certain medications and divalent or trivalent cations, such as iron, calcium, magnesium, zinc, or aluminum, and the absorption of drugs may be reduced by chelation with one of these metal ions. The antibiotics ciprofloxacin (Cipro) and tetracycline (Achromycin-V or Sumycin) form insoluble complexes with calcium in dairy products or calcium-fortified foods and beverages; calcium, magnesium, zinc, or iron supplements; or aluminum in antacids, thus preventing or reducing the absorption of both drug and nutrient (Neuhofel et al, 2002). The optimal approach to avoid this interaction is to stop noncritical supplements for the duration of the antibiotic prescription. If this is not possible, particularly with magnesium or with long-term antibiotic use, it is advisable to give the drug at least 2 hours before or 6 hours after the mineral.

Adsorption, or the adhesion to food or a food component, is another mechanism by which drug absorption is slowed or reduced. A high-fiber diet may decrease the absorption of tricyclic antidepressants such as amitriptyline (Elavil), leading to loss of therapeutic effect of the antidepressant because of the adsorption of the drug to the fiber. Likewise, the cardiovascular drug digoxin (Lanoxin) should not be taken with high-phytate food such as wheat bran or oatmeal.

Gastrointestinal pH is an important factor for the absorption of some drugs. Any situations resulting in changes in gastric acid pH, such as achlorhydria or hypochlorhydria, may reduce drug absorption. An example of such an interaction is the failure of ketoconazole (Nizoral) to clear a *Candida* infection in patients with human immunodeficiency virus (HIV) or in persons taking potent acid-reducing agents for gastroesophageal reflux disease (GERD). Ketoconazole achieves optimal absorption in an acid medium. Because of the high prevalence of achlorhydria in patients infected with HIV, dissolution of ketoconazole tablets in the stomach is reduced, leading to impaired drug absorption (Welage et al, 1995). This is also a concern with hypochlorhydria in persons receiving chronic acid suppression therapy, such as antacids, histamine 2 (H_2) receptor antagonists (e.g., famotidine [Pepcid]), or proton-pump inhibitors (e.g., omeprazole [Prilosec]). Ingestion of ketoconazole with an acidic liquid, such as cola or a dilute HCl solution, may improve bioavailability in these patients.

The presence of food in the stomach enhances the absorption of some medications, such as the antibiotic cefuroxime axetil (Ceftin) or the antiretroviral drug saquinavir (Fortovase or Invirase). These drugs are prescribed to be taken after a meal to reduce the dose that must be taken to reach an effective level. The bioavailability of cefuroxime axetil is substantially greater (52% versus 37%) when taken with food, compared with taking it in the fasting state. Maximum blood levels of saquinavir increased twofold in one study after the consumption of a heavy breakfast (940 to 1000 calories and 54 to 57 g of fat).

Medication and Enteral Nutrition Interactions

Continuous enteral feeding is an effective method of providing nutrients to patients who are unable to swallow or eat adequately (see Chapter 23). Use of the feeding tube to administer medication can cause problems, however. When liquid medications are mixed with enteral feeding formulas, incompatibilities may occur. Types of physical incompatibility include granulation, gel formation, and separation of the enteral product, frequently resulting in clogged feeding tubes and interruption of the delivery of nutrition to the patient. Examples of drugs that can cause granulation and gel formation are thioridazine (Mellaril) solution, chlorpromazine (Thorazine) concentrate, ferrous sulfate elixir, guaifenesin (Robitussin expectorant), and pseudoephedrine (Sudafed) cough syrup. Emulsion breakage also commonly occurs when acidic pharmaceutical syrups are added to enteral formulas. This reaction is more common in enteral formulas with intact protein and less common with hydrolyzed protein or free amino acids (Burns et al, 1988; Thomson and Rollins, 1991).

Most compatibility studies of medication and enteral products have focused on the effect of the drug on the integrity of the enteral product. More important is the effect of the enteral product on the bioavailability of the drug. This area requires much more research as the placement of feeding tubes becomes a more common practice. Bioavailability problems are common with phenytoin suspension (Dilantin suspension) and tube feeding. Because blood levels of phenytoin are routinely performed to monitor the drug, much information exists about the reduction of phenytoin bioavailability when given with enteral feedings, and individual variability is significant. Recommendations to separate phenytoin suspension from tube feeding formulas are common. Stopping the tube feeding before and after the phenytoin dose is generally suggested, but recommendations vary from 1- to 4-hour intervals. The most common is a 2-hour feeding–free interval before and after the dose of phenytoin is administered (Au Yeung and Ensom, 2000).

Information may not be readily available concerning a drug and enteral product interactions. Pharmaceutical manufacturers may have unpublished information about their product and enteral products. Checking with the manufacturer's medical information department may yield more information on this topic and a particular drug.

Drug Distribution

Albumin is the most important drug binding protein in the blood. Low serum albumin levels, often the result of inadequate protein intake and poor nutrition, provide fewer binding sites for highly protein-bound drugs. Fewer binding sites mean that a larger free fraction of drug will be present in the serum. Only the free fraction (unbound fraction) of a drug is able to leave the vasculature and exert a pharmacologic effect at the target organ. Patients with albumin levels below 3.0 g/dl are at increased risk for adverse effects from highly protein-bound drugs. Usual adult doses of highly protein-bound drugs in such persons may produce more pronounced pharmacologic effects than the same dose in persons with normal serum albumin levels. A lower dose of such drugs is often recommended for patients with low albumin levels. In addition, the risk for displacement of one drug from albumin binding sites by another drug is greater when albumin levels are less than 3.0 g/dl.

Anticoagulant warfarin, which is 99.9% serum protein bound, and anticonvulsant phenytoin, which is greater than 90% protein bound, are common drugs used in older patients. Low albumin levels tend to be more common in older patients. In the case of warfarin, higher levels of free drug lead to risk of excessive anticoagulation and bleeding. Phenytoin toxicity can result from higher levels of free phenytoin.

Drug Metabolism

Enzyme systems in the intestinal tract and the liver, although not the only sites of drug metabolism, account for a large portion of the drug metabolizing activity in the body. Food can both inhibit and enhance the metabolism of medication by altering the activity of these enzyme systems. A diet high in protein and low in carbohydrates can increase the hepatic metabolism of the antiasthma drug theophylline (Theo-Dur). The suspected mechanism of increased clearance of this drug is induction of the hepatic enzyme system responsible for metabolizing the drug (Walter-Sack and Klotz, 1996).

Conversely, a substance found in grapefruit and grapefruit juice can inhibit the intestinal metabolism of drugs such as calcium channel blockers that are dihydropyridine derivatives (felodipine [Plendil]) (Bailey et al, 1994) and/or some HMG CoA reductase inhibitors such as simvastatin (Zocor) (Lilja et al, 2000). Grapefruit inhibits the cytochrome P-450 3A4 enzyme system responsible for the oxidative metabolism of many orally administered drugs. This interaction appears to be clinically significant for drugs with low oral bioavailability, which are substantially metabolized and inactivated in the intestinal tract by the cytochrome P-450 3A4 enzyme in the intestinal wall. When grapefruit or grapefruit juice is ingested, the metabolizing enzyme is irreversibly inhibited, which reduces the normal metabolism of the drug. This reduction in metabolism allows more of the drug to reach the systemic circulation, and the increase in blood levels of unmetabolized drug results in a greater pharmacologic effect and possible toxicity. Unfortunately, the effects of grapefruit on intestinal cytochrome P-450 last up to 72 hours, until the body can reproduce the enzyme (Lilja et al, 2000). Therefore, separating the ingestion of the grapefruit and the drug does not appear to alleviate this interaction. Seville oranges (used in some marmelades, but not in commercial orange juice), pomelos, and tangelos may also cause similar reactions (Egashira et al, 2003; Malhotra et al, 2001). The interaction is not significant in drugs that are not metabolized by cytochrome P-4503A4 in the intestinal wall, such as the HMG CoA reductase inhibitors pravastatin (Pravachol) or fluvastatin (Lescol).

Competition between food and drugs such as propranolol (Inderal) and metoprolol (Lopressor) for metabolizing enzymes in the liver may alter the first pass metabolism of these medications. Drugs absorbed from the intestinal tract by the portal circulation are first transported to the liver before they reach the systemic circulation. Because many drugs are highly metabolized during this first pass through the liver, only a small percentage of the original dose is actually available to the systemic circulation and the target organ. In some cases, however, this percentage can be increased by concurrent ingestion of food with the drug. When food and drug compete for the same metabolizing enzymes in the liver, more of the drug is likely to reach the systemic circulation, which can lead to a toxic effect if the dose of the drug is titrated to an optimal level in the fasting state.

Drug Excretion

Food and nutrients can alter the reabsorption of drugs from the renal tubule. Reabsorption of the antimanic agent lithium is closely associated with the reabsorption of sodium. When sodium intake is low or when a patient is dehydrated, the kidneys will reabsorb more sodium. In the person treated with lithium, the kidney will reabsorb lithium as well as sodium under these conditions. Higher lithium levels and possible toxicity will result. When excess sodium is ingested, the kidneys will eliminate more sodium in the urine and likewise more lithium. This will produce lower lithium levels and possible therapeutic failure.

Drugs that are weak acids or bases are reabsorbed from the renal tubule into the systemic circulation only in the nonionic state. An acidic drug is largely in the nonionic state in urine with an acidic pH, whereas a basic drug is largely in a nonionic state in urine with an alkaline pH. A change in urinary pH by food may change the amount of drug existing in the nonionic state, thus increasing or decreasing the amount of drug available for tubular reabsorption. Foods such as milk, most fruits (including citrus fruits), and most vegetables are urinary alkalinizers. This change can affect the ionic state of a basic drug such as the antiarrhythmic agent quinidine gluconate (Quinaglute Dura-Tabs). In alkaline urine, the drug will be predominantly in the nonionic state and available for reabsorption from the urine into the systemic circulation, which may lead to higher blood quinidine levels and possible toxicity. This interaction is most likely to be clinically significant when the diet is composed exclusively of a single food or food group.

Patients should be cautioned against initiating fad diets without consulting their physician or dietitian.

Licorice, or glycyrrhizic acid, is an extract of glycyrrhiza root used in "natural" licorice candy. About 100 g of licorice (the amount in two or more twists of natural licorice) can increase cortisol concentration, resulting in pseudohyperaldosteronism. This causes increased sodium reabsorption, water retention, increased blood pressure, and greater excretion of potassium. The action of diuretics and antihypertensive drugs may be antagonized. The resultant hypokalemia may alter the action of some drugs (Pronsky, 2002).

EFFECTS OF DRUGS ON FOOD AND NUTRITION

Nutrient Absorption

Medication can decrease or prevent nutrient absorption (see Appendix 34). Chelation reactions between medications and minerals (metal ions) reduce the amount of mineral available for absorption. An example *is tetracycline* (Achromycin V or Sumycin) and ciprofloxacin, which will chelate calcium found in dairy products such as milk or yogurt or in supplements. This is also true for other divalent or trivalent cations such as iron, magnesium, and zinc found in individual mineral supplements or multivitamin or mineral supplements. Standard advice is to take the minerals at least 2 to 6 hours apart from the drug. For short-term antibiotic use, it may be more practical to discontinue the iron or calcium supplements during the course of the antibiotic.

Adsorption also can decrease nutrient absorption. Antihyperlipidemic, bile acid sequestrant cholestyramine (Questran) is also used to treat diarrhea. It adsorbs fat-soluble vitamins A, D, E, and K. Decreased absorption of folic acid has also been reported. Vitamin supplementation is recommended with long-term use of this drug, especially when it is taken more than once a day.

More than 2 tbsp (30 ml) of mineral oil per day decreases absorption of fat-soluble vitamins A, D, E, and K. It is advised to take the mineral oil in the morning and the vitamin(s) at least 2 hours later. This is not a clinically significant interaction with occasional use of mineral oil and consumption of a well-balanced diet (Clark et al, 1987).

Drugs can reduce nutrient absorption by influencing the transit time of food and nutrients in the gut. Cathartic agents and laxatives reduce transit time and may cause diarrhea, leading to losses of calcium and potassium. Diarrhea may be induced by drugs containing sorbitol, or by drugs that increase peristalsis such as the gastric mucosa protectant misoprostol (Cytotec).

A drug also can prevent nutrient absorption by changing the gastrointestinal environment. H_2-receptor antagonists, such as famotidine (Pepcid) or ranitidine (Zantac) and proton-pump inhibitors, such as omeprazole (Prilosec), are antisecretory drugs used to treat ulcer disease and GERD. They inhibit gastric acid secretion and raise gastric pH. These effects may impair absorption of vitamin B_{12} by reducing cleavage from its dietary sources. Cimetidine (Tagamet) is an antagonist that also reduces intrinsic factor secretion; this can be a problem for vitamin B_{12} absorption and can result in vitamin B_{12} deficiency with long-term use (Force and Nahata, 1992). Raising gastric pH to a more alkaline state is hypothesized to decrease the absorption of calcium, iron, zinc, folic acid, and β-carotene, but clinical studies have yielded contradictory results (Pelton et al, 2001).

Drugs with the greatest effect on nutrient absorption are those that damage the intestinal mucosa. Damage to the structure of the villi and microvilli inhibits the brush-border enzymes and intestinal transport systems involved in nutrient absorption. The result is general or varying degrees of specific malabsorption, which can alter the gastrointestinal tract's ability to absorb minerals, especially iron and calcium. Damage to the gut mucosa commonly results from chemotherapeutic agents, nonsteroidal anti-inflammatory drugs (NSAIDs), and long-term antibiotic therapy. NSAIDs may adversely affect the colon by causing a nonspecific colitis or by exacerbating a preexisting colonic disease (Faucheron and Parc, 1996). Patients with NSAID-induced colitis present with bloody diarrhea, weight loss, and iron deficiency anemia. The pathogenesis of this colitis is still controversial.

Drugs that affect intestinal transport mechanisms include (1) colchicine, an antiinflammatory agent used to treat gout; (2) paraaminosalicylic acid (PASA), an antituberculosis drug; (3) sulfasalazine (Azulfidine), used to treat ulcerative colitis; and (4) trimethoprim (antibiotic in Bactrim) and antiprotozoal agent pyrimethamine (Daraprim). The first two agents impair absorption of vitamin B_{12}; the others are competitive inhibitors of folate transport mechanisms.

Nutrient Metabolism

A drug may increase the metabolism of a nutrient(s), causing it to pass through the body faster, resulting in higher requirements; or a drug may cause vitamin antagonism by blocking conversion of a vitamin to the active form.

Anticonvulsants phenobarbital and phenytoin induce hepatic enzymes and increase the metabolism of vitamin D, vitamin K, and folic acid. Supplements of these vitamins are often prescribed with these drugs (Berg et al, 1995). Carbamazepine (Tegretol) has been reported to affect the metabolism of biotin, vitamin D, and folic acid, leading to possible depletion (Pelton et al, 2001).

The antituberculosis drug INH blocks the conversion of pyridoxine (vitamin B_6) to its active form pyridoxal 5-phosphate. Particularly in patients with low pyridoxine intake, this interaction may cause pyridoxine deficiency and peripheral neuropathy. Pyridoxine supplementation (25 to 50 mg/day) is generally recommended with the prescription of INH because it is prescribed for at least 6 months at a time. Some other drugs that function as pyridoxine antagonists are hydralazine (Apresoline), penicillamine, levodopa (Dopar), and cycloserine (Seromycin).

Methotrexate (MTX or Rheumatrex) is a folic acid antagonist used to treat cancer and rheumatoid arthritis. Without folic acid, DNA synthesis is inhibited, cell replication stops, and the cell dies. Pyrimethamine (Daraprim), used to treat malaria and ocular toxoplasmosis, is also a folic acid antagonist. These drugs bind to and inhibit the enzyme dihydrofolate reductase, preventing conversion of folate to its active form (see Chapter 4),which eventually can lead to megaloblastic anemia as a result of folate deficiency (see Chapter 34). Leucovorin (folinic acid, the reduced form of folic acid) is used with folic acid antagonists to prevent anemia and gastrointestinal damage, especially with chemotherapy such as high-dose methotrexate. Leucovorin does not require reduction by dihydrofolate reductase; thus, unlike folic acid, it is not affected by folic acid antagonists. Leucovorin therefore may "rescue" normal cells from MTX damage by competing for the same transport mechanisms into the cells. For patients with rheumatoid arthritis who are receiving low-dose MTX therapy, however, studies show that administration of daily folic acid supplements or folinic acid can lower toxicity without affecting efficacy of the drug (Ortiz et al, 1998).

Nutrient Excretion

Some drugs can either increase or decrease the urinary excretion of nutrients. Drugs can increase the excretion of a nutrient by interfering with nutrient reabsorption by the kidneys. For instance, most clinicians know that loop diuretics, such as furosemide (Lasix) or bumetanide (Bumex), increase the excretion of potassium; but these diuretics also increase the excretion of magnesium, sodium, chloride, and calcium. Potassium supplements are routinely prescribed with loop diuretics. In addition, clinicians need to consider supplements of magnesium and calcium, especially with long-term drug use, high doses of the diuretics, or poor dietary intake. Electrolyte and magnesium blood levels should be monitored. Prolonged use of high-dose diuretics, particularly by older patients on low-sodium diets, can cause sodium depletion. Hyponatremia may be overlooked in older patients because the mental confusion that is symptomatic of sodium depletion may be misdiagnosed as organic brain syndrome or senility. Thiazide diuretics, such as hydrochlorothiazide (HCTZ), increase the excretion of potassium and magnesium but reduce the excretion of calcium by enhancing renal reabsorption of calcium. High-dose HCTZ plus calcium supplementation may result in hypercalcemia.

Potassium-sparing diuretics, such as spironolactone (Aldactone) or triamterene (Dyrenium), increase excretion of sodium, chloride, and calcium. Blood levels of potassium can rise to dangerous levels if patients also take potassium supplements or suffer from renal insufficiency. Antihypertensive angiotensin-converting enzyme (ACE) inhibitors such as enalapril (Vasotec) or fosinopril (Monopril) decrease potassium excretion, leading to increased serum potassium levels. The combination of a potassium-sparing diuretic and an ACE inhibitor increases the danger of hyperkalemia.

Corticosteroids such as prednisone decrease sodium excretion, resulting in sodium and water retention. Conversely, enhanced excretion of potassium and calcium is caused by these drugs; so a low-sodium, high-potassium diet is recommended. Calcium and vitamin D supplements are generally recommended with long-term corticosteroid use, such as might be the case for a person with lupus or rheumatoid arthritis, to prevent osteoporosis. With corticosteroid use, this risk is important because it appears that not only is calcium lost in the urine, but corticosteroids may impair intestinal calcium absorption and the bone building activity of osteoblasts (Lems et al, 1998).

Phenothiazine-class antipsychotic drugs, such as chlorpromazine (Thorazine), increase excretion of riboflavin and can lead to riboflavin deficiency in those with poor dietary intake (Pinto and Rivlin, 1987).

A well-recognized complication associated with the use of cisplatin is the development of acute hypomagnesemia resulting from nephrotoxicity and renal magnesium wasting. Up to 90% of patients are affected (Lajer and Daugaard, 1999). Hypocalcemia, hypokalemia, and hypophosphatemia are also common. Both intravenous magnesium supplementation via rectal treatment or posttreatment hydration and oral magnesium supplements, taken between chemotherapeutic courses, have been used to prevent magnesium depletion. Results of the efficacy of each approach vary (Kibirige, Morris-Jones, and Addison, 1988; Sartori et al, 1993). Hypomagnesemia can result from cisplatin use even with high-dose magnesium replacement therapy. Hypomagnesemia can persist for months or even years after the final course of cisplatin.

MODIFICATION OF DRUG ACTION BY FOOD AND NUTRIENTS

Food or nutrients can alter the intended pharmacologic action of a medication by enhancing the medication effects or by opposing it. The classic example of an enhanced drug effect is the interaction between monoamine oxidase inhibitors (MAOI), such as tranylcypromine (Parnate) and pressor agents such as dopamine, histamine, and especially tyramine. These biologically active amines are normally present in many foods (see Box 19-2), but they rarely constitute a hazard because they are deaminated rapidly by MAO and diamine oxidases. Inhibition of MAO by medication prevents the breakdown of tyramine and other pressor agents. Tyramine is a vasoconstrictor that raises blood pressure. Significant ingestion of high-tyramine foods, such as aged cheeses and cured meats, while being treated with an MAOI antidepressant can cause a hypertensive crisis (increased heart rate, flushing, headache, stroke, and even death) (Gardner et al, 1997).

Caffeine in foods or beverages (see Appendix 43) increases the adverse effects of stimulant drugs such as amphetamines, methylphenidate (Ritalin, Concerta), or theophylline, causing nervousness, tremor, and insomnia. Conversely, caffeine's CNS stimulatory properties can oppose or counteract the antianxiety effect of tranquilizers such as lorazepam (Ativan).

Warfarin is an oral anticoagulant that reduces the hepatic production of four vitamin K–dependent clotting factors by inhibiting the conversion of vitamin K to a usable form. Because this is a competitive interaction, the ingestion of vitamin K in the usable form will oppose the action of warfarin and allow the production of more clotting factors. To achieve an optimal level of anticoagulation, a balance must be maintained between the dose of the drug and the ingestion of vitamin K. Counseling of a person taking oral anticoagulation therapy should include medical nutrition therapy to maintain a consistent dietary vitamin K intake rather than prohibiting all high–vitamin K foods, such as dark green, leafy vegetables (Booth et al, 1997) (see Appendix 50). Ingestion of other substances may enhance the anticoagulant effect of warfarin. These substances include onions, garlic, vitamin E supplements in doses greater than 400 IU, and certain herbal products such as dong quai, which contain coumarin-like substances or ginseng, which is a platelet inhibitor. Enhancement of the anticoagulation effects of warfarin may lead to serious bleeding events (Harris, 1995).

Alcohol

Ethanol combined with certain medications will produce additive toxicity, affecting various body organs and systems. Ethanol combined with CNS-depressant medications such as a benzodiazepine (e.g., diazepam [Valium]) or a barbiturate (e.g., phenobarbital) may produce excessive drowsiness, incoordination, and other signs of CNS depression.

In the gastrointestinal tract, ethanol acts as a stomach mucosal irritant. Combining ethanol with drugs that cause the same effect, such as aspirin or other NSAIDs (ibuprofen [Advil or Motrin]), may increase the risk of gastrointestinal ulceration and bleeding. Because of the hepatotoxic potential of ethanol, it should not be combined with medications that also exhibit a risk of hepatotoxicity, such as acetaminophen (Tylenol), amiodarone (Cordarone), or methotrexate (Rheumatrex) (Lieber, 1994).

Ethanol can inhibit gluconeogenesis, particularly when consumed in a fasting state. Inhibition of gluconeogenesis will prolong a hypoglycemic episode caused by insulin or an oral hypoglycemic agent such as glyburide (Diabeta, Micronase).

The combination of disulfiram (Antabuse) and ethanol produces a potentially life-threatening reaction characterized by flushing, rapid heartbeat, palpitations, and elevation of blood pressure. Disulfiram inhibits aldehyde dehydrogenase, an enzyme necessary for the normal catabolism of ethanol by the liver. As a result of this enzyme inhibition, high levels of acetaldehyde accumulate in the blood. Symptoms such as flushing, headache, and nausea appear within 15 minutes of alcohol ingestion. Because these symptoms are unpleasant, the drug is sometimes used as an aid to prevent alcoholics from returning to drinking. Because these symptoms may also be life threatening, however, candidates for this drug must be chosen carefully. Other medications, when ingested concurrently with ethanol, may produce disulfiram-like reactions. Some of these medications are the antibiotics metronidazole (Flagyl) and cefoperazone (Cefobid), the oral hypoglycemic agent chlorpropamide (Diabinese), and the antineoplastic agent procarbazine (Matulane).

EFFECTS OF DRUGS ON NUTRITIONAL STATUS

The desired effects of medications often are accompanied by effects that we consider undesirable or side effects. Side effects are often an extension of the desired effects, such as bacterial overgrowth, as a result of use of an antibiotic. Overgrowth of *Clostridium difficile* causes pseudomembranous colitis. Suppression of natural oral bacteria may lead to oral yeast overgrowth, or candidiasis.

Oral, Taste, and Smell

Many drugs affect the ability to taste or smell foods (Box 19-3). Drugs can cause an alteration in taste sensation (dysgeusia), reduced acuity of taste sensation (hypogeusia), or an unpleasant aftertaste, any of which may affect food intake. The mechanisms by which drugs alter the chemical senses are not well understood. They may alter the turnover of taste cells or interfere with transduction mechanisms inside taste cells. They may also alter neurotransmitters in the CNS that process chemosensory information (Schiffman, 1994). Common drugs that cause dysgeusia include the antihypertensive drug captopril (Capoten), the antiretroviral amprenavir (Agenerase), the antineoplastic cisplatin (Platinol-AQ), and the anticonvulsant phenytoin.

Captopril (Capoten) may cause a metallic or salty taste and the loss of taste perception. The antibiotic clarithromycin (Biaxin) enters the saliva. The drug itself has a bitter taste that stays in the mouth as long as the drug is present in the body.

Antineoplastic drugs, used in chemotherapy for cancer, affect cells that reproduce rapidly, including the mucous membranes. Inflammation of the mucous membranes, or mucositis, occurs and is manifest as stomatitis (mouth inflammation), glossitis (tongue inflammation), or cheilitis (lip inflammation and cracking). Mucositis can be extremely painful to the point that patients are not able to eat or even drink. Aldesleukin, also called interleukin-2 (Proleukin), paclitaxel (Taxol), and carboplatin (Paraplatin), are examples of antineoplastic agents that commonly cause severe mucositis.

Anticholinergic drugs (Box 19-4) compete with the neurotransmitter acetylcholine for its receptor sites, thereby inhibiting transmission of parasympathetic nerve impulses. This results in decreased secretions, including salivary secretions, causing dry mouth (xerostomia). Tricyclic antidepressants such as amitriptyline (Elavil), antihistamines such as diphenhydramine (Benadryl), and antispasmodic bladder control agents such as oxybutynin (Ditropan) are particularly problematic. Dry mouth immediately causes loss of taste sensation. Long-term dry mouth can cause dental caries and loss of teeth, gum disease, stomatitis and glossitis as well as nutritional imbalance and undesired weight loss.

Box 19-3. Examples of Drugs That Cause Altered Taste, or Dysgeusia

Cardiac Drugs

Acetazolamide (Diamox)
Captopril (Capoten)
Gemfibrozil (Lopid)
Quinidine (Quinaglute Dura, Quinidex Extentabs, Quinora)

Antiasthmatics

Beclomethasone (Beconase, Vancenase)
Terbutaline (Brethine, Bricanyl)

Antineoplastics

Carboplatin (Paraplatin)
Cisplatin (Platinol-AQ)
Dactinomycin (actinomycin-D)
Fluorouracil (5-FU) (Adrucil)
Interferon alfa 2a (Roferon-A)
Methotrexate (Methotrexate, Rheumatrex)

Antiinfectives

Amprenavir (Agenerase)
Cefuroxime (Ceftin, Zinacef)
Clarithromycin (Biaxin)
Clotrimazole (Mycelex)
Didanosine (Videx)
Ethionamide (Trecator-SC)
Metronidazole (Flagyl)
Pyrimethamine (Daraprim)
Pentamidine isethionate (NebuPent, Pentam 300)
Rifabutin (Mycobutin)

CNS Drugs

Clomipramine (Anafranil)
Levodopa (Dopar, Larodopa)
Phenytoin (Dilantin)
Phentermine (Adipex-P, Fastin, Ionamin)
Sumatriptan succinate (Imitrex)

Miscellaneous

Disulfiram (Antabuse)
Docusate sodium (Colace)
Etidronate disodium (Didronel)
Selenium (Se)

Data from Pronksy, ZM: *Food medication interactions*, ed 13, Birchrunville, Pa, 2004, Food Medication Interactions.
CNS, Central nervous system.

Gastrointestinal Effects

Gastrointestinal irritation and ulceration are serious problems with many drugs. The antiosteoporosis drug alendronate (Fosamax) is contraindicated in patients who are unable to sit upright for at least 30 minutes after taking it because of the danger of esophagitis. NSAIDs such as ibuprofen (Advil, Motrin) or aspirin can cause stomach irritation, dyspepsia, gastritis, ulceration, and sudden serious gastric bleeding, sometimes leading to fatalities (Box 19-5).

Antineoplastic drugs, used to treat cancer, often cause severe nausea and vomiting. Severe, prolonged nausea and vomiting, lasting as long as a week, have been reported with cisplatin (Platinol-AQ). Dehydration and electrolyte imbalances are of immediate concern. Weight loss and malnutrition are common long-term effects of these drugs, although it is often difficult to distinguish these effects from the complications of the disease itself (see Chapter 40).

Drugs can cause changes in bowel function that can lead to constipation or diarrhea (see Chapter 30). Narcotic agents such as codeine and morphine (MS Contin, MSIR) cause a nonproductive increase in smooth-muscle tone of the intestinal muscle wall, thereby decreasing peristalsis and causing constipation. Drugs with anticholinergic effects decrease intestinal secretions, slow peristalsis, and cause constipation (see Box 19-4). The atypical antipsychotic clozapine (Clozaril), tricyclic antidepressant amitriptyline (Elavil), and antihistamine diphenhydramine (Benadryl) cause constipation and possibly impaction. Deaths have been reported as a result of severe impaction with clozapine use (Gelenberg, 1997).

Destruction of intestinal bacteria leads to diarrhea (Box 19-6), possibly because of the overgrowth of *C. difficile*, causing pseudomembranous colitis. Some drugs are used to inhibit intestinal enzymes, such as the diabetic drugs acarbose (Precose) and miglitol (Glyset), which are α-glucosidase inhibitors. Such action leads to a delayed and reduced rise in postprandial blood glucose levels and plasma insulin responses. The major adverse effect is gastrointestinal intolerance,

Box 19-4. Examples of Drugs With Anticholinergic Effects

Psychotropics

Antipsychotics, Phenothiazines
Chlorpromazine (Thorazine)
Mesoridazine (Serentil)
Thioridazine HCl (Mellaril)

Antipsychotics, Atypical
Clozapine (Clozaril)
Olanzapine (Zyprexa)

Antipsychotics, Typical
Haloperidol (Haldol)
Perphenazine (Trilafon)
Thiothixene (Navane)

Antidepressants, Tricyclic
Amitriptyline (Elavil)
Clomipramine (Anafranil)
Doxepin (Sinequan)
Imipramine (Tofranil)

Antidepressants, MAOIs
Isocarboxazide (Marplan)
Phenelzine (Nardil)
Tranylcypromine (Parnate)

Antihistamines

Clemastine (Tavist)
Cyproheptadine (Periactin)
Diphenhydramine (Benadryl)
Hydroxyzine HCl (Atarax)
Hydroxyzine pamoate (Vistaril)
Promethazine (Phenergan)

GI Antispasmodics

Atropine
Dicyclomine (Bentyl)
Glycopyrrolate (Robinul)
L-Hyoscyamine (Levsin)
Propantheline (Pro-Banthine)

Antiemetics, Antivertigo Agents

Dimenhydrinate (Dramamine)
Meclizine (Bonine, Antivert)
Scopolamine (Transderm Scop)

Antiparkinson Agents

Benztropine (Cogentin)
Trihexyphenidyl (Artane)

Bladder Anticholinergics

Flavoxate (Uripas)
Oxybutynin (Ditropan)
Tolterodine (Detrol)

Inhalation Solution

Ipratropium (Atrovent)

Data from Pronsky ZM: *Food medication interactions*, ed 13, Birchrunville, Pa, 2004, Food Medication Interactions.
GI, Gastrointestinal; *MAOIs*, monoamine oxidase inhibitors.

Box 19-5. Examples of Drugs That Cause Gastrointestinal Bleeding and Ulceration

Antineoplastics

Aldesleukin interleukin-2 (Proleukin)
Fluorouracil (5-FU) (Adrucil)
Leuprolide acetate (Lupron)
Imatinib mesylate (Gleevec)
Mitoxantrone (Novantrone)
Methotrexate (Methotrexate, Rheumatrex)
Vinblastine sulfate (Velban)

NSAIDs, Analgesics, Antiarthritics

Aspirin/acetylsalicylic acid (Bufferin, Ecotrin)
Celecoxib (Celebrex)
Diclofenac sodium (Cataflam, Voltaren)
Etodolac (Lodine)
Ibuprofen (Advil, Motrin)
Indomethacin (Indocin)
Ketoprofen (Orudis)
Meloxicam (Mobic)
Nabumetone (Relafen)
Naproxen (Naprosyn, Anaprox, Aleve)
Rofexib (Vioxx)
Sulindac (Clinoril)

Immunosuppresants

Corticosteroids (Prednisone)
Myophenolate mofetil (CellCept)

Antiinfectives

Amphotericin B (Abelcet, Ambisome, Amphotec, Fungizone)
Ganciclovir sodium (Cytovene)

Miscellaneous

Bromocriptine (Parlodel)
Donepezil (Aricept)
Levodopa (Dopar)
Trazodone HCl (Desyrel)

Bisphosponates

Alendronate (Fosamax)
Risedronate (Actonel)

Data from Pronsky ZM: *Food medication interactions*, ed 13, Birchrunville, Pa, 2004, Food Medication Interactions.

Box 19-6. Examples of Drugs That Cause Diarrhea

Antibiotics

Amoxicillin (Amoxil)
Amphotericin B (Abelcet, AmBisome, Amphotec, Fungizone)
Ampicillin
Atovaquone (Mepron)
Azithromycin (Zithromax)
Cefdinir (Omnicef)
Cefixime (Suprax)
Cefuroxime (Ceftin Zinacef)
Cephalexin (Keflex)
Clofazimine (Lamprene)
Clindamycin (Cleocin)
Levofloxacin (Levaquin)
Linezolid (Zyvox)
Meropenem (Merrem I.V.)
Metronidazole (Flagyl)
Quinine sulfate (Quinine)
Rifampin (Rifadin)
Penicillin
Pyrimethamine (Daraprim)
Tetracycline HCl (Achromycin-V, Sumycin)

Antiviral Agents

Amprenavir (Agenerase)
Didanosine (Videx)
Lopinavir (Kaletra)
Nelfinavir (Viracept)
Ritonavir (Norvir)
Stavudine (Zerit)
Foscarnet (Foscavir)

Antineoplastics

Aldesleukin/interleukin-2 (Proleukin)
Capecitabine (Xeloda)
Carboplatin (Paraplatin)
Fluorouracil (5-FU) (Adrucil)
Imatinib mesylate (Gleevec)
Irinotecan (Camptosar)
Methotrexate (Methotrexate, Rheumatrex)
Mitoxantrone (Novantrone)
Paclitaxel (Taxol)

Oral Hypoglycemic Agents

Acarbose (Precose)
Metformin (Glucophage)
Miglitol (Glyset)

Gastrointestinal Agents

Lactulose (Chronulac)
Magnesium magonate (Milk of Magnesia)
Metoclopramide HCl (Reglan)
Misoprostol (Cytotec)
Casanthranol and docusate sodium (Peri-Colace)
Sorbitol
Orlitstat (Xenical)

Antigout Agents

Colchicine (Colchicine)

Data from Pronsky ZM: *Food medication interactions,* ed 13, Birchrunville, Pa, 2004, Food Medication Interactions.

specifically diarrhea, flatulence, and cramping secondary to both the osmotic effect and bacterial fermentation of undigested carbohydrates in the distal bowel.

Obviously, any of these problems, from dry mouth, to gastrointestinal irritation, to constipation or diarrhea, can negatively affect food intake and absorption and nutritional status.

Appetite Changes

Drugs can suppress appetite (Box 19-7), leading to undesired weight changes, nutritional imbalance, and growth retardation in children. Appetite suppression may be desired, such as with the use of the stimulant drug dextroamphetamine (Dexedrine), an appetite suppressant. Because of the potential for abuse, the use of amphetamines for appetite suppression is not recommended. Dexedrine is indicated for treatment of attention deficit disorder, attention deficit hyperactivity disorder (ADHD), and narcolepsy.

In general, most CNS stimulants, including the amphetamine mixture (Adderall) and methylphenidate (Ritalin), suppress appetite or cause frank anorexia. These drugs are used extensively to treat ADHD in children and may cause weight loss and inhibit growth (see Chapter 10).

Sibutramine (Meridia) and phentermine (Adipex-P, Ionamin), structurally related to amphetamines, are used as appetite suppressants. These drugs are indicated for short-term use, along with a reduced-calorie diet and exercise, in obese patients (i.e., patients with a body mass index [BMI] greater than 30) or in overweight patients (BMI greater than 25) if additional risk factors are present, such as hypertension, diabetes, or hyperlipidemia.

A major side effect of stimulant drugs is hypertension. Thus they are often contraindicated for hypertensive patients or those who have seizures or cardiac disease. Because hypertension is common among obese persons, these contraindications may limit the use of stimulants in obese or overweight hypertensive patients.

An alternative drug is orlistat (Xenical), a lipase inhibitor. Orlistat reduces the absorption of fat by binding to lipase in the intestine, thereby inhibiting its action. Consequently, fecal fat excretion is increased, a factor that contributes to the gastrointestinal complaints associated with the drug, specifically oily spotting, increased fecal urgency, and possible fecal incontinence. Because it acts peripherally, orlistat is not expected to have any adverse effects on cardiovascular function and thus has an advantage over centrally active agents. A low-fat diet of no more than 30% of calories from fat is essential, however. Fat intake should be distributed among all three meals. Orlistat is not an appetite suppressant, and some persons may find it difficult to maintain a low-fat diet.

Central nervous system side effects can interfere with the ability or desire to eat. Drugs that cause drowsiness, dizziness, ataxia, confusion, headache, weakness, tremor, or peripheral neuropathy can lead to nutritional compromise, particularly in older or chronically ill patients. Recognition of these problems as a drug side effect, rather than a consequence of disease or aging, is often overlooked.

Many medications stimulate appetite and lead to weight gain (Box 19-8). Antipsychotic drugs such as risperidone (Risperdal), olanzapine (Zyprexa), tricyclic antidepressant drugs such as amitriptyline (Elavil), and the anticonvulsant valproic acid (Depakote) often lead to weight gain. Patients complain of a ravenous appetite and the inability to "feel full." Weight gains of 40 to 60 pounds in a few months are not uncommon. Corticosteroid use is associated with dose-dependent body weight gain in many patients. Sodium and water retention as well as appetite stimulation cause the weight increases with corticosteroids. Medical nutrition therapy is essential, as is routine exercise.

Appetite stimulation is desirable for patients suffering from wasting (cachexia) resulting from disease states such as cancer (see Chapter 40) or HIV/AIDS (see Chapter 41) (Herrington et al, 1997). Drugs indicated as appetite stimulants or antiwasting agents are the hormone megestrol acetate (Megace), human growth hormone somatropin (Serostim), the anabolic steroid oxandrolone (Oxandrin), and the marijuana derivative dronabinol (Marinol). Drugs also used as appetite stimulants are the anabolic steroids oxymetholone (Anadrol-50) and nandrolone (Deca-Durabolin), the antihistamine cyproheptadine (Periactin), the hormone testosterone (Testoderm), and thalidomide (Thalomid).

With the successful advent of HAART (highly active antiretroviral therapy), lipodystrophy is now often a greater problem than wasting for HIV patients in the industrialized nations (see Chapter 41). Debate about an accurate definition of lipodystrophy is ongoing. Redistribution of body fat, fat wasting, glucose intolerance, and hyperlipidemia are common aspects of this syndrome. Antidiabetic drugs such as metformin (Glucophage) and rosiglitiazone (Avan-

Box 19-7. Examples of Drugs That Cause Anorexia

Antiinfectives

Amphotericin B (Abelcet, AmBisome, Amphotec, Fungizone)
Atovaquone (Mepron)
Cidofovir (Vistide)
Didanosine (ddI) (Videx)
Ethionamide (Trecator-SC)
Fomivirsen (Vitravene)
Foscarnet sodium (Foscavir)
Hydroxychloroquine sulfate (Plaquenil)
Metronidazole (Flagyl)
Pentamidine isethionate (NebuPent, Pentam 300)
Pyrimethamine (Daraprim)
Sulfadiazine
Zalcitabine (HIVID)

Antineoplastics

Aldesleukin/interleukin-2 (Proleukin)
Bleomycin sulfate (Blenoxane)
Capecitabine (Xeloda)
Carboplatin (Paraplatin)
Cytarabine (ara-C) (Cytosar-U)
Dacarbazine (DTIC-Dome)
Fluorouracil (Adrucil) (5-FU)
Hydroxyurea (Hydrea)
Imatinib mesylate (Gleevec)
Irinotecan HCl (Camptosar)
Methotrexate (MTX)
Vinblastine sulfate (Velban)
Vinorelbine tartrate (Navelbine)

Cardiovascular Drugs

Amiodarone HCl (Cordarone)
Acetazolamide (Diamox)
Hydralazine HCl (Apresoline)
Quinidine (Quinaglute Dura, Quinidex Extentabs, Quinora)

Bronchodilators

Albuterol sulfate (Proventil, Ventolin)
Theophylline (Elixophyllin, Slo-Phyllin Theo-24, Theobid, Theolair, Uniphyl)

Stimulants

Amphetamines (Adderall, Dexedrine)
Methylphenidate HCl (Ritalin)
Phentermine (Adipex-P, Fastin, Ionamin)

Miscellaneous

Fluoxetine (Prozac, Sarafem)
Galantamine (Reminyl)
Naltrexone HCl (ReVia)
Oxycodone (Oxycontin)
Rivastigmine (Exelon)
Sibutramine HCl (Meridia)
Sulfasalazine (Azulfidine)
Topiramate (Topamax)

Data from Pronsky ZM: *Food medication interactions*, ed 13, Birchrunville, Pa, 2004, Food Medication Interactions.

dia) are used to normalize glucose and insulin levels. Antihyperlipidemic drugs such as atorvastatin (Lipitor) or pravastatin (Pravachol) are used to control elevated triglycerides and cholesterol.

Organ System Toxicity

Drugs can cause specific organ system toxicity, such as hepatotoxicity, nephrotoxicity, pulmonary toxicity, neurotoxicity, ototoxicity, ocular toxicity, pancreatitis, or cardiotoxicity. Medical nutrition therapy may be indicated as part of the treatment of these toxicities. Although all toxicities are of concern, hepatotoxicity and nephrotoxicity are addressed here because drugs are eliminated from the body predominantly through the liver and the kidney.

Examples of drugs that cause hepatotoxicity (liver damage) leading to hepatitis, jaundice, hepatomegaly, or even liver failure are amiodarone (Cordarone), amitripyline (Elavil), lovastatin (Mevacor) and other "statin" antihyperlipidemic drugs, divalproex (Depakote), carbamazepine (Tegretol), kava, niacin, and sulfasalazine (Azulfidine). Monitoring of hepatic function through routine blood work for liver enzyme levels is generally prescribed with use of these drugs.

Nephrotoxicity (kidney damage) may change the excretion of specific nutrients (see *cisplatin*) or cause acute or chronic renal insufficiency, which may not resolve with cessation of drug use. Examples of drugs that often cause nephrotoxicity are antiinfectives amphotericin B (especially with intravenous desoxycholate form [Fungizone]) and cidofovir (Vistide) as well as antineoplastics cisplatin (Plaquinol-AQ), gentamicin (Garamycin), ifosfamide (Ifex), methotrexate, and pentamidine (Pentam 300). Adequate or extra prehydration, often administered intravenously, is prescribed to reduce renal toxicity. For example, with cidofovir, 1 L of intravenous normal saline (0.9% NaCl) is infused 1 to 2 hours before infusion of the drug. If tolerated, up to an additional liter may be infused after the drug infusion. Oral probenecid (Benemid) is also prescribed with cidofovir to reduce nephrotoxicity.

Glucose Levels

Many drugs affect glucose metabolism, causing hypoglycemia or hyperglycemia and, in some cases, frank diabetes (Box 19-9) (Pandit et al, 1993). The mechanisms of these effects vary from drug to drug and from individual to individual. Drugs may stimulate glucose production or impair glucose uptake. They may inhibit insulin secretion, decrease insulin sensitivity, or increase insulin clearance. Glucose levels may be affected by changes in other parameters, such as hypokalemia induced by diuretics or weight gain induced by antipsychotic medications. Cortiosteroids, particularly prednisone, prednisolone and

Box 19-8. Examples of Drugs That Increase Appetite

Psychotropics

Benzodiazepine Antianxiety Agents
Alprazolam (Xanax)
Chlordiazepoxide (Librium)

Antipsychotics, Typical
Haloperidol (Haldol)
Perphenazine (Trilafon)
Thiothixene (Navane)
Thioridazine HCl (Mellaril)

Antipsychotics, Atypical
Clozapine (Clozaril)
Olanzapine (Zyprexa)
Quetiapine Fumarate (Seroquel)
Risperidone (Risperdal)

Antidepressants, Tricyclic
Amitriptyline HCl (Elavil)
Clomipramine HCl (Anafranil)
Doxepin HCl (Sinequan)
Imipramine HCl (Tofranil)

Antidepressants, MAOI
Isocarboxazide (Marplan)
Phenelzine sulfate (Nardil)

Antidepressants, Other
Tranylcypromine sulfate (Parnate)
Mirtazapine (Remeron)
Paroxetine (Paxil)

Hormones

Corticosteroids (cortisone, methylprednisolone, prednisone)
Human growth hormone/somatropin (Serostim)
Medroxyprogesterone acetate (Provera, Depo-Provera)
Megestrol acetate (Megace)
Oxandrolone (Oxandrin)
Oxymetholone (Anadrol-50)
Testosterone (Androderm, Testoderm)

Anticonvulsants

Divalproex/valproic acid (Depakote/Depakene)
Gabapentin (Neurontin)

Miscellaneous

Cyproheptadine (Periactin)
Dronabinol (Marinol)
Thalidomide (Thalomid)

Data from Pronsky ZM: *Food medication interactions*, ed 13, Birchrunville, Pa, 2004, Food Medication Interactions.
MAOI, Monoamine oxidase inhibitor.

Box 19-9. Examples of Drugs That Affect Glucose Levels

Antidiabetics (Lower or Normalize Glucose Levels)

Acarbose (Precose)
Glimepiride (Amaryl)
Glipizide (Glucotrol)
Glyburide (DiaBeta)
Insulin (Humulin)
Metformin (Glucophage)
Miglitol (Glyset)
Neteglinide (Starlix)
Pioglitazone HCl (Actos)
Repaglinide (Prandin)
Rosiglitazone maleate (Avandia)

Drugs That Can Cause Hypoglycemia

Disopyramide (Norpace) Antiarrhythmic
Pentamidine isethionate (Pentam 300) Antiprotozoal
Quinine Antimalarial
Ethanol

Drugs That Can Increase Glucose Levels

Antiretroviral Agents, Protease Inhibitors
Amprenavir (Agenerase)
Nelfinavir mesylate (Viracept)
Ritonavir (Norvir)
Saquinavir (Invirase, Fortovase)

Diuretics, Antihypertensives
Furosemide (Lasix)
Hydrochlorothiazide (HCTZ, HydroDIURIL, Microzide)
Indapamide (Lozol)

Hormones
Corticosteroid (cortisone, prednisone)
Danazol (Danocrine)

Estrogen or Estrogen/Progesterone (Hormone Replacement Therapy)
Medroxyprogesterone (Cycrin, Provera, Depo-Provera)
Megestrol acetate (Megace)
Nandrolone decanoate (Deca-Durabolin)
Octreotide acetate (Sandostatin)

Oral Contraceptives
Oxandrolone (Oxandrin)
Oxymetholone (Anadrol-50)

Miscellaneous
Niacin (nicotinic acid) antihyperlipidemic
Baclofen (Lioresal) skeletal muscle relaxant
Caffeine (No-Doz) stimulant
Clofazimine (Lamprene) antibiotic
Olanzapine (Zyprexa) antipsychotic
Cyclosporine (Neoral, Sandimmune) immunosuppressant
Interferon alfa-2a (Roferon-A) antineoplastic

Data from Pronsky ZM: *Food medication interactions,* ed 13, Birchrunville, Pa, 2004, Food Medication Interactions.

hydrocortisone, are diabetogenic because of increased gluconeogenesis, but they also cause insulin resistance and therefore inhibit glucose uptake.

EXCIPIENTS AND FOOD-DRUG INTERACTIONS

An excipient is added to drug formulations for its action as a buffer, binder, filler, diluent, disintegrant, glidant, flavoring, dye, preservative, suspending agent, or coating. Excipients are also called inactive ingredients (Box 19-10). Hundreds of excipients are approved by the U.S. Food and Drug Administration (FDA) for use in pharmaceuticals. Several common excipients have potential for interactions in persons with an allergy or enzyme deficiency. Often just one brand of a drug, or one formulation or strength of a particular brand, may contain the excipient of concern. For example, tartrazine, listed as yellow dye No. 5, is used in Cleocin (brand of clindamycin) capsules in the 75- and 150-mg strengths but not in the 300-mg strength. Reglan (brand of metoclopramide) 5-mg tablets contain lactose, but the 10-mg tablets do not. Prometrium (micronized progesterone) capsules contain peanut oil and lecithin, whereas other progesterone forms do not. Prometrium labeling includes a warning that anyone allergic to peanuts should not use the drug.

Patients with celiac disease have gluten sensitivity and must practice life-long abstinence from wheat, barley, rye, and sometimes oats. They are particularly concerned with the composition and source of excipients, such as wheat starch or flour, which might contain gluten (see Chapter 30). Only a few pharmaceutical companies guarantee their products to be gluten free. Excipients such as dextrin and sodium starch glycolate are usually made from corn and potato, respectively, but can be made from wheat. The excipient dextrimaltose, a mixture of maltose and dextrin, is produced by the enzymatic action of barley malt on corn flour (Crowe and Falini, 2001; Kibbe, 2000). The source of each drug ingredient, if not specified, should be checked with the manufacturer.

Finally, some drug brands may contain enough excipient to be nutritionally significant (Table 19-1), such as vitamin E in Agenerase (amprenavir), mag-

Box 19-10. Examples of Potential Interactive Drug Excipients

Albumin (egg or human): May cause allergic reaction. Human albumin is a blood product.

Alcohol (ethanol): CNS depressant used as a solvent. All alcohol and alcohol-containing products and drugs must be avoided with medications such as disulfiram (Antabuse) or limited with other drugs to prevent additive CNS or hepatic toxicity. Elixirs contain 4% to 20% alcohol. Some solution, syrup, liquid, and parenteral forms contain alcohol.

Aspartame: A nonnutritive sweetener composed of the amino acids aspartic acid and phenylalanine. PKU (phenylketonuria) patients lack the enzyme phenylalanine hydroxylase. If aspartame is ingested in significant quantities by PKU patients, accumulation of phenylalanine causes toxicity to brain tissue.

Benzyl alcohol: Bacteriostatic agent used in parenteral solution. It causes allergic reactions in some people. Benzyl alcohol has been associated with a fatal "gasping syndrome" in premature infants.

Lactose: Lactose is used as a filler. The natural sweetener in milk, lactose is hydrolyzed in the small intestine by the enzyme lactase to glucose and galactose. Lactose intolerance (due to lactase deficiency) results in GI distress when lactose is ingested. Lactose in medications may cause this reaction.

Mannitol: The alcohol form of the sugar mannose, used as a filler. Mannitol is absorbed more slowly, yielding half as many calories per gram as glucose. Because of slow absorption, mannitol can cause soft stools and diarrhea.

Saccharin: Nonnutritive sweetener. Extensive human research has found no evidence of carcinogenicity.

Sorbitol: The alcohol form of sucrose. Absorbed more slowly than sucrose, sorbitol inhibits the rise in blood glucose. Because of slow absorption, sorbitol can cause soft stools or diarrhea.

Starch: Starch, from wheat, corn, or potato, is added to medication as a filler, binder, or diluent. Celiac disease patients have a permanent intolerance to gluten, a protein contaminant of wheat, barley, rye or oat starch. In celiac disease, gluten causes damage to the lining of the small intestine.

Sucrose: Sweetener. Significant source of simple carbohydrate and calories.

Sulfites: Sulfiting agents are used as antioxidants. Sulfites may cause severe hypersensitivity reactions in some people, particularly asthmatics. They include sulfur dioxide, sodium sulfite, and sodium and potassium metabisulfite. The FDA requires the listing of sulfites when present in foods or drugs.

Tartrazine: Tartrazine is yellow dye No. 5 color additive, which causes severe allergic reactions in some people (1 in 10,000). The FDA requires the listing of tartrazine when present in foods or drugs.

Vegetable oil: Soy, sesame, cottonseed, corn, or peanut oil is used in some parenteral drugs as a nonaqueous vehicle. Hydrogenated vegetable oil is a tablet/capsule lubricant. May cause allergic reactions in sensitive people.

Modified from Pronsky ZM: Potential interactive ingredients. In Pronsky ZM: *Food medication interactions,* ed 13, Birchrunville, Pa, 2004, Food Medication Interactions.

CNS, Central nervous system; *FDA,* U.S. Food and Drug Administration; *GI,* gastrointestinal.

TABLE 19-1 Examples of Drugs That Contain Nutritionally Significant Ingredients

TRADE NAME	GENERIC NAME	INGREDIENT	NUTRITIONAL SIGNIFICANCE
Accupril	Quinapril	Magnesium carbonate Magnesium stearate	Provides 50-200 mg magnesium daily
Accutane	Isotretinoin	Drug is related to vitamin A, Contains soybean oil	Avoid vitamin A or β-carotene May cause allergic reaction
Agenerase	Amprenavir	Vitamin E	1744 IU in adult daily dose
Atrovent (inhaler)	Ipratropium Bromide	Soya lecithin	May cause allergic reaction
Fibercon/ Fiber-Lax	Calcium Polycarbophil	Calcium polycarbophil	100-mg Ca/tablet up to 6 tablets/day = 600 mg calcium total
Marinol	Dronabinol	Sesame oil	May cause allergic reaction
Phazyme	Simethicone	Soybean oil in capsule	May cause allergic reaction
Prometrium	Micronized progesterone	Peanut oil	May cause allergic reaction
Diprivan	Propofol	10% soybean oil emulsion Egg yolk phospholipids	Oil is significant caloric source May cause allergic reaction
Videx	Didanosine	Sodium buffer in powder	≥2760 mg Na/adult daily dose
Zantac	Ranitidine	Sodium in *prescription* granules and tablets; Zantac 75 (nonprescription) is sodium free	350-730 mg Na/adult daily dose

Data from Pronsky ZM: *Food medication interactions,* ed 13, Birchrunville, Pa, 2004, Food Medication Interactions.

nesium in Accupril (quniapril), calcium in Fibercon or Fiber-Lax (calcium polycarbophil), and soybean oil lipid emulsion in propofol (Diprivan). Proprofol is commonly used long term for sedation of patients in the intensive care unit. Its formulation includes 10% emulsion, which contributes 1.1 kcal/ml. When infused at doses up to 9 mg/kg/hour in a patient weighing 70 kg, for instance, it may contribute an additional 1663 kcal/day from the emulsion. For a patient receiving total parenteral nutrition, elimination of lipids may be recommended while he or she is taking propofol (Mateu-de Antonio and Barrachina, 1997). Specific brands or formulation(s) of a specific brand provide significant amounts of sodium and therefore may be contraindicated for patients who need to limit sodium.

MEDICAL NUTRITION THERAPY

Medical nutrition therapy (MNT) can be divided into *prospective* and *retrospective*. *Prospective* includes all MNT offered when the patient first starts a drug. *Retrospective* concerns evaluation of symptoms to determine whether medical problems might be the result of food-drug interactions.

A diet history must be obtained, including information about the use of alcohol, vitamin and mineral supplements, and herbal or phytonutrient supplements. The patient should be evaluated for genetic problems (see Chapter 16), weight and appetite changes, altered taste, and gastrointestinal problems (see Chapter 17).

Prospective drug information and MNT include basic information about the drug: the name, purpose, and duration of prescription of the drug plus when and how to take the drug. This information includes whether to take the drug with or without food. Specific foods and beverages to avoid while taking the drug and potential interactions between drug and vitamin or mineral supplements need to be emphasized. For instance, the patient taking tetracycline (Achromycin-V or Sumycin) or ciprofloxacin (Cipro) should be warned not to combine the drug with milk, yogurt, or supplements containing divalent cations, calcium, iron, magnesium, zinc, or vitamin-minerals containing any of these cations.

Potential significant side effects must be delineated, and possible dietary suggestions to relieve the side effects should be described. For instance, information about a high-fiber diet with adequate fluids should be part of MNT about an anticholinergic drug, such as oxybutynin (Ditropan), that often causes constipation.

Conversely, diarrhea can be controlled by the use of psyllium (Metamucil) or probiotics, such as *Lactobacillus acidophilus* (Lactinex), particularly for antibiotic-associated diarrhea (Elmer, Surawicz, and McFarland, 1996) (see Chapter 30).

Patients should be warned about potential nutritional problems, particularly when dietary intake is inadequate, such as hypokalemia with a potassium-depleting diuretic. Dietary changes that may alter drug action should be included, such as the effect of an increase in foods high in vitamin K on warfarin action. Special diet information, such as a low-cholesterol, low-fat, limited sugar diet with atorvastatin (Lipitor), or other antihyperlipidemic drugs, is essential information. Written information should list medication ingredients such as nonnutrient excipients in the medication (see Box 19-10). Examples include lactose, starch, tartrazine, aspartame, and alcohol. Patients with lactose intolerance, celiac disease, allergies, phenylketonuria, or alcoholism need to avoid or limit one or more of these ingredients.

Retrospective MNT addresses the possibility of food-drug interactions. To determine whether a patient's symptoms are the result of a food-drug interaction, a complete medical and nutritional history is essential, including prescription and nonprescription

Clinical Scenario I

Henry is a 31-year-old man who began to suffer seizures after a head trauma injury from a motorcycle accident at the age of 18. For the first 2 years after the accident, he was prescribed various anticonvulsant regimens. The combination of phenytoin (Dilantin), 300 mg daily, and phenobarbital, 120 mg daily, has proven to be the most effective therapy to control his seizures. Henry has been stabilized on this regimen for the last 11 years.

Henry is a senior computer programmer for a large corporation. He is 6 feet 2 inches tall and weighs 182 lb. Henry admits to having an aversion for exercise and athletics. In his free time, he enjoys reading, playing computer games, and watching television. During the past year, Henry has broken his left femur and tibia on two separate occasions. He broke his femur when he missed the bottom step on the stairway in his office building. Several months later, he broke his tibia when he tripped over a broken branch in his yard. Henry recently complained to his orthopedic surgeon about hip and pelvic pain of several weeks' duration. An orthopedic examination with x-rays, bone scan, and DEXA scan revealed that Henry is suffering from osteomalacia. A review of Henry's typical diet reveals a nutritionally marginal diet that commonly includes fast foods and frozen dinners. His diet is generally deficient in fresh fruits, vegetables, and dairy products.

1. Is osteomalacia common in young men?
2. How does Henry's lifestyle contribute to the development of osteomalacia?
3. What vitamin or mineral deficiency may have contributed to the current state of Henry's bones?
4. Describe the food-drug interaction that has contributed to Henry's osteomalacia.
5. What medical nutritional therapy would you recommend for Henry?

Courtesy *Food medication interactions*, ed 13, Birchrunville, Pa, 2004, Food Medication Interactions.

drugs, vitamin-mineral supplements, and herbal or phytonutrient products. The date of beginning to take the drug(s) versus the date of symptom onset is significant information. It is important to identify the use of nutritional supplements, such as enteral products, or significant dietary changes, such as fad diets, during the course of drug prescription.

Finally, it is important to investigate the reported incidence of side effects (by percentage as compared with a placebo). For example, for omeprazole (Prilosec), vomiting occurs in 1.5% of those taking the drug compared with 4.7% of those taking a placebo. Therefore, in a patient treated with omeprazole, it would be appropriate to consider other causes for vomiting. A rare drug effect is less likely to be the reason for a negative symptom than an effect that is common.

Clinical Scenario 2

Emma is a 79-year-old woman who suffered an embolic stroke from previously undetected atrial fibrillation. In the hospital she was noted to have left-sided weakness, slurred speech, and minimal difficulty with word finding. Because Emma was still in atrial fibrillation on admission to the hospital, the decision was made to begin anticoagulation therapy with warfarin (Coumadin). The plan for Emma was to transfer her to the local rehabilitation hospital for physical, occupational, and speech therapy as soon as she was physically stable. Her prognosis was considered good for full recovery.

A psychosocial consult in the rehabilitation facility revealed a 5 feet 1 inches, 119-lb woman who was anxious to regain her independence and return to her home, where she lives alone. A son and daughter live within a 10-mile radius and are willing to participate in their mother's care once she returned home.

While Emma was hospitalized, her warfarin dose remained stable at 2.5 mg daily. Her international normalized ratio (INR) was measured consistently between 2 and 3 during the 3-week period in the hospital and the rehabilitation facility. Once Emma returned to her own home, she began having her blood drawn to monitor her INR a minimum of twice a week. At this point, however, her INR is constantly changing. Each change in INR necessitates a change in her dose of warfarin. At times the INR is higher than 3, and Emma is instructed to hold the warfarin until the next blood draw. At other times the INR is below 2, and the dose of warfarin is increased.

1. How do you account for the difference in the stability of Emma's state of anticoagulation before and after her discharge? What questions would you ask Emma to discover the reasons for the fluctuation in her anticoagulation state?
2. What instruction about warfarin and diet should Emma have received before her discharge?
3. List dietary factors that can affect the pharmacologic action of warfarin.
4. What vitamins or supplements can interact with warfarin?
5. Emma would like to take ginseng to try to improve her memory since her stroke. Is this a safe idea? What would you advise Emma to do?

Courtesy *Food medication interactions*, ed 13, Birchrunville, Pa, 2004, Food Medication Interactions.

SUMMARY

Because of the importance of food-drug interactions in the effectiveness of medication and the overall health care provided, various strategies have been undertaken at health care facilities to meet the JCAHO requirements for food-drug interaction counseling. A policy addressing this issue and a procedure describing the steps to conform to the policy should be included in the policy and procedure manual for the facility. An example of a policy statement is as follows: "Patients discharged on modified diets receive written instructions and individualized counseling before discharge, including food-drug interaction counseling if indicated." Educational materials on each medication, including food-drug interactions, should be available in each facility for distribution to patients and approved by the medical team, including pharmacists and dietitians. Documentation in the medical record is also required when instruction has been given, including assessment of the patient's comprehension, ability, and willingness to follow instructions.

Relevant Web Sites

Access to MedLine
www.ncbi.nlm.nih.gov/entrez/query.fcgi
DRUGFACTS.com
www.factsandcomparisons.com/
FDA Center for Drug Evaluation and Research
www.fda.gov/cder/
Food and Nutrition Information Center
www.nal.usda.gov/fnic/
Food Medication Interactions
www.foodmedinteractions.com
Grapefruit-Drug Interactions
www.powernetdesign.com/grapefruit/
NIH Patient Handouts
www.cc.nih.gov/ccc/patient_education/drug_nutrient/
Project Inform's Drug Interactions (HIV/AIDS)
www.projinf.org/fs/drugin.html
RxList
www.rxlist.com/

Cited References

Au Yeung SCS, Ensom MHH: Phenytoin and enteral feedings: does evidence support an interaction? *Ann Pharmacother* 34:896, 2000.

Bailey DG et al: Grapefruit juice and drugs: how significant is the interaction? *Clin Pharm* 26(2):91, 1994.

Berg MJ et al: Folic acid improves phenytoin pharmacokinetics, *J Am Diet Assoc* 95:352, 1995.
Booth SL et al: Dietary vitamin K1 and stability of oral anticoagulation: proposal of a diet with constant vitamin K1 content, *Thromb Haemost* 77(3):504, 1997.
Burns P et al: Physical compatability of enteral formulas with various common medications, *J Am Diet Assoc* 88:1094, 1988.
Clark JH, et al: Serum beta-carotene, retinol, and alpha-tocopherol levels during mineral oil therapy for constipation, *Am J Dis Child* 141:1210, 1987.
Crowe JP, Falini NP: Gluten in pharmaceutical products, *Am J Health Syst Pharm* 58(5):396, 2001.
Duarte J et al: Efficiency of the protein redistribution diet in the anti-parkinsonian effect of L-dopa, *Neurologia* 8:248, 1993.
Egashira K et al: Pomelo-induced increase in the blood level of tacrolimus in a renal transplant patient, *Transplantation* 75:1057, 2003.
Elmer GW, Surawicz CM, McFarland LV: Biotherapeutic agents: a neglected modality for the treatment and prevention of selected intestinal and vaginal infections, *JAMA* 275(11):870, 1996.
Faucheron JL, Parc R: Non-steroidal anti-inflammatory drug induced colitis, *Int J Colorectal Dis* 11:99, 1996.
Force RW, Nahata MC: Effect of histamine H-2 receptor antagonists on vitamin B12 absorption, *Ann Pharmacother* 26:1283, 1992.
Fosamax package insert. West Point, Pa, Merck, September 2001.
Gardner DM et al: The making of a user friendly MAOI diet, *J Clin Psychol* 57(3): 99-104, 1996.
Gelenberg AJ: Severe CI reations to Clozapine, *Bio Ther Psych* 20(10):37-38, 1997.
Harris J: Interaction of dietary factors with oral anticoagulants: review and applications, *J Am Diet Assoc* 95:580, 1995.
Herrington AM et al: Pharmacologic options for the treatment of cachexia, *Nutr Clin Prac* 12(3):101, 1997.
Kibbe AH, editor: *Handbook of pharmaceutical excipients*, ed 3, Washington, DC, 2000, American Pharmaceutical Association.
Kibirige MS, Morris-Jones PH, Addison GM: Prevention of cisplatin-induced hypomagnesemia, *Pediatr Hematol Oncol*; 5(1):1, 1988.
Lajer H, Daugaard G: Cisplatin and hypomagnesemia, *Cancer Treat Rev* 35(1):47, 1999.
Lems WK et al: Pharmacological prevention of osteoporosis in patients on corticosteroid medication, *Ned Tijdschr Geneeskd* 142 (34):1904-1908, 1998.
Lieber CS: Mechanisms of ethanol-drug nutrition interactions, *J Toxicol Clin Toxicol* 32(6):631-681, 1994.
Lilja JJ et al: Duration of effect of grapefruit juice on the pharmacokinetics of the CYP3A4 substrate simvastatin, *Clin Pharmacol Ther* 68:384-390, 2000.
Malhotra S et al: Seville orange juice-felodipine interactions: comparison with dilute grapefruit juice and involvement of furocoumarins, *Clin Pharm Ther* 89(1):14-22, 2001.
Mateu-de Antonio J, Barrachina F: Propofol infusion and nutritional support, *Am J Health Syst Pharm* 54(21):2515-2516, 1997.
Neuhofel AL et al: Lack of bioequivalence of ciprofloxacin when administered with calcium-fortified orange juice: a new twist on an old interaction, *J Clin Pharmacol* 42:461, 2002.
Ortiz Z et al: The efficacy of folic acid and folinic acid in reducing methotrexate gastrointestinal toxicity in rheumatoid arthritis: a metaanalysis of randomized clinical trials, *J Rheumatol* 25 (1):36-43, 1998.
Pandit MK et al: Drug-induced disorders of glucose tolerance, *Ann Intern Med* 118:529-539, 1993.
Pelton R et al: *Drug-induced nutrient depletion handbook*, ed 2, Hudson, Ohio, 2001, Lexi-Comp.
Pinto JT, Rivlin RS: Drugs that promote renal excretion of riboflavin, *Drug Nutr Inter* 5:143-151, 1987.
Pronsky ZM: Food medication interactions, ed 13, Birchrunville, Pa, 2004, Food Medication Interactions.
Rees DC, Kelsey H, Richards JD: Acute haemolysis induced by high dose ascorbic acid in glucose-6-phosphate dehydrogenase deficiency, *BMJ* 306(6881):841, 1993.
Ritschel WA, Kearns GL: *Handbook of basic pharmacokinetics*, ed 5, Washington DC, 1999, American Pharmaceutical Association.
Roth JA. Drug metabolism. In Smith CM, Reynard AM, eds: *Essentials of pharmacology*, 1995, Philadelphia, W.B. Saunders.
Sartori S et al: Changes in intracellular magnesium concentrations during cisplatin chemotherapy, *Oncology* 50:230, 1993.
Schiffman S: Changes in taste and smell: drug interactions and food preferences, *Nutr Rev* 52(suppl 8):S11, 1994.
Thomson C, Rollins C: Enteral feedings and medication incompatibilities, *Support Line* 113(3):9, 1991.
Tischio JP: Pharmacogenetics. In Gennaro AR, ed: Remington: *The science and practice of pharmacology*, ed 19, Easton, Pa, 1995, Mack Publishing Co.
Walter-Sack I, Klotz U: Influence of diet and nutritional status on drug metabolism, *Clin Pharmacokinet* 31(1):47, 1996.
Welage LS et al: Alterations in gastric acidity in patients infected with HIV, *Clin Infect Dis* 21:1431, 1995.

Additional References

De Abajo FJ et al: Association between selective serotonin reuptake inhibitors and upper gastrointestinal bleeding: population based case-control study, *BMJ* 319:1106-1109, 1999.
Fava M et al: Fluoxetine versus sertraline and paroxetine in major depressive disorder: changes in weight with long-term treatment, *J Clin Psychiatry* 61 (11):863-867, 2000.
Garg SK et al: Effect of grapefruit juice on carbamazepine bioavailability in patients with epilepsy, *Clin Pharmacol Ther* 64 (3):286-288, 1998.
Herr SM: *Herb-drug interaction handbook*, ed 2, Nassau, NY, 2002, Church Street Books.
Holden K: *Parkinson's disease guidelines for medical nutrition therapy for use by nutrition professionals.* Fort Collins, Colo, 2000, Five Star Living.
Kanazawa S et al: The effects of grapefruit juice on the pharmacokinetics of erythromycin, *Eur J Clin Pharmacol* 56(11):799-800, 2001.
Murray JS, Healy MD: Drug-mineral interactions: a new responsibility for the hospital dietitian, *J Am Diet Assoc* 91:66, 1991.
Pronsky ZM et al: *HIV medication food interactions, and so much more*, ed 2, Birchrunville, Pa, 2001, Food Medication Interactions.
Thomas JA: Drug-nutrient interactions, *Nutr Rev* 53:271, 1995.

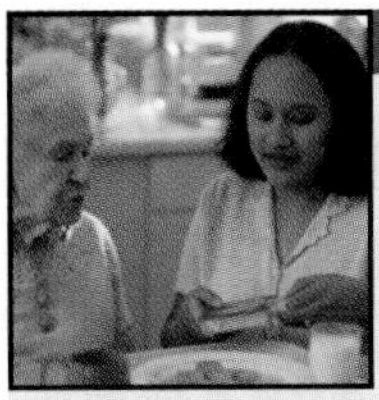

CHAPTER 20

Integrative Medicine and Phytotherapy

RUTH M. DEBUSK, PhD, RD

CHAPTER OUTLINE

- Integrative Therapies
- Commonly Used Botanicals
- Guidelines for Working With Clients Who Use Botanicals

KEY TERMS

acupuncture–use of thin needles inserted into points on the meridians to stimulate the body's vital energy

allicin–a sulfur compound contained in garlic that is responsible for garlic's odor and thought to be the active component

botanicals–plants (including their leaves, flowers, stems, rhizomes, or roots) that are used for medicinal purposes

***chi* (Qi)**–a term in traditional Oriental medicine that means life-force energy; the center of the body's functions

chiropractic–a healing system that involves manual manipulation of the musculoskeletal parts of the body to improve the normal functioning of the nervous system, which in turn is thought to promote health

Commission E monographs–therapeutic monographs on phytomedicines developed in Germany by an expert commission of scientists and health care professionals

Dietary Supplement Health and Education Act of 1994 (DSHEA)–a law that defines dietary supplements with provisions related to the marketing of these products

echinacea–a botanical that may be used to strengthen the immune system and that has adjunctive application for reducing the duration and severity of symptoms of colds and influenza

Sections of this chapter were written by Kimberly Mathai, RD, for the previous edition of this text.

garlic–a botanical that appears to have health benefits for the cardiovascular system

ginger–a botanical that has adjunctive therapeutic use as an antiemetic

ginkgo biloba–a botanical from an ancient tree used as an adjunctive treatment for vascular insufficiency and dementia

ginseng–a botanical that has a normalizing effect, affecting the whole organism in a positive way

hawthorn–a botanical containing flavonoids, particularly oligomeric procyanidins, that affect the cardiovascular system through vasodilation

holistic therapies–treatments that emphasize the healing force of nature and the body's ability to self-heal

homeopathy–a medical system based on the theory that substances in large doses that produce symptoms of a disease in healthy people will cure the same symptoms when administered in very dilute amounts

integrative medicine–a holistic approach to health that combines complementary and alternative therapies with conventional medicine

meridian–a concept in traditional Chinese medicine relating to channels of energy

milk thistle–a botanical that has silymarin as its principal active constituent and is known for its hepatoprotective characteristics

moxibustion–the application of heat along meridian acupuncture points to affect chi (Qi) and blood to balance the substances and organs

naturopathy–a therapeutic system that uses natural methods of healing (i.e., light, heat, air, water, and

KEY TERMS—Continued

massage); modalities of naturopathy include phytomedicines, nutrition, nutritional supplements, and natural forces

pharmacognosy–the science of natural drugs and their physical, botanical, and biochemical properties and applications

phytotherapy–the science of using plant-based medicines to prevent or treat illness

saw palmetto–a plant from which lipophilic extracts of berries are used as an adjunctive treatment for benign prostatic hyperplasia

silymarin–a bioflavonoid compound that is the active constituent in milk thistle; used as an adjunctive therapy for chronic inflammatory liver conditions and cirrhosis and as a liver protective agent

St. John's wort–a botanical that is sometimes used as an antidepressant, with applications for mild to moderate depression; also used as an antiviral agent

subluxation–the dislocation of part of the body, which is thought to interfere with normal nerve function; chiropractic focuses on identifying and removing these interferences

traditional Oriental medicine–a form of medicine based on the concept that energy, also termed *chi (Qi)* or life-force energy, is the center of body functions; wellness is a function of the balanced and harmonious flow of *chi;* illness or disease results from disturbances in this flow

valerian–a botanical that acts on the central nervous system and has adjunctive therapeutic application as a sleep aid

Complementary, alternative, or adjunctive health care practices refer to those practices that are not presently an integral part of conventional medicine. The list of what constitutes such therapies is changing rapidly as practices are investigated for their safety and effectiveness. Integrative medicine is the integration of these various approaches into conventional medicine, with the goal of deriving the best health care options for the consumer. Increasingly, health care practitioners are using an integrative approach.

The use of integrative therapies such as phytotherapy, chiropractic, naturopathy, homeopathy, and acupuncture to enhance conventional medical practices has been increasing in the United States since the 1960s. Two national surveys conducted by researchers at Harvard Medical School in 1990 and 1997 found that significant numbers of Americans visit providers of complementary and alternative therapies. In 1997 more than 40% of Americans used some form of alternative or complementary therapy. In both survey years, more Americans visited complementary care providers than U.S. primary care physicians (Eisenberg et al, 1993, 1998).

More recently, surveys of the use of integrative therapies in children and in adults ages 65 and older found significant use of these therapies (Foster et al, 2000; Simpson and Roman, 2001). A variety of complementary and alternative modalities are being used (Eisenberg et al, 2001; Kaptchuk and Eisenberg, 2001a, 2001b; Kessler et al, 2001). Those who use these therapies believe these options are more congruent with their beliefs and values about health and life than are conventional therapies (Astin, 1998). Of those who use both conventional and complementary and alternative therapies, many appear to value both for their perceived benefits (Eisenberg et al, 2001).

INTEGRATIVE THERAPIES

Complementary, alternative, or adjunctive therapies are not new. In fact, their roots can be traced to early Greek and Chinese cultures. Although natural therapies are often described as being "cutting edge," they are actually much older than conventional Western interventions. Experts estimate that herbal remedies and *ayurveda,* the traditional medicine of India, are more than 5000 years old.

As a result of the increased interest in these therapies, the Office of Alternative Medicine of the National Institutes of Health (NIH) was created in 1992 to evaluate their effectiveness. As of 1998, this office had grown significantly from an original budget of $2 million to a budget of $114 million (NCCAM, 2003). It was elevated in stature when it was designated a *center* and renamed the *National Center for Complementary and Alternative Medicine (NCCAM).* The mandate of this federal center is to investigate and evaluate alternative therapies and their effectiveness. Table 20-1 provides an overview of the institution-affiliated centers of research on integrative medicine that exist throughout the United States.

Complementary and alternative therapies are considered holistic. Holistic therapies, derived from the Greek word *holos,* meaning a "whole," are based on the theory that health is a vital dynamic state, reflecting a profound will and wisdom to maintain wellness rather than the absence of disease. *Vis mediatrix naturae,* the healing force of nature, is the underlying precept of holistic medicine. According to this precept, all living things can self-heal and organisms have inherent self-defense mechanisms against illness. Naturopathy, chiropractic, homeopathy, traditional Oriental medicine, acupuncture, and phytotherapy are based on these concepts.

TABLE 20-1 CAM* Specialty Centers of Research

SPECIALTY OF CENTER	NAME OF CENTER	LOCATION
Addictions	Center for Addiction and Alternative Medicine Research www.mmrfweb.org/research/addicton&alt_med/index.html	Minneapolis Medical Research Foundation Minneapolis, MN
Aging and women's health	Center for CAM Research in Aging and Women's Health cpmcnet.columbia.edu/dept/rosenthal	Columbia University College of Physicians and Surgeons New York, NY
Arthritis	Center for Alternative Medicine Research on Arthritis www.compmed.ummc.umaryland.edu	University of Maryland School of Medicine Baltimore, MD
Botanical†	Botanical Center for Age-Related Diseases	Purdue University West Lafayette, IN
	Botanical Dietary Supplements for Women's Health	University of Illinois at Chicago Chicago, IL
	UCLA Center for Dietary Supplements Research: Botanicals	University of California at Los Angeles Los Angeles, CA
	Arizona Center for Phytomedicine Research	University of Arizona College of Pharmacy Tucson, AZ
Cancer	Johns Hopkins Center for Cancer Complementary Medicine	Johns Hopkins University Baltimore, MD
	Specialized Center of Research in Hyperbaric Oxygen Therapy	University of Pennsylvania Philadelphia, PA
Cardiovascular diseases	Center for Complementary and Alternative Medicine Research in CVD www.med.umich.edu/camrc/index.html	The University of Michigan Ann Arbor, MI
Cardiovascular and aging in African Americans	Center for Natural Medicine and Prevention	Maharishi University of Management Fairfield, IA
Chiropractic	Consortial Center for Chiropractic Research www.palmer.edu	Palmer Center for Chiropractic Research Davenport, IA
Craniofacial disorders	Center for Health Research	Kaiser Foundation Hospitals Portland, OR
Neurologic disorders	Oregon Center for Complementary and Alternative Medicine in Neurological Disorders	Oregon Health Sciences University Portland, OR
Neurodegenerative diseases	Center for CAM in Neurodegenerative Diseases emory.edu/WHSC/MED/NEUROLOGY/CAM/index.html	Emory University School of Medicine Atlanta, GA
Pediatrics	University of Arizona Health Sciences Center Department of Pediatrics	University of Arizona Tucson, AZ

*CAM, Complementary and alternative medicine.
†The botanical research centers are funded in conjunction with the Office of Dietary Supplements, National Institutes of Health.
From the National Center for Complementary and Alternative Medicine, National Institutes of Health; information about each of the specialty centers is available at www.nccam.nih.gov/fi/research/desc.html.

Naturopathy (Natural Medicine)

The first precept of naturopathy is based on this concept of the healing force of nature, which emphasizes the prevention of disease and the maintenance of health. A second principle is derived from the Hippocratic precept, "First do no harm." Naturopathic physicians avoid therapies that weaken the body's innate ability to self-heal or that take over a function of the body. Instead, naturopathic practice emphasizes the concepts of wellness, prevention, and the role of the health care provider as a teacher (Bradley, 1999; Cody, 1999; Kratz, 1999).

As defined by the Department of Labor, naturopathic physicians diagnose and treat patients based on natural laws. Naturopaths are trained to diagnose and treat at the primary care level and may prescribe some drugs and do minor surgery. Their modalities include phytotherapy (treatment with plant-based preparations), electrotherapy, physiotherapy, minor surgery, mechanotherapy, and therapeutic manipulation. Other treatments include nutrition, with an emphasis on whole foods and nutritional supplements used for the prevention of disease. Naturopathic physicians do not perform major surgery or use radiography or radium modalities therapeutically.

Training for a degree in naturopathic medicine is conducted in 4-year postgraduate institutions. Classes in medical sciences include pathology, microbiology, histology, and physical and clinical diagnosis. Clinical training in botanical medicine (pharmacognosy), hydrotherapy, physiotherapy, therapeutic nutrition, and homeopathy are included in the curriculum of naturopathic medical schools.

Although not all states require naturopathic practitioners to be licensed, those that do require a resident course of study in naturopathic medicine of at least 4 years' duration as well as 4100 hours of study in a college or university recognized by the state examining board. Licensure examinations test students in the areas of basic sciences, diagnostic and therapeutic subjects, and clinical sciences. States that currently license naturopathic doctors include Alaska, Arizona, Connecticut, Hawaii, Maine, Montana, New Hampshire, Oregon, Utah, Vermont, and Washington.

Chiropractic

Chiropractic embraces many of the same principles as naturopathy, particularly the belief that the body has the ability to heal itself and that the practitioner's role is to assist the body in doing so. Like naturopathy, chiropractic focuses on wellness and prevention and favors noninvasive treatments. Chiropractors do not prescribe drugs or perform surgery. Instead they focus on locating and removing interferences to the body's natural ability to maintain health, called subluxations, specifically musculoskeletal problems that lead to interference with the nervous system functioning properly (Phillips and Mootz, 1992).

Chiropractic comes from the Greek word *chiropraktikos,* which means "effective treatment by hand." The central approach of chiropractic care is the manual manipulation of the body, such as spinal adjustment and muscle work, with support from physiologic approaches to healing, such as lifestyle modification. Correct alignment of the spine enables the body's nervous system to function appropriately, which in turn promotes health.

Many people seek out chiropractors for help with chronic pain, particularly low back pain, neck pain, and headache. According to the NIH, chiropractic is the most widely used of the complementary and alternative treatment modalities, particularly for low back pain.

The chiropractic philosophy toward health care has two fundamental precepts: (1) that the structure and condition of the body influences how well the body functions and (2) that the mind-body relationship is important in maintaining health and in promoting healing (Cherkin and Mootz, 1997). Although chiropractic has been in existence for some 100 years and is quite popular with consumers, it has only recently begun to be accepted by mainstream medicine. The idea that manipulating the spine can positively affect the body's ability to heal has been met with much skepticism by conventional health care practitioners.

Fortunately, this aspect of chiropractic is readily testable using today's standard research protocols, and a number of clinical trials are in progress. A typical study is one supported by the NIH that compares the effectiveness of managing acute low back pain by conventional approaches with management by chiropractic, acupuncture, or massage therapy. The NCCAM has established the Consortial Center for Chiropractic Research, which brings together faculty and administrators from five chiropractic institutions and two universities. The focus of the center is to conduct research designed to investigate the validity of chiropractic as an effective treatment modality. (Creating the Consortial Center for Chiropractic Research, www.clinicaltrials.gov).

Chiropractors are licensed and regulated in all 50 states and in some 30 countries. Practitioners must complete a 4-year program from a federally accredited college of chiropractic and, like other licensed practitioners, successfully pass an examination administered by a national certifying body.

Homeopathy

The root words of homeopathy are derived from the Greek *homios,* meaning "like" and *pathos,* meaning "suffering." Homeopathy is a medical theory and practice that was advanced to counter the conventional medical practices of 200 years ago; it endeavors to help the body heal itself by treating like with like, commonly known as the *law of similars.* The law of similars is based on the theory that if a large amount of a substance causes symptoms in a healthy person, a smaller amount of the same substance can be used to treat an ill person (Lange, 1999; Vickers et al, 1999).

Samuel Hahnemann, an eighteenth-century German physician, is credited with founding homeopathy. The law of similars is the concept that Hahnemann devised based on his own experience with quinine as a remedy for malaria. He observed that the remedy produced symptoms of the disease itself. Hahnemann called these tests, performed on himself and others, *provings.*

The amounts of the remedies used in homeopathic medicines are extremely diluted. According to homeopathic principles, the remedies are *potentized;* that is, they become more powerful through shaking. The healing power of the remedy is ascribed to the transfer of the remedy's vibrational pattern into a substrate, typically water or alcohol. A tincture is made directly from the source material. One drop of the tincture is then mixed with 99 drops of water or alcohol to make the first potency. The mixture is vigorously shaken more than 100 times, a process called *succussion,* which is thought to make the remedy more potent. One drop of the succussion mixture is then combined with 99 drops of water or alcohol, and the process is repeated. Potentized remedies are taken as tinctures and are used to make pills and creams. The minimum-dose principle means that many homeopathic remedies are so dilute that no actual molecules of the healing substance can be detected by chemical tests.

Homeopathic practitioners emphasize that assessment of all aspects of the physical, mental, and spiritual life of a patient is essential for the prescription of appropriate remedies. The goal of homeopathy is to select a remedy that will bring about a sense of well-being on all levels—physical, mental, and emotional—and that will alleviate physical symptoms and restore the patient to a state of wellness and creative energy. A wide range of physicians and other health care providers practice homeopathy.

Clinical evidence on the efficacy of homeopathy is highly contradictory. In recent years attempts have been made to subject homeopathy to standard research protocols to determine whether it is effective as a treatment modality. In a recent annotated bibliography of existing studies comparing homeopathy with conventional approaches, the results are equivocal (Linde et al, 2001c). Existing data suggest that homeopathy has more than a placebo effect, but the nature of that effect and the underlying scientific basis remain elusive (Riley et al, 2001). Most homeopathic remedies are considered relatively safe.

Traditional Oriental Medicine

Traditional Oriental medicine is based on the concept that energy, also termed *chi* (Qi) or life-force energy, is the center of body functions. *Chi* is the intangible force that animates life and enlivens all activity. Wellness is a function of the balanced and harmonious flow of *chi,* whereas illness or disease results from disturbances in its flow. Wellness also requires preserving equilibrium between the contrasting states of *yin* and *yang* (the dual nature of all things). The underlying principle of traditional Oriental medicine is preventive in nature, and the body is viewed as a reflection of the natural world.

Four substances—blood, *jing* (essence, substance of all life), *shen* (spirit), and fluids (body fluids other than blood)—constitute the fundamentals of Oriental medicine. The nutritional modality of Oriental medicine has several components: food as a means of obtaining nutrition, food as a tonic or medicine, and the abstention from food (fasting). Foods are classified according to taste (sour, bitter, sweet, spicy, and salty) and property (cool, cold, warm, hot, and plain) to regulate yin, yang, *chi,* and blood.

Within this framework of traditional Chinese medicine, the meridians are channels that carry *chi* and blood throughout the body. These are not channels per se, but rather they are invisible vertical networks that act as energy circuits, unifying all parts of the body and connecting the inner and the outer body. In traditional Oriental medicine, organs are not viewed as anatomic concepts but as energetic fields.

Acupuncture is the use of thin needles, inserted into points on the meridians, to stimulate the body's *chi,* or vital energy. Related to the concept of acupuncture is moxibustion, the application of heat along meridian acupuncture points for the purpose of affecting *chi* and blood so as to balance substances and organs. This therapy is used to treat disharmony in the body, which leads to disease (Linde et al, 2001a; Nolting, 1999). Disharmony, or loss of balance, is caused by a weakening of the yin force in the body, which preserves and nurtures life, or a weakening of the yang force, which generates and activates life. The concept of yin and yang expresses the dual nature of all things, the opposing but complementary forces that are interdependent on each other and must exist in equilibrium.

Acupuncture has also been used to produce regional anesthesia. Its method of action appears to be through needle stimulation, which triggers the release of opioids (natural, morphine-like substances) into the body. In 1997 a panel of experts convened by the NIH found that, although many studies have investigated the potential usefulness of acupuncture, these studies often have yielded equivocal results because of design, sample size, or other factors. One problem in designing appropriate studies is related to the issue of controls (e.g., placebo or sham acupuncture). Areas in which acupuncture has been shown to be efficacious include adult postoperative management, chemotherapy-induced nausea and vomiting, and postoperative dental pain. The panel also found that acupuncture may be useful as a complementary or alternative therapy for the treatment of other conditions, including addiction, stroke rehabilitation, headache, menstrual cramps, tennis elbow, fibromyalgia, myofascial pain, osteoarthritis, low back pain, carpal tunnel syndrome, and asthma (NIH Consensus Conference, 1998).

The use of Chinese herbs is integral to the practice of traditional Oriental medicine. The Chinese pharmacopoeias, published as early as the third century BC, contain herbs and minerals as well as animal products. Typically, a Chinese medicinal formula incorporates multiple substances. In a clinical trial, a formulation of seven Chinese herbs was given to patients with cirrhosis, along with the conventional drugs for their condition. The incidence of liver cancer development and the survival rate of the patients were followed for 5 years. Those who received the herbal formula had a lower rate of developing liver cancer and a higher survival rate than patients who received the drugs only (Oka et al, 1995). In another clinical trial, patients who were treated with a standard Chinese herbal medicine for irritable bowel syndrome (IBS) showed significant improvement in bowel symptom scores, and the degree of interference in life caused by IBS symptoms was significantly reduced (Bensoussan et al, 1998).

Phytotherapy

Phytotherapy (from *phyto,* the Greek word for "plant") is the science of using plant-derived substances to treat and prevent illness. Technically these plants—including their leaves, flowers, stems, rhizomes, and roots—are called botanicals, but the terms *herb* and *botanical* are often used interchangeably. Herb technically refers only to a plant with a nonwoody stem that dies back in the winter. Botanicals come in a variety of forms, for example as bulk herbs, extracts, tinctures, and as capsules or tablets (Table 20-2).

Botanicals can be used as therapeutic agents, and in other cultures have a long history of use (Linde et al, 2001b; Murray and Pizzorno, 1999). In Europe botanicals have a significant history of research and clinical use. As mentioned, Chinese herbs are an integral part of traditional Oriental medicine.

For many botanical products, the active ingredients and the mode of action have been defined; others are still being researched. The scientific basis for botanical medicine can be investigated with the same scientific tools as prescription drugs (e.g., double-blind, placebo-controlled clinical trials). Research information on phytotherapy as a modality of complementary medicine is burgeoning.

Clinical Assessment

Popular interest in the use of botanical products for health applications is widespread in the United States (Brevoort, 1998; Ernst, 2002). Health care professionals should be aware that the therapeutic action of many botanical products is similar to that of drugs, so the potential for harmful interactions exists. A helpful safety rating classification has been developed by the American Herbal Products Association and is listed in Table 20-3 (McGuffin et al, 1997). Health care professionals should also be aware that people typically do not inform their health care practitioners of their use of botanicals or other dietary supplements (Eisenberg et al, 1993, 1998; Foster, 2000). It is particularly important that dietary supplement use be revealed before surgery (Ang-Lee et al, 2001). Table 20-4 lists recommended discontinuation times before surgery for eight popular botanicals.

To facilitate obtaining critical information, health care providers should ask the following types of questions:

- What allergies, if any, do you have to plant materials?
- Are you currently pregnant or breast-feeding?
- Which prescription drugs are you currently taking?
- Which over-the-counter (OTC) drugs are you taking?
- Are you taking any dietary supplements (including botanicals)?

Intake and follow-up information about these therapies provides important pharmacologic and treatment information for the health care provider. In particular, botanicals that have similar actions to prescription and OTC medications should not be combined because the effects can be additive and cause harm (DeBusk and Treadwell, 2000). Conversely, botanicals that counter the effect of prescription and OTC medications should not be combined, such as taking a blood pressure–lowering medication along with a botanical that can raise blood pressure. The funding of studies that evaluate botanical-drug interactions is a priority of the NCCAM.

TABLE 20-2 Botanical Formulations

TYPE	FORM
Bulk herbs	Sold loose to be used as teas, in cooking, and to prepare capsules; rapidly lose potency; should be stored in opaque containers, away from heat and light
Beverages	
Teas	Beverage weak in concentration; steep fresh or dried herbs in a cup of hot water for a few minutes, strain, and drink
Infusions	More concentrated than teas; steep fresh or dried herbs for approximately 15 min to allow more of the active ingredients to be extracted than for teas
Decoction	Most concentrated of the beverages, made by boiling the root, rhizome, bark or berries for 30-60 min to extract the active ingredients
Extracts	Herbs are extracted with an organic solvent to dissolve the active components; forms a concentrated form of the active ingredients
Tinctures	Extract in which the solvent is alcohol
Glycerite	Extract in which the solvent is glycerol or a mixture of glycerol, propylene glycol, and water; more appropriate for children than a tincture
Pill Forms	Pills should be taken with at least 4-8 oz of water to avoid leaving residue in the esophagus
Capsules	Herbal material is enclosed in a hard shell made from animal-derived gelatin or plant-derived cellulose
Tablets	Herb material is mixed with filler material to form the hard tablet; may be uncoated or coated with films
Lozenges	Also called *troches;* method of preparation allows the active components to be readily released in the mouth when chewed or sucked
Soft gels	Soft capsule used to encase liquid extracts, such as omega-3 fatty acids or vitamin E
Essential oils	Fragrant, volatile plant oils; used for aromatherapy, bathing; concentrated form and not to be used internally unless specifically directed (such as enteric-coated peppermint oil)

Data from DeBusk RM: A practical guide to herbal supplements for nutrition practitioners, *Top Clin Nutr* 16:53, 2001.

Regulation

Botanical products are regulated in the United States as dietary supplements. The Dietary Supplement Health and Education Act of 1994 (DSHEA) is a law that clarifies marketing regulations for botanicals and reclassifies them as dietary supplements, distinct from food or drugs. Under DSHEA dietary supplements, which include plant extracts, enzymes, vitamins, minerals, and hormonal products that are available to consumers without prescription, may carry "structure/function" claims. That is, the physiologic effects of a product can be noted, but no claims about prevention or cure of specific conditions can be made. For example, a product manufacturer cannot claim that a dietary supplement "prevents heart disease"; however, it can be said that a product "helps to increase blood flow to the heart." All products must display the following disclaimer: "This statement has not been evaluated by the Food and Drug Administration. This product is not intended to diagnose, treat, cure, or prevent any disease." (See Chapter 14.)

Compared with their regulation in the United States, European regulation of herbal products is distinctly different. In the European market, especially in Germany, botanicals are considered drugs and are prescribed by physicians and dispensed by pharmacists. In Germany, an Expert Commission for Phytopharmaceuticals at the Federal Health Agency in Germany was established in 1978. Botanical products were reviewed by this expert commission of professionals, which was drawn from a variety of health care and scientific disciplines. This group, known as the Commission E, developed 330 therapeutic monographs on botanicals until it was disbanded in 1993. These Commission E monographs include information on the pharmacologic properties and toxicology of botanicals and outline their uses, contraindications, side effects, dosages, and administration, in addition to noting any special warnings for use (Blumenthal et al, 1998, 2000).

In the United States, DSHEA provides consumers with ready access to dietary supplements but does not require stringent premarket safety and efficacy evaluations or uniform manufacturing standards for these products. It is therefore the responsibility of consumers to educate themselves about the appropriate application of each dietary supplement they choose to use and how to select a quality product. Among the more common problems that have been reported since the passage of DSHEA are misrepresentation of product contents; variable potency and recommended dosages among products; inadequate information about how a company's herbs are grown and processed; and poor standards of quality, product safety, or activity of ingredients (Edzard, 1998; U.S. General Accounting Office, 2000). Although rare, herb contamination and misidentification do occur (Slifman et al, 1998). Presently, governmental and industry entities are working to develop high-quality manufacturing guidelines for all dietary supplements, including botanical products. It is essential that users and their health care providers be knowledgeable about botanical products and their modes of action and quality of manufacture to ensure their safe and effective use, particularly with reference to the potential interactions between botanicals and prescription and OTC medications. Guidelines for evaluating botanical products are given in Box 20-1.

TABLE 20-3 The American Herbal Products Association's Botanical Safety Rating Classification

SAFETY CLASSIFICATION	CLASS DEFINITION
Class 1	Herbs that can be safely consumed when used appropriately
Class 2	Herbs for which the following use restrictions apply unless otherwise directed by an expert qualified in the use of the described substance: (2a) For external use only (2b) Not to be used during pregnancy (2c) Not to be used while nursing (2d) Other specific use restrictions as noted
Class 3	Herbs for which significant data exist to recommend the following labeling: "To be used only under the supervision of an expert qualified in the appropriate use of this substance." Labeling must include proper use information: dosage, contraindications, potential adverse effects and drug interactions, and any other relevant information related to the safe use of the substance
Class 4	Herbs for which insufficient data are available for classification

From McGuffin M et al, eds: *American Herbal Products Association's botanical safety handbook: guidelines for the safe use and labeling for herbs of commerce,* Boca Raton, Fla, 1997, CRC Press.

TABLE 20-4 Recommended Preoperative Discontinuation Times for Some Common Botanicals

BOTANICAL	RECOMMENDED DISCONTINUATION TIME BEFORE SURGERY
Echinacea	Insufficient data
Ephedra	At least 24 hr
Garlic	At least 7 days
Ginkgo	At least 36 hr
Ginseng*	At least 7 days
Kava	At least 24 hr
St. John's wort	At least 5 days
Valerian	Insufficient data

Data from Ang-Lee MK et al: Herbal medicines and perioperative care, *JAMA* 286:208, 2001.

*American ginseng, Asian ginseng, Chinese ginseng, Korean ginseng.

Box 20-1. Guidelines for Choosing Botanical Products

- Be sure the choice of a botanical is appropriate to the health care goals and compatible with any prescription and over-the-counter medications or other dietary supplements the patient may be taking. The help of a nutrition professional or other health care professional knowledgeable about dietary supplements can be invaluable in this education process. Information is available at www.consumerlab.com for specific validation of products on the market.
- Investigate the quality of the manufacturer whose product is being considered. At a minimum, it is important to know that the retail suppliers carry only manufacturers that adhere to high-quality standards or that the health care professional recommending a product is knowledgeable about the quality of dietary supplements. One of the questions to ask is how herbs are grown, selected, stored, and processed to ensure absence of microbial contamination, proper identification, and potency. The risk of pesticide contamination can be minimized by choosing organically grown herbs whenever possible.
- Investigate the claims being made about the products and avoid products with exaggerated claims associated with them.
- Use the dietary supplement label to obtain important information, such as the following:
  - The complete botanical name of the product and confirm that this is the appropriate botanical
  - The part of the plant used to prepare the product, confirming that it is the part that contains the active components
  - The concentration of the botanical and whether the concentration is appropriate for obtaining the reported benefits of the product, neither too weak nor too strong
  - The daily dosage needed to obtain the desired effect
  - The list of ingredients used to confirm that no animal by-products, fillers, dyes or other colorings, preservatives, or potential allergens have been added
  - A lot number, which is helpful if problems arise because it allows the product to be tracked through each stage of the manufacturing process and permits recalls of the product, if needed
  - An expiration date
  - A recognized seal of approval that indicates Good Manufacturing Practices have been used in the production of the product and that the product has passed independent analyses confirming that the label accurately represents the product
  - A toll-free number for contacting the manufacturer in the event of adverse reactions
- After determining that a manufacturer and its product meet these standards, compare prices among products of similar quality. Prices can vary widely.

Data from DeBusk RM: A practical guide to herbal supplements for nutrition practitioners, *Top Clin Nutr* 16:53, 2001.

COMMONLY USED BOTANICALS

General information about each of the following botanicals can be found in several key resources (see Additional References). Current research varies by botanical and is indicated with the appropriate reference from the scientific literature. The information given is for adults. Knowledge of the safety and efficacy of botanical products during pregnancy, lactation, or childhood continues to be limited.

Echinacea

Echinacea is a genus of plants related to the daisy family and is native to the midwestern United States (Figure 20-1, *A*). Echinacea was the most commonly used herb of the Plains Native Americans. They used the root of the plant externally for healing wounds, burns, and insect bites and internally for treating infections, toothache, joint pains, and rattlesnake bites (Blumenthal et al, 1998). Introduced to American medicine in the late 1800s, echinacea was widely used as an antiinfective. With the subsequent introduction of antibiotics, however, echinacea's use waned.

Echinacea purpurea, Echinacea angustifolia, and *Echinacea pallida* are the most commonly used of the nine species of the plant. *Echinacea purpurea* is the most widely cultivated species, and its medicinal properties have been studied more than the others.

Indications and Common Uses

At present, the most common adjunctive use of echinacea is for the prevention or moderation of the symptoms of colds and influenza. In Germany *E. purpurea* was approved by the Commission E as supportive therapy for colds and chronic infections of the upper respiratory tract. Clinical trials in Europe using the expressed juice of *E. purpurea* have shown that patients with colds who received the preparation had colds of shorter duration and less severity and had longer intervals between infections (Hoheisel et al, 1997; Schulten et al, 2001). In another clinical trial in healthy volunteers, however, echinacea showed no prophylactic effect (Melchart et al, 1998).

Mechanisms of Action and Active Constituents

Many components may be responsible for echinacea's immune-stimulating activity, including high-molecular-weight polysaccharides such as arabinogalactan and low-molecular-weight flavonoids and caffeic acid derivatives; however, no single compound has been identified as being responsible for the immune properties of this herb.

Contraindications, Side Effects, and Toxicity

Echinacea is rated as a class 1 botanical according to the American Herbal Products Association's Botanical Safety Rating Classification, which suggests that this botanical can be safely consumed when used appropriately (McGuffin et al, 1997) (see Table 20-3).

Echinacea products are available in many different forms: crude plant in ground, powdered, or freeze-dried form; alcohol-based tinctures and liquid extracts; aqueous tinctures and liquid extracts; and dry powdered alcoholic or aqueous extracts. The dosage of echinacea depends on the potency of the particular formulation. Safe dosages for long-term use are up to 1 tsp of the liquid (expressed juice of the herb stabilized at 22% alcohol) or one capsule of dried juice (88.5 mg/capsule) three times daily. Other dosage forms for echinacea include dried root (1 to 2 g), tincture (0.75 to 1 tsp), fluid extract (0.25 to 0.5 tsp), and solid (dry powdered) extract (300 mg of 3.5% echinacoside [compounds in the plant used as chemical markers for standardization]). A common caution with echinacea is to use it for an 8-week course of therapy followed by 1 week's rest because of its immune-stimulating effect, but the necessity for this precaution has not been verified.

Potential Adverse Interactions

Echinacea is well tolerated. Those hypersensitive to other members of the daisy family may have allergic reactions to echinacea. The herb has not been demonstrated to interact with drugs or other supplements in humans. Theoretically, it may have an additive effect with other immunostimulant drugs and interfere with the therapeutic effect of immunosuppressive drugs.

Garlic

Garlic, *Allium sativum,* is a member of the botanical family Liliaceace, which includes onions, leeks, and shallots. Garlic grows wild almost everywhere in the world. As a medicinal herb, garlic has been used since the earliest days of recorded history. The Greek physician Galen (130-200 AD) considered garlic a panacea.

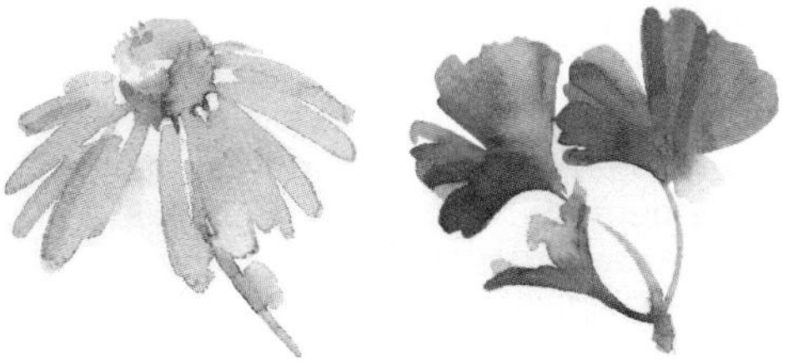

FIGURE 20-1 • **A,** Echinacea. **B,** Ginkgo biloba. (Courtesy Pharmanex Provo, Utah.)

Indications and Common Uses

Garlic is a popular botanical in the United States and is among the most researched of the herbs. The most frequent uses of garlic are to treat hyperlipidemia and hypertension (DeBusk, 2000). Garlic may also be useful against bacterial, fungal, and viral infections; studies investigating these applications are needed.

Mechanisms of Action and Active Constituents

The main chemical constituents of garlic are sulfur-containing compounds and S-allyl cysteine (SAC), a water-soluble amino acid. Whole garlic bulbs or cloves contain an odorless, sulfur-containing amino acid derivative, alliin. When garlic is crushed or macerated, alliin comes into contact with the enzyme alliinase and is converted to allicin. Allicin (the compound responsible for garlic's characteristic odor) in turn yields a variety of other compounds, including diallyl disulfides, methyl allyl sulfides, and dimethyl sulfides, dithiins, and ajoenes.

One measure of garlic's total activity is its allicin formation. In fresh garlic, allicin is developed when the garlic is chewed in the mouth. Most dried dietary supplements of garlic contain allicin potential; that is, they contain alliin and the enzyme alliinase, but most of the alliinase is thought to be inactivated by stomach acids so that little to no allicin is developed in the stomach. Therefore, dried garlic preparations appear to be most effective if they are enteric coated. Typically, commercial garlic products are standardized for allicin potential, but some standardized for SAC are also available. At recommended doses of garlic, a commercial preparation should deliver a minimum of 10 mg of alliin or a total allicin potential of 5000 μg in an enteric-coated form. Suggested raw garlic dose is one clove, equal to 4 g.

The health benefits attributed to garlic include moderate reductions in blood pressure, modest reductions in blood cholesterol levels, and inhibition of blood clot formation. In a metaanalysis of studies of patients with cholesterol levels exceeding 200 mg/dl, ingestion of a garlic supplement of 900 mg daily (equivalent to 0.5 to 1 clove of garlic per day) decreased total serum cholesterol levels by about 9% (Warshafsky et al, 1993). More recently, a double-blind placebo-controlled trial of persons with elevated cholesterol levels for whom drug therapy had not been effective were treated with 9.6 mg of enteric-coated allicin–releasing–potential garlic powder supplements for 12 weeks, along with a low-fat diet (Kannar et al, 2001). The garlic supplement group had modest decreases in total cholesterol (4.2%) and low-density lipoprotein (LDL)-cholesterol (6.6%). Garlic is thought to produce its modest reduction of high blood pressure by relaxing the smooth muscle of blood vessels (Pedraza-Chaverri et al, 1998).

Although many studies have investigated garlic's therapeutic effects, no clear picture has yet emerged. The confusion is thought to be due to the many different types of garlic compounds that are used, which range from powdered garlic to garlic oil. When studies using the same dried garlic preparation are compared, garlic appears to be effective in lowering cholesterol. In at least 17 randomized, double-blind, placebo-controlled trials, 900 mg of garlic powder standardized for alliin and allicin content lowered total cholesterol and LDL cholesterol and, when measured, triglycerides (Mader, 1990; Silagy and Neil, 1994). Two trials that presumably used the same garlic preparation failed to confirm these results (Issacsohn et al, 1998; McCrindle et al, 1998). Subsequent analysis of these preparations, however, found that they released only about one third the amount of allicin as the preparations used in the earlier trials (Lawson 1998). Garlic oil preparations in another study showed no significant cholesterol-lowering activity (Berthold et al, 1998). It may be that the allyl sulfides in the garlic oil preparation are less active than allicin (Lawson, 1998). Another possible confounding variable is the recent finding that garlic oil's effect on plasma cholesterol differs in men and women. In a randomized clinical trial of normal lipidemic men and women, the women had reductions in total cholesterol after 11 weeks' treatment with garlic oil, but the men did not (X.H. Zhang et al, 2001).

Contraindications, Side Effects, and Toxicity

Garlic is rated as a class 2c botanical according to the American Herbal Products Association's Botanical Safety Rating Classification (see Table 20-3), which suggests that this herb should not be used while breast-feeding (McGuffin et al, 1997); however, the editors qualify this rating by stating that the concerns for this herb are based on therapeutic use and dosage and that garlic has a long history of safety when consumed as a food.

Garlic is considered safe for normal persons who consume moderate amounts. Consumption of garlic in amounts of five or more cloves per day may produce heartburn or flatulence, mild allergic reactions, dermatitis, and gastrointestinal symptoms.

Potential Adverse Interactions

Garlic reduces clotting time and should be used with caution when using aspirin or other anticoagulant drugs, such as warfarin, antiplatelet aggregation drugs, and dietary supplements such as *Ginkgo biloba* and omega-3 fatty acid supplements that have blood-thinning effects. Garlic supplements also appear to be effective in lowering cholesterol levels and blood pressure and should be used with caution by those taking lipid-lowering and antihypertensive medications or dietary supplements. Multiple agents with similar actions should be used only under the direction of a knowledgeable health care professional.

The major adverse interaction of garlic appears to be with the human immunodeficiency virus (HIV) medication saquinavir, a protease inhibitor. In a recent study, garlic supplements (4.64 mg allicin/capsule, the equivalent of two cloves of garlic/day) decreased blood levels of saquinavir by 51% (Piscitelli et al, 2002).

Ginger

Ginger *(Zingiber officinale)* is native to the Orient. The plant has green-purple flowers, resembles an orchid, and is also known as Jamaican ginger, African ginger, Cochin ginger, black ginger, and race ginger. The rhizome (underground stem) contains the active components.

Indications and Common Uses

Ginger's most popular therapeutic application is as a prophylactic treatment for digestive system problems, especially nausea, motion sickness, and hyperemesis gravidarum (excessive vomiting during pregnancy). Because it suppresses the production of inflammatory mediators such as prostaglandins, thromboxanes, and leukotrienes, ginger is often used to ease symptoms in disorders such as arthritis, cardiovascular disease, and other inflammatory disorders.

The Commission E monograph on ginger recommends ginger for both indigestion and the prevention of symptoms of motion sickness (Blumenthal et al, 1998). One study found ginger to be as effective as dimenhydrinate (Dramamine) in reducing symptoms of motion sickness (Mowrey and Clayson, 1982), but other studies have not confirmed this effect. Poor-quality ginger may have been used in the studies that reported negative results (Schulz et al, 1997).

Ginger has also traditionally been used as a remedy for nausea and vomiting in the first trimester of pregnancy. In a review of drug therapy during pregnancy, ginger and vitamin B_6 have both been recognized as effective treatments for nausea and vomiting in early pregnancy (Niebyl, 1992). Ginger is usually taken in the form of capsules, each containing 500 mg of powdered ginger. When used as an antiemetic, 1 to

2 g of ginger is taken in two divided doses. For maximum effect on motion sickness, ginger should be used several days before travel, with continuous use during the trip.

Mechanisms of Action and Active Constituents

The characteristic pungent odor of ginger is due to volatile oils in the rhizome, called gingerols, which are also responsible for its pharmacologic properties. Galanolactone and shogaol, which are derived from the gingerols, also appear to have pharmacologic activity and may be responsible for the antiemetic properties of ginger because of their action at the serotonin (5HT-3) receptors in the ileum. These are the same receptors acted on by antinausea prescription medications.

The antiinflammatory properties may be due to ginger's ability to inhibit the cyclooxygenase and lipoxygenase enzymes that are involved in producing proinflammatory eicosanoids. A recent study found that a standardized extract of ginger was moderately effective in reducing symptoms of osteoarthritis of the knee (Altman and Marcussen, 2001).

Contraindications, Side Effects, and Toxicity

Ginger is rated as a class 1 botanical, which suggests that the botanical can be safely consumed when used appropriately (McGuffin et al, 1997). Ginger is usually well tolerated, but sensitive persons may develop gastrointestinal upset, dermatitis, or heartburn. The use of ginger is considered safe at the levels found in food and when used orally for medicinal purposes, if used appropriately. The use of ginger during pregnancy and lactation is controversial because its safety has not been established. The German Commission E advises persons with gallstones not to use ginger unless under the supervision of a health care practitioner (Blumenthal et al, 1998).

Potential Adverse Interactions

Adverse interactions of ginger with prescription medications, OTC medications, or other dietary supplements have not been documented. Theoretically ginger may increase the risk of bleeding when combined with blood-thinning agents and may interfere with blood pressure–and blood sugar–regulating drugs also, so ginger should be combined with these agents only under the direction of a knowledgeable health care professional (Verma, 1994).

Ginkgo

Ginkgo biloba is the oldest living species of tree and can be traced back more than 200 million years to the fossils of the Permian period (see Figure 20-1, *B*). It is now a popular ornamental tree throughout the world and has been used medicinally in China for hundreds of years. Ginkgo biloba extract (GBE) is the term for standardized preparations made from the leaf of the ginkgo tree.

Indications and Common Uses

Ginkgo has a wide range of physiologic actions, including vasodilation, inhibition of platelet aggregation, improved peripheral circulation, and antioxidant activity. GBE is widely used in Europe for the treatment of cardiovascular disease and peripheral vascular disease, including intermittent claudication. GBE is used to treat age-related decline in mental function secondary to cerebrovascular insufficiency (short-term memory loss, poor concentration, tinnitus, possibly dementia) and early-stage senility of the Alzheimer's type may also be improved by the use of GBE (LeBars et al, 1997; McKenna et al, 2001).

Mechanisms of Action and Active Constituents

The extract of *Ginkgo biloba* leaf, GBE, is derived from green-picked ginkgo leaves that have been developed specifically for pharmaceutical purposes. The leaves are extracted with an acetone-water mixture, the organic solvent is removed, and the extract is processed, dried, and standardized. Standardized preparations of ginkgo typically contain 24% ginkgo flavone glycosides (including bioflavonoids, such as quercetin, kaempferol, isorhamnetine, and proanthocyanidins) and 6% terpene lactones (ginkgolides and bilobalide, compounds unique to ginkgo).

The flavone glycosides in the standardized extract exert antioxidant activity and protect cells against free radical damage, particularly damage to the lipid layer of the cell membrane. The flavone glycosides also inhibit platelet aggregation. The ginkgolides act as platelet-activating factor (PAF) antagonists. PAF promotes aggregation of blood platelets, which leads to blood clot formation, and is involved in many effects of allergic response. The ginkgolides appear to block these actions, thereby increasing blood fluidity and enhancing circulation.

In a systematic review of more than 50 clinical studies, Oken and colleagues concluded that GBE was effective for treating dementia and other cognitive declines associated with Alzheimer's disease (Oken et al, 1998). LeBars and colleagues essentially confirmed this conclusion in a double-blind, placebo-controlled study (LeBars et al, 2000). In a metaanalysis of double-blind, placebo-controlled studies in which GBE was used for different types of dementia, Ernst and Pittler (1999) concluded that GBE improved symptoms and delayed further deterioration. It is not yet clear whether GBE is helpful in preventing the onset of dementia. A study of 230 adults over the age of 60 with healthy cognitive functioning did not show any measurable benefit in memory after administration of 120 mg of *ginkgo biloba* daily for 6 weeks (Solomon et al, 2002).

In addition, GBE is effective for the treatment of peripheral vascular disease, in which there is blockage in the blood vessels that often leads to pain upon walking. In a multicenter controlled trial, GBE increased the pain-free walking distance when measured at regular intervals throughout the 24-week trial (Peters et al, 1998).

Ginkgo biloba was studied as a treatment for sudden deafness and for tinnitus, and the results are promising. In a randomized, prospective, double-blind study comparing GBE with the standard drug pentoxifylline for treatment of sudden deafness, GBE was equally effective (Reisser and Weidauer, 2001).

Most clinical studies using GBE have been conducted using the EGb 761 extract, produced in Germany by Schwabe GmbH and Company. The efficacy of other products is not yet known. Studies have typically used 120 to 240 mg daily as the adult dose, which has been found to be modestly effective for microvascular improvement and dementia. For cerebrovascular insufficiency and early-stage Alzheimer's disease, 240 to 480 mg daily is commonly used.

Contraindications, Side Effects, and Toxicity

Ginkgo is rated as a class 2d botanical because it may potentiate pharmaceutical monoamine oxidase inhibitors [MAOIs] (McGuffin et al, 1997) (see Table 20-3). These drugs increase neurotransmitters by preventing their degradation, and ginkgo can potentially enhance this effect and raise the level of neurotransmitters undesirably high.

Side effects reported with GBE use include mild gastrointestinal complaints, headache, and allergic skin reactions, but these reactions are rare. Whole ginkgo plant, particularly the plant pulp, however, has been associated with severe allergic reactions. Spontaneous bleeding has been reported in two cases (Rosenblatt and Mindel, 1997; Rowin and Lewis, 1996).

Potential Adverse Interactions

Ginkgo has blood-thinning activity and should not be combined with medications and dietary supplements that also can cause prolonged bleeding. These medications include the anticoagulant warfarin and the antiplatelet aggregation drugs such as aspirin, ticlopidine, clopidogrel, indomethacin, and others. Ginkgo also should not be combined with dietary supplements that have a blood-thinning effect, such as the omega-3 fatty acids, fenugreek, feverfew, ginger, garlic, licorice, panax ginseng, horse chestnut, white willow, and others. Ginkgo may interfere with diabetes management. Blood sugar levels should be closely monitored, and medications may need to be adjusted (Kudolo, 2000).

Botanicals can potentially enhance the effects of prescription medications and also decrease their side effects when used appropriately and properly supervised by a knowledgeable health care professional. As an example, GBE can enhance the effectiveness of the antipsychotic haloperidol used to treat schizophrenia and can decrease the magnitude of undesirable side effects (X.Y. Zhang et al, 2001).

Ginseng

Ginseng is a yellowish, radishlike herb and a slow-growing plant that takes at least 6 years of cultivation to produce a marketable product. Ginseng has a rich history in Eastern medicine; in China, ginseng has been in continuous use for more than 4000 years.

Almost all of the numerous varieties of ginseng are cultivated. The most common is panax ginseng, also called Korean, Chinese, or Asian ginseng, and it is the form that has been researched most extensively. The American variety of ginseng, *Panax quinquefolium,* has been declared an endangered species and is subject to stringent requirements governing its collection. A related species of the ginseng family is commonly known as Siberian ginseng, but it is actually *Eleutherococcus sentiocosus* and contains active constituents that differ from those of *panax ginseng* and *quinquifolium.* The trend now is to refer to Siberian ginseng as *eleuthero.*

The colors of ginseng indicate how the herb has been processed. White ginseng is the dried root. Red ginseng means that the ginseng root has been sterilized and preserved through steam treatment—hence its red color. The two varieties have no significant chemical differences, simply a color variation.

Indications and Common Uses

The name *panax,* from a Greek word meaning "all healing," implies the many suggested uses for ginseng, including antifatigue and antistress actions, mental performance improvements, immune system enhancement, cardiovascular effects, and supportive therapy for diabetes.

In Chinese medicine, ginseng's traditional use is as a tonic to help the body cope with stress of all types. Ginseng is also known as an *adaptogen,* a substance that reduces excesses, stimulates deficient states, exerts a balancing action, and is nontoxic. An adaptogen helps the body with normal functions, essentially supporting the body and strengthening it. In the United States, ginseng is often used to counter stress; improve energy levels; increase circulation; treat fatigue and reduced work capacity; and increase alertness, concentration, and the ability to grasp abstract concepts.

Mechanisms of Action and Active Constituents

Ginseng species differ in their composition and mechanisms of action. Panax ginseng is the most complex, with multiple ginsenosides, which are steroidlike compounds known as *saponin glycosides.* Because of the interaction of the ginsenosides, which are all in the root of the plant and occur in small amounts, the whole root is used in herbal preparations. The interaction of the ginsenosides is evidenced by the actions of ginsenosides Rb1 and Rg1, which exert different yet harmonizing influences on the body. Rb1 has a hypoactive effect on blood pressure and a mildly sedative effect, whereas Rg1 is thought to exert a mildly stimulatory action on the central nervous system.

The adaptogenic effect of ginseng has not been documented in humans in terms of scientific studies, but ginseng has a long history of traditional use, with apparent success. Much of the investigation of ginseng's ability to improve physical and mental performance or to counter physical or mental fatigue has been performed in animal or laboratory studies.

Ginseng may be beneficial for persons with type 2 diabetes. One study showed reduced fasting blood glucose levels and improvements in glycated hemoglobin (HbA1C) in persons with diabetes who received 200 mg doses of Asian ginseng (Sotaniemi et al, 1995). Combining ginseng with konjac-mannan (glucomannan), which forms a viscous gel in the digestive tract and appears to work by a mechanism different from ginseng, appears promising for improving blood sugar control for type 2 diabetes (Vuksan, 2001).

In a pilot study that examined Panax ginseng's ability to support maximal physical performance output by healthy volunteers, there was no benefit of ginseng (Engels et al, 2001). However, immune system enhancement may be a benefit of consistent use (for 8 weeks). Healthy volunteers who received 100 mg of a standardized extract of ginseng in a clinical study showed enhanced natural killer cell activity, interferon production, and macrophage activity (Scaglione et al, 1990).

Contraindications, Side Effects, and Toxicity

Both Asian and American ginsengs are classified as class 2d botanicals and are contraindicated in people with hypertension (McGuffin et al, 1997) (see Table 20-3).

Ginseng is generally regarded as safe at the recommended dosage of 100 mg of a preparation of 4% to 7% ginsenosides used once or twice per day. Cycled use of ginseng in 2- to 3-week intervals with 1- to 2-week rest periods is advised. Reported side effects of ginseng use include overstimulation and possible insomnia, which may diminish after continual use or after dosage reduction; however, ginseng consumption with caffeine may cause overstimulation and gastrointestinal distress.

No long-term safety data are available concerning the use of ginseng during pregnancy, lactation, or childhood. Therefore, ginseng is not recommended for use during these life stages.

Potential Adverse Interactions

As an adaptogen, ginseng could potentially enhance or reduce the effectiveness of a number of medications and dietary supplements. Special care should be taken with agents that affect blood sugar or blood pressure regulation, act as stimulants, interfere with blood coagulation, or affect the heart rate.

Hawthorn

Hawthorn *(Crataegus oxyacantha)* is a small to medium-sized tree native to Europe; other species include *C. monogyna* and *C. pentagyna.* The leaves, blossoms, and fruits are used in modern standardized extracts. Only the leaf and blossom formulations are approved for use in Germany, where much research on hawthorn has been conducted using proprietary formulas.

Indications and Common Uses

Hawthorn is used to improve blood flow in circulatory disorders, such as congestive heart failure and peripheral vascular disease, and to improve the symptoms and risk of heart disease, such as irregularities of the heartbeat and elevated cholesterol levels.

Mechanisms of Action and Active Constituents

Hawthorn leaves, berries, and blossoms contain oligomeric procyanidins and other flavonoids. Hawthorn appears to act on the cardiovascular system in two ways: (1) it directly dilates the coronary vessels to lower blood pressure, and (2) it improves the metabolic processes of the heart through its inotropic (strength of contraction) and chronotropic (heart rate) effects, increasing nerve conductivity and heart muscle contractability. Hawthorn apparently inhibits angiotensin-converting enzyme (ACE), which converts angiotensin I to angiotensin II, a powerful blood vessel constrictor. In a clinical trial, 900 mg of a proprietary hawthorn extract compared favorably with the ACE inhibitor captopril in increasing capacity to withstand exercise-induced stress, reducing post-exercise shortness of breath, and reducing fatigue in study participants (Tauchert et al, 1994).

Hawthorn extracts are typically standardized to 20% procyanidins or 2.2% flavonoid content, with typical daily doses of 160 mg. Higher doses of hawthorn should not be self-prescribed (Schulz et al, 1997).

Contraindications, Side Effects, and Toxicity

Hawthorn is rated as a class 1 botanical according to the American Herbal Products Association's Botanical Safety Rating Classification, which suggests that hawthorn can be safely consumed when used appropriately (McGuffin et al, 1997) (see Table 20-3).

Side effects of hawthorn are rare; however, persons with heart disease should be advised to consult health care professionals for appropriate treatment. Because insufficient information is available about the safety of hawthorn use during pregnancy, lactation, or childhood, use is not recommended during these life stages.

Potential Adverse Interactions

No adverse reactions of hawthorn with medications or dietary supplements have been reported. Hawthorn's effect on the heart and blood vessels, however, suggests that caution should be exercised when considering combining hawthorn with cardioactive drugs or supplements, such as digoxin, digitoxin, or natural cardiac glycosides, or with blood pressure–lowering medications or supplements.

Milk Thistle

Milk thistle *(Silybum marianum)* is a tall plant with prickly leaves and a milky sap, and it belongs to the daisy family (Figure 20-2, *A*). It is native to the Mediterranean region and is naturalized to the eastern United States, California, and other parts of North America. Milk thistle was enjoyed as a vegetable in earlier years, used in salads and eaten much as we eat broccoli today. Since the sixteenth century, milk thistle has been used to enhance liver function, and that use continues today.

Indications and Common Uses

Milk thistle is known as the liver herb because of its apparent hepatoprotective characteristics. In Europe intravenous preparations of the active constituent in milk thistle—silymarin—are used clinically to counter the overdose effects of the death cap mushroom *(Amanita phalloides)*, primarily because it protects the liver cells from damage secondary to the action of phalloidine, a toxic liver poison in the mushroom.

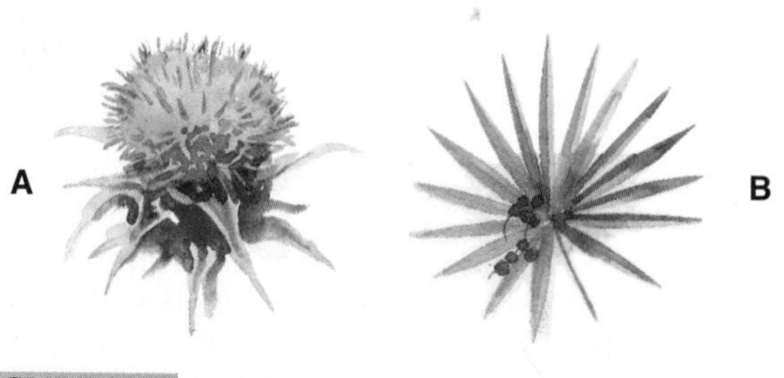

FIGURE 20-2 • **A,** Milk thistle. **B,** Saw palmetto. (Courtesy Pharmanex, Provo, Utah.)

Adjunctive uses for silymarin, approved by the German Commission E, include treatment of inflammatory liver damage secondary to cirrhosis, hepatitis, or fatty infiltration caused by alcohol or other toxins (Blumenthal et al, 1998). Silymarin has also been used to regenerate hepatocytes in persons with chronic viral hepatitis B or alcoholic cirrhosis, provided the liver cells have not been damaged irreversibly.

Mechanisms of Action and Active Constituents

The active constituent of milk thistle is silymarin, found in highest concentrations in the seeds of the plant. Silymarin consists of flavonolignans, unique forms of flavonoids, and silibinin, considered the most important component of silymarin. Silymarin supports the liver by protecting hepatocytes from toxins and increasing the ability of liver cells to regenerate by stimulating protein synthesis (Hobbs, 1992). In addition, silymarin has antioxidant and free-radical scavenging properties, which may be beneficial in protecting against cancer (Schulz et al, 1997). In a review of various types of trials to date, Saller and colleagues (2001) found silymarin to be moderately effective in treating alcoholic liver cirrhosis.

Silymarin is poorly soluble in water, making water-based extractions (e.g., teas) less effective than other preparations. Milk thistle extracts are typically standardized to 70% to 80% silymarin. In the United States, the botanical is available in capsule form, usually containing 200 mg of concentrated extract equal to 140 mg of silymarin, which is taken up to three times daily.

Contraindications, Side Effects, and Toxicity

Milk thistle is rated as a class 1 botanical according to the American Herbal Products Association's Botanical Safety Rating Classification, which suggests that the botanical can be safely consumed when used appropriately (McGuffin et al, 1997) (see Table 20-3).

There are no known contraindications to the use of milk thistle extract at recommended dosages. A mild laxative effect may be experienced in the first few days of use. Milk thistle is a member of the daisy family, and persons hypersensitive to members of this family may have an allergic reaction. The Commission E monograph indicates that those with gallstones should be cautious with its use (Blumenthal et al, 1998).

Potential Adverse Interactions

Milk thistle is widely considered safe and unlikely to interact with other medications or dietary supplements; however, a recent report of silymarin extract's effects on human liver cells in culture suggests that the botanical may reduce the activity of cytochrome

P450 3A4, a major drug-metabolizing enzyme in the intestines and liver (Venkataramanan et al, 2000). If this report is confirmed in clinical trials, particular care will need to be exercised when using milk thistle along with drugs metabolized by this enzyme, which include immunosuppressants used to prevent the rejection of transplanted organs, protease inhibitors such as those used as therapy for HIV and acquired immunodeficiency syndrome (AIDS), oral contraceptives, and the statin drugs used to lower blood cholesterol levels. Disclosing botanical product use to a knowledgeable health care professional is more important than ever when an interaction of this type is possible because the consequences are particularly dangerous.

Saw Palmetto

Saw palmetto (*Serenoa repens*) is a shrublike palm tree that is native to the southeastern United States (see Figure 20-2, *B*). Its fruits were used during the early 1900s as a mild diuretic and for enlarged prostate.

Indications and Common Uses

Saw palmetto acts to reduce the incidence of benign prostatic hyperplasia (BPH), which is a nonmalignant abnormal growth of the prostate gland. This condition affects 50% to 60% of men beginning in midlife, and by 80 years of age more than 90% of men are affected. BPH increases urinary frequency, which can have a significant impact on lifestyle and overall quality of life.

Saw palmetto extract compares favorably with the pharmaceutical drug finasteride (Proscar) in the management of BPH, although the mechanisms of action are believed to be different. In a clinical trial that compared the efficacy of a commercial saw palmetto extract with that of finasteride, both products relieved symptoms in two thirds of the men (Carraro et al, 1996). The saw palmetto extract, however, had fewer adverse side effects, such as impotence and decreased libido. Saw palmetto reduced the symptoms of BPH, but it did not significantly reduce the size of the enlarged prostate. Despite these suggestive results, the safety and efficacy of using phytotherapy for the management of BPH is not yet proven (Lowe, 2001).

Mechanisms of Action and Active Constituents

Despite the popularity of saw palmetto use for BPH symptoms, only a limited number of clinical trials have been conducted to date. Few have been double-blinded, placebo-controlled, or longer than 6 months' duration. All, however, appear to support the successful use of saw palmetto extract for improving the symptoms of mild BPH (Gerber et al, 2001; Marks et al, 2000; Wilt et al, 2000). Clearly, additional carefully conducted trials are warranted, particularly given the prevalence of BPH and the fact that saw palmetto extract appears equivalent to finasteride, but without the side effects.

The active constituents of saw palmetto are derived from the herb's berries that contain free fatty acids and sterols. The berries contain about 1.5% of an oil (beta-sitosterol) that contains saturated and unsaturated fatty acids and sterols. A purified fat-soluble extract of the berries containing the fatty acids and sterols is used medicinally.

The mechanism of action of saw palmetto is not yet clear. A primary challenge in identifying the active components of saw palmetto and their mechanism of action is the fact that manufacturers use different extraction procedures, which yield different mixtures of components in the final product (Lowe, 2001).

For stage I or II BPH, a dosage of 160 mg of the lipophilic extract (standardized to 85% to 95% fatty acids and sterols) twice a day has been used in clinical trials. To assess efficacy, 6 to 8 weeks of continuous use is advised; however, to assess clinical efficacy, a minimum 6-month trial is required (Blumenthal et al, 1998). Tea made from saw palmetto is of little value because few of the active ingredients are water-soluble.

Contraindications, Side Effects, and Toxicity

Saw palmetto is rated as a class 1 botanical according to the American Herbal Products Association's Botanical Safety Rating Classification, which suggests that the botanical can be safely consumed when used appropriately (McGuffin et al, 1997).

The Commission E monograph on saw palmetto lists rare cases of stomach problems as a side effect, but it lists no contraindications (Blumenthal et al, 1998). Because no current evidence exists that saw palmetto has any effect on prostate-specific antigens (PSA), it does not mask prostate carcinoma (Braeckman et al, 1997).

Potential Adverse Interactions

Saw palmetto contains phytoestrogens, compounds that mimic the effects of the animal hormone estrogen, and potentially could interfere with drug therapies such as estrogen therapy, oral contraceptives, progesterone therapy, and postmenopausal hormone replacement therapy and with other phytohormone-containing herbs such as black cohosh, licorice, red clover, Siberian ginseng, wild yam, and vitex. Similarly, soy foods, which are rich in phytoestrogens, would be expected to have an additive effect with saw palmetto. These effects may be interfering or beneficial, depending on the therapeutic intent. Multiple agents with similar actions should only be used under the direction of a knowledgeable health care professional.

St. John's Wort

St. John's wort *(Hypericum perforatum)* is an aromatic perennial with small yellow, five-petaled flowers. It has been used since the Middle Ages to calm the nerves, improve mood, and decrease inflammation during wound healing.

Indications and Common Uses

St. John's wort has long been used in Europe, where it is a popular remedy for mild to moderate depression. Numerous studies have validated its use for this purpose, including a recent double-blind, placebo-controlled multicenter clinical trial of persons with mild to moderate major depressive disorder (Kalb et al, 2001). St. John's wort has not been validated for use in severe depression, however (Kasper, 2001; Shelton et al, 2001). St. John's wort also has documented pharmacologic effects as an antiviral and antibacterial agent (Barnes et al, 2001).

Mechanisms of Action and Active Constituents

The two components that appear to be responsible for the pharmacologic effects of St. John's wort are hypericin and hyperforin, which are found in the flowering tops of the plant. Hypericin was originally thought to be the major active constituent, but it now appears that hyperforin is responsible for the antidepressant effects of St. John's wort. Hypericin is suspected of being the primary component responsible for the antiviral properties of St. John's wort and perhaps its antibacterial effects, but a recent study found hyperforin to be quite effective against methicillin-resistant strains of *Staphylococcus aureus,* a medically significant antibiotic-resistant bacterium (Reichling et al, 2001).

A number of actions have been proposed for the antidepressant activity of St. John's wort. These actions involve inhibition of the reuptake of the neurotransmitters serotonin, norepinephrine, and dopamine, possibly through weak inhibition of monoamine oxidase-A and oxidase-B activities (Calapai et al, 2001; Muller et al, 1997; Nathan, 2001).

Numerous clinical trials have confirmed the efficacy of St. John's wort as an antidepressant. In a recent metaanalysis of 22 randomized controlled trials, St. John's wort was significantly more effective than placebo and comparable to standard antidepressants (Whiskey et al, 2001). In a large randomized controlled trial that was carefully designed and conducted, St. John's wort was found to be equivalent to imipramine, a tricyclic antidepressant, in relieving mild to moderate depression and slightly better in relieving the anxiety that often accompanies depression (Woelk, 2000).

The recommended daily dosage for St. John's wort, based on clinical studies involving the management of mild to moderate depression, is 900 mg of extract standardized to 0.3% hypericin, given with meals in three divided doses of 300 mg each.

Contraindications, Side Effects, and Toxicity

St. John's wort is rated as a class 2d botanical according to the American Herbal Products Association's Botanical Safety Rating Classification because it may potentiate pharmaceutical MAOIs (McGuffin et al, 1997) (see Table 20-3). These drugs increase neurotransmitters by preventing their degradation, and St. John's wort can potentially enhance this effect and raise the level of neurotransmitters to an undesirably high level.

Reported side effects of St. John's wort include emotional vulnerability, fatigue, pruritis, and weight increase, but side effects are reported to be milder and less frequent than those associated with prescription antidepressant drugs (Kasper, 2001). Photosensitivity is possible with large doses (i.e., 3 to 5 g/day, equivalent to 5 to 10 mg hypericin), particularly for persons with fair skin; so caution is advised if exposure to the sun is anticipated (Schulz, 2001).

Potential Adverse Interactions

St. John's wort increases the amount of, and thereby activity of, cytochrome P450 3A4 (CYP3A4), an important drug-metabolizing enzyme in the intestine and liver. The impact of increased CYP3A4 activity is to decrease the amount of drug that enters the circulation. For drugs with narrow ranges of concentrations in which they are effective or drugs of a critical nature, insufficient amounts of these drugs may be available when St. John's wort is also taken. St. John's wort was first found to interact with cyclosporine, an immunosuppressant, which led to heart-transplant rejections, and with indinavir, a protease inhibitor used by persons with HIV/AIDS, which led to lowered antiviral activity of the drug (Piscitelli et al, 2000; Ruschitzka et al, 2000). Subsequently, the mechanism of action was identified whereby hyperforin interacts with a transcription factor, the pregnane X receptor, which promotes the increased synthesis of the CYP3A4 enzyme (Moore et al, 2000). Among the drugs affected by this action are oral contraceptives and the HMGCoA-reductase inhibitors that help to lower LDL cholesterol levels. One report stated that St. John's wort may also increase thyroid-stimulating hormone levels (Ferko and Levine, 2001). The importance of disclosing herbal supplement use to health care practitioners and of not using multiple drugs or supplements except under the direction of a knowledgeable health care professional cannot be overemphasized.

Valerian

Valerian, *Valeriana officinalis,* is a tall perennial herb whose hollow stem bears leaves with white or reddish flowers. Valerian preparations are made from the dried rhizome and roots; the vertical rhizome and its numerous rootlets are harvested in the autumn in the second year of growth. These parts possess the volatile, essential oil that contains the distinctive odor of valerian.

Indications and Common Uses

Valerian has a 1000-year history of use as a minor tranquilizer and sleep aid. Nervous system disorders, including anxiety and insomnia, are conditions for which valerian may be useful.

Mechanisms of Action and Active Constituents

At present the specific ingredients responsible for the sedative effects of valerian remain unknown; however, the identified major components of the volatile oil include the monoterpene bornyl acetate and the sesquiterpene valerenic acid and are thought to be important for valerian's action as a sedative (Reichert, 1998). Other sesquiterpenes and additional, nonvolatile, monoterpenes such as the valepotriates are also being studied for their effects on the central nervous system (Houghton, 1999). The chemical variability of the volatile oils resulting from growing and harvesting conditions and genetic variation in the strains used has made characterization of components and association with valerian's activities difficult.

The mechanism of action of valerian appears to be similar to that of benzodiazepines and barbiturates, which bind to gamma-aminobutyric acid-A (GABA-A) receptor sites to depress central nervous system activity. Because valerian weakly binds to these receptor sites, sedation results without adverse effects, such as addiction or dependence. However, valerian may also have other actions not related to GABA binding (Reichert, 1998).

Clinical studies with valerian have demonstrated that this botanical improves the quality of sleep time and reduces the time required to fall asleep, even in older persons and in poor or irregular sleepers, without producing morning sleepiness. In a study that compared the efficacy of a combination preparation of valerian and lemon balm with benzodiazepine in shortening sleep latency and increasing sleep quality, the valerian combination (160 mg of valerian combined with 80 mg of lemon balm [*Melissa officinalis*]) compared favorably with 0.125 mg of triazolam (Halcion). Patients treated with this combination experienced no daytime sedation or loss of concentration (Dressing et al, 1992). In a small but carefully designed study that examined how valerian affected sleep quality, the researchers found valerian to be effective for insomnia (Donath et al, 2000). Persons suffering from stress-induced insomnia appeared to benefit from the use of valerian in terms of time to fall asleep, hours slept, and their mood upon waking (Wheatley, 2001). Overall, however, the evidence for valerian's effectiveness for insomnia is promising but inconclusive (Stevinson and Ernst, 2000).

The recommended dosage of valerian for treatment of insomnia is 300 to 400 mg of standardized valerian root extract (containing not less than 0.5% essential oil), administered 1 hour before bedtime. Persons suffering from anxiety may also benefit from an added morning dose of 200 to 300 mg.

Contraindications, Side Effects, and Toxicity

Valerian is rated as a class 1 botanical according to the American Herbal Products Association's Botanical Safety Rating Classification, which suggests that valerian can be safely consumed when used appropriately (McGuffin et al, 1997) (see Table 20-3). At recommended dosages, use of valerian has not been associated with side effects or contraindications. In fact, a common experience with valerian is the lack of side effects on waking, in contrast to prescription sleep medications. Use of valerian does not appear to impair reaction time, alertness, or concentration (Kuhlmann et al, 1999). There is concern that abrupt discontinuation may precipitate withdrawal symptoms similar to those seen on withdrawal of the benzodiazepine sedatives (Garges et al, 1998).

Potential Adverse Interactions

Valerian could potentially enhance the action of agents that depress the central nervous system, such as alcohol, antidepressants, sedating antihistamines, barbiturates, benzodiazepines, narcotics, and other prescription sedatives as well as herbs such as German chamomile, goldenseal, kava, passion flower, skullcap, and St. John's wort that have sedating effects. Multiple agents with similar actions should be used only under the direction of a knowledgeable health care professional.

GUIDELINES FOR WORKING WITH CLIENTS WHO USE BOTANICALS

The goal is to determine which botanicals a client is using and the health goals they hope to achieve through the use of these botanicals. Typically people do not divulge their use of dietary supplements to their health care practitioners, so it is imperative that the practitioner establish rapport with the client and is nonjudgmental of the client's practices in order to foster a constructive dialogue. The role of the health care practitioner is one of coach who helps clients assess the need for supplements and helps them to become more knowledgeable about their options.

As the basis for an educational discussion of dietary supplement use, clients should bring with them all the prescription, OTC, and dietary supplements they are using. Each supplement should be discussed in terms of what the client hopes to achieve by using that supplement, whether the preparation is appropriate for the client's health goals, and whether the dosage being taken provides levels that have been found to be safe and effective in clinical trials. The quality of the particular preparation and how to recognize a quality preparation; any known safety or contraindication concerns; and whether there are any known or potential interactions between each supplement and prescription or OTC medications, other dietary supplements, or foods should also be reviewed. The client should be instructed to use the dosage commonly recommended for that botanical and should be given guidance on locating credible resources for obtaining this type of information. A low starting dosage, even less than the recommended dosage, should be encouraged and the response monitored to minimize the chances of an adverse reaction. Lastly, dietary supplement use by clients provides an excellent platform for teaching consumers analytical skills that will serve them well in their pursuit of increased self-management of their health.

SUMMARY

Complementary and alternative medicine such as acupuncture, moxibustion, chiropractic, naturopathy, and phytotherapy are commonly practiced in the United States. Most of these therapies emphasize a holistic approach to health and promote the body's ability to heal itself. Phytotherapy, with the use of botanical medicines, is growing in popularity, but self-treatment with botanicals is generally appropriate only for minor, self-limiting conditions or as preventive measures against certain chronic diseases. For ongoing education in this area, see the Relevant Web Sites sites section, which lists web sites that present credible information regarding integrative medicine and phytotherapy.

Relevant Web Sites

American Botanical Council
www.herbalgram.org
American Herbal Pharmacoepeoia
www.herbal-ahp.org
American Herbal Products Association
www.ahpa.org
Clinical Trials.gov
www.clinicaltrials.gov
Dietary Supplements Database (IBIDS)
www.dietary-supplements.info.nih.gov
Food and Drug Administration (FDA)
www.fda.gov
Healthfinder
www.healthfinder.gov
Herb Research Foundation
www.herbs.org
National Center for Complementary and Alternative Medicine
www.nccaam.nih.gov
National Institutes of Health
www.nih.gov
National Nutritional Foods Association
www.nnfa.org
Natural Medicines Comprehensive Database
www.naturaldatabase.com
NSF International, Inc.
www.nsf.org
U.S. Pharmacopeial Convention
www.usp.org

Clinical Scenario 1

Ellen is 66 years old and has been diagnosed as having hypertension, hypercholesterolemia, and type 2 diabetes (non–insulin-dependent diabetes mellitus). She has been referred by her physician for nutritional counseling, with a specific request from the referring physician that you evaluate any herbal preparations she is taking. At the initial consult, Ellen tells you she is taking the following dietary supplements: garlic pills, ginseng, ginkgo, and St. John's wort, along with the following medications: warfarin, a tricyclic antidepressant, and blood pressure–lowering medication.

1. What recommendations would you make about Ellen's diet?
2. What additional questions would you ask regarding Ellen's supplements?
3. List potential adverse interactions between the botanicals and the prescription drugs. How would you counsel Ellen?

Clinical Scenario 2

Matthew is a 43-year-old highly successful sales representative for a major medical company. He enjoys the competitive nature of his job, travels a lot, and is knowledgeable about health care. Matthew "eats healthy," is at a normal weight, jogs daily, and takes a number of dietary supplements to improve his energy level, to manage his stress, to help him sleep, and to protect against heart disease. (His father had a heart attack in his fifties.) He takes a high-potency daily multivitamin/multimineral with extra B vitamins for stress, a caffeine-containing supplement to give him energy, St. John's wort and kava for anxiety, valerian at night to help him sleep, and vitamin E and omega-3 fatty acids to protect against heart disease.

1. Which foods would you recommend to help Matthew achieve his health goals?
2. What questions would you ask Matthew about the supplements he's taking?
3. Which other complementary approaches might be appropriate to help Matthew accomplish his health goals?
4. How would you counsel Matthew?

■ Cited References

Altman RD, Marcussen KC: Effects of a ginger extract on knee pain in patients with osteoarthritis, *Arthritis Rheum* 44:2531, 2001.

Ang-Lee MK et al: Herbal medicines and perioperative care, *JAMA* 286:208, 2001.

Astin JA: Why patients use alternative medicine: results of a national study, *JAMA* 279:1548, 1998.

Barnes J et al: St. John's wort (*Hypericum perforatum* L.): a review of its chemistry, pharmacology and clinical properties, *J Pharm Pharmacol* 53:583, 2001.

Bensoussan A et al: Treatment of irritable bowel syndrome with Chinese herbal medicine: a randomized controlled trial, *JAMA* 280:1585, 1998.

Berthold HK et al: Effect of a garlic oil preparation on serum lipoproteins and cholesterol metabolism: a randomized controlled trial, *JAMA* 279:1900, 1998.

Blumenthal M et al, eds: *The complete German Commission E monographs: therapeutic guide to herbal medicines,* Austin, Tex, 1998, American Botanical Council, and Boston, Integrative Medicine Communications.

Blumenthal M et al, eds: *Herbal medicine: expanded commission E.,* Austin, Tex, 2000, American Botanical Council.

Bradley RS: Philosophy of naturopathic medicine. In Pizzorno JP, Murray M: *Textbook of natural medicine,* ed 2, New York, 1999, Churchill Livingstone.

Braeckman J et al: Efficacy and safety of the extract of *Serenoa repens* in the treatment of benign prostatic hyperplasia: therapeutic equivalence between twice and once daily dosage forms, *Phytother Res* 11:558, 1997.

Brevoort P: The booming U.S. botanical market: a new overview, *Herbal-Gram* 44:33, 1998.

Calapai G et al: Serotonin, norepinephrine and dopamine involvement in the antidepressant action of *Hypericum perforatum, Pharmacopsychiatry* 34:45, 2001.

Carraro JC et al: Comparison of phytotherapy (Permixon) with finasteride in the treatment of benign prostate hyperplasia: a randomized international study of 1,098 patients, *Prostate* 29:231, 1996.

Cherkin DC, Mootz RD, eds: Chiropractic in the United States: training, practice, and research. Agency for Health Care Policy and Research Report, AHCPR Publication No 98-N002; 1997; complete report downloadable from www.chiroweb.com/archives/ahcpr/uschiros.htm.

Cody G: History of naturopathic medicine. In Pizzorno JP, Murray M, editors: *Textbook of natural medicine,* ed 2, New York, 1999, Churchill Livingstone.

Creating the Consortial Center for Chiropractic Research, www.clinicaltrials.gov.

DeBusk RM: Dietary supplements and cardiovascular disease, *Curr Athero Rep* 2:508, 2000.

DeBusk RM: A practical guide to herbal supplements for nutrition practitioners, *Top Clin Nutr* 16:53, 2001.

DeBusk RM, Treadwell PR: *Herbs as medicine: what you should know.* Tallahassee, Fla, 2000, DeBusk Communications.

Dietary Supplement Health and Education Act of 1994, Public law 103-417, October 25, 1994.

Donath F et al: Critical evaluation of the effect of valerian extract on sleep structure and sleep quality, *Pharmacopsychiatry* 33:47, 2000.

Dressing H et al: Insomnia: are valerian/lemon balm combinations of equal value to benzodiazepine? *Therapiewoche* 42:726, 1992.

Edzard E: Harmless herbs? A review of the recent literature, *Am J Med* 104:170, 1998.

Echinacea, *Altern Med Rev* 6:411, 2001.

Eisenberg DM et al: Unconventional medicine in the United States: prevalence, costs, and patterns of use, *N Engl J Med* 328:246, 1993.

Eisenberg DM et al: Trends in alternative medicine use in the United States, 1990-1997: results of a follow-up national survey, *JAMA* 280:1569, 1998.

Eisenberg DM et al: Perceptions about complementary therapies relative to conventional therapies among adults who use both: results from a national survey, *Ann Intern Med* 135: 344-351, 2001.

Engels HJ et al: Effects of ginseng supplementation on supramaximal exercise performance and short-term recovery, *J Strength Cond Res* 15:290, 2001.

Ernst E: The risk-benefit profile of commonly used herbal therapies: ginkgo, St. John's wort, ginseng, echinacea, saw palmetto, and kava, *Ann Intern Med* 136:42, 2002.

Ernst E, Pittler MH: *Ginkgo biloba:* dementia: a systematic review of double-blind, placebo-controlled trials, *Clin Drug Invest* 17:301, 1999.

Ferko N, Levine MA: Evaluation of the association between St. John's wort and elevated thyroid-stimulating hormone, *Pharmacotherapy* 21:1574, 2001.

Foster DF et al: Alternative medicine use in older Americans, *J Am Geriatr Soc* 48:1560, 2000.

Garges HP et al: Cardiac complications and delirium associated with valerian root withdrawal, *JAMA* 280:1566, 1998.

Gerber GS et al: Randomized, double-blind, placebo-controlled trial of saw palmetto in men with lower urinary tract symptoms, *Urology* 58:960, 2001.

Hobbs C: *Milk thistle: the liver herb,* ed 2, Capitola, Calif, 1992, Botanica Press.

Hoheisel O et al: Echinagard treatment shortens the course of the common cold: a double-blind, placebo-controlled clinical trial, *Eur J Clin Res* 9:261, 1997.

Houghton PJ: The scientific basis for the reputed activity of valerian, *J Pharm Pharmacol* 51:505, 1999.

Isaacsohn JL et al: Garlic powder and plasma lipids and lipoproteins: a multicenter, randomized, placebo-controlled trial, *Arch Intern Med* 158:1189, 1998.

Kalb R, et al: Efficacy and tolerability of hypericum extract WS5572 versus placebo in mildly to moderately depressed patients: a randomized double-blind multicentre clinical trial, *Pharmacopsychiatry* 34:96, 2001.

Kannar D et al: Hypocholesterolemic effect of an enteric-coated garlic supplement, *J Am Coll Nutr* 20:225, 2001.

Kaptchuk TJ, Eisenberg DM: Varieties of healing. 1. Medical pluralism in the United States, *Ann Intern Med* 135:189, 2001a.

Kaptchuk TJ, Eisenberg DM: Varieties of healing. 2. A taxonomy of unconventional healing practices, *Ann Intern Med* 135:196, 2001b.

Kasper S: *Hypericum perforatum*—a review of clinical studies. *Pharmacopsychiatry* 34:S51, 2001.

Kessler RC et al: Long-term trends in the use of complementary and alternative medical therapies in the United States. *Ann Intern Med* 135:262, 2001.

Kratz AM: Contemporary homeopathy. In Pizzorno JP, Murray M: *Textbook of natural medicine,* ed 2, New York, 1999, Churchill Livingstone.

Kudolo GB: The effect of 3-month ingestion of Ginkgo biloba extract on pancreatic beta-cell function in response to glucose loading in normal glucose tolerant individuals, *J Clin Pharmacol* 40:647, 2000.

Kuhlmann J et al: The influence of valerian treatment on "reaction time, alertness and concentration" in volunteers, *Pharmacopsychiatry* 32:235, 1999.

Lange A: Homeopathy. In Pizzorno JP, Murray M: *Textbook of natural medicine,* ed 2, New York, 1999, Churchill Livingstone.

Lawson LD: Garlic powder for hyperlipidemia—analysis of recent negative results, *Q Rev Nat Med* 5:187, 1998.

LeBars PL et al: A placebo-controlled, double-blind, randomized trial of an extract of Ginkgo biloba for dementia, *JAMA* 278:1327, 1997.

LeBars PL et al: A 26-week analysis of a double-blind, placebo-controlled trial of the Ginkgo biloba extract EGb 761 in dementia, *Dement Geriatr Cogn Disord* 11:230, 2000.

Linde K et al: Systematic reviews of complementary therapies—an annotated bibliography. 1. Acupuncture, *BMC Complement Altern Med* 1:3, 2001a.
Linde K et al: Systematic reviews of complementary therapies—an annotated bibliography. 2. Herbal medicine, *BMC Complement Altern Med* 1:5, 2001b.
Linde K et al: Systematic reviews of complementary therapies—an annotated bibliography. 3. Homeopathy, *BMC Complement Altern Med* 1:4, 2001c.
Lowe FC: Phytotherapy in the management of benign prostatic hyperplasia, *Urology* 58:71, 2001.
Mader FH: Treatment of hyperlipidemia with garlic-powder tablets: evidence from the German Association of General Practitioners' multicentric placebo-controlled double-blind study, *Arzneimittelforschung* 40:111, 1990.
Marks LS et al: Effects of a saw palmetto herbal blend in men with symptomatic benign prostatic hyperplasia, *J Urol* 163:1451, 2000.
McCrindle BW et al: Garlic extract therapy in children with hypercholesterolemia, *Arch Pediatr Adolesc Med* 152:1089:1998.
McGuffin M et al, eds: *American Herbal Products Association's botanical safety handbook: guidelines for the safe use and labeling for herbs of commerce,* Boca Raton, Fla, 1997, CRC Press.
McKenna DJ et al: Efficacy, safety, and use of Ginkgo biloba in clinical and preclinical applications, *Altern Ther Health Med* 7:70, 2001.
Melchart D et al: Echinacea root extracts for the prevention of upper respiratory tract infections: a double-blind, placebo-controlled randomized trial, *Arch Fam Med* 7:541, 1998.
Moore LB et al: St. John's wort induces hepatic drug metabolism through activation of the pregnane X receptor, *Proc Natl Acad Sci USA* 97:7500, 2000.
Mowrey D, Clayson DL: Motion sickness, ginger, and psychophysics, *Lancet* 1:655, 1982.
Muller WE et al: Effects of hypericum extract (LI 160) in biochemical models of antidepressant activity, *Pharmacopsychiatry* 30(suppl):102, 1997.
Murray MT, Pizzorno Jr JE: Botanical medicine—a modern perspective. In Pizzorno JP, Murray M, eds: *Textbook of natural medicine,* ed 2, New York, 1999, Churchill Livingstone.
Nathan PJ: *Hypericum perforatum* (St. John's wort): a non-selective reuptake inhibitor? A review of the recent advances in its pharmacology, *J Psychopharmacol* 15:47, 2001.
National Center for Complimentary and Alternative Medicine (NCCAM): NCCAM funding: appropriations history, accessed June 15, 2003, www.nccam.nih.gov.
National Institutes of Health Consensus Conference: Acupuncture. *JAMA* 280:1518, 1998. Consensus statement available at odp.od.nih.gov/consensus/cons/107/107_intro.htm
Niebyl J: Drug therapy during pregnancy, *Curr Opin Obstet Gynecol* 4:43, 1992.
Nolting MH: Acupuncture. In Pizzorno JP, Murray M, eds: *Textbook of natural medicine,* ed 2, New York, 1999, Churchill Livingstone.
Oka H et al: Prospective study of chemoprevention of hepatocellular carcinoma with Sho-saiko-to (TJ-9), *Cancer* 76:743, 1995.
Oken BS et al: The efficacy of *Ginkgo biloba* on cognitive function in Alzheimer disease, *Arch Neurol* 55:1409, 1998.
Pedraza-Chaverri J et al: Garlic prevents hypertension induced by chronic inhibition of nitric oxide synthesis, *Life Sci* 62:PL 71, 1998.
Peters H et al: Demonstration of the efficacy of *Ginkgo biloba* special extract EGb 761 on intermittent claudication—a placebo-controlled, double-blind multicenter trial, *Vasa* 27:106, 1998.
Phillips RB, Mootz RD: Contemporary chiropractic philosophy. In Haldeman S, eds: *Principles and practice of chiropractic,* ed 2, Norwalk, Conn, 1992, Appleton & Lange.
Piscitelli SC et al: Indinavir concentrations and St. John's wort, *Lancet* 355:547, 2000.
Piscitelli SC et al: The effect of garlic supplements on the pharmacokinetics of saquinavir, *Clin Infect Dis* 34:234, 2002.
Reichert RG: Valerian clinical monograph, *Q Rev Natl Med* Fall:207, 1998.
Reichling J et al: A current review of the antimicrobial activity of *Hypericum perforatum* L, *Pharmacopsychiatry* 34:116, 2001.
Reisser CH, Weidauer H: *Ginkgo biloba* extract EGb 761 or pentoxifylline for the treatment of sudden deafness: a randomized, reference-controlled, double-blind study, *Acta Otolaryngol* 121: 579, 2001.
Riley D et al: Homeopathy and conventional medicine: an outcomes study comparing effectiveness in a primary care setting, *J Altern Compl Med* 7:149, 2001.
Rosenblatt M, Mindel J: Spontaneous hyphema associated with ingestion of Ginkgo biloba extract [Letter], *N Engl J Med* 336:1008, 1997.
Rowin J, Lewis S: Spontaneous bilateral subdural hematomas associated with chronic *Ginkgo biloba* ingestion, *Neurology* 46: 1775, 1996.
Ruschitzka F et al: Acute heart transplant rejection due to Saint John's wort, *Lancet* 355:548, 2000.
Saller R, et al: The use of silymarin in the treatment of liver diseases, *Drugs* 61:2035, 2001.
Scaglione F et al: Immunomodulatory effects of two extracts of *Panax ginseng,* C.A. Meyer. *Drugs Exp Clin Res* 16:537, 1990.
Schulten B, et al: Efficacy of *Echinacea purpurea* in patients with a common cold: a placebo-controlled, randomised, double-blind clinical trial, *Arzneimittelforschung* 51:563, 2001.
Schulz V: Incidence and clinical relevance of the interactions and side effects of Hypericum preparations, *Phytomedicine* 8:152, 2001.
Schulz V et al: *Rational phytotherapy: a physician's guide to herbal medicine.* New York, 1997, Springer-Verlag.
Serenoa repens. Monograph, *Altern Med Rev* 3:227, 1998.
Shelton RC et al: Effectiveness of St. John's wort in major depression: a randomized controlled trial, *JAMA* 285:1978, 2001.
Silagy CA, Neil HA: A meta-analysis of the effect of garlic on blood pressure, *J Hypertens* 12:463, 1994.
Simpson N, Roman K: Complementary medicine use in children: extent and reasons: a population-based study, *Br J Gen Pract* 51:914, 2001.
Slifman N et al: Contamination of botanical dietary supplements by *Digitalis lanata, N Engl J Med* 339:806, 1998.
Solomon PR et al: Ginkgo for memory enhancement: a randomized controlled trial, *JAMA* 288:835, 2002.
Sotaniemi E et al: Ginseng therapy in non–insulin-dependent diabetic patients, *Diabetes Care* 8:1373, 1995.
Stevinson C, Ernst E: Valerian for insomnia: a systematic review of randomized clinical trials, *Sleep Med* 1:91, 2000.
Tauchert M et al: Effectiveness of hawthorn extract LI 132 compared with the ACE inhibitor captopril: multicenter double-blind study with 132 NYHA stage II, *Muench Med Wochenschr* 136 (suppl):S27, 1994.
U.S. General Accounting Office: Report to congressional committees, Food safety: improvements needed in overseeing the safety of dietary supplements and "functional foods," GAO/RCED-00-156, 2000.
Venkataramanan R et al: Milk thistle, a herbal supplement, decreases the activity of CYP3A4 and uridine diphosphoglucouronosyl transferase in human hepatocyte cultures, *Drug Metab Dispos* 28:1270, 2000.
Verma SK et al: Effect of ginger on platelet aggregation in man, *Indian J Med Res* 98:240, 1994.
Vickers A et al: Homeopathy, *BMJ* 319:1115, 1999.
Vuksan V: Konjac-mannan and American ginseng: emerging alternative therapies for type 2 diabetes mellitus, *J Am Coll Nutr* 20:370S, 2001.
Warshafsky S et al: Effect of garlic on total serum cholesterol: a meta-analysis, *Ann Intern Med* 119:599, 1993.
Wheatley D: Kava and valerian in the treatment of stress-induced insomnia, *Phytother Res* 15:549, 2001.
Whiskey E et al: A systematic review and meta-analysis of *Hypericum perforatum* in depression: a comprehensive clinical review, *Int Clin Psychopharmacol* 16:239, 2001.
Wilt TJ et al: Phytotherapy for benign prostatic hyperplasia, *Public Health Nutr* 3:459, 2000.

Woelk H: Comparison of St John's wort and imipramine for treating depression: randomised controlled trial, *BMJ* 321:536, 2000.

Zhang XH et al: Gender may affect the action of garlic oil on plasma cholesterol and glucose levels of normal subjects, *J Nutr* 131:1471, 2001.

Zhang XY et al: A double-blind, placebo-controlled trial of extract of Ginkgo biloba added to haloperidol in treatment-resistant patients with schizophrenia, *J Clin Psychiatry* 62:878, 2001.

■ Additional References

Fabrega H Jr: Medical validity in Eastern and Western traditions, *Perspect Biol Med* 45:395, 2002.

Herr SM: *Herb-drug interaction handbook,* ed 2, Nassau, NY, 2002, Church Street Books.

Jellin JM et al: Pharmacists letter/prescribers letter natural medicines comprehensive database, Stockton, CA, 2002, Therapeutic Research Faculty, updated daily online at www.naturaldatabase.com.

Kumar NB et al: Use of complementary/integrative nutritional therapies during cancer treatment: implications in clinical practice, *Cancer Control* 9:236, 2002.

Miller LG, Murray WJ, eds: *Herbal medicinals: a clinician's guide,* Binghamton, NY, 1998, Pharmaceutical Products Press.

Moyad MA: The placebo effect and randomized trials: analysis of alternative medicine, *Urol Clin North Am* 29:135, 2002.

Newall CA, Anderson LA, Phillipson JD: *Herbal medicines: a guide for health-care professionals,* London, 1996, The Pharmaceutical Press.

Pizzorno JP, Murray M: *Textbook of natural medicine,* ed 2, New York, 1999, Churchill Livingstone.

Robbers JE, Tyler VE: *Tyler's herbs of choice: the therapeutic use of phytomedicinals,* Binghamton, NY, 1999, The Haworth Herbal Press.

Sarubin A: *The health care professional's guide to dietary supplements,* Chicago, 2002, American Dietetic Association.

Schulz V, Hänsel R, Tyler VE: *Rational phytotherapy: a physician's guide to herbal medicine,* New York, 1997, Springer-Verlag.

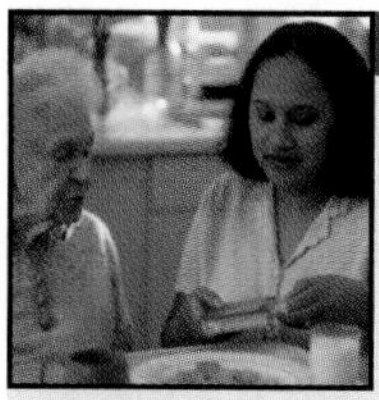

CHAPTER 21

The Nutrition Care Process

CYNTHIA M. BRYLINSKY, MS, RD, LDN

CHAPTER OUTLINE

- Nutrition Care Process and Medical Nutrition Therapy
- Nutritional Care Record
- Charting and Documentation
- Influences on Nutritional Care
- Nutritional Intervention and Diet Modification
- Nutritional Care for the Hospitalized Patient
- Nutritional Care of the Terminally Ill or Hospice Patient
- Discharge Planning and Home Care

KEY TERMS

advance directives–guidelines established by a patient allowing a designated person(s) to make medical decisions if the patient loses decision-making capabilities; may include items such as use of mechanical ventilation or feeding tubes

case management–process to ensure timely, efficient, cost-effective achievement of patient goals

diet prescription–designates the type, amount, texture, and frequency of feeding; may limit or increase amounts of carbohydrate, protein, fat, fluid, vitamins, and minerals

discharge planning–team planning for necessary education, counseling, and resources needed by the patient following hospitalization

disease management–a disease-specific standardized approach to patient care, primarily used in an outpatient setting

evidence-based medical nutrition therapy (MNT) guides for practice–MNT protocols that include a more stringent review of research summarized in evidence tables and conclusion statements that reflect the strength of the evidence

Health Information Portability and Accountability Act (HIPAA)–federal regulations promoting medical record rights by the patients

Joint Commission on Accreditation of Healthcare Organizations (JCAHO)–a peer review organization that evaluates health care institutions and ensures their compliance with established minimum standards

managed care organizations (MCOs)–mechanism for financing and organizing health care delivery in which providers and payers have predetermined payments for care provided

medical nutrition therapy (MNT)–the use of specific nutritional interventions to treat an illness, injury, or condition

medical nutritional therapy protocols–preestablished, standardized guidelines that incorporate current professional knowledge and available research and provide step-by-step instructions for providing nutritional care

nutrition care process–the process of planning for and meeting the nutritional needs of an individual

nutritional care record–written documentation of the nutrition care process, including the interventions and activities used to meet the nutritional objectives

patient-centered objective–a goal that is stated in terms of what the patient will achieve or will be able to do when the objective is met

patient-focused care–care that is organized around the patient as the central focus of the team, the "customer" of health services

preferred provider organization (PPO)–an organization that has negotiated a contract that specifies a favored status in providing health care services for a specific population group

standards of care–practice guidelines established by a facility to ensure that, at a minimum, reasonable care is rendered

standards of professional practice–standards for how an individual practitioner provides service; developed by the American Dietetic Association

utilization management–cost-efficient patient care management with a focus on reducing excessive use of diagnostic or therapeutic tests, procedures, or services

Nutritional care is an organized group of activities allowing identification of nutritional needs and provision of care to meet these needs. The nutrition care process consists of (1) assessing nutritional status and analyzing data to identify nutrition-related problems, (2) nutrition diagnosis, (3) planning and prioritizing nutrition intervention to meet these needs, and (4) evaluating the nutritional care outcomes. The care provided as a result of following this process is called medical nutrition therapy (MNT). This process could also be used to provide other types of nutritional care (e.g., community nutrition program). A standardized nutrition care process has been developed by the American Dietetic Association; Appendix 56 details this model.

NUTRITION CARE PROCESS AND MEDICAL NUTRITION THERAPY

The type of nutritional care provided for an individual depends on the presence of disease or potential disease, the environment, the stage of growth and development, and socioeconomic issues. It may include an assessment of the adequacy of nutritional intake, manipulation of the diet, provision of enteral or parenteral support, and intervention in the form of counseling or education. In most cases, institutions will have established standards of care or practice guidelines that describe recommended steps in the nutrition care process (Table 21-1). These standards often serve as a basis for assessing the quality of care provided to the patient.

Comprehensive nutritional care involves many disciplines: the physician, dietitics professional, nurse, pharmacist, physical or occupational therapist, social worker, speech therapist, case manager, and other care providers may all be integral in achieving desired outcomes, depending on the care setting. The patient is also an integral part of the nutrition care process. A collaborative approach helps to ensure that care is coordinated and that all team members and the patient are aware of goals and priorities. Coordinating the activities of health care professionals requires documentation of the process as well as regular discussions to allow the communication and interaction necessary for complete nutritional care. Patients benefit from interdisciplinary decision-making regarding nutritional and medical concerns. Team conferences, formal or informal, are useful in all settings, whether the patient or client is receiving care in the home, in the community, in a nursing home, in a long-term care facility, in a clinic, or in a hospital (Figure 21-1).

Nutritional Assessment

Nutritional assessment involves the gathering and evaluation of medical, social, nutritional, and medication histories; physical examination; and biochemical data. The identification of nutritional problems (both present and potential) evolves from a thorough assessment of these factors. Both overnutrition and undernutrition have been shown to impact negatively a patient's response to medical treatment. For example, malnutrition increases morbidity, length of hospital stay, and mortality; and infections and other complications resulting from malnutrition can significantly increase health care costs.

Nutritional screening, using simple assessment techniques, helps to identify patients who would benefit from more intensive nutritional assessment. The Joint Commission on Accreditation of Health Care Organizations (JCAHO) requires that nutritional risk be identified in hospitalized patients within 24 hours of admission, but it does not mandate a standardized method to accomplish this task. In the hospital setting, nutritional screening must be designed efficiently so that it can be accomplished within 24 hours of each patient's admission. Different personnel administer the screen, depending on the setting, and the information will vary according to the type of patient being screened. Patients identified as being "at risk" during the initial screening process should have their nutritional status reviewed by a dietetics professional. Box 21-1 lists information that is frequently included in a nutritional screening.

In a hospital setting, screening should be repeated during the course of the patient's stay because nutritional risk increases in patients who are hospitalized for 10 days or longer. Reassessment is important in all care settings to determine whether changes in diagnosis or condition have occurred that alter the patient's nutritional risk. A screening program can be a valuable tool in providing appropriate and cost-effective care to patients regardless of the setting. Chapters 17 and 18 provide detailed information

TABLE 21-1 Sample Standard of Care for the General Patient

THRESHOLD (%)*	DATABASE	PLAN	DOCUMENTATION	EXCEPTIONS
100	1. Complete nutrition screen within 24 hr		(a) Document results of screen	Data unavailable
100	2. Review medical record within 24-48 hr if nutritional intervention indicated by screen			
95	(a) Diet Order 1. Diet prior to admission 2. Appetite or % intake	(a1) Assess appropriateness of diet order (a2) Evaluate adequacy of intake/acceptance of diet if appropriate	(a) Document if diet order inappropriate	Data unavailable
	(b) Physical data 1. Height 2. Weight history 3. Usual weight (c) Diagnosis-med history (d) Lab values as appropriate (e) Medications affecting nutritional status	(b-e) Evaluate appropriate data in terms of patient's nutrition status	(b-e) Document evaluation of data if needed for intervention	
100	3. Determine need for further intervention in conjunction with health care team			Patient refuses intervention
	(a) Education	(a) Provide basic information; schedule for outpatient visit if in-depth counseling needed	(a-c) Document intervention and outcome	
	(b) Poor intake	Recommend if appropriate: (b1) Supplementation (b2) Calorie count (b3) Alternate feeding route	Refer to calorie count and TF/TPN policies	
	(c) No intervention needed	(c) Rescreen in 7 days		
100	4. Review patient's nutritional status and response to changes in data and/or patient condition	Evaluate and adjust accordingly	Document evaluation and adjustments in care plan	

(Courtesty Barnes-Jewish Hospital, St. Louis, Mo.)
*Threshold is the level below which services are considered to be substandard.
TF, Tube feeding; *TPN*, total parenteral nutrition.

about the screening process and a complete review of nutritional assessment techniques.

Nutrition Diagnosis

Once the assessment process has been completed, the dietetics professional, through synthesis of information obtained in the assessment process, makes a "nutrition diagnosis." This diagnosis is unique to the patient's nutritional status and takes into account the medical diagnosis. For instance, a patient may have the diagnosis of coronary artery disease, but his nutrition diagnosis may be "excessive intake of high fat, high cholesterol foods." A sample that illustrates this further follows.

Many facilities use standardized formats to facilitate communication of this information (see Figure 21-3 for a form used for this purpose in a clinic setting).

Nutrition Intervention

Identification of nutritional problems leads to formulation of a plan for dealing with each problem individually, with greatest attention being paid to the problem(s) of highest priority. If complete nutritional information is not available, the first objective is to collect the data necessary to complete the plan. Once the plan is completed, the dietetics professional implements the plan.

Implementation is the component of the nutrition care process that translates assessment data into strategies, activities, or interventions that will enable the patient or client to meet the established objectives. Implementation can begin once the objectives are determined. Sample steps may include changing the diet prescription, counseling the patient, providing food or nutritional supplements, initiating a tube feeding for a patient who cannot eat, or providing information on financial or food resources. The care process is a continuous one; the initial plan may change as the condition of the patient changes, as new needs are identified, or if the patient does not respond to the interventions that are implemented.

Interventions should be specific; they are the "what, where, when, and how" of the care plan. For example, for the patient with malnutrition, an objective might be to increase caloric intake. This could be implemented through provision of high-calorie, high-protein foods via small, frequent meals and snacks or through provision of a supplement or milk-

Practice Clinical Scenario

John is a 70-year-old white male admitted for bypass surgery. A review of his health record, laboratory data, anthropometric data, and nutritional history reveals the need for further nutritional intervention. Chart review reveals the following objective data:

Laboratory Data and Medications
- Glucose and electrolytes: normal range; albumin: −2.5 g/dL; cholesterol/triglycerides: normal
- Medications: Inderal

Anthropometric Data
- Height: 70 inches
- Weight: 130 lb (down in 3 months from usual weight of 145 lb in 3 months)

Nutrition Interview Findings
- Caloric intake: 1200 kcal/day (less than energy needs)
- Meals: irregular throughout the day; drinks coffee frequently

Medical History
- History of hypertension, thyroid dysfunction, asthma, prostate surgery

Psychosocial Data
- John lives alone in his own home. His wife died 3 months ago, and he rarely has a cooked meal.

Nutritional Assessment
John was admitted for a cardiac condition, but he also has some nutritional issues. He has been consuming fewer calories than he requires and has little interest in eating. These facts might be referred to as his *nutritional diagnosis.* This nutritional diagnosis may be quite different from his medical problem list because it is specific to the patient's nutritional status. John's nutritional problems consist of (1) unintentional weight loss and (2) poor appetite and inadequate intake (possibly because of the death of his spouse).

shake between meals. Plans should be communicated to the health care team and the patient to ensure understanding of the plan and its rationale. Thorough communication by the dietitics professional increases the likelihood of adherence to the plan.

In the education process, the client and the counselor must jointly establish goals, and they should be achievable. For example, one objective in dealing with a client being counseled on weight loss would be to agree on both an initial and an ultimate goal weight. Objectives should be expressed in behavioral terms and stated in terms of what the patient will do or achieve if the objectives are met. They should consider the educational level and the economic and social resources available to the patient and his or her family. Objectives should also be stated in quantifiable terms to facilitate evaluation. For example, a patient-centered objective in the sample case above would be as follows: "John will be able to identify nutrient-dense foods after instruction." This is more appropriate than "I will teach John how to identify nutrient-dense foods," which states the objective but

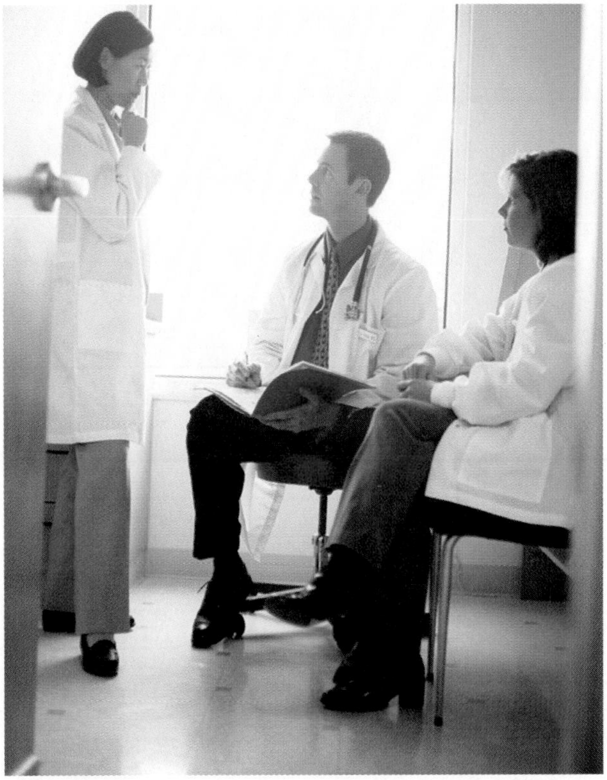

FIGURE 21-1 • Team conference. (Courtesy: PhotoDisc.)

Box 21-1. Nutritional Screening Information

Age
Height
Usual weight
Ideal weight
Present weight
Percentage weight change from the ideal or usual weight
Change in appetite
Dysphagia or difficulty with chewing
Presence of nausea, vomiting, or diarrhea
Serum albumin level
Hemoglobin and hematocrit values
Total lymphocyte count

does not make John responsible for learning and behavioral change.

The objectives for the two nutritional problems identified in the sample case could be stated as follows:

Problem 1: Weight loss
Objectives: (1) John will stop losing weight and begin to gain weight slowly, up to a target weight of 145

CLINIC NOTES
NUTRITION SERVICES

Date: ____________
Referring Physician: ____________ Service: ____________
Primary Care Physician (if different): ____________

S: ____________
____
____

Weight, Hx: ____________ Weight Goal: ____________
Activity: ____________ Supplements: ____________
Prior Nutrition Counseling: ____________

O: Age/Sex: ______ Height: ______ Weight: ______ Body Mass Index: ______
Ideal Body Weight: ______ % Ideal Body Weight: ______
Energy needs: ____________
Diagnosis: ____________ PMH: ____________
Medications: ____________ Other Significant Information: ____________
Labs: ____________ ____________
Diet Instruction: ____________ Videos: ____________
Handouts: ____________

A: ____________
____
____

Patient's Comprehension:
- ☐ Poor: Demonstrated limited understanding.
- ☐ Basic: Can explain rationale of diet; can identify foods to limit.
- ☐ Comprehensive: Can plan sample menus using diet modifications; can effectively evaluate how to incorporate changes into lifestyle.

Expected Outcome:
- ☐ Demonstrated no interest in learning; expect minimal changes.
- ☐ Expect attempts at changing eating habits.
- ☐ Patient very motivated. Expect adherence to diet.

Patient Goals: ____________
____

P: Nutrition Services phone number was made available to patient.
- ☐ Return appointment recommended but patient declined.
- ☐ No return appointment necessary.
- ☐ Return in ______ to review ____________
- ☐ Other ____________

Signature/Title: ____________

FIGURE 21-2 • Sample form to facilitate communication. (Courtesy Geisinger Health System, Danville, Pa.)

lb; (2) John will modify his diet to include adequate calories and protein through the use of nutrient-dense foods.

Problem 2: Inadequate intake/poor appetite

Objectives: (1) John will attend a local senior center for lunch on a daily basis to help improve his socialization and caloric intake; (2) he will include nutrient-dense foods in his diet, especially when his appetite is limited.

To facilitate change, goals must be agreeable to those involved. In the case presented, John must concur with the approach taken. It is often helpful to offer several choices to the patient to empower him or her to decide which choice is most suitable.

In the instance where a patient is not able to be involved, for example, a patient being fed by nasogastric tube, the dietitian and physician may need to discuss the amount of fluid that can be provided by the tube feeding. If the dietitian were to establish this goal without a thorough review of the patient's medical status, and perhaps consulting with the physician, a recommendation might be made that would not be appropriate.

Referring again to the sample case, the nutritional interventions for each objective might be stated as follows:

For unintentional weight loss: John and the dietitian will determine the likely cause of his weight loss.

- Intervention: John will make an effort to eat three meals a day plus a bedtime snack.
- Intervention: John will include at least one nutrient-dense supplement per day in his diet.
- Intervention: John will increase his energy intake to 1800 kcal per day and complete a 3-day food record for analysis of adequacy.

For inadequate intake/poor appetite: John will recognize the impact of his poor appetite on his weight and nutritional status.

- Intervention: John will include nutrient-dense foods with meals, especially when his appetite is minimal.
- Intervention: John will attend the senior center for lunch daily to improve socialization/appetite.

This process of defining interventions is continued for every objective of each problem. In the case being discussed, care must be taken to not overwhelm the patient but rather to implement changes incrementally as success is achieved. Focusing on high-priority objectives and formulating short-term and long-term goals can help to make the problem list more manageable. The interventions just described would be implemented over several sessions to allow the patient to focus his efforts on the items of highest priority. Once a high-priority intervention has been successfully accomplished, additional changes may be pursued.

Nutrition care plans are often based on standards in the profession, such as **MNT Protocols** and **Evidence-Based Guides for Practice,** which summarize the evidence for a given medical condition (see *Focus On:* Evidence-Based Medicine in Nutrition Practice).

Monitoring and Evaluation of Nutritional Care

The last step in the nutrition care process is to evaluate the care provided. This step makes the nutritional care plan dynamic and responsive to the patient's needs. If objectives have been written in measurable behavioral terms, evaluation is relatively easy because new behavior is being measured against a behavior that has already been defined. For example, an evaluation might be that "John was not able to include a supplement in his daily diet because of cost." A revision in the care plan at this point might include the following: "John will be provided a list of low-cost supplements and recipes for boosting intake in foods typically eaten." This new intervention is then implemented and evaluated to determine whether the objective was met.

The goal of nutritional care is to meet the nutritional needs of the patient; thus the objectives must be reviewed frequently to ensure that unmet objectives are addressed and that care is evaluated and modified as needed. When the evaluation reveals that objectives are not being met or that new needs have arisen, the process begins again with reassessment, identification of new needs, and formulation of a new nutrition intervention.

For example, during John's hospitalization, supplements have been provided. Evaluation of this intervention reveals that the patient has developed a dislike of the current supplement and has stopped drinking it. A taste test of products available in the facility is conducted, and the patient agrees to change to a different supplement and to receive smaller, more frequent portions. Further review will be needed to ascertain whether the change in supplement or method of delivery improves intake.

All steps in the nutrition care process require critical thinking by the dietetics professional. Documentation is also an integral part of the process and is discussed in more detail in the following section. The nutrition care process is summarized in Figure 21-6. Details of the steps are included in Appendix 56.

NUTRITIONAL CARE RECORD

Medical nutrition therapy or nutritional care provided must be documented in the health or medical record. The medical record is a legal document; if interventions are not recorded, it is assumed that they

TABLE 21-2 Sample Nutritional Steps in Care

STEPS	COMPONENTS	FACTORS TO CONSIDER
1. Nutritional Assessment	Diet history Biochemical data Clinical examination findings Medical history Anthropometric data Psychosocial data Exercise/activity level Assess the educational level of the patient and family and readiness to learn Identify available resources Organize and evaluate available information	The information should be accurate, pertinent to the patient, and appropriately interpreted. The problems identified should be the same as those in the medical record, be given priority ratings in the order of their importance, be related to assessment data, and include present and potential problems. Professional judgment must be used to analyze information.
2. Nutritional Diagnosis	Consider protocol, care map, and clinical practice guidelines	Use standardized nutrition language for the profession
3. Nutritional Intervention	Collect additional necessary information Establish goals and define strategies to reach goals Identify measures to enable patient to meet nutritional requirements Modify diet, as required, to make it acceptable to the patient Supplement nutrient intake Counsel/educate the patient/family Provide necessary nutritional supplements and alternative forms of nutrition support Resolve health problems Referral to other health care/community agencies Schedule follow-up visit Use format appropriate for the setting. Focus on desired outcomes	Objectives should be patient-centered, stated in behavioral terms, realistic, measurable, and designated as short- or long-term. Involve patient and health care team in goal development. Interventions should specifically relate to the problem and objective, be individualized for each patient, and be specific in describing what, how, why, when, and where.
4. Monitoring and Evaluation of Nutritional Care	Monitor food and fluid intake; evaluate intake for adequacy in meeting patient's nutritional needs Assess nutritional knowledge of the patient/family as reflected by behavioral (food choice) change. Monitor biochemical and anthropometric data Monitor the patient's progress. Adjust goals as needed	Evaluation should include a comparison between observed behavior and expected behavior, a determination of the effectiveness of intervention in meeting objectives, an explanation of the effectiveness or ineffectiveness of intervention, and suggestions for revising the care plan based on evaluation.

have not occurred. Documentation affords the following advantages:

1. It helps to ensure that nutritional care will be relevant, thorough, and effective by providing a record that identifies the problems and sets criteria for evaluating the care.
2. It allows the entire health care team to understand the rationale for nutritional care, the means by which it will be provided, and the role each team member must play to reinforce the plan and assure its success.
3. Notes in the medical record serve as a communication tool, verifying important information for evaluation of health care delivery, as well as for accreditation and peer review (see *Focus On:* Joint Commission on Accreditation of Healthcare Organizations [JCAHO]).

Much of the information needed to develop a nutritional care plan is collected routinely by health professionals other than the dietitian. For example, a physician completes a medical history, including information about the gastrointestinal tract, medications, weight loss, and other relevant factors; a nurse typically weighs and measures the patient and asks about allergies (to include food allergies). Social workers may ask about the economic issues related to food availability and the patient's living conditions. The nutritional care record ensures that all aspects relating to nutritional care are summarized in one place as part of the total health record.

The clinical dietitian may keep a detailed record of the patient's assessment, plan, and outcomes that is separate from the medical record. The information contained in it should be summarized periodically in the medical record. The medical record and the information it contains are important for hospital care audits, professional standards reviews, patient education, and other efforts to maintain quality health care. The record kept by the dietitian may be useful when patients are frequently readmitted

FOCUS ON

Evidence-Based Medicine in Nutrition Practice

Evidence-based medicine is described as the use of current "best evidence" in making decisions about the care of individual patients. "Best evidence" may include research, a consensus statement, and other evidence to support the practice. *Medical Nutrition Therapy (MNT) Evidence-Based Nutrition Guides for Practice and Protocols* are available through the American Dietetic Association (ADA) to assist dietetic practitioners in providing nutrition care (ADA, 1998).

Information is organized by background, rationale, and intended use of each protocol. The MNT process and the expected outcomes can be communicated to Managed Care Organizations, insurance companies, administrators, and other health care providers. A *summary page* summarizes the entire MNT process and includes the number of encounters typically needed, the expected length of time for each encounter, and the length of the intervals between encounters.

Outcomes are defined as the result of the performance (or nonperformance) of a function or process, specifically "what" happened to the client. Outcome assessment factors include three elements: (1) clinical assessment factors (anatomic and physiologic elements, such as biochemical parameters, anthropometric parameters, and clinical signs and symptoms); (2) behavioral assessment factors or therapeutic lifestyle changes (changes in the client's behavior related to food selection, preparation, and physical activity that ultimately may result in changes in clinical or functional outcomes); and (3) expected outcomes (type of change anticipated, such as improvement in abnormal laboratory values, decreasing blood pressure, or decreasing weight).

An *Ideal/Goal Value* section lists values for control or improvement of the disease/conditions as defined and supported in the literature. The *flowchart* provides a one-page visual overview of the process, including specific information to be obtained before the initial encounter, data to be assessed, self-management training expectations, and communications to the primary care provider or other appropriate health care provider.

The *Encounter Process* section provides details of the MNT protocol by encounter with specific factors outlined, such as nutrient calculations, self-management training materials, and appropriate communications to other health care providers. The information is extremely valuable for staff orientation, competence verification, and training.

Nutrition Progress Notes are specific to the diagnosis and are designed to document the intervention and outcomes of MNT as outlined in the encounter process. This standardized form includes *Expected Outcome; Intervention Provided to Meet Goal; and Goals Reached.* The *Compliance Potential* is recorded for each encounter and includes evaluation for comprehension, receptivity, and adherence potential. The *Conclusion Statements Worksheets* summarize the evidence and reflect how strong the evidence is for that particular nutrition care recommendation.

Use of the evidence-based guides for practice for the profession will establish standardized, predictable practice. They also may create research questions for obtaining information needed in the profession (Meyers, et al, 2001). The ADA Web site can be accessed at www.eatright.org for further information on these protocols.

Data from Meyers EF et al: Evidence-based pratice guides vs. protocols: what's the difference? *J Am Diet Assoc* 101:1085, 2001; American Dietetic Association: *MNT Evidence-based guides for practice: nutrition practice guidelines for type 1 and 2 diabetes mellitus*, CD-ROM, 2001; and Splett, PL: *Developing and validating evidence-based guides for dietetics practice: a tool kit for dietetics professionals*, Chicago, 2000, American Dietetic Association.

or when a patient is transferred to a different unit (and hence to a different dietitian). Figure 21-3 is an example of a nutritional care record that may be used by a dietitian.

CHARTING AND DOCUMENTATION

The medical record serves as a tool for communication among members of the health care team. It typically includes sections for physician orders, medical history and physical examinations, laboratory test results, consults, progress reports on the actual care being delivered to the patient, and the patient's prognosis. The format of records may vary from institution to institution, but they all contain the basic information necessary to document the care provided and provide a record of compliance with acceptable standards of professional practice. Many facilities are converting to electronic medical records to streamline charting and to facilitate storage and retrieval of patient data.

The medical record also serves as the basis for evaluating the care delivered. The dietitian provides information relative to nutritional status, assessment regarding nutrition support or education for patients and family, and the goals of nutritional therapy. Information shared should be useful to the health care team. Notes should be structured to allow routine documentation of the following JCAHO standards: reassessment of status, adequacy of intake, appropriateness of the route of delivery, complications of the therapy, presence of measurable outcome goals, and multidisciplinary nutrition care plans that consider education and discharge needs (Klein et al, 1997). The record is a legal, confidential document. The following are general guidelines for documentation in the hospital setting; Health Information Portability and Accountability Act (HIPAA) guidelines must be followed:

- Medical records are permanent legal documents; therefore all entries should be written in black pen or typewritten. Soft felt pens, multicolored pens, and pencils should not be used.
- Documentation should be complete, clear, concise, objective, legible, and accurate.
- Entries should include date, time, and service. Each page should include the patient's name and hospital number (most facilities use a stamp for this purpose).
- Entries should be in chronologic order and consecutive, consistent and noncontradictory.
- The first word of every statement should be capitalized, with periods placed at the end of each thought. Complete sentences are not necessary, but grammar and spelling should be correct.
- Abbreviations with multiple meanings should be avoided. Each institution typically defines acceptable abbreviations.
- Personal opinions and comments criticizing or casting doubt on the professionalism of others should never be included in the chart.
- Documentation must be done at the time of the actual procedure or service. Entries never should be made in advance of performance of a task.
- All entries must be signed at the end and should include credentials (e.g., J.Wilson, RD).
- No one should ever chart or sign the medical record for another person.
- Late entries should be identified as such, including the actual date and time of the entry and the date and time it should have been recorded.

Medical record entries should always be legible. If an error is made, apply the following guidelines:

I. When making a correction, do not:
   A. Use White-Out, correction tape, or self-adhesive labels.
   B. Obliterate an entry by use of a thick marker or pen strokes.

FOCUS ON

Joint Commission on Accreditation of Healthcare Organizations (JCAHO)

The Joint Commission on Accreditation of Healthcare Organizations (JCAHO) is the predominant accrediting body that sets standards for health care. It seeks to improve the quality of patient care in various health settings, such as hospitals, long-term care organizations, health care networks, home care organizations, ambulatory care organizations, assisted living facilities, and organizations offering mental health services. This is accomplished through a set of standards, adherence to which is measured by formal facility surveys and evaluations. Accreditation by JCAHO is voluntary but is highly regarded in terms of its impact on third-party payment and its effect on confidence rating by the community, physician recruitment, and fulfillment of portions of state or federal licensure and certification requirements. To earn and maintain accreditation, an organization must undergo and pass an on-site survey by a JCAHO survey team at least every 3 years.

Accreditation focuses on the facility's actual performance of important governance, managerial, clinical, and support functions (i.e., those functions that directly affect the delivery of quality patient care). It also focuses on the continual improvement in an organization's performance of these functions. Standards are provided in an *Accreditation Manual for Hospitals* document, which is updated and revised on a yearly basis. This document consists of three sections: (1) patient-focused functions, (2) organization-focused functions, and (3) structures with functions. Its approach is a functional one, and all departments and disciplines must be familiar with relevant issues found in applicable chapters. Most chapters contain standards that affect the care provided by a dietitian.

The Care of the Patient section contains standards that apply specifically to medication use, rehabilitation, anesthesia, operative and other invasive procedures, and special treatments as well as nutritional care standards. The focus of nutritional care standards is the provision of appropriate nutritional care in a timely and effective manner using an interdisciplinary approach (i.e., involvement of physicians, registered dietitians, nurses, pharmacists, and other disciplines as appropriate).

Appropriate care is considered to include screening of patients for nutritional need, assessment and reassessment of patient needs, development of a nutritional care plan, ordering and communication of the diet order, preparation and distribution of the diet order, monitoring of the process, and continual reassessment and improvement of the nutrition care process. A facility can define who, when, where, and how the process is accomplished, but JCAHO specifies that a qualified dietitian must be involved in establishing this process. A plan for the delivery of nutritional care may be as simple as providing a regular diet for a patient who is not at nutritional risk or as complex as managing tube feedings in a ventilator-dependent patient, which involves the collaboration of multiple disciplines.

The accreditation process typically involves an on-site survey that lasts for several days. During this survey, adherence to standards is ascertained through interviews, review of documents (including patient medical records), and visits to patient care and other areas. Dietitians are actively involved in the survey process. Standards set by JCAHO play a large role in influencing the standards of care delivered to patients in all health care disciplines.

NUTRITION CARE RECORD

Name: Rm#:

MR#:

Age: Sex: Adm. Date: DOB:

MDs:

Consulting MD: Corrected age:

Ht: Adm. Wt: IBW: %IBW:

UBW: %UBW: ABW:

HC: NCHS% Wt: Ht: Wt/Ht: HC:

Wt Δ PTA:

Diet Rx PTA: Appetite:

Food allergies/Intolerances:

Adm Dx:

Current problems:

Current procedures/Surgery:

PmHx:

PSurgHx:

Current meds: IVF:

Home meds:

Miscellaneous: Constipation Diarrhea

Dentures ↓ ↑ Normal BM pattern ______________ Illiterate

Poor denture fit/teeth Date last BM PTA ______________ Ø speak Eng.

Blind Nursing home resident ______________ Lang. ______________

HOH Deaf Social Hx: ______________

Mobility ______________

Date	Task	Date	Task

Date	Comments	Diet

See Box 2-1, Chapter 2.

Protein ______________ gm/day

Fluid ______________ cc/day

Date	WBC / PLT	H/H	NA / K	CL / CO_2	BUN / CR	Gly / Hgb / Glu	OSMO	Ionized Ca / Ca	Mg / Phos	PAB / Alb	Chol / Trig	Bili / Alk Phos	AST / ALT	NH_3 / LDH	Amy / Lip			I/Os	Wt

Calorie Count Results															
	Date														
	Kcals														
	Protein														

#1058 (R 09/00) (1 of 2)

FIGURE 21-3 • The nutritional care record shows assessment data, the nutritional care plan, intervention strategies, and monitoring and evaluation data. *MR,* Medical record; *DOB,* date of birth; *IBW,* ideal body weight; *UBW,* usual body weight; *ABW,* adjusted body weight; *HC,* head circumference; *PTA,* prior to admission; *Dx,* diagnosis; *PmHx,* past medical history; *IVF,* intravenous fluid; *I/O,* intake/output. (Courtesy St. John's Hospital, Springfield, Ill.)

C. Add notes after the fact without accurately authenticating, dating, and referencing the original entry.
D. Remove the original and replace it with a copy.

II. Corrections at the time an entry is in progress should be handled as follows:
   A. Minor errors in transcription, spelling, one word, etc.: draw a single line through the error; then enter the correction, initial it, and date it.
   B. Other errors (e.g., an entry in the wrong chart)
      1. Draw a single line through the entry, or mark an "X" through the paragraph or page in error.
      2. Note "error" plus the date and time. Initial the correction.
         • Example: "~~The patient would not respond to questions regarding alcohol use.~~ Error 10/19/03 0900 JW"
   C. Omitted information
      1. Note "See addendum," beside the original entry, enter the date, and initial.
      2. Write the addendum in chart sequence. Identify it as an addendum and reference the original entry (e.g., "10/19/03 0900 Addendum to (progress) note of 10/18/03"). Continue entry and sign.

III. Corrections performed after the original entry (e.g., because an interval of time has elapsed during which the chart has been out of the recorder's possession) should follow the following guidelines:
   A. Minor errors in transcription, spelling, one word, etc.: draw a single line through the error, followed by the correction, date, time, and signature.
   B. Other errors, test results, misquoted orders, entry in wrong chart:
      1. Draw one line through the entry, or an "X" through the section or page.
      2. Note "error" plus the date and time. Sign the correction.

Format for Medical Record Charting

A tool frequently used for medical record documentation is the problem-oriented record. This record is organized according to the patient's primary problems. Entries into the medical record can be done in many styles. One of the most common forms is the SOAP note (**S**ubjective, **O**bjective, **A**ssessment, and **P**lan). Items to be included in each section are listed in Table 21-3.

TABLE 21-3 SOAP FORMAT

Subjective	Information provided by patient, family, or significant other Significant nutritional history Pertinent socioeconomic, cultural information Level of physical activity Current dietary intake (in terms of nutrients)
Objective	Factual, reproducible observations (e.g., anthropometric and laboratory data) Diagnosis Height, weight, and age Weight loss or weight gain patterns Desirable weight or realistic goal weight Pertinent clinical data (nausea, vomiting, diarrhea) Diet order Pertinent medications Calculation of nutrient needs
Assessment	Interpretation of the patient's status based on subjective and objective data Evaluation of the nutritional history as it pertains to medical condition Assessment of laboratory data as they apply to nutrition/hydration status Assessment of medications as they affect nutritional status Assessment of patient's comprehension and motivation, if appropriate Assessment of the diet order or feeding modality Anticipated problems or difficulties affecting patient compliance or adherence
Plan	Diagnostic studies needed Suggestions for gaining further pertinent data Further workup, data gathering, consultations to other health care providers, etc. Medical nutrition therapy goal Recommendations for nutritional care Discharge planning

An example of a SOAP note follows:

10/19/03 0900 NUTRITION SERVICES
S—Patient states that she "never eats fish and is allergic to milk." Some questions regarding eating at restaurants and sick days.
O—45-year-old white female; hx type 1 diabetes mellitus × 20 years. Admission dx: gastroparesis and GI discomfort. Ht. 65 inches, wt. 125 lb, fasting blood glucose—122 mg/dl; BUN 16. No other labs.
A—Patient is at a desirable weight. Demonstrates strong knowledge of diet related to diabetes and to milk allergy; uses nondairy sources of calcium. Would benefit from review of eating-out guidelines and sick days.
P—Review foods appropriate at restaurants or when traveling and on sick days.
J Wilson, RD

Other documentation styles include DAP (diagnosis, assessment, plan), PIE (problem, intervention, evaluation), PES (problem, etiology, symptoms), IER (intervention, evaluation, and revision), HOAP (history, observation, assessment, plan), SAP (screen, assess, plan), SOAPIER (subjective, objective, analysis/assessment, plan, intervention, evaluation and revisions), focus/DAR charting (a positive instead of negative perspective on a problem with data, action, response), and diagnostic charting (a clinical judgment about a patient that describes an actual or potential nutrition diagnosis but not a diagnosis of a

FOCUS ON

Coding for Malnutrition

Malnourished patients require nutritional attention to improve their medical outcomes and responsiveness to other therapies. By documenting malnutrition in a patient's medical record, the dietitian or other health care professional can bring attention to potential nutritional deficits or complications that may help the physician decide how, when, and where to intervene. The use of International Classification of Diseases (ICD-9) codes enables multiple practitioners to gather the requisite data and to identify the diagnoses and conditions to be addressed in the overall plan of care. Commonly, pulmonary, gastrointestinal, endocrine, mental disorders, and cancer can lead to malnutrition as a comorbidity factor. Codes frequently used to classify malnutrition include the following:*

260—kwashiorkor (severe protein deficiency; marked by changes in skin and hair pigment)
261—nutritional marasmus (severe tissue wasting or loss of subcutaneous fat)
262—other severe protein-calorie malnutrition (nutritional edema without mention of dyspigmentation of skin and hair)
263—other and unspecified protein-calorie malnutrition
263.0—malnutrition of a moderate degree
263.1—malnutrition of a mild degree
263.2—arrested development following protein-calorie malnutrition (nutritional dwarfism)
263.8—other protein-calorie malnutrition
263.9—unspecified protein-calorie malnutrition

Coordinated nutritional care and coding for malnutrition are important elements in patient services. Use of MNT guides, established by the ADA, may improve client outcomes. Identification of malnutrition leads to improved, cost-efficient treatment of patients and may also positively affect hospital reimbursement.

*Modified from the World Health Organization's International Classification of Diseases, ICD-9 at www.cdc.gov/nchs/htm.

disease). Outcome-focused documentation has been recognized for its ability to create outcome-oriented monitoring and evaluation, an important aspect for nutrition professionals.

The important factor is the content of the documentation, not necessarily the style. All entries made by the dietitian should address the issues of nutritional status and needs. Notes must be written efficiently, and they must be able to engage the physician and other health care team members to take action to achieve the desired nutrition care outcomes. MNT protocols and evidence-based guides for practice offer an alternative for charting that incorporates assessment and outcome data facilitating evidence of progress toward goals. *Focus On:* Coding for Malnutrition highlights key information that is helpful to include to ensure that malnutrition is adequately addressed in the patient's medical record (see also Appendix 3).

Electronic charting has been in existence for some time, but its use is rapidly becoming more common. Computer documentation can reduce duplication and repetition of information, save time, and offer new tools for decision making, such as providing prescription renewal reminders or potential drug interaction alerts for care providers. Brevity in charting, regardless of the style used, is important. In one study of the use of abbreviated charting style, physicians were found to implement brief dietitian recommendations more readily than lengthy ones (Grace-Farfaglia and Rosow, 1995). Figure 21-4 shows a format that documents both screening and assessment notes in an abbreviated style.

One last consideration for charting and use of medical records is the Health Information Portability and Accountability Act of 1996 (HIPAA), which states that all health care providers ensure the protection of patient privacy with HIPAA compliance (required by April 14, 2003). Patients must be notified if their medical information is to be shared in various places with different practitioners, insurance companies, or facilities.

INFLUENCES ON NUTRITIONAL CARE

The health care environment has undergone considerable change related to the provision of care and reimbursement in the past decade. Governmental influences, cost-containment issues, changing demographics, and the changing role of the patient as a "consumer" have influenced the health care arena. These changes in the delivery of health care have resulted in new parameters that affect the provision of MNT. Managed care organizations (MCOs) have changed health care reimbursement from a fee-for-service system to one in which fiscal risk is borne by health care organizations and physicians.

Managed Care Organizations

Managed care organizations (MCOs) finance and deliver care through a contracted network of providers

NUTRITION RISK ASSESSMENT

Date ____________ O. Admit date ____________ Diagnosis ____________

Time ____________ Ht. ________ Wt. ________ Sex: F M %IBW ____________

Albumin (date) ____________ Other pertinent labs: ____________

Diet order ____________

A. Nutritional Status

- ________ Insufficient data to complete risk assessment.
- ________ No detectable risk at this time.
- ________ At risk based on available data.
- ________ Potential for nutritional risk 2° to ____________ .
- ________ ____________ .

P.

- ________ Will reattempt reassessment within the next 5 days.
- ________ No identified need for nutrition intervention at this time. Patient will be reassessed in 7-10 days.
- ________ Patient will be assessed according to department standards (see below), and care plan recommendations and goals will be placed in the progress notes. (See Progress Notes Section.)

________ ____________

________ ____________ , R.D.

Followup Risk Assessment (See P. above)

Date	Not at Risk	At Risk	Comments	R.D.	Date	Not at Risk	At Risk	Comments	R.D.

COMPREHENSIVE NUTRITION ASSESSMENT

Date ____________ S. Usual wt. ____________ % Wt. change/time ____________

Time ____________ Diet PTA ____________ Previous diet educ. ____________

Eating/Digestive related problems: ____________

Other: ____________

O. PMH ____________

Pertinent labs ____________

Pertinent meds ____________

Other ____________

A. Assessment of visceral protein stores:

adequate ________ unable to assess ________

mild depletion ________ moderate depletion ________

severe depletion ________

Estimate needs: KCAL = ____________

protein = ____________

other nutrients ____________

Additional comments ____________

P. **See Nutrition Note in Progress Notes Section**

____________ , R.D.

CAROLINAS MEDICAL CENTER

DEPARTMENT OF DIETETICS
ADULT NUTRITION ASSESSMENT/REASSESSMENT

ADDRESSOGRAPH PLATE

FIGURE 21-4 • A nutritional chart format that includes both screening and assessment information. *PTA,* Prior to admission; *PMH,* past medical history; *HB,* Harris-Benedict; *SF,* stress factor. (Courtesy Carolinas Medical Center, Charlotte, N.C.)

in exchange for a monthly premium. Preferred provider organizations (PPOs), health maintenance organizations (HMOs), and MCOs have changed the face of health care in recent years.

Strategies of Managed Care Systems

Strategies used by MCOs, PPOs, and HMOs are intended to contain health care costs while providing efficient and effective care that is of consistently high quality. To accomplish this, practice guidelines (or standards of care) are often used. These sets of recommendations serve as a guide for defining appropriate care for a patient with a specific diagnosis or medical problem. They help to ensure consistency and quality for both providers and clients in a health care system and as such are specific to an institution or health care organization.

Case management is a process that strives to promote the achievement of patient care goals in a cost-effective, efficient manner. It is an essential component in MCO and HMO efforts toward delivering care in a manner that provides a positive experience for the patient and ensures achievement of clinical outcomes while using resources wisely. Case management involves assessing, evaluating, planning, implementing, coordinating, and monitoring care, especially in patients with chronic disease or those who are at high risk. Case management is most appropriate for patients who present a complex picture in terms of their health; economic status; and social, emotional, and psychological care, not necessarily in terms of the acuity or severity of their condition (Laramee, 1995).

Critical pathways are a key component in case management systems. They identify essential elements that should occur in the patient's care and define a time frame in which each activity should occur to maximize patient outcomes. Disease management is a disease-specific approach to patient care that focuses on the outpatient setting (Biesemeier, 1997). The goal is to prevent disease progression or exacerbations and to reduce the frequency and severity of disease symptoms and complications.

Education is an important component, as are other strategies that maximize compliance with disease treatment. Provision of education to a patient with type 1 diabetes regarding control of blood glucose levels would be an example of a disease management strategy; it is aimed at decreasing the complications associated with the disease (nephropathy, neuropathy, and retinopathy) and the frequency with which the client needs to access the care provider, especially on an emergent basis. Decreasing the number of emergency room visits related to hyperglycemic episodes would be a sample goal.

Utilization management is a system that strives for cost efficiency by eliminating or reducing unnecessary tests, procedures, and services. A manager is usually assigned to a group of patients and is responsible for ensuring adherence to preestablished criteria.

Payment Systems

One of the largest influences on health care delivery in the past decade has been the change in the method of payment for services provided. Several common methods of reimbursement exist: cost-based reimbursement, negotiated bids, and diagnostic related groups (DRGs). Under the DRG system, a facility receives payment for a patient's admission based on the principal diagnosis, secondary diagnosis (comorbid conditions), surgical procedure (if appropriate), and the age and sex of the patient.

About 500 DRGs cover the entire spectrum of medical diagnoses and surgical treatments. DRGs allow a hospital to receive the same amount for a specific stay regardless of the number of studies, procedures, or the length of stay. It is to the advantage of the facility to manage patient care prudently in these cases. Nutrition screening can be important in identifying patients who are malnourished or nutritionally compromised. Early identification of these factors allows timely intervention and helps to prevent the comorbidities often seen with malnutrition, which may cause the length of stay (and thus cost) to increase.

Patient-Focused Care

Patient-focused care (PFC) changes how care is delivered to a patient by focusing on the patient's needs and perspective rather than the caregiver's assumptions. It drastically reduces the number of persons with whom the patient comes in contact by decentralizing services and cross-training personnel in efforts to increase the continuity and quality of care provided. Hospitals have moved to PFC to overcome the fragmentation in care that has occurred as health care has become more specialized.

How PFC is delivered varies from institution to institution, but its basic elements focus on the patient's needs, cost-effectiveness of care, reduction in work steps, and more direct patient care. Team membership varies, but it usually includes both skilled (licensed) and unskilled (unlicensed) personnel. Cross-training is important in making the model work. Typically, only patient care services that require highly specialized expertise remain centralized.

Clinical dietitians may be centralized (part of a core nutrition department) or decentralized (individual dietitians are part of a specialized unit or service), depending on the model adopted by a specific institution. Certain departments, such as food service, accounting, and human resources, remain centralized in most models because some of the functions for which these departments are responsible are not directly related to patient care. Dietitians should be involved in the planning and instituting of patient care to ensure that MNT is considered part of any redesign of services.

NUTRITIONAL INTERVENTION AND DIET MODIFICATION

Therapeutic diets are based on a general, adequate diet, which has been modified as necessary to provide for individual requirements, such as digestive and absorptive capacity, alleviation or arrest of a disease process, and psychosocial factors. In general, the therapeutic diet should vary as little as possible from the patient's normal diet. Personal eating patterns and food preferences should be recognized, along with socioeconomic conditions, religious practices, and any environmental factors that influence food intake, such as where the meals are eaten and who prepares them (see Cultural Aspects of Dietary Planning in Chapter 15).

A nutritious and adequate diet can be planned in many ways. One foundation of such a diet is the Food Guide Pyramid (see Chapter 15). This is a basic plan; additional foods or more of the foods listed are included to provide additional energy and increase the intake of required nutrients for the individual. The *Dietary Guidelines for Americans* are also used in meal planning and to promote wellness. The latest revision includes seven key components related to health maintenance (see Chapter 15).

The dietary reference intakes (DRIs) and specific nutrient recommended dietary allowances (RDAs) are formulated for healthy persons, but they are also used as a basis for evaluating the adequacy of therapeutic diets. Nutrient requirements specific to a particular disease state or disorder must always be kept in mind during diet planning.

The Diet Prescription

The diet prescription designates the type, amount, and frequency of feeding based on the patient's disease process and disease management goals. The prescription may specify a caloric level to be implemented. It may also limit or increase various components of the diet, such as carbohydrate, protein, fat, specific vitamins or minerals, fiber, or water.

Energy Allowance

Appetite regulates body weight with surprising accuracy in most normally active people; however, it is not always valid or reliable in disease. Energy needs may be calculated by a variety of methods. When necessary, actual measurement of the basal or resting metabolic rate using a metabolic cart and indirect calorimetry can be very useful (see Chapter 2).

A person's energy requirement can be calculated by either (1) calculating the required number of kilocalories per day or (2) calculating the percentage increase over basal metabolic demands. To make these determinations, the patient's desirable weight, based on sex, age, height, and body build (frame), is determined. The weight parameter that should be used for calculating nutritional needs is often debated. Desirable weight is generally used rather than actual weight because it may result in miscalculation of needs due to undernutrition or overnutrition. An exception is made, however, for extremely malnourished patients. In these cases, actual weight is used because overfeeding could occur if desirable weight is used.

The basal energy expenditure (BEE) is calculated by using one of the methods described in Chapter 2. A physical activity factor then is added based on the specific needs of the patient. Also, a factor may be added if the patient is under physiologic stress (see Chapter 42).

Patients with mild stress, such as those undergoing uncomplicated surgery, may require additional energy, up to 20% over their REE. Those with multiple fractures or trauma are considered to be under moderate stress and may require additional calories. Acute major infections or burns may increase the need for energy intake to 100% over basal requirements. When calculating needs, it should be remembered that even the most hypermetabolic patients usually do not require more than 35 to 40 kcal per kilogram of body weight for anabolism. Sections of this text dealing with disease states review energy needs related to specific conditions or illnesses.

Protein Allowance

The RDA for protein for age is usually considered adequate for previously well-nourished persons who are ambulatory or who require only brief periods of hospitalization. The minimum level of protein needed to maintain nitrogen balance in healthy adults is 0.5 g per kilogram of body weight daily. In the presence of malabsorption or protein loss from burns, exudates, or ascites, an increase in protein allowance is required. Infection, fever, trauma, burns, and surgery also increase protein catabolism and may necessitate provision of additional protein. Sections of this text dealing with disease states review protein needs related to specific conditions and illnesses.

Minerals and Vitamins

Appropriate levels of vitamins and minerals for stressed patients are difficult to accurately determine. In times of stress, inadequacies of nutrients may be countered with mobilization of body stores, decreased losses, increased absorption, or improved utilization. Individual responses vary, and true deficiencies with clinical signs and symptoms may take weeks, months, or even years to develop. Biochemical measurements for identifying inadequacies at early stages are still being developed (see Chapter 18).

To determine appropriate levels of vitamin and mineral intakes, the following should be considered: (1) requirements for healthy persons; (2) the nature of the disease or injury; (3) body stores of specific nutrients; (4) normal and abnormal losses through the skin, urine, or intestinal tract; and (5) drug-nutrient interactions (see Chapter 19). These factors are discussed further in the chapters relating to nutritional care for various disease states.

Fluids

A healthy adult at rest who is not perspiring needs 1800 to 2500 ml daily (2+ quarts) of water (or approximately 1 ml per kilocalorie consumed) to provide for urinary excretion and replace insensible fluid losses. Optimal convalescence demands adequate tissue hydration. Additional fluids must be given to replace water lost by excessive perspiration, vomiting, diarrhea, tube drainage, or other conditions marked by increased water loss. If sufficient water cannot be taken in orally, it must be supplied parenterally, usually along with electrolytes (see Chapter 6).

Modifications of the Normal Diet

Normal nutrition is the foundation on which therapeutic diet modifications are based. Regardless of the type of diet prescribed, the purpose of the diet is to supply needed nutrients to the body in a form it can handle. Adjustment of the diet may take any of the following forms:

1. Change in consistency of foods (liquid diet, soft diet, low-fiber diet, high-fiber diet)
2. Increase or decrease in energy value of diet (weight-reduction diet, high-calorie diet)
3. Increase or decrease in the type of food or nutrient consumed (sodium-restricted diet, lactose-restricted diet, high-fiber diet, high-potassium diet)
4. Elimination of specific foods (allergy diet, gluten-free diet)
5. Adjustment in the level, ratio, or balance of protein, fat, and carbohydrate (diet for diabetes, ketogenic diet, renal diet, cholesterol-lowering diet)
6. Rearrangement of the number and frequency of meals (diet for diabetes, postgastrectomy diet)
7. Change in the route of delivery of nutrients (enteral or parenteral nutrition)

Foods as Nutrient Sources

Evaluation of general and modified diets requires knowledge of the nutrients contained in different foods. In particular, it is helpful to be aware of nutrient-dense foods that contribute to dietary adequacy. (Chapters 4 and 5 provide more detailed information about specific minerals and vitamins and the foods that contain them.) Often, a vitamin-mineral supplement is necessary to meet the patient's needs when the diet is limited.

NUTRITIONAL CARE FOR THE HOSPITALIZED PATIENT

Food is an important part of nutritional care. Attempts should be made to honor patient preferences (including cultural preferences), provide a pleasant atmosphere, and arrange for assistance with eating when needed. Imagination and ingenuity in menu planning are essential when planning meals acceptable to a varied patient population. Attention to color, texture, composition, and temperature of the foods, coupled with a sound knowledge of therapeutic diets, is required for menu planning. To the patient, however, good taste and attractive presentation are the most important elements. When it is possible, patient selection of menus results in the delivery of food that will most likely be consumed. The ability to make food selections gives the patient an option in an otherwise limiting environment.

Standard Hospital or Health Care Diets

All hospitals and health care institutions have basic, routine diets designed for uniformity and convenience of service. These standard diets are based on the foundation of an adequate diet pattern, with nutrient levels as derived from the RDAs. The diets should be as realistic as possible and yet ensure that nutritional needs of patients are met. The most important consideration of the type of diet offered is providing foods that the patient is willing and able to eat and that fit in with any required dietary restrictions (if any). The shortened lengths of stay in many health care settings often result in the need to optimize intake of calories and protein and often translate into a relatively liberal approach to therapeutic diets. This is especially true when the therapeutic restrictions might compromise intake and subsequent recovery from surgery, stress, or illness. More specific modifications for diets are found in the respective chapters.

Types of standard diets vary but can be categorized as general, soft or modified consistency, or liquid. These diets are used routinely for patients and serve as a foundation for more diversified therapeutic diets. Table 21-4 summarizes the basic hospital or health care facility diets and their components.

Regular Diet

In some institutions, a diet that has no restrictions is referred to as the "regular" or "house" diet. It is used when the patient's medical condition does not warrant any limitations. This diet is a basic, adequate, general diet of approximately 1600 to 2200 kcal; it usually contains 60 to 80 g of protein, 80 to 100 g of fat, and 180 to 300 g of carbohydrate. Although this diet has no particular food restrictions, some facilities have instituted regular diets that are low in fat, saturated fat, cholesterol, sugar, and salt to follow the dietary recommendations for the general population (Singer et al, 1996). In other facilities, the diet focuses on providing foods the patient is willing and able to eat, with less focus on restriction of nutrients. Many institutions have a selective menu that allows the patient certain choices; the adequacy of the diet will vary based on the patient's selection.

Soft Diet

The soft diet, described in Table 21-5, is used as a transition between a liquid and regular diet. It is moderately low in cellulose and connective tissue and low in residue. The soft diet can be prescribed for postoperative patients or for those with gastrointestinal problems. It is not appropriate for patients whose dentition is poor; these patients require a mechanically altered diet. The soft diet is most useful when the selection of food is guided by the patient's tolerance.

The average composition of the soft diet is 1800 to 2000 kcal; however, energy levels as well as protein, fat, and carbohydrate levels will vary based on menu selection, patient preferences, and other restrictions that may be imposed.

Liquid Diets

Liquid diets are sometimes ordered for patients with conditions that require nourishment that is easily digested and consumed or that has minimal residue. Such diets are often prescribed for a brief period for patients undergoing diagnostic tests or in preparation for, or immediately following, surgery. Chewing or swallowing difficulties or dental wiring may also necessitate a liquid diet. The two varieties of oral liquid diets are the clear liquid diet and the full liquid diet.

TABLE 21-4 Summary of Basic Hospital Diets

FOOD	GENERAL, ADEQUATE, OR "HOUSE" DIET	SOFT DIET	FULL LIQUID DIET	CLEAR LIQUID DIET
Milk, cream, buttermilk	Included	Included	Included	Not included
Eggs	Pasteurized or cooked	Included	In beverages (eggnog)	Not included
Cheese	All varieties	Cottage, cream, mildly flavored cheeses	Not included	Not included
Fats	All kinds	Butter, margarine, oil, mayonnaise, and mildly seasoned dressings	Butter, margarine, oil	Not included
Meat, fish, poultry	All included	Tender beef, lamb, veal; liver, bacon, fish and poultry	Not included	Not included
Vegetables	All included	Cooked or canned vegetables of low fiber; tender lettuce; vegetable juices	Vegetable juices, vegetable purée used in soups	
Fruits	All included	Fruit juices, ripe bananas, cooked fruit without skin or seeds	Fruit juices, fruitades	Strained fruit juices, fruitades
Breads	All varieties	Refined grain products, rye without seeds, refined crackers	Not included	Not included
Cereals	All varieties	Refined cereals	Cooked, refined cereals	Not included
Cereal products	All varieties	Cooked macaroni, spaghetti, noodles, white rice	Not included	Not included
Soups	All varieties	Clear broth, consommé; cream and vegetable soups containing allowed items	Clear broth, consommé; strained vegetable and cream soups	Clear broth, consommé
Beverages	All kinds	All kinds	Tea, decaffeinated or regular coffee, carbonated beverages, eggnog	Tea, decaffeinated coffee, carbonated beverages
Desserts	All kinds	Plain puddings, yogurt, simple cakes and cookies, frozen desserts without nuts, custard, gelatin	Plain gelatin dessert, ice cream or yogurt without nuts and seeds, ices, sherbets, soft custard, pudding	Plain gelatin desserts and ices
Other			Liquid supplements	Elemental liquids

Clear Liquid Diet

The clear liquid diet (Table 21-6) is occasionally used as preparation for endoscopic or colonscopic evaluations and in acute gastrointestinal disturbances (ADA Manual of Clinical Dietetics, 1998). This diet furnishes fluids, some electrolytes, and small amounts of energy; it consists of clear liquids, such as tea, broth, carbonated beverages, clear fruit juices, and gelatin. Milk and liquids prepared with milk are omitted, as are fruit juices that contain pulp. Carbonated beverages, such as ginger ale, and hot beverages, such as tea and broth, are usually well tolerated. The average clear liquid diet contains 500 to 600 kcal, 5 to 10 g of protein, minimal fat, 120 to 130 g of carbohydrate, and small amounts of sodium and potassium. It is inadequate in calories, fiber, and all other essential nutrients and should be used only for short periods.

The clear liquid diet is not sufficient to replace the electrolytes lost in vomitus and diarrheal fluid. Electrolytes are often replaced via intravenous fluids until the diet can be advanced to a more nutritionally adequate one. Although little scientific evidence has been established to support the use of clear liquid diets as transition diets immediately postoperatively (Jeffery et al, 1996), they are often used in that capacity. When a clear liquid is ordered for prolonged periods, an appropriate commercially prepared low-residue, lactose-free or elemental formula with added vitamins and minerals can be selected from the formulas presented in Appendixes 36 through 41 to improve the adequacy of the diet.

Full Liquid Diet

The full liquid diet, presented in Table 21-7, is comprised of foods that are liquid or semiliquid at room or body temperature. For example, ice cream and gelatin are both included in a full liquid diet. The diet is used for patients who are unable to chew, swallow, or digest solid foods because it is easily consumed and digested. With proper design, the diet can be adequate for maintenance requirements, except for fiber. The average full liquid diet contains 1000 to 1500 kcal, with 45 to 50 g of protein, 50 to 65 g of fat, and 150 to 170 g of carbohydrates; if snacks are included, nutrients can be increased significantly. With careful planning, the diet can be increased in protein and caloric value to equal a regular or even a high-calorie diet. These changes are necessary when the diet must be continued for a protracted period. Protein and vitamin supplements can be added to increase the nutrient content. Because this diet is inadequate in fiber, constipation may result from prolonged use. A fiber-containing formula or a fiber supplement may be useful for some patients. Full liquid diets can be planned to meet the needs of a patient with diabetes, renal disease, or other disorders. Lactose-free products are available for patients requiring a lactose-free liquid diet (see Appendixes 36-41).

TABLE 21-5 Soft Diet

MEAL PLAN	SAMPLE MENU	SERVING SIZE
Breakfast		
Fruit	Orange juice	½ cup
Cereal	Cooked farina	½ cup (cooked weight)
Egg	Poached egg	1
Bread	Toast	1 slice
Butter	Butter or margarine	1 pat
Milk	Milk (2%)	1 cup
Sugar	Sugar	3 tsp
Coffee	Coffee	2 cups
Lunch		
Soup	Tomato consommé	½ cup
Entrée	Baked macaroni and cheese	1 cup
Vegetables	Cooked asparagus tips	½ cup
Bread	White bread	1 slice
Butter	Butter or margarine	1 pat
Fruit	Applesauce	½ cup
Milk	Milk (2%)	1 cup
Dinner		
Meat	Chicken breast	3 oz
Potato	Mashed potato	½ cup
Vegetable	Buttered spinach	½ cup
Bread	White bread	1 slice
Butter	Butter or margarine	1 pat
Dessert	Chocolate ice cream, ice milk, or frozen yogurt	½ cup
Milk	Milk (2%)	1 cup

Nutrient content: kcal: 1850; pro(g): 92; CHO(g): 228; fat(g): 65.

TABLE 21-6 Clear Liquid Diet

MEAL PLAN	SAMPLE MENU	SERVING SIZE
Breakfast		
Fruit juice	Apple juice	½ cup
Beverage	Coffee (decaffeinated)	2 cups
Sugar	Sugar	2 tsp
AM Snack		
Fruitade	Lemonade	1 cup
Lunch		
Soup	Beef broth	½ cup
Fruit juice	Grape juice	½ cup
Tea	Tea	2 cups
Sugar	Sugar	2 tsp
Fruit ice	Cherry fruit ice	½ cup
PM Snack		
Carbonated beverage	Gingerale	1 cup
Dinner		
Fruit juice	Fruit punch	½ cup
Soup	Chicken broth	½ cup
Gelatin	Raspberry gelatin	¼ cup
Tea	Tea	2 cups
Sugar	Sugar	2 tsp
Evening Snack		
Fruit juice	Cranberry juice	1 cup

Nutrient content: kcal: 785; pro(g): 5; CHO(g): 193; fat(g): <2.

TABLE 21-7 Full Liquid Diet

MEAL PLAN	SAMPLE MENU	SERVING SIZE
Breakfast		
Fruit	Orange juice	½ cup
Cereal	Cooked farina	1 cup (cooked weight)
Supplement	Commercial eggnog	1 cup
Butter	Butter or margarine	2 tsp
Milk	Milk (2%)	1 cup
Sugar	Sugar	2 tsp
Coffee or tea	Coffee or tea	1 cup
AM Snack		
Supplement	Commercial milkshake (chocolate)	1 cup
Lunch		
Soup	Cream of potato soup (strained) with margarine/butter	1 cup
Fruit	Pineapple juice	½ cup
Milk	Milk (2%)	1 cup
	Vanilla pudding	½ cup
Coffee or tea	Coffee or tea	1 cup
Sugar	Sugar	2 tsp
PM Snack		
Supplement	Commercial milkshake (strawberry)	1 cup
Dinner		
Fruit	Apple juice	½ cup
Soup	Cream of mushroom (strained) with margarine/butter	1 cup
Supplement	Commercial milkshake	1 cup
Milk	Ice cream	½ cup
Coffee or tea	Coffee or tea	1 cup
Sugar	Sugar	2 tsp
Bedtime (h.s.) Snack		
Gelatin	Gelatin, strawberry	½ cup
Supplement	Commercial milkshake (vanilla)	1 cup

Nutrient content: kcal: 2850; pro(g): 77; CHO(g): 422; fat(g): 99.

Consistency Modifications

Further modifications in consistency may be needed for patients who have limited chewing or swallowing ability. Chopping, mashing, pureeing, or grinding food will modify its texture. (See Chapter 43 for more information on consistency modifications.)

Food Intake

Food as served does not necessarily match the actual intake of the patient. Prevention of iatrogenic malnutrition in the health care setting requires observation and monitoring of the adequacy of patient intake. If food intake is inadequate, measures should be taken to provide foods or supplements that may be better accepted or tolerated. Regardless of the type of diet prescribed, both the food served and the amount actually eaten must be considered to obtain an accurate determination of the patient's energy and nutrient intake. Nourishments and calorie-containing beverages consumed between meals are also considered in the overall intake. Calorie counts or diet analyses are often ordered in hospitalized patients to quantify the actual food and nutrient intake of the patient. Good records of intake require a systemized data collection procedure that typically involves nursing and nutrition and food service personnel.

Psychological Factors

Meals and between-meal nourishments are often highlights of the day and are anticipated with pleasure by the patient. Mealtime should be as positive an experience as possible. Whatever setting the patient is eating in should be comfortable for the patient. Food intake in a pleasant room is encouraged, with the patient in a comfortable eating position in bed or sitting in a chair located away from unpleasant sights or odors. Eating with others often promotes better intake.

Arrangement of the tray should reflect consideration of the patient's needs. Dishes and utensils should be in a convenient location. Independence should be encouraged in those who require assistance with eating. The caregiver can accomplish this by asking patients to specify the sequence of foods to be eaten and having them participate in eating, if only by holding their bread. Even visually impaired persons can eat unassisted if they are told where to find foods on the tray. Patients who require feeding assistance should be fed when the foods are still at an optimal temperature. The feeding process requires about 20 minutes as a general rule.

Rejection of meals or the prescribed diet frequently reflects a negative patient attitude toward the illness and hospitalization. Other reasons for poor acceptance may be unfamiliar foods, a change in eating schedule, improper food temperatures, the patients' medical condition, or the effects of medical therapy. Food acceptance is improved when personal selection of menus is encouraged. Patients should be given the opportunity to share concerns regarding meals; this may improve acceptance and intake.

In encouraging acceptance of a therapeutic diet, the attitude of the caregiver is important. The nurse who understands that the diet contributes to the restoration of the patient's health will communicate this conviction by actions, facial expressions, and conversation. Patients who understand that the diet is important to the success of their recovery and therapy usually accept it more willingly.

When the patient must adhere to a therapeutic dietary program indefinitely, an interdisciplinary approach will help the patient achieve nutritional goals. Because they have frequent contact with patients, nurses have an important role in a patient's acceptance of nutritional care. Ensuring that the nursing staff is aware of the nutrition care plan can greatly improve the probability of success.

Nutritional Counseling

Nutritional counseling is an important part of the MNT provided to many patients. The goal of counseling is to help the patient acquire the knowledge and skills needed to make changes, including modifying behavior to facilitate sustained change. Nutritional counseling and resultant dietary changes implemented by the patient result in many benefits. One of the most important benefits is the control of the disease or symptoms, but others, such as improved health status, improved quality of life, and decreased health care costs, may also result when dietary changes are successful. As the average length of hospital stays has decreased, the role of the dietitian in counseling inpatients has changed to providing "survival" skills. These survival skills include basic types of foods to limit, timing of meals, and portion sizes. Follow-up outpatient counseling regarding details of the diet should reinforce the basic counseling given during hospitalization. See Chapter 22 for detailed information on counseling.

NUTRITIONAL CARE OF THE TERMINALLY ILL OR HOSPICE PATIENT

Maintenance of comfort and quality of life are most typically the goals of nutritional care for the terminally ill patient. Dietary restrictions are rarely appropriate. Nutritional care should be mindful of strategies that facilitate symptom and pain control. Recognition of the various phases of dying—denial, anger, bargaining, depression, and acceptance—will help the health care practitioner understand the patient's response to food and nutrition support.

The decision about when life support should be terminated often involves the issue of whether to continue enteral or parenteral nutrition. With advance directives, the patient can advise family and health care team members of his or her individual preferences with regard to end-of-life issues. Food and hydration issues may be discussed, such as whether or not tube feeding should be initiated or discontinued and under what circumstances. Nutrition support should be continued as long as the patient is competent to make this choice (or if specified in the patient's advance directives).

Palliative care encourages the alleviation of physical symptoms, anxiety, and fear while attempting to maintain the patient's ability to function independently. Hospice home care programs allow the patient to stay at home and delay or avoid hospital admission. Quality of life is the critical component. A dietitian's intervention may benefit the patient and family as they adjust to issues related to the approaching death. Families who might be accustomed to a modified diet should be reassured if they are uncomfortable about easing dietary restrictions. Ongoing communication and explanations to the family are important and helpful.

DISCHARGE PLANNING AND HOME CARE

Nutritional care continues as a part of discharge planning when the patient returns home or goes to a long-term care facility or rehabilitation center. Education, counseling, and mobilization of resources to provide home care and nutrition support are included as components of discharge procedures. Completing a discharge nutritional summary for the next caregiver is imperative for optimal care. Appropriate discharge documentation includes a summary of nutritional therapies and outcomes; pertinent information such as weights, laboratory values, and dietary intake; potential drug-nutrient interactions; expected progress or prognosis; and recommendations for follow-up services (Figure 21-5). The amount and type of instruction given, the patient's comprehension of the instruction, and the expected degree of adherence to the prescribed diet must be included. An effective discharge plan increases the likelihood of a positive outcome for the patient.

A variety of resources, including home health care agencies, are available to provide services related to nutrition, including enteral or parenteral nutrition at

Clinical Scenario

Bill, a 47-year-old man, 6 feet 2 inches tall and weighing 200 lb, is admitted to the hospital with chest pain. Three days after admission, during the nutrition screening process, it is discovered that Bill has gained 30 lb over the past 2 years. Review of the medical record reveals the following laboratory data: low-density lipoprotein (LDL) 240 (desirable <130), high-density lipoprotein (HDL) 30 (desirable >65), and triglycerides 350 (desirable <200). Blood pressure is 120/85. Current medications: multivitamin/mineral daily. Cardiac catherization is scheduled for tomorrow.

1. What other information do you need to develop a nutritional care plan?
2. Was nutrition screening completed in a timely manner? Discuss the implications of timing of screening versus implementing care.
3. Develop a SOAP note based on the preceding information and the interview with the patient.
4. What nutrition care goals would you develop for this patient during his hospital stay?
5. What goals would you develop for this patient after discharge? Discuss how the type of health care insurance coverage the patient has might influence this plan.

DISCHARGE SUMMARY

Name ____________________ Discharge date ____________________

Hospital number ____________________ Admission date ____________________

Age ________ Sex ________ Diagnosis ____________________

Anthropometrics: Ht. ________ Wt.: ________ Admit Wt.: ________ DC Wt.: ________

Usual Wt. ____________ Activity level ____________________

Laboratory Albumin: ____________ Prealbumin: ____________________

Other ____________________

Diet: Estimated needs: ____________ kcal ________ g pro

____________ kcal/kg ________ g/kg

Current diet: ____________________ Nutritional supplements ____________________

Major nutritional problems:

Ongoing: Follow-up recommendations:

Resolved:

FIGURE 21-5 • Discharge summary. (Courtesy University of Washington Medical Centers, Seattle, Wash.)

FOCUS ON

A Standardized Model for Providing Nutrition Care

In 1998 the ADA formed the Health Services Research (HSR) task force to explore research on the outcomes and effectiveness of medical nutrition therapy (MNT). The HSR task force found that the lack of a specified nutrition care process and lack of a common definition for nutrition care were obstacles that needed to be overcome to move forward. In 1999 a model of nutrition care was formulated and a core set of outcome measures that could be used in outcomes research was identified. This Nutrition Care Model has three components: (1) trigger event—the "where" and "how" of identification of a patient or client as a candidate for nutrition care; (2) nutrition care process—the essential components of nutrition care are identified; and (3) nutrition-related outcomes—results noted after the provision of nutrition care; these results may be produced by or influenced by the care (Splett and Myers, 2001).

In this model, the nutrition care process includes MNT as provided by registered dietitians. It stresses interaction with the patient or client with the goal of optimizing nutritional status, health, and well-being.

The proposed model (Figure 21-6) will continue to evolve, but it sets the stage for a universal model of care that guides the dietetics profession.

home. Follow-up monitoring may be needed to provide continuity of care in the new setting or to ensure a smooth transition back to the original health care site, if readmission becomes necessary.

Regardless of the setting the patient is discharged to, effective discharge planning begins on day 1 of a hospital or nursing home stay and continues throughout the institutionalization. The patient should be included in every step of the planning process whenever possible to ensure that the decisions made by the health care team reflect the desires of the patient.

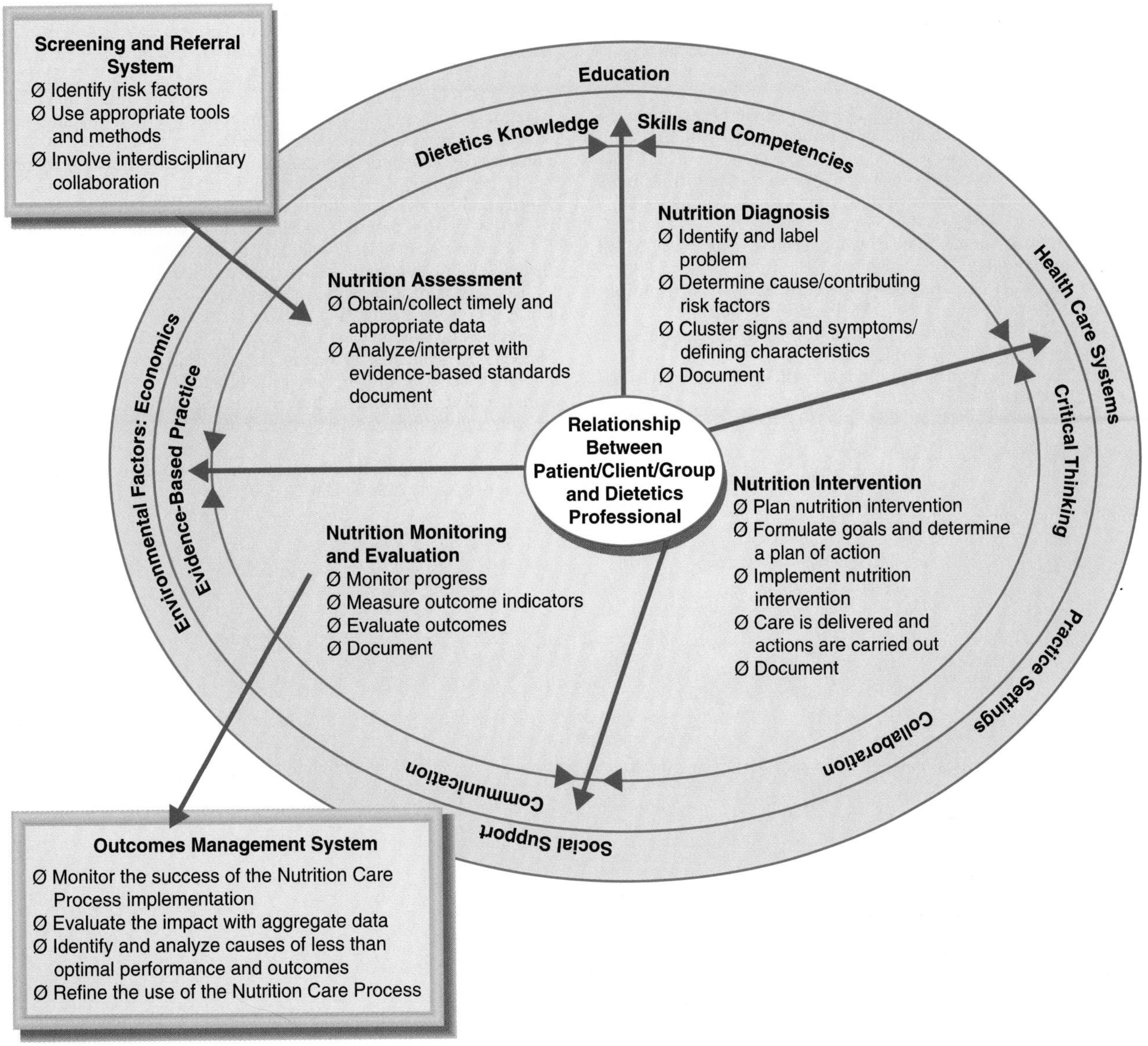

FIGURE 21-6 • Nutrition care model. (From American Dietetic Association: Nutrition care process and model: ADA adopts roadmap to quality care and outcomes management, *J Am Diet Assoc* 103:1061, 2003.)

SUMMARY

The astute dietetics professional provides nutrition care in a predictable, stepwise manner to provide services that meet the needs of clients. A standardized model is required by federal law for MNT that is reimbursed. Use of the model will help to achieve the best possible outcomes for all parties (see *Focus On:* A Standardized Model for Providing Nutrition Care).

Relevant Web Sites

American Dietetic Association
www.eatright.org
Benedictine University Nutrition Department
www.nutrition4living.org
Joint Commission on Accreditation
www.jchao.org
Managed Care Information Center
www.themcic.com/
Tufts University Nutrition
www.navigator.tufts.edu

Cited References

American Dietetic Association: *Medical nutrition therapy protocols,* ed 2, Chicago, 1998, American Dietetic Association.

American Dietetic Association: *Manual of clinical dietetics,* ed 5, Chicago, 1998, American Dietetic Association.

Biesemeier C: Case manager/registered dietitian partnerships: teaming up to achieve positive patient outcomes, *J Care Manage* 3:72, 1997.

Grace-Farfaglia P, Rosow P: Automating clinical dietetics documentation, *J Am Diet Assoc* 95:688, 1995.

Grant A, DeHoog S: *Nutrition assessment support and management,* ed 5, Seattle, 1999, Grant-DeHoog.
International Classification of Diseases: Clinical Modification Tabular List, ed 9, Washington, DC, 1980, U.S. Department of Health and Human Services.
Jeffery KM et al: The clear liquid diet is no longer necessary in the routine postoperative management of surgical patients, *Am J Surg* 62:167, 1996.
Klein CJ et al: Physicians prefer goal-oriented note format more than three to one over other outcome focused documentation, *J Am Diet Assoc* 97:1306, 1997.
Laramee S: Case management: an overview, *Clin Nutr Mgmt Newslett* 14 (4):1, 1995.
Meyers EF et al: Evidence-based practice guides vs. protocols: what's the difference? *J Am Diet Assoc* 101:1085, 2001.
Singer AJ et al: The nutritional value of university-hospital diets [Letter], *N Engl J Med* 335:1466, 1996.
Splett P, Meyers E: A proposed model for effective nutrition care, *J Am Diet Assoc* 101:357, 2001.

Additional References

American Dietetic Association: Position on management of health care food and nutrition services, *J Am Diet Assoc* 97:1427, 1997.
Biesemeier C, Chima C: Computerized patient record: are we ready for our future practice? *J Am Diet Assoc* 97:1099, 1997.
Escott-Stump S: *Nutrition and diagnosis-related care,* ed 5, Philadelphia, 2002, Lippincott Williams & Wilkins.
Lacey K, Cross N: A problem-based nutrition care model that is diagnostic driven and allows for monitoring and managing outcomes, *J Am Diet Assoc* 102:578, 2002.
Laramee SH: Nutrition services in managed care: new paradigms for dietitians, *J Am Diet Assoc* 96:335, 1996.
Moreland K et al: Development and implementation of the clinical privileges for dietitian nutrition order writing program at a long-term acute-care hospital, *J Am Diet Assoc* 102:72, 2002.
Page G et al: Developing key-feature problems and examinations to assess clinical decision-making skills, *Acad Med* 70:194, 1995.
Rosal MC et al: Facilitating dietary change: the patient-centered counseling model, *J Am Diet Assoc* 101:332, 2001.
Sandrick K: Is nutritional diagnosing a critical step in the nutrition care process? *J Am Diet Assoc* 102:427, 2002.
Simko MD et al: *Nutrition assessment: a comprehensive guide for planning intervention,* ed 2, Gaithersburg, Md, 1995, Aspen Publishers.
Vickery CE et al: Use and barriers to use of laboratory data by clinical dietitians, *Hosp Top* 79:13, 2001.

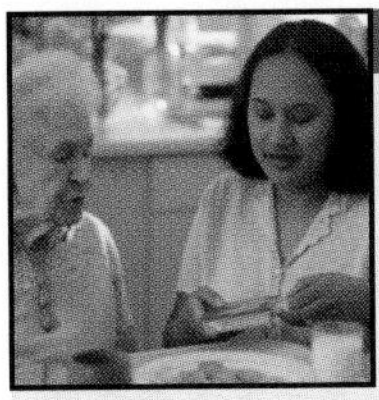

CHAPTER 22

Counseling for Change

LINDA G. SNETSELAAR, BS, MS, PhD, RD

CHAPTER OUTLINE

- Counseling Techniques
- Stages of Change
- Activities That Facilitate Behavior Change
- Intervention Model
- Not-Ready-to-Change Counseling Sessions
- Ready-to-Change Counseling Sessions
- Resistance Behaviors and Potential Strategies to Modify Them

KEY TERMS

affirming–telling a patient that what he or she is doing is normal and understandable given the circumstances; supporting the patient's change efforts

alignment–supportive statement telling a patient that the counselor understands and is with him or her in difficult times

ambivalence–when a patient has mixed feelings about change-modifying behaviors that are difficult

cognitive-behavioral therapy–therapy in which maladaptive thoughts (cognitions) are modified; problem-solving and coping skills are enhanced

discrepancy–strategy that identifies conflicting feelings when change results in both positive and negative consequences

double-sided reflection–statement from the counselor describing a discrepancy between the patient's current and previous words that provides ideas for open discussion to facilitate change

empathy–technique by which the counselor accepts a patient's feelings of turmoil about making changes

motivational interviewing–counseling style designed to achieve the willingness to change within a patient; responsibility is assigned to the patient, but counselor style is persuasive and supportive

negotiation–strategy whereby the patient and counselor interaction allows compromise designed to achieve a specific goal

normalization–statement indicating that the patient's behavior is perfectly within reason and normal; validates the patient's reaction to a given situation

reflective listening–given information from the patient, the counselor comments on how he or she feels; promotes understanding on the part of the counselor

reframing–strategy whereby the counselor changes the patient's interpretation of the same basic data that he or she has given and offers a new viewpoint

self-efficacy–when a patient believes in his or her ability to carry out change

self-management–strategy whereby the counselor facilitates the ability to change through the patient's decisions

self-monitoring–recording by the patient of behavior changes

social marketing–application of commercial marketing techniques to programs with intent to influence the voluntary behavior of target audiences

stages of change or transtheoretical model–describes behavior change as a process in which individuals progress through a series of six distinct stages: precontemplation, contemplation, preparation, action, maintenance, and relapse

Every person comes from a "community." Within the community, health behaviors and responses are often programmed by family and peers. The concept of social marketing goes beyond the individual, using the concept of traditional marketing to "sell" healthy behaviors to groups. Some behaviors are affected by demographics, geographic location, usual behaviors, attitudes and beliefs, and psychographic factors of lifestyle, values, and perceived norms.

Behavior does not occur in a vacuum. When a person makes a lifestyle change, he or she is giving up something; adapting new behaviors entails "costs" and "benefits." In communities where individual health care providers and the mass media promote healthy habits, there may be more impetus for people to make changes (Hunt et al, 2001; Seigel and Donner, 1998). Despite considerable variability, nutrition advice is given in about one fourth of all office visits to family physicians; efforts to focus nutrition counseling on high-risk patients may increase the impact (Eaton et al, 2002).

Knowing which methods are most effective is a step in the right direction for the nutrition counselor. For purposes of this text, the models for behavioral change will emphasize individual internal change processes rather than sociocultural and physical environmental influences. The individual patient's or client's expectations, beliefs, self-perception, and goals give shape to the counseling session.

COUNSELING TECHNIQUES

People are motivated to change through their ability to self-manage behaviors. The nutrition counselor sets up an environment that is a transient support system to prepare the patient to handle social and personal demands more effectively while providing favorable conditions for change. Different strategies may be used to offer guidance. One style is cognitive-behavioral therapy (Dobson, 1998), which assumes that thinking affects behavior; that relevant beliefs may be identified and altered; and that desired behavior change may be achieved through changes in thinking (cognition).

Motivational interviewing, initially developed for addiction counseling, has increasingly been applied in public health, medical, and health promotion settings (Resnicow et al, 2002). By using motivational interviewing techniques, the counselor can help the patient move from the precontemplation stage, through the contemplation stage, to the preparation stage, where plans for change can be made (Mallin, 2002). Motivational interviewing helps the client recognize and do something about concerns and problems (Miller and Rollnick, 2002). The client is responsible for making the change. The goal is to increase the client's intrinsic motivation so that he or she can express the rationale for the changes. Persuasion and support are key elements of this style of counseling.

The following concepts are important to consider in facilitating dietary changes (Miller and Rollnick, 2002):

- People make behavioral changes only when they are ready to change.
- The nutrition intervention, including both the content and nutritionist's style, is a powerful determinant of resistance and denial, as well as motivation, in persons who want to make changes in their diet.
- People cycle through different phases of changing and maintaining their dietary modifications.
- Different interventions are needed for persons who are in different phases of motivation.
- Ambivalence is a key block that can be resolved through intervention.
- Resistance and denial get in the way of meeting behavioral goals.

STAGES OF CHANGE

The transtheoretical model, also referred to as the stages of change model, describes behavior change as a process in which individuals progress through a series of six distinct stages of change, as shown in Figure 22-1: (1) precontemplation, (2) contemplation, (3) preparation, (4) action, (5) maintenance, and (6) relapse (Prochaska and DiClemente, 1982, 1984; Sigman-Grant, 1996). The counselor should learn the steps to identify the patient's readiness to change; these techniques have been successful in other behavioral models, as with smoking cessation (Mallin, 2002; Spencer et al, 2002) (see *Clinical Insight:* Stages of Change).

Research data have shown that the value of the transtheoretical model is in determining which stage a person is in and then using change processes matched to that stage (Prochaska et al, 1992). Behavior change is more successful when using this approach rather than the traditional approach of assigning the same intervention techniques to everyone, regardless of the readiness or stage of change (Prochaska et al, 1994).

Traditional nutrition counseling focuses on the change process matched to the action and maintenance stages. This works well for persons who are actively trying to make behavior change; however, most persons who have problem dietary behavior are in a preaction stage that includes one of the following: precontemplation, contemplation, or preparation. These persons are not yet ready to change (Sandoval et al, 1994; Sporny and Contento, 1995). The traditional approach, which assumes that the patient is already in the action or maintenance stage, does not meet the needs of many and may be one of the reasons for lack of success in long-term maintenance of many intervention programs (Brownell, 1982; National Cholesterol Education Program, 1993; Ockene et al, 1988; Prochaska et al, 1994).

ACTIVITIES THAT FACILITATE BEHAVIOR CHANGE

A variety of principles are important when determining what facilitates behavior change. The following are important when working with persons struggling with behavior change:

1. Expressing empathy
2. Understanding cultural factors
3. Developing discrepancy
4. Avoiding arguments or defensiveness
5. Rolling with resistance
6. Supporting self-efficacy

Expressing Empathy

Counselor acceptance of what a patient feels in times of turmoil can often result in change. Acceptance facilitates change. A woman wrote a letter to her nutritionist saying that she wanted to stop working on her dietary changes. Life was too complicated, and the dietary changes were more than she could master. The nutritionist reviewed several scenarios in approaching this problem. One certainly would be to take the woman's word seriously and allow her to drop out of the diet intervention process. Another would be to call the woman immediately to discuss the letter, always indicating acceptance of the woman's concerns.

Beyond this, acceptance would be a skillful form of reflective listening, which would allow the woman to describe her thoughts and feelings while the nutri-

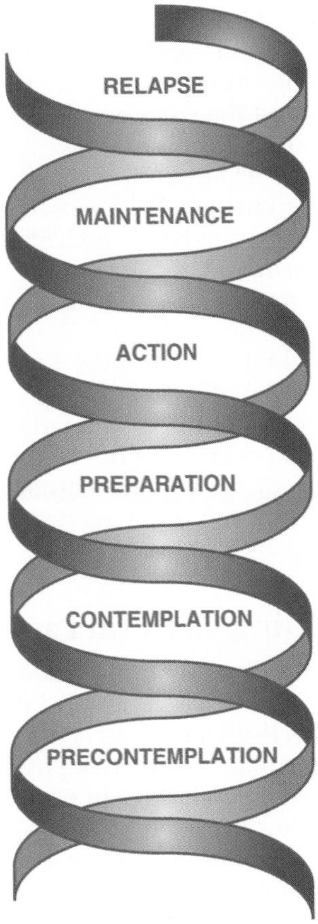

FIGURE 22-1 • A spiral model of the stages of change. In changing, a person moves up this spiral to maintenance. If relapse occurs, he or she must reenter the spiral again at any point.

CLINICAL INSIGHT

Stages of Change

Precontemplation
This is the point at which the patient has not even contemplated having a problem or needing to make a change. A person in the precontemplative stage needs information and feedback to raise his or her awareness of the problem and possibility of change. Nutrition advice for eating changes is counterproductive at this point.

Contemplation
Once some awareness of the problem arises, the person enters a period of ambivalence: the contemplation stage. The contemplator seesaws between reasons to change and reasons to stay the same. At this stage, the counselor works with the patient on advantages and disadvantages of making dietary changes.

Preparation
The preparation stage is a window of opportunity that allows the patient either to move forward or to fall back into contemplation. At this point, the patient needs help in finding a change strategy or goal that is acceptable, achievable, and appropriate.

Action
The patient engages in actions that bring about change. At this point, the goal is to produce a change in the problem area.

Maintenance
During this stage, the challenge is to sustain the change accomplished by previous action and to prevent relapse.

Relapse
If relapse occurs, the individual's task is to start the change process again rather than become stuck in this stage. Slips and relapses are normal, expected occurrences as a person seeks to change any long-standing pattern of behavior. The goal is to resume action efforts.

Data from Prochaska JO, Di Clemente CC: Transtheoretical therapy: toward a more integrative model of change, *Psychother Theory Res Pract* 20:161, 1982.

tionist reflected back understanding. Many people have no one to talk to about problems in their lives. This opportunity to have someone listen and really try to understand the emotions behind the words is crucial to eventual dietary change.

As most people talk about their lives and a lack of time for dietary changes, the counselor will hear ambivalence. On the one hand, patients want to make changes; on the other hand, they want to pretend that change is not important. Ambivalence is normal.

Patient: I feel totally worthless. On the one hand I want to follow this new eating pattern, and on the other I want to eat spontaneously, not worrying about decreasing my fat intake.

Counselor: Your feelings are normal. You are having a difficult time merging new and old habits. This happens to many people.

Understanding Cultural Factors

Effective culturally specific nutrition counseling is dependent on sensitive communication strategies. Randall-David (1989) identified how the values of the American white majority are in opposition to those of many other cultures. Changes in eating habits can be affected by what we value in Anglo-American culture: mastery over nature, personal control over the environment, doing (activity), the domination of time, human equality, individualism and privacy, youth, self-help, competition, orientation to the future, informality, directness, openness and honesty, practicality, efficiency, and materialism. Other ethnocultural groups value harmony with nature, fate, being, personal interaction, rank or status, group welfare, elders, birthright inheritance, cooperation, past or present orientation, formality, indirectness, idealism, and spiritualism. A patient's view of the world can guide verbal and nonverbal approaches that may be more effective (USDA and USDHHS, 1987).

The nutrition counselor should be familiar with cultural norms regarding indirect or direct questioning; formality or informality; eye contact; individual space; and touching (Sucher and Kittler, 1996). In Hispanic culture touching, shaking hands, backslapping, and embracing are important. Native Americans may be insulted when counselors try to direct their lives to change eating habits. An Asian client might agree with whatever the dietitian says because it would be impolite to question professional expertise. African Americans may be uncomfortable with prolonged eye contact and look away while talking or listening. A Mexican American woman might need her husband's approval before implementing any changes. Finally, the Vietnamese find touching inappropriate.

Developing Discrepancy

An awareness of consequences is important. Identifying the advantages and disadvantages of modifying a behavior or developing discrepancy is a crucial process in making changes.

Patient: I want to follow the new eating pattern, but so many things get in the way.

Counselor: Let's make a list of the positives and negatives of following this new eating pattern.

Avoiding Arguments or Defensiveness

Arguments are counterproductive. A counselor's urges may lead in the direction of defending one's own ideas, but the result is frequently defensiveness on the part of the patient. When a patient resists, this is the signal to the counselor to change strategies.

Patient: I just cannot do everything right now. I just can't.

Counselor: You are the best judge of what you can do. Perhaps we need to step back and wait for things in your life to calm down. Let's talk about what you can do and eliminate those things that are too difficult at this time. We can look at ways to meet your goals in the future. Now is the time to take care of pressing issues.

Rolling With Resistance

The counselor can invite new perspectives without imposing them. The patient is a valuable resource in finding solutions to problems. Perceptions can be shifted, and the counselor's role is to help with this process. For example, a patient who is wary of describing why he or she is not ready to change may become much more open to change when seeing openness to his or her resistive behaviors. When it becomes acceptable to discuss resistance, the rationale for its original existence may seem less important.

Patient: I just feel that my level of enthusiasm for following the diet is low. It all seems like too much effort.

Counselor: I appreciate your concerns. Many people at this point in following a new diet feel the same way. Tell me more about your concerns and feelings.

Supporting Self-Efficacy

Belief in the possibility of change is an important motivator. The patient is responsible for choosing and carrying out personal change. Hope exists when there are alternative approaches to a problem.

Patient: I just feel hopeless sometimes when I try to follow the diet.

Counselor: Look at the progress you have made from 6 months ago. Your food records are a testimony to how much you have been able to change your eating habits. You can learn from your setbacks and do better in the future.

These concepts, along with other intervention models, shape the content of each contract described in the motivational intervention model that follows. This model comprises an integration of the following theories: stages of change (Prochaska and DiClemente, 1982, 1986), motivational interviewing (Miller and Rollnick, 1991), brief negotiation (Watson and Tharp, 1989), and behavioral self-management.

INTERVENTION MODEL

To be effective, interventions require careful planning by the counselor. The first step in an intervention is interviewing. Skills in knowing how to elicit information about eating habits are important as the assessment of the patient's diet proceeds. The key to obtaining vital information that will later dictate treatment strategies involves initially establishing a counseling relationship.

Interviewing

The purpose of the client interview is to obtain information. A series of questions are asked in a nonthreatening manner to obtain background information that will guide the session. The session is opened with appropriate introductions of all individuals to one another. The client should state why he or she is there. The counselor usually begins with broad, open-ended questions and closes the interview with close-ended follow-up questions.

First Session

The first session is an important time to establish the counseling relationship. The environment should be conducive to privacy, and there should be a plan for reduction of interruptions (no telephone calls, staff or other patients knocking on the door, or other interruptions). The counselor should be seated in a manner that reflects interest in the client, such as sitting directly across from one another in chairs, without a desk as a barrier. Communication skills and body language are also important. A firm handshake and appropriate eye contact are important elements (see *Clinical Insight:* Body Language and Communication Skills).

In an initial visit the counselor introduces the subject of the session. The following are samples:

- "The purpose of this visit is to see how you are doing in covering your dietary carbohydrate intake with insulin."
- "In looking at your monitoring tools, it seems that you have had excellent progress at some times and that at other times it may have been more difficult."
- "Could we talk about your diet records to identify problems that we could solve?"

The following approaches might be used during a follow-up contact:

- "I talked to you about a month ago to see how you were doing with your carbohydrate levels for each meal and insulin dosage."

CLINICAL INSIGHT

Body Language and Communication Skills

Active listening forms the basis for effective nutrition counseling. The two aspects to effective listening are nonverbal and verbal. *Nonverbal listening skills* consist of varied eye contact, attentive body language, a respectful but close space, adequate silence, and encouragers. Eye contact is direct, yet varied. Lack of eye contact implies that the counselor is too busy to spend time with the client. When the counselor leans forward slightly and has a relaxed posture and avoids fidgeting and gesturing, the client will be more at ease. Showing the client respectful but close space is another important nonverbal message. Silence can give the client time to think and provide positive time for the counselor to contemplate what the client has said. Shaking one's head in agreement can be a positive encourager, leading to more conversation. Moving forward slightly toward the client is an encourager that allows more positive interaction.

Verbal components of listening include keeping the focus on the client by demonstrating a willingness to listen. Often the nutritionist feels obligated to solve a problem or give advice. These two desires can decrease the time left for active listening. Questions that are open to detailed descriptions are preferred. Questions that begin with *what, how, why,* and *could* should be emphasized.

Two types of encouragers are important in counseling: paraphrasing and summarizing. Paraphrasing is a brief repeat of the essence of what the speaker has said using fresh and concise wording. It is not parroting or word swapping. Paraphrasing is not easy and requires careful listening and caring. Summarizing is more lengthy than paraphrasing because it uses more information and summarizes what has been said over a period of time.

In general, it is important to accomplish these as the basis for the interactive relationship before beginning the actual process of nutrition counseling.

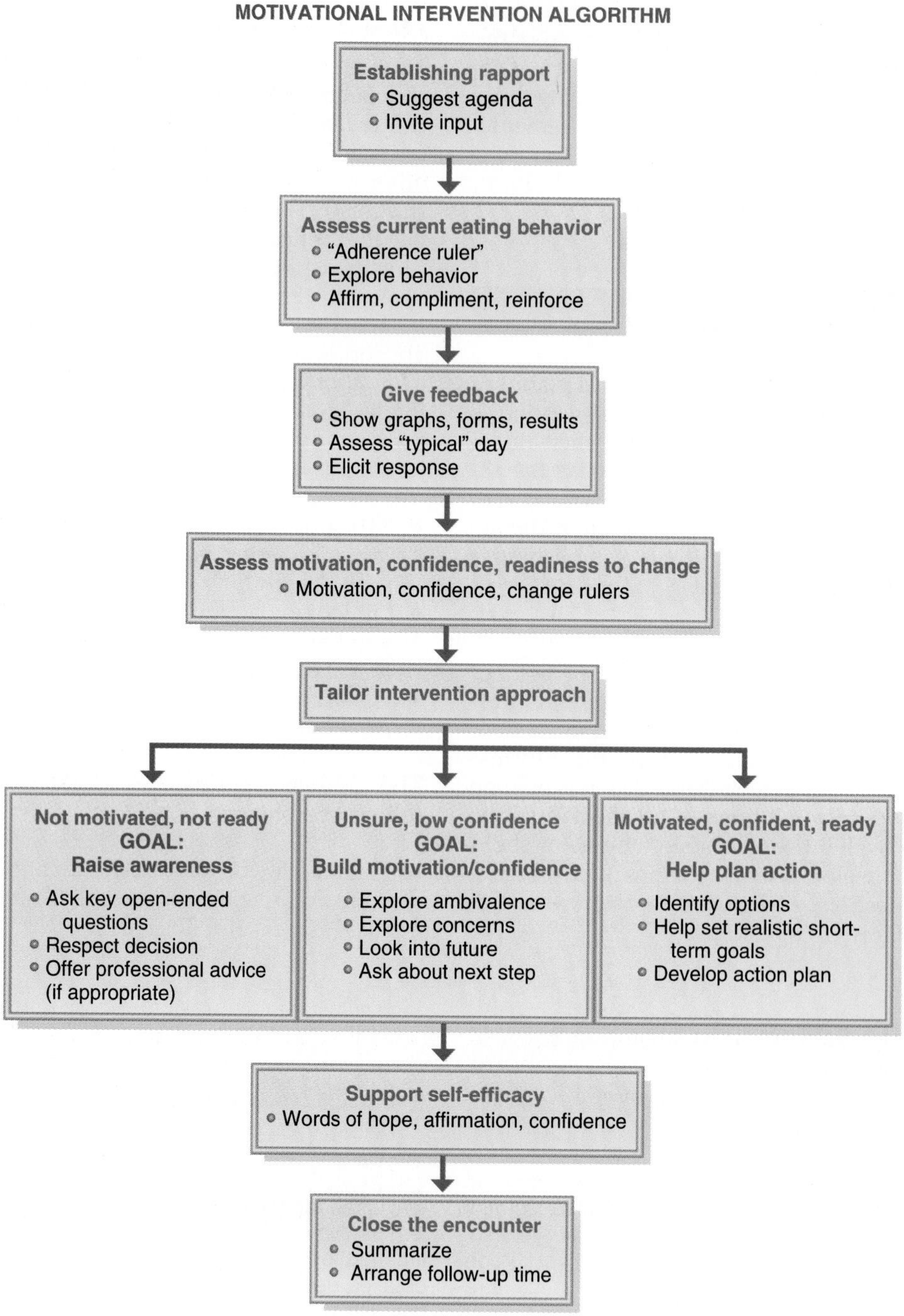

FIGURE 22-2 • Algorithm of motivational intervention. (Data from Miller WR, Rollnick S, eds: *Motivational interviewing: preparing people for change,* ed 2, New York, 2002, Guilford Press.)

- "I'd like to see if you have made any changes or had any further thoughts on meeting your fat intake goals."

To make the stages of change model less complicated, an alternative is to view the stages in terms of three phases: stage 1—not ready to change; stage 2—considering meeting goals; and stage 3—ready to change. To identify which of these three stages a patient is in, it is important to assess the patient's situation (Figure 22-2).

Assessment

The purpose of assessment is to identify what stage of change the patient is in and to provide appropriate help in facilitating change. The assessment should be completed in the first visit, if possible. If conversation extends beyond the designated time for the session, the assessment steps should be completed at the next session. The stage of readiness for change should be assessed and documented.

Establishing Rapport

To build rapport, one begins by asking one or two questions that are relevant to important aspects of the participant's life.

- Tell me about how __________ (e.g., hobby or interest) is going?
- We have about __________ minutes to meet today. I thought we might talk about how you're doing with your dietary changes. How does this sound to you?

Assessment of Current Eating Behavior

Determining present eating habits provides ideas about how to change in the future. The following questions can be used to assess current eating behavior:

- How do you limit the amount of saturated fat in your diet now?
- Would you say that you are eating a low-fat diet now?
- During the past 6 months, have you thought about changes that you could make to reduce the amount of saturated fat in your diet?
- In the next month, do you plan to make any changes to reduce the amount of fat in your diet?

It is important to review self-monitoring tools to assess where the patient sees his or her adherence level. Food diaries help to identify eating habits and potential modifications. Using a ruler that allows the patient to select his or her level of adherence to the diet is one method of allowing patient participation in the discussion of dietary adherence. You might say, "The ruler will help us see where you are in terms of changing your diet. On a scale of 1 to 12, to what extent would you say you are meeting your goal of changing your diet in the past month? (1 = absolutely never; 12 = absolutely always)."

Explore eating behaviors by using the following statements:

- Tell me about your progress so far.
- Why did you choose that number on the ruler? Why did you not choose 1? Why did you not choose 12?
- How do you generally feel about following this new eating pattern?

Provide positive confidence-building statements:

- It is great that you __________.
- You've worked really hard at this.

To elicit responses from the patient on ideas about where changes in the diet need to occur, it is helpful to provide feedback on the patient's progress toward a goal, for example, by showing the patient an example of his or her progress. After indicating what the goal is and what the average score for the targeted nutrient is, the counselor can ask, "What do you think about this?"

Assessment of Readiness to Change

At this point, it is important to assess readiness to make additional changes. A ruler works well here also. Up to this point, discussions have focused on changes the patient has already made. The counselor then asks the patient, "On a scale of 1 to 12, how ready are you right now to make any new changes to eat less fat? (1 = not ready to change; 12 = very ready to change)." At this point, the intervention becomes specific to the readiness to change. Three possibilities for readiness exist: (1) not ready to change, (2) unsure about change, and (3) ready to change. These three concepts of readiness have condensed the six distinct stages of changes described in this chapter to assist the counselor in determining the level of patient readiness.

Many concepts must be remembered when working with patients in whom readiness to change is an issue, and readiness to change may fluctuate during the course of the discussion. The counselor must be ready to move back and forth between the phase-specific strategies. If the patient seems confused, detached, or resistant during the discussion, the counselor should return and ask about readiness to change. If readiness has lessened, tailoring the intervention is necessary. Every counseling session does not have to end with patient agreement to change; even a decision to think about change can be a useful conclusion.

NOT-READY-TO-CHANGE COUNSELING SESSIONS

To approach the not-ready-to-change stage of intervention, three goals are the focus: (1) to facilitate the patient's ability to consider change, (2) to identify and reduce the patient's resistance and barriers to change, and (3) to identify behavioral steps toward change that are tailored to each patient's needs.

To achieve these goals, several communication skills are important to master: asking open-ended questions, listening reflectively, affirming, summarizing, and eliciting self-motivational statements.

Asking Open-Ended Questions

Open-ended questions allow the patient to express a wider range of ideas. Closed questions can help in targeting concepts and eliminating tangential discussions. For the person who is not ready to change, targeted discussions around difficult topics can help focus the session.

The counselor asks questions that must be answered by explaining and discussing, not by one-word answers. This is particularly important for someone who is not ready to change because it opens the discussion to problem areas that keep the patient from being ready. The following statements and questions are examples that create an atmosphere for discussion:

- We are here to talk about your dietary change experiences up to this point. Could you start at the beginning and tell me how it has been for you?
- What are some things you would like to discuss about your dietary changes so far? What do you like about them? What don't you like about them?

Reflective Listening

Nutrition counselors not only listen but also try to tag those feelings that surface as a patient is describing difficulties with an eating pattern. Listening is not simply hearing the words spoken by the patient and paraphrasing them back. Reflective listening involves a guess at what the person feels and is phrased as a statement, not a question. By stating a feeling, the counselor communicates understanding. One also more fully understands the patient by labeling a feeling. Figure 22-3 shows a nutrition counselor listening reflectively to her patient. The following are examples of listening reflectively:

Example 1

Patient: I really do try, but I am retired and my husband always wants to eat out. How can I stay on the right path when that happens?

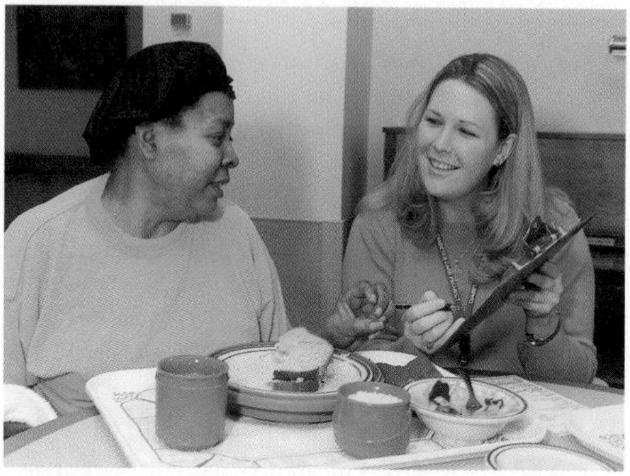

FIGURE 22-3 • This nutrition counselor is using reflective listening techniques with her patient.

Counselor: You feel frustrated because you want to follow the diet, but at the same time you want to be spontaneous with your husband. Is this correct?

Example 2

Patient: I feel like I let you down every time I come in to see you. We always discuss plans, and I never follow them. I almost hate to come in.

Counselor: You are feeling like giving up. You haven't been able to modify your diet, and it is difficult for you to come in for our visits when you haven't met the goals we set. Is this how you are feeling?

Example 3

Patient: Some days I just give up. It is on those days that I do very badly in following my diet.

Counselor: You just lose the desire to try to eat well on some days, and that is very depressing for you.

Example 4

Patient: I just don't want to do this any more!

Counselor: You sound hassled by other priorities and feel that the changes in your eating habits just get in the way.

Affirming

Counselors often understand the idea of supporting a patient's efforts at following a new eating style but do not put those thoughts into words. When the counselor affirms someone, alignment and normalization of the patient's issues occur. In alignment the counselor tells the patient that he or she understands and is with him or her in understanding difficult times. Normalization means telling the patient that he or she is perfectly within reason and that it is typical to have such reactions and feelings. Below are some statements that indicate affirmation:

- I know that it is hard for you to tell me this. But, thank you.
- You have had amazing competing priorities. I feel that you have done extremely well given your circumstances.
- Many people I talk with express the same problems. I can understand why you are having difficulty.

Summarizing

The counselor periodically summarizes the content of what the patient has said by covering all the key points. Simple and straightforward statements are most effective, even if they involve negative feelings. If conflicting ideas arise, the counselor can use the strategy "on the one hand you . . ." to remind both persons about the issues; this ensures greater clarity.

Eliciting Self-Motivational Statements

The four communication strategies (asking open-ended questions, listening reflectively, affirming, and summarizing) are important for eliciting self-motivational statements. The goal here is for the patient to realize that a problem exists, that concern exists about it, and that positive steps in the future can be taken to correct the problem. The goal is to use these realizations to set the stage for later efforts at dietary change. The following are examples of questions to use in eliciting the self-motivational feeling statements:

Problem Recognition

- What things make you think that eating out is a problem?
- In what ways has following your diet been a problem?

Concern

- How do you feel when you cannot follow your diet?
- In what ways does not being able to follow your diet concern you?
- What do you think will happen if you don't make a change?

Intention to Change

- The fact that you are here indicates that at least a part of you thinks it's time to do something. What are the reasons you see for making a change?
- If you were 100% successful and things worked out exactly as you would like, what would be different?
- What things make you think you should keep eating the way you have been? And, on the opposite side, what makes you think it is time for a change?
- What would be the advantages of making a change?

Optimism

- What makes you think that if you decide to make a change you could do it?
- What encourages you that you can change if you want to?
- What do you think would work for you, if you decided to change?

Patients in this "not-ready-to-change" category have already told the counselor they are not doing well at making changes. Usually, if a tentative approach is used by asking permission to approach the problem, the patient will not refuse. One asks permission by saying, "Would you be willing to continue our discussion and talk about the possibility of change?"

At this point, it is helpful to discuss thoughts and feelings about the current status of dietary change by asking open-ended questions, such as the following:

- Tell me why you picked ______ on the ruler. (Refer to previous discussion on the use of a ruler.)
- What would have to happen for you to move from a ______ to a ______ (referring to a number on the ruler). How could I help get you there?
- What would need to be different for you to consider making new or additional changes in your eating?
- If you did start to think about changing, what would be your main concern?

To show real understanding about what the patient is saying, summarizing the statements about his or her progress, difficulties, possible reasons for change, and what needs to be different to move forward is beneficial. This paraphrasing will allow the patient to rethink his or her reasoning about readiness to change. The mental processing provides new ideas that can promote actual change.

Ending the Session

Counselors often expect a decision and at least a goal-setting session when working with a patient; however, it is important at this stage to realize that traditional goal setting will result in feelings of failure on the part of both the patient and the nutritionist. If the patient is not ready to change, respectful acknowledgment of this decision is important. The counselor might say, "I can understand why making a change right now would be very hard for you. The fact that you are able to indicate this as a problem is very important, and I respect your decision. Our lives do change; if you feel differently later on, I will always be available to talk with you. I know when the time is right for you to make a change, you will find a way to do it."

When the session ends, the counselor will let the patient know that the issues will be revisited after he or she has had time to think. Expression of hope and confidence in the patient's ability to make changes in the future, when the time is right, will be beneficial. Arrangements for follow-up contact can be made at this time.

With a patient who is not ready to change, it is easy to become defensive and authoritarian. At this point, it is important to avoid pushing, persuading, confronting, coaxing, or telling the patient what to do. It is reassuring to a nutritionist to know that change at this level will often occur outside the office. The patient is not expected to be ready to do something during the visit.

Unsure-About-Change Counseling Sessions

The only goal in this stage of change is to build readiness to change. This is the point at which big changes can occur. This "unsure" stage is a transition from not being ready to deal with a problem eating behavior to preparing to continue the change. It involves summarizing the patient's perceptions of what is going on, including self-motivational statements that the participant has made. It includes the process of identifying the participant's ambivalence. The counselor can restate any statements that the participant has made about intentions or plans to change or do better in the future.

One crucial aspect of this stage is the process of discussing thoughts and feelings about current status. Use of open-ended questions will help the participant discuss dietary change progress and difficulties and will help him or her to discuss possible reasons for change, that is, what would need to be different to move forward.

This stage is characterized by feelings of ambivalence. The counselor should encourage the patient to explore ambivalence to change by thinking about "pros" and "cons." The following are some questions that can be asked:

- What are some of the things you like about your current eating habits?
- What concerns you about your current eating habits?
- What are some of the good things about making a new or additional change?
- What are some of the things that are not so good about making a new or additional change?

By trying to look into the future, one can help patients see new and often positive scenarios. The counselor helps to tip the balance away from being ambivalent about change toward considering change by guiding the patient to talk about what life might be like after a change, anticipating the difficulties as well as the advantages. An opening to generate discussion with the patient might go like this: "I can see why you're unsure about making new or additional changes in your eating. Imagine that you decided to change. What would that be like? What would you want to do?" The counselor then summarizes the patient's statements about the "pros" and "cons" of making a change and includes any statements about wanting, intending, or planning to change.

The next step is to negotiate a change. The negotiation process has three parts. The first is setting goals, broad goals at first, holding more specific nutritional goals until later. For example, ask: "How would you like things to be different from the way they are?" and "What is it that you would like to change?"

The second step is to consider options. The counselor asks about alternative strategies and options and then asks the patient to choose from among them. This is effective because if the first option does not work, the patient has other choices.

The third step is to arrive at a plan. This should be a plan that has been devised by the patient. The counselor touches on the key points and the problems and then writes down the plan.

To end the session, the counselor asks about the next step, allowing the patient to bring up the topic. The following questions provide some ideas for questions that might promote discussion:

- Where do you think you will go from here?
- What do you plan to do between now and the next visit?
- Where does this leave you now?

Arranging for the Next Contact

Clinicians always want to jump ahead. Instead, the counselor must take this process slowly and not assume that the patient is ready to change. In a rush to help, counselors often give advice too soon. An astute counselor will avoid giving advice about change and will not feel bad if the patient does not agree to change. One might say the following: "You say you're unsure about what to do. I will not push you into a decision. It is up to you. Take your time to think about it. Let me know if you want to talk about it again. You have made changes in the past, and you are the best judge of when is the best time to consider change."

READY-TO-CHANGE COUNSELING SESSIONS

The major goal in this stage of change is to collaborate with the patient to set goals for change that include a plan of action. The nutrition counselor provides the patient with the tools to use in meeting nutritional goals.

When a counseling session begins, the patient is most often assumed to be in this state of change. To assume erroneously that the patient is in this stage means that all the strategies used to make a change are misused. The assumption that the patient is in this stage often results in a lack of adherence on the part of the patient and discouragement on the part of the nutritionist.

Initially, it is important to discuss thoughts and feelings about where the patient stands relative to current dietary change status. Use of open-ended questions helps the patient confirm and justify the decision to make a change. The following questions may elicit information about feelings toward change:

- Tell me why you picked _______ on the ruler.
- Why did you pick _______ instead of 1 or 12?
- Give me some ideas for why you think you are ready to change.

Helping the patient to identify change options by asking whether he or she would like to change and what a first step might be is an effective method. The following questions might help the patient identify options:

- What could you do to change your eating habits?
- Is this feasible?
- How do you see things turning out if you make these changes?

In this stage, goal setting is extremely important. Here the counselor helps the patient to set a realistic and achievable short-term goal. "Let's do things gradually. What is a reasonable first step?"

Action Plan

After goal setting, an action plan is set to help the patient map out the specifics of what must be done to achieve a goal. Having supportive people around to help with dietary adherence is important. What can others do to help? Early identification of barriers to adherence is important. If barriers are identified, plans can be formed to help eliminate those roadblocks to adherence.

Many patients fail to notice when a plan is working. Make sure that the patient knows when an action plan is a success by asking the patient to summarize the plan. The counselor then documents the plan for discussion at future sessions and ensures that the patient also has the plan in writing.

The session should be closed with an encouraging statement and reflection about how the patient identified this plan personally. An indication that each person is the expert on his or her own behavior is important. The patient should be complimented on carrying out the plan. The following are ways of expressing these ideas to patients:

- You are working very hard at this, and it's clear that you're the expert on what is best for you. You can do this!
- Keep in mind that change is gradual and takes time. If this plan doesn't work, there will be other plans to try.

Arranging for the Next Contact

The key point to remember for this stage is to avoid telling the patient what to do. Clinicians often want to provide advice; however, it is critical that the patient express ideas of what will work best. "There are a number of things you could do, but what do you think will work best for you?"

RESISTANCE BEHAVIORS AND POTENTIAL STRATEGIES TO MODIFY THEM

Resistance to change is the most consistent emotion or state that will be faced when dealing with poor performers. Following are examples of resistance to change. In one type of resistance, the patient contests the accuracy, expertise, or integrity of the nutrition counselor. In another type, the patient directly challenges the accuracy of what the nutrition counselor has said. In a third type, the patient discounts what the nutrition counselor has said by questioning the therapist's personal authority and expertise. Finally, the nutrition counselor may be confronted with a hostile patient.

Resistance may also surface as interrupting, as when the patient breaks in during a conversation in a defensive manner. The patient speaks while the nutrition counselor is still talking without waiting for an appropriate pause or silence. The patient may also break in with words obviously intended to cut off the nutrition counselor's discussion.

When patients express an unwillingness to recognize problems, cooperate, accept responsibility, or take advice, they may be denying a problem. Some patients blame other people for problems; a wife may blame her husband for her inability to follow a diet.

Patients may disagree with the nutrition counselor when a suggestion is offered, but they frequently provide no constructive alternative. This includes the familiar "Yes, but . . . ," which explains what is wrong with the suggestion.

Patients try to excuse their behavior. They may say, "I want to do better, but my life is always in a turmoil since my husband died 3 years ago." An excuse that was once acceptable is reused beyond the point that it actually is a factor in the woman's life.

Some patients will make pessimistic statements about themselves or others. "My husband will never help me." "I have never been good at sticking with a goal. I'm sure I won't do well with it now."

Some patients are reluctant to accept advice. They express reservations about information or advice given. "I just don't think that will work for me."

Some patients will express a lack of willingness to change or an intention not to change. They make it clear that they want to stop the dietary regimen.

Often patients show evidence of not following the nutrition counselor's advice. Clues that this is happening include using a response that does not answer the question, providing no response to a question, or changing the direction of the conversation.

A variety of strategies are available to assist the nutrition counselor in dealing with these problem situations. These strategies include reflecting, double-sided reflecting, shifting focus, agreeing with a twist, emphasizing personal choice, and reframing. Each of these options is described as follows.

Reflecting

In reflecting, the counselor identifies the patient's emotion or feeling and reflects it back. This allows the patient to stop and think about what was said. An example of this type of counseling skill is: "You seem to be very frustrated by what your husband says about your food choices."

Double-Sided Reflection

In double-sided reflection, the counselor will use ideas that the patient has expressed previously to show the discrepancy between the patient's current words and the previous ones. For example:

Patient: I am doing the best I can. (Previously this patient stated that she sometimes just gives up and does not care about following the diet.)

Counselor: On the one hand you say you are doing your best, but on the other hand I believe I recall a time when you said you just felt like giving up and didn't care about following the diet. Do you remember that? Was that point in time different from now?

Shifting Focus

Patients may hold onto an idea that they feel is getting in the way of their progress. If this really is not the problem, the counselor should state that. For example:

Patient: I will never be able to follow this low-fat diet as long as my grandchildren come to my house and want snacks.

Counselor: Are you sure this is really the problem? Is part of the problem that you like those same snacks?

Patient: Oh, you are right. I love them.

Counselor: Could you compromise? Ask your grandchildren which of this long list of low-fat snacks they like and buy them.

Agreeing With a Twist

This strategy involves offering agreement but then moving the discussion in a different direction. The counselor agrees with a piece of what the patient says but then offers another perspective on his or her problems. This allows the opportunity to agree with the patient's statement and feelings but then to redirect the conversation onto a key topic. For example:

Patient: I really like eating out, but I always eat too much and my blood sugars go sky high.

Counselor: You are in the majority when you say you like eating out. Now that you are retired, it is easier to eat out than to cook. I can understand that. What can we do to make you feel great about eating out so that you can still follow your eating plan and keep your blood glucose values in the normal range?

Emphasizing Personal Choice

Counselors should always emphasize that any future action belongs to the patient. Any advice given can be taken or avoided. This emphasis on personal choice helps patients avoid feeling trapped and confined by the discussion.

Reframing

With reframing the counselor changes the patient's interpretation of the same basic data by offering a new one from another person's perspective. The counselor repeats the basic observation that the participant has provided and then offers a new hypothesis for interpreting the data. For example:

Patient: I gave up trying to meet my dietary goals because I was having some difficulties when my husband died, and I have decided now that I just cannot meet those strict goals.

Counselor: I remember how devastated you were when he died and how just cooking meals was an effort. Do you think this happened as a kind of immediate response to his death and that you might have just at that time decided that all of the goals were too strict? (Pause)

Patient: Well, you are probably right.

Counselor: Could we look at where you are now and try to find things that will work for you now to help you in following the goals we have set?

SUMMARY

In summary, facilitating dietary self-management in patients involves knowledge of where they are in regard to their willingness to change. In facilitating change, nutrition counselors should tailor strategies to each stage of change. Successful change interventions lead to satisfying outcomes for both counselor and client.

■ Relevant Web Site

Counseling Relationships Code of Ethics
www.apa.org/ethics/code.html

Clinical Scenario 1

Over the past several months, Jane has struggled with changing her dietary fat intake and keeping her carbohydrate intake consistent. She is concerned that she has not been doing well and wants to stop following the new style of eating and forget that she has type 2 diabetes. She has just stated to you, "I never get it right. It is so hard having diabetes! I just want to quit having this condition and go back to my old self."

1. Reword this statement to indicate your own thoughts about the patient's preceding statement.
2. What summarizing statements might you say?
3. What other open-ended questions could you ask to determine her readiness to change? This is just one way to elicit self-motivational statements. It sends the counseling session in a positive direction with focus on a specific type of problem.
4. What does Jane's initial statement indicate about her stage of change?
5. In what other directions might you take this interview to elicit self-motivational statements?
6. What are some problem recognition questions?
7. What questions would you ask to elicit patient concerns?

Clinical Scenario 2

Lee is originally from mainland China. She has been living in your area for several years but has numerous health problems, including high blood pressure and glaucoma. You have been asked to counsel her about making changes in her diet. Because her vision is poor, she will not be able to use printed materials that you have in your office that have been translated into Chinese.

1. What steps should you take to make her comfortable with this session?
2. Should you invite family members to attend the counseling session? Why or why not?
3. What tools might help Lee to understand portions or types of food that she should select?
4. Would a supermarket tour be useful? Why or why not?
5. What other types of information will be needed to help Lee?

Cited References

Brownell KD: Obesity: understanding and treating a serious, prevalent, and refractory disorder, *J Consult Clin Psychol* 50:829, 1982.

Dobson KS: *Handbook of cognitive-behavioral therapies,* New York, 1998, Guilford Press.

Eaton C et al: Direct observation of nutrition counseling in community family practice, *Am J Prev Med* 23:174, 2002.

Hunt MK et al: Process evaluation of a clinical preventive nutrition intervention, *Prev Med* 33:82, 2001.

Mallin R: Smoking cessation: integration of behavioral and drug therapies, *Am Fam Physician* 65:1107, 2002.

Miller W, Rollnick S, eds: *Motivational interviewing: preparing people for change,* ed 2, New York, 2002, Guilford Press.

National Cholesterol Education Program: *Hearty habits don't eat your heart out,* NIH Publication No. 93-3102. Washington, DC, 1993, National Heart, Lung, and Blood Institute.

Ockene J et al: *The Coronary Artery Smoking Intervention Study.* Worcester, Mass, 1988, National Heart, Lung, and Blood Institute.

Prochaska JO, DiClemente CC: Transtheoretical therapy: toward a more integrative model of change, *Psychother Theory Res Pract* 20:161, 1982.

Prochaska JO, DiClemente CC: *The transtheoretical approach: crossing traditional boundaries of change,* Homewood, Ill, 1984, Dorsey Press.

Prochaska J, DiClemente C: Toward a comprehensive model of change. In Miller WR, Heather N, eds: *Treating addictive behaviors: processes of change,* New York, 1986, Plenum.

Prochaska JO et al: In search of how people change, *Am Psychol* 47:1102, 1992.

Prochaska JO et al: *Changing for good,* New York, 1994, William Morrow.

Randall-David E: *Strategies for working with culturally diverse communities and clients,* Bethesda, Md, 1989, Association for the Care of Children's Health.

Resnicow K et al: Motivational interviewing in health promotion: it sounds like something is changing, *Health Psychol* 21:444, 2002.

Sandoval WM et al: Stages of change: a model for nutrition counseling, *Top Clin Nutr* 9:64, 1994.

Seigel M, Doner L: *Marketing public health: strategies to promote social change,* Gaithersburg, Md, 1998, Aspen Publishers.

Sigman-Grant M: Stages of change: a framework for nutrition interventions, *Nutr Today* 31:162, 1996.

Spencer L et al: Applying the transtheoretical model to tobacco cessation and prevention: a review of literature, *Am J Health Promot* 17:7, 2002.

Sporny LA, Contento IR: Stages of change in dietary fat reduction: social psychological correlates, *J Nutr Educ* 27:191, 1995.

Sucher KP, Kittler PG: Cultural considerations in diabetes nutrition therapy. In Powers MA, ed: *Handbook of diabetes medical nutrition therapy,* Gaithersburg, Md, 1996, Aspen Publishers.

U.S. Department of Agriculture, U.S. Department of Health and Human Services: *Cross-cultural counseling: a guide for nutrition and health counselors,* Washington, DC, 1987, U.S. Department of Agriculture/U.S. Department of Health and Human Services.

Watson DL, Tharp RG: *Self-directed behavior: self-modification for personal adjustment,* ed 5, Pacific Grove, Calif, 1989, Brooks/Cole.

Additional References

AbuSha R, Achterberg C: Review of self-efficacy and locus of control for nutrition- and health-related behavior, *J Am Diet Assoc* 10:1122, 1997.

Baldwin T, Falciglia G: Application of cognitive behavioral theories to dietary change in clients, *J Am Diet Assoc* 95:1315, 1995.

Blissmer B, McAuley E: Testing the requirements of stages of physical activity among adults: the comparative effectiveness of stage-matched, mismatched, standard care, and control interventions, *Ann Behav Med* 24:181, 2002.

Coulston AM: Diabetes mellitus in 2002, *Nutr Today* 37:163, 2002.

Danish S et al: The anatomy of a dietetic counseling interview, *J Am Diet Assoc* 75:626, 1979.

Greene G, Rossi S: Stages of change for reducing dietary fat over 18 months, *J Am Diet Assoc* 98:529, 1998.

Humphreys AS et al: Assessment of breastfeeding intention using the Transtheoretical Model and the Theory of Reasoned Action, *Health Educ Res* 13:331, 1998.

Johnson JL et al: Testing stage effects in an ethnically diverse sample, *Addict Behav* 27:605, 2002.

Marlatt GA: Mindfulness and metaphor in relapse prevention: an interview with G. Alan Marlatt, *J Am Diet Assoc* 94:846, 1994.
Rollnick S et al: Negotiating behavior change in medical settings: the development of brief motivational interviewing, *J Ment Health* 1:25, 1992.
Snetselaar L: *Nutrition counseling skills,* ed 3, Baltimore, 1997, Aspen Publishers.
Suminski RR, Petosa R: Stages of change among ethnically diverse college students, *J Am Coll Health* 51:26, 2002.
Willey C et al: Public health and the science of behavior change, *Curr Issues Public Health* 2:18, 1996.

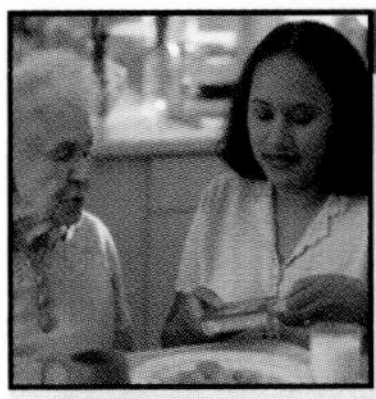

CHAPTER 23

Enteral and Parenteral Nutrition Support

ABBY S. BLOCH, PhD, RD, FADA
CHARLES MUELLER, PhD, MS, RD, CNSD, CDN

CHAPTER OUTLINE

- Rationale and Criteria for Appropriate Nutrition Support
- Enteral Nutrition
- Parenteral Nutrition
- Transitional Feeding
- Pharmacologic Use of Nutrients
- Nutrition Support in Long-Term and Home Care
- Ethical Issues
- Interdisciplinary Nutrition Support Services

KEY TERMS

aspiration of gastric residuals–withdrawal of the stomach's fluid volume to check for adequate gastric emptying

bacterial translocation–the potential for passage of enteric pathogens or endotoxin through the epithelial mucosa of an impaired gastrointestinal tract into the blood or lymphatic system

bolus feeding–infusion of up to 500 ml of enteral formula into the stomach over 5 to 20 minutes, usually with a large-bore syringe

catheter–a fine tube that can be threaded into the lumen of a blood vessel for infusion of fluids or withdrawal of blood

continuous drip infusion–enteral formula administration into the gastrointestinal tract via pump, usually over 8 to 24 hours per day

cyclic total parenteral nutrition–administration of total parenteral nutrition solution for 12 to 18 consecutive hours, usually at night, followed by a 6- to 12-hour period of no infusion

enteral nutrition–provision of nutrients into the gastrointestinal tract through a tube when oral intake is inadequate

gastric decompression–prevention of gaseous inflation (distention) of the gastrointestinal tract by the application of intermittent or continuous negative pressure (suction) through a nasogastric tube

gastroparesis–hypomotility of the stomach resulting in impeded gastric emptying

hemodynamic stability–the ability of a patient to maintain adequate blood pressure

intermittent drip feeding–enteral formula administered at specified times throughout the day; generally in smaller volume and at a slower rate than a bolus feeding but in larger volume and faster rate than continuous feedings

lumen–the interior area of a tube, catheter, or blood vessel

monomeric–when referring to protein and carbohydrate, the form in which the nutrient has been hydrolyzed into its smaller parts

nasoenteric tube–a tube inserted through the nasal passage into the stomach, duodenum, or jejunum

needle catheter jejunostomy–feeding tube used to provide small-bore needle insertion into the jejunum at time of surgery

KEY TERMS—Continued

parenteral nutrition–provision of nutrients directly into the bloodstream intravenously

percutaneous endoscopic gastrostomy (PEG)–feeding tube, the insertion of which into the stomach involves using an endoscope and pulling the tube through a small incision in the abdominal wall

percutaneous endoscopic jejunostomy (PEJ)–feeding tube inserted into the jejunum using an endoscopic technique

peripheral parenteral nutrition (PPN)–delivery of nutrients into a smaller peripheral vein

polymeric–when referring to protein and carbohydrate, the form in which the molecules appear intact or as an isolate

pulmonary aspiration–inadvertent inspiration into the lungs of body fluids, such as vomitus, from the stomach

rebound hypoglycemia–low blood sugar resulting from abrupt cessation of total parenteral nutrition solutions

refeeding syndrome–low serum levels of potassium, magnesium, and phosphorus with severe, potentially lethal outcome that results from the too rapid infusion of substrates, particularly carbohydrate, into the plasma with the consequent release of insulin and shift of electrolytes into the intracellular space as glucose moves into the cells for oxidation and reduction in salt and water excretion

stoma–artificially created opening between a body cavity and the body's surface that has healed

total parenteral nutrition (TPN)–delivery of nutrients into a large central vein, usually the superior vena cava

transitional feeding–the process of progressing from one method of nutrition support to another or to oral feeding

Nutrition support is the delivery of formulated enteral or parenteral nutrients to appropriate patients for the purpose of maintaining or restoring nutritional status. Enteral nutrition refers to the provision of nutrients into the gastrointestinal tract through a tube or catheter when oral intake is inadequate. In certain instances, enteral nutrition may include the use of formulas as oral supplements or meal replacements. In this chapter, *enteral nutrition* refers to the delivery of nutrients via a tube or catheter into the gastrointestinal tract. Parenteral nutrition is the provision of nutrients intravenously.

Historically, the use of enteral nutrition for acutely ill, postoperative, or posttrauma patients rested on evidence of bowel function as indicated by bowel sounds and flatus. These signs verify colonic motility. Small bowel motility returns much sooner, however, within hours of surgery and trauma and is the primary site of nutrient absorption. The feeding technique described by Abbott and Rawson (1939) required small bowel motility but not colonic and gastric motility. Using this technique, which requires gastric decompression with concomitant small bowel feeding, enteral nutrition is now implemented in patients with small bowel function who previously were supported parenterally because their gastrointestinal function was assumed to be inadequate. Most practitioners agree that enteral nutrition presents fewer risks than parenteral nutrition and provides advantages to the patient that parenteral nutrition does not.

RATIONALE AND CRITERIA FOR APPROPRIATE NUTRITION SUPPORT

The theory that enteral nutrition is better for a patient than parenteral nutrition provides the rationale for justifying its use whenever feasible. This theory is based on the hypothesis that parenteral nutrition or bowel rest, rather than enteral nutrition, during critical illness causes a breakdown of the gastrointestinal mucosal barrier and increases its permeability to bacteria and endotoxins (bacterial translocation), in turn contributing to sepsis syndrome and multiple organ dysfunction syndrome (Alexander, 1990; Deitch, 1992) (see Chapter 42). A major component of the gastrointestinal mucosa, gut-associated lymphoid tissue (GALT), is also compromised by bowel rest or parenteral nutrition (Mosenthal et al, 2002). GALT comprises half of total body immunity; immunoglobulin production is secreted across the gastrointestinal mucosa to defend against pathogenic substances in the gastrointestinal lumen (see Chapter 12).

Research that forms the basis for evidence that parenteral feeding can compromise the gastrointestinal barrier and immune function has used animal models, not human trials. Additional studies investigated gastrointestinal permeability in humans but not the ability of bacteria and endotoxins to move across the gastrointestinal mucosa. Harmless substances such as lactose and mannitol have been used in the studies; these substances are not comparable to bacteria and endotoxins. Nevertheless, compelling indirect data indicate that bowel rest via parenteral feeding is associated with higher infection rates in trauma or surgical patients (Moore et al, 1992). There is no recent evidence suggesting that stable patients who are dependent on parenteral nutrition automatically translocate bacteria, become septic, or develop organ dysfunction (Jeejeebhoy, 2001). Such patients usually have less than 2 to 3 ft (60 to 100 cm) of functioning small bowel available for absorption of nutrients. For these persons, parenteral nutrition is life-sustaining therapy, and the risks of bacterial translocation are outweighed by the benefit.

The following criteria can be applied to select appropriate candidates for nutrition support (Table 23-1). Enteral nutrition should be used in patients who have at least 2 to 3 ft of functional gastrointestinal tract, who are or will become malnourished, and in whom oral intake is inadequate to restore or maintain optimal nutritional status. Parenteral nutrition should be used in patients who are or will become malnourished and who do not have sufficient gastrointestinal function to be able to restore or maintain optimal nutritional status (Matarese and Gottschlich, 2002). Figure 23-1 presents an algorithm for selecting enteral and parenteral nutrition routes.

These guidelines would seem to make the selection of the best type of nutrition support an easy decision; however, this is not always the case. For example, not all access methods reviewed in this chapter are universally available in all health care settings. Therefore, if a specific type of small bowel access is not available for enteral nutrition, parenteral nutrition may be the only realistic option. Often parenteral nutrition is used temporarily until adequate gastrointestinal function can support either enteral nutrition or oral intake. In this situation, a combination of feeding methods is used (see Transitional Feeding in this chapter).

TABLE 23-1 Conditions That Often Require Nutrition Support

RECOMMENDED ROUTE OF FEEDING	CONDITION	TYPICAL DISORDERS
Enteral nutrition	Impaired nutrient ingestion	Neurologic disorders HIV/AIDS Facial trauma Oral or esophageal trauma Congenital anomalies Respiratory failure Cystic fibrosis Traumatic brain injury
	Inability to consume adequate nutrition orally	Hyperemesis of pregnancy Hypermetabolic states such as with burns Comatose states Anorexia in congestive heart failure, cancer, COPD, ED Congenital heart disease Impaired intake after orofacial surgery or injury Spinal cord injury
	Impaired digestion, absorption, metabolism	Severe gastroparesis Inborn errors of metabolism Crohn's disease Short bowel syndrome with minimal resection
	Severe wasting or depressed growth	Cystic fibrosis Failure to thrive Cancer Sepsis Cerebral palsy Myasthenia gravis
Parenteral nutrition	Gastrointestinal incompetency	Short bowel syndrome—major resection Severe acute pancreatitis Severe inflammatory bowel disease Small bowel ischemia Intestinal atresia Severe liver failure Major gastrointestinal surgery
	Critical illness with poor enteral tolerance or accessibility	Multiorgan system failure Major trauma or burns Bone marrow transplantation Acute respiratory failure with ventilator dependency and gastrointestinal malfunction Severe wasting in renal failure with dialysis Small bowel transplantation, immediate postoperatively

AIDS, Acquired immunodeficiency syndrome; *COPD*, chronic obstructive pulmonary disease; *ED*, eating disorder; *HIV*, human immunodeficiency virus.

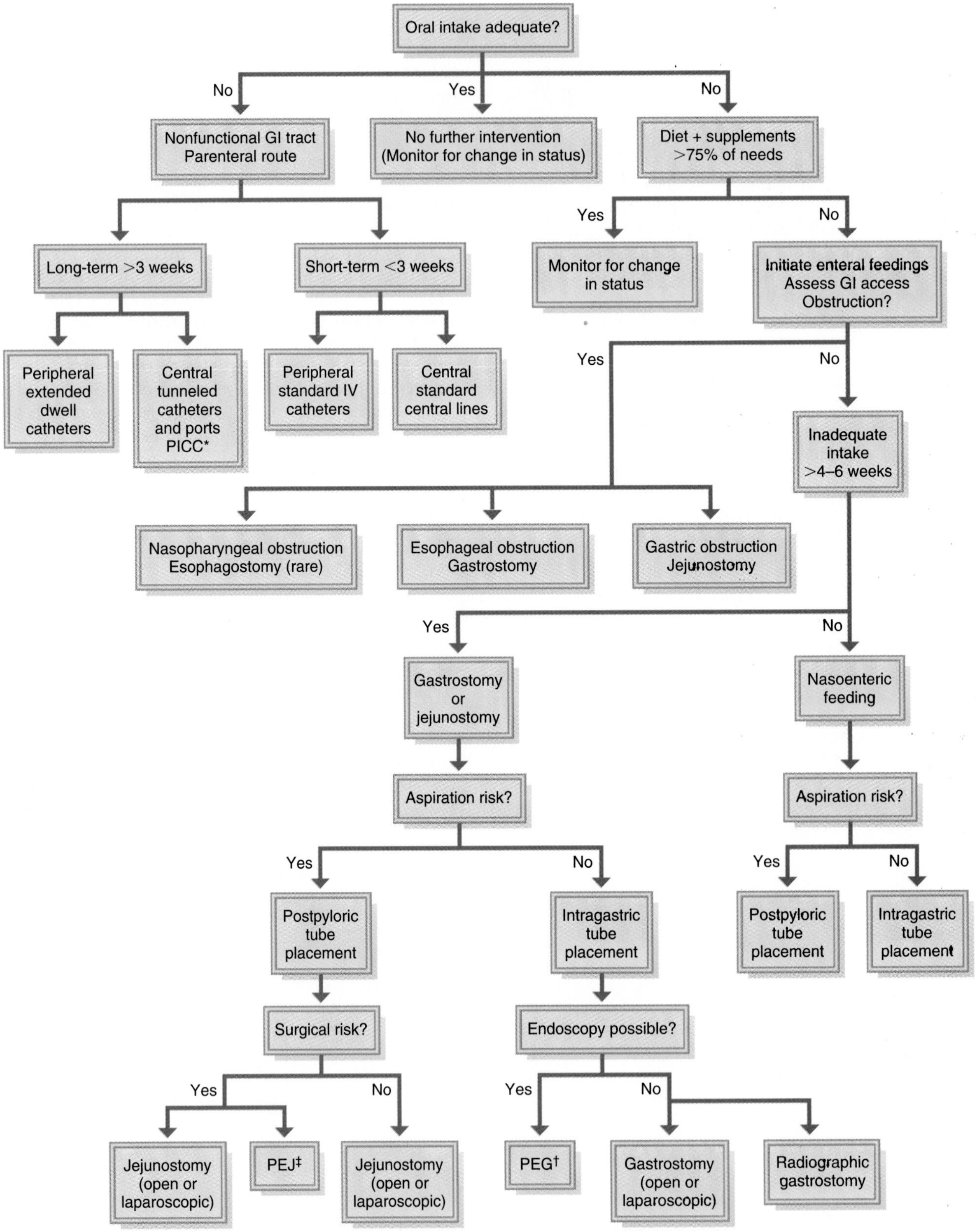

**PICC*, Peripherally inserted central catheter
†*PEG*, Percutaneous endoscopic gastrostomy
‡*PEJ*, Percutaneous endoscopic jejunostomy

FIGURE 23-1 • Algorithm for route selection. (Modified from Gorman RC, Morris JB: Minimally invasive access to the gastrointestinal tract. In Rombeau JL, Rolandelli RH, editors: *Clinical nutrition: enteral and tube feeding,* Philadelphia, 1997, WB Saunders; and Ali A et al: Nutrition support services, *Nutrition Support Algorithms* 8[7]:13, 1988.)

Although methods of nutrition support can be standardized for the course of certain disease states or treatments, it is important to note that every patient presents an individual challenge, and nutrition support must often be adapted to unanticipated developments or complications. The optimal treatment plan requires interdisciplinary input and is closely aligned with the overall patient care plan. In a few instances, nutrition support may be warranted but physically impossible to implement within the overall care plan. Conversely, nutrition support may be achievable but may not be warranted because of the prognosis, unacceptable risk, or the patient's right to self-determination.

ENTERAL NUTRITION

By definition, *enteral* means "within or by the way of the gastrointestinal tract." In practice, enteral nutrition is generally considered tube feeding. The consensus of nutrition experts is that the gastrointestinal tract is more physiologically and metabolically effective than the intravenous route for nutrient utilization (Klein et al, 1997; Lord et al, 1998). Once the patient has been assessed and found to be a good candidate for enteral nutrition, the clinician selects the appropriate tube and route of access for tube placement (see Figure 23-1). Enteral access selection depends on several factors: (1) anticipated length of time enteral feeding will be required, (2) degree of risk for aspiration or tube displacement, (3) presence or absence of normal digestion and absorption, (4) whether or not there is a planned surgical intervention, and (5) administration issues such as formula viscosity and volume.

Enteral Access

Nasogastric Route

For short-term enteral nutrition of 3 to 4 weeks, a nasogastric tube passed through the nose into the stomach is appropriate. Patients with normal gastrointestinal function and gag reflex tolerate this method, which takes advantage of normal digestive, hormonal, and bactericidal processes in the stomach. Feedings can be administered by bolus injection or intermittent or continuous infusions (see Administration). Soft, flexible, and well-tolerated polyurethane or silicone tubes of various diameters, lengths, and design features may be used, depending on formula characteristics and feeding requirements. For a more complete description of feeding tube characteristics, many resources are available. Tube placement is verified by aspirating gastric contents in combination with auscultation of air insufflation into the stomach or radiographic confirmation of the tube tip location. Techniques for placement verification have been described elsewhere (Guenter et al, 1997; Kirby et al, 1998; Levy, 1998). When soft, small-bore tubes are used, aspiration of gastric contents must be performed cautiously to prevent the tube from collapsing.

Nasoduodenal or Nasojejunal Route

For short-term enteral nutrition support of 3 to 4 weeks in patients with gastric motility disorders, esophageal reflux, or persistent nausea and vomiting nasoenteric tubes placed postpylorically (into the small bowel) are appropriate. These tubes have various design features, such as weighted or nonweighted tips and stylets to guide placement. The tube is passed through the nose and esophagus and inserted into the stomach. The tip of the tube migrates into the small bowel via peristaltic activity. In critically ill patients, tube migration can take several days, causing feeding delays. Radiologic verification of tube placement is the preferred method of confirmation to ensure safety. Tubes can also be placed with endoscopic or fluoroscopic guidance (Metheny, 1996; Shike and Bloch, 1998).

Percutaneous Endoscopic Gastrostomy or Jejunostomy

The percutaneous endoscopic gastrostomy (PEG) is a nonsurgical technique for placing a tube directly into the stomach through the abdominal wall, performed using an endoscope and with the patient under local anesthesia. Tubes are endoscopically guided into the stomach or the jejunum and then brought out through the abdominal wall to provide the access route for enteral feedings. The PEG is the preferred access route for patients requiring tube feeding for more than 3 to 4 weeks because of its short procedural time required for insertion, limited need for anesthesia, and minimal wound complications. After the initial PEG tube has been used successfully and the abdominal stoma site healed, it can be replaced with a "low-profile" device that allows the patient more freedom of movement and convenience, such as ease in showering or wearing tight clothing. It is also possible to place a percutaneous endoscopic jejunostomy (PEJ) tube percutaneously; however, this procedure carries a higher degree of risk (Kirby et al, 1998; Shike and Bloch, 1998).

Other Minimally Invasive Techniques

High-resolution video cameras have made percutaneous radiologic and laparoscopic gastrostomy and jejunostomy enteral access an option for patients in whom endoscopic procedures are contraindicated. Using fluoroscopy, a radiologic technique, tubes can be guided visually into the stomach or the jejunum and then brought out through the abdominal wall to provide the access route for enteral feedings (Georgeson and Owings, 1998). Neither laparoscopic nor fluoroscopic techniques are widely used at this time but offer potential options for enteral access in the future (Gorman and Morris, 1997; Shike and Bloch, 1998).

Surgically Placed Enterostomies

Surgical gastrostomies and jejunostomies are placed in patients requiring enteral support who are undergoing a surgical procedure or in whom endoscopic and radiologic techniques are not possible. The simplest surgical procedures for placing a gastrostomy tube are the Stamm and Witzel techniques. A more permanent method is the Janeway procedure. Surgical gastrostomy tubes have virtually the same use as PEGs (Ideno, 1992; Kirby et al, 1998; Shike and Bloch, 1998).

The Witzel jejunostomy and needle-catheter jejunostomy are short-term small bowel access methods. They are usually used for early postoperative enteral nutrition in combination with gastric decompression. The small lumen size of the needle-catheter jejunostomy can be problematic because it is easily dislodged and not all formulas flow readily through the catheter. Surgical jejunostomies provide the same decreased benefits as nasojejunal and PEJ feeding techniques.

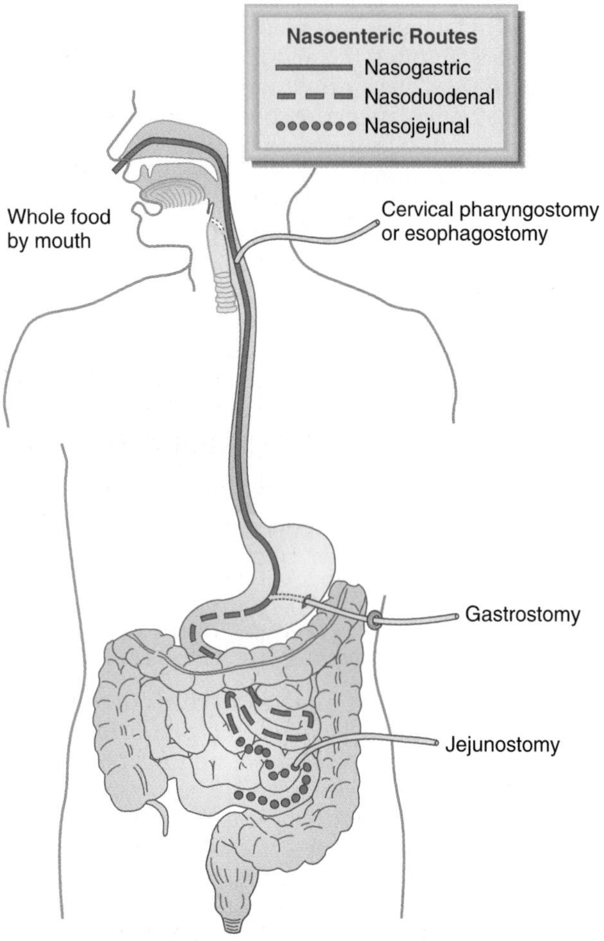

FIGURE 23-2 • Diagram of enteral tube placement.

Multiple Lumen Tubes

Gastrojejunal dual tubes are available for either endoscopic or surgical placement. These tubes are designed for patients in whom prolonged gastric decompression is anticipated. The tube has one lumen for decompression, and the other lumen is used to feed into the small bowel. These tubes are used for early postoperative feeding. For a summary of access sites, see Figure 23-2.

Enteral Formula Composition

A wide variety of enteral feeding products are commercially available. Evaluation of the suitability and efficacy of products, whether for individual use or for institutional use, is increasingly complex. As more products become available, with claims for pharmacologic effects, clinical trial evidence for each new product must be carefully evaluated by the clinician before a decision is made to use a formula (Matarese, 1998).

The suitability of a feeding formula for a patient should be evaluated based on the following characteristics: (1) functional status of the patient's gastrointestinal tract; (2) physical characteristics of the formula, such as osmolality, fiber content, caloric density, and viscosity; (3) macronutrient ratios; (4) digestion and absorption capability of the patient; (5) specific metabolic needs; (6) contribution of the feeding to fluid and electrolyte needs or restrictions; and (7) cost-effectiveness. Small bowel feeding requires careful selection of formula because of the sensitivity to osmolality and absorptive function of the small bowel. See Chapter 9 for a similar discussion for feeding infants. Figure 23-3 presents an algorithm for formula selection.

Formulas are classified in a variety of ways, usually based on protein or overall macronutrient composition. Table 23-2 presents one method of categorizing enteral formulas (see also Appendixes 36 through 41). General-purpose formulas are tolerated by most patients, and most of these formulas provide 1.0 kcal/ml. General formulas that provide 1.5 to 2.0 kcal/ml are used when it is necessary to restrict fluid for patients with cardiopulmonary, renal, and hepatic failure. High-nitrogen formulas are used for patients with increased protein requirements, such as those with burns, fistulas, sepsis, or trauma. Disease-specific formulas are available for patients who have renal, hepatic, or cardiopulmonary disease; metabolic stress; immunosuppression; or glucose intolerance. The efficacy of disease-specific formulas is controversial (Gottschlich et al, 1997).

Protein

Protein in enteral formulas provides 4% to 32% of total kilocalories (Olree et al, 1998). Polymeric formulas contain biologically complete, intact proteins such as caseinate, lactalbumin, beef, and soy protein isolate. Formulas containing peptide fragments (dipeptides, tripeptides, or oligopeptides) and amino acids derived from hydrolysis of casein, whey, lactalbumin, or soy are available for patients with maldigestion or malabsorption. These formulas have higher osmolalities because of the hydrolyzed protein. The form of protein (intact or hydrolyzed) that is most efficiently digested and absorbed by the gastrointestinal tract remains controversial (Olree et al, 1998). High-protein formulas increase nitrogenous waste excretion by the kidneys; this process requires adequate amounts of fluid for efficient excretion, which is particularly important in patients who cannot communicate thirst.

Carbohydrate

Carbohydrate contributes 40% to 90% of total kilocalories in enteral formulas. Carbohydrate sources used in formulas are pureed fruits and vegetables, corn syrup solids, corn and tapioca starch hydrolysates, maltodextrins, sucrose, fructose, and glucose. Similar to protein, the carbohydrate source and degree of hydrolysis affect osmolality. Lactose is not used as a carbohydrate source in most formulas

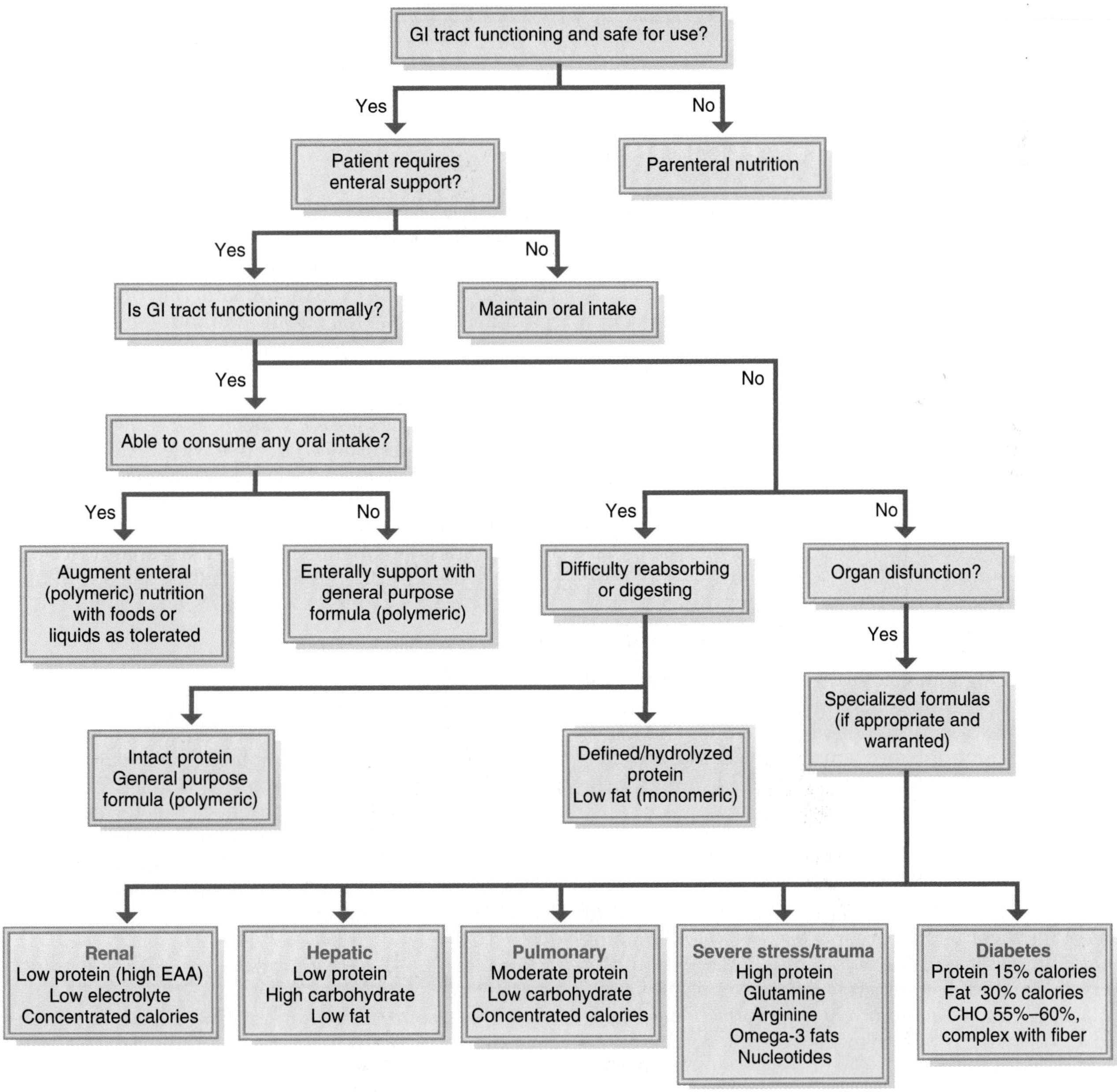

FIGURE 23-3 • Algorithm for enteral formula selection. (Modified from Ali A et al: Nutrition support services, *Nutrition Support Algorithms* 8[7]:13, July 1988.)

TABLE 23-2 Enteral Formula Categories

General purpose/intact (polymeric)	For use in patients with normal or minimally impaired digestion; absorption required; contains intact protein; can be instituted at full strength; low viscosity; 300-500 mOsm/kg; 1-1.2 kcal/ml; lactose free; 30-40 protein/L; inexpensive; also known as "house," general, meal replacement.
Defined/hydrolyzed (monomeric)	For patients with GI compromise who require hydrolyzed nutrients for improved digestion; osmolality depends on hydrolysis; 1-1.2 kcal/ml; lactose free; 30-45 g protein/L; is more expensive than general purpose formula; also known as chemically defined, peptide-based, elemental formula.
Semielemental	For use in patients with limited GI function; contains free amino acids, minimal fat, and minimal residue; hyperosmolar; low viscosity; 1 kcal/ml, 40 g protein/L; expensive; also known as free amino acid formula.
Disease-specific	Designed for specific organ dysfunction or metabolic abnormality; may not be nutritionally complete; most are hyperosmolar; products specific for hepatic, renal, and pulmonary diseases, glucose intolerance, impaired immune function, and trauma (BCAA); expensive; available data should be evaluated carefully for efficacy and benefits.
Rehydration	For patients requiring an optimal ratio of simple carbohydrates to electrolytes for the purpose of maximizing fluid and electrolyte absorption and rehydration.
Modular	Formula providing protein, fat, or carbohydrate as single nutrients to alter the nutrient composition of commercial formulas or food; may also contribute electrolytes and increase osmotic or renal solute load; increase cost, require labor and safe mixing technique; also known as *modular formula.*

Modified from Olree K et al: Enteral formulations. In *The ASPEN nutrition support practice manual,* Silver Spring, Md, 1998, American Society for Parenteral and Enteral Nutrition; Gottschlich MM et al: Defined formula diets. In Rombeau JL, Rolandelli RH, editors: *Clinical nutrition: enteral and tube feeding,* Philadelphia, 1997, WB Saunders; and Ideno KT: Enteral nutrition. In Gottschlich MM et al, editors: *Nutrition support dietetics core curriculum,* Silver Spring, Md, 1992, American Society for Parenteral and Enteral Nutrition.

because lactase deficiency is common among acutely ill patients.

Lipid

Lipid provides 1.5% to 55% of the total kilocalories of enteral formulas. General-purpose formulas have between 30% and 40% of their total kilocalories provided by lipids, usually from corn, soy, sunflower, or safflower oils. Defined or monomeric formulas usually have minimal amounts of lipid. About 2% to 4% of the daily calories in the form of linoleic acid is necessary to prevent essential fatty acid deficiency. Research suggests that high dosages of linoleic acid may suppress immune function. Short-chain and medium-chain saturated fatty acids, monounsaturated fatty acids, and omega-3 polyunsaturated fatty acids have been included in disease-specific formulas as alternatives to the high linoleic acid-containing vegetable oil in formulas. Formulas high in lipid that are intended to prevent excess carbon dioxide retention and facilitate weaning from mechanical ventilation are also available (Gottschlich et al, 1997), even though they are not commonly necessary or used in practice.

Vitamins, Minerals, and Electrolytes

Most, but not all, available formulas are designed to meet the dietary reference intakes (DRIs) for vitamins and minerals if a sufficient volume is taken. It should be noted that these recommendations are for healthy populations, not for acute or chronically ill populations. Electrolytes are provided in relatively modest amounts compared with the oral diet and may require supplementation when diarrhea or drainage losses occur. Patients with compromised cardiopulmonary, renal, or hepatic function often require electrolyte restriction.

Fluid

Fluid needs for adults can be estimated at 1 ml of water/kcal, or 30 to 35 ml per kilogram of usual body weight (Lord et al, 1998). Without an additional source of fluid, tube-fed patients may not get enough free water to meet their needs, particularly when nutrient-dense formulas are used. Standard formulas contain 80% to 85% free water. Calorie-dense formulas may have as little as 60% free water. All sources of fluid being given to a patient receiving enteral nutrition, including feeding tube flushes, medications, and intravenous fluids, should be considered when determining a patient's intake. Additional water can be provided through the feeding tube as needed (see Chapter 6).

Osmolality

The size and number of the nutrient particles in a solution define its osmolality (see Chapter 6). General-purpose formulas have osmolalities between 300 and 500 mOsm, which is close to the osmolality of body fluids. Osmolalities of nutrient-dense formulas are higher, ranging from 400 to 700 mOsm. Hydrolyzed formulas are as high as 900 mOsm per kilogram of water. Box 23-1 summarizes factors to consider when selecting an enteral formula.

Administration

The three common methods of tube feeding administration are bolus feeding, intermittent drip, and continuous drip. Method selection is based on the patient's clinical status and quality of life considerations. One method can serve as a transition to another method as the patient's status changes.

Box 23-1. Factors to Consider When Choosing an Enteral Formula

Gastrointestinal function
The type of protein, fat, carbohydrate, and fiber in the formula as related to the patient's digestive and absorptive capacity
Caloric and protein density of the formula (i.e., kcal/ml, g protein/ml, and kcal:nitrogen ratio)
Ability of the formula, taken in the amounts tolerated, to meet the patient's nutritional requirements
Sodium, potassium, magnesium, and phosphorus content of the formula, especially for patients with cardiopulmonary, renal, or hepatic failure
Viscosity of the formula related to tube size and method of feeding

Bolus

The feeding modality of choice when patients are clinically stable with a functional stomach is the syringe bolus method. Syringe bolus feedings are more convenient and less expensive than pump or gravity bolus feedings and should be encouraged when tolerated. A 60-ml syringe is used to infuse the formula. If bloating or abdominal discomfort develops, the patient is encouraged to wait 10 to 15 minutes before proceeding with the remainder of formula allocated for that feeding. The patient with normal gastric function can usually tolerate 500 ml of formula at each feeding. Three or four bolus feedings per day can provide the daily nutritional requirements for most patients (Lord et al, 1998).

Intermittent Drip

Quality of life issues are often the reason for the initiation of intermittent drip feeding regimens, which allow mobile patients more free time and autonomy compared with continuous drip infusions. These feedings can be given by pump or gravity drip. A schedule is based on four to six feedings per day administered for 20 to 60 minutes. Formula administration is initiated at 100 to 150 ml per feeding and increased incrementally as tolerated. Success with this method of feeding depends largely on the degree of mobility, alertness, and motivation of the patient to tolerate the regimen. Intermittent feedings as well as bolus feedings should not be used with patients at high risk for pulmonary aspiration.

Continuous Drip

Continuous drip infusion of formula requires a pump. This method is appropriate for patients who do not tolerate large-volume infusions such as those occurring with bolus or intermittent methods. Patients with compromised gastrointestinal function because of disease, surgery, antineoplastic therapy, or other physiologic impediments are candidates for continuous drip infusion. Patients with small bowel access should also be fed by continuous drip infusion. The feeding-rate goal, in milliliters per hour, is set by dividing the total daily volume by the number of hours per day of administration (usually 18 to 24 hours). Feeding is started at one quarter to one half the goal rate and advanced every 8 to 12 hours to the final volume. Formulas with osmolalities between 300 and 500 mOsm/kg can be started at full strength. Hyperosmolar formulas should be advanced conservatively to ensure tolerance. Dilution of formulas is not necessary (Lord et al, 1998).

Modern enteral pumps are small and easy to handle. Many pumps are battery operated for up to 8 hours in addition to being electrically powered, allowing flexibility and mobility for the patient. Most pumps have a complete delivery system available, including bags and tubing compatible with proper pump operation.

Complications and Monitoring

Complications

Box 23-2 provides a comprehensive list of complications associated with enteral nutrition and possible solutions. Aspiration of formula into the airway is a major concern for patients receiving enteral nutrition. To reduce the risk of aspiration, patients should be positioned with their heads and shoulders above their chests during and immediately after feeding. There is confusion in the literature as to the efficacy of checking gastric residuals. Stable patients, especially those on long-term feeding, do not need residuals checked regularly. Also, it is difficult to aspirate the stomach contents, and the residuals may contain more secretions and gastric fluids than feeding. Aspiration of gastric residuals is most relevant in critically ill patients and others at risk for gastroparesis. In these patients, residuals are usually checked every 4 hours or as needed (Lord et al, 1998).

For many years clinicians have used blue dye in enteral formulas to detect aspiration of formula; however, this practice has become controversial. Reports indicate that some critically ill patients have discoloration of the skin, urine, serum or other body fluids after ingestion of the blue dye. Blue dye may also cause a falsely positive reading on guaiac tests, causing unnecessary follow-up procedures or laboratory tests. Although several deaths have been reported with the use of blue dye, the mechanisms are still unknown (Maloney et al, 2001). Many hospitals have discontinued the use of blue dye.

Abdominal leakage of gastric contents from a gastrostomy site can cause skin erosion and skin breakdown, leading to infection and peritonitis; however, fewer than 10% of patients experience serious complications. The remaining complications are minor and can be prevented with careful patient monitoring (Farwell et al, 2002; Gorman and Morris, 1997; Hamaoui and Kodsi, 1997).

Diarrhea is a common complication frequently associated with enteral nutrition. The most likely causes of diarrhea among enterally fed patients are bacterial overgrowth, antibiotic therapy, and gastrointestinal motility disorders associated with acute and critical illness. Hyperosmolar medications such as magnesium-containing antacids, sorbitol-containing elixirs, and electrolyte replacement supplements can also contribute to diarrhea. Adjustment of medications or administration methods can frequently correct the diarrhea. The addition of soy polysaccharide, pectin, and other fibers, bulking agents, and antidiarrheal medications can also help.

Among stable patients receiving enteral nutrition, constipation may be a problem. Fiber-containing formulas or stool-bulking medication may be helpful, and adequate fluid must be provided. Gastrointestinal motility should be assessed. Diarrhea can coexist with constipation, usually when a patient has impaction.

Box 23-2. Complications of Enteral Nutrition

Access Problems

Pressure necrosis/ulceration/stenosis
Tube displacement/migration
Tube obstruction
Leakage from ostomy/stoma site

Administration Problems

Regurgitation
Aspiration
Microbial contamination

Gastrointestinal Complications

Nausea/vomiting
Distention/bloating/cramping
Delayed gastric emptying
Constipation
High gastric residuals
Diarrhea
- Osmotic
- Secretory
- Medications
- Treatment/therapies
- Hypoalbuminemia
- Maldigestion/malabsorption
- Formula choice/rate of administration

Metabolic Complications

Refeeding syndrome
Drug–nutrient interactions
Glucose intolerance/hyperglycemia/hypoglycemia
Hydration status—dehydration/overhydration
Hyponatremia
Hyperkalemia/hypokalemia
Hyperphosphatemia/hypophosphatemia
Micronutrient deficiencies

Modified from Hamaoui E, Kodsi R: Complications of enteral feeding and their prevention. In Rombeau JL, Rolandelli RH, editors: *Clinical nutrition: enteral tube feeding,* Philadelphia, 1997, WB Saunders; and Ideno KT: Enteral nutrition. In Gottschlich MM et al, editors: *Nutrition support dietetics core curriculum,* Silver Spring, Md, 1992, American Society for Parenteral and Enteral Nutrition.

Monitoring

Patients receiving enteral nutrition are monitored to prevent and correct complications. In addition, monitoring of the patient's actual intake and tolerance is necessary to ensure that nutritional goals are achieved and maintained. During routine patient care, actual feeding time is commonly lost from the patient's prescribed feeding schedule. One study showed that fewer than half of tube-fed patients receive their entire prescribed intake on any given day. The most common reasons continue, as they have for many years, to be (1) dislodged tube, (2) gastrointestinal intolerance, (3) medical procedures requiring discontinuation of feeding, and (4) difficulties with the feeding tube position (Abernathy et al, 1989).

Monitoring of metabolic and gastrointestinal tolerance, hydration status, and nutritional status is extremely important for the tube-fed patient, and Box 23-3 gives guidelines. Practice guidelines, institutional protocols, and standardized ordering procedures are helpful to ensure optimal, safe provision of enteral nutrition support. Figure 23-4 displays an enteral nutrition order form.

Box 23-3. In-Patient Enteral Nutrition Monitoring

Weight (at least 3 times/wk)
Signs and symptoms of edema (daily)
Signs and symptoms of dehydration (daily)
Fluid intake and output (daily)
Adequacy of enteral intake (at least 2 times/wk)
Nitrogen balance (24-hr urine urea nitrogen) (weekly), if appropriate
Gastric residuals (every 4 hr) if appropriate
Serum electrolytes, blood urea nitrogen (BUN), creatinine, (2-3 times/wk)
Serum glucose, calcium, magnesium, phosphorus, (weekly or as ordered)
Stool output and consistency (daily)

ENTERAL NUTRITION SUPPORT ORDER
Date: ____________Time: ______________________
DX: ______________________________
Reason for TF: ______________________

ENTERAL NUTRITION SUPPORT ORDERS:

1. ROUTE: Check tube type
   ( ) NGT ( ) PEG/G-TUBE ( ) PEG/JTUBE

2. FORMULA: Check the desired formula

Formula	kcal/cc	Formula	kcal/cc
( ) General purpose	1.0	( ) Fiber enriched	1.0
( ) General purpose High Nitrogen	1.2-1.4	( ) Monomeric	1.0

3. METHOD OF FEEDING: Check the desired schedule.

( ) Schedule A: Bolus Feeding Via Syringe/Gravity Bag
1. 8:00 PM 240 cc formula
   12:00 PM 240 cc formula
   4:00 PM 240 cc formula
   8:00 PM 240 cc formula
2. Water can be added to gravity bag pending hydration needs.
3. As tolerated, registered dietitian to advance feeding and adjust water to meet goal rates.
4. Formula progression to goal: ______________

( ) Schedule B: Pump
1. Begin full strength 30 cc/hr × 8 hr.
2. If tolerated after 8 hr, advance to 50cc/hr × 24 hr.
3. As tolerated, registered dietitian to advance feeding and adjust water to meet goal rates.
4. Formula progression to goal: ______________

( ) Schedule C: Tube Feeding Protocol Via Gravity Bag
1. Schedule: 6:00 AM, 10:00 AM, 2:00 PM, 6:00 PM, 10:00 PM
2. Initial feeding - 240 cc water.
   At next scheduled time - 240 cc Formula + 240 cc water.
3. As tolerated, registered dietitian to advance feeding and adjust water to meet goal rates.
4. Formula progression to goal:

4. ( ) ALTERNATE ORDERS:
   CONSULT REGISTERED DIETITIAN TO DETERMINE FORMULA AND SCHEDULE:
   1. Formula: ______________
   2. Schedule: ______________

REGISTERED DIETITIAN:

1. NUTRITIONAL GOAL:

Formula: ______________
Calories: ______________
Protein: ______________
Vitamins/Minerals: ______________

2. RECOMMENDATIONS:
____

Registered Dietitian: ______________

ENTERAL NUTRITION SUPPORT GUIDELINES:

PHYSICIAN:

1. PLACEMENT: Confirm placement of NGT by abdominal x-ray.
2. MEDICATIONS: Identify via enternal feeding tube:
   A. Consult pharmacist to verify appropriate form of medication.
   B. 30 cc water flush before and after each medication.
   C. Administer each medication separately.
3. FLUID BALANCE: Patient fluid requirements and intake should be assessed, include IV, water flush, and water available from tube feeding (formula is approximately 80% free water).
4. LABORATORY WORK-UP:
   A. Initial: Na, K, CO_2, C1, BUN, Creat, Mg, Ca, Phos.
   B. Thereafter: As needed.

FIGURE 23-4 • Enteral nutrition order form. (Courtesy Memorial-Sloan Kettering Cancer Center, New York, N.Y.)

PARENTERAL NUTRITION

Parenteral nutrition is the provision of nutrients directly into the bloodstream intravenously. Assuming a patient is an appropriate candidate for parenteral nutrition, it is then necessary to choose between central and peripheral access (see Figure 23-1). Central access refers to catheter tip placement in a large, high-blood-flow vein such as the superior vena cava; this is total parenteral nutrition (TPN). Peripheral access refers to catheter tip placement in a small vein typically in the arm. Many clinicians do not use peripheral parenteral nutrition (PPN) because they argue that it is short-term therapy with minimal impact on nutritional status. Therefore, they believe that central access is required for effective parenteral nutrition. Others argue that PPN can be used as a supplemental feeding or in a transitional phase to enteral or oral feeding.

Newer peripheral devices have made it possible to infuse PPN with a single catheter placed for up to a month. Peripheral veins cannot tolerate concentrated solutions; therefore, diluted larger-volume infusions are often necessary to meet nutritional requirements. Volume-sensitive patients such as those with cardiopulmonary, renal, or hepatic failure are not good candidates for PPN.

Additional helpful information for appropriate access selection is previous access history, edema or skin damage at the access site, medical and medication history, coagulation time, need for additional infusions, peripheral vein condition, functional status, and lifestyle (Krzysda and Edmiston, 1998). See Chapter 9 for discussion related to feeding low-birth-weight infants.

Parenteral Access

Peripheral Access

Nutrient solutions not exceeding 800 to 900 mOsm per kilogram of solvent can be infused through a routine peripheral intravenous catheter placed in a vein in good condition. Protocols for dressing changes and rotation of the site are used to prevent the principal complication of peripheral catheters—thrombophlebitis.

A more recent development in peripheral catheter technology is the extended dwell catheter. These catheters are sometimes called *midline* or *midclavicular* catheters, depending on their position. Extended dwell catheters require a vein large enough to advance the catheter 5 to 7 inches into the vein. These catheters can remain at the original site for 3 to 6 weeks and have made PPN a more feasible option in patients with veins that are large enough to tolerate the catheter (Krzysda and Edmiston, 1998).

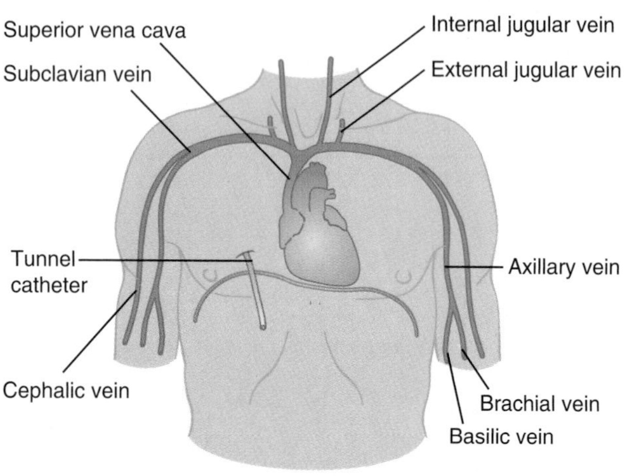

FIGURE 23-5 • Venous sites from which the superior vena cava may be accessed.

Short-Term Central Access

Catheters used for central or TPN ideally consist of a single lumen. If central access is needed for other reasons, such as hemodynamic monitoring, drawing blood samples, or giving medications, multiple-lumen catheters are available. To reduce the risk of infection, the catheter lumen used to infuse TPN should be reserved for only that purpose. Catheters are most commonly inserted into the subclavian vein and advanced until the catheter tip is in the superior vena cava, using strict aseptic technique. Alternatively, an internal or external jugular vein catheter can be used with the same catheter tip placement. The motion of the neck, however, makes this site much more difficult for maintaining the sterility of a dressing. Radiologic verification of the tip site is necessary before infusion of nutrients can begin. Strict infection control protocols should be used for catheter placement and maintenance (Krzysda and Edmiston, 1998). Figure 23-5 shows alternative venous access sites for TPN; femoral placement is also possible.

Long-Term Central Access

A commonly used long-term catheter is a "tunneled" catheter. These single- or multiple-lumen catheters are placed in the cephalic, subclavian, or internal jugular veins and fed into the superior vena cava. A subcutaneous tunnel is created so that the catheter exits the skin several inches away from its venous entry site. Another type of long-term catheter is a port device that is implanted under the skin where the catheter would normally exit at the end of the subcutaneous tunnel. A special needle must access the entrance port. Ports can be single or double; an individual port is equivalent to a lumen. The latest development in catheter technology is a peripherally inserted central catheter, or PICC. This catheter is inserted into a vein in the antecubital area of the arm and threaded into the subclavian vein with the catheter tip placed in the superior vena cava. Trained professionals can insert PICCs, whereas placement of a tunneled catheter is a surgical procedure (Krzysda and Edmiston, 1998).

Both tunneled catheters and PICCs can be used for extended therapy in the hospital and are frequently used for home infusion therapy. Their greatest advantage for patients is better mobility and time away from infusion, which can be cycled at intervals. They also minimize risk of infection because the tunnel creates a barrier between the entry of the catheter into the skin and into the vein. Care of long-term catheters requires specialized handling and extensive patient education (see Home Care).

Parenteral Nutrition Solutions

Protein

Commercially available standard solutions are composed of both essential and nonessential crystalline amino acids. Specialized solutions with adjusted amino acid content are available for patients with hypermetabolism or renal or liver disease. These products are used on a limited basis because of their expense and the lack of conclusive research data supporting the efficacy of their use.

The concentration of amino acids in these solutions ranges from 3% to 15%. Thus, a 10% solution of amino acids supplies 100 g of protein per liter. The percentage of a solution is usually expressed at its final concentration after dilution with other nutrient solutions, but it is sometimes described by initial concentration. The caloric content of amino acid solutions is approximately 4 kcal/g protein provided. About 15% to 20% of total energy intake should come from protein (Strausburg, 1998).

Carbohydrate

Carbohydrate is supplied as dextrose monohydrate in concentrations ranging from 5% to 70%. The dextrose monohydrate yields 3.4 calories/g. As with amino acids, a 10% solution yields 100 g of carbohydrate per liter of solution. The use of carbohydrate (100 g daily for a 70-kg person) ensures that protein is not catabolized for energy. Maximal rates of carbohydrate administration should not exceed 5 mg/kg/min. Excessive administration can lead to hyperglycemia, hepatic abnormalities, and increased ventilatory drive. Calculation of osmolarity of a parenteral solution may be useful to ensure venous tolerance (Strausburg, 1998). (See *Clinical Insight:* Calculating the Osmolarity of a Parenteral Nutrition Solution.)

Lipid

Lipid emulsions, available in 10% and 20% concentrations, are composed of aqueous suspensions of soybean or safflower oil with egg yolk phospholipid as the emulsifier. The three-carbon molecule, glycerol, which is water soluble, is added to the emulsion to provide osmolarity. Glycerol is oxidized and yields 4.3 kcal/g. A 10% emulsion provides 1.1 kcal/ml; a 20% emulsion provides 2.0 kcal/ml. About 10% of calories per day from fat emulsions provide the 2% to 4% of calories from linoleic acid required to prevent essential fatty acid deficiency. Linoleic acid alters prostaglandin metabolism when it is a major source of energy and therefore can decrease immune function (Bell et al, 1991). Because soybean and safflower oils are rich sources of linoleic acid, lipid infusions that provide significantly more than 1 g of lipid/kg per 24 hours may be immunosuppressive. In addition, slow and continuous 24-hour infusion, as opposed to short (less than 10 hours) infusion, can improve hepatic reticuloendothelial function (Jensen et al, 1990). Sometimes, however, clinicians will provide more than 30% of total calories as lipid to help hyperglycemic patients control serum glucose levels or pulmonary-compromised patients to decrease carbon dioxide production and to improve respiratory function. Maximal dosage of lipid should not exceed 2.0 g/kg of body weight daily.

Electrolytes, Vitamins, and Trace Elements

General guidelines for daily requirements are given for electrolytes (Table 23-3), vitamins (Table 23-4), and trace elements (Table 23-5). Because parenterally administered vitamins and trace elements do not go through the digestive and absorptive processes, these recommendations are lower than the DRIs. Parenteral solutions also represent a significant portion of total daily fluid and electrolyte intake. Once a solution is prescribed and initiated, minor to major adjustments for proper fluid and electrolyte balance

CLINICAL INSIGHT

Calculating the Osmolarity of a Parenteral Nutrition Solution

1. Multiply the grams of dextrose per liter by 5. Example: 50 g of dextrose × 5 = 250 mOsm/L
2. Multiply the grams of protein per liter by 10. Example: 30 g of protein × 10 = 300 mOsm/L
3. Fat is isotonic and does not contribute to osmolarity.
4. Electrolytes further add to osmolarity. Total osmolarity = 250 + 300 = 550 mOsm/L + mOsm of electrolytes.

(See also Chapter 6.)

may be necessary, depending on the stability of the patient. The choice of the salt form of electrolytes (e.g., chloride, acetate) has an impact on acid–base balance. Iron is also not normally part of parenteral infusions because it is not compatible with lipids and may enhance certain bacterial growth. When needed, it is given separately to stable home care patients as iron dextran.

Fluid

Fluid needs for parenteral and enteral nutrition are calculated similarly. Maximum volumes of TPN rarely exceed 3 L, with typical prescriptions of 1.5 to 3 L daily. In critically ill patients, volumes of prescribed TPN should be closely coordinated with the overall care plan. The administration of other medical therapies requiring fluid administration, such as intravenous medications and blood products, necessitates careful monitoring. Patients with cardiopulmonary, renal, and hepatic failure are especially sensitive to fluid administration.

TABLE 23-3 Daily Electrolyte Requirements During Total Parenteral Nutrition—Adults

ELECTROLYTE	PARENTERAL EQUIVALENT OF RDA	STANDARD INTAKE
Calcium	10 mEq	10-15 mEq
Magnesium	10 mEq	8-20 mEq
Phosphate	30 mmol	20-40 mmol
Sodium	N/A	1-2 mEq/kg + replacement
Potassium	N/A	1-2 mEq/kg
Acetate	N/A	As needed to maintain acid–base balance
Chloride	N/A	As needed to maintain acid–base balance

From National Advisory Group on Standards and Practice Guidelines for Parenteral Nutrition, ASPEN: Safe practices for parenteral nutrition formulations, *JPEN J Parenter Enteral Nutr* 22(2):49, 1998.

Compounding Methods

Parenteral nutrition prescriptions require preparation or compounding by competent pharmacy personnel under laminar airflow hoods using aseptic techniques. Prescriptions are compounded in two general ways. One method compounds all components except the fat emulsion, which is infused separately. Solutions are usually mixed in one bag at a 1:1 dextrose-to-amino acid volume ratio. The second method combines the lipid emulsion with the dextrose and amino acid solution and is referred to as a *total nutrient admixture* or 3-in-1 solution. Institutions frequently use standardized solutions, which are compounded in batches, thus saving labor and lowering costs; however, flexibility for individualized compounding should be available when warranted (Strausburg, 1998). Standard order forms are often useful (Table 23-6).

It is possible to include medications with TPN, including antibiotics, vasopressors, narcotics, diuretics, and many other commonly administered drugs. In fact, this occurs infrequently because it requires specialized knowledge of physical compatibility or incompatibility of the solution contents. The most common drug additives are insulin for persistent hyperglycemia and histamine-2 antagonists to avoid gastroduodenal stress ulceration (Klang, 1998). Heparin and exogenous albumin have been added to parenteral nutrition solutions; however, this practice is controversial (Foley et al, 1990).

Administration

Parenteral nutrition administration issues are addressed after the goal infusion rate based on calculations (see considerations in Box 23-4) has been

TABLE 23-4 Adult Parenteral Multivitamins: Comparison of Guidelines and Products

VITAMIN	"OLD" NAG-AMA GUIDELINES	FDA REQUIREMENTS	MVI-12	MVI-13 (INFUVITE) BAXTER
A (retinol)	3300 IU (1 mg)	3300 IU (1 mg)	3300 IU (1 mg)	3300 IU (1 mg)
D (ergocalciferol or cholecalciferol)	200 IU (5 μg)	200 IU (5 μg)	200 IU (5 μg)	200 IU (5 μg)
E (α-tocopherol)	10 IU (10 mg)	10 IU (10 mg)	10 IU (10 mg)	10 IU (10 mg)
B_1 (thiamin)	3 mg	6 mg	3 mg	6 mg
B_2 (riboflavin)	3.6 mg	3.6 mg	3.6 mg	3.6 mg
B_3 (niacinamide)	40 mg	40 mg	40 mg	40 mg
B_5 (dexpanthenol)	15 mg	15 mg	15 mg	15 mg
B_6 (pyridoxine)	4 mg	6 mg	4 mg	6 mg
B_{12} (cyanocobalamin)	5 μg	5 μg	5 μg	5 μg
C (ascorbic acid)	100 mg	200 mg	100 mg	200 mg
Biotin	60 μg	60 μg	60 μg	60 μg
Folic acid	400 μg	600 μg	400 μg	600 μg
Vitamin K		150 μg	0	150 μg

From *Federal Register* 66(77): April 20, 2000.
NAG, National Advisory Group; *AMA*, American Medical Association; *FDA*, U.S. Food and Drug Administration; *MVI-12* and *MVI-13*, multivitamin supplements.

established. Parenteral nutrition calculations and orders are inherently complex. Protocols for ordering parenteral nutrition vary considerably among institutions. Nevertheless, general considerations as listed in Box 23-4 can be applied to almost any protocol.

Continuous Infusion

Parenteral solutions are usually initiated below the goal infusion rate via a volumetric pump and then increased incrementally over a 2- or 3-day period to attain the goal infusion rate. Some practitioners start parenteral nutrition based on the amount of dextrose, with initial prescriptions containing 100 to 200 g daily and advancing over a 2- or 3-day period to a final goal. With high dextrose concentrations, abrupt cessation of TPN should be avoided, particularly if the patient's glucose tolerance is abnormal. If TPN is to be stopped, it is prudent to taper the rate of infusion in an unstable patient to prevent rebound hypoglycemia. For most stable patients, however, this is not necessary.

TABLE 23-5 Daily Trace Element Supplementation for Adult Total Parenteral Nutrition Formulations*

TRACE ELEMENT	INTAKE
Chromium	10-15 μg
Copper	0.3-0.5 mg
Manganese	60-100 μg
Zinc	2.5-5.0 mg

From National Advisory Group on Standards and Practice Guidelines for Parenteral Nutrition, ASPEN: Safe practices for parenteral nutrition formulations, *JPEN J Parenter Enteral Nutr* 22(2):49, 1998.
*Assumes normal organ function.

Cyclic Infusion

Cyclic total parenteral nutrition can be infused for 8- to 12-hour periods, usually at night, to permit a free period of 12 to 16 hours each day and improve the quality of life. The goal cycle for infusion time is established incrementally when a higher rate of infusion or a more concentrated solution is required. Cycled infusions should not be attempted if glucose intolerance or fluid tolerance is a problem.

Complications and Monitoring

As with enteral feeding, routine monitoring of actual intake is necessary to ensure compliance with the treatment plan. Administration time may be decreased because of patient ambulation and bathing, tests or other treatments, intravenous administration of medications, or other therapies.

Box 23-5 lists complications that can occur with parenteral nutrition. The primary associated complication is infection. Therefore, strict adherence to protocols and monitoring for signs of infection, such as chills, fever, tachycardia, sudden hyperglycemia, or elevated white blood cell count, are necessary to prevent infection. Monitoring of metabolic tolerance is critical to parenteral nutrition therapy. Electrolytes, acid-base balance, glucose tolerance, renal function, and cardiopulmonary and hemodynamic stability

TABLE 23-6 Sample Parenteral Nutrition Formulations

ADULT PATIENT* INSTITUTION/PHARMACY NAME, ADDRESS AND PHARMACY PHONE NUMBER		
Name	Dosing weight: 70 kg	Location
Administration date/time		Expiration date/time
Basic formula	Amount/day	(Amount/L)
Dextrose	400 g	(166.7 g/L)
Amino acids†	100 g	(41.7 g/L)
Lipid†	65 g	(27.1 g/L)
Electrolytes		
Sodium chloride	80 mEq	(33.3 mEq/L)
Sodium acetate	80 mEq	(33.3 mEq/L)
Potassium chloride	40 mEq	(16.7 mEq/L)
Potassium phosphate	30 mmol of P	(12.5 mmol/L)
	(45 mEq of K)	(18.8 mEq/L)
Calcium gluconate	10 mEq	(4.2 mEq/L)
Magnesium sulfate		
Vitamins, trace elements, and medications		
Multiple vitamins†	10 ml	
Multiple trace elements†	1-3 ml‡	
Infusion rate 100 ml/hr	Volume 2400 ml	Infuse over 24 hr
	Admixture contains 2400 ml plus 100 ml overfill	
	Central Line Use Only	

*From National Advisory Group on Standards and Practice Guidelines for Parenteral Nutrition, ASPEN: Safe practices for parenteral nutrition formulations, *JPEN J Parenter Enteral Nutr* 22(2):49, 1998.
†Specify product name.
‡Volume dependent on specific product used.

Box 23-4. Calculation Considerations For Enteral and Parenteral Nutrition

Enteral

1. Clinical status
2. Fluid requirement*
3. Energy (kcal) requirement†
4. Protein requirement†
5. Carbohydrate/lipid considerations
6. Micronutrient considerations
7. Formula selection
   a. Concentration (osmolarity)
   b. Protein content
   c. Carbohydrate/lipid content
   d. Micronutrient content
   e. Special formula considerations
8. Calculation
   a. Energy: use kcal/ml formula
   b. Protein: use g/1000 ml
   c. Fat and micronutrient considerations: units/1000 ml
   d. Fluid considerations: extra water, IV fluids (including medications)

Parenteral

1. Clinical status
2. Fluid requirement†
3. Energy (kcal) requirement†
4. Protein requirement†
5. Carbohydrate/lipid considerations
6. Micronutrient considerations
7. Solutions considerations
   a. Osmolarity (peripheral versus central infusion)
   b. "3 in 1" (amino acid, dextrose, lipid) versus "2 in 1" (amino acid, dextrose) plus piggyback lipid infusion
8. Calculation
   a. Energy
      i. Carbohydrate: g/100 ml, e.g., D20 = 20 g/100 ml, maximum 24-hr infusion
         • (Maximum 24-hr infusion: 5 mg/kg
      ii. Lipid: 10% = 1.1 kcal/ml, 20% = 2 kcal/ml
         • (Optimal infusion 1 g/kg/24 hr, maximum 2 g/kg/hr
   b. Amino acid: g/100 ml, e.g., 10% amino acid = 10 g/100 ml
   c. Micronutrient considerations (see Tables 23-3, 23-4, and 23-5)
9. Medications
   a. Insulin
   b. Histamine-2 antagonists

Modified from the American Society for Parenteral and Enteral Nutrition: Safe practice for parenteral nutrition formulations, *JPEN J Parenter Enter Nutr* 22(2):56, 1998.
*Maximum or minimum based on clinical status.
†Energy and protein requirements are disease and condition specific.

Box 23-5. Parenteral Nutrition Complications

Mechanical Complications

Pneumothorax
Hemothorax
Hydrothorax
Tension penumothorax
Subcutaneous emphysema
Brachial plexus injury
Subclavian artery injury
Subclavian hematoma
Central vein thrombophlebitis
Arteriovenous fistula
Thoracic duct injury
Hydromediastinum
Air embolism
Catheter fragment embolism
Catheter misplacement
Cardiac perforation
Endocarditis

Infection and Sepsis

Catheter entrance site
  Contamination during insertion
  Long-term catheter placement
Catheter seeding from bloodborne or distant infection
Solution contamination

Metabolic Complications

Dehydration from osmotic diuresis
Hyperosmolar, nonketotic, hyperglycemic coma
Rebound hypoglycemia on sudden cessation of parenteral nutrition in patient with unstable glucose levels
Hypomagnesemia
Hypocalcemia
Hypercalcemia
Hyperphosphatemia
Hypophosphatemia
Hyperchloremic metabolic acidosis
Uremia
Hyperammonemia
Electrolyte imbalance
Trace mineral deficiencies
Essential fatty acid deficiency
Hyperlipidemia

Gastrointestinal Complications

Cholestasis
Hepatic abnormalities
Gastrointestinal villous atrophy

TABLE 23-7 In-Patient Parenteral Nutrition Monitoring*

VARIABLE TO BE MONITORED	SUGGESTED FREQUENCY INITIAL PERIOD*	LATER PERIOD*
Weight	Daily	Weekly
Serum electrolytes	Daily	1-2/wk
Blood urea nitrogen	3/wk	Weekly
Serum total calcium or ionized Ca^{++}, inorganic phosphorus, magnesium	3/wk	Weekly
Serum glucose	Daily	3/wk
Serum triglycerides	Weekly	Weekly
Liver function enzymes	3/wk	Weekly
Hemoglobin, hematocrit	Weekly	Weekly
Platelets	Weekly	Weekly
WBC count	As indicated	As indicated
Clinical status	Daily	Daily
Catheter site	Daily	Daily
Temperature	Daily	Daily
I & O	Daily	Daily

*Initial period refers to that period in which a full glucose intake is being achieved. Later period implies that the patient has achieved a steady metabolic state. In the presence of metabolic instability, the more intensive monitoring outlined under initial period should be followed.
I & O, Intake and output; refers to all fluids going into the patient: oral, intravenous, medication; and all fluid coming out: urine, surgical drains, suctioning, vomitus, diarrhea.
WBC, White blood cell.

can be affected by parenteral nutrition and should be monitored carefully. Table 23-7 lists parameters that should be monitored routinely.

The TPN catheter site is a potential source for introduction of microorganisms into a major vein. Protocols to prevent infection vary. A common recommendation is to change dressings at the catheter site every 48 to 72 hours; the Centers for Disease Control and Prevention (CDC) has proposed recommendations for changes every 7 days in stable patients. Tubing is usually changed every 24 to 72 hours, depending on lipid content of the solution. With signs of infection, the catheter should be removed and the catheter tip cultured.

Refeeding Syndrome

Patients who require parenteral nutrition therapy are often moderately to severely malnourished. Aggressive administration of nutrition, particularly via the intravenous route, can precipitate the complication known as refeeding syndrome with severe, potentially lethal electrolyte fluctuations involving metabolic, hemodynamic, and neuromuscular problems. Refeeding syndrome occurs when energy substrates, particularly carbohydrates, are introduced into the plasma of anabolic patients.

Proliferation of new tissue requires increased amounts of glucose, potassium, phosphorus, magnesium, and other nutrients essential for tissue growth. If intracellular electrolytes are not supplied in sufficient quantity to keep up with tissue growth, low serum levels of potassium, phosphorus, and magnesium develop. Low levels of these electrolytes are the hallmark of refeeding syndrome. Carbohydrate metabolism by cells also causes a shift of electrolytes to the intracellular space as glucose moves into cells for oxidation. Rapid infusion of carbohydrate stimulates insulin, which reduces salt and water excretion and increases the chance of cardiac and pulmonary complications from fluid overload.

Patients just starting parenteral nutrition who have received no form of nutrition for a significant period should be monitored for electrolyte fluctuation and fluid overload. They should receive conservative amounts of carbohydrate and be given adequate amounts of intracellular electrolytes. The syndrome may also be seen and should be closely monitored in enterally fed patients; however, the digestive and absorptive processes somewhat mediate a rapid impact from refeeding syndrome. In the early phase of refeeding, nutrient prescriptions should be moderate in carbohydrate, lactose-free, and supplemented with phosphorus, potassium, and magnesium (Hamaoui and Kodsi, 1997).

TRANSITIONAL FEEDING

All nutrition support care plans strive to use the gastrointestinal tract when possible, either with enteral nutrition or by a total or partial return to oral intake. Therefore, care plans frequently involve transitional feeding, moving from one type of feeding to another with multiple feeding methods being used simultaneously. The challenge to clinicians is to maintain adequate feeding to meet nutritional requirements throughout the transition period. This requires careful monitoring of patient tolerance and quantification of intake from parenteral, enteral, and oral routes. Most experts advise that oral diets be initially low fat, lactose free, and low in other simple carbohydrates. These provisions will make digestion easier and minimize the possibility of an osmotic-type diarrhea. Attention to individual tolerance and food preferences will help maximize intake.

Parenteral to Enteral Feeding

To begin the transition from parenteral to enteral feeding, the initial step is to introduce a minimal amount of enteral feeding at a low rate of 30 to 40 ml/hr to establish gastrointestinal tolerance. Once this has been established over a period of hours, the parenteral rate can be decreased to keep the nutrient levels at the same prescribed amount. As the enteral rate is increased by 25- to 30-ml/hr increments every 8 to 24 hours, the parenteral prescription is reduced accordingly. Once it is established that the patient tolerates about 75% of nutrient needs by the enteral route, the parenteral solution can be discontinued. This process ideally takes 2 to 3 days; however, it may become more complicated, depending on the degree of gastrointestinal function. At times, this weaning process may not be practical, and parenteral therapy can be stopped sooner. This will depend on overall treatment decisions and likelihood for tolerance of enteral feeding.

Parenteral to Oral Feeding

Once again, this transition is ideally accomplished by monitoring oral intake and concomitantly decreasing the parenteral infusion to maintain a stable nutrient intake until about 75% of the nutrient needs can be met consistently by oral intake. This process is often less predictable than the transition to enteral feeding and depends on the patient's appetite, motivation, and general well-being. It is important to continue monitoring the patient for adequate oral intake once parenteral nutrition has been stopped and to initiate alternate nutrition support if necessary.

Enteral to Oral Feeding

A stepwise decrease is also used in the transition from tube feeding to oral feeding. It is usually more effective to move from continuous feeding to a 12- and then an 8-hour formula administration cycle during the night. This reestablishes hunger and satiety cues during daytime oral intakes. In practice, oral diets are often tried after inadvertent or deliberate removal of a nasoenteric tube. This type of interrupted transition should be monitored closely for adequate oral intake. Patients receiving enteral nutrition who desire to eat, and for whom it is safe to eat, can be encouraged to do so. Patients who cannot meet their needs by the oral route can be maintained by a combination of enteral nutrition and oral intake. Often oral supplements are useful.

Oral Supplements

The most common type of oral supplements are commercially available formulas meant primarily to augment the intake of solid foods. They generally provide approximately 250 kcal/8-oz or 240-ml portion and approximately 8 to 14 g of intact protein. Fat sources are most commonly long-chain triglycerides, although some contain medium-chain triglycerides. More concentrated, and thus more nutrient-dense, formulas are also available, as well as a variety of flavors, consistencies, and modifications of nutrients for various disease states. Some oral supplements theoretically provide a nutritionally complete diet if taken in sufficient volume.

The form of carbohydrate is a key factor to patient acceptance and tolerance. Supplements with appreciable amounts of simple carbohydrate taste sweeter and have higher osmolarities, which may contribute to gastrointestinal intolerance. Individual taste preferences vary widely, and normal taste is altered by certain drug therapies, most commonly chemotherapy. More concentrated formulas or greater volumes can contribute to taste fatigue, and satiety. It is wise to monitor the intake of food as well as the actual intake of prescribed supplement. Oral supplements that contain hydrolyzed protein and free amino acids such as those developed for renal, liver, and malabsorptive diseases tend to be mildly to markedly unpalatable, and acceptance by the patient depends on motivation. Some of these formulas also lack sufficient vitamins and minerals.

Although commercially available supplements are most commonly used for convenience, modules of protein, carbohydrate, or fat or commonly available food items can produce highly palatable additions to a diet that needs nutritional bolstering. As examples, liquid or powdered milk, yogurt, tofu, or protein powders can be used to enrich cereals, casseroles, soups, or milk shakes. Thickening agents are now used to add variety, texture, and aesthetics to pureed foods, which are used when swallowing ability is limited (see Chapters 40, 41, and 43). Imagination and individual tailoring can sometimes do much to increase oral intake, avoiding the necessity for more complex forms of nutrition support.

PHARMACOLOGIC USE OF NUTRIENTS

Nutrition is entering an era in which ongoing research suggests a therapeutic role for specific nutrients and other food substances. This research shows promise for the future as researchers learn more about specific metabolic pathways in disease, stress, and trauma and begin to be able to manipulate these pathways with the use of specific nutrients.

Nutrients that have been supplemented in commercially available nutrition support products for a therapeutic effect have been limited primarily to adult enteral nutrition formulas. In the United States these formulas are the equivalent of medical foods. Parenteral solutions containing these nutrients are regulated as drugs and therefore must undergo prior approval for demonstration of safety and efficacy before becoming clinically available.

Some of these nutrients and substances are recognized by the government as dietary supplements and have relatively flexible regulations governing product claims for health and well-being (Mueller and Nestle, 1995). In 1994 Congress passed the Dietary Supplement Health and Education Act (see Chapter 14). This legislation provides flexible guidelines for health claims and exempts dietary supplements from

Box 23-6. Substances Being Investigated for Potential Therapeutic Effects in Enteral or Parenteral Solutions

Antioxidants such as β-carotene, vitamin C, vitamin E, vitamin A, zinc, copper, manganese, and selenium have specific roles in deactivating free radicals.
Arginine is an amino acid that may enhance nitrogen retention, wound healing, and immune function.
Carnitine is a nitrogenous compound synthesized from lysine and methionine that is required for oxidation of long-chain fatty acids.
Choline is an amine that is required for phospholipid synthesis and very-low-density lipoprotein production; choline deficiency has been associated with hepatic abnormalities in patients receiving parenteral nutrition.
Glutamine is an amino acid that plays a pivotal role in metabolic processes; it is utilized by intestinal and immune cells as fuel.
Medium-chain triglycerides (MCT) do not require bile acids for digestion and are absorbed directly into hepatic portal circulation; they also do not require carnitine for oxidation.
Omega-3 fatty acids are precursors of prostaglandins that may enhance immune function and decrease the risk of cardiovascular disease.
Phytochemicals are active chemical compounds found in foods of plant origin that play a potential beneficial role in the prevention and treatment of disease. Some classes of phytochemicals include organosulfur compounds (allium), polyphenols including flavonoids and isoflavones, and terpenes, which include carotenoids.
Short-chain fatty acids are derived from dietary fiber after digestion by colonic bacteria; they provide fuel for intestinal cells and maintain healthy gastrointestinal mucosa.
Structured lipids are artificially produced lipids comprised of both long-chain and medium-chain fatty acids on the same glycerol moiety.
Taurine is an amino acid synthesized from cysteine that may be conditionally essential in metabolic stress.

premarket approval regulations such as those that exist for food additives (Bartels and Miller, 1998). Box 23-6 presents nutrients and substances that are being investigated for their potential therapeutic effects. Some of them are classified as dietary supplements.

NUTRITION SUPPORT IN LONG-TERM AND HOME CARE

Long-Term Care

Long-term care generally refers to the nursing home setting and health care provided to the large proportion of older residents who reside in these facilities. Health care provided to long-term care residents focuses on quality of life and self-determination in addition to the management of acute and chronic disease. Indications for enteral and parenteral nutrition are generally the same for older patients as they are for younger adults. Legal documents that state resident preferences about aspects of care, including those regarding the use of nutrition support, are important to help guide interventions on behalf of long-term care residents when they are no longer able to participate in decision making. Differentiation between the effects of advanced age and malnutrition in older adults is beginning to receive research attention, as is the influence that nutrition support has on the quality of life among long-term care residents (Somogyi-Zalud et al, 2002).

Home Care

Resources and technology for safe and effective management of long-term enteral or parenteral therapy are now widely available for the home care setting (Ireton-Jones, 1997a, 1997b, Nelson et al, 1998; Nutrition Intervention in Home Care, 1998). The elements needed to implement home nutrition successfully include identification of appropriate candidates, a choice of a suitable nutrition support regimen, training of the patient and family, and a plan for medical and nutritional follow-up visits. These objectives are achieved through coordinated efforts of an interdisciplinary team.

Home nutrition therapy organizations provide nutrients, medications, supplies, equipment, and professional clinical services to patients at home in accordance with standards developed by professional organizations (American Society for Parenteral and Enteral Nutrition, 1992). Commercial companies manage nutrition support therapy alone or in combination with other home therapies and may be affiliated with acute care facilities or private subcontractors. Criteria for selecting a home care company to provide nutrition support should be based on the company's ability to provide ongoing nutritional assessment, monitoring, and care plan revision (American Dietetic Association, 1994).

Although home management has been available for over 20 years, little outcome data have been generated. Because mandatory reporting requirements

Box 23-7. Selecting Appropriate Candidates for Home Nutrition Support

Considerations

1. Potential improvement in the patient's quality of life
2. Benefit of long-term nutrition support for the patient's nutritional status
3. Patient's or family's ability to handle the financial commitment
4. Patient's or caretaker's ability to learn the protocol for administration
5. Ability to comply with the standards for safety
6. Patient's or caretaker's physical limitations that influence the ability to administer nutrition support safely

Data from Matarese L: Nutrition support: enteral nutrition. In Lysen LK, editor: *Quick reference to clinical dietetics,* Gaithersburg, Md, 1997, Aspen Publishers; and Weckwerth J et al: Home nutrition support. In Gottschlich MM et al: *Nutrition support dietetic core curriculum,* Silver Spring, Md, 1992, American Society for Parenteral and Enteral Nutrition.

do not exist in the United States for patients receiving home nutrition support, the exact number of patients receiving home nutrition support is unknown (Howard et al, 1998).

The key factors in successful home nutrition support therapy are careful and coordinated discharge planning as well as patient and caregiver education (Evans and Czopek, 1995). Box 23-7 presents criteria to be considered when selecting candidates for home nutrition support. Patients can successfully manage their home care with the support of their families and an interdisciplinary team consisting of the physician, nurse, dietitian, pharmacist, social worker, or discharge planner or case manager, working in conjunction with the home care provider (Nelson et al, 1998; Nutrition Intervention in Home Care, 1998).

ETHICAL ISSUES

Whether to provide or withhold nutrition support is often a central issue in "end of life" decision making. For patients who are terminally ill or in a persistent vegetative state, nutrition support can extend life to the point that issues of quality of life and the patient's right to self-determination come into play. Often surrogate decision makers are involved in treatment decisions. The nutrition support practitioner has a responsibility to know whether documentation, such as a living will regarding the patient's wishes for nutrition support, is in the medical record and whether counseling and support resources for legal and ethical aspects of patient care are available to the patient and his or her significant others (American Dietetic Association, 1992).

INTERDISCIPLINARY NUTRITION SUPPORT SERVICES

Optimal nutrition support requires the dedication and involvement of multiple disciplines. Organizational structure at the institutional level is necessary for the quality, safety, and cost-effectiveness of nutrition support. Often this structure begins with a nutrition committee charged with setting or suggesting policy and standards of care. Historically, in institutions where patients required complex and sophisticated nutrition support, nutrition support teams or services were often developed with patient care provided by a team consisting of physician, dietitian, pharmacist, and nurse specialist. These teams became models for interdisciplinary care. In fact, the Joint Commission on Accreditation of Healthcare Organizations (JCAHO) and the Health Care Financing Administration (HCFA) both emphasize effective, efficient, collaborative and consistent action from an interdisciplinary team (Comprehensive Accreditation Manual for Hospitals, 1998; Health Care Financing Administration, 1998).

Some experts believe standards of care and practice guidelines for optimal nutrition support have reduced the need for nutrition support teams and services (American Society for Parenteral and Enteral Nutrition, 1998). Cost containment has resulted in the dismantlement of teams, although conversely some institutions have justified the interdisciplinary team approach to help control costs (ChrisAnderson et al, 1996; Wesley, 1994). This apparent contradiction highlights the importance of documenting outcomes affected by health care interventions such as nutrition support.

Clinical Scenario I

Lindy is a 24-year-old Native American who has newly diagnosed diabetes mellitus and Crohn's disease. She has had recent surgery for removal of one third of her ileum. She is 75% of her usual weight, which is 125 lb; she is 65 inches tall. She will require specialized nutrition support for several months until her body adapts to the shortened bowel.

1. What immediate nutrition support method would be recommended?
2. What long-term nutrition support plan is likely to be designed? What specialty products, if any, might be beneficial to Lindy?
3. What other factors should be identified as part of your nutritional assessment?

Clinical Scenario 2

Jerome is a 44-year-old man admitted to the emergency room after a motor-vehicle accident. After being stabilized, he was transferred to the operating room, where he underwent a splenectomy, Whipple procedure, ascending colectomy including the ileocecal valve, and a needle catheter jejunostomy as a result of blunt abdominal trauma. He also underwent a left thoracotomy for chest tube placement because of a perforated lung and placement of a triple lumen right internal jugular (IJ) catheter for central venous access. After stabilization in the postanesthesia care unit, Jerome was transferred to the intensive care unit (ICU) with an endotrachial tube in place for mechanical ventilation. He had a nasogastric tube in place for gastric decompression and bilateral Jackson Pratt tubes in place for postoperative abdominal wound drainage.

Jerome has an unremarkable medical history. He is 5 feet 10 inches tall and weighs 180 lb on admission to the ICU. He had +1 pitting edema in his arms and legs on admission to the ICU.

Parenteral nutrition was started on postoperative day 2 in the ICU via the IJ catheter because the surgeons were concerned that the small bowel was not yet functional, although there was no abdominal distention. On postoperative day 4, enteral formula at 20 ml/hr, formula was started via the needle catheter jejunostomy with concomitant intermittent nasogastric decompression. By postoperative day 8, the jejunostomy enteral nutrition infusion was at 40 ml/hr, providing close to half the amount of protein and energy that Jerome requires. The parenteral nutrition infusion was decreased by half. On postoperative day 11, the parenteral nutrition was stopped because the jejunostomy infusion had been advanced to 80 ml/hr. On postoperative day 12, the endotracheal tube was removed because Jerome had been successfully weaned from mechanical ventilation. An antiaspiration pureed diet was started.

1. What are Jerome's fluid and electrolyte requirements in the first 5 days postoperatively?
2. What is the maximum amount of carbohydrate (per 24 hours) that could be given to Jerome parenterally?
3. What is the maximum amount of fat over 24 hours that should be given parenterally to avoid adverse effects?
4. What is the rationale for starting enteral nutrition through the needle catheter jejunostomy even though Jerome was on gastric decompression?
5. What kind of enteral formula would you recommend for Jerome and why?
6. At what point in the transition from enteral nutrition to an oral diet would you recommend stopping the enteral nutrition?
7. What is the nutritional significance of Jerome's resection of the ascending colon and ileocecal valve?

SUMMARY

Health care outcomes research represents a significant trend in nutrition support research. Indeed, the JCAHO and HCFA have made outcomes the standard by which all health care is evaluated. The goal of this type of research is to identify medical care that is effective, and there is tremendous pressure on nutrition support clinicians to prove that enteral and parenteral nutrition are effective interventions (August, 1996). Research investigating the metabolic and physiologic differences between parenteral and enteral nutrition, as mentioned in the introduction of this chapter, is ongoing. Another important area of research focuses on the use of nutrients and other substances normally occurring in foods as pharmacologic or preventive agents for specific diseases and conditions. Nutrition support provides many opportunities to offer life-saving nutrition. Careful planning, implementation, and follow-up are needed to provide excellent care.

■ Relevant Web Site

American Society for Enteral and Parenteral Nutrition
http://clinnutr.org/

■ Cited References

Abbott WO, Rawson AJ: Tube for use in postoperative care of gastroenterostomy patients, *JAMA* 112:2414, 1939.

Abernathy GB et al: Efficacy of tube feeding in supplying energy requirements of hospitalized patients, *JPEN J Parenter Enteral Nutr* 13(4):387, 1989.

Alexander JW: Nutrition and translocation, *JPEN J Parenter Enteral Nutr* 14:170s, 1990.

Ali A et al: nutrition support services, *Nutrition Support Algorithms* 8(7):13, 1988.

American Dietetic Association: Position of the American Dietetic Association: issues in feeding the terminally ill adult, *J Am Diet Assoc* 92: 996, 1992.

American Dietetic Association: Position of the American Dietetic Association: nutrition monitoring of the home parenteral and enteral patient, *J Am Diet Assoc* 94:664, 1994.

American Society for Parenteral and Enteral Nutrition Board of Directors and The Clinical Guidelines Task Force: Guidelines for the use of parenteral and enteral nutrition in adult and pediatric patients, *JPEN J Parenter Enteral Nutr* 26:1(S), 2002.

American Society for Parenteral and Enteral Nutrition: Standards of practice: standards for home nutrition support, *Nutr Clin Pract* 7:65, 1992.

American Society for Parenteral and Enteral Nutrition: *The ASPEN nutrition support practice manual.* Silver Spring, Md, 1998, American Society for Parenteral and Enteral Nutrition.

August DA: Creation of a specialized nutrition support outcomes research consortium: if not now, when? *JPEN J Parenter Enteral Nutr* 20:394, 1996.

Bartels CL, Miller SJ: Herbal and related remedies, *Nutr Clin Pract* 5:211, 1998.

Bell SJ et al: Alternative lipid sources for enteral and parenteral nutrition: long- and medium-chain triglycerides, structured triglycerides and fish oils, *J Am Diet Assoc* 91(1):74, 1991.

ChrisAnderson D et al: Metabolic complications of total parenteral nutrition: effects of a nutrition support service, *JPEN J Parenter Enteral Nutr* 20(3):206, 1996.

Comprehensive accreditation manual for hospitals: the official handbook, Oakbrook Terrace, Ill, 1998, Joint Commission on Accreditation of Healthcare Organizations.

Deitch EA: Multiple organ failure, *Ann Surg* 216:117, 1992.

Evans MA, Czopek S: Home nutrition support materials, *Nutr Clin Pract* 10:37, 1995.

Farwell DG et al: Predictors of perioperative complications in head and neck patients, *Arch Otolaryngol Head Neck Surg* 128:505, 2002.

Foley EF et al: Albumin supplementation in the critically ill, *Arch Surg* 125:739, 1990.

Georgeson K, Owings E: Surgical and laparoscopic techniques for feeding tube placement. In Shike M, Bloch AS, editors: *Gastrointestinal endoscopy clinics of North America,* Philadelphia, 1998, WB Saunders, 1998:581.

Gorman RC, Morris JB: Minimally invasive access to the gastrointestinal tract. In Rombeau JL, Rolandelli RH, editors: *Clinical nutrition: enteral and tube feeding,* Philadelphia, 1997, WB Saunders.

Gottschlich MM et al: Defined formula diets. In Rombeau JL, Rolandelli RH, editors: *Clinical nutrition: enteral and tube feeding.* Philadelphia, 1997, WB Saunders.

Guenter P et al: Delivery systems and administration of enteral nutrition. In Rombeau JL, Rolandelli RH, editors: *Clinical nutrition: enteral and tube feeding,* Philadelphia, 1997, WB Saunders.

Hamaoui E, Kodsi R: Complications of enteral feeding and their prevention. In Rombeau JL, Rolandelli RH, editors: *Clinical nutrition: enteral and tube feeding,* Philadelphia, 1997, WB Saunders.

Health Care Financing Administration (HCFA): Medicare and Medicaid programs; hospital conditions of participation; provider agreements and supplier approval: proposed rule, *Federal Register* 62:66726, 1998.

Howard L et al: Outcome of long-term enteral feeding. In Shike M, Bloch AS, editors: *Gastrointestinal endoscopy clinics of North America,* Philadelphia, 1998, WB Saunders.

Ideno KT: Enteral nutrition. In Gottschlich MM et al, editors: *Nutrition support dietetics core curriculum,* Silver Spring, Md, 1992, American Society of Parenteral and Enteral Nutrition.

Ireton-Jones C: Nutrition management of the patient outside the hospital setting. In Lysen L, editor: *Quick reference to clinical dietetics,* Gaitherburg, Md, 1997a, Aspen Publishers.

Ireton-Jones C et al: Clinical pathways in home nutrition support, *J Am Diet Assoc* 97:1003, 1997b.

Jeejeebhoy KN: Enteral and parenteral nutrition: evidence-based approach, *Proc Nutr Soc* 60:399, 2001.

Jensen GL et al: Parenteral infusion of long- and medium-chain triglycerides and reticuloendothelial system function in man, *JPEN J Parenter Enteral Nutr* 14(5):467, 1990.

Kirby DF et al: Enteral access and infusion equipment. In *The ASPEN nutrition support practice manual,* Silver Spring, Md, 1998, American Society for Parenteral and Enteral Nutrition.

Klang MC: Drug-nutrient considerations-parenteral nutrition. In *The ASPEN nutrition support practice* manual, Silver Spring, Md, 1998, American Society for Parenteral and Enteral Nutrition.

Klein S et al: Nutrition support in clinical practice: review of published data and recommendations for future research directions, *JPEN J Parenter Enteral Nutr* 21(3):133, 1997.

Krzysda EA, Edmiston CE: Parenteral access and equipment. In *The ASPEN nutrition support practice* manual, Silver Spring, Md, 1998, American Society for Parenteral and Enteral Nutrition.

Levy H: Nasogastric and nasoenteric feeding tubes. In Shike M, Bloch AS, editors: *Gastrointestinal endoscopy clinics of North America,* Philadelphia: WB Saunders, 1998.

Lord L et al: Enteral nutrition implementation and management. In *The ASPEN nutrition support practice manual,* Silver Spring, Md, 1998, American Society for Parenteral and Enteral Nutrition.

Maloney JP et al: FD&C blue no. 1 food dye is a mitochondrial poison that can be absorbed from enteral tube feedings in sepsis: a report of 3 deaths linked to systemic absorption, *JPEN J Parenter Enteral Nutr* 25:S25, 2001.

Matarese LE: Enteral feeding solutions. In Shike M, Bloch AS, editors: *Gastrointestinal endoscopy clinics of North America,* Philadelphia, 1998, WB Saunders.

Matarese LE, Gottschlich MM: *Contemporary nutrition support practice,* ed 2, St Louis, 2002, Elsevier.

Metheny N: Verification of feeding tube placement. In *Ross current issues in enteral nutrition support: report of the first Ross Conference on Enteral Devices,* Columbus, Ohio, 1996, Ross Products Division, Abbott Laboratories.

Moore FA et al: Early enteral feeding compared with parenteral reduces postoperative septic complications, *Ann Surg* 216:172, 1992.

Mosenthal AC et al: Elemental and intravenous total parenteral nutrition diet-induced gut barrier failure is intestinal site specific and can be prevented by feeding nonfermentable fiber, *Crit Care Med* 30:396, 2002.

Mueller C, Nestle M: Regulation of medical foods: toward a rational policy, *Nutr Clin Pract* 10:8, 1995.

Nelson JK et al: Considerations for home nutrition support. In *The ASPEN nutrition support practice manual,* Silver Spring, Md, 1998, American Society for Parenteral and Enteral Nutrition.

Nutrition Intervention in Home Care: New paradigms for quality patient care. In *Ross roundtables on medical issues,* vol 18, Columbus, Ohio, 1998, Ross Products Division, Abbott Laboratories.

Olree K et al: Enteral formulations. In *The ASPEN nutrition support practice manual,* Silver Spring, Md, 1998, American Society for Parenteral and Enteral Nutrition.

Shike M, Bloch AS: Enteral nutrition, *Gastrointest Endosc Clin North Am* 8(3):529, 1998.

Somogyi-Zalud E et al: The use of life-sustaining treatments in hospitalized persons aged 80 and older, *J Am Geriatr Soc* 50:930, 2002.

Strausburg KM: Parenteral nutrition admixture. In *ASPEN nutrition support practice manual,* Silver Spring, Md, 1998, American Society for Parenteral and Enteral Nutrition.

Wesley JR: Nutrition support teams: past, present, and future, *Nutr Clin Pract* 9:165, 1994.

Additional References

Aihara R et al: Guidelines for improving nutritional delivery in the intensive care unit, *J Health Qual* 24:22, 2002.

Bistrian BR: Update on total parenteral nutrition, *Am J Clin Nutr* 74:153, 2001.

Bower R et al: Early enteral administration of a formula (impact) supplemented with arginine, nucleotides, and fish oil in intensive care unit patients: results of a multicenter, prospective, randomized clinical trial, *Crit Care Med* 23:436, 1995.

Braga M et al: Early postoperative enteral nutrition improves gut oxygenation and reduces costs compared with total parenteral nutrition, *Crit Care Med* 29:242, 2001.

Chima C et al: Relationship of nutritional status to length of stay, hospital costs, and discharge status of patients hospitalized in the medicine service, *J Am Diet Assoc* 97:975, 1997.

Choban P et al: Hypoenergetic nutrition support in hospitalized obese patients: a simplified method for clinical application, *Am J Clin Nutr* 66:546, 1997.

Dietscher JE et al: Nutritional response of patients in an intensive care unit to an elemental formula vs. a standard enteral formula, *J Am Diet Assoc* 98:335, 1998.

Dorner B et al: To "feed or not to feed" dilemma, *J Am Diet Assoc* 97:S172, 1997.

Dudrick SJ et al: Management of the short bowel syndrome, *Surg Clin North Am* 71:625, 1991.

Eisen GM et al: Role of endoscopy in enteral feeding, *Gastrointest Endosc* 55:794, 2002.

Heyland DK et al: Should immunonutrition become routine in critically ill patients? A systematic review of the evidence, *JAMA* 286:944, 2001.

Marik PE, Zaloga G: Early enteral nutrition in acutely ill patients: a systematic review, *Crit Care Med* 29(12):2264-2270, 2001.

Matarese L: Nutrition support: enteral nutrition. In Lysen LK, editor: *Quick reference to clinical dietetics,* Gaithersburg, Md, 1997, Aspen Publishers.

McCamish MA et al: History of enteral feeding: past and present perspectives. In Rombeau JL, Rolandelli RH, editors: *Clinical nutrition: enteral and tube feeding,* Philadelphia, 1997, WB Saunders.

Metheny N et al: PH concentrations of pepsin and trypsin in feeding tube aspirates as predictors of tube placement, *JPEN J Parenter Enteral Nutr* 21:279, 1997.

Mueller C et al: Order writing for parenteral nutrition by registered dietitians, *J Am Diet Assoc* 96:764, 1996.

National Advisory Group on Standards and Practice Guidelines for Parenteral Nutrition, ASPEN: Safe practices for parenteral nutrition formulations, *JPEN J Parenter Enteral Nutr* 22(2):49, 1998.

Reynolds J et al: Does the role of feeding modify gut barrier function and clinical outcome in patients after major upper gastrointestinal surgery? *JPEN J Parenter Enteral Nutr* 21:196, 1997.

Rhodes JE, Dudrick SJ: History of intravenous nutrition. In Rombeau JL, Caldwell MD, editors: *Parenteral nutrition*, Philadelphia, 1993, WB Saunders.

Schloerb P, Henning J: Patterns and problems of adult total parenteral nutrition use in U.S. academic medical centers, *Arch Surg* 133:7, 1998.

Seldinger SI: Catheter replacement of needle in percutaneous arteriography: a new technique, *Acta Radiol* 39:368, 1953.

Shronts E: Essential nature of choline with implications for total parenteral nutrition, *J Am Diet Assoc* 97:639, 1997.

Silver HJ, Wellman NS: Family caregiver training is needed to improve outcomes for older adults using home care technologies, *J Am Diet Assoc* 102:831, 2002.

Swails W et al: Effect of a fish oil structured lipid-based diet on prostaglandin release from mononuclear cells in cancer patients after surgery, *JPEN J Parenter Enteral Nutr* 21:266, 1997.

Upperman JS et al: Post-hemorrhagic shock mesenteric lymph is cytotoxic to endothelial cells and activates neutrophils, *Shock* 10:415-416, 1998.

Weckwerth J et al: Home nutrition support. In Gottschlich MM et al, editors: *Nutrition support dietetics core curriculum,* Silver Spring, Md, 1993, American Society for Parenteral and Enteral Nutrition.

Wilmore DW, Dudrick SJ: Growth and development of an infant receiving all nutrients exclusively by vein, *JAMA* 203:869, 1968.

Xu DZ et al: The effect of hypoxia/reoxygenation on the cellular function of intestinal epithelial cells, *J Trauma* 46:280-285, 1999.

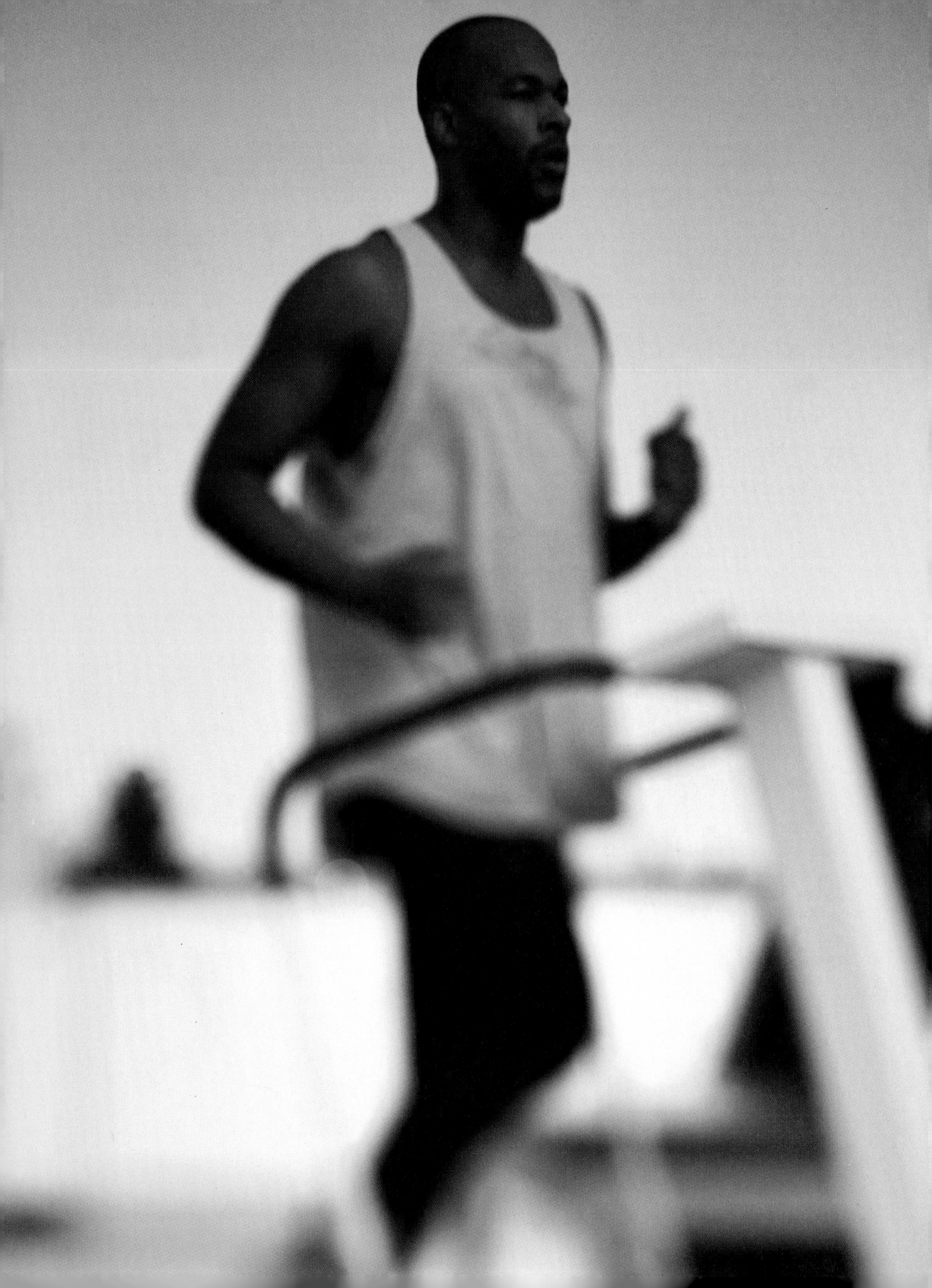

PART 4

NUTRITION FOR HEALTH AND FITNESS

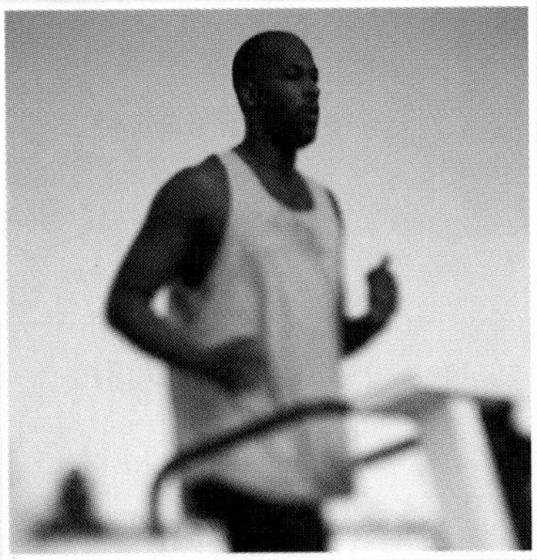

The chapters in this section reflect the evolution of nutritional science, from the identification of nutrient requirements and the practical application of this knowledge to the more recent concepts that relate nutrition to the prevention of degenerative disease.

The relationship between nutrition and dental disease has long been recognized. In more recent decades, the possibility of reducing the incidence of cancer, atherosclerotic heart disease, hypertension, and osteoporosis by emphasizing appropriate nutrition has continued to accumulate supportive evidence.

Government agencies have traditionally assumed responsibility for ensuring the safety of the food supply and for making adequate nutrients available to high-risk segments of the population. The recommended dietary allowances have been a part of the nutrition scene for almost 50 years; new revisions are expanded and called dietary reference intakes (DRIs). However, setting nutritional goals appropriate to health and fitness and specifically to prevention of degenerative diseases is a relatively new role for government.

The first federal guidelines on the identification, evaluation, and treatment of overweight and obesity in adults were released in the summer of 1998. The opportunities for an affluent society to choose from a great variety of foods can easily lead to an overabundant intake of energy, and efforts to reduce body weight, widely pursued with varying degrees of enthusiasm and diligence, are seldom successful. The prevention, or at least postponement, of various degenerative diseases is closely associated with physical fitness and is achieved in part through exercise and management of body weight.

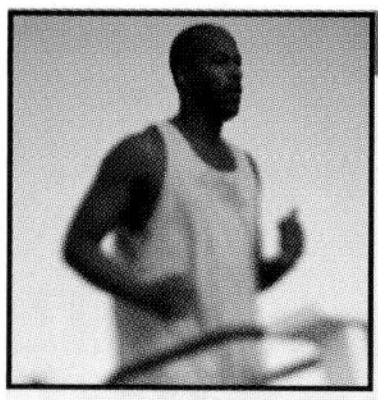

CHAPTER 24

Nutrition for Weight Management

IDAMARIE LAQUATRA, PhD, RD

CHAPTER OUTLINE

- Body Weight Components
- Regulation of Body Weight
- Weight Management Throughout Life
- Weight Imbalance: Overweight and Obesity
- Management of Obesity in Adults
- Common Problems Encountered in Obesity Management
- Weight Management in Children
- Weight Imbalance: Excessive Leanness

KEY TERMS

adipocyte–a cell that synthesizes and stores triglyceride; fat cell

android fat deposition–deposition of fat around the waist and upper abdomen; "apple-shape" fat distribution

bariatrics–branch of medicine concerned with weight control, including gastroplasty and other types of surgical procedures

body mass index (BMI)–a mathematical formula that correlates with body fat and is expressed as weight in kilograms divided by height in meters squared ($BMI = kg/m^2$)

brown adipose tissue (BAT)–fat located in the scapular area that is involved in heat production for cold adaptation and possibly burning off excess energy

catecholaminergic–referring to the brain neurotransmitters norepinephrine, epinephrine, and dopamine

comorbidity–any condition associated with obesity that usually worsens as the degree of obesity increases and often improves as the obesity is successfully treated

essential fat–the body fat located in specific sites that is necessary for survival; about 3% to 12% of body weight

gastric bypass–a surgical procedure in which the size of the stomach is reduced by a stapling procedure and the small intestine is connected to the smaller stomach pouch through a new opening

gastroplasty–a surgical procedure in which the size of the stomach is reduced with a row of staples across the top half of the stomach with a small opening left into the distal stomach

gynoid fat distribution–deposition of fat in the thighs and buttocks; "pear-shape" fat distribution

hormone-sensitive lipase (HSL)–an enzyme in the adipose cell that is responsible for the hydrolysis of triglyceride into fatty acids and glycerol, which then leave the adipose cell and enter the circulation

hyperphagia–a period of overeating

hyperplasia–increase in tissue size by an increase in the number of cells

hypertrophy–increase in tissue size by an increase in cell size

hypophagia–a period of undereating

lean body mass (LBM)–the total of all body components except storage lipid and bone

lifestyle modification–change in the antecedents, behaviors, and consequences associated with eating habits, exercise, or thinking patterns

lipogenesis–the conversion of glucose and intermediates to fat

lipoprotein lipase (LPL)–an enzyme on the luminal side of the capillary that facilitates transport of lipid from the blood into the adipose cell

liposuction–aspiration of fat deposits by means of a small incision through which a tube is fanned out into the adipose tissue

metabolic syndrome–a condition associated with glucose intolerance, insulin resistance, hyperlipidemia, and hypertension; strongly linked to abdominal obesity

morbid obesity–a state of adiposity in which body weight is 100% above the ideal body weight; a body mass index of 45 or greater

obesity–a state of adiposity in which body fatness is above the ideal; a body mass index of 30 to 39.9

overweight–a state in which weight exceeds a standard based on height; having a body mass index of 25 to 29.9 or greater

sensory-specific satiety–a decline in the pleasantness of a food as it is consumed

storage fat–the fat that accumulates under the skin and around internal organs

underweight–a body weight 15% to 20% below the accepted weight standard; a body mass index of less than 18.5

very-low-calorie diet (VLCD)–a diet providing 800 kcal or less per day

visceral obesity–fat accumulation predominantly in the intraabdominal cavity

white adipose tissue–repository for triglycerides; a cushion to protect body organs and an insulator to preserve body heat

yo-yo effect–the process of losing and gaining weight several times throughout a lifetime; often characterized by increased fatness with each cycle

Body weight is the sum of bone, muscle, organs, body fluids, and adipose tissue. Some or all of these components are subject to normal change as a reflection of growth, reproductive status, variation in exercise levels, and the effects of aging. Maintaining a constant body weight is orchestrated by a complex system of neural, hormonal, and chemical mechanisms that keeps the balance between energy intake and energy expenditure within fairly precise limits. Abnormalities of these mechanisms, many of which are not completely understood, result in exaggerated weight fluctuations. Of these, the most common are overweight and obesity. The obesity "epidemic," as many health professionals label it, is now pervasive throughout the United States. As shown in Figure 24-1, only four states had obesity rates of 15% or higher in 1991. By 2000, all states except Colorado had these rates (Mokdad et al, 2001). The inability to gain weight can be a problem, although this is usually secondary to another disease state; underweight is discussed briefly at the end of this chapter.

BODY WEIGHT COMPONENTS

Body weight is often described in terms of its composition, and different models have been advanced to estimate body fat. Traditionally, a two-compartment model has been used, dividing the body into the fat mass and the fat-free mass (FFM) or fat-free body (FFB). Fat mass combines the fat from all body sources, including fat in the brain, skeleton, and adipose tissue; FFM is tissue devoid of all extractable fat. FFM can be further divided into water, protein, and mineral components (Wagner and Heyward, 2000). FFM is often used interchangeably with lean body mass (LBM), but it is not the same. LBM is the part of the body free of adipose tissue (Jensen, 1992) and includes the skeletal muscles, water, bone, and a small amount of essential fat in the internal organs, bone marrow, and nerve tissues. FFM is higher in men than in women, increases with exercise, and is lower in older adults. It is the major determinant of the resting metabolic rate. Water, which makes up 60% to 65% of body weight, is the most variable component of FFM, and the state of hydration can induce fluctuations of several pounds. Muscle and even skeletal mass adjust to some extent to support the changing burden of adipose tissue. Studies on the composition of excess weight gained showed that the FFM of the body accounts for an average of 29% of the excess weight (Pierson et al, 1997).

Body Fat

Fat in the body is categorized as either "essential" or "storage." Essential fat, which is necessary for normal physiologic functioning, is stored in small amounts in the bone marrow, heart, lung, liver, spleen, kidneys, muscles, and lipid-rich tissues in the nervous system. In men, about 3% of body fat is considered essential. In women essential fat is higher, about 12%, because it also includes sex-specific body fat in the breasts, pelvic regions, and thighs. The primary energy reserve of the body is the fat stored as triglyceride in depots made up of adipose tissue. This storage fat accumulates under the skin and around the internal organs to protect them from trauma. Most storage fat is considered "expendable." The totality of fat stores in adipocytes is capable of extensive variation, thus allowing for changing requirements of growth, reproduction, and aging as well as fluctuations in environmental and physiologic circumstances such as the availability of food and the demands of physical exercise. The range of total body fat (essential fat plus storage fat) associated with optimum health is 8% to 24% in males and 21% to 35% in females (Gallagher et al, 2000), although

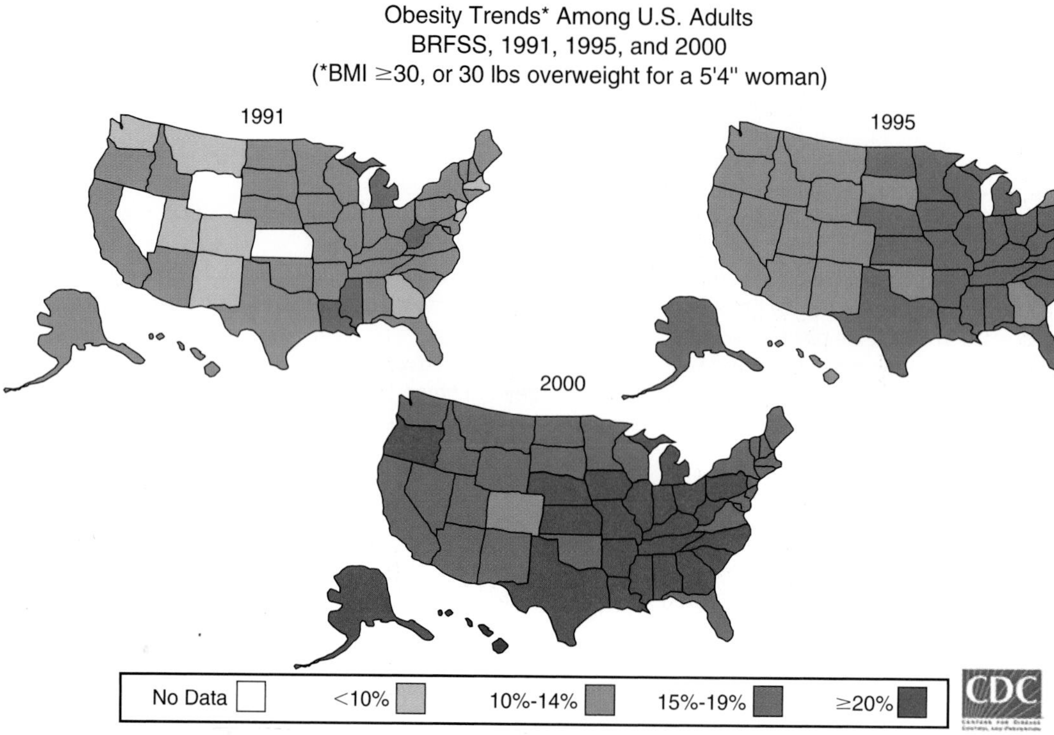

FIGURE 24-1 • Prevalence of obesity among U.S. adults. (Redrawn from the Centers for Disease Control and Prevention [CDC], Behavior Risk Factor Surveillance System [BRFSS], based on data from Mokdad AH et al: The continuing epidemics of obesity and diabetes in the United States, *JAMA* 286:1195, 2001.)

professional and elite athletes have body fats much lower than those of the average person (Figure 24-2).

Adipose Tissue Structure

Adipose tissue is located primarily under the skin, in the mesenteries and omentum, and behind the peritoneum. Although it is primarily fat, adipose tissue is also composed of small amounts of protein and water (Jensen, 1992). White adipose tissue serves as a repository for triglycerides, a cushion to protect abdominal organs, and an insulator to preserve body heat. Carotene gives it a slight yellow color. Brown adipose tissue (BAT), seen in infants and in very small amounts in adults, occurs primarily in the scapular and subscapular areas. The brown color is due to extensive vascularization. It has been studied most extensively in animals, where it appears to be involved in heat production as a means of adapting to cold and possibly of dissipating excess energy. Its function in adults remains poorly understood.

Adipocytes, Hypertrophy, and Hyperplasia

The mature adipocyte consists of a large central lipid droplet surrounded by a thin rim of cytoplasm, which contains the nucleus and the mitochondria; these cells store fat in quantities equal to 80% to 95% of their volume. Adipose tissue increases either by increasing the size of cells already present when lipid is added (hypertrophy) or by increasing the number of cells (hyperplasia). Weight gain may be the result of hypertrophy, hyperplasia, or a combination of the two. Obesity is always characterized by hypertrophy, but only some forms of obesity also involve hyperplasia (Bray, 1990).

The fat depots can expand as much as 1000 times through hypertrophy alone, a process that can occur at any time as long as space is available in the adipocytes. Hyperplasia occurs primarily as a part of the growth process during infancy and adolescence, but it can also occur in adulthood, when the fat content of existing cells has reached capacity. When weight is reduced as a result of trauma, illness, starvation, or changes in diet and exercise, fat cell size decreases.

Fat Cell Development

The greatest level of fatness in normal growth (about 25%) occurs at the age of 6 months. In lean children, fat cell size then decreases; however, this decrease does not occur in obese children. At the age of 6 years in lean children, increase in fatness occurs ("adiposity rebound"), with the increase being greater in girls

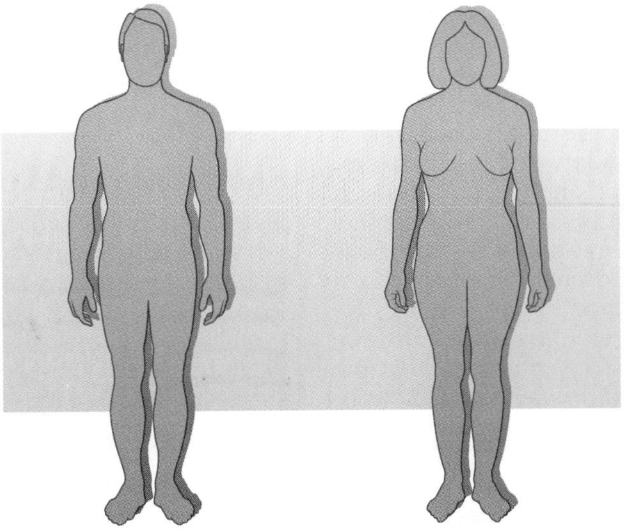

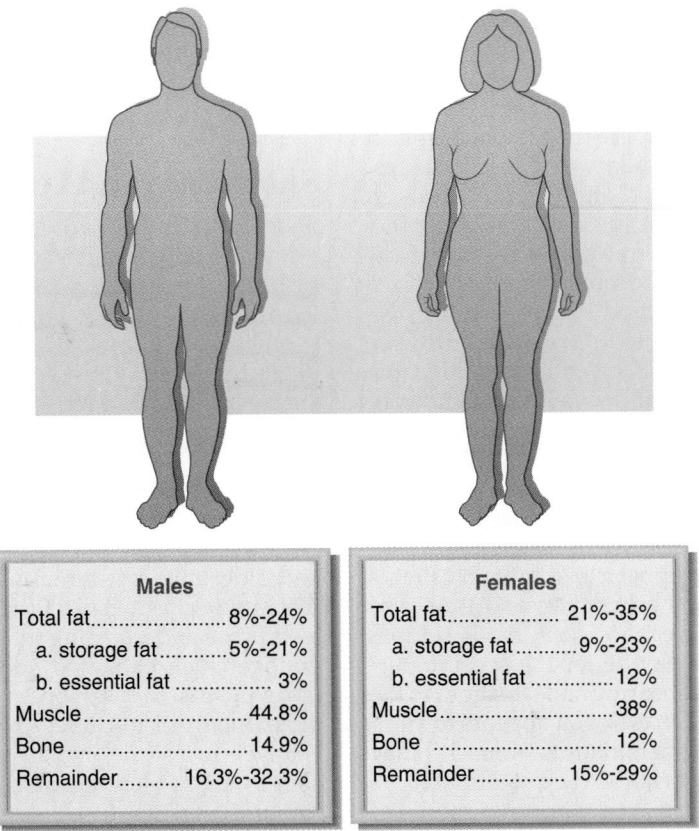

Males	
Total fat	8%-24%
a. storage fat	5%-21%
b. essential fat	3%
Muscle	44.8%
Bone	14.9%
Remainder	16.3%-32.3%

Females	
Total fat	21%-35%
a. storage fat	9%-23%
b. essential fat	12%
Muscle	38%
Bone	12%
Remainder	15%-29%

FIGURE 24-2 • Behnke's theoretical body composition model for a man and a woman with healthy percentage body-fat ranges. (Data from Gallagher D et al: Healthy percentage body-fat ranges: an approach for developing guidelines based on body mass index, *Am J Clin Nutr* 72:694, 2000.)

than in boys. An early adiposity rebound occurring before 5.5 years is predictive of a higher level of adiposity at 16 years of age and in adulthood, a relationship that appears to occur regardless of the child's adiposity at 1 year of age. A later rebound is correlated with normal adult weight (Rolland-Cachera et al, 1984, 1990).

Cell number increases in both lean and obese children throughout childhood into adolescence, but the number increases faster in obese children than in lean children. After adolescence, increases in body fat occur primarily by an increase in fat cell size. Contrary to old theories, the number of fat cells can increase throughout life. Cell numbers do not increase until maximal cell size is reached. The number of cells does not decrease with weight loss. Prevention is the key because once fat is gained and maintained over time, it is more difficult to lose.

Fat Storage

Most depot fat comes directly from dietary triglycerides, evidenced by the fact that fatty acid composition of adipose tissue mirrors the fatty acid composition of the diet. Excess dietary carbohydrate and protein are also converted to fatty acids in the liver by means of a comparatively inefficient process, lipogenesis.

Composition of the diet has been the focus of intense study. Dietary fat provides a metabolizable energy value often greater than 9 kcal/g, in a range of 10.9 to 11.2 kcal/g (Dattilo, 1992). Under normal feeding conditions, little dietary carbohydrate is used to produce adipose tissue, and it requires about three times as much energy to convert excess energy from carbohydrate to fat storage as it does to convert excess energy from dietary fat. When high-carbohydrate diets are fed, however, in particular, when the carbohydrate is in the form of simple sugars, lipogenesis does occur (Hirsch, 1995) but does not represent a significant contribution to fat stores (McDevitt et al, 2001). Surplus carbohydrate energy will make individuals fatter, however, not by lipogenesis but by suppressing fat oxidation (Hellerstein, 2001). Data from several sources indicate that Americans eat too many calories, even though they eat less fat than was consumed 30 years ago (Foreyt and Poston, 1997). Therefore, recommendations simply to reduce dietary fat are inappropriate; total calories remain critical as the variable for weight management.

Lipoprotein Lipase

Dietary triglyceride is transported to the liver as a part of chylomicrons and is removed from the blood by the enzyme lipoprotein lipase (LPL), which sits on the luminal side of the capillary and facilitates removal of lipid from the blood and its entry through the capillary wall into the adipose cell. Triglyceride, synthesized in the liver from free fatty acids, travels as part of very-low-density lipoprotein (VLDL) particles and is removed from the blood in the periphery by LPL. The enzyme hydrolyzes triglyceride into free fatty acids and glycerol. Glycerol proceeds to the liver; fatty acids enter the adipocyte, where they are reesterified into triglyceride. When needed by other cells, the latter are hydrolyzed once again to fatty acids and glycerol through the action of hormone-sensitive lipase (HSL) and they reenter the circulation.

Hormones affect LPL activity in different adipose tissue regions. Estrogens appear to stimulate LPL activity in the gluteofemoral adipocytes and thus promote fat storage in this area, an effect that is seldom seen in obese men. This may be for the specific purpose of providing for childbearing and lactation. In the abdominal region, however, estrogen appears to stimulate lipolysis. The "postmenopausal stomach" may thus have a hormonal association (Ley et al, 1992).

Lipoprotein lipase increases during periods of weight gain in both the obese and nonobese (Pi-Sunyer et al, 1994). After weight is lost, LPL returns to normal levels in nonobese persons; however, in reduced-obese persons (i.e., obese persons who have lost weight), the LPL does not decrease but in fact increases. This increase is one of the factors contributing to the rapid weight regain that is so common.

Smoking is associated with lower body weight, and the cessation of smoking is associated with weight gain. During 10 years of follow-up, a weight gain of 4.4 kg (about 10 lb) for men and 5.0 kg (11 lb) for women may be observed after smoking cessation (Flegal et al, 1995). The physiologic mechanisms by which cigarette smoking reduces body weight and smoking cessation increases body weight are uncertain. In fact, some research indicates that smoking cessation does not favor fat deposition (Hellerstein et al, 1994). Despite the weight gain that occurs after an individual stops smoking, the health benefits of smoking cessation are greater (U.S. Department of Health and Human Services, 1990).

REGULATION OF BODY WEIGHT

Regulatory systems such as neurochemicals, body-fat stores, protein mass, hormones, and postingestion factors all play a role in regulating intake and weight. Some evidence suggests that regulation takes place on both a short-term and a long-term basis. Short-term regulation governs consumption of food from meal to meal; long-term regulation is controlled by the availability of adipose stores (Bray, 1987). Total calories are more important than any singular nutrient alone.

Short-Term and Long-Term Regulation

Short-term controls are concerned primarily with factors governing hunger, appetite, and satiety. Satiety is associated with the postprandial state when excess food is being stored. Hunger is associated with the postabsorptive state when those stores are being mobilized. Physical triggers for hunger are much stronger than those for satiety, and it is easier to override the signals for satiety (Blundell et al, 1993).

A study investigated the effects of aging on the mechanisms of body energy regulation in an attempt to determine the causes of unexplained weight loss in older persons (Roberts et al, 1994). Healthy younger and older men of normal weight consumed a typical diet and performed usual activities. When either overfeeding or underfeeding interventions were made, the younger men exhibited spontaneous hypophagia or hyperphagia to alter body weight accordingly. The older men did not have the same responsiveness to changes in caloric intake. Findings from this study suggest that older persons are more vulnerable to unexplained weight losses or gains because of their inability to control spontaneous short-term changes in food intake. Yet age alone should not preclude weight loss treatment in older adults; careful evaluation of risks and benefits is needed (NIH, 1998).

Long-term regulation seems to involve a feedback mechanism in which a signal from the adipose mass is released when "normal" body composition is disturbed, as when weight loss occurs. This factor may play a greater role in younger persons than in older adults.

Set-Point Theory

Fat storage in nonobese adults appears to be regulated in a manner that preserves a specific body weight. In both animals and humans, deliberate efforts to starve or overfeed are followed by a rapid return to the original body weight, as though the latter constitutes a "set point" that is amenable to physiologic influences. If this is true, then some forms of obesity could be the result of an abnormally established set point; however, data are not conclusive in this area of research.

Body weight remains remarkably stable despite variations, possibly from internal regulatory mechanisms that are genetically determined (Rosencrans, 1994). In a study of obese and nonobese subjects, a 10% increase or decrease in usual body weight was accompanied by a 16% increase or 15% decrease in 24-hour total energy expenditure corrected for body composition (Leibel et al, 1995). Some studies suggest that body weight can be displaced only temporarily and that resting metabolic rate lowers, resulting in body weight returning (Liebel et al, 1995). Other studies do not show an adaptive metabolic response to weight loss. Instead, a transient reduction in energy expenditure is observed with energy restriction that normalizes on return to energy balance conditions (Weinsier et al, 2000). This controversy is far from settled; indeed, the same data can be interpreted to support or reject the set-point theory (Astrup et al, 1999; Hill and Wyatt, 1999).

Factors Regulating Energy Intake and Body Weight

Thermogenesis and the Thermogenic Effect of Food

The components of energy expenditure are the resting energy expenditure (REE), expressed as resting metabolic rate (RMR); the energy expended in voluntary activity; and the thermogenic effect of food (TEF) or diet-induced thermogenesis, discussed in detail in Chapter 2. Meal size, meal composition, the nature of the previous diet, insulin resistance, physical activity, and aging influence TEF. The TEF is made up of an obligatory component related to the energy value of the food consumed and an additional adaptive component that presumably responds to overeating by eliminating the excessive energy in the form of heat. There is support for the hypothesis of a defect in TEF in obese persons, but it is not clear whether this defect causes the obesity or results from the obesity (de Jonge and Bray, 1997).

Workers who work at night and eat snacks that provide about 20% of daily kilocalorie intake during their shifts may have a different metabolic efficiency. Diet-induced thermogenesis is higher after a morning snack than after afternoon or night snacks, suggesting that the effect of thermogenesis declines as the evening progresses (Romon et al, 1993).

Resting Metabolic Rate

The RMR explains 60% to 70% of total energy expenditure but less than 50% of the variation in total energy expenditure among healthy children, young adults, and older adults (Carpenter et al, 1995). RMR declines with age and with restriction of energy intake. When the body is suddenly deprived of adequate energy, such as with involuntary or deliberate starvation or semistarvation, the RMR adapts to conserve energy against an unpredictable future by dropping rapidly, by as much as 15% in 2 weeks. When adequate food intake is restored, the RMR returns to baseline levels (Ravussin and Swinburn, 1992).

Energy Expended in Voluntary Activity

The energy expended in voluntary activity is the most variable component of energy expenditure. Under normal circumstances, physical activity accounts for 15% to 30% of total energy expenditure (McArdle et al, 1999). Data indicate that persons who do not restrict calories require an increasing amount of physical activity to maintain body weight as they age to offset declines in FFM and, consequently, RMR (Williams, 1997).

Brain Neurotransmitters

Regulatory systems involving neurotransmitters in the brain govern feeding activities in response to signals originating in affected body tissues. Norepinephrine and dopamine are released by the sympathetic nervous system (SNS) in response to dietary intake. These neurotransmitters mediate the activity of areas in the hypothalamus that govern feeding behavior. Fasting and semistarvation lead to decreased SNS activity and increased adrenal medullary activity with a consequent increase in epinephrine, which fosters substrate mobilization (Katzeff et al, 1986; Vasselli and Maggio, 1988). Dopaminergic pathways in the brain are thought to play a role in the reinforcement properties associated with food.

Serotonin, neuropeptide Y, and endorphins are other neurochemicals thought to be involved in feeding behaviors. Decreases in serotonin and increases in neuropeptide Y have been associated with an increase in carbohydrate appetite. The level of neuropeptide Y increases during food deprivation, suggesting that it may be a factor leading to an increase in appetite after dieting. Preferences and cravings for sweet high-fat foods observed among obese and bulimic patients may involve the endorphin system (Drewnowski et al, 1992).

Corticotropin-releasing factor (CRF) is produced in the brain and is involved in controlling adrenocorticotropic hormone release from the pituitary gland. CRF is a potent anorexic agent. It decreases food intake on its own and weakens the feeding response produced by norepinephrine and neuropeptide Y. CRF is released during exercise, and increased levels of CRF have been noted in depressed patients and during starvation (Morley et al, 1992; Richard, 1989).

Gut Peptides

Mechanical contact of food with the mucosa of the stomach and small intestine muscles stimulates secretion of gut peptides, which have an immediate effect on satiety (see Chapter 1). Among those that have been identified is cholecystokinin (CCK), which is released by the intestinal tract when fats and proteins reach the small intestine. Receptors for CCK have been found in the gastrointestinal tract and in the brain. CCK causes the gallbladder to contract and stimulates the pancreas to release enzymes. At the brain level, CCK inhibits food intake.

Released by the nerve cells of the gut, bombesin is another gut peptide. Bombesin reduces food intake and enhances the release of CCK. Another peptide produced by the intestine is enterostatin, which seems to be involved specifically with the satiety following the consumption of fat.

Apolipoprotein A-IV is synthesized and secreted by the intestine in the process of the lymphatic secretion of chylomicrons. After entering the circulation, a small portion of apolipoprotein A-IV enters the central nervous system (CNS) and suppresses food consumption.

Hormones

Thyroid hormones modulate the tissue responsiveness to the catecholamines secreted by the SNS. A decrease in triiodothyronine lowers the response to SNS activity and consequently diminishes adaptive thermogenesis. Such a subtle defect could be one of the factors predisposing some obese persons to excessive weight gain. Women should be tested for hypothyroidism, particularly after menopause, because it is more common than once thought. It has been suggested that weight regain after weight loss may be a function of a hypometabolic state. Research in this area confirmed that energy restriction produced a hypothyroid, hypometabolic state. This state was transient, however, and normalized once energy-balanced conditions returned (Weinsier et al, 2000).

Insulin acts in the CNS and the periphery nervous system to regulate food intake. Insulin's effect on the CNS is to inhibit intake while in the periphery; insulin is involved in the synthesis and storage of fat. Impaired insulin activity may lead to reduced SNS activity and thus to impaired thermogenesis. It is possible that obese persons with insulin resistance or deficiency have a defective glucose disposal system and a depressed level of thermogenesis (Pi-Sunyer et al, 1994). In addition, the greater the insulin resistance, the lower the TEF. Fasting insulin levels increase proportionately with the degree of obesity; however, many obese persons demonstrate insulin resistance because of a lack of response by insulin receptors, impaired glucose tolerance, and associated hyperlipidemia. These sequelae can usually be corrected with weight loss.

Leptin is a hormone secreted by the adipose tissue that is correlated with the percent of body fat. Compared with men, women have significantly higher concentrations of serum leptin. The gender difference in Hispanic and non-Hispanic white adults 34 to 87 years of age was explained by percent of body fat and lean mass (Marshall et al, 2000). Studies support a role for leptin in the complex system of body weight regulation, including actions in the CNS with neuropeptides. Animal studies established the involvement of leptin in increasing satiety and energy expenditure (Flier and Maratos-Flier, 1998).

Weight loss is associated with a reduction in leptin, as are long-term changes in diet and exercise (Reseland et al, 2001). After weight loss, during a maintenance period, serum leptin concentrations increased slightly despite no changes in body weight. This finding suggests that leptin secretion is regulated by other factors in addition to adipose tissue size. Factors proposed include energy intake and insulin levels (Considine et al, 1996). Energy restriction reduces leptin levels and has been found to coincide with self-reported hunger, desire to eat, and prospective consumption (Keim et al, 1998). These observations suggest a role for leptin in regulating appetite.

Resistin is a newly described hormone expressed primarily in adipocytes. Resistin caused considerable excitement when animal studies showed that it antagonized insulin action (Janke et al, 2002). Researchers were hopeful that this hormone provided the link between obesity and diabetes in humans. Unfortunately, excitement about resistin has waned in light of recent studies that demonstrated (1) inconsistent expression and regulation of resistin in different animal models; (2) a total lack or only very low levels of expression in human fat cells; and (3) the absence of a relationship between resistin expression and degree of insulin resistance or presence of diabetes (Smith, 2002).

Ghrelin, a hormone produced primarily by the stomach, acts on the hypothalamus to stimulate feeding and on other tissues to slow metabolism and reduce fat oxidation. Ghrelin levels are highest in lean individuals and lowest in the obese. Increased levels are seen in people who are dieting, and markedly suppressed levels are noted after gastric bypass (Cummings et al, 2002). These findings support ghrelin's role in the long-term regulation of body weight (see *New Directions:* The Role of New Hormones).

WEIGHT MANAGEMENT THROUGHOUT LIFE

Balancing energy intake and energy expenditure is the basis of weight management throughout life. The 2000 *Dietary Guidelines for Americans* clearly acknowledge this relationship, specifically stating that calories eaten should be balanced with physical activity. Although it may sound simple, this feat can be extraordinarily difficult. Researchers in the area of weight management believe that part of the reason for the failure of many persons to balance energy intake and expenditure is the lack of tools that accurately assess either one (Hill, 2000). It is hoped that future technologic progress will allow people ready access to tools that clearly demonstrate the impact of their behaviors on energy balance. Lack of completely accurate tools does not imply that nothing can or should be done. Patterns of healthful eating and regular physical activity should begin in childhood and continue throughout adulthood. The aging process introduces special challenges to the energy balance equation. As a result of a lower RMR caused in part by a loss of fat-free mass, intake must be re-

NEW DIRECTIONS

The Role of New Hormones

The process of discovery of the controls on energy balance has been compared to "peeling back the layers of an onion," with new molecules being uncovered as we learn more about the system (Schwartz and Morton, 2002). The latest discovery is the hormone peptide YY_{3-36} (PYY_{3-36}). A member of the neuropeptide Y (NPY) family, PYY_{3-36} is secreted by endocrine cells lining the small bowel and colon in response to food. A recent study showed that when nonobese men and women were infused with a physiologic dose of PYY_{3-36}, eating was significantly inhibited for up to 12 hours, resulting in a decrease of 33% in total calorie intake for a 24-hour period (Batterham et al, 2002). No side effects were noted. PYY_{3-36} appears to work in the hypothalamus as a "middleman," binding to a receptor and inhibiting NPY production. This inhibition then allows the production of appetite-decreasing peptides. Drugs targeting the PYY_{3-36} system may hold promise for the future treatment of obesity.

duced and output increased if weight is to be maintained as individuals age.

Weight and Longevity

There is no biologic reason to suggest that persons should increase their body weight as they age; there is more evidence to the contrary (Langseth, 1991). Energy restriction in genetically obese animals greatly increases longevity and slows signs of aging, even when animals remain obese. Typically, a 40% reduction in food intake below that of animals eating freely increases the length of life in rodents by 50% (Masoro, 1994). Studies on rhesus monkeys suggest that the antiaging effects of calorie restriction in rodents can also occur in longer-lived species (Lane et al, 1997). These studies strengthen the possibility that calorie restriction will also prove beneficial in humans. Strong evidence suggests that longevity is affected by energy intake, not necessarily just fat calories. Plasma glucose and insulin levels are markedly lower when energy intake is reduced, and stress-protective glucocorticoids are higher.

WEIGHT IMBALANCE: OVERWEIGHT AND OBESITY

Overweight is a state in which weight exceeds a standard based on height; obesity is a condition of excessive fatness, either generalized or localized. It is possible to be obese at a weight within normal limits according to standard tables, just as it is possible to be overweight without being obese. In most people, however, overweight and obesity tend to parallel each other.

Assessment

Underweight and obesity are assessed in a variety of ways, depending on the necessity for accuracy. The tables of the Metropolitan Life Insurance Company were once widely used to establish a standard of ideal body weight (IBW). The more preferred methods include body mass index (BMI) or Quetelet Index (W/H^2), in which W is weight in kilograms and H is height in meters), and waist circumference. Waist-to-hip ratio is now seldom used.

Waist circumference over 40 inches in men and over 35 inches in women signifies increased risk to those with BMIs of 25 to 34.9 (NIH, 1998). These and other body fatness assessment methods are discussed in detail in Chapter 17. Tables for determining BMI are presented in the Appendix 17.

The National Institutes of Health (NIH) clinical guidelines classify individuals with a BMI of 25 as overweight. Although the risk for some comorbidities increases at a BMI of less than 25, mortality does not significantly increase until BMI reaches 27 (Manson et al, 1995). Persons who have a BMI of 30 or higher are classified as obese (NIH, 1998). Overweight and obesity as defined by the National Institutes of Health (NIH) are shown in Table 24-1.

TABLE 24-1 Classification of Overweight and Obesity

CLASSIFICATION	BMI kg/m²
Underweight	<18.5
Normal	18.5-24.9
Overweight	25.0-29.9
Obesity, class I	30.0-34.9
Obesity, class II	35.0-39.9
Extreme obesity, class III	≥40

From National Institutes of Health, National Heart, Lung, and Blood Institute: *Clinical guidelines on the identification, evaluation, and treatment of overweight and obesity in adults—the evidence report*, NIH Publication No. 98-4083.

Prevalence

The 2000 Behavioral Risk Factor Surveillance System (BRFSS), a random-digit telephone survey conducted in all states by the Centers for Disease Control and Prevention, indicated that a majority of U.S. adults

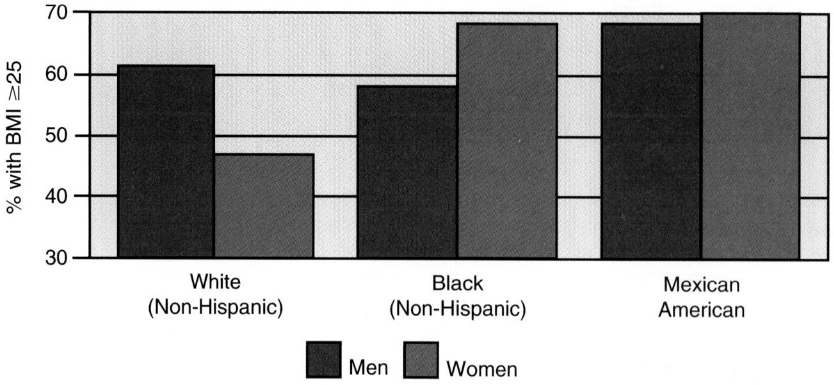

FIGURE 24-3 • Age-adjusted prevalence of overweight or obesity in selected groups (National Health and Nutrition Examination Survey [HANES] III, 1994-1998). (Modified from U.S. Department of Health and Human Services: *The Surgeon General's call to action to prevent and decrease overweight and obesity,* Rockville, Md, 2001, U.S. Department of Health and Human Services, Public Health Service, Office of the Surgeon General; and Centers for Disease Control and Prevention [CDC], National Center for Health Statistics [NCHS], and National Health and Nutrition Examination Survey [NHANES].)

ages 18 years and older are overweight or obese. About 56.4% of all participants had a BMI of 25 or higher. Of these, 19.8% were considered obese, a 61% increase in obesity since 1991 (Mokdad et al, 2001). The BRFSS self-report statistics are grimly supported by the clinical height and weight measurements in the 1999 National Health and Nutrition Examination Survey (NHANES), in which 61% of the adult population 20 to 74 years of age were classified in the overweight/obese category, with 34% in the overweight category and an additional 27% in the obese category (NCHS, 1999). The higher percentage in NHANES compared with that in BRFSS is due most likely to underestimation in the self-report data of BRFSS.

Obesity affects males and females, all races and ethnicities, and all age groups. Disparities do exist, however, and the prevalence of overweight and obesity is higher in women who are members of racial and ethnic minorities compared with non-Hispanic white women (Figure 24-3). Gender differences are also evident. Mexican American and non-Hispanic black women have a higher prevalence of overweight and obesity compared with men of the same race. This picture reverses in non-Hispanic white men and women, with men having a higher prevalence of overweight and obesity compared with women. Of interest, however, is the fact that, when looking at obesity alone (BMI ≥ 30), the prevalence in non-Hispanic white women was 23% and in non-Hispanic white men, 21% (Eberhart et al, 2001). Poverty also exerts its impact on weight status. In all racial and ethnic groups, women of lower socioeconomic status (SES) are about 50% more likely to be obese compared with those with higher SES (USDHHS, 2001).

Etiology

The nature and causes of obesity are the subject of intensive and continuing research. Both environmental and genetic factors are involved in a complex interaction of variables, which include psychological and cultural influences as well as physiologic regulatory mechanisms.

Over the years many hypotheses have evolved to explain why some people become fat whereas others remain lean and why it is so difficult for reduced-obese persons to maintain the weight loss that was so painstakingly achieved. The fact that no single theory can completely explain all manifestations of obesity, or apply consistently to all persons, underscores the complex nature of this condition. Theories suggesting imbalances of energy input are generally related to factors influencing hunger and appetite or satiety. Theories relating to imbalances of energy output are concerned primarily with TEF, physical activity, and RMR. Heredity and environment influence both the input and output of energy.

Heredity

Many of the hormonal and neural factors involved in normal weight regulation are determined genetically. These include the short- and long-term signals that determine satiety and feeding activity. Small defects in their expression or interaction could contribute significantly to weight gain. Number and size of fat cells, regional distribution of body fat, and RMR are also determined genetically.

The first studies of the role of inheritance in obesity estimated it to be from 66% to 80%. A more reasonable estimate is a heritability of the BMI of about 33% (Stunkard, 1996). The number of genes, markers, and chromosomal regions associated with obesity phenotypes is currently above 250 (Pérusse et al, 2001). In fact, the 2000 human obesity gene map includes genes on every chromosome except the Y chromosome (Pérusse et al, 2001). Still remaining is the task of identifying the combination of genes and mutations that contribute most to human obesity and defining the environmental circumstances that result in obesity when these genes and mutations are present (Foreyt and Poston, 1997).

Although numerous genes are involved in obesity, two have received much attention—the *ob* gene and the β3-adrenoreceptor gene. The *ob* gene produces leptin, and mutations in the mouse *ob* gene result in obesity. Mechanisms are being explored to explain leptin activities in humans, but some scientists believe it is unlikely that the *ob* gene plays a major role in human obesity (Foreyt and Poston, 1997).

The β3-adrenoreceptor gene, located primarily in the adipose tissue, is thought to regulate RMR and fat oxidation in humans. It was hypothesized that persons with a mutation of the gene for the β3-adrenergic receptor may have an increased capacity to gain weight (Clement et al, 1995); however, not all reports demonstrated a significant association with obesity. Therefore, the gene is not likely to be a major determinant of obesity, but it may contribute to weight gain in some persons. In fact, none of the gene variants identified to date plays a major role in obesity. It has been suggested that typical obesity is so heterogeneous and polygenic that there will be no major genes; rather, 20 or more common gene variants may each contribute a small genetic burden (Shuldiner and Sabra, 2001). Further, whereas genes appear to increase vulnerability to obesity, other determinants must be present for obesity to occur (Foreyt and Poston, 1997). A major factor is the environment.

Factors Affecting Weight Gain

Evidence strongly suggests that dietary and activity patterns are the primary causes of weight problems in industrial societies and that there is a mismatch between how we live and our genetic makeup (Foreyt and Poston, 1997). Excessive energy intake can be active or passive. Active overeating in Western societies is partly the result of the excessive portion sizes that are accepted as the norm. The portions and calories that restaurants and fast food outlets offer for one meal can often exceed a person's caloric needs for the entire day. In fact, the number of large-sized portions has increased dramatically since the 1970s (Young and Nestle, 2002). Passive overeating refers to eating energy-dense diets. In passive overeating, the amount of food may not be excessive, but the calorie content is (Prentice, 2001). Data from NHANES III suggest that intake of energy-dense, nutrient-poor foods result in an increased risk of overeating (Kant, 2000).

Research supports that food and its taste elements evoke pleasure responses (Van Horn et al, 1998). The endless variety of food available at any time at a reasonable cost can contribute to higher calorie intake because people eat more when offered a variety of choices than when a single food is available. Normally, as foods are consumed, they become less pleasant. This decline is known as sensory-specific satiety and is associated with a shift to other food choices during the meal (Rolls and Drewnowski, 1996). An example of this principle in action is an all-you-can-eat buffet. Although sensory-specific satiety can promote the intake of a more varied and nutritionally balanced diet, it can also lead to overconsumption of calories.

The effect of eating more calories than needed is compounded by low energy expenditure. The sedentary nature of the American society is a factor in the growing problem of obesity. Fewer Americans are exercising, and more time is being spent in low-energy activities such as watching television and using the computer (see *Focus On:* Do Americans Understand Weight Management?).

Health Risks

Obesity has been directly linked with mortality and many chronic ailments (NIH, 1998). The relative risk for mortality among overweight and obese women (BMI ≥27) was one and one-half to two times that of the leanest women (BMI <19) enrolled in the Nurses' Health Study, a prospective study established in 1976 that follows the health of registered nurses in 11 states. Furthermore, a weight gain of 10 kg or more after age 18 years was predictive of increased mortality (Manson et al, 1995). In a large prospective study of more than one million adults in the United States, a high BMI was associated with an increased risk of death from all causes among both men and women in all age groups.

The optimal BMI for longevity was within the range of 20.5 to 24.9 (Calle et al, 1999). In this study, the risk associated with a high BMI was greater for whites than for blacks. Figure 24-4 shows mortality risks at various BMIs.

A subset of obese persons who are metabolically normal seems to exist. This subgroup has uncomplicated obesity and appears to have early-onset obesity, hyperplasia of normal adipocytes, and normal quantities of visceral fat (Sims, 2001). In general, however, obesity can be viewed as metabolically unhealthy. Chronic diseases such as heart disease, type 2 diabetes, hypertension, stroke, gallbladder disease, sleep apnea, certain cancers, and osteoarthritis are associated with obesity and tend to worsen as the degree of obesity increases (NIH, 1998; Pi-Sunyer, 1993; Shape Up America! and American Obesity Association, 2001). An increasingly recognized condition associated with obesity is nonalcoholic fatty liver disease, which may progress to end-stage liver disease (Angulo, 2002). Genetically obese experimental animals show reductions in various aspects of cell-mediated immunity and decreased resistance to bacterial and viral infections (Stallone, 1994). Obesity is also a risk factor for cancer, poor wound healing, and poor antibody response to hepatitis B vaccine. The costs of obesity are staggering. Health economists,

FOCUS ON

Do Americans Understand Weight Management?

For years, the media, health organizations, and the government have sent an important message to American consumers: "Fat intake should be reduced to 30% or less of calories." The Surgeon General, the National Academy of Sciences, the American Heart Association, and the American Dietetic Association (ADA) all advocate this reduction in dietary fat. The food nutrition labels implemented in 1994 are based on the 30% fat-intake level.

The message has taken hold—somewhat. A survey conducted by the National Center for Health Statistics (NCHS) shows that in 1990, the average American diet contained 34% of total calories from fat, down 2% from 36% in 1978. Although this still does not meet the standards set by the government, it is an encouraging decrease from the 40% level of the 1960s.

The new dilemma that challenges food manufacturers is that many people in the world are getting heavier. The proportion of U.S. adults who are overweight continues to increase. The NIH conducted a study indicating that in 1992 through 1993, the average body weight of Americans 25 to 30 years of age was 171 lb. In 1985 through 1986, the average weight was 161 lb for the same age group (see Figure 24-4). If the percentage of fat in the diet is decreasing, why are Americans getting heavier? Experts believe a number of factors contribute to the increase in body weight, especially continued lack of exercise.

Physical activity trends indicate that the majority of the U.S. population gets insufficient levels of physical activity or none at all. Data from the BRFSS (MMWR, 2001) show that in 1998, of adults 18 years of age and older:

- 25.4% engaged in recommended levels of activity
- 45.9% reported insufficient activity
- 28.7% reported no physical activity

Excess energy intake is also a factor. According to the latest National Health and Nutrition Examination Survey (NHANES III), total average energy intake by adults increased from 1969 calories in 1978 to 2200 calories in 1990. Merely controlling grams of fat consumed, which is popular nutrition advice, does not necessarily result in a reduction in calories and therefore does not always lead to weight control.

The ADA position on weight management for adults states that it "requires a lifelong commitment to healthful lifestyle behaviors emphasizing eating practices and daily physical activity that are sustainable and enjoyable" (American Dietetic Association, 2002). Although Americans often hear that they need to balance food intake with output, is the message really understood? Do Americans have the knowledge and skills necessary to manage their weight? Is it a problem of wanting instant gratification rather than future rewards? Is it a belief that an effortless solution exists (a pill, cream, drink, a new diet)? Is it a combination of factors? (Pfizer, 1994.)

using prospective studies and national health statistics, pegged the cost for obesity at $99.2 billion in 1995 (Wolf and Colditz, 1998).

Healthy People 2010 objectives recognize the public health implications of overweight and obesity in our society. The objectives include ambitious targets to increase the proportion of adults who are at a healthy weight and to reduce the proportion of adults, children, and adolescents who are obese. Underscoring the concern that overweight and obesity increase the risk for heart disease, diabetes, certain types of cancer, and other chronic health problems, the Surgeon General released in 2001 a "Call to Action." Dr. Satcher's urgent call acknowledged the consequences of canceling the gains made in other areas of public health if overweight and obesity increases are not reversed (USDHHS, 2001).

In April 2002, the Internal Revenue Service issued a new ruling qualifying obesity as a disease and allowing taxpayers to claim weight-loss expenses as a medical deduction if undertaken at a physician's direction to treat an existing disease. Although not all obese persons who have weight-loss expenses will qualify for the deduction, experts believe the significance of the new ruling is the government's recognition of obesity's immense impact on the health and financial well-being of the country.

Regional Distribution of Fat and Metabolic Syndrome

Regional patterns of fat deposit are controlled genetically and differ between and among men and women. Two major types of fat deposition are currently recognized: excess subcutaneous truncal–abdominal fat *(android)* and excess gluteofemoral fat *(gynoid)*. Excess subcutaneous fat on the trunk, particularly in the abdominal area, is android or "apple-shape" obesity and is more common among men. Aging is also an important factor in visceral obesity and fat accumulation. Studies indicate that this type of obesity is highly correlated with insulin resistance (NIH, 1998). Visceral fat component is strongly correlated with risk factors such as glucose intolerance, hyperlipidemia, and hypertension (Matsuzawa et al, 1994).

When the chronic disorders of glucose intolerance, insulin resistance, hyperlipidemia, and hypertension are linked together, they are known as the metabolic

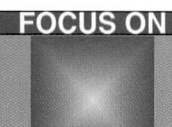

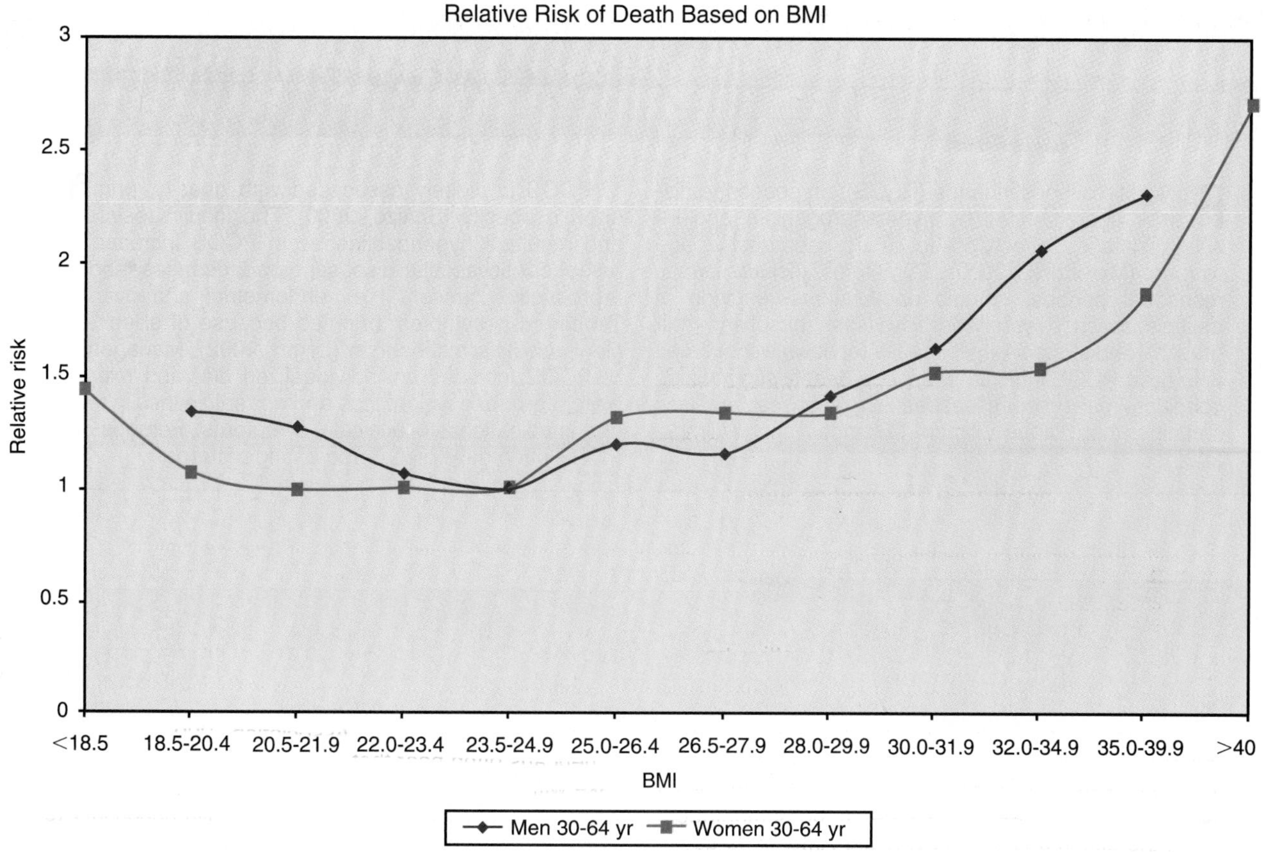

FIGURE 24-4 • Body mass index and mortality risk. (Data from Callee EE et al: Body mass index and mortality in a prospective cohort of U.S. adults, *N Engl J Med* 341:1097, 1999.)

syndrome (Reaven, 1988). The Third Report of the National Cholesterol Education Program Expert Panel on the Detection, Evaluation, and Treatment of High Blood Cholesterol in Adults (ATP III) defined the metabolic syndrome as having three or more of the following abnormalities: waist circumference >102 cm in men and >88 cm in women, serum triglycerides of at least 150 mg/dl, high-density lipoprotein (HDL) level <40 mg/dl in men and <50 mg/dl in women, blood pressure ≥135/85 mm Hg, or serum glucose ≥110 mg/dl. Findings from NHANES III indicated that the metabolic syndrome is highly prevalent, with 23.7% of the population or about 47 million U.S. residents, based on 2000 census data, having the syndrome (Ford et al, 2002). Risks are also associated with polycystic ovary syndrome (see *Focus On:* Polycystic Ovary Syndrome; see also Chapters 12 and 35).

Gynoid fat distribution, characterized by the "pear shape," is created by heavier deposits of fat around the thighs and buttocks. Gynoid obesity is more common in women, and the fat deposits are presumably energy reserves to support the demands of pregnancy and lactation. Women with the gynoid type of obesity do not develop the impairments of glucose metabolism seen in obese women of the same weight who carry their fat in the abdominal area.

Combinations of abdominal fat accumulation and gluteofemoral fat accumulation are also seen, particularly in women. Postmenopausal women more closely follow the male pattern of abdominal fat stores. As a result, these women are at increased risk for blood glucose, lipid, and pressure abnormalities. In both men and women who were obese during adolescence, rates of cardiovascular disease and diabetes are increased (Dietz, 1998a). Regional fat distribution defines the risk of hyperlipidemia and hyperinsulinemia in children, as it does in adults (Goran, 1998).

Discrimination

Perhaps equally devastating is the negative image of obesity in current society, which fosters the widespread attitude that obesity is a disgrace. Young children, 6 to 9 years of age, have already adopted the disparaging attitudes of their parents toward the obese (Feldman et al, 1988). Although society is gradually being exposed to the concept that fatness is a more complex issue than a matter of self-control, the obese—particularly women, adolescent girls, and the morbidly obese—continue to encounter discrimination (see *Focus On:* Fat Discrimination).

FOCUS ON

Polycystic Ovary Syndrome

Polycystic ovary syndrome (PCOS), an endocrine disorder characterized by hyperandrogenism and insulin resistance, affects 5% to 10% of reproductive age women (McKittrick, 2000). Symptoms include erratic menstrual periods, chronic anovulations resulting in multiple ovarian cysts, infertility, acne, hirsutism (hair growth), and alopecia (hair loss). Interviews with women who have PCOS indicate that it is a deeply stigmatizing condition, making them feel freakish, abnormal, and less feminine than other women (Kitzinger and Willmott, 2002).

PCOS is closely associated with obesity, primarily android obesity (Scalzo, 2000). The insulin resistance and resultant hyperinsulinemia in PCOS increase the risk of cardiovascular disease, type 2 diabetes, and the reproductive cancers (i.e., endometrial and ovarian). Treatment is symptom oriented because of a lack of a clear etiologic mechanism (Legro, 2002). Management of PCOS includes an individualized diet and exercise plan to promote weight loss and normalize insulin levels and medications to alleviate symptoms. Persons with PCOS often have disordered eating patterns.

FOCUS ON

Fat Discrimination

Obese people, particularly women, are socially stigmatized. This negative perception adversely affects their educational, socioeconomic, marital, and employment status (Enzi, 1994). Obese high school students, despite comparable grades, test scores, attendance, and extracurricular activities as their nonobese counterparts, are less likely to be accepted into college (Wing and Greeno, 1994). Overweight women are found to have lower household incomes, a higher incidence of household poverty, and are more likely to be single (Enzi, 1994). Many employers are unwilling to hire overweight persons. Research confirms that diverse groups, including children, adults, and medical personnel, hold negative stereotypes of obese persons (Wing and Greeno, 1994). These negative attitudes may stem from the belief that obese persons are weak willed and self-indulgent (Stunkard, 1996).

The Council on Size and Weight Discrimination works to end discrimination based on standards for body size and weight or shape through public policy and opinions. Another organization working to overcome this stigma is the American Obesity Association. Founded in 1995, this nonprofit corporation is dedicated to encouraging obese persons to obtain the best possible medical care for their condition; achieving greater research of obesity as a disease; and urging health insurance companies and government agencies responsible for programs to treat obesity as they do other diseases.

Data from Council on Size and Weight Discrimination, P.O. Box 305, Mt. Marion, NY 12456 (www.cswd.org); and American Obesity Association, 1250 24th St. NW, Washington, DC 20037.

MANAGEMENT OF OBESITY IN ADULTS

The management of obesity has evolved over the years as more research has increased knowledge of weight regulation. Initially, clinicians focused entirely on weight loss, and little was known about weight maintenance. It was assumed that if people could just lose the weight, maintenance would easily follow. It soon became clear that focusing on weight loss without attention to weight maintenance was inappropriate, unfair, and possibly harmful to anyone trying to manage his or her weight.

Treatment has also evolved. Years ago, an energy-restricted diet represented the only treatment. Eventually, lifestyle modifications were added after research supported their inclusion. Finally, the importance of physical activity was recognized, not just as a component for weight loss but also as an essential ingredient for weight maintenance after weight loss.

Today a chronic disease-prevention model that involves both lifestyle interventions and interdisciplinary team therapies from physicians, dietitians, exercise specialists, and behavior therapists offers the best treatment opportunity (Rippe et al, 1998). Weight-reduction programs with the most promise of success integrate healthier food choices, exercise, and lifestyle modification. Pharmacologic treatment and surgical intervention are appropriate in some circumstances but are not a substitute for the necessary changes in eating and physical activity patterns. Figure 24-5 presents an algorithm for the management of obesity.

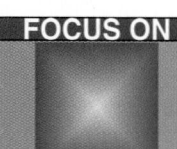

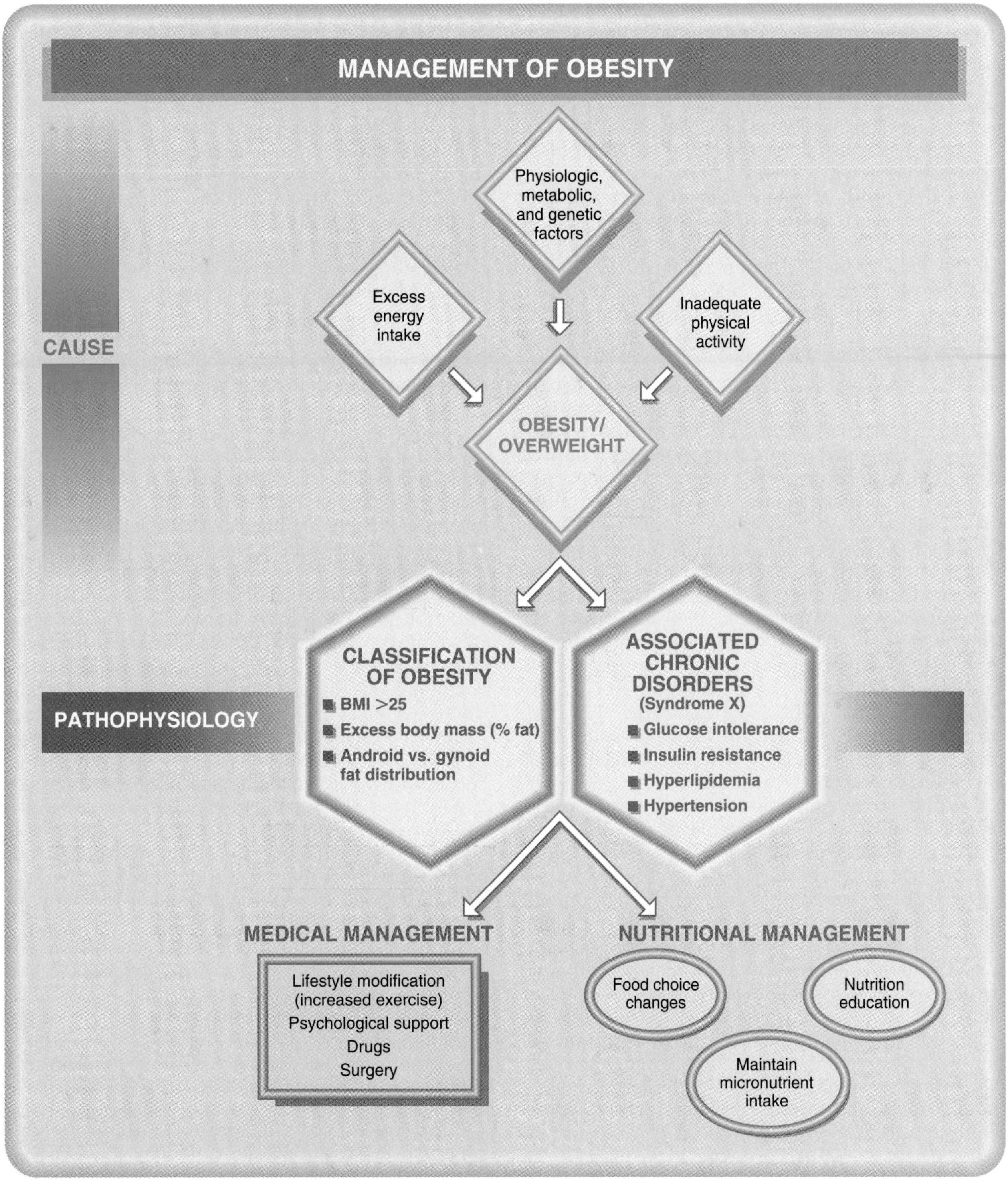

FIGURE 24-5 • Pathophysiology algorithm: management of obesity. (Algorithm content developed by John Anderson, PhD, and Sanford C. Garner, PhD, 2000.)

Goals of Treatment

The ADA has taken the position that the goal of obesity treatment should be refocused from weight loss alone to weight management, defined as attaining the best weight possible in the context of overall health (ADA, 2001). Achieving ideal body weight or percentage of body fat is not always realistic or desirable, and under some circumstances it may not be appropriate at all.

Depending on the type and severity of the existing obesity and on the age and lifestyle of the individual, successfully reducing body weight varies from a relatively simple matter to being virtually impossible. Maintaining present body weight or achieving a moderate loss is beneficial. Obese persons who lose even small amounts of weight (5% to 10% of initial body weight) are likely to improve their health in the short run by reducing the severity of the comorbidities associated with obesity (Anderson and Konz, 2001; NIH, 1998). A review of studies in which patients experienced about a 10% or less weight reduction showed that they also had improved glycemic control, reduced blood pressure, and reduced cholesterol levels. Weight loss of 10% of initial weight in one study resulted in significant improvements in serum lipids even though patients remained more than 20 kg overweight (Andersen et al, 1995). In addition, it also appears to increase longevity (Goldstein, 1992).

The critical question of whether modest weight losses, if maintained, would have a long-term impact is beginning to be answered. A study of obese patients with diabetes mellitus who experienced more than a 5% reduction in body weight and maintained the loss, showed that they had significant improvements in glycosylated hemoglobin values at 1 year compared with patients losing less weight and those who gained weight (Wing et al, 1987). The initial effects on glycemic control were greater than the long-term effects, supporting the role of energy restriction as well as weight loss in glycemia improvement (Anderson and Konz, 2001). The maintenance of improvements at 1 year supported the prediction that long-term improvements in body weight could have a long-term effect on glycemic control.

Despite the recognition that modest weight loss is beneficial and may be more achievable, it has been found that obese persons have self-defined goal weights that differ considerably from the goals suggested by professionals (Foster et al, 1997). Their personal weight-loss goals and expectations are often unrealistic and not achievable. Health professionals must therefore intervene to help patients accept more modest weight loss and understand what can realistically be achieved with current treatment methods.

In addition to developing realistic goals, a comprehensive assessment is needed for any patient who is 40% or more above ideal body weight; medical evaluation is also warranted (Brownell and Wadden, 1991; Rippe et al, 1998). Psychosocial, behavioral, and biologic factors should be assessed in the plan.

Rate and Extent of Weight Loss

Reduction of body weight involves the loss of both protein and fat, in amounts determined to some degree by the rate of weight reduction. A drastic reduction in calories resulting in a high rate of weight loss can mimic the starvation response. Tissue response to starvation, or even semistarvation of the kind encountered in many weight-loss programs, is one of adaptation to an anticipated period of deprivation. The classic starvation studies done by Keys (1950) found that during the first 10 days of a fast and after utilization of glycogen stores, about 8% to 12% of the energy expenditure is from protein and the balance is from fat. As starvation progresses, up to 97% of energy expenditure is from stored triglyceride. Use of fat, with more than twice the kilocalories of protein, is not only more efficient but also spares vital protein tissues. Even when the body has adjusted completely, however, 5% of weight loss is still from protein in muscle supporting adipose tissue (Bray and Gray, 1988a). Metabolic aberrations that occur during starvation cause a host of negative effects, including bradycardia, hypotension, dry skin and hair, easy fatigue, constipation, nervous system abnormalities, depression, and death (Callaway, 1988) (see Chapters 25 and 42).

Steady weight loss over a longer period favors reduction of fat stores, limits the loss of vital protein tissues, and avoids the sharp decline in RMR that accompanies rapid weight reduction. NIH treatment recommendations outline calorie deficits that result in a loss of about 0.5 to 1 lb per week for persons with a BMI of 27 to 35 and 1 to 2 lb per week for those with BMIs greater than 35. This rate of loss should continue for about 6 months, leading to a reduction of 10% of body weight. For the next 6 months, the focus changes from weight loss to weight maintenance. Following this phase, further weight loss may be considered (NIH, 1998).

Final goals should be individualized and chosen realistically with reduction of body fat as the focus. For example, neither the hyperplastic obese nor the gynoid types will be able to maintain a large weight loss. Female role models of dress sizes 6 to 10 and male models with 30-inch to 34-inch waists "may not be appropriate for the obese population," and in fact even BMIs of 25 are unreasonable goals for many dieters (Blackburn, 1988).

Even with the same caloric intake, rates of weight reduction vary. Men reduce weight faster than women of similar size because of their higher LBM and RMR. The heavier person, who because of the higher weight expends more energy than one who is less obese, loses faster on a given calorie intake than a lighter person. Some obese persons who fail to lose weight on a diet they state is low in calories actually consume more energy than they report and overestimate their physical activity levels (Lichtman et al, 1992).

Lifestyle Modification

Lifestyle modification or behavior modification interventions rely on analyzing behavior to identify events that are associated with inappropriate as well as appropriate eating, exercise, or thinking habits (Wadden and Sarwer, 1998). Antecedents, behaviors, and consequences are analyzed to determine how to modify the situation. For example, if an individual finds that he or she overeats when angry, steps are taken to help the person deal with anger in more constructive ways. In addition to nutrition and exercise, the principal components of treatment include self-monitoring, problem solving, stimulus control, slowing of eating, and cognitive restructuring (Wadden and Sarwer, 1998).

Self-monitoring with daily records of place and time of food intake, as well as accompanying thoughts and feelings, helps identify the physical and emotional settings in which eating occurs. It also provides feedback on progress and places the responsibility for change and accomplishment on the patient. Self-monitoring also gives clues to the occurrence of relapses and consequent guilt and how they can be prevented.

Problem solving is a process for defining the eating or weight problem, generating possible solutions, evaluating the solutions, choosing the best one, implementing the new behavior, evaluating the outcome, and reevaluating alternative solutions if the one selected is not successful.

Stimulus control involves modification of (1) the settings or the chain of events that precede eating, (2) the kinds of foods consumed when eating does occur, and (3) the consequences of eating. Patients are taught to slow their rate of eating to become mindful of satiety cues and reduce food intake. Strategies such as putting down the utensils between bites, pausing during meals, and chewing for a minimum number of times are some ways to slow the eating process.

Cognitive restructuring teaches patients to identify, challenge, and correct the negative thoughts that frequently undermine their efforts. For example, excessive self-criticism in response to a dietary lapse could lead to total abandonment of effort. Positive self-talk, such as "I had a piece of cake. One slice is not going to increase my weight. I will continue eating in a healthful way," can sometimes help patients deal more constructively with such incidents. Some lifestyle modification strategies are listed in Box 24-1. A program of this type that appears to be successful is The Solution (see Table 24-3). In this program, participants learn how to set limits and to nurture healthful behaviors.

Comprehensive lifestyle modification in weight control appears to be most effective for the mildly obese (20% to 40% overweight). Patients can lose 20 to 25 lb and successfully maintain the weight loss if they continue to practice the techniques and exercise regularly. It also appears that longer programs are more successful (Buckmaster and Brownell, 1988). Most programs usually last for 15 weeks and result in an average weight loss of 1.2 lb per week.

A review of lifestyle modification studies from 1985 to 1995 indicated that patients treated by behavior therapy combined with a 1200-calorie daily diet regained 30% to 35% of their weight loss in the year following treatment. Five years after treatment, subjects had, on average, returned to their baseline weight (Wadden and Sarwer, 1998). Weight regain is a problem regardless of the type of program.

Dietary Modification

Weight-loss programs with any degree of success integrate food-choice changes with exercise, frequently with behavior modification, nutritional education, and psychological support. When these approaches fail to bring about the desired reduction in body fat,

Box 24-1. Lifestyle Modification Strategies

Elimination of Eating Cues

- Eat only sitting down at one designated place.
- Sit in a different seat at the table.
- Leave the table as soon as eating is done.
- Do not combine eating with other activities, such as reading or watching television.
- Do not put bowls of food on the table.
- At a restaurant, limit intake from the bread basket to one roll with no or a small amount of butter.
- Stock home with healthier food choices.
- Keep all food in cupboards where it cannot be seen.
- Shop for groceries from a list after a full meal.
- Limit the amount of money taken when shopping.
- Plan meals and snacks.
- Plan for special events, parties, and dinners.
- Immediately place leftovers in storage containers and refrigerate or freeze them for another meal.
- Negotiate with the family to eat healthier foods.
- Ask others to monitor eating patterns and provide positive feedback.
- Substitute other activities for snacking.
- Snack on fresh vegetables and fruit.

Behaviors to Prolong Eating and Reduce the Amount of Food Eaten

- Eat slowly and savor each mouthful.
- Put down the fork between bites.
- Delay eating for 2 to 3 min and converse with others.
- Postpone a desired snack for 10 min.
- Serve food on a smaller plate.
- Leave 1 or 2 bites of food on the plate.
- Divide portions in half so that another portion can be permitted.

Modified from Holli BB: Using behavior modification in nutrition counseling, *J Am Diet Assoc* 88:1530, 1988.

medication may be added to the program and, in the case of morbid obesity, surgical intervention may be required.

Recommendations

Weight-loss programs should combine a nutritionally balanced dietary regimen with exercise and lifestyle modification at the least possible expense (NIH, 1992, 1998). Selecting the appropriate treatment strategy depends on the goals of the patient as well as his or her health risks. Treatment options include the following:

- A low-calorie diet, increased physical activity, and lifestyle modification
- The preceding plus pharmacotherapy
- Surgery plus an individually prescribed dietary regimen, physical activity, and lifestyle modification program
- Prevention of weight gain through energy balance

Restricted-Energy Diets

A balanced energy-restricted diet is the most widely prescribed method of weight reduction. The diet should be nutritionally adequate except for energy, which is decreased to the point where fat stores must be mobilized to meet daily energy needs. A caloric deficit of 500 to 1000 kcal daily usually meets this goal. The energy level varies with the individual's size and activities, usually ranging from 800 to 1500 kcal daily. Regardless of the level of calorie restriction, healthful eating should be taught and emphasized, and recommendations for increasing physical activity should be included (Shape Up America! and American Obesity Association, 2001).

The low-calorie diet should be relatively high in carbohydrates (50% to 55% of total kilocalories), using sources such as vegetables, fruits, and whole grains. The diet should also include generous protein, about 15% to 25% of kilocalories, to prevent conversion of dietary protein to energy. Fat content should not exceed 30%. The inclusion of extra fiber is recommended to reduce caloric density, to promote satiety by delaying stomach-emptying time, and to decrease to a small degree the efficiency of intestinal absorption.

Calculating fat grams has become a trend in recent years. One simple rule is to divide ideal calorie level by 4 for a 25% fat intake (e.g., an 1800-kcal intake would need to include 450 kcal from fat, or about 50 g of fat). Giving the person license to distribute fat grams as desired throughout the day makes the approach more appealing, involves the person in the treatment process, and results in lower energy intake without hunger. Total calories must also be considered, however (see *Focus On:* Do Americans Understand Weight Management?).

Alcohol and foods high in sugar should be limited as unnecessary sources of energy; however, small amounts can be included for palatability. Alcohol makes up 10% of the diet for many regular drinkers and contributes 7 kcal per gram. Alcohol behaves like a fat because it spares fat from being oxidized. Ethanol increases 24-hour energy expenditure and decreases lipid oxidation when added to the diet or substituted for other foods (Suter et al, 1992). Heavy drinkers (who consume 50% or more of daily calories from alcohol) may have a depressed appetite to the point of weight loss, emaciation, and even malnutrition, but moderate users tend to gain weight with the alcohol calories added to their usual diet. Habitual use of ethanol in excess of energy requirements most likely favors lipid storage and weight gain and should be considered a risk factor for obesity.

Artificial sweeteners (discussed in Chapter 33) and fat substitutes (discussed in Chapter 3) may improve the acceptability of limited food intakes for some people. There is no evidence that using artificial sweeteners reduces food intake or results in weight loss.

Vitamin and mineral supplements that meet age-related requirements are usually recommended with weight-reduction programs that provide less than 1200 kcal for women or 1800 kcal for men.

Exchange System Diets

A popular and easily manipulated method for planning a diet program tailored to the individual is the exchange system, which is described in Appendix 53. A 1200-kcal diet based on this system is shown in Table 24-2. The energy content of the diet can be increased by adding midafternoon and evening snacks or by increasing the number of servings from various groups. Nonnutritious, high-energy foods, such as sweets, desserts, or alcohol, can be added sparingly.

Formula Diets and Meal Replacement Programs

Formula diets or meal replacement programs come in a variety of forms. The good ones contain high-quality protein, sugar as fructose, and a moderate amount of monounsaturated fat. Total calories range from 1000 to 1600 calories daily with the meal replacement drink or bars replacing two meals (for weight loss) or one meal (for weight maintenance) each day. The recommended daily quantity of the drink or powder supplies approximately 900 kcal distributed as 20% protein, 30% fat, and 50% carbohydrate. At this energy level, and with vitamins and minerals to meet daily requirements, these formulas are considered safe. Quantities of the meal replacement equivalent to a single meal can also be used successfully as substitutes for a meal at times when it is difficult to obtain foods appropriate to a weight-reduction program. A 4-year follow-up of patients originally instructed on the use of meal replacements for weight loss and weight maintenance demon-

TABLE 24-2 1200-kcal Diet—22% of Kilocalories From Fat

FOOD	FOOD EXCHANGES* (NO.)	CARBOHYDRATE (G)	PROTEIN (G)	FAT (G)
Milk, skim	2	24	16	—
Vegetables	3	15	6	
Fruits	4	60		
Bread	5	75	10	
Meat,† lean	5		35	15
Fat	3			15
	TOTALS	174	67	30

Sample Meal Plan

Breakfast
Fruit, 1 exchange
Bread, 2 exchanges
Milk, skim, 1 exchange

Lunch or supper
Vegetables, 1 exchange
Bread, 2 exchanges
Meat, lean, 2 exchanges
Fruit, 1 exchange
Milk, skim, 1 exchange

Dinner or supper
Meat, lean, 3 exchanges
Vegetable, 2 exchanges
Bread, 1 exchange
Fat, 1 exchange
Fruit, 2 exchanges

Sample Menu

Breakfast
½ grapefruit
1 slice of whole-wheat toast
1 glass (8 oz) of skim milk
¾ cup of dry cereal
Coffee or tea as desired

Lunch
Sandwich:
2 slices of rye bread
2 oz of sliced turkey
2 stalks of celery
1 carrot
1 peach (medium)
1 glass (8 oz) of skim buttermilk

Dinner
Bouillon
1 parsley potato (2-inches in diameter)
3 oz of roast veal, lean
½ cup of peas and carrots
1 green salad
2 tsp salad dressing
½ cup applesauce (unsweetened)
1 small banana
Tea or coffee as desired

*From exchange lists, see Appendix 53.
†Lean meat with visible fat removed is used, reducing the fat content from 5 to 3 mg per meat exchange.

strated that they were able to maintain weight loss and sustain improvements in disease risk factors (Flechtner-Mors et al, 2000).

Commercial Programs

Millions of Americans use commercial weight-loss programs to lose weight, and new programs enter the marketplace regularly (Table 24-3). Most offer diets that are balanced. Programs can be evaluated by comparing them with sound nutritional practices. Programs have begun to collect data on the effects of treatment, including dropout rates, success rates, and maintenance data.

As Table 24-3 illustrates, the programs vary considerably. Some require the use of proprietary prepackaged low-fat meals. Some provide classes on self-introspection, behavior modification, and nutrition. Prepackaged diets appeal to some people because they allow them to avoid making choices about food. Use of the Internet has spawned a new generation of commercial programs as shown in Table 24-3. A randomized, controlled trial of overweight adults with BMIs of 25 to 36 indicated that the Internet can be used successfully to deliver a weight-loss program if it includes behavioral therapy with weekly contact and individualized feedback (Tate et al, 2001).

Extreme Energy Restriction

Extreme energy-restricted diets provide fewer than 800 kcal per day, and starvation or fasting diets provide fewer than 200 kcal per day.

Fasting

Fasting is seldom prescribed as a treatment; however, it is frequently invoked as a part of religious or protest regimens or in a personal effort to lose weight. Under these circumstances, it is seldom continued long enough to produce the serious neurologic, hormonal, and other side effects that accom-

TABLE 24-3 Popular Commercial Diet Programs

NAME	FOODS OR PRODUCTS	EDUCATION	TEACHERS/COUNSELORS	MAINTENANCE
VLCD Programs				
Health Management Resources (HMR) www.yourbetterhealth.com	Special drink, multidisciplinary team	1½-hr weekly group meetings w/RD and midweek phone calls	Physicians, health educators, registered nurses, registered dietitians, exercise physiologists	Weekly meetings for 18 mo
Medifast www.med.fast.net	Special drink; physician supervised	Weekly individual sessions Weekly group meetings	Supervised by physicians	Weekly meetings for 5 mo
Optifast www.optifast.com	Special drink; physician supervised	Weekly individual sessions w/MD 1½-hr weekly group meetings 1 meeting w/RD	Physicians, registered nurses, registered dietitians, and psychologists at most locations	No time limit, begins at 20th week
Diet Programs				
Diet Center www.dietcenter.com	Regular food	Daily individual sessions	Trained staff	Maintenance—weekly meetings for the first 3 mo; biweekly for months 4-6; monthly for months 6-12
Jenny Craig www.jennycraig.com	Prepackaged foods	14 1-hr video group classes; weekly individual sessions	Registered dietitians and psychologists	Monthly meetings for 6 mo or 1 yr
Nutri/System www.nutrisystem.com	Prepackaged foods	30-min weekly group meetings; 10-min weekly individual sessions	College graduates	1-yr transition diet—program and regular foods
Weight Watchers www.weightwatchers.com	Regular food	45-min weekly group meetings	Program graduates	Weekly meetings for 6 wk; free meetings if maintain goal weight
The Solution www.shapedown.com	Regular food	Weekly 2-hr group meetings	Registered dietitians and psychologists certified by the program	Continuation with weekly meetings as necessary; no time limit
Internet-Based Diets				
Cyberdiet www.DietWatch.com and www.Cyberdiet.com	Regular food	Personal and Professional eCounseling provide weekly meal plans and nutrition and fitness report cards. Professional eCounseling provides biweekly chats with an RD. Chat rooms, bulletin boards, e-newsletter also available.	Registered dietitians; also uses the expertise of physiologists, fitness trainers, culinary chefs, MDs, and psychologists	Maintenance program available once personal goals are met
eDiets www.ediets.com	Regular food	Weekly meal plan and exercise routines. Chat rooms, bulletin boards, e-newsletter available.	Registered dietitian, registered nurse, fitness trainer, counselors, psychologists	Maintenance meal plans are available
Nutrio www.nutrio.com	Regular food	Daily and weekly meal plans; exercise and nutrition logs, community message boards and e-newsletter.	Registered dietitians, exercise physiologists, and psychologists	Maintenance meal plans are available

VLCD, very-low-calorie diet.

pany prolonged starvation. More than 50% of the rapid weight reduction is fluid, which often leads to serious hypotension problems. Accumulation of uric acid can precipitate episodes of gout; gallstones can also occur.

Very-Low-Calorie Diets

Diets providing 200 to 800 kcal are classified as very-low-calorie diets (VLCDs). Little evidence suggests that intakes of fewer than 800 calories daily are of any advantage (NIH, 1993). Most VLCDs have the following characteristics: they are hypocaloric but relatively rich in protein (0.8-1.5 g/kg IBW per day); they are designed to include a full complement of vitamins, minerals, electrolytes, and essential fatty acids, but not calories; they are given in a form that completely replaces usual food intake; and they are usually given for a period of 12 to 16 weeks (NIH, 1993). Their major advantage is rapid weight loss. Because of potential side effects, prescription of these diets is reserved for persons with a BMI above 30 for whom other diet programs with psychotherapy have been unsuccessful. Occasionally, VLCDs may be indicated for persons with a BMI of 27 to 30 who have comorbidities or other risk factors.

The VLCD that first became popular in the early 1970s resulted in several deaths; however, improved formulation with respect to protein quality has led to acceptability for those whose obesity is potentially life-threatening (see *Focus On:* History of Protein-Sparing Modified Fast Diets).

Most VLCDs are in one of two forms. The PSMF contains 1.5 g of protein per kilogram of IBW in the form of lean meat, fish, and poultry; no carbohydrates; and only the fat contained in the protein sources. In PSMF, nitrogen excretion is high at 11 to 23 g daily, declining steeply in the first few days to obligate levels; simply adding 100 g of carbohydrate to the diet may prevent further losses of nitrogen (Pi-Sunyer, 1994).

The second and more common form of the VLCD uses commercially formulated liquid diets based on milk or egg protein. These typically contain 33 to 70 g of protein, 30 to 45 g of carbohydrate, and a small amount of fat. Patients who follow a VLCD (400-800 kcal daily) lose 20 kg in 12 to 16 weeks and maintain 33% to 50% of this loss in the following year (Wadden, 1993). Cardiac complications, including risk of sudden death, are still a concern. Risks include potassium loss as well as loss of body protein, which is proportionately greater (20 g/kg of weight lost) in the less obese than in the more obese (Forbes, 1987). Serum electrolytes need to be monitored and supplemented when necessary.

The VLCDs can lead to an increase of urinary ketones that interfere with the renal clearance of uric acid, resulting in increased serum uric acid levels, often manifested as gout. Higher serum cholesterol levels resulting from mobilization of adipose stores pose

FOCUS ON

History of Protein-Sparing Modified Fast Diets

The first protein-sparing modified fast (PSMF) diets were developed after observing that during total fasts, which were popular for weight reduction in the late 1950s and early 1960s, dieters lost large amounts of potassium and protein. The first PSMF diets were developed to add protein to the fasting regimen. Protein in the early formulas was exclusively in the form of hydrolyzed collagen, a protein lacking the essential amino acid tryptophan. The formulas were not supplemented with vitamins, minerals, or electrolytes and were not necessarily supported by medical supervision. The products were used by more than 100,000 people, among whom 60 diet-related deaths had been reported to the Centers for Disease Control and Prevention by the end of 1977.

The diet was directly implicated as the basis for the cardiac dysrhythmia causing 17 deaths (Isner et al, 1979). Of these 17 deaths, those with the highest percentage of body fat before the diet began were better able to preserve body protein, especially that in the myocardium (Van Itallie and Yang, 1984).

Sudden death during dieting presents with a classic prolonged QT interval on the electrocardiogram. The highest risk for sudden death syndrome is during weight loss with total fasting, with VLCDs, or following obesity surgery (Berg, 1994). Causes may include nutritional inadequacies, depletion of myocardial proteins, excessive β-adrenergic sensitivity of the myocardium, electrolyte abnormalities leading to ventricular fibrillation, ingestion of medications, or predisposition to aggravation of cardiac dysrhythmia. The heart is usually small in children or adults who die from protein-energy malnutrition or anorexia, although it may be enlarged in some patients who are starving. Patients should be made aware of the risks for sudden death syndrome with restrictive dieting.

The hazardous products were removed from the market. PSMF formulas currently contain complete protein and some carbohydrate; are supplemented with vitamins, minerals, and electrolytes; and are usually included as part of a complete multidisciplinary program. Patients must be carefully screened before they start these programs and then must be closely monitored.

a risk of gallstones. Additional adverse reactions that are common include cold intolerance, fatigue, lightheadedness, nervousness, euphoria, constipation or diarrhea, dry skin, thinning reddened hair, anemia, and menstrual irregularities. Some of these are typical of triiodothyronine (thyroid) deficiency.

In 1998, the NIH recommended against using VLCDs for weight-loss therapy because the deficits are too great, and nutritional inadequacies will occur unless VLCDs are supplemented with vitamins and minerals (NIH, 1998). Although the NIH cited clinical trials demonstrating that LCDs were just as effective as VLCDs in producing weight loss after 1 year, a recent metaanalysis showed that VLCD participants maintained significantly greater weight losses compared with those who followed LCDs 5 years after completing a structured weight-loss program (Anderson et al, 2001).

Nondiet Approach

The nondiet paradigm maintains that the body will attain its natural weight if the individual eats healthfully, becomes attuned to hunger and satiety cues, and incorporates physical activity. This approach focuses on achieving health rather than attaining a certain weight. Advocates for the nondiet approach promote size acceptance and maintaining respect for the diversity of body shapes and sizes. Given the evidence that a 5% to 10% loss of initial weight can result in health benefits, that many persons set weight-loss goals that are unrealistic, and that fat discrimination continues to plague society, this approach may help some persons to develop a better relationship with food and a healthier perspective about their bodies.

Popular Diets and Practices

A continuous supply of new approaches to weight reduction is available to the consumer through the popular press. Some of the programs are sensible and appropriate, whereas others emphasize fast results with minimal effort. Some of the proposed diets would lead to nutritional deficiencies over an extended period; however, the potential health risks are seldom realized because the diets are usually abandoned after a few weeks. Diets that emphasize fast results with minimal effort encourage unrealistic expectations, setting the dieter up for failure, subsequent guilt, and feelings of helplessness at ever managing the weight problem.

The U.S. Department of Agriculture Research Education and Economics supported a scientific review of popular diets to assess their efficacy for weight loss and weight maintenance as well as their effect on metabolic parameters, psychological well-being, and reduction of chronic disease (Freedman et al, 2001). Diets were divided into categories based on their macronutrient content and included high-fat, low-carbohydrate; moderate-fat, balanced nutrient reduction; and low- and very-low-fat diets. A summary of the overall results of the review is shown in Table 24-4.

TABLE 24-4 Results of U.S. Department of Agriculture Scientific Review of Popular Diets

AREA	FINDING
Weight loss	Diets that reduce caloric intake result in weight loss; all popular diets result in short-term weight loss if followed.
Body composition	All low-calorie diets result in a loss of body fat. In the short term, high-fat, low-carbohydrate ketogenic diets cause a greater loss of body water than body fat.
Nutritional adequacy	• High-fat, low-carbohydrate diets are low in vitamins E, A, thiamin, B_6, and folate, and the minerals calcium, magnesium, iron, and potassium. They are also low in dietary fiber. • Very-low-fat diets are low in vitamins E and B_{12} and the mineral zinc. • With proper food choices, a moderate-fat, balanced nutrient reduction diet is nutritionally adequate.
Metabolic parameters	• Low-carbohydrate diets cause ketosis and may significantly increase blood uric acid concentrations. • Blood lipid levels decline as body weight decreases. • Energy restriction improves glycemic control. • As body weight declines, blood insulin and plasma leptin levels decrease. • As body weight declines, blood pressure decreases.
Hunger and compliance	No diet was optimal for reducing hunger.
Effect on weight maintenance	Controlled clinical trials of high-fat, low-carbohydrate, low-fat, and very-low-fat diets are lacking; therefore, no data are available on weight maintenance after weight loss or long-term health benefits or risks.

From Freedman M et al: Popular diets: a scientific review, *Obes Res* 9(suppl 1):1S, 2001.

The low-carbohydrate, high-fat diet restricts carbohydrate to less than 20% of calories (≤100 g), and fat constitutes 55% to 65% of calories, with protein making up the balance. Protein obtained from animal sources means that fat, saturated fat, and cholesterol intakes are high. Although these diets feature high ketone production, they suppress appetite to only a minor degree. The initial rapid weight loss from diuresis is secondary to the carbohydrate restriction. Examples of carbohydrate-restricted diets include *Dr. Atkins' New Diet Revolution* and *The Carbohydrate Addict's Diet.*

One popular regimen (the "Zone" diet) restricts carbohydrate to no more than 40% of total calories,

Box 24-2. Tips for Evaluating Popular Diets and Practices

1. Stay current in the medical and nutrition literature. Read professional journals regularly to stay on the cutting edge; read more than one reliable reference.
2. Teach consumers to make healthy choices wherever they are—at home, at a restaurant, in other homes for holidays and special events.
3. Think first before advancing the latest diet trend; review the content of the proposed diet first.
4. Stick to logical nutrition principles, such as maintaining an intake of 15%-20% protein and ≤30% fat. Calculate the individual's needs accordingly.
5. Keep language simple for the consumer's benefit.
6. Evaluate fads and trends using the following principles:
   - Does the diet exclude any major food groups (using the Food Guide Pyramid as a guideline)? For example, a high-meat diet would be too low in breads and cereals. A high-fat diet would be higher than recommended amounts to match current standards (i.e., ≤30% calories from fat).
   - Does the diet propose use of supplements, pills, or drugs to the exclusion of normal foods? This may be a dangerous practice.
   - Does the diet suggest avoiding certain foods because they "cause" certain diseases (such as cancer, arthritis, heart disease)? No individual food has been verified as the cause of disease at this time.
   - Does the diet suggest including certain foods because they "cure" certain diseases? No singular food cures disease. Foods and nutrients in combination have been suggested as being beneficial in preventing some forms of cancer, but focusing on any given food should not exclude other foods or food groups.
   - Food forms (frozen versus fresh, etc.) should not be highlighted. It is not necessary to use only raw fruits and vegetables to the exclusion of canned and frozen foods.
   - Beware of sweeping statements—"salty foods cause weight gain in everyone." Not everyone is sensitive to sodium.
   - More is not always better. Too much of one food to the exclusion of others is a tip-off that a diet is unbalanced.
7. Analyze for total content, including a balance of vitamins, minerals, protein, carbohydrate, and fat, using current guidelines.

with fat and protein providing 30% of calories each. This particular diet composition is claimed to keep insulin in check, which is blamed for fat storage. The diet includes generous amounts of fiber and fresh fruits and vegetables. Weight loss ensues not because insulin is kept in a narrow range, but because calories are restricted. Calculations have shown that at most the diet provides 1700 calories daily (Gladwell, 1998).

Moderate-fat, balanced nutrient reduction diets contain 20% to 30% of calories from fat, 15% to 20% of calories from protein, and 55% to 60% of calories from carbohydrate (Freedman et al, 2001). *Volumetrics,* a program in this category, focuses on the energy density of foods. Foods high in water content have a low energy density. These include fruits, vegetables, low-fat milk, and cooked grains as well as lean meats, poultry, fish and beans. Low-water-containing foods that are energy dense, such as potato chips, crackers, and fat-free cookies, are restricted.

Very-low-fat diets are those containing less than 10% of calories from fat, and low-fat diets contain 10% to 19% of calories from fat (Freedman et al, 2001). *Dr. Dean Ornish's Program for Reversing Heart Disease* and *The Pritikin Program* fall into this category. These diets produce rapid weight loss and are very restrictive. A popular variation limits fat to 20% of total energy intake. Because fat provides more than two times the energy per gram as protein or carbohydrate (9 kcal versus 4 kcal), an effective diet can be one that includes extensive controls on this nutrient.

A study at Vanderbilt University investigated the effects of a low-fat diet with ad lib carbohydrate versus a low-fat/calorie-restricted diet (Schlundt et al, 1993). The "low-fat only" group lost an average of 4.6 kg compared with 8.3 kg in the low-fat/low-calorie group. Although not as dramatic a loss, a "low-fat" program may be appropriate for persons who (1) are discouraged by other programs, (2) do not mind a more gradual loss, and (3) have sufficient self-control to avoid compensating with low-nutrient, fat-free products for calories saved through fat restriction.

Box 24-2 provides some guidelines for evaluating popular diets. Although hypnosis and acupuncture are popular with some, there is no definitive support for these practices.

To help consumers find their way through the maze of programs available for weight loss, several initiatives have been undertaken. In 1996, Shape Up America! and the American Obesity Association released the first edition of *Guidance for Treatment of Adult Obesity,* an educational resource for physicians. It provides the tools needed to identify and intervene as appropriate and gives treatment guidance and support for patients; the Web site is www.shapeup.org. In 1997, the Federal Trade Commission convened a conference to better understand the problem of obesity and to explore ways to improve the information that consumers routinely receive about the nature of obesity and weight-loss products and programs. It marked the first time that representatives of the weight-loss industry, members of the scientific and academic community, agencies from state and federal government, and public interest and consumer groups met together to explore voluntary approaches and to address issues regarding weight-loss products and programs (Gross and Daynard, 1997).

In 1998, the NIH released *Clinical Guidelines on the Identification, Evaluation, and Treatment of Overweight and Obesity in Adults—The Evidence Report.* The intent of the guidelines is to provide evidence for the effects of treatment on overweight and obesity. The guidelines are directed to physicians and associated health professionals in clinical practice, health care policy makers, and clinical investigators (NIH, 1998). In October 2000, the National Heart, Lung, Blood Institute (NHLBI) in cooperation with the North American Association for the Study of Obesity (NAASO) released *The Practical Guide: Identification, Evaluation, and Treatment of Overweight and Obesity in Adults* based on the *1998 Clinical Guidelines* publication. The practical guide provides tools for the clinician to manage overweight and obese adults (NIH and NAASO, 2000).

Exercise

Exercise is an extremely important part of a weight-management program. By increasing LBM in proportion to fat, exercise helps to balance the loss of LBM and reduction of RMR that inevitably accompany even a well-managed weight-reduction program. Numerous positive side effects include strengthening cardiovascular integrity as well as increasing sensitivity to insulin.

A combination of aerobic and resistance training is recommended. Resistance training increases LBM, adding to the resting metabolic rate and the ability to utilize more of the energy intake, and increases bone mineral density, which is especially important for women (see Chapter 27). In addition to the physiologic benefits of exercise are the relief of boredom, increased sense of control, and improved sense of well-being (Figure 24-6).

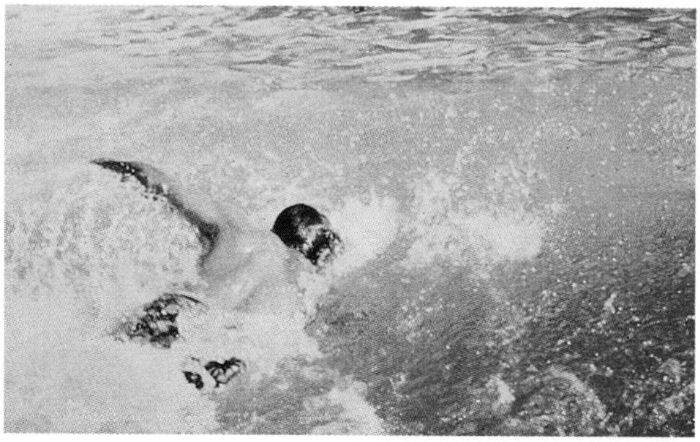

FIGURE 24-6 • Swimming is an excellent aerobic activity to include in a weight-reduction program.

Increased exercise can result in an energy deficit; and even without diet, exercise alone can be expected to lower weight around 2 to 3 kg, depending on the intensity, duration, and type of exercise (Blair, 1993.) Dieters with hypertrophic obesity lose more fat during an exercise program than the very obese with hyperplastic obesity (Bjorntorp, 1983). This may account for the observation that although the moderately obese lose body fat during physical training, it is difficult to demonstrate this result in the massively obese.

Some studies of programs combining diet and exercise have shown that although there is no increase in weight loss in the exercising group over diet alone, an increased loss of body fat does occur (Hill et al, 1987; Van Dale et al, 1987). A decrease in body fat does not necessarily mean a decrease in body weight. Initially, physical exercise increases muscle mass, and because LBM is denser than the fat it replaces, body weight may not change. With continued exercise, the limited capacity of muscle mass to increase is overcome by the decrease in fat, resulting in a net decrease in body weight. A minimum of 2 months is needed to obtain any reduction of adipose tissue with training programs.

The RMR is elevated during aerobic exercise. Except after fairly high levels of intensity or large amounts of exercise, RMR returns to resting levels within an hour or so following exercise (Brehm and Keller, 1990). Energy expenditure during this period represents replacement of muscle glycogen as well as the effects of hormonal changes and the increase in metabolic processing of fuel stores. Whether or not exercise has an effect on TEF remains unresolved. Increases in lean body mass result in 8% to 14% higher daily energy expenditures in moderately and highly active men compared with sedentary men (Horton and Geissler, 1994); however, this study did not find that habitual exercise leads to prolonged stimulation of metabolic rate per unit of active tissue.

Contrary to popular belief, spot reduction, that is, reducing fat in one area of the body, is not possible with exercise; fat is burned from the largest concentrations of adipose tissue. Another misconception is that exercise is counterproductive because it increases the desire to eat.

Consistency is key to realizing the health and weight-management benefits of exercise. Previous exercise recommendations for health called for 20 to 60 minutes of moderate- to high-intensity endurance exercise performed three or more times weekly. It now appears that the majority of health benefits can be gained by physical activity of moderate intensity (enough to expend 200 kcal daily) accumulated in intermittent short bouts. "The current recommendation to maintain cardiovascular health at maximum level, regardless of weight, is at least one hour per day of moderately intense physical activity or 20 to 30 minutes of high-intensity activity 4 to 7 days per week" (Institute of Medicine, 2002).

Programs that involve supervision or regular participation within a social group appear to be more successful in the long term. Socioeconomic circumstances can be an important factor. Many exercise programs are expensive, and it is not always possible, or even safe, to indulge in brisk walking in some neighborhoods.

Only 10% of Americans meet the exercise requirements thought to be needed to reduce disease risks. In one recent study, 82% of overweight adults believed they failed to maintain healthy weight because they did not exercise, even though they were aware of the benefits (Miller, 1994). This society tends to view the barriers to exercise as outweighing its benefits. Whatever the selected exercise, it should be readily available, pleasant, affordable, and easy to do.

Exercise also helps the individual maintain weight loss. It has been demonstrated that weight regain is significantly less likely to occur when physical activity is combined with any weight-reduction method (Blair, 1993).

Pharmaceutical Management

In patients with BMIs of 30 and above, or 27 and above with other risks, pharmaceutical agents can be a helpful addition to a diet and exercise program. They cause an energy deficit through a number of mechanisms, including acting on the brain to suppress appetite; producing bulk to fill the stomach, thereby suppressing appetite; possibly increasing thermogenesis; increasing metabolism; and selectively interfering with fat absorption. Medications have side effects, however, and the benefits and risks must be weighed carefully for each individual.

Medications currently available can be categorized as CNS-acting agents and non–CNS-acting agents. The CNS-acting agents fall into the categories of catecholaminergic agents, serotoninergic agents, and combination catecholaminergic-serotoninergic agents. Common side effects of CNS-acting agents are dry mouth, headache, insomnia, and constipation.

Catecholaminergic drugs act on the brain, increasing the availability of norepinephrine. Table 24-5 lists catecholaminergic agents. Drug Enforcement Agency (DEA) Schedule II anorexic agents, such as amphetamines, have a high potential for abuse and are not recommended for obesity treatment. DEA Schedule III agents also pose abuse potential that should be carefully considered. Commonly used DEA Schedule IV catecholaminergic agents such as phentermine have a low potential for abuse. Because of its effects on blood pressure, phentermine is prescribed with caution in patients with even mild hypertension. The over-the-counter medication phenylpropanolamine (PPA) was used for many years as an appetite suppressant. In May 2000, scientists at Yale University released a report linking exposure to PPA with hemorrhagic stroke in women. Because so few men were exposed to PPA, no definitive conclusions could be

TABLE 24-5 Available Catecholaminergic Agents

AGENT	TRADE NAME	DAILY DOSAGE (mg)*
Schedule II Agents		
amphetamine	Biphetamine	10-15
phenmetrazine HCl	Preludin	75
Schedule III Agents		
benzphetamine HCl	Didrex	25-50 to 75-150
phendimetrazine tartrate	Bontril	105
	Slow-Release Bontril	105
	Prelu-2	105
	Plegine	105
	X-Trozine	105
	Extended Release X-Trozine	105
Schedule IV Agents		
diethypropion HCl (amfepramone)	Tenuate	75
	Tenuate dospan	75
mazindol HCl	Sanorex	1-3
	Mazanor	1-3
phentermine HCl	Adipex-P	37.5*
	Fastin	30
	Obenix	37.5
	Oby-Cap	30
	Oby-Trim	30
	Zantryl	30
phentermine resin	Ionamin	30†

From Shape Up America! and American Obesity Association: *Guidance for treatment of adult obesity,* ed 3, Bethesda, Md, 2001, Shape Up America! and American Obesity Association.
OTC, Over the counter.
*Represents recommended daily intake. Ranges represent initial dose to maximum dose. Titration may be indicated depending on each patient's therapeutic response.
†Usual dosage. Some patients may respond to half this dosage.

made about the risk in men. The U.S. Food and Drug Administration (FDA) was concerned because of the seriousness of a stroke and the inability to predict persons at risk. As a result, in November 2000, the FDA asked firms that market drugs containing PPA to discontinue them voluntarily.

Serotoninergic agents act by increasing serotonin levels in the brain. Two drugs in this category, fenfluramine hydrochloride (HCl) and dexfenfluramine HCl, were removed from the market in September, 1997, after concerns were raised regarding the possible side effect of cardiac valvulopathy and regurgitation (Connolly et al, 1997). In this disease, the heart valves have a glistening white appearance that is plaque-like, and regurgitation is present. These drugs had also been associated with primary pulmonary hypertension, a rare, often fatal disease (Abenhaim et al, 1996). Further studies clarified the relationship between fenfluramine and dexfenfluramine and valvular abnormalities (Jick et al, 1998; Khan et al, 1998; Weissman et al, 1998).

Combination of catecholaminergic and serotoninergic agents include sibutramine (Meridia), which inhibits the reuptake of serotonin and norepinephrine. The drug was initially developed to counteract depression. Classified as a DEA Schedule IV agent, it has a low potential for abuse; however, careful observation of blood pressure and heart rate of patients using sibutramine has been recommended (Lean, 1997). Caution is needed in patients with hypertension; use is not recommended for patients with coronary heart disease, arrhythmias, stroke, or congestive heart failure (Aronne, 1998).

Orlistat, a non–CNS-acting agent, is not an appetite suppressant. It acts directly on the gastrointestinal tract to inhibit fat absorption (Guerciolini, 1997). Orlistat (Xenical) is taken with mildly hypocaloric meals, resulting in a 30% reduction in fat absorption. Inhibiting fat absorption raises concern about fat-soluble vitamins; However, fat-soluble vitamins generally remain within the normal range in patients treated with orlistat (James et al, 1997). A small percentage of patients showed reductions in blood levels of vitamins D and E and β-carotene, which were corrected with vitamin supplementation (James et al, 1997). Side effects are gastrointestinal in nature: oily spotting, fecal urgency, and flatus with discharge. Health benefits include reduced LDL cholesterol and elevated HDL cholesterol, improved glycemic control, and reduced blood pressure (Aronne, 1998).

Not all individuals respond to pharmacotherapy, but for patients who do respond, a weight loss of about 1 lb per week can be expected. Most studies conducted for less than 24 weeks show continued weight loss for the duration of the study. Long-term studies show most weight loss occurs during the first 6 months of therapy. Significant maintenance of loss has been shown at 1 year or more as long as the drug treatment is continued. After medication is stopped, most patients regain weight.

Natural weight-loss aids hold varying degrees of promise for weight-loss results (see *Focus On:* Natural Weight-Loss Aids).

Surgical Procedures

Morbid obesity is sometimes treated surgically. This treatment is preferably reserved for those with a BMI of 40 or greater, or a BMI of 35 or greater with other risk factors (NIH, 1998; Shape Up America! and American Obesity Association, 2001). Various surgical procedures have been used to decrease the amount of food entering or being absorbed from the gastrointestinal tract. These include esophageal banding, gastric restrictive surgery, and jejunoileal bypass. Gastric restrictive surgery includes gastric banding, or gastroplasty, and gastric bypass. The current surgery of choice, gastric bypass, is a gastric restrictive surgery with malabsorption. New surgical treatments in bariatrics will likely continue to emerge.

Before any morbidly obese person is considered for surgery, failure of a comprehensive program that includes calorie restriction, exercise, lifestyle modification, psychological counseling, and family involvement should be demonstrated. *Failure* is defined as an inability of the patient to reduce body weight by one third and body fat by one half and an inability to maintain any weight loss achieved. Such patients have intractable morbid obesity and should be considered for surgery. Before surgery the patient should be evaluated extensively with respect to physiologic and medical complications, psychological problems such as depression and poor self-esteem, and the extent of motivation.

Postoperative follow-up includes evaluation at regular intervals by the surgical team and a registered dietitian. In addition, behavioral or psychological support is necessary. Lifelong follow-up on the part of the patient and surgeon, including involvement of the patient's primary physician, is essential (Choban et al, 1996; NIH, 1998).

Gastric Restriction (Gastric Bypass and Gastroplasty)

Gastric restriction, which surgically reduces the reservoir capacity of the stomach by closing off a part of it, is successful in achieving weight reduction in people who are morbidly obese and is a well-accepted bariatric surgery for that purpose. Gastroplasty reduces the size of the stomach by applying rows of stainless-steel staples to partition the stomach and creating a small gastric pouch, leaving only a small opening (0.8-1.0 cm) into the distal stomach. This opening may be banded by a piece of mesh to prevent it from enlarging during the years after surgery. The most popular gastroplasty is the vertical banded gastroplasty (Figure 24-7). Gastric bypass involves reducing the size of the stomach with the sta-

FOCUS ON

Natural Weight-Loss Aids

Americans are constantly being told that "diets don't work." The lure of a quick and easy solution to the challenge of weight management is strong, and the market for natural weight-loss aids is booming. What are the claims and what are the facts?

Chromium: According to the claims, chromium should promote fat loss and increase lean body mass. Chromium potentiates the action of insulin in carbohydrate, lipid, and protein metabolism, although the exact mechanism is not known. Dietary surveys indicate that most persons consume less than the recommended amounts of chromium (Anderson and Kozlovsky, 1985). Also, participating in strenuous physical activity results in increased acute losses of chromium (Anderson et al, 1988).

Findings suggest that indiscriminate use of chromium supplements has no effect on body composition. When sensitive methods of human body composition are used, data indicate that chromium supplementation during strength training does not promote an increase in muscle mass and fat loss in men (Clancy et al, 1994; Lukaski et al, 1996).

Chromium competes with iron for binding on transferrin. Researchers hypothesized that significant increases in serum chromium concentration as a result of chromium supplementation, particularly as chromium picolinate, may adversely affect iron transport and distribution (Lukaski et al, 1996). A recent study examined the effects of chromium picolinate supplementation on iron status in older men who participated in resistance training; chromium did not affect changes in iron transport and did not compromise iron status in the men (Campbell et al, 1997).

Dehydroepiandrosterone (DHEA): Among other claims, DHEA is supposed to promote weight loss. Unfortunately, only animal work has been completed for testing the effects of DHEA on weight loss. Problems noted with DHEA include liver cancer, which occurred in rats. In addition, supplementation can lead to increased insulin resistance, the growth of unwanted hair, and a drop in high-density lipoprotein cholesterol, increasing the risk for heart disease (see Chapter 35).

Ma huang: Ma huang (ephedra) promoters claim benefits such as weight loss, increased energy, performance enhancement, and increased LBM. Studies demonstrated that ma huang given alone does not result in weight loss; however, when combined with caffeine plus a calorie-restricted diet, greater weight loss can be achieved than with calorie-restricted diets alone (Astrup et al, 1992; Breum et al, 1994; Daly et al, 1993). Ma huang is a CNS stimulant; it increases blood pressure and heart rate. Ma huang is hazardous to those with heart ailments, diabetes, hypertension, and thyroid conditions. When combined with caffeine-containing herbs (kola nut, guarana, and mat), ma huang can be especially hazardous. The FDA has received more than 100 reports of adverse reactions ranging from heart attacks to hepatitis and several deaths among people who used supplements containing a ma huang–kola nut combination. Common, less severe side effects of ma huang–caffeine combinations are insomnia, dizziness, and tremor. When individuals discontinue treatment, they can experience headache and fatigue.

Senna: Senna leaves are the dried leaflets of plants found in Egypt and India. Senna is a potent cathartic (Tyler, 1993). Use of this herb, which induces diarrhea, can lead to low potassium levels. Three deaths have been associated with senna use.

Chitosan: This indigestible compound extracted from crustacean shells is an over-the-counter weight-loss agent. Claims are that chitosan blocks fat absorption. A controlled study showed no effect of chitosan on fecal fat excretion (Guerciolini et al, 2001).

Garcinia cambogia: Hydroxycitric acid is the active ingredient in garcinia cambogia, and it is promoted to reduce the body's ability to store fat. Citric acid is a component of the TCA (tricarboxylic acid) (krebs) cycle. Studies have been limited to animals, and there is no evidence that it promotes weight loss.

pling procedure but then connecting a small opening in the upper portion of the stomach to the small intestine by means of an intestinal loop (see Figure 24-7). Mason and Ito developed the original operation in the late 1960s (Mason and Ito, 1969). Numerous improvements of the original operation occurred, and the most successful modification is the Greenville Gastric Bypass, also known as the Roux-en-Y gastric bypass (see Figure 24-7).

Both gastroplasty and gastric bypass procedures have the effect of reducing the amount of food that can be eaten at one time and producing early satiety. The new stomach capacity may be as small as 20 to 30 ml. In addition to the greater absolute weight loss observed, the gastric bypass tends to have safe and sustainable results with significant resolution of serious comorbidities (Rubenstein, 2002).

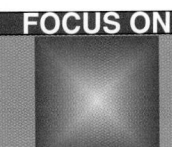

The most frequent complications of gastric restriction are bloating of the pouch, nausea, and vomiting. A postsurgical food record noting the tolerance for specific foods in particular amounts helps in devising a program to avoid these episodes. A careful postoperative feeding regimen progresses from liquids to solid foods with a focus on protein intake. Attention to vitamin and mineral supplementation, particularly calcium, folate, iron, and vitamin B_{12} (in gastric bypass) is advised. Patients should be counseled to eat slowly, chew food well, and avoid swallowing chunks of meat or other food that cannot be completely liquefied and that could block the pouch opening. Frequent small meals are important. Patients tend to choose liquids; however, weight loss can be deterred by drinking too much calorically-dense liquid, such as milk shakes and soft drinks. Eventually, the pouch expands to accommodate 4 to 5 oz at a time.

Because use of the lower part of the stomach is omitted, the gastric bypass patient may also have dumping syndrome (see Chapter 29). The symptoms of tachycardia, sweating, and abdominal pain are so negative that they can further motivate the patient to make the appropriate behavior changes and refrain from overeating.

Completion of the surgery does not end the obesity treatment; in fact, the procedure is considered to create malnutrition, and lifelong follow-up and regular monitoring by a multidisciplinary team of health care professionals is needed (Consensus Development Conference Panel, 1991). Monitoring should include an assessment of body-fat loss, potential anemia, and deficiencies of potassium, magnesium, folate, and vitamin B_{12}, especially in patients with gastric bypass. The results of gastric surgery are favorable and are attended by fewer complications than with the intestinal bypass surgery practiced during the 1970s. On average, the reduction of excess body weight after gastric restriction surgery correlates to about 30% to 40% of initial body weight (Brolin et al, 1994).

In most patients, surgically induced weight loss will correct hypertension, type 2 diabetes mellitus (Pories et al, 1995), sleep apnea, obesity hypoventilation syndrome, gastroesophageal reflux, venous stasis disease, urinary incontinence, female sexual hormone dysfunction, and degenerative joint disease pains, as well as improve self-image and employability (Sugerman, 2001) and decrease long-term mortality rate from cardiovascular disease (MacDonald et al, 1997). A review of more than 5000 patients from 12

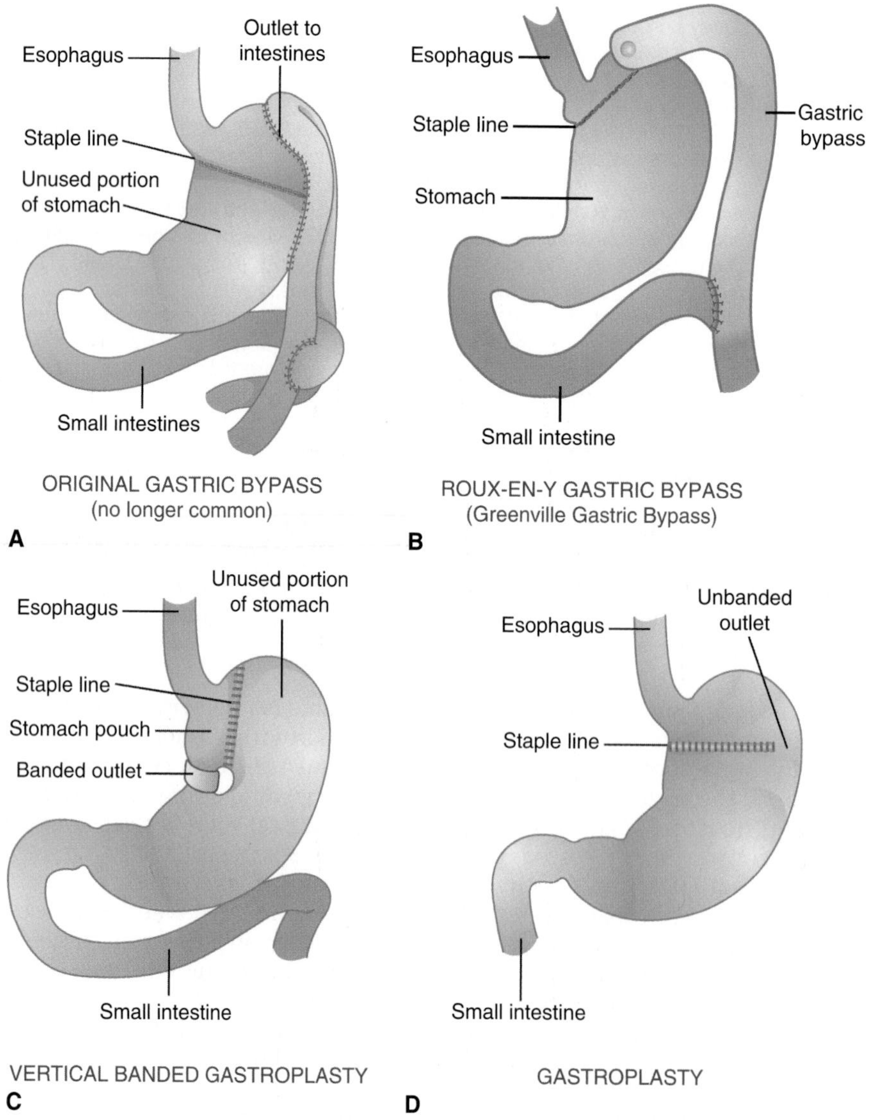

FIGURE 24-7 • Gastric surgeries for obesity.

centers showed a mortality rate after gastric restriction surgery one fourth that of morbidly obese patients and equivalent to that in normal-weight patients of the same age (Forse et al, 1989).

Jaw Wiring (Maxillomandibular Fixation)

Wiring the jaws closed restricts eating to liquids that can be taken through a straw. Dental attention before wiring as well as oral hygiene and nutritional care while the jaws are wired are important. Counseling should include recommendations for combinations of liquids and supplements that will provide adequate nutrients. The patient should also be taught how to cut the wires if necessary and how to deal with any episode of vomiting.

This technique has been effective in producing weight reduction; however, without education and ongoing support, body weight generally returns to pretreatment levels after the wires are removed. New behaviors need to be internalized, and a sense of control must be established to maintain weight loss.

Liposuction

Liposuction (or lipo-sculpture) involves aspiration of fat deposits by means of a 1- to 2-cm incision through which a tube is fanned out into the adipose tissue. The most successful operations are performed on younger persons with only small amounts of fat to be removed, where the elastic properties of the skin are able to allow tightening over the aspirated areas. It is not a weight-reduction technique but rather a cosmetic surgery because only 5 lb of fat can be removed at a time; not all cases provide the anticipated outcome. Deaths (Rao et al, 1999), severe infectious cellulitis (Vermeulen et al, 1999), and hemorrhage (Talmore and Barie, 1999) have been noted to occur with liposuction.

Maintenance of Reduced Body Weight

Prognosis for maintaining the status of the reduced-obese is typically reported as poor. Of those who do reduce weight, only 5% manage to keep from gaining weight by the end of 5 years (National Task Force on Prevention and Treatment of Obesity, 1994). This population may not represent all those who reduce weight because many do not present themselves to a medical program and are therefore not available for follow-up or inclusion in the statistics. The typical picture, however, is one of recidivism. Continued dieting, with repeated ups and downs, leads gradually to a net increase in body fat and thus to a health risk for hyperlipidemia, hypertension, and diabetes.

Energy requirements for weight maintenance after weight reduction appear to be 25% lower than at the original weight. The net effect is that reduced-obese persons are faced with the necessity of maintaining a reduced energy intake even after the desired weight has been lost. Whether this reduced intake must be maintained for an indefinite period is not known.

Lifestyle modification appears to be a key to weight maintenance. The National Weight Control Registry (NWCR), the largest study of individuals successful at long-term maintenance of weight loss, reported that long-term weight maintainers consume a diet with 24% of energy from fat, restrict total energy intake, and participate in regular physical activity (Klem et al, 1997). Permanent modification of lifestyle is required because obesity is a chronic disease, and its management requires continuous treatment (modification of unacceptable behaviors) as with other chronic diseases (e.g., insulin for diabetes or medication for hypertension). A shift from the medical model to empowerment of the individual (healthy living) encourages choice and positive expressions and self-awareness (Dalton, 1998).

Regular, planned physical activity has been a consistent factor in maintaining the reduced obese state over the long term. In a study of previously obese women, an average of 80 minutes per day of moderate activity or 35 minutes daily of vigorous activity added to a sedentary lifestyle was necessary to minimize weight gain for 1 year after weight loss (Schoeller et al, 1997).

Support groups are invaluable for the obese who are trying to lose weight and for reduced-obese persons who are maintaining a new lower weight. They help individuals facing similar problems to learn about ways to stay with their programs. Two large networks of self-help support groups are Overeaters Anonymous and Take Off Pounds Sensibly (TOPS). These groups are inexpensive, continuous, include a "buddy system," and encourage participation on a regular basis or as often as needed. The Weight Watchers program offers free lifelong maintenance classes for those who have reached and are maintaining their goal weights.

COMMON PROBLEMS ENCOUNTERED IN OBESITY MANAGEMENT

Plateau Effect

A common experience in weight-reduction programs is arrival at a weight plateau, when weight remains at the same level for a while. Eventually, weight loss halts completely. One theory is that interim plateaus reflect a reduction of lipid in individual adipocytes to some signal that demands metabolic adjustment and weight maintenance.

Any weight loss, whether fast or slow, results in a loss of the extra muscle that has developed to support the excess adipose tissue. Because this extra LBM has contributed to an increased metabolic rate, RMR decreases as LBM is lost. The fact that RMR decreases rapidly at the onset of a weight-reduction diet, by as much as 15% within 2 weeks, indicates that other adaptations to the lower weight as well as to the threat of deprivation are taking place.

Other factors join to decrease RMR and limit effectiveness of the restricted energy intake. A decrease in the total kilocalories ingested results in a decrease in TEF. Because a body that weighs less requires less energy expenditure to move around, the cost of physical activity is also less. A state of equilibrium is eventually reached at which the energy intake is equal to energy expenditure. Unless a change is made in either nutritional intake or physical activity, weight loss stops at this point.

Weight Cycling

Many obese people lose and gain weight several times over their lifetimes (i.e., the yo-yo effect). With each turn of the cycle, it takes longer to lose the same amount of weight and, conversely, less time to regain it. Reasons for this are unclear and may be metabolic or behavioral or both, that is, lower compliance with each try. The Framingham Study (Lissner et al, 1991) suggests that variability in weight contributes to health risks, but other studies have not shown the same results (Jeffrey et al, 1992; Wing, 1992). Moderate weight loss followed by weight gain does not increase visceral fat accumulation compared with body fatness before the loss. There is a slight tendency for accumulation of subcutaneous fat at the expense of visceral fat. Weight cycling takes its toll on the individual in many ways, including loss of money and damaged self-esteem.

WEIGHT MANAGEMENT IN CHILDREN

About 25% of children and adolescents 6 to 17 years of age are overweight or obese. Obese children are often the targets of discrimination. Childhood obesity increases the risk of obesity in adulthood. For the child who is obese after 6 years of age, the probability of obesity in adulthood exceeds 50% and the risks are significantly greater if either the mother or the father is obese (Whitaker et al, 1997). Obesity in adults that began in childhood tends to be more severe (Dietz, 1998b). New BMI tables for determining childhood obesity are available for use by health care practitioners. (See Appendixes 18 and 19).

Childhood obesity is linked to abnormalities in blood pressure, lipid, lipoprotein, and insulin levels in adults (Rocchini, 2002). In addition, the increasing incidence of type 2 diabetes in children parallels the increasing prevalence of obesity (Rocchini, 2002).

Children should not be put on "diets." The treatment goal for the child who is overweight should be weight maintenance or a slowing of the rate of weight gain. This gives the child time to "grow into" his or her weight. If the weight appropriate for the child's anticipated adult height has already been reached, then maintenance at that weight should be the lifetime goal (see *Clinical Insight:* Determining Appropriate Rate of Weight Gain in the Obese Child).

CLINICAL INSIGHT

Determining Appropriate Rate of Weight Gain in the Obese Child

From the history of family growth patterns and review of the prior growth pattern of the obese child, determine the predicted adult height of the child. He or she will probably maintain his or her present height growth channel. For example, an 8-year-old girl on the 75th percentile for height will probably maintain that growth channel and will achieve 67 in. as an adult height.

First, determine a rough estimation of the appropriate weight for the anticipated adult height. Using the Hamwi equation, for women the rule is 100 lb for the first 5 ft of height and an additional 5 lb for each inch in height over 5 ft. For men, it is 106 lb for the first 5 ft and an additional 6 lb for each inch over 5 ft. An appropriate range is 10% on either side of this weight. Then subtract the child's present weight from the calculated appropriate adult weight. The remainder is the number of pounds the child should gain throughout the rest of his or her growth period. This amount, divided by the number of years remaining of linear growth, is the appropriate yearly rate of weight gain for the child to achieve a normal adult weight. The number of years of growth remaining is based on the parental report of their own growth patterns and assessment of the present channel of height gain and the Tanner stage of adolescent development (see Chapter 11). In the case of the 8-year-old girl, if her mother reports reaching adult height at age 15, then probably her daughter will do the same. Thus, the daughter has 7 years of growth remaining.

Example: An 8-year-old girl who presently weighs 90 lb (over 95th percentile) and is 52 in. tall (75th to 90th percentile).

Eventual adult height = 67 in.

Appropriate weight for adult height = 100 lb + 35 lb = 135 lb (±13 lb)

Number of years of growth remaining = 15 years (age when the mother reached adult height) − 8 years (present age) = 7 years

(122-148 lb) − 90 lb (present weight) = 32 to 58 lb to be gained over next 7 years

Approximate rate of weight gain = 5 to 8 lb per year for the next 7 years

The child who already exceeds his or her optimal adult weight can safely experience a slow weight loss of 10 to 12 lb per year until the optimal adult weight is reached. Obviously, the child who needs to reduce weight is going to require more attention from family and health professionals and effort on his or her part. This attention should be directed to all the areas mentioned previously with family modification of eating habits and increased physical activity. The program should be long term over the entire growth period and perhaps longer (Mahan, 1987).

Increased physical activity is extremely important in a weight-management program for children. Inactivity usually coupled with excessive TV watching or sitting in front of a computer must be changed for the child to eventually reach the long-term weight goal. Studies have monitored the effects of television watching on children. Measurements of energy expenditure are lower during television watching than during rest in children 8 to 12 years of age, especially in obese children (Klesges et al, 1993). The conclusion that sedentary hobbies have a profound inclination toward obesity in children is significant for nutrition counselors and physicians who work with this population.

Expert recommendations for managing obesity in children and adolescents are found in *Clinical Insight:* Evaluation and Treatment of Childhood and Adolescent Obesity.

WEIGHT IMBALANCE: EXCESSIVE LEANNESS

Almost eclipsed by the attention focused on obesity is the effort of some people to gain weight. The term *underweight* is applicable to those who are 15% to 20% or more below accepted weight standards. Because underweight is often a symptom of disease, it should be assessed medically (Egbert, 1996). A low BMI is associated with greater mortality risk than that of normal individuals, especially with aging (Grabowski and Ellis, 2001). Undernutrition may lead to underfunction of the pituitary, thyroid, gonads, and adrenals. Other risk factors include loss of energy and susceptibility to injury and infection, as well as a distorted body image and other psychological problems.

Etiology

Underweight can be caused by (1) an intake insufficient in quantity to meet activity needs; (2) excessive activity, such as in the case of compulsive athletes in training; (3) poor absorption and utilization of the food consumed; (4) a wasting disease, such as cancer or hyperthyroidism, that increases the metabolic rate and energy needs; and (5) psychological or emotional stress.

CLINICAL INSIGHT

Evaluation and Treatment of Childhood and Adolescent Obesity

The Maternal and Child Health Bureau, Health Resources and Services Administration, and the Department of Health and Human Services convened a committee of pediatric obesity experts in 1997, which issued recommendations for identifying obese children, evaluating them medically, and treating them.

The Committee identified the following cutoff points for evaluation and possible treatment: children with a BMI greater than or equal to the 85th percentile with complications of obesity or with a BMI greater than or equal to the 95th percentile with or without complications. These children should be carefully assessed for any underlying syndromes (genetic, endocrinologic, or psychologic) or secondary complications such as hypertension, dyslipidemias, sleep apnea, and orthopedic problems. If the complications are found to cause serious morbidity and require rapid weight loss, referral to a pediatric obesity specialist is recommended. Otherwise, parent and child readiness to make changes should be evaluated along with a careful assessment of eating and activity patterns.

Once assessment is complete, treatment can begin. The primary goal of treatment is to achieve healthy eating and activity, not to achieve an ideal body weight. The group outlined the use of weight maintenance versus weight loss depending on the patient's age, baseline BMI percentile, and presence of medical complications. The following guidelines were issued: For children 7 years of age and younger, prolonged weight maintenance, which allows for a gradual decline in BMI as children grow in height, is an appropriate goal in the absence of any secondary complications of obesity; however, if secondary complications are present, children in this age group may benefit from weight loss if their BMI is at the 95th percentile or higher. For children older than 7 years, prolonged weight maintenance is appropriate if their BMI is between the 85th and 95th percentile and if they have no secondary complications. If a secondary complication is present, or if BMI is at the 95th percentile or above, weight loss (about 1 lb per month) is advised. Treatment recommendations call for family involvement, gradual changes in activity and eating patterns, and ongoing family support because obesity is chronic and may require lifelong attention.

Data from Barlow SE, Dietz WH: Obesity evaluation and treatment: expert committee recommendations, *Pediatrics* 102:3, 1998.

Assessment

Assessing the cause and extent of underweight before starting a treatment program is important. A thorough history and pertinent medical tests usually determine whether underlying disorders are causing the underweight. From anthropometric data such as arm muscle and fat areas, it is possible to determine whether health-endangering underweight really exists. Assessment of body fatness is useful, especially in dealing with the patient who has an eating disorder and needs to begin the body acceptance process (see Chapter 25). Biochemical measurements will indicate whether malnutrition accompanies the underweight.

Management

Any underlying cause of underweight must be dealt with as a first priority. A wasting disease or malabsorption requires treatment. Activity should be modified, and psychological counseling should be started if necessary. Nutritional support and dietary change are effective along with or after treatment of the underlying disorder or when the cause of the underweight is merely inappropriate or inadequate food intake.

High-Energy Diets for Weight Gain

A careful history before planning a dietary program may reveal inadequacies in dietary habits and nutritional intakes. Meals are advised to be at scheduled hours instead of hastily planned and quickly eaten. Because nervous tension often contributes to underweight in some individuals, mealtimes should be relaxed.

In addition to the kilocalories needed to meet total energy requirements, an allowance of 500 to 1000 extra kilocalories per day should be planned. Daily energy requirements can be calculated on the basis of the individual's present weight. If 2400 kcal is normally needed to maintain present weight, 2900 to 3400 kcal would be required to achieve weight gain. The intake should be increased gradually to these levels to avoid gastric discomfort and periods of discouragement and, more seriously, electrolyte imbalances and heart dysfunction. A 500-kcal step-up program is outlined in Table 24-6 and Figure 24-8.

The energy distribution of the diet should be about 30% of the kilocalories from fat, with the majority from monounsaturated or polyunsaturated sources and at least 12% to 15% of the kilocalories from protein. A basic vitamin and mineral supplement may be necessary, depending on nutritional status revealed by the initial assessment.

The underweight person frequently must be encouraged to eat, even when not hungry. The secret is to individualize the program with readily available foods that the individual really enjoys and with a plan for regular eating times throughout the day. In addition to larger meals, snacks are usually necessary to adequately increase the energy intake. Often a liquid supplement taken with meals or between meals is effective because it is easy to prepare and consume. This is important when it is necessary to overcome a lack of interest in food and eating.

TABLE 24-6 Suggestions for Increasing Energy Intake

ADDITIONAL FOODS	kcal	PROTEIN (G)
Plus 500 kcal (Served Between Meals)		
1. 1 cup (c) dry cereal	110	2
1 banana	80	
1 c whole milk	159	8
1 slice toast	60	2
1 T peanut butter	86	4
	495	16
2. 8 saltine crackers	99	3
1 oz cheese	113	7
1 c ice cream	290	6
	502	16
3. 6 graham cracker squares	165	3
2 T peanut butter	172	8
1 c orange juice	122	
2 T raisins	52	
	511	11
Plus 1000 kcal (Served Between Meals)		
1. 8 oz fruit flavored yogurt	240	9
1 slice bread	60	2
2 oz cheese	226	14
1 apple	87	
¼ of 14-inch cheese pizza	306	16
1 small banana	81	1
	1000	42
2. Instant Breakfast with whole milk	280	15
1 c cottage cheese	239	31
½ c pineapple	95	
1 c apple juice	117	
6 graham cracker squares	165	3
1 pear	100	1
	996	50
Plus 1500 kcal (Served Between Meals)		
1. 2 slices bread	120	4
2 T peanut butter	172	8
1 T jam	110	
4 graham cracker squares	110	2
8 oz fruit-flavored yogurt	240	9
¾ c roasted peanuts	628	28
1 c apricot nectar	143	1
	1523	52
2. 1 baked custard	285	13
Instant Breakfast with whole milk	280	15
1 c dry cereal	110	2
1 banana	80	
1 c whole milk	159	8
1 c orange juice	122	
4 T raisins	104	
1 bagel	165	6
2 T cream cheese	99	2
2 T jam	110	
	1514	46

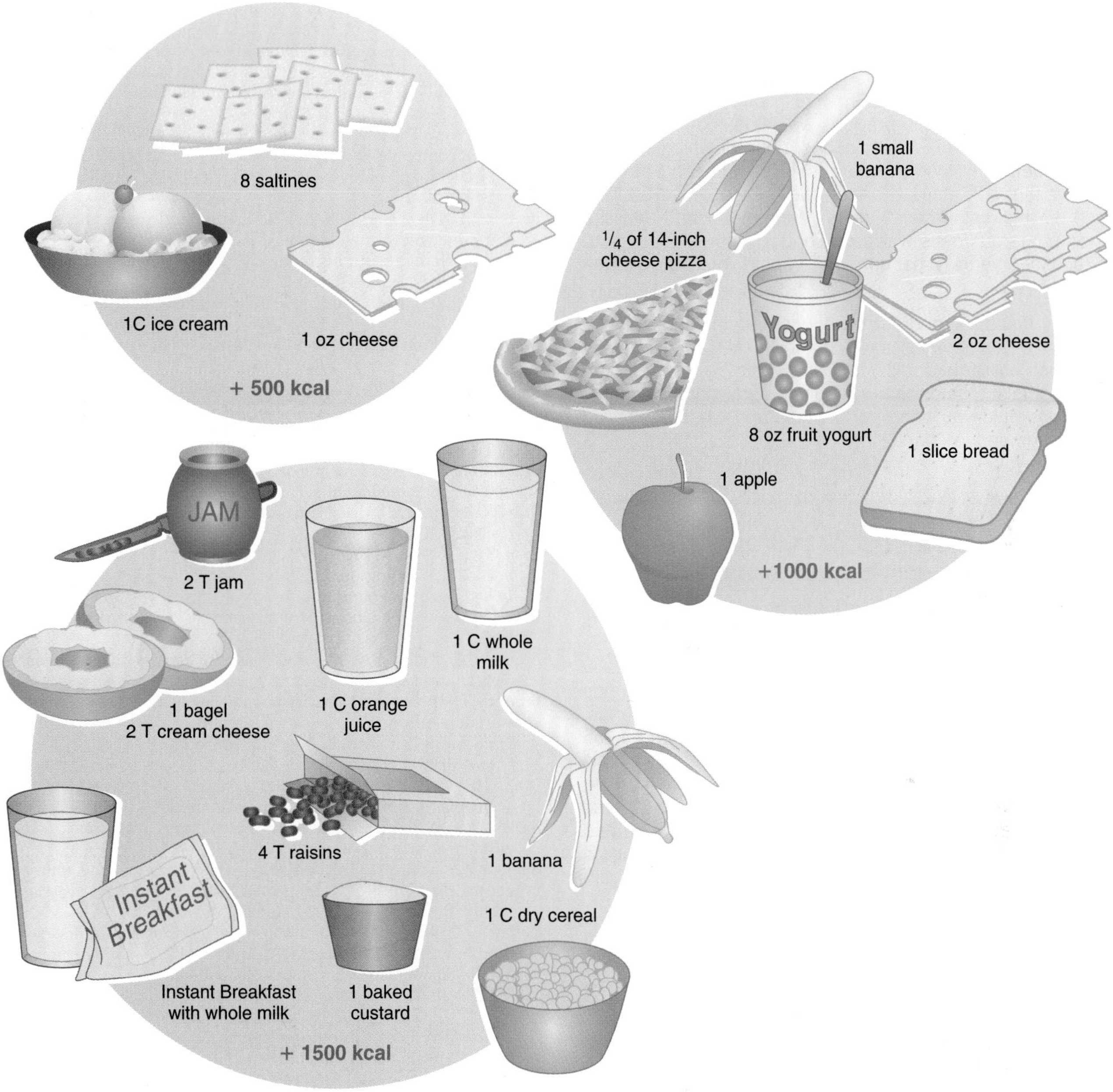

FIGURE 24-8 • Each circle illustrates the total amount of food that can be added to the diet to increase the intake by either 500 kcal, 1000 kcal, or 1500 kcal.

■ Relevant Web Sites

American Obesity Association
www.obesity.org
Centers for Disease Control (CDC)
www.cdc.gov
Council on Size and Weight Discrimination
www.cswd.org
Food and Drug Administration
www.fda.gov
International Obesity Task Force
www.iotf.org/
National Institutes of Health, National Institute of Diabetes and Digestive and Kidney Disease:
Weight Control Network
www.niddk.nih.gov/health/nutrit/nutrit.htm
National Heart, Lung, and Blood Institute and the North American Association for the Study of Obesity's *The Practical Guide: Identification, Evaluation, and Treatment of Overweight and Obesity in Adults*
www.nhlbi.nih.gov/guidelines/obesity/ob_home.htm
www.nhlbi.nih.gov/guidelines/obesity/practgdc.htm
ShapeUp America
www.shapeup.org/
Weight Watchers
www.weightwatchers.com/

Clinical Scenario 1: Weight Loss

Maria is a 45-year-old white woman who has tried numerous weight-loss programs. She has followed strict diets and has never exercised in previous weight-loss attempts. She takes several cardiac medications, none of which she can remember. Her blood pressure is 160/90, she is 5 ft 4 in., and weighs 195 lb. Her lowest body weight was 130 lb at age 30, maintained for 2 years. Maria mentioned that she tried numerous diets while a teenager, when she weighed 170 lb for 3 years. What guidelines would you offer to Maria at this time?

1. How would you address the concern about medications?
2. What types of exercise would you be likely to discuss?
3. Which nutrients would you discuss with Maria, for example, total fat, saturated fat, sodium, potassium, calcium?
4. How would you bring up exercise and what would you recommend for Maria?
5. What would be the goals of her treatment?

Clinical Scenario 2: Weight Gain

Jim, a 26-year-old man, has had trouble maintaining his weight. He is physically active, cycling three times each week for at least an hour each time. He also strength-trains twice each week. He is 5 ft 9 in. tall and weighs 134 pounds. He states that he feels best when his weight is between 155 and 160 pounds. Jim works as a hairdresser and is on his feet all day. On busy days, he cannot take a full lunch break, so he often skips lunch. At least once each week, he works late, and when he gets home, he is too tired to make and eat dinner. He does have 5 to 10 minutes between some appointments. He is willing to do what he can to gain weight. He does not have any medical problems.

1. What seems to be the major problem with Jim's eating patterns?
2. How would you help him structure an eating plan?
3. What are the goals of his treatment?

Cited References

Abenhaim L et al: Appetite-suppressant drugs and the risk of primary pulmonary hypertension, *N Engl J Med* 335:609, 1996.

American Dietetic Association: Position of the American Dietetic Association: weight management, *J Am Diet Assoc* 101:1145, 2002.

Andersen RE et al: Relation of weight loss to changes in serum lipids and lipoproteins in obese women, *Am J Clin Nutr* 62:350, 1995.

Anderson JW, Konz EC: Obesity and disease management: effects of weight loss on comorbid conditions, *Obes Res* 9(suppl 4): 326S, 2001.

Anderson JW et al: Long-term weight-loss maintenance: a meta-analysis of US studies, *Am J Clin Nutr* 74:579, 2001.

Anderson RA, Kozlovsky AS: Chromium intake, absorption, and excretion of subjects consuming self-selected diets, *Am J Clin Nutr* 41:1177, 1985.

Anderson RA et al: Exercise effects on chromium excretion of trained and untrained men consuming a constant diet, *J Appl Physiol* 64:249, 1988.

Angulo P: Nonalcoholic fatty liver disease, *N Engl J Med* 346:1221, 2002.

Aronne L: Modern medical management of obesity: the role of pharmaceutical management, *J Am Diet Assoc* 98:23, 1998.

Astrup A et al: Meta-analysis of resting metabolic rate in formerly obese subjects, *Am J Clin Nutr* 69:1117, 1999.

Astrup A et al: The effect and safety of an ephedrine/caffeine compound compared with ephedrine, caffeine and placebo in obese subjects on an energy restricted diet: a double blind trial, *Int J Obes* 16:269, 1992.

Barlow SE, Dietz WH: Obesity evaluation and treatment: expert committee recommendations, *Pediatrics* 102:3, 1998.

Batterham RL et al: Gut hormone PYY_{3-36} physiologically inhibits food intake, *Nature* 418:650, 2002.

Berg F: Sudden death syndrome continues to chill treatment centers, *Healthy Weight J* 8(3):51, 1994.

Bjorntorp P: Physiological and clinical aspects of exercise in obese persons, *Exerc Sport Sci Rev* 11:159, 1983.

Blackburn GL: *Weight management.* Presentation at the American Dietetic Association Annual Meeting, 1988, San Francisco.

Blair SN: Evidence for success of exercise in weight loss and control, *Ann Intern Med* 119(7 pt 2):702, 1993.

Blundell JE et al: Mechanisms of appetite control and their abnormalities in obese patients, *Horm Res* 39(suppl 3):72, 1993.

Bray GA: Obesity: a disease of nutrient or energy balance? *Nutr Rev* 45:33, 1987.

Bray GA: Obesity. In Brown ML, editor: *Present knowledge in nutrition,* ed 6, Washington, DC: International Life Sciences Institute, 1990, Nutrition Foundation.

Bray GA, Gray DS: Obesity. I. Pathogenesis, *West J Med* 149:429, 1988.

Brehm BA, Keller BA: Diet and exercise factors that influence weight and fat loss, *Idea Today* October:33, 1990.

Breum L et al: Comparison of an ephedrine/caffeine combination and dexfenfluramine in the treatment of obesity: a double-blind multi-centre trial in general practice, *Int J Obes Rel Metab Disord* 18:99, 1994.

Brolin RE et al: Weight loss and dietary intake after vertical banded gastroplasty and Roux-en-Y bypass, *Ann Surg* 220:782, 1994.

Brownell K, Wadden T: Matching weight control programs to individuals: how to find the best fit, *Weight Control Dig* 1(5):65, 1991.

Buckmaster L, Brownell KD: Behavior modification: the state of the art. In Frankle RT, Yang M-U, editors: *Obesity and weight control,* Rockville, Md, 1988, Aspen Publishers.

Callaway CW: Biologic adaptations to starvation and semistarvation. In Frankle RT, Yang M-U, editors: *Obesity and weight control,* Rockville, Md, 1988, Aspen Publishers.

Calle EE et al: Body-mass index and mortality in a prospective cohort of U.S. adults, *N Engl J Med* 341:1097, 1999.

Campbell WW et al: Chromium picolinate supplementation and resistive training by older men: effects on iron-status and hematologic indexes, *Am J Clin Nutr* 66:944, 1997.

Carpenter WH et al: Influence of body composition and resting metabolic rate on variation in total energy expenditure: a meta-analysis, *Am J Clin Nutr* 61:4, 1995.

Choban PS et al: Obesity treatment: the role of surgery, *Medical Update for Psychiatrists* 1:21, 1996.

Clancy SP et al: Effects of chromium picolinate supplementation on body composition, strength and urinary chromium loss in football players, *Int J Sports Nutr* 4:142, 1994.

Clement K et al: Genetic variation in the β3-adrenergic receptor and an increased capacity to gain weight in patients with morbid obesity, *N Engl J Med* 333:352, 1995.

Connolly H et al: Valvular heart disease associated with fenfluramine-phentermine, *N Engl J Med* 337:581, 1997.

Consensus Development Conference Panel: Gastrointestinal surgery for severe obesity: consensus development conference statement, *Ann Intern Med* 115:956, 1991.

Considine RV et al: Serum immunoreactive-leptin concentrations in normal-weight and obese humans, *N Engl J Med* 334:292, 1996.

Cummings DE et al: Plasma ghrelin levels after diet-induced weight loss or gastric bypass surgery, *N Engl J Med* 346(21): 1662, 2002.

Dalton S: The dietitians' philosophy and practice in multidisciplinary weight management, *J Am Diet Assoc* 98:49, 1998.
Daly PA et al: Ephedrine, caffeine and aspirin: safety and efficacy for treatment of human obesity, *Int J Obes Relat Metab Disord* 17(suppl 1):S73, 1993.
Datillo A: Dietary fat and its relationship to body weight? *Nutr Today* 27(1):13, 1992.
de Jonge L, Bray GA: The thermic effect of food and obesity: a critical review, *Obes Res* 5:622, 1997.
Dietz WH: Childhood weight affects adult morbidity and mortality, *J Nutr* 128(25):411, 1998a.
Dietz WH: Childhood obesity: the contribution of diet and inactivity, Childhood Obesity: Causes & Prevention. Symposium Proceedings, October 27, 1998b. Washington, DC, Center for Nutrition Policy and Promotion, U.S. Department of Agriculture.
Drewnowski A et al: Taste responses and preferences for sweet high-fat foods: evidence for opioid involvement, *Phys Behav* 51:371, 1992.
Eberhardt MS et al: *Urban and rural health chartbook:* health, United States, 2001, Hyattsville, Md, 2001, NCHS.
Egbert A: The dwindles: failure to thrive in older patients, *Nutr Rev* 54(1):S25, 1996.
Enzi G: The socioeconomic consequences of obesity: the effect of obesity on the individual, *Pharm Econ* 5(suppl 1):54, 1994.
Feldman W et al: Culture vs. biology: children's attitudes toward thinness and fatness, *Pediatrics* 81:190, 1988.
Flechtner-Mors M et al: Metabolic and weight loss effects of long-term dietary intervention in obese patients: four-year results, *Obes Res* 8:399, 2000.
Flegal KM et al: The influence of smoking cessation on the prevalence of overweight in the United States, *N Engl J Med* 333:1165, 1995.
Flier JS, Maratos-Flier E: Obesity and the hypothalamus: novel peptides for new pathways, *Cell* 92:437, 1998.
Forbes GB: Lean body mass-body fat interrelationships in humans, *Nutr Rev* 45:225, 1987.
Ford ES et al: Prevalence of the metabolic syndrome among U.S. adults: findings from the third National Health and Nutrition Examination Survey, *JAMA* 287:356, 2002.
Foreyt JP, Poston WSC II: Diet, genetics, and obesity, *Food Technol* 51:70, 1997.
Forse A et al: Morbid obesity: weighing the treatment options—surgical options, *Nutr Today* 24(5):10, 1989.
Foster GD et al: What is a reasonable weight loss? Patients' expectations and evaluations of obesity treatment outcomes, *J Consult Clin Psychol* 65:79, 1997.
Freedman M et al: Popular diets: a scientific review, *Obes Res* 9(suppl 1):1S, 2001.
Gallagher D et al: Healthy percentage body fat ranges: an approach for developing guidelines based on body mass index, *Am J Clin Nutr* 72:694, 2000.
Gladwell M: The Pima paradox, *The New Yorker,* Feb 2:44, 1998.
Goldstein DJ: Beneficial health effects of modest weight loss, *Int J Obes* 16:397, 1992.
Goran M: Obesity and health risk in children. Childhood Obesity: Causes and Prevention. Symposium Proceedings, October 27, 1998. Washington, DC, Center for Nutrition Policy and Promotion, U.S. Department of Agriculture.
Grabowski DC, Ellis JE: High body mass index does not predict mortality in older people: analysis of the Longitudinal Study of Aging, *J Am Geriatr Soc* 49:968, 2001.
Gross WC, Daynard MD, editors: Commercial weight loss products and programs: what consumers stand to gain and lose. Report of the Presiding Panel, Federal Trade Commission, 1977, Washington, DC.
Guerciolini R: Mode of action of orlistat, *Int J Obes* 21(suppl 3):S12, 1997.
Guerciolini R et al: Comparative evaluation of fecal fat excretion induced by orlistat and chitosan, *Obes Res* 9:364, 2001.
Healthy People 2010: Nutrition and Overweight. www.health.gov/healthypeople/Document/HTML/Volume2/19Nutrition.htm.
Hellerstein MK: No common energy currency: de novo lipogenesis as the road less traveled, *Am J Clin Nutr* 74:707, 2001.
Hellerstein MK et al: Effects of cigarette smoking and its cessation on lipid metabolism and energy expenditure in heavy smokers, *J Clin Invest* 93:265, 1994.
Hill JO: Monitoring tools in the new millennium: technology solutions for weight management, *Obes Res* 9(suppl 5):359S, 2000.
Hill JO, Wyatt HR: Relapse in obesity treatment: biology or behavior? *Am J Clin Nutr* 69:1064, 1999.
Hill JO et al: Effects of exercise and food restriction on body composition and metabolic rate in obese women, *Am J Clin Nutr* 46:622, 1987.
Hirsch J: Role and benefits of carbohydrate in the diet: key issues for future dietary guidelines, *Am J Clin Nutr* 61:996S, 1995.
Holli BB: Using behavior modification in nutrition counseling, *J Am Diet Assoc* 88:1530, 1988.
Horton T, Geissler C: Effect of habitual exercise on daily energy expenditure and metabolic rate during standardized activity, *Am J Clin Nutr* 59:13, 1994.
Institute of Medicine, Food and Nutrition Board: *Dietary reference intakes for energy, carbohydrate, fiber, fat, fatty acids, cholesterol, protein, and amino acids,* Washington, DC, 2002, National Academy Press.
Isner JM et al: Sudden, unexpected death in avid dieters using the liquid-protein-modified-fast diet, *Circulation* 60:1401, 1979.
James WPT et al: A one-year trial to assess the value of orlistat in the management of obesity, *Int J Obes* 21(suppl 3):S24, 1997.
Janke J et al: Resistin gene expression in human adipocytes is not related to insulin resistance, *Obes Res* 10:1, 2002.
Jeffery R et al: Weight cycling and cardiovascular risk factors in obese men and women, *Am J Clin Nutr* 55:641, 1992.
Jensen MD: Research techniques for body composition assessment, *J Am Diet Assoc* 92:454, 1992.
Jick H et al: A population-based study of appetite-suppressant drugs and the risk of cardiac valve regurgitation, *N Engl J Med* 339:719, 1998.
Kant AK: Consumption of energy-dense, nutrient-poor foods by adult Americans: nutritional and health implications: the third National Health and Nutrition Examination Survey, 1988-1994, *Am J Clin Nutr* 72:929, 2000.
Katzeff HL et al: Metabolic studies in human obesity during overnutrition and undernutrition: thermogenic and hormonal responses to norepinephrine, *Metabolism* 35:166, 1986.
Keim NL et al: Relation between circulating leptin concentrations and appetite during a prolonged, moderate energy deficit in women, *Am J Clin Nutr* 68:794, 1998.
Keys A: *The biology of human starvation,* Minneapolis, 1950, University of Minnesota Press.
Khan MA et al: The prevalence of cardiac valvular insufficiency assessed by transthoracic echocardiography in obese patients treated with appetite-suppressant drugs, *N Engl J Med* 339:713, 1998.
Kitzinger C, Willmott J: "The thief of womanhood": women's experience of polycystic ovarian syndrome, *Soc Sci Med* 54(3):349, 2002.
Klem ML et al: A descriptive study of individuals successful at long-term maintenance of substantial weight loss, *Am J Clin Nutr* 66:239, 1997.
Klesges R et al: Effects of television on metabolic rate: potential implications for childhood obesity, *Pediatrics* 91:281, 1993.
Lane MA et al: Beyond the rodent model: calorie restriction in rhesus monkeys, *Age Aging* 20:45, 1997.
Langseth L, editor: Body weight: editorial condemns new weight guidelines, *Nutr Res Newsletter* X(6):63, 1991.
Lean MEJ: Sibutramine—a review of clinical efficacy, *Int J Obes* 21(suppl 1):S30, 1997.
Legro RS: Polycystic ovary syndrome; the new millennium, *Mol Cell Endocrinol* 186(2):219, 2002.
Leibel RL et al: Changes in energy expenditure resulting from altered body weight, *N Engl J Med* 332:621, 1995.
Lew EA, Garfinkle L: Variations in mortality by weight among 750,000 men and women, *J Chronic Dis* 32:563, 1979.
Ley CJ et al: Sex- and menopause-associated changes in body-fat distribution, *Am J Clin Nutr* 55:950, 1992.
Lichtman SW et al: Discrepancy between self-reported and actual caloric intake and exercise in obese subjects, *N Engl J Med* 327(27):1893, 1992.

Lissner L et al: Variability of body weight and health outcomes in the Framingham population, *N Engl J Med* 324:1839, 1991.

Lukaski HC et al: Chromium supplementation and resistance training: effects on body composition, strength, and trace element status of men, *Am J Clin Nutr* 63:954, 1996.

MacDonald KG et al: The gastric bypass operation reduces the progression and mortality of non-insulin-dependent diabetes mellitus, *J Gastrointest Surg* 1:213, 1997.

Mahan LK: Family-focused behavioral approach to weight control in children, *Pediatr Clin North Am* 34:983, 1987.

Manson JE et al: Body weight and mortality among women, *N Engl J Med* 333:677, 1995.

Marshall JA et al: Percent body fat and lean mass explain the gender difference in leptin: analysis and interpretation of leptin in Hispanic and Non-Hispanic white adults, *Obes Res* 8:543, 2000.

Mason EE, Ito C: Gastric bypass, *Ann Surg* 170:329, 1969.

Masoro E: Energy intake and the aging process: clues from the laboratory, *Nutr MD* 20:1, 1994.

Matsuzawa Y et al: Pathophysiology and pathogenesis of visceral fat obesity, *Diabetes Res Clin Pract* 24(suppl):S111, 1994.

McArdle WD et al: *Sports and exercise nutrition,* Philadelphia, 1999, Lippincott Williams & Wilkins.

McDevitt RM et al: De novo lipogenesis during controlled overfeeding with sucrose or glucose in lean and obese women, *Am J Clin Nutr* 74:737, 2001.

McKittrick M: Case problem: dietary recommendations to combat obesity, insulin resistance, and other concerns related to polycystic ovary syndrome [Response], *J Am Diet Assoc* 100:958, 2000.

Miller W: Exercise: Americans don't think it's worth it! *Obes Health* 8(2):29, 1994.

Mokdad AH et al: The continuing epidemics of obesity and diabetes in the United States, *JAMA* 286:1195, 2001.

Morbidity and Mortality Weekly Report: Physical activity trends—United States, 1990-1998, *MMWR* 50(9):166, 2001.

Morley JE et al: Effects of peripheral hormones on memory and ingestive behaviors, *Psychoneuroendocrinology* 17:391, 1992.

National Center for Health Statistics: Prevalence of overweight and obesity among adults: United States, 1999, www.cdc.gov/nchs/products/pubs/pubd/hestats/obese/obse99.htm.

National Institutes of Health, National Heart, Lung, and Blood Institute: *Clinical guidelines on the identification, evaluation, and treatment of overweight and obesity in adults—the evidence report,* NIH Publication No. 98-4083, 1998.

National Institutes of Health, National Heart, Lung, and Blood Institute, North American Association for the Study of Obesity: The practical guide: identification, evaluation, and treatment of overweight and obesity in adults, NIH Publication No. 00-4084, October 2000.

National Institutes of Health, National Task Force on Prevention and Treatment of Obesity: very low calorie diets, *JAMA* 270: 967, 1993.

National Task Force on Prevention and Treatment of Obesity: towards prevention of obesity, research directions, *Obes Res* 2:571, 1994.

NIH Technology Assessment Conference Panel: Methods for voluntary weight loss and control, *Ann Intern Med* 116:942, 1992.

Pérusse L et al: The human obesity gene map: the 2000 update, *Obes Res* 9:135, 2001.

Pfizer Food Science Group: Americans are getting the message on fat, *Food Forum* 4(4):2, 1994.

Pierson RN Jr et al: Body composition and metabolic rate. In: Dalton S, editor: *Overweight and weight management,* Gaithersburg, Md, 1997, Aspen Publishers.

Pi-Sunyer FX: Medical hazards of obesity, *Ann Intern Med* 119:655, 1993.

Pi-Sunyer FX et al: Obesity. In Shils ME et al, editors: *Modern nutrition in health and disease,* Philadelphia, 1994, Lea & Febiger.

Pories WJ et al: Who would have thought it? An operation proves to be the most effective therapy for adult-onset diabetes mellitus, *Ann Surg* 222:339, 1995.

Prentice AM: Overeating: the health risks, *Obes Res* 9(suppl 4): 234S, 2001.

Rao RB et al: Deaths related to liposuction, *N Engl J Med* 340:1471, 1999.

Ravussin E, Swinburn BA: Effect of caloric restriction and weight loss on energy expenditure. In Wadden TA, Van Itallie TB, editors: *Treatment of the seriously obese patient,* New York, 1992, Guilford Press.

Reaven GM: Role of insulin resistance in human disease, *Diabetes* 37:1595, 1988.

Reseland JE et al: Effect of long-term changes in diet and exercise on plasma leptin concentrations, *Am J Clin Nutr* 77:240, 2001.

Richard D: Involvement of corticotropin-releasing factor in the control of food intake and energy, *Ann N Y Acad Sci* 575:155, 1989.

Rippe J et al: Obesity as a chronic disease: modern medical and lifestyle management, *J Am Diet Assoc* 98:9, 1998.

Roberts S et al: Control of food intake in older men, *JAMA* 272:1601, 1994.

Rocchini AP: Childhood obesity and a diabetes epidemic, *N Engl J Med* 346:854, 2002.

Rolland-Cachera M-F, Bellisle F: Letter to the Editor, *Lancet* 335:918, 1990.

Rolland-Cachera M-F et al: Adiposity rebound in children: a simple indicator for predicting obesity, *Am J Clin Nutr* 39:129, 1984.

Rolls BJ, Drewnowski A: Diet and nutrition, *Encyclopedia Gerontol* 1:429, 1996.

Romon M et al: Circadian variation of diet-induced thermogenesis, *Am J Clin Nutr* 57:476, 1993.

Rosencrans K: Does the body defend weight at a set-point? *Healthy Weight J* 8(3):47, 1994.

Rubenstein RB: Laparoscopic adjustable gastric banding at a U.S. center with up to 3-year follow-up, *Obes Surg* 12:380, 2002.

Scalzo K: Case problem: dietary recommendations to combat obesity, insulin resistance, and other concerns related to polycystic ovary syndrome [Response], *J Am Diet Assoc* 1000:957, 2000.

Schlundt D et al: Randomized evaluation of a low fat ad libitum carbohydrate diet for weight reduction, *Int J Obes Relat Metab Disord* 17:623, 1993.

Schoeller DA et al: How much physical activity is needed to minimize weight gain in previously obese women? *Am J Clin Nutr* 66:551, 1997.

Schwartz MW, Morton GJ: Keeping hunger at bay, *Nature* 418:595, 2002.

Shape Up America! and American Obesity Association: *Guidance for treatment of adult obesity,* Bethesda, Md, 2001, Shape Up America! and American Obesity Association.

Shuldiner AR, Sabra M: TRp64Arg β3-adrenoceptor: when does a candidate gene become a disease-susceptibility gene? *Obes Res* 9:806, 2001.

Sims EA: Are there persons who are obese, but metabolically healthy? *Metabolism* 50:1499, 2001.

Smith U: Resistin-resistant to defining its role, *Obes Res* 10:61, 2002.

Stallone D: The influence of obesity and its treatment on the immune system, *Nutr Rev* 52(2 pt 1):37, 1994.

Stunkard AJ: Current views on obesity, *Am J Med* 100:230, 1996.

Sugerman HJ: Bariatric surgery for severe obesity, *J Assoc Acad Minor Phys* 12:129, 2001.

Suter P et al: The effect of ethanol on fat storage in healthy subject, *N Engl J Med* 326:983, 1992.

Talmore M, Barie, PS: Deaths related to liposuction [Letter to the Editor], *N Engl J Med* 341:1001, 1999.

Tate DF et al: Using Internet technology to deliver a behavioral weight loss program, *JAMA* 285:1172, 2001.

Tyler VE: *The honest herbal.* New York, 1993, Pharmaceutical Products Press.

U.S. Department of Health and Human Services: *The health benefits of smoking cessation: a report of the Surgeon General, 1990,* Washington, DC, 1990, U.S. Government Printing Office.

U.S. Department of Health and Human Services: *The Surgeon General's call to action to prevent and decrease overweight and obesity.* Rockville, Md, 2001, U.S. Department of Health and Human Services, Public Health Service, Office of the Surgeon General.

Van Dale D et al: Does exercise give an additional effect in weight reduction regimens? *Int J Obes* 11:367, 1987.

Van Horn L et al: The dietitian's role in developing and implementing the first federal obesity guidelines, *J Am Diet Assoc* 98:1115, 1998.

Van Itallie TB, Yang M: Cardiac dysfunction in obese dieters: a potentially lethal complication of rapid, massive weight loss, *Am J Clin Nutr* 39:695, 1984.
Vasselli JR, Maggio CA: Mechanisms of appetite and body-weight regulation. In Frankle RT, Yang M, editors: *Obesity and weight control,* Rockville, Md, 1988, Aspen Publishers.
Vermeulen C et al: Deaths related to liposuction [Letter to the Editor], *N Engl J Med* 341:1000, 1999.
Wadden T: Treatment of obesity by moderate and severe caloric restriction: results of clinical research trial, *Ann Intern Med* 119:688, 1993.
Wadden T, Sarwer DB: Behavioral treatment of obesity: new approaches to an old disorder. In Goldstein D, editor: *The management of eating disorders,* Totowa, NJ, 1998, Humana Press.
Wagner DR, Heyward VH: Measures of body composition in blacks and whites: a comparative review, *Am J Clin Nutr* 71:1392, 2000.
Weinsier RL et al: Do adaptive changes in metabolic rate favor weight regain in weight-reduced individuals? An examination of the set-point theory, *Am J Clin Nutr* 72:1088, 2000.
Weissman NJ et al: An assessment of heart valve abnormalities in obese patients taking dexfenfluramine, sustained-release dexfenfluramine, or placebo, *N Engl J Med* 339:725, 1998.
Whitaker RC et al: Predicting obesity in young adulthood from childhood and parental obesity, *N Engl J Med* 337:869, 1997.
Williams PT: Evidence for the incompatibility of age-neutral overweight and age-neutral physical activity standards from runners, *Am J Clin Nutr* 65:1391, 1997.
Wing R: Weight cycling in humans: a review of the literature, *Ann Behav Med* 14:113, 1992.
Wing RR, Greeno GC: Behavioural and psychosocial aspects of obesity and its treatment, *Baillieres Clin Endocrinol Metab* 8:689, 1994.
Wing RR et al: Long-term effects of modest weight loss in type II diabetic patients, *Arch Intern Med* 147:1749, 1987.
Wolf AM, Colditz GA: Current estimates of the economic cost of obesity in the United States, *Obes Res* 6:97, 1998.
Young LR, Nestle M: The contribution of expanding portion sizes to the US obesity epidemic, *Am J Public Health* 92:246, 2002.

Additional References

Abdallah L: Cephalic phase responses to sweet taste, *Am J Clin Nutr* 65:737, 1997.
Abu Sabha R, Achterberg C: Review of self-efficacy and locus of control for nutrition and health-related behavior, *J Am Diet Assoc* 97:1122, 1997.
Bouchard C et al: The response to long-term overfeeding in identical twins, *N Engl J Med* 322:1477, 1990.
Bray GA, Gray DS: Obesity. II. Treatment, *West J Med* 149:555, 1988b.
Dulloo A et al: Poststarvation hyperphagia and body fat overshooting in humans: a role for feedback signals from lean and fat tissues, *Am J Clin Nutr* 65:717, 1997.
Loube D et al: Continuous positive airway pressure treatment results in weight loss in obese and overweight patients and obstructive sleep apnea, *J Am Diet Assoc* 97:896, 1997.
Naslund E et al: Reduced food intake after jejunoileal bypass: a possible association with prolonged gastric emptying and altered gut hormone patterns, *Am J Clin Nutr* 66:26, 1997.
National Institutes of Health: First federal obesity clinical guidelines released. Press release. June 17, 1998, www.nhlbi.nih.gov/nhlbi/news/obere14f.htm.
National Task Force on the Prevention and Treatment of Obesity: Long term pharmacotherapy in the management of obesity [Review], *JAMA* 276:1907, 1996.
Pekkarinen T, Mustajoki P: Comparison of behavior therapy with and without very-low-energy diet in the treatment of morbid obesity, *Arch Intern Med* 157:1581, 1997.
Ronnemaa T et al: Relation between plasma leptin levels and measures of body fat in identical twins discordant for obesity, *Ann Intern Med* 126:26, 1997.
St Jeor S: New trends in weight management, *J Am Diet Assoc* 97:1096, 1997.
St Jeor S et al: A classification system to evaluate weight maintainers, gainers and losers, *J Am Diet Assoc* 97:481, 1997.

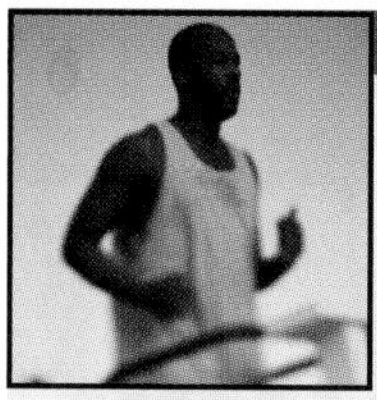

CHAPTER 25

Nutrition in Eating Disorders

JANET E. SCHEBENDACH, MA, RD
PAMELA REICHERT-ANDERSON, MA, RD

CHAPTER OUTLINE

- Diagnostic Criteria
- Etiology
- Pathophysiology
- Nutritional Assessment
- Psychological Management
- Nutritional Care
- Nutrition Education
- Prognosis

KEY TERMS

amenorrhea–absence of three consecutive menstrual periods when otherwise expected to occur

anorexia nervosa (AN)–a disease characterized by (1) refusal to maintain a minimally normal body weight, (2) intense fear of gaining weight, (3) body image distortion, and (4) amenorrhea in postmenarcheal females; it may be one of two subtypes: restricting or binge eating/purging

binge–an episode of eating marked by three particular features: (1) the amount of food eaten is larger than most persons would eat under similar circumstances; (2) the excessive eating occurs in a discrete period, usually less than 2 hours; and (3) the eating is accompanied by a subjective sense of loss of control

binge eating disorder (BED)–a disorder characterized by the occurrence of binge eating episodes at least twice a week for a 6-month period

body image distortion–a significant disturbance in the perception of body shape or size

bulimia nervosa (BN)–an illness characterized by repeated episodes of binge eating followed by inappropriate compensatory methods such as purging, including self-induced vomiting or misuse of laxatives, diuretics, or enemas, or nonpurging, including fasting or engaging in excessive exercise

Diagnostic and Statistical Manual of Mental Disorders (DSM)–a manual published by the American Psychiatric Association that establishes diagnostic criteria for anorexia nervosa, bulimia nervosa, eating disorder not otherwise specified, and binge eating disorder

Eating disorder not otherwise specified (EDNOS)–a diagnostic category for eating disorders that fail to meet full criteria for either anorexia nervosa or bulimia nervosa

hypercarotenemia–an elevation of serum carotene, frequently encountered in patients with eating disorders; most likely attributable to an acquired defect in carotene metabolism, secondary to semistarvation

low T3 syndrome–a low metabolic state characteristic of AN, in which thyroid hormone production tends to be normal but the peripheral deiodination of thyroxin favors formation of the less metabolically active reduced triiodothyronine (rT3) rather than T3; resolves with refeeding

marasmus–a starvation state characterized by maintenance of the circulatory pool of visceral proteins at the expense of somatic protein stores

purging–methods intended to reverse the effects of binge eating; self-induced vomiting is the most common purging method, but additional methods include laxative, enema, and diuretic abuse

Anorexia nervosa (AN) and bulimia nervosa (BN) are eating disorders that affect primarily adolescents and young adult women. Weight preoccupation is a primary symptom in both disorders. At the end of the seventeenth century, Morton described a condition that would later be defined as anorexia. One hundred seventy years later, Gull in England and Laseque in France gave the condition its current name (Russell, 1985).

DIAGNOSTIC CRITERIA

Criteria for the establishment of a diagnosis of AN were first published in 1972 by Feighner. In 1980 the American Psychiatric Association (APA) published the criteria for diagnosis of AN, but it was not until 1987 that the APA recognized AN and BN as two separate and distinct clinical entities. The most current diagnostic criteria are listed in Box 25-1 (APA, 2000a).

Box 25-1. American Psychiatric Association Diagnostic Criteria

Anorexia Nervosa (AN)

A. Refusal to maintain body weight at or above a minimally normal weight for age and height (e.g., weight loss leading to maintenance of body weight less than 85% of that expected; or failure to make expected weight gain during period of growth, leading to body weight less than 85% of that expected).
B. Intense fear of gaining weight or becoming fat, even though underweight.
C. Disturbance in the way in which one's body weight or shape is experienced; undue influence of body weight or shape on self-evaluation; or denial of the seriousness of the current low body weight.
D. In postmenarcheal females, amenorrhea, i.e., the absence of at least three consecutive menstrual cycles.
   1. *Restricting type:* During the current episode of AN, the person has not regularly engaged in binge eating or purging behavior.
   2. *Binge eating/purging type:* During the current episode of AN, the person has regularly engaged in binge eating and purging behavior.

Bulimia Nervosa (BN)

A. Recurrent episodes of binge eating. An episode of binge eating is characterized by both of the following:
   1. Eating, in a discrete period of time (e.g., within any 2-hour period), an amount of food that is definitely larger than most people would eat during a similar period of time and under similar circumstances.
   2. A sense of lack of control over eating during the episode (e.g., a feeling that one cannot stop eating or control what or how much one is eating).
B. Recurrent inappropriate compensatory behavior in order to prevent weight gain, such as self-induced vomiting, misuse of laxatives, diuretics, enemas, or other medications; fasting; or excessive exercise.
C. The binge eating and inappropriate compensatory behaviors both occur, on average, at least twice a week for 3 months.
D. Self-evaluation is unduly influenced by body shape and weight.
E. The disturbance does not occur exclusively during episodes of AN.
   1. *Purging type:* During the current episode of BN, the person has regularly engaged in self-induced vomiting or the misuse of laxatives, diuretics, or enemas.
   2. *Nonpurging type:* During the current episode of BN, the person has used other inappropriate compensatory behaviors, such as fasting or excessive exercise, but has not regularly engaged in self-induced vomiting or the misuse of laxatives, diuretics, or enemas.

Eating Disorder Not Otherwise Specified (EDNOS)

This category is for disorders of eating that do not meet criteria for any specific eating disorder. For example:
1. For females, all of the criteria for AN are met except that the individual has regular menses.
2. All of the criteria for AN are met except that, despite significant weight loss, the individual's current weight is in the normal range.
3. All of the criteria for BN are met except that the binge eating and inappropriate compensatory mechanisms occur at a frequency of less than twice a week or for a duration of less than 3 months.
4. The regular use of inappropriate compensatory behavior by an individual of normal body weight after eating small amounts of food.
5. Repeatedly chewing and spitting out, but not swallowing, large amounts of food.
6. Binge Eating Disorder (BED): Recurrent episodes of binge eating in the absence of the regular use of inappropriate compensatory behaviors characteristic of BN.

From American Psychiatric Association: *Diagnostic and statistical manual of mental disorders,* DSM-IV-TR, ed 4, (text revision) Washington, DC, 2000, Task Force on DSM-IV, APA Press.

Anorexia Nervosa

Anorexia nervosa (AN) is a condition characterized by voluntary self-starvation and emaciation. Weight loss is viewed as a sign of extraordinary achievement and self-discipline. Weight gain is perceived as an unacceptable loss of self-control. The reported lifetime prevalence of AN among women is 0.5% to 3.7%, depending on how strictly the diagnostic criteria are defined (APA, 2000b). Among males, estimated prevalence is about one tenth that of females (APA, 2000). The diagnosis of AN requires a weight deficit. Although Feighner and colleagues' (1972) and the *Diagnostic and Statistical Manual of Mental Disorders* (DSM) criteria required a weight loss of at least 25% of original body weight, the DSM-III, DSM-IV, and DSM-IV test revision (TR) all specify a body weight less than 85% of expected. If AN develops during childhood or early adolescence, failure to make expected weight gains (while growing in height) instead of weight loss may occur. Stunting also may occur in prepubertal children afflicted with this disorder, and it is essential that growth records be obtained. If stunting has occurred, the weight deficit should be calculated using the patient's premorbid height percentile.

Anorexia nervosa appears to be more prevalent in industrialized countries that embrace and idealize a thin body type, including the United States, Canada, Europe, Australia, Japan, New Zealand, and South Africa (APA, 2000b). Whereas some non-Western societies still embrace a more corpulent female body shape, a recent review suggests that AN is increasing even in developing Third World countries (Miller and Pumariega, 2001).

Patients with AN have body image distortion, causing them to feel fat despite their often cachectic state. Some individuals feel overweight all over, whereas others are overly concerned about the fatness of a specific body part, such as the abdomen, buttocks, or thighs.

The DSM criterion of amenorrhea is the absence of at least three consecutive menstrual cycles in postmenarcheal women, but this criterion may not be useful for diagnosis in younger patients. If AN develops before early puberty, sexual maturation may be arrested and menarche may be delayed. Furthermore, even healthy adolescent girls have periods of amenorrhea during the first 1 to 2 years after menarche (Fisher et al, 1995).

Patients with AN manifest symptoms of depression that may be due, in part, to the psychological stress of starvation. In a study of physical and psychological effects of semistarvation conducted in the 1940s, healthy male volunteers developed symptoms of psychological deterioration and depression during a 6-month period of restricted caloric intake (50% of maintenance energy requirements). Patients with AN also exhibit obsessive-compulsive features, particularly with regard to food. Participants in the Minnesota Study also developed obsessive behaviors during the semistarvation period, and many of these behaviors did not reverse immediately on refeeding (Keys et al, 1950), which suggests that food-related obsessive–compulsive behaviors may be caused or exacerbated by malnutrition. The APA recommends that in AN (1) depressive symptoms should be reassessed after partial or complete weight restoration, and (2) patients exhibiting non–food-related obsessive-compulsive behaviors should be evaluated for a comorbid diagnosis of obsessive-compulsive disorder (APA, 1994). Comorbid personality disorders are also common in AN, particularly in patients with the binge and purge subtype. Poor impulse control, substance abuse, mood swings, and suicide tendencies may be exhibited (APA, 2000b).

Bulimia Nervosa

Bulimia nervosa (BN) is a disorder characterized by recurring episodes of binge eating followed by one or more inappropriate compensatory behaviors to prevent weight gain. These behaviors include self-induced vomiting, laxative abuse, diuretic abuse, excessive fasting, or compulsive exercise. The lifetime prevalence of BN among young adult women is 1.4 % to 4.2%. The rate of occurrence in males is approximately one tenth that in females (APA, 2000b).

Unlike AN patients with binge and purge subtype, patients with BN are typically within the normal weight range, although some may be slightly underweight or overweight. Like their AN counterparts, these individuals place considerable importance on body shape and size, and they are often frustrated by their inability to attain an underweight state.

It is commonly thought that vomiting is the predominant feature of BN; however, it is the binge eating behavior that is central to the diagnosis. A binge is consumption of an unusually large amount of food in a discrete period (usually ≤2 hours). There is a sense of lack of control over the eating episode. A binge may start in one setting and continue in another. Although continuous ingestion of small amounts of food throughout the day may result in excessive caloric intake, this would not constitute a binge.

The most commonly used compensatory behavior is self-induced vomiting, seen in 80% to 90% of persons with BN. Patients stimulate the gag reflex with a finger or instrument (e.g., toothbrush, eating utensil), and some can vomit at will. Syrup of ipecac is occasionally used to induce vomiting, a dangerous practice that can result in cardiomyopathies and sudden death. About one third of patients abuse laxatives, and a few also abuse enemas (APA, 2000b). Compulsive exercise is described as that which significantly interferes with life activities or occurs at inappropriate times or in inappropriate settings. Despite injury or other medical complications, these individuals often continue to exercise compulsively.

Comorbid mood, anxiety, and personality disorders are often diagnosed in patients with BN. Although their onset may precede the development of BN, in some instances, symptoms of mood lability and anxiety actually improve after successful treatment of BN.

Although patients with AN typically reject treatment interventions, patients with BN are more distressed by their symptoms and seek relief from their disorder. One of the chief psychological characteristics is guilt over the cycle of binge eating and purging that is carried out in secret, even while their lives may seem ideal to those around them.

Eating Disorder Not Otherwise Specified

Patients diagnosed with an eating disorder not otherwise specified (EDNOS) constitute about 50% of the population with eating disorders. These patients have partial symptoms of either AN or BN. For example, this may be the patient who meets all criteria for AN except amenorrhea. Another example would be a person of normal weight who does not binge but self-induces vomiting after an average-size meal. If left untreated, patients with an EDNOS may develop eating disorders that meet the full criteria for AN or BN.

Binge Eating Disorder

Binge eating disorder (BED) has been described and proposed as a new eating disorder. Research criteria for BED are listed in Box 25-1. Binge eating, similar to that seen in BN, is characteristic of BED; however, there are no inappropriate compensatory behaviors after the binge. Binge episodes must occur at least 2 days per week for a period of 6 months. Persons with BED experience a feeling of powerlessness over their eating similar to that felt by BN patients. Significant emotional distress, characterized by feelings of disgust, guilt, and depression, occurs after the binge. The onset of BED generally occurs in late adolescence or in the early twenties, with women being 1.5 times more likely to develop this disorder than men. Community samples suggest that most patients with this disorder are overweight, with a 15% to 50% prevalence among participants in weight-control programs (APA, 1994).

Childhood Eating Disorders

The use of DSM criteria in childhood eating disorders is problematic because clinical presentation differs from that seen in older adolescents and young adults. Although the exact prevalence is unknown, it appears to be lower than that seen in older patients. BN is more common than AN in adolescents and young adults, but the reverse is true in children and young adolescents. Documented cases of AN have been reported in children as young as 8 years of age, whereas BN is considered rare in childhood. The ratio of boys to girls with AN is higher than that seen in older patients. Multiethnic, multicultural presentation also occurs (Robin, Gilroy, and Dennis, 1998).

Symptoms of childhood eating disorders vary. Complaints of nausea, abdominal pain, and difficulty in swallowing may coexist with concerns about weight, shape, and body fatness. Food avoidance, self-induced vomiting, and excessive exercise may occur. Laxative abuse is uncommon. Any child or adolescent practicing unhealthy weight-control practices or exhibiting obsessional thoughts about food, weight, shape, or exercise may be a candidate for an eating disorder (Kreipe et al, 1995). Depression and obsessive-compulsive disorder may coexist in these children as well.

Woodside (1995) suggests five warning signs of a childhood and early adolescent eating disorder. These include dieting associated with (1) a decreasing weight goal, (2) increasing criticism of the body, (3) increasing social isolation, (4) disruption of menstruation, and (5) reports of purging in the context of dieting. The term *eating disturbance* versus *eating disorder* is suggested by Bryant-Waugh (2000), and a description of childhood eating disturbances treated at London's Great Ormond Street Hospital for Children is given in Table 25-1.

The relationship between problematic childhood eating behaviors and subsequent development of eating disorders in later life is of concern. In a 17-year longitudinal study of 800 children, Kotler and colleagues (2001) found that eating conflicts, struggles with food, and unpleasant meals were risk factors for the development of an eating disorder in adolescence or young adulthood. Other childhood eating problems, however, such as not eating, disinterest in food, picky eating, eating too little, and eating too slowly, failed to predict subsequent development of an eating disorder. There is an obvious need for developmentally appropriate diagnostic criteria, screening instruments, and validated treatments for children and younger adolescents.

Eating Disorders in Athletes

Athletes tend to be highly competitive, high-achieving, and self-disciplined persons. Similar personality traits are seen in patients with AN. A lean body type is associated with enhanced strength and performance in many competitive sports, and this is true for both male and female athletes. In addition, female athletes have to deal with westernized values equating a thin body type with physical attractiveness. To attain low body weights, athletes may increase training and decrease food intake.

In females the drive for thinness may result in excessive training, disordered eating, and menstrual dysfunction or amenorrhea. Osteopenia and osteoporosis develop thereafter. This drive for both performance and appearance thinness has been identified in the Female Athlete Triad (see Chapter 26).

TABLE 25-1 Childhood Eating Disturbances

EATING DISTURBANCE	CHARACTERISTICS
Anorexia nervosa	Determined food avoidance Weight loss or failure to gain weight during the period of preadolescent growth (10-14 yr) in the absence of any physical or other mental illness Any two or more of the following: Preoccupation with body weight Preoccupation with energy intake Distorted body image Fear of fatness Self-induced vomiting Extensive exercising Laxative abuse
Bulimia nervosa	Binge eating followed by purging, restricting, excessive exercise, or laxative abuse Rarely seen in childhood
Food avoidance emotional disorder	A primary emotional disorder resulting in avoidance of food Weight loss, or failure to gain developmentally appropriate amounts of weight No preoccupation with weight and shape Absence of body image distortion May have comorbid medical disorders/diseases
Selective eating	Food intake limited to a very small number of foods May be rigid about the brand of food, or its place of purchase Food choices tend to be carbohydrates Selective eating hinders participation in social situations that include eating Attempts to increase variety in diet are met with extreme resistance Age-appropriate gains in weight and height No preoccupation with weight and shape Absence of body image distortion No fear of choking or gagging (see functional dysphagia)
Restrictive eating	Characteristically eats a smaller than normal amount of food Disinterested in eating No intentional food restriction Normal balance of carbohydrates, protein, and fats in diet Absence of mood disorder Height and weight within normal limits but at the lower end of percentiles May have difficulty meeting increased energy requirement during puberty No preoccupation with weight and shape Absence of body image distortion
Food refusal	Episodic, situational, or intermittent food refusal No preoccupation with weight and shape Absence of body image distortion Emotional issues, such as unhappiness or worry, may be the underlying cause
Functional dysphagia	Food avoidance, particularly foods of a certain type or texture Fearful of swallowing, vomiting, choking An aversive event may precipitate the disorder No preoccupation with weight and shape Absence of body image distortion
Pervasive refusal syndrome	Profound and pervasive refusal to eat, drink, walk, talk, or engage in self-care May be underweight and dehydrated May be a form of post traumatic stress disorder Rare but potentially life threatening Usually requires hospitalization

From Bryant-Waugh R: Overview of eating disorders. In Lask B, Bryant-Waugh R, editors: *Anorexia nervosa and related eating disorders in childhood and adolescence,* ed 2, East Sussex, UK, 2000, Psychology Press.

Performance thinness refers to the commonly held belief that achieving a lower weight and lower percentage of body fat will enhance performance, particularly in endurance sports. *Appearance thinness* refers to the trend over the past several decades to reward thinner athletes in adjudicated sports, such as gymnastics and figure skating (Ryan, 1995).

Identifying the eating-disordered athlete can be challenging. Signs may include excessive training, exercise associated with injury, increased frequency of injury, restrictive eating patterns, frequent self-weighing, and excessive concern with body size and shape. Female gymnasts, figure skaters, dancers, runners, swimmers and divers, as well as male wrestlers and body builders, are at high risk for eating disorders (Sundjot-Borgen, 1994).

Eating Disorders in People With Diabetes

Because of the requirements for long-term awareness and control of eating behavior, persons with diabetes are at risk for developing eating disorders. Whether an eating disorder develops seem to depend on the person's psychological sense of control and is related to metabolic control (Surgenor et al, 2002). This is especially true in young women, for whom there is the added psychological pressure for body thinness.

ETIOLOGY

The etiology of AN is multifactorial, with biologic, genetic, intrapersonal, familial, and sociocultural precipitants to the development and maintenance of the disorder. Onset of AN, most common during adolescence, is often viewed as biopsychological developmental arrest. Pubertal changes in body habitus heighten concern about body shape and size. Patients are typically introverted, obsessional, and perfectionistic in nature. They are overachievers but feel ineffective. Low self-esteem is common. Family pathology is characterized by enmeshment, overprotectiveness, rigidity, and lack of conflict resolution. Development of the disorder may be viewed as an attempt to gain control and autonomy. Comorbid anxiety disorders, depressive disorders, and personality disorders may be present. There is an increased risk of AN among first-degree biological relatives of persons with the disorder and a higher concordance in monozygotic twins compared with dizygotic twins (APA, 2000b).

Several etiologic models have been proposed for the development of BN, including addictive, family, sociocultural, cognitive-behavioral, and psychodynamic. The addiction model suggests food and behavioral addiction, with treatment similar to that used in alcohol and substance-abuse patients (i.e., 12-step programs). The family model focuses on the identification and treatment of family dysfunction. The sociocultural model attributes development of BN to cultural pressures for thinness. Because this body type cannot be naturally attained by all persons, susceptible persons resort to bulimic behaviors when conventional methods of dieting fail. The cognitive-behavioral model attributes the development of BN to irrational thoughts and beliefs concerning body weight, dieting, and self-esteem. Treatment is aimed at identification and behavioral treatment of dysfunctional beliefs. The psychodynamic model is one of the strongest etiologic models. Here BN represents the patient's attempt to control, avoid, or minimize the impact of distressful feelings, impulses, and anxieties. Comorbid mood disorders, anxiety disorders, personality disorders, and substance abuse may occur in BN.

PATHOPHYSIOLOGY

Although eating disorders are classified as psychiatric illnesses, they are associated with significant medical complications, morbidity, and mortality rates between 5% and 15%. Even though the primary dysfunction is related to deficiencies in the sense of self, identity, and autonomy, the physical and psychological consequences of malnutrition dominate the clinical picture.

Numerous physiologic changes result from the weight-control habits of patients with AN and BN (Table 25-2). Some are minor changes that occur secondarily to a reduced energy intake; some are pathologic alterations that may have long-term consequences; and a few represent potentially life-threatening conditions.

Clinical Characteristics and Medical Complications: Anorexia Nervosa

Patients with AN have a typical and distinctive appearance (Figure 25-1). Their cachectic and prepubescent body habitus often makes them look younger than their age. Common physical characteristics include lanugo; brittle, listless hair; cyanosis of the extremities; and dry skin that may have a yellow cast because of hypercarotenemia. Bradycardia below 60 beats per minute and hypotension below 70 mm Hg (systolic) are frequently present. Patients with AN will often ascribe their low heart rates and low blood pressures to their exercise regimen and proclaim physical fitness; however, cardiovascular testing has shown altered cardiovascular response to exercise in AN (Nudel et al, 1984). Patients are hypothermic and often wear more clothing than is environmentally appropriate.

Cardiovascular complications have been associated with death in AN. Reduction in heart mass is associated with reduced blood pressure and pulse rate. Mitral valve prolapse may be related to hypovolemia or cardiomyopathy. Unlike chronically ill adults with AN, adolescents have relatively well-preserved cardiac output; however, death from congestive heart failure may occur in AN patients of any age (Fisher et al, 1995).

The gastrointestinal tract may be profoundly affected in AN. Complications secondary to starvation include delayed gastric emptying, decreased small bowel motility, and constipation. These complications may result in complaints of abdominal bloating and a prolonged sensation of abdominal fullness, which can last several hours after eating.

Major changes in the central nervous system occur in AN. Although controlled studies provide evidence of structural abnormalities in the brains of adults, less is known about the long-term effect of these structural changes in adolescents with AN (Fisher et al, 1995).

Bone marrow hypoplasia, found in 50% of AN patients, results in varying degrees of leukopenia, anemia, and thrombocytopenia (Hardoff et al, 1991). Gelatinous bone marrow transformation and hypoplasia secondary to dietary restriction of protein, fat, and carbohydrate have been documented in AN (Lambert et al, 1997; Wang et al, 2001). Low erythrocyte sedimentation rates are common and may result from decreased fibrinogen production by the malnourished liver (Fisher et al, 1995).

TABLE 25-2 Medical Complications of Eating Disorders

	AN		BN	
	RESTRICTING	BINGE-EATING PURGING	PURGING	NONPURGING
Fluid and Electrolyte Imbalance				
Hypokalemia		√	√	
Hyponatremia		√	√	
Hypochloremic alkalosis		√	√	
Elevated BUN	√	√	√	√
Inability to concentrate urine	√	√		
Decreased glomerular filtration rate	√	√		
Ketonuria	√	√	√	√
Cardiovascular				
Bradycardia	√	√		
Orthostatic hypotension	√	√	√	√
Dysrhythmias	√	√	√	√
Electrocardiographic abnormalities				
Prolonged QT interval	√	√	√	
T wave abnormalities	√	√	√	
Conduction defects	√	√	√	
Ipecac cardiomyopathy		√	√	
Mitral valve prolapse	√	√		
Congestive cardiac failure	√	√		
Pericardial effusion	√	√		
Gastrointestinal				
Parotid hypertrophy		√	√	
Perimolysis and increased incidence of dental caries		√	√	
Constipation	√	√	√	√
Bloody diarrhea		√	√	
Delayed gastric emptying	√	√	√	√
Intestinal atony	√	√	√	√
Esophagitis		√	√	
Mallory-Weiss tears		√	√	
Esophageal or gastric rupture		√	√	
Perforation/rupture of stomach		√	√	
Barrett esophagus		√	√	
Fatty infiltration and focal necrosis of liver	√	√		
Superior mesenteric artery syndrome	√	√		
Gallstones	√	√	√	√
Skeletal				
Osteopenia	√	√	?	?
Fractures	√	√	?	?
Dermatologic				
Acrocyanosis	√	√		
Yellow dry skin (hypercarotenemia)	√	√		
Brittle hair and nails	√	√		
Lanugo	√	√		
Russell sign (calluses over the knuckles)		√	√	
Pitting edema	√	√	√	√
Endocrine				
Growth retardation and short stature	√	√		
Delayed puberty	√	√		
Amenorrhea	√	√		
Low T_3 syndrome	√	√		
Decreased capacity to concentrate urine 2° to	√	√		
↓ vassopressin secretion	√	√		
Hypercortisolism	√	√		
Hematologic				
Bone marrow suppression				
Mild anemia	√	√		
Leukopenia	√	√		
Thrombocytopenia	√	√		
Low sedimentation rate	√	√		
Impaired cell-mediated immunity	√	√		
Neurologic				
Seizures	√	√	√	√
Myopathy	√	√	√	
Peripheral neuropathy	√	√		
Cortical atrophy	√	√		

From Fisher M et al: Eating disorders in adolescents: a background paper, *J Adolesc Health* 16:420, 1995.
AN, Anorexia nervosa; *BN,* bulimia nervosa; *BUN,* blood urea nitrogen; T_3 triiodothyronine.

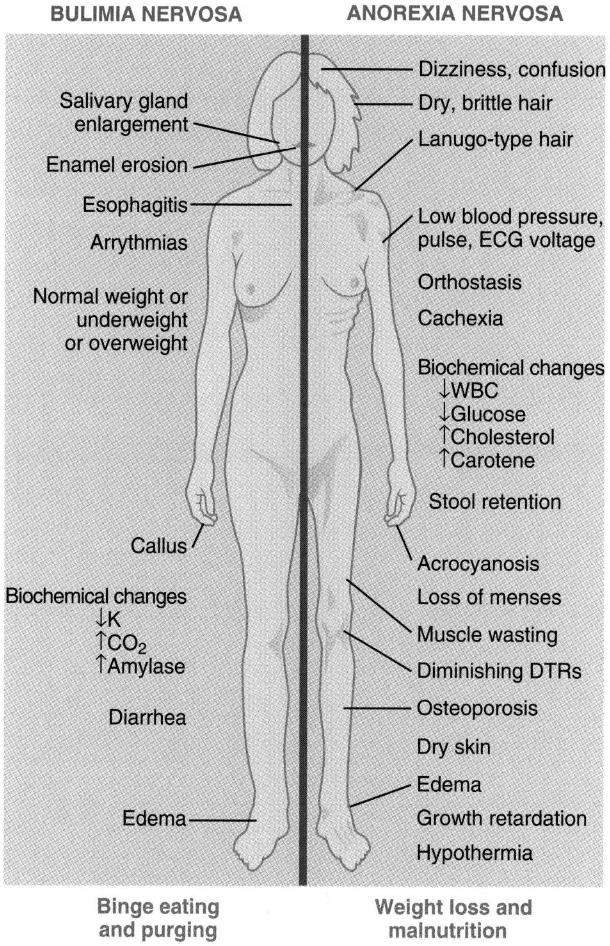

FIGURE 25-1 • Physical and clinical signs and symptoms of bulimia nervosa and anorexia nervosa. *DTRs,* Deep tendon reflexes; *ECG,* electrocardiographic; *WBC,* white blood cell.

Osteopenia, which may result in vertebral compression and pathologic fractures, is one of the most serious medical complications of AN. Estrogen deficiency, elevated glucocorticoid levels, malnutrition, and reduced body mass may all contribute to this state (see Chapter 27) Males with AN are also at significant risk for the development of osteopenia and osteoporosis (Anderson et al, 2000). Hormone imbalance, including testosterone deficiency, must be evaluated in these patients (Anderson, 1999).

Children and adolescents with AN develop unique medical complications that affect normal growth and development. Complications include pubertal delay or interruption, reduction in peak bone mass, and structural abnormalities in the brain (Katzman and Zipursky, 1997; Nicholls et al, 2000).

Clinical Characteristics and Medical Complications: Bulimia Nervosa

Clinical signs and symptoms of BN are more difficult to detect because patients are usually of normal weight and are secretive in behavior. When vomiting occurs, there may be clinical evidence, such as (1) scarring of the dorsum of the hand used to stimulate the gag reflex, known as *Russell's sign;* (2) parotid gland enlargement; and (3) erosion of dental enamel with increased dental caries resulting from the frequent presence of gastric acid in the mouth (Russell, 1985).

Chronic vomiting can result in dehydration, alkalosis, and hypokalemia. Common clinical manifestations include sore throat, esophagitis, mild hematemesis, abdominal pain, and subconjunctival hemorrhage. More serious gastrointestinal complications include Mallory-Weiss esophageal tears, rare occurrence of esophageal rupture, and acute gastric dilatation or rupture. Laxative abuse may lead to dehydration, elevation of serum aldosterone and vasopressin levels, rectal bleeding, intestinal atony, and abdominal cramps. Diuretic abuse may lead to dehydration and hypokalemia. Cardiac arrhythmias can occur secondary to electrolyte and acid-base imbalance caused by vomiting, laxative, and diuretic abuse. Ipecac, used to induce vomiting, may cause irreversible myocardial damage and sudden death. Although the profound amenorrhea associated with AN is uncommon in BN, menstrual irregularities may occur (see Figure 25-1).

NUTRITIONAL ASSESSMENT

Nutritional assessment routinely includes a diet history as well as the assessment of biochemical, metabolic, and anthropometric indices of nutritional status (Figure 25-2) (see Chapters 17 and 18).

Diet History

Guidelines should include assessment of energy intake, macronutrient and micronutrient consumption, eating attitudes, and eating behaviors (Box 25-2) (see Chapter 17).

Inadequate caloric intake, generally less than 1000 kcal per day, is common in AN (Fernstrom et al, 1994). In BN, however, daily caloric intake is unpredictable. The caloric content of a binge, the degree of caloric absorption after a purge, and the extent of calorie restriction between binge episodes make assessment of total energy intake quite challenging. In a study of 54 female BN patients, Weltzin and colleagues (1991) reported a mean 24-hour intake of 4446 (±584) kcal, but they also noted a wide range of caloric intake, with 44% overeating and 19% undereating compared with controls. Bulimic patients assume that vomiting is an efficient mechanism for eliminating calories consumed during binge episodes; however, study of the caloric content of food ingested and purged in a feeding laboratory revealed that, as a group, 17 BN subjects consumed a mean of 2131 (±1154) kcal during a binge and vomited only 979 (±1003) kcal afterward (Kaye et al, 1993). There was, however, an apparent ceiling on caloric retention, regardless of whether binges were smaller or larger (see *Clinical Insight:* Can Dieting Cause Eating Disorders?).

Inadequate energy intake results in decreased consumption of carbohydrate, protein, and fat. Patients with AN were historically described as carbohydrate avoiders (Crisp, 1965) but now appear to restrict dietary fat preferentially (Fernstrom et al, 1994; Schebendach et al, 1977). Indeed, severe dietary fat restriction resulting in essential fatty acid deficiency has been reported in AN (Holman et al, 1995). Percent of calories contributed by protein may be in the average to above-average range, but the adequacy of intake will be relative to total caloric consumption. For example, one study revealed that although the

EATING DISORDER ASSESSMENT

Date of birth: ______

DIAGNOSIS:
- ☐ Anorexia Nervosa
- ☐ Bulimia Nervosa
- ☐ Eating Disorder NOS

Hospitalizations for eating disorder:
- ☐ In-patient
- ☐ Day patient
- ☐ Out-patient
- ☐ Intensive out-patient

WEIGHT HISTORY
Wt. loss: # lb______ From ______ To______
Minimum weight at current height ______
Maximum weight at current height ______
IBW:______ %IBW:______ %Wt loss:______ BMI%:______

ANTHROPOMETRIC PROFILE
Skinfolds (mm): ______
Triceps:______ Biceps:______ Subscapular:______
Suprailiac:______
Sum of sites (mm):______ % Body fat:______ TSF%:______
MAC (cm):______ MAMC (cm):______ MAMC%:______

BODY IMAGE: ______

FOOD ALLERGIES: ______

24-HOUR RECALL: ______

FLUID INTAKE: ______

VITAMIN/MINERAL SUPPLEMENTS: ______

OTHER SUPPLEMENTS: ______

SUGAR AND FAT SUBSTITUTES: ______

MISCELLANEOUS: Chewing gum: ______
Hard candy: ______
Condiments: ______

BINGES: # per day # per week
Duration per episode: ______
Binge foods: ______

Approximate kcal/binge: ______

SELF-INDUCED VOMITING:
Times per day:______ Method:______

LAXATIVES:
Type/brand:______ Amount:______
Duration of use:______ Frequency of use:______

DIURETICS:
Type:______ Amount:______
Duration of use:______ Frequency of use:______

EXERCISE:
Type:______
Minutes/day:______ Times/week:______
Purpose of exercise:______

MENSTRUAL HISTORY:
Age of menarche:______
Last menstrual period:______

MEDICATIONS (prescription and over-the-counter): ______

BOWEL FUNCTION: ______

FIGURE 25-2 • Sample nutritional assessment form for eating disorders.

mean percentage of calories provided by protein was 22% in early illness and 21% in late illness, actual protein intake was only 38 and 17 g per day, respectively, in patients with AN (Beaumont et al, 1981).

Many patients with AN claim to be vegetarians (Bakan et al, 1993). This may be a covert method of limiting foods, particularly those containing fat. It may be helpful to determine when the adoption of vegetarian food choices occurred relative to the development of AN.

Box 25-2. Assessment of Nutrient Intake

1. Calories
   A. Compare intake with DRI (Table 15-2)
   B. Estimate typical intake
   C. Determine range of intake in BN
   D. Determine hidden sources: gum, hard candy, etc.
2. Macronutrients
   A. Carbohydrate
      (1) Determine percent kcal intake
      (2) Compare intake to DRI intake (Table 15-2)
      (3) Simple
      (4) Complex
      (5) Fiber: water soluble versus insoluble
   B. Protein
      (1) Determine percent kcal intake
      (2) Compare intake with DRI (Table 15-2)
      (3) Evaluate vegetarian diet for high biologic value sources
   C. Fat
      (1) Determine percent kcal intake
      (2) Source of essential fatty acid
      (3) Compare intake to DRI (Table 15-2)
3. Micronutrients
   A. Vitamins
      (1) Water soluble
      (2) Fat soluble
      (3) Identify supplements
   B. Minerals
      (1) Calcium
      (2) Iron
      (3) Zinc
      (4) Identify supplements
4. Fluid
   A. Determine total daily consumption
   B. Identify sources
5. Miscellaneous
   A. Alcohol
   B. Caffeine
   C. Amount and type of nonnutritive sweeteners and fat substitutes
   D. Other nutritional supplements (i.e., herbal supplements)

Modified from Luder E, Schebendach J: Nutrition management of eating disorders, *Top Clin Nutr* 8:53, 1993.
RDA, Recommended dietary allowance; *BN*, bulimia nervosa.

When BN patients are not binge eating, they often restrict their intake of carbohydrate and fat. In a study of eating behavior, Walsh and colleagues (1989) found that the bulimic group consumed a smaller percentage of total fat calories at a nonbinge meal than the control group.

Inadequate caloric intake, limited variety in the diet, and poor food group representation result in inadequate vitamin and mineral consumption in eating-disordered patients (Hadigan et al, 2000). Vitamin and mineral supplements may be used, and patients must be queried about use.

When obtaining a diet history, typical fluid intake should also be determined. Some patients severely restrict intake, being intolerant of the feeling of fullness after fluid ingestion. Others drink excessive amounts, attempting to stave off hunger. Abnormalities in fluid balance are prevalent in this population. Extremes in fluid restriction or consumption may require monitoring of urine specific gravity and serum electrolytes.

Eating Behavior

Characteristic attitudes, behaviors, and eating habits seen in AN and BN are shown in Box 25-3. Food aversions, common in this population, include red meat, baked goods, desserts, added fats, and fried foods. Patients with eating disorders often regard specific foods or groups of foods as absolutely "good" or absolutely "bad" for them. Irrational beliefs and dichotomous thinking about food choices should be identified and challenged throughout the treatment process.

In the assessment, it is important to determine unusual or ritualistic behaviors, which may include the ingestion of food in an atypical manner or with nontraditional utensils, unusual food combinations, or the excessive use of spices, vinegar, or lemon juice. Meal spacing and length of time allocated for a meal should also be determined. Many patients will save their self-allotted food ration until late in the day, and yet others are fearful of eating past a certain time of day. Setting time limits for completion of meals and snacks is important. Many BN patients eat quickly, reflecting their difficulties with satiety cues. Many AN patients eat in an excessively slow manner, often playing with their food and cutting it into small pieces. This is sometimes regarded as a tactic to avoid food intake, and yet it may also represent a starvation effect (Keys et al, 1950). In addition, BN patients may identify foods they fear will trigger a binge episode. The patient may have an all-or-nothing approach to "trigger" foods. Although the patient may prefer avoidance, assistance with reintroduction of controlled amounts of these foods may be helpful.

Laboratory Data

The often marked cachexia of AN may lead one to expect biochemical indices of malnutrition, but this is rarely the case. Compensatory mechanisms are re-

CLINICAL INSIGHT

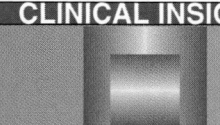

Can Dieting Cause Eating Disorders?

In a review of five studies with 3037 participants, Hsu (1997) concluded that ". . . longitudinal studies point unanimously to the role of dieting behavior in the pathogenesis of an eating disorder." In bulimia nervosa, patients may diet in response to a binge; however, current research suggests that dieting may actually precipitate binge eating in biologically predisposed persons.

Animal and human studies suggest that serotonin, a central nervous system neurotransmitter, is involved in the control of feeding. Serotonin contributes to satiety after eating, and research suggests that decreased serotonin function may lead to impaired satiety and weight gain. The synthesis of serotonin in the brain depends on the availability of its amino acid precursor, tryptophan, in plasma. When the effect of a liquid diet devoid of the serotonin precursor tryptophan was compared in 10 recovered female subjects with a history of BN and 12 healthy controls, the recovered bulimic subjects exhibited a significant decrease in mood and an increase in body image concern as well as subjective loss of control of eating 7 hours after ingestion of the tryptophan-free formula, an occurrence not noted in the healthy subjects (Smith et al, 1999). A 1000-kcal, low-carbohydrate diet has been shown to decrease plasma tryptophan levels and alter brain serotonin function in healthy women (Smith et al, 1997). These investigators suggest that persistent dieting may result in chronic depletion of plasma tryptophan and brain serotonin and subsequent development of eating disorder symptoms in a biologically vulnerable person.

Box 25-3. Assessment of Eating Attitudes, Behaviors, and Habits

1. Eating attitudes
   A. Food aversions
   B. "Safe" foods
   C. Magical thinking
   D. Binge trigger foods
   E. Ideas on appropriate amounts of food
2. Eating behaviors
   A. Ritualistic behaviors
   B. Unusual food combinations
   C. Atypical seasoning of food
   D. Atypical use of eating utensils
3. Eating habits
   A. Intake pattern
      (1) Number of meals and snacks
      (2) Time of day meals and snacks are consumed
      (3) Duration of feedings
      (4) Eating environment—where and with whom
      (5) How consumed—sitting or standing
   B. Avoidance of particular food groups
   C. Variety of foods consumed
   D. Fluid intake—restricted or excessive

Modified from Schebendach J, Nussbaum M: Nutrition management in adolescents with eating disorders, *Adolesc Med State Art Rev* 3(3):545, 1992.

markable, and laboratory abnormalities may not be observed until the illness is far advanced.

In AN, serum albumin levels are generally within normal limits. Although true levels may be masked by dehydration in early treatment, significant alterations in visceral protein status are uncommon. Indeed, adaptive phenomena that occur in chronic starvation are aimed at the maintenance of visceral protein metabolism at the expense of the somatic compartment (see Chapters 18 and 42).

Despite consumption of low-fat, low-cholesterol diets, patients with AN often have elevated serum cholesterol levels and abnormal lipoprotein profiles. The cause of these lipoprotein abnormalities is unknown, but several mechanisms have been postulated. These include mild hepatic dysfunction, decreased bile acid secretion, hypothalamic dysfunction, and abnormal eating patterns (Arden et al, 1990). Values that are elevated in the acute phase may normalize during a chronic course of illness (Mehler, 1998). An elevated blood cholesterol or lipid value does not warrant the prescription of a low fat-diet, low-cholesterol diet. If hyperlipidemia predated the development of AN, or if a strong family history of hyperlipidemia is identified, the patient should be reassessed after weight restoration has occurred.

Patients with BN may also have abnormal lipid levels. In a study of 126 bulimic women, 67% exhibited elevated serum cholesterol levels, which were attributed to the fat and cholesterol content of foods consumed during binge-eating episodes (Sullivan et al, 1998). Patients with BN are prone to eating low-fat, low-energy foods during the restriction phase and high-fat, high-sugar foods during binge episodes. Premature prescription of a low-fat, low-cholesterol diet may only reinforce their dichotomous approach to eating. Care must be taken to balance extremes in the types and amounts of foods consumed. An accurate lipid profile can be obtained only after a period of dietary stabilization. Patients with BN may also have difficulty complying with the fast required for an accurate lipid profile.

Low serum glucose results from a deficit of precursors needed for gluconeogenesis and glucose production. Thyroid hormone production tends to be normal, but the peripheral deiodination of thyroxin favors formation of the less metabolically active reduced triiodothyronine (rT_3) rather than triiodothyronine (T_3). This metabolic state, known as the low T3 syndrome, is characteristic of AN but resolves with refeeding (Fisher et al, 1995).

Vitamin and Mineral Abnormalities

Hypercarotenemia is a common finding in AN, particularly in the restrictor subgroup. Etiology is attributed to mobilization of lipid stores, catabolic changes caused by weight loss, and metabolic stress. Excessive dietary intake of carotenoids is less suspect. Normalization of serum carotene occurs during the course of nutritional rehabilitation.

Despite obviously deficient diets, reports of clinical and biochemical findings of true deficiency diseases are rare in AN and BN. The decreased need for micronutrients in a catabolic state, use of vitamin supplements (Rock and Yager, 1987), and judicious selection of micronutrient-rich foods may be protective. Documented cases of riboflavin, vitamin B_6, thiamin, γ-tocopherol, and α-tocopherol deficiencies have been reported in lower-weight patients with AN (Langan and Farrell, 1985; Rock and Vasantharajan, 1995).

Likewise, iron deficiency anemia is also uncommon in AN. Iron requirements are decreased secondary to amenorrhea and the overall catabolic state. The true hematologic picture may be masked by hemoconcentration resulting from dehydration in early treatment (Lucas, 1977).

Zinc deficiency resulting from suboptimal intake (7 to 8 mg daily) has been documented in both AN and BN (Bakan et al, 1993) and its etiology attributed to inadequate energy intake, avoidance of red meat, and the adoption of vegetarian food choices. Zinc's relationship to altered taste and poor appetite has led some researchers to investigate whether zinc deficiency perpetuates poor food intake in this population (Casper et al, 1980).

Anorexia nervosa, past and present, is associated with a high prevalence of osteopenia and osteoporosis in both males and females. Whereas low estrogen and testosterone levels and weight loss are the primary causes, concurrent dietary deficiencies of calcium, magnesium, and vitamin D contribute to the overall pathogenesis. Dual x-ray absorptiometry to determine the degree of impaired bone mineralization is recommended (see Chapter 27).

Fluid and Electrolyte Abnormalities

Vomiting and laxative and diuretic use can result in significant fluid and electrolyte imbalances in patients with eating disorders. Laxative use may result in hypokalemia, and diuretic use can lead to dehydration and hypokalemia. Vomiting may result in dehydration, hypokalemia, and alkalosis with hypochloremia. Hyponatremia is a serious complication that is seen less frequently.

Urine concentration is decreased, and urine output is increased in semistarvation. Starvation edema may present initially, and refeeding edema may develop during nutritional rehabilitation (Barbosa-Saldivar and Van Itallie, 1979) (see Chapters 23 and 42). Fluid consumption varies from restricted to excessive intake. Depletion of glycogen and lean tissue is accompanied by obligatory water loss that reflects characteristic hydration ratios. For example, the obligatory water loss associated with glycogen depletion may be in the range of 600 to 800 ml.

Metabolic Changes

Malnourished patients with AN have characteristically low metabolic rates (Table 25-3). Weight loss, decreased lean body mass, energy restriction, and decreased leptin levels have been implicated in the pathogenesis of this hypometabolic state. Consistent refeeding results in progressive increases in resting energy expenditure (REE) with a trend toward normalization.

An elevated diet-induced thermogenesis (DIT) has also been reported in AN (de Zwann et al, 2002). This elevated DIT, along with progressive increases in REE, may result in the need for high-calorie prescriptions during the course of nutritional rehabilitation in AN.

Patients with BN can have unpredictable metabolic rates. Dietary restraint between episodes of binge eating may place bulimic patients in a state of semistarvation (de Zwann et al, 2002), which can result in a hypometabolic rate (Detzer MJ et al, 1994; Schebendach et al, 1995). Binge eating followed by purging, however, also can increase the metabolic rate secondary to a preabsorptive release of insulin, which activates the sympathetic nervous system (de Zwann et al, 2002).

Anthropometric Assessment

Patients with AN have protein energy malnutrition characterized by significantly depleted adipose and somatic protein stores but a relatively intact visceral protein compartment. These patients meet the criteria for a diagnosis of marasmus (see Appendix 33). A goal of nutritional rehabilitation is restoration of body fat and fat-free mass. Although these compartments do regenerate, the extent and rate vary.

An accurate body fat percent can be obtained from underwater weighing or bone mineral densitometry (DXA) equipped with body composition software; however, these methods are not generally available in an office or clinic setting (see Chapter 17). Bioelectrical impedance analysis (BIA) is commercially available but of questionable validity because of shifts in intracellular and extracellular fluid compartments in patients with severe eating disorders (Birmingham et al, 1996; Scalfi et al, 1993). Percent body fat can be estimated from the sum of four skin-fold measure-

TABLE 25-3 Measured Versus Predicted Energy Expenditure in Anorexia Nervosa

INVESTIGATORS	N	AGE (yr)	MEASURED RESTING ENERGY EXPENDITURE (kcal/24 hr)	% HARRIS-BENEDICT PREDICTED ENERGY EXPENDITURE (kcal/24 hr)
Schebendach et al (1995)*	21	17.1 ± 4.0	781 ± 263	62 ± 18
Schebendach et al (1997)*	50	16.3 ± 3.2	895 ± 24.5	72 ± 2
Vaisman et al (1988)*	18	15.8 ± 1.5	832 ± 151	62 ± 17
Vaisman et al (1991)*	24	15.5 ± 1.2	817 ± 176	69 ± 10
Obarzanek et al (1994)†	10	23.3 ± 1.9	742 ± 38	
Melchior et al (1989)†	11	21.4 ± 5.1	831 ± 172	69.5
Polito et al (2000)*	16	25 ± 5	939 ± 127	

*Results reported as mean ± SD.
†Results reported as mean ± SEM.

ments (triceps, biceps, subscapular, and suprailiac crest) using the calculations of Durnin and colleagues (Durnin and Rahaman, 1967; Durnin and Wormersley, 1974) (see Appendix 56). This method has been validated against underwater weighing in adolescent girls with AN (Probst et al, 1996, 2001).

Sophisticated measures of lean tissue can be obtained from DXA equipped with body composition software, total body nitrogen measured by neutron activation analysis (NAA), and total body potassium using a whole-body counter. These methods are used exclusively in research studies. For practical purposes, the midarm muscle circumference, derived from midarm circumference and triceps skin-fold measurements, can be easily obtained and compared with sex- and age-matched population standards (see Chapter 17 and Appendixes 27 through 29 and 31). Baseline and follow-up measurements should be obtained during nutritional rehabilitation.

Body weight is assessed and routinely monitored in patients with eating disorders. In AN, weight gain is necessary. In BN the short-term goal should be weight maintenance. Although weight loss may be warranted, this cannot be addressed until chaotic eating patterns are stabilized.

Rate of weight gain in AN may be affected by hydration status, glycogen stores, metabolic factors, and changes in body composition (Box 25-4). Rehydration and replenished glycogen stores contribute to weight gain during the first few days of refeeding. Thereafter, weight gain results from increased lean and fat stores. It is generalized that one needs to increase or decrease caloric intake by 3500 kcal to affect a 1-lb change in body weight, but the true energy cost depends on the type of tissue gained. More energy is required to gain fat versus lean tissue, and actual weight gain may be a mix of both.

Variables that affect the type of tissue gained include the stage of growth and development, the degree of baseline malnutrition, genetics, physical activity, and possibly the type and rate of refeeding. There may be different patterns of body fat distribution after weight restoration in recovered adolescents vs. in adult females with AN (Misra et al, 2003; Grinspoon et al, 2001).

Box 25-4. Factors Affecting Rate of Weight Gain in Anorexia Nervosa

1. Fluid balance
   - A. Polyuria seen in semistarvation
   - B. Edema
     - (1) Starvation
     - (2) Refeeding
   - C. Hydration ratios in tissues
     - (1) Glycogen: 3-4:1
     - (2) Protein: 3-4:1
2. Metabolic rate
   - A. Resting energy expenditure
   - B. Postprandial energy expenditure
3. Energy cost of tissue gained
   - A. Adipose tissue
   - B. Lean body mass
4. Previous obesity
5. Physical activity

Modified from Schebendach J, Nussbaum M: Nutrition management in adolescents with eating disorders, *Adolesc Med State Art Rev* 3(3):545, 1992.

The anthropometric status of patients with eating disorders should be assessed and monitored regularly (Box 25-5) (see Chapter 17). The patient's goal weight can be determined by various methods, none of which are perfect. The height, weight, and body mass index tables of the National Center for Health Statistics (NCHS) should be used to assess boys and girls up to 18 years of age (see Appendixes 8, 11, 18, and 19). A bone age can be obtained in adolescents with stunted height to determine catch-up growth potential.

If a patient is hospitalized, a daily preprandial, early morning weight should be obtained. On an outpatient basis, a gowned weight should be obtained on the same scale, at approximately the same time of day, at least once a week in early treatment. Before weigh-in, the patient should void, and urine specific gravity should be checked for dehydration or fluid

Box 25-5. Patient Monitoring

1. Body weight
   A. Establish goal weight
   B. Determine
      (1) Acceptable rate of weight gain in AN
      (2) Maintenance weight range in BN
   C. Monitor
      (1) Inpatient
         a. Daily
         b. Gowned
         c. Preprandial
         d. Postvoid
         e. Obtain urine specific gravity
         f. Obtain additional, random, afternoon, or evening weight if fluid loading is suspected
      (2) Day treatment
         a. May vary depending on diagnosis, age of patient, and treatment setting (i.e., daily; several times per week; once per week)
         b. Gowned
         c. Postvoid
         d. Same time of day
         e. Same scale
         f. Obtain urine specific gravity
      (3) Outpatient
         a. Once every 1-2 wk in early treatment, less frequently in mid- to late treatment
         b. Gowned
         c. Postvoid
         d. Same time of day
         e. Same scale
         f. Obtain urine specific gravity
2. Height
   A. Obtain baseline: (NCHS percentile for children and adolescents)
   B. Monitor: every 1-2 mo in patients with growth potential
3. Anthropometric measurements
   A. Obtain baseline
      (1) Skinfolds; triceps, biceps, subscapula, suprailiac
      (2) Midarm circumference
      (3) Midarm muscle circumference
   B. Monitor
      (1) Inpatient: as medically indicated
      (2) Outpatient: as medically indicated
4. Resting and postprandial energy expenditure
   A. Obtain baseline indirect calorimetry if available
   B. Monitor
      (1) Inpatient: every 2 wk
      (2) Outpatient: as medically indicated
5. Outpatient diet monitoring
   A. Anorexia nervosa
      Daily food record to include:
      (1) Food
      (2) Fluid: caloric and noncaloric, alcohol
      (3) Artificial sweeteners and fat substitutes
      (4) Eating behavior: time, place, how eaten, with whom
      (5) Exercise
   B. Bulimia nervosa
      Daily food record to include:
      (1) Food
      (2) Fluid: caloric and noncaloric, alcohol
      (3) Artificial sweeteners and fat substitutes
      (4) Eating behavior: time, place, how eaten, with whom
      (5) Emotions/feelings when eating
      (6) Foods eaten at a binge
      (7) Time and method of purge
      (8) Exercise

Modified from Luder E, Schebendach J: Nutrition management of eating disorders, *Top Clin Nutr* 8:48, 1993.
AN, Anorexia nervosa; *BN*, bulimia nervosa; *NCHS*, National Center for Health Statistics.

loading. If the patient claims to be unable to provide a urine specimen, the physician should examine the patient to see whether the bladder is full. Patients may resort to deceptive tactics (water loading, hiding heavy objects on their person, and withholding urine and bowel movements) to make a mandated weight goal (Ammerman et al, 1966).

PSYCHOLOGICAL MANAGEMENT

Management of patients with eating disorders is best performed by a multidisciplinary team consisting of physicians, nutritionists, and psychotherapists experienced in working with this patient population. Treatment settings vary and may include inpatient medical or psychiatric hospitalization, partial (full-day outpatient) hospitalization, and residential treatment, intensive outpatient, or outpatient programs. Level-of-care criteria for patients with eating disorders were developed by the APA (2000b).

Practice guidelines of the APA (2000) and the Society for Adolescent Medicine (Kreipe et al, 1995) include nutritional rehabilitation; however, nutrition professionals should not attempt to treat these patients without the support of a comprehensive, multidisciplinary team. Severe malnutrition seen in AN is associated with serious psychological problems. Refeeding may precipitate potentially life-threatening medical and psychiatric complications.

Nutritional rehabilitation includes a nutritional assessment, diet therapy, and nutrition education (Figure 25-3). Although AN and BN are distinct illnesses,

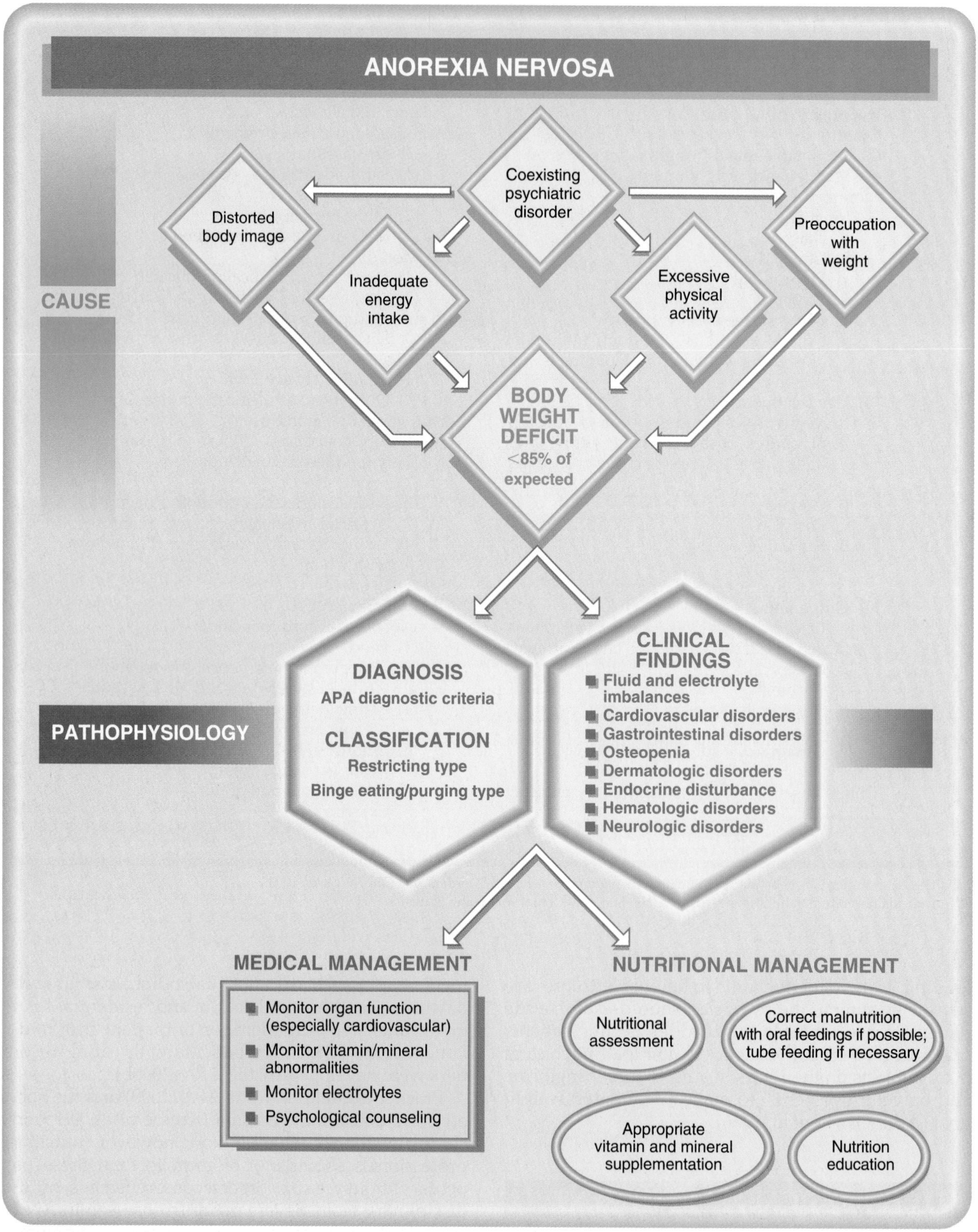

FIGURE 25-3 • Pathophysiology algorithm: anorexia nervosa. (Algorithm content developed by John Anderson, PhD, and Sanford C. Garner, PhD, 2000.)

similarities exist in both the nutritional consequences and nutritional management of the two disorders.

NUTRITIONAL CARE

Anorexia Nervosa

Patients with AN often require hospitalization to begin the refeeding process. Nasogastric tube feedings are occasionally needed, but most AN patients cooperate with oral feedings. The goal of nutritional rehabilitation is positive energy balance that results in weight gain. To accomplish this, energy intake must be gradually increased while energy expenditure is minimized. To improve compliance, "privileges" such as being out of bed, using the telephone, or visiting with friends and family may be combined with weight gain as contingencies in a behavior modification program.

Initial calorie prescriptions are typically in the range of 1000 to 1600 kcal per day or 30 to 40 kcal per kilogram of body weight per day (APA, 2000b). Thereafter, 100- to 200-calorie increases every 2 to 3 days will promote controlled weight gain. The desired rate of weight gain varies among treatment programs and settings. A weight gain of 2 to 3 lb per week is reasonable for hospitalized patients, whereas a gain of 1 lb per week is more attainable in outpatient treatment.

Refeeding malnourished patients with AN can be associated with life-threatening hypophosphatemia, cardiac arrhythmia, and delirium. Patients weighing less than 70% ideal body weight are at particular risk. Initial caloric prescriptions must be low, with small increases thereafter. Supplemental phosphorus may be required immediately on refeeding, and serum phosphorus levels must be closely monitored (Kohn et al, 1998). Cases of refeeding syndrome precipitated by high-calorie prescriptions during inpatient and outpatient treatment have been reported (Fisher et al, 2000). Those who treat severely malnourished patients with AN must be vigilant for the development of this life-threatening complication (see Chapters 23 and 42).

During the course of refeeding, about 70 to 100 kcal per kilogram of body weight daily may be needed for continued weight gain (APA, 2000b). Changes in REE, DIT, and type of tissue gained are all factors. In addition, energy cost of physical activity must be considered. Even though they are markedly underweight and hypometabolic, the total energy expenditure (TEE) of AN patients may be similar to that of normal weight controls (1972 versus 1985 kcal daily). This is attributed to the fact that AN patients expend more energy in physical activity than do control subjects, and they also require more calories for weight maintenance, a mean of 2899 in one study (Pirke et al, 1991), again as a result of excessive activity levels (Casper et al, 1991; Kaye et al, 1988). Anorectics required 8301 ± 2272 kcal (mean ± SD) to gain 1 kg of body weight, and 73% of AN patients had higher levels of physical activity compared with normal volunteers (Kaye et al, 1988). These levels of activity tend to continue after recovery and dictate the need for more calories to maintain the new weight at least in the first few weeks after recovery (Kaye et al, 1988).

In general, caloric prescriptions in the range of 3000 to 4000 kcal per day may be needed later in the course of weight restoration. Patients who require higher energy intakes should be evaluated for discarding food, vomiting, exercising, and increased motor activity (i.e., fidgeting). Metabolic resistance may also contribute to unusually high-energy requirements. To elucidate metabolic causes, indirect calorimetry measurement of both fasting and postprandial metabolic rate can be determined. Once goal weight is attained, an intake of 40 to 60 kcal per kilogram of body weight daily should promote weight maintenance as well as continued growth and development in adolescents (APA, 2000b).

Once the caloric prescription is calculated, a reasonable distribution of macronutrients must be determined (Box 25-6). Patients may express multiple food aversions. Extreme avoidance of dietary fat is common, but continued omission will make it difficult to provide concentrated sources of energy needed for weight restoration. A dietary fat intake in the range of 25% to 30% of calories is recommended. Some patients will accept small amounts of added fat, such as salad dressing or butter. Others do better when the fat source is less obvious, such as in whole milk or peanut butter.

A protein intake in the range of 15% to 20% of total calories is recommended. To ensure adequacy, the minimum protein prescription should equal the recommended dietary allowance (RDA) for age and sex in grams per kilogram of *ideal* body weight (see Table 15-2). Vegetarian diets are often requested but should be discouraged during nutritional rehabilitation.

Carbohydrate intake in the range of 50% to 55% of calories is well tolerated. Sources of insoluble fiber should be included for optimal health but also to relieve the constipation frequently seen in this population.

Although vitamin and mineral supplements are not universally prescribed, the potential for increased needs during anabolic processes must be considered. A vitamin and mineral supplement providing 100% of the RDA is recommended, but iron-containing preparations may aggravate constipation in some patients. Care must be taken throughout the refeeding process to ensure a reasonable variety of intake. Particular attention to the inclusion of calcium-rich foods is recommended because of the increased risk of osteopenia and osteoporosis.

Delayed gastric emptying with complaints of abdominal distention and discomfort after eating are common in AN. In early treatment, caloric intake is generally low and can be tolerated in three meals per day. Snacking may relieve some physical discomfort

Box 25-6. Guidelines for Diet Therapy in Anorexia Nervosa

1. Caloric prescription:
   A. Initial weight gain:
      (1) Start at 30 to 40 kcal/kg/day (approximately 1000 to 1600 kcal/day)
      (2) Assess risk for refeeding syndrome
   B. Controlled weight gain phase:
      (1) Increase prescription in small, progressive increments to promote expected rate of controlled weight gain (e.g., 2-3 lb/wk for inpatients, 0.5-1 lb/wk for outpatients)
      (2) Up to 70 to 100 kcal/kg/day may be required
      (3) If patient requires a higher kcal prescription, evaluate for vomiting, discarding food, increased exercise, increased motor activity, increased REE/DIT
   C. Weight maintenance phase:
      (1) Adults: 40 to 60 kcal/kg/day
      (2) Ongoing growth and development in children/adolescents: 40-60 kcal/kg/day
2. Macronutrients
   A. Protein
      (1) Minimum intake = RDA in g/kg ideal body weight
      (2) 15%-20% kcal
      (3) High biologic value sources
   B. Carbohydrate
      (1) 50%-55% kcal
      (2) Encourage insoluble fiber for treatment of constipation
   C. Fat
      (1) 25%-30% kcal
      (2) Encourage small increases in fat intake until goal can be attained
      (3) Provide source of essential fatty acid
3. Micronutrients
   A. 100% RDA multivitamin with minerals supplement
   B. Note that iron-containing preparations may aggravate constipation

Modified from Luder E, Schebendach J: Nutrition management of eating disorders, *Top Clin Nutr* 8:48, 1993.
RDA, Recommended dietary allowance.

but may result in guilt feelings for indulging between meals. As the caloric prescription increases in late treatment, multiple feedings become unavoidable. At this point, defined formula liquid supplements may be useful (see Appendixes 36 through 39), and products containing 30 to 45 calories per fluid ounce may be prescribed once or twice a day. Because patients are fearful that they will become accustomed to the large amount of food required to fulfill late treatment caloric requirements, liquid feeding is appealing because it can easily be discontinued when goal weight is attained.

Bulimia Nervosa

Bulimia nervosa is described as a state of dietary chaos, characterized by periods of uncontrolled, poorly structured eating, often followed by a period of restrained food intake. The nutritionist's role is to help develop a plan for controlled eating while assessing the patient's need and tolerance for structure.

In bulimia, much of the patient's eating and purging behavior is aimed at weight loss, and he or she will often ask for help in attaining this goal. Although long-term weight loss may be reasonable, the immediate goal should be interruption of the binge-and-purge cycle with stabilization of body weight. Unlike the AN population, patients with BN are hospitalized less frequently, and when hospitalization does occur, it may be a brief admission for the purpose of correcting dehydration and electrolyte imbalance.

Although most patients with bulimia are normal to overweight, they may be hypometabolic, and this must be considered when prescribing the caloric intake. A study of Harris and Benedict–predicted REE versus indirect calorimetry measurement of REE revealed good correlation between predicted and measured values in the AN group but poor correlation in the BN group (Harris and Benedict, 1919; Schebendach et al, 1995).

If a measured REE is obtained, maintenance calories should be prescribed at 120% to 130% of the measured REE. If a measured REE is not available, the patient must be assessed for clinical signs of a hypometabolic state. These may include a history of chronic dieting, a low T_3 level, and cold intolerance. If a low metabolism is suspected, an initial caloric prescription may be equal to 100% of the Harris Benedict–predicted REE. This would cover basal metabolic requirements plus sedentary activity. Typically, this is around 1500 kcal daily.

Body weight should be monitored with a goal of stabilization. If the patient's weight is stabilized on a lower than average caloric intake, small but consistent increases in the caloric prescription should be attempted over time. This may tease up the metabolic rate to a more appropriate level. BN patients need a great deal of encouragement to follow weight-maintenance versus weight-loss diets. They must be reminded that attempts to restrict caloric intake significantly may only increase the risk of binge eating and that their pattern of restrained intake followed by binge eating has not facilitated weight loss in the past (Box 25-7).

A balanced macronutrient intake should be encouraged in patients with BN. This should include sufficient carbohydrate to prevent craving and adequate protein and fat to promote satiety. In general, a balanced diet providing 50% to 55% of the calories

Box 25-7. Guidelines for Nutrition Management of Bulimia Nervosa

1. Caloric prescription: weight maintenance
   A. 1.2-1.3 × measured REE for sedentary activity
   B. If indirect calorimetry measurement is not available, prescribe diet at 100% Harris-Benedict predicted REE as follows:
   Females: 655 + (9.6 × wt in kg) + (1.85 × ht in cm) − (4.7 × age in yr)
   Males: 66 + (13.7 × wt in kg) + (5.0 × ht in cm) − (6.8 × age in yr)
   C. Monitor anthropometric status and adjust caloric prescription for weight maintenance.
   D. Avoid weight reduction diets until eating patterns and body weight are stabilized.
   E. Initial prescriptions are generally around 1500 kcal/day.
2. Macronutrients
   A. Protein
      (1) Minimum intake = RDA in g/kg ideal body weight
      (2) 15%-20% kcal
      (3) High biologic value sources
   B. Carbohydrate
      (1) 50%-55% kcal
      (2) Encourage insoluble fiber for treatment of constipation.
   C. Fat
      (1) 25%-30% kcal
      (2) Provide source of essential fatty acids.
3. Micronutrients
   A. 100% RDA multivitamin with minerals supplement
   B. Note that iron-containing preparation may aggravate constipation.

Modified from Luder E, Schebendach J: Nutrition management of eating disorders. *Top Clin Nutr* 8:48, 1993.
RDA, Recommended dietary allowance; *REE*, resting energy expenditure.

from carbohydrate, 15% to 20% from protein, and 25% to 30% from fat is reasonable. Small amounts of dietary fat should be encouraged at each meal. As is the case with AN, this may be better tolerated when provided in a less obvious manner, such as in peanut butter, cheese, or whole milk.

Bulimic patients are likely to remain on low-calorie intakes for longer periods than their anoretic counterparts. Adequacy of micronutrient intake relative to the caloric prescription and variety of intake should be assessed. A multivitamin–multimineral preparation may be prescribed to ensure adequacy, particularly in the initial phase of treatment.

Bingeing, purging, and restrained intake often impair recognition of hunger and satiety cues in bulimic patients. The cessation of purging behavior, coupled with a reasonable daily distribution of calories at three meals and prescribed snacks, can be instrumental in strengthening these biologic cues. Many patients with BN are afraid to eat earlier in the day, however, fearful that these calories will only contribute to caloric excess if they binge later. Patients may also digress from their meal plan after a binge, attempting to restrict intake to balance out the binge calories. Patience and support are essential in the process of helping bulimic persons to make positive changes in their eating habits.

Monitoring

Guidelines for monitoring the nutritional management of patients with eating disorders are indicated in Box 25-5. The treatment team, patient, and family must be realistic about treatment, which is often a long-term process. Care may be provided in inpatient, day hospital, or outpatient settings. Although outcomes may be favorable, the course of treatment is rarely smooth, and the clinician must be prepared to monitor progress carefully.

NUTRITION EDUCATION

Patients with eating disorders appear quite knowledgeable about nutrition. Despite this, nutrition education is an essential component of their treatment plan. Indeed, some patients spend significant amounts of time reading nutrition-related information, but their sources may be unreliable and their interpretation potentially distorted by their illness. Malnutrition may impair the patient's ability to assimilate and process new information. Early- and mid-adolescent development is characterized by the transition from concrete to abstract operations in problem-solving and directed thinking, and normal developmental issues must be considered when teaching adolescents with eating disorders (see Chapter 11).

Although the interactive process of a group setting may have advantages, these topics can be incorporated effectively into individual counseling sessions as well. Topics for nutrition education are suggested in Box 25-8.

PROGNOSIS

Early and more effective treatment of AN has led to decreased mortality, but follow-up studies suggest that two thirds of patients will have enduring morbid food and weight preoccupation (APA, 2000b). After 6

Box 25-8. Topics for Nutrition Education

1. Impact of malnutrition on growth and development
2. Impact of malnutrition on behavior
3. Set-point theory
4. Metabolic adaptation to dieting
5. Restrained eating and disinhibition
6. Causes of bingeing and purging
7. What does "weight gain" mean?
   A. Glycogen storage
   B. Fluid balance
   C. Lean body mass
   D. Adipose tissue
8. Impact of exercise on caloric expenditure
9. Ineffectiveness of vomiting, laxatives, and diuretics in long-term weight control
10. Portion control
11. Food exchange system
12. Social dining and holiday dining
13. Food Guide Pyramid
14. Hunger and satiety cues
15. Interpreting food labels
16. Nutrition misinformation

Modified from Schebendach J, Nussbaum MP: Nutrition management in adolescents with eating disorders, *Adolesc Med State Art Rev* 3(3):545, 1992.

years of intensive treatment for BN, outcome was reported as good (60%), intermediate (29%), and poor (10%), with death reported in 1% of patients (APA, 2000b). Outcome criteria that include dietary habits; weight and shape ideation; adequate weight for height; menstrual function; and adjustment of sexual, psychological, and social attitudes must be assessed for several years after onset of treatment to identify the extent of recovery.

Nutrition management should promote health, support growth and development, and decrease food conflicts in patients with eating disorders. Although correction of some pathophysiologic consequences (i.e., hypometabolic rate) is well documented, less is known about restoration of others (i.e., loss of brain tissue, osteopenia). It is hoped that nutritional rehabilitation will restore complete health.

When refeeding occurs in an outpatient setting, the treatment team (psychotherapist, nutritionist, physician) should advise both the patient and family about the appropriate degree of parental or spousal involvement. This is critical for maintenance of appropriate boundaries, the containment of manipulative behaviors, and the avoidance of power struggles and control issues. During treatment, both the patient and family benefit from education about all aspects of the disease. Nutrition education may help the patient make more rational and scientifically based decisions regarding food choices. Developmental issues, cognitive abilities, and psychological readiness all must be considered in the design of nutrition education programs.

Clinical Scenario 1: Anorexia Nervosa

Sara is a 13-year-old girl. Her height is 61 inches and her weight is 72 lb. Sara began menstruating at age 12 but has not menstruated for the past 5 months.

Laboratory data: Glucose, 62 mg/dl; albumin, 4.6 g/dl; cholesterol, 240 mg/dl; phosphorus, 2.3 mg/dl; T3-RIA (radioimmune assay), 78 ng/dl; ESR, 2 mm/hr

Anthropometric status: Skin folds: triceps, 4 mm; biceps, 2 mm; subscapular, 5 mm; suprailiac, 4 mm; midarm circumference, 18.0 cm; midarm muscle circumference, 16.7 cm.

Sara's maximum weight was 103 lb 8 months ago. She was concerned that her hips and thighs were fat and started to eliminate snacks and desserts from her diet. Sara was pleased with her "willpower." She then decided to eat heart healthy and excluded all sources of dietary fat. About 5 months ago, Sara eliminated red meat, poultry, and seafood, claiming that a vegetarian diet was a healthier option. As she lost weight, Sara became increasingly more concerned about her body shape and size. Her diet became more restricted in the amount and variety of intake, providing about 650 kcal per day. Sara's family expressed concern about her eating behaviors. She would ritualistically cut small portions of food into many pieces and spend up to an hour consuming one small meal. After eating, Sara expressed considerable guilt about overeating and often cried. Some days she barely ate at all, consuming only large amounts of water and diet soda. Despite her limited caloric intake, Sara's parents were amazed at her energy level. She continued to play soccer (1 to 2 hours daily, 5 days a week), did regular calisthenics (leg lifts and sit-ups, 30 minutes daily), and went running each morning (5 to 7 miles).

1. What are some possible medical complications that Sara may develop secondary to self-starvation?
2. Discuss laboratory values and what you might expect to happen to these indices during refeeding.
3. Determine Sara's ideal body weight, goal weight for treatment, and recommended rate of weight gain.
4. Calculate Sara's initial caloric prescription and discuss how you arrived at this. How might this change over time and why?
5. Plan a sample menu.

SUMMARY

Both AN and BN must be understood to be appreciated as chronic disorders. Family expectation of a quick cure should be dispelled. Likewise, professional staff can also become frustrated by the patient's lack of progress, relapse, and seemingly self-

Clinical Scenario 2: Bulimia Nervosa

Jennifer is a 19-year-old woman. Her height is 65 in. and her weight is 138 lb.

Laboratory data: Glucose, 82 mg/dl; albumin, 4.2 g/dl; cholesterol, 180 mg/dl; potassium, 2.7 mmol/L; serum CO_2, 31 mmol/L

Anthropometric status: Skin folds: triceps, 20 mm; biceps, 7 mm; subscapular, 10 mm; suprailiac, 13 mm; midarm circumference, 26.7 cm; midarm muscle circumference, 20.4 cm.

Jennifer has always been unhappy with her weight. She went on every fad diet throughout high school and lost some weight but always regained it. About 1 year ago, Jennifer began binge eating. Binge episodes now occur three to four times per week. During these binges, Jennifer consumes about 1500 to 2000 kcal in a 2-hour period. Binge foods include ice cream, cookies, potato chips, and other foods. Jennifer describes them as "fattening and unhealthy." After binge eating, Jennifer feels extremely guilty, and vomiting is immediately self-induced. Jennifer always tries to eat as little as possible the next day, sometimes consuming only 700 or 800 kcal. Three months ago, Jennifer started to overdose on laxatives about three times a week. She occasionally uses over-the-counter diet pills, but they never really help. Jennifer feels fat in her abdomen, buttocks, and thighs. Her physical activity includes 100 sit-ups and 100 leg lifts three or four times per week.

1. What are some possible medical complications that Jennifer may develop secondary to binge eating and her compensatory behaviors?
2. Discuss her laboratory values and what you might expect to happen to these indices during rehabilitation.
3. Determine Jennifer's ideal body weight and goal weight for short-term and long-term treatment.
4. Calculate Jennifer's initial caloric prescription and discuss how you arrived at this.
5. Plan a sample menu.
6. Discuss how you would handle those foods Jennifer considers binge "trigger" foods.
7. What would you suggest for Jennifer to help control her episodes of vomiting, laxative use, and diet pill use?

destructive behaviors. Learning to anticipate and accept relapse in the natural course of treatment and recovery may enable the patient, family, and treatment team to maintain a unified effort and optimistic attitude. It is hoped that this will improve outcome.

Relevant Web Sites

Academy for Eating Disorders: For Professionals Working in the Area of Eating Disorders
www.aedweb.org
Association of Anorexia Nervosa and Associated Disorders
www.ANAD.org
National Eating Disorders Association
www.edap.org

Cited References

American Psychiatric Association: *Diagnostic and statistical manual of mental disorders,* ed 3, Washington, DC, 1980, APA Press.

American Psychiatric Association: *Diagnostic and statistical manual of mental disorders,* ed 3, Revised. Washington, DC, 1987, APA Press.

American Psychiatric Association: *Diagnostic and statistical manual of mental disorders,* ed 4, Washington, DC, 1994, APA Press.

American Psychiatric Association: *Diagnostic and statistical manual for mental disorders,* ed 4, text revision, Washington, DC, 2000, APA Press.

American Psychiatric Association: *Practice guideline for the treatment of patients with eating disorders,* ed 2, Washington DC, 2000b, APA Press.

Ammerman S et al: Unique considerations for treating eating disorders in adolescents and preventive intervention, *Top Clin Nutr* 12(1):79, 1996.

Anderson AE: Gender-related aspects of eating disorders: a guide to practice, *J Gender-Spec Med* 2(1): 47, 1999.

Anderson AE et al: Osteoporosis, and osteopenia in men with eating disorders, *Lancet* 355:1967, 2000.

Arden MR et al: Effect of weight restoration on the dyslipoproteinemia of anorexia nervosa, *J Adolesc Health* 11:199, 1990.

Bakan R et al: EM: dietary zinc intake of vegetarian and nonvegetarian patients with anorexia nervosa, *Int J Eating Disord* 13:229, 1993.

Barbosa Saldivar JL, Van Itallie TB: Semistarvation: an overview of an old problem, *Bull NY Acad Med* 55:774, 1979.

Beaumont PJ et al: The diet composition and nutritional knowledge of patients with anorexia nervosa, *J Hum Nutr* 35:265, 1981.

Birmingham CL et al: The reliability of bioelectrical impedance analysis for measuring changes in the body composition of patients with anorexia nervosa, *Int J Eating Disord* 19:311, 1996.

Bryant-Waugh R: Overview of the eating disorders. In Lask B, Bryant-Waugh R, editors: *Anorexia nervosa and related eating disorders in childhood and adolescence,* ed 2, East Sussex, UK, 2000, Psycholology Press.

Casper RC et al: An evaluation of trace metals, vitamins, and taste function in anorexia nervosa, *Am J Clin Nutr* 33:1810, 1980.

Casper RC et al: Total daily energy expenditure and activity level in anorexia nervosa, *Am J Clin Nutr* 53:1143, 1991.

Crisp AH: Some aspects of the evolution, presentation and follow-up of anorexia nervosa, *Proc R Soc Med* 58:814, 1965.

de Zwann M et al: Research on energy expenditure in individuals with eating disorders: a review, *Int J Eating Disord* 31361, 2002.

Detzer MJ et al: Resting metabolic rate in women with bulimia nervosa: a cross-sectional and treatment study, *Am J Clin Nutr* 60:327, 1994.

Durnin JVGA, Rahaman MM: The assessment of the amount of the amount of body fat in the human body from measurements of skinfold thickness, *Br J Nutr* 21:681, 1967.

Durnin JVGA, Womersley J: Body fat assessed from total body density and its estimation from skinfolds thickness: measurements of 481 men and women aged from 16 to 72 years, *Br J Nutr* 32:77, 1974.

Feighner JP et al: Diagnostic criteria for use in psychiatric research, *Arch Gen Psychiatry* 26:57, 1972.

Fernstrom MH et al: Twenty-four hour intake in patients with anorexia nervosa and in healthy control subjects, *Biol Psychiatry* 36:696, 1994.

Fisher M et al: Eating disorders in adolescents: a background paper, *J Adolesc Health* 16:420, 1995.

Fisher M et al: Hypophosphatemia secondary to oral feeding in anorexia nervosa, *Int J Eat Disord* 28:181, 2000.

Grinspoon S et al: Changes in regional fat distribution and the effects of estrogen during spontaneous weight gain in women with anorexia nervosa, *Am J Clin Nutr* 73:865, 2001.

Hadigan CM et al: Assessment of macronutrient and micronutrient intake in women with anorexia nervosa, *Int J Eat Disord* 28(3):284, 2000.

Hardoff D et al: Pathological consequences of eating disorders, *Children's Hospital Quarterly* 3:17, 1991.

Harris JA, Benedict FG: *A biometric study of basal metabolism in man,* Washington, DC, 1919, Carnegie Institute.
Holman RT et al: Patients with anorexia nervosa demonstrate deficiencies of selected fatty acids, compensatory changes in nonessential fatty acids and decreased fluidity of plasma lipids, *J Nutr* 125:901, 1995.
Hsu LKG: Can dieting cause an eating disorder? *Psycol Med* 27:509, 1997.
Katzman DK, Zipursky RB. Adolescents with anorexia nervosa: the impact of the disorder on bones and brains. In Jacobson MS, Rees JM, Golden NH, editors: *Adolescent nutritional disorders,* New York, 1997, New York Academy of Sciences.
Kaye WH et al: Relative importance of calorie intake needed to gain weight and level of physical activity in anorexia nervosa, *Am J Clin Nutr* 47:989, 1988.
Kaye WH et al: Amounts of calories retained after binge eating and vomiting, *Am J Psychiatry* 150:969, 1993.
Keys A et al: *The biology of human starvation,* vols 1 and 2, Minneapolis, 1950, University of Minnesota Press.
Kohn MR et al: Cardiac arrest and delirium: presentations of the refeeding syndrome in severely malnourished adolescents with anorexia nervosa, *J Adolesc Health* 22:239, 1998.
Kotler LA et al: Longitudinal relationships between childhood, adolescent, and adult eating disorders, *J Am Acad Child Adolesc Psychiatry* 40(12):1434, 2001.
Kreipe R et al: Eating disorders in adolescents: a position paper of the Society for Adolescent Medicine, *J Adolesc Health* 16:475, 1995.
Lambert M et al: Hematological changes in anorexia nervosa are correlated with total body fat mass depletion, *Int J Eating Disord* 21:329, 1997.
Langan SM, Farrell PM: Vitamin E, vitamin A and essential fatty acid status of patients hospitalized for anorexia nervosa, *Am J Clin Nutr* 41:1054, 1985.
Lucas A: On the meaning of laboratory values in anorexia nervosa, *Mayo Clin Proc* 52:748, 1977.
Luder E, Schebendach J: Nutrition management of eating disorders, *Top Clin Nutr* 8(3):48, 1993.
Mehler PS et al: Lipid levels in anorexia nervosa, *Int J Eat Disord* 24:217, 1998.
Melchior JC et al: Energy expenditure economy induced by decrease in lean body mass in anorexia nervosa, *Eur J Clin Nutr* 43:793, 1989.
Miller MN, Pumariega AJ: Culture and eating disorders: a historical and cultural review, *Psychiatry* 64(2):93, 2001.
Misra S et al: Regional body composition in adolescents with anorexia nervosa and changes with weight recovery, *Am J Clin Nutr* 77:1361, 2003.
Nicholls D et al: Physical assessment and complications. In Lask B, Bryant-Waugh R, editors: *Anorexia nervosa and related eating disorders in childhood and adolescence,* ed 2, East Sussex, UK, 2000, Psycholology Press.
Nudel DB et al: Altered exercise performance in patients with anorexia nervosa, *J Pediatr* 105:34, 1984.
Obarzanek E et al: Resting metabolic rate of anorexia nervosa patients during weight gain, *Am J Clin Nutr* 60:666, 1994.
Pirke KM et al: Average total energy expenditure in anorexia nervosa, bulimia nervosa, and healthy young women, *Biol Psychiatry* 30:711, 1991.
Polito A et al: Basal metabolic rate in anorexia nervosa: relation to body composition and leptin concentrations, *Am J Clin Nutr* 71:1495, 2000.
Powers PS et al: Athletes and eating disorders: the National Collegiate Athletic Association study, *Int J Eat Disord* 26(20):179, 1996.
Probst M, et al. Body composition in female anorexia nervosa patients, *Br J Nutr* 76:639, 1996.
Probst M et al: Body composition of anorexia nervosa patients assessed by underwater weighing and skin-fold thickness measurements before and after weight gain, *Am J Clin Nutr* 73:190, 2001.
Robin AL, Gilroy M, Dennis AB: Treatment of eating disorders in children and adolescents, *Clin Psychol Rev* 18(4):421, 1998.
Rock CL, Vasantharajan S: Vitamin status of eating disorder patients: relationship to clinical indices and effect of treatment, *Int J Eating Disord* 18:257, 1995.
Russell GFM: The changing nature of anorexia nervosa, *J Psychiatr Res* 19:101, 1985.
Ryan J: *Little girls in pretty boxes: the making and breaking of elite gymnasts and figure skaters,* New York, 1995, Doubleday.
Scalfi L et al: Bioimpedance and resting energy expenditure in undernourished and refed anorectic patients, *Eur J Clin Nutr* 47:61, 1993.
Schebendach J, Nussbaum M: Nutrition management in adolescents with eating disorders. *Adolesc Med State Art Rev* 3(3):545, 1992.
Schebendach J et al: Use of indirect calorimetry in the nutritional management of eating disorders, *Int J Eating Disord* 1:59, 1995.
Schebendach J et al: The metabolic responses to starvation and refeeding in adolescents with anorexia nervosa. In Jacobson MS et al, editors: *Adolescent nutritional disorders: prevention and treatment.* New York: NY Academy of Sciences, 817:110, 1997.
Schebendach J et al: Nutrient quality of diets of adolescents with anorexia nervosa (abst), *J Adolesc Health* 20:151, 1997.
Smith KA et al: Relapse of depression after rapid depletion of tryptophan, *Lancet* 349:915, 1997.
Smith KA et al: Symptomatic relapse in bulimia nervosa following acute tryptophan depletion, *Arch Gen Psychiatry* 56:171, 1999.
Sullivan PF et al: Elevated total cholesterol in bulimia nervosa, *Int J Eating Disord* 23:425, 1998.
Sundgot-Borgen J: Risk and trigger factors for the development of disorders in female elite athletes, *Med Sci Sports Exerc* 26:414, 1994.
Surgenor LJ et al: Links between psychological sense of control and disturbed eating behavior in women with diabetes mellitus: implications for predictors of metabolic control, *J Psychosom Res* 52(3):121, 2002.
Vaisman N et al: Energy expenditure and body composition in patents with anorexia nervosa, *J Pediatr* 113:919, 1988.
Vaisman N et al: Effect of refeeding on the energy metabolism of adolescent girls who have anorexia nervosa, *Eur J Clin Nutr* 45:527, 1991.
Walsh BT et al: Eating behavior of women with bulimia, *Arch Gen Psychiatry* 46:54, 1989.
Wang C et al: Gelatinous transformation of bone marrow from a starch-free diet, *Am J Hematol* 68(1):58, 2001.
Weltzin TE et al: Feeding patterns in bulimia nervosa, *Biol Psychiatry* 30:1093, 1991.
Woodside DB: A review of anorexia nervosa and bulimia nervosa, *Curr Prob Pediatr* 25:67, 1995.

Additional References

American Dietetic Association: Position paper: nutrition intervention in the treatment of anorexia nervosa, bulimia nervosa, and eating disorders not otherwise specified, *J Am Diet Assoc* 101: 810, 2000.
AAP Committee on Sports Medicine and Fitness, *Pediatrics* 106(3): 610, 2000.
Forbes GB et al: Body composition changes during recovery from anorexia nervosa: comparison of two dietary regimens, *Am J Clin Nutr* 40:1137, 1984.
Gwirtsman HE et al: Energy intake and dietary macronutrient content in women with anorexia nervosa and volunteers, *J Am Diet Assoc* 89:54, 1989.
Gwirtsman H et al: Decreased caloric intake in normal weight patients with bulimia: comparison with female volunteers, *Am J Clin Nutr* 49:86, 1989.
Hetherington MM, Rolls BJ: Dysfunctional eating in the eating disorders, *Psychiatr Clin North Am* 24(2):235, 2001.
Iketani T et al: Altered body fat distribution after recovery of weight in patients with anorexia nervosa, *Int J Eat Disord* 26(3):275, 1999.
Jeejeebhoy KN: Nutritional management of anorexia nervosa, *Semin Gastrointest Dis* 9(4):183, 1998.

Kaye W et al: Nutrition, serotonin and behavior in anorexia and bulimia nervosa, *Nestle Nutr Workshop Ser Clin Perform Programme* 5:153, 2001.
Keel PK et al. Long-term outcome of bulimia nervosa, *Arch Gen Psychiatry* 56:63, 1999.
Krahn DD et al: Changes in resting energy expenditure and body composition in AN patients during refeeding, *J Am Diet Assoc* 93:434, 1993.
Levine RL: Endocrine aspects of eating disorders in adolescents, *Adolesc Med* 13:129, 2002.
Lucas AR et al: 50-year trends in the incidence of anorexia nervosa in Rochester, Minn: a population-based study, *Am J Psychiatry* 148:917, 1991.
Mordasini R et al: Secondary type II hyperlipoproteinemia in patients with anorexia nervosa, *Metabolism* 27:71, 1978.
Moyano D et al: Plasma total-homocysteine in anorexia nervosa, *Eur J Clin Nutr* 52:172, 1998.
Piaget J, Inhelder B: *The growth of logical thinking from childhood to adolescence,* New York, 1958, Basic Books.
Sedlet KJ, Ireton Jones CS: Energy expenditure and the abnormal eating pattern of a bulimic: a case report, *J Am Diet Assoc* 89:74, 1989.
Stordy BJ et al: Weight gain, thermic effect of glucose and resting metabolic rate during recovery from anorexia nervosa, *Am J Clin Nutr* 30:138, 1977.
Vaisman N et al: Energy expenditure and body composition in patients with anorexia nervosa, *J Pediatr* 113:919, 1988.
Walker J et al: Caloric requirements for weight gain in anorexia nervosa, *Am J Clin Nutr* 32:1396, 1979.

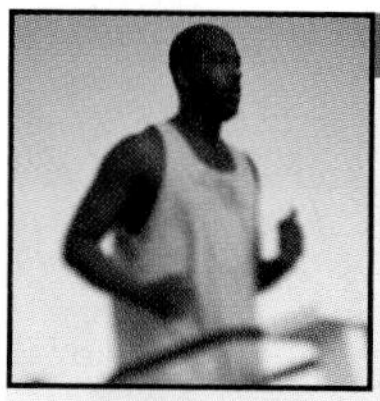

CHAPTER 26

Nutrition for Exercise and Sports Performance

JACQUELINE R. BERNING, PhD, RD

CHAPTER OUTLINE

KEY TERMS

actomyosin–a complex of the proteins actin and myosin occurring in muscle

adenosine diphosphate (ADP)–a nucleotide involved in energy metabolism; it is produced by the hydrolysis of ATP and converted back to ATP by the processes of oxidative phosphorylation

adenosine triphosphate (ATP)–a nucleotide occurring in all cells; it is involved in energy transfer

aerobic metabolism–the transfer of usable energy through oxidative phosphorylation in the respiratory chain in the presence of oxygen

anaerobic metabolism–the production of energy from glucose without the presence of oxygen

creatine phosphate (CP)–an important temporary storage form of high-energy phosphate in muscle cells

ergogenic aid–a substance or practice that increases energy or work output

female athlete triad–a pattern in strenuously exercising athletes of estrogen deficiency and athletic amenorrhea, disordered eating and low body fat, and loss of bone mass

glycemic index–the ratio of the area under the blood glucose curve resulting from ingestion of a given quantity of a carbohydrate and the area under the glucose curve after the ingestion of the same quantity of carbohydrate as glucose or white bread

glycogen–the form of carbohydrate storage in animals

glycogen loading (glycogen supercompensation)–a combination of exercise and high-carbohydrate diet that enables muscles to store glycogen beyond their normal capacity

glycogenolysis–the hydrolysis of glycogen to yield glucose

glycolysis–the breaking down of glucose with or without the presence of oxygen into simpler compounds, chiefly pyruvate or lactate

lactic acid–a product of anaerobic glucose metabolism

mitochondria–spherical components in the cytoplasm of cells that are the principal sites of the generation of energy in the form of ATP; they contain the enzymes of the Krebs and fatty acid cycles and the respiratory pathway

myoglobin–a ferrous protoporphyrin protein similar to hemoglobin but with only one iron atom per molecule instead of four; contributes to the color of muscle and acts as a store of oxygen

respiratory exchange ratio (RER)–the amount of CO_2 produced by the body divided by the amount of O_2 consumed by the body in metabolizing the dietary intake

sports anemia–a transient anemia seen in heavily training athletes characterized by a decrease in the red blood cell count, hemoglobin concentration, and packed cell volume, but with normal red blood cell morphology

thermoregulation–the body's system for maintaining appropriate temperatures by transferring heat from the body core to the skin, where it is dissipated through convection, radiation, sweat production, and evaporation

Vo_2max–a measure of maximal oxygen uptake; liters of O_2 consumed per kilogram of body weight per minute

Now more than ever, the need for accurate sports nutrition information is increasing. Whether the athlete's performance is recreational or elite, it will be influenced by what he or she eats and drinks. Unfortunately, there is much misinformation regarding a proper diet for physically active persons. In the quest for success, many health- and fitness-conscious persons will try any dietary regimen or nutritional supplement in the hope of reaching a new level of wellness or physical performance.

ENERGY PRODUCTION

The human body must be supplied continuously with energy to perform its many complex functions. As a person's energy demands increase with exercise, the body must provide additional energy or the exercise will cease. Two metabolic systems supply energy for the body—one dependent on oxygen (aerobic metabolism) and the other independent of oxygen (anaerobic metabolism). Both systems provide energy; however, the use of one system over the other depends on the duration, intensity, and type of physical activity.

Adenosine Triphosphate

The body obtains its continuous supply of fuel through an energy-rich compound called adenosine triphosphate, or simply ATP, which is the fuel used for all the energy-requiring processes found within the cells of the body. ATP has been called the energy currency of the cell.

The energy produced from the breakdown of ATP provides the fuel that activates the processes of muscle contraction. The energy from ATP is transferred to the contractile filaments (myosin and actin) in the muscle, which form an attachment of actin to the cross-bridges on the myosin molecule, thus forming actomyosin. Once activated, the myofibrils slide past each other and cause the muscle to contract.

Resynthesizing ATP

Although ATP is the main currency for energy in the body, it is stored in limited amounts. In fact, only about 3 oz of ATP is stored in the body at any one time. This provides only enough energy for several seconds of exercise. ATP must continually be resynthesized to provide a constant energy source during exercise. When ATP loses a phosphate, thus releasing energy, the resulting adenosine diphosphate (ADP) is enzymatically combined with another high-energy phosphate from creatine phosphate (CP) to resynthesize ATP. The concentration of high-energy CP in the muscle is five times that of ATP.

Creatine kinase is the enzyme that catalyzes the reaction of CP with ADP and inorganic phosphate to produce creatine and regenerate ATP. It is the fastest and most immediate means of replenishing ATP, and it does so without the use of oxygen *(anaerobic)*. Although this system has great power, it is limited because of the concentration of CP found in the muscles (see *Creatine* on p. 635).

The energy released from this ATP-CP system will sustain an all-out exercise effort for about 5 to 8 seconds, such as in a power lift, tennis serve, or sprint. If the all-out effort continues for longer than 8 seconds, or if moderate exercise is to proceed for longer periods, an additional source of energy must be provided for the resynthesis of ATP (Figure 26-1). The production of ATP carries on within the muscle cells through two important pathways: anaerobic or aerobic metabolism.

Anaerobic or Lactic Acid Pathway

Another rapid pathway for supplying ATP for more than a few seconds is the process of anaerobic glycolysis. In this pathway the energy in glucose is released without the presence of oxygen. Lactic acid is the end product of anaerobic glycolysis. Without the production of lactic acid, glycolysis would shut down. A coenzyme called nicotinic acid dehydrogenase (NAD) is in limited supply in this pathway. When NAD is limited, the glycolytic pathway cannot provide constant energy. By converting pyruvic acid to lactic acid, NAD is freed to participate in further ATP synthesis. The amount of ATP furnished is relatively small (the process is only 30% efficient). This pathway contributes energy during an all-out effort lasting up to 60 to 120 seconds. Examples would be a 440-yard sprint and many sprint swimming events.

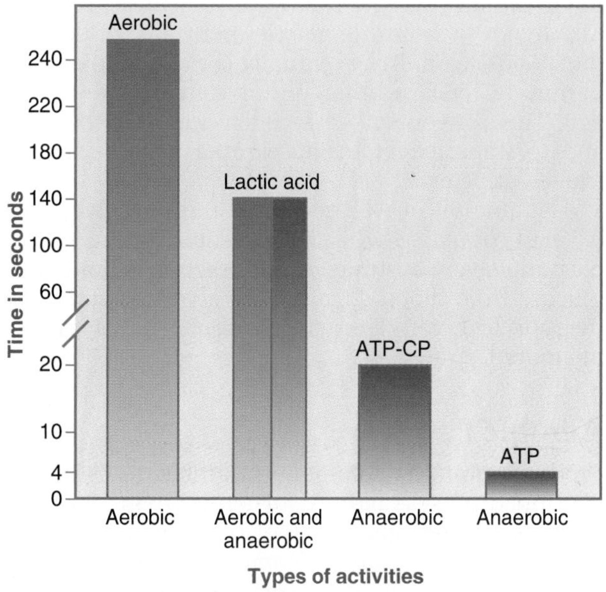

FIGURE 26-1 • Classification of activities based on duration of performance and the predominant pathways of energy production.

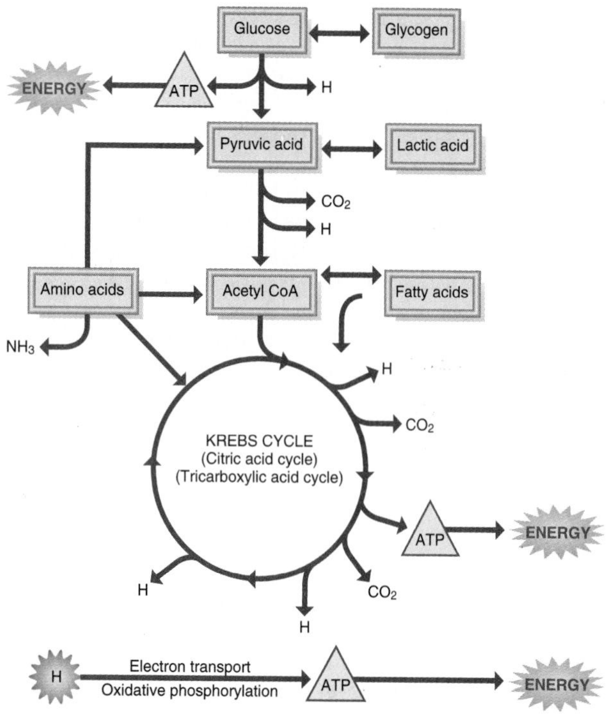

FIGURE 26-2 • Pathways of energy production. *H*, Hydrogen atoms; *ATP*, adenosine triphosphate; *CoA*, coenzyme A.

Although this process provides immediate protection from the consequences of insufficient oxygen, it cannot continue indefinitely. When exercise continues at intensities beyond the body's ability to supply oxygen and convert lactic acid to fuel, lactic acid accumulates in the blood, eventually lowering the pH to a level that interferes with enzymatic action, leading to fatigue. Research shows that lactic acid is rapidly removed from the muscle and transported into the bloodstream. It is eventually converted to energy in muscle, liver, or brain, or it is converted to glycogen. This conversion to glycogen occurs in the liver and to some extent in muscle, particularly among trained athletes.

The amount of ATP produced through glycolysis is small compared with that available through aerobic pathways. Substrate for this reaction is limited to glucose from blood sugar or the glycogen stored in the muscle. Liver glycogen contributes but is limited in amount.

Aerobic Pathway

Production of ATP in amounts sufficient to support continued muscle activity for longer than 90 to 120 seconds requires the input of oxygen. If sufficient oxygen is not present to combine with hydrogen, in the electron transport chain, then no further ATP is forthcoming. Therefore, the oxygen furnished through the process of respiration is of vital importance.

In the aerobic pathway, glucose can be broken down far more efficiently for energy, producing 18 to 19 times more ATP. In the presence of oxygen, pyruvate is converted to acetyl coenzyme A (CoA), which enters the mitochondria. In the mitochondria, acetyl CoA goes through the Krebs cycle, which generates 36 to 38 ATP per molecule of glucose (Figure 26-2).

The aerobic pathway can also provide ATP by metabolizing fats and proteins. Beta-oxidation of fatty acids derived from lipolysis provides a large amount of acetyl CoA, which enters the Krebs cycle and provides enormous amounts of ATP. Proteins may be catabolized into acetyl CoA or Krebs cycle intermediates, or they may be directly oxidized as another source of ATP.

Aerobic metabolism is limited by the availability of substrate, a continuous and adequate supply of oxygen, and the availability of coenzymes. At the onset of exercise and with the increase in exercise intensity, the capability of the cardiovascular system to supply adequate oxygen becomes a limiting factor, and this is largely due to the level of conditioning.

Energy Continuum

Although each of the preceding systems produces ATP for the exercising muscle, a person who is exercising may use one or more energy pathways for the physical activity. For example, at the beginning of any physical activity, ATP is produced anaerobically. As exercise continues, the lactic acid system is producing ATP for exercise. If the person continues to exercise and does so at a moderate intensity for a prolonged period, the aerobic pathway will become the dominant pathway for fuel. On the other hand, the anaerobic pathway provides most of the energy for short-duration, high-intensity exercise, such as sprinting; the 200-m swim; or high-power, high-intensity moves in basketball, football, or soccer.

The production of ATP for exercise is on a continuum that depends on the availability of oxygen. Other factors that influence oxygen capabilities, and thus energy pathways, are the capacity for intense exercise and its duration. These two factors are inversely related. For example, an athlete cannot perform high-power, high-intensity moves over a prolonged period. To do this, he or she would have to decrease the intensity of the exercise to increase the duration (Figure 26-3).

The aerobic pathway cannot tolerate the same level of intensity as the duration increases because of the decreased availability of oxygen and accumulation of lactic acid. As the duration of exercise increases, power output decreases. The contribution of energy-yielding nutrients must be considered also. As the duration of exercise lengthens, the contribution of fats as an energy source becomes greater. The opposite is true for high-intensity exercise. As intensity increases, the body relies increasingly on carbohydrate as its fuel source.

Duration of maximal exercise	Seconds			Minutes						
	10	30	60	2	4	10	30	60	120
Anaerobic (%)	90	80	70	50	35	15	5	2	1
Aerobic (%)	10	20	30	50	65	85	95	98	99

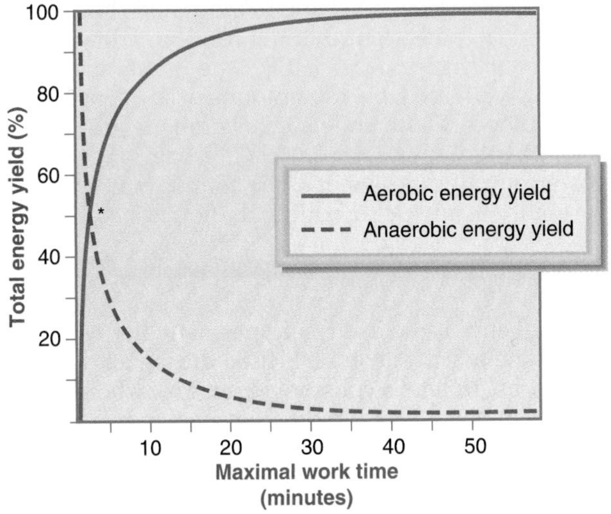

FIGURE 26-3 • Relative contribution of aerobic and anaerobic energy during maximal physical activity of various durations. Note that 90 to 120 seconds of maximal effort requires 50% of the energy from each of the aerobic and anaerobic processes. This will also be the point when the lactic acid pathway for energy production will be at its maximum.

FUELS FOR CONTRACTING MUSCLES

Sources of Fuel

Proteins, fats, and carbohydrates are all possible sources of fuel for muscle contraction. The glycolytic pathway is restricted to glucose, which can originate in dietary carbohydrates or stored glycogen, or it can be synthesized from the carbon skeletons of certain amino acids through the process of gluconeogenesis. The Krebs cycle is fueled by three-carbon fragments of glucose; two-carbon fragments of fatty acids; and carbon skeletons of specific amino acids, primarily alanine and the branched-chain amino acids. All these substrates can be used during exercise; however, the intensity and duration of the exercise determine the relative rates of substrate utilization.

Substrate Choice

A variety of factors determine which type of fuel the muscle will use during exercise. These include the intensity and duration of the exercise, the fitness level of the individual, and the dietary intake.

Intensity

The intensity of the exercise is particularly important in determining what fuel will be used by contracting muscles. High-intensity, short-duration exercise has to rely on anaerobic production of ATP. Because oxygen is not available for aerobic pathways, only glucose and glycogen can be broken down anaerobically for fuel. When glycogen is broken down anaerobically, it is used 18 to 19 times faster than when glucose is broken down aerobically. Persons who are performing in high-intensity workouts or competitive races may run the risk of running out of muscle glycogen before the event or exercise is done as a result of its high utilization.

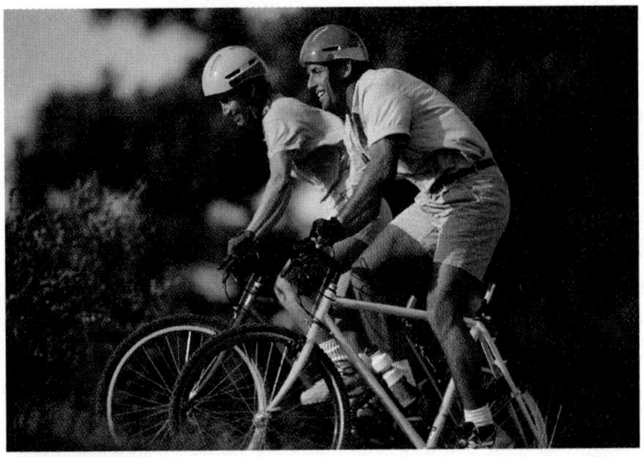

FIGURE 26-4 • Cycling is a moderate form of exercise that uses both carbohydrate and fat as fuel sources. (From PhotoDisc.)

Sports that use both the anaerobic and aerobic pathways also have a higher glycogen utilization rate and, like anaerobic athletes, athletes in these sports also run the risk of running out of fuel before the race or exercise is finished. Sports like basketball, football, soccer, and swimming are good examples of activities in which athletes have a higher glycogen utilization rate because of their intermittent bursts of high-intensity sprints and running drills. In moderate-intensity sports or exercise like jogging, hiking, aerobic dance, gymnastics, cycling (Figure 26-4), and recreational swimming, about half of the energy for these activities comes from the aerobic breakdown of muscle glycogen, whereas the other half comes from circulating blood glucose and fatty acids.

Moderate- to low-intensity exercise, such as walking, is fueled entirely by the aerobic pathway; thus, a greater proportion of fat can be used to create ATP for energy. Fatty acids cannot supply ATP during high-intensity exercise because fat cannot be broken down fast enough to provide the energy. Also, fat provides less energy per liter of oxygen consumed than does glucose (4.65 kcal/L of O_2 versus 5.01 kcal/L of O_2). Therefore, when less oxygen is available in high-intensity activities, there is a definite advantage for the muscles to be able to use glycogen because less oxygen is required to produce energy from glycogen.

In general, both glucose and fatty acids provide fuel for exercise in proportions depending on the intensity and duration of the exercise and the fitness of the athlete. Exertion of extremely high-intensity and short duration draws primarily on reserves of ATP and CP. High-intensity exercise that continues for more than a few seconds depends on anaerobic glycolysis. During exercise of low to moderate intensity (≤60% of maximal oxygen uptake, $\dot{V}O_2max$), energy is derived mainly from fatty acids. Carbohydrate becomes a larger fraction of the energy source as intensity increases until, at an intensity level of 85% to 90% $\dot{V}O_2max$, carbohydrate from glycogen is the principal energy source and the duration of activity is limited (Figure 26-5).

Duration

How long the activity lasts also determines what substrate is used during the exercise bout. For example, the longer the time spent exercising, the greater the contribution of fat as the fuel. Fat can supply up to 60% to 70% of the energy needs for ultraendurance events lasting 6 to 10 hours. As the duration of exercise increases, the reliance on aerobic metabolism becomes greater and a greater amount of ATP can be produced from fatty acids. It must be noted, however, that fat cannot be metabolized unless carbohydrate is available. Therefore, muscle glycogen and blood glucose are the limiting factors in human performance of any type of intensity or duration.

Effect of Training

The length of time an athlete can oxidize fatty acids as a fuel source is related to the athlete's conditioning as well as the exercise intensity. In addition to improving cardiovascular systems involved in oxygen delivery, training increases the number of mitochondria and the levels of enzymes involved in the aerobic synthesis of ATP, thus increasing the capacity for fatty acid metabolism. Increases in mitochondria with aerobic training are seen mainly in the type IIA (intermediate fast-twitch) muscle fibers. These fibers quickly lose their aerobic capacity with the cessation of aerobic training, reverting to the genetic baseline.

These changes from training result in a lower respiratory exchange ratio (RER), the amount of CO_2 produced divided by the amount of O_2 consumed; lower blood lactate and catecholamine levels, and a breakdown of lower net muscle glycogen at a certain power output. These metabolic adaptations enhance the ability of muscle to oxidize all fuels, especially fat.

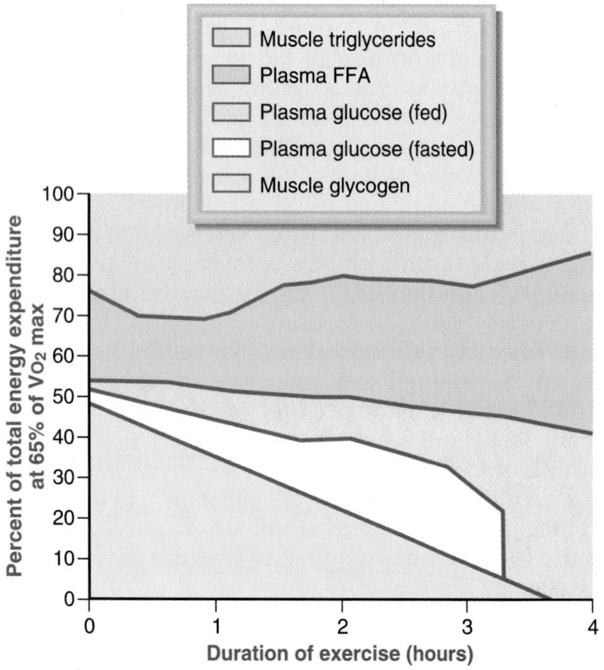

FIGURE 26-5 • Sources of energy during 4 hours of exercise.

Diet

The makeup of the exercising person's diet will also determine which substrate is used during an exercise bout. If an athlete is consuming a high-carbohydrate diet, he or she will use more glycogen as fuel for the exercise. If the diet is high in fat, more fat will be oxidized as a fuel source. This does not mean the athlete or exercising person should consume a high-fat diet. Even the leanest athlete has more than enough fat stored in his or her body to fuel any long or endurance exercise (see *Focus On:* The 40-30-30 Diet).

Eating more fat, especially saturated fat, can increase a person's risk for heart disease and other lifestyle diseases associated with high-fat diets. The goal is to increase the availability of fat as a fuel during exercise. The proper way to do that is by training, not by consuming a high-fat diet. Persons who have tried to perform on high-fat diets find that their performance suffers because of lower glycogen stores. Glycogen stores are limited because the amount of carbohydrate consumed in the diet is limited. Low muscle glycogen stores limit endurance and the ability of the athlete to perform high-intensity exercise, which may occur during a competition.

NUTRITIONAL REQUIREMENTS OF EXERCISE

Fluid

Proper fluid balance maintains blood volume, which in turn supplies blood to the skin for body temperature regulation. Because exercise produces heat, which must be eliminated from the body to maintain appropriate body temperatures, regular fluid intake is essential for maintaining a body temperature that maximizes performance.

The human body is not efficient at converting potential energy from oxygen and nutrients into mechanical energy. During exercise only about one fourth of this potential energy is converted into mechanical energy, resulting in about 75% of the energy turnover generated as heat. Most of the heat gener-

FOCUS ON

The 40-30-30 Diet

A popular sports nutrition dietary fad revolves around the myth that high-carbohydrate diets impair athletic performance and make athletes fat. Proponents of this dietary regimen believe that food has a tremendous impact on the complex hormonal systems that help control physiologic processes within the body—processes such as cellular oxygen transfer, maintenance of blood glucose, and regulation of body fat.

Athletes must supposedly eat the perfect ratio of protein, carbohydrate, and fat at each meal and snack to control these hormonal systems and thus reach their maximum performance and ideal weight. This "perfect ratio" consists of 40% carbohydrate, 30% protein, and 30% fat at each meal and snack. Proponents claim that this diet promotes optimal athletic performance and health by altering the production of eicosanoids so that the body makes more "good" eicosanoids than "bad" ones. A balanced production of eicosanoids regulates the local tissue response to stimulatory events (see Chapters 3 and 44 for a discussion of eicosanoids).

The carbohydrate/protein/fat ratio of the 40-30-30 diet allegedly maintains the proper balance between the hormones insulin and glucagon. The correct insulin-glucagon balance in turn supposedly increases the production of "good" eicosanoids that inhibit platelet aggregation, promote vasodilation, and are antiinflammatory. Proponents of the diet recommend limiting carbohydrate to keep the body from producing too much insulin because high insulin levels allegedly increase the production of "bad" eicosanoids. Prostaglandin-E_2, thromboxanes, and leukotrienes are supposedly "bad" eicosanoids because they promote platelet aggregation and vasoconstriction and are proinflammatory. "Bad" eicosanoids and high insulin levels purportedly impair athletic performance by reducing oxygen transfer to the cells, lowering blood glucose levels, and interfering with body fat utilization.

Proponents of the 40-30-30 diet also claim that insulin makes it hard for people to stay or become thin. Basically, insulin is treated as the "monster" hormone that makes people fat. Insulin supposedly does this by taking carbohydrate and storing it as fat rather than allowing the body to use it for energy.

Protein supposedly increases glucagon levels, and glucagon helps to increase the production of "good" eicosanoids by opposing the effect of insulin. Protein then, along with carbohydrate in a meal or snack, promotes this "glucagon favorable diet," which supposedly maintains blood glucose, increases endurance by increasing fatty acid utilization, and reduces body fat by increasing the utilization of stored fat.

The scientific basis for this diet for athletes can be faulted on many fronts, beginning with the claim that high-carbohydrate diets increase insulin levels, thereby causing low blood glucose and suppressing fat mobilization. During exercise, serum glucose levels increase while serum insulin levels fall. This occurs because of the exercise-induced rise in the catecholamines (epinephrine and norepinephrine) and growth hormone, which inhibits the release of insulin from the pancreas. This enhances liver glucose output by making the liver more sensitive to the effects of glucagon and epinephrine. The hormonal changes that occur during exercise prompt greater fat oxidation.

Endurance training also causes several major adaptations in the muscles that increase fat utilization. First, endurance training increases the number of capillaries in the trained muscles so that the muscles receive more blood and oxygen. Second, endurance training increases the activity of the specific muscle enzymes that are responsible for burning fat. Third, endurance training increases tissue insulin sensitivity, resulting in lower plasma insulin levels.

The claim that a high-carbohydrate diet promotes greater body fat storage is also unfounded. Insulin is not a "monster" hormone—it is required for the transport of glucose into the body's cells, where it is used to fuel all activities. Insulin-mediated glucose uptake is also necessary for muscle and liver glycogen synthesis—the primary fuel for endurance exercise.

The 40-30-30 diet does not improve access to the body's fat stores so that more fat is burned during exercise. Carbohydrate, not fat, is the preferred energy source during exercise at or above 70% of $\dot{V}O_2max$—the intensity at which most endurance athletes train and compete. Athletes do not usually work out long enough to burn significant amounts of fat during exercise. Rather, it is the caloric deficit resulting from the exercise session that promotes body fat utilization; and, as for gradual loss of body fat, that comes from burning more calories than are consumed at the table, not from some special dietary ratio. Because endurance training already creates a metabolic milieu favorable for fat metabolism, the best way to crank up the body's fat-burning ability is to keep working out.

A small study of male athletes following the 40-30-30 (Zone) diet for 7 days showed that besides a significant reduction in energy intake (about 400 kcal) in those following the diet compared with controls, the time to exhaustion was significantly decreased in performance trials. The authors of the study conclude that based on their work, this nutritional strategy should not be adopted by athletes (Jarvis et al, 2002).

No doubt, what a person eats and drinks can affect his or her health, body weight, recovery, and ultimately human performance. By obtaining sound credible sports nutrition advice from a qualified nutrition expert in the field, athletes and active persons can maximize their athletic potential.

Content developed by Ellen Coleman, MS, MPH, RD.

ated by exercising muscle transfers to the blood, circulates through the body, and raises core temperature. The amount of heat produced during exercise, even in physically fit persons, is enough to raise core body temperatures by 1° C every 5 to 8 minutes. Without effective means to dissipate this heat, moderate-intensity exercise could raise body temperatures to lethal levels in 15 to 30 minutes.

The body maintains appropriate temperatures by means of a system referred to as thermoregulation. As heat is generated in the muscles during exercise, it is transferred via the blood to the body's core. Increased core temperature results in increased blood flow to the skin, where, in cool to moderate ambient temperatures, heat is transferred to the environment by convection, radiation, and evaporation.

Environmental conditions have a large impact on thermoregulation. When ambient temperatures range from warm to hot, the body must dissipate the heat generated from exercise as well as the heat absorbed from the environment. When this occurs, the body relies solely on the evaporation of sweat to maintain appropriate body temperatures. Thus, maintaining hydration becomes crucial when ambient temperatures reach or exceed 36° C. The hotter the temperature, the more important sweating is for body heat dissipation.

Humidity also affects the body's ability to dissipate heat to a greater extent than air temperatures. As humidity increases, the rate at which sweat evaporates decreases, which means more sweat drips off the body without transferring heat from the body to the environment. Combining the effects of a hot, humid environment with a large metabolic heat load produced during exercise taxes the thermoregulatory system to its maximum. Ensuring proper and adequate fluid intake is key to reducing the risk of heat stress.

Fluid Balance

The body fluid of healthy persons is conserved on a daily basis by factors that control the intake and output of both water and electrolytes. *Antidiuretic hormone* (vasopressin; ADH) and the renin–angiotensin–aldosterone system are hormonal control mechanisms that maintain the osmolality, sodium content, and volume of extracellular fluids and play a major role in the regulation of fluid balance.

There is loss of water from the skin and respiratory tract that is continuous, plus losses from the kidneys and gastrointestinal tract, which are intermittent. When fluid is lost from the body in the form of sweat, plasma volume decreases and plasma osmolality increases. The kidneys, under hormonal control, regulate water and solute excretion in excess of the obligatory urine loss. However, when the body is subjected to hot environments, whether the heat load is imposed internally or externally, certain hormonal adjustments occur to maintain body function. The body begins by trying to conserve both water and sodium. The pituitary gland releases ADH to increase water absorption from the kidneys, which causes the urine to become more concentrated, thus conserving fluid and making the urine a dark gold color.

This feedback process helps to conserve body water and blood volume. At the same time, *aldosterone* is released from the adrenal cortex and acts on the renal tubules to increase the reabsorption of sodium, which helps maintain the correct osmotic pressure. These reactions also activate thirst mechanisms in the body. However, in situations where water losses are increased acutely, such as in athletic workouts or competition, the thirst response can be delayed, making it difficult for athletes to trust their thirst to ingest enough fluid to offset the volume of fluid lost during training and competition. A loss of 1.5 to 2 L of fluid is necessary before the thirst mechanism kicks in, and this level of water loss already has a serious effect on temperature control. Athletes need to rehydrate on a timed basis rather than as a reaction to thirst, and it should be enough to maintain the preexercise weight.

It appears that plain water is not the best beverage to consume following exercise to replace the water lost as sweat. The replacement of electrolytes, particularly sodium, as well as water is essential for effective rehydration. If sufficient amounts of sodium and water are ingested, plasma osmolality and sodium concentration do not decline, as may occur if plain water is ingested. As a result, the circulating levels of vasopressin and aldosterone are maintained, and the excess urine output that would otherwise occur, even though the body is still in net negative fluid balance, is prevented.

Also, when there are no restrictions on fluid intake, maintenance of the plasma osmolality and the circulating sodium concentration plays an important role in maintaining the drive to drink, thus ensuring that an adequate volume of fluid is consumed. Several researchers (Costill and Sparks, 1973; Gonzalez-Alonso, Heaps, and Coyle, 1992; Nose et al, 1988) have found that rehydration with water alone dilutes the blood rapidly, increases its volume, and stimulates urine output. Blood dilution lowers both sodium and the volume-dependent part of the thirst drive, thus removing much of the drive to drink and replace fluid losses.

Another electrolyte that is involved with maintaining body fluids is potassium. Potassium is the major ion of the intracellular fluid. As the major electrolyte inside the body's cells, potassium works in close association with sodium and chloride in the maintenance of body fluids and in the generation of electrical impulses in the nerves and the muscles, including the heart. Potassium balance, like sodium balance, is also regulated by aldosterone. Potassium regulation in the body is precise, and deficiencies are rare, although they may occur during fasting, episodes of diarrhea, and diuretic use.

Most researchers agree that there is little loss of potassium through sweat. Nevertheless, it has been suggested that inclusion of potassium in beverages consumed after sweat loss may aid in the movement of water into the intracellular spaces in rehydration (Cunningham, 1997; Nadel et al, 1990).

Fluid Absorption

Most athletes believe that as soon as they ingest a fluid, it is rehydrating their system; however, the speed at which fluid is absorbed depends on a number of different factors, including the amount, type and osmolality of the fluid consumed and the rate of gastric emptying.

The proximal small intestine (duodenum and jejunum) is the primary site of fluid absorption. About 50% to 60% of any given fluid load is absorbed. The colon absorbs about 80% to 90% of the fluid it receives but accounts for only about 15% of the total fluid load. Intestinal fluid absorption is a passive process and can occur against an osmotic gradient. The intestinal mucosa is a semipermeable membrane with relatively large aqueous channels. Thus, in the presence of an osmotic gradient, there is a large and rapid movement of water across the duodenojejunum, compared with only a modest water flux across the colon (Gisolfi et al, 1990).

Water-soluble electrolytes such as sodium can also move rapidly across the proximal intestines. Water movement occurs passively and generally depends on solute absorption. For example, if solute absorption is zero, water absorption is zero. Leiper and Maughan (1986b), however, found that the perfusion of a hypotonic solution through the jejunum increases water absorption with increasing solute absorption. This finding suggests that the greater the osmotic gradient, the greater the water movement from the intestinal lumen to the blood. It is also true that, although water movement is usually passive, water can be absorbed against a concentration gradient.

Glucose and Sodium

Because glucose is actively absorbed in the intestines, it can markedly increase both sodium and water absorption. It has been known for more than 70 years that the small intestine absorbs certain hexoses faster than it absorbs others. The first suggestion of selectivity of the intestinal membrane for simple sugars was made by Cori (1926), who found that sugars disappeared from the intestine at strikingly different rates (e.g., galactose ≥ glucose ≥ fructose ≥ mannose ≥ xylose ≥ arabinose).

It has been established that galactose and glucose are actively absorbed against a concentration gradient and that fructose, mannose, xylose, and arabinose are not. The glucose and sodium associate with a carrier in the microvilli on the intestinal cell. The complex travels to the inner side of the membrane, where it disassociates, releasing the glucose and sodium. The sodium is then actively transported out of the cell, and the glucose is emptied into the bloodstream. It appears that the sodium ion attaches to the carrier first, changing the configuration of the carrier and allowing the glucose molecule to attach for transfer across the membrane; then it assumes another shape when the site accommodates potassium going out of the cell.

Early studies indicate that water absorption is maximized when luminal glucose concentrations range from 1% to 3% (55 to 140 mM) (Malawer, 1965); however, most sport drinks contain two to three times this quantity without causing adverse gastrointestinal symptoms. If the concentration of glucose in the lumen reaches 10% (550 mOsm), it can cause fluid secretions and gastrointestinal distress (Gisolfi, 2000).

A recent comparison of the rates of absorption of popular sport drinks with water showed that fluid absorption rates for water and a 6% carbohydrate sport drink were similar (Ryan et al, 1998). Sport drinks with higher concentrations of carbohydrate (8% or 9%) had slower absorption rates and should not be used. To determine the concentration of carbohydrate in a sport drink, the grams of carbohydrate or sugar in a serving is divided by the weight of a serving of the drink, which is usually 240 g, the approximate weight of 1 cup of water. A 6% carbohydrate drink contains 14 to 16 g of carbohydrate per 8 oz (1 cup) of drink (Figure 26-6).

Osmolality

Sport drinks are hypertonic, isotonic, or hypotonic. Some evidence indicates that hypotonic solutions are more efficacious in maximizing water absorption than isotonic solutions (Leiper and Maughn, 1986a, b). Although exercise produces a condition of hypertonic dehydration that may favor fluid absorption from a hypotonic solution, this concept requires further investigation in human subjects.

Fluid Requirements

Short-Duration Events

Athletes who participate in short-duration events often believe they are not exposed to the heat stress to which endurance athletes are exposed and that they do not need to worry about fluid consumption or hydration. However, athletes who participate in short-duration activities, such as sprint running in track and field or stop-and-go sports like basketball, volleyball, or baseball, are just as likely to develop dehydration as are distance runners or ultramarathoners. Although many athletes, like sprinters, have short-duration events, they may have to run several heats before making a championship event, thus exposing themselves to both environmental and internal heat stresses. All participants in physical activity or sports should be educated about the guidelines of drinking fluids to prevent dehydration.

It was once thought that if the physical activity were less than an hour, water would be the best choice for fluid replacement; however, researchers

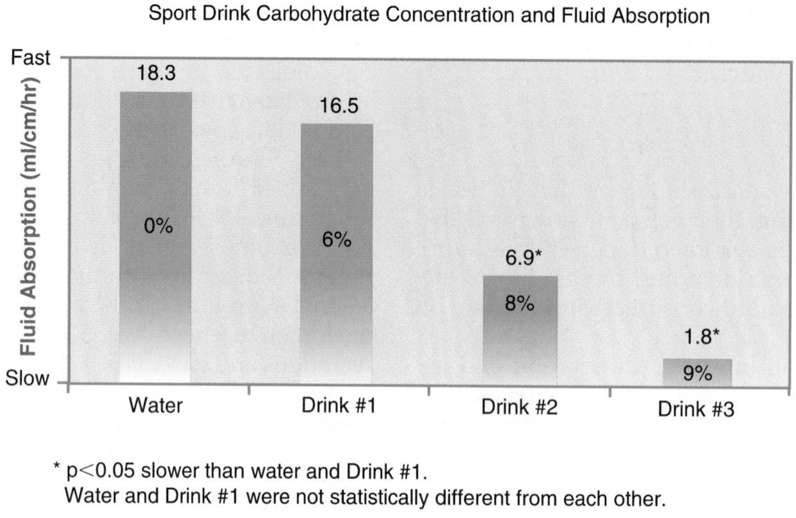

FIGURE 26-6 • Intestinal absorption of sports drinks based on carbohydrate concentration. (Modified from Ryan AJ et al: Effect of hypohydration on gastric emptying and intestinal absorption during exercise, *J Appl Physiol* 84:1581, 1998.)

(Jackson et al, 1995) are finding that using a sport drink during high-intensity stop-and-go sports like basketball, volleyball, and sprint cycling helps delay fatigue and maintains hydration. Unfortunately, athletes who just consume water as a fluid replacement, even for short-term exercise, risk the chance of diluting the blood and increasing urine output, thus shutting off the drive to drink and becoming dehydrated.

Young children are more likely to participate in physical activities that are less than 60 minutes in duration. Many youth soccer, t-ball, and basketball games are less than 60 minutes in duration. Children, like adults, do not drink enough when offered fluids ad libitum during exercise in hot and humid climates; but children differ from adults in that for any given level of dehydration, children's core temperatures rise faster than those of adults, putting them at far greater risk for heat stress. Children who participate in sports activities must be taught to prevent dehydration by drinking above and beyond thirst and drinking at frequent intervals, for example, every 20 minutes (Bar-Or, 2001).

A rule of thumb is that a child 10 years of age or younger should drink until he or she does not feel thirsty and then should drink an additional half a glass (⅓ to ½ cup). Older children and adolescents should follow the same guidelines; however, they should consume an additional cup of fluid (8 oz). When relevant, regulations for competition should be modified to allow children to leave the playing field periodically to drink.

Other concerns with children are the palatability of the drink and its ability to stimulate further thirst. Prepubertal and early pubertal girls and boys prefer grape flavor to apple and orange flavors in sport drinks. This preference is apparent at rest, following a maximal exercise bout, and during rehydration after prolonged exercise in hot, dry conditions (Meyer et al, 1994). One of the hurdles to getting children to consume fluids is to provide fluids they like. Providing them a sport drink that will maintain the drive to drink and rehydrate them is the key to preventing active children from becoming dehydrated.

Box 26-1. Guidelines for Proper Hydration

Monitor fluid losses: Weigh in before and after practice, especially during hot weather and the conditioning phase of the season.

For each pound lost during exercise, drink 3 c of fluid.

Do not restrict fluids before, during, or after the event.

Do not rely on thirst as an indicator of fluid losses.

Before Exercise

Drink 400-600 ml (14-22 oz) of fluid at least 2 hr before the start of exercise.

During Exercise

Drink 150-350 ml (6-12 oz) of fluid every 15-20 min

After Exercise

Drink 450-675 ml (16-24 oz) of fluid for every pound of body weight lost during exercise.

If an athlete is participating in multiple workouts in 1 day, then 80% of fluid loss must be replaced before the next workout.

Data from American Dietetic Association, Dietitians of Canada, and the American College of Sports Medicine: Nutrition and athletic performance—Position statement, *J Am Diet Assoc* 100:1543, 2000; Casa DJ et al: National Atheletic Trainers Association: Position statement—Fluid replacement for athletes, *J Athletic Training* 35:212, 2000.

Box 26-1 gives the fluid recommendations from the American Dietetic Association (ADA) position paper on Sports Nutrition as well as the position paper on fluids and hydration from the National Athletic Trainers (Casa et al, 2001). These guidelines emphasize the importance of an aggressive fluid-replacement plan designed to prevent even slight dehydration during training and competition and also suggest the use of a 6% to 8% carbohydrate concentration sport drinks in events lasting longer than 30 minutes.

Endurance Events

Marathoners talk of "hitting the wall." Cyclists speak of "bonking." Both groups attribute their fatigue in long events to drained fuel stores. Along with replacing fluids, athletes who participate in activities that last longer than an hour also need to be concerned about supplying the brain and muscles with a continuous supply of carbohydrate for energy.

When exercise lasts longer than an hour, blood glucose levels start to dwindle. After 1 to 3 hours of continuous cycling, running, or swimming at 65% to 80% of maximum effort, or after repeated bouts of intense sprinting at 85% or more of maximum effort, muscle glycogen stores may become depleted. In addition, if only water is being consumed, blood glucose levels may be extremely low *(hypoglycemia)*, and this will result in higher use of muscle glycogen. When muscle glycogen levels are low and blood glucose levels have dropped, no matter how fast an athlete wants to go, the body cannot respond, and the athlete "hits the wall" or runs out of available fuel.

The liver generally supplies glucose to maintain blood sugar for proper functioning of the central nervous system. As muscles run out of glycogen, they begin to take up glucose that is available in the blood, placing a drain on the liver glycogen stores. The longer the exercise bout, the greater the utilization of blood glucose by the muscles for energy. It appears that carbohydrate feedings improve performance by maintaining blood glucose levels at a time when muscle glycogen stores are diminished. This allows carbohydrate utilization and energy production to continue at high rates.

Athletes can help maintain the supply of energy by consuming about 26 to 30 g of carbohydrate every half-hour during exercise. Because most 8- to 12-oz servings of sport drinks provide about 15 to 20 g of carbohydrate, drinking 8 to 12 oz every 15 minutes should help to fight off the fatigue that occurs when the muscles and liver run out of glycogen.

Macronutrient Distribution

An athlete's energy and nutrient requirements vary with weight, height, age, sex, and metabolic rate and with the type, frequency, intensity, and duration of training. Because the emotional and physical stress of training and competition, combined with hectic travel schedules, affects dietary intake, adequate caloric and essential nutrient intake must be planned carefully to meet the requirements for training and fitness.

Depending on the training regimen, athletes need to consume at least 50%, but ideally 60% to 70%, of their total calories from carbohydrate. The remaining calories should be obtained from protein (10%-15%) and fat (20% to 30%). These percentages are only guidelines for estimating macronutrient requirements; however, specific guidelines with respect to carbohydrates, proteins, and fat should be used when counseling an active individual or athlete. When energy intake is high (>4500 calories), even a diet containing only 50% of the calories from carbohydrate would provide 500 g of carbohydrate, which is sufficient to maintain muscle glycogen stores. Similarly, if protein intake in this high-calorie diet were low, at 10% of calories, absolute protein intake would still exceed the recommendation for a 70-kg athlete. Thus, specific recommendations based on an individual's body size, body composition, sport, and gender may be more useful than using a guideline based on a proportion. Calories and nutrients should come from a wide variety of foods on a daily basis (ADA and others, 2000).

Carbohydrate

The first source of glucose for the exercising muscle is its own glycogen store. When this is depleted, glycogenolysis and then gluconeogenesis (both in the liver) maintain the glucose supply. During endurance exercise that exceeds 90 minutes, such as marathon running, muscle glycogen stores become progressively lower. When they drop to critically low levels, high-intensity exercise cannot be maintained. In practical terms, the athlete is exhausted and must either stop exercising or drastically reduce the pace.

Glycogen depletion may also be a gradual process, occurring over repeated days of heavy training, in which muscle glycogen breakdown exceeds its replacement, as well as during high-intensity exercise that is repeated several times during competition or training. For example, a distance runner who averages 10 miles per day, but does not take the time to consume enough carbohydrates in his or her diet, or the swimmer who completes several interval sets at above his or her maximal oxygen consumption can both deplete glycogen stores rapidly.

In a classic study Costill and associates (1977b) compared glycogen synthesis on a 40% carbohydrate diet with that on a 70% carbohydrate diet during repeated days of 2-hour workouts. On the low-carbohydrate diet, the muscle glycogen stores dropped lower with each successive day of training. After several days of the diet and exercise regimen, the athletes had low muscle glycogen stores and could not exercise at even a moderate intensity. The high-carbohydrate diet provided nearly maximal repletion of the muscle glycogen stores after the strenuous training. The high-carbohydrate or glycogen loading (glycogen supercompensation) diet provided the athletes with muscle glycogen values that remained above 100 mmol/kg, and they were able to continue the heavy training. This study and others suggest that athletes who fail to consume enough carbohydrate on a daily basis while training will possibly decrease endurance as well as exercise performance.

It is recommended that athletes in heavy training should consume a carbohydrate intake of 6 to 10 g/kg of body weight daily to help prevent daily carbohydrate and glycogen depletion. The amount required depends on the athlete's total daily energy expenditure, type of sport, gender, and environmental conditions. For example, a 70-kg (154-lb) athlete would consume 350 to 700 g of carbohydrate daily. Table 26-1 lists several products that could be consumed during or after exercise for the maintenance of blood glucose or for glycogen resynthesis.

Types of Carbohydrate

The optimal type of carbohydrate for the athlete is still debatable. One study by Costill and colleagues (1981) compared the effects of simple and complex carbohydrate consumption during a 48-hour period after a glycogen-depleting exercise. During the first 24 hours, no differences were found in muscle glycogen synthesis; however, at 48 hours, the complex carbohydrates resulted in significantly greater muscle glycogen synthesis than the simple carbohydrates. Kiens and colleagues (1990), however, reported that increases in muscle glycogen content were significantly greater during the first 6 hours after exercise with simple rather than complex carbohydrates and that plasma insulin levels were greater after the intake of simple carbohydrates.

The question of which type of carbohydrate is better for athletic performance may be better understood if the carbohydrate is classified by its physiologic reaction in the body or by its glycemic index rather than by its structure. Glycemic index represents the ratio of the area under the blood glucose curve resulting from the ingestion of a given quantity of carbohydrate and the area under the glucose curve resulting from the ingestion of the same quantity of white bread or glucose (see Appendix 54 and Chapter 12). Coyle and Hargreaves both recommend that carbohydrates with a moderate to high glycemic index be consumed after exercise (Coyle, 1991; Hargreaves, 1991). Indeed, preliminary work has demonstrated that a diet based on high–glycemic index carbohydrate foods promoted greater glycogen storage in the first 24 hours of recovery after strenuous exercise than an equal amount of carbohydrate eaten in the form of low–glycemic index foods. Current data

TABLE 26-1 Recommendations for Use of Sport Foods

		GUIDELINES FOR CONSUMPTION IN EXERCISE		
SPORT FOOD	CHARACTERISTICS	BEFORE	DURING	AFTER
Sport drink	CHO: 5%-7% by volume (about 14 g/8 oz) Sodium: 20-30 mEq/L (110-165 mg/8 oz) Multiple carbohydrates with high glycemic indices	0.5 L (16 oz) 1 hr before exercise	150-300 ml every 15-20 min (20-40 oz/hr)	24 oz/lb of body weight lost
High CHO energy drink	CHO: >13% by volume (more than 50 g/8 oz) Optional B vitamins: thiamin, niacin, and riboflavin at 10%-40% of RDA	0.5 L (16 oz) 2-5 hr before exercise	Typically not advised for use during the event	Immediately after and at 1-hr intervals to deliver 1 g CHO/kg body weight
Sport bar	CHO: >70% of total kcal High glycemic index Fat: low (1-2 g/bar) or absent Vitamins and minerals not critical components	One bar 2 hr before exercise	Usually not advised except for those desiring solid foods during long-duration events	One to two bars immediately after exercise and with daily meals as desired
Sport shake	CHO: >65% of total kcal (>18 g/100 ml) High glycemic index Fat: not to exceed 25% of total kcal Protein: 15%-20% of total kcal Vitamins and minerals: optional at low levels (10%-40% of RDA)	0.5 L (16 oz) 2-5 hr before exercise	Not recommended	Immediately after to deliver 1 g CHO/kg body weight and as a supplement to daily meals
Energy gel	CHO: >50% by volume (>50 g/100 ml or 15 g/oz) Vitamins and minerals: trace or absent Avoid those with herbs	1 packet before exercise; consume adequate fluid to promote absorption	If overall fluid intake is adequate, enough to supply 30-60 g CHO/hr	Immediately after exercise and at 1-hr intervals to deliver 1 g CHO/kg body weight

Modified from Gatorade Sports Science Exchange Roundtable: *Sport foods for athletes: what works?* vol 9, No. 2, Chicago, 1998, Gatorade Sports Science Institute.
CHO, Carbohydrate.

are mixed concerning whether the glycemic index of carbohydrate in the preexercise meal affects performance (DeMarco et al, 1999; Wee et al, 1999). Appendix 54 lists the glycemic indexes and glycemic loads for several foods.

Carbohydrate Intake Before, During, and After Exercise

Preexercise meal. The preevent or pretraining meal serves two purposes. It keeps the athlete from feeling hungry before and during the exercise bout, and it maintains optimal levels of blood glucose for the exercising muscles. A preexercise meal can improve performance compared with exercising in a fasted state (Wright, Sherman, and Dernback, 1991). Athletes who train early in the morning before eating or drinking risk developing low liver glycogen stores, and this can impair performance, particularly if the exercise regimen involves endurance training.

Carbohydrate feedings before exercise can help to restore suboptimal liver glycogen stores, which may be called on during prolonged training and high-intensity competition. While allowing for personal preferences and psychological factors, the pre-event meal should be high in carbohydrate, nongreasy, and readily digested. Fat should be limited because it delays stomach emptying time and takes longer to digest. A meal eaten 3.5 to 4 hours before competition can have as much as 25% of the kilocalories from fat. Closer to the event, the fat content should be less than 25% of the kilocalories. Exercising with a full stomach also may cause indigestion, nausea, and vomiting.

The pregame meal should be eaten 3 to 4 hours before an event and should provide 200 to 350 g of carbohydrate (4 g/kg). Evidence indicates that eating within 4 hours of an event benefits performance compared with competing on an empty stomach (Sherman et al, 1989). Allowing time for partial digestion and absorption provides a final addition to muscle glycogen, additional blood sugar, and also relatively complete emptying of the stomach. To avoid gastrointestinal distress, the carbohydrate content of the meal should be reduced the closer the meal is to the exercise. For example, 4 hours before the event it is suggested that the athlete consume 4 g of carbohydrates per kilogram of body weight, whereas 1 hour before the competition the athlete would consume 1 g of carbohydrate per kilogram of body weight (Coleman, 1998).

Commercial liquid formulas providing an easily digested high-carbohydrate fluid, intake are popular with athletes and probably do leave the stomach faster. Other appropriate pregame meals are toast with jelly, a baked potato, spaghetti with tomato sauce, cereal with skim milk, or low-fat yogurt with fruit-sugar flavorings.

Within 15 minutes before a long event, the athlete should drink 4 to 8 oz of water or fluid. This prehydration allows for maximal absorption of fluid without urination. After exercise begins, the kidney slows down urine production to compensate for water loss. Box 26-2 suggests preevent meals based on time of competition.

Twenty-five years ago, Costill and colleagues (1977a) suggested that preexercise glucose intake could be associated with hypoglycemia and increased muscle glycogen utilization during exercise; however, more recent studies report either no effect or beneficial effects of preevent feeding on performance (Coyle, 1995; Horowitz and Coyle, 1993). Although these guidelines for preevent eating work well for the average athlete, individual needs must be emphasized. The more recent studies suggest that individuals differ in their susceptibility to lowering blood glucose from sugar consumption before exercise. The physiologic and biochemical bases for these differ-

Box 26-2. Examples of Pre-event Meals

For athletes who compete in events all day such as with track or swimming meets or soccer, basketball, volleyball, and wrestling tournaments, nutritious food choices may be a problem. The athlete should consider the amount of time between eating and performance when choosing foods during all-day events. Suggested precompetition menus include the following:

1 Hr or Less Before Competition—about 100 kcal

Fresh fruit such as apples, watermelon, peaches, grapes, oranges, or a sport energy bar

or

1½ c of a commercial sport drink

2-3 Hr Before Competition—about 300-400 kcal

Fresh fruit and fruit and vegetable juices

and/or

Breads, bagels, English muffins with limited amounts of butter or margarine or cream cheese, or low-fat yogurt, oatmeal, pancakes with limited amounts of butter and syrup, or a sports bar

or

4 c of a commercial sport drink or 1 can of a sport nutritional supplement

3-4 Hr Before Competition—about 700 kcal

Fresh fruit and fruit and vegetable juices

and

Breads, bagels, baked potatoes, cereal with low-fat milk, low-fat yogurt, sandwiches with a small amount of peanut butter or lean meat or low-fat cheese, or spaghetti with a tomato sauce,

or

7½ c of a commercial sport drink or 1-2 cans of a sport nutritional supplement

ences have not been determined. Athletes should always practice and use what works best for them by experimenting with foods and beverages during practice sessions and planning ahead to ensure they have these foods available when they compete.

Carbohydrate intake during exercise. Carbohydrate consumed during endurance exercise lasting longer than 1 hour ensures the availability of sufficient amounts of energy during the later stages of exercise and improves performance (Jeukendrump and Jentjens, 2000; Sugiura and Kobayashi, 1998). Thus, consuming an exogenous carbohydrate during endurance exercise helps to maintain blood glucose and improve performance. The form of carbohydrate does not seem to matter; some athletes prefer to use a sports drink, whereas others prefer to eat a solid or gel and consume water. If a sports drink with carbohydrate is consumed during exercise, the rate of carbohydrate ingestion should be about 26 to 30 g every 30 minutes, an amount equivalent to 1 cup of a 6% to 8% carbohydrate solution taken every 15 to 20 minutes (Harkins et al, 1993). This ensures that 1 g of carbohydrate will be delivered to the tissues per minute at the time fatigue sets in (Butterfield and Gates, 1994). It is unlikely that a carbohydrate concentration of less than 5% is enough to help performance, but solutions with a concentration greater than 10% are often associated with abdominal cramps, nausea, and diarrhea.

Carbohydrate feeding does not prevent fatigue; rather, it simply delays fatigue. During the final minutes of exercise, when muscle glycogen is low and athletes rely heavily on blood glucose for energy, their muscles feel heavy, and they must concentrate to maintain exercise at intensities that are ordinarily not stressful when muscle glycogen stores are filled.

Carbohydrate intake after exercise. On average, only 5% of the muscle glycogen used during exercise is resynthesized each hour following exercise. Accordingly, at least 20 hours will be required for complete restoration after exhaustive exercise, provided about 600 g of carbohydrate is consumed. When carbohydrate at 1.5 to 2 g/kg is consumed immediately after exercise, muscle glycogen synthesis is 15 mmol/kg. When the carbohydrate feeding is delayed for 2 hours after exercise, muscle glycogen synthesis is cut by 66% to 5 mmol per kilogram of body weight. By 4 hours after exercise, total muscle glycogen synthesis from the delayed feeding is still 45% slower than for the feeding given immediately after exercise (Ivy, 2001).

This means that delaying carbohydrate intake for too long after exercise will reduce muscle glycogen resynthesis. Resynthesis is promoted when carbohydrates are consumed immediately after exercise, and the current recommendations are to consume about 100 g of carbohydrate within 30 minutes after exercise to maximize muscle glycogen synthesis. It also appears that the consumption of carbohydrates with a high glycemic index results in higher muscle glycogen levels 24 hours after exercise compared with the same amount of carbohydrates provided as foods with a low glycemic index (Burke, 1997).

Many athletes find it difficult to consume food immediately after exercise. Usually, when body or core temperature is elevated, appetite is depressed and it is difficult to consume carbohydrate-rich foods. Many athletes find it easier and simpler to drink their carbohydrates rather than eat them. For them a sports drink rich in carbohydrates after a hard practice will not only provide the necessary carbohydrate for glycogen synthesis but will also help with rehydration.

More than 10 years ago, Zawadski and colleagues (1992) found that adding about 5 to 9 g of protein with every 100 g of carbohydrate eaten after exercise increased the rate of glycogen resynthesis rate. It appears that this small amount of protein with 100 g of carbohydrate elicits a greater insulin response and therefore activates glycogen synthase, the enzyme responsible for glycogen storage. More recent studies show that when isocaloric amounts of carbohydrates or carbohydrates plus protein and fat are provided following endurance or resistance exercise, glycogen synthesis rates are similar. While adding protein may not appreciably enhance glycogen storage, protein may provide needed amino acids for muscle repair and promote a more anabolic hormonal profile (Burke et al, 1995).

Protein

Although it has long been a popular belief among athletes that additional protein increases strength and enhances performance, nutritionists and most exercise physiologists generally agree that research does not support this thesis. Noting that the small amount of protein required for muscle development during training is easily met by the average diet, the 2002 recommended daily allowances (RDAs) for protein do not specify intakes for work or training different from those indicated for adults. The RDA is 0.66 g per kilogram of body weight daily for 14 to 18 year olds, and 0.80 g per kilogram of body weight daily for adults, which is 12% to 15% of energy intake (Institute of Medicine, 2002) (see Table 15-2).

Protein Needs for Endurance Athletes

Early research showed a decrease in nitrogen balance in response to initiation of a moderate endurance exercise program, suggesting an increased need for protein under these conditions (Gontzea et al, 1974; Yoshimura, 1961). This decline corrected itself, however, within 2 weeks of the start of exercise without dietary change. Nitrogen balance was more positive after adaptation to the exercise than before, suggesting that the protein intake required for nitrogen equilibrium in persons performing moderate endurance exercise may actually be lower than that in a seden-

NEW DIRECTIONS

Should the Athlete Eat Protein During Exercise . . . and if so, How Much?

Recent research in athletic performance is looking at the issue of whether protein consumed during exercise, usually in a sport drink or right before or right after exercise, will improve performance or enhance muscle protein synthesis. Typically protein is consumed at meals and snacks, away from activity, leaving a carbohydrate or carbohydrate and electrolyte beverage as the drink of choice during exercise. Several studies have already shown that adding protein or amino acids to a carbohydrate supplement is no more effective for muscle glycogen synthesis than taking the same amount of calories as carbohydrate. Research, however, is suggesting that some benefit for muscle protein synthesis may be gained from the consumption of small amounts of protein (as little as 6 g) after weight training exercise (Tipton et al, 1999). Newer research suggests that muscle protein synthesis is stimulated even more when a carbohydrate drink is consumed immediately before the weight training exercise (Rasmussen et al, 2000). As yet, no advantage to consuming protein during exercise has been established because only a few amino acids can be used by muscles for energy during exercise, and even during intense exercise this only accounts for 2% to 5% of the total energy expenditure. It has been hypothesized, however, that consuming a protein-carbohydrate will raise the blood insulin to higher levels than carbohydrate alone, thus increasing the use of carbohydrate in muscle to better delay fatigue; but this has not been proven (Roy and Tamopolsky, 1998). In fact, amino acid ingestion during exercise may result in excess ammonia accumulation, which could contribute to fatigue. In summary, the search continues, but at present there are no good data to support adding protein along with carbohydrate to drinks taken during endurance exercise.

tary population, provided energy intake is adequate (Butterfield and Tremblay, 1994).

More recent work suggests that persons who exercise at a higher intensity have protein needs that might be greater (Tarnopolsky et al, 1988, 1992). A classic nitrogen balance regression assessment of trained male runners exercising daily at 75% of their VO_2max estimated protein requirements of 0.94 g per kilogram of body weight daily (Meredith et al, 1989).

The need for protein in exercise depends on energy intake. Butterfield (1987) demonstrated that feeding as much as 2 g of protein per kilogram of body weight daily to men running 5 or 10 miles a day at 65% to 75% of their VO_2max is insufficient to maintain nitrogen balance when energy intake is inadequate by as little as 100 kcal daily. Delvin et al (1990) observed an increase in whole-body protein degradation during 2 hours of 75% of VO_2max exercise, returning to baseline levels within 2 hours after exercise.

Another indicator that endurance athletes may require higher protein intake than the recommended intake is that muscle contractile proteins are broken down during prolonged exercise (Dohm et al, 1987; Synder et al, 1984). These studies point out the important role that calories play in sparing protein. Protein will be used as an energy source if calories are insufficient (see *New Directions:* Should the Athlete Eat Protein During Exercise . . . and if so, How Much?).

Protein Needs for Resistance Exercise

For body builders or persons interested in increasing body mass, the mythology of increased protein needs is rampant. Weight lifters consume anywhere from 1.0 to 3.5 g of protein per kilogram of body weight per day, and most of this protein is in the form of supplements. The basis for this practice is word of mouth and traditions that have not been substantiated by scientific studies. The traditional thinking among body builders and weight lifters is the more protein consumed, the bigger the muscles.

Sufficient data have established that the study of protein needs with resistance exercise is divided into two areas: the need for maintenance (minimum protein required to accomplish nitrogen equilibrium) and the need for increasing lean tissue (positive nitrogen balance).

Experienced body builders can maintain nitrogen equilibrium on intakes similar to those required by sedentary controls (Tarnopolsky et al, 1991). The requirements for maintenance of nitrogen balance, under circumstances of initiation of a resistance exercise program, however, may depend on the intensity of the exercise. Protein requirements in young novice male body builders exercising 6 days a week for 1.5 hours a day were estimated to be 1.5 g per kilogram of body weight daily (Tarnopolsky et al, 1988). Energy intake was not reported, however. In another study, Tarnopolsky et al (1992) found that whole-body protein synthesis was increased in strength athletes consuming 1.4 g of protein per kilogram of body weight per day compared with those consuming 0.9 g of protein per kilogram of body weight per day. When intake was increased to 2.4 g of protein per kilogram of body weight daily, protein synthesis did not increase above that achieved when consuming the 1.4 g protein per kilogram of body weight daily.

On the other hand, Hickson et al (1990) found no change in nitrogen excretion with the initiation of a program of 30 minutes of lifting three times a week at an intensity of about 50% of maximum capacity when subjects were consuming 0.8 g of protein per kilogram of body weight daily, the RDA for protein for adult males.

In an attempt to establish the relevance of added protein in the accretion of lean tissue in recreational weight lifters, it was observed that when energy intake exceeded the need by 400 kcal per day, increasing the nitrogen intake from the requirement (mean = 10 g N/day) to 1.5 times the requirement (mean = 15 g N/day) had no significant effect on nitrogen retention. Any improvement in nitrogen balance seen with increased energy and protein intake was explained by the energy contribution of the protein (Butterfield, 1991).

Nutritional Implications

If the need for protein during exercise is slightly elevated above that for sedentary persons, the usual protein intake of the population will more than meet these needs. Reports of food intake in athletes and nonathletes consistently indicate that protein represents from 12% to 20% of total energy intake or 1.2 to 2 g of protein per kilogram of body weight daily. The exception to the rule will be small, active women who may consume a low-energy intake in conjunction with an exercise or training program. These women may consume close to the RDA for protein, and if the data of Butterfield are correct, this value in conjunction with the restricted energy intake may be inadequate to maintain lean body mass.

Consuming more protein than the body can use is not necessary and should be avoided. When athletes consume diets that are high in protein, they compromise their carbohydrate status and may therefore affect their ability to train and compete at peak levels. High-protein intakes can also result in diuresis and potential dehydration. Protein foods are often also high in fat, and consumption of excess protein can create difficulty in maintaining a low-fat diet. In addition, the hypercalciuric effect of high-protein diets is still considered by some a significant factor in calcium balance, and until the controversy is settled, a conservative approach is advised (see Chapter 27).

Amino Acid Supplementation

Protein or amino acid supplementation in the form of powders or pills is not necessary and should be discouraged. Taking large amounts of protein or amino acid supplements can lead to dehydration, hypercalciuria, weight gain, and stress on the kidney and liver (Synder and Naik, 1998). Taking single amino acids or in combination, such as arginine and lysine, may interfere with the absorption of certain other essential amino acids (Wardlaw, 1999). An additional concern is that substituting amino acid supplements for food may cause deficiencies of other nutrients found in protein-rich foods such as iron, niacin, and thiamin.

Athletes and coaches need to realize that amino acid supplements taken in large doses have not been tested in human subjects, and no margin of safety is available. It is important for the health professional to develop a strategy to approach and discuss supplement use effectively with both athletes and coaches (Berning, 1998).

Table 26-2 estimates the requirements of the athlete whose protein needs are greatest—a growing male adolescent in rigorous training in a warm climate. This liberal allowance is for about 104 g per day of protein or 1.5 g per kilogram of body weight. Although greater than the RDA of 0.85 g/kg for the male adolescent, this is still easily within the range of intake of most male teenagers and athletes. Many studies of athletes' diets indicate that their protein intakes are two to three times higher than the RDA. In meeting his or energy needs, the athlete described would probably be consuming at least 3500 kcal. Considering the usual composition of diets in the United States, this would provide 10% to 15% protein, or 87 to 131 g daily. Thus, there is generally no need to recommend additional protein unless this nutrient makes up less than 12% of adequate energy intake for weight maintenance.

In the case of young or small female athletes, protein needs calculated as a percentage of energy intake may be inadequate; a better calculation is based on 1 to 1.5 g per kilogram of body weight. The same is true for athletes with exceptionally high-energy requirements. Protein needs based on 12% to 15% of energy results in an excessive protein intake.

Fat

Even though maximal performance is impossible without muscle glycogen, fat also provides energy for exercise. Fat is the most concentrated source of food energy and supplies more than twice as many

TABLE 26-2 Liberal Estimate of Protein Requirement for a 70-kg Male Adolescent Athlete

28.7 g	Replacement of obligatory nitrogen loss in urine, feces, skin, and other sites assuming largest loss
8.6 g	30% allowance for individual variation
4.8 g	Allowance for growth, assuming most rapid growth
7.5 g	Replacement of nitrogen lost in sweat during 4 hr of vigorous exercise in the heat
6.3 g	Allowance for increased muscle mass, as during some kinds of training
8.6 g	Allowance for loss of efficiency of standard protein
39.5 g	Allowance for use of protein for energy during rigorous exercise*
104.0 g	Total estimated protein requirement = 1.5 g/kg

Data from Report of Joint FAO/WHO Ad Hoc Expert Committee: Energy and protein requirements, No. 522, Geneva, Switzerland, 1973, *WHO, Tech. Sys. Series*, and Durnin JVGA: *Nutrition, physical fitness, and health*, Baltimore, 1978, University Press.

*Determined using an energy expenditure during activity of an average of 12 kcal/min and exercising time daily of 240 min, and the assumption that 5.5% of the total energy expenditure during exercise is from protein.

calories (9 kcal/g) by weight as protein (4 kcal/g) or carbohydrate (4 kcal/g) (see Chapter 3). Fat provides essential fatty acids that are necessary for cell membranes, skin, hormones, and transport of fat-soluble vitamins. The body has total glycogen stores (both muscle and liver) equaling about 2600 calories, whereas each pound of body fat supplies 3500 calories. This means that an athlete weighing 74 kg (163 lb) with 10% body fat has 16.3 lb of fat, which equals 57,000 calories.

Fat is the major, if not most important, fuel for light- to moderate-intensity exercise. Although fat is a valuable metabolic fuel for muscle activity during longer aerobic exercise and performs many important functions in the body, no attempt should be made to consume more fat over the usual amount unless the athlete is eating less than 15% of calories from fat (Dreon et al, 1999). In addition, athletes who consume a high-fat diet typically consume fewer calories from carbohydrate.

Simonsen et al (1991) had elite rowers consume either 40% of their calories from fat or 20% of their calories from fat and then compared the power output and speed of the rowers. After performing a biopsy of the muscle, they found that the rowers who consumed the low-fat, high-carbohydrate diet had more muscle glycogen. Rowers on the high-fat, low-carbohydrate diet had moderate levels of muscle glycogen and actually were able to complete the workout sets. When it came to power output and faster speeds, however, athletes who consumed the lower-fat, higher-carbohydrate diets had significantly higher power and speed. This has significant implications for athletes in muscular endurance sports, for which they need a burst of power, such as rowing, swimming, gymnastics, figure skating, judo, boxing, or any sport that will need to have some energy generated by the anaerobic pathway. Some studies have proposed a positive effect of relatively high-fat diets (more than 70% of energy intake) on athletic performance (Lambert et al, 1994; Muoio et al, 1994). Careful review of these studies show some design flaws, however, and little evidence supports the concept of consuming a high-fat diet for athletes. Long-term use of such a diet has been well documented as having negative health effects. Following a low-fat, high-carbohydrate diet is also important for health reasons because a high-fat diet is associated with cardiovascular disease, obesity, diabetes, and some types of cancers.

Athletes should consume 20% to 30% of their calories from fat. Aside from decreasing overall calories, limiting consumption of dietary fat is the first step toward losing excess body fat. Doing so eliminates excess calories, but not nutrients. Severe fat restriction (≤15% of energy intake) may limit performance by hindering intramuscular triglyceride storage, which provides a significant proportion of energy at all intensities of exercise as well as negative effects on blood lipid profiles in some people when total dietary fat intake is less than 15% of total energy (Butterfield and Tremblay, 1994; Dreon et al, 1999).

Vitamins and Minerals

It has usually been assumed that if the athlete meets requirements for increased energy, the vitamin and mineral requirements will also be satisfied. Although this may be true in most cases, one study of triathletes indicates low intakes of selenium, molybdenum, iron, copper, and biotin, even though the athletes were consuming energy at levels two to three times the RDA (Green et al, 1989). The authors of the study speculate that because of training and work schedules, athletes seldom eat three balanced meals, but they rely heavily on snacking to maintain their energy levels, and these snacks may be less nutrient dense than the meals they replace. The poor nutritional status of some athletes may be due to their training and work schedules. Some athletes have low-energy intakes because of concerns about body weight and appearance, which makes the likelihood of them having inadequate intakes of vitamins and minerals even greater (Bishop et al, 1999).

The need for vitamins and minerals in exercise has been reviewed by Haymes and Clarkson (1998) with the consensus that unless an individual is deficient in a given nutrient, supplementation with that nutrient does not have a major effect on performance. Several nutrients are of concern in athletes, however, including folate, the B vitamins, calcium, and zinc. Because many women athletes are also vegetarians, iron and specifically vitamin B_{12} may be of additional concern in this subgroup.

Iron

Iron performs several functions vital to muscle activity. As a component of hemoglobin, it is instrumental in transporting oxygen from the lungs to the tissues. It performs a similar role in myoglobin, which acts within the muscle as an oxygen acceptor to hold a supply of oxygen readily available for use by the mitochondria. Iron is also a vital component of the cytochrome enzymes involved in the production of ATP.

It thus follows that iron deficiency anemia limits aerobic endurance and the capacity for work; however, partial depletion of iron stores in the liver, spleen, and bone marrow, as evidenced by low serum ferritin levels, can have a detrimental effect on exercise performance, even when anemia is not present.

Although iron deficiency anemia is not frequently seen among athletes, suboptimal iron stores as assessed by serum ferritin levels are relatively common. Athletes at risk for developing low iron stores are the rapidly growing male adolescent, the female athlete with heavy menstrual losses, the athlete with an energy-restricted diet, distance runners who may have increased gastrointestinal iron loss, and those training heavily in hot climates with heavy sweating. All athletes, especially female long-distance runners and vegetarians, should be screened periodically to assess their iron status (ADA and others, 2000).

Heavy training can cause a transient decrease in serum ferritin and hemoglobin that may be experienced by some athletes, especially in the conditioning phase of the sport. (Spodaryk, 2002). This was once called sports anemia, but erythrocyte morphology remains normal, and performance does not appear to deteriorate. These decreases in serum ferritin and hemoglobin are a result of an increase in plasma volume, which causes a hemodilution and appears to have no effect on performance (see Chapter 34).

Some athletes, especially long-distance runners, experience gastrointestinal bleeding. Iron loss through gastrointestinal bleeding can be detected by fecal hemoglobin assays. The percentage of runners who experience gastrointestinal bleeding is significant and is related to the intensity and duration of the exercise, the ability of the athlete to stay hydrated, how well the athlete is trained, and whether he or she has taken nonsteroidal antiinflammatory medication (NSAID), particularly ibuprofen, before the competition (Peters et al, 2001; Smetanka et al, 1999).

The iron concentration of sweat during exercise ranges from 0.13 to 0.42 mg/L. Waller and Haymes (1996) observed that the iron concentration in sweat is lower in a hot environment (35° C) than in a thermoneutral environment (26° C). Because sweating is greater in the heat, the same amount of sweat iron was lost during 1 hour of exercise in both environments, with male athletes losing three times as much sweat iron as female athletes. They also found that as the exercise time continued, less iron was lost in the sweat. Sweat iron concentration decreased significantly from 30 to 60 minutes, which suggests that much of the iron lost in sweat is done early in the exercise bout. Iron supplementation can be beneficial in improving iron stores of athletes who are iron depleted, but the effects on aerobic performance of nonanemic athletes are equivocal. Because large doses of iron (75 mg/day) may be toxic in persons with the genetic disorder hemochromatosis (see Chapter 34), such supplements should be used only by those diagnosed as iron depleted or anemic (Haymes and Clarkson, 1998). At present the data do not support the value of iron supplementation for either treating or preventing sports anemia; however, testing serum ferritin may be useful in assessing iron stores in athletes. If true iron depletion is present, iron supplementation along with vitamin C to enhance its absorption is appropriate. Oral iron therapy is effective and maintains performance in runners who are deficient in iron but not anemic (see Chapter 34).

Calcium

Osteoporosis is a major health concern, especially for women. Although the disease has been regarded as a problem of older women, young women, especially those who have had interrupted menstrual function, may be at risk for decreased bone mass. Although there is still much to be discovered about the cause of osteoporosis, three major risk factors have been identified: hormonal status, particularly estrogen deficiency; deficient calcium consumption; and physical inactivity (see Chapter 27).

Bone mass is attained until the age of 30 to 35 years; however, peak rate of bone mass accumulation is between the ages of 14 and 24 years. The amount of bone mass a woman has by age 35 strongly influences her susceptibility to fractures in later years. Therefore, it is important that young women consume calcium throughout the peak bone mass years and throughout early adulthood. Unfortunately, the National Health and Nutrition Examination Survey (NHANES) found that 50% of all women age 15 and older consume less than 75% of the RDA of 1200 mg and that three fourths of women over 35 years of age consume less than the DRI of 1000 mg (Alaimo et al, 1994).

In 1997 the American College of Sports Medicine (ACSM) identified the female athlete triad as a disturbing pattern emerging in women's athletics (Otis et al, 1997). It is characterized by estrogen deficiency, evidenced as athletic amenorrhea, disordered eating and low body fat, and loss of bone mass. Some women who exercise strenuously stop menstruating, a condition known as *athletic amenorrhea.* Unfortunately, the exact cause of amenorrhea has not been fully determined, but probably many factors are involved. The two most current theories are that the excessive exercise is an "energy drain" that may lead to a hypothalamic dysfunction or that excess cortisol levels inhibit the release of gonadotropins (Loucks, 2001). Regardless of the cause, the lack of estrogen has a negative impact on bone, and if the estrogen deficiency persists, bone loss may be substantial and bone may never be regained (Drinkwater et al, 1986; Jonnavithula et al, 1993; Warren and Stiehl, 1999).

Strategies to promote the resumption of menses include estrogen replacement therapy, weight gain, and reduced training. Diet changes modification to include more calcium, vitamin D, and magnesium are also instituted. Regardless of menstrual history, most female athletes need to increase their calcium intake to meet the RDA for calcium (Turner and Bass, 2001). Low-fat and nonfat dairy products, calcium-fortified fruit juices, calcium-fortified soy milk, and tofu made with calcium sulfate are all good sources. Amenorrheic athletes who need 1500 mg of calcium daily may require supplementation with calcium and vitamin D (see Chapter 27).

Antioxidant Vitamins and Beta-Carotene

The antioxidant nutrients—such as vitamins A, E, and C and beta-carotene and selenium—play an important role in protecting the cell membrane from oxidative damage. Exercise can increase the oxidative processes in the muscle, leading to increased generation of lipid peroxides and free radicals. In animals it has been shown that there is a twofold to threefold increase in free radical concentrations in the muscle and liver following exercise to exhaustion (Davies et al, 1982). Kanter (1998), however, questions the fact that this study was published more than 15 years ago and that these results have never been replicated.

Most studies that investigate free radical formation during exercise actually determine indirect measures of lipid peroxidation, not free radical production. Despite the lack of specificity, sensitivity, and reproducibility, much of our understanding about exercise and free radicals is based on these methodologies. A few recent studies have looked at the effect of exercise on the susceptibility of low-density lipoprotein to oxidation. The results suggest that strenuous exercise does indeed promote free radical formation (Sanchez-Quesada et al, 1995).

Vitamins with antioxidant activity, particularly vitamin C, vitamin E, and beta-carotene, neutralize free radicals. The question is whether they enhance recovery from exercise (Konig et al, 2001). Results from studies in humans show that when 10 mg (33,333 IU) of beta-carotene, 800 IU of vitamin E, and 1000 mg of vitamin C were added to the diets of moderately trained runners for 3 to 4 weeks, levels of creatine phosphokinase and lactic dehydrogenase (both indices of muscle damage) were significantly lower, plasma glutathione did not increase, and recovery after exercise was faster (Viguie et al, 1989). Another study showed that these same three nutrients, when given in high amounts, decreased elevated serum malondialdehyde and breath pentane (measures of lipid oxidation) in individuals at rest and during exercise (Singh, 1992). Antioxidant nutrients may have a role in enhancing recovery from exercise and maintaining optimal immune response, but there is no consistent evidence that they improve performance per se. The available evidence suggests that antioxidant supplementation has favorable effects on markers of lipid peroxidation after exercise. Although the physiologic implications of this effect remain to be elucidated, the prudent use of an antioxidant supplement may provide insurance against a suboptimal diet and the increased demand of physical activity.

Athletes need to understand that more is not always better. The National Academy of Sciences has established the dietary reference intakes (DRIs) for vitamins and minerals as a guide for determining nutritional needs. The DRIs are the daily amounts of nutrients recommended for practically all healthy persons to promote optimal health (see Chapter 15). Although it has been shown that a severely inadequate intake of certain vitamins can impair performance, it is unusual for an athlete to have such deficiencies. Even marginal deficiencies do not appear to affect the ability to exercise efficiently.

Vitamin C

The effect of vitamin C supplementation on performance has received considerable attention, mainly because athletes consume vitamin C in large quantities, often because of the volume of food they consume. In studies where athletes were deficient in vitamin C, supplementation improved physical performance, but a thorough analysis of these studies supports the general conclusion that vitamin C supplementation does not increase physical performance capacity in subjects with normal body levels of vitamin C (Keith, 1994). On the other hand, because exercise is a stressor to the body, some nutritionists recommend that the active individual may need slightly more vitamin C than the RDA. Keith suggests vitamin C supplementation may be beneficial for heat acclimation, an idea that merits more research.

Vitamin E

Vitamin E is used widely as a supplement by athletes who hope to improve performance. Recent research is showing vitamin E to have a protective effect against exercise-induced oxidative injury and the acute immune response changes that exercise produces. Researchers found that supplementation with vitamin E enhances the immune response, preventing changes similar to those of infectious disease seen after exercise (Cannon et al, 1990; Meydani et al., 1993). Over the course of an exercise season with intense workouts and competition, vitamin E supplementation at the level of 200 to 450 IU daily may help to prevent oxidative injury (Cooper, 1994). Further studies are recommended, however.

Whether this vitamin has a protective effect during exercise in polluted environmental conditions is unclear (Dillard et al, 1978). The positive effect of vitamin E may be due to protection against oxidative injury caused by inhalation of pollutants.

Although research has shown that exercise can increase levels of lipid peroxidation, and that certain antioxidants can help prevent oxidative injury, habitual exercise has been shown to result in an augmented antioxidant system and a reduction of lipid peroxidation (Clarkson, 1995). Thus, persons and athletes who train daily may have a more developed endogenous antioxidant system compared with a sedentary person. The recommendation for athletes to supplement their diet with antioxidants remains equivocal and controversial. To date there is no clear consensus on whether supplementation of antioxidants is necessary; however, athletes at greatest risk for poor antioxidant intakes are those who limit fat or restrict energy intake and restrict or limit their intake of fruits and vegetables.

B Vitamins

Increased energy metabolism creates a need for more of the B vitamins that serve as part of coenzymes involved in the energy cycles (see Chapters 3 and 4). When dietary intakes are expanded to meet increased energy needs, however, the extra foods consumed usually provide enough B vitamins to enable the release of that energy. There is no evidence that supplementing the well-nourished athlete with B vitamins will increase performance (Keith, 1994).

Studies have shown, however, that athletes can become depleted in some B vitamins, and in these athletes, dietary change or supplementation will improve exercise performance (Belko et al, 1983). A deficiency of vitamin B_{12}, found only in animal foods, could develop in a vegetarian athlete after several years of a strict vegan intake (see Chapter 34); a vitamin B_{12} supplement is warranted for these individuals. Vitamin B_{12} metabolism may also be altered in ultraendurance athletes (Singh et al, 1993).

The intake of folic acid is marginal for a large portion of the U.S. population and could be low in an athlete whose consumption of whole fruits and vegetables is low. If diets of athletes reflect those of the general population, they could easily not contain the recommended number of fruits and vegetables. The NHANES studies have found that 90% of the study participants fail to ingest the recommended minimum of five servings of fruits and vegetables daily (Patterson et al, 1990) (see Chapters 12, 14, and 15). A folate supplement to meet the RDA is recommended for such athletes. For some athletes, such as wrestlers, gymnasts, or rowers, who consume low-calorie diets for long periods, a B vitamin supplement to meet the RDA may be appropriate.

WEIGHT MANAGEMENT

In efforts to maximize performance, many athletes alter normal energy intake to either gain or lose weight. For example, 41% of college wrestlers surveyed have weight fluctuations of 11 to 20 lb every week during the competitive season (Steen and Brownell, 1990). Although such efforts are sometimes appropriate, weight-reduction programs may involve elements of risk. For some young athletes, achievement of unrealistically light weights may jeopardize growth and development (Pugliese et al, 1983; Strauss et al, 1985). Chronic dieting of female athletes, many of whom are dancers and gymnasts, can lead to eating disorders, delayed menarche, amenorrhea, and potential osteoporosis (Harber, 2000) (see Chapters 25 and 27).

The goal weight of an athlete should be based on body fatness (see Chapters 17 and 24). Adequate time should be allowed for a slow, steady weight loss of about 1 to 2 lb each week over several weeks. Weight loss should be achieved before the competitive season begins to ensure maximal strength. In addition, the exercise should be of moderate intensity because at this level a greater proportion of energy is derived from fat than carbohydrate, and the exercise can be sustained longer.

Weight gain should be achieved through a gradual increase in energy intake combined with a strength training program to maximize muscle weight gain over fat gain. A realistic goal is ½ to 1 lb weekly. Fat intake should not exceed 30% of kilocalories from fat, and protein should be 1 to 1.5 g per kilogram of body weight.

Appropriate programs for modifying the weight of athletes and others are discussed in Chapter 24. Because pressure to have the perfect body for a sport, which for many sports (e.g., gymnastics, track, swimming, diving, rowing, dancing, and figure skating) means leanness for both performance and appearance, unrealistic dieting and eating disorders are common. The pursuit of thinness leading to calorie restriction is especially evident in women involved in college athletics, where the pressure to perform, contribute to the team, and maintain scholarships is great (Lindeman, 1994). The professional working with an elite athlete with an eating disorder must remember the tremendous motivation supplied by the desire to perform well in the sport (see Chapter 25).

OTHER CONSIDERATIONS

Alcohol

Alcohol consumption has a detrimental effect on athletic performance, even though by reducing feelings of insecurity, tension, and discomfort, it may cause the athlete to feel that he or she is performing better. Many athletes incorrectly believe that because alcohol contains carbohydrates, they can load on beer to improve their performance. Perceptual motor performance is affected; however, except for some deleterious effects on prolonged endurance performance, alcohol has no effect on the physiologic processes of maximal exercise. Light social drinking (one or two drinks) during the day before a competition will probably not influence athletic performance the following day.

Caffeine

Caffeine contributes to endurance performance, apparently because of its ability to enhance mobilization of fatty acids and thus conserve glycogen stores. Caffeine may also directly affect muscle contractility, possibly by facilitating calcium transport. It could reduce fatigue as well by reducing plasma K^+ accumulation, which contributes to fatigue (Lindinger et al, 1993). Probably some ergogenic effects occur at doses of 6.5 mg per kilogram of body weight taken before endurance exercise; however, caffeine does not seem to offer any benefits before high-intensity exercise (Tarnopolsky, 1994).

Presently, caffeine is listed as a restricted drug by the International Olympic Committee (IOC) and is considered a doping agent if the intake results in urine concentrations above 12 mg/L. To have ergogenic benefits, caffeine must therefore be taken at doses (about 6.5 mg/kg) that do not exceed the IOC urine limit (Tarnopolsky, 1994). In a 70-kg man, this would be 455 mg of caffeine, the amount in 4 to 5 cups of coffee.

Caffeine's diuretic action could be a negative effect for athletes with excessive water needs or for those in long-distance events who do not want to have to urinate during the event.

ERGOGENIC AIDS

Many athletes use nutritional ergogenic aids because they are bombarded with advertisements and testimonials from other athletes and coaches about their effects on performance. Many believe that ergogenic aids will improve their performance and assist in recovery. As in the past, and probably in the future, many of these ergogenic aids are not supported by scientific studies. In fact, many act only as placebos.

Their increased visibility has occurred primarily because of the passage of the Dietary Supplement Health and Education Act (DSHEA) in 1994 (Bass and Young, 1996) (see Chapter 20). Under this act, the Food and Drug Administration (FDA) no longer has regulatory control of supplements, including vitamin, mineral, amino acid, herbal, and other botanical preparations. This has led to an increased number of nutritional ergogenic aids on the market (Table 26-3).

Nutritional supplements are now classified as foods, not as food additives or drugs. Another interesting and somewhat controversial section of the act allows manufacturers to publish limited information about the benefits of dietary supplements in the form of statements of support as well as so-called structure and function claims. The result is a great deal of printed material at the points of sale of nutritional products.

β-Hydroxy-β-Methylbutyrate

β-Hydroxy-β-methylbutyrate (HMB) is an important compound made in the body and is a metabolite of the essential amino acid leucine. Several studies done with both animals and humans have found that subjects supplemented with HMB have less stress-induced muscle protein breakdown (Abumrad and Flakoll, 1991). In one study, the volunteers supplemented with HMB had greater strength gains compared with the control group (Nissen et al, 1996). It is interesting, however, to point out that the control group started out much stronger than the HMB-supplemented group; therefore it is not surprising that the control group, who were more highly trained, had lesser strength gains from the same exercise protocol than the lesser-trained experimental HMB group.

Creatine

Creatine, in the form of phosphocreatine and ATP, supplies most of the energy for short-term, maximal exercise like base running and stealing, swinging the bat, and throwing. When creatine stores in the muscles are depleted, ATP synthesis is prevented and energy can no longer be supplied at the rate required by the working muscle. Creatine is a naturally occurring compound that can be found in considerable amounts in meat and fish. In normal healthy persons, muscle creatine is broken down to creatinine and excreted by the kidneys. For meat eaters, dietary intake of creatine is about 1 g daily. The body also synthesizes about 1 g of creatine per day for a total production of about 2 g daily. The normal daily excretion of creatine is about 2 g for most persons. It appears that vegetarians may be at the highest risk of not having enough creatine. Vegetarian athletes with lower stores of creatine demonstrate a greater uptake of creatine after supplementation than athletes with higher stores.

Creatine supplementation elevates muscle creatine levels and facilitates the regeneration of phosphocreatine, which in turn helps regenerate ATP. Ingesting 20 g daily (four 5-g doses per day) for 5 days can produce a 20% increase in muscle creatine levels (Greenhaff et al, 1994). Human muscle appears to have an upper limit of creatine storage; thus, creatine will presumably be of little benefit to someone with an already high concentration of muscle creatine or to one who has been ingesting high doses of creatine for many weeks. Once creatine is taken up by the muscles, it is trapped within the muscle tissue. It is estimated that muscle creatine stores decline slowly and will still be elevated 2 to 3 months after ingestion of 20 g for 5 days. Whereas the original loading of creatine used the regimen of 20 g for 5 days, current thought is to do away with the loading phase and simply consume creatine at a lower dose of 2 to 5g daily.

Creatine supplementation does not enhance endurance activities, but it is associated with an increase in body weight and lean body mass of around 2 to 6 lb, which is due either to fluid retention or enhanced skeletal muscle synthesis. This weight gain might interfere with the performance of some athletes. Although there are no scientific reports of dangerous side effects, there have been anecdotal descriptions of athletes who have had muscle strains and pulls as well as dehydration problems while taking creatine supplements. This is a bigger problem for athletes who play in hot, humid environments and for those who do not drink enough water.

Because the safety of long-term creatine use has not been studied, and because excess creatine cannot be stored in the muscles and must be excreted by the kidneys, it is recommended that a maintenance dose be no more than 5 g daily.

TABLE 26-3 Unproven Ergogenic Aids

ERGOGENIC AID	DESCRIPTION	CLAIM	ADVERSE SIDE EFFECTS/CAUTION
Amino acid supplements	Arginine, ornithine, glycine plus lysine, predigested amino acids, branch-chain amino acids	Promotes muscle development	
Bee pollen	Mixture of bee saliva, plant nectar, and pollen	Increases energy levels, enhances physical fitness	Reports anecdotal; not proven; allergic reactions in bee-sensitive individuals most common adverse side effect; because of content of nucleic acids, should be avoided by those with gout
Boron	Nonmetallic trace element that influences calcium and magnesium metabolism	Increases testosterone	Intakes of 50 mg/day may be toxic
Brewer's yeast	By-product of beer brewing; rich source of B vitamins and bioavailable chromium	Increases energy levels	Claims of blood glucose improvement due to chromium content are documented (see Chapters 5 and 33)
Carnitine	A compound synthesized in the body from lysine and methionine	Improves cardiovascular function and muscle strength; delays fatigue; decreases muscle pain; decreases body fat	Although necessary for fat metabolism (see Chapter 3), appears that body synthesizes adequate amounts
Choline	Precursor of the neurotransmitter acetylcholine	Improves performance	Should be avoided by athletes with gout
Chromium	Essential component of the glucose tolerance factor	Improves insulin sensitivity and carbohydrate metabolism during exercise	Prolonged or excessive supplementation may lead to chromium accumulation in the body to levels at which chromosomal damage has been observed in animals and in vitro
Conjugated linoleic acid (CLA)	Structured lipid	Antioxidant; addition of lean body mass and reduction of body fat; modulates serum glucose	No human studies have been published in peer-reviewed journals
DNA/RNA	Deoxyribonucleic acid, ribonucleic acid	Tissue regeneration	
Ephedra/ ma huang	Amphetamine-like stimulant	Enhances performance	Banned by the NFL, NCAA, and IOC; can cause dizziness, irregular heartbeat, heart attack, stroke, or death in individuals sensitive to its effects
Ginkgo	From the leaves of the Chinese ginkgo tree; has biologically active compounds	Improves cognitive function	Delays blood clotting time so should not be used by those using anticoagulants (see Chapter 16)
Ginseng	Extract of ginseng root	Protects against tissue damage	Ginseng products (teas, powders, extracts) are of variable quality and strength because of expense of the authentic product (see Chapter 16)
Glycine	An amino acid that is a phosphorcreatine precursor	Improves muscle contraction	
Guarana	Derived from seeds of a South American shrub that contains twice the caffeine of coffee beans	Enhances performance	Risks associated with caffeine
Kelp	Seaweed	Vitamin/mineral source, especially iodine	Monitor for iodine allergy
Lecithin	Phosphatidylcholine	Decreases triglyceride and cholesterol levels	
Medium-chain triglycerides	Fatty acids with shorter carbon chain lengths (8-12)	Improves performance by sparing muscle glycogen; promotes muscularity and lower body fat	Gastric distress in some subjects
Octacosanol	Alcohol isolate extracted from wheat germ oil	Supplies energy and improves performance	
Pangamic acid	Also referred to as vitamin B_{15}; varied composition depending on the supplier	Increases delivery of oxygen	
Spirulina	Microscopic blue-green algae; excellent source of beta-carotene	Protein source	Probably does not function as protein source, but supplies beta-carotene, a powerful antioxidant for which athletes may have increased need
Superoxide dimutase	Antioxidant enzyme system	Protects body against oxidative cell damage incurred from aerobic metabolism	Antioxidant protection provided may affect recovery from athletic endeavors
Yohimbine/ yohimbe bark	Nitrogen-containing alkaloid from the bark of the yohimbe tree	Functions as a alpha 2-adrenoreceptor blocker, increasing blood levels of norepinephrine; stimulant	Can cause anxiety, insomnia, hypertension, dizziness, and headaches

DHEA

Dehydroepiandrosterone (DHEA) is a product of dehydroandrosterone-3-sulfate (DHEA-S) and is a precursor of at least two hormones: testosterone and estradiol. Although DHEA-S is the most abundant circulating adrenal hormone in humans, its physiologic role and that of DHEA are poorly understood.

Dehydroepiandrosterone has been labeled the "youth hormone" because its levels peak during early adulthood. Several studies have suggested a positive correlation between increased plasma levels of DHEA and improved vigor, health, and well-being in persons who ranged in age from 40 to 80 years (Morales et al, 1994). Is DHEA anabolic? By modifying cortisol output, DHEA may indeed exert an anabolic effect. Scientists originally thought that DHEA may competitively bind to cortisol cell receptors in a manner analogous to anabolic steroids, but studies failed to prove this hypothesis (Regelson and Kalimi, 1994). Other studies involving DHEA and liver cortisol receptors show that the DHEA directly decreases cortisol in the liver by 50% (Regelson et al, 1994). If this were to occur in muscle tissue as well, the anabolic effect would be comparable to that of anabolic steroids; however, no proof of this currently exists, and yet DHEA is a precursor to testosterone and estrogen.

Because DHEA can take several different hormonal pathways, the one that it follows depends on several factors, including existing levels of other hormones. It can take several routes in the body and interact with certain enzymes along the sex-steroid pathway. Thus, it can turn into less desirable byproducts of testosterone including dehydrotestosterone, which is associated with male pattern baldness, prostate enlargement, and acne.

Until recently, DHEA was a prescription drug. Because of the 1994 DSHEA, it is now sold over the counter. The benefits of taking DHEA for sports performance have not been clearly established, and the effects of chronic DHEA ingestion are not known. Long-term safety has not been established. DHEA is not recommended for athletic use and has been banned by the U.S. Olympic Committee, the National Football League (NFL), and the National Collegiate Athletic Association (NCAA).

Recently a "safe" alternative to DHEA has been touted—Mexican yam. Although Mexican yams contain a DHEA precursor (a plant sterol used in the semisynthetic production of DHEA in the laboratory), the idea that the body can convert this plant sterol to testosterone is a complete scam.

Androstenedione

Androstenedione (andro) has about one seventh the activity of testosterone and is a precursor that directly converts to testosterone by a single reaction. It is naturally produced in the body from either DHEA or 17-α-hydroxyprogesterone. Researchers have found that taking androstenedione elevates testosterone more than DHEA does; however, the induced increase lasts only several hours and remains at peak levels for just a few minutes (Mahesh and Greenblatt, 1962). The results of this single, 42-year-old study remain the basis for marketing androstenedione as a muscle-building supplement for athletes, and no scientific evidence has been found to support using androstenedione to improve athletic performance.

Athletes in the former East Germany used androstenedione as an anabolic energy-enhancing supplement, but few details are available about its use and dosages. Because of its short half-life, athletes would need to take androstenedione several times a day or on a nearly continual basis to maintain a substantial blood level. To get around this, several companies are now marketing time-release forms of androstenedione; however, no scientific proof has been established to show that these formulations are effective or safe. If it does in fact increase testosterone levels, it has the potential to cause the same side effects as androgenic anabolic supplements such as steroids and growth hormones.

Details of the doping program in the former East Germany reveal a litany of adverse reactions in male and female athletes, including muscle tightness and cramps, increased body weight, acne, gastrointestinal problems, changes in libido, amenorrhea, liver damage, and stunted growth in adolescents (Franke and Berendonk, 1997). Men between 35 and 65 years of age who consumed androstenedione or androstenediol for 12 weeks had significant increases in androstenedione concentrations and had higher testosterone concentrations at months 1 and 2, but returned to baseline after 12 weeks. In addition, estrogen concentrations were significantly higher in the androstenedione group at all measurement periods, whereas only the week 12 values for the androstenediol group were statistically greater than baseline. Luteinizing hormone was suppressed 33% in the androstenedione group at week 4 and remained suppressed at week 12. These findings provide further support that consumption of a prohormone supplement can alter a patient's hypothalamic-pituitary-gonadal axis (Broeder et al, 2000).

Weindruch of the University of Wisconsin–Madison states: "Epidemiological data suggest that diet and serum androstenedione levels may influence the progression of latent forms of prostate cancer into more aggressive prostate cancer." He adds that one prospective study linked high androstenedione levels with later development of prostate cancer. Selling androstenedione may be irresponsible because of the potential risks associated with long-term use (Weindruch, 1997).

Until there is scientific support for its use, androstenedione should not be sold under the assumption that it is either an effective or safe athletic ergogenic aid. Clearly, adolescents and women of childbearing age should not use it. In 1998 androstenedione was

Clinical Scenario 1

Lisa is a 35-year-old single mother of two children. She is a dedicated marathon runner. Her daily 3:30 AM workout during the week includes 1 hour of running 7 to 8 miles on her treadmill and 15 to 20 minutes of stretching and strength building with free weights. On weekends, when her children are with their father, she does a long run of 10 to 15 miles. She has a marathon coming up in 2 months.

Lisa works as a stockbroker; and because she lives on the West Coast, she must be in her office by 6:00 AM at the latest. She is a vegetarian. She often skips breakfast and eats lunch at her desk. Dinner is hurried between her children's sports, homework, and housework.

Within the past 6 months, Lisa has had a weight gain of 8 lb that she would like to lose before the marathon. She is not sure why she gained the weight because she claims to eat a low-fat diet (10% to 15% of kilocalories from fat). She has come to you for a nutritional program to accompany her training for this event.

1. Is it reasonable to expect Lisa to meet her weight goal before the marathon? Explain.
2. What would you recommend for fat intake for Lisa and why?
3. Is calcium a concern for Lisa? How could you find out, and if it is, what would you advise?
4. What protein intake would you recommend, and how would you find out if Lisa is getting enough?
5. What vitamins might be of concern, and how would you advise Lisa to optimize her intake?
6. Lisa has asked you specifically about her premarathon diet, both right before and a few days ahead. What would you recommend?

Clinical Scenario 2

Bill, a 25-year-old professional football player, wants to bulk up and lose fat weight. At the time of consultation, he weighs 300 lb (height 6 ft 3 in.). He wants to lose about 15 to 20 lb while maintaining muscle mass. A 24-hour recall reveals that he is eating 10 microwaved chicken breasts for breakfast with a glass of skim milk. For lunch he consumes 15 microwaved chicken breasts and sometimes a cup of vegetables. For dinner he might eat 20 chicken breasts with two glasses of milk. He states that this is the diet he usually goes on to lose weight and gain lean tissue. He complains of being able to only last 15 to 20 minutes in the weight room and has trouble staying alert and awake in the afternoon. His 40-yard sprint times are slipping, and he has not lost any weight in the past 2 weeks on his current diet. He believes that by eating more protein and taking a protein supplement, he will add bulk to his muscles and at the same time lose fat weight. Bill has been told that by taking certain amino acids, his fat would "melt away" while his muscles would begin to grow.

1. How many grams of protein is Bill consuming? What is his protein per kilogram of body weight consumption?
2. Why is Bill so tired in the afternoon, and why are his sprint times decreasing?
3. Bill believes that he needs to take a protein supplement to maintain his competitiveness. What would you tell him?
4. What level of protein intake would you recommend for him?
5. How would you advise Bill to lose weight?
6. What other dietary changes would you recommend for Bill?

added to the list of banned substances by the IOC and several amateur and professional organizations, including the NFL and the NCAA.

SUMMARY

Nutrition not only plays a role in performance, but it can also help to prevent injuries, enhance recovery from exercise, help maintain body weight, and improve overall health. It is important for professionals in the field to have a good working knowledge and understanding of exercise science and sports nutrition so that they can help their clients perform close to their potential, whether they are competitive athletes or weekend warriors just trying to maintain health.

Relevant Web Sites

American College of Sports Medicine
www.acsm.org
ConsumerLab.com
www.consumerlab.com
Gatorade Sports Science Institute
www.gssiweb.com
SupplementWatch, Inc.
www.supplementwatch.com

Cited References

Abumrad N, Flakoll P: *The efficacy and safety of CaHMB (beta-hydroxy-beta-methylbutyrate) in humans,* Annual report: MTI, Memphis, 1991, Vanderbilt University Medical Center.

Alaimo K et al: Dietary intake of vitamins, minerals, and fiber of persons ages 2 months and over in the United States: third National Health and Nutrition Examination Survey, Phase I, 1988-1991, *Advanced Data* 14(258):1-28, 1994.

American College of Sports Medicine: Position on exercise and fluid replacement, *Med Sci Sports Exerc* 28:I, 1996.

American Dietetic Association, Dietitians of Canada, and the American College of Sports Medicine: Nutrition and athletic performance—position statement, *J Am Diet Assoc* 100:1543, 2000.

Bar-Or O: Nutritional considerations for the child athlete, *Can J Appl Physiol* 26(suppl):S186, 2001.

Bass IS, Young AL: *The Dietary Supplement Health and Education Act: a legislative history and analysis,* Washington DC, 1996, Food and Drug Law Institute.

Belko AZ et al: Effects of exercise on riboflavin requirements of young women, *Am J Clin Nutr* 37:509, 1983.

Berning JR: Eating while traveling. In Berning JR, Steen S, editors: *Nutrition for sport and exercise,* Gaithersburg, Md, 1998, Aspen Publishers.

Bishop NC et al: Nutritional aspects of immunosuppression in athletes, *Sports Med* 28(3):151, 1999.

Broeder CE et al: The Andro Project: the physiological and hormonal influences of androstenedione supplementation in men 35-65 years old participating in a high intensity resistance training program, *Arch Intern Med* 160(20):3093, 2000.

Burke LM: Nutrition for post-exercise recovery, *Aust J Sci Med Sport* 29(1):3, 1997.

Burke LM et al: Effect of coingestion of fat and protein with carbohydrate feedings on muscle glycogen storage, *J Appl Physiol* 78:2187, 1995.

Butterfield GE: Whole body protein utilization in humans, *Med Sci Sports Exerc* 19:S157, 1987.

Butterfield GE: Amino acids and high protein diets. In Lamb DR, Williams MH, editors: *Perspectives in exercise science and sports medicine,* vol 4, *Ergogenic enhancement of performance in exercise and sport,* Ann Arbor, Mich, 1991, Brown and Benchmark.

Butterfield GE, Gates JE: Fueling activity: current concepts. In *Topics in nutrition and food safety,* Hershey, Pa, 1994, Hershey Foods Corporation.

Butterfield GE, Tremblay A: Physical activity and nutrition in the context of fitness and health. In Bouchard C et al, editors: *Physical activity, fitness and health: international proceedings and consensus statement,* Champaign, Ill, 1994, Human Kinetics Publishers.

Cannon JG et al: Acute phase response in exercise: interaction of age and vitamin E on neutrophils and muscle enzyme release, *Am J Physiol* 269(28):R1214, 1990.

Casa DJ et al: National Athletic Trainers Association, Position statement: Fluid replacement for athletes, *J Athletic Training* 35:212, 2000.

Clarkson PM: Antioxidants and physical performance, *Crit Rev Food Sci Nutr* 35(1&2):13, 1995.

Coleman E: Carbohydrate—the master fuel. In Berning JR, Steen SN, editors: *Nutrition for sport and exercise,* Gaithersburg, Md, 1998, Aspen Publishers.

Cooper K: *Cooper's antioxidant revolution,* Nashville, Tenn, 1994, Thomas Nelson Publishers.

Cori CF: The fate of sugar in the animal body. I. The rate of absorption of hexoses and pentoses from the intestinal tract, *J Biol Chem* 66:7691, 1926.

Costill DL, Sparks KE: Rapid fluid replacement following thermal dehydration, *J Appl Physiol* 34:299, 1973.

Costill DL et al: Effects of elevated plasma FFA and insulin on muscle glycogen usage during exercise, *J Appl Physiol* 43:695, 1977a.

Costill DL et al: Muscle glycogen utilization during prolonged exercise on successive days, *J Appl Physiol* 31:834, 1977b.

Costill DL et al: The role of dietary carbohydrate in muscle glycogen resynthesis after strenuous running, *Am J Clin Nutr* 34: 1831, 1981.

Coyle EF: Timing and method of increased carbohydrate intake to cope with heavy training, competition, and recovery, *J Sport Sci* 9:29, 1991.

Coyle EF: Substrate utilization during exercise in active people, *Am J Clin Nutr* 61(suppl):S157, 1995.

Cunningham JJ: Is potassium needed in sports drinks for fluid replacement during exercise? *Int J Sports Nutr* 7(2):154, 1997.

Davies KJA et al: Free radical and tissue damage produced by exercise, *Biochem Biophys Res Commun* 107:1198, 1982.

Delvin J et al: Amino acid metabolism after intense exercise, *Am J Physiol* 268:E249, 1990.

DeMarco HM et al: Pre-exercise carbohydrate meals: application of glycemic index, *Med Sci Sports Exerc* 31:164-170, 1999.

Dillard CJ et al: Effects of exercise, vitamin E, and ozone on pulmonary function and lipid peroxidation, *J Appl Physiol Respir Environ Exerc Physiol* 45:927, 1978.

Dohm G et al: Protein degradation during endurance exercise and recovery, *Med Sci Sports Exerc* 19:5166, 1987.

Dreon DM et al: A very lowfat diet is not associated with improved lipoprotein profiles in men with a predominance of large low density lipoproteins, *Am J Clin Nutr* 69:411, 1999.

Drinkwater BL et al: Bone mineral density after resumption of menses in amenorrheic athletes, *JAMA* 266:380, 1986.

Franke WW, Berendonk B: Hormonal doping and androgenization of athletes: a secret program of the German Democratic Republic government, *Clin Chem* 43:1262, 1997.

Gisolfi CV: Is the GI system built for exercise? *News Physiol Sci* 15:114, 2000.

Gisolfi CV et al: Human intestinal water absorption: direct vs. indirect measurements, *Am J Physiol* 268:G216, 1990.

Gontzea I et al: The influence of muscular activity on nitrogen balance and on the need of man for protein, *Nutr Rep Int* 10:35, 1974.

Gonzalez-Alonso J, Heaps CL, Coyle EF: Rehydration after exercise with common beverages and water, *Int J Sports Med* 13:399, 1992.

Green DR et al: An evaluation of dietary intakes of triathletes: are RDAs being met? *J Am Diet Assoc* 89:1653, 1989.

Greenhaff PL et al: The effect of oral creatine supplementation on skeletal muscle ATP degradation during repeated bouts of maximal voluntary exercise in man, *Am J Physiol* 266(SPTI): E726, 1994.

Harber VJ: Menstrual dysfunction in athletes: an energetic challenge, *Exerc Sport Sci Rev* 28:19, 2000.

Hargreaves M: Carbohydrate and exercise, *J Sport Sci* 9:17, 1991.

Harkins C et al: Protocols for developing dietary prescriptions. In Benardot D, editor: *Sports nutrition: a guide for the professional working with active people,* ed 2, Chicago, 1993, American Dietetic Association.

Haymes EM, Clarkson PM: Minerals and trace minerals. In Berning JR, Steen SN, editors: *Nutrition for sport and exercise,* Gaithersburg, Md, 1998, Aspen Publishers.

Hickson JF et al: Repeated days of body building exercise do not enhance urinary excretions from untrained young adult males, *Nutr Res* 10:723, 1990.

Horowitz JF, Coyle EF: Metabolic responses to pre-exercise meals containing various carbohydrates and fat, *Am J Clin Nutr* 58:235-241, 1993.

Institute of Medicine, Food and Nutrition Board: *Dietary reference intakes (DRIs) for energy and the macronutrients, carbohydrate, fiber, fat, fatty acids, cholesterol, protein and amino acids,* Washington, DC, 2002, National Academy Press.

Ivy JL: Dietary strategies to promote glycogen synthesis after exercise, *Can J Appl Physiol* 26:(suppl):S236, 2001.

Jackson D et al: Effects of carbohydrate feedings on fatigue during intermittent high-intensity exercise in males and females, *Med Sci Sports Exer* 27:S223, 1995.

Jarvis M et al: The acute 1-week effects of the Zone diet on body composition, blood lipid levels, and performance in recreational endurance athletes, *J Strength Cond Res* 16(1):50, 2002.

Jonnavithula S et al: Bone density is compromised in amenorrheic women despite return of menses: a 2 year study, *Obstet Gynecol* 81:669, 1993.

Juenkendrump AE, Jentjens R: Oxidation of carbohydrate feedings during prolonged exercise: current thoughts, guidelines and directions for future research, *Sports Med* 29(6):407, 2000.

Kanter M: Antioxidant supplementation for persons who are physically active. In Berning JR, Steen SN, editors: *Nutrition for sport and exercise,* Gaithersburg, Md: Aspen Publishers, 1998.

Keith RE: Vitamins and physical activity. In Wolinsky I, Hickson JF, editors: *Nutrition in exercise and sport,* Boca Raton, Fla, 1994, CRC Press.

Kiens B et al: Benefit of dietary simple carbohydrates on the early post exercise muscle glycogen repletion in athletes, *Med Sci Sports Exerc* 22(S4):88, 1990.

Konig D et al: Exercise and oxidative stress: significance of antioxidants with reference to inflammatory, muscular, and systemic stress, *Exerc Immunol Rev* 7:108, 2001.

Lambert EV et al: Enhanced endurance in trained cyclists during moderate intensity exercise following 2 weeks adaptation to a high fat diet, *Eur J Appl Physiol* 69:287, 1994.

Leiper JB, Maughn RJ: Absorption of water and electrolytes from hypotonic, isotonic and hypertonic solutions, *J Physiol* 373:90P, 1986a.

Leiper JB, Maughn RJ: The effect of luminal tonicity on water absorption from a segment of the intact human jejunum, *J Physiol* 378:95P, 1986b.

Lindeman AK: Body image and college women athletes, *Top Clin Nutr* 10(1):58, 1994.
Lindinger MI et al: Caffeine attenuates the exercise-induced increase in plasma [K^+] in humans, *J Appl Physiol* 74:1149, 1993.
Loucks AB: Physical health of the female athlete: observations, effects, and causes of reproductive disorders, *Can J Appl Physiol* 26(suppl):S176, 2001.
Mahesh VB, Greenblatt RB: The in vivo conversion of dehydroepiandrosterone and androstenedione to testosterone in the human, *Acta Endocrinol* 41:400, 1962.
Malawer SJ: Interrelationship between jejunal absorption of sodium, glucose, and water in man, *Am Soc Clin Invest* 44:1072, 1965.
Meredith CN et al: Dietary protein requirements and body protein metabolism in endurance trained men, *J Appl Physiol* 66:2850, 1989.
Meydani M et al: Protective effect of vitamin E on exercise-induced oxidative damage in young and older adults, *Am J Physiol* 264:R992, 1993.
Meyer FO et al: Hypohydration during exercise in children: effect on thirst, drink preferences and rehydration, *Int J Sports Nutr* 1:22, 1994.
Morales AJ et al: Effects of replacement dose of DHEA in men and women of advancing age, *J Endocrinol Metab* 78:1360, 1994.
Muoio DM et al: Effect of dietary fat on metabolic adjustments to maximal V_{O_2} and endurance in runners, *Med Sci Sports Exerc* 26:81, 1994.
Nadel ER et al: Influence of fluid replacement beverages on body fluid homeostasis during exercise and recovery. In Gisolfi CV, Lamb DR, editors: *Perspectives in exercise science and sports medicine,* vol 3, *Fluid homeostasis during exercise,* Indianapolis, 1990, Benchmark Press.
Nissen S et al: Effect of leucine metabolite beta hydroxy beta methylbutyrate on muscle metabolism during resistance training, *J Appl Physiol* 81:2095, 1996.
Nose H et al: Role of osmolality and plasma volume during rehydration in humans, *J Appl Physiol* 65:326, 1988.
Otis CL et al: American College of Sports Medicine position stand on the female athlete triad, *Med Sci Sports Exerc* 29(5):i, 1997.
Patterson BH et al: Fruit and vegetables in the American diet: data from the NHANES II survey, *Am J Public Health* 80:1443, 1990.
Peters HP et al: Potential benefits and hazards of physical activity and exercise on the gastrointestinal tract, *Gut* 48:435, 2001.
Pugliese MT et al: Fear of obesity: a cause of short stature and delayed puberty, *N Engl J Med* 309:513, 1983.
Rasmussen B et al: An oral essential amino acid–carbohydrate supplement enhances muscle protein anabolism after resistance exercise, *J Appl Physiol* 88:386, 2000.
Regelson W, Kalimi M: Dehydroepiandrosterone (DHEA)—the multifunctional steroid. II. Effects on the CNS, cell proliferation, metabolic and vascular, clinical, and other effects, *Ann N Y Acad Sci* 719:564, 1994.
Regelson W et al: Dehydroepiandrosterone (DHEA)—the mother steroid. I. Immunological action, *Ann N Y Acad Sci* 719:553, 1994.
Roy BD, Tarnopolsky MA: Influence of differing macronutrient intakes on muscle glycogen resynthesis after resistance exercise, *J Appl Physiol* 84:890, 1998.
Ryan AJ et al: Effect of hypohydration on gastric emptying and intestinal absorption during exercise, *J Appl Physiol* 84:1581, 1998.
Sanchez-Quesada JL et al: Increase of LDL susceptibility to oxidation occurring after intense, long duration aerobic exercise, *Atherosclerosis* 118:297, 1995.
Sherman WM et al: Effect of 4 h pre exercise carbohydrate feedings on cycling performance, *Med Sci Sports Exerc* 21:598, 1989.
Simonsen JC et al: Dietary carbohydrate, muscle glycogen, and power output during rowing training, *J Appl Physiol* 70:1500, 1991.
Singh A et al: Dietary intakes and biochemical profiles of nutritional status of ultramarathoners, *Med Sci Sport Exerc* 26:328, 1993.
Singh VN: A current perspective on nutrition and exercise, *J Nutr* 122:760, 1992.
Smetanka RD et al: Intestinal permeability in runners in the 1996 Chicago marathon, *Int J Sports Nutr* 9:426, 1999.
Spodaryk K: Iron metabolism in boys involved in intensive physical training, *Physiol Behav* 75(1-2):201, 2002.
Steen SN, Brownell KD: Patterns of weight loss and regain in wrestlers: has the tradition changed? *Med Sci Sports Exerc* 22:762, 1990.
Strauss RH et al: Weight loss in amateur wrestlers and its effect on serum testosterone levels, *JAMA* 264:3337, 1985.
Sugiura K, Kobayashi K: Effect of carbohydrate ingestion on sprint performance following continuous and intermittent exercise, *Med Sci Sports Exerc* 30:1624, 1998.
Synder AC, Naik J: Protein requirement of athletes. In Berning JR, Steen SN, editors: *Nutrition for sport and exercise,* Gaithersburg, Md, 1998, Aspen Publishers.
Synder AC et al: Myofibrillar protein degradation after eccentric exercise, *Experientia* 40:69, 1984.
Tarnopolsky MA: Caffeine and endurance performance, *Sports Med* 18:109, 1994.
Tarnopolsky MA et al: Influence of protein intake and training status on nitrogen balance and lean body mass, *J Appl Physiol* 64:187, 1988.
Tarnopolsky MA et al: Effect of body building exercise on protein requirements, *Can J Sports Sci* 15:226, 1991.
Tarnopolsky M et al: Evaluation of protein requirements for trained strength athletes, *J Appl Physiol* 73:1986, 1992.
Tipton K et al: Postexercise net protein synthesis in human muscle from orally administered amino acids, *Am J Physiol* 276:E628, 1999.
Turner LW, Bass MA: Osteoporosis knowledge, attitudes, and behaviors of female collegiate athletes, *Int J Sport Nutr Exerc Metab* 11:482, 2001.
Viguie CA et al: Antioxidant supplementation affects indices of muscle trauma and oxidant stress in human blood during exercise, *Med Sci Sports Exerc* 21:S16, 1989.
Wardlaw GM: *Perspectives in nutrition,* ed 4, New York, 1999, WCB–McGraw Hill.
Waller MF, Haymes EM: The effects of heat and exercise on sweat iron loss, *Med Sci Sport Exerc* 28:197, 1996.
Warren MP, Stiehl AL: Exercise and female adolescents: effects on the reproductive and skeletal systems, *J Am Med Womens Assoc* 54(3):115, 138, 1999.
Wee SL et al: Influence of high and low glycemic index meals on endurance running capacity, *Med Sci Sports Exerc* 31:393, 1999.
Weindruch R: National Institute of Aging, Grant Number 5RC1AG10536-05 CRISP, 1997.
Wright DA, Sherman WM, Dernback AR: Carbohydrate feedings before, during or in combination improve cycling performance, *J Appl Physiol* 71:1082-1088, 1991.
Yoshimura H: Adult protein requirements, *Fed Proc* 20:103, 1961.
Zawadski KM et al: Carbohydrate-protein complex increases the rate of muscle glycogen storage after exercise, *J Appl Physiol* 72:1854, 1992.

Additional References

Beals K, Manore M: Nutritional status of female athletes with subclinical eating disorders, *J Am Diet Assoc* 98:419, 1998.
Below PR et al: Fluid and carbohydrate ingestion independently improve performance during 1 hour of intense exercise, *Med Sci Sports Exerc* 27:200, 1994.
Bosch A et al: Fuel substrate kinetics of carbohydrate loading differs from that of carbohydrate ingestion during prolonged exercise, *Metabolism* 45:415, 1996.
Burke LM: Energy needs of athletes, *Can J Appl Physiol* 26(suppl): S202, 2001.
Clarkson P: Antioxidants and physical performance, *Crit Rev Food Sci Nutr* 35(1&2):131, 1995.
Coombes JS, Hamilton KL: The effectiveness of commercially available sports drinks, *Sports Med* 29(3):181, 2000.
Feldman EB: Creatine: a dietary supplement and ergogenic aid, *Nutr Rev* 57:45, 1999.

Hargreaves M, Cameron-Smith D: Exercise, diet, and skeletal muscle gene expression, *Med Sci Sports Exerc* 34:1505, 2002.

Haymes EM: Vitamin and mineral supplementation to athletes, *Int J Sports Med* 1:146, 1991.

Kirschner E et al: Bone mineral density and dietary intake of female college gymnasts, *Med Sci Sports Exerc* 27:543, 1995.

Lawrence ME, Kirby DF: Nutrition and sports supplements: fact or fiction, *J Clin Gastroenterol* 35(4):299, 2002.

Leddy J et al: Effect of a high or a low fat diet on cardiovascular risk factors in male and female runners, *Med Sci Sports Exerc* 29:17, 1997.

Maughan R: The athlete's diet: nutritional goals and dietary strategies, *Proc Nutr Soc* 61(1):87, 2002.

Murray R: Fluid needs of athletes. In Berning JR, Steen SN, editors: *Nutrition for sport and exercise,* Gaithersburg, Md, 1998, Aspen Publishing.

Oppliger R et al: The Wisconsin wrestling minimum weight project: a model for weight control among high school wrestlers, *Med Sci Sports Exerc* 27:1220, 1995.

Ryan M: Sports drinks: research asks for reevaluation of current recommendations, *J Am Diet Assoc* 97:S197, 1997.

Stewart JG et al: Gastrointestinal blood loss and anemia in runners, *Ann Intern Med* 100:843, 1984.

Tegelman R et al: Influence of a diet regimen on glucose homeostasis and serum lipid levels in male elite athletes, *Metabolism* 45:435, 1996.

Thompson J, Manore M: Predicted and measured resting metabolic rate of male and female endurance athletes, *J Am Diet Assoc* 96:30, 1996.

Volek J et al: Creatine supplementation enhances muscular performance during high-intensity resistance exercise, *J Am Diet Assoc* 97:765, 1997.

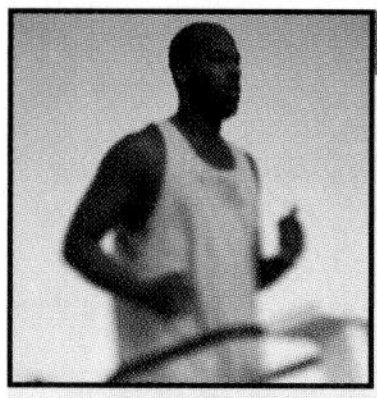

CHAPTER 27

Nutrition and Bone Health

JOHN J.B. ANDERSON, PhD

CHAPTER OUTLINE

- Bone Structure and Bone Physiology
- Bone Mass and Bone Density
- Nutrition and Bone
- Osteopenia and Osteoporosis

KEY TERMS

age-related osteoporosis (type II)–loss of bone mineral density in both cortical and trabecular bone that occurs in older persons of both sexes after 70 years of age; characterized by hip and vertebral fractures, the latter may lead to back pain, loss of height, and "dowager's hump"

bisphosphonates–drugs that act on osteoclasts to inhibit their resorption of bone tissue; examples include etidronate, alendronate, and pamidronate

bone densitometry–measurement of bone using tissue absorption of x-rays (photons) by an instrument called a dual–x-radiographic absorptiometer (DXA)

bone markers–molecules or portions of molecules derived from bone tissue that can be measured in blood serum or urine; matrix markers include portions of collagen molecules, whereas bone cell markers include enzymes such as alkaline phosphatase

bone mineral content (BMC)–bone accumulated before the end of growth cessation; expressed in grams of mineral per centimeter of bone

bone mineral density (BMD)–a measurement of bone mass after development is complete; expressed in grams per centimeter squared

bone modeling–the process by which bones grow in size and change their longitudinal and cross-sectional dimensions; bone formation by osteoblasts precedes bone resorption by osteoclasts; formation and resorption are usually spatially separated

bone remodeling–the process by which bone is continually dismantled and reformed to repair itself, grow, adapt to external strains, and furnish calcium for other body needs; resorption and formation involve the same bone space

calcium homeostasis–the process of maintenance of a constant serum calcium concentration, that is, at a set level; bone furnishes calcium ions for other tissue needs by calcium ion transfer from bone fluid to blood and by resorption of bone tissue via osteoclasts

cortical bone–the compact bone of the shaft that surrounds the medullary cavity of the long bones

estrogen receptor (ER)–cellular molecule that binds to estrogens, SERMS, and phytoestrogens before delivering these molecules to nuclear DNA for initiation of events typical of estrogen stimulation of the cell; ERs are important in osteoblasts of both sexes

estrogen replacement therapy (ERT)–administration of estrogen molecules to replace the natural hormone, which declines drastically after menopause; similar to hormone replacement therapy (HRT)

hydroxyapatite–a crystalline structure composed of calcium phosphate and calcium carbonate in an organic collagen matrix that gives strength and rigidity to bones

intermittent parathyroid hormone (PTH) therapy–action of PTH (as a drug) at low concentrations on osteoblasts to increase cell proliferation and stimulate new bone formation, which results in increased BMD

matrix–the organic matrix (osteoid) of bone, consisting mainly of collagen, gives both strength and flexibility to bones

osteoblast–a bone cell responsible for the formation of bone

osteocalcin–a vitamin K–dependent bone-specific protein that is released into blood from the resorbed matrix as well as from the osteoblast cells that make it

osteoclast–a bone cell responsible for the resorption and removal of bone

osteocyte–a bone cell derived from an osteoblast that gets buried in mineralized bone after the bone forms; it maintains communication with osteoblasts on bone surfaces

osteomalacia–a condition of impaired mineralization caused by vitamin D and calcium deficiency

osteopenia–too little bone mass at any stage of the life cycle

osteoporosis–a loss of bone tissue to the point that the specific skeletal site is unable to sustain ordinary strains where a fracture may develop

peak bone mass (PBM)–the greatest amount (mass) of bone accumulated at any age; typically PBM occurs by approximately 30 years of age, but in some individuals PBM may accrue at an earlier or even a later age

phytoestrogens–estrogen-like molecules derived from soybeans, clover, and other plant sources; isoflavone and lignin molecules act on estrogen receptors more like SERMs than true estrogens

postmenopausal osteoporosis (type I)–a loss of bone mineral density after significant declines of sex hormones, especially estrogens in women; involves primarily the trabecular bone tissue and characterized by fractures of the distal radius and ulna and crush fractures of the lumbar vertebrae

secondary osteoporosis–a loss of bone density secondary to another disease, such as liver disease or renal disease

selective estrogen receptor modulator (SERM)–molecules, including a specific class of drugs, that act on ERs in osteoblasts to promote the maintenance of bone tissue but without having the undesirable effects on reproductive tissues that lead to breast or uterine cancers; examples include tamoxifen and raloxifene

trabecular bone (cancellous bone)–the spongy bone found primarily in the knobby ends of the long bones, the iliac crest, scapula, and vertebrae

Adequate nutrition is essential for the development and maintenance of the skeleton, that is, bone health. Although diseases of the bone, such as osteoporosis and osteomalacia, have complex etiologies, the development of these diseases can be minimized by providing adequate nutrients in all periods of the life cycle. Of these diseases, osteoporosis is the most common and destructive of productivity and quality of life. The number of older adults (over age 65 years) in the United States is projected to reach almost 25% by 2020, a doubling since 1988 (Schneider and Guralnik, 1990), greatly increasing the numbers in the population at risk for osteoporosis. The average life expectancy in the United States early in the twenty-first century is almost 81 years for women and 74 for men. As a result of the increasing numbers of older adults, osteoporosis, as manifested by hip fractures, is becoming more significant in both morbidity and mortality as well as in cost.

The provision of bone-building nutrients is necessary even after the onset of osteoporosis. The benefits of adequate intakes of calcium and other nutrients during adulthood and older adulthood remain as significant as during the early period of bone growth and development.

BONE STRUCTURE AND BONE PHYSIOLOGY

Bone is a term used to mean both an organ, such as the femur, and a tissue, such as trabecular bone tissue. Each bone (organ) contains bone tissues of two major types: trabecular and cortical (Figure 27-1). These tissues undergo bone modeling during growth (height) and bone remodeling after growth ceases.

Composition of Bone

Bone consists of an organic matrix or osteoid, primarily collagen fibers, in which salts of calcium and phosphate are deposited in combination with hydroxyl ions in crystals of hydroxyapatite. The tensile strength of collagen and the hardness of hydroxyapatite combine to give bone its great strength. Other components of the bone matrix include osteocalcin, osteopontin, and several other matrix proteins.

Types of Bone Tissue

About 80% of the skeleton consists of compact or cortical bone tissue. Shafts of the long bones are primarily cortical bone. The remaining 20% of the skeleton is trabecular or cancellous bone tissue, which exists in the knobby ends of the long bones, the iliac crest of the pelvis, the wrists, scapulas, vertebrae, and the regions of bones that line the marrow.

Trabecular bone (cancellous bone) tissue is less dense than cortical bone tissue as a result of an open structure of interconnecting bony spicules that resemble a sponge in appearance (thus trabecular bone is also called *spongy bone* or *spongiosa*). The elaborate interconnecting components (columns and struts) of trabecular bone tissue add support to the cortical bone tissue shell of the long bones as well as provide a large surface area that is exposed to circulating fluids from the marrow and lined by a disproportionately

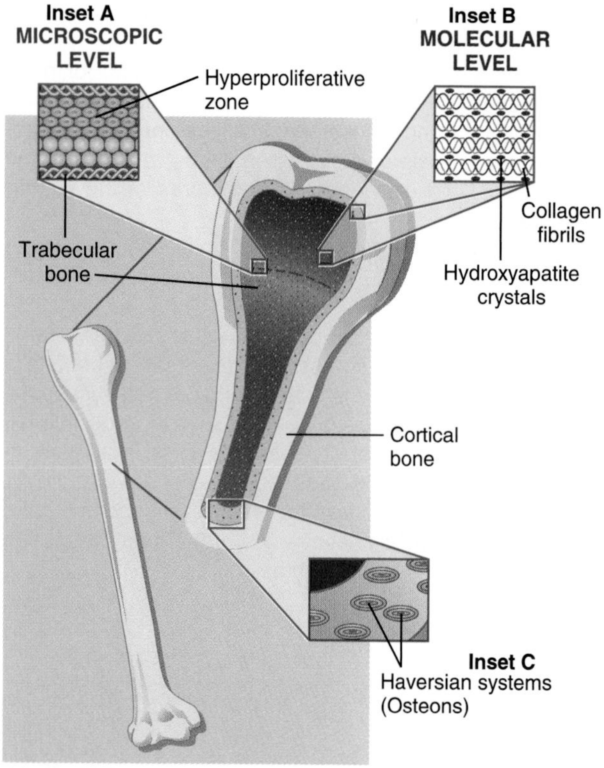

FIGURE 27-1 • Schematic diagram of the structure of a long bone (hemisection of a long bone, such as the tibia). The ends of the long bones contain high percentages of trabecular (cancellous) bone tissue, whereas the shaft contains predominantly cortical bone tissue. **A,** An enlarged section (approximately 100-fold) of the growth plate (epiphysis) and the subjacent hyperproliferative zone containing cartilage cells stacked like coins. Mineralization in this zone produces the primary spongiosa, which is subsequently modeled by osteoblasts and osteoclasts to form the mature trabecular bone tissue. (Cartilage is replaced by bone in this region.) **B,** Section of collagen molecules (triple helices) surrounded by mineralized deposits (dark spheroids) at a magnification of approximately one million. These collagen-mineral complexes exist in both trabecular and cortical bone tissues in association with other matrix proteins (not shown). **C,** Cross-section of half of the midshaft of a long bone (magnification approximately tenfold). This section of cortical bone tissue contains vertical Haversian systems (osteons) that run in parallel with the shaft axis (many are required to extend this system from one end of the shaft to the other). At the center of each osteon is a canal that contains an artery that supplies bone tissues with nutrients and oxygen, a vein for removing wastes, and a nerve for returning afferent relays to the brain. The lamellar structure of Haversian systems not only adds strength to the bone, but these units also undergo remodeling, which permits both repair of microfractures and adaptation to loads (strains) of the body bearing on the bone. (Copyright of John J. B. Anderson and Sanford C. Garner.)

larger number of cells than cortical bone tissue. Trabecular bone tissue is therefore much more responsive to estrogens or the lack of estrogens than cortical bone tissue (see Figure 27-1). The loss of trabecular bone tissue late in life is largely responsible for the occurrence of fractures.

TABLE 27-1 Functions of Osteoblasts and Osteoclasts

OSTEOBLASTS	OSTEOCLASTS
Bone Formation	**Bone Resorption**
Synthesis of matrix proteins	Degradation of bone tissue via enzymes and acid (H^+) secretion
Collagen type 1 (90%)	
Osteocalcin and others (10%)	
Mineralization	
Communication	Communication
Secretion of cytokines that act on OCs	Secretion of cytokines that act on OBs

OBs, Osteoblasts; *OCs,* osteoclasts.

Bone Cells

Two cells are responsible for the formation and maintenance of bone: osteoblasts, which form bone, and osteoclasts, which resorb bone. Osteoblasts contain estrogen receptors (ERs). The functions of these two cell types are listed in Table 27-1. Two other important cell types also exist in bone tissue: osteocytes and bone-lining cells, both of which are derived from osteoblasts. The origin of the osteoblasts and osteoclasts is from primitive precursor cells found in bone marrow.

Calcium Homeostasis

Bone tissue serves as a reservoir of calcium and other minerals that are used by other tissues of the body. Calcium homeostasis is almost totally reliant on this source of calcium when the diet is inadequate. Bone tissue is also dynamic, although a slow dynamic, because it undergoes both modeling early in life and remodeling after skeletal growth (height) ceases.

Although 99% of the body calcium is found in the skeleton, the remaining 1% is critical to a great variety of indispensable life processes. The concentration of calcium in blood and other extracellular fluids is regulated by complex mechanisms that balance calcium intake and excretion with bodily needs. When calcium intake is not adequate, homeostasis is maintained by drawing on mineral from the bone to keep the serum calcium ion concentration at its set level, that is, about 10 mg/dl or 2.5 mmol. Depending on the amount of calcium required, homeostasis can be accomplished by drawing from two major skeletal sources: readily mobilizable calcium ions in the bone fluid or, through the process of osteoclastic resorption, from the bone tissue itself (see Chapter 5).

Adaptation of the homeostatic mechanism regulating blood calcium concentration is achieved through two calcium-regulating hormones, parathyroid hormone (PTH) and 1,25-dihydroxyvitamin D (calcitriol). This calcium-regulatory system works more efficiently early in life, especially during the first few decades, but the efficiency undergoes a gradual decline in later life. For example, within a few years after menopause, urinary calcium losses from the body increase, but intestinal absorption of calcium does not increase enough to balance the losses. PTH activity, which directly contributes to bone loss, increases in most persons beginning in their sixties, even though PTH measurements typically remain within normal range-albeit at the high end. Calcium supplements help to reduce serum PTH.

The hormonal form of vitamin D, calcitriol, also plays an adaptational role by increasing the efficiency of intestinal calcium absorption in the upper half of the small bowel when dietary calcium is inadequate. This hormone is especially critical in the prepubertal and postpubertal growth years of girls and boys who have less than recommended intakes of calcium. Calcitriol, however, is much less effective in improving intestinal calcium absorption in women a decade or so after the onset of the menopause, even though serum calcitriol concentrations are elevated (Ebeling et al, 1992).

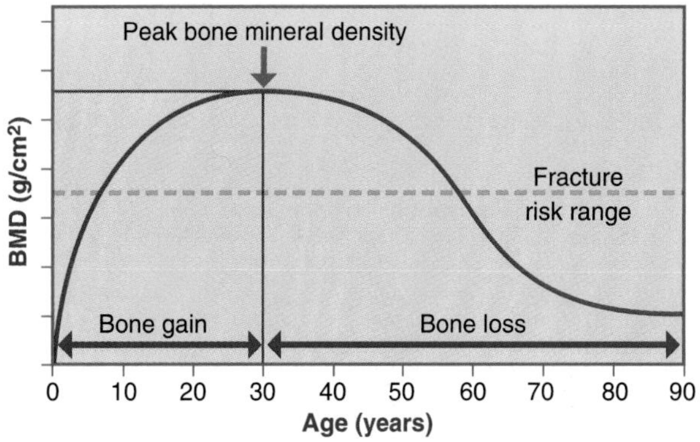

FIGURE 27-2 • Early gain and later loss of bone in females. Peak bone mineral density (BMD) is typically achieved by age 30. Menopause occurs at approximately age 50 or within a few years thereafter. Postmenopausal women typically enter the fracture risk range after age 60. Men have a more gradual decline in BMD, which starts at 50 years of age. (Copyright of John J. B. Anderson and Sanford C. Garner.)

Bone Modeling

Bone modeling is the term applied to the growth of the skeleton until mature height is achieved. For example, during bone modeling, long bones elongate and widen by undergoing great internal changes as well as external expansions in their structures. In modeling, the process of formation of new bone tissue occurs first and is followed by the resorption of old tissue.

Growth occurs at *epiphyses* (growth plates that undergo hyperproliferation) and circumferentially, where at each location cells undergo division and contribute to the formation of new bone tissue (see Figure 27-1).

Bone modeling is typically completed in girls by 16 to 18 years of age and in boys by age 18 to 20. After growth (height) ceases, gains in bone tissue may continue by the process known as *bone consolidation* (see later section, Peak Bone Mass). The major event in the skeleton in early life is growth, whereas in later life it is the loss of bone. This concept underlines the inevitable decline of bone mass in the late stages of life, at least in the U.S. population (Looker et al, 1995, 1997). A way to think of these bone processes is early gain and later loss (Garn, 1970) (Figure 27-2).

Bone Remodeling

After skeletal growth is completed, there is continuous bone remodeling in response to strains on the skeleton, adaptation to changes in lifestyle factors and dietary intakes, maintenance of set calcium concentration in extracellular fluids, and repairs of microscopic fractures that occur over time. About 4% of the total bone surface is involved in remodeling at any given time as new bone is renewed continually at specific loci throughout the skeleton. Even in the mature skeleton, bone remains a dynamic tissue. Normal bone turnover is illustrated in Figure 27-3.

Bone remodeling is a process in which bone is continuously resorbed through the action of the osteoclasts and reformed through the action of the osteoblasts. After activation by specific hormones and cytokines, osteoclasts resorb both the mineral and organic components of bone by forming small cavities on bone surfaces. The resorptive process is rapid and it is completed within a few days, whereas the refilling of these cavities by osteoblasts is slow, that is, on the order of 3 to 6 months or even longer in older persons.

Trabecular bone especially declines after menopause because of unopposed osteoclastic activity; that is, there is insufficient osteoblastic bone formation (Eriksen et al, 1990). In normal young adults, the resorption and formation phases are tightly coupled and the amount of bone mass is maintained. In older persons, bone loss involves an uncoupling of the phases of bone remodeling with an increase of resorption over formation. As a result of the uncoupled bone remodeling, bone loss occurs.

The remodeling process is initiated by the *activation* of preosteoclastic cells in the bone marrow. Interleukin-1 and other cytokines released from bone-lining cells, that is, inactive osteoblasts, are considered to act as the triggers in the activation process. The preosteoclast cells migrate to the surfaces of bone while differentiating into mature osteoclasts. The osteoclasts then cover a specific area of trabecular or cortical bone tissue. Acids and proteolytic enzymes released by the osteoclasts *resorb* both bone mineral and matrix on the surface of trabecular bone or cortical bone. The *rebuilding or formation* stage

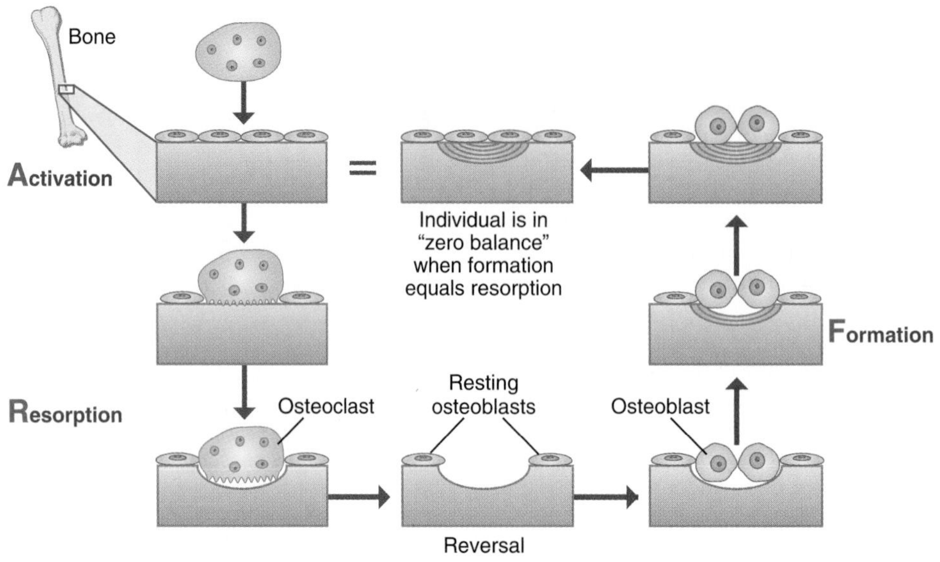

FIGURE 27-3 • Bone turnover in healthy adults. (Copyright of John J. B. Anderson and Sanford C. Garner.)

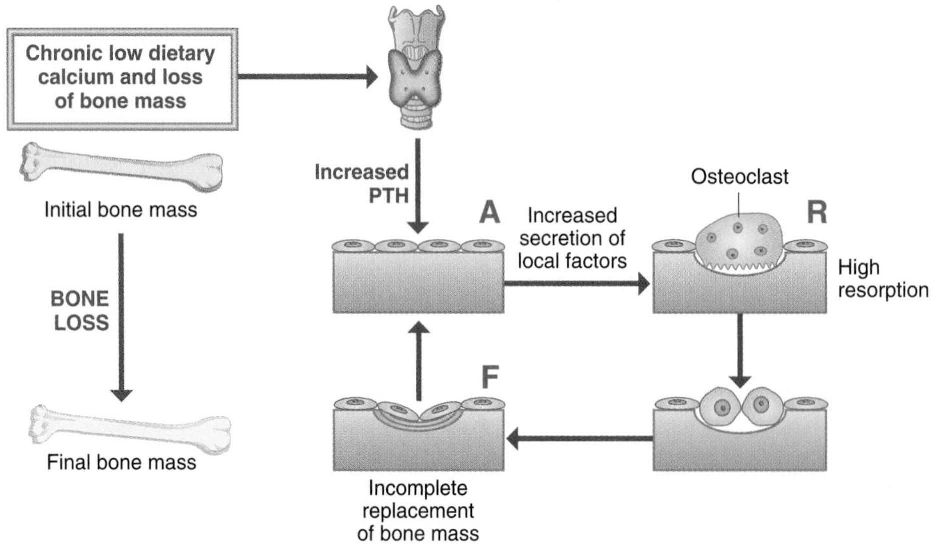

FIGURE 27-4 • Effects of persistently elevated parathyroid hormone (PTH) on bone mass. (Copyright of John J. B. Anderson and Sanford C. Garner.)

involves secretion of collagen (type I) and other matrix proteins by the osteoblasts. Collagen polymerizes to form mature triple-stranded fibers. In a few days, salts of calcium and phosphate begin to precipitate on the collagen fibers, developing into crystals of hydroxyapatite.

When the resorption and formation phases are in balance, the same amount of bone tissue exists at the completion of the formation phase (see Figure 27-3). The benefit to the skeleton of this remodeling is the renewal of bone, that is, new bone, without any microfractures. When dietary calcium is low, however, osteoclastic resorption becomes greater than formation by osteoblasts because of a persistently elevated PTH concentration in blood (Figure 27-4).

The action of PTH in promoting activity of the osteoclasts is countered by estrogen, which reduces the response of osteoblasts to PTH. Then PTH acts directly on osteoblasts, which increase the production of interleukin-6 (IL-6) and other cytokines that in turn stimulate osteoclasts to resorb bone. Estrogen helps to block the production of PTH-stimulated IL-6 and other cytokines (Chen et al, 2002; Jilka et al, 1992). These steps of bone remodeling are illustrated in Figure 27-5. *Calcitonin* directly inhibits osteoclast activity, that is, resorption, but the significance of its physiologic role in humans is not clear. Impaired production of this hormone could occur in older adults, which could contribute to age-related bone loss, but no data have been published in support of this possibility.

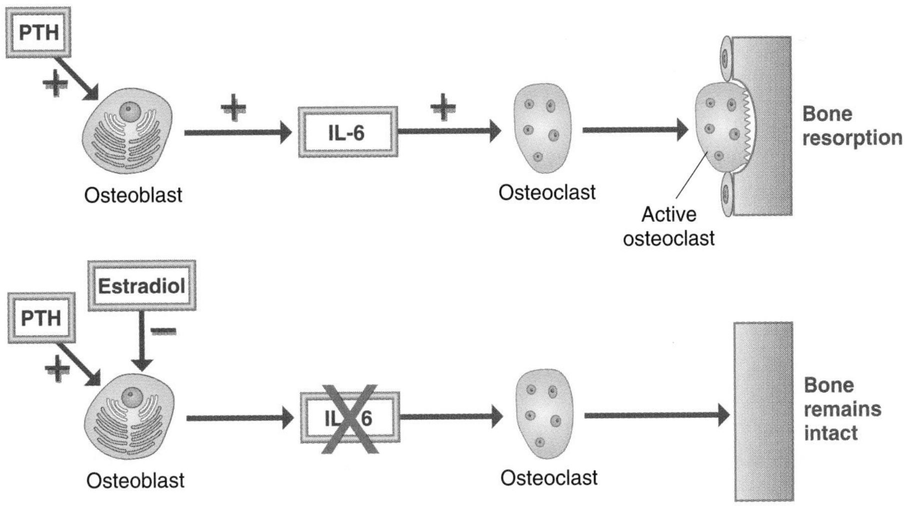

FIGURE 27-5 • Interaction between osteoblasts and osteoclasts in bone remodeling. The role of parathyroid hormone (PTH) in stimulating osteoclasts to resorb bone *(upper)* is contrasted with the inhibitory action of estrogens on osteoblasts, which negates the action of PTH *(lower)*. (Copyright of John J. B. Anderson and Sanford C. Garner.)

Bone Markers

Bone markers exist for both bone formation and bone resorption. Plasma bone-specific alkaline phosphatase is a marker of bone formation, although total plasma alkaline phosphatase may also be used. Markers of bone resorption include plasma cross-linked collagen telopeptides, urinary N-telopeptides (NTXs), and plasma tartrate-resistant acid phosphatase (TRAP). Osteocalcin, considered a bone formation marker, is also released from resorbed bone matrix, and therefore interpretation of its blood values is not as clear under most conditions.

BONE MASS AND BONE DENSITY

Bone mass is a generic term that refers to bone mineral content but not to bone mineral density. Bone mineral content (BMC) is more appropriate in assessing the amount of bone accumulated before the cessation of growth (height), whereas bone mineral density (BMD) is used to describe bone after the developmental period is completed. These measurements are often used interchangeably, but BMD is more useful in studies of adults.

Measurement of Bone Mineral Content and Bone Mineral Density

Bone densitometry measures bone mass on the basis of tissue absorption of photons produced by one or two monoenergetic x-ray tubes. Dual-energy x-ray absorptiometry (DXA) is available in most hospitals and many clinics for the measurement of the total body and regional skeletal sites of interest, such as the lumbar vertebrae and the proximal femur (hip). Results of bone mineral content (BMC) measurements are expressed as grams of mineral per centimeter, and bone mineral density (BMD) in grams per centimeter squared is calculated from the BMC divided by the width of the bone at the measurement site.

Computerized tomography may also be used to measure bone mineral density (a true volumetric density) of the spine, but this technique has not yet been developed to measure the limb bones.

Ultrasound Measurements

Quantitative ultrasound measurements of the heel bone (calcaneus) and the kneecap are now possible. Measurements by ultrasound machines provide information on two properties, the elasticity and strength of bone, that cannot be assessed by DXA. The ultrasound values are not equivalent to the BMD measurements because ultrasound assesses the properties of collagen in the organic matrix especially well rather than the mineral phase of bone tissue. Ultrasound instruments actually measure the velocity of sound waves transmitted through bone and broadband ultrasound attenuation (BUA). Measurements at the calcaneus correlate well with BMD measurements at this same skeletal site, meaning that low values by DXA are typically mirrored by low values of BUA. Therefore ultrasound is about as good as DXA in predicting the risk of fracture (Baran et al, 1991).

Accumulation of Bone Mass

During the growth periods of childhood and puberty and beyond into early adulthood, formation exceeds the resorption of bone. The long bones stop growing in length before age 18 in females and age 20 in males, but bone mass continues to accumulate for a few more years by a process known as *consolidation.* The age when bone mineral content acquisition ceases will vary, depending not only on diet but also on physical activity and strain loading on the skeleton (Bradney, 2000; Wosje et al, 2000). The consumption of both calcium supplements and calcium-enriched foods contributes to increased bone accumulation (Bonjour et al, 1997).

Peak Bone Mass

Peak bone mass (PBM) is reached by 30 years of age or soon thereafter (see Figure 27-2). PBM is greater in men than in women because of their larger frame size. BMC, but not necessarily BMD, is typically lower in women. Both the lean and fat components of body composition contribute to these differences in bone mass. BMD is also greater in blacks and Hispanics than in whites and Asians, a factor that may be related to larger muscle mass (Anderson and Pollitzer, 1994).

A strong *hereditary component* is also related to the development of bone mass. The contribution of heredítable factors to bone is estimated to be about 60%, which means the estimated contribution from environmental factors is only about 40%. Premenopausal daughters of osteoporotic mothers have demonstrated reduced bone mass in the spine and femoral neck compared with daughters of mothers within the normal range of bone measurements (Seeman et al, 1989).

Peak bone mass is related to both dietary calcium intakes and weight-bearing physical activity (Snow-Harter et al, 1990; Wosje et al, 2000). *Calcium intake* appears to be a critical factor in the early postmenarcheal growth of girls (Jackman et al, 1997), as well as in the few years before menarche (Bonjour, 2001). The contribution of *weight-bearing exercise* to PBM during the growth and development period may be greater than that of calcium (Welten et al, 1994). Whether an interaction exists between these two variables is not yet clear, but a positive interaction between them appears to affect favorably measurements of BMD (Wosje et al, 2000). *Oral contraceptive use* for several years during early adulthood may also increase bone mass, especially in the lumbar spine and femoral neck (Kritz-Silverstein and Barrett-Connor, 1993).

Finally, *body weight* (or body mass index [BMI]) is a good indicator of greater BMC and BMD. Studies that adjusted for other factors reported that body weight was the most consistent factor related to bone mass, both in older women (Edelstein and Barrett-Connor, 1993) and in young adult women (Halioua and Anderson, 1990). The component of body composition more closely associated with bone mass is the fat compartment, although the lean body mass (muscle especially) also contributes to bone mass during adulthood (Hla et al, 1996).

Loss of Bone Mass

Age is an important determinant of BMD. If the age of a woman is known, her vertebral bone mass can be predicted within 10% (see *Clinical Insight:* Women at High Risk for a Hip Fracture).

At about age 40, BMD begins to diminish gradually in both sexes, but bone loss increases greatly in

CLINICAL INSIGHT

Women at High Risk for a Hip Fracture

At present no safe and effective treatment exists to replace bone that is already lost. It is nevertheless important to identify women who are at risk of developing osteoporosis as early as possible so that measures can be taken to prevent further bone loss. Because low BMD is a major risk factor for osteoporosis, its assessment is clinically useful.

Assessment of bone status based on the existence of one or more risk factors, such as age, height, weight, smoking status, alcohol consumption, calcium intake, exercise, frame size, and selected bone markers, is not sufficiently accurate. BMD, as measured by bone densitometry, is more clinically useful. The machines that make these measurements are now readily available. Fees for the measurements are reasonable, and the procedures are safe, providing low radiation exposure. In addition, the measurements are both precise and accurate. Low BMD itself is a risk factor for osteoporotic fractures (see p. 655).

A committee of the National Osteoporosis Foundation recommends several situations in which bone densitometry is appropriate, two of which are (1) estrogen deficiency and (2) long-term glucocorticosteroid therapy (Johnston et al, 1991). A BMD measurement of an at-risk woman entering the menopause, that is, before becoming estrogen deficient, serves as a baseline for subsequent measurements as the woman becomes increasingly estrogen deficient and develops low bone mass, especially osteoporosis, according to the WHO definition. This information helps physicians and patients make decisions about the need for and use of drug therapy, such as estrogen-replacement therapy (ERT), bisphosphonates, and SERMS. In persons taking long-term glucocorticosteroid therapy, male or female, a BMD measurement can indicate the need for treatment with a bone-preserving medication and also calcitonin.

Typically total body BMD is measured, as well as the regional sites, such as the proximal femur and lumbar vertebrae. In addition, an evaluation of the skeletal status of a woman at age 50 may also include the measurement of bone markers and assessment of calcium, vitamin D, magnesium, boron, and vitamin K intakes.

women after age 50 or at menopause. A continuous loss thereafter in postmenopausal women occurs at the rate of 1% to 2% per year over the next decade. Men continue to have bone loss but at a much lower rate than for women of the same age until 70 years of age, when the loss rates are about the same for both genders. Loss of bone mass is the result of changes in the hormone-directed mechanisms that govern bone remodeling. The processes of resorption and formation are uncoupled to a degree that interferes with the ability of osteoblastic activity to keep pace with the resorptive activities of osteoclasts, that is, maintain balance. In the older persons, the bone mass become so low that these individuals are at greatly increased risk of fragility fractures that result from minimal trauma.

Cortical bone tissue and trabecular bone tissue have different patterns of aging. Loss of cortical bone eventually plateaus and may even cease late in life (Riggs and Melton, 1986). Trabecular bone begins to diminish in both sexes at as early as 40 years of age. Premenopausal loss of trabecular bone in women is much greater than that of cortical bone. Loss of both kinds of bone accelerates in women after the menopause, although trabecular bone is also lost at a much higher rate than cortical bone (Figure 27-6).

The accelerated bone loss rate of 2% to 3% per year continues for between 5 and 10 years after menopause, and then the rate declines gradually to 0.5% to 1% per year; however, a subgroup of postmenopausal women lose bone at an even faster rate (Christiansen, Riis, Rodbro, 1987) (Figure 27-7). A woman who reaches 80 years of age will lose up to 45% to 50% of her PBM, and a similarly aged man will lose about 30% of his PBM (Riggs and Melton, 1986).

The typical bone loss in older women amounts to about 300 mg of calcium per day lost in both the urine and the stool. If calcium balance is to be maintained, this amount must be replaced by absorbed calcium from the diet each day. Older women without estrogen lose more calcium in their urine than premenopausal women: as much as 100 mg more per day.

Calcium absorption is governed to a large extent by need. The vitamin D hormone allows the body of an older person theoretically to adapt to reduced intakes of calcium to maintain calcium balance, and therefore homeostasis, but at the expense of a loss of bone tissue. The vitamin D adaptive mechanism, however, typically becomes less efficient with late age. In older women not receiving ERT or other drug therapy, the achievement of calcium balance seldom occurs, even though calcium homeostasis can be maintained. This slightly negative calcium balance results because the action of hormones and other factors responsible for maintaining calcium balance, as well as the absorption of calcium, become less efficient with age. The decreased intestinal calcium absorption in women after 65 years of age, and presumably in similarly aged men also, invariably leads to a negative calcium balance.

The normal bone loss that occurs with aging in both sexes is related to the decline of osteoblastic function, such as the reduced production of type I collagen, osteocalcin, osteopontin, and other matrix proteins. As a result of the uncoupling of the remodeling process, osteoclastic resorption exceeds formation with an increasing differential. Bone loss in men accelerates in later years, typically in the sixties and seventies, as other body functions begin to decline as well. The reason for bone loss in men is presumed to result from a decline in gonadal androgen production, that is, testosterone.

Age-related changes leading to age-related osteoporosis (type II) in both men and women are not well understood. Impaired calcitriol activity in the small intestine of older women (Ebeling et al, 1992) is one

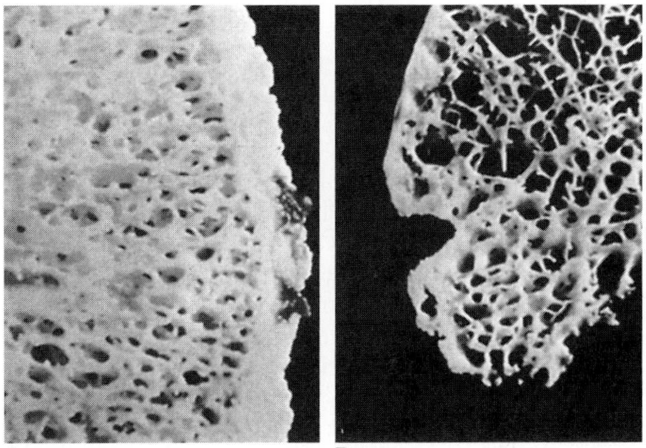

FIGURE 27-6 • Difference between normal bone **(A)** and osteoporotic bone **(B)**. (From Maher AB, Salmond SW, Pellino TA: *Orthopaedic nursing*, Philadelphia, 1994, WB Saunders.)

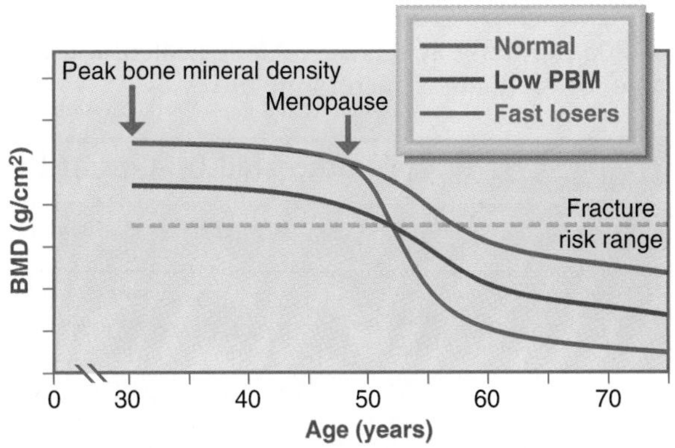

FIGURE 27-7 • Variable patterns of bone loss of women following the onset of the menopause at approximately 50 years of age. The rapid loss of bone mineral density (BMD) in some women, referred to as "fast losers," is contrasted to the loss of "slow losers." Women who develop low-peak BMD have less bone mass than women with normal BMD, but they also can lose BMD either as slow or fast losers. (Copyright of John J. B. Anderson and Sanford C. Garner.)

important factor, and decreased levels of local growth factors, such as insulin-like growth factor 1 (IGF-1), that stimulate osteoblasts to increase bone formation are another (Bauer et al, 1998). In addition, some evidence suggests that the loss of estrogens from menopause also permits an increase in the loss of urinary calcium; this loss continues into late adulthood (Nordin et al, 1991).

NUTRITION AND BONE

Not only are calcium, phosphate, and vitamin D essential for normal bone structure and functions, but several other micronutrients also have essential roles in bone. Nonnutrient plant molecules, such as phytoestrogens, may improve the status of bone tissues, but the roles of these dietary components are still uncertain.

Calcium

Calcium From Foods

Calcium intake in the primary prevention of osteoporosis has received much attention. Recommendations for the intakes of calcium and several bone-related nutrients were made in 1997 by the Institute of Medicine (Food and Nutrition Board, 1997). These recommendations are given in Table 27-2. The new recommendations for calcium, vitamin D, and a few other nutrients are given as adequate intakes (AIs) because the board did not consider that the mean requirements for calcium and vitamin D during the stages of the life cycle could be quantified. The board expressed its concern that maximizing bone mass during the adolescent growth period was extremely important by increasing the AI from preadolescence (age 11 years) through adolescence (up to age 19 years) to 1300 mg daily (Food and Nutrition Board, 1997), which exceeds the previous RDA for calcium of 1200 mg daily at this age. AIs for calcium are the same for each gender across the life cycle.

Calcium intakes typically do not meet the recommended AI for all ages beyond 11 years, especially for females. According to the U.S. Department of Agriculture (USDA) Household Food Consumption Survey (USDA, 1994), teenage females and adult women consume considerably less than the current AIs; males are more likely to consume more than females, but they do not meet the recommended levels either. These deficits translate, on average, into the need for an additional 500 mg daily for teenage females and adult women. Although it is recommended that calcium should be supplied by foods because of the coingestion of other essential nutrients, many persons, especially older women, may need to increase their intakes of calcium with supplements.

A major concern among nutritionists is that a large percentage of girls beyond age 11 are not consuming sufficient amounts of calcium. The importance to adolescents of an adequate calcium intake is unquestioned even though the precise requirements may not be known. Reaching AI levels of calcium from foods should be the first goal, but if insufficient amounts of calcium from foods are consumed, supplements of calcium salts should then be ingested to reach the age-specific AI.

Calcium From Supplements

Studies that have increased calcium intakes with supplements typically have shown significant increases in spinal and total body bone density in prepubertal and adolescent girls, which may translate into later protection against osteoporosis. The use of calcium supplements from pills, chewable tablets, and other formulations has increased in the United States because so many females have become concerned about calcium insufficiency.

Calcium consumption during childhood and adolescence is beneficial for the acquisition of peak bone mass. An 18-month double-blind study was conducted on the BMD of 70 pairs of identical twins to determine the impact of additional calcium from supplements (Johnston et al, 1992). The twins who

TABLE 27-2 Recommended Intakes of Bone-Related Nutrients

AGE (yr)	CALCIUM (mg/day)	PHOSPHORUS (mg/day)	MAGNESIUM (mg/day)		VITAMIN D (μg/day)	FLUORIDE (mg/day)	
	AI	RDA	RDA		AI	AI	
1-3	500	460	80		5	0.7	
4-8	800	500	130		5	1.1	
			M	F		M	F
9-13	1300	1250	240	240	5	2.0	2.0
14-18	1300	1250	410	360	5	3.2	3.9
19-30	1000	700	400	310	5	3.8	3.1
31-50	1000	700	420	320	5	3.8	3.1
51-70	1200	700	420	320	10	3.8	3.1
>70	1200	700	420	320	15	3.8	3.1

Modified from the Food and Nutrition Board, Institute of Medicine, National Academy of Sciences: *Dietary reference intakes,* Washington, DC, 1998, National Academies Press.
AI, Adequate intake; *RDA,* Recommended Dietary Allowance; *M,* male; *F,* female.
5 Micrograms = 200 IU.

were given calcium supplements had significantly greater BMD at all sites after 18 months than those who were given placebo. Mean daily calcium intakes were 908 mg for those taking placebo and 1612 mg in those taking the supplement. The gain in BMD of the supplemented group, however, did not persist after an additional period of 12 months with no supplementation. So even the twins consuming the lower intake of calcium from foods alone achieved the same BMD after about 3 years of observation in the study.

Supplementation studies of postmenopausal women—at least 5 years beyond the menopause—have demonstrated that an additional 500 to 1000 mg of calcium per day yielded improvements in BMD in the calcium-treated group (less steep rate of loss) compared with a placebo-treated group in which loss of BMD continued at a greater rate.

In general, calcium bioavailability from supplements containing various anions with calcium is good, but from a few that contain citrate as an anion, the bioavailability may be slightly higher. Calcium bioavailability from foods is similar to that from supplements (see Chapter 5).

Calcium Bioavailability

Calcium bioavailability from selected foods may be low and adversely affect calcium nutritional status. Wheat bread may be a good source of calcium for those who consume a lot of bread; green leafy vegetables such as broccoli, kale, and bok choy have good bioavailability; and calcium from soybeans is also well absorbed. Spinach and a few other high–oxalate-containing vegetables, however, have low calcium bioavailability (Weaver et al, 1991).

The consumption of dairy products, especially high-calcium milks and yogurts, appears to be the best way for most persons to meet their daily calcium requirements (Randall, 1992). The amount of calcium in major food sources is listed in Table 27-3. An additional benefit of meeting calcium requirements from foods alone is that the foods containing calcium are also rich in several other nutrients needed for health in general, for bone health in particular, and that the consumption of a calcium-rich diet from foods is also a marker of a balanced intake with respect to practically all micronutrients (Barger-Lux ET AL, 1992).

Although increasing calcium intake for the first several years after menopause has little effect on slowing the high rate of BMD loss, 1% to 2% per year, it remains important to maintain an adequate calcium intake for this potentially small benefit (Dawson-Hughes et al, 1990). Beyond these early postmenopausal years, however, BMD has been shown to be retained when calcium supplements are taken (Reid et al, 1993).

The major benefit of the additional calcium from supplements is the suppression of PTH secretion and hence the retention of bone (McKane et al, 1996). Older women respond especially well in terms of BMD and PTH to calcium supplements (Riggs et al, 1998). Men are thought to respond to adequate intakes of calcium in a similar way as women. The guideline of meeting the current AIs seems reasonable at all ages and for both sexes, including during the older years.

Bioavailability of Calcium From Supplements

The bioavailability of calcium from calcium supplements depends on the anion used, but practically all calcium-containing supplements on the market today have good bioavailability. Calcium citrate malate supplements appear to be absorbed slightly more efficiently than calcium carbonate and other calcium supplements, but the difference is typically only a couple of percentage points (Weaver et al, 1991). Calcium carbonate can have a constipating effect that may be minimized by dividing the dose and taking more fluids and fiber. High-dose calcium supplements may reduce the absorption of non-heme iron, and possibly zinc, magnesium, and other divalent cations, but additional evidence is needed to substantiate these potentially adverse interactions. Box 27-1 lists potential risks of excessive calcium supplementation.

Although peak bone mass is determined by a number of factors, calcium intake from birth through adolescence is a major contributor. The BMD attained at the time growth is complete determines to a great extent how much bone a woman will have as she enters the menopause. The BMD that is lost after the menopause depends on many factors, but drug therapy is far more effective in limiting this loss than supplements of calcium or any other dietary factor. Evidence indicates that those with a lifetime history of adequate calcium intake will be at a lower risk of osteoporosis as they age (Nieves et al, 1995), and it is

TABLE 27-3 Calcium in Selected Foods

FOOD/PORTION	CALCIUM (mg)
Yogurt, part skim, 1 c	415
Sardines, in oil, drained, 3 oz	372
Collard greens, cooked, 1 c	357
Ricotta cheese, ½ c	337
Nonfat milk, 1 c	302
Pudding, vanilla 1 c	298
Custard, 1 c	297
Whole milk, 1 c	291
Buttermilk, 1 c	286
Ice milk, soft serve, 1 c	274
Swiss cheese, 1 oz	272
Turnip greens, cooked, 1 c	249
Rhubarb, cooked, 1 c	212
Cheddar cheese, 1 oz	204
Spinach, cooked, 1 c	200
Pumpkin pie, 4 inch section	166
Refried beans, canned, 1 c	141

Source: *Home and Garden Bulletin* No. 72, Human Nutrition Information Service, U.S. Deptartment of Agriculture, 1985, http://www.nal.usda.gov/fnic/foodcomp/data/index.html#HG-72.

Box 27-1. Potential Risks Associated With Excessive Calcium Intake

Contamination of bone meal or dolomite supplements with cadmium, mercury, arsenic, or lead
Hypercalcemia from extremely high intakes (4000 mg/day or more)
Milk alkali syndrome from extremely high intakes (4000 mg/day or more)
Deficiency of iron and other mineral divalent cations resulting from decreased absorption
Exacerbation of constipation

Modified from Committee on Dietary Guidelines, Institute of Medicine, National Academy of Sciences, 1998.

apparently never too late to start taking calcium supplements or eating calcium-fortified foods.

Phosphate

Phosphates are available in practically all foods, whereas calcium is not as available in the food supply. The simple act of eating provides a rather constant amount of phosphate, roughly 1000 to 1200 mg per day for women and 1200 to 1400 for men. Proportionate amounts of calcium are not consumed unless a conscious effort is made to select enough servings of the few calcium-rich foods, but both calcium and phosphate ions in proportionate amounts are needed for the mineralization of bone. Excessive phosphorus intake as phosphate can greatly alter the calcium-to-phosphate ratio, especially if calcium intakes are low (see Chapter 5). Too much phosphate compared with calcium lowers the serum calcium ion concentration, which then stimulates PTH, and, if this pattern of intake becomes chronic, bone loss is thought to follow (see Figure 27-4).

Vitamin D

Adequate vitamin D intake is important, but excess should be avoided. Use of excessive vitamin D supplementation may be toxic because high doses induce hypercalcemia and raise the risk of soft tissue calcification, especially in the kidneys. The AIs for vitamin D across the life cycle are given in Table 27-2 (see Chapter 4).

Sunlight exposure for skin biosynthesis of vitamin D may be a critical source for older subjects who commonly obtain little vitamin D from their foods and who live far from the equator. Not only is the skin of older persons less efficient in producing vitamin D after exposure to ultraviolet (UV) light, but older adults have thinner skin and fewer cells that can synthesize vitamin D. In addition, older subjects living in nursing homes and similar institutions typically have little exposure to sunlight. Those who live at northern latitudes in the United States and Canada may also be at increased risk of osteomalacia and osteoporosis during the winter and spring months because of limited UV light during these seasons (Holick, 1994, 1996).

Vitamin D deficiency is associated with secondary hyperparathyroidism and increased bone turnover (see Chapter 4). Low levels of 25 (OH)-hydroxyvitamin D have been found in free-living older women as well as those living in nursing homes (Kinyamu et al, 1997). In a study of high–calcium-consuming Dutch adults, vitamin D treatment of older subjects had no effect on BMD (Lips et al, 1996).

Calcium and vitamin D supplements are often given together to older adults to reduce the circulating concentration of PTH when it is at the upper end of the normal range (or possibly beyond this limit in a small percentage of older hyperparathyroid subjects). In a report by Dawson-Hughes and colleagues (1997) both calcium (500 mg) and vitamin D (700 IU) supplementation for older women and men for 3 years resulted in significantly improved BMD and reduced fracture rates.

Magnesium

More than 50% of the magnesium in the body is found in bone tissue, but the role of this mineral in bone functions is poorly understood. The largest percentage of the magnesium ions in bone exists in the bone fluids, but a smaller fraction of these ions is bound in the bone crystals, probably at the surfaces only. A small percentage of the magnesium ions is located within bone cells, where they serve as enzyme cofactors, as in all other cells (Rude, 1998). The AIs for magnesium across the life cycle are given in Table 27-2.

Vitamin K

Vitamin K is an essential micronutrient for bone health. Its role in posttranslational modification of several matrix proteins, including osteocalcin, is now well established. Osteocalcin, a bone-specific protein made by osteoblasts, requires vitamin K for its posttranslational carboxylation, that is, maturation. This molecule is secreted into the bone matrix, where the roles of osteocalcin are not well characterized except that it appears to be involved in the mineralization process, perhaps acting to stop the formation of crystals to prevent overmineralization. Some osteocalcin is also secreted by osteoblasts directly into the circulating blood. A second way that osteocalcin enters blood is following bone resorption and the release of these molecules; in this way, osteocalcin serves as a serum bone marker for predicting the risk of a fracture. For example, older women had a significant increase in risk of hip fracture when they had low intakes of vitamin K and inadequate availability of osteocalcin (Liu and Peacock, 1998).

Many older persons, perhaps as many as 50%, have inadequate intakes of vitamin K, primarily because their consumption of dark green leafy vegetables is so low. In addition to its role in the modification of osteocalcin and other matrix proteins, vitamin K may have other functions that relate to calcium regulation, specifically reducing urinary calcium excretion and improving intestinal calcium absorption, functions that are well established for vitamin D but not for vitamin K. Persons who consume suboptimal amounts of vitamin K may be at increased risk of fractures (Booth et al, 2000; Kohlmeier et al, 1997). Therefore an optimal intake of this fat-soluble vitamin, especially later in life, may be important for calcium homeostasis, bone health, and the reduction of fractures.

Vitamin A (Retinol)

Vitamin A consumption is generally considered beneficial to bone growth and maintenance. Recent epidemiologic findings, however, suggest that excessive consumption of retinol (not derived from carotenoids) may contribute to hip fractures (Fescanich et al, 2002). The concern expressed by the authors of this report is that vitamin supplementation fortification may be too high, especially in postmenopausal white women. If this report is confirmed by prospective trials, the window of safe consumption of vitamin A may be fairly narrow, at least for the health of bone tissue of the proximal femur.

Trace Minerals

Trace minerals, especially fluoride, iron, zinc, copper, manganese, and boron, function in bone metabolism, but in general their roles in preventing bone loss are not well established. In one study, the administration of several trace elements (copper, fluoride, manganese, and zinc) along with calcium for 1 year resulted in a smaller loss of lumbar BMD compared with a control group who received calcium only (Strause et al, 1994).

Fluoride

Fluoride enters the hydroxyapatite crystals of bone and, within narrow limits, increases the hardness of bone mineral without any adverse effects. At intakes of 2 ppm or greater, fluoride is considered to produce bone that is subject to increased microfractures because of the change in the properties of the hydroxyapatite crystals. Water containing 1 ppm fluoride does not help bone like it does tooth surfaces; to get an increase in BMD from fluoride in addition to that in the usual diet requires several ppm. However, this also increases the risk of fluorosis and poorly mineralized bone (Palmer and Anderson, 2000). The AIs for fluoride across the life cycle are given in Table 27-2.

Copper

Copper is needed for the cross-linking of collagen and elastin molecules, and it may have roles in other enzymes of bone cells.

Manganese

Manganese is required for the biosynthesis of mucopolysaccharides in bone matrix formation, and it acts as a cofactor in energy-generating reactions.

Iron

Iron serves as a catalytic cofactor for the vitamin C–dependent hydroxylations of proline and lysine in collagen maturation. Iron also has other roles in osteoblasts and osteoclasts related to mitochondrial oxidative phosphorylation as well as in other enzymes, similar to the needs of other cells in the body.

Zinc

Zinc is essential for enzymes in osteoblasts that are responsible for collagen synthesis. In addition, an important enzyme in osteoblasts, alkaline phosphatase, requires zinc for its activity.

Boron

Boron appears to be utilized by osteoblasts for bone formation, as demonstrated in both rodent and human studies (Nielsen et al, 1992), but whether boron is absolutely required for human bone formation has not been determined (see Chapter 5).

Other Nutrients

Several other dietary factors associated with bone health have been identified. It is not yet clear how quantitatively important any of these factors are in the typical North American diet.

Dietary Fiber

Excessive *dietary fiber intake* may interfere with calcium absorption, but any interference is considered extremely small in the typical low-fiber U.S. diet. Vegans, who may consume as much as 50 g of fiber a day, would be the most likely persons to have a significant depression in intestinal calcium absorption.

Protein

Excessive protein consumption may lead to increased urinary calcium excretion. Whereas high calcium intakes are not significantly affected by a high protein intake, low calcium intakes are generally not sufficient to offset a high protein intake (Heaney, 1993). Also important is total protein in the diet; low levels of serum albumin negatively affect serum calcium. Fracture patients may be especially vulnerable.

According to one report, protein intake needs to be at least 1.0 g per kilogram of body weight to keep the serum PTH concentration from becoming elevated (Kerstetter et al, 2000). This interesting finding, which requires confirmation, goes counter to previous explanations of high-protein effects on calcium retention. Also, a clear mechanism of action is needed to explain how this phenomenon occurs.

Animal protein increases urinary losses of calcium acutely, that is, with each meal containing large amounts of animal protein; soy protein has little effect on urinary calcium losses (Anderson, Thomsen, and Christiansen, 1987).

Sodium

High sodium intakes, particularly in association with a low calcium intake, can contribute to osteoporosis because they result in increased calcium excretion (Nordin, 1991, 1993).

Potassium Bicarbonate

In postmenopausal women, an oral dose of potassium bicarbonate sufficient to neutralize endogenous acid improves calcium balance and bone. Decreased bone resorption and an increased rate of bone formation result. The skeleton serves as a buffer to help regulate acid-base balance, and a high-acid diet may contribute to the progressive decline in bone mass and development of osteoporosis (Barzel, 1995; Kraut and Coburn, 1994; Reddy et al, 2002).

Vegetarian Diets

Vegetarian diets may be more beneficial for bone than animal diets for proteins, but they typically provide less calcium than animal diets (Weaver and Plawecki, 1994). Vegetarian diets may also contribute to a lower lifetime exposure to estrogens, which could increase the risk of osteoporotic fractures (Anderson and Garner, 1999).

Isoflavones

The isoflavones in soybeans, which function both as estrogen agonists and antioxidants in bone cells, may result in the inhibition of bone resorption (Anderson and Garner, 1999; Chen and Anderson, 2002; Lee et al, 2001). Populations with low calcium intakes from dairy products, such as Asians, may have some protection against osteoporosis and hip fractures when the intake of soy foods is high (Ho et al, 2001). Isoflavones, such as genistein, may act like selective estrogen receptor modulators (SERMs) because they promote bone health without stimulating proliferation of reproductive tissues.

Caffeine

The relationship of moderate consumption of caffeine to osteoporosis has not been clearly established, but studies suggest that excessive caffeine intake may have a deleterious effect on the BMD of women, even if they consume adequate amounts of calcium (Massey and Whiting, 1993). In older women who do not compensate for their less effective intestinal absorption of calcium with sufficient amounts of calcium-rich dairy products, caffeine may have an adverse effect on calcium balance (Harris and Dawson-Hughes, 1994). Another study, however, showed that BMD was not affected by lifetime coffee intake if the subjects drank milk (one glass) daily during adulthood (Barrett-Connor, 1994).

Alcohol

Alcohol (ethanol) intake has adverse effects on the skeleton. Several reports have implicated alcohol as a major contributor to bone loss (Moniz, 1994). Heavy alcohol consumption, however, is typically accompanied by poor dietary intake and cigarette smoking, especially in women.

OSTEOPENIA AND OSTEOPOROSIS

Osteoporosis, a disease that manifests itself late in life, may have its origin in early life during the period of skeletal growth and PBM accumulation (see earlier sections on skeletal growth). Although women have almost twice the hip fracture rate as men, the rate for men will catch up as the average life span of males continues to increase. Practically everyone over 80 years of age can be said to be osteoporotic (Table 27-4) and at risk for a hip fracture. This section reviews the

TABLE 27-4 World Health Organization Definitions of Osteopenia and Osteoporosis*

Osteopenia	1-2.5 SD
Osteoporosis	>2.5 SD

From Kanis JA et al: The diagnosis of osteoporosis, *J Bone Miner Res* 9:1137, 1994.

*Extent below mean bone mineral density *(BMD)* of 20- to 29-year-old subjects. *SD,* Standard deviation.

prevalence and types of osteoporosis as well as risk factors and treatment options. Osteoporosis is defined in terms of decline in BMD in Table 27-4.

Definitions of Osteopenia and Osteoporosis

The bone loss that begins in midadult life, that is, after age 40 in women and later in men, and continues into old age, is a normal process. Bone composition remains unchanged, but both the BMC and BMD decrease with age. When BMD falls sufficiently below healthy values (1 standard deviation [SD] according to WHO standards), osteopenia, or too little bone, exists. Osteoporosis occurs when the BMD becomes so low (greater than 2.5 SD below healthy values) that the skeleton is unable to sustain ordinary strains, a condition marked by the occurrence of fractures or the strong likelihood of a fracture. Deterioration of bone tissue, especially trabecular bone tissue, results in microfractures, an index of poor architectural quality, another component of the definition of osteoporosis. Fragility fractures result from poor quality tissue.

Table 27-4, the WHO definitions, are based on measurements of BMD by DXA (Kanis et al, 1994). The standard BMD values for comparison are the 20- to 29-year-old means, because this age group is considered to represent the healthiest adults and to have essentially achieved peak bone density. Osteopenia, low BMD, is a precursor state to the more severe osteoporosis.

A study of 200,000 women 50 years or older who have had BMD measurements (or related measurements) at routine office visits showed that roughly 40% were classified as osteopenic and 7% as osteoporotic according to WHO values (Siris et al, 2001). This alarming finding suggests that many perimenopausal women are at risk of fractures because of low BMD, which is the single most predictive risk factor for fractures.

Prevalence of Osteoporotic Fractures

Although it is difficult to estimate rates of osteoporosis, about 25 million women and 12 million men are classified as osteoporotic. More than 1.5 million fractures occur annually in osteoporotic subjects, which represents a cost of more than an estimated $15 billion in health care and rehabilitation services. Half of these osteoporosis-related fractures involve the vertebrae; 250,000 are fractures of the hip, which typically result in incapacitation, long-term nursing care, and a 20% death rate within a year of the fracture. Although incidence rates of fractures in the United States are not expected to increase substantially, the actual numbers (prevalence) are predicted to increase greatly until 2030 (Melton, 1997).

Statistics indicate that women are about four times more likely than men to develop osteoporosis, although with aging both genders gradually lose bone mass and become more vulnerable, especially to hip fractures, as they age. Reported data on low femoral BMD for men and women in the United States have been compiled from analyses of the findings of the National Health and Nutrition Examination Survey (NHANES III) (Looker, 2003; Looker et al, 1997).

Types of Osteoporosis

In the past, the types of osteoporosis were distinguished by sex, the age at which fractures occur, and the kinds of bone involved (Riggs and Melton, 1986). Today osteoporosis should be considered a disease with a broad spectrum of variant forms of the disorder. Primary osteoporosis results from postmenopausal or senile causes; secondary osteoporosis occurs from endocrine changes, medications, chronic diseases, including renal failure or hepatic insufficiency. Box 27-2 lists the disorders associated with osteopenia, a forerunner of osteoporosis.

Estrogen- or androgen-deficient or postmenopausal osteoporosis (type I) occurs in women within a few years of menopause, and it primarily involves loss of trabecular bone tissue because of a cessation of ovarian production of estrogens. (Men may also develop type I osteoporosis during adulthood if they have a significant decline in androgen production, but in practice such cases are rare.) Type I osteoporosis is characterized by fractures of the distal radius (Colles' fractures) and "crush" fractures of the lumbar vertebrae, which are often painful and deforming. Acceleration of the process that occurs in women after menopause is directly related to the lack of estrogen. BMC and BMD measurements of the lumbar spine of women with postmenopausal osteoporosis may fall to as low as 25% to 40% of that in age-matched

TABLE 27-5 Characteristics of Primary Osteoporosis: Types I and II

	TYPE I	TYPE II
Gender	Females, rare in males	Female and male
Age/period of life cycle	Menopause (~50 yr)	Beyond 65 yr of age
Bone tissue	Trabecular	Trabecular and cortical
Fracture sites	Lumbar vertebrae	Hips and vertebrae; any other bone in the skeleton
Etiology	Loss of estrogens or androgens	Aging—otherwise poorly understood

Data from in Riggs BL, Melton LJ III: Involutional osteoporosis, *N Engl J Med* 314:1676, 1986.

Box 27-2. Disorders Associated With Osteopenia

Primary osteoporosis
- Postmenopausal or senile osteoporosis
- Juvenile osteoporosis (genetic)

Secondary osteoporosis
- Endocrine causes (Cushing's syndrome, hypogonadism, hypopituitarism, diabetes mellitus, hyperthyroidism, hyperparathyroidism)
- Blood disorders (myeloma, leukemia, sickle cell anemia)
- Drugs (corticosteroids, heparin; anticonvulsants, immunosuppressants)
- Alcohol in excess
- Diseases (chronic renal or liver disease; GI malabsorption)
- Chronic immobilization
- Nutrient deficiencies (vitamin D, calcium, scurvy, general malnutrition)
- Inborn errors of metabolism (osteogenesis imperfecta, homocystinuria)

Data from Genant H: Radiology of osteoporosis and other metabolic bone diseases. In Kanis J, editor: *Textbook of osteoporosis*, Sheffield, England, 1996, World Health Organization Collaborating Centre for Metabolic Bone Disease.

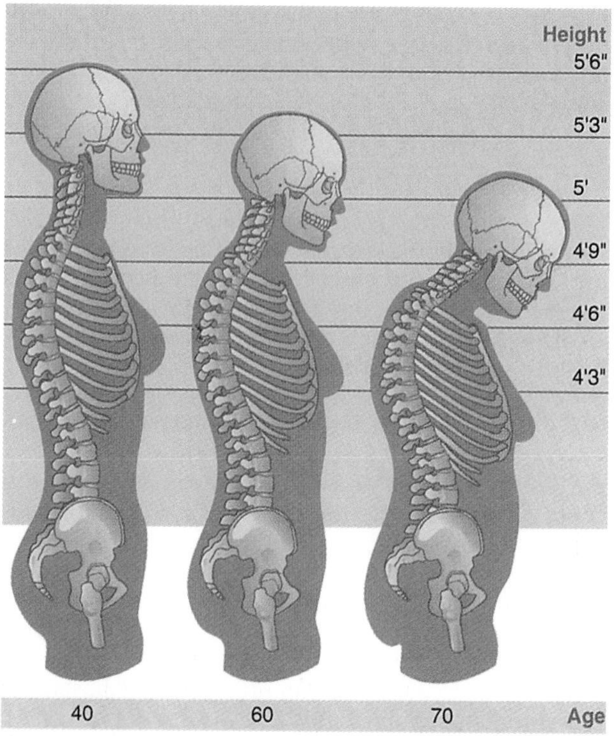

FIGURE 27-8 • Normal spine at 40 years of age and osteoporotic changes at 60 and 70 years of age. These changes can cause a loss of as much as 6 to 9 inches in height and result in the so-called dowager's hump *(far right)* in the upper thoracic vertebrae. (From Ignatavicius D, Bayne MV: *Medical-surgical nursing: a nursing process approach*, Philadelphia, 1991, WB Saunders.)

nonosteoporotic control women. Other bone sites with a preponderance of trabecular bone, such as the pelvis, the ribs, and the proximal femur, also display low BMD in postmenopausal osteoporosis.

Age-related osteoporosis (type II) occurs around age 70 and beyond, and it affects both sexes; older men are increasingly at risk for hip fractures. Both types of bone tissue, cortical and trabecular, undergo remodeling, but the greater degree of remodeling occurs in trabecular tissue. In the older period of life, the processes of bone resorption and bone formation become uncoupled. Fractures of the hips characterize type II osteoporosis, but vertebral fractures continue to increase with age. A dramatic increase in hip fractures occurs late in life, and almost all women older than 80 years of age are at risk for hip fracture. Wedge fractures of vertebrae typically lead to back pain, loss of height, spinal deformity, and kyphosis or "dowager's hump" (Figure 27-8). Many women lose several inches in height between 50 and 80 years of age. Fractures may occur during ordinary activities, such as lifting a sack of groceries or stepping over a shower opening, but a large percentage of hip fractures result from a fall.

Although age-associated osteoporosis affects both sexes, women are more severely affected because they have a smaller skeletal mass than men have and because they live longer. According to the American Association of Clinical Endocrinologists, one out of every two women over the age of 50 will experience an osteoporosis-related fracture in her lifetime. Another 20% will die each year because of osteoporosis-related complications, such as hip fracture (www.aace.com/pub/stand/ss-factsheet.php.).

Secondary osteoporosis results when an identifiable drug (Box 27-3) or disease process (Box 27-4) causes loss of bone tissue (see Chapter 19).

Etiology

Osteoporosis is a complex heterogeneous disorder of unknown etiology, but many risk factors over a lifetime are thought to contribute to this condition. Although the fracture-precipitating condition of low BMD is common to all types of osteoporosis, the process by which this condition is reached, that is, an imbalance between resorption and formation, results from an array of etiologic factors characteristic of each type or form of this disease.

Loss of bone mass to a degree that produces fractures can result from (1) an excessive acceleration of resorption, especially after the menopause, or (2) a suboptimal peak bone mass that results in bone after the menopause (or later in life in men) that becomes fragile and susceptible to fracture. The algorithm in Figure 27-9 illustrates different scenarios of older or younger postmenopausal women that lead to osteoporotic fractures. Several risk factors are listed in Figure 27-9.

Box 27-3. Common Drugs That Increase Calcium Loss

Phenytoin (Dilantin)	Lithium
Phenobarbital	Tetracycline
Thyroid hormone	Aluminum-containing antacids
Corticosteroids	Heparin
Methotrexate	Phenothiazine derivatives
Cyclosporine	

Box 27-4. Diseases or Conditions That Result in Negative Calcium Balance and Possible Osteoporosis

Hyperthyroidism
Diabetes
Chronic renal failure
Chronic diarrhea or malabsorption
Hyperparathyroidism
Chronic obstructive lung disease
Subtotal gastrectomy
Hemiplegia

Risk Factors

Risk factors for osteoporosis include age, race, gender, body weight or size, family history, premature menopause, nulliparity, dietary factors, limited exercise, use of cigarettes, excessive alcohol consumption, and prolonged use of certain medications that adversely affect bone or calcium metabolism (Box 27-5).

Race and Ethnicity

Caucasians and Asians suffer more osteoporotic fractures than African-Americans and Hispanics, who have a greater bone density (Siris et al, 2001). However, hypovitaminosis D with secondary hyperparathyroidism (see Figure 27-9) occurs more often in the black population. Thin women, particularly of Northern European extraction, are at greater risk of osteoporosis than heavier women (Edelstein and Barrett-Conner, 1993).

Menstrual Status

Loss of menses at any age is a major determinant of osteoporosis risk in women. Acceleration of bone loss coincides with the menopause, either natural or surgical, at which time the ovaries stop producing estrogen. ERTs has been shown to conserve BMD and reduce fracture risk following the menopause, at least in short-term studies. The skeleton of young amenorrheic women, especially runners and dancers, may also benefit from the use of oral contraceptive agents.

Any interruption of menstruation for an extended period results in bone loss. The amenorrhea that accompanies excessive weight loss seen in patients with anorexia nervosa or in persons who participate in high-intensity sports, dance, or other forms of exercise has the same adverse effect on bones as the menopause. BMD in amenorrheic athletes has been measured at levels 25% to 40% below control levels. When menses were resumed in these athletes, bone mass increased but eventually plateaued at a level lower than that of sedentary women. Young women with the "athlete triad" of disordered eating, amenorrhea, and low BMD are at increased risk of having fractures while involved in athletics (Thrash and Anderson, 2000) (see Chapter 26).

Lactation

Sufficient calcium and vitamin D intake is essential during this time for the mother to replete her own serum and storage levels, but repletion typically does not occur until several months after peak lactation. The recovery of bone is complete for most women and occurs even with shortly spaced pregnancies. Epidemiologic studies have found that pregnancy and lactation are not associated with an increased risk of osteoporotic fractures (Kalkwarf and Specker, 2002.)

Limited Exercise

Immobility in varying degrees is well recognized as a cause of bone loss (Figure 27-10). Maintenance of healthy bone requires exposure to weight-bearing pressures.

Stresses from muscle contraction and maintaining the body in an upright position against the pull of gravity stimulate osteoblast function. Bones not subjected to normal use rapidly lose mass. Invalids confined to bed or persons unable to move freely are commonly affected. Astronauts living in conditions of zero gravity for only a few days experience so much bone loss, especially in the lower extremities, that appropriate exercise is a feature of their daily routines. To a lesser degree, lack of exercise and a sedentary lifestyle that continue over a lifetime also contribute significantly to bone loss, although their most important influence is probably on inadequate accumulation of bone mass (see Figure 27-10).

Physical activity, especially upper-body activities, may also contribute to an increase in bone mass or density, although the evidence for skeletal benefit is limited (Karlsson et al, 2001). A few studies of post-

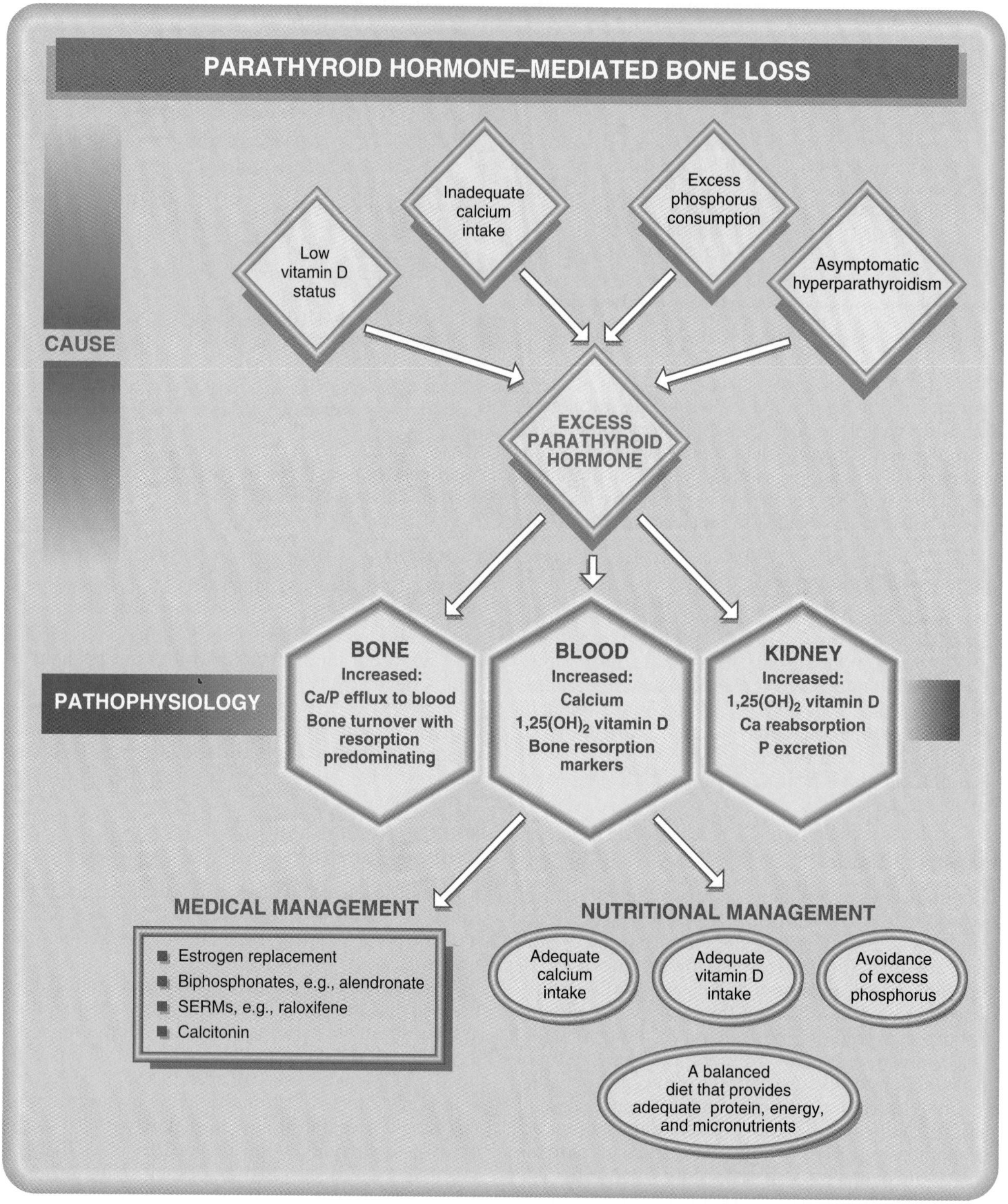

FIGURE 27-9 • Pathophysiology algorithm: parathyroid hormone–mediated bone loss. *SERMs,* Selective estrogen receptor modulators. (Algorithm content developed by John Anderson, PhD, and Sanford C. Garner, PhD, 2000.)

menopausal women have shown that a shift from relative inactivity to a high-activity regimen may increase bone measurements by a significant amount, whether or not a woman is receiving ERT (Figure 27-11) (Kohrt et al, 1995).

Reduced activities in daily life may also contribute to bone loss. For example, Asian women who migrate to urban areas and change their lifestyles from more agrarian to less active ones also have increased risk of hip fractures (Lau et al, 2001).

Box 27-5. Risk Factors for Developing Osteoporosis

Family history of osteoporosis
Female
Caucasian or Asian
Slight body build
Estrogen depletion
- Menopause
- Early oophorectomy in women
- Hypogonadism in men
- Hypogonadism in women with excessive exercise

Age: especially after age 60 yr
Lack of exercise
Prolonged use of certain medications (see Box 27-3)
Diseases or conditions that affect calcium and bone metabolism (see Box 27-4)
Underweight or underfat
Cigarette smoking
Excessive alcohol consumption
Excessive fiber consumption
Excessive caffeine consumption
Inadequate calcium or vitamin D intake

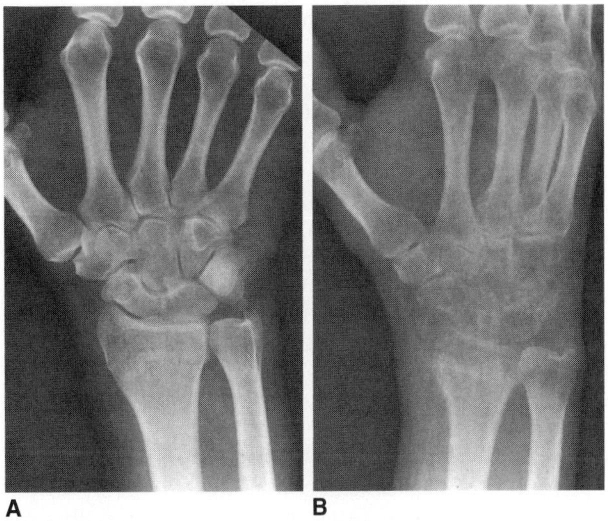

FIGURE 27-10 • **A,** Roentgenogram of the carpal area shortly after fracture of the distal radius. The part was immobilized by a plaster cast. **B,** Roentgenogram of the same area several weeks after immobilization. Note the disuse atrophy of the carpal bones. (From Aegerter EE, Kirkpatrick JA: *Orthopedic diseases: physiology, pathology, radiology,* ed 4, Philadelphia, 1975, WB Saunders.)

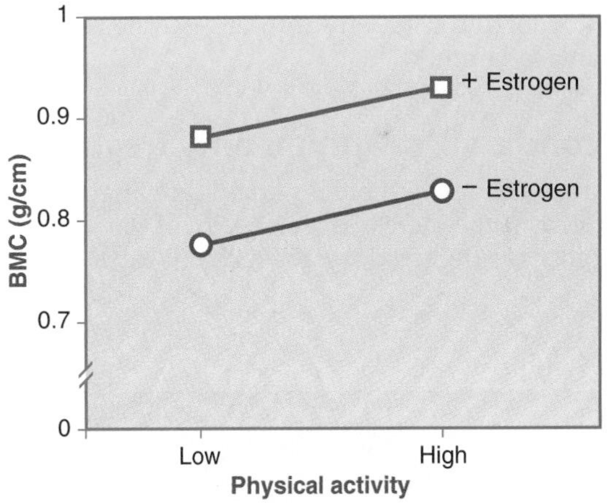

FIGURE 27-11 • Effects of physical activity and estrogen treatment on trabecular bone mineral content (BMC) of postmenopausal women. Estrogen (either estrogen-replacement therapy [ERT] or hormone-replacement therapy [HRT]) improves BMC whether women are exercising at a high or low level. (Copyright of John J. B. Anderson and Sanford C. Garner.)

Body Weight

Body weight (mass) is an important factor that affects BMC and BMD. The greater the body mass, the greater the BMD; and the converse is also true: the lower the body mass, the lower the BMD. For example, young girls, who are typically premenarchal, may incur fractures with minimal trauma (Goulding et al, 1998, 2000), in part because of low BMC and BMD related to rapid growth (height) that is not accompanied by a proportionate increase in weight. Young overweight males with low bone mass may also suffer fractures (Goulding et al, 2001). Fractures in preteens and early teenagers have previously been rare events, but they are now more frequent because of less play and more TV or computer time.

Weight loss in dieting persons is also typically associated with bone loss (Fogelholm et al, 2001; Pluijm et al, 2001). The reason for the greater BMD in heavier adult persons relates largely to the load (weight) that is borne by the different skeletal sites. The non–weight-bearing bones of the arms are less affected by body weight than they are by repetitive use in physical activities.

Dietary Factors

Many nutrients and several nonnutrients have been implicated as etiologic risk factors for osteoporosis. These nutrients have been largely covered in the previous section, but a few points about calcium need to be stated. Vitamin D deficiency, widely reported at northern latitudes in North America and Europe, may also be more common at latitudes closer to the equator in the Northern Hemisphere than previously thought (Lamberg-Allardt et al, 2001). Older persons in the United States and elsewhere, both men and women, may benefit from a diet with 1000 or more mg of calcium, preferably from foods or alternatively from a combination of foods and supplements. Such a high intake of calcium may keep serum PTH concentration within the normal range, and it may also maintain a healthier vitamin D status. Finally, such an intake probably reduces fractures at all skeletal sites (Cumming et al, 1997).

The nonnutrients like dietary fiber, phytoestrogens (isoflavones and lignans), and many other plant molecules may also play important roles in either maintaining bone or contributing to bone loss. Compared with omnivores, vegan diets may contribute to lower lifetime estrogen exposure of the skeleton, contribute to lower bone mass, and possibly increase the risk of osteoporosis (Anderson, 1999).

Another benefit of plant-rich diets is the reduced generation of acid (hydrogen ions) with the metabolism of plant proteins.

Medications

A number of *medications* contribute adversely to osteoporosis, either by interfering with calcium absorption or by actively promoting calcium loss from bone (see Box 27-3).

Use of Alcohol and Cigarettes

Cigarette smoking and excessive alcohol consumption are risk factors for developing osteoporosis. Excesses should be avoided (see *Focus On:* The Impact of Alcohol and Cigarette Smoking on the Skeleton: A Double Whammy!)

Secondary Prevention and Treatment

Because virtually all older persons are affected by osteoporosis, the increasing longevity of the population emphasizes the need for prevention, especially after menopause and later in life. Secondary prevention is a form of treatment following the development of osteoporosis, either sex-hormone deficient (type I) or age-related (type II). Primary prevention applies to persons who have no osteoporotic disease, typically adults younger than 50 years of age.

Because bone health is influenced by three major interacting factors—diet, exercise, and estrogen—it is never too early or too late to prevent or lessen the onset and severity of osteoporosis by ensuring adequate intakes of calcium from foods (and supplements), engaging in regular weight-bearing exercises, and, if necessary, taking bone-conserving drugs. Weight-bearing exercise and estrogens may have additive effects on BMD of older women (Kohrt et al, 1995).

All the recommended bone-conserving drugs except intermittent PTH therapy have antiresorptive effects; only intermittent PTH and growth hormone are bone-forming drugs. All drugs are recommended to be taken along with calcium supplements (500 to 1500 mg of calcium per day) for the purpose of meeting the needs of bone formation.

Estrogen Replacement Therapy

Estrogen replacement therapy (ERT), or hormone-replacement therapy (HRT), is a treatment previously used for reducing bone resorption and arresting early postmenopausal bone loss in women. Even if estrogen therapy was instituted several years after the onset of menopause, bone resorption could be slowed and fractures reduced. Combined ERT and high calcium supplementation may also improve BMD.

FOCUS ON

The Impact of Alcohol and Cigarette Smoking on the Skeleton: A Double Whammy!

Cigarette smoking is a risk factor for vertebral, forearm, and hip fractures, especially in slender women (Daniell, 1976). In a cross-sectional study of bone density at the lumbar spine and the femoral neck and shaft in 41 pairs of twins, bone density was 0.9% to 2% lower for every 10 pack-years of smoking (Hopper and Seeman, 1994). Smoking was also associated with higher follicle-stimulating hormone (FSH) and luteinizing hormone (LH) levels and lower serum PTH levels, serum calcium levels, and urinary calcium concentrations, markers for bone resorption. Conclusions of this study suggest that women who smoke about one pack of cigarettes daily will have an average deficit of 5% to 10% in bone density, which increases the risk of fracture. The strong correlation between reproductive function and bone mass and density appears to be affected by smoking through a decrease in estrogen. Women who smoke enter menopause 1 to 2 years earlier and lose bone more rapidly than nonsmokers (Slemenda, 1994). Female consumers who smoke need to be educated about the risk of a decrease in BMD, which may lead to an increase in fractures.

Alcohol, especially excessive consumption (more than two drinks a day) for an extended period, results in bone loss. Bone loss is thought to occur because the metabolism of alcohol generates additional acid that is buffered, in part, by the skeleton. The combination of smoking and alcohol, so common among young women, places them at increased risk for osteoporosis because both these risk factors operate to reduce BMD. Men are affected similarly.

A high calcium intake alone, however, will not substitute for ERT in blunting postmenopausal bone loss.

Recently, HRT has been reduced greatly because of concerns about increased risks for cancer (Harris, 2002). Other drugs are rapidly replacing estrogens for the prevention and treatment of osteoporosis. Recently many women have been exploring the use of phytoestrogens and other plant products as substitutes for estrogens.

Bisphosphonates

Bisphosphonates act on osteoclasts to reduce their resorptive activities. Chemically, bisphosphonates resemble pyrophosphate, which is present at the surfaces of bone crystals. The bisphosphonates act by inhibiting osteoclast-mediated bone resorption. Examples include etidronate, a first-generation drug used seldom today, and several second-generation bisphosphonates, such as alendronate and pamidronate.

Etidronate

Cyclic administration of etidronate to women with postmenopausal osteoporosis provided greatly increased vertebral bone mineral content and reduced fractures. Continued treatment provided long-term beneficial effects on the maintenance of BMD (Miller et al, 1997).

Alendronate

The skeletal benefits of alendronate have been similar to those of etidronate, but alendronate has been more effective in fracture reduction (Black et al, 2000). Although this drug has become widely accepted in the United States and other nations, it may result in esophageal reflux, a side effect that makes it difficult for a small subset of the population to continue this oral therapy. Alendronate may be used in combination with a SERM (see later discussion) or another bone-conserving drug in an effort to protect the skeleton.

Risedronate

This drug has effects similar to alendronate, but it seems to be tolerated better by some subjects (Harris et al, 1999).

Selective Estrogen Receptor Modulators

Drugs that positively affect estrogen receptors (ERs) in bone tissue, but have little effect on reproductive tissues of the breast or uterus, are known as selective estrogen receptor modulators (SERMs) (Sadovsky and Adler, 1998). Two examples of these drugs in the marketplace are tamoxifen and raloxifene. Genistein, a phytoestrogen found in soy foods, may act as a SERM.

Tamoxifen

Tamoxifen was developed as an antiestrogen to help prevent breast cancer, and it was found by chance to conserve bone. This drug has not been prescribed, however, for preventing bone loss.

Raloxifene

Raloxifene, a drug recently approved by the U.S. Food and Drug Administration (FDA) for the express purpose of maintaining bone and reducing fractures, has been found to be effective (Ettinger et al, 1999).

Intermittent Parathyroid Hormone Therapy

Intermittent parathyroid hormone PTH therapy uses low doses of a modified PTH (1-34) molecule to improve both bone mass and density. For example, BMD of the lumbar vertebrae may be increased by as much as 15% after 1 year of treatment, and total-body BMD may be increased by 5% to 10%. Unfortunately BMD of the hip (proximal femur) does not increase much, although it does not decrease. Reports of the few human investigations approved by the FDA suggest that intermittent PTH therapy will be a boost to the therapeutic arsenal because it increases osteoblastic formation of new bone tissue, especially in trabecular bone, and it reduces fractures (Dempster et al, 2001; Neer et al, 2001). Calcium also needs to be taken along with this anabolic therapy. If approved by the FDA for regular prescription use, this drug may become the major one used that positively increases bone formation; that is, it is anabolic. Only growth hormone, insulin-like growth factor-1, and a few other agents are anabolic.

Other Drug Treatments

These treatment options are less often used for the prevention or treatment of osteoporosis, but each one may be effective under special conditions or in certain persons.

Calcitonin

Calcitonin, a hormone, is a powerful inhibitor of osteoclast activity that exerts a rapid, transient, and reversible inhibition of bone resorption (Body, 2002). Calcitonin therapy decreases the rate of bone loss in osteoporotic women; however, it is most effective if given early after the menopause. Calcitonin can be administered by subcutaneous injection or nasal spray. Prolonged administration of parenteral calcitonin, by injections of 100 IU every 1 or 2 days, can prevent postmenopausal or postoophorectomy bone loss and is also able to increase trabecular bone mass among patients presenting an established osteoporosis (Body, 2002).

Sodium Fluoride

Increases in bone mass, especially in trabecular bone, follow treatment with sodium fluoride, but the quality of the bone may not be normal. Fluoride ions become incorporated at the surfaces of hydroxyapatite crystals, and thereby the size and structure of the crystals become so altered that the mechanical competence of the bone declines. Fluoride therapy is not likely to be approved by the FDA because of these concerns, and the use of fluoride must still be regarded as experimental (Palmer and Anderson, 2000).

Vitamin D

The AI for vitamin D intakes of older adults have been greatly increased (see Table 27-2), but supplements are most likely necessary because it is almost impossible for older adults to consume this amount from foods. Maintenance of an adequate dietary intake of vitamin D (400-600 IU or 20-30 mg of cholecalciferol) is important for healthy younger adults, but it is inadequate for the many housebound older persons who fail to get adequate exposure to sunlight.

Calcitriol

Calcitriol, or 1,25-dihyroxyvitamin D, without calcium, has had little use in the treatment of osteoporosis because of its potential toxicity. Calcium plus calcitriol may be useful, however, with high-dose corticosteroid therapy, during which vertebral fractures are common. Other investigators have also shown the benefits of countering the adverse effects of glucocorticoids on bone with calcium or calcitriol (Reid, Veale, and France, 1994).

Growth Hormone and Insulin-Like Growth Factors

Treatment with human growth hormone may improve bone through its anabolic effects (Rosen and Bilezekian, 2001). Similarly, insulin-like growth factor-1 (IGF-1) may improve bone BMC and BMD in human subjects by increasing bone formation (Bauer et al, 1998; Rosen and Bilezekian, 2001).

Osteoprotegerin

A natural cytokine, osteoprotegerin (OPG), is secreted by osteoblasts as well as other cell types. OPG, which can be detected in human serum, acts by inactivating another cytokine that affects osteoclasts, thereby inhibiting osteoclast activation and bone resorption. When given to postmenopausal women, OPG exerts long-lasting inhibition of bone resorption (Bekker et al, 2001). Results of clinical trials examining the effects of OPG on bone mass and fracture risk are awaited because this therapy may be effective against osteoporosis in older subjects.

Dietary Treatment

Calcium, vitamin D, and other micronutrients have been previously covered. A novel approach to the dietary treatment of patients recovering from hip fractures, however, has been shown to be effective. Older patients with hip fracture may benefit from protein supplements coupled with adequate amounts of micronutrients. In one study clinical outcomes and BMD were improved in patients who were given a protein supplement enriched with other nutients (Schurch et al, 1998). The high-quality protein was shown to increase serum IGF-1 concentrations.

Isoflavones improve or maintain BMD in perimenopausal or postmenopausal women when ingested with soy protein as an isoflavone-enriched supplement (Alekel et al, 2000; Potter et al, 1998). These soy-derived molecules may have not only estrogen-like effects in bone but also antioxidant actions (Chen and Anderson, 2002).

Other Treatment Modalities

Several other approaches to prevent fractures have been examined; despite their demonstrated benefits in small study populations, they have not been utilized in any institution for older adults in the United States, insofar as is known. These approaches include exercise, strength activities, fall-prevention education, UV lamps, and special hip-padding girdles (NIH, 2001).

Exercise

Physical activities such as regular walking and swimming appear to have little or no skeletal benefits for older persons, but more active participation, such as weight-bearing exercises and intensive walking, have positive effects on BMD (Karlsson et al, 2001). Although most exercise studies have been conducted with healthy young adults, those that have been performed on older adult men and women have generated some impressive data (Wallace and Cumming, 2000). The difficulty with these studies is in keeping up participation of older subjects, who are slower to respond to loads or forces.

Strength Activities

In terms of prevention, strength activities have been underused. In very old men (nonagenarians), strength exercises of the thigh muscles resulted in significant improvement of strength and possibly of BMD of the femur, although the latter was not measured (Fiatarone et al, 1990). Exercise helps to improve and maintain lumbar spine BMD in postmenopausal women (Kelley et al, 2002).

Clinial Scenario 1

Annie, a 70-year-old white woman of Northern European ancestry, developed lactose intolerance during her early fifties when she had a serious gastrointestinal infection. She currently is retired, lives alone, and stays indoors most of each day watching television. Approximately 3 years earlier at 67 years of age, she had DXA measurements that showed that she had low BMD values of her proximal femur and lumbar vertebrae (both values would be classified as osteoporotic according to WHO definitions). Her physician recommended that she start taking supplements of calcium (1000 mg per day) and vitamin D (600 IU per day) because of her lactose intolerance and her lack of consumption of any dairy products. Annie took the supplements regularly for a year; when a second set of DXA measurements revealed that she had maintained her BMD values of 1 year earlier rather than having any loss. The continuing low measurements, however, concerned her physician, and he ordered laboratory tests of calcium-regulatory hormones to see whether she had any hormonal complications. These tests showed that her PTH and 25-hydroxyvitamin D concentrations fell in the upper half of the normal range for each variable. Other routine measurements, such as serum calcium and phosphate, were normal. Her physician, in consultation with Annie, decided to place her on a bisphosphonate (alendronate) because she refused to consider taking an estrogen.

After 1 year on the new therapy plus continuing the calcium and vitamin D, her BMD values (her third set of DXA measurements) actually increased a few percentage points, even though they remained within the classification of osteoporosis. She was then instructed by her physician to continue on this therapeutic regimen.

1. How would you classify Annie's calcium intake at the initial visit with her physician (who did not take a diet history or estimate her calcium intake)? Her vitamin D intake? Her exposure to sunlight?
2. What would you have recommended to improve her calcium intake from foods so that she could reduce her supplemental calcium to 500 mg per day? Why would you recommend foods to provide calcium rather than supplements?
3. Design a set (3 days minimum) of daily menus that provide approximately 800 mg of calcium from foods alone, which, when coupled with a 500-mg supplement, would provide a total of 1300 mg, the current AI for calcium.

Prevention of Falls

Fractures of the humerus, wrist, pelvis, and hip are considered to be age related, resulting from a combination of osteoporosis and falling. Although only a small percentage of falls result in fractures, preventing falls through education and attention to the living environment of the very old is an important measure.

Hip-Protector Girdles

The wearing of girdles with built-in pads to protect the hips during a fall has been demonstrated to reduce the rate of fractures within a selected population at high risk (Parker et al, 2000).

Clinical Scenario 2

Laura is a 50-year-old white woman who had a hysterectomy last year. She drinks milk and eats dairy foods in sufficient quantity each day; however, she recently had a DEXA scan, which revealed osteopenia in her femur and lumbar spine. She is experiencing signs and symptoms of menopause. Laura is 5 ft 0 in. tall and weighs 110 lb. She has the following questions for you, her nutrition counselor:

1. Will diet make any difference for Laura? Should she start taking supplements of vitamin D and calcium? If so, how much?
2. She walks 3 miles a week. Should she increase her activity level?
3. What else do you need to know before you make any recommendations?

Ultraviolet Lamps

The development of new ultraviolet (UVB) lamps with built-in safety against excessive skin damage may be a potential way to improve vitamin D status of older adults, especially those living in nursing homes and similar institutions.

SUMMARY

Bone health is dependent on numerous factors, including genetics, dietary intake of specific nutrients, exercise, management of chronic diseases, and use of medications. Whether young or old, any person can make improvements in lifestyle, which can protect skeletal integrity.

Fracture prevention is the primary goal in the treatment of patients with osteoporosis. Several treatments have been shown to reduce the risk of osteoporotic fractures: therapies that enhance bone mass and reduce the risk or consequences of falls. Adults with vertebral, rib, hip, or distal forearm fractures should always be evaluated for the presence of osteoporosis and given appropriate therapy (NIH, 2001).

■ Relevant Web Sites

American Association of Clinical Endocrinologists
www.aace.com
Menopause and Osteoporosis
www.menopause.org/
National Osteoporosis Foundation
www.nof.org/
Osteoporosis On-Line
www.osteoporosis.ca/OSTEO/D02-01.html

Cited References

Alekel DL et al: Isoflavone-rich soy protein isolate attenuates bone loss in the lumbar spine of perimenopausal women, *Am J Clin Nutr* 72:844, 2000.

Anderson JJB: Plant-based diets and bone health: nutritional implications, *Am J Clin Nutr* 70:539S, 1999.

Anderson JJB, Garner SC: Phytoestrogens and bone, *Ballieres Clin Endocrinol Metab* 282:1344, 1999.

Anderson JJB, Pollitzer WS: Ethnic and genetic differences in susceptibility to osteoporotic fractures. In Draper HH, editor: *Advances in nutritional research,* vol 9, New York, 1994, Plenum Press.

Anderson JJB, Thomsen K, Christiansen C: High protein meals, insular hormones and urinary calcium excretion in human subjects. In Christiansen C et al, editors: *Osteoporosis 1987,* Copenhagen, 1987, Osteopress ApS.

Baran DT et al: Broadband ultrasound attenuation of the calcaneus predicts lumbar and femoral neck density in Caucasian women: a preliminary study, *Osteoporosis Int* 1:110, 1991.

Barger-Lux MJ et al: Nutritional correlates of low calcium intake, *Clin Appl Nutr* 2(4):39, 1992.

Barrett-Connor E: Coffee-associated osteoporosis offset by daily milk consumption: the Rancho Bernardo Study, *JAMA* 271:280, 1994.

Barzel US: The skeleton as an ion exchange system: implications for the role of acid-base imbalance in the genesis of osteoporosis, *J Bone Miner Res* 10:1431, 1995.

Bass S et al: Exercise before puberty may confer residual benefits in bone density in adulthood, *J Bone Miner Res* 13:500, 1998.

Bauer DC et al: Low serum IGF-1 but not IGFBP-3 predicts hip and spine fracture: the study of osteoporotic fractures, *J Bone Miner Res* 23:S561, 1998.

Bekker PJ et al: The effect of a single dose of osteoprotegerin in postmenopausal women, *J Bone Miner Res* 16:348, 2001.

Black DM et al: Fracture risk reduction with alendronate in women with osteoporosis: the Fracture Intervention Trial, *J Clin Endocrinol Metab* 85:4118, 2000.

Body JJ: Calcitonin for the long-term prevention and treatment of postmenopausal osteoporosis, *Bone* 30:75, 2002.

Bonjour J-P et al: Calcium-enriched foods and bone mass growth in prepubertal girls: a randomized double-blind, placebo-controlled trial, *J Clin Invest* 99:1287, 1997.

Bonjour J-P et al: Gain in bone mineral mass in prepubertal girls 3-5 years after discontinuation of calcium supplementation: a follow-up study, *Lancet* 358:1208, 2001.

Booth SL et al: Dietary vitamin K intakes are associated with hip fracture but not with bone mineral density in elderly men and women, *Am J Clin Nutr* 71:1201, 2000.

Bradney M, Karlsson MK, et al. Heterogeneity in the growth of the axial and appendicular skeleton in boys: implications for the pathogenesis of bone fragility in men, *J Bone Miner Res* 10:1871, 2000.

Chen XW, Anderson JJB: Isoflavones and bone: animal and human evidence of efficacy, *J Musculoskel Neuron Interact* 2002 (in press.)

Chen XW et al: Isoflavones regulate interleukin-6 and osteoprotegerin synthesis during osteoblast cell differentiation via an estrogen-receptor-dependent pathway, *Biochem Biophys Res Commun* 295:417, 2002.

Christiansen C, Riis BJ, Rodbro P: Prediction of rapid bone loss in postmenopausal women, *Lancet* 1:1105, 1987.

Cumming RG et al: Calcium intake and fracture risk: results from the Study of Osteoporotic Fractures, *Am J Epidemiol* 145: 926, 1997.

Daniell HW: Osteoporosis of the slender smoker, *Arch Intern Med* 136:298, 1976.

Dawson-Hughes B et al: A controlled trial of the effect of calcium supplementation on bone density in postmenopausal women, *N Engl J Med* 323:878, 1990.

Dawson-Hughes B et al: Effect of calcium and vitamin D supplementation on bone density in men and women 65 years of age or older, *N Engl J Med* 337:670, 1997.

Dempster DW et al: Effects of daily treatment with parathyroid hormone on bone microarchitecture and turnover in patients with osteoporosis: a paired biopsy study, *J Bone Miner Res* 16:1846, 2001.

Ebeling PR et al: Evidence of an age-related decrease in intestinal responsiveness to vitamin D: relationship between serum 1,25-dihydroxyvitamin D_3 and intestinal vitamin D receptor concentrations in normal women, *J Clin Endocrinol Metab* 75:176, 1992.

Edelstein S, Barrett-Connor E: Relation between body size and bone mineral density in elderly men and women, *Am J Epidemiol* 138:160, 1993.

Eriksen EF et al: Cancellous bone remodeling in type I (postmenopausal) osteoporosis: quantitative assessment of rates of formation, resorption, and bone loss at tissue and cellular levels, *J Bone Miner Res* 5:311, 1990.

Ettinger B et al: Reduction of vertebral fracture risk in postmenopausal women with osteoporosis treated with raloxifene, *JAMA* 282:1344, 1999.

Feskanich D et al: Vitamin A intake and hip fractures among postmenopausal women, *JAMA* 287:47, 2002.

Fiatarone MA et al: High-intensity strength training in nonagenarians, *JAMA* 263:3029, 1990.

Fogelholm GM et al: Bone mineral density during reduction, maintenance and regain of body weight in premenopausal, obese women, *Osteoporos Int* 12:199 2001.

Food and Nutrition Board, Institute of Medicine, National Academy of Sciences: dietary reference intakes, 1997, Washington, DC, National Academy Press.

Garn SM: *The earlier gain and the later loss of cortical bone,* Springfield, Ill, 1970, Charles C Thomas.

Goulding A et al: Bone mineral density in girls with forearm fractures, *J Bone Miner Res* 13:143, 1998.

Goulding A et al: More broken bones: a 4-year double cohort study of young girls with and without distal forearm fractures, *J Bone Miner Res* 15:2011, 2000.

Goulding A et al: Bone mineral density and body composition in boys with distal forearm fractures: a dual-energy x-ray absorptiometry study, *J Pediatr* 139:509, 2001.

Halioua L, Anderson JJB: Age and anthropometric determinants of radial bone mass in premenopausal Caucasian women: a cross-sectional study, *Osteoporos Int* 1:50, 1990.

Harris PF. Medical issues and hormone replacement therapy, *Curr Womens Health Rep* 2:373, 2002.

Harris S, Dawson-Hughes B: Caffeine and bone loss in healthy postmenopausal women, *Am J Clin Nutr* 60:573, 1994.

Harris ST et al: Effects of risedronate treatment on vertebral and non-vertebral fractures in women with postmenopausal osteoporosis, *JAMA* 282:1344, 1999.

Heaney RP: Protein intake and the calcium economy, *J Am Diet Assoc* 93:1259, 1993.

Hla MM et al: A multicenter study of the influence of fat and lean mass on bone mineral content: evidence for differences in their relative influence at major fracture sites, *Am J Clin Nutr* 64:354, 1996.

Ho SC et al: Soy intake and the maintenance of peak bone mass in Hong Kong Chinese women, *J Bone Miner Res* 16:1363, 2001.

Holick MF: McCollum Award Lecture, 1994: vitamin D—new horizons for the 21st century, *Am J Clin Nutr* 60:619, 1994.

Holick M: Vitamin D and bone health, *J Nutr* 126:1159S, 1996.

Hopper J, Seeman E: The bone density of female twins discordant for tobacco use, *N Engl J Med* 330:387, 1994.

Jackman LA et al: Calcium retention in relation to calcium intake and postmenarcheal age in adolescent females, *Am J Clin Nutr* 66:327, 1997.

Jilka RL et al: Increased osteoclast development after estrogen loss: mediation by interleukin-6, *Science* 257:88, 1992.

Johnston CC Jr, et al: Calcium supplementation and increases in bone mineral density in children, *N Engl J Med* 327(2):82, 1992.

Johnston CC et al: Clinical use of bone densitometry, *N Engl J Med* 324:1105, 1991.

Kanis JA et al: The diagnosis of osteoporosis, *J Bone Miner Res* 9:1137, 1994.

Karlsson M et al: The evidence that exercise during growth or adulthood reduces the risk of fragility fractures is weak, *Best Pract Res Clin Rheumatol* 15:429, 2001.

Kalkwarf HJ, Specker BL: Bone mineral changes during pregnancy and lactation, *Endocrine* 17:49, 2002.

Kelley GA et al: Exercise and lumbar spine bone mineral density in postmenopausal women: a meta-analysis of individual patient data, *J Gerontol A Biol Sci Med Sci* 57:599, 2002.

Kerstetter JE et al: A threshold for low-protein-induced elevations in parathyroid hormone, *Am J Clin Nutr* 72:168, 2000.

Kinyamu HK et al: Serum vitamin D metabolites and calcium absorption in normal young and elderly free-living women and in women living in nursing homes, *Am J Clin Nutr* 65:790, 1997.

Kohlmeier M et al: Bone health of adult hemodialysis patients is related to vitamin K status, *Kidney Int* 51:1218, 1997.

Kohrt WM et al: Additive effects of weight-bearing exercise and estrogen on bone mineral density in older women, *J Bone Miner Res* 10:1303, 1995.

Kraut J, Coburn J: Bone, acid and osteoporosis, *N Engl J Med* 330:1821, 1994.

Kritz-Silverstein D, Barrett-Connor E: Bone mineral density in postmenopausal women as determined by prior oral contraceptive use, *Am J Public Health* 83:100, 1993.

Lamberg-Allardt CJE et al: Vitamin D deficiency and bone health in healthy adults in Finland: could this be a concern in other parts of Europe? *J Bone Miner Res* 16:2066, 2001.

Lau ERMC et al: The incidence of hip fractures in four Asian countries: the Asian Osteoporosis Study (AOS), *Osteoporos Int* 12:239, 2001.

Lee Y-S et al: Physiological concentrations of Genistein stimulate the proliferation and protect against free-radical induced oxidative damage of MC3Ts-E1 osteoblast-like cells, *Nutr Res* 21:1287, 2001.

Lips P et al: Vitamin D supplementation and fracture incidence in elderly persons: a randomized, placebo-controlled clinical trial, *Ann Intern Med* 124:400, 1996.

Liu G, Peacock M: Age-related changes in serum undercarboxylated osteocalcin and its relationship with bone density, bone quality, and hip fracture, *Calcif Tissue Int* 62:286, 1998.

Looker AC: Interaction of science, consumer practices and policy: calcium and bone health as a case study, *J Nutr* 133(6):1987, 2003.

Looker AC et al: Prevalence of low femoral bone density in older US adults from NHANES III, *J Bone Miner Res* 12:1761, 1997.

Massey L, Whiting S: Caffeine, urinary calcium, calcium metabolism and bone, *J Nutr* 123:1611, 1993.

McKane WR et al: Role of calcium intake in modulating age-related increases in parathyroid function and bone resorption, *J Clin Endocrinol Metab* 81:1699, 1996.

Melton LJ III: The prevalence of osteoporosis [Editorial], *J Bone Miner Res* 12:1769, 1997.

Miller PD et al: Cyclical etidronate in the treatment of postmenopausal women: efficacy and safety after seven years of treatment, *Am J Med* 103:468, 1997.

Moniz C: Alcohol and bone, *Br Med Bull* 50:67, 1994.

Neer RM et al: Effect of parathroid hormone (1-34) on fractures and bone mineral density in postmenopausal women with osteoporosis, *N Engl J Med* 344:1434, 2001.

Nielsen FH et al: Boron enhances and mimics some effects of estrogen therapy in postmenopausal women, *J Trace Elem Exp Med* 5:237, 1992.

Nieves JW et al: Teenage and current calcium intake are related to bone mineral density of the hip and forearm in women aged 30-39, *Am J Epidemiol* 141:342, 1995.

NIH Consensus Development Panel on Osteoporosis Prevention, Diagnosis, and Therapy: Osteoporosis prevention, diagnosis, and therapy, *JAMA* 285:785, 2001.

Nordin BEC et al: Evidence for a renal calcium leak in postmenopausal women, *J Clin Endocrinol Metab* 74:401, 1991.

Nordin BEC et al: The nature and significance of the relationship between urinary sodium and urinary calcium in women, *J Nutr* 123:1615, 1993.

Palmer CA, Anderson JJB: Position of the American Dietetic Association: the impact of fluoride on health, *J Am Diet Assoc* 200:1208, 2000.

Parker MJ et al: Hip protectors for preventing hip fractures in the elderly, *Cochrane Database Syst Rev* (2):CD001255, 2000.

Pluijm SMF et al: Determinants of bone mineral density in older men and women: body composition as a mediator, *J Bone Miner Res* 16:2142, 2001.

Potter SM et al: Soy protein and isoflavones: their effects on blood lipids and bone density in postmenopausal women, *Am J Clin Nutr* 68:1375S, 1998.

Randall T: Longitudinal study pursues questions of calcium, hormones, and metabolism in life of the skeleton, *JAMA* 268:2357, 1992.

Reddy ST et al: Effect of low-carbohydrate high protein diets on acid-base balance, stone-forming propensity, and calcium metabolism, *Am J Kidney Dis* 40(2):265, 2002.

Reid IR, Veale AG, France JT: Glucocorticoid osteoporosis, *J Asthma* 31:7, 1994.

Reid I et al: Effect of calcium supplementation on bone loss in postmenopausal women, *N Engl J Med* 328:460, 1993.

Riggs BL, Melton LJ III: Involutional osteoporosis, *N Engl J Med* 314:1676, 1986.

Riggs BL et al: Long-term effects of calcium supplementation on serum parathyroid hormone level, bone turnover and bone loss in elderly women, *J Bone Miner Res* 13:168, 1998.

Rosen CJ, Bilezekian JP: Anabolic therapy for osteoporosis, *J Clin Endocrinol Metab* 86:957, 2001.

Rude RK: Magnesium deficiency: a cause of heterogenous diseases in humans, *J Bone Miner Res* 13:749, 1998.

Sadovsky Y, Adler S: Selective modulation of estrogen receptor action, *J Clin Endocrinol Metab* 83:3, 1998.

Schneider EL, Guralnik JM: The aging of America: impact on health care costs, *JAMA* 263:2335, 1990.

Schurch MA et al: Protein supplements increase serum insulin-like growth factor-1 levels and attenuate proximal femur bone loss in patients with recent hip fracture, *Ann Intern Med* 128:801, 1998.

Sebastian A: Improved mineral balance and skeletal metabolism in postmenopausal women treated with potassium bicarbonate, *N Engl J Med* 330:1776, 1994.

Seeman E et al: Reduced bone mass in daughters of women with osteoporosis, *N Engl J Med* 320:554, 1989.

Siris ES et al: Identification and fracture outcomes of undiagnosed low bone mineral density in postmenopausal women: results from the National Osteoporosis Risk Assessment, *JAMA* 286: 2815, 2001.

Slemenda CW: Cigarettes and the skeleton [Editorial], *N Engl J Med* 330:430, 1994.

Slemenda CW, Christian JC, et al: Long-term bone loss in men: effects of genetic and environmental factors, *Ann Intern Med* 117(4):286, 1992.

Snow-Harter C et al: Muscle strength as a predictor of bone mineral density in young women, *J Bone Miner Res* 5:589, 1990.

Strause L et al: Spinal bone loss in postmenopausal women supplemented with calcium and trace minerals, *J Nutr* 124:1060, 1994.

Thrash LE, Anderson JJB: The female athlete triad, *Nutr Today* 35:168, 2000.

U.S. Department of Agriculture: *continuing survey of food intake by individuals (CSFII): diet and health knowledge survey 1991,* National Technical Information Service, Springfield, Va, 1994.

Wallace BA, Cumming RG: Systematic review of randomized trials of the effect of exercise on bone mass in pre- and postmenopausal women, *Calcif Tissue Int* 67:10, 2000.

Weaver CM, Plawecki KL: Dietary calcium: adequacy of a vegetarian diet, *Am J Clin Nutr* 59:1238S, 1994.

Weaver CM et al: Calcium absorption from foods. In Burckhardt P, Heaney RP, editors: *Nutritional aspects of osteoporosis*, Serono Symposium No. 85, New York, 1991, Raven Press, 1991.

Welten DC et al: Weight-bearing activity during youth is a more important factor for peak bone development than calcium intake, *J Bone Miner Res* 9:1089, 1994.

Wosje KS et al: High bone mass in Hutterite women, *J Bone Miner Res* 15, 2000.

Additional References

Anderson JJB: The important role of physical activity in skeletal development: how exercise may counter low calcium intake, *Am J Clin Nutr* 71:1384, 2000.

Anderson JJB et al: Phosphorus. In Bowman BA, Russell RM, editors: *Present knowledge in nutrition,* ed 8, Washington, DC, 2001, ILSI Press.

Baker VL et al: Reproductive endocrine and endometrial effects of raloxifene hydrochloride, a selective estrogen receptor modulator, in women with regular menstrual cycles, *J Clin Endocrinol Metab* 83:6, 1998.

Dawson-Hughes B: Osteoporosis. In Bowman BA, Russell RM, editors: *Present knowledge in nutrition,* ed 8, Washington, DC, 2001, ILSI Press.

Heaney RP: Calcium, dairy products, and osteoporosis, *J Am Coll Nutr* 12:835, 2000.

Hodgson SF et al: American Association of Clinical Endocrinologists 2001 medical guidelines for clinical practice for the prevention and management of postmenopausal osteoporosis, *Endocr Pract* 7(4):293, 2001.

Nordin BEC: Calcium requirement as a sliding scale, *Am J Clin Nutr* 71:1381, 2000.

Orwoll E, editor: *Osteoporosis in men,* vol 1, San Diego, 1999, Academic Press.

Pak C et al: Slow-release sodium fluoride in the management of postmenopausal osteoporosis: a randomized controlled trial, *Ann Intern Med* 120:625, 1994.

Roughead ZK et al: Controlled high meat diets do not affect calcium retention or indices of bone status in healthy postmenopausal women, *J Nutr* 133(4):1020, 2003.

Sayegh RA, Stubblefield PG: Bone metabolism and the perimenopause overview, risk factors, screening, and osteoporosis preventive measures, *Obstet Gynecol Clin North Am* 29:495, 2002.

Seeman E. Genetic and environmental determinants of variance in bone size, mass, and volumetric density of the proximal femur. In Econs MJ, editor: *The genetics of osteoporosis and metabolic bone diseases,* Totowa, NJ, 2001, Humana Press.

Snow-Harter C et al: Muscle strength as a predictor of bone mineral density in young women, *J Bone Miner Res* 5:589, 1990.

Steiner PD et al: Influence of a low calcium and phosphorus diet on the anabolic effect of human parathyroid hormone (1-38) in female rats, *Bone* 29:344, 2001.

Weaver C: Calcium. In Bowman BA, Russell RM, editors: *Present knowledge in nutrition,* ed 8, Washington, DC, 2001, ILSI Press.

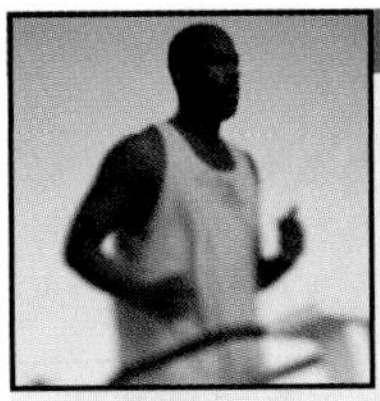

CHAPTER 28

Nutrition for Oral and Dental Health

RIVA TOUGER-DECKER, PhD, RD, FADA

CHAPTER OUTLINE

- Nutritional Factors in Tooth Development
- Dental Caries
- Fluoride
- Preventive Care
- Periodontal Disease
- Early Childhood Caries
- Tooth Loss and Dentures
- Oral Manifestations of Systemic Disease
- Polypharmacy

KEY TERMS

anticariogenic–suppressing the development of caries by preventing plaque from recognizing an acidogenic food

calculus–a hard, stonelike concretion that forms on the teeth as a result of calcification of dental plaque

candidiasis–an infection caused by the yeastlike fungus *Candida,* usually *Candida albicans*

cariogenic–containing fermentable carbohydrates that can cause a decrease in salivary pH to <5.5 and demineralization when in contact with microorganisms in the mouth; promoting caries development

cariogenicity–caries-promoting properties of a food

cariostatic–having the characteristic of not being metabolized by microorganisms in plaque to cause a drop in salivary pH to <5.5

demineralization–the dissolution of enamel or the loss of minerals from the hydroxyapatite, the principal component of the enamel

dental caries–an oral infectious disease in which acid produced by bacterial metabolism of fermentable carbohydrates leads to bacterial invasion, causing demineralization of enamel and destruction of the tooth structure

dentin–the chief organic tissue of the tooth that surrounds the pulp and is covered by enamel on the crown and by cementum on the roots

early childhood caries (ECC)–caries pattern in infants or children, also known as baby bottle tooth decay; generally caused by prolonged exposure to sweetened beverages

enamel–an inorganic, white, crystalline, compact, and very hard substance that covers and protects the dentin of the tooth; the principal component is hydroxyapatite

fermentable carbohydrate–any carbohydrate that is susceptible to the actions of salivary amylase

fluoroapaptite–the form in which the fluoride ion, along with calcium and phosphorus, is incorporated into dentin and enamel

fluorosis–a condition caused by exposure of the tooth enamel to excessive amounts of fluoride during enamel development before tooth eruption.

gingiva–the part of the oral mucosa overlying the crowns of unerupted teeth and encircling the necks of those that have erupted; the gums

gingival sulcus–a shallow, V-shaped space around the tooth that is bounded by the tooth surface on one side and the epithelium lining the gingiva on the other

KEY TERMS—Continued

periodontal disease (PD)–oral infectious disease characterized by inflammation and destruction of the attachment apparatus of the teeth, including the ligamentous attachment of the tooth to the surrounding alveolar bone

plaque–a sticky, colorless film of microorganisms, salivary proteins, inorganic components, and polysaccharides that adheres to teeth and gums

remineralization–the process of mineral restoration to the hydroxyapatite in the dental enamel

stomatitis–inflammation of the oral mucosa

Streptococcus mutans–an oral bacteria implicated in the formation of dental caries

xerostomia–mouth dryness secondary to insufficiency or lack of saliva

Diet and nutrition play key roles in tooth development, gingival and oral tissue integrity, bone strength, and the prevention and management of diseases of the oral cavity. Diet has a local effect on tooth integrity; that is, the type, form, and frequency of foods and beverages consumed have a direct effect on teeth and the oral microbe environment. Nutrition, by contrast, has a systemic effect. The impact of nutrient intake systemically affects the development, maintenance, and repair of the teeth and oral tissues. Deficiencies of the B vitamins riboflavin, folate, and B_{12}, along with vitamin C and the minerals iron and zinc along with other nutrients, can be detected in the mouth because of the rapid tissue turnover rate of the oral mucosa.

Nutrition and diet affect the oral cavity, but the reverse is also true; that is, the status of the oral cavity affects one's ability to consume an adequate diet and thus to achieve nutrient balance. Oral diseases extend beyond dental caries. Tooth loss, *edentulism,* is common in persons older than 65 years of age and can have a significant impact on intake and continues to be a significant influence on overall and nutritional well-being of this segment of the population. The following sections detail the known roles of nutrients in the growth, development, and maintenance of the oral cavity structure, bones, and tissues.

Periodontal disease (PD) is a local and systemic disease. Select nutrients, including vitamins A, C, E, folate, β-carotene, and the minerals calcium, phosphorus, and zinc, play a role in this disease.

Oral cancer, often secondary to tobacco and alcohol abuse, can have a significant impact on eating ability and nutritional status. This problem is compounded by the increased caloric and nutrient needs of persons with oral carcinomas. Surgery, radiation therapy, and chemotherapy are modalities used to treat oral cancer that can also affect dietary intake, appetite, and the integrity of the oral cavity.

Several chronic and acute diseases have oral sequelae that affect eating ability. Poorly controlled diabetes can result in burning tongue syndrome, candidiasis, and xerostomia, which in turn compromise a person's eating ability and appetite. Oral manifestations of immunosuppressive diseases, such as acquired immunodeficiency syndrome (AIDS), also have an impact on appetite, intake, and nutrient needs (Touger-Decker and Mobley, 2003).

NUTRITIONAL FACTORS IN TOOTH DEVELOPMENT

Primary tooth development begins at 2 to 3 months of gestation. Mineralization begins at about 4 months' gestation and continues through the preteen years. Maternal nutrients must therefore supply the preeruptive teeth with the appropriate building materials. Table 28-1 details the effects of nutrient deficiencies on tooth development. Figure 28-1 shows the parts of a tooth.

Teeth are formed by the mineralization of a protein matrix. In dentin, protein is present as collagen, which depends on vitamin C for normal synthesis. Vitamin D is essential to the process by which calcium and phosphorus are deposited in crystals of hydroxyapatite. Fluoride, added to the hydroxyapatite, provides unique caries-resistant properties in both prenatal and postnatal developmental periods.

Diet and nutrition are important in all phases of tooth development, eruption, and maintenance. Posteruption, diet and nutrient intake continue to affect tooth development and mineralization, enamel development and strength, as well as eruption patterns of the remaining teeth. The local effects of diet, particularly fermentable carbohydrates and eating frequency, affect the production of organic acids by oral bacteria and the rate of decay. Throughout the life span, diet and nutrition continue to affect tooth, bone, and oral mucosal integrity, resistance to infection, and tooth longevity.

DENTAL CARIES

Dental caries is one of the most common infectious diseases. According to the Surgeon General's 2000 Report on Oral Health, caries is seven times more

TABLE 28-1 Effects of Nutrient Deficiencies on Tooth Development

NUTRIENT	EFFECT ON TISSUE	EFFECT ON CARIES	HUMAN DATA
Protein/calorie malnutrition	Delayed tooth eruption Decreased tooth size Decreased enamel solubility Salivary gland dysfunction	Yes	Yes
Vitamin A	Decreased epithelial tissue development Tooth morphogenesis dysfunction Decreased odontoblast differentiation Increased enamel hypoplasia	Yes	Yes
Vitamin D/calcium/phosphorus	Lowered plasma calcium levels Hypomineralization (hypoplastic defects) Compromised tooth integrity (decreased mineral concentration) Delayed eruption patterns	Yes	Yes
Ascorbic acid	Dental pulpal alterations Odontoblastic degeneration Aberrant dentin	No	No
Fluoride	Increased stability of enamel crystal (enamel formation) Inhibition of demineralization Stimulation of remineralization Mottled enamel (excess) Inhibition of bacterial growth	Yes	Yes
Iodine	Delayed tooth eruption Altered growth patterns Malocclusions?	No	Yes
Iron	Slow growth Salivary gland dysfunction	Yes	No

Modified from DePaola D, Faine MP, Vogel RI: Nutrition in relation to dental medicine. In Shils ME, Olson JA, Shike M, editors: *Modern nutrition in health and disease*, vol 2, ed 8, Philadelphia, 1994, Lea & Febiger.

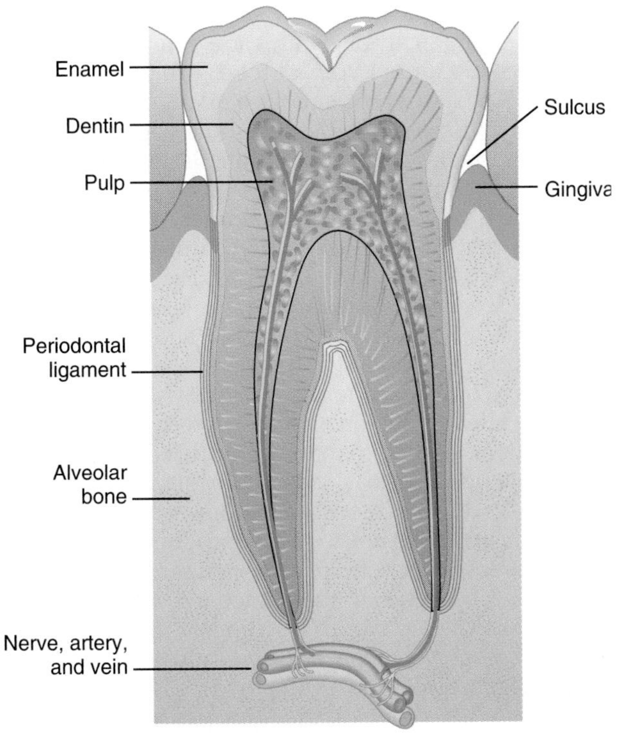

FIGURE 28-1 • Anatomy of a tooth.

common than hay fever and five times more common than asthma. Unfortunately, approximately 20% to 25% of U.S. children have 80% of the dental caries. Trends in dental caries have demonstrated that children who come from homes where parents have at least a college education have fewer caries than children from homes where parents have less than a college education (US DHHS, 2000).

Pathophysiology

Dental caries is an oral infectious disease in which organic acid metabolites produced by the metabolism of oral microorganisms lead to gradual demineralization of tooth enamel, followed by rapid proteolytic destruction of the tooth structure (Figure 28-2). Caries can occur on any tooth surface.

The etiology of dental caries is multifactorial. Four factors must be present simultaneously: (1) a susceptible host or tooth surface; (2) microorganisms, such as *Streptococcus mutans* or *Lactobacillus*, in the dental plaque or oral cavity; (3) fermentable carbohydrates in the diet, which serve as the substrate for bacteria; and (4) time (duration) in the mouth for bacteria to metabolize the fermentable carbohydrates, produce acids, and cause a drop in salivary pH to less than 5.5. Once the pH falls below 5.5, oral bacteria can initiate the demineralization process. Plaque pH can fall

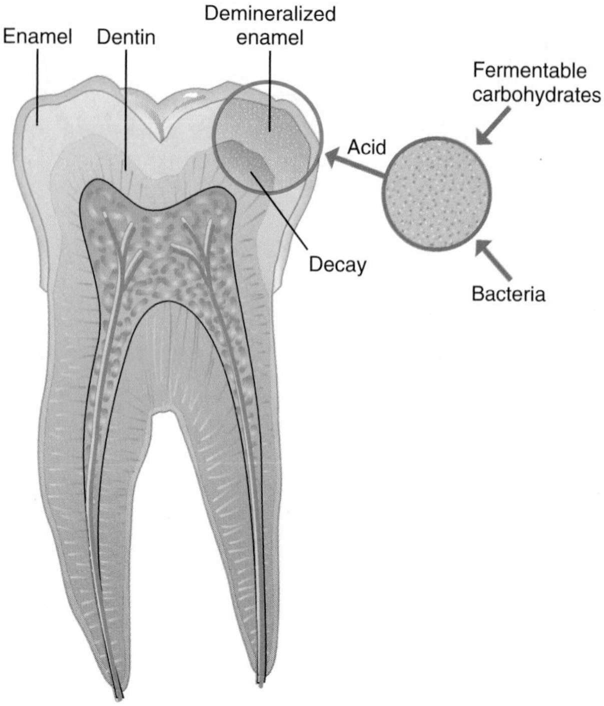

FIGURE 28-2 • Formation of dental caries.

in as little as 5 minutes and take up to 2 hours to return to neutral levels if no oral hygiene measures are introduced.

Susceptible Tooth

The development of dental caries requires the presence of a tooth that is vulnerable to attack. The composition of enamel and dentin, location of teeth, quality and quantity of saliva, and the presence and extent of pits and fissures in the tooth crown are some of the factors that govern susceptibility. The composition of the saliva is also important. Alkaline saliva may have a protective effect, whereas an acidic saliva increases susceptibility to decay. Lifestyle can also affect caries risk. It is difficult to separate the effects of family factors of food selection, eating patterns, and oral hygiene from possible genetic influences.

Microorganisms

Bacteria are an essential part of the decay process. Several microorganisms are capable of fermenting dietary carbohydrate. *Streptococcus mutans* is the most prevalent, followed by *Lactobacillus casein* and *Streptococcus sanguis.* All three contribute to the process because they metabolize carbohydrates and produce acid at levels sufficient to cause decay.

Box 28-1. Factors Affecting Food Cariogenicity

Frequency of consumption of fermentable carbohydrates
Food form (e.g., liquid, solid, slowly dissolving)
Sequence of eating foods and beverages
Combination of foods
Nutrient composition of foods and beverages
Duration of exposure of teeth to food and beverages

Substrate

Fermentable carbohydrates are the ideal substrate for bacterial metabolism. The acids produced by their metabolism cause a drop in salivary pH to less than 5.5, creating the environment for decay. In light of the *Dietary Guidelines for Americans* and the Food Guide Pyramid, both of which support a diet high in carbohydrate, it is important to be aware of the myriad of factors that can affect the potential for bacterial action on fermentable carbohydrates and to guide individuals in integrating positive diet and oral hygiene habits to improve oral health status. Factors that affect the cariogenicity of substrates are listed in Box 28-1.

Fermentable carbohydrates are found in four of the six Food Guide Pyramid food groups: (1) grains, (2) fruits, (3) dairy products, and (4) the added sugars and fats and sweets. Although some vegetables may contain fermentable carbohydrate, little has been reported about the cariogenicity, or caries-promoting properties, of vegetables. Examples of grains and starches that are cariogenic by nature of their fermentable carbohydrate composition, which can cause a decrease in salivary pH to less than 5.5, include crackers, chips, pretzels, hot and cold cereals, and breads. All fruits (fresh, dried, and canned) and fruit juices may be cariogenic. Fruits with high water content, such as melons, have a lower cariogenicity than others, such as bananas and dried fruits. Fruit drinks, sodas, ice teas, and other sugar-sweetened beverages, desserts, cookies, candies, and cake products may be cariogenic. Dairy products sweetened with fructose, sucrose, or other sugars can also be cariogenic because of the added sugars; however, dairy products are rich in calcium, so that their alkaline nature may have a positive influence, reducing the cariogenic potential of the food.

Sucrose, like other sugars (glucose, fructose, maltose, and lactose), stimulates bacterial activity. All dietary forms of sugar, including honey, molasses, brown sugar, and corn syrup solids, have cariogenic potential and can be used by bacteria to produce organic acid by-products of metabolism. Maltose, found in candies, doughnuts, potato chips, crackers, and other snack foods, also contributes to a food's cariogenic potential. Kashket and colleagues (1996) demonstrated increases in concentrations of maltose and sucrose in saliva with longer durations of exposure in the oral cavity. Salivary amylase was able to break down the dietary sugars over time.

Cariogenicity of Individual Foods

It is important to differentiate between cariogenic, cariostatic, and anticariogenic foods. Sophisticated testing methods have enabled an evaluation of the cariogenicity of specific foods. Results of such studies have demonstrated that the amount of acid formed from a food as a result of fermentation by salivary bacteria is not proportional to its sugar content, nor does the amount of demineralization necessarily parallel the amount of acid produced from the food. These observations may reflect the formation of different types of fermentation products or the presence of substances in the food that reduce, reverse, or accentuate a sugar's caries-producing action. Cariogenicity is also influenced by the volume and quality of saliva a person produces; the sequence, consistency, and nutrient composition of the foods eaten; plaque buildup; and the genetic predisposition of the host to decay. Cariogenic foods are those that contain fermentable carbohydrates, which, when in contact with microorganisms in the mouth, can cause a drop in salivary pH to 5.5 or less and stimulate the caries process.

Cariostatic foods, or foods that do not contribute to decay, are not metabolized by microorganisms in plaque and do not cause a drop in salivary pH to 5.5 or less within 30 minutes. Examples of cariostatic foods are protein foods, such as eggs, fish, meat, and poultry; most vegetables; fats; and sugarless gums. Noncarbohydrate sweeteners, such as saccharin, cyclamate, and aspartame, are cariostatic. Some evidence supports the idea that aspartame and saccharin may inhibit bacterial action because neither provides a usable substrate for streptococcus bacteria (Grenby et al, 1989).

Anticariogenic foods are those that prevent plaque from recognizing an acidogenic food when it is eaten first. The five-carbon sugar alcohol, xylitol, is considered anticariogenic. It is not broken down by salivary amylase and is not subject to bacterial degradation. Its mechanisms of action include antimicrobial activity against *Streptococcus mutans* (SM) (Hildebrandt and Sparks, 2000) and the impact of gum chewing on salivary stimulation. Salivary stimulation leads to increased buffering activity of the saliva and subsequently increased clearance of fermentable carbohydrates from tooth surfaces. Sugarfree chewing gum may help to reduce decay potential because of its ability to increase saliva flow and is recommended after meals and snacks to reduce the caries risk.

Remineralization capabilities are subsequently enhanced. Another anticariogenic mechanism of xylitol gum is that it replaces fermentable carbohydrates in the diet. SM cannot metabolize xylitol; it actually inhibits the SM. Other anticariogenic foods are cheeses, such as aged cheddar, Monterey jack, and Swiss cheese.

Factors Affecting Cariogenicity of Food

Foods contain fermentable carbohydrate, the basis for bacterial action, which, in turn, stimulates caries development. Cariogenicity refers to the caries-promoting properties of a diet or food, and the cariogenicity of a food varies depending on the form in which it occurs, its nutrient composition, when it is eaten in relation to other foods and fluids, the duration of its exposure to the tooth, and the frequency with which it is eaten (see Box 28-1).

Form and Consistency

A food's form and consistency have a significant impact on its cariogenic potential and pH-lowering or buffering capacity. Food form determines the duration of exposure or retention time of a food in the mouth, which, in turn, affects how long the decrease in pH or the acid-producing activity will last. Liquids are rapidly cleared from the mouth and have low adherence (or retentiveness) capabilities. Solid foods, such as crackers, chips, pretzels, dry cereals, and cookies, can stick between the teeth (in the interproximal spaces) and have high adherence (or retention) capability. Consumption of hard candies, lollipops, and sugared breath mints results in prolonged sugar exposure in the mouth.

Consistency also affects adherence. Chewy foods, such as gum drops and marshmallows, although high in sugar content, stimulate saliva production and have a lower adherence potential than solid, sticky foods, such as pretzels, snack crackers, or chips. The last of these, although lower in sucrose, have a longer duration of exposure. High-fiber foods with little to no fermentable carbohydrate, such as popcorn and raw vegetables, are cariostatic.

Exposure

The duration of exposure may be best explained with starchy foods, which are fermentable carbohydrates subject to the action of salivary amylase. The longer starches are retained in the mouth, the greater their cariogenicity (Kashket et al, 1996). Given sufficient time, such as when food particles become lodged between the teeth, salivary amylase makes additional substrate available as it hydrolyzes starch to simple sugars. Processing techniques make some starches rapidly fermentable, either by partial hydrolysis or by reducing particle size, thus increasing availability for enzyme action. Although sugar-containing candies cause a rapid increase in the amount of sugars available in the oral cavity to be hydrolyzed by bacteria, their effect is short lived. By comparison, simple carbohydrate-based snacks and dessert foods (e.g., potato chips, pretzels, cookies, cakes, and doughnuts) provide gradually increasing oral sugar concentrations for a longer duration because these foods often adhere to the tooth surfaces and are retained for longer periods than candies (Kashket et al, 1996).

Nutrient Composition

Nutrient composition contributes to the substrate's ability to produce acid and to the duration of acid exposure. Dairy products, by virtue of their calcium- and phosphorus-buffering potential, are considered to have low cariogenic potential. Studies have shown that cheese and milk, when consumed with cariogenic foods, help to buffer the acid pH produced by cariogenic foods. Cheeses—in particular, cheddar cheese—have anticariogenic properties and stimulate an alkaline saliva, which reduces plaque bacteria (Jenkins and Hargreaves, 1989). Eating cheese with a fermentable carbohydrate, such as dessert at the end of a meal, may decrease the cariogenicity of the meal. Nuts, which do not contain a significant amount of fermentable carbohydrates and are high in fat and dietary fiber, are cariostatic. Protein foods, such as seafood, fish, meats, eggs, and poultry, along with other fats, such as oils, margarine, butter, and seeds, are also cariostatic.

Sequence and Frequency of Eating

Eating sequence and combination of foods also affect the caries potential of the substrate. Bananas, which are cariogenic because of their fermentable carbohydrate content and adherence capability, have less potential to contribute to decay when eaten with cereal and milk than when eaten alone as a snack. Milk, as a liquid, reduces the adherence capability of the fruit. Crackers eaten with cheese are less cariogenic than when eaten alone. The buffering capacity of cheese and milk makes them desirable foods to eat at the end of a meal or in combination with other fermentable carbohydrates to reduce potential cariogenicity.

The frequency with which a cariogenic food or beverage is consumed determines the number of opportunities for acid production. Every time a fermentable carbohydrate is consumed, a decline in pH, causing caries-promoting activity, is initiated within 5 to 15 minutes and lasts up to 30 minutes. Small, frequent meals and snacks, often high in fermentable carbohydrate, increase the cariogenicity of a diet considerably more than a diet consisting of three meals and minimal snacks. Eating several cookies at once, followed by brushing the teeth or rinsing the mouth with water, is less cariogenic than eating one cookie several times throughout a day.

The Decay Process

The carious process begins with the production of acids as a by-product of bacterial metabolism taking place in the dental plaque. Decalcification of the surface enamel continues until the buffering action of the saliva is able to raise the pH above the critical level (see Figure 28-2).

Plaque Formation

Plaque is a sticky, colorless mass of microorganisms and polysaccharides that forms around the tooth and adheres to teeth and gums. It harbors acid-forming bacteria and keeps the organic products of their metabolism in close contact with the enamel surface. As a cavity develops, the plaque shields the tooth, to some extent, from the buffering and remineralization action of the saliva. In time the plaque combines with calcium and hardens to form calculus.

Acid Production

Several beverage categories, such as soft drinks (diet and regular), sports beverages, citrus juices and "ades," and vitamin C supplements have high acid content and therefore can contribute to an acidic pH. In England a study using sports beverages documented that the four popular brands had pH levels of 2.52 to 4.46 (Milsevic, 1997). Although the study did not show a significant relationship between erosion patterns and consumption, it did demonstrate the critically low pH values of these products, which can contribute to demineralization of enamel. Diet soft drinks, which may not contain sugar, are also acidic by nature and therefore cause a drop in pH. Chewable vitamin C supplements provide an acidic food that directly contacts tooth surfaces, causing a drop in pH of the oral cavity.

In the absence of foods, beverages, or medications containing fermentable carbohydrates or acids, the plaque pH stays relatively constant. When food or drink containing fermentable carbohydrate is ingested, however, the pH of the plaque is reduced. At a pH of less than 5.5 (the critical pH), acid begins to dissolve tooth enamel. This process continues for at least 30 minutes and may last up to 120 minutes until the buffering effect of saliva neutralizes plaque acidity; however, constant or frequent acid challenges (such as sucking on a lemon or self-induced vomiting) cause enamel decalcification, demineralization, and erosion.

Saliva Function

Salivary flow clears food from around the teeth. By means of the bicarbonate-carbonic acid and phosphate buffer system, it also provides buffering action to neutralize bacterial acid metabolism. Chewing promotes saliva production and may account for the reduced cariogenicity of fermentable carbohydrates consumed with a meal.

Saliva is supersaturated with calcium and phosphorus. Once buffering action has restored plaque pH above the critical point, remineralization can occur. If fluoride is present in the saliva, the minerals are deposited in the form of fluoroapatite, which is resistant to erosion. Salivary production decreases during sleep as a result of diseases affecting salivary gland function (e.g., Sjögren's syndrome), as a side effect of fasting, as a result of radiation therapy to the head and neck, or with the use of certain medications associated with reduced salivary flow, or xerostomia (see Chapter 19).

Caries Patterns

Caries patterns describe the location and surfaces of the teeth affected. Although the overall incidence of decay in the United States has declined, up to 17% of children between 2 and 4 years of age have tooth decay (CDC, 2001). According to the National Health and Nutrition Examination Survey (NHANES) III, up to 50% of children have experienced some decay by age eight (US DHHS, 2000).

Root caries, occurring on the root surfaces of teeth secondary to gingival recession, affect a large portion of the older population. Josti and colleagues (1994) reported a 52% incidence of root caries in older adults in New England. In a study of 196 older Dutch adults (mean age, 79 years), root caries was reported in 52% of men and in 35% of women (Narhi et al, 1998). A primary factor in the development of root decay is gingival recession, often secondary to periodontal disease, which results in exposure of root surfaces to the oral environment. These surfaces lack an enamel layer and are therefore more vulnerable to rapid decay.

Other factors related to the increased incidence of this decay pattern are age, lack of fluoridated water, poor oral hygiene practices, and frequent eating of fermentable carbohydrates. Management of root caries includes dental restoration and nutrition counseling. Root caries is a dental infectious disease that is increasing in older adults, partly because this population is retaining their natural teeth longer (Shay, 1997).

Lingual caries, or caries on the lingual side (surface next to or toward the tongue) of the anterior teeth, are seen in persons with bulimia or anorexia-bulimia (see Chapter 25). Frequent intake of fermentable carbohydrates, combined with repeated episodes of induced vomiting of acidic stomach contents, results in a constant influx of acid into the oral cavity. The caries are the end result of tooth erosion characterized by erosion of the palatal and buccal surfaces of the maxillary anterior teeth and the lingual surfaces of the palatal surface of the maxillary posterior teeth (Robb et al, 1995). Lingual caries may also be seen in persons with gastroesophageal reflux disease as a result of repeated episodes of acid regurgitation.

FLUORIDE

Fluoride is a primary anticaries agent. Used systemically and locally, it is a safe, effective public health measure to reduce the incidence and prevalence of dental caries (ADA, 2000). Water fluoridation alone led to a 40% to 60% decline in caries prevalence from 1946 to 1979 in persons consuming fluoridated water from birth through adolescence. Fluoridation contributed to a 30% decline in caries incidence from 1979 to 1989 (Newbrun, 1989). The impact of fluoride on caries prevention continues with water fluoridation, fluoridated toothpastes, oral rinses, and dentrifices as well as beverages made with fluoridated water.

Optimal water fluoridation concentrations (0.7 to 1.2 ppm) can provide protection against caries development without causing tooth staining (ADA, 2000). *Fluoridation* is "the adjustment of fluoride in the water supply to an optimal concentration of 0.7-1.2 ppm" (ADA, 2000).

Mechanism of Action

The three primary mechanisms of fluoride action on teeth are as follows: First, when incorporated into enamel and dentin along with calcium and phosphorus, it forms fluoroapatite, a compound more resistant to acid challenge than hydroxyapatite. Fluoride also promotes repair and remineralization of tooth surfaces with incipient carious lesions. It helps to reverse the decay process while promoting the development of a tooth surface that has increased resistance to decay. Finally, fluoride may also help to deter the harmful effects of bacteria in the oral cavity by interfering with the formation and function of microorganisms.

Fluoride can be used topically and systemically. When consumed in food and drink, fluoride enters the systemic circulation and is deposited in bones and teeth. Systemic sources have a topical benefit as well by providing fluoride to the saliva. A small amount of fluoride enters the soft tissues; the remainder is excreted. The primary source of systemic fluoride is fluoridated water; food and beverages supply a smaller amount. Topical fluoride sources include toothpastes, gels, and rinses used by consumers daily, along with more concentrated forms applied by dental professionals in the form of gels, foams,

FOCUS ON

Water Fluoridation

Fluoride supplementation has been endorsed as a public health measure by the American Dental Association and American Dietetic Association (ADA, 2000). The *U.S. Surgeon General's Report on Oral Health* (US DHHS, 2000) also stresses the value of fluoridation in dental disease prevention and tooth protection. Despite this support, however, the widespread use of fluoride has been challenged by "antifluoridationists," who claim that fluoridation restricts individual freedom of choice and increases the risk of AIDS and cancer. Disease-associated risks of fluoride are unfounded. No epidemiologic studies have demonstrated any link between fluoride and cancer or AIDS. Fluoride has no adverse health effects, and the risk of toxicity is negligible (ADA, 2000). The American Dietetic Association endorses the use of systemic and topical fluoride and water fluoridation as a vital public health measure (ADA, 2000).

and rinses. Frequent fluoride exposure via topical fluorides, fluoridated toothpastes, rinses, and fluoridated water is important in maintaining a high concentration of fluoride on the tooth enamel (see *Focus on:* Water Fluoridation).

Sources of Fluoride

Most foods, unless prepared with fluoridated water, contain minimal amounts of fluoride except for brewed tea, with approximately 1.4 ppm (Kiritsky et al, 1997). Fluoride may be unintentionally added to the diet in a number of ways, including the use of fluoridated water in the processing of foods and beverages. Fruit juices and drinks, particularly white grape juice produced in cities with fluoridated water, may have increased fluoride content; however, because of the wide variation in fluoride content, it is difficult to estimate amounts consumed.

It is prudent for health professionals to consider a child's fluid intake as well as sources and the availability of fluoridated water in the community before prescribing fluoride supplements. Because bones are repositories of fluoride, bone meal, fish meal, and gelatin made from bones are potent sources of the mineral.

In communities without fluoridated water, dietary fluoride supplements are recommended for children ages 6 months to 16 years (Table 28-2). Causes of mild fluorosis include misuse of dietary fluoride supplements, ingestion of fluoridated toothpastes and rinses, and the "halo" effect (i.e., excessive fluoride intake secondary to fluoride in foods and beverages processed in fluoridated areas and transported to other areas) (ADA, 2000). It is now recommended that supplementation start at the age of 6 months if the level of fluoride in the water supply is less than 0.6 ppm (not 0.7 ppm as previously designated). Fluoride supplements are not recommended for breastfed infants living in fluoridated communities if these infants receive drinking water between feedings.

Topical fluorides, available as fluoridated toothpaste and mouthwashes, are effective sources of fluoride that can be used in the home, school, or dental office. Fluoride rinse programs in schools have resulted in a decrease in caries incidence. Children younger than 6 years of age should not use fluoridated mouthwashes, and older children should be instructed to rinse, but not swallow, mouthwash. No more than a pea-sized amount of toothpaste should be placed on a child's toothbrush to reduce the risk of accidental fluoride ingestion.

TABLE 28-2 Dietary Fluoride Supplement Schedule 1994 (3)

AGE	FLUORIDE ION LEVEL IN DRINKING WATER (ppm)*		
	<0.3 ppm	0.3-0.6 ppm	>0.6 ppm
Birth-6 mo	None	None	None
6 mo-3 yr	0.25 mg/day†	None	None
3-6 yr	0.50 mg/day	0.25 mg/day	None
6-16 yr	1.0 mg/day	0.50 mg/day	None

From ADA Council on Access Prevention and Interprofessional Relations: Caries diagnosis and risk assessment, *J Am Diet Assoc* 126(suppl):195, 1995. Copyright American Dental Association.
*1.0 part per million (ppm)=1 mg/l.
†2.2 mg sodium fluoride contains 1 mg fluoride ion.

Topical fluorides may be administered in the dental office. Fluoride gels are often prescribed for adults and older adults. Such gels are effective in reducing the risk of coronal and root decay and tooth loss. Fluoride is most effective when given from birth through age 12 to 13, the period when mineralization of unerupted permanent teeth occurs.

Fluorosis can occur secondary to excessive fluoride intake from diet and supplements, excessive topical fluoride, or ingestion of fluoridated toothpastes, rinses, or dentrifices during the early years of tooth development. Excessive dietary intake of fluoride can occur as a result of long-term use of infant formulas in powder form that are reconstituted with fluoridated water. Mild fluorosis starts with white patchy spots. Fluorosis progresses to dark brown stains on the teeth as it becomes severe. Mottling, which occurs in severe fluorosis, results in pitting of the enamel surface of the tooth.

PREVENTIVE CARE

Caries prevention programs focus on a balanced diet, modification of the sources and quantities of fermentable carbohydrates, and the integration of oral hygiene practices into individual lifestyles. Meals and snacks should be followed with brushing, rinsing the mouth with water, or chewing sugarless gum for 15 to 20 minutes. Positive habits should be encouraged, including snacking on anticariogenic or cariostatic foods, chewing sugarless gum after eating or drinking cariogenic items, and having sweets with meals rather than as snacks. Despite the potential for a diet that is based on the Food Guide Pyramid to be cariogenic, with proper planning and good oral hygiene, a balanced diet low in cariogenic risk can be planned (Figure 28-3).

Practices to avoid include sipping carbonated beverages over extended periods, frequent snacking, and harboring candy, sugared breath mints, or hard candies in the mouth for extended periods. Over-the-counter chewable or liquid medications and vitamin preparations may also contain sugar. Chewable vitamin C is one example of a sugar-containing acid product that may contribute to tooth decay. Careful label reading is important to avoid or minimize the use of such products. Box 28-2 provides caries prevention guidelines. Table 28-3 also provides guidelines on caries prevention.

Fermentable carbohydrates, such as candy, crackers, cookies, pastries, pretzels, snack crackers, and chips, should be eaten with meals. A piece of cheese at the end of a meal or with a snack is an example of a caries reduction strategy. The plethora of "fat-free" snack and dessert items has resulted in foods with a higher simple carbohydrate concentration. "Baked" chips and snack crackers tend to have a higher simple sugar concentration than their fat-containing counterparts. Although fruits and fruit juices are fermentable carbohydrates, oral hygiene practices, such as tooth brushing, rinsing with water, or chewing sugarless gum following these foods, can reduce potential caries risk. Combining fruits with cheese with meals helps reduce the cariogenic potential of these foods.

Growing evidence supports the use of xylitol-sweetened gum as an anticaries agent after meals and snacks (Hildebrandt and Sparks, 2000; Steinberg et al, 1992). Xylitol is a five-carbon sugar that cannot be metabolized by oral bacteria. Research has documented its ability to reduce caries incidence by reducing the levels of *S. mutans* in saliva. The current recommended dose is two pieces after each meal or snack containing fermentable carbohydrates. Twenty minutes of chewing appears to cause a rise in salivary pH to a level greater than 5.5. Table 28-3 provides a summary of oral health and nutrition messages for 3- to 10-year-old children. These messages apply for caries risk reduction across the life span.

Breakfast:	1 1/2 cups toasted oat cereal + 1 cup low-fat milk or 2 slices wheat toast with 1 oz melted cheese 1 cup fresh berries coffee + low-fat milk BRUSH TEETH
Lunch:	2 slices of mushroom pizza small salad with 2 Tbs Italian dressing 16 oz spring water banana FOLLOW WITH 2 pieces xylitol gum
Afternoon snack:	1 cup pretzels + 1 oz cheese FOLLOW WITH 2 pieces xylitol gum
Dinner:	tossed salad with 2 Tbs grated cheese 1 1/2 cups spaghetti + 1 cup marinara sauce + 1/2 cup sauteed peppers 1 cup fresh fruit salad 1 slice Italian bread with 1 pat margarine 1/2 cup ice cream 1 cup low-fat milk
Snack:	4 cups popcorn BRUSH TEETH BEFORE BED

FIGURE 28-3 • A balanced diet plan with low cariogenic risk.

Box 28-2. Caries Prevention Guidelines

Brush at least twice daily, preferably after meals.
Rinse mouth after meals and snacks when brushing is not possible.
Chew sugarless gum for 15 to 20 min after meals and snacks.
Floss twice daily.
Use fluoridated toothpastes.
Pair cariogenic foods with cariostatic foods.
Snack on cariostatic and anticariogenic foods, such as cheese, nuts, popcorn, and vegetables.
Limit between-meal eating and drinking of fermentable carbohydrates.

TABLE 28-3 Oral Health and Nutrition Messages for 3- to 10-Year-Old Children and Their Caregivers

MESSAGE	RATIONALE	AGE 3-5 yr	AGE 6-10 yr
Starchy, sticky, or sugary foods should be eaten with nonsugary foods.	The pH will rise if a nonsugary item that stimulates saliva is eaten immediately before, during, or after a challenge.	√	√
Combine dairy products with a meal or snack.	Dairy products (nonfat milk, yogurt) enhance remineralization and contain calcium.	√	√
Combine chewy foods like fresh fruits and vegetables with fermentable carbohydrates.	Chewy, fibrous foods induce saliva production and buffering capacity.	√	√
Space eating occasions at least 2 hours apart and limit snack time to 15-30 minutes.	Fermentable carbohydrates eaten sequentially one after another promote demineralization.	√	√
Limit bedtime snacks.	Saliva production declines during sleep.	√	√
Limit consumption of acidic foods like sports drinks, juices, and sodas.	Acidic foods promote tooth erosion that increases risk for caries.	√	√
Combine proteins with carbohydrates in snacks. Examples: Tuna and crackers; Apples and cheese	Proteins act as buffers and are cariostatic.	√	√
Combine raw and cooked or processed foods in a snack.	Raw foods encourage mastication and saliva production whereas cooked or processed foods may be more available for bacterial metabolism if eaten alone.	√	√
Encourage use of xylitol/sorbitol–based chewing gum and candies immediately following a meal or snack.	Five minutes of exposure is effective in increasing saliva production and dental plaque pH. Excessive use may cause gastrointestinal distress.	Gum not rec.	√
Sugar-free chewable vitamin/mineral supplements and syrup-based medication should be recommended.	Sugar-free varieties are available and should be suggested for high–caries risk groups.	√	√
Encourage children with pediatric Gastroesophageal reflux disease (GERD) to adhere to dietary guidelines.	GERD increases risk for dental erosion and thus increases risk for caries.	√	√

Modified from Mobley C: Frequent dietary intake and oral health in children 3 to 10 years of age, *Building Blocks* 25(1):17-20, 2001.
GERD, Gastroesophageal reflux disease.

PERIODONTAL DISEASE

Pathophysiology

Periodontal disease (PD) is an inflammation of the gingiva with destruction of the tooth attachment apparatus. *Gingivitis*, an early form of PD, is an inflammation and infection of the gingiva, the oral tissue component of the periodontium. Both are the result of infections caused by oral bacteria in the plaque. Periodontitis results in a gradual loss of tooth attachment to the bone. Progression is influenced by the overall health of the host and the integrity of the immune system.

The primary etiologic factor in the development of PD is plaque. Plaque in the gingival sulcus, a shallow, V-shaped space around the tooth, produces toxins that destroy tissue and permit loosening of the teeth. Important factors in the defense of the gingiva to bacterial invasion are (1) oral hygiene, (2) integrity of the immune system, and (3) optimal nutrition. The defense mechanisms of the gingival tissue, epithelial barrier, and saliva are affected by nutritional intake and status. Healthy epithelial tissue prevents the penetration of bacterial endotoxins into subgingival tissue.

Nutritional Care

Deficiencies of vitamin C, folate, and zinc increase the permeability of the gingival barrier at the gingival sulcus, increasing susceptibility to PD. Severe deterioration of the gingiva is seen in individuals with scurvy or vitamin C deficiency (see Figure 4-27). Although additional nutrients, including vitamins A, E, β-carotene, and protein, have a role in maintaining gingival and immune system integrity, there are little scientific data to support supplemental uses of any of these nutrients to treat PD.

Numerous studies have attempted to link nutrient deficits to PD; however, in societies where malnutrition and PD are prevalent, poor oral hygiene is also usually evident. In such instances, it is difficult to determine whether malnutrition is the cause of the disease or one of many contributing factors, including poor oral hygiene, heavy plaque buildup, insufficient saliva, or coexisting illness. The roles of calcium and vitamin D relate to the link between osteoporosis and PD, in which bone loss is the common denominator. The association between PD and systemic osteopenia and osteoporosis has been documented as has tooth loss and osteoporosis in postmenopausal women. (Krall, 2001). The inverse relationship between decreased calcium intake and increased risk of PD has also been demonstrated (Nishida et al, 2000; Tezel et al, 2000).

Beginning with a diet evaluation, including a several-day food diary or diet recall to determine eating frequency, food intake, and oral hygiene habits, a dental or dietetic professional can evaluate the overall eating pattern and nutritional adequacy of the diet. Individual dental nutrition risk factors that may contribute to oral disease are areas that can then be addressed in counseling the patient. Nutritional and dietary management of the patient with PD follows many of the guidelines listed in Box 28-2.

Diet adequacy is particularly important both before and after periodontal surgery, when adequate nutrients are needed to regenerate tissue and maintain an immune response to prevent infection. Adequacy of calories, protein, and micronutrients should be ensured. If the ability to consume one's regular diet will be altered, a diet modified in consistency can be individually designed for each patient. Oral supplements can be used, when necessary, to supplement meals.

EARLY CHILDHOOD CARIES

Early childhood caries (ECC), often called baby-bottle tooth decay (BBTD), is a term used to describe a caries pattern in the maxillary anterior teeth of infants and young children. Characteristics include rapidly developing carious lesions in the primary anterior teeth and the presence of lesions on tooth surfaces not usually associated with a high caries risk. Because tooth decay remains the preeminent oral disease of childhood and national data are available on dental office visits, caries are a primary marker for children's oral health.

Pathophysiology and Incidence

Often ECC occurs secondary to prolonged bottle-feeding, especially at night, of juice, milk, formula, or other sweetened beverages. The extended contact time with the fermentable carbohydrate–containing beverages, coupled with the position of the tongue against the nipple, which causes pooling of the liquid around the maxillary incisors, particularly during sleep, contributes to the decay process. The lower front teeth are usually spared as a result of the protective position of the lip and tongue (Figure 28-4).

Early childhood caries is particularly prevalent in Native American and Native Alaskan communities. A study of 3- to 5-year-old children in Head Start programs in five southwestern states demonstrated a 24% incidence of ECC (Barnes et al, 1992). Native Americans had the highest incidence of ECC (35.1%), followed by Hispanics (23.8%), whites (22.2%), and blacks (20.5%). Rural children had more maxillary anterior caries than city children, independent of water fluoridation. A recent study found that maternal or caretaker fear and displeasure related to the dental experiences of adults and children affect parenting practice (Weinstein et al, 1999). It is important to provide positive dental experiences to support more appropriate practices.

Health habits that contribute to this problem include poor oral hygiene, failure to brush a child's teeth at least daily, frequent use of bottles filled with

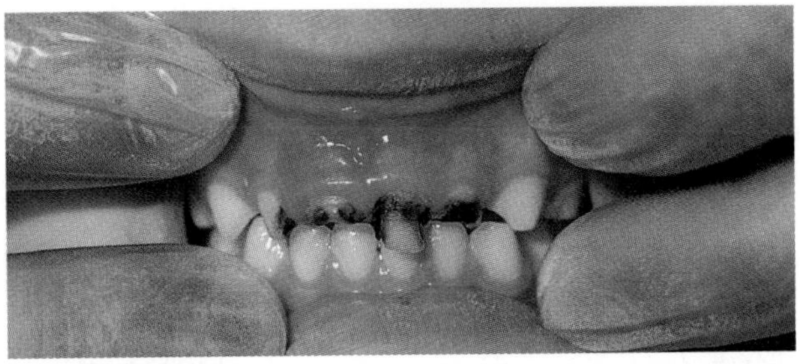

FIGURE 28-4 • Early childhood caries. (From Swartz MH: *Textbook of physical diagnosis, history, and examination*, ed 3, Philadelphia, 1998, WB Saunders.)

sweetened beverages, lack of fluoridated water, and infrequent toothbrushing (Levy et al, 2003).

In a study of the incidence of ECC in multicultural children in Texas, 72.2% of Hispanics and 37% of black children were found to have ECC. Children who were weaned from a bottle after 14 months of age had a greater incidence of ECC than those who were weaned at a younger age (Febres et al, 1997). Children with maxillary anterior caries at ages 3 to 4 years had a greater incidence of future caries than those who were caries-free at an earlier age (O'Sullivan and Tinanoff, 1996).

Generally, low-income, undereducated groups are at high risk for ECC as well as other dental diseases. In a study of the nutrition and oral health habits of infants and young children in Iowa, a 23% incidence of decay was noted (Levy et al, 2003). In a study of more than 1600 children in Manhattan, the level of untreated decay was 91%, significantly higher than the U.S. national population, which is 76% overall and 76% for blacks and Mexican Americans within the population (Albert et al, 2002). In general, children from low-income families experience the greatest amount of oral disease, the most extensive disease, and the most frequent use of dental services for pain relief, yet these children have the fewest overall dental visits (Edelstein, 2002). Enhanced dental services targeting the very young are needed in these communities (Albert et al, 2002).

Nutritional Care

Management of ECC includes diet and oral hygiene education for parents, guardians, and caregivers. Dietary guidelines include removal of the bedtime bottle and modification of the frequency and content of the daytime bottles. Bottle contents should be limited to water, formula, or milk. Infants and young children should not be put to bed with a bottle. Teeth and gums should be cleaned with a gauze pad or washcloth after all bottle feedings. All efforts should be made to wean children from a bottle by 1 year of age. Juice can be provided in a diluted form in a cup.

Educational efforts should be positive and simple, focusing on oral hygiene habits and promotion of a balanced, healthy diet. Between-meal snacks should include cariostatic foods or, when foods are cariogenic, should be followed by tooth brushing or rinsing the mouth. Parents and caregivers need to understand the causes of ECC and how it can be avoided.

TOOTH LOSS AND DENTURES

Tooth loss, edentulism, and removable prostheses can have a significant impact on dietary habits, masticatory function, olfaction, and nutritional adequacy. Compromised masticatory function, from partial or complete edentulism or complete dentures, tends to have a negative impact on food choices, resulting in decreased intake of whole grains, fruits, and vegetables (Krall et al, 1998). This results in an inadequate intake of dietary fiber and vitamins A and C, as well as other vitamins and minerals (Joshipura et al, 1996). As dentition status declines, masticatory performance, as measured by biting force, is significantly compromised (Krall et al, 1998).

Poor diet quality can have a negative impact on nutritional and overall health in dentate, as well as edentulous, individuals. This problem is more pronounced in older adults, whose appetite and intake may be compromised further by chronic disease, social isolation, and the use of multiple medications. An inverse relationship between the number of natural teeth and fruit and vegetable intake was identified in a study of free-living subjects ages 40 to 80 years old (Joshipura and Willet, 1994).

Unfortunately, dentures do not fully solve the problem. As demonstrated in a longitudinal study of individuals both before and after denture placement, many individuals continued to experience eating difficulty (biting and chewing) after denture insertion (Garrett et al, 1997). The foods that were found to cause the greatest difficulty for persons who wore complete dentures included fresh whole fruits and vegetables (e.g., apples and carrots), corn on the cob, hard-crusted breads, and steak.

Nutritional Care

Dietary assessment and counseling related to oral health should be provided to the denture wearer. Simple guidelines should be provided for cutting and preparing fruits and vegetables to minimize the need for biting and reduce the amount of chewing. Changing the dentition does not consistently result in improved eating habits. Studies have shown that, despite improving objective and subjective chewing ability, significant changes in eating habits may be difficult to make (Ettinger, 1998). The importance of positive eating habits needs to be stressed as a component of preventive health. Overall, health guidelines that reinforce the importance of a balanced diet based on the Food Guide Pyramid should be part of the routine health counseling given to all patients. Consumers can be guided to peel and chop fruits, vegetables, and other foods to reduce the need for biting and chewing. Foods can be cooked to a softer consistency, and meats and vegetables can be cut across the fibers into bite-size pieces to make eating easier. Sticky foods such as soft white breads, caramels, chewing gum, toffees, and chewy candies should be avoided. Patients can be encouraged to use their knife and fork as their "teeth" initially, cutting food into small pieces.

ORAL MANIFESTATIONS OF SYSTEMIC DISEASE

Acute systemic diseases, such as cancer and AIDS, as well as chronic diseases, such as diabetes mellitus, autoimmune diseases, and end-stage renal disease, are characterized by oral manifestations that may alter the diet and nutritional status. Cancer therapies, including irradiation of the head and neck region, chemotherapy, and surgeries to the oral cavity, have a significant impact on the integrity of the oral cavity and on an individual's eating ability and consequently can affect nutritional status (see Chapter 40).

Manifestations of HIV/AIDS

Viral and fungal infections, stomatitis, xerostomia, PD, and Kaposi's sarcoma are oral manifestations of human immunodeficiency virus (HIV) that can cause limitations in nutrient intake and result in weight loss and compromised nutritional status. These infections are often compounded by a compromised immune response, preexisting malnutrition, and gastrointestinal sequelae of HIV infection. Viral diseases, including herpes simplex and cytomegalovirus, result in painful ulcerations of the mucosa. Candidiasis on the tongue, palate, or esophagus can make chewing, sucking, and swallowing painful *(odynophagia)*, thus compromising intake. Table 28-4 outlines the impact of associated oral infections in the upper gastrointestinal tract (see Chapter 41).

Fungal Infections

Oropharyngeal fungal infections may cause a burning, painful mouth and dysphagia. The ulcers that accompany viral infections, such as herpes simplex and cytomegalovirus, cause pain and reduced oral intake. Kaposi's sarcoma compromises oral intake and increases nutrient needs. Very hot and cold foods or beverages, spices, and sour or tart foods also may cause pain and should be avoided. Consumption of temperate, moist foods without added spices should be encouraged. Small, frequent meals followed by rinsing with lukewarm water or brushing to reduce the risk of dental caries are helpful. Once the type and extent of oral manifestations are identified, a nu-

TABLE 28-4 Impact of Oral Infections

LOCATION	PROBLEM	EFFECT	DIET MANAGEMENT
Oral cavity	Candidiasis, KS, herpes, stomatitis	Pain, infection, lesions, altered ability to eat, dysgeusia	Increase kcal and protein intake Administer oral supplements Provide caries risk reduction education
	Xerostomia	Increased caries risk, pain, no moistening power, tendency of food to stick, dysgeusia	Moist, soft, nonspicy foods; "smooth" cool/warm foods and fluids; caries risk reduction education
Esophagus	Candidiasis, herpes, KS, cryptosporidiosis	Dysphagia, odynophagia	Try oral supplementation first. If that is unsuccessful, initiate NG feedings using silastic feeding tube or PEG
	CMV CMV + ulceration	Dysphagia, food accumulation	PEG

KS, Kaposi's sarcoma; *CMV*, cytomegalovirus; *NG*, nasogastric; *PEG*, percutaneous endoscopic gastrostomy.

trition care plan can be developed. Oral high calorie–high protein supplements in liquid or pudding form may be needed to meet calorie requirements.

Other Painful Mouth Problems

Stomatitis, or inflammation of the oral mucosa, causes severe pain and ulceration of the gingiva, oral mucosa, and palate, which makes eating painful. Xerostomia, or dry mouth, is seen in poorly controlled diabetes mellitus, Sjögren's syndrome, several autoimmune diseases, and as a consequence of radiation therapy and certain medications (Box 28-3). Xerostomia from radiation therapy may be more permanent than that from other causes (Garg and Malo, 1997). Efforts to stimulate saliva production using pilocarpine and citrus-flavored, sugar-free candies may ease eating difficulty.

Individuals without any saliva at all have the most difficulty eating; artificial salivary agents may not offer relief. Lack of saliva impedes all aspects of eating, including chewing, swallowing, and the sensation of taste; causes pain; and increases the risk of dental caries and infections. Dietary guidelines focus on the use of moist foods without added spices, increased fluid consumption with and between all meals and snacks, and judicious food choices. Problems with chewy (steak), crumbly (cake, crackers), dry (chips), and sticky (peanut butter) foods are common in persons with severe xerostomia, and avoiding these foods may help a great deal with eating. Water with a lemon or lime twist, citrus-flavored seltzers, or sucking on frozen grapes or sugar-free candies may help. Good oral hygiene habits are important in reducing the risk of tooth decay and should be practiced after all meals and snacks. Xylitol-flavored gums and mints may help to reduce the risk of associated decay.

Box 28-3. Medications That May Cause Xerostomia

- Antianxiety agents
- Anticonvulsants
- Antidepressants
- Antihistamines
- Antihypertensives
- Diuretics
- Narcotics
- Sedatives
- Serotonin uptake inhibitors
- Tranquilizers

Diabetes Mellitus

Diabetes is associated with several oral manifestations, many of which occur only in periods of poor control. These include burning mouth syndrome, PD, candidiasis, dental caries, and xerostomia (Finney et al, 1997; Touger-Decker and Sirois, 1995). The microangiopathies seen in diabetes, along with altered responses to infection, contribute to PD risk in affected persons. Besides blood glucose control, dietary management of the diabetic patient after any surgical procedures and or placement of dentures should include modifications in the consistency, temperature, and texture of food to increase eating comfort, reduce oral pain, and prevent infections or decay.

Head and Neck Cancers

Head, neck, and oral cancers can alter eating ability and nutrition status by virtue of the surgeries and therapies used to treat these cancers. Surgery, depending on the location and extent, may alter eating or swallowing ability as well as the capacity to produce saliva. Radiation therapy of the head and neck area as well as chemotherapeutic agents can affect the quantity and quality of saliva and the integrity of the oral mucosa. A thick, ropey saliva is often the result of radiation therapy to the head and neck area causing xerostomia. Dietary management focuses on the recommendations described earlier for xerostomia, along with modifications in food consistency following surgery.

POLYPHARMACY

Several categories of medications can alter the integrity of the oral mucosa, taste sensation, and salivary production (see Chapter 19). Phenytoin (Dilantin) may cause severe gingivitis. Many of the protease inhibitor drugs used to treat AIDS are associated with altered taste and dry mouth. Care should be taken to assess the effects of medication on the oral cavity and how these effects can be minimized by alterations in diet or drug therapy.

Clinical Scenario 1

Shelly is a 51-year-old single mother of two teenage daughters who works full-time as a real estate agent. She goes to the dentist for the first time in 5 years because she just got dental insurance. Her chief complaint is "all my teeth hurt." She further states that she spends 50% of her time in her car traveling between appointments. She has no significant medical history; her family history reveals that her mother has type 2 diabetes. She quit smoking 1 pack per day 6 months ago and at that time went on a diet. She is presently 5 ft 6 in. tall and weighs 135 lb. Six months ago she weighed 165 lb. Since then she has been on a fruit-based vegetarian diet. She has always chewed sugar gum but since quitting smoking has increased her gum chewing and reports chewing three jumbo packs (18 sticks per pack) of cinnamon-flavored sugar gum daily.

On examination the dentist determines that she has periodontal disease, extensive dental caries, two broken teeth, and a broken three-unit bridge (a bridge that supports three teeth). She needs root canal surgery in three teeth. To restore her smile aesthetically, she will either need a removable partial denture or implants.

Diet History

7:30 AM	1 banana
7:45 AM	½ large cantaloupe
8:00 AM	2 c watermelon
8:15 AM	1 banana and 1 apple
10:00 AM	2 bite-size chocolate mint patties
Noon	sandwich: 2 slices wheat bread with 1 tsp mustard, ½ c alfalfa sprouts, 1 c sliced tomatoes and cucumbers, ¼ c avocado
	15 minipretzels
12:45 PM	½ c vanilla custard
Between 2 and 6 PM	1 each apple and banana, 2 chocolate mint patties
6:30 PM	3 c mixed salad, 1 c japanese noodles
9:00 PM	4 bite-size chocolates

She drinks 2-3 L of water throughout the day.

1. What are the social, lifestyle, and environmental influences that are affecting Shelly's dental and nutritional health?
2. What are her nutritional and dietary risk factors?
3. What are appropriate diet counseling recommendations for this patient?

SUMMARY

As the gateway to the human body, the oral cavity can have a significant effect on nutritional and overall health and well-being. Diet and nutrition are important in the phases of managing oral health and disease. The integrity of the oral cavity and surrounding structures can affect functional and sensory components of normal dietary intake and subsequent nutrition status. Similarly, compromised nutrition status resulting from poor diet or disease can affect the integrity of the oral cavity.

In planning nutrition care, the dietetics professional is encouraged to incorporate questions about the patient's oral health status as a component of nutritional screening and assessment, including prob-

Clinical Scenario 2

Nathan, a 3-year-old African-American, is brought to the local health clinic by his grandmother because his front teeth are "turning black." Nathan seems small for his age; his height is measured at 35.5 in., and his weight is 25 lb. According to the growth charts, he is in the 10th percentile for height, and 5th percentile for weight, and below the 5th percentile of weight for height.

On examination by the dentist, the child is found to have eight decayed surfaces on his four anterior teeth (the two central incisors and the two lateral incisors). The dentist recommends that Nathan have metal crowns put on the decayed teeth. She also recommends that the grandmother have the child's diet and nutritional status evaluated by the clinic's registered dietitian.

The grandmother agrees, and the dietary history taken by the dietitian reveals the following:

- A diet high in simple sugar with small, frequent meals
- Continued use of a bottle filled with fruit drink, soda, or strawberry-flavored milk three times a day, including at naptime
- Suboptimal calorie and protein intake (70% and 75% of estimated needs, respectively)
- Lack of vitamin-mineral and fluoride supplements
- Nonrenewal of WIC (Women, Infants, and Children) checks within the last 6 months because the grandmother does not like traveling to the area where the clinic is located
- Inconsistent toothbrushing (The grandmother reports brushing the child's teeth three to four times per week. She does not think care of baby teeth is important, as "they fall out anyway.")

1. What are the cultural, educational, and environmental influences affecting Nathan's dental and nutritional health?
2. What type of dental condition does Nathan have? What are the diet counseling recommendations for this condition?
3. What are the nutritional and dietary risk factors?
4. Design a nutrition care plan to improve this youngster's dental health and growth.

lems with biting, chewing, or swallowing; dry mouth; or the presence of sores in the mouth that interfere with eating comfort. Such questions can be routinely incorporated into nutrition screening and assessment strategies. Diet guidelines to facilitate masticatory function can be integrated into nutrition care plans.

Relevant Web Sites

American Dental Association
www.ada.org/
American Dental Hygienists Association
www.adha.org/
American Academy of Periodontology
www.perio.org/
Colgate Kids
www.colgate.com/cp/oralcare.class/kids/kids_home.jsp
HIV Dent
www.hivdent.org/
National Institute of Dental and Craniofacial Research
www.nidr.nih.gov/
Proctor and Gamble Dental Resources
www.pg.com/frameset_fs.jhtml?frameURL=http%3A//www.dentalcare.com/

Cited References

Albert DA et al: Dental caries among disadvantaged 3- to 4-year-old children in northern Manhattan, *Pediatr Dent* 24(3):229, 2002.

American Dietetic Association (ADA): Position of the American Dietetic Association (ADA): oral health and nutrition, *J Am Diet Assoc* 96:184, 1996.

American Dietetic Association (ADA): Position of the ADA: the impact of fluoride on dental health, *J Am Diet Assoc* 100:1208, 2000.

Barnes GP et al: Ethnicity, location, age and fluoridation factors in baby bottle tooth decay and caries prevalence of Head Start children, *Public Health Rep* 107(2):167, 1992.

Centers for Disease Control and Prevention: Improving oral health: preventing unnecessary disease among all Americans. www.cdc.gov/nccdphp/oh/ataglanc.htm, accessed 1/25/02, last updated July 2001.

Edelstein BL: Disparities in oral health and access to care: findings of national surveys, *Ambul Pediatr* 2(2 suppl):141, 2002.

Ettinger RI: Changing dietary patterns with changing dentition: how do people cope? *Spec Care Dentistry* 18 (1):33, 1998.

Febres C et al: Parental awareness, habits, and social factors and their relationship to baby bottle tooth decay, *Pediatr Dent* 19(1):22, 1997.

Finney LS et al: What the mouth has to say about diabetes: careful examinations can avert serious complications, *Postgrad Med* 102:117, 1997.

Garg AK, Malo M: Manifestations and treatment of xerostomia and associated oral effects secondary to head and neck radiation therapy, *J Am Dent Assoc* 97:1128, 1997.

Garrett NR et al: Veterans Administration Cooperative Dental Implant Study—comparisons between fixed partial dentures supported by blade-vent implants and removable partial dentures. Part V: Comparisons of pretreatment and posttreatment dietary intakes, *J Prosthet Dent* 77:153, 1997.

Grenby TH et al: Laboratory studies of the dental properties of soft drinks, *Br J Nutr* 62:451, 1989.

Hildebrandt G, Sparks B: Maintains Mutans Stretocci suppression with xylitol chewing gum, *J Am Dent Assoc* 131:909, 2000.

Jenkins GN, Hargreaves JA: Effect of eating cheese on Ca and P concentrations of whole mouth saliva and plaque, *Caries Res* 23:159, 1989.

Josti A et al: The distribution of root caries in community dwelling elders in New England, *J Public Health Dent* 54:15, 1994.

Kashket S et al: Accumulation of fermentable sugars and metabolic acids in food particles that become entrapped on the dentition, *J Dent Res* 75:1885, 1996.

Kiritsky MC et al: Assessing fluoride concentration of juices and juice-flavored drinks, *J Am Dent Assoc* 127:895, 1997.

Koenigsberg S et al: Incidence of baby bottle tooth decay in young inner city children, Unpublished report, 1994.

Krall E: The periodontal-systemic connection: implications for treatment of patients with osteoporosis and periodontal disease, *Ann Periodontol* 6(1):209, 2001.

Krall E et al: How dentition status and masticatory function affect nutrient intake, *J Am Dent Assoc* 129:1261, 1998.

Levy SM et al: Flouride, beverages and dental caries in the primary dentition, *Caries Res* 37:157, 2003.

Milsevic A et al: Sports supplement drinks and dental health in competitive swimmers and cyclists, *Br Dent J* 182:303, 1997.

Mobley C: Frequent dietary intake and oral health in children 3-10 years of age, *Building Blocks for Life: Pediatric Nutrition Practice Group Newsletter* 25(1):20, 2001.

Narhi TO et al: Salivary findings, daily medication and root caries in the elderly, *Caries Res* 32(1):5, 1998.

Newbrun E: Effectiveness of water fluoridation, *J Pubic Health Dent* 49(special issue):279, 1989.

Nishida M et al: Calcium and the risk for periodontal disease, *J Periodontal* 71(7):1057, 2000.

Robb ND et al: The distribution of erosion in the dentitions of patients with eating disorders, *Br Dent J* 178:171, 1995.

Shay K: Root caries in the older patient: significance, prevention and treatment, *Dent Clin North Am* 41(4):763, 1997.

Tezel M et al: The relationship between bone mineral density and periodontitis in postmenopausal women, *J Periodontol* 71(9):1492, 2000.

Touger-Decker R, Mobley CC: Position of the American Dietetic Association: Oral health and nutrition, *J Am Diet Assoc* 103:615, 2003.

Touger-Decker R, Sirois D: Dental care of the person with diabetes. In Powers M, editor: *Handbook of diabetes nutrition management*, ed 2, Gaithersburg, Md, 1995, Aspen Publishers.

U.S. Department of Health and Human Services: CDC's oral health program at-a-glance 1996-1997, Washington, DC, US DHHS Public Health Service, 1997.

U.S. Department of Health and Human Services: *Oral health in America: a report of the Surgeon General*, Rockville Md, 2000, U.S. Department of Health and Human Services, National Institute of Dental Orofacial Research, National Institute of Health.

Weinstein P et al: Dental experiences and parenting practices of Native American mothers and caretakers: what we can learn for the prevention of baby bottle tooth decay, *SCD J Dent Child* 66:120, 1999.

Additional References

American Dental Association ONLINE: Fluorides and fluoridation, www.ada.org/consumer/fluoride.

Faine M: The role of dietetics professionals in preventing early childhood caries, *Building Blocks for Life: Pediatric Nutrition Practice Group Newsletter* 25(1):1, 2001.

Garrett NR et al: Effects of improvements of poorly fitting dentures and new dentures on masticatory performance, *J Prosthet Dent* 75:269, 1996.

Joshipura KJ, Willet WC: Effect of edentulousness on diet and nutrition, [IADR abstr] *J Dent Res* 73:207, 1994.

Joshipura KJ et al: The impact of edentulousness on food and nutrient intake, *J Am Dent Assoc* 127:459, 1996.

National Institute of Dental Health: Results of National Oral Health Survey released March 12, 1996, Available: www.nidr.nih.gov/news.

O'Sullivan DM, Tinanoff N: Social and biological factors contributing to caries of the maxillary anterior teeth, *Pediatr Dent* 15:41, 1993.

O'Sullivan DM, Tinanoff N: The association of early dental caries patterns with caries incidence in preschool children, *J Public Health Dent* 56(2):81, 1996.

Pappas AS et al: The effects of denture status on nutrition, *Spec Care Dent* 18(1):17, 1998.

Sebring NG et al: Nutritional adequacy of reported intake of edentulous subjects treated with new conventional or implant-supported mandibular dentures, *J Prosthet Dent* 74: 358, 1995.

Shinkai RSA et al: Oral function and diet quality in a community-based sample, *J Dent Res* 80(7):1625, 2001.

Slavkin H: Maturity and oral health: Live longer and better, National Institute of Dental and Craniofacial Research, National Institute of Health, www.nidr.nih.gov/slavkin/slav0600.asp; accessed January 9, 2002.

Steinberg LM et al: Remineralizing potential, antiplaque and antigingivitis effects of xylitol and sorbitol sweetened chewing gum, *Clin Prev Dent* 14(5):31, 1992.

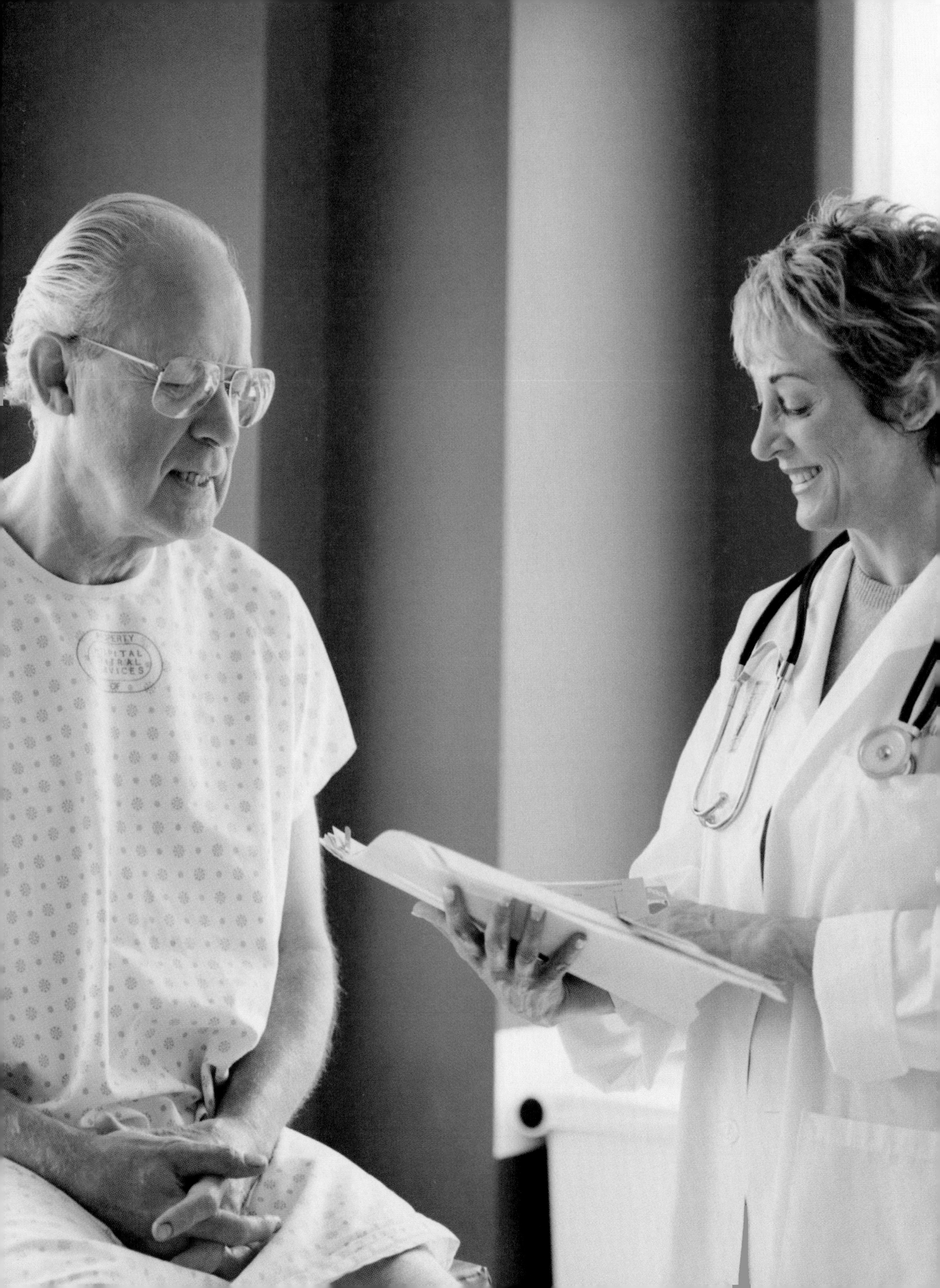

PART 5

MEDICAL NUTRITION THERAPY

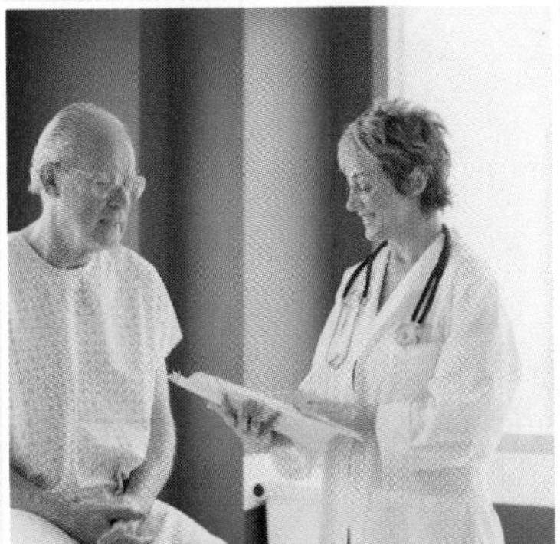

Nutrition plays a primary role in growth, development, health, and fitness. As we have seen, maintaining appropriate nutrition throughout life can also prevent, or at least delay, the onset of some nutrition-related disease. This section covers the importance of medical nutrition therapy (MNT) in the treatment of established disease.

As the knowledge base expands, the list of diseases amenable to nutrition intervention increases. Availability of sophisticated feeding and nourishment procedures places increased responsibility on those who provide nutritional care. Most of the nutrition-related diseases included here are preventable by changes in dietary practices, at least on the basis of current knowledge. Exceptions, such as some forms of neoplastic disease, are discussed in terms of both the evidence for prevention and the appropriate nutritional care in disease.

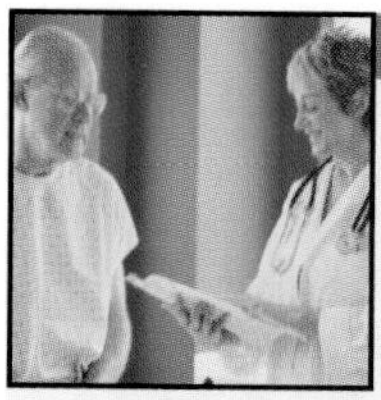

CHAPTER 29

Medical Nutrition Therapy for Upper Gastrointestinal Tract Disorders

PETER L. BEYER, MS, RD, LD

CHAPTER OUTLINE

- Disorders of the Esophagus
- Disorders of the Stomach

KEY TERMS

achlorhydria–absence of hydrochloric acid from maximally stimulated gastric secretions

achylia gastrica–absence of hydrochloric acid and pepsin in the gastric juice

alimentary hypoglycemia–low blood glucose manifesting as weakness, perspiration, hunger, nausea, anxiety, and tremors 1 to 2 hours after a meal

atrophic gastritis–chronic inflammation of the stomach with deterioration of the mucous membrane and glands, resulting in achlorhydria and loss of intrinsic factor

Barrett's esophagus–a condition in which cells lining the distal esophagus become abnormal and premalignant

dumping syndrome–a complex physiologic response to the rapid emptying of hypertonic contents into the duodenum and jejunum

duodenal ulcer–a peptic ulcer situated in the duodenum

dyspepsia (indigestion)–a general term used to describe epigastric discomfort following meals

endoscopy–a procedure used to view the esophagus, stomach, and upper part of the small intestine using a flexible tube with a camera

epigastric–referring to the upper middle region of the abdomen

esophagitis–inflammation of the esophagus

fundoplication–a surgical procedure for the treatment of reflux esophagitis that involves mobilizing the lower end of the esophagus and wrapping the fundus of the stomach around it

gastrectomy–removal of all (e.g., total gastrectomy) or part of the stomach (hemi-gastrectomy)

gastric ulcers–lesions that are associated with disruption of the gastric mucosal barrier

gastritis–inflammation of the stomach

gastroesophageal reflux disease (GERD)–backward flow of the stomach or duodenal contents into the esophagus; may occur normally or as a chronic pathologic condition

heartburn–a retrosternal burning related to reflux of acid fluid from the stomach into the esophagus

Helicobacter pylori–a type of bacteria that can chronically infect the stomach; thought to be a primary contributor to the development of gastritis, peptic ulcers, and even gastric cancer

hiatal hernia–an outpouching of a portion of the stomach into the chest through the esophageal hiatus of the diaphragm

lower esophageal sphincter (LES)–the last few centimeters of the esophagus, which prevents reflux of gastric contents into the esophagus

melena–black, tarry stools indicative of gastrointestinal bleeding

parietal cells–large cells, located on the margin of the peptic glands of the stomach, which secrete hydrochloric acid and produce intrinsic factor

parietal cell vagotomy–resection or removal of the portion of the vagus nerve innervating the parietal cells for the purpose of diminishing gastric acid secretion

peptic ulcer–an eroded lesion in either the esophageal, gastric, or duodenal mucosa resulting from the action of gastric acid

truncal vagotomy–resection or removal of portions of the vagus nerve to decrease the cholinergic stimulation of parietal cells and reduce the cellular response to stimulants, such as gastrin

vagus nerve–the tenth cranial nerve, which has many branches that supply sensory fibers to the ear, tongue, pharynx, and larynx; motor fibers to the pharynx, larynx, and esophagus; and parasympathetic and visceral afferent fibers to the thoracic and abdominal viscera

Digestive disorders persist to be among the most common problems in health care. About 30% to 40% of adults claim to have frequent indigestion, and more than 47 million visits are made annually to ambulatory care facilities for symptoms related to the digestive system. About 2.8 million endoscopies and 5 million surgical procedures involving the gastrointestinal (GI) tract are performed each year (Frank et al, 2000; Kozak and Owings, 1998; Schappert, 1998).

Dietary habits and specific food types can play a significant role in the onset, treatment, and prevention of many GI disorders. In many cases, diet can also play a role in improving patients' sense of well-being and quality of life and in decreasing pain, suffering, and the costs associated with GI disease (Beyer, 1998). Table 29-1 lists disorders of the upper GI tract that are described in this chapter and the typical symptoms and nutritional consequences.

DISORDERS OF THE ESOPHAGUS

The entire esophagus functions as one tissue during swallowing. As a bolus of food is moved voluntarily from the mouth to the pharynx, the upper sphincter relaxes, the food moves into the esophagus, and peristaltic waves move the bolus down the esophagus; the lower esophageal sphincter (LES) relaxes to allow the food bolus to pass into the stomach (Figure 29-1).

Disorders of the esophagus may be caused by derangement of the swallowing mechanism, obstruction, inflammation, or abnormal sphincter function. Because difficulty in swallowing *(dysphagia)* is often

TABLE 29-1 Upper GI Disorders and Nutritional Consequences

GI CONDITION	COMMON SYMPTOMS	POSSIBLE NUTRITIONAL CONSEQUENCES
Esophagitis and esophageal reflux disease (GERD)	Reflux of gastric contents Burning sensation in upper middle of chest after meals (heartburn); increased belching, and sometimes painful spasm	Possible discomfort during and after eating or change in eating habits, especially in evening; reduced intake
Esophageal stricture or tumor	Swallowing solid food causes discomfort; liquids are tolerated	Possible weight loss if intake is chronically inadequate
Hiatal hernia	Asymptomatic or prolonged heartburn after heavy meals, bending over, or reclining after a meal	Possible discomfort after eating, especially after large meals and with position changes; may worsen GERD symptoms
Cancer of oral cavity, esophagus	Asymptomatic or epigastric pain when eating (more likely with gastric tumor); difficulty chewing or swallowing; delayed gastric emptying	May lead to surgical procedures, radiation therapy, chemotherapy; difficulty chewing or swallowing; change in food textures; may require enteral feeding; weight loss is common
Indigestion/dyspepsia/gastritis	GI discomfort after eating	Abdominal discomfort; altered diet; decreased overall intake possible, increased food intolerances
Duodenal ulcer	Pain 2-5 hr after a meal; pain relief after eating	Abdominal discomfort; altered diet, decreased overall intake possible; increased food intolerances
Gastric ulcer	Vague epigastric discomfort or pain when eating	Abdominal discomfort that may lead to lowered food intake and weight loss
Gastrectomy, partial gastrectomy	Early satiety or symptoms of nausea, bloating, or diarrhea after eating (dumping syndrome)	Smaller, more frequent meals; decreased lactose tolerance; altered composition of foods; possible weight loss, malabsorption, and diarrhea

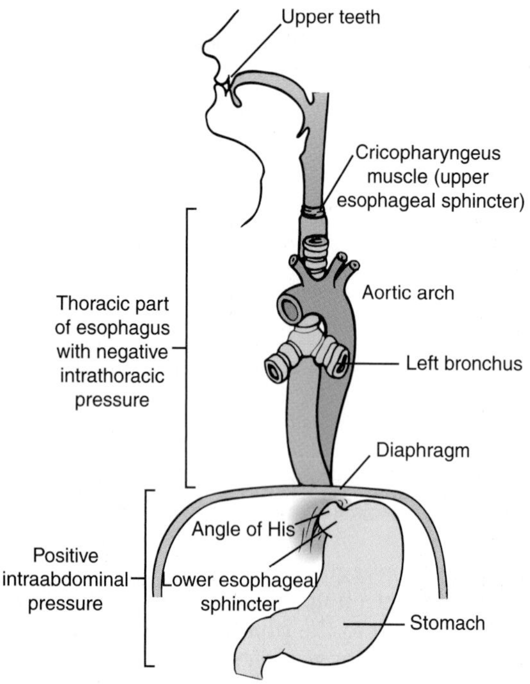

FIGURE 29-1 • Normal esophagus. (Modified from Price SA, Wilson LM: *Pathophysiology: clinical concepts of disease processes*, ed 5, St. Louis, 1997, Mosby.)

the result of a neurologic problem, it is discussed in Chapter 43.

Gastroesophageal Reflux and Esophagitis

Pathophysiology

Occasional reflux of gastric contents is not an entirely uncommon event in healthy persons; about 7% of the population experiences daily heartburn resulting from frequent reflux of gastric and sometimes duodenal contents into the esophagus. About 20% of adults report frequent symptoms of heartburn, and the lifetime prevalence of gastroesophageal reflux disease (GERD) in the United States is 25% to 35% (Frank et al, 2000; Scott and Gelhot 1999).

Persons with chronic esophageal reflux have increased episodes of substernal pain, belching, and esophageal spasm. Other symptoms may include pharyngeal irritation, hoarseness, and asthmatic symptoms. Prolonged severe disease can result in esophagitis, ulceration, scarring, stricture, and, in some cases, dysphagia (Figure 29-2). Symptoms often interfere with sleep, work, social events, and the overall quality of life. A major concern in persons with long-standing esophageal reflux is the development of Barrett's esophagus, a condition in which cells lining the distal esophagus become abnormal and become premalignant. Barrett's esophagus and the metaplasia that develops are responsible for the rising incidence of adenocarcinoma of the esophagus in the population (DeMeester and DeMeester, 1999; Katzka and Rustgi, 2000).

Acute esophagitis may be caused by ingestion of a corrosive agent, viral inflammation, or intubation. Risk of reflux is increased with hiatal hernia, reduced LES pressure, tobacco use, increased abdominal pressure (as in obstructive lung disease), delayed gastric emptying, recurrent vomiting, or other factors. The severity of the esophagitis resulting from gastroesophageal reflux is influenced by several factors. These include the composition, frequency, and volume of the gastric reflux; mucosal resistance; rate of clearance from the esophagus; and the rate of gastric emptying (Goyal, 1998).

Competency of the LES is also important. The pressure of this sphincter is influenced by many factors, including scleroderma-like disorders, smoking, diet, and smooth-muscle relaxants. LES pressures also decrease during pregnancy, in women taking progesterone-containing oral contraceptives, and even in the late stage of a normal menstrual cycle. Although most cases of esophagitis are related to reflux of gastric contents, esophagitis may also be related to viral and bacterial infection, ingestion of corrosive agents, and radiation. Smoking, large doses or chronic use of aspirin or the nonsteroidal anti-inflammatory drugs (NSAIDs), and several other oral medications can increase the risk of esophagitis in susceptible persons (Goyal, 1998).

Medical and Surgical Management

Primary medical treatment of esophageal reflux is directed toward reduction of acid secretion. Proton pump inhibitors, which decrease acid production by the gastric parietal cell, are considered the most effective treatments, but milder forms of reflux can be managed by H_2 receptor antagonists or antacids (Webb, 2000). Prokinetic agents may be used in persons who have delayed gastric emptying. Medications that raise LES pressure are currently being evaluated (Lanas and Santolaria, 2001). Activities that require frequent bending should be avoided, and to reduce the likelihood of nocturnal reflux, raising the head of the bed 4 to 6 inches can be beneficial.

The 5% to 10% of patients with severe gastroesophageal reflux who do not respond to medical therapy after 3 to 6 months may be treated surgically with fundoplication, a procedure in which the fundus of the stomach is wrapped around the lower esophagus to limit reflux (Kahrilas, 1999).

Because nicotine decreases LES pressure and the use of tobacco products compromises gastrointestinal integrity, their use is contraindicated (Gustafsson et al, 2000; Kabat, Ng, and Wynder, 1993; Mitchell, Sobel, and Alexander, 1999) (see *Clinical Insight:* Smoking and Gastrointestinal Function). Cigarette smoking has been studied most thoroughly, primarily because it is the main use of tobacco, and the ex-

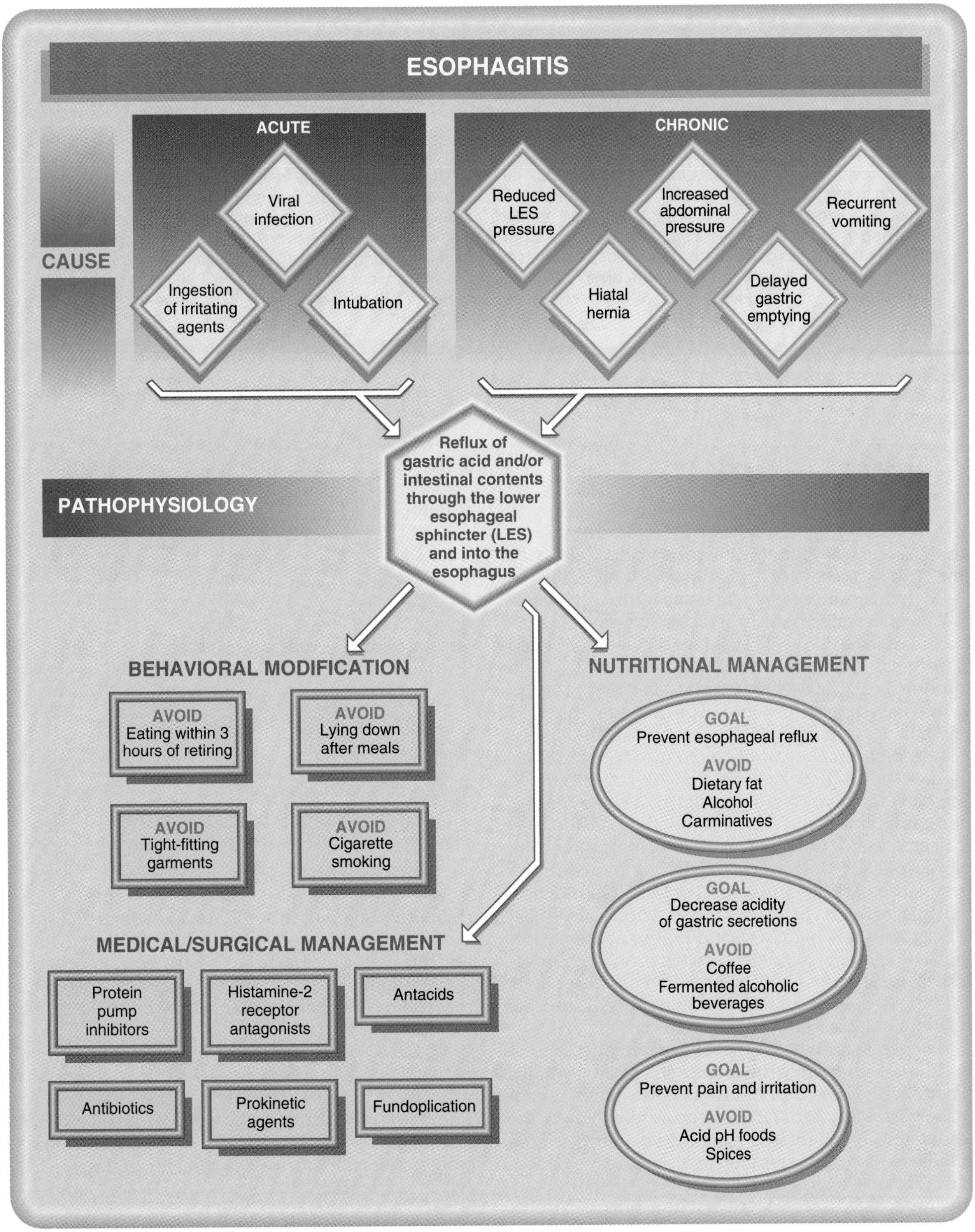

FIGURE 29-2 • Pathophysiology algorithm: esophagitis. (Algorithm content developed by John Anderson, PhD, and Sanford C. Garner, PhD, 2000. Updated by Peter L. Beyer, MS, RD, LD, 2002.)

CLINICAL INSIGHT

Smoking and Gastrointestinal Function

The GI effects of smoking include the reduction of LES and pyloric sphincter pressure, increased reflux, alteration of the nature of the gastric contents, inhibition of pancreatic bicarbonate secretion, accelerated gastric emptying of liquids, and lower duodenal pH. The acid secretory response to gastrin or acetylcholine is increased considerably. Smoking also impairs the ability of cimetidine and other drugs to lower the overnight acid secretion that is thought to play a key role in ulcerogenesis. Nicotine is responsible for many of the effects of tobacco use, but increased exposure to hydrocarbons, oxygen radicals, and a number of other substances is thought to also contribute to the overall effects. Finally, smoking impairs spontaneous healing and increases the risk and rapidity of ulcer recurrence as well as the likelihood that the ulcer will perforate and require surgery.

posure from direct smoke inhalation is considered greater than with other forms.

Medical Nutrition Therapy

The objectives of nutritional care are to (1) prevent esophageal reflux, (2) prevent pain and irritation of the inflamed esophageal mucosa, and (3) decrease the erosive capacity or acidity of gastric secretions.

Many measures help to manage reflux, but probably the most effective is to avoid eating several hours before retiring. Large, high-fat meals lower LES pressure, delay gastric emptying, and increase latent acid production, all of which increase the risk of reflux while the person is reclined. This measure might be difficult for some, especially because in the United States, nighttime meals are often the largest and are part of socialization or recreation. Most admit, however, that avoidance of foods in the evening reduces their symptoms.

The size and timing of meals also appear to be important. Lying down after consuming meals can increase the likelihood of reflux, especially if the meal is large or high in fat or protein. Large meals and desserts that are high in fat and protein stimulate significant amounts of gastric secretions, and rich meals slow gastric emptying. Persons with reflux, therefore, will have fewer problems if they consume little or no food for at least 3 hours before retiring.

For a person who has severe esophagitis, a low-fat liquid diet may be better tolerated initially. Foods with an acid pH, such as citrus juices, tomatoes, and soft drinks, may cause pain when the esophagus is inflamed. In rare circumstances, harsh foods may cause perforation (e.g., chips, crisp crackers, and husks). The role of spices in the pathology of upper GI disorders is not clear, but the use of foods that are highly seasoned with chili powder and black pepper may cause discomfort when the esophagus is inflamed (Marotta and Floch, 1991; Rodriguez et al, 1998).

Avoidance of certain foods and drugs that lower LES pressure may improve or prevent symptoms of reflux. Dietary fat, alcohol, and carminatives (peppermint and spearmint) lower LES pressure. Coffee and fermented alcoholic beverages (such as beer and wine) stimulate the secretion of gastric acid. Some medications, especially elixirs, may be acidic or may have an acid pH.

Obesity is likely be a contributing factor to hiatal hernia and reflux because it increases intragastric pressure, although partial weight loss has not been found to reduce reflux symptoms (Kjellin et al, 1996). Use of loose-fitting garments by obese or normal-weight persons, however, is thought to decrease the risk of reflux (Box 29-1).

Box 29-1. Nutritional Care Guidelines for Patients With Reflux and Esophagitis

1. Avoid large, high-fat meals, especially 3 to 4 hr before retiring.
2. Avoid smoking.
3. Avoid chocolate, alcohol, and caffeine-containing beverages, such as coffee.
4. Avoid peppermint and spearmint oils.
5. Stay upright and avoid vigorous activity soon after eating.
6. Avoid tight-fitting clothing, especially after a meal.
7. Avoid acidic and highly spiced foods when inflammation exists.

Hiatal Hernia

Pathophysiology

A common contributor to gastroesophageal reflux and esophagitis is hiatal hernia. The esophagus passes through the diaphragm by way of the esophageal hiatus or ring. The attachment of the esophagus to the hiatal ring may become incomplete, allowing the esophagus or a portion of the upper stomach to move above the diaphragm. The most common type of hiatal hernia is the sliding hernia, and the less common form is the paraesophageal hernia (Mittal and Balaban, 1997) (Figure 29-3).

The presence of hiatal hernia is not synonymous with reflux, but it increases the risk. The hiatal canal in the diaphragm serves as a "second sphincter" during abrupt increases in intraabdominal pressure (Kahrilas, 1999).

When the acid reflux occurs with a hiatal hernia, gastric contents may remain in the esophagus above the hiatus longer than if the canal were intact. Because increases in intragastric pressure force acidic stomach contents up into the esophagus, persons with hiatal hernia may experience difficulty when lying down or bending over and may experience more epigastric discomfort after large, calorically dense meals.

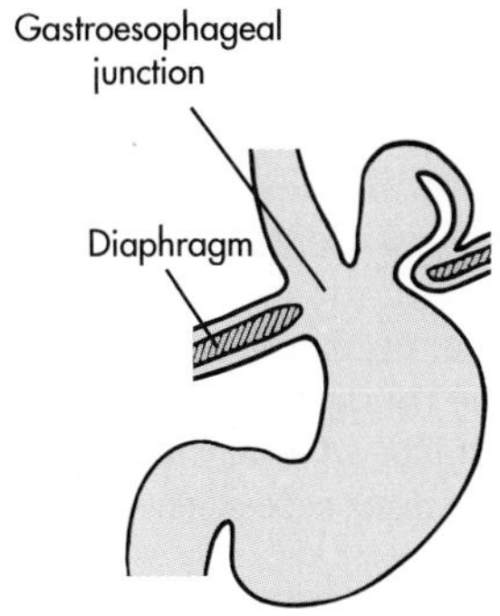

FIGURE 29-3 • Rolling or paraesophageal hernia. (Modified from Price SA, Wilson LM: *Pathophysiology: clinical concepts of disease processes*, ed 5, St. Louis, 1997, Mosby.)

Medical Nutrition Therapy

Diet therapy for hiatal hernia is aimed at decreasing symptoms in those who have reflux or esophagitis. Therapy is similar to that for GERD and esophagitis: consumption of smaller, low-fat meals and the avoidance of foods that may increase gastric secretions or reduce LES pressure. Surgery is not always indicated for hiatal hernia; symptom control through medications and diet is generally the preferred treatment.

Oral Cavity Cancer and Surgery

Pathophysiology

The patient diagnosed with cancer of the oral cavity, pharynx, or esophagus may initially manifest with existing nutritional problems and eating difficulties caused by the tumor mass, obstruction, oral infection and ulceration, or alcoholism, a coexisting condition that is frequently associated with these tumors. Nutritional deficits may be compounded by the treatment, which commonly involves surgical resection, regional irradiation, or chemotherapy. Chewing, swallowing, salivation, and taste acuity are often affected. Extensive dental decay, osteoradionecrosis, and infections may also occur. Chemotherapy can be expected to produce nausea, vomiting, and anorexia (see Chapter 40).

Surgery of the Mouth or Esophagus

After extensive surgery of the mouth or esophagus, it may be necessary to provide oral nutrition support in liquid form. Many nutritionally complete formulas are available (see Appendixes 36 through 41). To add variety to the diet, ordinary foods, such as fruits, can be puréed and mixed with water until liquefied. With more extensive oral involvement, it may be necessary to use a gastrostomy or jejunostomy tube for administering the formula. Enteral tube feedings may involve the use of ready-to-feed formulas or table foods put in a blender. If the GI tract is not functioning, nutritional support can be provided parenterally (see Chapter 23).

Tonsils are lymphatic tissue and part of the immune system. Tonsillectomy is less common today than in the past because mild inflammation of the tonsils is considered a natural part of the immune system's efforts to fight infection. When necessary, the doctor may remove the tonsils in an attempt to reduce the number and frequency of ear infections, tonsillitis, and sinusitis. The convalescent period following a tonsillectomy is short. Cold, mild-flavored, soft, moist foods bring the most comfort to the patient and offer the most protection against unexpected bleeding from the surgical area. During the first 24 hours after surgery, foods that are best accepted include dairy beverages, such as milk, malted milk, and eggnogs; ice cream or frozen yogurt; fruit ice; and pear, peach, or apricot nectars. By the second day, warm fluids and soft foods may be introduced; thereafter, hot foods can be introduced cautiously as healing progresses and as these foods are tolerated. The patient can be back to a normal diet within 3 to 5 days.

Medical Nutrition Therapy

If the patient with oral cancer is unable to eat for prolonged periods, nutritional support may be provided by tube-feeding if the remainder of the gastrointestinal tract is functional. Gastrostomy feedings can be used if long-term feeding by tube is necessary for total or supplemental support. If oral feeding is possible after surgery, general dietary recommendations include liquid or soft-textured, moist foods for easy mastication and swallowing, and small, frequent meals of relatively high caloric density. Complex carbohydrates are preferred over simple sugars.

Periodic use of an artificial saliva solution is also helpful, as is the frequent consumption of fluids to prevent dry mouth. Normal saline rinses may ameliorate mucositis, and topical anesthetics can be used to relieve pain. Necessary dental restorations, aggressive oral hygiene, and daily use of fluoride are recommended. Oral infections are usually fungal. Unfortunately, some of the medications used in treatment may leave a metallic taste in the mouth that can further compromise the patient's desire to eat (see Chapter 40).

DISORDERS OF THE STOMACH

Indigestion and Dyspepsia

Pathophysiology

Dyspepsia (indigestion) is a general term that is frequently used to describe common symptoms of upper GI discomfort. Symptoms of dyspepsia are reported in about one fourth of adults and may include vague abdominal pain, bloating, nausea, regurgitation, and belching. Dysphagia may be relatively benign and have little consequence, or it may be an indicator of more serious problems. Symptoms of prolonged dysphagia may be related to underlying problems, such as gastroesophageal reflux, gastritis, peptic ulcer disease, delayed gastric emptying, gallbladder disease, or cancer. Many persons have symptoms that persist despite lack of specific pathology (Robinson, 2001; Talley et al, 1998). In patients with dyspepsia unrelated to a specific pathologic process, diet, stress, and other lifestyle factors may contribute to the symptoms.

Medical Nutrition Therapy

Dietary indulgences—excessive volumes of food or high intake of fat, sugar, caffeine, spices, or alcohol—are commonly implicated in dyspepsia (Mishkin et al, 1997). Dietary management of uncomplicated dyspepsia is simple and probably has been passed on for generations: eat slowly, chew thoroughly, and do not eat or drink excessively. Reaction to life stresses may also contribute to abdominal distress, in which case behavioral management and emotional support may also help. If symptoms persist despite these strategies, further evaluation and diet therapy should be tailored to the underlying cause.

Gastritis and Peptic Ulcer Disease

Pathophysiology

Gastritis and peptic ulcers may result when infectious, chemical, or neural abnormalities disrupt mucosal integrity. The most common cause of gastritis and peptic ulcer is *Helicobacter pylori* infection. *H. pylori* infection is responsible for chronic inflammation of the gastric mucosa, for gastric and duodenal ulcers, and for some forms of atrophic gastritis and gastric cancer. Factors that affect the occurrence and severity of symptoms include the patient's age at onset of the initial infection, the concentration of organisms, the specific strain of the organism, and the lifestyle and overall health of the patient. The infection is typically confined to the mucosa of the stomach (Dunn et al, 1997).

H. pylori organisms are gram-negative bacteria with flagella that facilitate mobility. These organisms are somewhat resistant to the acidic medium of the stomach, but additional protection is provided by their colonization beneath the protective mucous layer and by significant urease production. Urease allows the generation of ammonia to facilitate alkalinization of the immediate surroundings. The size and shape of these organisms range from spirals to coils to rods, depending on the culture media of the stomach. The prevalence of *H. pylori* infection among the adult population ranges from about 50% in developed countries to greater than 90% of the population in developing countries. Only 10% to 15% of those infected by the organism develop symptomatic ulceration, however. The exposure and prevalence in the United States may be declining over time. Infection with *H. pylori* in young persons is now only about 10%, but the incidence in persons older than 60 years of age is about 50% (Laine and Fendrick, 1998).

Infection with the *H. pylori* organism results in a chronic inflammatory state. Infection induces inflammation from both humoral and systemic immune response, with damage resulting from cytotoxins produced by the organism during the inflammatory response by the host (Gomollon and Sicilia, 2001). Treatment typically involves combination therapy of three or four medications, including bismuth, antibiotics, and antisecretory agents. The degree of microbial resistance to specific agents in different parts of the world and the varying strains of the organism may necessitate the use of different protocols and combinations of medications. Eradication of the organism results in elimination of the inflammatory state and the symptoms (Dunn et al, 1997; Laine and Fendrick, 1998; see *New Directions:* The Genome of *Helicobacter pylori*).

Chronic use of aspirin or other NSAIDs, steroids, alcohol abuse, ingestion of erosive substances, tobacco use, or any combination of these factors may also compromise mucosal integrity (Abdel-Salam et al, 1995). Poor nutrition and general poor health may also contribute to the onset and severity of the symptoms and delay healing.

The mucosa of the stomach and duodenum is normally protected from the proteolytic actions of gastric acid and pepsin by a coating of mucus secreted by glands in the epithelial walls from the lower esophagus to the upper duodenum. The mucosal layer is also protected from bacterial invasion by the digestive actions of pepsin and hydrochloric acid and the mucus secretions. The mucus contains acid-neutralizing bicarbonates, and additional bicarbonates are provided by the pancreatic juice secreted into the intestinal lumen. Production of mucus is stimulated by the action of prostaglandins. Hydrochloric acid is secreted by the parietal cells in response to stimuli by gastrin, acetylcholine, and histamine (Hojgaard et al, 1996).

Acute gastritis refers to rapid onset of inflammation and symptoms. Chronic gastritis may occur over a period of months to decades, with waxing and waning of symptoms. Gastritis may manifest by a number of symptoms, including nausea, vomiting, malaise, anorexia, hemorrhage, and epigastric pain.

Chronic gastritis, which is common in older adults, results in atrophy and loss of stomach parietal cells, with a loss of secretion of hydrochloric acid (achlorhydria) and intrinsic factor (Baik and Russel, 1999). Patients may have a low or low normal serum B_{12} level or elevated serum homocystine levels. Many cases are considered to have an autoimmune origin, although a significant percent of cases may result from long-term *H. pylori* infection (Sipponen and Marshall, 2000).

Medical Treatment

Endoscopy is a common procedure used to identify problems (see *Focus on:* Endoscopy). Treatment of gastritis includes the eradication of pathogenic organisms (e.g., *H. pylori*) and withdrawal of any provoking agents. Antibiotics, antacids, H_2-receptor antagonists, and proton pump inhibitors may each play a role in the treatment of gastritis, depending on the precipitating cause.

Medical Nutritional Therapy

In persons with atrophic gastritis, vitamin B_{12} status should be evaluated because a lack of intrinsic factor and acid results in malabsorption of this vitamin (see the discussion on vitamin status assessment in Chapters 4, 18, and 34).

Peptic Ulcers

Pathophysiology

Normal gastric and duodenal mucosa is protected from the digestive actions of acid and pepsin by the secretion of mucus, the production of bicarbonate, the removal of excess acid by normal blood flow, and the rapid renewal and repair of epithelial cell injury. *Peptic ulcer* refers to an ulcer that occurs as a result of the breakdown of these normal defense and repair mechanisms. Typically, more than one of the mechanisms must be malfunctioning for symptomatic peptic ulcers to develop. Unlike damage from gastritis and other forms of superficial injury, classic peptic ul-

NEW DIRECTIONS

The Genome of *Helicobacter pylori*

The ability of robotic analyzers to sequence long lengths of DNA automatically and the rapidity with which computers can scan gene data banks have spawned a new discipline in the biomedical sciences: genomics. Sequencing genomes for microbial conditions offers an expeditious means of searching for novel treatments for infectious disease. *H. pylori* genome studies are important in this realm. *H. pylori* organisms live only in the human stomach, and the enzymatic pathways they need for survival in this harsh milieu are continually switched on. There are a number of antigenic variations that occur. Many genes have been found to code for iron-scavenging pathways, indicating a crucial role for iron in the survival of *H. pylori* in the stomach. The unlocking of the genome and the logical sequencing of key targets will allow the creation of novel inhibitory and bactericidal products against which no microbe has yet had the chance to become resistant (Lee, 1998).

FOCUS ON

Endoscopy

The mucosa of the upper GI tract can be viewed, studied, and even photographed by means of endoscopy, a procedure that involves passing a flexible tube with a light and an eyepiece through the esophagus and into the stomach or upper small bowel. Erosions, ulcerations, changes in the blood vessels, and destruction of surface cells can be identified. These changes can then be correlated with chemical, histologic, and clinical findings to formulate a diagnosis. Endoscopy is also important in the long-term monitoring of patients with chronic esophagitis and gastritis because of the possibility that they will develop premalignant lesions or carcinoma.

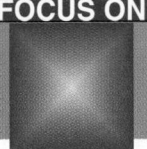

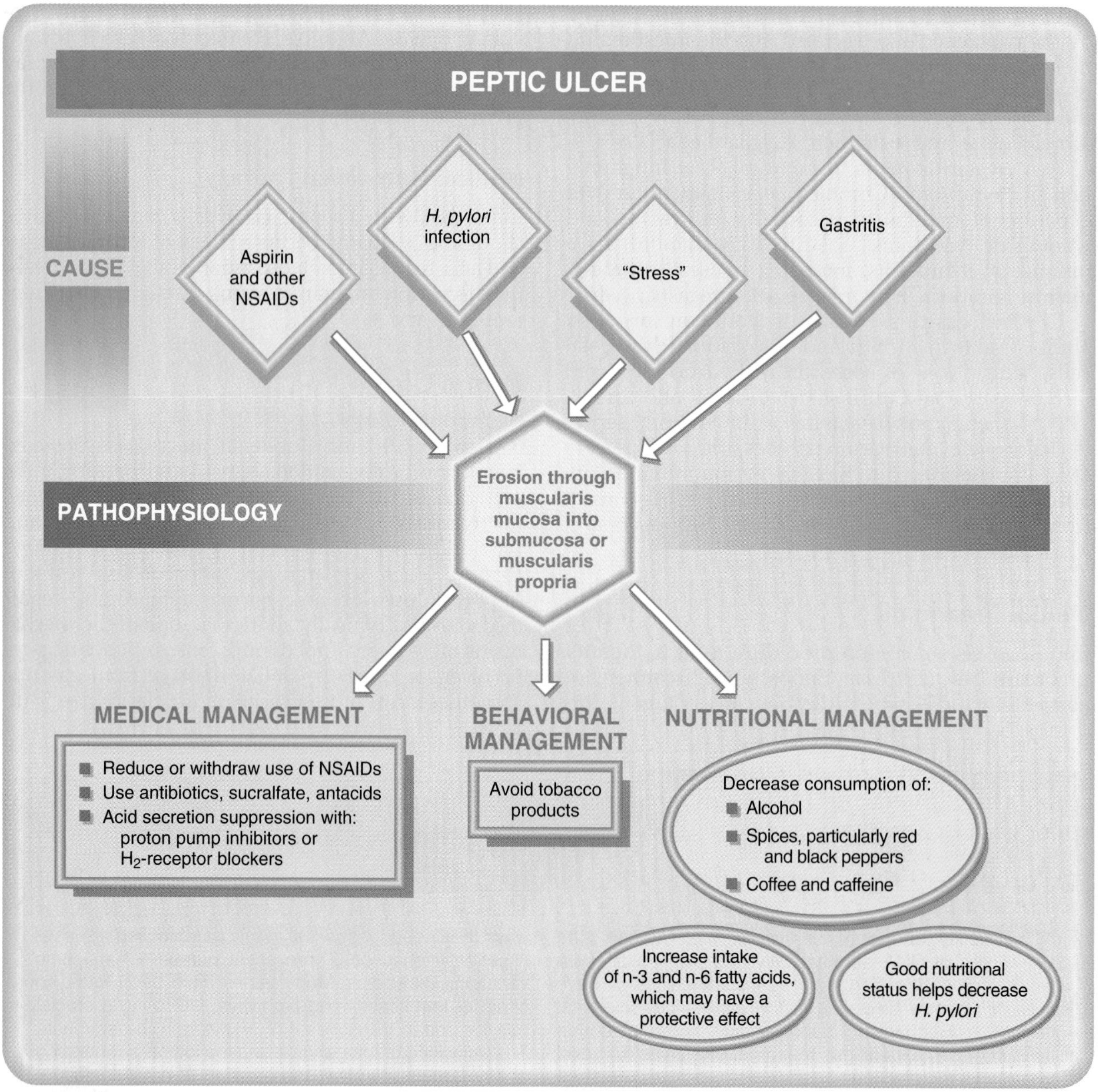

FIGURE 29-4 • Pathophysiology algorithm: peptic ulcer. (Algorithm content developed by John Anderson, PhD, and Sanford C. Garner, PhD, 2000. Updated by Peter L. Beyer, MS, RD, LD, 2002.)

cers erode through the muscularis mucosa into the submucosa or muscularis propria. Peptic ulcers typically show evidence of chronic inflammation and repair processes surrounding the lesion.

The primary causes of peptic ulcers are *H. pylori* infection, gastritis, the use of aspirin and other NSAIDs, corticosteroids (Figure 29-4), and so-called stress ulcers. Excessive use or concentrated forms of ethanol can damage gastric mucosa, worsen symptoms of peptic ulcer, and interfere with ulcer healing, but modest doses of alcoholic beverages in otherwise healthy persons do not appear to cause peptic ulcer. Consumption of beer and wine increases gastric secretions, whereas low concentrations of ethanol may not (Bujanda, 2000). Use of tobacco products decreases bicarbonate secretion, decreases mucosal blood flow, exacerbates inflammation, and is associated with additional complications of *H. pylori* infection.

As a result of the early recognition of the symptoms and associated causes of peptic ulcer, the incidence, prevalence of and number of surgical procedures related to peptic ulcer have decreased markedly in the last three decades. In particular, the eradication of *H. pylori* and the recognition of potential damage from NSAIDs have had a considerable impact on reducing the incidence of peptic ulcer.

Peptic ulcer normally involves two major regions: gastric and duodenal. Uncomplicated peptic ulcer in either region may present with signs similar to those associated with dyspepsia and gastritis. Abdominal pain or discomfort is characteristic of both gastric and duodenal ulcers, although anorexia, weight loss, nausea and vomiting, and heartburn may occur slightly more often in persons with gastric ulcer (Soll, 1998). In some patients, peptic ulcers are asymptomatic. Often complications of hemorrhage and perforation add to the significance of the presentation.

Complications

Although a chronic ulcer usually follows a typical course with characteristic symptoms, occasionally hemorrhage and perforation are the first signs of illness. Ulcers can perforate into the peritoneal cavity or penetrate into an adjacent organ (usually the pancreas), or they may erode an artery and cause massive hemorrhage. Melena, which refers to black, tarry stools, is a common finding associated with peptic ulcer disease in older adults. Melena may suggest either acute or chronic gastrointestinal bleeding.

Characteristics of and Comparisons Between Gastric and Duodenal Ulcers

Although gastric ulcers can occur anywhere in the stomach, most occur along the lesser curvature of the stomach (Figure 29-5). Gastric ulcers typically are associated with widespread gastritis, inflammatory involvement of oxyntic (acid-producing) cells, and atrophy of acid- and pepsin-producing cells with advancing age. In some cases, gastric ulceration develops despite relatively low acid output. Antral hypomotility, gastric stasis, and increased duodenal reflux are common in gastric ulcer and, when present, may increase the severity of the gastric injury. With a gastric ulcer, hemorrhage and overall mortality are higher than with a duodenal ulcer.

Duodenal ulcer is characterized by considerably increased acid secretion, nocturnal acid secretion, and decreased bicarbonate secretion. Most duodenal ulcers occur within the first few centimeters of the duodenal bulb, in an area immediately below the pylorus. Gastric outlet obstruction occurs more commonly with duodenal ulcers than with gastric ulcers, and gastric metaplasia may occur with duodenal ulcer related to *H. pylori* (i.e., replacement of duodenal villous cells with gastric-type mucosal cells). Suppression of acid with H_2-receptor blockers or proton pump inhibitors is used in management of duodenal ulcers.

Medical Management of Ulcers

Peptic Ulcers

Because the primary cause of gastritis and peptic ulcers is *H. pylori* infection, the primary focus of treatment in most cases is the eradication of this organism. Because of the presence of different strains of this organism and the relative resistance of the organism throughout the world, the drug protocol usually involves the use of two antibiotics plus bismuth or a proton pump inhibitor. Although new antibiotic protocols will continue to be introduced and evaluated, treatment protocols involve combinations of tetracycline, metronidazole, amoxycillin, and clarithromycin (Gomollon and Sicilia, 2001; Miehlke, Bayerdorffer, and Graham, 2001). Bismuth and proton pump inhibitors, such as omeprazole or lansoprazole, have been shown to inhibit the growth of *H. pylori,* and their use has been found to be more effective in the treatment of *H. pylori* infection than antibiotics alone. Use of tobacco products, alcohol, NSAIDs, and aspirin interfere with several aspects of ulcer therapy and increase the likelihood of complications.

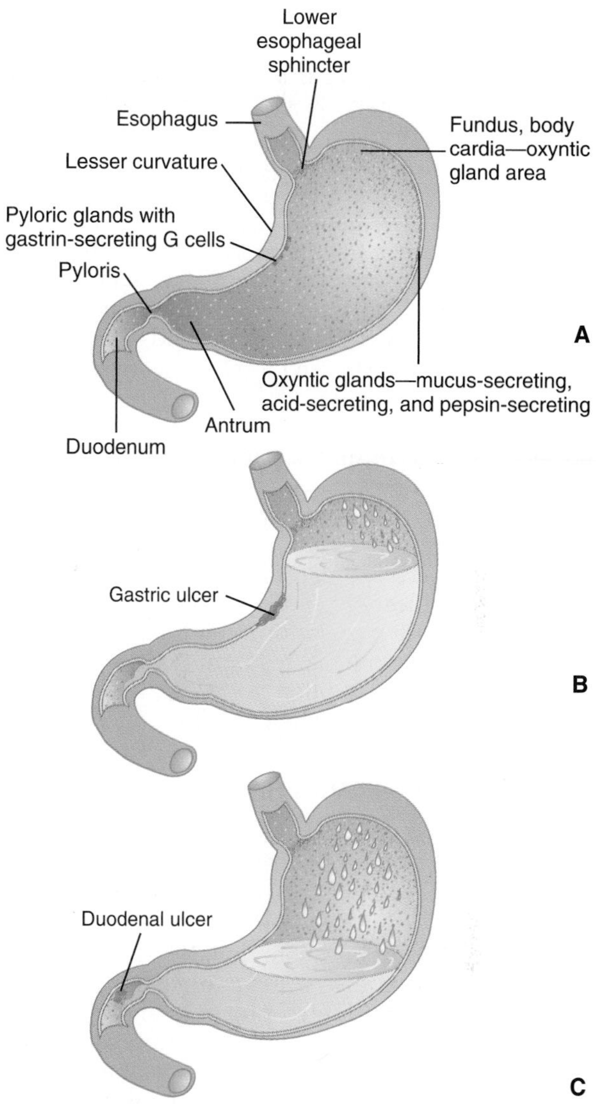

FIGURE 29-5 • Diagram showing **(A)** the stomach and duodenum with eroded lesions, **(B)** a gastric ulcer, and **(C)** a duodenal ulcer.

Stress Ulcers

Stress ulcers may occur as a complication of severe burns, trauma, surgery, shock, renal failure, or radiation therapy. A primary concern with stress ulceration is the potential for significant hemorrhage. Gastric ischemia is thought to be the underlying cause, but mucosal barrier changes and reflux of bile acid or pancreatic enzymes have also been implicated. The true mechanisms are not completely understood (Friedman and Peterson, 1998). Proton pump inhibitors, H_2-receptor blockers, antacids, and other medications have been used to prevent stress ulceration in high-risk patients.

Stress ulcers that bleed may be a significant cause of morbidity in critically ill patients, but our knowledge of effective prevention and treatment is still incomplete. Sucralfate, antacids, and acid secretion suppressors are still among the best drugs for these patients (Cook et al, 1996; Lasky et al, 1998). Efforts to prevent stress ulcers in "stressed" patients have focused on preventing or limiting conditions leading to hypotension and ischemia, respiratory disorders, and coagulopathies, in addition to avoidance of large doses of corticosteroids when possible.

Ulcers Associated With the Use of NSAIDs

The first mode of treatment for ulcers associated with NSAID use is to withdraw the drug or reduce the dosage when possible. Because a significant number of persons with NSAID-induced ulcers also have concurrent *H. pylori* infection (Soll, 1998), eradication of the organism is also a focus of therapy. Proton pump inhibitors and H_2-receptor antagonists are recommended for treatment. Methods for preventing ulcers in persons at risk (i.e., older adults, those with a past history of peptic ulcer, and those taking anticoagulants or corticosteroids) are currently being evaluated. Prostaglandins (misoprostol) and antisecretory agents may have some value in prevention, but few studies have been performed that show convincing protection in high-risk patients.

Medical Nutrition Therapy for Ulcers

For several decades, dietary factors have gained and lost favor as a significant component in the cause and treatment of dyspepsia, gastritis, and peptic ulcer disease. Since the identification of *H. pylori* as the major contributor to these disorders, the role of diet and nutritional status again must be reevaluated.

Protein foods temporarily buffer gastric secretions, but they also stimulate secretion of gastrin and pepsin. Milk or cream, which in the early days of peptic ulcer management was considered important in "coating" the stomach, is no longer considered medicinal. In animal studies, milk and cream were considered protective against peptic ulcer generation, but they were not tested against other foods (Dial et al, 1995).

The pH of a food before ingestion has little therapeutic importance except for patients with lesions of the mouth or the esophagus. Most foods are considerably less acidic than the normal gastric pH of 1 to 3. The pH of both orange juice and grapefruit is 3.2 to 3.6, and the pH of commonly used soft drinks ranges from approximately 2.8 to 3.5 (Flick, 1970). On the basis of their intrinsic acidity, fruit juices and soft drinks are not likely to cause peptic ulcer or appreciably interfere with healing. Some patients express discomfort with ingestion of acidic foods, but the response is not consistent among patients and, in some, symptoms may be related to heartburn.

Consumption of large amounts of alcohol from any source may cause at least superficial mucosal damage and may worsen existing disease or interfere with treatment of the peptic ulcer. Modest consumption of alcohol does not appear to be pathogenic for peptic ulcer unless coexisting risk factors are also present. On the other hand, beers and wines significantly increase gastric secretions and should be avoided in symptomatic disease.

Both coffee and caffeine stimulate acid secretion and may also decrease LES pressure; however, neither has been strongly implicated as a cause of peptic ulcer outside of the increased acid secretion and discomfort associated with their consumption.

When very large doses of certain spices are fed orally or placed intragastrically without other foods, they increase acid secretion and cause small, transient superficial erosions, inflammation of the mucosal lining, and altered GI permeability or motility. Most often incriminated are chili, cayenne, and black peppers (Jensen-Jarolim et al, 1998; Myers et al, 1987; Vasudevan et al 2000). Small amounts of chili pepper or its pungent ingredient, capsicum, may serve to increase mucosal protection by increasing production of mucus, but large amounts may cause superficial mucosal damage, especially when consumed with alcohol or other known irritants (Abdel-Salam et al, 1995). Despite the common association of spicy foods and abdominal discomfort and the evidence of mucosal changes with large amounts as single test agents, consumption of spicy foods in the typical Western diet has not been shown to cause or affect the healing of peptic ulcer (Marotta and Floch, 1991). At least a small percent of intolerances to spices may be related to specific allergic responses (Niinimake et al, 1989). The long-term use of spices, either as protective or harmful agents, has not been well studied in health or disease.

Because prostaglandins from omega-3 and omega-6 fatty acids are involved in inflammatory, immune, and cytoprotective physiology of the GI mucosa, they have been considered for use in management of *H. pylori* infection and peptic damage. In vitro and animal and human studies are conflicting, with some showing protective and others reporting harmful effects of both omega-3 (n-3) and omega-6 fatty acids. Omega-3 fatty acids, when protected from lipid peroxidation, have shown antiinflammatory properties and have been shown to be protective against mucosal injury evoked from drugs and *H. pylori* (Al-Shabanah, 1997; Manjari and Das, 2000; Olafsson et al, 2000; Shimizu et al, 2001). Long-term clinical trials have not been performed using specific fatty acids, and identification of the ideal dose or form of lipids to be used in the diet has not been established.

Animal and epidemiologic studies show some positive relationship between good dietary practices (adequate nutrient, fruit and vegetable, and fiber intakes) and decreased risk of complications from *H. pylori* infection (Aldoori et al, 1997; Hung and Neu, 1997). Malnutrition originating from either micronutrient deficiencies or generalized protein-calorie malnutrition affects rapidly dividing cells like those of the GI tract, and deficiencies could compromise wound healing. Overall a high-quality diet and avoidance of nutrient deficiencies may offer some protection from peptic ulcer disease and may play a role in healing.

From a practical perspective, persons being treated for gastritis and peptic ulcer disease may be advised to avoid the excessive use of specific spices, alcohol, and coffee (both caffeinated and decaffeinated); to eat a good-quality diet; and to use supplements to make up for dietary inadequacies as needed. Because some patients may have significant gastric outlet obstruction or bezoars, chewing thoroughly and avoiding foods with skins that are difficult to break down is advisable, especially in those persons with dentures or missing teeth (Cifuentes-Tebar et al, 1992; Escamilla et al, 1994).

Meal frequency is a controversial issue in the management of peptic ulcer disease. Frequent, small meals may increase comfort, decrease the chance for acid reflux, and stimulate gastric blood flow but also may increase net acid output. There is broad agreement that affected persons should avoid consuming large meals, especially before retiring, to reduce latent increases in acid secretion. In the case of stress ulcers, continuous enteral feeding and early postoperative feeding may help maintain the mucosal barrier and GI circulation, thus reducing the risk of stress ulceration. Factors that increase or decrease gastric acidity are listed in Box 29-2.

Carcinoma of the Stomach

Pathophysiology

Malignant neoplasms of the stomach can lead to malnutrition as a result of excessive blood and protein losses or, more commonly, because of obstruction and mechanical interference with food intake. Most cancers of the stomach are treated by surgical resection; thus the nutritional considerations are similar to those pertinent to partial or total gastrectomy.

Factors that appear to increase the risk of carcinoma of the stomach include chronic infection with *H. pylori* (see *Focus on:* Sulforaphane and *H. pylori*), smoking, heavy alcohol consumption, obesity, and consumption of a diet low in fibrous foods, highly

Box 29-2. Factors That Affect Gastric Acidity

Increased Gastric Acidity

Cephalic Phase of Digestion

Thought, taste, smell of food, and chewing and swallowing initiate vagal stimulation of the parietal cells in the fundic mucosa, resulting in secretion of gastric acid.

Gastric Phase of Digestion

Effect of food in the stomach:	Distention of the fundus stimulates the parietal cells to produce acid.
	Increased alkalinity of antrum causes the release of gastrin, which stimulates gastric acid secretion.
	Distention of the antrum causes release of gastrin.
	Substances in certain foods and digestive products increase acidity (e.g., coffee, both with or without caffeine; alcohol; polypeptides and amino acids [products of protein digestion]).

Decreased Gastric Acidity

Gastric Phase of Digestion

Acidification of the antrum reduces gastrin release and thus gastric acid secretion.
Food, especially protein, has an initial buffering effect.

Intestinal Phase of Digestion

Fat, acid, and protein in the small intestine stimulate release of one or more gastrointestinal hormones that inhibit gastric acid secretion.

FOCUS ON

Sulforaphane and *H. pylori*

Infection with *H. pylori* is common in developing regions where there is also a high prevalence of gastric cancer; therefore eradication of this organism is an important medical goal. Obstacles to this goal include resistance to conventional antimicrobial agents and economic and practical problems precluding the widespread use of antibiotics. Sulforaphane, an isothiocyanate abundant as its glucosinolate precursor in certain varieties of broccoli and broccoli sprouts, is a potent bacteriostatic agent against *H. pylori* in mice. There is hope that these mechanisms might function synergistically to provide diet-based protection against gastric cancer in humans.

Data from Fahey JW et al: Sulforaphane inhibits extracellular, intracellular, and antibiotic-resistant strains of *Helicobacter pylori* and prevents benzo[a]pyrene-induced stomach tumors, *Proc Natl Acad Sci U S A* 99:7610, 2002.

salted foods or pickled foods, or inadequate in micronutrients (Li and Mobarhan, 2000; Roth and Mobarhan, 2001). Because symptoms are slow to manifest themselves and the growth of the tumor is rapid, carcinoma of the stomach is frequently overlooked until it is too late for a cure. Loss of appetite, strength, and weight frequently precede other symptoms. In some cases, achylia gastrica (absence of hydrochloric acid and pepsin) or achlorhydria may exist for years before the onset of gastric carcinoma.

Medical Nutrition Therapy

The dietary regimen for carcinoma of the stomach is determined by the location of the cancer, the nature of the functional disturbance, and the stage of the disease. Gastrectomy is one of the possible therapies, and some patients may experience difficulties with nutrition postoperatively (see the section on dumping syndrome that appears later in this chapter). The patient with advanced, inoperable cancer should receive a diet that is adjusted to provide comfort. Anorexia is almost always present from the early stages. Any food preferences, unless definitely harmful, are granted, and the patient should be made as comfortable as possible. In the later stages of the disease, the patient may tolerate only a liquid diet, or it may be necessary to resort to parenteral nutrition. As long as other therapeutic procedures, such as surgery, radiation therapy, or chemotherapy, are being performed, the nutritional support for the patient should be equally aggressive (see Chapter 40 for further discussion of nutritional care during cancer treatment).

Gastric Surgery

Because of more effective medical treatment, gastric surgery and gastrectomy for peptic ulcer disease occur less frequently. Partial or total gastrectomy may still be necessary when peptic ulcer is complicated by hemorrhage, perforation, intractability, cancer, or obstruction, or when the patient is unable to follow the medical regimen.

Vagal denervation decreases cholinergic stimulation of parietal cells and reduces cellular response to stimulants, such as gastrin. A parietal cell vagotomy affects only the area of gastric acid secretion. As the antrum and pylorus remain innervated by the vagus nerve, gastric emptying can proceed normally; however, because the surgery is difficult and time consuming, patients who are at high risk for operative morbidity and mortality are not candidates for this procedure. A truncal vagotomy with pyloroplasty (enlargement of the pyloric sphincter) would probably be used in these circumstances (Figure 29-6).

The truncal vagotomy not only interrupts innervation of the gastric parietal cells, but it also results in antral and pyloric dysfunction and poor peristalsis. Incorporating pyloroplasty or gastrojejunostomy permits adequate gastric emptying; however, the postoperative side effects of dumping, diarrhea, and weight loss still occur at a rate of about 6%. Surgery for gastric ulcer consists of removing the ulcerated area, usually by a partial gastric resection.

Medical Nutrition Therapy After Gastric Surgery

After most types of gastric surgery, oral intake of foods and fluids is suspended until GI tract function returns. Once function is regained, liquids are initiated, after which the patient can progress to solids as tolerated based on volume and consistency. If the surgery requires an extended period for healing, the patient may be fed enterally through a tube, often placed as a jejunostomy. The use of total parenteral nutrition (TPN) is usually reserved for patients with postoperative complications that delay enteral feeding for an extended period (see Chapter 23).

The first type of fluid allowed by mouth is usually water, typically administered in the form of ice, given in small amounts and allowed to melt in the mouth, or as frequent sips of water. Some patients may toler-

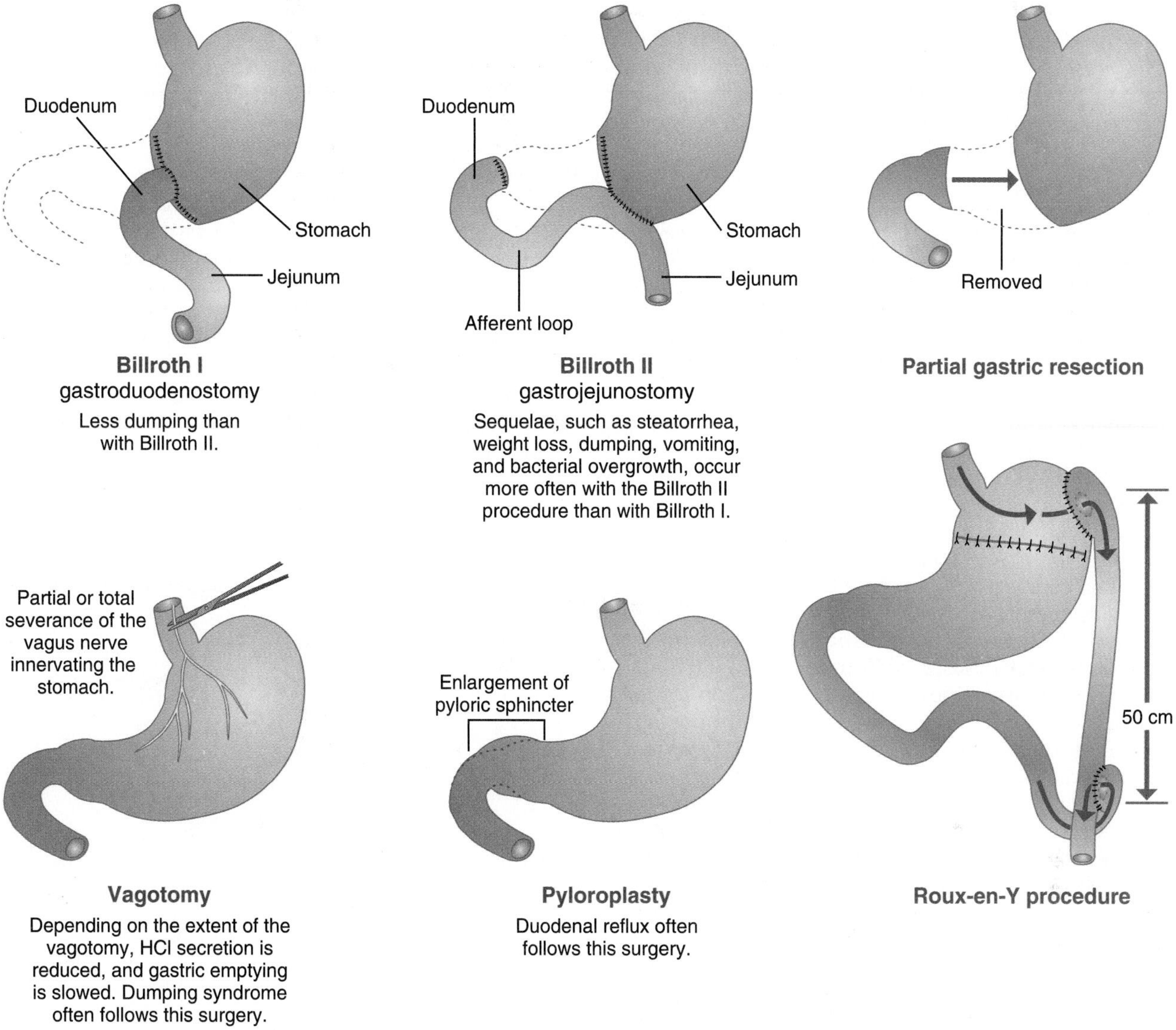
Duodenum
Stomach
Jejunum
Billroth I
gastroduodenostomy
Less dumping than with Billroth II.
Duodenum
Afferent loop
Stomach
Jejunum
Billroth II
gastrojejunostomy
Sequelae, such as steatorrhea, weight loss, dumping, vomiting, and bacterial overgrowth, occur more often with the Billroth II procedure than with Billroth I.
Removed
Partial gastric resection
Partial or total severance of the vagus nerve innervating the stomach.
Vagotomy
Depending on the extent of the vagotomy, HCl secretion is reduced, and gastric emptying is slowed. Dumping syndrome often follows this surgery.
Enlargement of pyloric sphincter
Pyloroplasty
Duodenal reflux often follows this surgery.
50 cm
Roux-en-Y procedure

FIGURE 29-6 • Gastric surgical procedures.

ate water at room temperature or warm water better than iced or cold water. Later, larger amounts and varieties of fluids can be offered, followed by small amounts of soft, starchy, and low-fat protein foods. Highly spiced, fatty, or hypertonic foods may not be well tolerated by the patient. Small, frequent meals or snacks are usually better tolerated than large meals. Many "full liquid" diets (see Table 21-7) are high in sugars and lactose. Low-lactose and more isotonic liquids might be substituted.

Nutritional impairment occurs in some patients after gastrectomy, and some have difficulty regaining normal preoperative weight because of (1) inadequate food intake related to anorexia or to symptoms related to dumping syndrome or (2) malabsorption of ingested food. Patients who have had total or almost total gastrectomy often have difficulty eating large amounts of food and may need to make a permanent habit of eating several small meals daily.

Dumping Syndrome

Pathophysiology

The dumping syndrome is a complex physiologic response to the presence of larger-than-normal amounts of food and liquid in the proximal small intestine. Dumping syndrome usually occurs as a result of a loss of normal regulation of gastric emptying and GI and systemic responses to a meal. Most of the symptoms can be reproduced in normal individuals by infusing a loading dose of glucose into the jejunum (Vecht et al, 1997).

The syndrome may occur as a result of total or subtotal gastrectomy, manipulation of the pylorus, or fundoplication (Bufler et al, 2001). The incidence of dumping ranges from about 5% after minor surgical procedures to as high as 40% after total gastrectomy (Vecht et al, 1997). After surgical procedures in which portions of the stomach remain, the size of the remaining stomach can increase somewhat over a period of several months. Newer surgical procedures that preserve proximal and distal segments of stomach or create small stomachlike reservoirs have helped to reduce dumping symptoms.

Medical Management

The severity of symptoms ranges from mild to relatively debilitating, depending on the nature of the surgery and the individual's dietary practices. Short-term and long-term implications are numerous, but dietary interventions can reduce or eliminate symptoms in most persons. Medications that slow motility may be advised for those whose symptoms persist after changing dietary habits.

Symptoms may occur in several stages; each is related to the "dumping" of foods and beverages into the small intestine, but the mechanisms vary. Not all patients suffer all consequences or to the same degree. In the first stage, patients may experience abdominal fullness and nausea within 10 to 20 minutes of eating a meal. This stage may be attributed to distention of the small bowel from foods and liquids, plus a modest fluid shift from systemic circulation into the small intestine as a result of ingestion of foods that become hypertonic from the action of digestive enzymes. Patients may, at the same time, experience flushing, rapid heartbeat, faintness, sweating, and the need to sit or lie down. This set of systemic symptoms was originally attributed to fluid loss from the vascular space into the mesenteric bed and GI tract. Fluid does shift from systemic circulation into the GI tract but apparently not enough to account for the magnitude of vascular symptoms. It is now thought that patients with these early dumping symptoms are experiencing a decrease in peripheral vascular resistance and, perhaps, splanchnic (visceral) pooling of blood.

In the intermediate stage, which can occur from 20 minutes to more than 1 hour after eating, patients may experience abdominal bloating, increased flatulence, crampy abdominal pain, and diarrhea. The "colonic" symptoms are likely related to the increased malabsorption of carbohydrates and other foodstuffs and the subsequent fermentation of the substrates entering the colon (see Chapter 1).

The late stage, occurring from 1 to 3 hours after a meal, is related to reactive hypoglycemia, sometimes referred to as alimentary hypoglycemia. Patients may perspire; feel anxious, weak, shaky, or hungry; and may have difficulty concentrating (Box 29-3). Rapid delivery, as well as hydrolysis and absorption of carbohydrate, produces an exaggerated rise in insulin level with a subsequent decline in blood glucose level. The rapid changes in blood glucose and the secretion of gut peptides, glucose insulinotropic polypeptide (GIP), and glucagon-like polypeptide-1 (GLP-1) appear to be at least partly responsible for the symptoms.

Complications

Patients who are symptomatic after gastric surgery often lose weight. The weight loss may be attributable to inadequate intake resulting from the fear and anxiety that is often associated with the confusing and often distressing symptoms. Some patients may associate the symptoms with the act of eating rather than attributing them to specific patterns, volumes, or types of foods consumed. Patients sometimes can correctly relate consumption of food types with distress, but they rarely can select appropriate foods based on their experiences with foods or meals.

Following some forms of gastric surgery, malabsorption and steatorrhea may occur in addition to dumping and hypoglycemia. About 10% of these patients have clinically significant steatorrhea secondary to rapid transit, loss of gastric lipase, or pancreatic or biliary insufficiency. Because of disturbances

Box 29-3. Nutritional Care Guidelines for Patients With Dumping Syndrome and Alimentary Hypoglycemia

1. Small meals, spread throughout the day, are likely to result in improved net absorption and less dramatic fluid shifts.
2. High-protein, moderate-fat foods are recommended, with sufficient calories for weight maintenance or gain as needed. Complex carbohydrates are included as tolerated.
3. Intake of fibrous foods slows upper GI transit and increases viscosity. However, to avoid obstruction, caution should be used with large particles and fiber supplements, especially with esophageal or gastric outlet narrowing or dysmotility.
4. Lying down and avoiding activity an hour after eating may help slow gastric emptying.
5. Taking large amounts of liquids with meals is thought to hasten GI transit, but adequate amounts of liquid should be consumed throughout the day, small amounts at a time.
6. Only very small quantities of hypertonic, concentrated sweets should be ingested. These include soft drinks, juices, pies, cakes, cookies, and frozen desserts (unless made with sugar substitutes).
7. Lactose, especially in milk or ice cream, may be poorly tolerated because of rapid transit and so may need to be avoided. Cheeses and yogurt are likely to be better tolerated.

in the timing of entry of food into the small intestine and the release of intestinal hormones and enzymes, efficiency of digestion may be reduced. Patients who were lactose tolerant before gastric surgery may experience relative lactase deficiency, either because food enters the small intestine further downstream or because the rate of transit through the proximal small intestine is increased.

Anemia, osteoporosis, and select vitamin and mineral deficiencies may occur as a result of long-term malabsorption or limited dietary intake. Iron deficiency may be attributable to loss of acid secretion, which normally facilitates the reduction of iron compounds, allowing their absorption; rapid transit; diminished contact with sites of iron absorption; or blood loss. Vitamin B_{12} deficiency may cause a megaloblastic anemia. If the amount of gastric mucosa is reduced, intrinsic factor may not be produced in quantities adequate to allow for complete vitamin B_{12} absorption, and pernicious anemia may result (see Chapter 34). Bacterial overgrowth in the proximal small bowel or in the afferent loop can contribute to vitamin B_{12} depletion because bacteria compete with the host for utilization of the vitamin. After gastrectomy, therefore, patients generally receive prophylactic vitamin B_{12} injections or reservoirs.

Because of the complications of reflux or dumping syndrome associated with traditional gastrectomies, other procedures are used, including truncal, selective, or parietal cell vagotomy, pyloromyotomy, antrectomy, Roux-en-Y esophagojejunostomy, loop esophagojejunostomy, and pouches made from jejunal or ileocecal segments (Okuyama et al, 1997; Tomita et al, 2001; Uras et al, 1997) (see Figure 29-6).

Somatostatin analogs are used to slow gastric emptying in patients with rapid emptying and dumping syndrome. Acarbose, an α-glucoside hydrolase inhibitor that is normally used to manage type 2 diabetes mellitus, has been used in some persons with dumping syndrome (Ng et al, 2001). Acarbose inhibits the digestion and absorption of starch, sucrose, and maltose. Acarbose may blunt the alimentary hyperglycemia or hypoglycemia related to dumping but has the potential to worsen the colonic gas and diarrhea. Table 29-2 lists some of the other common medications used in GI disorders.

Medical Nutrition Therapy

Because of the problems that accompany eating, patients with dumping syndrome frequently do not eat enough, have diarrhea from the increased intestinal activity, and become underweight, malnourished, and frustrated. The prime objective of nutritional care is to restore nutritional status and quality of life.

Proteins and fats are better tolerated than carbohydrates because they are hydrolyzed more slowly into osmotically active substances. Simple carbohydrates, such as lactose, sucrose, and dextrose, are hydrolyzed rapidly; so quantities should be limited, but complex carbohydrates (starches) can be included in the diet. Liquids enter the jejunum rapidly, and so some patients may have problems tolerating liquids with meals. Patients who have severe problems with dumping may fare better if they limit the amount of liquids taken with meals or if they take liquids only between meals, without solid food. Lying down immediately after meals may also decrease the severity of symptoms.

The use of fiber supplements can be beneficial in managing dumping syndrome because they reduce upper GI transit time and decrease the rate of glucose absorption, thus decreasing the insulin response (see Appendix 54). Pectin, the dietary fiber contained in fruits and vegetables, or gums (e.g., guar) may be useful in treating dumping syndrome. Caution must be exercised, however, with the use of bulk fiber sources. Several cases of obstruction have been reported with the use of guar gum and other viscous substances when large amounts have been taken, especially without adequate water.

Basically, a diet that aims to prevent symptoms of dumping syndrome is somewhat higher in fat content (35% to 45% of calories), low in simple carbohydrates, and high in protein (20% of calories). Such a diet will help the patient achieve and maintain optimal weight and nutritional status. The exchange lists given in Appendix 53 can be used to calculate carbohydrate intake and teach the patient about carbohydrate control.

After gastrectomy, patients often do not tolerate lactose and only small amounts (6 g or less per meal) can be eaten at a time. These patients do better with cheeses or unsweetened yogurt than with fluid milk. Vitamin D and calcium supplements may be needed when intake of dairy products is reduced. Commer-

TABLE 29-2 Common Drugs Used in the Treatment of Gastrointestinal Disorders

TYPE OF DRUG	EXAMPLE OF USE/APPLICATION
Antibiotics	Eradicate *Helicobacter pylori*, prevent or treat infection after abdominal wounds or surgery
Antacids	Neutralize gastric acid in acid reflux, peptic ulcer
Proton pump inhibitors (omeprazole, lansoprazole)	Decrease gastric acid secretion
Histamine-2 receptor antagonists (cimetidine, ranitidine)	Inhibit gastric acid secretion
Sucralfate (sulfated disaccharide)	Protects stomach lining and may increase mucosal resistance to acid or enzyme damage

FOCUS ON

Milestones in Dietary Management of Upper GI Disorders

The treatment of peptic ulcer disease has involved attempts to control gastric acid secretion to heal and to prevent recurrence of duodenal ulcers.

Before 1900: Surgeons began performing gastric resections. Early treatment attempted to heal by neutralizing gastric acid with diet modification and the milk and cream-based sippy diet.

1943: Dr. Lester Dragstedt performed the first truncal vagotomy to limit cholinergic stimulation of gastric acid secretion. This led to surgery that combined gastric resections with vagotomy.

1960s: The bland diet with four levels, starting with stage 1 as a sippy diet and progressing to stage 4, a liberal bland diet that omitted only chocolate, peppermint, black pepper and alcoholic beverages, was used to address various levels of healing. Antacids to neutralize acid and anticholinergics to reduce the amount of acid produced were widely used.

1970: The first parietal cell vagotomy was performed to limit vagal initiation of acid secretion while minimizing the impact on other gastrointestinal functions.

1976: Introduction of the first H_2-receptor antagonist, cimetidine. Ranitidine, the second H_2-receptor antagonist, produced greater acid suppression in the morning and at night with twice daily dosing than cimetidine with four doses each day. The bland diet was refined to have just two levels: restricted and liberal.

2000: Eradication of *H. pylori* via use of antibiotics, antacids, H_2-receptor antagonists, and proton pump inhibitors. Diet alterations are minimal and specific to the patient.

Modified from Warner CW, McIsaac RL: The evolution of peptic ulcer therapy: a role for temporal control of drug delivery, *Ann NY Acad Sci* 618:504, 1991.

cial lactase products are available for those with significant lactose malabsorption (see Chapter 30).

When steatorrhea is a problem, formulas whose fat content is derived primarily from medium-chain triglycerides may be better tolerated. Supplemental formulas are described in Appendixes 36 to 41. Box 29-3 provides general nutrition guidelines for patients with dumping syndrome after gastric surgery; however, each diet must be adjusted based on a careful dietary and social history from the patient.

SUMMARY

Treatment for disorders of the upper GI tract has changed drastically in the last century. For many years, patients were given "sippy diets" with high amounts of milk and cream because it was thought that this would coat the stomach lining and reduce pain. It was later discovered, however, that this diet was ineffective. The bland diet historically involved up to four stages of management, starting with stage 1 as the sippy diet and progressing to stage 4, a liberal bland diet that omitted only chocolate, peppermint, black pepper, and alcoholic beverages. Progress in the medical management of these disorders has mostly eliminated the need for this strict level of medical nutrition therapy (see *Focus on:* Milestones in Dietary Management of Upper GI Disorders).

Today, fortunately, nutritional care for patients with upper GI disorders is more specific, individualized, and far more effective than in the past because of increased knowledge of neuroendocrine mechanisms, pathogens, and environmental agents. The nutritional professional has far more tools and dietary manipulations available that can enhance surgery and overall treatment.

Clinical Scenario 1

Jim is a 45-year-old white man, an executive who travels extensively in his work. He is 6 ft tall and weighs 186 lb. He recently visited his doctor complaining about upper GI distress. He reports frequent bouts of heartburn in the middle of the night, and he has lost 15 lb over the last year without intentionally dieting. Jim also occasionally experiences heartburn soon after consumption of specific meals and foods. Jim's doctor diagnosed esophageal reflux, and x-ray studies revealed a hiatal hernia.

Jim has received a good deal of advice regarding specific foods and diets from a variety of sources, but he is confused about what he should eat. Jim is coming to you to discuss nutritional therapies.

1. What is heartburn? Does hiatal hernia have anything to do with it?
2. Why might Jim experience heartburn in the middle of the night?
3. Why might Jim experience burning after consumption of certain foods or meals?
4. Why do you suppose Jim lost weight?
5. Do you recommend that he regain the weight?
6. What recommendations would you give for reducing or preventing Jim's symptoms?

Relevant Web Sites

American Gastrointestinal Association
www.gastro.org/
GERD Information Center
www.gerd.com/

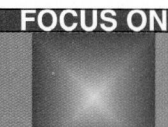

Clinical Scenario 2

Mr. Smith had his stomach removed as a result of gastric cancer and is having difficulty with bloating, nausea, and light-headedness soon after meals. Later, after the meal, he often experiences lower abdominal cramping and diarrhea.

1. What do you think could be responsible for the different symptoms Mr. Smith is experiencing?
2. Are there dietary measures that would prevent the postprandial discomfort?
3. Are there any medications that could help his situation?
4. Are there any surgical procedures that could reduce the likelihood that these symptoms do not occur after gastrectomy?

Cited References

Abdel-Salam OM et al: Studies on the effect of intragastric capsaicin on gastric ulcer and on the prostacyclin-induced effect, *Pharmacol Res* 32:209, 1995.

Aldoori WH et al: Prospective study of diet and the risk of duodenal ulcer in men, *Am J Epidemiol* 145:42, 1997.

Al-Shabanah OA: Effect of evening primrose oil on gastric ulceration and secretion induced by various ulcerogenic and necrotizing agents in rats, *Food Chem Toxicol* 35:769, 1997.

Baik HW, Russel RM: Vitamin B_{12} deficiency in the elderly, *Annu Rev Nutr* 19:357, 1999.

Beyer PL: Gastrointestinal disorders: roles of nutrition and the dietetics practitioner, *J Am Diet Assoc* 98:272, 1998.

Bufler P et al: Dumping syndrome: a common problem following Nissen fundoplication in young children, *Pediatr Surg Int* 17:351, 2001.

Bujanda L: The effects of alcohol consumption upon the gastrointestinal tract, *Am J Gastroenterol* 95:3374, 2000.

Cifuentes-Tebar J et al: Gastric surgery and bezoars, *Dig Dis Sci* 37:1694, 1992.

Cook DJ et al: Stress ulcer prophylaxis in critically ill patients: resolving discordant meta-analyses, *JAMA* 275:308, 1996.

DeMeester SR, DeMeester TR: The diagnosis and management of Barrett's esophagus, *Adv Surg* 33:29, 1999.

Dial EJ et al: Gastroprotection by dairy foods against stress-induced ulcerogenesis in rats, *Dig Dis Sci* 40:2295, 1995.

Dunn BE et al: *Helicobacter pylori, Clin Microbiol Rev* 10:720, 1997.

Escamilla C et al: Intestinal obstruction and bezoars, *J Am Coll Surg* 179:285, 1994.

Flick AL: Acid content of common beverages, *Am J Dig Dis* 15:317, 1970.

Frank L et al: Upper gastrointestinal symptoms in North America, *Dig Dis Sci* 45:809, 2000.

Friedman LS, Peterson WL: Peptic ulcer and related disorders. In Fauci AS et al, editors: *Harrison's principles of internal medicine,* ed 14, New York, 1998, McGraw-Hill.

Gomollon F, Sicilia B: Helicobacter pylori: strategies for treatment, *Expert Opin Investig Drugs* 10:1231, 2001.

Goyal RK: Diseases of the esophagus. In Fauci AS et al, editors: *Harrison's principles of internal medicine,* ed 14, New York, 1998, McGraw-Hill.

Gustafsson H et al: Peptic ulcer pathophysiology: acid, bicarbonate, and mucosal function, *Scand J Gastroenterol* 216(suppl):10, 1996.

Hojgaard et al: Peptic ulcer pathophysiology: acid, bicarbonate, and mucosal function, *Scand J Gastroenterol* 216(suppl):10, 1996.

Hung CR, Neu SL: Acid-induced gastric damage in rats is aggravated by starvation and prevented by several nutrients, *J Nutr* 127:630, 1997.

Jensen-Jarolim E et al: Hot spices influence permeability of the human intestinal epithelial monolayers, *J Nutr* 128:577, 1998.

Kabat GC, Ng SK, Wynder EL: Tobacco, alcohol intake and diet in relation to adenocarcinoma of the esophagus and gastric cardia, *Cancer Causes Control* 4:123, 1993.

Kahrilas PJ: The role of hiatus hernia in GERD, *Yale J Biol Med* 72:101, 1999.

Katzka DA, Rustgi AK: Gastroesophageal reflux disease and Barrett's esophagus, *Med Clin North Am* 84:1137, 2000.

Kjellin A et al: Gastroesophageal reflux in obese patients is not reduced by weight reduction, *Scand J Gastroenterol* 31:1047, 1996.

Kozak LJ, Owings MF: Ambulatory and inpatient procedures in the United States, 1995, National Center for Health Statistics, *Vital Health Stat* 13(135), 1998.

Laine L, Fendrick AM: *Helicobacter pylori* and peptic ulcer disease, *Postgrad Med* 103:231, 1998.

Lanas A, Santolaria S: Gastroesophageal reflux disease (GERD) current agents and future prospective, *Curr Pharm Des* 7:1, 2001.

Lasky MR et al: A prospective study of omeprazole suspension to prevent clinically significant gastrointestinal bleeding from stress ulcers in mechanically ventilated trauma patients, *J Trauma* 44:527, 1998.

Lee A: The *Helicobacter pylori* genome—new insights into pathogenesis and therapeutics, *N Engl J Med* 338:832, 1998.

Li SD, Mobarhan S: Association between body mass index and adenocarcinoma of the esophagus and gastric cardia, *Nutr Rev* 58:54, 2000.

McQuaid K: Dyspepsia. In Feldman M, Scharschmidt BF, Sleisenger MH, editors: *Gastrointestinal and liver disease,* ed 6, Philadelphia, 1998, WB Saunders.

Manjari V, Das UN: Effect of polyunsaturated fatty acids on dexamethasone-induced mucosal damage, *Prostaglandins Leukot Essent Fatty Acids* 62:85, 2000.

Marotta RB, Floch MH: Diet and nutrition in ulcer disease, *Med Clin North Am* 75:4, 1991.

Miehlke S, Bayerdorffer E, Graham DY: Treatment of *Helicobacter pylori* infections, *Semin Gastrointest Dis* 12:167, 2001.

Mishkin D et al: Fructose and sorbitol malabsorption in ambulatory patients with functional dyspepsia: comparison with lactose maldigestion/malabsorption, *Digest Dis Sci* 42:2591, 1997.

Mitchell BE, Sobel HL, Alexander MH: The adverse effects of tobacco and tobacco-related products, *Prim Care* 26:463, 1999.

Mittal RK, Balaban DH: The esophagogastric junction, *N Engl J Med* 336:924, 1997.

Myers BM et al: Effect of red pepper and black pepper on the stomach, *Am J Gastroenterol* 82:211, 1987.

Ng DD et al: Acarbose treatment of postprandial hypoglycemia in children after Nissen fundoplication, *J Pediatr* 139:877, 2001.

Niinimake A et al: Spice allergy: results of skin prick tests and RAST with spice extracts, *Allergy* 44:60, 1989.

Okuyama H et al: A comparison of the efficacy of pyloromyotomy and pyloroplasty in patients with gastroesophageal reflux and delayed gastric emptying, *J Pediatr Surg* 32:316, 1997.

Olafsson SO et al: Dietery cod liver oil decreases arachidonic acid in rat gastric mucosa and increases stress-induced gastric erosions, *Lipids* 35:601, 2000.

Robinson M: Dyspepsia: challenges in diagnosis and selection of treatment, *Clin Ther* 23:1130, 2001.

Rodriguez S et al: Meal type affects heartburn severity, *Dig Dis Sci* 43:485, 1998.

Roth J, Mobarhan S: Preventive role of dietary fiber in gastric cardia cancers, *Nutr Rev* 59:372, 2001.

Schappert SM: Ambulatory care visits to physician offices, hospital outpatient departments, and emergency departments: United States, 1996, National Center for Health Statistics, *Vital Health Stat* 13(134):1, 1998.

Scott M, Gelhot AR: Gastroesophageal reflux disease: diagnosis and management, *Am Fam Physician* 59:1161, 1999.

Shimizu T et al: Effects of n-3 fatty acids and vitamin E on colonic mucosal leukotriene generation, lipid peroxidation, and microcirculation in rats with experimental colitis, *Digestion* 63:49, 2001.

Sipponen P, Marshall BJ: Gastritis and gastric cancer: western countries, *Gastroenterol Clin North Am,* 29:579, 2002.

Soll H: Peptic ulcer and its complications. In Feldman M, Scharschmidt BF, Sleisenger MH, editors: *Gastrointestinal and liver disease,* ed 6, Philadelphia, 1998, WB Saunders.

Talley NJ et al: AGA technical review: evaluation of dyspepsia, *Gastroenterology* 114:582, 1998.

Tomita R et al: Operative technique on nearly total gastrectomy reconstructed by interposition of a jejunal J pouch with preservation of vagal nerve, lower esophageal sphincter, and pyloric sphincter for early gastric cancer, *World J Surg* 25:1524, 2001.

Uras C et al: Restorative caecogastroplasty reconstruction after pylorus-preserving near-total gastrectomy: a preliminary study, *Br J Surg* 84:406, 1997.

Vasudevan K et al: Influence of intragastric perfusions of aqueous spice extracts on acid secretion in anesthetized albino rats, *Indian J Gastroenterol* 19:53, 2000.

Vecht J et al: The dumping syndrome: current insights into pathophysiology, diagnosis and treatment, *Scand J Gastroenterol* 32(suppl 223):21, 1997.

Warner CW, McIsaac RL: The evolution of peptic ulcer therapy: a role for temporal control of drug delivery, *Ann N Y Acad Sci* 618:504, 1991.

Webb D: New therapeutic options in the treatment of GERD and other acid-peptic disorders, *Am J Manag Care* 6:S467, 2000.

Additional References

Peek RM, Blaser MJ: Pathophysiology of *Helicobacter pylori*–induced gastritis and peptic ulcer disease, *Am J Med* 102:200, 1997.

Perdikis G et al: Laparoscopic Nissen fundoplication: where do we stand? *Surg Laparosc Endosc* 7(1):17, 1997.

Pounder RE: New developments in *Helicobacter pylori* eradication therapy, *Scand J Gastroenterol* 223(suppl):43, 1997.

Spechler SJ: Barrett's esophagus, *N Engl J Med* 346:836, 2002.

Tomb J et al: The complete genome sequence of the gastric pathogen *Helicobacter pylori, Nature* 388:539, 1997.

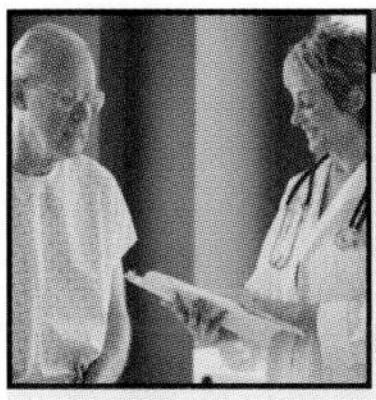

CHAPTER 30

Medical Nutrition Therapy for Lower Gastrointestinal Tract Disorders

PETER L. BEYER, MS, RD, LD

CHAPTER OUTLINE

- Common Intestinal Problems
- Diseases of the Small Intestine
- Intestinal Brush-Border Enzyme Deficiencies
- Inflammatory Bowel Diseases
- Disorders of the Large Intestine
- Intestinal Surgery

KEY TERMS

aerophagia–swallowing of air

blind loop syndrome–a disorder of bacterial overgrowth with resultant malabsorption secondary to alterations in the anatomy of the small intestine involving a loop that is disconnected from the main intestinal tract

borborygmus–intestinal rumbling

celiac disease–common term for gluten-sensitive enteropathy

colostomy–surgical creation of an opening into the colon through a stoma in the abdominal wall to permit defecation

constipation–a condition in which the frequency or quantity of stools is reduced

Crohn's disease–a chronic, granulomatous inflammatory disease of unknown etiology involving the small or large intestine that results in diarrhea, strictures, fistulas, malabsorption, and the need for surgical resection

dermatitis herpetiformis–a skin disorder that is a variant of celiac disease

diarrhea–abnormal volume and liquidity of stools

diverticulitis–inflammation of diverticula

diverticulosis–presence of herniations of the mucous membrane through the muscular layers of the colonic wall

fistula–an abnormal passage between two internal organs, or from an internal organ to the surface of the body

flatulence–excessive collection and passage of gas from the gastrointestinal tract

flatus–gas in the gastrointestinal tract that is expelled through the anus

glutamine–an amino acid and the preferred fuel of the enterocyte

gluten-sensitive enteropathy (celiac disease)–a syndrome precipitated by the immunologic interaction of gluten-containing foods and intestinal cells; characterized by flattening of the villi of the small intestine

high-fiber diet–a diet containing more than 25 g of dietary fiber

hypolactasia–a decrease in the amount of the intestinal enzyme lactase

ileostomy–surgical creation of an opening into the ileum through a stoma in the abdominal wall

ileal pouch–surgical creation of a small reservoir, using folds of the distal ileum, which is then attached to the rectum

inflammatory bowel disease (IBD)–a general term for inflammatory diseases of the bowel of unknown etiology, including Crohn's disease and ulcerative colitis

irritable bowel syndrome (IBS)–an abnormal stooling pattern associated with symptoms of intestinal dysfunction that persists for more than 3 months of the year

KEY TERMS—Continued

lactose intolerance–an inability to digest lactose to galactose and glucose because of a deficiency of the enzyme lactase

medium-chain triglycerides (MCTs)–triacylglycerols with fatty acids of 8 and 10 carbons in length—short enough to be absorbed directly into the portal blood

minimal-residue diet–a diet that results in decreased fecal volume

phytobezoars–stomach obstructions composed of partially digested plant foods

prebiotic–dietary substrates used to promote the growth of beneficial intestinal bacteria

probiotic–orally consumed source of bacteria used to reestablish the presence of beneficial intestinal flora

refractory sprue–celiac disease that persists even after adherence to a strict gluten-free diet

residue–the fecal contents, including bacteria and any remaining gastrointestinal secretions and foods not digested or absorbed

short-bowel syndrome (SBS)–a malabsorption syndrome resulting from major resections of the small bowel; characterized by diarrhea, steatorrhea, and malnutrition

steatorrhea–excessive amounts of fat in the feces, as seen in malabsorption syndromes

tropical sprue–a syndrome of unknown etiology that causes diarrhea and malabsorption but is not responsive to gluten-free diet therapy

ulcerative colitis–an inflammatory disease of the colonic mucosa

Dietary modifications in disorders of the intestinal tract are designed to alleviate symptoms, correct nutrient deficiencies, and, when possible, address the primary cause of difficulty. In disease, assessment of the nature and severity of the primary gastrointestinal problem precedes targeted medical, nutrition, and other forms of therapy. Increased intakes of energy, protein, vitamins, minerals, and electrolytes are frequently required to replace nutrients lost as a result of impaired digestive and absorptive capacity. Consistency, meal frequency, and other characteristics of the diet may be altered to fit the patient's needs. Medical nutrition therapy (MNT) for all patients with diseases of the intestines must be individualized. For this reason, the principles presented in the chapter are general guidelines.

COMMON INTESTINAL PROBLEMS

Intestinal Gas and Flatulence

Pathophysiology

Intestinal gases include nitrogen (N_2), oxygen (O_2), carbon dioxide (CO_2), hydrogen (H_2), and, in some persons, methane (CH_4). About 200 ml of gas is normally present in the gastrointestinal (GI) tract, and humans excrete an average of 700 ml each day. However, the difference in the amount of intestinal gas among individuals and from day to day varies greatly (Strocchi and Levitt, 1998). Considerable amounts of gas may be swallowed or produced within the GI tract and may be absorbed across the alimentary tract into the bloodstream and expired through the lungs, expelled through eructation (belching), or passed rectally.

When patients complain about "excessive gas," they may be referring to increased volume or frequency of passage of gas (flatulence). They may also be complaining about abdominal distention or cramping pain associated with the accumulation of gases in the upper or lower GI tract. The association between the amount of gas in the GI tract perceived by an individual and the amount actually measured is not always accurate (Levitt et al, 1996). Inactivity, decreased GI motility, aerophagia, dietary components, and GI disorders can all contribute to the amount of intestinal gas and an individual's gas-related symptoms.

Gas in the upper intestinal tract results primarily from swallowing air (aerophagia) and, to a lesser extent, from chemical reactions that occur during the digestion of foods. Normally, only small amounts of swallowed air or gases dissolved in foods make their way as far as the colon. High N_2 and O_2 concentrations in rectal gas, both of which are substances that are present in the atmosphere in high concentrations, may indicate aerophagia. Aerophagia can be avoided to some degree by eating slowly, chewing with the mouth closed, and refraining from drinking through straws.

Increased gas production may occur in the stomach and small intestine because of bacterial fermentation, particularly with the consumption of carbohydrate, and can result in abdominal discomfort and distention. Bacterial overgrowth may occur in the stomach or small intestine with partial obstruction, with dysmotility, in immune disorders, or after some GI surgical procedures.

Increased amounts of H_2 and CO_2—and sometimes, CH_4—in rectal gas with lowered fecal pH indicate excessive colonic bacterial fermentation and suggest malabsorption of a fermentable substrate. The amounts and types of gases produced may depend on the mix of microorganisms in the individual's colon. Consumption of large amounts of dietary fiber (especially soluble fiber), resistant starches, lactose in persons who are lactase deficient, or modest amounts of fructose or alcohol sugars (such as sorbitol) may result in increased gas production in the colon and increased flatulence.

Consumption of fructose in the United States, especially from fruit juices and fruit drinks and high-fructose corn syrup in soft drinks and confections, has increased significantly in recent years. The average level of fructose in the daily diet is in the range of 35 to 40 g, which is sufficient in many children and adults to result in malabsorption of fructose and evoke symptoms. Sucrose is normally well tolerated but in large quantities may also result in increased amounts of fecal substrate.

Medical Nutrition Therapy

In the assessment of the patient, one must ask whether the problem is increased production of gas or whether the patient has difficulty with cramping and distention because the gas is not being passed. Inactivity, dysmotility, or partial obstruction may be contributing to the inability to move normal amounts of gas produced. Movement or exercise may help expel gases through eructation or rectal passage.

The primary emphasis in dietary management is the reduction of carbohydrate foods that are likely to be malabsorbed and fermented, including legumes, soluble fiber, resistant starches, and simple sugars such as fructose and alcohol sugars. When undigested carbohydrates pass into the colon, they are fermented to varying degrees to short-chain fatty acids and gases. The primary gases include H_2, CO_2, and, in about one third of individuals, CH_4. The widely recognized propensity of legumes to produce **flatus** (gas) is related to the presence of not only ample amounts of fiber but also stachyose and raffinose—carbohydrates that are only partially digested in the small intestine.

Excess production of gas may also be related to the dose of carbohydrate consumed. Starches such as breads, baked goods, and starchy vegetables may be almost completely digested in normal portions but when consumed in large quantities may leave a considerable fraction of undigested or unabsorbed **residue** for bacterial action in the colon. The properties of some so-called gas-forming foods may be explained simply by the type and amount of sugar, starch, or fiber they contain.

Constipation

Pathophysiology

Constipation is one of the most common intestinal maladies in Western societies, and it occurs in 5% to more than 25% of the population, depending on the definition of the disorder (Candelli et al, 2001). Definitions of constipation tend to be highly subjective but usually include hard stools, straining with defecation, and infrequent bowel movements. At least in older patients, hard stools, incomplete evacuation, and difficulty passing stools may be more troublesome than the infrequency of bowel movements.

Normal stool weight is about 100 to 200 g daily, and normal frequency may range from one stool every 3 days to three times per day. Normal transit time through the GI tract ranges from about 18 to about 48 hours. Persons who consume a diet that contains the recommended amounts of dietary fiber in the form of fruits, vegetables, and whole-grain breads and cereals tend to have larger, softer stools that are relatively easy to pass. Some people who believe that it is necessary to have frequent bowel movements and who ignore dietary and other health recommendations may become disturbed when this does not occur and try to compensate with the use of medications and enemas.

The most common causes of constipation in otherwise healthy persons include repeated lack of response to the urge to defecate, lack of fiber in the diet, insufficient fluid intake, inactivity, and chronic use of laxatives. Nervous strain or anxiety may aggravate the condition. Chronic constipation may also result from a variety of causes, as outlined in Box 30-1.

Box 30-1. Causes of Constipation

Systemic/Neurogenic/Metabolic

- Side effect of medication
- Metabolic and endocrine abnormalities, such as hypothyroidism, uremia, and hypercalcemia
- Lack of exercise
- Ignoring the urge to defecate
- Vascular disease of the large bowel
- Systemic neuromuscular disease leading to deficiency of voluntary muscles
- Poor diet, low in fiber
- Pregnancy

Gastrointestinal

- Cancer
- Diseases of the upper gastrointestinal tract
- Diseases of the large bowel resulting in:
  - Failure of propulsion along the colon (colonic inertia)
  - Failure of passage through anorectal structures (outlet obstruction)
- Irritable bowel syndrome
- Anal fissure or hemorrhoid
- Laxative abuse

Data from Siddiqui MA, Castell DO: Gastrointestinal disorders in the elderly, *Comp Ther* 23:349, 1997; DeLillo AR and Rose S: Functional bowel disorders in the geriatric patient: constipation, fecal impaction and fecal incontinence, *Am J Coll Gastroenterol* 95:901, 2000.

Medical Treatment for Adults

The first approach to treatment of constipation is to ensure adequate dietary fiber, fluid, and exercise and heed the urge to defecate. Patients dependent on laxatives are usually encouraged to use milder products and reduce the dose until withdrawal is complete. When constipation is not amenable to conservative treatment, that is, the patient is unable to consume an adequate amount of fibrous foods or exercise, substances that promote regular evacuation of soft stools may be prescribed. Bulking agents, such as cellulose, hemicellulose derivatives, psyllium seed, flaxseed, and ispaghula, and osmotic agents, such as lactose, magnesium hydroxide, and sorbitol, can be used. Stool softeners such as Colace may also be used. Impactions of stool may require additional evaluation, more stringent oral medications, rapid consumption of large volumes of fluids, enemas, or digital evacuation (Candelli et al, 2001). In more extreme cases, such as toxic megacolon, surgery may be advised.

Medical Treatment for Infants and Children

About 3% to 5% of all pediatric outpatient visits are related to chronic constipation. In the most severe cases, there is a flaccid colon that is insensitive to distention and encopresis develops. After initial treatment with laxatives and lubricants, fiber intake is the next focus of care. A careful history and physical examination, followed by parent and child education, behavioral intervention, and appropriate use of laxatives, often leads to dramatic improvement (Loening-Baucke, 2002) (see Chapter 10).

Medical Nutrition Therapy

Primary nutrition therapy for constipation is adequate consumption of both soluble and insoluble dietary fiber. Fiber increases colonic fecal fluid, microbial mass, stool weight and frequency and the rate of colonic transit. Fiber also softens stools and makes them easier to pass. Most adults and children in the United States chronically consume only about half the amount of fiber recommended (Institute of Medicine, 2002). These recommendations need to be written out the first time.

The recommended amount of dietary fiber is about 14 g per 1000 kcal. For adult women the diet should contain 25 g of fiber daily, and for men about 38 g (Institute of Medicine, 2002). Fiber is best provided in the form of whole grains, fruits, vegetables, legumes, seeds, and nuts (Marlett et al, 2002). These foods are high in nutrients and healthful phytochemicals and may serve as prebiotics to maintain the desired colonic microflora. Brans and powdered fiber supplements may be helpful in persons who cannot or will not eat sufficient amounts of fibrous foods. When changes in diet and activity patterns do not improve constipation, further evaluation is warranted.

High-Fiber Diet

Dietary fiber refers primarily to edible plant materials not digested by the enzymes in the upper digestive tract of humans. It generally consists of cellulose, hemicelluloses, pectins, gums, and lignin. Newer definitions may include starchy materials and oligosaccharides that are at least partially resistant to digestive enzymes. Some forms of fiber and resistant starches may also be termed *prebiotics.* The term *roughage* tends to refer to vegetable matter, but it is not a quantitative term. *Residue* is not the same as fiber, and this term refers to the end result of digestive, secretory, absorptive, and fermentative processes. Thus, increasing dietary fiber may result in increased fecal output, but increasing dietary lactose (a fiber-free food) in a person who is a lactose malabsorber would also increase fecal weight (residue).

The high-fiber diet in Box 30-2 provides more than 25 g of dietary fiber, depending on the foods selected. A high-fiber therapeutic diet may exceed 25 to 38 g, but amounts greater than 50 g per day are not likely to be necessary and may increase abdominal distention and excessive flatulence in some persons. Appendix 42 provides a list of the fiber content of foods.

Ideally, fiber in the diet should be ingested in the form of foods such as fruits, vegetables, whole-grain breads and cereals, legumes, nuts, and seeds. These foods are not only rich in fiber but are excellent sources of vitamins, minerals, trace elements, antioxidants, and numerous protective phytochemicals. Fibrous powders or bran concentrates may be necessary to obtain the desired fiber level in some persons. Several of these concentrates available on the market are palatable and can be added to cereals, yogurts, fruit sauces, juices, or soups. The use of foods as the

Box 30-2. Guidelines for High-Fiber Diets*

1. Increase consumption of whole-grain breads, cereals, flours, and other whole-grain products (6-11 servings daily).
2. Increase consumption of vegetables, legumes, and fruits, nuts, and edible seeds (5-8 servings daily).
3. Consume high-fiber cereals, granolas, and legumes as needed to bring fiber intake to 25 g or more daily.
4. Increase consumption of fluids to at least 2 L (or about 2 qt) daily.

*May increase stool weight, fecal water, and/or gas. The amount that causes clinical symptoms varies among individuals. The age of the individual, the presence of gastrointestinal (GI) disease or malnutrition, any resection of the GI tract, and recent use of the GI tract all impact tolerance.

fiber source results in benefits from both the fiber content and the nutrients and protective phytochemicals included in the foods.

Cooking does not destroy fiber, although the structure may change. Consumption of eight 8-oz glasses (2 L) of fluids daily is recommended to facilitate the effectiveness of a high-fiber intake. Gastric obstruction and fecal impaction may occur when boluses of fibrous gels or bran are not consumed with sufficient fluid to disperse the fiber. Appropriate cautions are also warranted for persons with GI strictures or dysmotility syndromes. In these situations, the fiber content of the diet should be increased slowly, taking almost a month to reach intakes of 25 to 38 g of fiber per day (Institute of Medicine, 2002).

On initiation of a high-fiber diet, unpleasant side effects may occur, such as increased flatulence, borborygmus, cramps, or diarrhea. A gradual increase in fiber intake helps alleviate these symptoms. If fiber supplements are used, doses should be interspersed with meals, preferably in two or more small doses per day, and fluid intake may need to be increased at the same time. GI disturbances associated with initial fiber ingestion usually decrease within 4 to 5 days, but some increase in flatulence is normal with a high-fiber intake. The high-fiber diet is most effective when consumed continuously for several months.

Diarrhea

Pathophysiology

Diarrhea is characterized by the frequent evacuation of liquid stools, usually exceeding 300 ml, accompanied by an excessive loss of fluid and electrolytes, especially sodium and potassium. It occurs when there is excessively rapid transit of intestinal contents through the small intestine, decreased enzymatic digestion of foodstuffs, decreased absorption of fluids and nutrients, or increased secretion of fluids into the GI tract (Branski et al, 1996; Fine, 1998). Causes may be related to inflammatory disease; infections with fungal, bacterial, or viral agents; medications; the overconsumption of sugars; an insufficient or damaged mucosal absorptive surface; or malnutrition.

Osmotic diarrheas occur when osmotically active solutes are present in the intestinal tract and are poorly absorbed. Examples include the diarrhea that accompanies dumping syndrome and following lactose ingestion in the person with a lactase deficiency.

Secretory diarrheas are the result of active secretion of electrolytes and water by the intestinal epithelium. Bacterial exotoxins, viruses, and increased intestinal hormone secretion cause acute secretory diarrheas. Unlike osmotic diarrhea, fasting does not relieve secretory diarrhea.

Exudative diarrheas are always associated with mucosal damage, which leads to an outpouring of mucus, fluid, blood, and plasma proteins, with a net accumulation of electrolytes and water in the gut. Prostaglandin and cytokine release may be involved. The diarrheas associated with Crohn's disease, ulcerative colitis, and radiation enteritis are exudative.

Medications, especially antibiotics, can contribute to diarrhea in several ways. Antibiotics can reduce the usual "salvage" by colonic bacteria of the small amounts of foodstuffs that escape digestion and absorption. Broad-spectrum antibiotics can greatly reduce the numbers of colonic bacteria that normally convert osmotically active molecules (carbohydrate and amino acids) to gases and short-chain fatty acids (SCFAs). The SCFAs are normally absorbed from the lumen of the colon as long as the amount produced is close to normal. Absorption of the SCFAs also aids absorption of electrolytes and water from the colon (Cunha, 1998). Eradication of the bacteria from the colon results in accumulation of osmotically active molecules and reduced absorption of electrolytes and water.

If more substrates than usual are malabsorbed, as often occurs in acutely ill patients, the resulting rise in osmolality can cause considerable fluid loss. Antibiotics can also have direct effects on GI function (Bartlett, 2002; Kyne et al, 2001) (see Chapter 19). Erythromycin, for example, increases GI motility. Erythromycin, clarithromycin, and clindamycin may all increase GI secretions. Finally, some antibiotics allow opportunistic proliferation of pathogenic organisms normally suppressed by competitive organisms in the GI tract. The organisms or the toxins produced decrease absorption and increase secretion of fluid and electrolytes. *Clostridium difficile* is most commonly associated with antibiotic-related diarrhea and accounts for 10% to 25% of cases, but *Clostridium perfringens, Salmonella, Shigella, Campylobacter, Yersinia enterocolitica,* and *Escherichia coli* organisms have also been implicated in antibiotic-associated diarrhea (Bartlett, 2002; Job and Jacobs, 1997; Kyne et al, 2001). Clindamycin, penicillins, and cephalosporins are associated most often with the development of *C. difficile* infection, and its occurrence depends on the number of antibiotics used, the duration of exposure to antibiotics, and the patient's overall health.

With human immunodeficiency virus (HIV) and other immune deficiency states, several factors may contribute to the diarrhea, including the toxic effects of medications, proliferation of opportunistic organisms, and the GI manifestations of the disease itself (Fine, 1998; Mitra et al, 2001). Increased risk of opportunistic infection is also associated with use of antineoplastic agents (Fine, 1998; Kornblau et al, 2000) and with severe malnutrition. Antacids (especially magnesium salts), histamine H_2-receptor blockers, and proton pump inhibitors have also been implicated in cases of diarrhea.

Diarrhea caused by limited functional mucosa results from conditions of inadequate absorptive area or rapid transit of chyme, such as might occur in Crohn's disease or after extensive bowel resection. This type of diarrhea is often complicated by malabsorption of lipid (steatorrhea) and other macronutrients and micronutrients.

TABLE 30-1 Foods to Limit in a Low- or Minimal-Residue Diet

FOOD	COMMENTS
Lactose (in lactose malabsorbers)	6-12 g normally tolerated in healthy, lactase-deficient individuals
Fiber (excess; >20 g)	Modest amounts (10-15 g) may help maintain normal consistency of GI contents and normal colonic mucosa in healthy states and in GI disease
Resistant starch (especially raffinose and stachyose found in legumes)	
Sorbitol, mannitol, and xylitol (excess; >10 g/day)	
Fructose (excess; 20-25 g/meal)	
Sucrose (excess; >25-50 g/meal)	Well tolerated in moderate amounts; large amounts may cause hyperosmolar diarrhea or decreased fecal pH with fermentation to short-chain fatty acids
Caffeine	Increases GI secretions, colonic motility
Alcoholic beverages (especially wine and beer)	Increase GI secretions

Data from Rummessen JJ, Gudmand-Hoyer E: Functional bowel disease: malabsorption and abdominal distress after ingestion of fructose, sorbitol, and fructose-sorbitol mixtures, *Gastroenterology* 95:694, 1998; Gudmand-Hoyer E: The clinical significance of disaccharide maldigestion, *Am J Clin Nutr* 59:(suppl):735, 1994; Piche T et al: Colonic fermentation influences lower esophageal sphincter function in gastroesophageal reflux disease, *Gastroenterology* 124:894, 2003; and Rao SS et al: Is coffee a colonic stimulant? *Eur J Gastroenterol Hepatol* 10:113, 1998.

Medical Treatment

Because diarrhea is a symptom of a disease state, the first step in medical treatment is to identify and treat the underlying problem. The next priority is to manage fluid and electrolyte replacement. Losses of electrolytes, especially potassium and sodium, should be corrected early by using oral glucose electrolyte solutions with added potassium. With intractable diarrhea, especially in an infant or young child, parenteral feeding may be required. Parenteral nutrition may even be necessary if exploratory surgery is anticipated or if the patient is not expected to resume full oral intake within 5 to 7 days (see Chapter 23).

Medical Nutrition Therapy for Adults

Nutrition therapy for adults with diarrhea includes replacing lost fluids and electrolytes by adding broths and electrolyte solutions. In most cases of diarrhea, a minimum-residue diet (Table 30-1) may be started as the acute episode resolves. Modest amounts of fat may be used if digestive mechanisms for lipid are intact. Sugar alcohols, lactose, fructose, and large amounts of sucrose may worsen osmotic diarrheas and might need to be limited. Because the activity of the disaccharidases and transport mechanisms may be decreased during inflammatory and infectious intestinal disease, sugars may need to be limited (Rumessen and Gudmand-Hoyer, 1998).

Use of modest amounts of foods or dietary supplements containing prebiotic components, such as pectin, fructose, oligosaccharides, inulin, oats, banana flakes, and chicory, may help to control or treat diarrhea. They favor the maintenance of so-called friendly lactobacillus and bifidus microbes and may prevent the overgrowth of potentially pathogenic organisms (Gibson, 1999; Van Loo et al, 1999). SCFAs in physiologic quantities serve as substrate for colonocytes, facilitate the absorption of fluid and salts, and may help to regulate GI motility. Fibrous material and several types of prebiotic foods also tend to slow gastric emptying, moderate overall GI transit, and hold water.

Ingestion of some types of probiotics (sources of bacteria used to reestablish beneficial gut flora) in the form of cultured foods or supplements, with or without prebiotics, has been modestly successful in antibiotic-related diarrhea, traveler's diarrhea, bacterial overgrowth, and some pediatric diarrhea. Additional study is needed, but some products appear to have promise in specific applications (Madsen, 2001; Szajewska and Mrukowicz, 2001).

Severe and chronic diarrhea is accompanied by dehydration and electrolyte depletion. If also accompanied by prolonged infectious, immunodeficiency, or inflammatory disease, malabsorption of vitamins, minerals, and protein or lipid may also occur, and the nutrients may need to be replaced parenterally or enterally. The loss of potassium alters bowel motility, encourages anorexia, and can introduce a cycle of bowel distress. Loss of iron from GI bleeding may be severe enough to cause anemia. Nutrition deficiencies themselves cause mucosal changes, such as decreased villi height and reduced enzyme secretion, further contributing to malabsorption. As the diarrhea begins to resolve, the addition of more normal amounts of fiber to the diet may help to restore normal mucosal function, increase electrolyte and water absorption, and increase the firmness of the stool.

Food in the lumen is needed to restore the compromised GI tract after disease and periods of fasting. Early refeeding after rehydration reduces stool output and shortens the duration of illness. Micronutrient replacement or supplementation may also be useful for acute diarrhea, probably because it accelerates the normal regeneration of damaged mucosal epithelial cells.

Medical Nutrition Therapy for Infants and Children

Acute diarrhea is most dangerous in infants and small children, who are easily dehydrated by large fluid losses. In these cases, replacement of fluid and electrolytes must be aggressive and immediate. Standard oral rehydration solutions recommended by

TABLE 30-2 Oral Rehydration Solution: Composition and Recipe

ELEMENT	COMPOSITION
Glucose (g/100 ml)	20
Sodium (mEq/L)	90
Potassium (mEq/L)	20
Chloride (mEq/L)	80
Bicarbonate (mEq/L)	30
Osmolarity (mOsm/L)	330

Recipe*
To 1 L of water add the following:

3.5 g sodium chloride
2.5 g sodium bicarbonate
1.5 g potassium chloride
20.0 g glucose

Data from World Health Organization, 1986.
*The solution should be made fresh every 24 hr.

the World Health Organization (WHO) since 1986 and the American Academy of Pediatrics (AAP) contain a 2% concentration of glucose (20 g/L), 45 to 90 mEq/L of sodium, 20 mEq/L of potassium, and a citrate base (Table 30-2). Newer, reduced osmolarity solutions (osm ~ 130 to 200 mOsm/L) have been shown to be equally or more effective in treating persistent diarrhea in children (Hahn, Kim, and Garner, 2002).

Newer solutions such as Pedialyte, Infalyte, Lytren, Equalyte, and Rehydralyte typically contain less glucose and slightly less salt and are available in pharmacies, some without prescription. Oral rehydration therapy is less invasive and less expensive than intravenous rehydration and, when used with children, allows parents to assist with their children's recovery (Goepp and Katz, 1993).

A substantial proportion of children 9 to 20 months of age can maintain adequate intake when offered either a liquid or a semisolid diet continuously during bouts of acute diarrhea. Even during acute diarrhea, the intestine can absorb up to 60% of the food eaten. Some practitioners have been slow to adopt the practice of early refeeding after severe diarrhea in infants, despite evidence that "resting the gut" is actually more damaging (Booth, 1993). A recent report from the working group report of the First World Congress of Pediatric Gastroenterology, Hepatology, and Nutrition suggests that strategies must be cohesive and uniform to address the problems of pediatric diarrhea to reduce deaths worldwide (Davidson et al, 2002). Prescription of a high-sugar, clear liquid diet is inappropriate for recovery from diarrhea.

Steatorrhea

Pathophysiology

Steatorrhea, or excessive fat in the stool, is a consequence of disease, surgical resection of organs involved in digestion, and absorption of lipid. Normally, 90% to 98% of ingested fat is absorbed; but in steatorrhea, the percent remaining in the stool may increase to 20% or more. Diagnosis is usually based on a ratio of fecal fat to ingested fat or a coefficient of absorption. A diet containing 75 to 100 g of fat is usually fed for 72 hours, the amount of fat actually consumed is recorded, and the fecal fat content is analyzed. The upper limit of normal fecal fat is usually in the range of 7%. Steatorrhea may result from (1) inadequate bile secretion secondary to liver disease or biliary obstruction; (2) blind loop syndrome; (3) pancreatic insufficiency; (4) inadequate reabsorption of bile salts due to diseases involving the distal ileum (as in sprue, Crohn's disease, or GI irritation); or (5) decreased fat reesterification and decreased formation and transport of chylomicrons, as may be seen in abetalipoproteinemia and intestinal lymphangiectasia. Box 30-3 lists disorders associated with malabsorption.

Medical Treatment

Because steatorrhea is a symptom and not a disease, the underlying cause of malabsorption must be determined and treated. With pancreatic insufficiency, oral pancreatic enzymes can be used to increase lipid digestion.

Medical Nutrition Therapy

Steatorrhea can result in chronic weight loss and may require compensatory increased energy intake, primarily in the form of dietary protein and complex carbohydrate. Medium-chain triglycerides (MCTs) can be used in the diet because they have a short chain length, allowing easier absorption in the absence of bile acids. Medium-and short-chain fatty acids are able to enter the portal venous blood for direct transport to the liver without being resynthesized into triglycerides in the intestinal cell.

The MCTs are available in some enteral formulas and also as MCT oil (8.3 kcal/g; 1 T = 116 kcal). The oil is best used when it is incorporated into foods rather than administered by the spoonful. MCT can be used to make salad dressings, sandwich spreads, or confections, and it can be substituted for fats in most recipes. Normally, divided doses of less than 15 g of oil per feeding are better tolerated and absorbed than larger quantities. When steatorrhea is present, there is increased risk of vitamin deficiencies, especially fat-soluble vitamins and deficiencies of the minerals calcium, zinc, and magnesium.

Gastrointestinal Strictures and Obstruction

Pathophysiology

Inflammatory bowel disease (IBD), peptic ulcer disease, GI surgeries, tumors, or radiation enteritis may partially or completely obstruct the GI tract as can scarring or dysfunctional segments. Obstructions in the stomach that result from the ingestion of plant foods are called phytobezoars and are more common in patients who are edentulous, have poor dentition, or use dentures. Foods commonly incriminated in the formation of phytobezoars include potato skins, oranges, and grapefruit, but many foods that are consumed in large segments or that have skins that are difficult to chew may be problematic. When obstructions occur in the intestine, the patient usually experiences prolonged bloating, abdominal distention and pain, and sometimes nausea and vomiting.

Medical Nutrition Therapy

Because fiber is not digested to any significant degree (except by fermentation in the colon), and because chewing is not a reliable way of reducing the size of fibrous foods, both the amount and size of fibrous material usually must be controlled. A restricted-fiber diet typically restricts fruits, vegetables, and coarse grains and usually provides less than 10 to 15 g of dietary fiber, usually in the form of particulate matter. Particularly with distal obstructions or strictures, it may be beneficial to keep the stool soft by including modest amounts of fiber but of small particle size.

Some intestinal obstruction cases may require clear liquids or total restriction of food and parenteral nutrition and fluid used as needed. Working with the physician is necessary to determine the nature, site, and duration of the obstruction so that nutrition therapy can be individualized.

Box 30-3. Diseases and Conditions Associated With Malabsorption

- Inadequate digestion
  - Pancreatic insufficiency
  - Gastric acid hypersecretion
  - Gastric resection
- Altered bile salt metabolism with impaired micelle formation
  - Hepatobiliary disease
  - Interrupted enterohepatic circulation of bile salts
  - Bacterial overgrowth
  - Drugs that precipitate bile salts
- Abnormalities of mucosal cell transport
  - Biochemical or genetic abnormalities
    - Disaccharidase deficiency
    - Monosaccharide malabsorption
    - Specific disorders of amino acid malabsorption
    - Abetalipoproteinemia
    - Vitamin B_{12} malabsorption
    - Celiac disease
  - Inflammatory of infiltrative disorders
    - Crohn's disease
    - Ulcerative colitis
    - Amyloidosis
    - Scleroderma
    - Tropical sprue
    - Gastrointestinal allergy
    - Infectious enteritis
    - Whipple's disease
    - Intestinal lymphoma
    - Radiation enteritis
    - Drug-induced enteritis
  - Endocrine and metabolic disorders
  - Short-bowel syndrome
- Abnormalities of intestinal lymphatics and vascular system
  - Intestinal lymphangiectasia
  - Mesenteric vascular insufficiency
  - Chronic congestive heart failure

Data from Beyer PL: Short bowel syndrome. In Coulston AM, Rock CL, Monson ER, editors: *Nutrition in the prevention and treatment of disease*, ed 1, San Diego, 2001, Academic Press; Sundarum A et al: Nutritional management of short bowel syndrome in adults, *J Clin Gastroenterol* 34:207, 2002; Podolsky DK: Inflammatory bowel disease, *N Engl J Med* 347:417, 2002; Mitra AD et al: Management of diarrhea in HIV-infected patients, *Int J STD AIDS* 12:630, 2001; Branski D et al: Chronic diarrhea and malabsorption, *Pediatr Clin North Am* 43:307, 1996; and Fine KD: Diarrhea. In Feldman M, Sleisenger MH, Scharschmidt BF, editors: *Gastrointestinal and liver disease*, ed 6, Philadelphia, 1998, WB Saunders.

DISEASES OF THE SMALL INTESTINE

Celiac Disease (Gluten-Sensitive Enteropathy)

Pathophysiology

Celiac disease, or gluten-sensitive enteropathy, results from an inappropriate T-cell–mediated immune response caused by ingested gluten by people who are genetically predisposed. The prevalence of the disease may have been underestimated in the past and now is considered to be about 1 in 133 persons in the United States. Prevalence is higher in relatives of persons with celia disease (Fasano et al, 2003). Onset is usually from infancy to young adulthood, but about 20% of cases occur in adults over 60 years of age (Farrell and Kelley, 2002).

Gluten refers to specific peptide fractions of proteins found in wheat, rye, and barley. These peptide molecules are modified during absorption to a form that triggers a local and in many cases systemic immune response. In untreated cases, the overzealous immune and inflammatory response eventually results in damage to the intestinal mucosa, altered neuropeptide secretion, and decreased digestive and absorptive functions. Cells of the villi become deficient in the disaccharidases and peptidases needed for digestion and also in the carriers needed to transport nutrients into the bloodstream. The extent of villous changes varies greatly, but sufficient atrophy and flattening of the villi eventually occur to compromise micronutrient and macronutrient absorption (Figure 30-1).

Decreased release of peptide hormones from the small intestine results in reduced secretions from the gallbladder and pancreas, further contributing to maldigestion. The disease primarily affects the proximal and midportions of the small bowel, although the more distal segments may also be involved. Because the symptoms are nonspecific and vary greatly, celiac disease may be misdiagnosed for years as irritable bowel or other GI disorders.

The disease may also be associated with other inflammatory states such as dermatitis herpetiformis (a variant of celiac disease that involves the skin), muscle and joint pain, and other autoimmune diseases such as thyroiditis and type 1 diabetes. Celiac disease is normally considered chronic and requires life-long omission of gluten from the diet. Morbidity and mortality rates may be increased in persons who are undiagnosed until late or in persons who are unable to comply with the diet (Seraphin and Mobarin, 2002). Increased risk of lymphomas and other malignancies influences overall morbidity, and the risk of malignancies appears to be increased in those who continue to eat gluten-containing foods (Troncone et al, 1996). Box 30-4 lists the extraintestinal manifestations.

The diagnosis of celiac disease is made by a combination of clinical, laboratory, and histologic evaluations, but small bowel biopsy is the final diagnostic end point. The disease may become apparent when an infant begins eating gluten-containing cereals, or it may not appear until middle age, when it may be triggered or unmasked by GI surgery, stress, pregnancy, or viral infection. The presentation in young children is more likely to include the more "classic" symptoms of diarrhea and steatorrhea, malodorous stools, abdominal bloating, apathy, and poor weight gain. In late onset, the first manifestation is more varied and may include other inflammatory and autoimmune disorders, generalized fatigue, failure to gain or maintain weight, or the consequences of nutrient malabsorption, including anemias, osteoporosis, or vitamin K–related coagulopathy. Fifty percent of celiac patients, however, have few or no obvious symptoms, and some may be overweight at presentation (Fasano and Catassi, 2001; Hill et al, 2002).

Persons in whom celiac disease is suspected are further evaluated for the overall pattern of symptoms and family history and then are typically screened using serologic tests, which include the presence of antien-

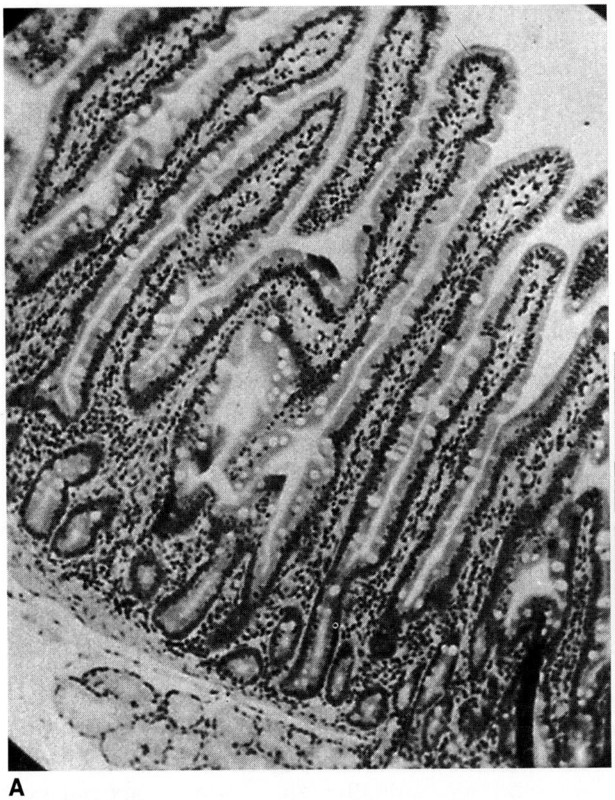

A

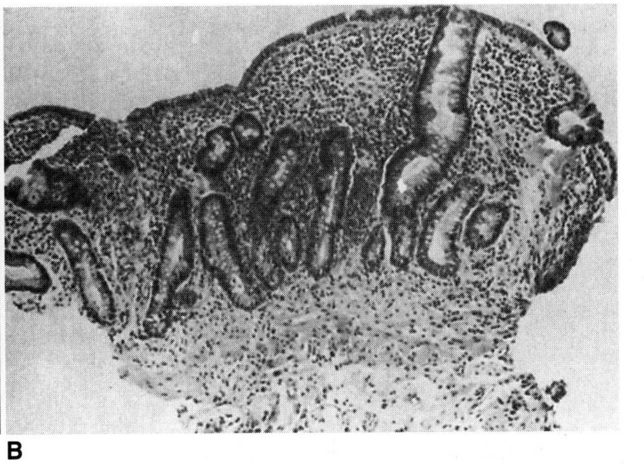

B

FIGURE 30-1 • **A,** Low-power photomicrograph (×100) of a normal human duodenal mucosa. Note the long, thin villi. **B,** Low-power photomicrograph (×100) of a peroral small-bowel biopsy specimen from a patient with gluten enteropathy. Note the complete loss of villi and the heavy infiltrate of white blood cells in the lamina propria. (From Floch MH: *Nutrition and diet therapy in gastrointestinal disease,* New York, 1981, Plenum Medical.)

Box 30-4. Extraintestinal and Associated Manifestations of Celiac Disease

Extraintestinal

- Anemia (iron or folate, rarely, B_{12})
- Lassitude, malaise (sometimes despite lack of anemia), arthritis, arthralgia
- Dermatitis herpetiformis
- Osteomalacia, osteopenia, fractures (vitamin D deficiency, inadequate calcium absorption)
- Dental enamel hypoplasia
- Coagulopathies (vitamin K deficiency)
- Infertility, increased risk of abortion, delayed puberty, delayed growth
- Hepatic steatosis, hepatitis
- Neurologic symptoms (ataxia, poly-neuropathy, seizures)
- Psychiatric syndromes

Associated Disorders

- Autoimmune diseases—type 1 diabetes, thyroiditis, hepatitis, collagen vascular disease
- Malignancies
- IgA deficiencies

Data from Hill ID et al: Celiac disease: working group report of the first world congress of pediatric gastoenterology, hepatology and nutrition, *J Pediatr Gastroenterol Nutr* 35:785, 2002; Fasano A, Catassi C: Current approaches to diagnosis and treatment of celiac disease: an evolving spectrum, *Gastroenterology* 120:636, 2001.
IgA, Immunoglobulin.

domysial antibodies (AEAs), immunoglobulin A (IgA) or IgG-AGA antibodies (antigliadin antibodies), or the autoantigen that appears to trigger the immune response (IgA tissue transglutaminase [tTG]) (Hill et al, 2002; Mustalahi et al, 2002; Petaros et al, 2002). Some persons thought to have celiac disease may be IgA deficient, and so IgA levels are normally done first. The serologic tests may also be used for monitoring the progress of persons with confirmed celiac disease.

The serologic tests are highly specific and sensitive for celiac disease, but the gold standard for final diagnosis is still the intestinal mucosal biopsy (Farrell and Kelly, 2002). Because intestinal biopsy is relatively expensive and must be performed by upper GI endoscopy, it is not usually used for initial screening. Because dietary change would alter the diagnostic results, initial diagnostic evaluation should be done before the patient has withdrawn gluten-containing foods from the diet.

Major clinical symptoms usually abate in most patients 2 to 8 weeks after consuming a gluten-free diet, but for some patients it may take longer. With strict dietary control, levels of the specific antibodies usually become undetectable in 3 to 6 months in most persons, but in some the recovery may be slower (Farrell and Kelley, 2002; Hill et al, 2002). A small percentage of patients may be refractory to dietary therapy because of inadvertent gluten intake, pancreatic insufficiency, irritable bowel, bacterial overgrowth, fructose intolerance, or other coexisting GI maladies (Abdulkarim et al, 2002).

Medical Treatment

Institution of a gluten-free diet greatly diminishes the autoimmune process, and the intestinal mucosa usually reverts to normal; however, some patients may require months or even years of diet therapy for maximal recovery. The toxic peptide fractions of the respective cereals must be avoided for life. Refractory sprue may not respond entirely to the removal of gluten, or it may respond only temporarily. Many of these patients, however, do show a response to steroids, azathioprine, cyclosporine, or other medications classically used in inflammatory or immunologic reactions. For some, treatment of other underlying disease may further resolve symptoms (Figure 30-2).

A new study has identified the peptide fraction from gliadin that causes the problem (see *New Directions:* Bacterial Endopeptidase—A New Treatment for Celiac Disease?).

Medical Nutrition Therapy

Complete withdrawal of gluten results in clinical improvement. The diet requires a major life change on the part of the patient to adhere to it sufficiently to bring about remission. Insofar as possible, the diet omits all dietary wheat (gliadin), rye (secalin), and barley (hordein), sources of the prolamin fractions (Thompson, 2001) (Table 30-3).

The diet should initially be supplemented with vitamins, minerals, and extra protein to remedy deficiencies and replenish nutrient stores. Anemia should be treated with iron, folate, or vitamin B_{12}, depending on the nature of the anemia. Calcium and vitamin D administration may be necessary to correct osteoporosis or osteomalacia. Vitamins A and E may be necessary to replenish stores depleted by steatorrhea. Vitamin K may be prescribed for purpura, bleeding, or prolonged prothrombin time. Electrolyte and fluid replacement is essential for those dehydrated from severe diarrhea.

Those who continue to have malabsorption should take a multiple vitamin and mineral supplement to at least meet dietary reference intakes (DRIs). MCT may help provide calories, especially in persons with steatorrhea. Lactose and fructose intolerance sometimes occurs secondary to celiac disease. A low-lactose or low-fructose diet may be useful in controlling symptoms, at least initially. Once the GI tract returns to more normal function, lactase activity may also return and a trial of lactose ingestion can be tried.

In the traditional diet, wheat, rye, barley, and oats are normally excluded. Recently, the need for exclu-

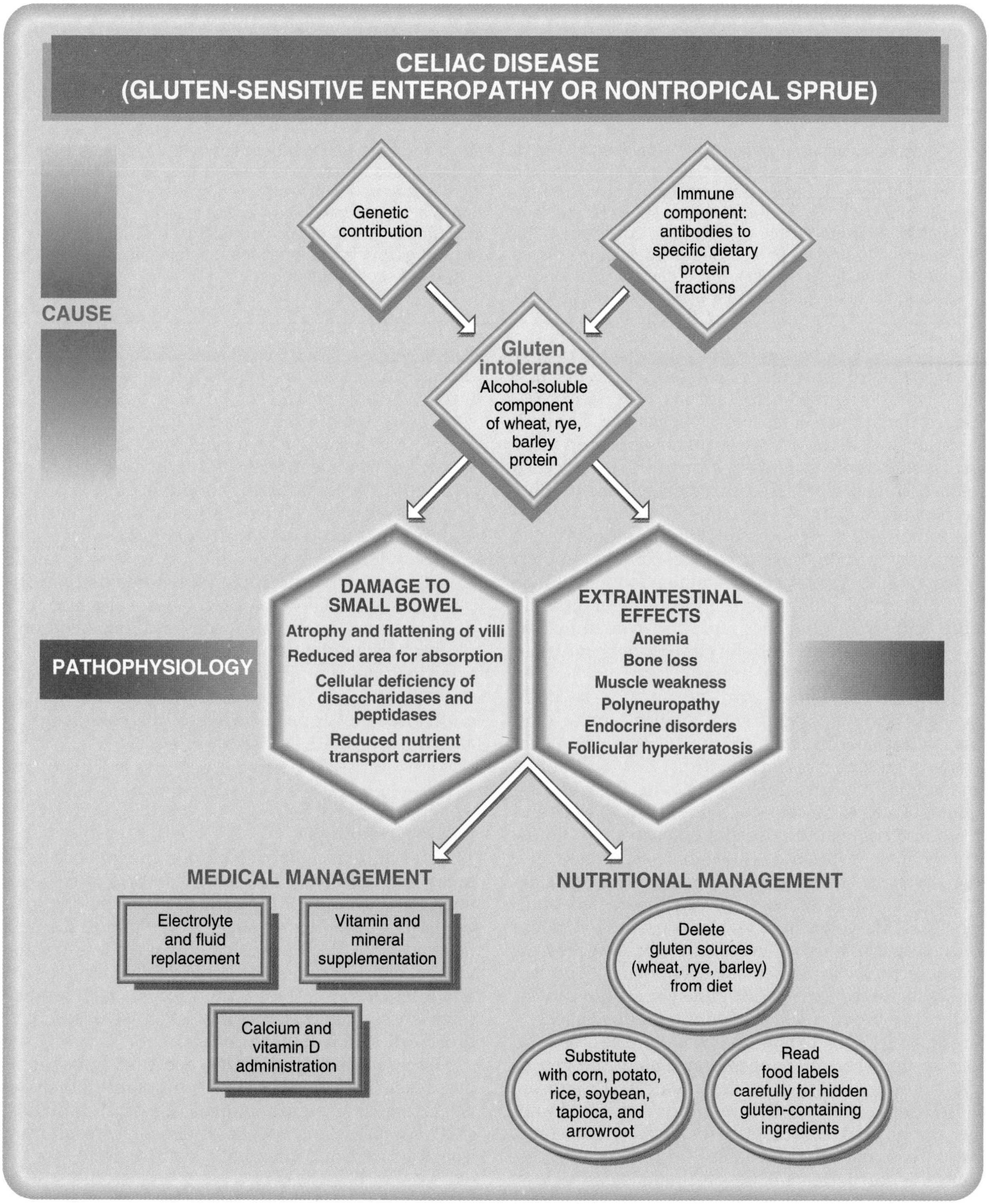

FIGURE 30-2 • Pathophysiology algorithm: celiac disease (gluten-sensitive enteropathy or nontropical sprue). (Algorithm content developed by John Anderson, PhD, and Sanford C. Garner, PhD, 2000. Updated by Peter L. Beyer, MS, RD, LD, 2002.)

NEW DIRECTIONS

Bacterial Endopeptidase—A New Treatment for Celiac Disease?

Recently scientists identified a 33-amino acid peptide fraction from the 266-amino acid gliadin that triggers the destructive inflammatory response in celiac disease (Shan et al, 2002). The fragment appears to be the same one in other grains that contain gluten. It appears that this peptide fraction is resistant to digestion by normal human digestive enzymes, but it can be degraded by bacterial endopeptidases. In preliminary studies, destruction of the peptide fragment by the addition of the endopeptidase enzyme prevented the typical immunologic response seen with celiac disease. The hope is that oral endopeptidase enzymes can be used as an oral supplement to digest and destroy the specific fragment of gliadin in the foods that contain gluten, thus allowing their consumption.

sion of oats from the diet of persons with celiac disease and dermatitis herpetiformis has been challenged (Janatuinen et al, 2002). Clinical and GI manifestations of gluten sensitivity do not appear to recur in evaluations of oat intake lasting from 6 months to 5 years or longer. Until larger numbers of patients have been evaluated, however, some clinicians and patients may still be reluctant to add oat products to the diet. Many oat products may be contaminated with wheat or other grains, and contamination may not be easily detected. Long-term study in larger populations and strict guidelines regarding contamination of gluten-containing grains in oat products may help to resolve the issue in the future.

Products made from corn, potato, rice, soybean, tapioca, arrowroot, amaranth, quinoa, millet, and buckwheat can be substituted in food products. When using the flours, it is important that they also not be contaminated with gluten-containing flour during milling. Patients can expect differences in textures and flavors of common foods using the substitute flours, but the new recipes can also be quite acceptable once the adjustment is made. In some countries, specially processed wheat starch has been considered sufficiently low in gluten to be safe for consumption, but in other countries the protein fraction remaining after extraction may be expressed only as nitrogen or protein rather than the more specific gluten or gliadin content of the final product. When reading a product label listing only nitrogen content, one would not be able to be certain that the source of the remaining nitrogen or protein was gliadin or another protein (Thompson, 2001). Celiac organizations in North America do not yet recommend consumption of these wheat starch products or oat products. Table 30-4 provides suggestions for incorporating flour substitutions into recipes.

The diet for celiac disease requires a major change in the types of foods normally consumed in the Western diet. Foods made from wheat, in particular (breads, cereals, pastas, and baked goods), are consumed as staples in the U.S. diet. A truly gluten-free diet requires careful scrutiny of the labels of all bakery products and packaged foods. Gluten-containing grains are not only used as a primary ingredient but may also be added during processing or preparation of foods. Hydrolyzed vegetable protein can be made from wheat, soy, corn, or mixtures of these grains (Table 30-5).

Freedom from symptoms after eating gluten does not necessarily mean that cells of the GI tract are undamaged. The precipitating condition usually continues to exist, and gluten causes mucosal changes within hours; however, overt symptoms may take 8 weeks or longer to reappear or may remain latent. Adults who start and stop a gluten-free diet numerous times eventually may reach a state at which they do not respond to the diet. Complications of chronic ulcerative jejunoileitis and extraintestinal manifestations may develop. Risk of malignant disease, especially lymphoma, is increased, and adherence to a gluten-free diet appears to reduce the risk (Saraphin and Mobarin, 2002; Troncone, 1996).

Tropical Sprue

Pathophysiology

Tropical sprue is a diarrheal syndrome that occurs in many tropical areas. The diarrhea appears to be an infectious type, and the intestinal organism identified may differ from one region of the tropics to the next (Farthing, 1998). As in celiac disease, the intestinal villi are shortened, but the surface cell alterations are much less severe. The gastric mucosa may be atrophied and inflamed, with diminished secretion of hydrochloric acid and intrinsic factor.

Symptoms include diarrhea, anorexia, and abdominal distention as well as symptoms of nutritional deficiency, such as night blindness, glossitis, stomatitis, cheilosis, pallor, and edema. Anemia may result from iron, folic acid, and vitamin B_{12} deficiencies.

Medical Treatment

Treatment involves restoration of fluids, electrolytes, and nutrients. Tropical sprue typically responds promptly to broad-spectrum antibiotics and folate therapy. Along with other nutrients as needed, folate is given orally, 5 mg daily, along with intramuscular vitamin B_{12} (1000 mg/month) until symptoms subside.

TABLE 30-3 Gluten-Free Diet by Food Groups

FOOD PRODUCTS	FOODS ALLOWED	FOODS TO QUESTION	FOODS NOT ALLOWED
Milk products	Milk, cream, most ice cream, buttermilk, plain yogurt, cheese, cream cheese, processed cheese, processed cheese foods, cottage cheese	Milk drinks, flavored yogurt, frozen yogurt, sour cream, cheese sauces, cheese spreads	Malted milk, ice cream made with ingredients not allowed
Grain products	**Breads:** Bread and baked products containing amaranth, arrowroot, buckwheat, corn bran, corn flour, cornmeal, cornstarch, flax, legume flours (bean, garbanzo or chickpea, fava, lentil, pea), millet, potato flour, potato starch, quinoa, rice bran, rice flours (white, brown, sweet), sago, sorghum flour, soy flour, sweet potato flour, tapioca and teff	Buckwheat flour	Bread and baked products containing wheat, rye, triticale, barley, oats, wheat germ, wheat bran, graham flour, gluten flour, durum flour, wheat starch, oat bran, bulgur, farina, wheat-based semolina, spelt, kamut, einkorn, emmer, farro, imported foods labeled "gluten-free," which may contain ingredients not allowed, e.g., wheat starch
	Cereals: **Hot:** Amaranth flakes, cornmeal, cream of buckwheat, cream of rice (brown, white), hominy grits, rice flakes, quinoa flakes, soy flakes and soy grits **Cold:** Puffed amaranth, puffed buckwheat, puffed corn, puffed millet, puffed rice, rice flakes and soy cereals	Rice and corn cereals, rice and soy pablum	Cereals made from wheat, rye, triticale, barley and oats; cereals with added malt extract or malt flavoring
	Pastas: Macaroni, spaghetti, and noodles from beans, corn, pea, potato, quinoa, rice, soy and wild rice flours	Buckwheat pasta	Pastas made from wheat, wheat starch and other ingredients not allowed
	Miscellaneous: Corn tacos, corn torillas	Rice crackers, some rice cakes and popped corn cakes	Wheat flour tacos, wheat tortillas
Meats and alternatives	**Meat, fish, poultry:** Fresh	Deli or processed meats such as luncheon meat, ham, bacon, meat and sandwich spreads, meat loaf, frozen meat patties, sausages, pâté, wieners, bologna, salami, imitation meat or fish products, meat product extenders	Fish canned in vegetable broth containing HVP/HPP* Turkey basted or injected with HVP/HPP* Frozen chicken containing chicken broth (made with ingredients not allowed)
	Eggs: Eggs	Egg substitutes, dried eggs	
	Others: Lentils, chickpeas (garbanzo beans), peas, beans, nuts, seeds, tofu	Baked beans, dry roasted nuts	
Fruits and vegetables	**Fruits:** Fresh, frozen, and canned fruits and juices **Vegetables:** Fresh, frozen, dried and canned	Fruit pie fillings, dried fruits, fruits or vegetables with sauces French-fried potatoes (e.g., those in restaurants)	Scalloped potatoes (containing wheat flour) Battered dipped vegetables
Soups	Homemade broth, gluten-free bouillon cubes, cream soups and stocks made from allowed ingredients	Canned soups, dried soup mixes, soup bases and bouillon cubes	Soups made with ingredients not allowed, bouillon and bouillon cubes containing HVP or HPP* or wheat
Fats	Butter, margarine, lard, vegetable oil, cream, shortening, homemade salad dressing with allowed ingredients	Salad dressings, some mayonnaise	Packaged suet
Desserts	Ice cream, sherbet, whipped toppings, egg custards, gelatin desserts; cakes, cookies, pastries made with allowed ingredients; gluten-free ice cream cones, wafers, and waffles	Milk puddings, custard powder, pudding mixes	Ice cream made with ingredients not allowed; cakes, cookies, muffins, pies and pastries made with ingredients not allowed; ice cream cones, wafers and waffles made with ingredients not allowed
Miscellaneous	**Beverages:** Tea, instant or ground coffee (regular or decaffeinated), cocoa, soft drinks, cider; distilled alcoholic beverages such as rum, gin, whiskey, vodka, wines and pure liqueurs; some soy and rice beverages	Instant tea, flavored and herbal teas, flavored coffees, coffee substitutes, fruit-flavored drinks, chocolate drinks, chocolate mixes	Beer, ale and lager; cereal and malted beverages; soy or rice beverages made with barley or oats

Modified by Case S, Molloy M, and Zarkadas M. From Canadian Celiac Association: *Celiac disease needs a diet for life,* October 2000. Further revisions by Case S, April 2002 and June 2003.

*If the plant source in HVP/HPP (hydrolyzed vegetable protein/hydrolyzed plant protein) is not identified or if the source is from wheat protein, HVP/HPP must be avoided.

Continued

TABLE 30-3 Gluten-Free Diet by Food Groups—cont'd

FOOD PRODUCTS	FOODS ALLOWED	FOODS TO QUESTION	FOODS NOT ALLOWED
Miscellaneous—cont'd	**Sweets:** Honey, jam, jelly, marmalade, corn syrup, maple syrup, molasses, sugar (brown and white), icing sugar (confectioner's)	Spreads, candies, chocolate bars, chewing gum, and lemon curd	Licorice and other candies made with ingredients not allowed
	Snack foods: Plain popcorn, nuts, and soy nuts	Dry roasted nuts, flavored potato chips, tortilla or taco (corn) chips, and soy nuts	Pizza, unless made with ingredients allowed
	Condiments: Plain pickles, relish, olives, ketchup, mustard, tomato paste, pure herbs and spices, pure black pepper, vinegars (apple or cider, distilled white, grape or wine, spirit), gluten-free soy sauce	Seasoning mixes, Worcestershire sauce	Soy sauce (made from wheat), mustard pickles (made from wheat flour), malt vinegar
	Other: Sauces and gravies made with ingredients allowed, pure cocoa, pure baking chocolate, carob chips and powder, chocolate chips, monosodium glutamate (MSG), cream of tartar, baking soda, yeast, brewer's yeast, aspartame, coconut, vanilla, gluten-free communion wafers	Baking powder	Sauces and gravies made from ingredients not allowed, hydrolyzed vegetable/plant protein (HVP/HPP)*, communion wafers

Modified by Case S, Molloy M, and Zarkadas M. From Canadian Celiac Association: *Celiac disease needs a diet for life*, October 2000. Further revisions by Case S, April 2002 and June 2003.

*If the plant source in HVP/HPP (hydrolyzed vegetable protein/hydrolyzed plant protein) is not identified or if the source is from wheat protein, HVP/HPP must be avoided.

TABLE 30-4 Substitutions

Substitutions for 1 tbsp (15 ml) Wheat Flour			
	½ tbsp	Cornstarch	7 ml
	½ tbsp	Potato starch	7 ml
	½ tbsp	White rice flour	7 ml
	½ tbsp	Arrowroot starch	7 ml
	2 tsp	Quick-cooking tapioca	10 ml
	2 tsp	Tapioca starch	10 ml
	2 tbsp	Uncooked rice	30 ml
Substitutions for 1 c (250 ml) Wheat Flour*			
Mix A:	2 c	Brown rice flour	500 ml
	2 c	Sweet rice flour	500 ml
	2 c	Rice polish	500 ml
Mix B:	4 c	White rice flour	1 L
	1⅓ c	Potato starch	325 ml
	1 c	Tapioca starch	250 ml
Other Substitutions for 1 c (250 ml) Wheat Flour*			
	⅝ c	Potato starch	150 ml
	⅞ c	White or brown rice flour	215 ml
	1 c	Cornmeal	250 ml
	1 c	Fine cornmeal	250 ml
	¾ c	Coarse cornmeal	175 ml
	⅝ c	White or brown rice flour	150 ml
		PLUS	
	⅓ c	Potato starch	75 ml
	1 c	Soy flour	250 ml
		PLUS	
	¼ c	Potato starch	50 ml
	¾ c	Rice flour	175 ml
		PLUS	
	¼ c	Cornstarch	50 ml
	⅞ c	Whole bean flour	215 ml

*Store in an airtight container and use ⅞ c (215 ml) of mix A or 1 c (250 ml) of mix B for 1 c (250 ml) wheat flour. A combination of flours and starches gives a better gluten-free product. For specific flour mixes see recipes in gluten-free cookbooks using a variety of gluten-free flours.

Modified from Case S: *Gluten-free diet: a comprehensive resource guide*, ed 2, Saskatchewan, 2003, Case Nutrition Consulting.

Medical Nutrition Therapy

It is important to correct the related anemias (see Chapter 34). Nutritional deficiency may increase susceptibility to infectious agents, further aggravating the condition.

INTESTINAL BRUSH-BORDER ENZYME DEFICIENCIES

Intestinal enzyme deficiency states involve deficiencies of the brush-border disaccharidases that hydrolyze disaccharides at the mucosal cell membrane. Disaccharidase deficiencies may occur as (1) rare congenital defects, such as the sucrase, isomaltase, or lactase deficiencies seen in the newborn; (2) generalized forms secondary to diseases that damage the intestinal epithelium (e.g., Crohn's disease or celiac disease); or, most commonly, (3) a genetically acquired form (e.g., lactase deficiency) that usually appears after childhood but can appear as early as 2 years of age. For purposes of this chapter, only lactose maldigestion is described in detail (see Chapter 45 for a discussion of metabolic disorders).

Lactose Maldigestion and Lactose Intolerance

Pathophysiology

Lactose intolerance is the most common carbohydrate intolerance, and it affects persons of all age groups. Lactose maldigestion and intolerance to lac-

TABLE 30-5 Notes on "Foods to Question"

CATEGORY	FOOD PRODUCTS	NOTES
Milk products	Milk drinks	Chocolate milk and other flavored drinks may contain wheat starch or barley malt.
	Cheese spreads or sauces (e.g., nacho)	May be thickened or stabilized with wheat. Flavorings and seasonings may contain wheat.
	Flavored or frozen yogurt	May be thickened or stabilized with a gluten source. May contain granola or cookie crumbs.
	Sour cream	Some low-fat or fat-free may contain modified food starch.
Grains	Buckwheat flour	Pure buckwheat flour is gluten-free. Sometimes buckwheat flour may be mixed with wheat flour.
	Rice cereals	May contain barley malt extract.
	Corn cereals	May contain oat syrup or barley malt extract.
	Buckwheat pasta	Some "soba" pastas contain pure buckwheat flour, which is gluten-free, but others may also contain wheat flour.
	Rice cakes, corn cakes, rice crackers	Multigrain often contains barley and/or oats. Some contain soy sauce (may be made from wheat).
Meats/alternatives	Baked beans	Some are thickened with wheat flour.
	Imitation crab	May contain fillers made from wheat starch.
	Dry-roasted nuts	May contain wheat.
	Processed meat products	May contain fillers made from wheat. May contain HPP or HVP made from wheat.
	Imitation meats	Often contain wheat or oats.
Fruits and vegetables	Dried fruits	Dates and other dried fruits may be dusted with wheat flour to prevent sticking.
	Fruits/vegetables with sauces	Some may be thickened with flour.
	Fruit pie fillings	
	French fries	May contain wheat as an ingredient.
Soups	Canned soups, dried soup mixes, soup bases and bouillon cubes	May contain noodles or barley. Cream soups are often thickened with flour. May contain HPP or HVP (from wheat). Seasonings may contain wheat flour, wheat starch or hydrolyzed wheat protein.
Fats	Salad dressings	Seasonings may contain wheat flour or wheat starch.
Desserts	Milk puddings/mixes	Starch source may be from wheat.
Miscellaneous	Beverages	Some instant teas, herbal teas, coffee substitutes and other drinks may have grain additives. Nondairy substitutes (e.g., rice drinks and soy drinks) may contain barley, barley malt extract or oats.
	Lemon curd	Usually thickened with flour.
	Potato, tortilla chips, and soy nuts	Some potato chips contain wheat. Seasoning mixes may contain wheat flour, wheat starch or hydrolyzed wheat protein.
	Baking powder	Contains starch, which may be from wheat.
	Seasoning mixes	May contain wheat flour, wheat starch or hydrolyzed wheat protein.
	Worcestershire sauce	May contain malt vinegar which is not gluten-free.

From Case S: *Gluten-free diet: a comprehensive resource guide,* ed 2, Saskatchewan, 2003, Case Nutrition Consulting.
HPP, Hydrolyzed plant protein; *HVP,* hydrolyzed vegetable protein.

tose are caused by a deficiency of lactase, the enzyme that digests the sugar in milk. Lactose that is not hydrolyzed into galactose and glucose in the upper small intestine passes into the colon, where bacteria ferment the lactose to SCFAs and gases, carbon dioxide, and hydrogen gas. Consumption of small amounts should be of little consequence because both the SCFAs are readily absorbed and the gases can be absorbed or passed. Larger amounts, usually greater than 12 g, consumed in a single food (the amount typically found in 240 ml of milk), may result in more substrate entering the colon than can be disposed of by normal processes. As is the case with any malabsorbed sugar, the lactose may act osmotically and increase fecal water, and rapid fermentation by intestinal bacteria may result in bloating, flatulence, and cramps. In some cases loose stools or diarrhea may occur.

Seventy percent of the adult worldwide population, especially blacks, Asians, and South Americans, are lactase deficient, which implies that decline of the lactase enzyme after early childhood is the more normal state and lactase sufficiency is abnormal. Although it has been suggested that lactase persistence is induced by the continuation of milk in the diet after weaning, no evidence has been found to support this theory. It is more likely that the maintenance of lactase throughout adulthood reflects the continuation of an ancient genetic mutation (see *Focus on:* Lactose Tolerance—An Uncommon Anomaly?).

Typically, lactase activity declines exponentially at weaning to about 10% of the neonatal value. Even in adults who retain a high level of lactase levels (75% to 85% of white adults of Western European heritage), the quantity of lactase is about half that of other saccharidases, such as sucrase, α-dextrinase, or glucoamylase

(Gray, 1993). The decline of lactase is commonly known as hypolactasia; the adult form is the most common type of lactase deficiency (Srinivasan and Minocha, 1998).

Secondary lactose intolerance can also develop as a consequence of infection of the small intestine, inflammatory disorders, HIV, or malnutrition. In children, it is typically secondary to viral or bacterial infections. Lactase activity may also be slow to return after prolonged parenteral nutrition. Lactose maldigestion with all its symptoms may also occur in adults with irritable bowel syndrome or in children with recurrent abdominal pain, even though they have normal lactase activity (Srinivasan and Minocha, 1998).

Lactase deficiency is typically diagnosed on the basis of (1) a history of GI symptoms occurring after milk ingestion, (2) a test for abnormal hydrogen levels in the breath, or (3) an abnormal lactose tolerance test. The lactose tolerance test was originally based on an oral dose of lactose equivalent to the amount in 1 quart of milk (50 g). If the patient has insufficient lactase enzyme, blood glucose produced from the lactose increases less than 25 mg/100 ml of serum above the fasting level, and GI symptoms may appear. Because hydrogen production in the colon increases significantly if lactose is not digested in the small intestine, hydrogen absorbed into the bloodstream and exhaled through the lungs can be used as another test of malabsorption. The breath hydrogen test shows increased levels 60 to 90 minutes after ingestion. Recently, doses lower than 50 g of lactose have been used to approximate more closely the usual consumption of lactose from milk products.

Medical Nutrition Therapy

Management of lactase insufficiency requires dietary changes. The symptoms of lactose intolerance are alleviated by reduced consumption of lactose-containing foods. Persons who avoid dairy products should take calcium supplements and should read ingredient labels carefully (Srinivasan and Minocha, 1998). A completely lactose-free diet is not necessary in lactase-deficient persons. Most lactose maldigesters can consume some lactose (6 to 12 g) without major symptoms, especially when taken with meals or in the form of cheeses or cultured dairy products. Many adults with intolerance to moderate amounts of milk can ultimately adapt to and tolerate 12 g or more of lactose in milk (equivalent to 240 ml of full-lactose milk) when introduced gradually, in increments, over several weeks (Srinivasan and Minocha, 1998).

Apparently, incremental or continuous exposure to increasing quantities of fermentable sugar can lead to improved tolerance, not as a consequence of increased lactase enzyme production but perhaps by altered colonic flora. This has been shown with lactulose, a nonabsorbed carbohydrate that is biochemically similar to lactose (Bezkorovainy, 2001). Individual differences in tolerance may relate to the state of

FOCUS ON

Lactose Tolerance—An Uncommon Anomaly?

When lactose intolerance was first described in 1963, it appeared to be an infrequent occurrence, arising only occasionally in the white population. Because the capacity to digest lactose was measured in people from a wide variety of ethnic and racial backgrounds, it soon became apparent that disappearance of the lactase enzyme shortly after weaning, or at least during early childhood, was actually the predominant (normal) condition in most of the world's population. With a few exceptions, the intestinal tracts of adult mammals produce little, if any, lactase after weaning. (The milk of pinnipeds—seals, walruses, and sea lions—does not contain lactose.)

The exception of lactose tolerance has attracted the interest of geographers and others concerned with the evolution of the world's population. A genetic mutation favoring lactose tolerance appears to have arisen around 10,000 years ago, when dairying was first introduced. Presumably, it would have occurred in places where milk consumption was encouraged because of some degree of dietary deprivation and in groups in which milk was not fermented before consumption. (Fermentation breaks down much of the lactose into monosaccharides.) The mutation would have selectively endured, because it would promote greater health, survival, and reproduction of those who carried the gene.

It is proposed that the mutation occurred in more than one location and then accompanied migrations of populations throughout the world. It continues primarily among whites from northern Europe and in ethnic groups in India, Africa, and Mongolia. The highest frequency (97%) of lactose tolerance occurs in Sweden and Denmark, suggesting an increased selective advantage in those able to tolerate lactose related to the limited exposure to ultraviolet light typical of northern latitudes. (Lactose favors calcium absorption, which is limited in the absence of vitamin D produced by skin exposure to sunlight.) (See Chapter 4.)

Dairying was unknown in North America until the arrival of Europeans. Thus, Native Americans and all of the non-European immigrants are among the 90% of the world's population who tolerate milk poorly, if at all. This has practical implications with respect to group feeding programs, such as school breakfasts and lunches. Fortunately, most lactose-intolerant people are able to digest milk in small to moderate amounts.

colonic adaptation. Regular consumption of milk by lactase-deficient persons may increase the threshold at which diarrhea occurs.

Often solid or semisolid milk products, such as aged cheeses, are well tolerated because gastric emptying of these foodstuffs is slower than for liquid milk beverages, and the lactose content is low. Tolerance of yogurt may be the result of a microbial β-galactosidase in the bacterial culture that facilitates lactose digestion in the intestine. The presence of galactosidase depends on the brand and processing method. Because this microbial enzyme is sensitive to freezing, frozen yogurt may not be as well tolerated, but the addition of probiotics may change this in the future (Davidson et al, 2000).

Lactase enzyme and milk products treated with lactase enzyme (e.g., Lactaid) are available for lactase maldigesters who have discomfort with milk ingestion. Commercial lactase preparations may differ somewhat in their effects on both hydrogen breath excretion and symptom reduction (Ramirez et al, 1994) and in their effectiveness (Srinivasan and Minocha, 1998).

INFLAMMATORY BOWEL DISEASES

The two major forms of inflammatory bowel disease (IBD) are Crohn's disease and ulcerative colitis. The onset of IBD occurs most often in patients 15 to 30 years of age, but some persons have first onset of the disease later in adulthood. Both sexes are equally affected. The cause of IBD is not fully known, but it appears to involve the interaction of environmental factors, host microflora, genetic predisposition, and an abnormal immune or autoimmune response in the intestinal wall. At least part of the susceptibility (and perhaps behavior and complications) of IBD have been mapped to gene mutations on different chromosomes. The specific genes and their roles, however, have not been completely elaborated (Ahmad et al, 2001; Hugot et al, 2001).

The overzealous inflammatory response with local and systemic involvement of leukocytes results in the release of proteases, prostaglandins, leukotrienes, eicosanoids, and oxygen free radicals. The exaggerated immune response appears to be largely responsible for the GI tissue damage incurred (Laroux and Grisham, 2001; van Dullemen et al, 1997).

Triggers for the initial onset and subsequent exacerbations likely include an exaggerated inflammatory response to a specific microbe or combinations of microbes in the lumen of the GI tract (Beutler, 2001; Podolsky, 2002) (Figure 30-3).

Food allergies and other immunologic reactions to specific foods may have been considered in the pathogenesis of IBD and certainly its symptoms; however, the incidence of documented food allergies, compared with food intolerances, is relatively small. In one objective evaluation of 375 patients with GI disease, adverse reactions to foods occurred in 32% of patients, allergies were suspected in 14.4%, and allergies were confirmed in 3.2% of patients (Bischoff et al, 1996). The permeability of the intestinal wall to molecules of food and cell fragments is likely increased in inflammatory states, allowing heightened interaction of antigens with host immune systems.

Food intolerances of various types occur more than twice as often in persons with IBD than in the population at large (Ballegaard et al, 1997). Except for a small increase in the occurrence of lactose intolerance, however, the patterns are not consistent among individuals, or even from one time to the next. Reasons for specific and nonspecific food intolerances are abundant and are likely related to the stage, location, and manifestations of the disease process. Partial GI obstructions, malabsorption, diarrhea, altered GI transit, increased secretions, food aversions, and associations are but a few of the problems experienced by persons with IBD (Reif et al, 1997). Neither food allergies nor intolerances, however, fully explain the onset or overall pathologic or clinical manifestations in all patients (see Chapter 32).

Normally, when an antigenic challenge or trauma occurs, the immune response rises to the occasion; it is then turned off (and continues to be held in check) after the challenge resolves. In IBD, either the regulatory mechanisms are defective or the factors stimulating the immune and acute-phase response are enhanced, leading to tissue fibrosis and destruction. The clinical course of the disease may be mild and episodic, or severe and unremitting.

Both Crohn's disease and ulcerative colitis share some clinical features. For example, food intolerances, diarrhea, fever, weight loss, anemias, malnutrition, growth failure, and extraintestinal manifestations (arthritic, dermatologic, and hepatic) occur in both diseases. The diseases, however, also have distinctive features in terms of their genetic characteristics, clinical presentation, and treatment (Table 30-6).

Persons with IBD are at risk for several forms of malnutrition, and nutrition is a major consideration in each stage of the disease. Although malnutrition can occur in both forms of IBD, it is more likely to be a major and lifelong concern in patients with Crohn's disease. In both forms of IBD, the risk of malignant disease is increased with long-standing disease. The reasons for the increased risk are not firmly established but may be associated with the increased proliferative state and nutritional factors.

Crohn's Disease

Pathophysiology

Crohn's disease may involve any part of the GI tract, from mouth to anus. The most common pattern of involvement (about 50% to 60% of cases) is the combination of both the distal ileum and the colon; 15% to 25% of cases involve only the small intestine or only

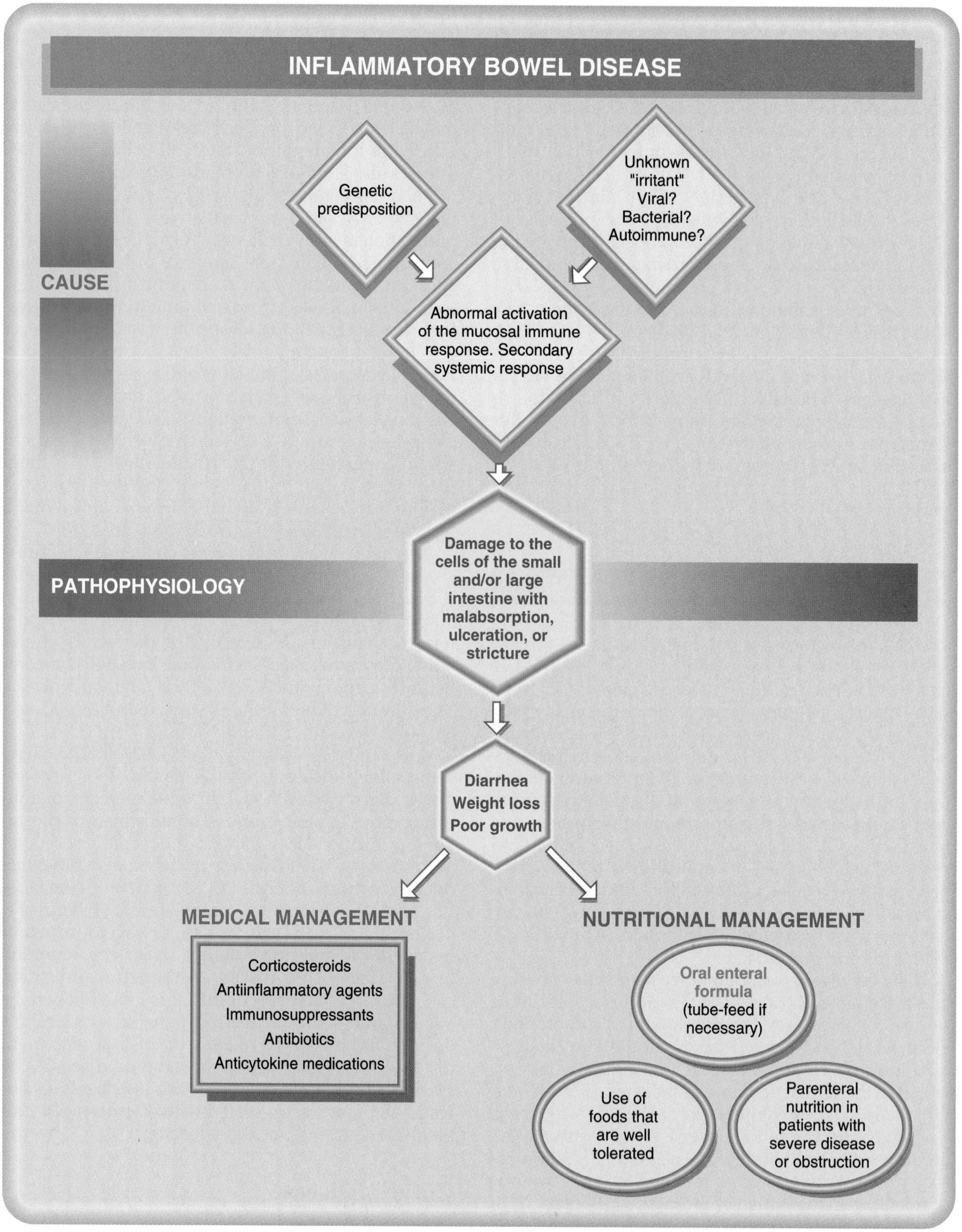

FIGURE 30-3 • Pathophysiology algorithm: inflammatory bowel disease. (Algorithm content developed by John Anderson, PhD, and Sanford C. Garner, PhD, 2000. Updated by Peter L. Beyer, MS, RD, LD, 2002.)

TABLE 30-6 Differences Between Crohn's Disease and Ulcerative Colitis

CHARACTERISTIC	REGIONAL ENTERITIS (CROHN'S DISEASE)	ULCERATIVE COLITIS
General Description		
Age at onset	Young	Young to middle-aged
Pathology and Anatomy		
Depth of involvement	Transmural (all layers of submucosa)	Mucosa and submucosa
Rectal involvement	50%	95%
Right colon involvement	Frequent	Occasional
Small bowel involvement	Involved; ileum narrowed	Usually normal
Distribution of disease	Segmental	Continuous
Inflammatory mass	Chronic and extensive	Rare (crypt abscess)
Cobblestone-like mucosa and granuloma	Common	Absent
Mesentery lymph involvement	Edema and hyperplasia	Not involved
Toxic megacolon	Occasional	Occasional
Steatorrhea	Frequent	Absent
Malignant disease	Rare	After 10 yr
Fibrous stricture	Common	Absent
Clinical Manifestations		
Course of disease	Slowly progressive	Remissions and relapses
Rectal bleeding	Occasional	Common (90%-100%)
Abdominal pain	Colicky (45%)	Predefecation (60%-70%)
Hematochezia	Unusual or absent	Almost always present
Diarrhea	Present (65%-85%)	Early and frequent (80%-95%)
Vomiting	Present (35%)	Present (15%)
Nutritional deficit	Common	Common
Weight loss	Present (60%-70%)	Present (20%-50%)
Fever	Present (35%)	Present (10%)
Anal abscess	Common (75%)	Occasional (10%)
Fistula and anorectal fissure fistula	Common (80%)	Rare (10%-20%)
Systemic Manifestations		
Arthritis	Present (20%)	Uncommon (10%)
Peripheral sacroiliitis	18%	18%-20%
Hepatobiliary involvement	Uncommon	15% cholestatic dysfunction 19%-38% fatty liver 30%-50% pericholangitis
Skin: erythema nodosum, pyoderma gangrenosum	Common	Present (5%-10%)
Nephrolithiasis	Occasional	Rare

Modified from Black J, Matassarin-Jacobs E, editors: *Luckmann & Sorensen's medical-surgical nursing,* ed 4, Philadelphia, 1993, WB Saunders.

the colon (Kornbluth et al, 1998). In the portions of intestine involved, the inflammation may skip areas, and so these healthy segments of bowel separate inflamed portions. Mucosal involvement in Crohn's disease is transmural in that it affects all layers of the mucosa. As inflammation, ulceration, abscesses, and fistulas resolve, fibrosis, submucosal thickening, and scarring may result, leading to narrowed segments of bowel, localized strictures, and partial or complete obstruction of the intestinal lumen.

Medical Treatment

Surgery may be necessary to repair strictures or remove portions of the bowel when medical management fails. About 50% to 70% of persons with Crohn's disease will undergo surgery related to the disease (Hyams, 1996; Patel et al, 1997). Surgery does not cure the disease; recurrence often occurs within 1 to 3 years of surgery, and the chance of reoperation sometime in the patient's life is about 30% to 70%, depending on the type of surgery and the age at first operation. Major resections of the intestine may result in varying degrees of malabsorption of fluid and nutrients. In extreme cases, patients may have extensive or multiple resections, resulting short-bowel syndrome, and dependence on parenteral nutrition to maintain adequate nutrient intake and hydration.

Ulcerative Colitis

Pathophysiology

Ulcerative colitis involves only the colon, and the disease always extends from the rectum. Microscopic examination shows diffusely inflamed mucosa, usually with small ulcers. Continuous disease (rather than skipped areas) is characteristic. Serosal involvement, strictures, and significant narrowing are uncommon, but rectal bleeding or bloody diarrhea is relatively common (Jenkins, 2001; Jewell, 1998) (see Table 30-6 and Figure 30-4).

Ulcerative colitis occurs most commonly in young people 15 to 30 years of age, with a secondary peak at 50 to 60 years of age, although no age group is ex-

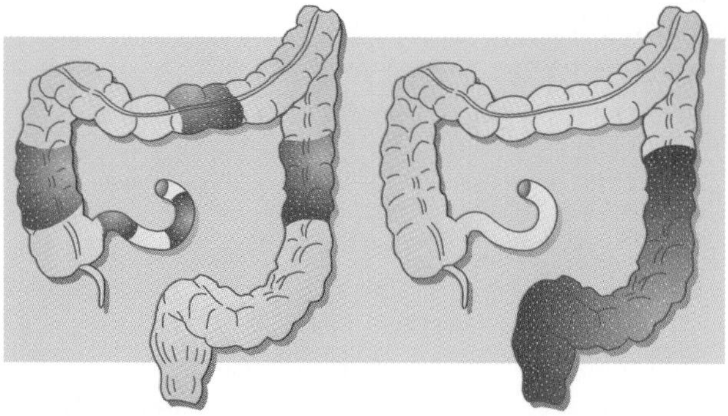

FIGURE 30-4 • Crohn's disease *(left)* and ulcerative colitis *(right)*. Whereas Crohn's disease typically involves the small and large intestine in a segmental manner, with intervening "skip" areas, ulcerative colitis is generally a contiguous disease process that starts in the rectum and progresses in a retrograde fashion to involve varying lengths of the colon. (Modified from Cotran KS, Kumar V, Robbins SI: *Robbins' pathologic basis of disease*, ed 4, Philadelphia, 1989, WB Saunders.)

empt. Persons with long-standing disease are at increased risk for cancer. In severe disease and with increased risk of cancer, complete removal of the colon is recommended, with creation of an ileostomy, ileal pouch, or ileoanal anastomosis.

Medical Management

The goals of treatment in IBD are to induce and maintain remission and to maintain nutritional status. Treatment of the primary GI manifestations appears to correct most of the extraintestinal features of the disease as well. The most effective medical agents during the acute stages of the disease are corticosteroids, although antiinflammatory agents (aminosalicylates), immunosuppressive agents (cyclosporine, azathioprine, mercaptopurine), and antibiotics (metronidazole) may be used for maintaining remission. Each carries the potential for medical and nutritional consequences (Regueiro, 2000). One of the newest therapeutic agents is monoclonal anti–tumor necrosis factor (anti-TNF) (infliximab), an agent that inactivates one of the primary inflammatory cytokines. It is normally used in more severe cases of Crohn's disease and in the management of fistulas, but it has not been shown to be effective in ulcerative colitis. Figure 30-5 shows an algorithm for reversing pediatric growth failure.

Investigations of various treatment modalities for the acute and chronic stages of IBD are ongoing and include new forms of existing drugs as well as new agents targeted to regulate cytokines, eicosanoids, or other mediators of the inflammatory/acute-phase cascade response (Holtmann et al, 2001; Panes, 2001; Regueiro, 2000). Use of prebiotics and probiotic cultures have been considered plausible because each has the potential to alter the GI microflora as well as the immunologic response at the gut level (Madsen, 2001).

Medical Nutrition Therapy

Persons with IBD are at increased risk of nutrition problems for a host of reasons related to the disease and its treatment, so the primary goal is to restore and maintain the nutritional status of the individual patient (Box 30-5). Foods, dietary and micronutrient supplements, enteral and parenteral nutrition may all be used to accomplish that mission. Diet and the other means of support may change during remissions and exacerbations of the disease. Persons with IBD often have fears and misconceptions regarding the significance of minor or major GI symptoms and the role of foods and nutrition. Patients are also often confused by advice from associates, various media, and health care providers. Education is a key form of therapy.

Diet and specific nutrients may play a role in maintaining or bringing on the remission of IBD. The ability of parenteral or enteral nutrition to induce remission of IBD has been debated for several years, and the issue is still not entirely resolved. At least in theory, the use of low-residue, low-fiber liquid diets can decrease the antigenic load or reduce microbial populations in the colon. Clinical trials with parenteral and enteral nutrition and other supplements have been confounded by small numbers of patients, differences in study design, severity and location of the disease, differences in the nutritional formulas, and whether an oral diet was continued. Evaluation is further confounded by the fact that the natural course of IBD is one of exacerbations and remissions.

Results of reviews and metaanalyses of several studies have generally concluded that (1) "bowel rest" with parenteral nutrition is not a major requirement for achieving remission, (2) enteral nutrition may be the preferred means of nutritional support, and (3) at least in some cases, enteral nutrition is more successful at inducing remission than parenteral nutrition (Han et al, 1999; Messori et al, 1996). Commitment from the patient and caretaker to the sole use of oral enteral formulas must be high, or the formula must be fed by tube; however, current enteral or parenteral nutrition formulas do not appear to be as consistently effective as corticosteroids or combination medical therapy in inducing remission.

Regardless of whether or not current forms of parenteral or enteral nutrition induce remission, timely nutritional support is a vital component of therapy to restore and maintain nutritional health (Beyer, 2001). Currently available parenteral solutions are not as complete or well suited as enteral nutrition, but parenteral nutrition may be required to restore nutrition in patients with obstructions, fistulas, severe disease, and major GI resections.

Malnutrition itself compromises digestive and absorptive function and may increase the permeability of the GI tract to potential inflammatory agents (Han et al, 1999). Energy needs of patients with IBD are not greatly increased (unless weight gain is desired), but

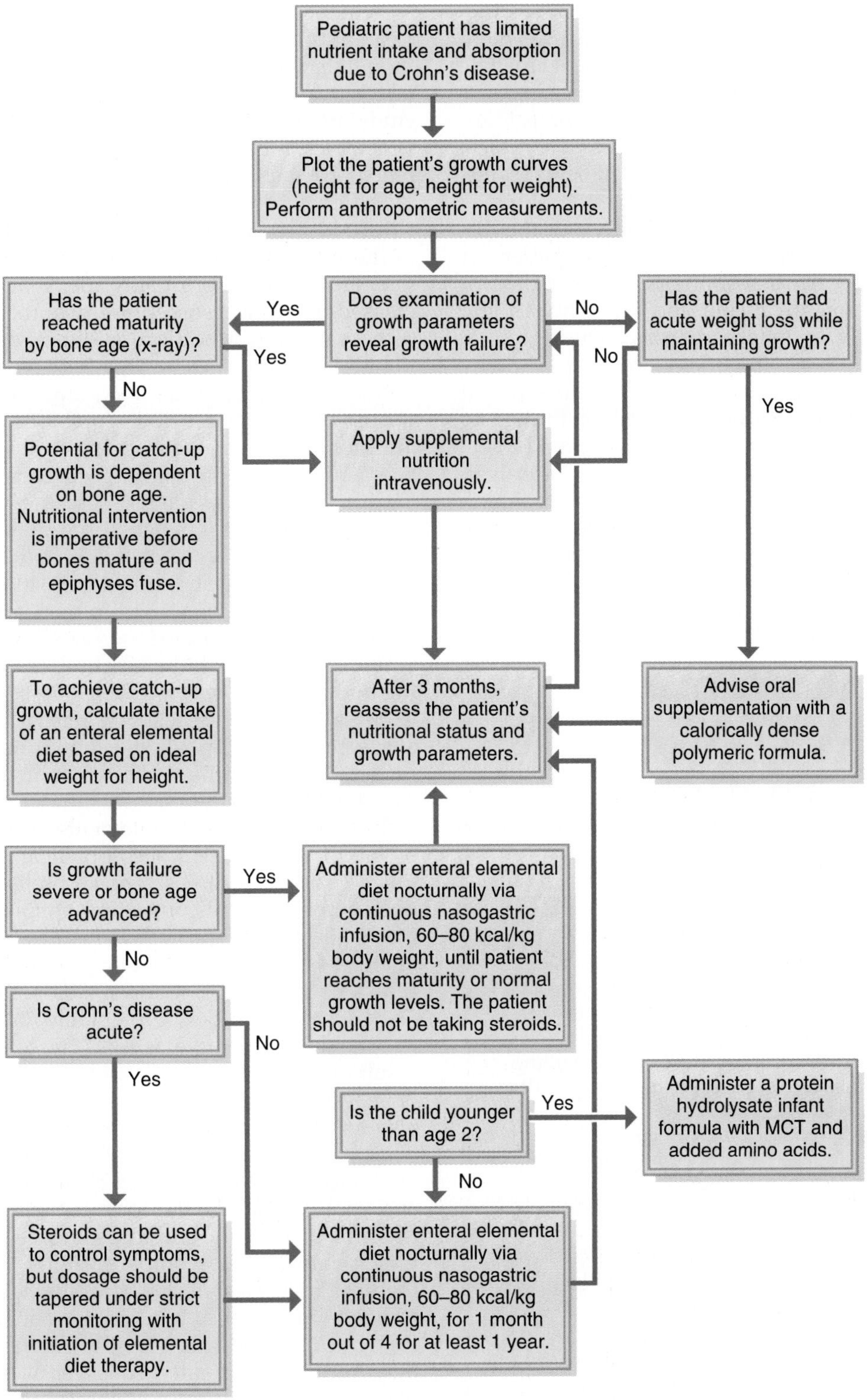

FIGURE 30-5 • Algorithm for reversing growth failure in pediatric patients with Crohn's disease. *MCT,* Medium-chain triglycerides. (Modified from RD 11:5, 1991, Norwick-Eaton Pharmaceuticals, New York, N.Y.)

protein requirements may be increased by 50%, especially during active stages of the disease. Supplemental vitamins and minerals and trace elements may be needed to replace stores or for maintenance because of maldigestion, malabsorption, drug-nutrient interactions, or because the patient cannot eat a complete diet. Diarrhea can aggravate losses of zinc, potassium, and selenium stores in particular.

During acute and severe exacerbations of the disease, the diet is tailored to the individual patient. A minimal-residue diet that limits poorly absorbed or hyperosmolar sugars, caffeine, and excess fiber might be used initially to reduce diarrhea. During either acute or chronic stages, inflammation or scarring may result in a partially obstructed bowel; and, in that case, fiber may have to be restricted or limited to minute particles to pass through the narrowed lumen. Small, frequent feedings may be tolerated better than large meals, and small amounts of isotonic, liquid, oral supplements may be valuable in restoring intake without provoking symptoms. In cases in which fat malabsorption is likely, supplementation with foods made with MCT may be valuable in adding calories and serving as a vehicle for fat-soluble nutrients.

Box 30-5. Potential Nutrition-Related Problems Associated With Inflammatory Bowel Disease

- Anemias related to blood loss and poor food intake
- Gastrointestinal (GI) narrowing and strictures leading to bloating, nausea, bacterial overgrowth, and diarrhea
- Inflammation and surgical resections resulting in diarrhea and malabsorption of bile salts and micronutrients and macronutrients
- Increased GI secretions with inflammation and increased transit leading to diarrhea and malabsorption
- Abdominal pain, nausea, vomiting, bloating, diarrhea
- Food aversions, anxiety, and fear of eating related to experiences with abdominal pain, bloating, nausea, or diarrhea
- Associations of foods, or the simple ingestion of foods, with adverse symptoms of the disease (leading to anxiety and avoidance of food, which further limits intake)
- Drug-nutrient interactions
- True and perceived food allergies
- Dietary restrictions, both iatrogenic and self-imposed
- Growth failure, weight loss, micronutrient deficiencies, and protein-calorie malnutrition

Whether dietary factors cause exacerbations is not clear, but they certainly can aggravate symptoms. Although study results are inconsistent, the dietary factors commonly noted before exacerbations include increased sucrose intake, lack of fruits and vegetables, a low intake of dietary fiber, and altered omega-6/omega-3 fatty acid ratios (Reif et al, 1997; Shoda et al, 1996). In a small number of patients, specific food allergies may be identified. The significance of these factors is not clear, but they may simply reflect an overall poor-quality diet that may have increased the overall susceptibility of the GI tract to the disease process. Modification of oral diets and nutritional formulas with omega-3 fatty acids, specific amino acids (e.g., glutamine), and antioxidants and the use of fermentable fibers (prebiotics) or probiotics are therapeutic strategies being evaluated for management of IBD (Han et al, 1999; Jacobasch et al, 1999; Madsen, 2001; Panes, 2001).

In everyday life, patients may have intermittent "flares" of the disease characterized by partial obstructions, nausea, abdominal pain, bloating, or diarrhea. Patients can be taught to manage their disease by selecting appropriate foods and beverages. For example, patients might be taught to restrict foods during bouts of diarrhea (see Table 30-1) or to limit fiber (especially large particles) if partial obstruction is suspected. They can also be shown how to increase omega-3 fats with food choices and supplements so as to benefit from their antiinflammatory effect.

Probiotic foods or supplements may hold promise by modifying the microbial flora. In animal models of inflammatory GI disease and in preliminary studies of humans with IBD, ingestion of specific strains or mixtures of probiotic organisms has been shown to alter the GI flora and to prolong periods of remission (Linskins et al, 2001; Madsen, 2001). Prebiotic foods (e.g., oligosaccharides, fermentable fibers, and resistant starches) can serve as fuels for colonic flora and result in altered microflora and increased production of SCFAs. The altered flora and SCFAs produced may also serve to attenuate the inflammatory process, especially in ulcerative colitis. Additional study continues to identify the dose and most effective prebiotic and probiotic foods, the form in which they can be used for therapeutic and maintenance purposes, and their relative value compared with other forms of therapy (Fukuda et al, 2002; Jacobasch et al, 1999).

Food intolerances are common in patients with IBD, but the foods are variable among patients and may not be incriminated consistently from one time to the next. Patients are sometimes advised simply to eliminate the foods that they suspect are responsible for the intolerance. Often, however, the patient becomes increasingly frustrated as the diet becomes more and more limited, and symptoms may not resolve. One study (Pearson et al, 1993) revealed no significant differences in the duration of remission between patients who did or did not identify food sensitivities.

Confirming true allergic GI reactions to foods is a difficult and painstaking process (see Chapter 32). The patient must be willing to consume either an amino acid diet or a very restricted diet composed of only three or four foods, with the addition of each of the suspected foods one at a time. The allergen is identified on the basis of subjective and objective symptoms related to the repeated addition and elimination of the food. Circulating antibodies to food proteins have been considered a sign of allergy but may in fact be a sign of increased permeability rather than local GI allergy.

The same foods that are most consistently responsible for GI symptoms (gas, bloating, and diarrhea) in a normal healthy population are likely to be the triggers for at least the same symptoms in patients with mild stages of IBD or those in remission. Patients receive nutritional information from a variety of sources, including support groups, Internet news groups, the audio and printed media, well-meaning friends, and food supplement salespersons. The information is sometimes inaccurate or exaggerated, or it may pertain only to one individual's situation. The health care provider can help patients sort out the role of foods in normal everyday GI disturbances and the role of foods in IBD and teach them how to evaluate valid nutrition information from unproved or exaggerated claims. Patients' participation in the management of their disease may help to reduce not only the symptoms of the disease but the associated anxiety level as well.

DISORDERS OF THE LARGE INTESTINE

Irritable Bowel Syndrome

Pathophysiology

Irritable bowel syndrome (IBS) is not a disease but a common syndrome involving altered intestinal motility, increased sensitivity of the GI tract, and increased awareness and responsiveness of the viscera to enteral and external stimuli. The disorder likely involves more than the large intestine, but most of the early speculation regarding the pathology of IBS focused on the colon. In IBS no obvious tissue damage, no inflammation, and no immunologic involvement are present. In all persons, the enteric nervous system is sensitive to the presence, chemical composition, and volume of foods, and the GI tract receives various types of input from the brain and the autonomic nervous system (see Chapter 1).

Persons with IBS tend to overrespond to many of these stimuli (Mayer, 2001; Simren et al, 2001). The mediators may be abnormal secretion of peptide hormones or signaling agents (e.g., neurotransmitters secreted in response to the hormones). The syndrome typically involves one of three predominant symptom patterns (diarrhea, constipation, or abdominal pain), but patients may describe combinations of GI complaints. GI discomfort after meals or with psychosocial distress, bloating, gas, heightened gastrocolic response, lowered threshold for normal GI discomfort, and abnormal bowel movements are all common with IBS.

The diagnosis is based on international consensus criteria (ROME I or II criteria) and diagnostic algorithms that help to rule out other GI or surgical disorders that may manifest with similar symptoms (Drossman, 1997; Thompson et al, 1999). According to the criteria, symptoms of abdominal discomfort must be present for at least 12 weeks of the past year and include at least two of three features: discomfort relieved by defecation, onset associated with a change in frequency of stool, and onset associated with a change in form of the stool.

The diagnosis is usually further refined to categorize the syndrome into subtypes, such as predominant patterns of alternating constipation and diarrhea, painless diarrhea, or constipation. The most common symptoms are alternating diarrhea and constipation, abdominal pain (typically relieved by defecation), and bloating; but perception of excessive flatulence, sensation of incomplete evacuation, rectal pain, and mucus in the stool may also occur (Figure 30-6).

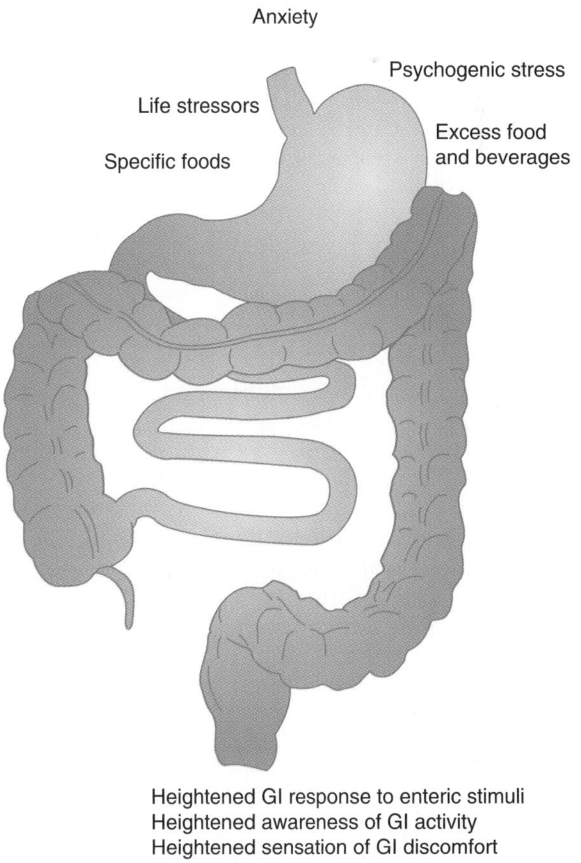

FIGURE 30-6 • Heightened gastrointestinal response to enteric stimuli.

Symptoms typically first occur between adolescence and the fourth decade of life, but many persons do not bring the problem to the attention of a physician. In the United States, IBS occurs in about 20% of women and 10% to 15% of men. It represents about 12% of visits to family medicine clinics and 20% to 40% of visits to gastroenterologists, and it is one of the most common reasons for which patients first seek medical care (Drossman et al, 1997; Olden and Schuster, 1998). Persons with IBD often have increased absenteeism from school and work, decreased productivity, increased health care costs, and decreased quality of life as a result of their symptoms.

Persons with IBS appear to have altered enteric sensitivity and motility in response to usual GI and environmental stimuli. They react more significantly than normal persons to intestinal distention, dietary indiscretions, and psychosocial factors (Drossman et al, 1997). Normal persons may experience mild GI disturbances in response to all the situations mentioned, but they appear to have a milder response. Life stressors, such as employment changes, travel, relocation, or uncomfortable social situations, may trigger the onset or worsen symptoms and may override many therapeutic efforts. A history of psychosocial trauma, such as physical or sexual abuse, has been reported in 32% to 44% of cases, but the higher estimate may be somewhat exaggerated as a result of sampling.

In addition to stress and dietary patterns, factors that may worsen symptoms include (1) excess use of laxatives and other over-the-counter medications, (2) antibiotics, (3) caffeine, (4) previous GI illness, and (5) lack of regularity in sleep, rest, and fluid intake. In patients with a strong family history of allergy, hypersensitivity to certain foods may be the cause of IBS (Bischoff et al, 1996). A trial of food elimination and challenge may be justified under these circumstances (see Chapter 32).

Medical Management

Management includes a combination of approaches to deal with the symptoms and the factors that may trigger them. Education, medications, counseling, and diet all play a role in the care. Depending on the predominant pattern and severity of the symptoms, medications may include antispasmodic, anticholinergic, antidiarrheal, prokinetic, or antidepressive agents. Newer agents are being evaluated to target specific neurotransmitters, peptides, or other mechanisms involved in the GI motility and enteric nervous system. Biofeedback, relaxation, and stress reduction techniques may also be useful (Drossman, 1997; Villanueva et al, 2001).

Medical Nutrition Therapy

Unlike IBD, IBS is not life threatening and does not result in maldigestion or malabsorption of nutrients. However, dietary practices of persons with IBS may result in a less than complete diet, insufficient nutrient intake, and less enjoyment of foods. Dietary selections and patterns are also important in controlling symptoms.

The aim of nutritional care is to ensure adequate nutrient intake, to guide the patient toward a diet that is not likely to contribute to symptoms, and to explain the role of ordinary dietary practices in producing or avoiding GI symptoms. The recommendations made for all persons for a good-quality diet are probably even more important in IBS. Excesses of dietary fat; caffeine; sugars such as lactose, fructose, and sorbitol (Rumessen and Gudmand-Hoyer, 1998); large meals; and alcohol are less well tolerated than in normal persons. Dietary fiber intake in adolescents and adults is typically about half that recommended. Excessive use of bran or coarse fibers is not needed or recommended, but increasing dietary fiber to the recommended 25 g or so per day may help to normalize bowel habit in all types of IBS patterns. If the patient is not able to consume fiber from food sources or does not respond adequately, fiber in the form of bulk laxatives (e.g., psyllium) may be helpful. Consumption of adequate fluid is recommended, especially when powdered fiber supplements are used. Large doses of wheat bran are no longer recommended and may exacerbate symptoms in some persons with IBS.

Foods with fiber, resistant starches, and oligosaccharides may also serve as prebiotic foods, which favor the maintenance of "healthy" microflora and resistance to pathogenic infections (Madsen, 2001; Nobaek et al, 2000). Results of initial studies on the use of prebiotic and probiotic supplements have been mixed, but additional studies with different products, doses, and subtypes of IBS are needed. The nutrition practitioner can work with the person with IBS to identify his or her concerns and perceptions, review the characteristics of the disease and the potential role of foods, and teach the client how to reduce the food-related symptoms associated with the syndrome. Sometimes clients become trapped in a vicious cycle in which anxiety about food, GI distress, and social embarrassment leave them with an unnecessarily restrictive diet, worsening nutritional status, increasing anxiety, and worsening symptoms. Calming reassurance and gradual return to a good diet with limitations of only items that likely will exacerbate symptoms will often greatly improve the quality of life.

Diverticular Disease

Pathophysiology

Diverticulosis is a situation of saclike herniations (diverticula) of the colonic wall, thought to result from long-term constipation and increased colonic pressures (Figure 30-7). The incidence of diverticulosis increases with age. Thirty percent of persons older than 50 years of age, 50% of those older than 70 years, and 66% of those 85 years of age and older develop diver-

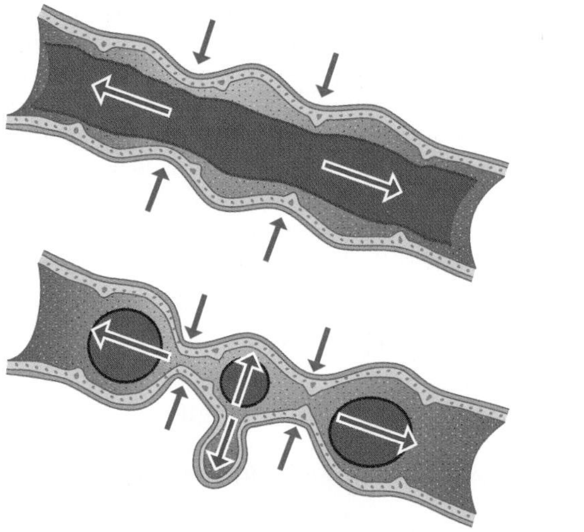

FIGURE 30-7 • Mechanism by which low-fiber, low-bulk diets might generate diverticula. Where the colon contents are bulky *(top)*, muscular contractions exert pressure longitudinally. If the fecal contents are small in diameter *(bottom)*, contractions can produce occlusion and exert pressure against the colon wall, which may produce a diverticular hernia.

ticulosis (Simmang and Shires, 1998). Sigmoid involvement occurs in almost all cases; right-sided colonic involvement occurs in Asians, but it is rare in whites).

The cause is not known for certain, but studies in animals and humans relate the disorder to constipation and lifelong increased intracolonic pressures. The pressures result from attempts to propel small, dry, hard fecal material through the lumen of the bowel. Theoretically, circular muscles completely close around the fecal material when the stools are small and longitudinal muscles contract, attempting to push the contents distally. Increased pressures result in the opportunity for herniations of the mucosal wall to develop through weaker segments of the colon (Simmang and Shires, 1998) (see Figures 30-7 and 30-8). This theory is supported by epidemiologic studies of populations consuming high- and low-fiber diets, prospective cohort studies in men, and experimental studies in animals fed low-fiber diets throughout their lifetimes (Scheppach et al, 2001). An abnormal pattern of excitatory innervation of the colon has been associated with intraluminal pressures and the presence of diverticulosis, but it is not known whether the pattern is a consequence of the disorder or related to the cause (Tomita et al, 1999).

In general, diverticular disease is (1) relatively rare in countries where a high-fiber diet is part of the lifelong pattern, and (2) increasing where "westernization" of the diet and increased intake of refined foods of the diet have begun (Camilleri et al, 2000; Scheppach et al, 2001). Lack of exercise may also contribute to the development of diverticular disease, presumably because of the more sluggish movement of GI contents (Peters et al, 2001).

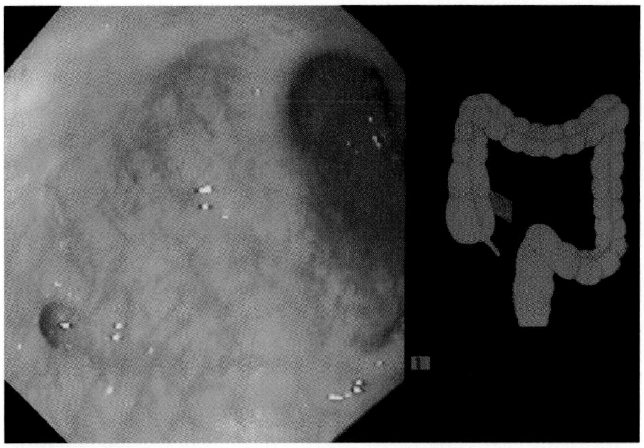

FIGURE 30-8 • Actual internal photograph of diverticular pouch. (Courtesy Pitt County Memorial Hospital, Greenville, N.C.)

Medical and Surgical Treatment

Complications of diverticular disease range from painless, mild bleeding and altered bowel habits to diverticulitis, which may include its own clinical spectrum of inflammation, abscess formation, acute perforation, acute bleeding, obstruction, and sepsis. About 10% to 25% of patients with diverticulosis develop diverticulitis, and about one third of those admitted to hospitals for diverticular disease require surgery. Death rates in patients requiring surgical intervention may be as high as 10% (Deckman and Cheskin, 1993).

Medical Nutrition Therapy

At one time it was thought that "roughage" (dietary fiber) aggravated diverticular disease, so the classic diet therapy was one that was low in fiber. It is now recognized that a high-fiber diet promotes soft, bulky stools that pass more swiftly, require less straining with defecation, and result in lower intracolonic pressures (Scheppach et al, 2001). High-fiber intakes have been found to relieve symptoms for most patients, and exercise appears to aid in both constipation and diverticular disease (Cheek and Radley, 1999; Peters, 2001; Sheppach et al, 2001).

Patients who have followed a low-fiber diet for years may require extensive encouragement to adopt the high-fiber approach. Fiber intake should be increased gradually because it may cause bloating or gas; however, these side effects usually disappear within 2 to 3 weeks. In cases in which the patient cannot consume the necessary amount of fiber, methylcellulose and psyllium fiber supplements have been used with good results. Adequate fluid intake (e.g., 2 to 3 L daily) should accompany the high-fiber intake.

For patients with an acute flareup of diverticulitis, a low-residue diet, elemental diet, or, in complicated cases, total parenteral nutrition may be required initially, followed by a gradual return to a high-fiber diet. Colonic smooth-muscle contractions, which intensify after a high-fat meal, may contribute to the discomfort felt by persons with diverticular disease (Snape, 1994). Therefore, a low-fat diet may be reasonable to suggest for these patients, at least initially.

The question of whether the consumption of seeds, nuts, or skins of plant matter should be avoided to prevent complications of diverticular disease or after bouts of diverticulitis to aid in healing remains unresolved. Common sense tends to favor avoiding consumption of very coarse materials such as husks (not necessarily seeds) like those surrounding sunflower seeds and peanuts. Whether seeds or normal fibrous materials play any role in the onset of symptoms or actually harm the diverticula has not been determined. In patients with clear cases of perforation or obstruction, large pieces of coarse plant matter might be restricted and patients should be encouraged to chew fibrous foods thoroughly.

Colon Cancer and Polyps

Pathophysiology

In the United States, colon cancer is the second most common cancer in adults (after lung cancer) and is also the second most common cause of death. The number of new cases of colorectal cancer in 2002 was estimated to be about 148,000 cases (American Cancer Society, 2002). Worldwide, it is the third most common malignant neoplasm and the second leading cause of cancer deaths. Colon cancer occurs more commonly in men than in women (52 versus 38 cases per 100,000 population, respectively). The highest rates are seen in whites of northern European origin. Rates in Africa and Asia are lower, but they tend to rise with migration and westernization.

Factors that increase the risk of colorectal cancer include family history, occurrence of IBD (both Crohn's disease and ulcerative colitis), familial polyposis, adenomatous polyps, and several dietary components. Polyps are considered precursors of colon cancers (see Chapter 40).

Use of aspirin and nonsteroidal antiinflammatory agents and exercise appear to be protective against colon cancer (Peters et al, 2001; Reddy, 2000; Slattery, 2000). Dietary risk factors may include increased meat or fat intake and inadequate intake of several micronutrients. Protective factors include intake of fruits, vegetables, several phytochemicals, high-fiber grains, omega-3 fatty acids, and carotenoids; maintenance of acceptable weight; the vitamins D, E, and folate; and the minerals calcium, zinc, and selenium (Garland et al, 1999; Reddy, 2000; Wollowske et al, 2001).

The role of dietary fat in colon carcinogenesis is not entirely clear because different dietary lipids may have different effects. Red meats, such as beef, pork, and lamb, along with their fats, may be incriminated more than other types of meats; poultry, fish, and dairy fats appear to have less of a role in carcinogenesis. Food preparation methods may also influence the carcinogenic potential of meats and fatty foods (Giovannucci and Goldin, 1997; Parodi, 1997) (see Chapter 40).

The use of prebiotics and probiotics alters colonic microflora, induces glutathione transferase, increases butyrate content of the stool, reduces toxic and genotoxic compounds, and in animal models reduces the development of some precancerous lesions (Brady et al, 2000; Wollowske et al, 2001).

Medical Management

Patients diagnosed with colorectal polyps or cancer may require moderate to significant interventions, including medications, radiation therapy, chemotherapy, colonic surgery, and parenteral nutritional support.

Medical Nutrition Therapy

Most Americans consume far less than the recommended amounts of fruits, vegetables, legumes, whole grains, and dairy products. Therefore the best advice for many patients might be to improve their diet based on recommendations from the American Cancer Society or the National Research Council or the *Dietary Guidelines for Americans.* These recommendations promote the consumption of adequate amounts of whole-grain breads and cereals, calcium-containing foods, fruits and vegetables, adequate micronutrient intake, and reasonable amounts of omega-3 fatty acids (from marine sources and other sources, such as flaxseed oil) along with adequate exercise. Cancer survivors should also be encouraged to follow these same nutrition and exercise guidelines.

INTESTINAL SURGERY

Small-Bowel Resections and Short-Bowel Syndrome

Short-bowel syndrome (SBS) refers to the malabsorption of fluid and nutrients associated with significant resections of the small intestine, which results in only 3 to 5 feet of intact small bowel remaining. The healthy small intestine has significant reserve, but resections of 40% to 60% may lead to several consequences of SBS, depending on the site of the resection and other factors. Resection of the distal ileum has the most significant impact on risk of SBS. Colonic resections alone do not produce SBS, but the risk of dehydration, electrolyte disorders, and malnutrition is increased after distal small-bowel resections or colon removal. The most common reasons for major resections of the intestine in adults include Crohn's disease, radiation enteritis, mesenteric infarct, malignant disease, and volvulus (Beyer, 2001). In the pediatric population, most cases of SBS result from congenital anomalies of the GI tract, atresia, volvulus, or necrotizing enterocolitis (Sigalet, 2001).

Obvious complications of short-bowel syndrome include malabsorption of micronutrients and macronutrients, fluid and electrolyte imbalances, weight loss, and growth failure (in children). Gastric hypersecretion, oxalate renal stones, cholesterol gallstones, and rarely *d*-lactic acidosis may also occur (Sundarum et al, 2002). The severity of malabsorption, the extent of complications, and the degree of dependence on parenteral nutritional support reflect the length and location of the resection, the age of the patient at the time of the operation, and the health of the remaining GI tract (Beyer, 2001; Wilmore et al, 1997) (Box 30-6).

Jejunal Resections

Normally most digestion and absorption of food and nutrients occurs in the first 100 cm of small intestine. What remains to be digested or fermented and absorbed are small amounts of sugars, resistant starch, fiber, lipids, dietary fiber, and fluids. After jejunal resections, the ileum is able to perform the functions of the jejunum, especially after a period of adaptation. The motility of the ileum is comparatively slow, and hormones secreted in the ileum and colon help to slow gastric emptying and secretions. Because jejunal resections result in reduced surface area and shorter intestinal transit than normal, the functional reserve for absorption of micronutrients, excess amounts of sugars (especially lactose), and lipids is reduced.

Ileal Resections

Significant resections of the ileum, especially the distal ileum, generally produce major nutritional and medical complications. The distal ileum is the only site for absorption of the vitamin B_{12}/intrinsic factor complex and bile salts, and the ileum normally absorbs a major portion of the several liters of fluid ingested and secreted into the GI tract (see Chapter 1). Although malabsorption of bile salts may appear to be a rather benign problem, it creates a potentially serious cascade of consequences (Beyer, 2001) (Box 30-7).

If the ileum cannot "recycle" bile salts secreted into the GI tract, hepatic production cannot maintain a sufficient bile salt pool or the secretions to emulsify lipids. The gastric and pancreatic lipases are capable of digesting some triglycerides to fatty acids and monoglycerides, but without adequate micelle formation facilitated by bile salts, lipids are poorly absorbed. This can result in significant malabsorption of fats and fat-soluble vitamins A, D, and E. In addition, malabsorption of fatty acids results in their combination with divalent cations, such as calcium, zinc, and magnesium, to form fatty acid–mineral "soaps." This results in malabsorption of these nutrients. To compound matters, colonic absorption of oxalate, which normally is bound to the divalent cations, is increased, leading to hyperoxaluria and increased renal oxalate stones. Relative dehydration and concentrated urine, which are common with ileal resections, may further increase the risk of stone formation.

If the patient has any colon left, malabsorption of what bile salts are secreted can act as irritants to the mucosa, resulting in increased fluid and electrolyte secretion and increased colonic motility rather than absorption. Consumption of high-fat diets with ileal

Box 30-6. Factors Affecting the Course of Short-Bowel Syndrome

- Length of remaining small intestine
- Loss of ileum, especially distal one third
- Loss of ileocecal valve
- Loss of colon
- Disease in remaining segment(s) of gastrointestinal tract
- Radiation enteritis
- Coexisting malnutrition
- Older age at surgery

Box 30-7. Consequences of Ileal Resection

- Rapid transit of intestinal contents
- Decreased fluid absorptive area
- Malabsorption of vitamin B_{12}/intrinsic factor complex
- Malabsorption of bile salts
- Inadequate bile salts for lipid solubilization, digestion, and absorption, leading to loss of fat and fat-soluble nutrients
- Loss of secreted bile salts into colon because of decreased reabsorption
- Formation of hydroxy fatty acids by colonic bacteria from malabsorbed fat, resulting in decreased fluid and electrolyte absorption
- Malabsorption of Ca^{2+}, Mg^{2+}, and Zn^{2+} because of formation of insoluble "soaps" with malabsorbed free fatty acids
- Increased risk of oxalate stones because of increased colonic absorption of oxalate, which normally binds to Ca^{2+}, Zn^{2+}, and Mg^{2+}

resections and retained colon may also result in the formation of hydroxy fatty acids, which also can increase fluid secretion. Cholesterol gallstones may occur more often because the ratio of bile acid, phospholipid, and cholesterol in biliary secretions is altered as a result of ileal resections. Dependence on parenteral nutrition may further increase the risk of biliary "sludge" secondary to decreased stimulus for evacuation of the biliary tract.

Lactic acidosis is a relatively rare complication that occurs only with severe SBS and remaining colon. The problem results from excessive intake and malabsorption of carbohydrate. Metabolic acidosis and production of *d*-lactate result from fermentation of carbohydrate, production of SCFAs, reduced colonic pH, and proliferation of acid-resistant colonic microbes that produce *d*-lactate (Bongaerts et al, 1997). The problem is resolved by treating the metabolic acidosis and reducing the intake of sugars and total carbohydrates.

Medical and Surgical Management of Resections

Medications are prescribed to retard gastric emptying, decrease secretions, slow GI motility, and treat bacterial overgrowth. Recently, somatostatin and somatostatin analogs and other hormones with antisecretory, antimotility, or trophic actions have been used to retard both motility and secretions (Drucker, 2002; Sundarum et al, 2002). Surgical procedures, including reversal of segments of bowel to slow transit of GI contents, creation of reservoirs ("pouches") to serve as a form of colon, intestinal lengthening, and intestinal transplant, have been performed to help patients with major GI resections (Pirenne et al, 2001). Intestinal transplant is still one of the most difficult organ transplants and is typically reserved for gut failure and when patients develop significant complications from TPN.

Medical Nutrition Therapy

Most patients who have significant bowel resections require TPN initially to restore and maintain nutritional status (Sundaram et al, 2002). The duration of TPN and subsequent nutrition therapy is based on the extent of the bowel resection, the health of the patient, and the condition of the remaining GI tract. In general, older patients with major ileal resections, patients who have lost the ileocecal valve, and patients with residual disease in the remaining GI tract do not fare as well. Some may require lifetime supplementation with parenteral nutrition to maintain adequate fluid and nutritional status.

The two general principles for resuming enteral nutrition after small-bowel resections are (1) to start enteral feedings early and (2) to increase feeding concentration and volume gradually over time (Beyer, 2001; Vanderhoof and Young, 2001). The role of enteral feedings is to provide a trophic stimulus to the GI tract; parenteral nutrition is used to restore and maintain nutrient status. The more severe the problem, the slower the progression. Small, frequent, minimeals (6 to 10 per day) are likely to be better tolerated than larger feedings. If enteral feedings are used, gradual introduction of feedings stimulates GI adaptation; TPN provides the major source of fluid and nutrients. More nutrients are gradually added enterally, and the volume or concentration of TPN decreases accordingly. Because of malnutrition and disuse of the GI tract, the digestive and absorptive functions of the remaining GI tract may be compromised, and malnutrition itself will delay adaptation (Cronk et al, 2000). The transition to more normal foods may take weeks to months, and some patients may never tolerate normal concentrations or volumes of foods.

Maximal adaptation of the GI tract may take up to a year after surgery. Adaptation improves function, but it does not restore the intestine to normal length or capacity. Whole foods are some of the most important stimuli to the GI tract, but other nutritional measures have been considered as a means of hastening the adaptive process and decreasing malabsorption. Glutamine, for example, is the preferred fuel for small intestinal enterocytes and so may be valuable in enhancing adaptation. Nucleotides may also enhance mucosal adaptation, but unfortunately they are often lacking in parenteral and enteral nutritional products. SCFAs (e.g., butyrate, propionate, acetate), produced from microbial fermentation of carbohydrate and fibers, are major fuels of the colonic epithelium (Mortensen and Clausen, 1996).

Patients with jejunal resections and an intact ileum and colon will likely adapt quickly to normal diets. A normal balance of protein, fat, and carbohydrate sources is satisfactory. Six small feedings, with avoidance of lactose, large amounts of concentrated sweets, and caffeine, may help to reduce the risk of bloating, abdominal pain, and diarrhea. Because the typical American diet may be nutritionally lacking and utilization of some micronutrients may be marginal, patients should be advised that the quality of their diet is of utmost importance. A multivitamin and mineral supplement may be required to meet nutritional needs.

Patients with ileal resections require increased time and patience in the advancement from parenteral to enteral nutrition. Because of losses, fat-soluble vitamins, calcium, magnesium, and zinc may need to be supplemented. Dietary fat may need to be limited, especially in those with remaining colon. Small amounts at each feeding are more likely to be tolerated and absorbed. MCT products add to the caloric intake and serve as a vehicle for lipid-soluble nutrients.

Because boluses of MCT oil (e.g., taken as a medication in tablespoon amounts) may add to the patient's diarrhea, it is best to divide the doses equally in feedings throughout the day. Fluid and electrolytes, especially sodium, should be provided in small amounts and frequently.

In patients with massive resections (e.g., when the duodenum and a few inches of jejunum are anastomosed to segments of colon), an oral diet will be able to nourish only partially. In some cases, overfeeding in an attempt to compensate for malabsorption results in further malabsorption, not only of ingested foods and liquids but also of the significant amounts of GI fluids secreted in response to food ingestion. Patients with an extremely short bowel are typically nutritionally dependent on parenteral solutions for at least part of their nutrient and fluid supply. Small, frequent snacks provide some oral gratification for these patients but typically can supply only a portion of their fluid and nutrient needs.

Blind-Loop Syndrome (Bacterial Overgrowth)

Pathophysiology

Blind-loop syndrome is a disorder characterized by bacterial overgrowth resulting from stasis of the intestinal tract as an outcome of obstructive disease, radiation enteritis, fistula formation, or surgical repair of the intestine. Bacteria deconjugate bile salts, which besides being cytotoxic in this form, are also less effective as micelle formers. Poor fat absorption and steatorrhea result. Carbohydrate malabsorption occurs because of injury to the brush border secondary to the toxic effects of the products of bacterial catabolism and consequent enzyme loss. The expanding numbers of bacteria use the available vitamin B_{12} for their own growth.

Medical Treatment

Treatment is directed toward the removal of the blind loop or control of the bacterial growth with antibiotics.

Medical Nutrition Therapy

Use of a lactose-free diet, along with MCT and parenteral vitamin B_{12}, may be useful.

Fistula Repair

Pathophysiology

Fistulas occur as a result of prenatal developmental error, trauma, or inflammatory or malignant disease processes. Fistulas of the intestinal tract can be serious threats to nutritional status because large amounts of fluid and electrolytes are lost, and malabsorption and infection can occur.

Medical Treatment

Fluid and electrolyte balance must be restored; infection must be brought under control; and aggressive nutritional support is mandatory to permit spontaneous or surgical closure of the fistula and wound.

Medical Nutrition Therapy

Either TPN or defined liquid formula diets have been used successfully in patients with fistulas (see Chapter 23). The success rate of either method depends on the location and the cause of the fistula and the patient's overall condition.

Ileostomy or Colostomy

Pathophysiology

Patients with severe ulcerative colitis, Crohn's disease, colon cancer, or intestinal trauma frequently require the surgical creation of an opening from the body surface to the intestinal tract to permit defecation from the intact portion of the intestine. When the entire colon, rectum, and anus must be removed, an ileostomy, or opening into the ileum, is performed. If only the rectum and anus are removed, a colostomy can provide entrance to the colon. In some cases, a temporary opening may be made to allow surgery and healing of more distal parts of the intestinal tract.

The opening, or stoma, eventually shrinks to the size of a nickel. The output from the stoma depends on its location, as shown in Figure 30-9. The consistency of the stool from an ileostomy is liquid, whereas that from a colostomy ranges from mushy to fairly well formed. Stool from a colostomy on the left side of the colon is firmer than that from a colostomy on the right side. Odor is a major concern of the patient with an ileostomy or colostomy; however, an ileostomy stool usually has a weakly acidic odor that is not unpleasant.

Medical Treatment

Patients with a permanent colostomy or ileostomy require sympathetic understanding from the entire health care team. Acceptance of the condition and the problems involved in maintaining bowel regularity is usually difficult. Nursing personnel, especially ostomy specialists, can play a major role in supporting and teaching patients with ostomies. Having these patients meet other people who have undergone similar surgery may help with the adjustment. Eventually, they may be encouraged by the realization that, in the future, they will not have the multiple hospitalizations or chronic disabilities that accompanied their intestinal disease.

Medical Nutrition Therapy

Malodorous stool is usually caused by steatorrhea or bacteria acting on particular foodstuffs to produce odorous gas. Because an individual patient may have different flora, types and amounts of gases and odors may differ among patients and with different dietary practices. Patients learn to observe their stools to de-

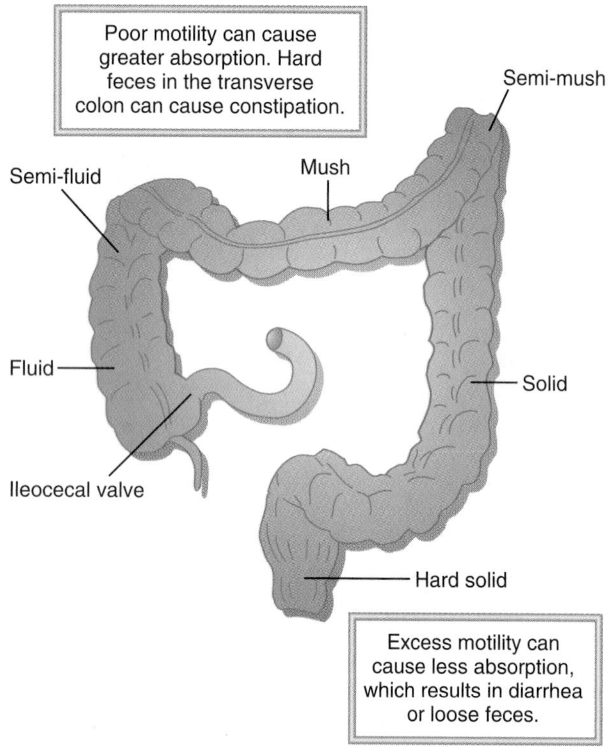
Poor motility can cause greater absorption. Hard feces in the transverse colon can cause constipation.
Semi-mush
Semi-fluid
Mush
Fluid
Solid
Ileocecal valve
Hard solid
Excess motility can cause less absorption, which results in diarrhea or loose feces.

FIGURE 30-9 • As the feces move from the ileocecal valve to the anus, water is absorbed and the feces become more solid. The characteristics of the output from a colostomy depend on its location in the colon.

termine which foods to eliminate, and this differs from one patient to the next. Foods that tend to cause odor from a colostomy are legumes, onions, garlic, cabbage, highly spiced foods, fish, antibiotics, and some vitamin and mineral supplements. Persistent odor may be attributable to poor stoma hygiene or to an ileostomy complication that allows bacterial overgrowth in the ileum. Deodorants are available, and modern pouch appliances are odor proof. Gas production may cause the pouch to become tense and distended, and accidental dislodgment is likely. The nutritional recommendations for reducing flatulence, presented at the beginning of this chapter, may be helpful for patients with colostomies.

The normal output from the ileum to the colon is in the range of 750 to 1.5 L in the intact GI tract. After a colectomy and creation of an ileostomy, adaptation occurs within 1 to 2 weeks. Fecal output will lessen and stools will become less liquid. Reduction in stool volume may not occur to the same extent in patients who have had an ileal resection in addition to a colectomy. Depending on the amount of ileum resected, their ileal output may be 1.5 to 5 times greater than that of the patient who has had only a colectomy. Patients with ileostomies have an above-average need for salt and water to compensate for excessive losses in stool. Inadequate water intake can result in small urine volumes and a predisposition for renal calculi. A normal diet provides adequate sodium, and patients should be instructed to drink at least 1 L more than their ostomy output daily.

The patient with a normal, functional ileostomy usually does not become nutritionally depleted. Surgical procedures, such as ileostomy, may require specific dietary changes but no greater energy intake; caloric expenditures in these patients are similar to those of normal subjects. Those who also undergo resection of the terminal ileum need vitamin B_{12} supplementation or intravenous injections. Patients with an ileostomy may have low vitamin C and folate intakes because of low fresh vegetable and fruit intakes, and they require supplementation. Patients with ileostomies should be guided by physiologic reasons for intolerance of foods, not by anecdotal reports. Because it is possible for a food bolus to get caught at the point where the ileum narrows as it enters the abdominal wall, it is important to warn the patient to avoid very fibrous vegetables and to chew all food well. Other than this, patients with either an ileostomy or a colostomy should be encouraged to follow their normal diet, omitting only those foods known to cause problems.

Ileal Pouch After Colectomy

Pathophysiology

As an alternative to creation of an ileostomy for persons who have had their colons removed, surgeons can create a reservoir using a portion of the distal ileum (ileal pouch). Folds of the ileum are joined together to create a small pouch, which is then connected to the rectum and ileum. This is called an *ileal pouch–anal anastomosis* (IPAA). The most common pouch is the J pouch, but S and W pouches are sometimes created using additional folds of ileum (Pemberton and Phillips, 1998). Like the colon, the pouch develops a microflora capable of at least partially fermenting fiber and carbohydrate (Alles et al, 1997). Because the reservoir is smaller than the colon, bowel movements are likely to occur more frequently than normal, between four and eight times daily.

Medical Treatment

Vitamin B_{12} injections are usually required because, as in blind loop syndrome, the microbes may compete for and bind intraluminal vitamin B_{12}. Other problems commonly reported include obstruction, "pouchitis," and increased stool output, frequency, and gas (Thompson-Fawcett et al, 1997; Pemberton and Phillips, 1998).

The incidence of obstruction may be lessened with attention to particle size of fibrous foods, chewing thoroughly, and consuming small meals frequently throughout the day. Stool frequency and volume do not return to normal, however. The normal, intact colon absorbs 80% to 90% of the liter or so of fluid entering from the ileum, leaving only 100 to 200 ml. After surgery, the remaining ileum does adapt to a small degree by increasing efficiency of fluid absorption, but even after adaptation, fluid output is always in the range of 300 to 600 ml.

Pouchitis, as implied by the name, is an inflammation of the mucosal tissue forming the pouch. The associated pathologic changes have been described as being somewhat similar to that of IBD (e.g., ulcerative colitis) (Goldstein et al, 1997). The cause of pouchitis is not entirely clear, but it may be related to selected bacterial overgrowth, bile salt malabsorption, or insufficient SCFA production. Antibiotics are the primary form of therapy, but experiments with different types of dietary fiber, prebiotics and probiotics, and other nutrient components are being investigated (Alles et al, 1997; Sandborn et al, 2000).

Medical Nutrition Therapy

The same dietary measures that are used by others to reduce excessive stool output (reduced caffeine, lactose avoidance in lactose-intolerant persons, avoidance of sorbitol) will likely reduce stool volume and frequency in persons with pouches. Adequate fluid and electrolyte intake are especially important because of the increase in intestinal losses.

Rectal Surgery

Nutritional care after rectal surgery, such as hemorrhoidectomy, should be directed toward maintaining an intake that will allow wound repair and prevent infection of the wound by feces. The frequency of stools is minimized by the use of constipating drugs and a minimal-residue diet (see Table 30-1). Chemically defined diets are low in residue, and their use can reduce stool volume and frequency to as little as 50 g every 6 days, making the surgical construction of a temporary colostomy unnecessary. A normal diet is resumed after healing is complete, and the patient is instructed about the benefits of eating a high-fiber diet to avoid constipation in the future (see Table 30-1).

SUMMARY

The GI tract is one of the largest sites of exposure to the outside environment. The function of the GI tract in monitoring and sealing the host interior (gut barrier) plays an important role in health maintenance. Disruptions in the gut barrier following injury from nonsteroidal antiinflammatory drugs and oxidative stress have been linked to multiorgan system failure in sepsis and immune dysregulation (DeMeo et al, 2002). Contribution of gut barrier dysfunction to GI disease is an evolving concept. As evidence for the role of gut barrier dysfunction in disorders such as Crohn's disease, celiac disease, food allergy, and related disorders mounts, new treatments and medical nutrition therapies will be developed.

Clinical Scenario 1

Suzanne is a 33-year-old teacher with Crohn's disease who has been referred for evaluation because of abdominal pain, bloating, and occasional nausea and diarrhea. The physician suspects a distal small-bowel stricture. Suzanne is seeking information about what to eat to prevent the problem from worsening during the 3-day period before her appointment at the clinic.

1. What information would be appropriate to gather about this patient before you advise her about a nutritional plan?
2. What, in terms of Suzanne's symptoms, makes the physician suspect a stricture?
3. What kind of dietary advice, based solely on her presumed problem, might be warranted?

Clinical Scenario 2

Mrs. Smith has IBS with a pattern of alternating constipation and diarrhea. She comes to you requesting dietary advice for (1) day-to-day management and (2) what might be "safest" to eat when she is getting ready to present weekly to biweekly reports to the executives in her large consulting company.

1. What do you want to know about Mrs. Smith's diet, perspectives, and lifestyle?
2. What foods or eating patterns would be best (or best to avoid) for Mrs. Smith for her day-to-day activities?
3. Why might she be asking for advice during stressful periods?

Relevant Web Sites

Celiac Disease
www.niddk.nih.gov/health/digest/pubs/celiac/
Crohn's Colitis Foundation
www.ccfa.org/
Gastrointestinal Disorders and Treatment
www.niddk.nih.gov/health/digest/digest.htm
Gluten Enteropathy Resources
www.gluten.net
www.glutenfreediet.com
www.niddk.nih.gov/health/digest/pubs/celiac/

Cited References

Abdulkarim AS et al: Etiology of nonresponsive celiac disease: results of a systematic approach, *Am J Gastroenterol* 97:2016, 2002.

Ahmad et al: Review article: the genetics of inflammatory bowel disease, *Aliment Pharmacol Ther* 15:731, 2001.

Alles MS et al: Bacterial fermentation of fructooligosaccharides and resistant starch in patients with an ileal pouch–anal anastomosis, *Am J Clin Nutr* 66:1286, 1997.

American Cancer Society: *Cancer facts and figures,* 2002, www.cancer.org/downloads/STT/CancerFacts&Figures2002TM.pdf.

Ballegaard M et al: Self-reported food intolerance in chronic inflammatory bowel disease, *Scand J Gastroenterol* 32:569, 1997.

Bartlett JG: Antibiotic associated diarrhea, *N Engl J Med* 346:334, 2002.

Beutler B: Autoimmunity and apoptosis: the Crohn's connection, *Immunity* 15:5, 2001.

Beyer PL: Short bowel syndrome. In Coulston AM, Rock CL, Monson ER, editors: *Nutrition in the prevention and treatment of disease,* ed 1, San Diego, 2001, Academic Press.

Bezkorovainy A: Probiotics: determinants of survival and growth in the gut, *Am J Clin Nutr* 73:399S, 2001.

Bischoff SC et al: Prevalence of adverse reactions to food in patients with gastrointestinal disease, *Allergy* 51:811, 1996.

Bongaerts GP et al: Role of bacteria in the pathogenesis of short bowel syndrome associated *d*-lactic acidemia, *Microb Pathog* 22:285, 1997.

Booth I: Dietary management of acute diarrhea in childhood [Commentary], *Lancet* 341:966, 1993.

Brady LJ et al: The role of probiotic cultures in the prevention of colon cancer, *J Nutr* 130S:410, 2000.

Branski D et al: Chronic diarrhea and malabsorption, *Pediatr Clin North Am* 43:307, 1996.

Camilleri M et al: Insights into the pathophysiology and mechanisms of constipation, irritable bowel syndrome and diverticulosis in older people, *Am Geriatr* Soc 48:1142, 2000.

Candelli M et al: Idiopathic chronic constipation: pathophysiology, diagnosis and treatment, *Hepatogastroenterology* 48:1050, 2001.

Case S: *Gluten-free diet: a comprehensive resource guide,* ed 2, Saskatchewan, 2003, *Case Nutrition Consulting.*

Cheek C, Radley S: Diverticulosis: fiber is the key, *Practitioner* 243:321, 1999.

Cronk DR et al: Malnutrition impairs postresection intestinal adaptation, *J Parenter Enteral Nutr* 24:76, 2000.

Cunha BA: Nosocomial diarrhea, *Crit Care Clin* 14:329, 1998.

Davidson G et al: Infectious diarrhea in children: working group report of the first world congress of pediatric gastroenterology, hepatology, and nutrition, *J Pediatr Gastroenterol Nutr* 35:143S, 2002.

Davidson RH et al: Probiotic culture survival and implications in fermented frozen yogurt characteristics, *J Dairy Sci* 83:666, 2000.

Deckman R, Cheskin L: Diverticular disease in the elderly, *J Am Geriatr Soc* 40:986, 1993.

DeLillo AR and Rose S: Functional bowel disorders in the geriatric patient: constipation, fecal impaction, and fecal incontinence, *Am J Coll Gastroenterol* 95:901, 2000.

DeMeo MT, et al: Intestinal permeation and gastrointestinal disease, *J Clin Gastroenterol* 34:385, 2002.

Drossman DA et al: Irritable bowel syndrome: a technical review for practice guideline development, *Gastroenterology* 112:2120, 1997.

Drucker DJ: Gut adaptation and the glucagon-like peptides, *Gut* 59:428, 2002.

Farrell RJ, Kelly CP: Celiac sprue, *N Engl J Med* 346:180, 2002.

Farthing MJG: Tropical malabsorption and tropical diarrhea. In Feldman M, Sleisenger MH, Scharschmidt BF, editors: *Gastrointestinal and liver disease,* ed 6, Philadelphia, 1998, WB Saunders.

Fasano A, Catassi C: Current approaches to diagnosis and treatment of celiac disease: an evolving spectrum, *Gastroenterology* 120:636, 2001.

Fasano A et al: Prevalence of celiac disease in at-risk and not at-risk groups in the United States: a large multicenter study, *Arch Intern Med* 163(3):286, 2003.

Fine KD: Diarrhea. In Feldman M, Sleisenger MH, Scharschmidt BF, editors: *Gastrointestinal and liver disease,* ed 6, Philadelphia, 1998, WB Saunders.

Fukuda M et al: Prebiotic treatment of experimental colitis with germinated barley foodstuff: a comparison with probiotic or antibiotic treatment, *Int J Mol Med* 9:65, 2002.

Garland CF et al: Calcium and vitamin D: their potential roles in colon and breast cancer prevention, *Ann NY Acad Sci* 889:107, 1999.

Gibson GR: Dietary modulation of the human gut microflora using the prebiotics oligofructose and inulin, *J Nutr* 129:1438S, 1999.

Giovannucci E, Goldin B: The role of fat, fatty acids, and total energy intake in the etiology of human colon cancer, *Am J Clin Nutr* 66:1564S, 1997.

Goepp J, Katz S: Oral rehydration therapy, *Am Fam Physician* 47:843, 1993.

Goldstein NS et al: Crohn's like complications in patients with ulcerative colitis after total proctocolectomy and ileal pouch–anal anastomosis, *Am J Surg Pathol* 21:1343, 1997.

Gray G. Intestinal lactase: what defines the decline? [Editorial], *Gastroenterology* 105:931, 1993.

Gudmand-Hoyer E: The clinical significance of disaccharide maldigestion, *Am J Clin Nutr* 59:(suppl):735, 1994.

Hahn S, Kim S, Garner P: Reduced osmolarity oral rehydration solution for treating dehydration caused by acute diarrhoea in children, *Cochrane Database Syst Rev* 1:CD002847, 2002.

Han P et al: Nutrition and inflammatory bowel disease, *Gastroenterol Clin North Am* 28:423, 1999.

Hill ID et al: Celiac disease: working group report of the first world congress of pediatric gastroenterology, hepatology and nutrition, *J Pediatr Gastroenterol Nutr* 35:S78, 2002.

Holtmann MH et al: Immunotherapeutic approaches to inflammatory bowel diseases, *Expert Opin Biol Ther* 1:455, 2001.

Hugot JP et al: Association of NOD2 leucine-rich repeat variants with susceptibility to Crohn's disease, *Nature* 411:599, 2001.

Hyams JS: Crohn's disease in children, *Pediatr Clin North Am* 43:255, 1996.

Institute of Medicine: Dietary reference intakes for energy, carbohydrate, fiber, fatty acids, cholesterol, protein and amino acids, Washington, DC, National Academies Press, 2002.

Jacobasch G et al: Dietary resistant starch and chronic inflammatory bowel diseases, *Int J Colorectal Dis* 14:201, 1999.

Janatuinen EK et al: No harm from five year ingestion of oats in coeliac disease, *Gut* 50:332, 2002.

Jenkins HR: Inflammatory bowel disease, *Arch Dis Child* 85:435, 2001.

Jewell DP: Ulcerative colitis. In Feldman M, Sleisenger MH, Scharschmidt BF, editors: *Gastrointestinal and liver disease,* ed 6, Philadelphia, 1998, WB Saunders.

Job ML, Jacobs NF: Drug induced *Clostridium difficile*–associated disease, *Drug Saf* 17:37, 1997.

Kornblau S et al: Management of cancer treatment–related diarrhea: issues and therapeutic strategies, *J Pain Symptom Manage* 19:118, 2000.

Kornbluth A et al: Crohn's disease. In Feldman M, Sleisenger MH, Scharschmidt BF, editors: *Gastrointestinal and liver disease,* ed 6, Philadelphia, 1998, WB Saunders.

Kyne L et al: *Clostridium difficile, Gastroenterol Clin North Am* 30:753, 2001.

Laroux FS, Grisham MB: Immunological basis of inflammatory bowel disease: role of microcirculation, *Microcirculation* 8:283, 2001.

Levitt MD et al: The relation of passage of gas and abdominal bloating to colonic gas production, *Ann Intern Med* 124:422, 1996.

Linskens RK et al: The bacterial flora in inflammatory bowel disease: current insights in pathogenesis and the influence of antibiotics and probiotics, *Scand J Gastroenterol* 234S:29, 2001.

Loening-Baucke V: Encopresis, *Curr Opin Pediatr* 14:570, 2002.

Madsen KL: Use of probiotics in gastrointestinal disease, *Can J Gastroenterol* 15:817, 2001.

Marlett JA et al: Position of the American Dietetic Association: health implications of dietary fiber, *J Am Dietet Assn* 102:993, 2002.

Mayer EA et al: Basic pathophysiologic mechanisms in irritable bowel syndrome, *Dig Dis* 19:212, 2001.

Messori A et al: Defined-formula diets versus steroids in the treatment of active Crohn's disease: a meta-analysis, *Scand J Gastroenterol* 31:267, 1996.

Mitra AD et al: Management of diarrhea in HIV-infected patients, *Int J STD AIDS* 12:630, 2001.

Mortensen PB, Clausen MR: SCFA in the human colon, *Scand J Gastroenterol* 216(suppl):132, 1996.

Mustalahti K et al: Coeliac disease among healthy members of multiple case celiac disease families, *Scand J Gastroenterol* 37:161, 2002.

Nobaek S et al: Alteration of intestinal microflora is associated with reduction in abdominal bloating and pain in patients with irritable bowel syndrome, *Am J Gastroenterol* 95:1231, 2000.

Olden KW, Schuster MM: Irritable bowel syndrome. In Feldman M, Sleisenger MH, Scharschmidt BF, editors: *Gastrointestinal and liver disease,* ed 6, Philadelphia, 1998, WB Saunders.

Panes J: Inflammatory bowel disease: pathogenesis and targets for therapeutic interventions, *Acta Physiol Scand* 173:159, 2001.

Parodi PW: Cows' milk fat components as potential anticarcinogenic agents, *J Nutr* 127:1055, 1997.

Patel HI et al: Surgery for Crohn's disease in infants and children, *J Pediatr Surg* 32:1063, 1997.

Pearson M et al: Food intolerance and Crohn's disease, *Gut* 34:783, 1993.

Pemberton JH, Phillips SF: Ileostomy and its alternatives. In Feldman M, Sleisenger MH, Scharschmidt BF, editors: *Gastrointestinal and liver disease,* ed 6, Philadelphia, 1998, WB Saunders.

Petaros P et al: Prevalence of autoimmune disorders in relatives of patients with celiac disease, *Dig Dis Sci* 47:1427, 2002.

Peters HP et al: Potential benefits and hazards of physical activity and exercise on the gastrointestinal tract, *Gut* 48:435, 2001.

Piche T et al: Colonic fermentation influences lower esophageal sphincter function in gastroesophageal reflux disease, *Gastroenterology* 124:894, 2003.

Pirenne J et al: Recent advances and future prospects in intestinal and multivisceral transplantation, *Pediatr Transplant* 5:452, 2001.

Podolsky DK: Inflammatory bowel disease, *N Engl J Med* 347:417, 2002.

Ramirez F et al: All lactase preparations are not the same: results of a prospective, randomized placebo-controlled trial, *Am J Gastroenterol* 89:566, 1994.

Rao SS et al: Is coffee a colonic stimulant? *Eur J Gastroenterol Hepatol* 10:113, 1998.

Reddy BS: The forth De Witt S. Goodman lecture: novel approaches to the prevention of colon cancer by nutritional manipulation and chemoprevention, *Cancer Epidemiol Biomarkers Prev* 9:239, 2000.

Regueiro MD: Update in medical treatment of Crohn's disease, *J Clin Gastroenterol* 31:282, 2000.

Reif S et al: Pre-illness dietary factors in inflammatory bowel disease, *Gut* 40:754, 1997.

Rumessen JJ, Gudmand-Hoyer E: Functional bowel disease: malabsorption and abdominal distress after ingestion of fructose, sorbitol, and fructose-sorbitol mixtures, *Gastroenterology* 95:694, 1998.

Sandborn W et al: Pharmacotherapy for inducing and maintaining remission in pouchitis, *Cochrane Database Syst Rev* 2:CD001176, 2000.

Saraphin P, Mobarin S: Mortality in patients with celiac disease, *Nutr Rev* 60:116, 2002.

Scheppach W et al: Beneficial health effects of low-digestible carbohydrate consumption, *Br J Nutr* 1S:23, 2001.

Shan L et al: Structural basis for gluten intolerance in celiac sprue, *Science* 297:2275, 2002.

Shoda R et al: Epidemiologic analysis of Crohn's disease in Japan: increased dietary intake of n-6 polyunsaturated fatty acids and animal protein relates to the increased incidence of Crohn disease in Japan, *Am J Clin Nutr* 63:741, 1996.

Sigalet DL: Short bowel syndrome in infants and children: an overview, *Semin Pediatr Surg* 10:49, 2001.

Simmang CL, Shires GT: Diverticular disease of the colon. In Feldman M, Sleisenger MH, Scharschmidt BF, editors: *Gastrointestinal and liver disease,* ed 6, Philadelphia, 1998, WB Saunders.

Simren M et al: An exaggerated sensory component of the gastrocolonic response in patients with irritable bowel syndrome, *Gut* 48:20, 2001.

Simren M et al: Food related gastrointestinal symptoms in the irritable bowel syndrome, *Digestion* 63:108, 2001.

Slattery ML: Diet, lifestyle, and colon cancer, *Semin Gastroentest Dis* 11:142, 2000.

Snape W: Nutrition and colonic diverticular disease, *Nutrition and the MD* 20:1, 1994.

Srinivasan R, Minocha A: When to suspect lactose intolerance: symptomatic, ethnic, and laboratory clues, *Postgrad Med* 104:109, 1998.

Strocchi A, Levitt MD: Intestinal gas. In Feldman M, Sleisenger MH, Scharschmidt BF, editors: *Gastrointestinal and liver disease,* ed 6, Philadelphia, 1998, WB Saunders.

Sundarum A et al: Nutritional management of short bowel syndrome in adults, *J Clin Gastroenterol* 34:207, 2002.

Szajewska H, Mrukowicz JZ: Probiotics in the treatment of acute infectious diarrhea in infants and children: a systematic review of published randomized, double blind placebo-controlled trials, *J Pediatr Gastroenterol Nutr* 2S:17, 2001.

Thompson T: Wheat starch, gliadin and the gluten-free diet, *J Am Diet Assoc* 101:1456, 2001.

Thompson WG et al: Functional bowel disorders and functional abdominal pain, *Gut* 45S:1143, 1999.

Thompson-Fawcett MW et al: Ileoanal reservoir dysfunction: a problem-solving approach, *Br J Surg* 84:1351, 1997.

Tomita R et al: Physiological studies on nitric oxide in the right sided colon of patients with diverticular disease, *Hepatogastroenterology* 46:2839, 1999.

Troncone R et al: Gluten-sensitive enteropathy, *Pediatr Clin North Am* 43:355, 1996.

van Dulleman H et al: Mediators of mucosal inflammation: implications for therapy, *Scand J Gastroenterol* 223(suppl):92, 1997.

Van Loo J et al: Functional food properties of non-digestible oligosaccharides: a consensus report from the ENDO project, *Br J Nutr* 81:121, 1999.

Vanderhoof JA, Young RJ: Enteral nutrition in short-bowel syndrome, *Semin Pediatr Surg* 10:65, 2001.

Villanueva A et al: Update in the therapeutic management of irritable bowel syndrome, *Dig Dis* 19:244, 2001.

Wilmore DW et al: Factors predicting a successful outcome after pharmacological bowel compensation, *Ann Surg* 226:288, 1997.

Wollowske et al: Protective role of probiotics and prebiotics in colon cancer, *Am J Clin Nutr* 73S:451, 2001.

World Health Organization: *World Health Organization guidelines for cholera control,* WHO/COD/Ser/80.4, Rev. 1, Geneva, 1986.

Additional References

American Gastroenterology Association: Medical position statement: irritable bowel syndrome, *Gastroenterology* 112:2118, 1997.

Beyer P: Gastrointestinal disorders: roles of nutrition and the dietetic practitioner, *J Am Diet Assoc* 98:272, 1998.

Horwitz BJ, Fisher RS: The irritable bowel syndrome, *N Engl J Med* 344:1846, 2001.

Hyams JS: Diet and gastrointestinal disease, *Curr Opin Pediatr* 14:567, 2002.

Inman-Felton A: Overview of gluten-sensitive enteropathy (celiac sprue), *J Am Diet Assoc* 99:352, 1999.

Inman-Felton A: Overview of lactose maldigestion (lactose nonpersistence), *J Am Diet Assoc* 99:481, 1999.

Kemppainen TA et al: Nutritional status of newly diagnosed celiac disease patients before and after the institution of a celiac disease diet—association with the grade of mucosal villous atrophy, *Am J Clin Nutr* 67:482, 1998.

Lagares-Garcia JA et al: Colonoscopy in octogenarians and older patients, *Surg Endosc* 15:262, 2001.

Singh J et al: Dietary fat and colon cancer: modulating effect of types of amount of dietary fat on ras-p21 function during promotion and progression stages of colon cancer, *Cancer Res* 57:253, 1997.

Suarez F, Saviano D: Diet, genetics, and lactose intolerance, *Food Technol* 51:74, 1997.

Tramonte SM et al: The treatment of chronic constipation in adults: a systematic review, *J Gen Intern Med* 12:15, 1997.

Udall JN Jr et al: Malnutrition and diarrhea: working group report of the first world congress of pediatric gastroenterology, hepatology, and nutrition, *J Pediatr Gastroenterol Nutr* 35:173S, 2002.

Wolfsdorf J, Crigler J: Cornstarch regimens for nocturnal treatment of young adults with type I glycogen storage disease, *Am J Clin Nutr* 65:1507, 1997.

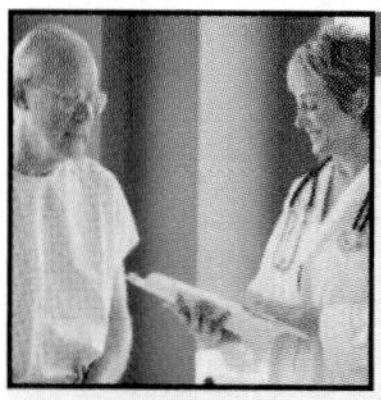

CHAPTER 31

Medical Nutrition Therapy for Liver, Biliary System, and Exocrine Pancreas Disorders

JEANETTE M. HASSE, PhD, RD, LD, CNSD, FADA
LAURA E. MATARESE, MS, RD, LD, CNSD, FADA

CHAPTER OUTLINE

- Physiology and Functions of the Liver
- Laboratory Assessment of Liver Function
- Diseases of the Liver
- Liver Resection and Transplantation
- Physiology and Functions of the Gallbladder
- Diseases of the Gallbladder
- Physiology and Functions of the Exocrine Pancreas
- Diseases of the Exocrine Pancreas

KEY TERMS

alcoholic liver disease–disease resulting from excessive alcohol ingestion, characterized by fatty liver (hepatic steatosis), hepatitis, or cirrhosis

aromatic amino acids (AAAs)–the amino acids phenylalanine, tryptophan, and tyrosine

ascites–accumulation of fluid, serum protein, and electrolytes within the peritoneal cavity caused by increased pressure from portal hypertension and decreased production of albumin (which maintains serum colloidal osmotic pressure)

balloon tamponade–stoppage of blood flow by using pressure from an inflated tube or balloon

bile–thick, viscous fluid secreted from the liver, stored in the gallbladder, and released into duodenum when fatty foods enter the duodenum; emulsifies fats in the intestine and forms compounds with fatty acids to facilitate their absorption

branched-chain amino acids (BCAAs)–the amino acids valine, isoleucine, and leucine

cholangitis–inflammation in the bile ducts; may be acute or sclerosing

cholecystectomy–removal of the gallbladder

cholecystitis–inflammation of the gallbladder

choledocholithiasis–presence of gallstones in the common bile duct

cholelithiasis–presence or formation of gallstones

cirrhosis–chronic liver disease due to diffuse necrosis and regeneration leading to an increase in fibrous tissue formation disrupting the normal liver structure

fasting hypoglycemia–low blood glucose due to decreased availability of glucose from glycogen due to depressed liver function

fatty liver–a condition (hepatic steatosis) characterized by the accumulation of excess fat in the liver commonly caused by alcohol abuse but also associated with obesity, starvation, intestinal bypass, parenteral alimentation, and diabetes mellitus

fulminant liver disease–absence of preexisting liver disease with development of hepatic encephalopathy within 2 months of onset of illness

hepatic encephalopathy–a clinical syndrome developing in advanced liver disease, characterized by impaired mentation, neuromuscular disturbances, and altered consciousness; four stages of progression

hepatic failure–condition in which liver function is diminished to 25% or less

hepatic osteodystrophy–a complication of chronic liver disease where bone mass declines

hepatic steatosis–fatty liver

hepatitis–widespread inflammation of the liver; usually viral in origin

hepatorenal syndrome–functional renal failure without anatomic or histopathologic renal changes associated with cirrhosis and ascites or with obstructive jaundice

jaundice (icterus)–a syndrome characterized by hyperbilirubinemia and deposition of bile pigment, resulting in yellowing of skin, mucous membranes, and sclera

Kayser-Fleischer ring–greenish yellow pigmented ring encircling the cornea just within the corneoscleral margin formed by copper deposits in Descemet's membrane of the cornea; occurs in patients with Wilson's disease

Kupffer cells–fixed phagocytes in the sinusoids of the liver

pancreaticoduodenectomy (Whipple procedure)–excision of the head of the pancreas along with the encircling loop of the duodenum; may include partial gastrectomy

pancreatitis–inflammation of the pancreas caused by autodigestion of pancreatic tissue by its own enzymes

paracentesis–a procedure during which fluid from the abdomen (ascites) is removed through a needle

portal hypertension–abnormally increased blood pressure in the portal venous system due to the obstruction of blood flow through the liver

portal systemic encephalopathy–another term for hepatic encephalopathy

primary biliary cirrhosis (PBC)–an immune-mediated chronic cirrhosis of the liver due to obstruction or infection of the small and intermediate-sized intrahepatic bile ducts while the extrahepatic biliary tree and larger intrahepatic ducts are normal; 90% of patients are women

steatorrhea–presence of excess fat in the stool

varices–low-pressure veins that become distended from increased pressure; most commonly develop in the lower esophagus and upper stomach

Wernicke's encephalopathy–condition of damage to the central nervous system from thiamin deficiency; common with alcoholism

Wilson's disease–autosomal recessive disorder of copper metabolism in which excessive accumulation of copper occurs in the liver, central nervous system, and kidney

The liver is an organ of primary importance to the body. One cannot survive without a liver. The pancreas and liver play an important part in digestion and metabolism. Although it is important, the gallbladder can be removed and the body will adapt comfortably to its absence. Knowledge of the structure and functions of these organs is vital, and when they are diseased, the necessary medical nutrition therapy is complex.

PHYSIOLOGY AND FUNCTIONS OF THE LIVER

Structure

The liver is the largest gland in the body, weighing about 1500 g. The liver has two main lobes—the right and left. The right lobe is further divided into the anterior and posterior segments; the right segmental fissure, which cannot be seen externally, separates the segments. The externally visible falciform ligament divides the left lobe into the medial and lateral segments. The liver is supplied with blood from two sources: the hepatic artery, which supplies about one third of the blood from the aorta, and the portal vein, which supplies the other two thirds and collects blood drained from the digestive tract.

About 1500 ml of blood per minute circulates through the liver and exits via the right and left hepatic veins into the inferior vena cava. Just as there is a system of blood vessels throughout the liver, there also exists a series of bile ducts. Bile, which is formed in the liver cells, exits the liver through a series of bile ducts that increase in size as they approach the common bile duct.

Functions

The liver has the ability to regenerate itself. Only 10% to 20% of functioning liver is required to sustain life, although removal of the liver will result in death within 24 hours. The liver is integral to most metabolic functions of the body and performs more than 500 tasks. The main functions of the liver include metabolism of carbohydrate, protein, and fat; storage and activation of vitamins and minerals; formation and excretion of bile; conversion of ammonia to urea; metabolism of steroids; and action as a filter and flood chamber.

The liver plays a major role in carbohydrate metabolism. Galactose and fructose, products of carbohydrate digestion, are converted into glucose in the hepatocyte or liver cell. The liver stores glucose as glycogen *(glycogenesis)* and then returns it to the blood when glucose levels become low *(glycogenolysis)*. The liver also produces "new" glucose *(gluconeogenesis)* from precursors such as lactic acid, glycogenic amino acids, and intermediates of the tricarboxylic acid cycle (see Chapter 3).

Important protein metabolic pathways occur in the liver. Transamination and oxidative deamination are two such pathways that convert amino acids to substrates that are used in energy and glucose production as well as in the synthesis of nonessential amino acids. Blood-clotting factors such as fibrinogen and prothrombin and serum proteins, including albumin, α-globulin, β-globulin, transferrin, ceruloplasmin, and lipoproteins, are formed by the liver.

Fatty acids from the diet and adipose tissue are converted in the liver to acetyl-coenzyme A (CoA) by the process of β-oxidation to produce energy. Ketone bodies are also produced. The liver synthesizes and hydrolyzes triglycerides, phospholipids, cholesterol, and lipoproteins as well.

The liver is involved in the storage, activation, and transport of many vitamins and minerals. It stores all the fat-soluble vitamins in addition to zinc, iron, copper, magnesium, and vitamin B_{12}. Hepatically synthesized proteins transport vitamin A, iron, zinc, and copper. Carotene is converted to vitamin A, folate to 5-methyl tetrahydrofolic acid, and vitamin D to its active form by the liver.

In addition to functions of nutrient metabolism and storage, the liver forms and excretes bile. Bile salts are metabolized and used for the digestion and absorption of fats and fat-soluble vitamins. Bilirubin is a metabolic end product from red blood cell destruction; it is conjugated and excreted in the bile.

Hepatocytes detoxify ammonia by converting it to urea, 75% of which is excreted by the kidneys. The remaining urea finds its way back to the gastrointestinal tract.

The liver also metabolizes steroids. It inactivates and excretes aldosterone, glucocorticoids, estrogen, progesterone, and testosterone. It is responsible for the detoxification of substances including drugs and alcohol.

Finally, the liver acts as a filter and flood chamber by removing bacteria and debris from blood through the phagocytic action of Kupffer cells located in the sinusoids and by storing blood backed up from the vena cava as in right heart failure.

LABORATORY ASSESSMENT OF LIVER FUNCTION

Biochemical laboratory markers are used to evaluate and monitor patients having or suspected of having liver disease. Enzyme assays measure the release of liver enzymes, and other tests measure liver function. Screening tests for hepatobiliary disease include serum levels of bilirubin, alkaline phosphatase, aspartate amino transferase, and alanine aminotransferase. Table 31-1 elaborates common laboratory tests for liver disorders (see also Appendix 33).

DISEASES OF THE LIVER

Diseases of the liver can be acute or chronic, inherited or acquired. Liver disease is classified in various ways: acute viral hepatitis, fulminant hepatitis, chronic hepatitis, alcoholic hepatitis and cirrhosis, cholestatic liver diseases, inherited disorders, and other liver diseases.

Acute Viral Hepatitis

Acute viral hepatitis is a widespread inflammation of the liver and is caused by hepatitis viruses A, B, C, D, and E (Figures 31-1 and 31-2). Minor agents such as Epstein-Barr virus, cytomegalovirus, herpes simplex, yellow fever, and rubella can also cause an acute hepatitis.

Hepatitis A (HAV) is transmitted by the fecal-oral route and is contracted through contaminated drinking water, food, and sewage. Anorexia is the most frequent symptom, and it can be severe. Other common symptoms include nausea, vomiting, right upper quadrant abdominal pain, dark urine, and jaundice (icterus). Recovery is usually complete, and long-term consequences are rare. Serious complications may occur in high-risk patients; subsequently, great attention must be given to adequate nutritional intake.

Hepatitis B (HBV) and hepatitis C (HCV) can lead to chronic and carrier states. HBV and HCV are transmitted via blood, blood products, semen, and saliva. For example, they can be spread from contaminated needles, blood transfusions, open cuts or wounds, splashes of blood into the mouth or eyes, or sexual contact. Chronic active hepatitis can also develop, leading to cirrhosis and liver failure.

The hepatitis D virus (HDV) is dependent on the HBV for survival and propagation in humans. HDV may be a coinfection (occurring at the same time as HBV) or a superinfection (superimposing itself on the HBV carrier state) (Seeff, 1996). This form of hepatitis usually becomes chronic.

Hepatitis E virus (HEV) is rare in the United States, but it is reported more frequently in many countries of southern, eastern, and central Asia; northern, eastern, and western Africa; and Mexico. HEV is transmitted via the oral-fecal route. Contaminated water appears to be the source of infection, which usually afflicts people living in crowded and unsanitary conditions. Hepatitis E is generally acute rather than chronic.

The general symptoms of acute viral hepatitis are divided into four phases. The first phase, the early *prodromal* phase, affects about 25% of patients, causing fever, arthralgia, arthritis, rash, and angioedema. This is followed by the *preicteric* phase, in which malaise, fatigue, myalgia, anorexia, nausea, vomiting, *dysgeusia* (taste changes), and *dysosmia* (partial loss of speech) occur. Some patients complain of epigastric or right upper quadrant pain. The third phase is the *icteric* phase, in which jaundice appears. Finally, during the *convalescent* phase, jaundice and other symptoms begin to subside. Complete recovery is expected in 95% of HAV cases, in 90% of acute HBV cases, but in only 15% to 30% of acute HCV cases (Seeff, 1996). Chronic hepatitis does not usually develop with HEV, and symptoms and liver function tests usually normalize within 6 weeks (Hoofnagle and Lindsay, 2000).

TABLE 31-1 Common Laboratory Tests Used to Test Liver Function

LABORATORY TEST	COMMENT
Hepatic Excretion	
Total serum bilirubin	When increased, may indicate bilirubin overproduction or defect in hepatic uptake or conjugation
Indirect serum bilirubin	Unconjugated bilirubin; increased with excessive bilirubin production (hemolysis), immaturity of enzyme systems, inherited defects, drug effects
Direct serum bilirubin	Conjugated bilirubin; increased with depressed bilirubin excretion, hepatobiliary disease, intrahepatic or extrahepatic cholestasis, benign postoperative jaundice and sepsis, and congenital conjugated hyperbilirubinemia
Urine bilirubin	More sensitive than total serum bilirubin; confirms if liver disease is the cause of jaundice
Urine urobilinogen	Used when obstructive jaundice is expected; rarely used
Serum bile acids	Reflects efficacy of ileal reabsorption and hepatic extraction of bile acids from portal circulation; levels increase with liver disease; little clinical utility
Cholestasis Tests	
Serum alkaline phosphatase	Enzyme widely distributed in liver, bone, placenta, intestine, kidney, leukocytes; mainly bound to canalicular membranes in liver; increased levels suggest cholestasis but can be increased with bone disorders, pregnancy, normal growth, and some malignancies
5′-Nucleotidase (5′ NT)	Enzyme present in canalicular and plasma membranes of hepatocytes; also in heart and pancreas; increases with liver disease
Leucine aminopeptidase (LAP)	Cellular peptidase; usually increased in cholestasis and suggests hepatobiliary origin of elevation of alkaline phosphatase; may also increase with pregnancy
γ-Glutamyl transpeptidase (GGT)	Enzyme associated with microsomes and plasma membranes in hepatocytes; also present in kidney, pancreas, heart, brain; increased with liver disease but also after myocardial infarction, in neuromuscular disease, pancreatic disease, pulmonary disease, diabetes mellitus, and during alcohol ingestion
Hepatic Enzymes	
Alanine aminotransferase (ALT, formerly SGPT)	Located in cytosol of hepatocyte; found in several other body tissues but highest in the liver; increased with liver cell damage
Aspartate aminotransferase (AST, formerly SGOT)	Located in cytosol and mitochondria of hepatocyte; also in cardiac and skeletal muscle, brain, pancreas, kidney, and leukocytes; increased with liver cell damage
Serum lactic dehydrogenase	Located in liver, red blood cells, cardiac muscle, kidney; increased with liver disease but lacks sensitivity and specificity because it is found in most other body tissues
Serum Proteins	
Prothrombin time (PT)	Most blood coagulation factors are synthesized in the liver; vitamin K deficiency and decreased synthesis of clotting factors increase prothrombin time and risk of bleeding
Partial thromboplastin time (PTT)	Assesses the "intrinsic" clotting mechanism; reflects activity of all clotting factors except platelet factor e, factors VII and XII; complementary to PT
Serum albumin	Main export protein synthesized in the liver and most important factor in maintaining plasma oncotic pressure; decreased synthesis occurs with liver dysfunction, thyroid and glucocorticoid hormone dysfunction, abnormal plasma colloid osmotic pressure, and toxins; increased losses occur with protein-losing enteropathy, nephrotic syndrome, burns, gastrointestinal bleeding, exfoliative dermatitis
Serum globulin	α_1 and α_2-globulins are synthesized in the liver; levels increase with chronic liver disease; limited diagnostic use in hepatobiliary disease
Mitochondrial antibody	90% of patients with PBC have antibodies in their serum against a lipoprotein component of the inner mitochondrial membrane; also present in 25% of patients with chronic active hepatitis and postnecrotic cirrhosis
Antinuclear and smooth-muscle antibodies	May be positive in patients with chronic active hepatitis (usually not associated with hepatitis B or C virus) and in a minority of patients with PBC; not organ or species specific
Markers of Specific Liver Diseases	
Serum ferritin	Major iron storage protein; increased level sensitive indictor of genetic hemochromatosis
Ceruloplasmin	Major copper-binding protein synthesized by the liver; decreased in Wilson's disease
α-Fetoprotein	Major circulating plasma protein; increased with hepatocellular carcinoma
α_1-Antitrypsin	Main function is to inhibit serum trypsin activity; decreased levels indicate α_1-antitrypsin deficiency, which can cause liver and lung damage
Specific Tests for Viral Hepatitis	
IgM anti-HAV	Marker for hepatitis A; indicates current or recent infection or convalescence
IgG anti-HAV	Marker for hepatitis A; indicates current or previous infection and immunity
HBsAG	Marker for hepatitis B; positive in most cases of acute or chronic infection
HBeAg	Marker for hepatitis B; transiently positive during active virus replication; reflects concentration and infectivity of virus

Data from Baker AL: Liver chemistry tests. In Kaplowitz N, editor: *Liver and biliary diseases,* ed 2, Baltimore, 1996, Williams & Wilkins; Hoofnagle JH, Lindsay KL: Acute viral hepatitis. In Goldman L, Bennett JC, editors: *Cecil textbook of medicine,* ed 21, Philadelphia, 2000, WB Saunders; Kamath PS: Clinical approach to the patient with abnormal liver test results, *Mayo Clin Proc* 71:1089, 1996; Lindsay KL, Hoofnagle JH: Serologic tests for viral hepatitis. In Kaplowitz N, editor: *Liver and biliary diseases,* ed 2, Baltimore, 1996, Williams & Wilkins; Weisiger RA: Laboratory tests in liver disease. In Goldman L, Bennett JC, editors: *Cecil textbook of medicine,* ed 21, Philadelphia, 2000, WB Saunders.

IgG, Immunoglobin G; *IgM,* immunoglobulin M; *HAV,* hepatic A virus; *HBsAG,* hepatitis B surface antigen; *HBeAG,* hepatitis B antigen; *PBC,* primary biliary cirrhosis.

Continued

TABLE 31-1 Common Laboratory Tests Used to Test Liver Function—cont'd

LABORATORY TEST	COMMENT
Specific Tests for Viral Hepatitis—cont'd	
IgM or IgG anti-HBc	Marker for hepatitis B; positive in all acute and chronic cases; positive in carriers; not protective
Anti-HBe	Marker for hepatitis B; transiently positive during convalescence and in some chronic cases and carriers; not protective; reflects low infectivity
Anti-HBs	Marker for hepatitis B; positive late in convalescence; protective
Anti-HCV	Marker for hepatitis C; positive 5-6 weeks after onset of hepatitis C virus; not protective; reflects infectious state
HCV-RNA	Marker for hepatitis C
IgM or IgG anti-HDV	Marker for hepatitis D; indicates infection; not protective
IgM anti-HEV	Marker for hepatitis E; indicates current or recent infection; not protective
IgG anti-HEV	Marker for hepatitis E; indicates current or previous infection and immunity
Miscellaneous Tests	
Ammonia	Liver converts ammonia to urea; may increase with hepatic failure and portal-systemic shunts

Data from Baker AL: Liver chemistry tests. In Kaplowitz N, editor: *Liver and biliary diseases*, ed 2, Baltimore, 1996, Williams & Wilkins; Hoofnagle JH, Lindsay KL: Acute viral hepatitis. In Goldman L, Bennett JC, editors: *Cecil textbook of medicine*, ed 21, Philadelphia, 2000, WB Saunders; Kamath PS: Clinical approach to the patient with abnormal liver test results, *Mayo Clin Proc* 71:1089, 1996; Lindsay KL, Hoofnagle JH: Serologic tests for viral hepatitis. In Kaplowitz N, editor: *Liver and biliary diseases*, ed 2, Baltimore, 1996, Williams & Wilkins; Weisiger RA: Laboratory tests in liver disease. In Goldman L, Bennett JC, editors: *Cecil textbook of medicine*, ed 21, Philadelphia, 2000, WB Saunders.

IgG, Immunoglobin G; *IgM*, immunoglobulin M; *HAV*, hepatic A virus; *HBsAG*, hepatitis B surface antigen; *HBeAG*, hepatitis B antigen; *PBC*, primary biliary cirrhosis.

HBc, Hepatis B core; HCV, hepatitis C virus; *HDV*, hepatitis D virus; *HEV*, hepatitis E virus.

Fulminant Hepatitis

Fulminant hepatitis is a syndrome in which severe liver dysfunction is accompanied by hepatic encephalopathy. Fulminant liver disease is defined by the absence of preexisting liver disease and the development of hepatic encephalopathy within 8 weeks of the onset of illness. The causes of fulminant hepatitis include viral hepatitis (about 75% of cases), chemical toxicity (e.g., acetaminophen, drug reactions, poisonous mushrooms, industrial poisons), and other causes (e.g., Wilson's disease, fatty liver of pregnancy, Reye's syndrome, hepatic ischemia, hepatic vein obstruction, and disseminated malignancies). Extrahepatic complications of fulminant hepatitis are cerebral edema, coagulopathy and bleeding, cardiovascular abnormalities, renal failure, pulmonary complications, acid-base disturbances, electrolyte imbalances, sepsis, and pancreatitis (Douglas and Rakela, 1996).

Chronic Hepatitis

To be defined as chronic hepatitis, a patient must have at least a 6-month course of hepatitis or biochemical and clinical evidence of liver disease with confirmatory biopsy findings of unresolving hepatic inflammation (Lindsay and Hoofnagle, 2000). Chronic hepatitis can have autoimmune, viral, metabolic, or toxic etiologies. Autoimmune hepatitis is diagnosed when other forms of liver disease caused by viruses, hepatotoxic agents, and metabolic diseases are excluded. The patient may exhibit serum antinuclear and smooth-muscle antibodies, hypergammaglobulinemia, and other autoimmune disorders. This condition usually responds to corticosteroid administration.

Hepatic viruses, especially HCV, can also become chronic conditions. Metabolic diseases such as Wilson's disease, hemochromatosis, and a_1-antitrypsin deficiency can cause chronic hepatitis. Finally, some drugs such as methyldopa, nitrofurantoin, papaverine, dantrolene, clometacin, and ticrynafen can cause chronic hepatitis.

Alcoholic Liver Disease, Alcoholic Hepatitis, and Cirrhosis

Alcoholic liver disease is the most common liver disease in the United States and is the fourth leading cause of death among middle-age Americans (Carithers, 1996). According to the National Institute on Alcohol and Alcohol Abuse, nearly 14 million people in the United States (1 in every 13 adults) abuse alcohol or are alcoholic. Alcohol problems are highest among young adults 18 to 29 years of age and lowest among adults ages 65 and older (www.niaaa.nih.gov). Acetaldehyde, a toxic by-product of alcohol metabolism, causes damage to mitochondrial membrane structure and function. Acetaldehyde is produced by multiple metabolic pathways, one of which involves alcohol dehydrogenase (see *Focus on:* Metabolic Consequences of Alcohol Consumption).

Several variables may predispose some persons to alcoholic liver disease. These include genetic polymorphisms of alcohol-metabolizing enzymes, gender (female more than male), simultaneous exposure to other drugs, infections with hepatotropic viruses, immunologic factors, and poor nutritional status (McCullough and O'Connor, 1998).

The pathogenesis of alcoholic liver disease progresses in three stages (Figure 31-3): hepatic steatosis (Figure 31-4), alcoholic hepatitis, and cirrhosis. Fatty infiltration or hepatic steatosis or fatty liver is caused by a culmination of these metabolic disturbances: (1) an increase in the mobilization of fatty acids from adipose tissue, (2) an increase in hepatic synthesis of

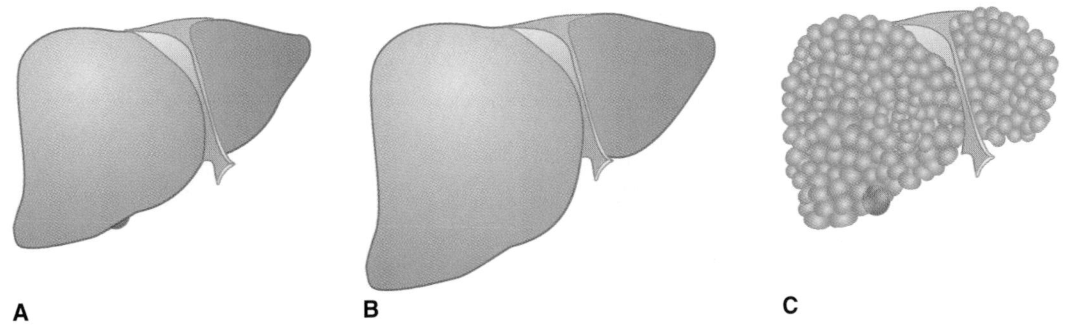

FIGURE 31-1 • **A,** Normal liver. **B,** Liver with viral hepatic damage. **C,** Cirrhotic liver.

FOCUS ON

Metabolic Consequences of Alcohol Consumption

Ethanol is metabolized primarily in the liver by alcohol dehydrogenase (ADH). This results in acetaldehyde production with the transfer of hydrogen to nicotinamide adenine dinucleotide (NAD), reducing it to NADH. The acetaldehyde then loses hydrogen and is converted to acetate, most of which is released into the blood.

$$\underset{\text{ethanol}}{C_2H_2OH} + NAD \xrightarrow[\text{alcohol dehydrogenase}]{} NADH + \underset{\text{acetaldehyde}}{CH_3\text{—}CHO}$$

$$\underset{\text{acetaldehyde}}{CH_3\text{-}CHO} + NADH + H_2O \xrightarrow[\text{alcohol dehydrogenase}]{} : NAD + H^+ + \underset{\text{acetate}}{CH_3\text{-}CHOOH}$$

Many metabolic disturbances occur because of the excess of NADH, which overrides the cell's ability to maintain a normal redox state. These include hyperlacticacidemia, acidosis, hyperuricemia, ketonemia, and hyperlipemia. The tricarboxylic acid (TCA) cycle is depressed because it requires NAD. The mitochondria, in turn, use hydrogen from ethanol rather than from the oxidation of fatty acids, to produce energy via the TCA cycle, which leads to a decreased fatty acid oxidation and accumulation of triglycerides. In addition, NADH may actually promote fatty acid synthesis. Hypoglycemia can also occur in early alcoholic liver disease secondary to the suppression of the TCA cycle, coupled with decreased gluconeogenesis due to ethanol.

fatty acids, (3) a decrease in fatty acid oxidation, (4) an increase in triglyceride production, and (5) a trapping of triglycerides in the liver. Hepatic steatosis is reversible with abstinence from alcohol. Conversely, if alcohol abuse continues, cirrhosis can develop.

Alcoholic hepatitis is characterized by hepatomegaly, modest elevation of transaminase levels, increased serum bilirubin concentrations, normal or depressed serum albumin concentrations, and possibly anemia and thrombocytopenia (Carithers, 1996). Patients may also have abdominal pain, anorexia, nausea, vomiting, weakness, diarrhea, weight loss, or fever. If patients discontinue alcohol intake, hepatitis may resolve; however, the condition often progresses to the third stage.

Clinical features of the third stage of alcoholic cirrhosis vary. Symptoms can mimic those of alcoholic hepatitis, or patients can develop ascites, gastrointestinal bleeding, portal hypertension, hepatic encephalopathy, and other symptoms of liver disease. A liver biopsy usually reveals micronodular cirrhosis, but it can be macronodular or mixed (Carithers, 1996). Prognosis depends on abstinence from alcohol and the degree of complications already developed. Ethanol ingestion creates specific and severe nutritional abnormalities (see *Clinical Insight:* Malnutrition in the Alcoholic).

Cholestatic Liver Diseases

Primary Biliary Cirrhosis

Primary biliary cirrhosis (PBC) is a chronic cholestatic disease caused by progressive destruction of small and intermediate-sized intrahepatic bile ducts. The extrahepatic biliary tree and larger intrahepatic ducts are normal. Ninety percent of patients with PBC are women, and this disease progresses slowly, eventually resulting in cirrhosis and portal hypertension and liver transplantation or resulting in death. Primary biliary cirrhosis is an immune-mediated disease in which serum autoantibodies, elevated immunoglobulin levels, circulating immune complexes, and depressed cell-mediated immune response are present. Several nutritional complications from cholestasis can occur with PBC, including osteope-

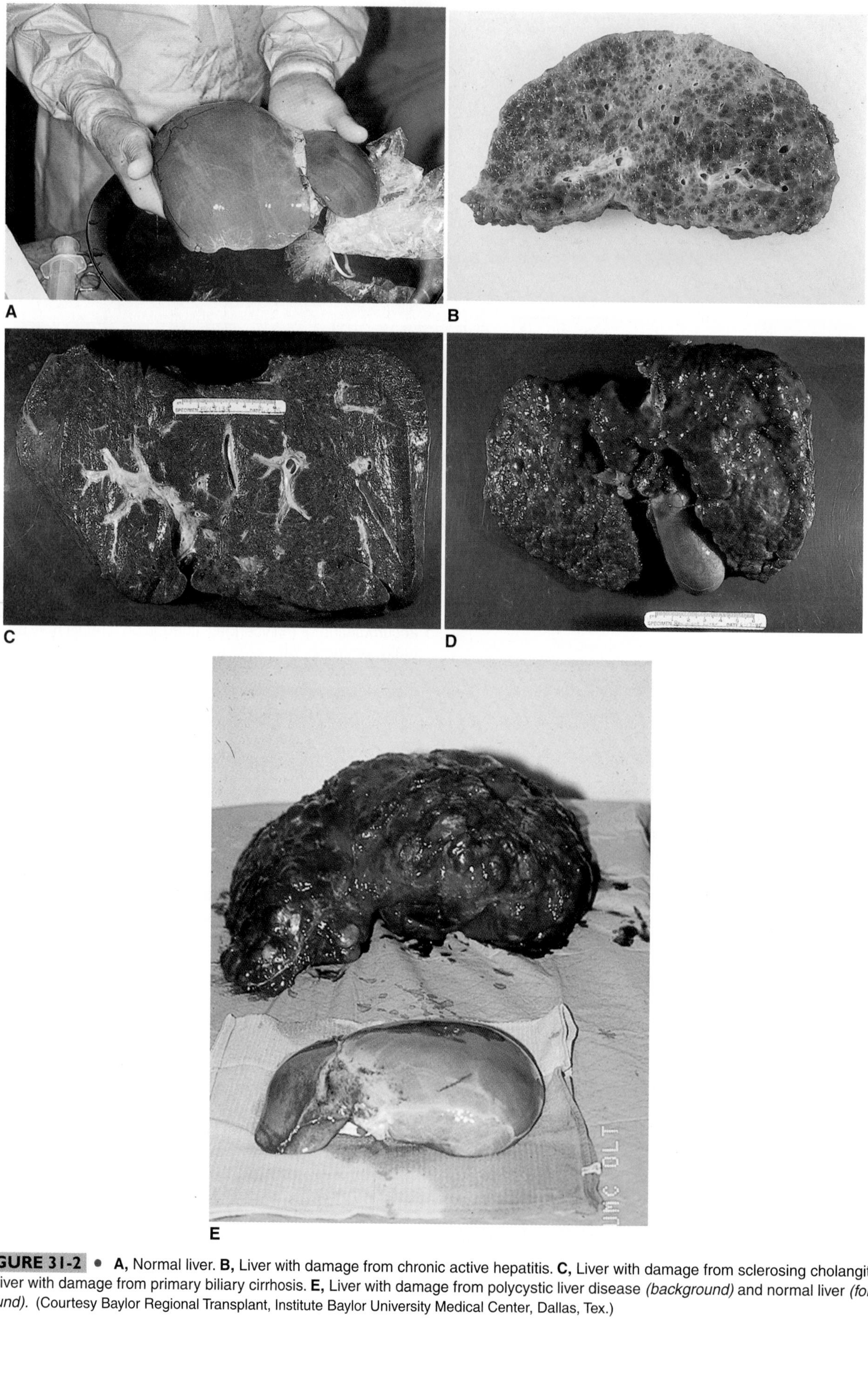

FIGURE 31-2 • **A,** Normal liver. **B,** Liver with damage from chronic active hepatitis. **C,** Liver with damage from sclerosing cholangitis. **D,** Liver with damage from primary biliary cirrhosis. **E,** Liver with damage from polycystic liver disease *(background)* and normal liver *(foreground).* (Courtesy Baylor Regional Transplant, Institute Baylor University Medical Center, Dallas, Tex.)

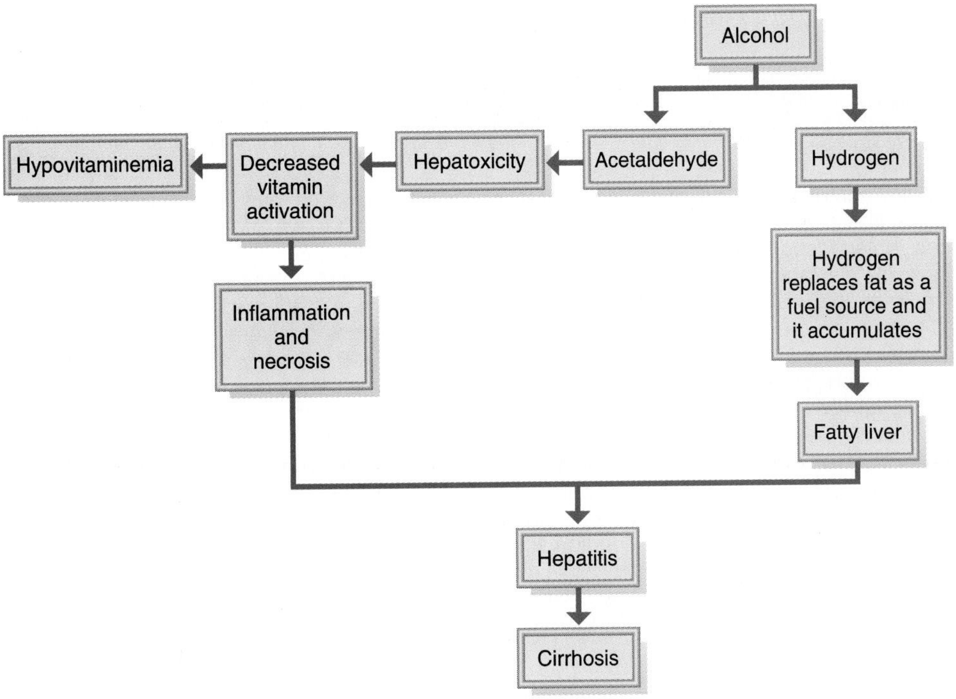

FIGURE 31-3 • Complications of excessive alcohol consumption stem largely from excess hydrogen and from acetaldehyde. Hydrogen produces fatty liver and hyperlipemia, high blood lactic acid, and low blood sugar. The accumulation of fat, the effect of acetaldehyde on liver cells, and other factors as yet unknown lead to alcoholic hepatitis. The next step is cirrhosis. The consequent impairment of liver function disturbs blood chemistry, notably causing a high ammonia level that can lead to coma and death. Cirrhosis also distorts liver structure, inhibiting blood flow. High pressure in vessels supplying the liver may cause ruptured varices and accumulation of fluid in the abdominal cavity. There are individual differences in response to alcohol; in particular, not all heavy drinkers develop hepatitis and cirrhosis.

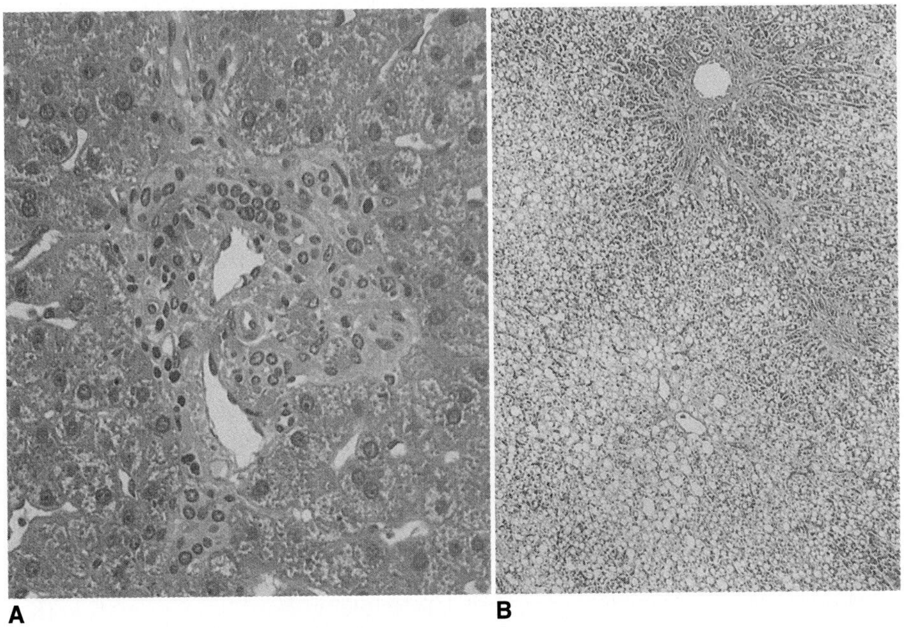

FIGURE 31-4 • **A,** Microscopic appearance of a normal liver. A normal portal tract consists of the portal vein, hepatic arteriole, one to two interlobular bile ducts, and occasional peripherally located ductules. **B,** Acute fatty liver. This photomicrograph on low power exhibits fatty change involving virtually all the hepatocytes, with slight sparing of the liver cells immediately adjacent to the portal tract *(top).* (From Kanel G, Korula J: *Atlas of liver pathology,* Philadelphia, 1992, WB Saunders.)

CLINICAL INSIGHT

Malnutrition in the Alcoholic

Several factors contribute to the malnutrition that is common in chronic alcoholics with liver disease:

1. Alcohol can replace food in the diet of moderate and heavy drinkers, displacing the intake of adequate calories and nutrients. In light drinkers it is usually an additional energy source (Lieber, 1988), also called "empty calories." Although alcohol yields 7.1 kcal/g, when it is consumed in large amounts, it is not utilized efficiently as a fuel source (Mezey, 1991).
2. In the alcoholic, impaired digestion and absorption are related to pancreatic insufficiency, as well as deficiency of brush-border enzymes such as lactase (Mezey, 1991). In particular, malabsorption of thiamin, vitamin B_{12}, folic acid, *d*-xylose, zinc, and amino acids is seen. Steatorrhea resulting from bile acid deficiency is also common in alcoholic liver disease. Ethanol itself has a direct effect on digestion and absorption, which is reversed by abstinence from ethanol.
3. Metabolism is altered in alcoholic liver disease. Micronutrients affected include folate, thiamin, pyridoxine, vitamin A, vitamin D, zinc, and selenium (McClain et al, 1991; Mezey, 1991). For example, ethanol metabolites can cause increased degradation of the active form of pyridoxine or interfere with the formation and release of the active form of folate. Wernicke-Korsakoff syndrome from thiamin deficiency is common and is related to deranged metabolism. Magnesium and phosphorus can also be added to the list of micronutrients deficient in alcoholics (Shronts and Fish, 1993).

nia, hypercholesterolemia, and fat-soluble vitamin deficiencies (Friedman, 2000).

Sclerosing Cholangitis

Primary sclerosing cholangitis (PSC) is another chronic cholestatic liver disease. Fibrosing inflammation of segments of extrahepatic bile ducts, with or without involvement of intrahepatic ducts, characterizes the disease. Progression of the disease leads to complications of portal hypertension, hepatic failure, and cholangiocarcinoma. Like PBC, PSC may be an immune disorder because of its strong association with human leukocyte antigen haplotypes, autoantibodies, and multiple immunologic abnormalities. Fifty to 75% of patients with PSC also have inflammatory bowel disease (especially ulcerative colitis), and 60% to 70% of persons with PSC are men. Patients with PSC are also at increased risk of fat-soluble vitamin deficiencies resulting from steatorrhea associated with this disease (Vierling, 1996). Hepatic osteodystrophy may occur from vitamin D and calcium malabsorption, resulting in secondary hyperparathyroidism and osteomalacia or rickets (Klein et al, 2002). Treatment often involves use of ursodeoxycholic acid (UDCA) and immunosuppressants such as prednisone, budesonide, and azathioprine, which can delay the need for transplantation (Holtmeier and Leuschner, 2001).

Inherited Disorders

Inherited disorders of the liver include hemochromatosis, Wilson's disease, α_1-antitrypsin deficiency, and others. Hemochromatosis is an inherited disease of iron overload. Patients with hereditary hemochromatosis may store 20 to 40 g of iron compared with 0.3 to 0.8 g in normal persons (see Chapter 34). Hepatomegaly, esophageal varices, ascites, impaired hepatic synthetic function, abnormal skin pigmentation, glucose intolerance, cardiac involvement, hypogonadism, arthropathy, and hepatocellular carcinoma may develop. Early diagnosis includes clinical, laboratory, and pathologic testing, including elevated serum transferrin levels. Life expectancy is normal if phlebotomy is initiated before the development of cirrhosis or diabetes mellitus (Brandhagen et al, 2002).

Wilson's disease is an autosomal recessive disorder associated with impaired biliary copper excretion. Copper accumulates in various tissues, including the liver, brain, cornea, and kidneys. Low serum ceruloplasmin levels and the presence of Kayser-Fleischer rings confirm the diagnosis, although patients with this disease may consult a physician before these confirming symptoms develop (Maher, 2000). Patients can present with acute, fulminant, or chronic active hepatitis secondary to Wilson's disease. Often neurologic signs may be the first indication of illness (Sokol, 1996). Copper-chelating agents and possibly zinc supplementation (to inhibit intestinal copper absorption and binding in the liver) are used to treat Wilson's disease once it is diagnosed. A low-copper diet is implemented if other therapies are unsuccessful (Table 31-2). If this disease is not diagnosed until onset of fulminant failure, survival is not possible without transplantation (Kayler et al, 2002).

α_1-Antitrypsin deficiency is another inherited disorder, and it can cause both liver and lung disease (Maher, 2000). α_1-Antitrypsin is a glycoprotein found in serum and body fluids; it inhibits several proteolytic enzymes. Cholestasis or cirrhosis is caused by this deficiency (Whitington, 1996), and there is no treatment except liver transplantation.

TABLE 31-2 Copper Content of Commonly Used Foods*

FOOD GROUPS	HIGH (>0.2 mg/PORTION COMMONLY USED†) (AVOID)	MODERATE (0.1-0.2 mg/PORTION) (NO MORE THAN 6 SERVINGS/DAY)	LOW (<0.1 mg/PORTION COMMONLY USED†) (MAY BE EATEN AS DESIRED)
Meat and meat substitutes	Lamb; pork; pheasant; quail; duck; goose; squid; salmon; all organ meats including liver, heart, kidney, brain; all shellfish, including oysters, scallops, shrimp, lobster, clams, and crab; meat gelatin; soy protein meat substitutes; tofu; all nuts and seeds	All other fish (3 oz), dark meat turkey (3 oz), peanut butter (2 tbsp)	Beef, cheese, cottage cheese, eggs, light meat turkey; cold cuts and frankfurters that do not contain pork, dark turkey, or organ meats; all others not listed on high or moderate list
Fats and oils	Avocado	Olives (2 medium); cream (½ c)	Butter; cream; margarine; mayonnaise; nondairy cream substitutes; oils; sour cream; salad dressings (made from allowed ingredients); all others not listed on high or moderate list
Milk	Chocolate; cocoa; soy milk		All other dairy products; milk flavored with carob
Starch	Dried beans including soybeans, lima beans, baked beans, garbanzo beans, pinto beans, dried peas; lentils; millet; barley; wheat germ; bran breads and cereals; cereals with >0.2 mg copper per serving (check label); soy flour; soy grits; sweet potatoes (fresh)	Whole-wheat bread (1 slice); potatoes in any form (½ c or 1 small); pumpkin (¾ c); melba toast (4); whole-wheat crackers (6); parsnips (⅔ c); winter squash (½ c); green peas (½ c); instant oatmeal (½ c); instant Ralston (½ c); cereals with 0.1-0.2 mg of copper per serving (check labels); dehydrated and canned soups (1 c)	Breads and pasta from refined flour; canned sweet potatoes; rice; regular oatmeal; cereals with <0.1 mg of copper per serving (check label); all others not listed on high or moderate list
Vegetables	Mushrooms; vegetable juice cocktail	Bean sprouts (1 c); beets (½ c); spinach (½ c cooked, 1 c raw); tomato juice and other tomato products (½ c); broccoli (½ c); asparagus (½ c)	All others, including fresh tomatoes
Fruits	Nectarines; dried fruits including raisins, dates, and prunes (dried fruits are permitted if dried at home)	Mango (½ c); pears (1 medium); pineapple (½ c); papaya (¼ average)	All others
Desserts	Desserts that contain significant amounts of any foods high in copper		All others
Sugar and sweets	Chocolate; cocoa	Licorice (1 oz); syrups (1 oz)	All others including jams, jellies, and candies made with allowed fruits; carob; flavoring extracts
Miscellaneous	Brewer's yeast	Ketchup	
Beverages‡	Instant breakfast beverages; mineral water; alcohol§	Postum and other cereal beverages	All others including fruit-flavored beverages; lemonade

From Pemberton CM et al: *Mayo Clinic diet manual: a handbook of nutrition practices*, ed 7, St. Louis, 1994, Mosby.

*Data that are available on the average copper content of foods vary greatly. There is disagreement on the copper content of the usual American diet, with estimates that range from 1 mg of copper a day to 5 mg/day. The concentration of copper in foods is affected by many factors, including soil conditions, geographic location, species, diet, processing method, and contamination in processing. The exact copper content of foods is difficult to verify. It is estimated that avoidance of high-copper foods and restriction of moderate-copper foods results in a diet of approximately 1 mg/day. For practical purposes, diets are designed to limit foods with a higher copper content than other foods, and not to achieve a specific level of copper in the diet.

†Portions commonly used are those generally accepted as typical portion sizes in various nutrient data source manuals.

‡A water sample from the patient's home water supply should be analyzed for copper content. Demineralized water should be used if the water contains more than 100 μg/L.

§Although not necessarily high in copper, alcoholic beverages are discouraged because of their action as a hepatotoxin.

Other Liver Diseases

Liver disease has several other causes. Liver tumors can be primary or metastatic, benign or malignant. The liver can be affected in the presence of systemic diseases such as rheumatoid arthritis, systemic lupus erythematosus, polymyalgia, rheumatic or temporal arteritis, polyarteritis nodosa, systemic sclerosis, and Sjögren's syndrome (Bonacini, 1996). Liver disease can also occur as a result of nonalcoholic steatohepatitis caused by obesity, diabetes mellitus, parenteral nutrition (PN), and jejunoileal bypass.

When hepatic blood flow is altered as in acute ischemic and chronic congestive hepatopathy, Budd-Chiari syndrome, and hepatic venoocclusive disease, hepatic dysfunction occurs (Bacon et al, 1996). Parasitic, bacterial, fungal, and granulomatous liver diseases also occur. Finally, cryptogenic cirrhosis is any cirrhosis for which the etiology is unknown.

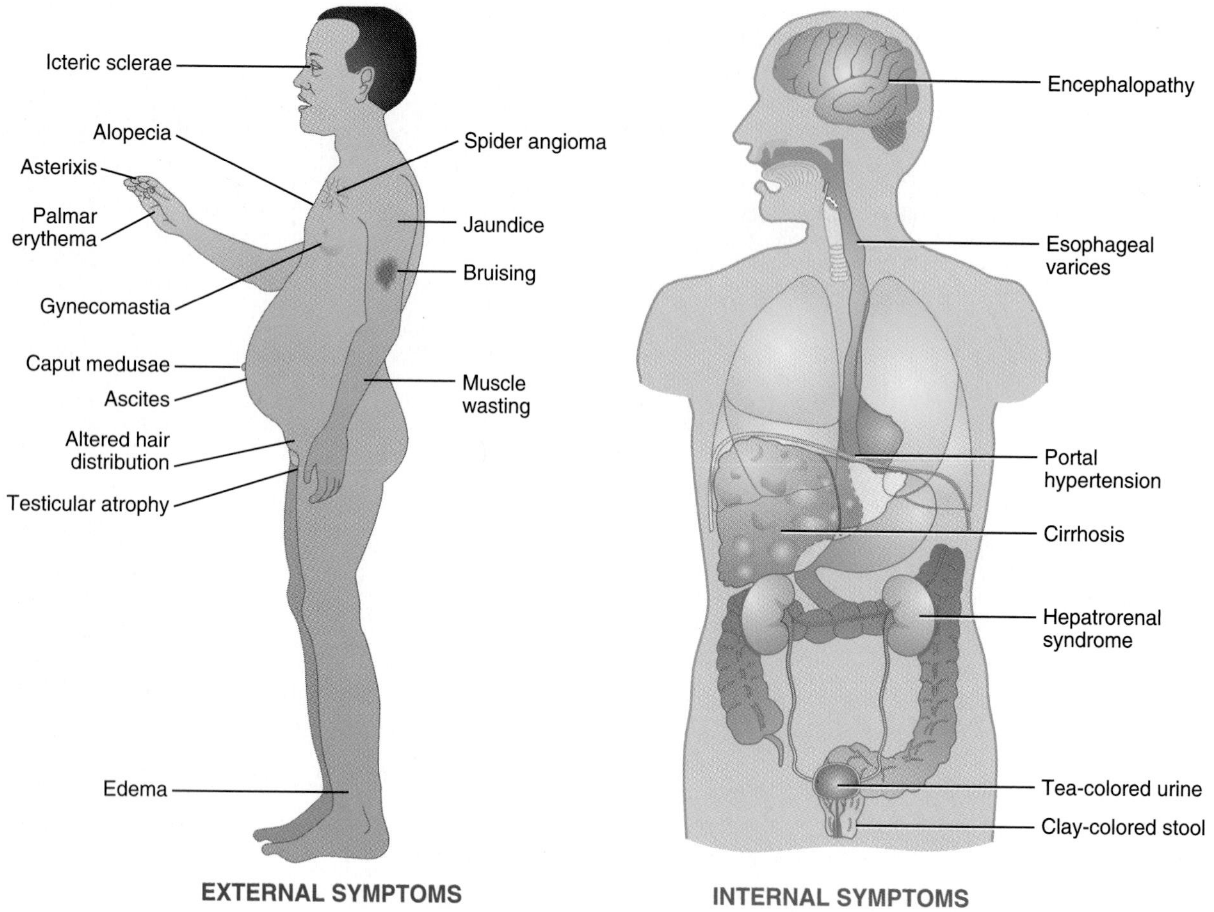

FIGURE 31-5 • Clinical manifestations of cirrhosis.

Cirrhosis

Medical Nutrition Therapy

Cirrhosis has many clinical manifestations, as illustrated in Figure 31-5. Several major complications of end-stage liver disease (ESLD), including malnutrition, ascites, hyponatremia, hepatic encephalopathy, glucose alterations, fat malabsorption, hepatorenal syndrome, and osteopenia, have nutritional implications. When appropriate nutrition therapy is provided to patients with liver disease, malnutrition can be reversed and clinical outcomes improved. Studies to date have been able to show positive outcomes with parenteral and enteral nutrition in malnourished patients with cirrhosis, including improvement in nutritional status and clinical complications of cirrhosis such as ascites, encephalopathy, and infection, in addition to decreased mortality (Campillo et al, 1995).

Before appropriate nutrition therapy can be implemented, a nutritional assessment must be performed to determine the extent and cause of malnutrition. Many traditional markers of nutritional status are affected by liver disease and its consequences, making assessment difficult. Table 31-3 summarizes the factors that affect interpretation of nutritional assessment parameters in patients with liver dysfunction.

Objective parameters that may be helpful when monitored serially include anthropometric measurements and dietary intake (Hasse, 2001; McCullough et al, 1998; Plauth et al, 1997). The best way to perform a nutritional assessment may be to combine these parameters with the subjective global assessment (SGA) approach.

The SGA has been used in liver disease and transplantation and has demonstrated an acceptable level of reliability and validity (Detsky et al, 1987; Hasse et al, 1993; Stephenson et al, 2001). This method uses a few readily available parameters obtained by an experienced clinician (see Chapter 17). The SGA gives a broad perspective, but it is not sensitive to changes in nutritional status. Other available parameters should also be reviewed for their impact on the patient's overall health status. The elements of SGA in evaluating nutritional status are summarized in Box 31-1.

Malnutrition

Moderate to severe malnutrition is a common finding in patients with advanced liver disease (McCullough et al, 1998) (Figure 31-6). This is extremely significant considering that malnutrition plays a major role in the pathogenesis of liver injury and has a profound negative impact on prognosis (Donaghy, 2002).

Box 31-1. Subjective Global Assessment (SGA) Parameters for Nutritional Evaluation of Liver Disease Patients

History

Weight change (consider fluctuations resulting from ascites and edema)
Appetite
Taste changes and early satiety
Dietary recall (calories, protein, sodium)
Persistent gastrointestinal problems (nausea, vomiting, diarrhea, constipation, difficulty chewing or swallowing)

Physical

Muscle wasting
Fat stores
Ascites or edema

Existing Conditions

Disease state and other problems that could influence nutritional status such as hepatic encephalopathy, gastrointestinal bleeding, renal insufficiency, infection

Nutritional Rating (Based on Results of Above Parameters)

Well nourished
Moderately (or suspected of being) malnourished
Severely malnourished

From Hasse J: Nutritional aspects of adult liver transplantation. In Busuttil RW, Klintmalm GB, editors: *Transplantation of the liver,* Philadelphia, 1996, WB Saunders.

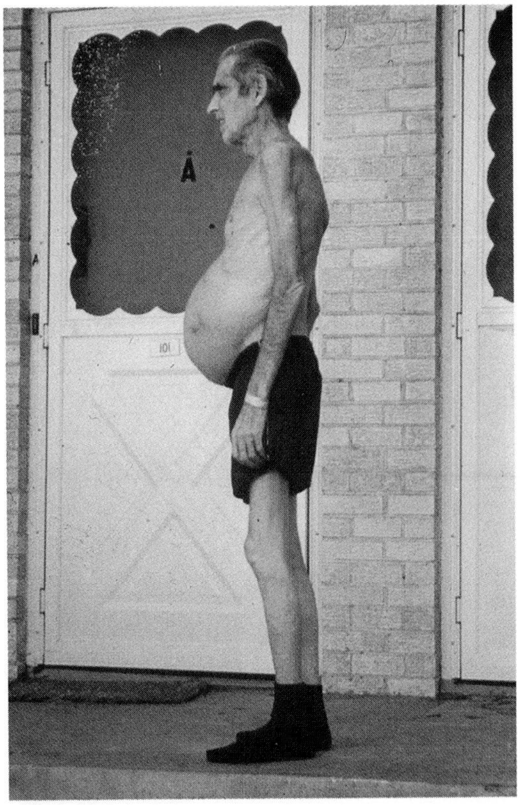

FIGURE 31-6 • Severe malnutrition and ascites in a man with end-stage liver disease.

Numerous coexisting factors are involved in the development of malnutrition in liver disease (Figure 31-7). Inadequate oral intake, a major contributor, is caused by anorexia, dysgeusia, early satiety, nausea, and vomiting associated with liver disease and the drugs used to treat it, including diuretics, bile acid sequestrants, neomycin, and lactulose (Francisco-Ziller

TABLE 31-3 Factors That Affect Interpretation of Objective Nutrition Assessment Tests in Patients With End-Stage Liver Disease

PARAMETER	FACTORS AFFECTING INTERPRETATION
Body weight	Affected by edema, ascites, and diuretic use
Anthropometric measurements	Questionable sensitivity, specificity, and reliability
	Multiple sources of error
	Unknown if skinfold measurements reflect total body fat
	References do not account for variation in hydration status and skin compressibility
Creatinine-height index	Affected by malnutrition, aging, decreased body mass, and protein intake
	Affected by renal function
	Creatinine is a metabolic end product of creatine synthesized in the liver; therefore, severe liver disease alters creatinine synthesis rates
Nitrogen balance studies	Nitrogen is retained in the body in the form of ammonia
	Hepatorenal syndrome can affect the excretion of nitrogen
3-Methyl histidine excretion	Affected by dietary intake, trauma, infection, and kidney function
Visceral protein levels	Synthesis of visceral proteins is decreased
	Affected by hydration status, malabsorption, and kidney insufficiency
Immune function tests	Affected by liver failure, electrolyte imbalances, infection, and kidney insufficiency

Modified from Hasse J: Nutritional aspects of adult liver transplantation. In Busuttil RW, Klintmalm GB, editors: *Transplantation of the liver,* Philadelphia, 1996, WB Saunders.

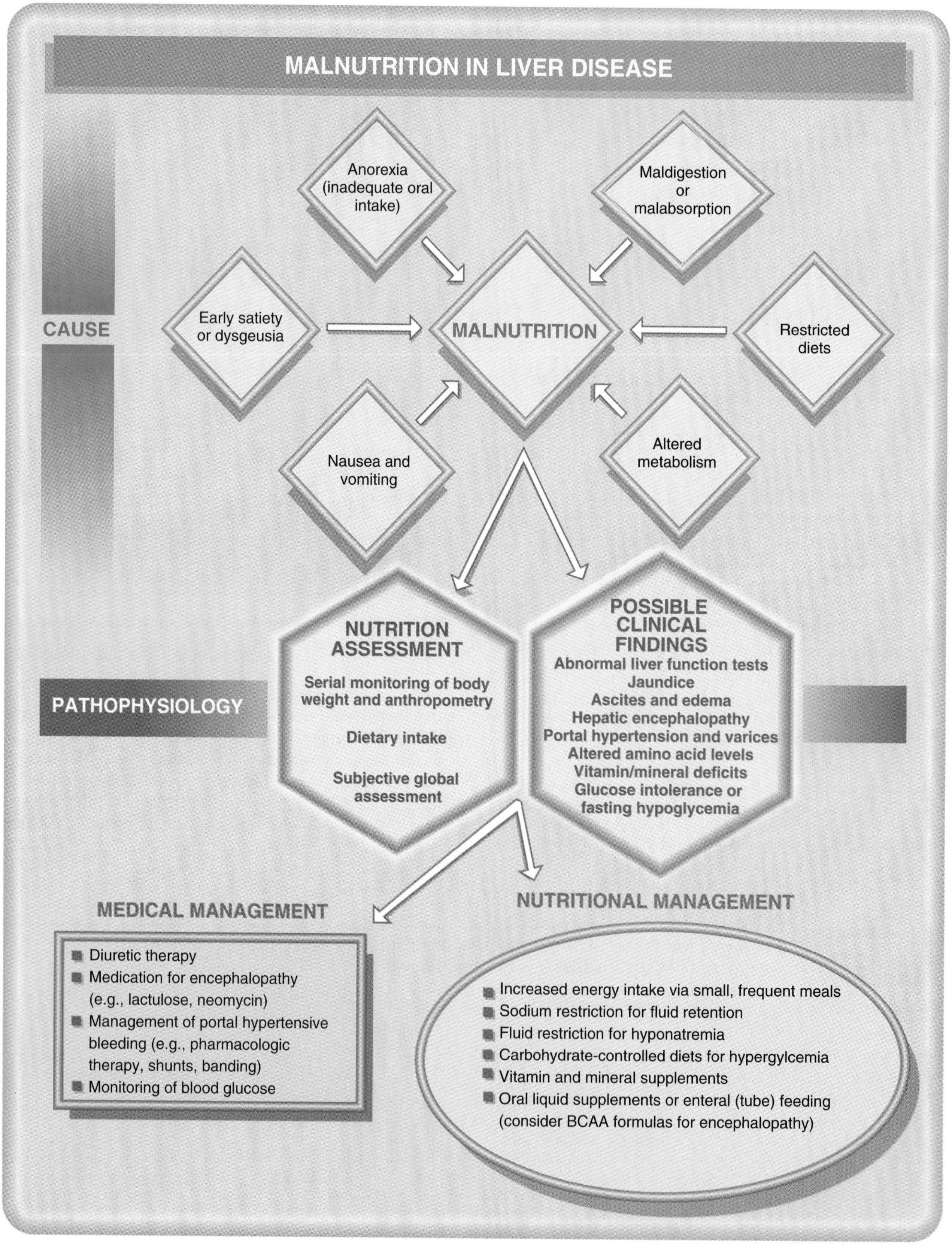

FIGURE 31-7 • Pathophysiology algorithm: malnutrition in liver disease. (Algorithm content developed by John Anderson, PhD, and Stanford C. Garner, PhD, 2000; updated by Jeanette Hasse, PhD, RD, LD, CNSD, FADA, and Laura E. Matarese, MS, RD, LD, CNSD, FADA, 2002.)

and DiCecco, 1998; Hasse et al, 1997; McCullough et al, 1998). Other causes of inadequate intake are related to dietary restrictions and unpalatable hospital diets.

Maldigestion and malabsorption also play a role in the malnutrition of liver disease. Steatorrhea is common in cirrhosis, especially if there is disease involving bile duct injury and obstruction. The medications previously mentioned may also cause specific malabsorptive losses. In addition, altered metabolism secondary to liver dysfunction causes malnutrition in various ways. Micronutrient function is affected by altered storage in the liver, decreased transport by liver-synthesized proteins, and renal losses associated with alcoholic and advanced liver disease. Abnormal macronutrient metabolism and increased energy expenditure can also contribute to malnutrition. Finally, protein losses can occur from large-volume paracentesis (Hasse et al, 1997).

Problems in Feeding

Because anorexia, nausea, dysgeusia, and other gastrointestinal symptoms are common, adequate nutrition intake is difficult to achieve. With ascites, early satiety is also a frequent complaint. Smaller, more frequent meals are better tolerated than three traditional meals. In addition, evidence suggests that frequent feedings also improve nitrogen balance and prevent hypoglycemia. Oral liquid supplements should be encouraged and, when necessary, enteral tube feedings used. Adjunctive nutrition support should be given to malnourished patients with liver disease if their intake is less than 0.8 g of protein and less than 30 calories per kilogram of body weight daily and if they are at risk for fatal complications of disease (Kondrup and Müller, 1997). Esophageal varices are usually not a contraindication for tube feeding.

Nutrient Requirements

Energy

Energy requirements vary among patients with cirrhosis. Several studies have measured resting energy expenditure (REE) in patients with liver disease to determine energy requirements. Some found patients with ESLD to be normometabolic and others hypometabolic or hypermetabolic. Although several studies concluded that patients with cirrhosis did not require any more calories than did healthy controls, Dolz and colleagues (1991) determined that ascites increases energy expenditure slightly. Other studies have found inverse relationships between severity of liver disease and energy expenditure without a significant increase in REE (Kondrup and Müller, 1997).

In general, energy requirements for patients with ESLD and without ascites are about 120% to 140% of the resting energy expenditure (REE) (McCullough et al, 1998). Requirements increase to 150% to 175% of REE if ascites, infection, or malabsorption is present or if nutritional repletion is necessary (Hasse et al, 1997). This equates to about 25 to 35 calories per kilogram. Estimated dry body weight should be used in calculations to prevent overfeeding.

Carbohydrate

Determining carbohydrate needs is often challenging in liver failure because of the liver's primary role in carbohydrate metabolism. Liver failure reduces glucose production and peripheral glucose utilization. The rate of gluconeogenesis is decreased, with preference for lipids and amino acids for energy (McCullough and Tavill, 1991; Plauth et al, 1997). Alterations in the hormones insulin, glucagon, cortisol, and epinephrine are responsible in part for the preference for alternative fuels.

Lipid

In cirrhosis, plasma free fatty acids, glycerol, and ketone bodies are increased in the fasting state. The body prefers lipids as an energy substrate, and lipolysis is increased with active mobilization of lipid deposits, but the net capacity to store exogenous lipid is not impaired. A range of 25% to 40% of calories as fat is generally recommended (Plauth et al, 1997).

Protein

Protein is by far the most controversial nutrient in liver failure, and its management also the most complex. Cirrhosis has long been thought of as a catabolic disease with increased protein breakdown and inadequate resynthesis, resulting in depletion of visceral protein stores and muscle wasting. Protein kinetic studies have been able to demonstrate increased nitrogen losses only in patients with fulminant hepatic failure or decompensated disease, but not in patients with stable cirrhosis (McCullough and Tavill, 1991). Patients with cirrhosis also have increased protein utilization (Nielsen et al, 1995).

At least one study (Nielsen et al, 1995) suggests that 0.8 g protein per kilogram per day is the mean protein requirement to achieve nitrogen balance in patients with stable cirrhosis. This is higher than the requirement to achieve nitrogen balance for normal persons (0.66 g/kg) (Kondrup and Müller, 1997). Therefore, in uncomplicated hepatitis or cirrhosis without encephalopathy, protein requirements range from 0.8 to 1.0 g per kilogram of dry weight per day to achieve nitrogen balance. To promote nitrogen accumulation or positive balance, at least 1.2 to 1.3 g per kilogram daily is needed (Nielsen et al, 1995). In situations of stress, such as alcoholic hepatitis or decompensated disease (sepsis, infection, gastrointestinal bleeding, severe ascites), at least 1.5 g of protein per kilogram, per day should be provided.

TABLE 31-4 Vitamin and Mineral Deficits in Severe Hepatic Failure

VITAMIN OR MINERAL	PREDISPOSING FACTORS	SIGNS OF DEFICIENCY
Vitamin A	Steatorrhea, neomycin, cholestyramine, alcoholism	Dermatitis, night-blindness
Vitamin D	Steatorrhea, glucocorticoids, cholestyramine	Osteomalacia
Vitamin E	Steatorrhea, cholestyramine	Edema, peripheral neuropathy
Vitamin K	Steatorrhea, antibiotics, cholestyramine	Bleeding
Vitamin B_6	Alcoholism	Mucous membrane lesions, dermatitis
Vitamin B_{12}	Alcoholism, cholestyramine	Megaloblastic anemia, glossitis, CNS dysfunction
Folate	Alcoholism	Megaloblastic anemia, glossitis, irritability
Niacin	Alcoholism	Dermatitis, dementia, diarrhea, inflammation of mucous membranes
Thiamin	Alcoholism, high CHO diet	Neuropathy, ascites, edema, CNS dysfunction
Zinc	Diarrhea, diuretics, alcoholism	Immunodeficiency, impaired taste acuity, wound healing, protein synthesis
Magnesium	Alcoholism, diuretics	Neuromuscular irritability, hypokalemia, hypocalcemia
Iron	Chronic bleeding	Stomatitis, microcytic anemia, malaise
Potassium	Diuretics, anabolism, insulin use	Muscular weakness, malaise, respiratory or cardiac arrest
Phosphorus	Anabolism, alcoholism	Anorexia, weakness, cardiac failure, glucose intolerance

Modified from Shronts EP: Nutritional assessment of adults with end-stage hepatic failure, *Nutr Clin Prac* 3:113, 1988.
CHO, Carbohydrate; *CNS*, central nervous system.

Vitamins and Minerals

Vitamin and mineral supplementation is needed in all patients with ESLD because of the liver's intimate role in nutrient transport, storage, and metabolism, in addition to the side effects of drugs (Table 31-4). Vitamin deficiencies can contribute to complications. For example, folate and vitamin B_{12} deficiencies can lead to macrocytic anemia. Deficiency of pyridoxine, thiamin, or vitamin B_{12} can result in neuropathy. Confusion, ataxia, and ocular disturbances can result from a thiamin deficiency, and impaired dark adaptation can occur from vitamin A deficiency (McCullough et al, 1998).

Deficiencies of fat-soluble vitamins have been found in all types of liver failure, especially in cholestatic diseases in which malabsorption and steatorrhea occur. Therefore, supplementation is necessary, using water-soluble forms. Intravenous or intramuscular vitamin K is often given for 3 days to rule out vitamin K deficiency as the cause of a prolonged prothrombin times. Water-soluble vitamin deficiencies associated with alcoholic liver disease include thiamin (which can lead to Wernicke's encephalopathy), pyridoxine (B_6), cyanocobalamin (B_{12}), folate, and niacin (B_3). Large doses (100 mg) of thiamin are given daily for a limited time if deficiency is suspected.

Mineral nutriture is also altered in liver disease. Iron stores may be depleted in patients experiencing gastrointestinal bleeding; however, iron supplementation should be avoided by persons with hemochromatosis or hemosiderosis (see Chapter 34). Elevated serum copper levels are found in cholestatic liver diseases (i.e., PBC and PSC). Because copper and manganese are excreted primarily via bile, supplementation should not be given.

Wilson's disease is a disorder of abnormal copper metabolism in which urinary excretion is high, serum levels are low, and excess copper in various organs causes severe damage. Oral chelating agents such as zinc acetate or *d*-penicillamine are the primary treatment. A vegetarian diet may be useful as adjunctive therapy because copper is less available (Brewer et al, 1993). Dietary copper restriction (see Table 31-2) is not routinely prescribed unless other therapies are unsuccessful.

Zinc and magnesium levels are low in liver disease related to alcoholism, in part because of diuretic therapy. Calcium as well as magnesium and zinc may be malabsorbed with steatorrhea. Therefore, at least standard doses to meet the DRIs for these minerals should be provided.

Portal Hypertension

Portal hypertension increases collateral blood flow and can result in varices in the gastrointestinal tract. These varices often bleed, causing a medical emergency. Treatment includes administration of α-adrenergic blockers to decrease heart rate, endoscopic banding or variceal ligation, and radiologic or surgical placement of shunts. During an acute bleeding episode, somatostatin analog may be administered to decrease bleeding, or a nasogastric tube equipped with an inflatable balloon will be placed to tamponade bleeding vessels (Crippin, 1996).

Medical Nutrition Therapy

During acute bleeding episodes, nutrition cannot be administered enterally. PN is indicated if a patient will be taking nothing orally for at least 5 days. Repeated endoscopic therapies may cause esophageal strictures or impair a patient's swallowing. Finally, surgically or radiologically placed shunts may increase the incidence of encephalopathy and reduce nutrient metabolism because blood is shunted past the liver cells.

Ascites

Fluid retention is common, and ascites (accumulation of fluid in the abdominal cavity) is a serious consequence of liver disease. Portal hypertension, hypoalbuminemia, lymphatic obstruction, and renal retention of sodium and fluid contribute to fluid retention. Increased release of catecholamines, renin, angiotensin, aldosterone, and antidiuretic hormone secondary to peripheral arterial vasodilation causes renal retention of sodium and water.

Large-volume paracentesis may be used to relieve ascites. Diuretic therapy is often used and includes spironolactone and furosemide. These drugs are often used in combination for best effect. Furosemide, a loop diuretic, has a stronger natriuretic effect, but spironolactone is more effective in increasing sodium excretion in patients with ESLD (Gurk-Turner, 1997). Major side effects of loop diuretics include hyponatremia, hypokalemia, hypomagnesemia, hypocalcemia, and hypochloremic acidosis. Conversely, spironolactone is potassium sparing. Serum potassium levels must therefore be monitored carefully and supplemented or restricted if necessary because deficiency or excess can contribute to metabolic abnormalities. Weight, abdominal girth, urinary sodium concentration, and serum levels of urea nitrogen, creatinine, albumin, uric acid, and electrolytes should be monitored during diuretic therapy.

Medical Nutrition Therapy

Dietary treatment for ascites includes sodium restriction in addition to diuretic therapy. Sodium is commonly restricted to 2 g per day (see Chapter 36 for discussion of low-sodium diets). More severe limitations may be imposed; however, caution is warranted because of the limited palatability of these diets. Adequate protein intake is also important when a patient undergoes frequent paracentesis.

Hyponatremia

Hyponatremia often occurs because of decreased ability to excrete water because of the persistent release of antidiuretic hormone, sodium losses via paracentesis, excessive diuretic use, or overly aggressive sodium restriction. Fluid intake is usually restricted to 1 to 1.5 L per day, depending on the severity of the edema and ascites. Daily fluid intake may be restricted to as little as 500 to 750 ml plus urinary losses if hyponatremia is severe and persistent (Hasse et al, 1997). A moderate sodium intake should be continued because excessive sodium intake will worsen fluid retention and the dilution of serum sodium levels.

Hepatic Encephalopathy

Many conditions can cause hepatic encephalopathy. Gastrointestinal bleeding, fluid and electrolyte abnormalities, uremia, infection, use of sedatives, hyperglycemia or hypoglycemia, alcohol withdrawal, constipation, and acidosis can precipitate hepatic encephalopathy. Subclinical or overt hepatic encephalopathy occurs in 50% to 70% of patients with chronic hepatic failure (Diehl, 2000), but it is precipitated by excessive dietary protein intake in only about 7% to 9% of patients with liver failure (Leevy and Davison, 1967). Hepatic or portal systemic encephalopathy results in neuromuscular and behavioral alterations. Box 31-2 describes the four stages of hepatic encephalopathy.

Box 31-2. Four Stages of Hepatic Encephalopathy

Stage	Symptoms
I	Mild confusion, agitation, irritability, sleep disturbance, decreased attention
II	Lethargy, disorientation, inappropriate behavior, drowsiness
III	Somnolent but arousable, incomprehensible speech, confused, aggressive behavior when awake
IV	Coma

Just as there are multiple causes of hepatic encephalopathy, there are multiple theories as to the mechanism by which hepatic encephalopathy occurs. Ammonia is considered an important etiologic factor in the development of encephalopathy (Latifi et al, 1991). When the liver fails, it is unable to detoxify ammonia to urea, and ammonia is a direct cerebral toxin. Although serum and cerebrospinal fluid levels do not correlate well with the degree of hepatic encephalopathy, treatment is based on lowering these levels. Ammonia metabolites such as glutamine and α-ketoglutarate in cerebrospinal fluid have, however, correlated more closely with the severity of encephalopathy.

The main source of ammonia is the endogenous production by the gastrointestinal tract (i.e., from the degradation of bacteria and blood from gastrointestinal bleeding). Therefore, drugs such as lactulose and neomycin are given. Lactulose is a nonabsorbable disaccharide. It acidifies the colonic contents, retaining ammonia as the ammonium ion. It also acts as an osmotic laxative to remove the ammonia. Neomycin is a nonabsorbable antibiotic that helps decrease colonic ammonia production.

Exogenous protein is also a source of ammonia. Some clinicians suggest that dietary protein causes an increase in ammonia levels and subsequently hepatic encephalopathy, but this has not been proven in studies. One study even showed that patients with worsening hepatic encephalopathy often have decreased protein intakes and increased blood urea nitrogen and creatinine levels. Patients with improved encephalopathy had higher protein intakes

Box 31-3. Amino Acids Commonly Altered in Liver Disease

Aromatic amino acids (AAAs)
- Tyrosine
- Phenylalanine*
- Free tryptophan*

Branched-chain amino acids (BCAAs)
- Valine*
- Leucine*
- Isoleucine*

Ammoniogenic amino acids
- Glycine
- Serine
- Threonine*
- Glutamine
- Histidine*
- Lysine*
- Asparagine
- Methionine*

*Denotes essential amino acids.

and lower blood urea nitrogen and creatinine levels (Morgan et al, 1995).

Another major hypothesis for the pathogenesis of portal systemic encephalopathy has been termed the *altered neurotransmitter theory.* A plasma amino acid imbalance exists in ESLD in which branched-chain amino acids (BCAAs) are decreased and aromatic amino acids (AAAs) plus methionine, glutamine, asparagine, and histidine are increased (Box 31-3).

The BCAAs furnish as much as 30% of energy requirements for skeletal muscle, heart, and brain when gluconeogenesis and ketogenesis are depressed (Latifi et al, 1991). This causes serum BCAA levels to fall. At the same time, plasma AAAs and methionine are released into circulation by muscle proteolysis, but the synthesis into protein and liver clearance of AAAs is depressed (Hiyama and Fischer, 1988). This changes the plasma molar ratio of BCAA to AAA and may contribute to the development of hepatic encephalopathy; AAAs may limit the cerebral uptake of BCAAs because they compete for carrier-mediated transport at the blood–brain barrier (Latifi et al, 1991).

Several other substances have been implicated in the development of hepatic encephalopathy, such as short-chain fatty acids, mercaptans, phenols, and *a*-aminobutyric acid (Diehl, 2000). Another final dietary theory implicates zinc deficiency, types of fatty acids, or the amino acid tryptophan in the development of hepatic encephalopathy (Mullen and Weber, 1991).

Medical Nutrition Therapy

The practice of protein restriction in patients with low-grade hepatic encephalopathy is based on empiric evidence that protein intolerance causes hepatic encephalopathy, but it has never been proven in a study that it will improve mental state (Kondrup and Müller, 1997). Unnecessary protein restriction may only worsen body protein losses and therefore must be avoided. Patients with encephalopathy often do not receive adequate protein. More than 95% of patients with cirrhosis can tolerate mixed-protein diets up to 1.5 g per kilogram of body weight. True dietary protein intolerance is rare except in fulminant hepatic failure or in a rare patient with chronic endogenous hepatic encephalopathy (McCullough et al, 1998).

Studies evaluating the benefit of supplements enriched with BCAAs and restricted in AAAs have varied in study design, sample size, composition of BCAA-enriched formulas, level of encephalopathy, type of liver disease, duration of therapy, and control groups (Hasse et al, 1997). Even though it is difficult to compare the studies, most experts agree that BCAA-enriched formulas are indicated for patients with encephalopathy who do not tolerate standard proteins and who have not responded to lactulose and neomycin therapy (Ichida et al, 1996; Plauth et al, 1997).

Other theories postulate that vegetable proteins and casein may improve mental status compared with meat protein (Bianchi et al, 1993). Casein-based diets are lower in AAAs and higher in BCAAs than meat-based diets. The potential advantage of vegetable protein is that it is low in methionine and ammoniagenic amino acids and it is BCAA rich. The high-fiber content of a vegetable–protein diet may also play a role in the excretion of nitrogenous compounds.

Glucose Alterations

Glucose intolerance occurs in almost two thirds of patients with cirrhosis, and 10% to 37% of patients will develop overt diabetes. Glucose intolerance in patients with liver disease occurs because of insulin resistance in peripheral tissues. Hyperinsulinism also occurs in patients with cirrhosis, possibly because insulin production is increased, hepatic clearance is decreased, portasystemic shunting occurs, there is a defect in the insulin-binding action at the receptor site, or there is a postreceptor defect.

Fasting hypoglycemia can occur because of the decreased availability of glucose from glycogen in addition to the failing gluconeogenic capacity in ESLD. Hypoglycemia occurs more often in acute or fulminant liver failure than in chronic liver disease. Hypoglycemia may also occur after alcohol consumption in patients whose glycogen stores are depleted by starvation due to the block of hepatic gluconeogenesis by ethanol. Patients with hypoglycemia should eat frequently to prevent this condition (see *Clinical Insight:* Fasting Hypoglycemia).

Fat Malabsorption

Fat absorption may be impaired in liver disease. Possible causes include decreased bile salt secretion (as

CLINICAL INSIGHT

Fasting Hypoglycemia

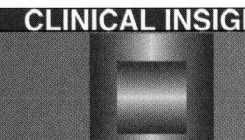

Two thirds of the glucose requirement in an adult is used by the central nervous system. During fasting, plasma glucose concentrations are maintained for use by the nervous system and the brain because liver glycogen is broken down, or new glucose is made from nonglucose precursors such as alanine (Polonsky, 1992). Fasting hypoglycemia occurs when there is reduced synthesis of new glucose or reduced liver glycogen breakdown.

Causes of fasting hypoglycemia include cirrhosis, consumption of alcohol, extensive intrahepatic cancer, deficiency of the hormones cortisol and growth hormone, or non–beta cell tumors of the pancreas. The method for detecting it involves measuring plasma insulin when plasma glucose is low. The diagnostic hallmark of an insulinoma is altered insulin secretion in the presence of hypoglycemia. Fasting hypoglycemia may also be caused by spontaneously produced antibodies. All patients with liver or pancreatic disease should be monitored for fasting hypoglycemia. Nutritional therapy involves balanced meals with small, frequent snacks to avoid periods of fasting. Monitoring of blood glucose and insulin levels is required.

in PBC, sclerosing cholangitis, and biliary strictures), administration of neomycin or cholestyramine, and pancreatic enzyme insufficiency. Stools may be greasy, floating, or light or clay colored, signifying malabsorption, which can be verified by a 72-hour fecal fat study (see Chapter 30).

Medical Nutrition Therapy

If significant steatorrhea is present, replacement of some of the long-chain triglycerides (LCTs) or dietary fat with medium-chain triglycerides (MCT) may be useful. Because MCTs do not require bile salts and micelle formation for absorption, they are readily taken up via the portal route (see Chapter 30). Some nutrition supplements contain MCT, which can be used in addition to liquid MCT oil (see Appendixes 36-41). Fifteen milliliters, three to four times per day, is recommended (15 ml provides 115 kcal, or about 7.7 kcal/ml).

Significant stool fat losses may warrant a trial of a low-fat (40 g) diet. If diarrhea does not resolve, the fat restriction should be discontinued because it decreases the palatability of the diet and severely hampers adequate calorie intake (Corish, 1997).

Renal Insufficiency and Hepatorenal Syndrome

Hepatorenal syndrome is renal failure associated with severe liver disease without intrinsic kidney abnormalities (Friedman, 2000). Hepatorenal syndrome is characterized by reductions in renal blood flow, cortical perfusion, and glomerular filtration rate (Friedman, 2000). If conservative therapies, including discontinuation of nephrotoxic drugs, optimization of intravascular volume status, treatment of underlying infection, and monitoring of fluid intake and output fail, dialysis may be required. In any case, renal insufficiency and failure may necessitate alteration in fluid, sodium, potassium, and phosphorus intake.

Osteopenia

Osteopenia has been identified as a problem particularly in patients with primary biliary cirrhosis, sclerosing cholangitis, and alcoholic liver disease. Depressed osteoblastic function and osteoporosis also can occur in patients with hemochromatosis, and osteoporosis is prevalent in patients who have had long-term treatment with corticosteroids. Corticosteroids increase bone resorption, suppress osteoblastic function, and affect sex hormone secretion, intestinal absorption of dietary calcium, renal excretion of calcium and phosphorus, and the vitamin D system (Epstein et al, 1995; Katz and Epstein, 1992).

Medical Nutrition Therapy

Prevention or treatment options for osteopenia include weight maintenance, ingestion of a well-balanced diet, adequate protein to maintain muscle mass, 1500 mg calcium per day, adequate vitamin D from the diet or supplements, avoidance of alcohol, and monitoring for steatorrhea, with diet adjustments as needed to minimize nutrient losses (Hasse et al, 1997).

LIVER RESECTION AND TRANSPLANTATION

Liver resection and thermal ablation are fairly common now that problem areas can be located by means of tomography and arteriography. As with any major surgery, protein and energy needs increase after liver resection. Needs are also increased to promote liver cell regeneration. Enteral nutrition is vital because of the role of portal hepatotrophic factors necessary for liver cell proliferation. Optimal nutrition is most important for patients with poor nutritional status before hepatectomy (e.g., patients with hepatocellular carcinoma or cholangiocarcinoma).

TABLE 31-5 Medications Commonly Used After Liver Transplantation

IMMUNOSUPPRESSANT DRUG	POSSIBLE NUTRITION SIDE EFFECTS	PROPOSED NUTRITION THERAPY
Azathioprine	Macrocytic anemia	Give folate supplements
	Mouth sores	Give foods if needed
	Nausea, vomiting, diarrhea, anorexia, sore throat, stomach pain, decreased taste acuity	Adjust food and meals as needed; monitor intake
Antithymocyte globulin	Nausea, vomiting	Adjust food and meals as needed; monitor intake
Basiliximab	None reported	
Cyclosporine	Sodium retention	Decrease sodium intake
	Hyperkalemia	Decrease potassium intake
	Hyperlipidemia	Limit fat and simple carbohydrate intake
	Hyperglycemia	Decrease simple carbohydrate intake
	Decreased serum magnesium level	Increase magnesium intake; give supplements
	Hypertension	Limit sodium intake
	Nausea, vomiting	Adjust food and meals as needed; monitor intake
Daclizumab	None reported	
Glucocorticoids	Sodium retention	Decrease sodium intake
	Hyperglycemia	Decrease simple carbohydrate intake
	Hyperlipidemia	Limit fat and simple carbohydrate intake
	False hunger	Avoid overeating
	Protein wasting with high doses	Increased protein intake
	Decreased absorption of calcium and phosphorus	Increase calcium and phosphorus intake; give supplements as needed
Muromonab-CD3	Nausea, vomiting, anorexia	Adjust food and meals as needed; monitor intake
Mycophenolate Mofetil	GI symptoms: nausea, vomiting, diarrhea	Adjust food and meals as needed; monitor intake
Sirolimus	Possible hyperglycemia	Decrease simple carbohydrate intake
	Possible GI symptoms	Adjust food and meals as needed; monitor intake
	Hyperlipidemia	Limit fat and simple carbohydrate intake
Tacrolimus	Hyperglycemia	Decrease simple carbohydrate intake
	Hyperkalemia	Decrease potassium intake
	Nausea, vomiting	Adjust food and meals as needed; monitor intake
15-Deoxysperagualin	GI symptoms	Adjust food and meals as needed; monitor intake

Modified from Hasse J: Role of the dietitian in the nutrition management of adults after liver transplantation, *J Am Diet Assoc* 91:473, 1991.

Liver transplantation has become an established treatment for ESLD. Malnutrition is common in liver transplant candidates. Dietary intake can often be enhanced if patients eat small, frequent, nutrient-dense meals; oral nutrition supplements may also be well tolerated. Enteral tube feeding is indicated when oral intake is inadequate or contraindicated. Varices are not an absolute contraindication for placement of a feeding tube. PN is reserved for patients without adequate gut function. Because PN can adversely affect liver function, enteral nutrition is preferred.

In the acute posttransplant phase, nutrient needs are increased to promote healing, deter infection, provide energy for recovery, and replenish depleted body stores (Hasse, 1998). Nitrogen requirements are elevated in the acute posttransplant phase and can be met with early postoperative tube feeding (Hasse et al, 1995; Wicks et al, 1994). Multiple medications used after transplant have nutritional side effects, such as anorexia, gastrointestinal upset, hypercatabolism, diarrhea, hyperglycemia, hyperlipidemia, sodium retention, hypertension, hyperkalemia, and hypercalciuria. Therefore, dietary modification is based on the specific side effects of drug therapy (Table 31-5). During the posttransplant phase, nutrient requirements are adjusted to prevent or treat problems of obesity, hyperlipidemia, hypertension, diabetes mellitus, and osteopenia (Hasse, 1997; Weseman and McCashland, 1998). Table 31-6 summarizes nutrient needs following liver transplantation.

PHYSIOLOGY AND FUNCTIONS OF THE GALLBLADDER

The gallbladder lies on the undersurface of the right lobe of the liver (Figure 31-8). The main function of the gallbladder is to concentrate, store, and excrete bile, which is produced by the liver. During the concentration process, water and electrolytes are reabsorbed by the gallbladder mucosa. The chief constituents of bile are cholesterol, bilirubin, and bile salts. Bilirubin, the main bile pigment, is derived from the release of hemoglobin from red blood cell destruction. It is transported to the liver, where it is conjugated and excreted via bile.

Bile salts, made by liver cells from cholesterol, are essential for the digestion and absorption of fats, fat-soluble vitamins, and some minerals (see Chapter 1). Excreted into the small intestine via bile, bile salts are then reabsorbed into the portal system (enterohepatic circulation). Bile also contains immunoglobulins that support the integrity of the intestinal mucosa. In addition, it is the primary excretory pathway for the minerals copper and manganese.

TABLE 31-6 Nutrition Care Guidelines for Liver Transplantation

	PRETRANSPLANTATION	IMMEDIATE POST-TRANSPLANTATION (FIRST 2 POSTTRANSPLANT MONTHS)	LONG-TERM POST-TRANSPLANTATION
Calories	High calorie (basal + 20% or more)	Moderate calorie (basal + 15%-30%)	Weight maintenance (basal + 10%-20%)
Protein*	Moderate protein (1-1.5 g/kg: minimize need for restriction)	High protein (1.2-1.75 g/kg)	Moderate protein (1 g/kg)
Fat	As needed	20%-30% of calories	Low fat (≤30% of calories)
Carbohydrate	High carbohydrate (complex and simple)	70% of calories	Reduced simple carbohydrate
Sodium	2-4 g (as indicated)	2-4 g (as indicated)	2-4 g (as indicated)
Fluid	Restrict to 1000-1500 ml (as indicated)	As needed	As needed
Calcium	800-1200 mg	800-1200 mg	1200-1500 mg
Vitamins	Multivitamin/mineral supplementation to DRI levels; additional water- and fat-soluble vitamins as indicated	Multivitamin/mineral supplementation to DRI levels; additional water- and fat-soluble vitamins as indicated	Multivitamin/mineral supplementation to DRI levels for first posttransplant year

Modified from Porayko MK et al: Impact of malnutrition and its therapy on liver transplantation, *Semin Liv Dis* 11(4):305, 1991.
*Use estimated dry or ideal weight.
RDA, Recommended dietary allowance.

Bile is removed by the liver via bile canaliculi that drain into intrahepatic bile ducts. The ducts lead to the left and right hepatic ducts, which leave the liver and join to become the common hepatic duct. The bile is directed to the gallbladder via the cystic duct for concentration and storage. The cystic duct joins the common hepatic duct to form the common bile duct. The bile duct then joins the pancreatic duct, which carries digestive enzymes. During the course of digestion, food reaches the duodenum, causing the release of intestinal hormones, such as cholecystokinin and secretin. This stimulates the gallbladder and pancreas and causes the sphincter of Oddi to relax, allowing pancreatic juice and bile to flow into the duodenum at the ampulla of Vater to assist in fat digestion. For this reason diseases of the gallbladder, liver, and pancreas are often interrelated.

DISEASES OF THE GALLBLADDER

Disorders of the biliary tract affect millions of people each year, causing significant suffering and even death by precipitating pancreatitis and sepsis. The common diseases of the biliary tract are cholelithiasis, choledocholithiasis, and cholecystitis. Other diseases include PSC, PBC, and bile duct cancer. Treatment may involve diet, medication, or surgery.

Cholelithiasis

Pathophysiology

The formation of gallstones (calculi) in the absence of infection of the gallbladder is called cholelithiasis. Virtually all gallstones form within the gallbladder. With rare exceptions, stones form behind biliary duct strictures as a result of stasis in bile ducts after cholecystectomy. Gallstone disease affects millions of Americans each year and causes significant morbidity. In most cases, gallstones are asymptomatic; however, symptomatic gallstone disease can have serious complications.

Gallstones that pass from the gallbladder into the common bile duct may remain there indefinitely without causing symptoms, or they may pass into the duodenum with or without symptoms. Choledocholithiasis develops when stones slip into the bile ducts, producing obstruction, pain, and cramps. If passage of bile into the duodenum is interrupted, cholecystitis can develop. In the absence of bile in the intestine, lipid absorption is impaired, and without bile pigments, stools become light in color *(acholic)*. If uncorrected, bile backup can result in jaundice and liver damage *(secondary biliary cirrhosis)*. Obstruction of the distal common bile duct can lead to pancreatitis if the pancreatic duct is blocked (see next section).

Most gallstones in people in the United States are unpigmented cholesterol stones, composed primarily of cholesterol, bilirubin, and calcium salts (Johnston and Kaplan, 1993). Risk factors for cholesterol stone formation include female gender, pregnancy, older age, family history, obesity and truncal body fat distribution, diabetes mellitus, inflammatory bowel disease, and drugs (lipid-lowering medications, oral contraceptives, and estrogens) (Everhart, 1993; Hoy et al, 1994). Certain ethnic groups are at greater risk of stone formation (i.e., Pima Indians, Scandinavians, Mexican Americans). Rapid weight loss (as with jejunoileal and gastric bypass and fasting or severe calorie restriction) is associated with a high incidence of biliary sludge and gallstone formation (Liddle et al, 1989; Marks et al, 1992).

Bacteria may also play a role in gallstone formation. Low-grade chronic infections produce changes in the gallbladder mucosa, which affect its absorptive capabilities. Excess water or excess bile acid may be absorbed as a result. Cholesterol may then precipitate out and cause gallstone formation (Johnston and Ka-

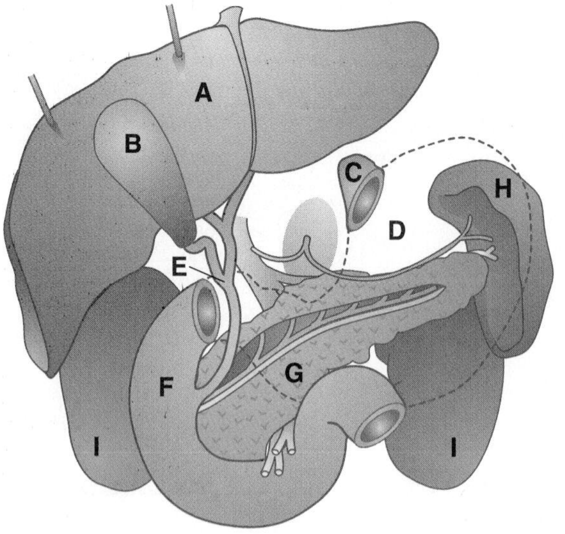

FIGURE 31-8 • Schematic drawing showing relationship of organs of the upper abdomen. *A*, Liver (retracted upward); *B*, gallbladder; *C*, esophageal opening of stomach; *D*, stomach (shown in dotted outline); *E*, common bile duct; *F*, duodenum; *G*, pancreas and pancreatic duct; *H*, spleen; *I*, kidneys. (Courtesy the Cleveland Clinic Foundation, Cleveland, Ohio, 2002.)

plan, 1993). High dietary fat intake over a prolonged period may predispose a person to gallstone formation because of the constant stimulus to produce more cholesterol for bile synthesis required in fat digestion.

Pigmented stones typically consist of bilirubin polymers or calcium salts. They are associated with chronic hemolysis. Risk factors associated with these stones are age, sickle cell anemia and thalassemia, biliary tract infection, cirrhosis, alcoholism, and long-term PN (Diehl, 1991).

Medical Management

Treatment of gallstone disease includes surgical removal of the gallbladder (cholecystectomy), especially if the stones are numerous, large, or calcified. The cholecystectomy may be done as a traditional open laparotomy or as a less invasive laparoscopic procedure. Chemical dissolution with the administration of bile salts, chenodeoxycholic acid, and ursodeoxycholic acid (litholytic therapy) or dissolution by extracorporeal shock-wave lithotripsy (ESWL) may also be used, but these are much less common than surgical techniques. Patients with gallstones that have migrated into the bile ducts may be candidates for endoscopic retrograde cholangiopancreatography (ERCP) techniques (Johnston and Kaplan, 1993).

Medical Nutrition Therapy

No specific dietary treatment is available to prevent cholelithiasis in susceptible persons. Nutrition-related factors include obesity and severe fasting, and these should be corrected when possible. In cholecystitis, dietary treatment includes a low-fat diet to prevent gallbladder contractions. Data are conflicting as to whether intravenous lipids stimulate gallbladder contraction (Priori et al, 1997).

After surgical removal of the gallbladder, oral feedings are usually resumed with the return of bowel sounds and after the patient can tolerate nasogastric drainage tube removal. The diet can be advanced as tolerated to a regular diet. In the absence of the gallbladder, bile is secreted directly by the liver into the intestine. The biliary tract dilates, forming a "simulated pouch" over time, to allow bile to be held in a manner similar to the original gallbladder.

Cholecystitis

Pathophysiology

Inflammation of the gallbladder is known as cholecystitis, and it may be chronic or acute. It is usually caused by gallstones obstructing the bile ducts (calculous cholecystitis), leading to the backup of bile. Bilirubin, the main bile pigment, gives bile its greenish color. When biliary tract obstruction prevents bile from reaching the intestine, it backs up and returns to the circulation. Bilirubin has an affinity for elastic tissues; therefore, when it overflows into the general circulation, it causes the yellow skin pigmentation and eye discoloration typical of jaundice.

Acute cholecystitis without stones (acalculous cholecystitis) may occur in critically ill patients or when the gallbladder and its bile are stagnant. Impaired gallbladder emptying in chronic acalculous cholecystitis appears to be due to diminished spontaneous contractile activity and decreased contractile responsiveness to the hormone cholecystokinin (CCK) (Merg et al, 2002). The walls of the gallbladder become inflamed and distended, and infection can occur. During such episodes, the patient experiences upper quadrant abdominal pain accompanied by nausea, vomiting, and flatulence.

Medical Management

Acute cholecystitis requires surgical intervention unless medically contraindicated. Without surgery, the condition may either subside or progress to gangrene.

Medical Nutrition Therapy

Acute Cholecystitis

In an acute attack, oral feedings are discontinued. PN may be indicated if the patient is malnourished and it is anticipated that he or she will not be taking anything orally for a prolonged period. When feedings are resumed, a low-fat diet is recommended to decrease gallbladder stimulation. A hydrolyzed low-fat formula (see Appendixes 36 through 41), or an oral diet consisting of 30 to 45 g of fat per day can be given. Studies have failed to show a relationship between dietary cholesterol and gallstone formation. Table 31-7 shows a combination of foods that provides this amount of fat.

TABLE 31-7 Fat-Restricted Diet*

FOODS ALLOWED	FOODS EXCLUDED
Beverages Skim milk or buttermilk made with skim milk; coffee, tea, Postum, fruit juice, soft drinks, cocoa made with cocoa powder and skim milk	**Beverages** Whole milk, buttermilk made with whole milk, chocolate milk, cream in excess of amounts allowed under fats
Bread and Cereal Products Plain, nonfat cereals, spaghetti, noodles, rice, macaroni; plain whole-grain or enriched breads, air-popped popcorn, bagels, English muffins	**Bread and Cereal Products** Biscuits, breads, egg or cheese bread, sweet rolls made with fat, pancakes, doughnuts, waffles, fritters, popcorn prepared with fat, muffins, natural cereals and breads to which extra fat is added
Cheese Cottage, ¼ c to be used as substitute for 1 oz of cheese, or low-fat cheeses containing less than 5% butterfat	**Cheese** Whole-milk cheeses
Desserts Sherbet made with skim milk; nonfat frozen yogurt; nonfat frozen nondairy desserts; fruit ice; sorbet; gelatin; rice, bread, cornstarch, tapioca, or pudding made with skim milk; fruit whips with gelatin, sugar, and egg white; fruit; angel food cake; graham crackers; vanilla wafers; meringues	**Desserts** Cake, pie, pastry, ice cream, or any dessert containing shortening, chocolate, or fats of any kind, unless especially prepared using part of fat allowance
Eggs 3 per week prepared only with fat from fat allowance; egg whites as desired; low-fat egg substitutes	**Eggs** More than 1/day unless substituted for part of the meat allowed
Fats Choose up to the limit allowed among the following (1 serving in the amount listed equals 1 fat choice): 1 tsp butter or margarine 1 tbsp reduced-fat margarine 1 tsp shortening or oil 1 tsp mayonnaise 2 tsp Italian or French dressing 1 tbsp reduced-fat salad dressing 1 strip crisp bacon ⅛ avocado (4-inch diameter) 2 tbsp light cream 1 tbsp heavy cream 6 small nuts 5 small olives	**Fats** Any in excess of amount prescribed on diet; all others
Fruits As desired	**Fruits** Avocado in excess of amount allowed on fat list
Lean Meat, Fish, Poultry, and Meat Substitutes Choose up to the limit allowed among the following: poultry without skin, fish, veal (all cuts), liver, lean beef, pork, and lamb, all with visible fat removed—1 oz cooked weight equals 1 equivalent; ¼ cup water packed tuna or salmon equals 1 equivalent; tofu or tempeh-3 oz equals 1 equivalent	**Meat, Fish, Poultry, and Meat Substitutes** Fried or fatty meats, sausage, scrapple, frankfurters, poultry skins, stewing hens, spareribs, salt pork, beef unless lean, duck, goose, ham hocks, pig's feet, luncheon meats (unless reduced fat), gravies unless fat-free, tuna and salmon packed in oil, peanut butter
Milk Skim, buttermilk, or yogurt made from skim milk	**Milk** Whole, 2%, 1%, chocolate, buttermilk made with whole milk
Seasonings As desired	**Seasonings** None
Soups Bouillon, clear broth, fat-free vegetable soup, cream soup made with skimmed milk, packaged dehydrated soups	**Soups** All others
Sweets Jelly, jam, marmalade, honey, syrup, molasses, sugar, hard sugar candies, fondant, gumdrops, jelly beans, marshmallows, cocoa powder, fat-free chocolate sauce, red and black licorice	**Sweets** Any candy made with chocolate, nuts, butter, cream, or fat of any kind
Vegetables All plainly prepared vegetables	**Vegetables** Potato chips; buttered, au gratin, creamed, or fried potatoes and other vegetables unless made with allowed fat; casseroles or frozen vegetables in butter sauce

*Fat content can be reduced further by reducing the fat exchanges. 1 Fat exchange = 5 g of fat.

Continued

TABLE 31-7 Fat-Restricted Diet—cont'd

Daily Food Allowances for 40-g Fat Diet

Food	Amount	Approximate Fat Content (g)
Skim milk	2 c or more	0
Lean meat, fish, poultry	6 oz or 6 equivalents	18
Whole egg or egg yolks	3 per week	2
Vegetables	3 servings or more, at least 1 or more dark green or deep yellow	0
Fruits	3 or more servings, at least 1 citrus	0
Breads, cereals	As desired, fat-free	0
Fat exchanges*	4-5 exchanges daily	20-25
Desserts and sweets	As desired from permitted list	0
	TOTAL FAT	38-43

*Fat content can be reduced further by reducing the fat exchanges. 1 Fat exchange = 5 g of fat.

Chronic Cholecystitis

Patients with chronic conditions may require a long-term low-fat diet that contains 25% to 30% of total kilocalories as fat. Stricter limitation is undesirable because fat in the intestine is important for some stimulation and drainage of the biliary tract. The degree of food intolerance varies widely among persons with gallbladder disorders; many complain of foods that cause flatulence and bloating. It is best to determine with the patient which foods should be eliminated for this reason. See Chapter 30 for a discussion of potential gas-forming foods. Administration of water-soluble forms of fat-soluble vitamins may be of benefit in patients with chronic gallbladder conditions or in those in whom fat malabsorption is suspected.

Acute Cholangitis

Pathophysiology and Medical Management

Inflammation of the bile ducts is known as cholangitis. Patients with acute cholangitis need resuscitation with fluids and broad-spectrum antibiotics. If the patient does not improve with conservative treatment, placement of a percutaneous biliary stent or cholecystectomy may be needed (Lee et al, 2002).

Sclerosing Cholangitis

Pathophysiology and Medical Management

Sclerosing cholangitis can result in sepsis and liver failure. Most patients have multiple intrahepatic strictures, which make surgical intervention difficult if not impossible. Patients are generally on broad-spectrum antibiotics. Percutaneous ductal dilatation may provide short-term bile duct patency in some patients. When sepsis is recurrent, patients may require chronic antibiotic therapy.

Cholestasis

Pathophysiology and Medical Management

Cholestasis is a condition of sludgelike buildup in the gallbladder as a result of stimulation or release of bile. This can occur in patients without oral or enteral feeding for a prolonged period, such as those requiring PN, and can predispose to acalculous cholestasis. Prevention includes stimulation of intestinal and biliary motility and secretions by at least minimal enteral feedings (Hager, 1994). If this is not possible, drug therapy is used.

PHYSIOLOGY AND FUNCTIONS OF THE EXOCRINE PANCREAS

The pancreas is an elongated, flattened gland that lies in the upper abdomen behind the stomach. The head of the pancreas is in the right upper quadrant below the liver within the curvature of the duodenum, and the tapering tail slants upward to the hilum of the spleen. This glandular organ has both an endocrine and exocrine function. Pancreatic cells manufacture glucagon, insulin, and somatostatin for absorption into the bloodstream *(endocrine function)* for regulation of glucose homeostasis. Other cells secrete enzymes and other substances directly into the intestinal lumen, where they aid in digesting proteins, fats, and carbohydrates *(exocrine function).*

In the vast majority of cases, the pancreatic duct, which carries the exocrine pancreatic secretions, merges with the common bile duct into a unified opening through which bile and pancreatic juices drain into the duodenum at the ampulla of Vater. Many factors regulate exocrine secretion from the pancreas. Neural and hormonal responses play a role, with the presence and composition of ingested foods being a large contributor. The two primary hormonal stimuli for pancreatic secretion are secretin and cholecystokinin (see Chapter 1).

Factors that influence pancreatic secretions during a meal can be divided into three phases: (1) the *cephalic phase* is mediated through the vagus nerve and is initiated by the sight, smell, taste, and anticipation of food, and it leads to the secretion of bicarbonate and pancreatic enzymes; (2) gastric distention with food initiates the *gastric phase* of pancreatic secretion, which stimulates enzyme secretion; and (3) the *intestinal phase* has the most potent effect on pancreatic secretions and is mediated by the release of cholecystokinin.

Box 31-4. Ranson's Criteria to Classify the Severity of Pancreatitis

At Admission or Diagnosis

Age >55 yr
White blood cell count >16,000/m^3
Blood glucose level >200 mg/100 ml
Lactic dehydrogenase >350 IU/L
Aspartate transaminase >250 U/L

During the Initial 48 hr

Hematocrit decrease of >10 mg/dl
Blood urea nitrogen increase of >5 mg/dl
Arterial Po_2 <60 mm Hg
Base deficit >4 mEq/L
Fluid sequestration >6000 ml
Serum calcium level <8 mg/ml

Modified from Ranson JH et al: Prognostic signs and the role of operative management in acute pancreatitis, *Surg Gynecol Obstet* 139:69, 1974.

DISEASES OF THE EXOCRINE PANCREAS

Pancreatitis

Pathophysiology and Medical Management

Pancreatitis is an inflammation of the pancreas and is characterized by edema, cellular exudate, and fat necrosis. The disease can range from mild and self-limiting to severe, with autodigestion, necrosis, and hemorrhage of pancreatic tissue. Ranson and colleagues (1974) identified 11 signs that could be measured during the first 48 hours of admission and that have prognostic significance (Box 31-4). By using these observations, one can determine the likely outcome of hospitalization. Surgical intervention may be necessary. Pancreatitis is classified as either acute or chronic, the latter with pancreatic destruction so extensive that exocrine and endocrine function are severely diminished, and maldigestion and diabetes may result.

The symptoms of pancreatitis can range from continuous or intermittent pain of varying intensity to severe upper abdominal pain, which may radiate to the back. Symptoms may worsen with the ingestion of food. Clinical presentation may also include nausea, vomiting, abdominal distention, and steatorrhea. Severe cases are complicated by hypotension, oliguria, and dyspnea. Laboratory evaluation will usually reveal elevations of serum amylase or lipase levels; however, the serum amylase test is nonspecific for pancreatitis and may be falsely negative or falsely positive. Serum lipase has the same degree of sensitivity as amylase but greater specificity. Severe cases of pancreatitis may lead to hemorrhage, shock, or death.

TABLE 31-8 Some Tests of Pancreatic Function

TEST	SIGNIFICANCE
Secretin stimulation test	Measures pancreatic secretion, particularly bicarbonate, in response to secretin stimulation
Glucose tolerance test	Assesses endocrine function of the pancreas by measuring insulin response to a glucose load
72-hr Stool fat test	Assesses exocrine function of the pancreas by measuring fat absorption that reflects pancreatic lipase secretion

Pancreatitis has numerous causes, including chronic alcoholism, biliary tract disease, gallstones, certain drugs, trauma, hypertriglyceridemia, hypercalcemia, and some infections such as viruses (Banks, 1998). Whereas alcohol is the leading cause of chronic pancreatitis in most Western societies (Strate et al, 2001), gallstones are the most common cause of acute pancreatitis (Steinberg and Tenner, 1994). Pancreatitis is associated with serious complications and significant mortality. For alcoholic pancreatitis, the overall mortality rate is about 5%; for gallstone-associated and idiopathic pancreatitis, it is 10% to 25% (de Beaux et al, 1995; Mann et al, 1994).

The exact mechanisms that lead to pancreatic injury have not been fully defined. One theory involves blockage or reflux of the ductal contents into the pancreatic duct (Calleja and Barkin, 1993). It appears that a common characteristic is premature activation of the enzymes within the pancreas, resulting in autodigestion within the pancreatic cells (Pisters and Ranson, 1992). The enzymes released by destroyed pancreatic cells eventually reach the bloodstream, causing elevated serum amylase and lipase levels. Usually a hallmark finding in acute pancreatitis, these markers alone are not always diagnostic, nor do they indicate the extent of pancreatic injury. Further evaluation of the extent or severity of pancreatic injury is best done with radiographic imaging (computed tomography, ultrasound) studies.

It should be noted that in cases of chronic pancreatitis involving extensive destruction of pancreatic tissue with subsequent fibrosis, enzyme production is diminished and serum amylase and lipase may appear normal. However, absence of enzymes to aid in the digestion of food leads to steatorrhea and malabsorption. Table 31-8 describes several tests used to determine the extent of pancreatic destruction.

Medical Nutrition Therapy

Acute Pancreatitis

Pain associated with pancreatitis is partially related to the secretory mechanisms of pancreatic enzymes and bile. The nutrition therapy is therefore adjusted to provide minimal stimulation of these systems (Figure 31-9).

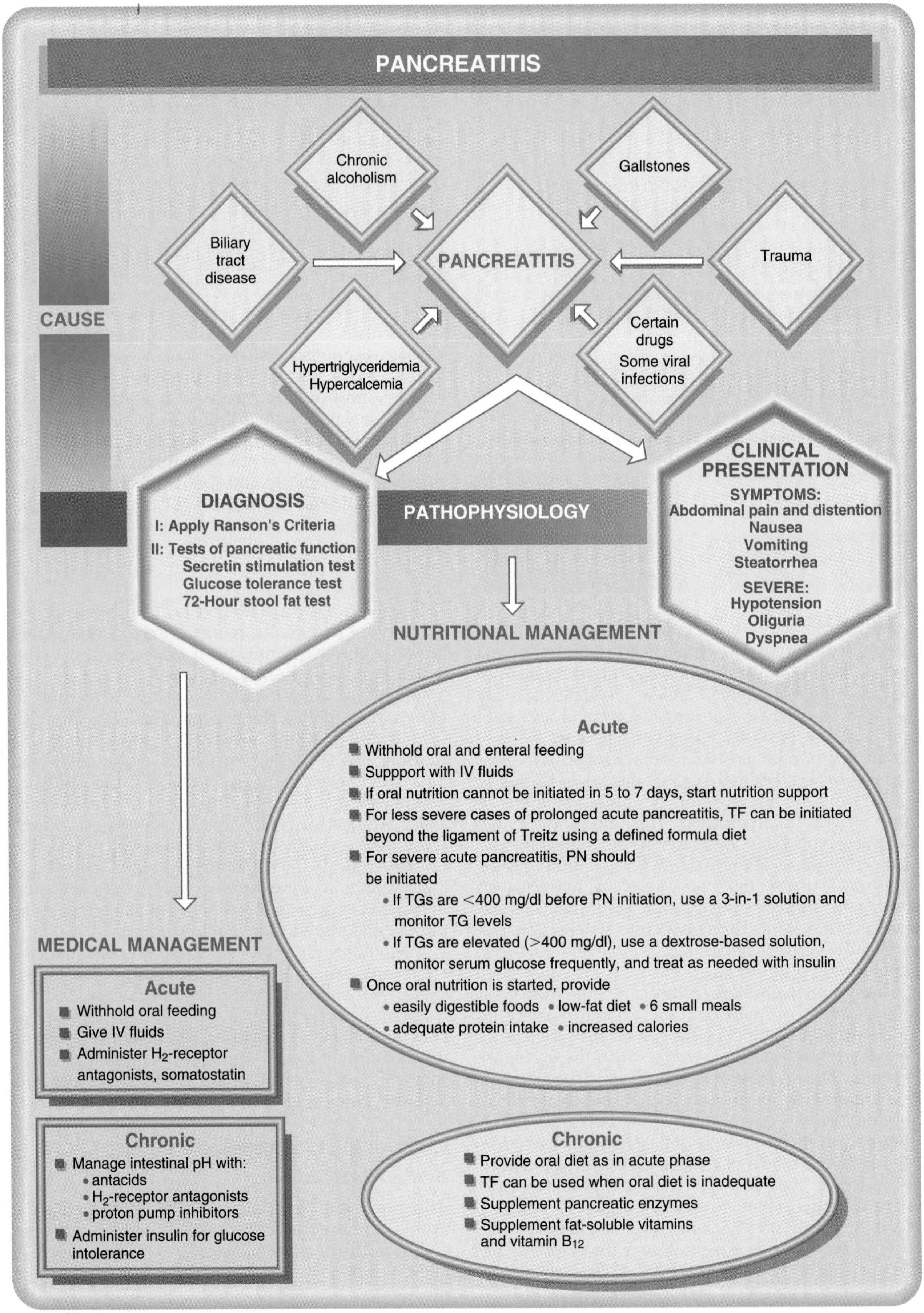
PANCREATITIS
CAUSE
Chronic alcoholism
Gallstones
Biliary tract disease
PANCREATITIS
Trauma
Hypertriglyceridemia
Hypercalcemia
Certain drugs
Some viral infections
DIAGNOSIS
I: Apply Ranson's Criteria
II: Tests of pancreatic function
Secretin stimulation test
Glucose tolerance test
72-Hour stool fat test
PATHOPHYSIOLOGY
CLINICAL PRESENTATION
SYMPTOMS:
Abdominal pain and distention
Nausea
Vomiting
Steatorrhea
SEVERE:
Hypotension
Oliguria
Dyspnea
NUTRITIONAL MANAGEMENT
Acute
Withhold oral and enteral feeding
Suppport with IV fluids
If oral nutrition cannot be initiated in 5 to 7 days, start nutrition support
For less severe cases of prolonged acute pancreatitis, TF can be initiated beyond the ligament of Treitz using a defined formula diet
For severe acute pancreatitis, PN should be initiated
• If TGs are <400 mg/dl before PN initiation, use a 3-in-1 solution and monitor TG levels
• If TGs are elevated (>400 mg/dl), use a dextrose-based solution, monitor serum glucose frequently, and treat as needed with insulin
Once oral nutrition is started, provide
• easily digestible foods • low-fat diet • 6 small meals
• adequate protein intake • increased calories
MEDICAL MANAGEMENT
Acute
Withhold oral feeding
Give IV fluids
Administer H2-receptor antagonists, somatostatin
Chronic
Manage intestinal pH with:
• antacids
• H2-receptor antagonists
• proton pump inhibitors
Administer insulin for glucose intolerance
Chronic
Provide oral diet as in acute phase
TF can be used when oral diet is inadequate
Supplement pancreatic enzymes
Supplement fat-soluble vitamins and vitamin B12

FIGURE 31-9 • Pathophysiology algorithm: pancreatic disorders. (Algorithm content developed by John Anderson, PhD, and Stanford C. Garner, PhD, 2000; updated by Jeanette Hasse, PhD, RD, LD, CNSD, FADA, and Laura E. Matarese, MS, RD, LD, CNSD, FADA, 2002.)

The pancreas is put "at rest." During acute attacks, all oral feeding is withheld and hydration is maintained intravenously. The average patient with uncomplicated pancreatitis is free from pain, nausea, and vomiting, usually within 2 to 3 days. In these less severe attacks, a clear liquid diet with negligible fat may be given in a few days. The patient should be monitored for any symptoms of pain, nausea, or vomiting. The diet should be progressed as tolerated to easily digested foods with a low fat content and then advanced as tolerated. Foods may be better tolerated if they are divided into six small meals. The low-fat diet described in Table 31-7 can be used.

Severe acute pancreatitis results in a hypermetabolic and catabolic state. Induction of severe acute pancreatitis results in immediate metabolic alterations in the pancreas, with rapid onset of metabolic disturbances, not only in the local, challenged organ (pancreas) but also in remote organs (Ederoth et al, 2002). Metabolic demands have been compared with those of a patient with sepsis (Pisters and Ranson, 1992). Amino acids are released from muscle and used for gluconeogenesis. These patients often exhibit signs of malnutrition such as decreased serum levels of albumin, transferrin, and lymphocytes. Attention should also be given to a nutrition regimen with adequate protein in an effort to achieve positive nitrogen balance. Energy expenditure has been shown to be up to 49% greater than predicted in these patients (Bouffard et al, 1989).

Oral nutrition must be delayed even longer when acute illness persists longer than a few days with persistent or recurrent elevation of serum amylase, continued abdominal pain, and ileus, or when cessation of nasogastric suction is followed by return of symptoms, the presence of a complication such as pancreatic abscess, pseudocyst, or obstruction to the main pancreatic ducts is suspected. In these severe, prolonged cases, PN may be necessary. Patients with mild to moderate stress can tolerate dextrose-based solutions, whereas patients with more severe stress require a mixed fuel system of dextrose and lipid to avoid complications of glucose intolerance. Lipid emulsion should not be included in a PN regimen if hypertriglyceridemia is the cause of the pancreatitis (Pisters and Ranson, 1992). A serum triglyceride level should be obtained before PN with lipids is initiated. Lipids may be given to patients with triglyceride values less than 400 mg/dl. Because of the possibility of pancreatic endocrine abnormalities as well as a relative insulin resistance, close glucose monitoring is also warranted. H_2-receptor antagonists may be prescribed to decrease hydrochloric acid production, which will reduce stimulation of the pancreas. Somatostatin is considered the best inhibitor of pancreatic secretion and may be added to the PN solution (Latifi and Dudrick, 1996).

Depressed serum calcium levels are often identified in patients with acute pancreatitis. Possible causes include hypoalbuminemia with subsequent third spacing of fluid. The calcium, which is bound to the albumin, is thus affected and may appear artificially low. Another possible explanation is a "soap" formation by the calcium and fatty acids created by the fat necrosis. Checking an ionized calcium level is a method of determining available calcium.

Aggressive nutrition support may also include attempts to use the gastrointestinal tract. The location of the feeding and the composition of the formula will determine the degree of pancreatic stimulation. In dogs, gastric infusion of an elemental formula increased the volume of pancreatic secretions as well as the bicarbonate and enzyme content (Ragins et al, 1973). Intraduodenal infusion of the same formula increased the volume of secretions, whereas infusion into the jejunum did not change basal pancreatic output. By feeding into the jejunum, the cephalic and gastric phases of exocrine pancreatic stimulation are eliminated.

Polymeric formulas infused at various sections of the gut stimulate the pancreas more than elemental and hydrolyzed formulas (Grant et al, 1987). It appears that the amino acids, short polypeptides, and deceased concentration of LCT in the elemental formulas minimize the neurohumoral response of the intestinal mucosa (Bodoky et al, 1991; Wolfe et al, 1975). Several prospective, randomized trials have shown that enteral nutrition into the jejunum is well tolerated in acute pancreatitis (Kalfarentzos et al, 1997; McClave et al, 1997). Close observation for patient tolerance is important. Chapter 23 discusses jejunal feedings in detail. When the patient is allowed to eat, supplemental pancreatic enzymes may be needed to treat steatorrhea.

Chronic Pancreatitis

In contrast to acute pancreatitis, chronic pancreatitis usually evolves insidiously over many years. Chronic pancreatitis is characterized by recurrent attacks of epigastric pain of long duration that may radiate into the back. The pain can be precipitated by meals. Associated nausea, vomiting, or diarrhea makes it difficult to maintain adequate nutritional status. Patients with chronic pancreatitis are at increased risk of developing protein calorie malnutrition because of pancreatic insufficiency and inadequate oral intake resulting from postprandial pain. In one study, patients with chronic pancreatitis admitted to a tertiary care center were found to have a 90% incidence of malnutrition, including weight loss, deficits of lean muscle and adipose tissue, visceral protein depletion, and impaired immune function (Matarese et al, 2000). There is also an increase in REE; weight loss may result (Hebuterne, et al, 1996).

The objective of therapy for patients with chronic pancreatitis is to prevent further damage to the pancreas, decrease the number of attacks of acute inflammation, alleviate pain, decrease steatorrhea and correct malnutrition. Dietary intake should be as liberal as possible, but modifications may be necessary to minimize symptoms (see *Clinical Insight:* Nutrition for Chronic Pancreatitis).

Substitution of dietary fat with MCT oil may relieve steatorrhea and lead to weight gain. Malabsorption of the fat-soluble vitamins may occur in patients with significant steatorrhea. Also, deficiency of pancreatic protease, necessary to cleave vitamin B_{12} from its carrier protein, could potentially lead to vitamin B_{12} deficiency. With appropriate supplemental enzyme therapy, vitamin absorption should be improved; however, the patient should still be monitored periodically for vitamin deficiencies. Water-soluble forms of the fat-soluble vitamins or parenteral administration of vitamin B_{12} may be necessary (see Chapter 34 for a discussion of B_{12} administration).

Because pancreatic bicarbonate secretion is frequently defective, medical management may also include maintenance of an optimal intestinal pH to facilitate enzyme activation. Antacids, H_2-receptor antagonists, or proton pump inhibitors that reduce gastric acid secretion may be used to achieve this effect.

In chronic cases with extensive pancreatic destruction, the insulin-secreting capacity of the pancreas decreases and glucose intolerance develops. Treatment with insulin and nutrition care similar to that used for a patient with diabetes mellitus is then required (see Chapter 33). Management is delicate and should focus on control of symptoms rather than normoglycemia as the goal (see *Clinical Insight:* Fasting Hypoglycemia).

Effort should be made to cater to the patient's tolerances and preferences for nutrition management; however, alcohol is prohibited because of the possibility of exacerbating the pancreatic disease. There is evidence that the progressive destruction of the pancreas will be slowed in the alcoholic patient who abstains from alcohol.

Pancreatic Surgery

A surgical procedure often used for pancreatic carcinoma is a pancreaticoduodenectomy (Whipple procedure). A cholecystectomy, vagotomy, or a partial gastrectomy may also be done during the surgery. The pancreatic duct is reanastamosed to the jejunum. Partial or complete pancreatic insufficiency can result, depending on the extent of the pancreatic resection. Most patients who have undergone pancreatic resection are at risk for vitamin and mineral deficiencies and will benefit from vitamin and mineral supplementation. Nutrition care is similar to that for chronic pancreatitis.

SUMMARY

The goals of nutrition care in diseases of the liver, biliary system, and exocrine pancreas are to improve nutritional status and to support the patient during the acute phases of illness. Understanding the physiology and function of these vital organs along with the pathology that results from disease will decrease patient morbidity and lead to better treatment and outcomes.

CLINICAL INSIGHT

Nutrition for Chronic Pancreatitis

The first goal of medical nutrition therapy is to provide optimal nutrition support, and the second is to decrease pain by minimizing stimulation of the exocrine pancreas. Because CCK stimulates secretion from the exocrine pancreas, one approach is to decrease CCK levels. If postprandial pain is a limiting factor, alternative enteral therapies that minimally stimulate the pancreas are warranted. Nutritional counseling, antioxidants, and pancreatic enzymes may play a role in effective management of CP as well (Shea et al, 2000).

Idiopathic CP is often associated with a cystic fibrosis gene mutation, and therapies directed toward cystic fibrosis may benefit these patients (Shea et al, 2000). When pancreatic function is diminished by about 90%, enzyme production and secretion are insufficient; maldigestion and malabsorption of protein and fat thus become a problem. Large meals with high-fat foods and alcohol should be avoided. The patient may present with weight loss despite adequate energy intake and will also give a history of bulky, greasy stools. Pancreatic enzyme replacement is mandatory at this time.

Pancreatic enzyme replacements are given orally with meals; the dosage should be at least 30,000 IU lipase with each meal. To promote weight gain, the level of fat in the diet should be the maximum a patient can tolerate without increased steatorrhea or pain. Additional therapies that may be tried to maintain nutritional status and minimize symptoms in patients with maximal enzyme supplementation include a lower fat diet (40 to 60 g/day) or substitution of some dietary fat with MCT oil to improve fat absorption and weight gain. Meals should be small and frequent.

Clinical Scenario 1

Frank is a 40-year-old man admitted to the hospital with chief complaints of right upper quadrant pain, anorexia, nausea, dysgeusia, and frequent loose stools. On physical examination he has mild peripheral edema with a slightly jaundiced appearance. No asterixis is noted. The patient's mental status is clear, but he appears lethargic. He reports no history of portal hypertension, ascites, or gastrointestinal bleeding. Muscle wasting is noted along with stomatitis. The patient has a significant alcohol abuse history spanning 15 years.

Abnormal laboratory values include elevated liver enzymes and total bilirubin; serum albumin, 2.5 g/dl; transferrin, 150 mg/dl; megaloblastic anemia profile; NH_3 = 55 mmol/L.

A preliminary diagnosis of alcoholic hepatitis with possible mild pancreatic insufficiency is made. On biopsy, steatosis and fibrosis are found.

Nutritional data include height, 177.8 cm; weight, 67 kg; ideal body weight (IBW), 75 kg ± 10%; usual body weight (UBW), 82 kg (5 years ago), 73 kg (6 months ago).

1. Based on available data, what vitamin or mineral deficiencies may exist?
2. What nutritional therapy would you prescribe?
3. What nutritional parameters are affected by the patient's liver dysfunction?
4. What is Frank's overall nutritional status?
5. What conditions may be leading to his frequent loose stools?
6. What further information would you require or obtain to complete your assessment?

Clinical Scenario 2

Michael is a 25-year-old white college student who was struck by a car 3 years ago. After the accident, his spleen was removed, and recovery seemed to be unremarkable; however, for about 6 months, Michael has been unable to eat meals with his friends and has noticed a weight loss of 25 lb. He is 6 ft 0 in. tall and weighs 160 lb; previously his usual weight was 185 lb. His physicians are puzzled but have identified chronic pancreatitis as a result of the injuries to his internal organs. Michael complains of postprandial pain and steatorrhea with every meal.

1. What dietary changes might be helpful?
2. If Michael were to try using pancreatic enzymes, what modifications in fat intake would you recommend?
3. Does Michael need nutritional support? If yes, what do you recommend?

Relevant Web Sites

Alcoholism
www.niaaa.nih.gov
Liver Foundation
www.liverfoundation.org
www.liver.org

Cited References

Bacon BR et al: Ischemia, congestive failure, Budd-Chiari syndrome, and veno-occlusive disease. In Kaplowitz N, editor: *Liver and biliary diseases,* ed 2, Baltimore, 1996, Williams & Wilkins.

Baker AL: Liver chemistry tests. In Kaplowitz N, editor: *Liver and biliary diseases,* ed 2, Baltimore, 1996, Williams & Wilkins.

Banks PA: Acute and chronic pancreatitis. In Feldman M et al, editors: *Sleisenger and Fordtran's gastrointestinal and liver disease,* Philadelphia, 1998, WB Saunders.

Bianchi GP et al: Vegetable versus animal protein diet in cirrhotic patients with chronic encephalopathy: a randomized crossover comparison, *J Intern Med* 233:385, 1993.

Bodoky G et al: Effect of enteral nutrition on exocrine pancreatic function, *Am J Surg* 161:144, 1991.

Bonacini M: Liver in systemic diseases. In Kaplowitz N, editor: *Liver and biliary diseases,* ed 2, Baltimore, 1996, Williams & Wilkins.

Bouffard YH et al: Energy expenditure during severe acute pancreatitis, *J Parent Enter Nutr* 13:26, 1989.

Brandhagen DJ et al: Recognition and management of hereditary hemochromatosis, *Am Fam Physician* 65:853, 2002.

Brewer G et al: Does a vegetarian diet control Wilson's disease? *J Am Coll Nutr* 12:527, 1993.

Calleja GA, Barkin JS: Acute pancreatitis, *Med Clin North Am* 77:1037, 1993.

Campillo B et al: Short-term changes in energy metabolism after 1 month of a regular oral diet in severely malnourished cirrhotic patients, *Metabolism* 44(6):765, 1995.

Carithers RL Jr: Alcoholic hepatitis and cirrhosis. In Kaplowitz N, editor: *Liver and biliary diseases,* ed 2, Baltimore, 1996, Williams & Wilkins.

Corish C: Nutrition and liver disease, *Nutr Rev* 55 (1):17, 1997.

Crippin JS: Monitoring and care of the patient before transplantation. In Busuttil RW, Klintmalm GB, editors: *Transplantation of the liver,* Philadelphia, 1996, WB Saunders.

de Beaux AC et al: Factors influencing morbidity and mortality in acute pancreatitis: an analysis of 279 cases, *Gut* 37:121, 1995.

Detsky AS et al: What is subjective global assessment? *J Parent Enter Nutr* 11:8, 1987.

Diehl AM: Epidemiology and natural history of gallstone disease, *Gastroenterol Clin North Am* 20:1, 1991.

Diehl AM: Acute and chronic liver failure and hepatic encephalopathy. In Goldman L, Bennett JC, editors: *Cecil textbook of medicine,* ed 21, Philadelphia, 2000, WB Saunders.

Dolz C et al: Ascites increases the resting energy expenditure in liver cirrhosis, *Gastroenterology* 100:738, 1991.

Donaghy A: Issues of malnutrition and bone disease in patients with cirrhosis, *J Gastroenterol Hepatol* 17:462, 2002.

Douglas DD, Rakela J: Fulminant hepatitis. In Kaplowitz N, editor: *Liver and biliary diseases,* ed 2, Baltimore, 1996, Williams & Wilkins.

Ederoth P et al: Experimental pancreatitis causes acute perturbation of energy metabolism in the intestinal wall, *Pancreas* 25: 270, 2002.

Epstein S et al: Organ transplantation and osteoporosis, *Curr Opin Rheumatol* 7:255, 1995.

Everhart J: Contributions of obesity and weight loss to gallstone disease, *Ann Intern Med* 119:1029, 1993.

Francisco-Ziller N, DiCecco S: Nutritional care of the pretransplant patient, *Top Clin Nutr* 13(2):1, 1998.

Friedman SL: Alcoholic liver disease, cirrhosis, and its major sequelae. In Goldman L, Bennett JC, editors: *Cecil textbook of medicine,* ed 21, Philadelphia, 2000, WB Saunders.

Grant JP et al: Effect of enteral nutrition on human pancreatic secretions, *J Parent Enter Nutr* 11:302, 1987.

Gurk-Turner C: Management of the metabolic complications of liver disease: an overview of commonly used pharmacologic agents, *Support Line* 19(4):17, 1997.

Hager LA: Hepatic complications associated with total parenteral nutrition, *Support Line* 16(3):1, 1994.

Hasse J: Role of the dietitian in the nutrition management of adults after liver transplantation, *J Am Diet Assoc* 91:473, 1991.

Hasse J: Nutritional aspects of adult liver transplantation. In Busuttil RW, Klintmalm GB, editors: *Transplantation of the liver*, Philadelphia, 1996, WB Saunders.

Hasse JM: Diet therapy for organ transplantation, *Nurs Clin North Am* 32(4):863, 1997.

Hasse JM: Recovery after organ transplantation in adults: the role of postoperative nutrition therapy, *Top Clin Nutr* 13(2):15, 1998.

Hasse JM: Nutrition assessment and support of organ transplant recipients, *J Parent Enter Nutr* 25:120, 2001.

Hasse J et al: Subjective global assessment—alternative nutritional assessment technique for adult liver transplant candidates, *Nutrition* 9:330, 1993.

Hasse JM et al: Early enteral nutrition support in patients undergoing liver transplantation, *J Parent Enter Nutr* 19:437, 1995.

Hasse J et al: Nutrition therapy for end-stage liver disease: a practical approach, *Support Line* 19(4):8, 1997.

Hebuterne X et al: Resting energy expenditure in patients with alcoholic chronic pancreatitis, *Dig Dis Sci* 41:533, 1996.

Hiyama DT, Fischer JE: Nutritional support in hepatic failure, *Nutr Clin Pract* 3:96, 1988.

Holtmeier J, Leuschner U: Medical treatment of primary biliary cirrhosis and primary sclerosing cholangitis, *Digestion* 64:137, 2001.

Hoofnagle JH, Lindsay KL: Acute viral hepatitis. In Goldman L, Bennett JC, editors: *Cecil textbook of medicine,* ed 21, Philadelphia, 2000, WB Saunders.

Hoy M et al: Reduced risk of liver-function-test abnormalities and new gallstone formation with weight loss on 3350-kj (800-kcal) formula diets, *Am J Clin Nutr* 60:249, 1994.

Ichida T et al: Clinical study of an enteral branched-chain amino acid solution in decompensated liver cirrhosis with hepatic encephalopathy, *Nutrition* 11(suppl 2):238, 1996.

Johnston D, Kaplan M: Pathogenesis and treatment of gallstones, *N Engl J Med* 328:412, 1993.

Kalfarentzos F et al: Enteral nutrition is superior to parenteral nutrition in severe acute pancreatitis: results of a randomized prospective trial, *Br J Surg* 84:1665, 1997.

Kamath PS: Clinical approach to the patient with abnormal liver test results, *Mayo Clin Proc* 71:1089, 1996.

Katz IA, Epstein S: Posttransplant bone disease, *J Bone Miner Res* 7:12, 1992.

Kayler LK et al: Long-term survival after liver transplantation in children with metabolic disorders, *Pediatr Transplant* 6:295, 2002.

Klein GL et al: Hepatic osteodystrophy in chronic cholestasis: evidence for a multifactorial etiology, *Pediatr Transplant* 6:136, 2002.

Kondrup J, Müller MJ: Energy and protein requirements of patients with chronic liver disease, *J Hepatol* 27:239, 1997.

Latifi R, Dudrick S: Nutrition support of acute pancreatitis. In: Latifi R, Dudrick S, editors: *Current surgical nutrition,* New York, 1996, Chapman & Hall.

Latifi R et al: Nutritional support in liver failure, *Surg Clin North Am* 71:567, 1991.

Lee DW et al: Biliary decompression by nasobiliary catheter or biliary stent in acute suppurative cholangitis: a prospective randomized trial, *Gastrointest Endosc* 56:361, 2002.

Leevy CM, Davison E: Portal hypertension and hepatic coma, *Postgrad Med J* 41:84, 1967.

Liddle RA et al: Gallstone formation during weight reduction dieting, *Arch Intern Med* 149:1750, 1989.

Lieber CS: The influence of alcohol on nutritional status, *Nutr Rev* 46:241, 1988.

Lindsay KL, Hoofnagle JH: Serologic tests for viral hepatitis. In Kaplowitz N, editor: *Liver and biliary diseases,* ed 2, Baltimore, 1996, Williams & Wilkins.

Lindsay KL, Hoofnagle JH: Chronic hepatitis. In Goldman L, Bennett JC, editors: *Cecil textbook of medicine,* ed 21, Philadelphia, 2000.

Maher JJ: Inherited, infiltrative, and metabolic disorders involving the liver. In Goldman L, Bennett JC, editors: *Cecil textbook of medicine,* ed 21, Philadelphia, 2000, WB Saunders.

Mann DV et al: Multicentre audit of death from acute pancreatitis, *Br J Surg* 81:890, 1994.

Marks JW et al: The sequence of biliary events preceding the formation of gallstones in humans, *Gastroenterology* 103:566, 1992.

Matarese LE et al: Nutritional status of patients with chronic pancreatitis admitted to a tertiary care center, *Am J Gastroenterol* 95:A2481, 2000.

McClain CJ et al: Trace metals in liver disease, *Semin Liver Dis* 11:321, 1991.

McClave SA et al: Comparisons of the safety of early enteral versus parenteral nutrition in mild acute pancreatitis, *J Parent Enter Nutr* 21:14, 1997.

McCullough AJ, O'Connor JFB: Alcoholic liver disease: proposed recommendations for the American College of Gastroenterology, *Am J Gastroenterol* 93:2022, 1998.

McCullough AJ, Tavill AS: Disordered energy and protein metabolism in liver disease, *Semin Liver Dis* 11:265, 1991.

McCullough AJ et al: Guidelines for nutritional therapy in liver disease. In *The A.S.P.E.N. Nutrition support practice manual,* Silver Springs, 1998, ASPEN.

Merg AR et al: Mechanisms of impaired gallbladder contractile response in chronic acalculous cholecystitis, *J Gastrointest Surg* 6:432, 2002.

Mezey E: Interaction between alcohol and nutrition in the pathogenesis of alcoholic liver disease, *Semin Liver Dis* 11:340, 1991.

Morgan TR et al: Protein consumption and hepatic encephalopathy in alcoholic hepatitis, *J Am Coll Nutr* 14:152, 1995.

Mullen KD, Weber FL: Role of nutrition in hepatic encephalopathy, *Semin Liver Dis* 11 (4):292, 1991.

Nielsen K et al: Long-term oral refeeding of patients with cirrhosis of the liver, *Br J Nutr* 74:557, 1995.

Pisters PWT, Ranson JHC: Nutritional support for acute pancreatitis, *Surg Gynecol Obstet* 175:275, 1992.

Plauth M et al: ESPEN guidelines for nutrition in liver disease and transplantation, *Clin Nutr* 16:43, 1997.

Polonsky K: A practical approach to fasting hypoglycemia, *N Engl J Med* 326:1020, 1992.

Porayko MK et al: Impact of malnutrition and its therapy on liver transplantation, *Semin Liver Dis* 11(4):305, 1991.

Priori P et al: Stimulation of gallbladder emptying by intravenous lipids, *J Parent Enter Nutr* 21(6):350, 1997.

Ragins H et al: Intrajejunal administration of an elemental diet at neutral pH avoids pancreatic stimulation: studies in dog and man, *Am J Surg* 126:606, 1973.

Ranson JH et al: Prognostic signs and the role of operative management in acute pancreatitis, *Surg Gynecol Obstet* 139:69, 1974.

Seeff LB: Acute viral hepatitis. In Kaplowitz N, editor: *Liver and biliary diseases,* ed 2, Baltimore, 1996, Williams & Wilkins.

Shea JC et al: Advances in nutritional management of chronic pancreatitis, *Curr Gastroenterol Rep* 2:323, 2000.

Shronts EP: Nutritional assessment of adults with end-stage hepatic failure, *Nutr Clin Pract* 3:113, 1988.

Shronts EP, Fish J: Hepatic failure. In Gottschlich MM, et al, editor: *Nutrition support dietetics—core curriculum,* Silver Spring, Md, 1993, ASPEN.

Sokol RJ: Copper storage diseases. In Kaplowitz N, editor: *Liver and biliary diseases,* ed 2, Baltimore, 1996, Williams & Wilkins.

Steinberg W, Tenner S: acute pancreatitis, *N Engl J Med* 330:1198, 1994.

Stephenson GR et al: Malnutrition in liver transplant patients: preoperative subjective global assessment is predictive of outcome after liver transplantation, *Transplantation* 72:666, 2001.

Strate T et al: Pathogenesis and the natural course of chronic pancreatitis, *Eur J Gastroenterol Hepatol* 14:929, 2002.

te Boekhorst T et al: Etiological factors of jaundice in severely ill patients, *J Hepatol* 7:111, 1988.

Vierling JM: Hepatobiliary complications of ulcerative colitis and Crohn's disease. In Zakim D, Boyer TD, editors: *Hepatology: a textbook of liver disease,* Philadelphia, 1996, WB Saunders.

Weisiger RA: Laboratory tests in liver disease. In Goldman L, Bennett JC, editors: *Cecil textbook of medicine,* ed 21, Philadelphia, 2000, WB Saunders.

Weseman RA, McCashland TM: Nutritional care of the chronic posttransplant patient, *Top Clin Nutr* 13(2):27, 1998.

Whitington PF: Metabolic liver diseases of childhood. In Kaplowitz N, editor: *Liver and biliary diseases,* ed 2, Baltimore, 1996, Williams & Wilkins.

Wicks C et al: Comparison of enteral feeding and total parenteral nutrition after liver transplantation, *Lancet* 344:837, 1994.

Wolfe BM et al: The effect of intraduodenal elemental diet on pancreatic secretion, *Surg Gynecol Obstet* 140:241, 1975.

Additional References

Angulo P: Nonalcoholic fatty liver disease, *N Engl J Med* 16:1221, 2002.

Colantoni A et al: Hepatic estrogen receptors and alcohol intake, *Mol Cell Endocrinol* 193:101, 2002.

Hasse JM, Weseman RA: Solid organ transplantation. In Gottschlich MM, editors: *The science and practice of nutrition support: a case-based core curriculum,* Silver Springs, Md, 2001, ASPEN.

Kalfarentzos FE et al: Total parenteral nutrition in severe acute pancreatitis, *J Am Coll Nutr* 10:156, 1991.

Lieber CS: Herman Award lecture, 1993: a personal perspective on alcohol, nutrition, and the liver, *Am J Clin Nutr* 58:430, 1993.

Teran JC, McCullough AJ: Nutrition in liver diseases. In Gottschlich MM, editors: *The science and practice of nutrition support: a case-based core curriculum,* Silver Springs, Md, 2001, ASPEN.

Yabuki K et al: Extensive hemorrhagic erosive gastritis associated with acute pancreatitis successfully treated with a somatostatin analog, *J Gastroenterol* 37:737, 2002.

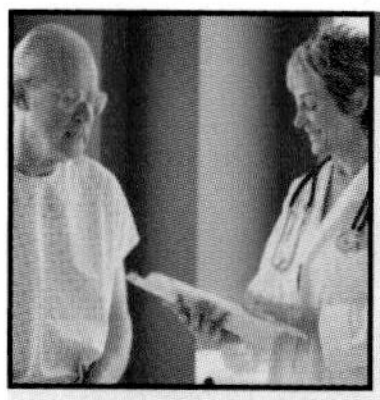

CHAPTER 32

Medical Nutrition Therapy for Food Allergy and Food Intolerance

SHERRY K. HUBBARD, RD, LD

CHAPTER OUTLINE

- Immunologic Basis
- Symptoms
- Risk Factors for the Development of Food Allergy
- Food Intolerances
- Diagnosis
- Treatment
- Natural History of Food Allergy
- Food Allergy in Infancy
- Diet and Prevention of Allergic Disease

KEY TERMS

adverse food reaction–any undesired response to a food regardless of mechanism

allergen–substance foreign to the body that on interaction with the immune system, causes an allergic reaction

antigen–usually a foreign substance (e.g., protein, cells, bacteria, polysaccharides) that stimulates antibody production

anaphylaxis–an acute, often severe, and sometimes fatal immune response that can affect one or more organ systems

antibodies–immunoglobulins produced in response to an antigen or allergen

atopic dermatitis (eczema)–a skin rash characterized by small red and white bumps that itch; often a symptom of allergy

atopic march–the presence of atopic characteristics, events, or conditions that develop into more permanent disease

atopy–tendency toward allergies, determined genetically

cap FEIA (fluroscein-enzyme immunoassay)–a blood test, more sensitive than the radioallergosorbent test (RAST), that provides quantitative assessment of food-specific IgE antibodies

cell-mediated immunity–immunity that is mediated by T lymphocytes, either through the release of lymphokines or by direct cytotoxicity

cross-reactivity–an allergic response to a food or substance either within a given group (e.g., crustacea, legumes) or with unrelated substances (e.g., banana, kiwi, or chestnuts with latex)

double-blind, placebo-controlled food challenge (DBPCFC)–a test of reaction to a food in which the food is disguised such that neither the patient nor the researcher knows it is being given; the "gold standard" for establishing food allergy

elimination diet–an investigational short-term or possible lifelong eating plan that omits one or more foods suspected or known to cause an adverse food reaction or allergic response

food allergy (hypersensitivity)–an adverse food reaction that is mediated by an immunoglobulin E (IgE) immunologic mechanism; induced by cell-mediated or immune-complex disease; the reaction occurs consistently after ingestion, inhalation, or touch of a particular food causing functional changes in target organs

food challenge–presenting a food to a patient with or without knowledge of when the food is being ingested using tolerated food vehicles to hide the food as necessary to prove or disprove a food-symptom relationship (open-, single-blind placebo-controlled, and double-blind placebo-controlled food challenges)

food intolerance–an adverse reaction to a food caused by toxic, pharmacologic, metabolic, or idiosyncratic reactions to the food or chemical substances in the food

food and symptom diary–a subjective tool for recording food and drink consumed, and onset, intensity, and duration of symptoms

humoral immunity–immunity mediated by antibodies produced by B lymphocytes

immunoglobulin E (IgE)–mediated reaction–rapid onset of symptoms occurring after ingestion of a specific allergen that cross-links the antigen-specific IgE molecule to mast cells and basophils

mast cells–tissue cells that release histamine or other substances causing allergic symptoms

oral allergy syndrome (OAS)–a mild to severe itch, tingle, or burning sensation affecting the mouth, tongue, or throat; throat tightness, or lip swelling after ingesting a food protein (e.g., melons) known to cross-react with a pollen (e.g., ragweed)

probiotics–a microbial dietary supplement affecting the intestinal tract that may modify immune response

radioallergosorbent test (RAST)–a test that measures specific IgE antibodies in serum; used as an alternative to skin tests

sensitization–exposure to an antigen or allergen that results in the development of hypersensitivity

skin test–a test in which an antigen is applied directly to the skin and then pricked or scratched through with a needle or a specifically designed prick or scratch implement to observe the histamine response

thymus and tonsils–tissues of lymphoid material that contribute to immunity

Food allergy prevalence among the pediatric population is perceived to be increasing by both allergists and pediatricians. Parents are requesting more food allergy evaluations as public awareness increases (Sampson et al, 2001). Increased public awareness of food allergies does not dissolve the frequent misconception that all reactions to food are allergy based. Until actual food allergy is properly diagnosed, the term adverse food reaction, an umbrella term used for any undesired food reaction, should be emphasized.

IMMUNOLOGIC BASIS

Definitions

The term *adverse food reaction* encompasses food intolerance and food hypersensitivity. Food intolerance is an adverse reaction to a food caused by toxic, pharmacologic, metabolic, idiosyncratic, or non-immunoglobulin E (IgE) reactions to food or chemical substances in the food. Food hypersensitivity, or food allergy, is an IgE-mediated reaction that occurs when the immune system reacts to a normally harmless food protein that the body has erroneously identified as harmful. This immunopathologic IgE-mediated process is reproducible through a "cause-and-effect relationship" (Taylor et al, 1999). IgE reactions usually occur instantly or within 2 hours of exposure, with severity ranging from mild to life threatening. Exposure includes inhalation, ingestion, and skin contact. Reactions to foods are not limited to ingestion reactions (Bahna, 2001; Belen, 2001).

Any person, especially a child, who has a genetic predisposition to atopic disease, or atopy, has an increased probability of developing food allergies (Zeiger, 2000). Allergic disease includes allergies to airborne particles (pollen, molds, grasses, weeds), food allergy, atopic dermatitis (eczema), and atopic-induced asthma (Wahn, 2001; Zeiger, 2000). Children with atopic dermatitis are 35% more likely to develop food allergies than other atopic children (Eigenmann, 1998). The incidence of food allergy appears to decrease with age. Infants younger than 2 years of age are more likely to develop food allergies than are older children or adults. Older children and adults are more likely to develop inhalant allergies than food allergies. Incidence estimates of food allergy indicate population ranges from 5% to 8% in children to 1.5% in adults (Sampson, 1999; Zeiger, 2000).

Immune System

The immune system functions to clear the body of foreign substances or antigens, such as viruses, bacteria, blood cells, and tissue cells. Normally, when antigens interact with cells of the immune system, they are cleared from the body without an adverse reaction. Allergy is different in that sensitization occurs. This happens on the first exposure of the immune cells to the allergen, when the immune cells are changed so that they subsequently recognize the allergen at the next exposure to it. Three types of cells respond to antigens presented: B lymphocytes, T lymphocytes, and macrophages. The lymphocytes arising from stem cells in the bone marrow, along with T cells originating from stem cells in the thymus, function as the basis for the two branches of the immune system: the humoral pathway and the cell-mediated pathway.

Humoral immunity involves antibodies (immunoglobulins) and has an important role in food allergy. Antigen-specific antibodies are produced by the B lymphocytes (B cells) in response to the antigen presented. The union of an antigen and its antibody results in the production of chemical mediators by the mast cells or direct cellular damage, which, in turn, causes symptoms. Five classes of antibodies have been identified: IgA, IgD, IgE, IgG, and IgM. They protect the body against bacteria and viruses. Secretory IgA antibodies in breast milk provide breast-fed infants with local intestinal protection against viruses and bacteria. IgA antibodies, present in saliva and intestinal secretions, block the absorption of antigens. IgE antibodies help to eliminate parasites from the body and are also responsible for classic allergic reactions: the immunoglobulen E (IgE-mediated reactions. IgD is involved in immunoglobulin class switching, but its other functions remain elusive.

Cellular or cell-mediated immunity involves the action of T lymphocytes (T cells). T cells do not produce antibodies, but they do recognize antigens. When an antigen stimulates T-cell growth, the T cells produce lymphokines and cytokines, substances that help regulate the activities of the B cells, or that cause direct cellular damage to target cells, resulting in the destruction of antigens. Cellular immunity has an important role in resistance to viruses, fungi, tumor cells, and other foreign cells through its production of the controller lymphocytes identified as Th1 and Th2 cells. Both Th1 and Th2 cells may work together. Cell-mediated immunity is stimulated by Th1-like cells linked to specific lymphokine profiles. IgE antibody formation is associated with Th2 type cells. Th2 stimulation produces eosinophils and mast cells, and the result is atopic disease. The Th1 cells linked to lymphokines stimulate cell-mediated immunity, and yet they suppress IgE antibody formation (Kay, 2001). The balance between antigen-specific Th1 and Th2 cells may have a significant effect on the antigen-specific IgE immune response. Future allergy prevention in high-risk newborns may include manipulating the immune response to change from Th2 to Th1 in character (Zeiger, 1999).

Tissue macrophages, derived from monocytes in the blood, also have important roles in the recognition, clearance, and presentation of antigens. Through the process of phagocytosis, the macrophage engulfs and destroys antigens. B cells, T cells, mast cells, and macrophages are all thought to interact (Figure 32-1).

The thymus and tonsils also play a role in immunity. The thymus is a ductless, glandlike organ that, because of its T-cell production, is essential to the development of peripheral lymphoid tissue. Although the thymus is largest and most active before puberty, the mature T cells it exports exert their effect into adulthood. Removal of the thymus during adulthood has little effect on a person's resistance to disease.

The tonsils consist of two small, rounded masses of lymphoid tissue that lie in the path of inspired air and all ingested food and liquids. Foreign material that is inspired into the airways and becomes trapped in the tonsillar crypts comes in contact with antigen-processing cells. Surgical removal of the tonsillar and adenoid tissue, especially during childhood, may impair or delay the development of a person's immunity to disease.

Allergic Reactions

Allergic reactions are unusual responses of the immune system and represent altered reactivity to an antigen. The antigens involved in allergic reactions are called allergens. Immune reactions are classified into four types: types I, II, and III, which are antibody-dependent, and type IV, which is T cell dependent (Table 32-1).

Immediate hypersensitivity (type I), involving IgE, is the most common allergic reaction and has the most clearly understood mechanism. The combination of an allergen with allergen-specific IgE fixed to tissue mast cells or circulating basophils causes the release of chemical mediators, including histamine, cytokines, lipid-derived prostaglandins, interleukins, and others. When released, these inflammatory mediators can cause itching, contraction of smooth muscle, vasodilation, and secretion of mucus. Manifestations, which are most often systemic, may involve the skin, gastrointestinal tract, or respiratory system (see Figure 32-1).

The contribution of non–IgE-mediated immunologic reactions to food hypersensitivity is not as clear. Circulating food-specific antibodies (IgA, IgG, and IgM) occur commonly. It has also been postulated that antigen-antibody complexes (type III reaction) may have a role in several food-related inflammatory diseases. These include various forms of colitis, enteritis with bleeding, malabsorptive disorders, ulceration, and chronic pneumonitis (Heiner's syndrome). Cell-mediated hypersensitivity (type IV reaction) may have a role in celiac disease, protein-losing enteropathies, eosinophilic gastroenteritis, and inflammatory bowel disorders, such as ulcerative colitis.

SYMPTOMS

A wide range of symptoms has been attributed to food allergy (Box 32-1). Skin, respiratory, cardiovascular, and gastrointestinal symptoms may express during an allergic reaction. Most frequently affected are the skin and respiratory systems (Sampson, 1999) (Figure 32-2).

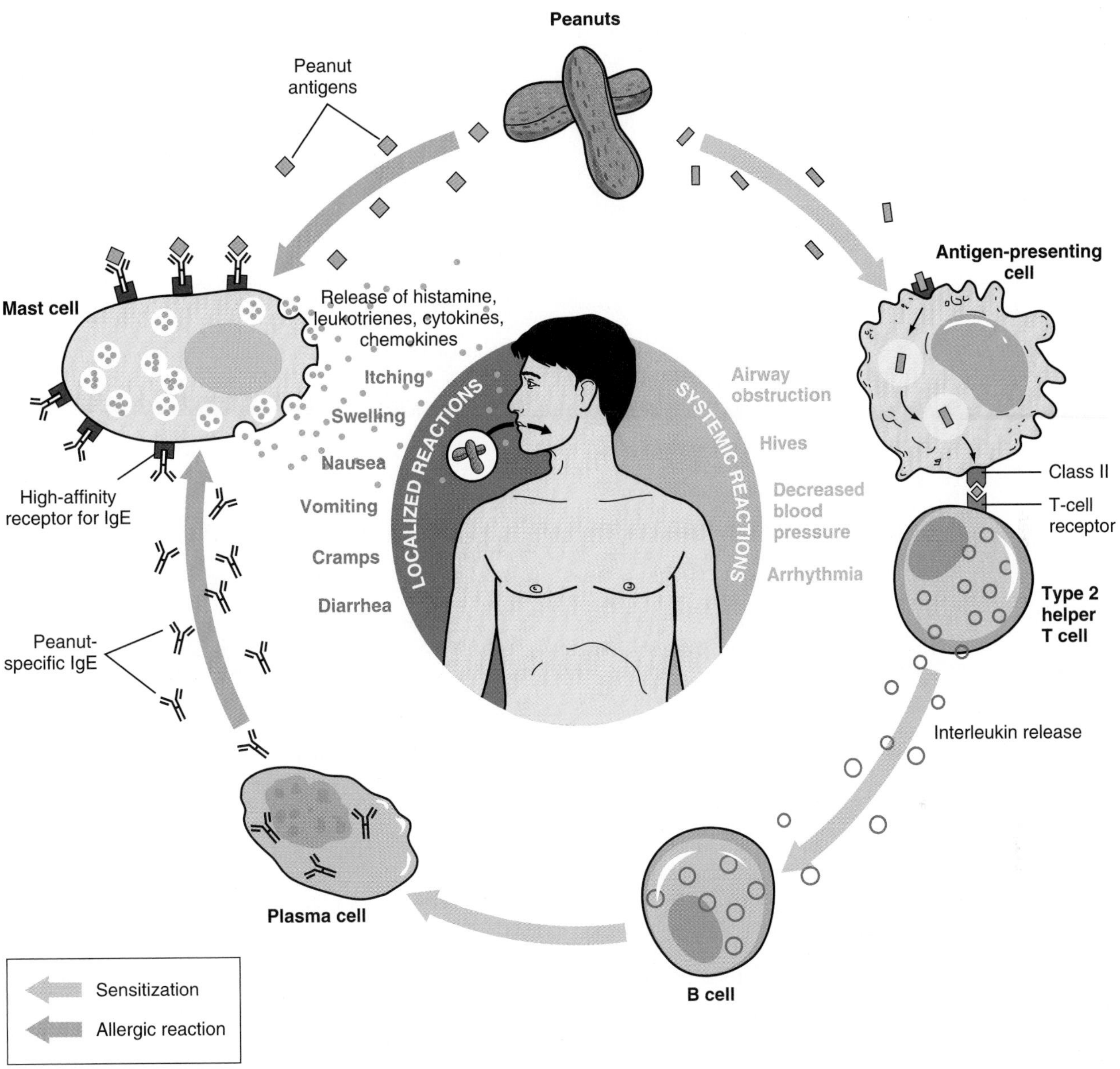

FIGURE 32-1 • Sensitization process and allergic reaction.

Food-induced anaphylaxis is an acute, often severe, and sometimes fatal immune response that usually occurs within a limited time following exposure to an antigen. Systemic anaphylaxis is the most dangerous allergic reaction and can include abdominal pain, nausea, vomiting, cyanosis, a drop in blood pressure, angioedema, chest pain, urticaria, diarrhea, shock, and death. A recent review of 32 fatal anaphylactic reactions to foods identified peanuts and tree nuts as causing the majority of deaths. Milk and fish were identified as causing 2 of the 32 deaths (Bock et al, 2001). People with known anaphylactic reactions to any food allergen should carry epinephrine (such as an Epi-Pen), the drug of choice to reverse an allergic reaction, at all times.

Food-dependent, exercise-induced anaphylaxis (FEIAn) is a distinct form of physical allergy. FEIAn may occur within 2 hours after rigorous activity when it is followed by the ingestion of one or more specific foods that are normally well tolerated. The pathophysiology is unknown (Vilke, 2002).

Unclear or Unproven Relationships

The role of food allergy in behavioral, psychological, neurologic, and musculoskeletal disorders remains largely unproved. When suspect symptoms not normally considered IgE mediated can be objectively measured without relying on the report of subjective symptoms, a double-blind, placebo-controlled food

TABLE 32-1 Types of Allergic Reactions

REACTION/CLASSIFICATION	MECHANISM	COMMENTS
Type I Immediate hypersensitivity, anaphylactic IgE-mediated, or reaginic reaction	The allergen binds with sensitized IgE antibody on mast cells (specialized granular cells in the intestines, skin, and respiratory tract) or basophils (similar cells in blood). This results in release of mediators (histamine, eosinophilic chemotactic factor, bradykinin, etc.). IgG has also been identified as being involved in this type of reaction.	Applies to hay fever, anaphylaxis, most food allergies, atopic dermatitis, asthma. Symptoms occur within seconds or up to 2 hr. Symptoms of food reactions may include laryngeal edema, nausea, vomiting, severe abdominal pain, bloating, diarrhea, angioedema, eczema, erythema, itching, hoarseness, wheezing, cough, chest tightness, hypotension, bronchospasm, and shock.
Type II Cytotoxic	IgG antibody reacts with the cell membrane or an antigen associated with the cell membrane.	Results from transfusion of incompatible blood types. No food reactions have been demonstrated.
Type III Antigen-antibody complex Arthus reaction	Antigen and antibodies (IgG and IgM) form a complex called a "precipitating antibody." The antigen-antibody complex is known as an Arthus reaction when it occurs in soft tissues, like blood vessels, lungs, or kidneys, and as serum sickness when the complex circulates. Complement is also activated in some cases.	Occurs in some food reactions. Milk precipitins have been found in the lungs of some children with chronic respiratory infection and in the gastrointestinal tract of those with gastroenteropathy. Reactions usually take 6 hr or more to appear and may take several days to become clinically apparent.
Type IV Delayed or cell-mediated hypersensitivity	T cells interact directly with antigen.	Usual mechanism of graft rejection. Possibly involved in some food allergies, such as protein-losing enteropathies.

Modified from Butkus SN, Mahan LK: Food allergies: immunological reactions to foods, *J Am Diet Assoc* 86:601, 1986.
IgG, Immunoglobulin G; *IgE,* immunoglobulin E.

challenge can help to determine whether a food-symptom relationship exists. This could apply to hyperactivity, tension fatigue syndrome, and migraine headaches. Measuring identifiable objective symptoms may take several disciplines and specialists, depending on the equipment needed to prove or disprove a food-symptom relationship. Even if a food-symptom relationship is not proved, but food avoidance is perceived as necessary for an investigation or because of personal choice, appropriate nutritional intervention may prevent or reduce nutritional risk.

RISK FACTORS FOR THE DEVELOPMENT OF FOOD ALLERGY

The risk of developing food allergy depends on heredity, exposure to a food (antigen), gastrointestinal permeability, and environmental factors, such as microbial exposure. Heredity is thought to play a major role in the development of atopic disease. Ironically, reduced childhood infections and exposures to microbes are perceived as a cause for the increased incidence of atopic disease in the population, thus initiating the atopic march, a collection of conditions, events, and characteristics preceding developing permanent atopic (allergic) disorders (Kalliomaki et al, 2001; Zeiger, 1999; Zeiger and Schatz, 2000). Infants who develop food allergies and atopic dermatitis are considered at risk for developing allergic rhinitis and asthma.

Exposure to an antigen is a prerequisite for the development of food allergy. The initial exposure can occur prenatally or postnatally (Frank et al, 1999; Vadas et al, 2001; Zeiger, 1999). Postnatal sensitization may occur with exposure to food allergens by inhalation, skin contact, or ingestion. Food allergen sensitization can happen with a food antigen in breast milk. Remembering this when taking a medical nutrition history can be very useful and may explain an allergic reaction that occurs at what appears to be the first time an infant eats the antigen in food (Isolauri et al, 1999). Gastrointestinal permeability may allow antigen penetration and presentation to the lymphocytes. Gastrointestinal permeability is thought to be greatest in early infancy and to decline with intestinal maturation. Other conditions, such as gastrointestinal disease, malnutrition, prematurity, and immunodeficiency states, may also be associated with increased permeability and risk of developing food allergy (Figure 32-3).

The amount of antigen present and environmental factors can also influence the development of food allergy. The effects of foods and other antigens may be

Box 32-1. Symptoms of Food Allergy

Gastrointestinal Manifestations

Abdominal pain
Nausea
Vomiting
Diarrhea
Gastrointestinal bleeding
Protein-losing enteropathy
Oral and pharyngeal pruritus

Cutaneous Manifestations

Urticaria (hives)
Angioedema
Eczema
Erythema (skin inflammation)
Itching
Flushing

Respiratory Manifestations

Rhinitis
Asthma
Cough
Laryngeal edema
Milk-induced syndrome with respiratory disease (Heiner's syndrome)
Airway tightening

Systemic Manifestations

Anaphylaxis
Hypotension
Dysrhythmias

Controversial or Unproven Manifestations

Behavioral disorders
Tension-fatigue syndrome
Attention-deficit and hyperactivity disorder (ADHD)
Otitis media
Psychiatric disorders
Neurologic disorders
Musculoskeletal disorders
Migraine headache

additive. Clinical symptoms of food allergy may increase when inhalant allergies are exacerbated by seasonal or environmental changes. Similarly, the effects of environmental factors, such as early exposure to microbes, tobacco smoke, stress, exercise, and cold, may enhance the clinical symptoms of food allergy.

FOOD INTOLERANCES

Food intolerances are adverse reactions to foods caused by nonimmunologic or non-IgE mechanisms, including toxic, pharmacologic, metabolic, or idiosyncratic reactions (Table 32-2). Symptoms caused by food intolerances include gastrointestinal, cutaneous, and respiratory disorders and are often similar to those of food allergy. Therefore, food intolerances must be considered in the differential diagnosis of food allergy. Although symptoms of food intolerance may be similar to those of food allergy, treatment may be different depending on the mechanism involved. Allergy skin or blood testing is not useful in the diagnosis and treatment of these conditions.

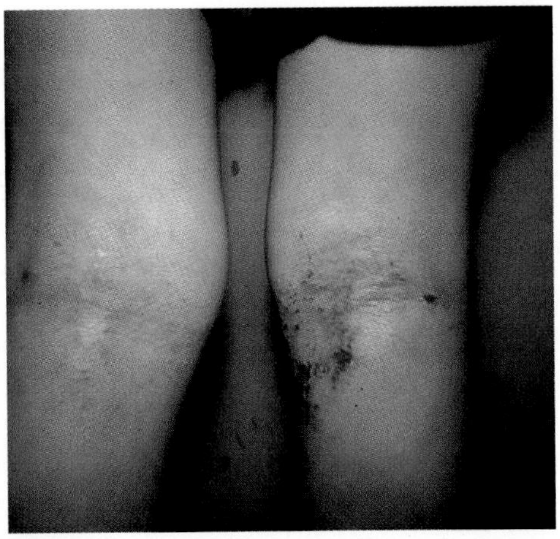

FIGURE 32-2 • Atopic eczema—an immunoglobulin E (IgE)–mediated skin reaction to a food allergen. Commonly seen on the back of knees and the inside of elbows.

Food Additives

Historically, food additives, such as preservatives, flavor enhancers, and coloring agents, have been linked to adverse reactions. Additives implicated include tartrazine (FD&C no. 5), carmine, azo dyes and other coloring agents, benzoic acid, sodium nitrate, butylated hydroxyanisole (BHA), butylated hydroxytoluene (BHT), monosodium glutamate (MSG), and sulfites (Reus et al, 2000) (see Table 32-2).

A recent study attempting to confirm symptoms perceived to be associated with food additives, including azo-dyes, benzoates, MSG, sorbates, BHT/BHA, and sulfites, found only sulfites to cause asthma and anaphylaxis (Reus et al, 2000); however, a documented case of nitrate causing anaphylaxis (Hawkins et al, 2000), an anaphylactic reaction to the color carmine (DiCello et al, 1999), and hives after ingestion of ice cream that contained acetylsalicylic acid (Bahna, 2001) have been reported. Adverse reactions to monosodium glutamate MSG are reported to include headache, nausea, flushing, abdominal pain, and asthma, and they generally occur 1 to 14 hours after ingestion (Raiten et al, 1995). The results from a study utilizing double-blind, placebo-controlled food challenges found symptoms perceived to be caused by MSG to be "neither persistent nor serious effects from MSG ingestion" (Geha et al, 2000). MSG is thought to be

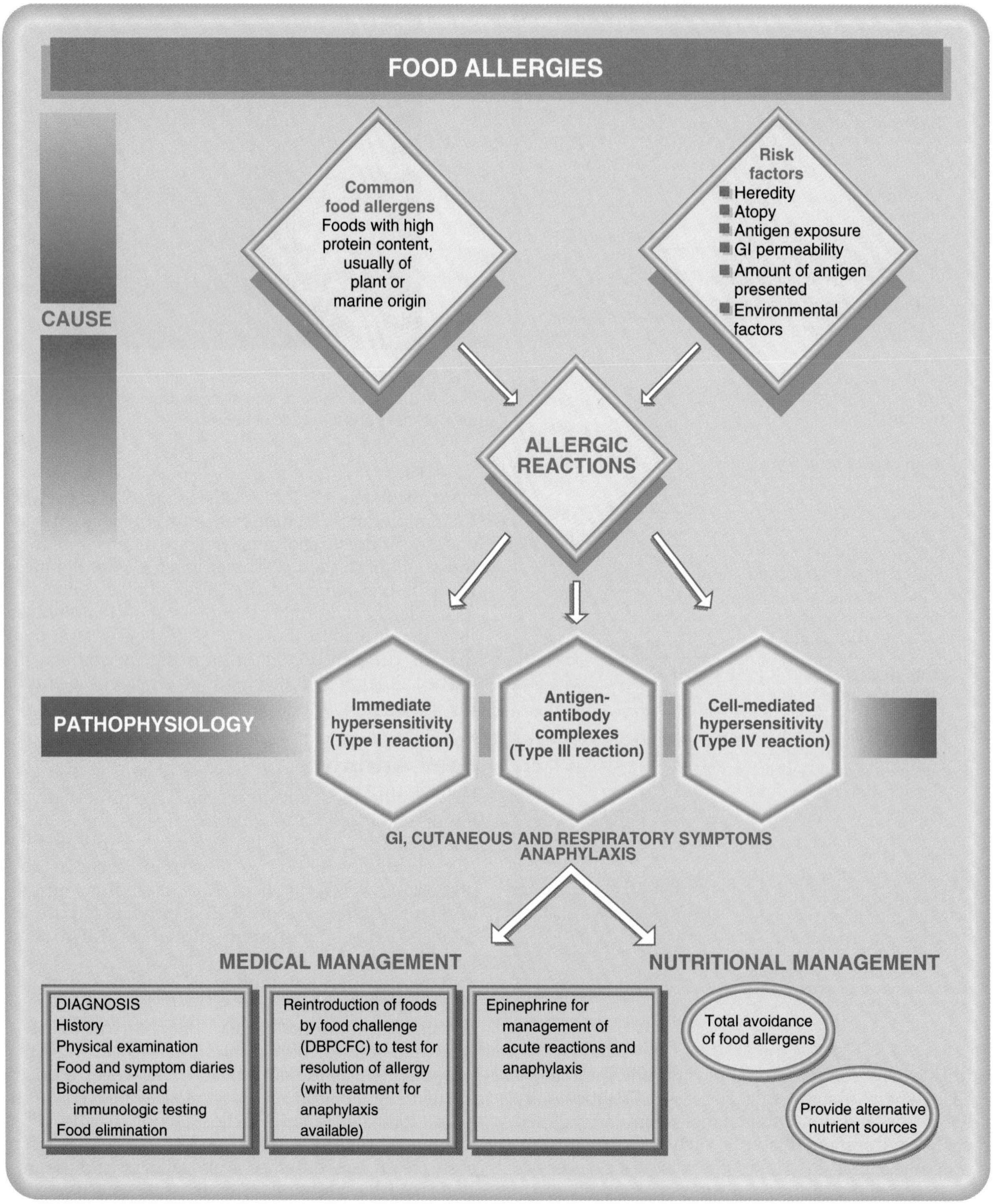

FIGURE 32-3 • Pathophysiology algorithm: food allergies. (Algorithm content developed by John Anderson, PhD, and Sanford C. Garner, PhD, 2000).

TABLE 32-2 Representative Nonimmunologic Reactions to Food

CAUSE	ASSOCIATED FOODS	SYMPTOMS
Gastrointestinal Disorders		
Enzyme deficiency		
Lactase	Foods containing lactose and milk	Bloating, flatulence, diarrhea, abdominal pain
Glucose-6-phosphate dehydrogenase	Fava or broad beans	Hemolytic anemia
Disease	Symptoms may be precipitated by many foods, especially high-fat foods or certain proteins	Bloating, loose stools, abdominal pain
Cystic fibrosis		
Gallbladder disease		
Enteropathies		
Inborn Errors of Metabolism		
Phenylketonuria	Foods containing phenylalanine	Elevated serum phenylalanine levels, mental retardation
Galactosemia	Foods containing lactose or galactose	Vomiting, lethargy, failure to thrive
Psychological Reactions	Symptoms may be precipitated by any food	Wide variety of symptoms involving any system
Reactions to Pharmacologic Agents in Foods		
Vasoactive amines		
Phenylethylamine	Chocolate, aged cheese, red wine	Migraine headaches
Tyramine	Cheddar cheese, French cheeses, brewers' yeast, Chianti wine, canned fish	Migraine headaches, cutaneous erythema, urticaria and hypertensive crisis in patients taking monoamine oxidase (MAO) inhibitors
Histamine	Fermented cheeses, fermented foods (e.g., sauerkraut, pork sausages, canned tuna, anchovies, sardines)	Erythema, headaches, decreased blood pressure
Histamine-releasing agents	Shellfish, chocolate, strawberries, tomatoes, peanuts, pork, wine, pineapple	Urticaria, eczema, pruritus
Reactions to Food Additives		
Tartrazine or FD&C Yellow No. 5	Yellow or yellow-orange colored foods, soft drinks, medicine	Hives, rash, asthma
Benzoic acid or sodium benzoate	Soft drinks and some cheeses, salt-free margarines, and processed potato products	Hives, rash, asthma
Sulfites		
Sodium sulfite, potassium sulfite, sodium metabisulfite, potassium metabisulfite, sodium bisulfite, potassium bisulfite, sulfur dioxide	Shrimp, many processed foods, avocado, instant potatoes, dried fruits, vegetables, acidic juices, wine, beer	Acute asthma and anaphylaxis, loss of consciousness
Reactions to Microbial Contamination of Foods		
Proteus causes histidine to break down to a histamine-like substance (anaphylactic type reaction)	Unrefrigerated scombroid fish (tuna, bonita, mackerel); heat-stable toxin produced	Scombroid fish poisoning (itching, rash, vomiting, diarrhea)
Gonyaulax catenella (red tide)	Mussels and clams that ingest the organism that produces saxitoxin, a heat-stable neurotoxin	Paralytic shellfish poisoning (progressive numbness from head to arms); frequently fatal

Modified from Butkus SN, Mahan LK: Food allergies: immunological reactions to foods, *J Am Diet Assoc* 86:601, 1986.

safe for most people. It is found naturally in tomatoes, Parmesan cheese, and mushrooms. Restaurant meals prepared with limited amounts or without MSG are usually available.

Multiple conditions are "blamed" on foods and environment without properly controlled studies and include behavior disorders, learning disabilities, depression, chronic fatigue, arthritis, and others (AAAAI, 1998). Improved behavior has been reported in preschool boys with attention-deficit and hyperactivity disorder (ADHD) who consume an additive-free and caffeine-free diet that is low in sugar; however, these effects may be related to other factors (Kaplan et al, 1989). Alternatively, it is possible that some food additives are related to behavioral changes in a subset of this population; however, elimination diets cannot be recommended for the routine management of hyperactivity. When families choose to pursue an altered diet in conjunction with recommended therapy, advice on implementing a nutritionally adequate and safe diet should be provided.

Sulfites

Adverse reactions to sulfites in foods have been well documented (Steinman, 1996; Taylor, 1992). Sulfiting agents are added to many foods and beverages to prevent browning, control microbial growth and spoilage, modify texture, and bleach certain foods.

Sulfites are also used as antioxidants in pharmaceuticals. The U.S. Food and Drug Administration (FDA) estimates that 1 of 100 persons is sulfite sensitive. Within that group, 5% are asthmatic (Papazian, 1996).

The diagnosis of sulfite sensitivity requires controlled, provocative challenge with sulfites. Guidelines for challenge have been outlined; most adverse reactions occur with doses of 20 to 50 mg of sulfite administered in solution (Simon, 1989). Reactions to the sulfites present in foods may differ, however. Sulfite-sensitive asthmatics may not always react after ingestion of sulfite-containing foods. The occurrence of reactions depends on the nature of the food, the level of residual sulfite, the sensitivity of the individual, and, perhaps, the form of residual sulfite and the mechanism of the sulfite-induced reaction (Lester, 1995).

Management of sulfite sensitivity requires avoidance of sulfite-containing foods. Foods that contain high levels of sulfites are listed in Table 32-2. Since 1986, the FDA regulations have banned the use of sulfites on fresh fruits and vegetables (other than potatoes) that are served raw. Current regulations of the FDA require disclosure when there is at least 10 parts per million concentration of a sulfiting agent. The smallest amount known to cause a reaction has yet to be identified (Papazian, 1996).

Carbohydrate Intolerance

Lactase deficiency is the most common enzyme deficiency worldwide. Persons who have a deficiency of the intestinal enzyme lactase have a decreased ability to digest lactose, the sugar in milk, and experience symptoms of abdominal cramping, flatulence, and diarrhea after its ingestion. Because the symptoms are similar, lactose intolerance is often confused with allergy to cow's milk. Deficiencies of lactase and other carbohydrate-digesting enzymes are discussed further in Chapter 30.

Gastrointestinal symptoms after the ingestion of fruit juice are commonly reported in infants and children, and they may be related to carbohydrate intolerance rather than to food allergy. Carbohydrate malabsorption has been documented following ingestion of pear, apple, and grape juices. A brief restriction of fruit juices may be useful in the evaluation of infants and children with chronic, nonspecific diarrhea (see Chapter 10).

DIAGNOSIS

No simple test can be used to diagnose food allergy. Diagnosis requires identification of the suspected food, proof that the food causes an adverse response, and verification of immunologic involvement. Nonallergic mechanisms must be ruled out. The omission of foods from the diet on the basis of improper diagnosis can and has threatened the nutritional status of the individual (Altman and Chiaramonte, 1996).

The first diagnostic tool is the clinical history. Gathered information should include a description of symptoms, the time of food ingestion relative to the onset of symptoms, a description of the most recent reactions, a list of suspected foods, and an estimate of the quantity of food required to cause a reaction. Food allergy may be linked to prenatal and postnatal exposures. The first exposure to suspect food allergens may occur during pregnancy, lactation, or in early childhood. The food does not have to be ingested by the infant directly. Introduction of highly allergenic foods (e.g., peanuts or other nuts) to the fetus during pregnancy or nursing can increase the likelihood of food allergy development (Sampson, 2002; Vadas et al, 2001). Eating peanuts more than once a week during pregnancy may increase peanut allergy risk. If peanut allergy already exists, there is a risk of the infant developing more food allergies (Frank et al, 1999; Sampson, 2002). Family history of atopic disease should be reviewed with both parents.

Physical examination includes measurements of weight, height, and body mass index (and head circumference for an infant) plotted on a growth chart and evaluated in relationship to earlier measurements. Decreased weight for height measurements may be related to malabsorption and potential food allergy. Therefore, patterns of growth and their relationship to the onset of symptoms should be explored. Clinical signs of malnutrition should be assessed, including the evaluation of fat and muscle stores (see Chapter 17). Malnutrition can affect skin test results and should be addressed before testing, when possible. Evidence of atopic march that includes atopic dermatitis or eczema (itchy rash with red and white bumps), allergic rhinitis, and asthma must be evaluated.

A 7- to 14-day food and symptom diary is useful if there is a perceived general food reaction with chronic symptoms but no specific suspect food(s) (Figure 32-4). This diary can also be used to identify possible nutrient deficiencies. A 24-hour recall is helpful when reactions occur less frequently. Both the food diary and the 24-hour recall should include the time the food is eaten, the quantity and type of food, all food ingredients identifiable, the time symptoms appear relative to the time of food ingestion, and any medications taken before or after the onset of symptoms because medications may alter the symptoms observed. The location where the reaction occurred can be informative, providing unexpected insights to possible food allergen exposure sources. Sometimes the information obtained indicates something other than a food reaction. A reaction that appears to be caused by a food allergen when the food allergen cannot be found may be caused by a different allergy source, such as a cat or dog. The more information obtained when a reaction occurs, the more useful the diary or recall. The 1- to 2-week diary record can also

Name ____________

	DAY 1 DATE ___	DAY 2 DATE ___	DAY 3 DATE ___	DAY 4 DATE ___	DAY 5 DATE ___	DAY 6 DATE ___	DAY 7 DATE ___
SYMPTOMS							
BREAKFAST							
SNACK SUPPLEMENTS							
SYMPTOMS							
LUNCH							
SNACK SUPPLEMENTS							
SYMPTOMS							
DINNER							
SNACK							
SYMPTOMS							
MEDICATION							

FIGURE 32-4 • Food and symptom diary.

serve as a baseline for future intervention. It is especially useful when reactions to food preservatives or additives are suspected.

Biochemical testing can rule out nonallergenic causes of symptoms. A complete blood count and differential; tests of stool for reducing substances, ova, parasites, or occult blood; and a sweat chloride test for the exclusion of cystic fibrosis are examples of tests that may be useful.

Immunologic testing is useful for screening patients and as a diagnostic tool. The Pharmacia CAP-FEIA (fluroscein-enzyme immunoassay) blood test is specific, with a 96% to 100% accuracy, in identifying children with milk, egg, fish, and peanut allergy. During a recent study, the predictability for wheat improved to 100% accuracy, whereas soy is still only 86% accurate. The blood test is being proven ef fective by testing known food allergic children whose food allergies had been previously proven with double-blind, placebo-controlled food challenges (DBPCFCs) (Sampson, 2001). Until test results are more accurate for more foods, however, skin testing and DBPCFCs will need to be used for the diagnostic process. The DBPCFC remains the "gold standard" for identifying food-induced symptoms (Sampson, 2001) (Table 32-3).

The radioallergosorbent test (RAST) and the enzyme-linked immunosorbent assay (ELISA) are diagnostic tools being replaced by the CAP FEIA blood test (see Table 32-3). The CAP FEIA blood test appears promising in the food allergy diagnostic process because it provides a quantitative assessment of allergen-specific IgE antibody, and higher levels of antibodies are predictors of clinical symptoms. Thus far, test accuracy has been approved for only six foods: egg, milk, peanut, fish, wheat, and soy, but soy is still not as predictive (Sampson, 2001).

Skin tests are the most economic and provide results within 15 to 30 minutes. Control comparisons using histamine skin-prick test results provide both positive and negative wheal diameters necessary for accurate readings (Figure 32-5). All skin-prick tests are compared with the control wheal. Test wheals that are 3 mm greater than the negative control indicate a positive result. Negative skin-prick skin tests have excellent negative predictive accuracy and suggest the absence of an IgE-mediated reaction. For children younger than 2 years of age, the skin test is reserved to confirm immunologic mechanisms after symptoms have been confirmed by a positive test result from a food challenge or when the history of the reaction is impressive (Sampson, 1999).

TABLE 32-3 Diagnostic Tests

TYPE OF TEST	DESCRIPTION	COMMENTS
Skin testing (scratch, prick, or puncture)	A drop of antigen is placed on the skin, and the skin is then scratched or punctured to allow penetration	Screening test; cannot be relied upon as sole diagnostic tool; a history of food-symptom relationship also important; must be followed by a DBPCFC
Radioallergosorbent test (RAST)	Serum is mixed with food on a paper disk and then washed with radioactively labeled IgE	No more accurate than the skin test, but more costly; may be useful in people who have skin disease
Enzyme-linked immunosorbent assay (ELISA)	This test is much like RAST, except no radioactive material is used	Same as for RAST
CAP-RAST fluroscein-enzyme immunoassay (FEIA)	Compared to RAST, this test binds more allergen	New test for food allergy; reliable for only six foods; shows promise as a component in diagnostic process for food allergy
Specific IgG, IgM, IgA antibody assays	Techniques: precipitation hemagglutination, complement fixation; requires special expertise	Best used in research only
Cytotoxic testing	Allergen is mixed with whole blood or serum leukocyte suspension; lysed leukocytes are then counted	Unreliable
Sublingual testing	Drops of allergen extract are placed under the tongue and symptoms are recorded	Unreliable
Provocation testing and neutralization	Subcutaneous injection of allergen extract elicits symptoms; this is then followed by injection of a weaker or stronger preparation to neutralize symptoms	Unreliable
Kinesiologic testing	Subject's arm is extended and foods to be tested are placed in the hand; test is considered to yield positive results if the arm moves more easily after the food has been placed in the hand	Unreliable
IgG4	Blood testing for food-specific IgG4	Not validated for diagnostic use
Change in leukocyte size Antigen leukocyte cellular antibody test (ALCAT)	Exposure to food allergen supposedly increases leukocyte diameter	Not validated for diagnostic use

Data from Bahna SL: *In vitro food allergy tests: the good, the bad, and the worst,* American College of Allergy, Asthma, and Immunology, Sixtieth Annual Meeting, San Antonio, Tex, November 19, 2001 and American Academy of Allergy, Asthma, and Immunology: Position statement.
Ig, Immunoglobulin.

Many children with atopic dermatitis have a food allergy that can be diagnosed using a skin-prick test for eight foods (milk, egg, peanut, soy, wheat, cod, catfish, and cashew) because these foods account for 89% of positive food challenge tests (Burks et al, 1998). Food allergies to egg, milk, and peanut now represent about 85% of children and adolescents with documented food allergy (Sampson, 2001). All foods that test positive must correlate with a strong exposure history (i.e. anaphylaxis) or be proven to cause allergic reactions through food challenges before they can be considered allergenic.

The following food allergy in vitro "diagnostic tests" are considered unproved or unreliable: IgG4 antibody assays; cytotoxicity testing (Bryran's testing); urine autoinjection; skin titration (Rinkel method); sublingual testing; provocative and neutralization testing; kinesiologic testing; change in leukocyte size test, called antigen leukocyte cellular antibody test (ALCAT); leukocyte cytotoxic test; neutrophil chemotaxis; lymphocyte proliferation; immune complexes; and basophil histamine release. These tests are considered to have no diagnostic validity. Specific IgG, IgM, and IgA antibody assays should be used for research purposes only (AAAAI, 1996; Bahna, 2001) (see Table 32-3). Sometimes laboratories that provide unproven or unreliable "diagnostic tests" are not appropriately regulated or are connected to products directed for the food allergic person's purchase.

Food elimination is another tool in the diagnosis process used for chronic symptoms, such as hives, angioedema, eczema. When a food is eliminated, all forms—cooked, raw, and protein derivatives of that food—must be removed from the diet (see Figure 32-4). A food record is kept during the elimination phase. This record is used to ensure that all forms of suspected foods have been eliminated from the diet and to evaluate the diet's nutritional adequacy. Vitamin and mineral supplementation should be considered when a severely limited diet continues for more than 7 to 14 days. A temporary elimination diet should be personalized, when possible, eliminating only one or two suspect foods at a time for each 2-week period. If multiple foods are suspected, a variation of the "strict" elimination diet shown in Table 32-4 should be used. Any food on the list that is suspect or that is eaten more often than once every 4 months should be substituted with a food that is rarely or almost never eaten.

If the individual or the health care provider continues to suspect foods, then an elemental diet, the most severe form of elimination diet, should be considered. An elemental diet prevents malnutrition but is expensive, not well accepted, and should be reserved for the most restrictive cases. Products such as EleCare, Neocate (infants), or Neocate One Plus for infants and young children, and Tolerex, L-Emental, Ultraclear, Biogenesis, and EO28 formulas for teenagers and adults are examples of formulas that can be used. Foods are returned to the diet one at a time while the patient is receiving the formula.

The elimination process will determine whether symptoms improve or resolve with avoidance. If symptoms persist with careful avoidance of suspect foods, other causes for the symptoms should be considered. If a positive result has been obtained on a skin test, and symptoms improve unequivocally with the elimination of the food, that food should be eliminated from the diet until an oral food challenge is appropriate. The oral food challenge will prove or disprove a food symptom relationship. If symptoms improve with only the elimination of multiple foods, multiple food challenges are necessary.

Food Challenge

A food challenge is conducted once symptoms have resolved and all antihistamines are stopped. Foods are challenged one at a time on different days, thus eliminating confusion while the person is carefully observed in a medical setting for the recurrence of symptoms. The three types of food challenges are as follows: open food challenge (OFC), which allows the food to be given openly; single-blind food challenge (SBPCFC), in which the food is hidden from the patient with at least one placebo; and double-blind, placebo-controlled food challenge (DBPCFC), in which the food is hidden from the patient and presented with at least one to three placebos. Increasing amounts of the offending food should be given every 15 to 60 minutes until there

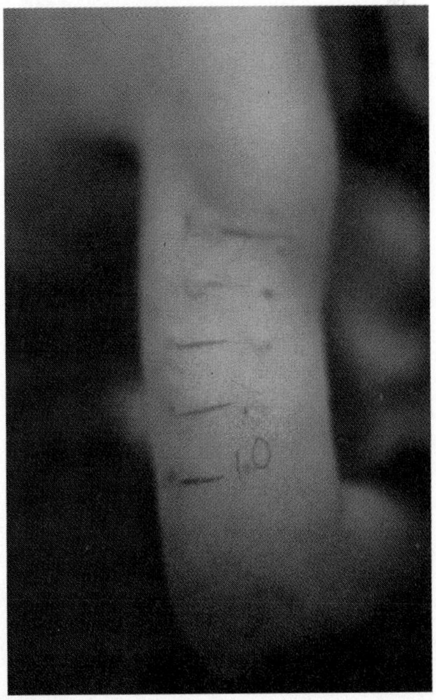

FIGURE 32-5 • A skin-prick test showing the wheal and flare of the reaction to the allergen as compared with the reaction to the histamine control at the bottom.

is a convincing but not life-threatening response. The goal is to ingest 60 to 100 g of food or 10 g of isolated suspect protein. Reactions have been observed in children after consumption of as little as 20 mg to as much as 8 g of dried food (Sampson, 1999). A person with a positive challenge must be given appropriate medications to stop symptoms and be observed for an additional 1 to 2 hours. Those who are observed to have a negative challenge should also be observed for an additional 1 to 2 hours. Occasionally a reaction may occur later than expected. The amount tolerated under observation can then be offered at home.

The DBPCFC, which provides objective results by eliminating outside influences, is considered the "gold standard" when attempting to establish a food and symptom relationship, and it is used to confirm a food

TABLE 32-4 Three Stages of Elimination Diets

	FOODS ALLOWED	FOODS TO AVOID
Elimination Diet Level 1: Milk-, Egg-, and Wheat-Free		
Animal protein sources	Lamb, chicken, turkey, beef, pork	Cow's milk, chicken eggs
Vegetable protein sources	Soy milk, soybeans, other beans, lentils	
Grains or alternative starches	White potato, sweet potato, yams, rice, tapioca, arrowroot, buckwheat, corn, barley, rye, millet, oats	Wheat
Vegetables	All vegetables	
Fruits	All fruits and juices	
Sweeteners	Cane or beet sugar, maple syrup, corn syrup	
Oils	Soy oil, corn oil, safflower oil, coconut oil, vegetable oil, olive oil, peanut oil, milk-free margarines	Butter and margarines that include milk
Other	Salt, all spices	
Elimination Diet Level 2: Stricter		
Animal protein sources	Lamb	All other animal protein, including meat, fish, poultry, eggs, and milk
Vegetable protein sources	None	Soy milk, soybeans, peas, other beans, lentils, peanuts, bean sprouts, all nuts
Grains or alternative starches	White potato, sweet potato, yams, rice, tapioca, buckwheat, arrowroot, corn	Wheat, oats, barley, millet, rye
Vegetables	Most vegetables	Peas, tomatoes
Fruits	Most fruits and juices	Citrus fruits, strawberries
Sweeteners	Cane or beet sugar, maple syrup, corn syrup	
Oils	Safflower oil, coconut oil, olive oil, sesame oil	Butter, margarine, vegetable oils, soy oil, corn oil, peanut oil, nonspecific shortening, or fats of animal origin
Other	Salt, pepper, all spices,* vanilla or lemon extract, baking soda, cream of tartar	Chocolate, coffee, tea, colas and other soft drinks, alcoholic beverages
Elimination Diet Level 3: Severe†		
	Rice in any form (rice cakes and rice cereal being especially helpful) Pineapple Apricots Cranberries Peaches Pears Apples including canned fruit and juices of these Lamb Chicken Asparagus Beets Carrots Lettuce Sweet potatoes White vinegar Olive oil Honey Cane or beet sugar Salt Safflower oil	All other foods

Modified from Bock SA: *Food allergy: a primer for people,* New York, 1988, Vantage Press.
*Suggest limiting number to five to minimize dietary variables.
†This is not a nutritionally complete diet and must only be used with the advice of a physician or nutritionist for short periods (2 weeks or less).

allergy. Each DBPCFC must be personalized. Single foods (applesauce, grape juice) or tolerated food combinations can "hide" a suspect food. The product must mask any hint of the flavor, color, or texture of the suspect food or allergen. The patient should not be able to detect the differences between the "active" food and the placebo food (Sampson, 1999). Because severe reactions can occur during a challenge, a physician must be in attendance with emergency supplies measured and ready to be administered.

After a negative DBPCFC, an open challenge should be given. In this challenge the patient is given a serving of the suspect food. Interestingly, reactions have occurred during the open challenge that did not occur in the blind challenge. Occasionally, symptoms may accompany the last presentation if the threshold is greater than indicated by the history. Most allergic reactions occur within 2 hours of the challenge. Non–IgE-mediated reactions may occur more than 24 hours after challenge. Monitoring of the patient should continue during this time (Sampson, 1999).

Although most food allergy reactions are not fatal, about 30,000 anaphylactic reactions, 2000 hospitalizations, and 200 deaths occur in the United States each year, and peanuts and tree nuts are believed to cause most of these near-fatal and fatal anaphylactic reactions (Sampson, 2002). If there is a clear history of a life-threatening anaphylactic reaction after eating a specific food, that food should not be challenged unless there is sufficient evidence that the person is no longer reacting to the allergen and skin test results are negative.

A single-blind food challenge, in which the person receiving the challenge does not know what has been offered, may be useful in similar situations and is easier to implement; however, challenges carried out for research purposes should be DBPCFC as specifically explained (Sampson, 1999).

TREATMENT

Total avoidance of a food allergen is the only proven treatment for food allergy (Joint Task Force on Practice Parameters, 1998; Sampson, 1999; Sicherer, 2001). Food immunotherapy vaccine is a possible future treatment meant to complement food allergen avoidance. The vaccine's purpose will be to prevent an allergic reaction or reduce its severity and prevent death in the event of accidental exposure. Food immunotherapy vaccines are still considered experimental. Although many food intolerances may allow some ingestion of the offending food, food hypersensitivities or allergies do not. Families and individuals need guidelines and suggestions for avoiding allergenic foods, substituting permissible foods for restricted foods in meal planning and preparation, and selecting nutritionally adequate replacement foods.

To help identify and avoid offending foods, allergy-specific lists that describe foods to avoid, list key words for ingredient identification, and present acceptable substitutes may be useful (Boxes 32-2 through 32-6). Caretakers and school personnel working with the food allergic child should be cau-

Box 32-2. Egg Allergy

Foods and Ingredients to Avoid*

Albumin	Egg yolk	Meringue
Apovitellin	Flavoprotein	Ovalbumin
Avidin	Frozen eggs	Ovogycoprotein
Bernaise sauce	Globulin	Ovomucin
Dried eggs	Hollandaise sauce	Ovomucoid
Eggnog	Imitation egg product	Ovomuxoid
Egg solids	Livetin	Powdered egg
Egg substitutes	Lysozyme	Simplesse
Egg white	Mayonnaise	

Egg Substitutes (Equivalent to 1 Egg)

Ener G Egg Replacer (ENERG-G Foods, Inc.) 1½ tsp + 1 tbsp of water	1 Packet plain gelatin + 2 tbsp warm water (Do not mix until ready to use.)
½ tsp Baking powder + 1 tbsp liquid + 1 tbsp vinegar	3 tbsp Puréed apple
1 tsp Yeast dissolved in ¼ c warm water	1 Medium banana
1 tbsp Apricot purée	
1½ tbsp Water + 1½ tbsp oil + 1 tsp baking powder	

Modified from Burns-Ogle G, Doerr J, Martin B, editors: *Manual of medical nutrition therapy,* ed 3, Oklahoma City, 1996, Oklahoma Dietetic Association.

*Eliminate the following foods, as well as any foods containing any of these ingredients, from your diet.

Box 32-3. Cow's Milk Allergy

Foods and Ingredients to Avoid*,†

Acidophilus milk
Artificial butter flavor
Butter
Butter fat
Butter oil
Caramel candy
Carob candies
Cheese (e.g., cheddar, Colby, cream, Edam, Gouda, Monterey Jack, mozzarella, Muenster, Neufchâtel, parmesan, provolone, ricotta, Romano, Swiss, cottage)
Chocolate milk
Creamed candies
Cultured buttermilk
Dry milk (whole, low-fat, nonfat)
Eggnog
Evaporated milk
Goat's milk‡
Half & half cream
Ice cream
Imitation milk, low-sodium
Light cream
Low-fat ice cream
Malted milk
Milk chocolate
Milk (whole, 2%, 1½%, 1%, ½%, skim, nonfat condensed milk)
Semisweet chocolate
Sherbet, most types
Sour cream
Sour cream dressings
Sour cream solids
Sour milk solids
Sweetened condensed milk
Whipping cream
Yogurt, frozen
Yogurt, regular

Ammonium caseinate
Calcium caseinate
Magnesium caseinate
Potassium caseinate
Sodium caseinate

Casein
Casein hydrolysate
Curds
Custard
Delactosed whey
Lactalbumin
Lactalbumin phosphate
Lactoglobulin
Lactose
Lactulose
Milk protein
Milk protein hydrolysates
Nougat
Protein hydrolysate
Pudding
Rennet casein
Sweet whey
Whey
Whey protein hydrolysate
Whey protein concentrate

Ingredients Potentially Made With Cow's Milk Products

Bavarian cream flavoring
Brown sugar flavoring
Butter flavoring
Caramel flavoring
Coconut cream flavoring
Natural flavoring
Simplesse

Milk Substitutes to Use in Recipes (Use to Replace 1 c of Cow's Milk)

1 c Light-colored fruit juice (e.g., apple, orange, white grape)
1 c Soy-based infant formula
1 c Soy milk (e.g., Edensoy, Westsoy, Vitasoy, Silk)
1 c Water

Milk-Free Infant Formulas

Elemental

Neocate One+ (Scientific Hospital Supplies International, Ltd.)
Neocate (Scientific Hospital Supplies International, Ltd.; 800-365-7354)

Protein Hydrolysates§

Alimentum (Ross Laboratories; 800-515-7677)
EleCare (Ross Laboratories)
Nutramigen (Mead Johnson; 415-474-2169)
Ultracare for Kids (Metagenics; 800-338-3948)

Modified from Burns-Ogle G, Doerr J, Martin B, editors: *Manual of medical nutrition therapy,* ed 3, Oklahoma City, 1996, Oklahoma Dietetic Association.
*Eliminate the following foods, as well as any foods containing any of these ingredients.
†Individuals who must avoid all cow's milk sources frequently need a calcium supplement.
‡Goat's milk protein is similar to cow's milk protein. Those with cow's milk allergy may experience similar symptoms with goat's milk ingestion. Goat's milk is not recommended as a cow's milk substitute.
§Protein hydrolysate–containing formulas may cause symptoms in some infants.

Box 32-4. Peanut Allergy

Foods and Ingredients to Avoid*

Beer nuts	Ground nuts	Peanut flakes
Chopped peanuts	High-protein food	Peanut flour
Cold-pressed peanut oil	Hydrolyzed plant protein	Peanut oil
Defattened peanuts	Hydrolyzed vegetable protein	Peanut soup
Egg rolls	Marzipan	Peanuts, roasted
Expelled or expressed peanut oil	Mixed nuts	Peanuts, shelled
Fresh peanuts	Nougat	Peanuts, whole, roasted in-shell
Granulated peanuts	Peanut butter	

Additional Products That May Contain Peanuts

Baked goods	Chocolate candy	Peanut meal
Candy	Hamster feed	Pie crusts
Cheesecake crusts	Ice cream	Sauces
Chili	Livestock feed	

Modified from Burns-Ogle G, Doerr J, Martin B, editors: *Manual of medical nutrition therapy,* ed 3, Oklahoma City, 1996, Oklahoma Dietetic Association.

*Eliminate all sources of peanuts from diet. DO NOT eat any food that has touched peanuts or use any utensils used in preparing peanut-containing dishes.

Remember that peanut powder, peanut butter, and peanuts may be used in casseroles, sprinkled on top of dishes, or used as an ingredient (e.g., in vegetable dishes, fruit dishes, cookies, cakes, pastries, desserts, chili, soups, stews, egg rolls, etc.). *Be careful when eating at social functions or when dining out! Take extra precautions when dining at Asian, Chinese, Thai, Mediterranean, and Indian restaurants, as these restaurants use many different peanut forms in multiple ways.*

When possible call the manager of a restaurant 2 or 3 days before dining out. Explain why peanuts must be avoided, and find out if any form of peanuts is used as a recipe ingredient or as garnish or if the food is cooked in peanut oil. Explain the severe reactions to peanuts. NEVER, NEVER assume a dish is peanut free just because the menu description does not mention peanuts. Many restaurant dishes are purchased prepared to heat and serve. This includes more expensive restaurants. Be sure to emphasize why this information is being requested.

Some sauces served in Mexican restaurants may contain peanuts. When dining at any restaurant, always ask your waitperson or the restaurant manager which dishes may contain peanuts. If not satisfied with the answer, choose a different dish or restaurant.

tioned to read labels carefully before purchasing or serving food. The Food Allergy and Anaphylaxis Network (FAAN), a nonprofit organization created to support the food allergic child, has developed through work with board-certified allergists and dietitians an excellent education program for day-care or school programs. Food substitutions can be challenging when working to stay within U.S. Department of Agriculture Child Nutrition Program Guidelines and state education departments should be contacted for specific information.

Foods to be avoided may be hidden in the diet in unfamiliar forms. When a food-sensitive person ingests a hidden allergen, the most common reason is that the "safe" food was contaminated. This may happen as a result of using common serving utensils, such as at an ice cream parlor, salad bar, or deli (where the meat slicer may be used to slice both meat and cheese). Manufacturing plants or restaurants may use the same equipment to produce two different products (e.g., peanut butter and almond butter), and despite cleaning, traces of an allergen may remain on the equipment between uses. Alternatively, a restaurant may use the same oil to fry both potatoes and fish (Box 32-7) (see *Clinical Insight:* Does "Pareve" Really Mean Milk Free?). Another situation that may lead to the unknowing ingestion of an allergenic food occurs when one product is used to make a second product, and only the ingredients of the second product are listed on the food label. An example would be the listing of mayonnaise as an ingredient in a salad dressing without specifically listing egg as an ingredient of the mayonnaise. Labels must be read often to ensure that ingredients have not changed in the processing of the food.

When foods are removed from the diet, alternative nutrient sources must be provided. Table 32-5 defines the levels of nutritional risk based on the types of food removed from the diet. For example, when dairy products are omitted, other foods must provide calcium, vitamin D, protein, riboflavin, and energy. The nutritional adequacy of the diet should be monitored on a regular basis by conducting an ongoing evaluation of the patient's growth, nutritional status, and food records. Malnutrition and poor growth have been documented in children who consume inadequate elimination diets (Isolauri et al, 1999). Vitamin and mineral supplementation is needed, especially when multiple foods are omitted.

Box 32-5. Soy Allergy

Foods and Ingredients to Avoid*

Chee-fan	Soy flour	Soybean sprouts
Deep-fried mature soy seed	Soy grits	Sufu
Fermented soybean paste	Soy protein concentrates	Tao-cho
Fermented soybeans	Soy protein isolates	Tao-si
Hamanatto	Soy protein shakes	Taotjo
Immature green soy seed	Soy sauce	Tempeh
Ketjap	Soybean curd	Textured soy protein
Metiauza	Soybean hydrolysates	Textured vegetable protein (TVP)
Miso	Soybean or soy lecithin†	Tofu
Natto	Soybean milk	Whey-soy drink
	Soybean oil	

Ingredients Potentially Made From Soybean Products

Hydrolyzed plant protein
Hydrolyzed soy protein
Hydrolyzed vegetable protein
Natural flavoring
Vegetable broth
Vegetable gum
Vegetable starch

Soy and Milk Substitutes

Fruit juices
Rice milk

Infant Formulas

Elemental
Neocate One+ (Scientific Hospital Supplies International, Ltd.)
Neocate (Scientific Hospital Supplies International, Ltd.; 800-365-7354)

Protein Hydrolysates‡
Alimentum (Ross Laboratories)
EleCare (Ross Laboratories; 800-515-7677)
Nutramigen (Mead Johnson; 415-474-2169)

Modified from Burns-Ogle G, Doerr J, Martin B, editors: *Manual of medical nutrition therapy,* ed 3, Oklahoma City, 1996, Oklahoma Dietetic Association.
*Eliminate the following foods, as well as any foods containing any of these ingredients, from your diet.
†Several studies indicate that soybean lecithin and soy oil are frequently tolerated by individuals who are soy-allergic.
‡*Note:* Protein hydrolysate–containing formulas may cause symptoms in some infants. Ask your allergist, physician, or dietitian to recommend the best formula for your infant.

Unless a clear diagnosis of food allergy is established, the patient may be well advised to return to a normal diet as tolerated. If symptoms persist or reappear, a review of intake will determine whether all forms of suspected foods have been omitted from the diet. If symptoms persist even with adherence to the diet, other causes for the allergy or other nonallergic causes for the symptoms should be investigated. Because food is an important part of a person's culture, the social aspects of eating can make adherence difficult. Continued support from health care providers is needed to minimize the impact of dietary changes on family and social life. The strategies listed in Box 32-8 can help families and individuals cope with food allergies.

NATURAL HISTORY OF FOOD ALLERGY

Food allergy, asthma, and atopic dermatitis (eczema) are atopic diseases that produce specific IgE antibodies (Zeiger, 1999), however test results that indicate high IgE levels (skin or blood) do not automatically point to allergy. Clinical symptoms occur in only 30% to 40% of those testing positive to a food. The development of food allergy may precede the development of the other atopic diseases such as atopic dermatitis and asthma. Infant gastroesophageal reflux may complicate asthma and food allergy symptoms. The process of developing any atopic disease is called

Box 32-6. Wheat Allergy

Foods and Ingredients to Avoid*

Atta	Laubina	Wheat bran
Bal ahar	Leche alim	Wheat bread
Bread flour	Malted cereals	Wheat bread crumbs
Bulgar	Minchin	Wheat flakes
Cake flour	Multi-grain breads	Wheat germ
Cereal extract	Multi-grain flours	Wheat gluten
Couscous	Puffed wheat	Wheat meal
Cracked wheat	Red wheat flakes	Wheat pasta
Durum flour	Rolled wheat	Wheat protein beverage
Durum	Semolina	Wheat protein powder
Enriched flour	Shredded wheat	Wheat starch
Farina	Soft wheat flour	Wheat tempeh
Gluten	Spelt	White flour
Graham flour	Superamine	Whole-wheat berries
High-gluten flour	Triticale	Whole-wheat flour
High-protein flour	Vital gluten	Winter wheat flour
Kamut flour	Vitalia macaroni	

Ingredients Potentially Made From Wheat Products

Gelatinized starch
Hydrolyzed vegetable protein
Modified food starch
Modified starch
Starch
Vegetable gum
Vegetable starch

Substitutions

When substituting any flour—either nongluten– or low-gluten–containing flour—use a recipe developed specifically for that flour. No nonwheat flour will produce an acceptable end product when substituted for wheat flour in a wheat flour–based recipe. A variety of recipes have been developed specifically for these particular grains as a replacement for wheat-containing products. More leavening is required in nongluten and low-gluten–containing flours. Try adding 2 to 2½ tbsp baking powder per cup of nongluten or low-gluten flours.

Modified from Burns-Ogle G, Doerr J, Martin B, editors: *Manual of medical nutrition therapy,* ed 3, Oklahoma City, 1996, Oklahoma Dietetic Association.
*Eliminate the following foods, as well as any foods containing any of these ingredients, from the diet.

the atopic march (Sicherer, 2002; Zeiger, 2000) and possibly has beginnings before birth (Jones et al, 2001).

There is indication that the improved hygiene of our society has caused changes in the neonatal gastrointestinal microflora, which directly affects the immune system's maturation process (Kalliomaki, 2001). The result is that with the greater cleanliness there is greater incidence of atopic disease, including food allergy. Probiotics are microbial dietary supplements that directly affect the intestinal tract by changing and adding to the gut flora, and this may prevent food allergy development (see Chapters 1 and 30). Lactobacillus GG, a probiotic supplement, has been found to improve gastrointestinal microflora, thus reducing the incidence of atopic dermatitis and possibly food allergy (Schneider, 2002). Currently, it is suspected that by supplementing the pregnant woman 1 month before delivery, or providing the infant with 6 months' treatment of probiotic therapy either from the nursing mother or with direct supplementation that infant food allergy–related atopic eczema can be reduced (Rautava et al, 2002; Schneider, 2002; Vanderhoof, 2001).

Breast-feeding continues to be the infant's best nutrition and protection against food allergy disease, but it does not eliminate the risk of developing food allergies (Rautava, 2002). When possible, nursing the infant exclusively for the first 3 months should be encouraged. Even as little as 3 months of exclusive breast-feeding reduces the potentially atopic infant's risk of food allergy development (Gdalevich et al, 2001). If the mother chooses to nurse her infant, she

CLINICAL INSIGHT

Does "Pareve" Really Mean Milk Free?

For many years, milk-allergic persons have used the kosher designation "pareve" to mean that the food is milk free and therefore "safe."

Pareve products are considered milk free from a religious standpoint and meet Jewish Dietary Law requirements; however, from a food allergy standpoint, pareve may NOT be 100% milk free. Equipment that has been cleaned to the Kosher Dietary Law specifications may contain trace amounts of milk or trace contamination from airborne dust in a food plant. These trace amounts of milk in products labeled "pareve" do not violate religious law, and these products can still be labeled as such; however, these products could present a problem to a milk-allergic person. Kosher labeling does help identify products that do have milk, such as kosher dairy (D) and dairy equipment (DE), but relying on pareve-labeled products as 100% milk free is *not* recommended.

The Food Allergy Network no longer recommends relying on pareve-labeled products for milk-free diets (Regenstein, 1998).

Content developed by Leila Beker, PhD, RD.

Box 32-7. Reasons Why Allergens May Contaminate a Food

- Common serving utensils used to serve different foods
- Manufacture of two different food products using the same equipment, but without proper cleansing in between
- Misleading labels (e.g., nondairy creamers that contain sodium caseinate)
- Ingredients added for a specific purpose are listed on the label only in general terms of their purpose, rather than as a specific ingredient (e.g., egg white that is simply listed as an "emulsifier")
- Addition of an allergenic product to a second product that bears a label listing only the ingredients of the second product (e.g., mayonnaise, without noting eggs)
- Switching of ingredients by food manufacturers (e.g., a shortage of one vegetable oil prompting substitution with another)
- An ingredient that is present in a food, but in such a low percentage that it does not *have* to be listed on a label

Modified from Steinman HA: Hidden allergens in foods, *J Allergy Clin Immunol* 98:241, 1996.

TABLE 32-5 Nutritional Risk in Food Allergy Management

LEVEL OF RISK	FOOD CHARACTERISTICS/EXAMPLES
Low risk	Any food that can easily be eliminated with minimal or no nutritional risk to the patient **Example:** Avoidance of a specific fruit or vegetable
Moderate risk	Any food that may be encountered frequently throughout the food supply, yet whose elimination does not significantly limit food choices or vital nutrient sources **Example:** Avoidance of fish, crustaceans, and tree nuts
Complex risk	Any food that permeates the food supply, providing a significant source of specific nutrients that are not readily available through other foods that are a part of the normal diet, whose elimination results in a significant lifestyle and dietary change because of the difficulty of avoiding that food and products containing that food **Example:** Avoidance of wheat, soy, egg, milk, peanuts, or multiple foods

Modified from Burns-Ogle G, Doerr J, Martin B, editors: *Manual of medical nutrition therapy*, ed 3, Oklahoma City, 1996, Oklahoma Dietetic Association.

should be encouraged to not eat peanuts while nursing because of the increased risk of developing peanut allergy on the part of the infant (Sampson, 2002). Once food allergy has developed, the only treatment continues to be total avoidance of the food allergen and its protein sources (Joint Task Force on Practice Parameters, 1998; Sampson, 1999; Sicherer, 2001).

Hypersensitivity to foods is most common in the first 1 to 2 years of life, and most infants outgrow their sensitivities by the age of 3 years. Because symptoms of food allergy tend to resolve with age, nutrient-dense allergenic foods such as wheat, soy, eggs, and cow's milk should be reintroduced by food challenge every 6 to 12 months to ensure that they are not being restricted unnecessarily. After two to three negative open challenges, blind challenges may be useful in overcoming any bias that has developed. It should be noted that RAST or skin testing results for IgE sensitization may remain positive even after the food can be eaten without symptoms.

Box 32-8. Strategies for Coping With Food Allergy

Food Substitutions

Try to substitute item-for-item at meals. For example, if the family is eating ice cream for dessert, substitution of another type of frozen dessert may be better accepted than a dissimilar dessert, such as cookies.

Dining Out and Eating Away From Home

Eating meals away from home can be risky for individuals with food allergies. Whether at a fancy restaurant or a fast-food establishment, inadvertent exposure to an allergen can occur, even among the most knowledgeable individuals. Here are some precautions to take:

- Bring "safe" foods along to make eating out easier. For breakfast, bring along soy milk if others will be having cereal with milk.
- Alert the waitstaff to the potential severity of your food allergy or allergies.
- Question the waitstaff carefully about ingredients.
- Always carry medications.

Special Occasions

Call the host family in advance to determine what foods will be served. Offer to provide an acceptable dish that all can enjoy.

Grocery Shopping

Be informed about what foods are acceptable, and read labels carefully. Product ingredients change over time; continue to read the labels on foods, even if they were previously determined to be "safe" foods. Allow for the fact that shopping will take extra time.

Label Reading

New labeling legislation makes it easier for individuals with food allergies to identify certain potential allergens from the ingredient list on food labels. For example, when food manufacturers use protein hydrolysates or hydrolyzed vegetable protein, they must now specify the source of protein used (e.g., hydrolyzed soy or hydrolyzed corn). Although reactions to food colors or food dyes are rare, individuals who suspect an intolerance will find them listed separately on the food label, rather than categorized simply as "food color."

Substitutions in Cooking

Milk: Use soy or rice milk, or fruit juice in recipes calling for milk. Use soy or rice milk for milk replacement. Use a 1:1 replacement ratio. Infant formulas, such as Neocate, Neocate One Plus, Nutramigen, or Alimentum, can also be used.

Egg: In baking, achieve the emulsifying effect of one egg by combining 2 tbsp whole-wheat flour, ½ tsp oil, ½ tsp baking powder, and 2 tbsp milk, water, or fruit juice. Egg-free substitutes are also available (see Box 32-2).

Chocolate: Use carob powder, measure for measure, when substituting for cocoa. As a substitute for one square of chocolate, use 3 tbsp carob powder plus 2 tbsp milk, water, butter, or margarine.

Wheat: Wheat flour replacements and tips for cooking without wheat are available from many sources.

FOOD ALLERGY IN INFANCY

Cow's milk protein (CMP) is the most common single allergen for infants. Prevalence of this allergy is about 2.5% in the first 3 years of life (Hoffman et al, 1997).

Recent studies suggest that some cases of constipation among infants and children may be related to cow's milk allergy. Hypersensitivity and constipation may have an allergenic pathogenesis in this population (Iacono et al, 1998). When constipation free, 21 of 27 infants and 44 of 65 children were consuming a diet free of CMP. An estimated 18% of infants have gastroesophageal reflux disease (GERD), which also might be related to cow's milk allergy (Faubion et al, 1998).

Recommendations for Infant Feeding

Human milk, the infant's best source of nutrition and protection against atopic disease, is the preferred food for all infants (Rautava et al, 2002; Zeiger, 1999). When the use of human milk is not possible, extensively hydrolysated cow's milk formulas are preferred alternatives to standard cow's milk formulas (Halken et al, 2000; Oldaeus et al, 1999; Zeiger, 1999). If symptoms continue, an amino-based formula may be offered. The American Academy of Pediatrics recommends the use of human milk or casein or whey protein hydrolysates with peptides having a molecular weight of less than 1200 Daltons for infants with clinical symptoms of cow's milk or soy allergy (AAP, 1989). Commercially available casein protein hydrolysate formulas (Nutramigen, Pregestimil, and

Alimentum) that meet this criterion have been used routinely to feed infants who are allergic to cow's milk protein, and adverse reactions have only rarely been reported; however, some partially hydrolysate whey proteins contain larger peptides and are not acceptable alternatives for these infants (AAP, 1989; Halken et al, 2000; Oldaeus et al, 1999).

The use of goat's milk as an alternative to cow's milk is not recommended because of the potential cross-reactivity with β-lactoglobulin in cow's milk. In addition, goat's milk is deficient in several nutrients and has a high renal solute load. It is especially low in folic acid, containing about one tenth the level present in whole cow's milk or human milk. Infants receiving goat's milk instead of infant formula require supplements of iron, folacin, and vitamins A, C, and D. Goat's milk must be diluted to three-quarters strength, and carbohydrates must be added to decrease the renal solute load.

Sensitivity to breast milk has been reported. Allergens in the mother's diet, such as cow's milk, eggs, and peanuts, can pass into the breast milk and cause sensitization and then an allergic reaction in the exclusively breast fed infant (Frank et al, 1999; Järvinen et al, 1999; Wahn et al, 2001; Vadas et al, 2001). Sometimes the reaction does not occur until the allergenic food is actually eaten by the infant. Infants with atopic dermatitis should be evaluated for possible food allergies. If the infant is still nursing, the mother should be placed on a 2-week diet free of milk, eggs, peanut, and soy to see whether her infant's symptoms improve. Food challenges to each food will determine food symptom relationships. The mother eats a suspect food before nursing, and the infant is observed for symptoms. If a food is judged to yield a positive test result through challenge, that food is eliminated from the mother's diet until the infant is weaned. If the mother is willing, continued breast-feeding is preferred while the offending food allergen is removed from her diet until the infant is weaned. The nutritional adequacy of the mother's diet should be monitored when foods, especially cow's milk, are omitted from her diet. A calcium supplement with vitamin D can help meet the adequate intake (AI) for calcium and vitamin D during lactation (Isolauri et al, 1999) (see Chapter 7).

Foods in the mother's diet may also be associated with nonallergic reactions, usually gastrointestinal upset. Implicated foods include caffeinated beverages, chocolate, some herbal teas, cabbage, onions, turnips, garlic, radishes, rhubarb, spinach, and spices. Avoidance of the problem food by the mother may alleviate her infant's symptoms, which is preferable to discontinuing breast-feeding, but in some cases the infant may need to be weaned from the breast (Isolauri et al, 1999).

Colic

The association between colic and food allergy remains controversial; however, persistent colic may warrant trial of an elimination diet for the breast-feeding mother, or a trial of a fiber-enriched casein hydrolysate formula for the infant receiving cow's milk or soy formula, or trial of an amino acid–based formula such as Neocate.

DIET AND PREVENTION OF ALLERGIC DISEASE

Early feeding of foods other than breast milk is believed to contribute to the increase in food allergy development among infants (Zeiger, 1999). Breast-feeding, together with maternal avoidance of allergens, may delay the development of allergic disease in high-risk infants (Zeiger, 1999). Reduced exposure to allergenic foods during infancy has been associated with a decreased prevalence of food allergy during the first year and a delay in the onset of atopic dermatitis (Isolauri et al, 1999; Zeiger et al, 1999, 2000). Breast-feeding the infant is strongly encouraged, even if only for the first few days of life. Breast milk is always best, but an extensively hydrolysated casein formula or an amino acid–based formula can be used for infants at risk for atopic disease. When possible, the infant should be exclusively breast-fed for the first 6 months of life. A protein hydrolysate or amino acid–based formula can be used to supplement as necessary. Withholding highly allergenic foods, such as milk, eggs, peanuts, tree nuts, and fish from children at high risk for allergy for the first 2 to 3 years of life is recommended (Cantani and Gagliesi, 1996).

Oral Allergy Syndrome

Patients with pollen allergy may experience a rapid onset of pruritis (itch) or angioedema (swelling) involving the lips, tongue, throat, and palate within moments of eating fresh fruits or vegetables (Sampson, et al, 2001; Sicherer 2000). Adults experience oral allergy syndrome (OAS) more frequently than children (Spergel and Pawlowski, 2002). Symptom intensity varies with patients, and the symptoms usually are not life threatening but may precede anaphylactic reactions (Sloane and Sheffer 2001). The cooked fruit or vegetable is usually tolerated. The response is believed to be a cross-reaction between common pollen allergens and fresh fruits or vegetables (Sampson et al, 2001; Sicherer, 2000) Patients with birch pollinosis may experience OAS symptoms with apples, carrots, celery, potatoes, and hazelnuts; ragweed pollinosis with melons and bananas; and brazil nut allergy with cherry, apricot, plum, and peach (Burks, 1999; Spergel and Pawlowski, 2002).

Latex Allergy

Repeated exposure to latex is considered the most potent cause of latex allergy. A recent review concluded that the greatest risk factor for developing latex allergy is occupational exposure (Charous et al, 2002). Symptoms include contact dermatitis (type IV) and immediate allergic reactions (type I), as manifested by rhinitis, asthma, conjunctivitis, angioedema, urticaria, anaphylaxis, and death. The recommendation is to reduce latex glove use and thus reduce latex exposure by reducing latex aeroallergens in the air. Several medical facilities were measured for latex aeroallergen, and in those facilities that switched to either nonpowdered latex gloves or nonlatex gloves, there was a significant reduction in latex aeroallergen levels (Charous et al, 2002). Food handling by workers wearing latex gloves is a source of oral ingestion of latex molecules, and latex gloves should not be worn while preparing foods to reduce allergic and non–latex allergic exposures (Beezhold et al, 2000).

Cross-reactivity between latex and one or more foods is now estimated to be at least 50% (Yagami et al, 2000). It should also be noted that persons with latex allergy could also have food allergies because between 30% and 80% of latex-allergic persons have also been found to have a food allergy (Yunginger, 2001). Latex allergy may develop before food allergy, or food allergy may develop before latex allergy. Sometimes food allergy appears probable when actually latex has contaminated the food. Parts of sandwiches eaten by latex-sensitive patients were found to contain latex protein, probably from the food handler using latex gloves. Documented latex-induced anaphylaxis has been seen during childbirth, dental procedures, gynecologic examinations, and surgical procedures (Yunginger, 2001). When working with either the latex- or food-allergic patient, a careful history is critical. Research continues to try to define this cross-reactivity and to identify whether foods should be avoided and, if so, which ones. The most frequent related latex-fruit dual allergies are banana, avocado, chestnuts, and kiwi (Condemi, 2002) (Box 32-9).

Box 32-9. Foods Known to Cross-React in Latex Allergy

Apple	Grape	Plum
Apricot	Hazelnut	Potato
Avocado*	Kiwi*	Rye
Banana*	Mango	Shellfish
Carrot	Melon	Strawberry
Celery	Nectarine	Tomato
Cherry	Papaya	Wheat
Chestnut*	Passion fruit	
Coconut	Peach	
Fig	Pear	
Fish	Pineapple	

*Most frequent.

Genetic Engineering

Genetic engineering can transfer a protein from one plant to another (see Chapter 16). The potential benefits are many to the consumer and food producer. Plants can be made more insect and disease resistant and climate tolerant with improved taste, texture, and appearance. Once a protein has been transferred, the allergenicity potential must be evaluated. The evaluation should include the gene source, how closely the new protein resembles known allergens, and how persons with known allergy to the protein transferred might react, if exposed. In addition, the food industry must consider the effect the new protein has on the plant's growth, functions within the plant, and physiochemical properties such as heat and digestion stability. Current potential transfer proteins will probably come from known allergenic sources (Taylor et al, 2001). Further engineering may someday be available to reduce levels of specific antigens in the food supply.

SUMMARY

Adverse reactions to foods are associated with different physical response mechanisms. Allergy is just one of these mechanisms. It is important for the nutrition professional to understand the differences between these reactions and the appropriate treatments so that foods are not limited or omitted unnecessarily and nutrient deficiencies can be avoided.

Clinical Scenario I

Sally is 18 months old. At birth, she was unable to tolerate cow's milk–based formulas. Each feeding brought diarrhea and vomiting. The pediatrician recommended that her mother switch to a casein hydrolysate formula, which Sally tolerated well. Within 2 months she developed eczema that was treated with steroid creams. Cow's milk was introduced when Sally was 12 months of age. Skin symptoms increased remarkably. When eggs and later peanut butter were introduced, she experienced immediate wheezing, watery swelling eyes, hives, increased skin itch, and diarrhea. Sally's parents are unaware of how to look for egg or peanut sources; thus, Sally experienced several trips to the emergency room. The last reaction was much more intense. Her family physician suspects egg and peanut allergies and has sent her to see a board-certified allergist and a nutritionist.

1. How many food allergen suspects are there and what are they? Why?
2. What measures will her mother need to take if Sally is to lose sensitivity to any of the food allergens?
3. What other circumstances may arise that may warrant special instructions to caregivers?
4. How often should Sally be checked for sensitivity changes?
5. What would you tell Sally's parents to look for on food labels?
6. What nutrient substitutions must be considered?

Clinical Scenario 2

Mrs. L. was recently diagnosed with diabetes. She is coming to see you, the nutritionist, for a medical nutrition assessment/evaluation to assist her with the multiple nutrition changes she knows she will have to make. She wishes to continue nursing Levi, her 6-month-old son. In the process of doing a history, you learn that Levi has several problems, including severe eczema since birth. He has had episodes of turning bright red head to toe and clawing at his skin, followed by intense sneezing and coughing. Symptoms have occurred on 6 different days, 30 minutes after either his 2:00 PM or 6:00 PM feeding, except the last episode occurred after his 10:00 AM feeding. Each episode lasts 12 hours and then begins to resolve. His pediatrician instructed the parents to give Levi ¼ teaspoon of Triaminic cough syrup every 4 to 6 hours for 48 hours once symptoms begin. Mom says that this helps his cough a little, but it does not relieve the other symptoms. With the most recent episode, a family friend suggested that the parents give Benadryl to Levi. Skin and respiratory symptoms improved within the hour. Mrs. L. has no idea what causes these dramatic, frightening episodes.

1. Do you suspect food allergies? More than one?
2. What are the most likely food allergen suspects without knowing exactly what Mrs. L. ate before nursing?
3. Would you consider putting Mrs. L. on an elimination diet or switching Levi to infant formula?
4. How would you personalize an elimination diet without confusing the end results?
5. How would you help Mrs. L. integrate the eating plan for managing her diabetes with what you would recommend for her to do to solve Levi's problem?
6. What recommendations are you going to make to the infant's pediatrician?

Relevant Web Sites

Allergy and Asthma Network/Mothers of Asthmatics, Inc.
www.podi.com/health/aanma
Allergy to Latex Education and Resource Team, Inc.
www.execpc.com/~alert
American Academy of Allergy, Asthma, and Immunology
www.aaaai.org
American College of Allergy, Asthma, and Immunology
www.allergy.mcg.edu
The American Dietetic Association
www.eatright.org
The Asthma and Allergy Foundation of America
www.aafa.org
The Food Allergy and Anaphylaxis Network
www.foodallergy.org
International Food Information Council (IFIC) Foundation
www.ificinfo.health.org

Cited References

Altman D, Chiaramonte L: Clinical aspects of allergic disease, *J Allergy Clin Immunol* 97:1247, 1996.

American Academy of Allergy, Asthma, and Immunology: Position statement: controversial techniques, *J Allergy Clin Immunol* 67:333, 1981.

American Academy of Allergy, Asthma, and Immunology: Position statement on anaphylaxis in school and other childcare settings, *J Allergy Clin Immunol* 102:173, 1998.

Bahna SL: In vitro food allergy tests: the good, the bad and the worst. American College of Allergy, Asthma and Immunology, Sixtieth Annual Meeting, San Antonio, Tex, November 19, 2001.

Beezhold DH et al: Latex protein: a hidden "food" allergen? *Allergy Asthma Proc* 21:301, 2000.

Belen M et al: Severe food allergies by skin contact, *Ann Allergy Asthma Immunol* 86:583, 2001.

Bock S et al: Fatalities due to anaphylactic reactions to foods, *J Allergy Clin Immunol* 107:1, 2001.

Burks A: Childhood food allergy, *Immunol Allergy Clin North Am* 19:2, 1999.

Burks A et al: Atopic dermatitis and food hypersensitivity reactions, *J Pediatr* 132:132, 1998.

Cantani A, Gagliesi D: Severe reactions to cow's milk in very young infants at risk of atopy, *Allergy Asthma Proc* 17:205, 1996.

Charous BL et al: Natural rubber latex allergy after 12 years: recommendations and perspectives, *J Allergy Clin Immunol* 109:31, 2002.

Condemi J: Allergic reactions to natural rubber latex at home, to rubber products, and to cross-reacting foods, *J Allergy Clin Immunol* 110:S107, 2002.

DiCello M et al: Anaphylaxis after ingestion of carmine colored foods: two case reports and a review of the literature, *Allergy Asthma Proc* 20:377, 1999.

Eigenmann PA et al: Prevalence of IgE-mediated food allergy among children with atopic dermatitis, *Pediatrics* 101:8, 1998.

Faubion WA et al: Gastroesophageal reflux in infants and children, *Mayo Clin Proc* 73(2):166, 1998.

Frank et al: Exposure to peanuts in utero and in infancy and the development of sensitization to peanut allergens in young children, *Pediatr Allergy Immunol* 10:1, 1999.

Gdalevich M et al: Breast-feeding and the onset of atopic dermatitis in childhood: a systematic review and metaanalysis of prospective studies, *J Am Acad Dermatol* 45:520, 2001.

Geha R et al: Multicenter, double-blind, placebo-controlled, multiple-challenge evaluation of reported reactions to monosodium glutamate, *J Allergy Clin Immunol* 106:973, 2000.

Halken S et al: Comparison of a partially hydrolyzed infant formula with two extensively hydrolyzed formulas for allergy prevention: a prospective, randomized study, *Pediatr Allergy Immunol* 11:149, 2000.

Hawkins C, Katelaris C: Nitrate anaphylaxis, *Ann Allergy Asthma Immunol* 85:74, 2000.

Hoffman KM et al: Evaluation of the usefulness of lymphocyte proliferation assays in the diagnosis of allergy to cow's milk, *J Allergy Clin Immunol* 99:360, 1997.

Iacono G et al: Intolerance of cow's milk and chronic constipation in children, *N Engl J Med* 339:1100, 1998.

Isolauri E et al: Breast-feeding of allergic infants, *J Pediatr* 134:27, 1999.

Järvinen K-M et al: Cow's milk challenge through human milk evokes immune responses in infants with cow's milk allergy, *J Pediatr* 135:506, 1999.

Joint Task Force on Practice Parameters (JTFPP) representing the American Academy of Allergy, Asthma and Immunology; American College of Allergy, Asthma and Immunology; and the Joint Council of Allergy, Asthma and Immunology: The diagnosis and management of anaphylaxis, *J Allergy Clin Immunol* 101 (pt 2): S488, 1998.

Jones CA et al: Costimulatory molecules in the developing human gastrointestinal tract: a pathway for fetal allergen priming, *J Allergy Clin Immunol* 108:235, 2001.

Kalliomaki M et al: Distinct patterns of neonatal gut microflora ininfants in whom atopy was and was not developing, *J Allergy Clin Immunol* 107:129, 2001.
Kaplan BJ et al: Dietary replacement in preschool-aged hyperactive boys, *Pediatrics* 83:7, 1989.
Kay AB: Allergy and allergic diseases, Part 1, *N Engl J Med* 344:30, 2001.
Lester MR: Sulfate sensitivity: significance in human health, *J Am Coll Nutr* 14:229, 1995.
Oldaeus G et al: Cow's milk IgE and IgG antibody responses to cow's milk formulas, *Allergy* 54:352, 1999.
Papazian R: Sulfites: safe for most, dangerous for some, U.S. Food and Drug Administration, *FDA Consumer,* December 1996.
Raiten D et al: Executive summary from the report: analysis of adverse reactions to monosodium gutamate (MSG), *J Nutr* 125:2892S, 1995.
Rautava S: Probiotics during pregnancy and breast-feeding might confer immunomodulatory protection against atopic disease in the infant, *J Allergy Clin Immunol* 109:119, 2002.
Regenstein JM: Are "Pareve" products really milk-free? *Food Allergy News* 17(6):1, 1998.
Reus K et al: Food additives as a cause of medical symptoms: relationship shown between sulfites and asthma and anaphylaxis: results of a literature review, *Nederlans Tijdschrift voor Geneeskunde* 144:38, 2000.
Sampson H: Food allergy. Pt 2. Diagnosis and management, *J Allergy Clin Immunol* 103:6, 1999.
Sampson H: Peanut allergy, *N Engl J Med* 346:17, 2002.
Sampson H: Utility of food-specific IgE concentrations in predicting symptomatic food allergy, *J Allergy Clin Immunol* 107:5, 2001.
Sampson H et al: AGA technical review on the evaluation of food allergy in gastrointestinal disorders, *Gastroenterology* 120:4, 2001.
Schneider LC: New treatment for atopic dermatitis, *Immunol Allergy Clin North Am* 22(1):141, 2002.
Sicherer S: Determinants of systemic manifestations of food allergy, *J Allergy Clin Immunol* 106:5, 2000.
Sicherer S: Clinical implications of cross-reactive food allergens, *J Allergy Clin Immunol* 108:6, 2001.
Sicherer S: The genetics of food allergy, *Immunol Allergy Clin North Am* 22:2, 2002.
Simon RA: Sulfite challenge for the diagnosis of sensitivity, *Allergy Proc* 10:357, 1989.
Sloane D, Sheffer A: Oral allergy syndrome, *Allergy Asthma Proc* 22:5, 2001.
Spergel J, Pawlowski N: Food allergy: mechanisms, diagnosis and management in children, *Pediatr Clin North Am* 49:1, 2002.
Steinman HA: Hidden allergens in foods, *J Allergy Clin Immunol* 98:241, 1996.
Taylor SL: Forty-Eighth Annual Meeting of the American Academy of Allergy and Immunology, *Food Safety Note* 3:13, 1992.
Taylor SL et al: Factors affecting the determination of threshold doses for allergenic foods: how much is too much? *J Allergy Clin Immunol* 109:24, 2002.
Taylor SL et al: Food allergies and avoidance diets, *Nutr Today* 34 (1):15, 1999.
Taylor SL et al: Will genetically modified foods be allergenic? *J Allergy Clin Immunol* 107:765, 2001.
Vadas P et al: Detection of peanut allergens in breast milk of lactating women, *JAMA* 285:13, 1746, 2001.
Vanderhoof J: Probiotics in primary prevention of atopic disease: a randomized placebo-controlled trial, *J Pediatr* 139:5, 2001.
Vilke GM: Food-dependent exercise-induced anaphylaxis, *Prehosp Emerg Care* 6(3):348, 2002.
Wahn U, Von Mutius E: Current reviews of allergy and clinical immunology, *J Allergy Clin Immunol* 107:4, 2001.
Yagami T et al: Digestibility of allergens extracted from natural rubber latex and vegetable foods, *J Allergy Clin Immunol* 106:752, 2000.
Yunginger JW: Latex-associated anaphylaxis, *Immunol Allergy Clin North Am* 21(4):669, 2001.
Zeiger R: Dietary aspects of food allergy prevention in infants and children, *J Pediatr Gastroenterol Nutr* 30(suppl):S77, 2000.
Zeiger R: Prevention of food allergy in infants and children, *Immunol Allergy Clin North Am* 19:3, 1999.
Zeiger RS, Schatz M: Effect of allergist intervention on patient-centered and societal outcomes: allergists as leaders, innovators, and educators, *J Allergy Clin Immunol* 106:995, 2000.

Additional References

Clinical management of latex allergy, *Nutr Clin Pract* 12:68, 1997.
Grote M et al: In situ localization of a high molecular weight cross-reactive allergen in pollen and plant-derived food by immunogold electron microscopy, *J Allergy Clin Immunol* 101:250, 1998.
Katsunama T et al: Wheat-dependent exercise-induced anaphylaxis: inhibition by sodium bicarbonate, *Am Allergy* 68:184, 1992.
Long A: The nuts and bolts of peanut allergy, *N Engl J Med.* 346:17, 2002.
Munoz-Furlong A: The food allergy network, *Top Clin Nutr* 9 (3):38, 1994.
Nordlee J et al: Identification of a brazil-nut allergen in transgenic soybeans, *N Engl J Med* 334:688, 1996.
Parker S et al: Foods perceived by adults as causing adverse reactions, *J Am Diet Assoc* 93:40, 1993.
Poley G et al: Latex allergy, *J Allergy Clin Immunol* 105:6, 2000.
Roesler TA et al: Factitious food allergy and failure to thrive, *Arch Pediatr Adolesc Med* 148:1150, 1994.
Sicherer S et al: The impact of childhood food allergy on quality of life, *Ann Allergy Asthma Immunol* 87:461, 2001.
Sussman G, Gold M: Guidelines for the management of latex allergies and safe latex use in health care facilities, Arlington Heights, Ill: American College of Allergy, Asthma, and Immunology, March 1996, www.allergy.meg.edu.
Vanderhoof JA: Intolerance to protein hydrolysate infant formulas: an underrecognized cause of gastrointestinal symptoms in infants, *J Pediatr* 131:741, 1997.

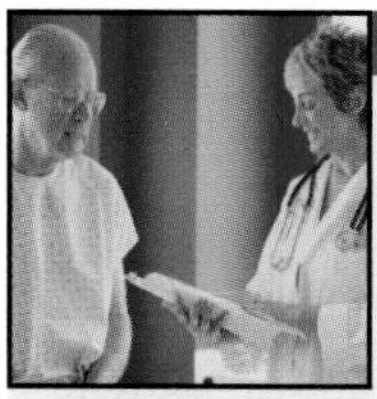

CHAPTER 33

Medical Nutrition Therapy for Diabetes Mellitus and Hypoglycemia of Nondiabetic Origin

MARION J. FRANZ, MS, RD, LD, CDE

CHAPTER OUTLINE

- Pathophysiology
- Diagnostic and Screening Criteria
- Management of Diabetes Mellitus
- Diabetes and Age-Related Issues
- Implementing Nutrition Self-Management
- Acute Complications
- Long-Term Complications
- Preventing Diabetes
- Hypoglycemia of Nondiabetic Origin

KEY TERMS

autonomic symptoms–symptoms of hypoglycemia that are adrenergically based and that arise from the action of the autonomic nervous system

combination therapy–a form of therapy for diabetes using combinations of oral medications or a combination of oral medication(s) and insulin injection(s)

counterregulatory (stress) hormones–hormones, including glucagon, epinephrine (adrenaline), norepinephrine, cortisol, and growth hormone, released during stressful situations, which have the opposite effect of insulin and cause the liver to release glucose from stored glycogen (glycogenolysis) and the adipose cells to release fatty acids for extra energy (lipolysis); these hormones counterbalance declining glucose levels

dawn phenomenon–a natural increase in morning blood glucose levels and insulin requirements that occurs in people with and without diabetes but tends to be more marked in people with diabetes; possibly caused by a diurnal variation in growth hormone, cortisol, or catecholamines

Diabetes Control and Complications Trial (DCCT)–a 10-year study in people with type 1 diabetes who were treated with either conventional therapy or intensive therapy; follow-up evaluations proved that tight blood glucose control reduces the risk of diabetic microvascular complications

diabetic ketoacidosis (DKA)–severe, uncontrolled diabetes, resulting from insufficient insulin, in which ketone bodies (acids) build up in the blood; if left untreated (with immediate administration of insulin and fluids), DKA can lead to coma and even death

fasting (food-deprived) hypoglycemia–low blood glucose concentrations in response to no food intake for 8 hours or longer

gestational diabetes mellitus (GDM)–glucose intolerance, the onset or first recognition of which occurs during pregnancy

glucagon–a hormone produced by the α-cells of the pancreas that causes an increase in blood glucose levels by stimulating the release of glucose from liver glycogen stores

glucotoxicity–pancreatic beta cells chronically exposed to hyperglycemia become progressively less efficient in responding to a glucose challenge

glycosylated hemoglobin–a blood test that reflects the blood glucose concentration over the life span of red blood cells (~120 days), expressed as a percentage of total hemoglobin with glucose attached; may also be called glycated hemoglobin or glycohemoglobin. Hemoglobin A1 (HbA1) is an evaluation of a combination of all fractions of the hemoglobin molecule. Hemoglobin A1c (HbA1c) is a measurement of the glycosylation of the "c" fraction and is the recommended assay method (simplified to A1c). An A1c of 6.0% reflects an average plasma glucose level of ~120 mg/dl. In general, each 1% increase in A1c is a reflection of an increase in average glucose levels of ~30 mg/dl

honeymoon phase–the period after the initial diagnosis of type 1 diabetes when there may be some recovery of β-cell function and a temporary decrease in exogenous insulin requirement

hyperglycemia–an excessive amount of glucose in the blood (generally ≥180 mg/dl or above) caused by too little insulin, insulin resistance, or increased food intake; symptoms include frequent urination, increased thirst, weight loss, and often tiredness or fatigue

hyperglycemic hyperosmolar state (HHS)–extremely high blood glucose levels with an absence of or only slight ketosis and profound dehydration

hypoglycemia (or insulin reaction)–low blood glucose level (usually ≤70 mg/dl), which can be caused by the administration of excessive insulin or insulin secretagogues, too little food, delayed or missed meals or snacks, increased amounts of exercise or other physical activity, or alcohol intake without food

hypoglycemia of nondiabetic origin–low levels of blood glucose that lead to neuroglycopenia symptoms that are ameliorated by the ingestion of carbohydrate

immune-mediated diabetes mellitus–a form of type 1 diabetes resulting from autoimmune destruction of the β-cells of the pancreas

impaired glucose homeostasis–metabolic stages of impaired glucose use (between normal glucose concentrations and diabetes), which are risk factors for future diabetes and cardiovascular disease

insulin–a hormone released from the β-cells of the pancreas that enables cells to metabolize and store glucose and other fuels

insulin resistance–an impaired biologic response (sensitivity) to either exogenous or endogenous insulin; insulin resistance and insulin deficiencies are involved in the etiology of type 2 diabetes

insulin secretagogues–oral medications that stimulate insulin release from the β-cell of the pancreas, such as sulfonylureas and nonsulfonylurea secretagogues (i.e., repaglinide and nateglinide)

insulin sensitizers–oral medications that enhance insulin action and include biguanides (metformin) and thiazolidinediones

macrovascular diseases–diseases of the large blood vessels, including coronary artery disease, cardiovascular disease, and peripheral vascular disease

metabolic syndrome–characterized by central obesity and insulin resistance with increased risk for cardiovascular disease and type 2 diabetes; associated risk factors include dyslipidemia (elevated triglycerides, low high-density lipoprotein [HDL] cholesterol, and high low-density lipoprotein [LDL] cholesterol), hypertension, prothrombotic factors, and impaired glucose tolerance

microvascular diseases–diseases of the small blood vessels, including retinopathy and nephropathy

neuroglycopenic symptoms–neurologic symptoms of hypoglycemia that are related to an insufficient supply of glucose to the brain

oral glucose-lowering medications–drugs, administered orally, that are used to control or lower blood glucose levels, including first- and second-generation sulfonylureas, nonsulfonylureas, secretagogues, biguanides, α-glucosidase inhibitors, and thiazolidinediones

polydipsia–excessive thirst

polyuria–excessive urination

postprandial (after a meal) blood glucose–blood glucose level 1 to 2 hours after eating

postprandial (reactive) hypoglycemia–low blood glucose within 2 to 5 hours after eating

pre-diabetes–blood glucose concentrations that are higher than normal but not yet high enough to be diagnosed as diabetes; sometimes referred to as impaired glucose tolerance (IGT) or impaired fasting glucose (IFG), depending on which test was used to detect it

preprandial (fasting) blood glucose–blood glucose level before eating

self-monitoring of blood glucose (SMBG)–a method whereby individuals can test their own blood glucose levels using a chemically treated strip and visually comparing the strip to a color chart or by inserting the strip into a meter that measures the glucose level; most blood glucose meters automatically convert capillary whole blood glucose values to plasma glucose values

Somogyi (rebound) effect–an episode of hypoglycemia usually caused by excessive exogenous insulin, which stimulates the overproduction of counterregulatory hormones, resulting in an excessive release of glucose from the liver and hyperglycemia; often caused by inappropriate evening insulin doses; evening insulin doses should not be increased in an attempt to improve glucose levels

target blood glucose goals–levels for capillary blood glucose tests that are as near normal as possible and that can be achieved without risk of serious hypoglycemia

type 1 diabetes–a type of diabetes that usually occurs in persons younger than 30 years of age but can occur at any age; previously known as insulin-dependent diabetes mellitus (IDDM) or juvenile-onset diabetes

type 2 diabetes–a type of diabetes usually occurring in persons older than 30 years of age, previously known as non–insulin-dependent diabetes mellitus (NIDDM) or maturity-onset diabetes; now also frequently diagnosed in youth and young adults; formerly called *maturity onset diabetes of youth (MODY)*

KEY TERMS—Continued

United Kingdom Prospective Diabetes Study (UKPDS)–a 20-year multicenter trial in the United Kingdom of subjects with type 2 diabetes who were randomized into intensive therapy or conventional therapy; lowering of A1c and aggressive treatment of hypertension significantly reduced the development of microvascular complications and lowered the risk for macrovascular complications

Whipple's triad–a triad of clinical features that includes (1) low blood glucose levels, (2) accompanied by symptoms, which are (3) relieved by administration of glucose

Diabetes mellitus is a group of diseases characterized by high blood glucose concentrations resulting from defects in insulin secretion, insulin action, or both. Abnormalities in the metabolism of carbohydrate, protein, and fat are also present. Persons with diabetes have bodies that do not produce or respond to insulin, a hormone produced by the β-cells of the pancreas that is necessary for the use or storage of body fuels. Without effective insulin, hyperglycemia (elevated blood glucose) occurs, which can lead to both the short-term and long-term complications of diabetes mellitus.

In 2000, about 15 million U.S. adults 18 years of age or older had diagnosed diabetes (6.3 million men and 8.7 million women), representing an increase from 4.9% of the adult population in 1990 to 7.3% in 2000. If undiagnosed diabetes is considered as well, it is likely that almost 10% of U.S. adults have diabetes (Mokdad et al, 2001). Much of the increase is because type 2 diabetes is no longer a disease that affects mainly older adults. Between 1990 and 1998, the prevalence of diabetes increased by 76% among people in their thirties (Mokdad et al, 2001). Among children with newly diagnosed diabetes, the prevalence of type 2 diabetes also increased dramatically in the past decade, growing from less than 4% in the years preceding 1990 to as high as 45% in certain racial/ethnic groups in recent years (American Diabetes Association [ADA], 2000).

Diabetes prevalence increases with increasing age, affecting 18.4% of those 65 years of age or older (ADA, 2001). Diabetes is particularly prevalent in minorities; indeed, the prevalence of type 2 diabetes is highest in ethnic minorities in the United States, such as African Americans, Hispanic populations (Latinos and Mexican Americans), Native Americans and Alaska Natives, Asian Americans, and Pacific Islanders (see *Focus on:* Diabetes Does Discriminate!).

Of great concern are the more than 20 million adults reported to have impaired glucose tolerance (IGT) (2-hour postchallenge glucose of 140-199 mg/dl), the 13 to 14 million with impaired fasting glucose (IFG) (fasting plasma glucose 110-125 mg/dl), and the 40 to 50 million with metabolic syndrome (ADA, 2001). Persons with IGT or IFG are now classified as having pre-diabetes, and they are at high risk for conversion to type 2 diabetes if lifestyle prevention strategies are not used and are at higher risk of cardiovascular disease compared with persons with normal blood glucose concentrations.

Diabetes mellitus contributes to a considerable increase in morbidity and mortality rates, which can be reduced by early diagnosis and treatment. In 2002 diabetes costs in the United States were $132 billion. Direct medical expenditures, such as inpatient care, outpatient services, and nursing home care, totaled $91.8 billion. Indirect costs, totaling $39.8 billion, were associated with lost productivity, including premature death and disability. Total medical expenditures incurred by people with diabetes totaled $91.8 billion, or an average annual total direct cost of medical care of $13,243 per person compared with $2560 per person without diabetes (ADA, 2003a).

PATHOPHYSIOLOGY

In 1997 new recommendations for the classification and diagnosis of diabetes mellitus were accepted and supported by the ADA, the National Institute of Diabetes and Digestive and Kidney Diseases (NIDDKD), and the Centers for Disease Control and Prevention, Division of Diabetes Translation. Recommendations were also made to eliminate the terms *insulin-dependent diabetes mellitus (IDDM)* and *non–insulin-dependent diabetes mellitus (NIDDM)* and to keep the terms *type 1* and *type 2* diabetes but to use Arabic rather than Roman numerals (Expert Committee on the Diagnosis and Classification of Diabetes Mellitus, 1997) (Table 33-1).

Type 1 Diabetes

At diagnosis, people with type 1 diabetes are usually lean and are experiencing excessive thirst, frequent urination, and significant weight loss. The primary defect is pancreatic β-cell destruction, usually leading to absolute insulin deficiency and resulting in hyperglycemia, polyuria (excessive urination), polydipsia (excessive thirst), weight loss, dehydration, electrolyte disturbance, and ketoacidosis. The rate of β-cell destruction is quite variable, proceeding rapidly in some persons (mainly infants and children) and slowly in others (mainly adults). The capacity of a healthy pancreas to secrete insulin is far in excess of what is needed normally; therefore, the clinical onset

FOCUS ON

Diabetes Does Discriminate!

Diabetes strikes particularly hard at minorities. Certain environmental or lifestyle factors may increase the risk of developing type 2 diabetes in susceptible populations. For example, an increase in the prevalence is observed in populations who have migrated to more urbanized locations compared with people of the same group who remained in their traditional home. Urbanization is usually related to major changes in diet, physical activity, and socioeconomic status as well as increased obesity.

One theory that might explain the increased prevalence of diabetes and insulin resistance among Native people is the "thrifty" gene. Years of subsistence living have created a thrifty genotype that allows Native people to extract a lot of energy and fat from small amounts of food. In an era of store-bought processed food, that gene backfires to induce obesity and diabetes. Adoption of a "Western" lifestyle (which may include a diet high in fat and a sedentary way of life) has been associated with a dramatically increased rate of type 2 diabetes in the Pima Indians of Arizona (ADA, 2001). Among the Pima Indians of Arizona, about 55% of adults older than 35 years of age have type 2 diabetes. This disease is increasingly being diagnosed in Native Americans younger than 30 years of age and has been diagnosed in some as young as 7 years of age.

Ravussin and colleagues (1994) surveyed a closely related population of Pima Indians living in Maycoba, a small village in a remote, mountainous region of northwestern Mexico. They found that individuals in this community ate a diet lower in fat than is typically consumed in Arizona, and both men and women were very physically active. The men and women of Maycoba weighed, on average, 50 lb less than a comparable group of Pimas from the Phoenix area. More important, diabetes was diagnosed in about 10% of the Maycoba Pimas compared with almost 50% of the Arizona Pimas.

The main staples of the Maycoba Pimas' diet are beans, corn (as tortillas), and potatoes. Several essential nutrients are lacking because of the relative absence of fruits and vegetables. Diet analysis reveals a diet composed of 13% protein, 23% fat, 63% carbohydrate, and less than 1% alcohol and containing more than 50 g of fiber. This is in sharp contrast to the present diet of the Arizona Pimas. Even more striking than the low-fat diet of the Maycoba population, however, was the high level of physical activity in this population; more than 40 hours a week were spent engaged in hard physical work (Ravussin et al, 1994).

Interventions involving increased physical activity and a reduced fat and energy diet slowed the progression to type 2 diabetes in high-risk populations (Diabetes Prevention Program Research Group, 2002). Health promotion activities through community-based exercise programs and a return to more traditional diets also may help to reduce the diabetes epidemic that affects many developing countries as well as the underprivileged in industrialized nations.

TABLE 33-1 Types of Diabetes and Prediabetes

CLASSIFICATIONS	DISTINGUISHING CHARACTERISTICS
Type 1 diabetes	Affected persons are usually lean, have abrupt onset of symptoms before the age of 30 yr (although it may occur at any age), and are dependent on exogenous insulin to prevent ketoacidosis and death.
Type 2 diabetes	Affected persons are often older than 30 yr at diagnosis, although it is now occurring frequently in young adults and children. Individuals are not dependent on exogenous insulin for survival; they may require it for adequate glycemic control.
Gestational diabetes mellitus (GDM)	A condition of glucose intolerance affecting pregnant women, the onset or discovery of which occurs during pregnancy.
Other specific types	Diabetes that results from specific genetic syndromes, surgery, drugs, malnutrition, infections, or other illnesses.
Pre-diabetes or impaired glucose homeostasis	Metabolic stage of impaired fasting glucose (IFG) or impaired glucose tolerance (IGT) that is between current definitions of normal glucose values and diabetes.

Modified from Report of the Expert Committee on the Diagnosis and Classification of Diabetes Mellitus, *Diabetes Care* 20:1183, 1997.

of diabetes may be preceded by an extensive asymptomatic period of months to years, during which β-cells are undergoing gradual destruction (Figure 33-1).

Type 1 diabetes accounts for 5% to 10% of all diagnosed cases of diabetes. Persons with type 1 diabetes are dependent on exogenous insulin to prevent ketoacidosis and death. Although it may occur at any age, even in the eighth and ninth decades of life, most cases are diagnosed in people younger than 30 years of age, with a peak incidence at around ages 10 to 12 years in girls and ages 12 to 14 years in boys.

Type 1 diabetes has two forms: immune-mediated diabetes mellitus and idiopathic diabetes mellitus. Immune-mediated diabetes mellitus results from an autoimmune destruction of the β-cells of the pancreas. *Idiopathic type 1 diabetes mellitus* refers to forms of the disease that have no known etiology. Although

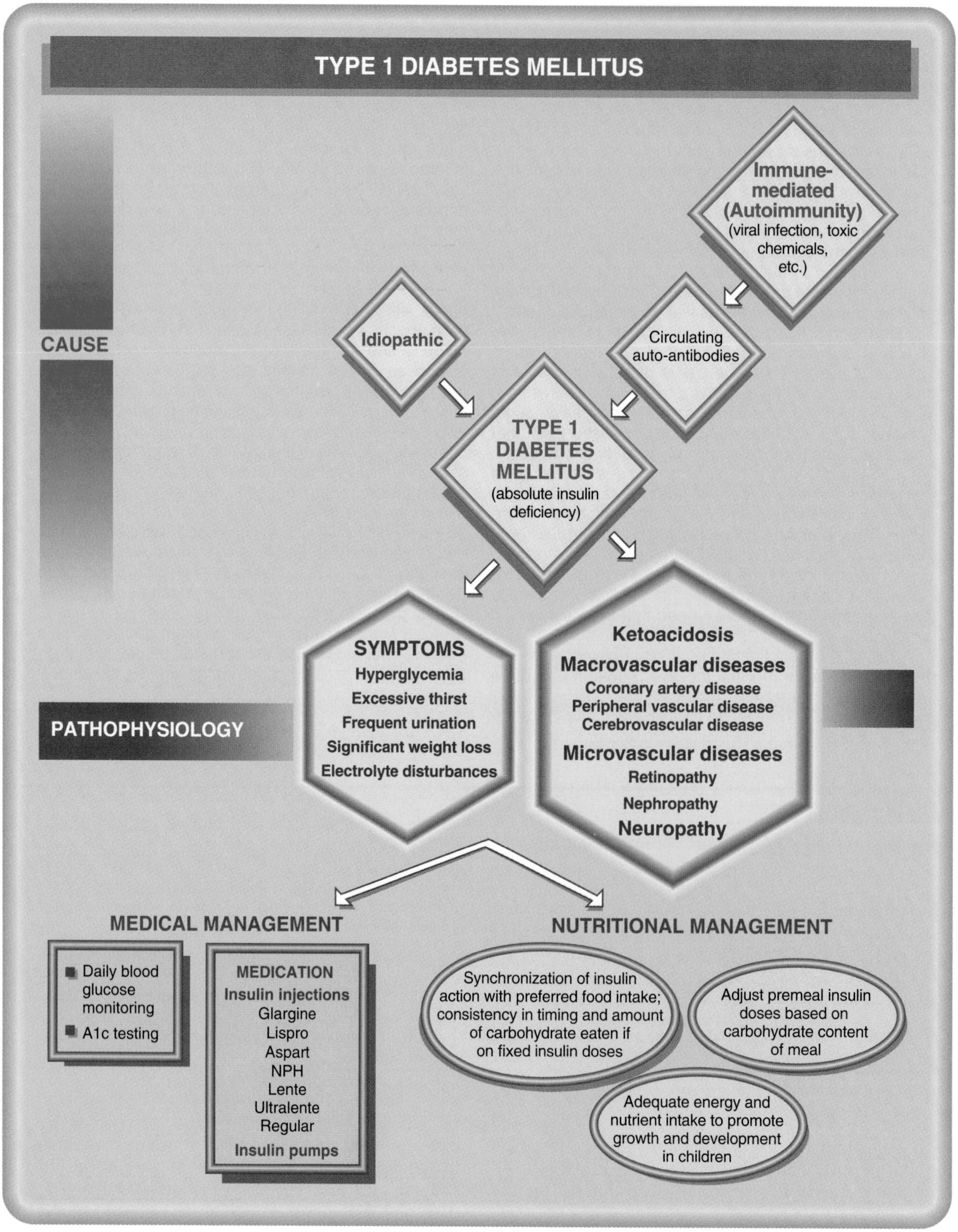

FIGURE 33-1 • Pathophysiology algorithm: type 1 diabetes mellitus. (Algorithm content developed by John Anderson, PhD, and Sanford C. Garner, PhD, 2000. Updated by Marion J. Franz, MS, RD, LD, CDE, 2002.)

only a minority of persons with type 1 diabetes fall into this category, of those who do, most are of African or Asian origin (Expert Committee on the Diagnosis and Classification of Diabetes Mellitus, 1997).

The etiology of immune-mediated diabetes involves a genetic predisposition and an autoimmune destruction of the islet β-cells that produce insulin. Genetic factors involve the association between type 1 diabetes and certain histocompatibility locus antigens (HLA), with linkage to the *DQA* and *DQB* genes and influenced by the *DRB* genes. These HLA-DR/DQ alleles can be either predisposing or protective (Expert Committee on the Diagnosis and Classification of Diabetes Mellitus, 1997).

At diagnosis, 85% to 90% of patients with type 1 diabetes have one or more circulating autoantibodies to islet cells, endogenous insulin, or other antigens that are constituents of islet cells. Antibodies identified as contributing to the destruction of β-cells are (1) islet cell autoantibodies (ICAs); (2) insulin autoantibodies (IAAs), which may occur in persons who have never received insulin therapy; and (3) autoantibodies to glutamic acid decarboxylase (GAD), a protein on the surface of β-cells. GAD autoantibodies appear to provoke an attack by the T cells (killer T lymphocytes), which may be what destroys the β-cells in diabetes.

Frequently, after diagnosis and the correction of hyperglycemia, metabolic acidosis, and ketoacidosis, endogenous insulin secretion recovers. During this honeymoon phase, exogenous insulin requirements decrease dramatically for up to 1 year; however, the need for increasing exogenous insulin replacement is inevitable, and within 8 to 10 years after clinical onset, β-cell loss is complete and insulin deficiency is absolute.

Type 2 Diabetes

Type 2 diabetes may account for 90% to 95% of all diagnosed cases of diabetes and is a progressive disease that, in many cases, is present long before it is diagnosed. Hyperglycemia develops gradually and is often not severe enough in the early states for the patient to notice any of the classic symptoms of diabetes. Although undiagnosed, these individuals are at increased risk of developing macrovascular and microvascular complications.

Risk factors for type 2 diabetes include genetic and environmental factors, including a family history of diabetes, older age, obesity, particularly intraabdominal obesity, physical inactivity, a prior history of gestational diabetes, impaired glucose homeostasis, and race or ethnicity. Total adiposity and a longer duration of obesity are established risks factors for type 2 diabetes. Nevertheless, type 2 diabetes is found in persons who are not obese, and many obese persons never develop type 2 diabetes. Obesity combined with a genetic predisposition may be necessary for type 2 diabetes to occur. Another possibility is that a similar genetic predisposition leads independently to both obesity and insulin resistance, which increases the risk for type 2 diabetes (ADA, 2001) (Figure 33-2).

In most cases, type 2 diabetes results from a combination of insulin resistance and β-cell failure, but the extent to which each of these factors contributes to the development of the disease is unclear (Ferrannini, 1998). Endogenous insulin levels may be normal, depressed, or elevated, but they are inadequate to overcome concomitant insulin resistance (decreased tissue sensitivity or responsiveness to insulin); as a result, hyperglycemia ensues. Insulin resistance is first demonstrated in target tissues, mainly muscle and the liver. Initially, there is a compensatory increase in insulin secretion, which maintains normal glucose concentrations, but as the disease progresses, insulin production gradually decreases. Hyperglycemia is first exhibited as an elevation of postprandial (after a meal) blood glucose caused by insulin resistance at the cellular level and is followed by an elevation in fasting glucose concentrations. As insulin secretion decreases, hepatic glucose production increases, causing the increase in preprandial (fasting) blood glucose levels. Compounding the problem is the deleterious effect of hyperglycemia itself—glucotoxicity—on both insulin sensitivity and insulin secretion (Yki-Jarvinen, 1997), hence the importance of achieving near-euglycemia in persons with type 2 diabetes.

Insulin resistance is also demonstrated at the adipocyte level, leading to lipolysis and an elevation in circulating free fatty acids. Increased fatty acids cause a further decrease in insulin sensitivity at the cellular level, impair pancreatic insulin secretion, and augment hepatic glucose production *(lipotoxicity)* (Bergman and Adler, 2000). The above defects contribute to the development and progression of type 2 diabetes and are also primary targets for pharmacologic therapy.

Persons with type 2 diabetes may or may not experience the classic symptoms of uncontrolled diabetes, and they are not prone to develop ketoacidosis. Although persons with type 2 diabetes do not require exogenous insulin for survival, about 40% or more will eventually require exogenous insulin for adequate blood glucose control. Insulin may also be required for control during periods of stress-induced hyperglycemia, such as during illness or surgery.

Gestational Diabetes Mellitus

Gestational diabetes mellitus (GDM) is defined as any degree of glucose intolerance with onset or first recognition during pregnancy. It occurs in about 7% of all pregnancies, resulting in more than 200,000 cases annually (ADA, 2001). Women with known diabetes mellitus before pregnancy are not classified as having GDM. GDM is usually diagnosed during the second or third trimester of pregnancy. At this point, insulin-antagonist hormone levels increase, and insulin resistance normally occurs.

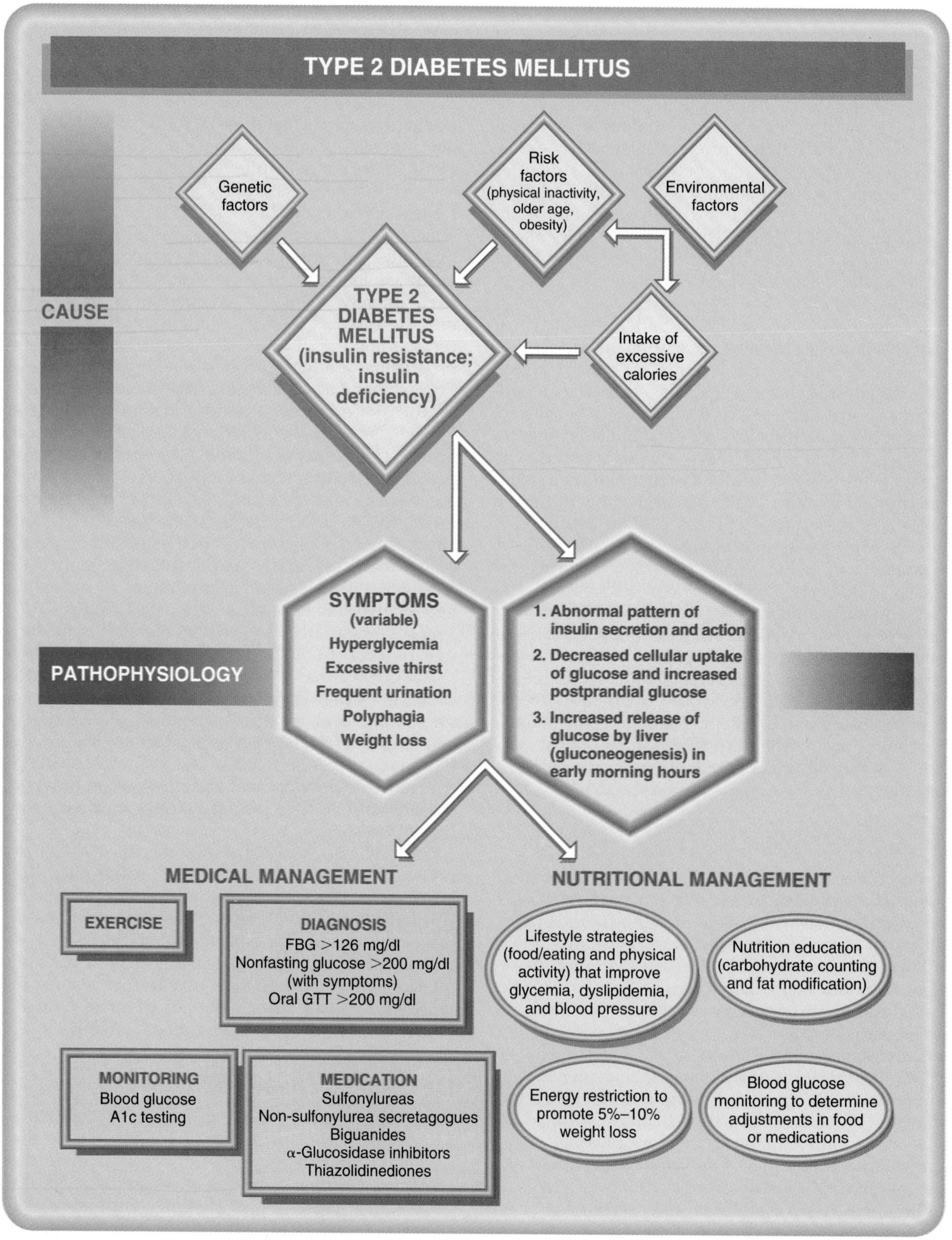

FIGURE 33-2 • Pathophysiology algorithm: type 2 diabetes mellitus. (Algorithm content developed by John Anderson, PhD, and Sanford C. Garner, PhD, 2000. Updated by Marion J. Franz, MS, RD, LD, CDE, 2002.)

Other Types of Diabetes

This category includes diabetes associated with specific genetic syndromes, surgery, drugs, malnutrition, infections, and other illnesses. Such types of diabetes may account for 1% to 2% of all diagnosed cases of diabetes.

Impaired Glucose Homeostasis

A stage of impaired glucose homeostasis includes IFG and IGT and is called pre-diabetes. This condition can be detected by either a fasting plasma glucose (FPG) test or an oral glucose tolerance (OGT) test. Individuals with pre-diabetes are at high risk for future diabetes and cardiovascular disease.

DIAGNOSTIC AND SCREENING CRITERIA

Diagnostic criteria for diabetes are summarized in Table 33-2. Three diagnostic methods may be used to diagnose diabetes; however, because of the ease, acceptability to the patient, and the cost, the FPG test is recommended (ADA, 2002a). At this time, hemoglobin A1c (A1C), is not recommended for diagnosis. In pregnant women, different criteria are applied in establishing the diagnosis of gestational diabetes. One of the following three tests can be used to diagnose diabetes but must be confirmed on a subsequent day:

- An FPG value equal to or greater than 126 mg/dl
- Symptoms of diabetes and a nonfasting plasma glucose (casual) value of greater than or equal to 200 mg/dl. *Casual* refers to any time of the day, without regard to the elapsed time since one's last meal. Symptoms of diabetes include the classic ones of polyuria, polydipsia, and unexplained weight loss.
- A 2-hour postprandial glucose equal to or greater than 200 mg/dl during an OGT test involving administration of 75 g of glucose

Testing or screening for diabetes should be considered in all patients 45 years of age and older; if normal, the test should be repeated at 3-year intervals. Testing should be considered at a younger age or be carried out more frequently in patients who:

- Have a family history of diabetes (i.e., parents or siblings with diabetes)
- Are overweight with a body mass index (BMI) ≥25 kg/m^2
- Are members of a high-risk ethnic population (e.g., African Americans, Hispanic Americans, Native Americans, Asian Americans, and Pacific Islanders)

TABLE 33-2 Diagnosis of Diabetes Mellitus and Impaired Glucose Homeostasis

DIAGNOSIS	CRITERIA
Diabetes	FPG ≥126 mg/dl (≥7.0 mmol/L) CPG ≥200 mg/dl (≥11.1 mmol/L) plus symptoms 2hPG ≥200 mg/dl (≥11.1 mmol/L)
Impaired glucose homeostasis	
Impaired fasting glucose	FPG ≥110 and <126 mg/dl (≥6.1 and <7.0 mmol/L)
Impaired glucose tolerance	2hPG ≥140 and <200 mg/dl (≥7.8 and <11.1 mmol/L)
Normal	FPG <110 mg/dl (<6.1 mmol/L) 2hPG <140 mg/dl (<7.8 mmol/L)

Modified from Expert Committee on the Diagnosis and Classification of Diabetes Mellitus: Report of the Expert Committee on the Diagnosis and Classification of Diabetes Mellitus, *Diabetes Care* 20:1183, 1997.

FPG, Fasting plasma glucose (preferred testing method); *CPG,* casual plasma glucose; *2hPG,* 2-hour plasma glucose level (measured 2 hours after an oral glucose tolerance test with administration of 75 g of glucose).

- Are women who have a history of GDM or a history of having infants weighing more than 9 lb at birth
- Are hypertensive (blood pressure ≥140/90 mm Hg)
- Have a high-density lipoprotein (HDL) cholesterol level ≤35 mg/dl or a triglyceride level ≥250 mg/dl
- Had IGT or IFG on previous testing
- Have polycystic ovary syndrome

The incidence of type 2 diabetes in children and adolescents is increasing dramatically and is consistent with screening recommendations for adults: children and youth at increased risk for type 2 diabetes should be tested. Youth who are overweight (body mass index [BMI] >85th percentile for age and sex) and who have two of the following risk factors should be screened: family history of type 2 diabetes, members of high-risk ethnic populations, signs of insulin resistance (such as acanthosis nigricans—gray-brown skin pigmentations). The age of initiation of screening is age 10 years or onset of puberty, and the frequency is every 2 years (ADA, 2002a).

Screening and diagnosis for GDM is discussed under Gestational Diabetes Mellitus in the Pregnancy section.

MANAGEMENT OF DIABETES MELLITUS

Optimal control of diabetes requires the restoration of normal carbohydrate, protein, and fat metabolism. Insulin is both anticatabolic and anabolic and facilitates cellular transport (Table 33-3). In general, the counterregulatory (stress) hormones (glucagon, growth hormone, cortisol, epinephrine, and norepinephrine) have the opposite effect of insulin.

Diabetes is a chronic disease that requires changes for a lifetime. The management of diabetes includes medical nutrition therapy (MNT), physical activity, blood glucose monitoring, medications, and self-management education. An important goal of treatment is to provide the patient with the necessary tools to achieve the best possible control of glycemia, lipidemia, and blood pressure to prevent, delay, or arrest the microvascular and macrovascular complications of diabetes while minimizing hypoglycemia and excess weight gain (ADA, 2002a).

Glycemic treatment goals for persons with diabetes are listed in Table 33-4. Achieving goals requires open communication and appropriate self-management education. Patients can assess day-to-day glycemic control by self-monitoring of blood glucose (SMBG) and measurement of urine and blood ketones.

Longer-term glycemic control is assessed from the results of glycosylated hemoglobin (simplified as A1C) tests. When hemoglobin and other proteins are exposed to glucose, the glucose becomes attached to the protein in a slow, nonenzymatic, and concentration-dependent fashion. Measurements of A1C reflect a weighted average of plasma glucose concentration over the preceding weeks, thereby complementing day-to-day testing. In nondiabetic persons, A1C values are 4.0% to 6.0%; these values correspond to mean blood glucose levels of about 90 mg/dl (or about 5 mmol/L). Lipid levels and blood pressure must also be monitored (Table 33-5). Lipids should be measured annually, and blood pressure at every diabetes management visit (ADA, 2002a).

Control and Outcomes

Evidence relating hyperglycemia and other metabolic consequences of insulin deficiency to the development of complications comes from a series of studies in Europe and North America; however, the Diabetes Control and Complications Trial (DCCT) demonstrated beyond a doubt the clear link between glycemic control and development of complications in persons with type 1 diabetes. The DCCT, sponsored by the National Institutes of Health, was a long-term, prospective, randomized, controlled, multicenter trial that studied approximately 1400 young adults (ages 13 to 39 years)

TABLE 33-3 Action of Insulin on Carbohydrate, Protein, and Fat Metabolism

EFFECT	CARBOHYDRATE	PROTEIN	FAT
Anticatabolic (prevents breakdown)	Decreases breakdown and release of glucose from glycogen in the liver	Inhibits protein degradation, diminishes gluconeogenesis	Inhibits lipolysis, prevents excessive production of ketones and ketoacidosis
Anabolic (promotes storage)	Facilitates conversion of glucose to glycogen for storage in liver and muscle	Stimulates protein synthesis	Facilitates conversion of pyruvate to free fatty acids, stimulating lipogenesis
Transport	Activates the transport system of glucose into muscle and adipose cells	Lowers blood amino acids in parallel with blood glucose levels	Activates lipoprotein lipase, facilitating transport of triglycerides into adipose tissue

TABLE 33-4 Recommendations for Glycemic Control*

BIOCHEMICAL INDEX	NORMAL	GOAL
Plasma Values		
Average preprandial glucose (mg/dl)	<110	90-130
Peak postprandial average plasma glucose (mg/dl) (measured within 1-2 hr after eating)	<140	<180
A1c (%)	<6	<7

Modified from American Diabetes Association: Standards of medical care for patients with diabetes mellitus, *Diabetes Care* 26(suppl 1):S37, 2003.
*Values are for nonpregnant individuals. A1c, glycosylated hemoglobin, is referenced to a nondiabetic range of 4.0%-6.0%.

TABLE 33-5 Lipid and Blood Pressure Goals*

LIPIDS (mg/dl)		BLOOD PRESSURE (mm Hg)	
Cholesterol	<200	Systolic	<130
LDL Cholesterol	<100	Diastolic	<80
HDL Cholesterol			
Men	>45		
Women	>55		
Triglycerides	<150		

Modified from American Diabetes Association: Standards of medical care for patients with diabetes mellitus [Postition Statement], *Diabetes Care* 25(suppl 1):S33, 2002.
*Values are for nonpregnant adults.
LDL, Low-density lipoprotein; *HDL,* high-density lipoprotein.

with type 1 diabetes who were treated with either intensive therapeutic regimens (multiple injections of insulin or use of insulin infusion pumps guided by blood glucose monitoring results) or conventional regimens (one or two insulin injections per day) (Diabetes Control and Complications Trial Research Group, 1995). Patients who achieved control similar to that of the intensively treated patients in the study could expect a 50% to 75% reduction in the risk of progression to retinopathy, nephropathy, and neuropathy after 8 to 9 years (DCCT Research Group, 1993).

Previously, small studies had demonstrated the relationship of blood glucose control to complications in type 2 diabetes (Kuusito et al, 1994; Ohkubbo et al, 1995). However, the reports of the United Kingdom Prospective Diabetes Study (UKPDS) in 1998 demonstrated conclusively that elevated blood glucose levels cause long-term complications in type 2 diabetes just as in type 1 diabetes (UKPDS, 1998a). The UKPDS recruited and followed up on 5102 newly diagnosed type 2 diabetic patients for an average of 10 to 11 years. Subjects were randomized into a group treated conventionally, primarily with nutrition therapy, and had an average HbA1c of 7.9% compared with subjects randomized into an intensively treated group, initially treated with sulfonylureas, and who had an average HbA1c of 7.0%. In the intensive therapy group, the microvascular complications rate decreased significantly by 25% and the risk of macrovascular disease decreased by 16%. Combination therapy (combining insulin or metformin with sulfonylureas) was needed in both groups to meet glycemic goals as loss of glycemic control was noted over the 10-year trial. Aggressive treatment of even mild-to-moderate hypertension was also beneficial in both groups (UKPDS, 1998b).

Before randomization into intensive or conventional treatment, subjects received individualized intensive nutrition therapy for 3 months. During this run-in period, the mean A1C decreased by 1.9% (~9% to ~7%) and patients lost an average of 3.5 kg (8 lb). UKPDS researchers concluded that a reduction of energy intake was at least as important, if not more important, than the actual weight lost in determining the FPG (UKPDS, 1990).

This study clearly illustrates the progressive nature of type 2 diabetes. An important lesson learned from the UKPDS is that therapy needs to be intensified over time and that as the disease progresses, MNT alone is not enough to keep most patients' A1C level at 7%. Medication(s), and for many patients, eventually insulin, needs to be added to the treatment regimen. It is not the "diet" failing; it is the pancreas failing to secrete enough insulin to maintain adequate glucose control.

Nutrition Therapy

Medical nutrition therapy is integral to total diabetes care and management. To integrate MNT effectively into the overall management of diabetes requires a coordinated team effort, including a dietitian who is knowledgeable and skilled in implementing current principles and recommendations for diabetes. MNT requires an individualized approach and effective nutrition self-management education. Monitoring glucose, A1C and lipid levels, blood pressure, weight, and quality-of-life issues is essential in evaluating the success of nutrition-related recommendations. If desired outcomes from MNT are not met, changes in overall diabetes care and management should be recommended (ADA, 2001).

The ADA's nutrition guidelines underscore the importance of individualizing nutrition care. Before 1994 nutrition recommendations attempted to define optimal percentages for macronutrient intake. Then, by determining a person's energy needs based on theoretic calorie requirements and using the ideal percentages for carbohydrate, protein, and fat, a nutrition prescription was developed—for example, 1800 calories, 225 g of carbohydrate (50%), 90 g of protein (20%), and 60 g of fat (30%). The problem with this approach is that the prescribed "diet" can not really be individualized, and it often lacks relevance to the patient's personal lifestyle, culture, or socioeconomic status. Furthermore, this approach is not supported by scientific evidence and usually does not produce successful outcomes. Beginning in 1994, the ADA recommended that an individualized nutrition prescription be based on metabolic profiles, treatment goals, and changes that the person with diabetes is willing and able to make, not on rigid, predetermined calorie levels and macronutrient percentages (Franz et al, 1994). This approach continues with the 2002 ADA nutrition principles and recommendations for persons with diabetes (ADA, 2002b; Franz, 2002).

Goals and Outcomes of Medical Nutrition Therapy for Diabetes

The goals for MNT for diabetes emphasize the role of lifestyle in improving not only glucose control but also lipid and lipoprotein profiles and blood pressure. Improving health through food choices and physical activity is the basis of all nutrition recommendations for the treatment and prevention of diabetes (Box 33-1).

Besides being skilled and knowledgeable in regard to assessing and implementing MNT, dietitians must also be aware of expected outcomes from nutrition therapy, when to assess outcomes, and what feedback, including recommendations, should be given to referral sources. Research supports MNT as an effective therapy in reaching diabetes treatment goals. Outcomes studies demonstrate that MNT provided by a registered dietitian

Box 33-1. Goals of Medical Nutrition Therapy for Diabetes Mellitus

Goals of Medical Nutrition Therapy That Apply to All Persons With Diabetes

1. Attain and maintain optimal metabolic outcomes including:
   - Blood glucose levels in the normal range or as close to normal as is safely possible to prevent or reduce risk or complications of diabetes.
   - A lipid and lipoprotein profile that reduces the risk for cardiovascular disease.
   - Blood pressure levels that reduce the risk for vascular disease.
2. Prevent and treat the chronic complications: Modify nutrient intake as appropriate for the prevention and treatment of obesity, cardiovascular disease, hypertension, and nephropathy.
3. Improve health through healthy food choices and physical activity.
4. Address individual nutritional needs, taking into consideration personal and cultural preferences and lifestyle while respecting the individual's needs and willingness to change.

Goals of Nutrition Therapy That Apply to Specific Situations

1. For youth with type 1 diabetes, provide adequate energy to ensure normal growth and development; integrate insulin regimen into usual eating and exercise habits.
2. For youth with type 2 diabetes, facilitate changes in eating and exercise habits that reduce insulin resistance and improve metabolic status.
3. For pregnant and lactating women, provide adequate energy and nutrients needed for successful outcomes.
4. For older adults, provide for the nutritional needs of an aging individual.
5. For individuals treated with insulin or insulin secretagogues, provide information on prevention and treatment of hypoglycemia and exercise-related blood glucose problems and how to manage acute illness.
6. For individuals at risk for diabetes, decrease risk by increasing physical activity and promoting food choices that facilitate moderate weight loss or at least prevent weight gain.

From American Diabetes Association: Evidence-based nutrition principles and recommendations for the treatment and prevention of diabetes and related complications [Position Statement], *Diabetes Care* 25:202, 2002.

(RD) is associated with a decrease of about 1.0% of A1C in patients with newly diagnosed type 1 diabetes (Kulkarni et al, 1998), a decrease of about 2.0% of A1C in patients with newly diagnosed type 2 diabetes (Franz et al, 1995; UKPDS Group, 1990), and a decrease of about 1.0% of A1C in patients with an average 4-year duration of type 2 diabetes (Franz et al, 1995). These outcomes are similar to those from oral glucose-lowering medications. Furthermore, the effect of MNT on A1C will be known by 6 weeks to 3 months, at which time the RD must assess whether the goals of therapy have been met by changes in lifestyle and whether changes or additions of medications are needed (ADA, 2001).

Prioritizing Nutrition Therapy for Type 1 Diabetes

The priority for anyone who requires insulin therapy is first to determine a food and meal plan and then to integrate an insulin regimen into his or her usual eating habits and physical activity schedule. With the many insulin options now available (new rapid-acting and long-acting insulins), an insulin regimen usually can be developed that will conform to an individual's preferred meal routines and food choices (ADA, 2002b; Franz et al, 2002). It is no longer necessary to create unnatural or artificial divisions of meals and snacks.

Flexible insulin regimens involve multiple injections (three or more insulin injections per day) or use of an insulin infusion pump. Half of the required insulin dose is given as a basal or background insulin, and the other half is divided and given before meals (bolus or premeal insulin). These types of insulin regimens allow increased flexibility in choosing when and what to eat. The total carbohydrate content of meals is the major determinant of the mealtime rapid-acting insulin dose and postprandial glucose response (Rabasa-Lhoret et al, 1999). Thus, individuals can be taught how to adjust mealtime insulin doses based on the carbohydrate content of the meal and how to delay mealtime insulin for late meals. Even with flexible insulin regimens, however, consistency in food intake facilitates improved glycemic control (Delahanty and Halford, 1993). For persons who receive fixed insulin regimens, such as with the use of premixed insulins, or those who do not adjust their mealtime insulin doses, day-to-day consistency in the timing and amount of carbohydrate eaten is recommended (Wolever et al, 1999).

Prioritizing Nutrition Therapy for Type 2 Diabetes

The priority for individuals with type 2 diabetes is to adopt lifestyle strategies that improve the associated metabolic abnormalities of glycemia, dyslipidemia, and hypertension (ADA, 2002b; Franz et al, 2002). Lifestyle strategies independent of weight loss that can improve glycemia include reducing energy intake, monitoring carbohydrate servings, limiting consumption of saturated fats, and increasing physical activity. These strategies should be implemented as soon as the diagnosis of diabetes (or prediabetes) is made.

In the short-term, small amounts of weight loss may improve insulin resistance and glycemia, but, because of the difficulty in maintaining weight loss long term, it is unknown whether this benefit continues. Short-term studies lasting 6 months or less demonstrate that modest amounts of weight loss improve metabolic abnormalities in many persons with type 2 diabetes (Markovic et al, 1998a; Wing et al, 1987) but not in all (Watts et al, 1990). Weight loss, especially of intraabdominal fat, reduces insulin resistance and helps to correct dyslipidemia (Markovic et al, 1998b); however, long-term data assessing the extent to which these improvements can be maintained in persons with diabetes are not available, probably because long-term weight loss is difficult to achieve. Long-term weight loss of 5% to 7% from baseline weight requires frequent, regular, and long-term follow-up of patients (Diabetes Prevention Program Research Group, 2002; Tuomilehto et al, 2001).

An energy-restricted diet, however, can have an important regulatory effect on glucose control in persons with type 2 diabetes, independent of any effects from weight loss (Kelley et al, 1993; Wing et al, 1994). When energy intake is restricted, hyperglycemia improves more rapidly than with weight loss. Furthermore, when calories are increased after weight reduction, glucose levels increase despite no regain of weight. This suggests that energy intake is more important than weight loss.

Physical activity improves insulin sensitivity, can acutely lower blood glucose in diabetic persons, and may also improve cardiovascular status; but by itself it has only a modest effect on weight. Physical activity is useful as an adjunct to other weight loss strategies and is essential for long-term maintenance of weight loss (Albright et al, 2000). It should be noted, however, that cardiorespiratory fitness appears to be more important than thinness in relation to all-cause and cardiovascular mortality (Lee et al, 1999). During an 8-year study of about 25,000 men, fit men had greater longevity than unfit men regardless of their body composition or risk factor status. No elevated mortality risk was observed in obese men if they were physically fit, and obese fit men had a lower risk of all-cause and cardiovascular mortality than lean unfit men.

Teaching which foods are carbohydrates (fruits, grains, starchy vegetables, milk, sweets), average portion sizes, how many servings to select at meals (and snacks, if desired), and how to limit fat and especially saturated fat intake; encouraging physical activity; and using blood glucose monitoring to adjust food and eating patterns and medications are important components of successful MNT for type 2 diabetes (Rickheim et al, 2002). Frequent follow-up with a dietitian as outlined in nutrition practice guidelines for type 2 diabetes can provide the problem-solving techniques, encouragement, and support that lifestyle changes require (Monk et al, 1995).

Carbohydrate

Sugars, starch, and *fiber* are the preferred terms for carbohydrates (Report of a Joint FAO/WHO Expert Consultation, 1998). Foods that contain carbohydrate from whole grains, fruits, vegetables, and low-fat milk are important components of a healthy diet for all Americans, including those with diabetes. They are excellent sources of vitamins, minerals, dietary fiber, and energy. Historically it was a long-held belief that sucrose must be restricted based on the assumption that sugars, such as sucrose, are more rapidly digested and absorbed than starches and thus aggravate hyperglycemia; however, scientific evidence does not justify restricting sugars or sucrose based on this belief. In approximately 20 studies in which sucrose was substituted for other carbohydrates, sucrose did not increase glycemia to a greater extent than isocaloric amounts of starch (Bantle et al, 1993; Peterson et al, 1986; Rickard et al, 1998). The glycemic effect of carbohydrate foods cannot be predicted based on their structure (i.e., starch versus sugar) owing to the efficiency of the human digestive tract in reducing starch polymers to glucose. Starches are rapidly metabolized into 100% glucose during digestion, in contrast to sucrose, which is metabolized into glucose and fructose. Fructose has a lower glycemic index, which has been attributed to its slow rate of absorption and its storage in the liver as glycogen (Nuttall et al, 1992) (see Chapters 3, 12, and 26).

Numerous factors influence glycemic responses of foods, including the amount of carbohydrate, type of sugar (glucose, fructose, sucrose, lactose), nature of the starch (amylose, amylopectin, resistant starch), cooking and food processing, particle size, and food form as well as the fasting and preprandial glucose concentrations, severity of the glucose intolerance, and the second meal or lente effect of carbohydrates. There is, however, strong evidence to state that the total amount of carbohydrate is more important than the source (sugar or starch) or the type (glycemic index) of carbohydrate. Numerous studies have reported that when subjects are allowed to choose from a variety of starches and sugars, the glycemic response is identical if the total amount of carbohydrate is similar (ADA, 2002b). Therefore, the first priority for food and meal planning is the total amount of carbohydrate that the person with diabetes chooses to have for meals or snacks. This is the basis of carbohydrate counting, whereby food portions contributing 15 g of carbohydrate (regardless of the source) are considered to be one carbohydrate serving.

Glycemic Index and Glycemic Load

Although different carbohydrates do have different glycemic responses (*glycemic index*), there is limited evidence to show long-term benefit when low glycemic index diets are compared with high glycemic index diets in studies lasting 2 weeks or longer. In subjects with type 1 diabetes (five studies in total, n = 48), no studies in which low versus high glycemic index diets are compared show a beneficial effect of the low glycemic index diet on A1c; three studies report the low glycemic index diet improved fructosamine (a short-term measure of overall control), whereas one study reported no improvement in fructosamine. In subjects with type 2 diabetes (nine studies in total, n = 129), one study reported beneficial effects of the low glycemic index diet on A1c, whereas four studies reported no beneficial effects on A1c. Three studies reported improvement in fructosamine from the low glycemic index diet, whereas three studies reported no improvement. FPG is reported in all studies; however, no studies in persons with type 1 or type 2 diabetes report improvements in FPG from the low glycemic index diets (Franz, 2001). Therefore, there is insufficient evidence to recommend low glycemic index diets as the primary strategy in food and meal planning for individuals with diabetes (ADA, 2002b). The concept of the glycemic index is perhaps best used for fine-tuning postprandial responses after focusing on total carbohydrate.

The glycemic load is a newer concept and incorporates both the number of grams of carbohydrate in a usual food serving or meal and the glycemic index (see Appendix 54). At this time, however, no intervention studies have been done that show benefit from using this technique in persons with diabetes.

g x glycemic index

Fiber

Early short-term studies using large amounts of fiber (>30 g daily) in small numbers of subjects suggested a positive effect on glycemia; however, results from later studies have shown mixed effects. In subjects with type 1 diabetes, a high-fiber diet (56 g daily) had no beneficial effects on glycemic control (Lafrance et al, 1998). Another study of subjects with type 1 diabetes showed positive effects from 50 g of fiber on glucose concentrations but no beneficial effects on lipids (Giacco et al, 2000). In persons with type 2 diabetes, increasing fiber from 11 to 27 g/1000 kcal did not improve glycemia, insulinemia, or lipemia (Hollenbeck et al, 1986), whereas another study comparing 24 g of fiber per day with 50 g of fiber reported improved glycemic control, reduced hyperinsulinemia, and decreased plasma lipids (Chandalia et al, 2000). Therefore, it appears that ingestion of large amounts of fiber (~50 g/day) is necessary to have beneficial effects on glycemia, insulinemia, and lipemia. It is unknown whether free-living individuals can maintain such high levels of fiber and whether this amount would be acceptable to most people (ADA, 2002b). Although the consumption of fiber is to be encouraged, just as it is for the general public, there is no reason to recommend that persons with diabetes eat a greater amount of fiber than other Americans.

Sweeteners

Even though sucrose restriction cannot be justified on the basis of its glycemic effect, it is still good advice to suggest that persons with diabetes be careful in their consumption of foods containing large amounts of sucrose. Besides often being high in total carbohydrate content, these foods may also contain significant amounts of fat. If sucrose is included in the food and meal plan, it should be substituted for other carbohydrate sources or, if added, be adequately covered with insulin or other glucose-lowering medications. Sucrose and sucrose-containing foods also should be eaten in the context of a healthy diet (ADA, 2002b).

There appears to be no significant advantage of alternative nutritive sweeteners over sucrose. Fructose provides 4 kcal/g, as do other carbohydrates, and even though it does have a lower glycemic response than sucrose and other starches, large amounts (15%-20% of daily energy intake) of fructose have an adverse effect on plasma lipids (Bantle et al, 1992, 2000). There is no reason, however, to recommend that persons with diabetes avoid fructose, which occurs naturally in fruits and vegetables as well as in foods sweetened with fructose (ADA, 2002b).

Sorbitol, mannitol, xylitol, isomalt, lactitol, and hydrogenated starch hydrolysates are common sugar alcohols that also have a lower glycemic response and lower caloric content than sucrose and other carbohydrates. Because they are not soluble in water, they are often combined with fat; therefore, foods sweetened with sugar alcohols may have a caloric content that is similar to that of the foods they are replacing. It is unlikely, however, that sugar alcohols in the amounts likely to be ingested in individual food servings or meals will contribute to significant reduction in total energy or carbohydrate intake (ADA, 2002b). Some patients report gastric discomfort after eating foods sweetened with these products, and consuming large quantities may cause diarrhea.

Saccharin (Sweet'N Low), aspartame (Equal and NutraSweet), acesulfame K, and sucralose are noncaloric sweeteners currently approved for use in the United States. Approval of the U.S. Food and Drug Administration (FDA) is being sought for alitame and cyclamates. All such products must undergo rigorous testing by the manufacturer and scrutiny from the FDA before they are approved and marketed to the public. For all food additives, including nonnutritive sweeteners, the FDA determines an acceptable daily intake (ADI), defined as the amount of a food additive that can be safely consumed on a daily basis over a person's lifetime without risk (see Chapter 14). The ADI includes a 100-fold safety factor and greatly exceeds average consumption levels. For example, aspartame actual daily intake in persons with diabetes is 2 to 4 mg per kilogram of body weight daily, well below the ADI of 50 mg/kg daily (Butchko and Stargel, 2001). All FDA-approved nonnutritive sweeteners can be used by persons with diabetes, including pregnant women (ADA, 2002b).

Protein

The rate of protein degradation and conversion of protein to glucose in type 1 diabetes depends on the state of insulinization and the degree of glycemic control. With less than optimal insulinization, conversion of protein to glucose can occur rapidly, adversely influencing glycemic control. In poorly controlled type 2 diabetes, gluconeogenesis is also accelerated and may account for most of the increased glucose production in the postabsorptive state (Henry, 1994). In those with controlled type 2 diabetes Gannon et al, 2001a; Nuttall et al, 1984) and well-controlled type 1 diabetes (Peters and Davidson, 1993), ingested protein did not increase plasma glucose concentrations. Although nonessential amino acids undergo gluconeogenesis, it is unclear why the glucose produced does not appear in the general circulation after ingestion of protein (Franz, 2000). Furthermore, protein does not slow the absorption of carbohydrate (Nordt et al, 1991; Nuttall et al, 1984), and adding protein to the treatment of hypoglycemia does not prevent subsequent hypoglycemia (Gray et al, 1996). In type 2 diabetic patients who are still able to produce insulin, ingested protein is just as potent a stimulant of insulin secretion as carbohydrate.

There is evidence that moderate hyperglycemia in persons with type 2 diabetes (Gougeon et al, 1994) and uncontrolled diabetes in persons with type 1 diabetes (Lariviere et al, 1994) cause increased protein catabolism. Protection against increased protein catabolism requires near-normal glycemia and an adequate protein intake (Brodsky and Devlin, 1996; Gougeon et al, 2000). Therefore, for persons with diabetes, the protein requirement may be greater than the recommended dietary allowance (RDA) but not greater than typical intake in the United States. No evidence has been found to suggest that typical protein intake (15%-20% of total daily energy) must be modified if renal function is normal (ADA, 2002b). In studies in which protein intake was in the range of usual intake and rarely exceeded 20% of energy intake, dietary protein intake was not associated with the development of diabetic nephropathy. In a cross-sectional study (Toeller et al, 1997), patients in whom protein intakes were 20% or greater of daily energy had a higher incidence of albuminuria. This finding suggests that it may be prudent to avoid protein intake that is more than 20% of total daily energy.

The long-term effects of weight-loss diets high in protein and low in carbohydrate are unknown. Although initially blood glucose levels may improve and weight may be lost, it is unknown whether weight loss is maintained better with these diets than with other low-calorie diets. Furthermore, protein is just as potent a stimulant of insulin as is carbohydrate. Because these diets are usually high in saturated fat, the long-term effect on LDL cholesterol is also a concern (ADA, 2002b) (see Chapters 24 and 35).

Dietary Fat

In all persons with diabetes, less than 10% of energy intake should be derived from saturated fats, and dietary cholesterol intake should be less than 300 mg daily. Some persons (i.e., those with LDL cholesterol ≥100 mg/dl) may benefit from lowering saturated fat intake to less than 7% of energy intake and dietary cholesterol to less than 200 mg daily. To lower plasma LDL cholesterol, saturated fat can be reduced if concurrent weight loss is desirable or replaced with carbohydrate or monounsaturated fat if weight loss is not a goal. Intake of *trans*-fatty acids should also be minimized (see Chapter 35).

If saturated fat contributes less than 10% of total daily energy, if about 10% of energy is from polyunsaturated fat, and if protein contributes 15% to 20% of energy, then 60% to 70% of total energy intake remains to be distributed between carbohydrate and monounsaturated fat. Diets high in monounsaturated fat or low in fat and high in carbohydrate result in improvement in glucose tolerance and lipids compared with diets high in saturated fat. Diets enriched with monounsaturated fats may also reduce insulin resistance (Parillo et al, 1992); however, other studies have reported high total dietary fat (regardless of the type of fat) to be associated with insulin resistance (Lovejoy and DiGirolamo, 1992). In metabolic studies in which energy intake is maintained so that subjects do not lose weight, diets high in either carbohydrate or monounsaturated fat lower LDL cholesterol equivalently, but the concern has been the potential of a high-carbohydrate diet (greater than 55% of energy intake) to increase triglycerides and postprandial glucose compared with a high–monounsaturated fat diet (Garg et al, 1994). If energy intake is reduced and a low-fat, high-carbohydrate diet is compared with a high–monounsaturated fat diet, no detrimental effects on triglycerides result from the high-carbohydrate diet (Heilbronn et al, 1999). Energy intake, therefore, appears to a factor in determining the effects of a high-carbohydrate versus high–monounsaturated fat diet.

Low-fat, high-carbohydrate diets over long periods have not been shown to increase triglycerides and have been shown to lead to modest weight loss (Kendall et al, 1991) and weight-loss maintenance (Carmichael et al, 1998). Thus, a person's metabolic profile and need to lose weight will determine nutrition recommendations. For persons who need to lose weight, a lower energy intake and a low-fat, moderate-carbohydrate approach can be used. For persons who do not need to lose weight, a high–monounsaturated fat approach may be recommended to improve triglycerides or postprandial glycemia (ADA, 2002b).

There is evidence from the general population that foods containing omega-3 fatty acids are beneficial, and two to three servings of fish per week are recommended. Although most studies in persons with diabetes have used omega-3 supplements and show beneficial lowering of triglycerides, an accompanying rise in LDL cholesterol also has been noted (Montori et al, 2000). If supplements are used, the effects on LDL cholesterol should be monitored. The omega-3 supplements may be most beneficial in the treatment of severe hypertriglyceridemia (Patti et al, 1999).

Fiber and Phytosterols

Evidence for the effects of fiber on lipids is provided by a metaanalysis of 67 controlled trials (Brown et al, 1999). Within the practical range of intake, the authors concluded that the effect of soluble fiber on total and LDL cholesterol is small. For example, daily intake of 3 g of soluble fiber from oats (three servings of oatmeal, 28 g each) or three apples can decrease total cholesterol by about 5 mg/dl, an approximate 2% reduction.

Intake of 2 to 3 g of plant stanols or sterols per day are reported to decrease total and LDL cholesterol levels by 9% to 20% (Hallikainen et al, 1999). Use of low-fat food and fat replacers or substitutes approved by the FDA are safe for use and may reduce total fat and energy intake.

Energy Balance and Obesity

Improved glycemic control with intensive insulin therapy is often associated with increases in body weight. Because of the potential for weight gain to affect lipids and blood pressure adversely, prevention of weight gain is desirable; however, the benefits of improved blood glucose control outweigh concerns about weight gain, at least initially (Chaturvedi et al, 1995). To prevent weight gain, insulin therapy should be integrated into usual eating and exercise habits and insulin doses adjusted accordingly. Overtreatment of hypoglycemia should be avoided; total protein, fat, and calories ingested must be accounted for; and adjustments in insulin should be made for exercise.

Many individuals with type 2 diabetes are overweight, with about 36% having a BMI of 30 kg/m^2 or greater (Cowie and Harris, 1995). The risk of obesity and excess mortality is controversial. Obesity in persons with type 2 diabetes was not related to mortality (Chaturvedi and Fuller, 1995) or to the long-term incidence of microvascular and macrovascular complications (Klein et al, 1997). Short-term studies that lasted 6 months or less, however, demonstrated that weight loss in subjects with type 2 diabetes is associated with improvement in insulin resistance, glycemia, serum lipids, and blood pressure. Long-term data assessing the extent to which these improvements can be maintained in people with type 2 diabetes are scarce, as already mentioned.

A genetic predisposition to obesity and possible impaired metabolic and appetite regulation as well as environmental factors make it difficult to lose and, more important, to maintain weight loss. Because of the psychological and physiologic impact of dieting, encouragement to attain and maintain a reasonable body weight is crucial. Emphasis should be on blood glucose control, improved food choices, increased physical activity, and moderate energy restriction rather than weight loss alone.

Standard weight-reduction diets, when used alone, are unlikely to produce long-term weight loss. Structured, intensive lifestyle programs are necessary to produce long-term weight loss of 5% to 7% of starting weight (Diabetes Prevention Program Research Group, 2002; Tuomilehto et al, 2001). Currently available weight-loss drugs have a modest beneficial effect in persons with diabetes and should be used only in people with a BMI greater than 27. Gastric reduction surgery can be an effective weight-loss treatment for severely obese patients with type 2 diabetes; however, it should be considered only in patients with a BMI greater than 35 because long-term data comparing the benefits and risks of gastric reduction surgery with medical therapy are not available (ADA, 2002b) (see Chapter 24).

Alcohol

The same precautions that apply to alcohol consumption for the general population apply to persons with diabetes. The effect of alcohol on blood glucose levels depends not only on the amount of alcohol ingested but also on its relationship to food intake. In the fasting state, alcohol may cause hypoglycemia in persons using exogenous insulin or insulin secretagogues. Alcohol is used as a source of energy, but it is not converted to glucose. It is metabolized in a manner similar to fat. It also blocks gluconeogenesis and augments or increases the effects of insulin by interfering with the counterregulation response to insulin-induced hypoglycemia. All these factors contribute to the development of hypoglycemia when alcohol is consumed without food (Franz, 1999).

If individuals choose to drink alcohol, daily intake should be limited to one drink for adult women and two drinks for adult men (1 drink = 12 oz beer, 5 oz of wine, or 1½ oz of distilled spirits [15 g alcohol]). For most persons, blood glucose levels are not affected by moderate use of alcohol when diabetes is well controlled (Koivisto et al, 1993). Alcoholic beverages should be considered an addition to the regular food and meal plan for all persons with diabetes. No food should be omitted given the possibility of alcohol-induced hypoglycemia and the fact that alcohol does not require insulin to be metabolized. Pregnant women and patients with medical problems such as pancreatitis, advanced neuropathy, severe hypertriglyceridemia, or alcohol abuse should avoid alcohol (ADA, 2002b).

Epidemiologic evidence in nondiabetic individuals suggests that light to moderate alcohol ingestion in adults is associated with decreased risk of type 2 diabetes and stroke and improved insulin resistance. In adults with type 2 diabetes, light to moderate alcohol ingestion is associated with decreased risk of coronary heart disease, perhaps because of the concomitant increase in HDL cholesterol. Long-term, prospective studies are needed to confirm these observations (ADA, 2002b) (see Chapter 35). Ingestion of light to moderate amounts of alcohol does not raise blood pressure, whereas excessive, chronic ingestions of alcohol does raise blood pressure and may be a risk factor for stroke (Joint National Committee on Prevention, Detection, Evaluation and Treatment of High Blood Pressure, 1997).

Micronutrients

No clear evidence has been established of benefits from routine vitamin or mineral supplements in persons with diabetes who do not have underlying deficiencies. Exceptions include folate for the prevention of birth defects and calcium for prevention of bone disease. Routine supplementation of the diet with antioxidants is not advised because of uncertainties related to long-term efficacy and safety (ADA, 2002b). Observational studies and several placebo-controlled clinical trials with small subject numbers have found beneficial effects of antioxidants, especially vitamin E, on physiologic and biochemical end points. Large placebo-controlled clinical trials have failed to show benefit from antioxidants and, in some instances, have suggested adverse effects (Omenn et al, 1996). Of interest is the Heart Outcomes Prevention Evaluation Trial, which included 9541 subjects, 38% of whom had diabetes (Yusuf et al, 2000). Supplementation with 400 IU daily of vitamin E for 4.5 years did not result in any significant benefit on cardiovascular outcomes.

Because the response to supplements is determined largely by a person's nutritional status, persons with micronutrient deficiencies are most likely to respond favorably. Although difficult to ascertain, if deficiencies of vitamins or minerals are identified, supplementation can be beneficial. Those at greatest risk of deficiency who may benefit from prescription of vitamin and mineral supplements include patients who consume extreme calorie-restricted diets, strict vegetarians, older adults, pregnant or lactating women, those taking medication known to alter micronutrient metabolism (see Chapter 19), patients in poor metabolic control (glycosuria), and patients in critical care environments.

Chromium deficiency in animal models is associated with elevated blood glucose, cholesterol, and triglyceride levels. It is unlikely, however, that most persons with diabetes are chromium deficient. In three double-blind crossover studies of chromium supplementation in individuals with diabetes, no improvement in blood glucose control was noted (Mooradian et al, 1994). In a randomized, placebo-controlled study in Chinese subjects with diabetes, chromium supplementation did have beneficial effects on glycemia (Anderson et al, 1997; Cheng et al, 1999); however, the study population may have had marginal baseline chromium status because the chromium status was not evaluated either at baseline or after supplementation. Therefore, before chromium supplementation can be recommended, placebo-controlled clinical trials need to be undertaken in which people with diabetes with known dietary intakes of chromium use chromium supplements that may be better absorbed than older supplements.

Exercise

Exercise should be an integral part of the treatment plan for persons with diabetes. Exercise helps all persons with diabetes improve insulin sensitivity, reduce cardiovascular risk factors, control weight, and bring about a healthier mental outlook. Given appropriate guidelines, people with diabetes can exercise safely. The exercise plan will vary depending on interest, age, general health, and level of physical fitness.

Despite the increase in glucose uptake by muscles during exercise, glucose levels change little in individuals without diabetes. Muscular work causes insulin levels to decline while counterregulatory hormones (primarily glucagon) rise. In this way, increased glucose utilization by the exercising muscle is matched precisely with increased glucose production by the liver. This balance between insulin and counterregulatory hormones is the major determinant of hepatic glucose production, underscoring the need for insulin adjustments in addition to adequate carbohydrate intake during exercise for people with diabetes.

In persons with type 1 diabetes, the glycemic response to exercise varies depending on overall diabetes control, plasma glucose, and insulin levels at the start of exercise; timing, intensity and duration of the exercise; previous food intake; and previous conditioning. An important variable is the level of plasma insulin during and after exercise. Hypoglycemia can occur because of insulin-enhanced muscle glucose uptake by the exercising muscle. In contrast, insulin deficiency in a poorly controlled (underinsulinized) exerciser results in increases in glucose concentrations and free fatty acids release continues with minimal uptake. This can result in large increases in plasma glucose and ketone levels (Wasserman and Zinman, 1994).

In persons with type 2 diabetes, blood glucose control can improve with exercise, largely because of decreased insulin resistance and increased insulin sensitivity, which results in increased peripheral use of glucose not only during but also after the activity. This exercise-induced enhanced insulin sensitivity occurs without changes in body weight. Exercise also decreases the effects of counterregulatory hormones; this, in turn, reduces the hepatic glucose output, contributing to improved glucose control. Exercise regimens at an intensity of 50% to 80% Vo_{2max} three to four times a week for 30 to 60 minutes a session can result in a 10% to 20% baseline improvement in A1c and are most beneficial in persons with mild type 2 diabetes and in those who are likely to be the most insulin resistant. Regular exercise also has consistently been shown to be effective in reducing triglyceride levels in persons with type 2 diabetes; however, the effect of exercise on HDL cholesterol levels is unclear. Reductions in blood pressure and improvements in impaired fibrinolysis have also been noted (ADA, 2002c).

Potential Problems With Exercise

Hypoglycemia is a potential problem associated with exercise in persons taking insulin or insulin secretagogues. Hypoglycemia can occur during, immediately after, or many hours after exercise. Hypoglycemia has been reported to be more common after exercise, especially after exercise of long duration, after strenuous activity or play, or after sporadic exercise, than during exercise (MacDonald et al, 1987). This is because of increased insulin sensitivity after exercise and the need to replete liver and muscle glycogen, which can take up to 24 to 30 hours (see Chapter 26). Hypoglycemia can also occur during or immediately after exercise. Blood glucose levels before exercise reflect only the value at that time, and it is unknown if this is a stable blood glucose level or a blood glucose level that is dropping. If blood glucose levels are dropping before exercise, adding exercise can contribute to hypoglycemia during exercise. Furthermore, hypoglycemia on the day before exercise is reported to increase the risk of hypoglycemia on the day of exercise as well (Davis et al, 2000).

Hyperglycemia can also result from exercise. When a person exercises at what for him or her is a high level of exercise intensity, there is a greater than normal increase in counterregulatory hormones. As a result, hepatic glucose release exceeds the rise in glucose utilization. The elevated glucose levels may also extend into the postexercise state (Mitchell et al, 1988; Purdon et al, 1993). Although not as likely, hyperglycemia and worsening ketosis can also result from insulin deficiency if exercise is done when fasting blood glucose levels are higher than 250 to 300 mg/dl. With elevated fasting blood glucose and ketones, exercise should be postponed until control improves (ADA, 2002b). The latter cause of hyperglycemia is not as likely to occur as the first.

Exercise Guidelines

The variability of glucose responses to exercise contributes to the difficulty in giving precise nutrition (and insulin) guidelines. Frequent blood glucose monitoring before, during, and after exercise helps individuals identify their response to physical activities. To meet their individual needs, patients must modify general guidelines to ingest carbohydrate after (or before) and to reduce insulin doses before (or after) exercise.

Carbohydrate for Insulin Users

During moderate-intensity exercise, glucose uptake is increased by 8 to 13 g per hour, and this is the basis for the recommendation to add 15 g carbohydrate for every 30 to 60 minutes of activity (depending on the intensity) over and above normal routines. Moderate exercise for less than 30 minutes rarely requires any additional carbohydrate or insulin adjustment; however, a small snack may be needed if the blood glucose level is less than 100 mg/dl (Franz, 2002).

In all persons, blood glucose levels decline gradually during exercise, and ingesting a carbohydrate feeding during prolonged exercise can improve performance by maintaining the availability and oxidation of blood glucose. For the exerciser with diabetes whose blood glucose levels may drop sooner and lower than the exerciser without diabetes, ingesting carbohydrate after 40 to 60 minutes of exercise is important and may also assist in preventing hypoglycemia. Drinks containing 6% or less of carbohydrate empty from the stomach as quickly as water and have the advantage of providing both needed fluids and carbohydrate (see Chapter 26). Consuming carbohydrate immediately after exercise optimizes repletion of muscle and liver glycogen stores. For the exerciser with diabetes, this takes on added importance because of increased risk for late-onset hypoglycemia (Franz, 2002).

Insulin Guidelines

It is often necessary to adjust the insulin dosage to prevent hypoglycemia. This occurs most often with moderate to strenuous activity lasting more than 45 to 60 minutes. For most persons, a modest decrease (of about 1 to 2 U) in the rapid- or short-acting insulin during the period of exercise is a good starting point. For prolonged vigorous exercise, a larger decrease in the total daily insulin dosage may be necessary. After exercise, insulin may also need to be decreased. In addition to these acute reductions in insulin dosages, individuals who participate in a regular, long-term fitness program often find their usual total dosage of insulin decreasing by as much as 15% to 20% (Wasserman and Zinman, 1994).

Insulin doses should be reduced in anticipation of exercise after a meal, depending on the duration and intensity of the exercise. In persons with type 1 diabetes, Rabasa-Lhoret and colleagues validated that exercise at 25% VO_{2max} for 60 minutes required a 50% reduction in mealtime rapid-acting insulin, and exercise at 50% VO_{2max} for 30 and 60 minutes required a 50% and 75% reduction in mealtime rapid-acting insulin, respectively. Such reductions in mealtime rapid-acting insulin for postprandial exercise resulted in a 75% decrease in exercise-induced hypoglycemia (Rabaca Lhoret et al, 2001).

Precautions for Persons With Type 2 Diabetes

Persons with type 2 diabetes may have a lower VO_{2max} and therefore need a more gradual training program. Rest periods may be needed; this does not impair the training effect from physical activity. Autonomic neuropathy or medications, such as for blood pressure, may not allow for increased heart rate, and individuals must learn to use perceived exertion as a means of determining exercise intensity. Blood pressure may also increase more in persons with diabetes than in those who do not have diabetes, and exercise should not be undertaken if systolic blood pressure is greater than 180 to 200 mm Hg.

Exercise Prescription

The type of exercise one chooses to perform should be tailored to his or her physical capacity and interests. A complete exercise program includes warm-up and cool-down periods. This not only prepares muscles for an aerobic workout, but it also improves range of motion. Cardiovascular conditioning is also helpful. Most people can at least undertake a walking program safely. Those with type 2 diabetes should strive to achieve a minimum cumulative total of 1000 kcal per week from physical activities, which equates to walking about 10 miles per week; 1 mile = ~100 kcal expenditure (Albright et al, 2000). Ideally, the aerobic portion of an exercise session should last a minimum of 20 minutes, with a goal of 30 to 40 minutes; however, even three sessions of 10 minutes of activity during the day can improve physical fitness (Pate et al, 1995). Muscle-strengthening exercises, such as lifting light weights, are also an important component of an exercise session. Because muscles dispose of glucose, this type of exercise can also improve glucose control.

Medications

Oral Glucose-Lowering Medications

The use of the newer oral glucose-lowering medications, alone or in combination, provides numerous options for achieving euglycemia in persons with type 2 diabetes. Some persons with hyperglycemia that is not adequately controlled by MNT alone can be treated with MNT, and oral medications—frequently combination therapy using two, and occasionally even three, oral medications may be needed. If glycemic control cannot be attained with MNT and oral medications, insulin, either alone or in combination with oral medications, is required. The transition to insulin often begins with an intermediate or long-acting insulin given at bedtime to control fasting glucose levels and oral medications given in the morning are to control daytime glucose levels. Eventually, however, many patients with type 2 diabetes will require two or more insulin injections daily to achieve control. If large doses of insulin are required, oral medications, such as insulin sensitizers, are often combined with the insulin regimen.

Currently, four classes of oral medications exist: (1) insulin secretagogues, which include the sulfonylureas (first and second generation) and the meglitinides (repaglinide and nateglinide); (2) biguanides (metformin); (3) thiazolidinediones (TZD; e.g., pioglitazone, rosiglitazone); and (4) α-glucosidase inhibitors (acarbose, miglitol). Each class has a different mechanism of action—in the pancreas, insulin secretion is stimulated; at the cellular level (muscle and adipose tissue), insulin resistance is decreased and glucose uptake enhanced; in the liver, hepatic glucose output is decreased, especially overnight, improving fasting glucose levels; or in the intestine, glucose absorption is slowed, improving postprandial glucose concentrations (Table 33-6). Because of the different sites of action, the medications can be used alone or in combination.

Insulin secretagogues (*sulfonylureas* and *meglitinides*) promote insulin secretion by the β-cells of the pancreas. First- and second-generation sulfonylurea drugs differ from one another in their potency, pharmacokinetics, and metabolism. Disadvantages of their use include weight gain and the potential to cause hypoglycemia. The meglitinides differ from the sulfonylureas in that they have short metabolic half-lives, which result in brief episodic stimulation of insulin secretion. As a result, a frequent dosing schedule is required with meals, postprandial glucose excursions are less, and because less insulin is secreted several hours after a meal, there is a decreased risk of hypoglycemia between meals and overnight. Nateglinide only works in the presence of glucose and is a somewhat less potent secretagogue (Inzucchi, 2002).

Insulin sensitizers enhance insulin action and include biguanides (metformin) and TZD. Both classes require the presence of insulin, exogenous or endogenous, to be effective. Metformin (Glucophage) sup-

TABLE 33-6 Oral Glucose-Lowering Medications for Type 2 Diabetes

CLASS AND GENERIC NAMES	RECOMMENDED DOSE	PRINCIPAL ACTION	MEAN DECREASE IN A1c
Sulfonylureas (Second Generation)		Stimulate insulin secretion from the β-cells	1%-2%
Glipizide (Glucotrol)	2.5-20 mg single or divided dose; single dose for XL		
Glipizide (Glucotrol XL)			
Glyburide (Glynase Prestabs)	12 mg once daily		
Glimepiride (Amaryl)	4 mg once daily		
Meglitinides		Stimulate insulin secretion from β-cells	1%-2%
Repaglinide (Prandin)	0.4-4.0 mg before meals		
Nateglinide (Starlix)	120 mg before meals		
Biguanides		Decrease hepatic glucose production	1.5%-2%
Metformin (Glucophage)	500-850 mg tid or 1000 mg bid		
Metformin Extended Release (Glucophage XR)	500-2000 mg once daily		
Metformin Glyburide (Glucovance) [1.25/250 mg]	2.5/500 mg to 5.0/500 mg once daily	Also increases insulin secretion	
Metformin/glipizide (Metaglip) [2.5 to 5./250 to 500 mg]	2.5/250 mg to 5.0/500 mg	Also increases insulin secretion	≈2%
Metformin/rosiglitazone (Avandamet) [1 to 4/500 mg]	2.5/250 mg to 2.5/500 mg	Improves insulin sensitivity and reduces hepatic glucose production	Unknown; no clinical trials yet
Thiazolidinediones		Improve peripheral insulin sensitivity	1%-2%
Pioglitazone (Actos)	15-45 mg daily		
Rosiglitazone (Avandia)	4-8 mg daily		
Alpha Glucosidase Inhibitors		Delay carbohydrate absorption	0.5%-1%
Acarbose (Precose)	25-100 mg tid		
Miglitol (Glyset)	25-100 mg tid		

From Franz MJ, Reader D, Monk A: *Implementing group and individual medical nutrition therapy for diabetes,* Alexandria, Va, 2002, American Diabetes Association.
bid, Twice daily; *tid,* three times daily.

presses hepatic glucose production and lowers insulin resistance, but it does not stimulate insulin secretion. It is not associated with hypoglycemia, may cause small weight losses when therapy begins, and improves lipid levels. Adverse effects include gastrointestinal distress, such as abdominal pain, nausea, and diarrhea, in up to 50% of patients. The frequency of these adverse effects can be minimized with food consumption and slow titration of dose. A rare side effect is severe lactic acidosis, which can be fatal. Acidosis usually occurs in patients who use alcohol excessively, have renal dysfunction, or have liver impairments (Inzucchi, 2002). Biguanides can be used alone or in combination with other diabetes medications. Other available agents include metformin extended release (Glucophage XR) and glyburide/metformin (Glucovance).

The TZDs decrease insulin resistance in peripheral tissues and thus enhance the ability of muscle and fat cells to take up glucose. TZDs also have certain lipid benefits. HDL cholesterol increases and triglycerides frequently decrease with TZD therapy. Although LDL cholesterol may increase because of a shift from small and dense to large and buoyant LDL particles, these types of particles are less atherogenic, and thus the increase in LDL cholesterol may not be a concern (Inzucchi, 2002). Adverse effects include weight gain and edema, and these effects are more common in patients who receive TZDs along with insulin. Patients with advanced forms of congestive heart disease or hepatic impairment should not receive TZDs. Troglitazone (Rezulin), the first approved TZD, was removed from the market because of hepatocellular injury. Rosiglitazone (Avandia) and pioglitazone (Actos) are the two TZD drugs currently available and have not been associated with liver injury.

α-Glucosidase inhibitors work in the small intestine to inhibit enzymes that digest carbohydrates, thereby delaying carbohydrate absorption and lowering postprandial glycemia. Acarbose (Precose) and miglitol (Glyset) are competitive inhibitors of intestinal brush-border α-glucosidases required for the breakdown of starches, dextrins, maltose, and sucrose to absorbable monosaccharides. They do not cause hypoglycemia or weight gain when used alone, but they can frequently cause flatulence, diarrhea, cramping, or abdominal pain. Symptoms may be alleviated by initiating therapy at a low dose and gradually increasing the dose to therapeutic levels (Coniff, 1995).

Insulin

Persons with type 1 diabetes depend on insulin to survive. In persons with type 2 diabetes, insulin may be needed to restore glycemia to near normal. Circumstances that require the use of insulin in type 2

TABLE 33-7 Action Times of Human Insulin Preparations

TYPE OF INSULIN	ONSET OF ACTION	PEAK ACTION	USUAL EFFECTIVE DURATION	MONITOR EFFECT IN:
Rapid-acting	<15 min	0.5-1.5 hr	2-4 hr	2 hr
Lispro				
Aspart				
Short-acting	0.5-1 hr	2-3 hr	3-6 hr	4 hr
Regular				
Intermediate-acting				
NPH	2-4 hr	6-10 hr	10-16 hr	8-12 hr
Lente	3-4 hr	6-12 hr	12-18 hr	8-12 hr
Long-acting				
Ultralente	6-10 hr	10-16 hr	18-20 hr	10-12 hr
Glargine (Lantus)	1.1 hr	—	24 hr	10-12 hr
Mixtures	0.5-1 hr	Dual	10-16 hr	
70/30 (70% NPH, 30% regular)				
50/50 (50% NPH, 50% regular)				
75/25 (75% neutral protamine lispro [NPL], 25% lispro)				
70/30 (75% neutral protamine aspart [NPA], 30% aspart)				

From Franz MJ, Reader D, Monk D: *Implementing group and individual medical nutrition therapy for diabetes*, Alexandria, Va, 2002, American Diabetes Association.
NPH, Neutral protamine Hagedorn.

diabetes include the failure to achieve adequate control with administration of oral medications; periods of acute injury, infection, or surgery; pregnancy; and allergy or serious reactions to sulfonylurea agents.

Insulin has four properties: action, concentration, purity, and source. These properties determine its onset, peak, and duration (Table 33-7). Most insulin now is made biosynthetically, purified, and then treated enzymatically to yield human insulin (Burge and Schade, 1997). A major advantage of human insulin is that it produces fewer antibodies and, as a result, can also be used for intermittent periods of insulin treatment, such as during surgery and pregnancy. U-100 is the concentration of insulin available in the United States. This refers to insulin activity per milliliter of insulin; therefore, U-100 means 100 U/ml of insulin. Pen injectors are now being used more frequently as an alternative to the traditional syringe-needle units.

Rapid-acting insulins include insulin lispro (Humalog) and insulin aspart (Novolog) and are used as bolus (mealtime) insulins. They are insulin analogs that differ from human insulin in amino acid sequence but bind to insulin receptors and thus function in a manner similar to human insulin. Both lispro and aspart have an onset of action within 15 minutes, a peak in activity at 60 to 90 min, and a duration of action of 3 to 5 hours. Both result in fewer hypoglycemic episodes compared with regular insulin. In the future, insulin administered via the pulmonary route (inhaled insulin) also may be used as bolus insulin.

Regular is a *short-acting* insulin with an onset of action 15 to 60 minutes after injection and a duration of action ranging from 5 to 8 hours. For best results, the slow onset of regular insulin requires it to be taken 30 to 60 minutes before meals.

Intermediate-acting insulins include NPH and lente. Their appearance is cloudy, and their onset, peak, and duration are similar. Their onset of action is about 2 hours after injection, and their peak effect is from 6 to 10 hours

Long-acting insulins are ultralente and glargine (Lantus). Ultralente has its peak activity 8 to 10 hours after injection and a duration of about 18 to 20 hours. Insulin glargine is the newest insulin on the market and is also an insulin analog. Slow dissolution of glargine at the site of the injection results in a relatively constant and peakless delivery over 24 hours. Glargine is clear in solution, similar to lispro, aspart, and regular, whereas NPH, lente, and ultralente are cloudy. Patients need to be sure they have their vial marked clearly. Glargine cannot be mixed with other insulins and is usually given at bedtime. However, glargine can also be given before any meal, but whichever time is chosen, glargine must be given consistently at that time. Clinical trials have demonstrated lower fasting glucose levels and less hypoglycemia with glargine than with NPH (Vajo et al, 2001). Detemir is a long-acting insulin still under development.

Premixed insulins are also available: 70/30, which is 70% NPH and 30% regular, and 50/50, which is 50% NPH and 50% regular. The addition of neutral protamine to lispro creates an intermediate-acting insulin that has been used in 75/25 combinations with lispro. Similarly, the addition of neutral protamine to aspart creates an immediate-acting insulin that has been used in 10/30 combination with aspart.

All persons with type 1 diabetes and those with type 2 diabetes who no longer produce adequate endogenous insulin need replacement of insulin that mimics normal insulin action. After individuals without diabetes eat, their plasma glucose and insulin concentrations increase rapidly, peak in 30 to 60 minutes, and return to basal concentrations within 2 to 3 hours. To mimic this, rapid-acting (or short-acting) insulin is given before meals, and this is referred to as *bolus* or *mealtime insulin.* Mealtime insulin doses are adjusted based on the amount of carbohydrate in the meal. An insulin-to-carbohydrate ratio can be established for an individual that will guide decisions on the amount of mealtime insulin to inject.

Basal or *background insulin* dose is that amount of insulin required in the postabsorptive state to restrain endogenous glucose output primarily from the liver. Basal insulin also limits lipolysis and excess flux of free fatty acids to the liver.

The type and timing of insulin regimens should be individualized, based on eating and exercise habits and blood glucose concentrations. For normal-weight persons with type 1 diabetes, the required insulin dosage is about 0.5 to 1.0 U per kilogram of body weight per day. About 50% of the total daily insulin dose is used to provide for basal or background insulin needs (such as NPH or glargine). The remainder (rapid-acting insulins, such lispro or aspart) is divided among the meals either proportionate to the carbohydrate content or by giving about 1.0 to 1.5 U insulin per 10 g carbohydrate consumed. The larger amount is usually needed to cover breakfast carbohydrate as a result of the presence in the morning of higher levels of counterregulatory hormones (Rabasa-Lhoret et al, 1999). Persons with type 2 diabetes may require insulin doses in the range of 0.5 to 1.2 U per kilogram of body weight daily. Large doses, even >1.5 U kg of body weight daily, may be required at least initially to overcome prevailing insulin resistance.

A single dose of insulin is seldom effective for optimal blood glucose control in either type of diabetes, although occasionally insulin is added at bedtime to suppress nocturnal hepatic glucose production and to normalize fasting glucose concentrations and oral medications are continued during the day (Yki-Jarvinen et al, 1992).

The administration of basal insulin twice a day may suffice for persons with type 2 diabetes who still have significant endogenous insulin production. A commonly used insulin regimen combines a short-acting (such as regular) or a rapid-acting (such as lispro or aspart) insulin and a basal insulin (such as NPH) given twice a day. The prebreakfast dose consists of about one third regular and two thirds NPH. The presupper dose is usually divided into equal amounts of NPH and regular insulin (Figure 33-3). Another option is to combine regular (or lispro or aspart) and NPH before breakfast, regular (or lispro or aspart) before supper, and NPH or ultralente at bedtime. The NPH (or ultralente) is administered at bedtime to control the early morning surge in blood glucose levels (dawn phenomenon).

For persons with type 1 diabetes and many patients with type 2 diabetes a *flexible insulin regimen* is preferred. Basal insulin, such as NPH, may be adminis-

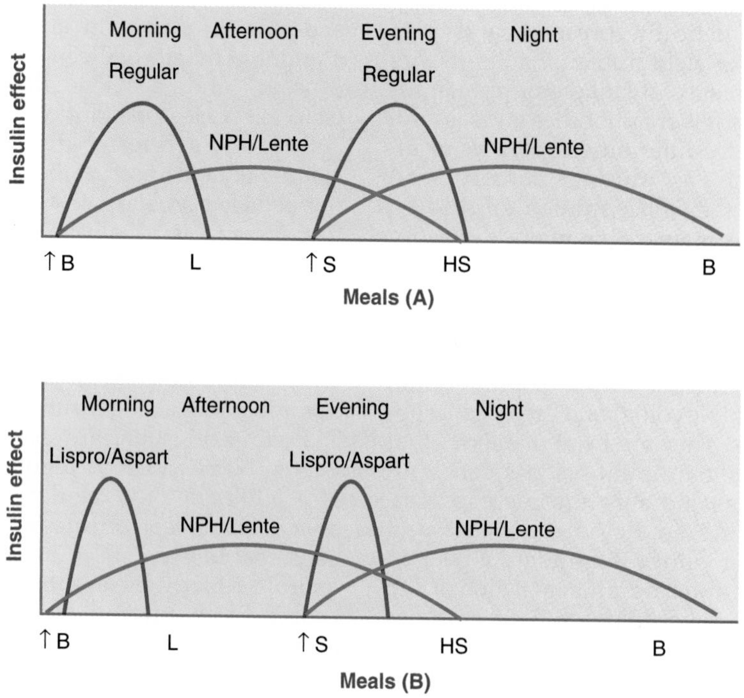

B, Breakfast; *L,* lunch; *S,* supper; *HS,* bedtime snack; *arrow,* time of insulin injection
Schematic representation only

FIGURE 33-3 • Time actions of two-injection insulin regimens.

tered twice a day, before breakfast and at bedtime. Meal insulin is provided by rapid-acting (lispro or aspart) insulin administered with each meal (Figure 33-4). Because of the peaking action of NPH, this regimen often results in erratic glucose levels. The introduction of glargine has provided a solution to many of these problems. With glargine as basal insulin at bedtime and rapid-acting insulin as bolus for meals, insulin doses can be identified more accurately, and initial dosing is simplified (Figure 33-5). These types of insulin regimens allow increased flexibility in the type and timing of meals.

Insulin pump therapy provides basal rapid-acting or short-acting insulin pumped continuously by a mechanical device in micro amounts through a subcutaneous catheter that is monitored 24 hours a day.

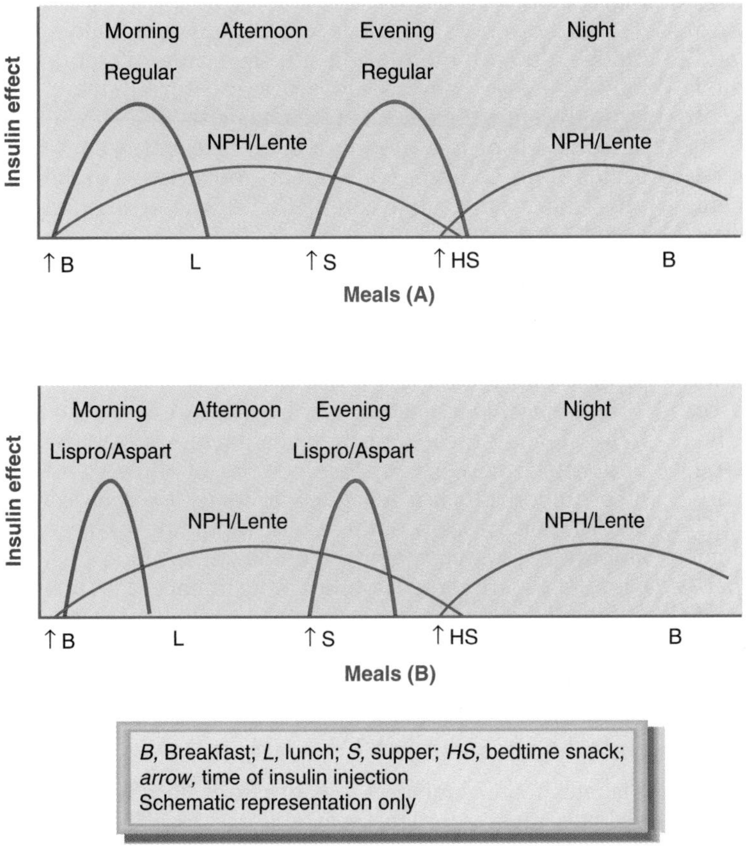

FIGURE 33-4 • Time actions of multiple-action insulin regimens. (Modified from Skyler US: *Medical management of type 1 diabetes,* ed 3, Alexandria, Va, 1998, American Diabetes Association.)

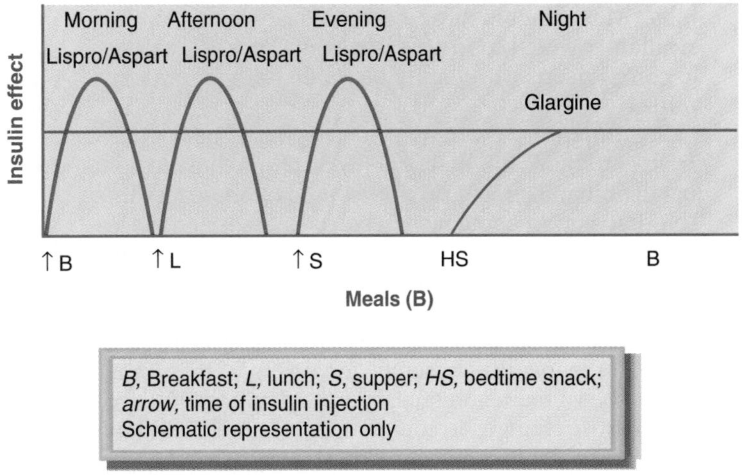

FIGURE 33-5 • Time actions of flexible insulin regimens. (Modified from Skyler US: *Medical management of type 1 diabetes,* ed 3, Alexandria, Va, 1998, Americam Diabetes Association.

Both lispro and aspart work well in insulin pumps, resulting in improved glycemia and less hypoglycemia than with regular insulin (Bode and Strange, 2001). Boluses of the insulin are given before meals. Pump therapy requires a committed and motivated person who is willing to do a minimum of four blood glucose tests per day, to keep blood glucose and food records, and to learn the technical features of pump use.

Blood Glucose Monitoring

Self-monitoring of blood glucose (SMBG) is used on a day-to-day basis to manage diabetes effectively and safely; however, laboratory measurement of glycated hemoglobin provides the best available index of overall diabetes control.

The health care team, including the individual with diabetes, should work together to implement blood glucose monitoring and establish individual target blood glucose goals (see Table 33-4 for a listing of these goals). The frequency of monitoring depends on the type of diabetes and overall therapy.

Patients can perform SMBG up to eight times per day—before breakfast, lunch, and dinner; at bedtime; 1 to 2 hours after meals; and during the night or whenever needed to determine causes of hypoglycemia or hyperglycemia. For most patients with type 1 diabetes, SMBG is recommended four or more times a day, before each meal and at bedtime. SMBG in patients with type 2 diabetes should be sufficient to facilitate reaching glucose goals and is often performed one to four times a day, often before breakfast and before and 2 hours after the largest meal but only 3 or 4 days per week. When adding to or modifying therapy, type 1 and type 2 patients with diabetes should test more often than usual (ADA, 2002d).

Because the accuracy of SMBG is instrument and user dependent, it is important for health care providers to evaluate each patient's monitoring techniques, both initially and at regular intervals thereafter. Comparisons between results from patient self-testing in the clinic and simultaneous laboratory testing are useful to assess the accuracy of patient results. Most meters now automatically convert the capillary whole-blood test to plasma glucose values so comparisons can readily be made with laboratory values.

It is important that the results of SMBG be written in a record book and that patients be taught how to adjust their management program based on these results. The first step in using such records is to learn how to identify patterns in blood glucose levels and how to adjust basic insulin doses. For example, if blood glucose levels are consistently (generally 3 days in a row) elevated at a specific testing time, adjustments are made in the insulin or medication acting at that time. After pattern management is mastered, algorithms for insulin dose changes to compensate for an elevated or low glucose value can be added.

In using blood glucose monitoring records, it should be remembered that factors other than food affect blood glucose concentrations. An increase in blood glucose can be the result of insufficient insulin or insulin secretagogue, too much food, or increases in glucagon and other counterregulatory hormones as a result of stress, illness, or infection. Factors that contribute to hypoglycemia include too much insulin or insulin secretagogue, not enough food, unusual amounts of exercise, and skipped or delayed meals. Urine glucose testing, frequently used in the past, has so many limitations that it should not used.

It is now possible to do continuous ambulatory blood glucose monitoring to determine 24-hour blood glucose patterns and to detect unrecognized hypoglycemia. One such system consists of a subcutaneous sensor that monitors interstitial glucose levels for up to 72 hours. Data can be downloaded in the physician's office after completion of the prescribed cycle. Another device is worn on the wrist and can provide up to three glucose readings each hour for a maximum of 12 hours. It works through a process called *reverse iontophoresis,* in which a low-level electric current passes through intact skin and extracts glucose molecules.

Urine or blood testing can be used to detect ketones. Testing for ketonuria or ketonemia should be performed regularly during periods of illness and when blood glucose levels consistently exceed 240 mg/dl. The presence of persistent, moderate, or large amounts of ketones, along with elevated blood glucose levels, requires insulin adjustments. Persons with type 2 diabetes rarely have ketosis; however, ketone testing should be done when the person is seriously ill.

Self-Management Education

Diabetes management is a team effort. Persons with diabetes must be at the center of the team because they have the responsibility for day-to-day management. Dietitians, nurses, physicians, and other health care providers contribute their expertise to developing therapeutic regimens that help the person with diabetes achieve the best metabolic control possible. The goal is to provide patients with the knowledge, skills, and motivation to incorporate self-management into their daily lifestyles.

For newly diagnosed patients, a staged approach to education should be used. Education initially focuses on the needed basic skills (Box 33-2). Optimal self-management of diabetes requires changes in existing behaviors in addition to the adoption of new ones. Successful behavioral change requires comprehensive education, skill development, and motivation (see Chapter 22). The knowledge and skills needed to implement nutritional recommendations cannot be acquired in one session; therefore, continued nutrition education is essential and must be an ongoing component of diabetes care (Box 33-3).

Box 33-2. Medical Nutrition Therapy Basic Self-Management Education Skills for Persons With Diabetes

- Basic food and meal planning guidelines
- Physical activity guidelines
- Self-monitoring of blood glucose levels
- For insulin or insulin secretagogue users, signs, symptoms, treatment, and prevention of hypoglycemia
- For insulin or insulin secretagogue users, guidelines for managing short-term illness
- Plans for follow-up and ongoing education

Modified from American Dietetic Association: *Medical nutrition therapy evidence-based guides for practice: nutrition practice guidelines for type 1 and type 2 diabetes,* CD-Rom, Chicago, Ill, 2001, American Dietetic Association.

Box 33-3. Essential Self-Management Nutrition Education Skills*

- Sources of carbohydrate, protein, fat
- Understanding nutrition labels
- Modification of fat intake
- Alcohol consumption guidelines
- Use of blood glucose monitoring data for problem solving related to food choices and physical activity options
- Use of blood glucose monitoring data to identify blood glucose patterns and need for medication changes
- Adjustments in carbohydrate or insulin for exercise
- Grocery shopping guidelines
- Guidelines for eating out: restaurant, cafeteria, school lunch
- Snack choices
- Mealtime adjustments
- Use of sugar-containing foods and nonnutritive sweeteners
- Recipes, menu ideas, cookbooks
- Behavior modification techniques
- Problem-solving tips for birthdays, special occasions, holidays
- Travel, schedule changes
- Vitamin, mineral, and botanical supplements
- Work shift rotation, if needed

Modified from American Dietetic Association: *Medical nutrition therapy evidence-based guides for practice: nutrition practice guidelines for type 1 and type 2 diabetes,* CD-Rom, Chicago, Ill, 2001, American Dietetic Association.

*Topics emphasized based on patient's lifestyle, level of nutrition knowledge, and experiences in planning, purchasing, and preparing food and meals.

DIABETES AND AGE-RELATED ISSUES

Children and Adolescents

Involvement of a multidisciplinary team, including a physician, dietitian, nurse, and behavioral specialist, all trained in pediatric diabetes, is the best means of achieving optimal diabetes management in youth. The most important team members, however, are the child or adolescent and his or her family.

A complete nutrition assessment, which is the basis for the food and meal plan for youth with diabetes, includes anthropometric measurements, nutrition assessment and food history, biochemical indices, assessment of feelings and family concerns related to nutrition and diabetes, and typical activity patterns (see Chapters 17 and 18).

A major nutrition goal for children and adolescents with type 1 diabetes is maintenance of normal growth and development. Possible causes of poor weight gain and linear growth include poor glycemic control, inadequate insulin, and overrestriction of calories. The last may be a consequence of the common erroneous belief that restricting food, rather than adjusting insulin, is the way to control blood glucose. Other reasons unrelated to diabetes management include thyroid abnormalities and malabsorption syndromes. Excessive weight gain can be due to excessive caloric intake, overtreatment of hypoglycemia, or overinsulinization. Other causes include low physical activity levels and hypothyroidism (accompanied by poor linear growth) (Drash, 1993).

The nutrition prescription is based on the nutrition assessment. Newly diagnosed children often present with weight loss and hunger; as a result, the initial meal plan must be based on adequate calories to restore and maintain appropriate body weight. In about 4 to 6 weeks, the initial caloric level may need to be modified to meet more usual caloric requirements. Children have a natural ability to know how much to eat for normal growth and development. Table 33-8 lists a formula that can be used to confirm that a child or adolescent is receiving the minimum number of calories necessary for growth and development. Height and weight should be recorded on growth charts every 3 to 6 months to make sure children are growing normally. If not, the overall diabetes management plan needs to be assessed. For growth charts see Appendixes 6 to 11, 18, and 19. Caloric needs in children change continuously, and so food intake should be evaluated every 3 to 6 months.

Individualized food and meal plans, insulin regimens using basal (background) and bolus (mealtime) insulins, and insulin algorithms can provide flexibility for children with type 1 diabetes and their families. This approach accommodates irregular meal times and schedules and varying appetites and activity levels (ADA, 2002b).

Daily eating patterns in young children generally include three meals and two or three snacks, depending on the length of time between meals and the child's physical activity level. Children often prefer smaller meals and snacks. Snacks can prevent hypoglycemia between meals and provide adequate calories. Older children and teens may prefer only three meals. Blood glucose monitoring data are then used to integrate an insulin regimen into the meal, snack, and exercise schedules.

Realistic blood glucose goals should be determined and discussed with the youth and family. Youth with diabetes are also more likely than their age- and sex-matched nondiabetic peers to be at risk for cardiovascular disease. It is therefore essential to reduce the risk factors in youth with type 1 diabetes. Lipid levels should be monitored regularly, and National Cholesterol Education Program treatment guidelines for children and adolescents should be followed (ADA, 2003b) (see Chapter 35).

After the appropriate nutrition prescription has been determined, the meal planning approach can be selected. Most pediatric educators agree that it is better to start with a more precise meal plan and then teach flexibility than to start with flexibility and try to teach precise planning later. A number of meal planning approaches can be used. Carbohydrate counting for food planning provides youth and their families with guidelines that facilitate glycemic control while still allowing the choice of many common foods that children and adolescents enjoy. Whatever approach to food planning is used, however, the youth and family must find it understandable and applicable to their lifestyle. Blood glucose records are essential to assist the dietitian and other team members in making appropriate changes in insulin regimens.

TABLE 33-8 Estimating Minimum Energy Requirements for Youth

Base energy requirements on food and nutrition assessment
Validate energy needs

AGE	ENERGY REQUIREMENTS
1 yr	1000 kcal for the first year
Toddler	
2-11 yr	Add 100 kcal/yr to 1000 kcal; up to 2000 kcal at age 10
Girls	
12-15 yr	2000 kcal plus 50-100 kcal/yr per year after age 10
>15 yr	Calculate as for an adult
Boys	
12-15 yr	2000 kcal plus 200 kcal/yr per year after age 10
>15 yr	Sedentary: 16 kcal/lb (30-35 kcal/kg) Moderate physical activity: 18 kcal/lb (40 kcal/kg) Very physically active: 23 kcal/lb (50 kcal/kg)

Data from Franz MJ, Reader D, Monk D: *Implementing group and individual medical nutrition therapy for diabetes,* Alexandria, Va, 2002, American Diabetes Association.

Type 2 Diabetes in Youth

Childhood obesity has been accompanied by an increase in the prevalence of type 2 diabetes among children and adolescents. Impaired glucose tolerance has been shown to be highly prevalent in obese youth, irrespective of ethnic group, and is associated with insulin resistance. Once type 2 diabetes develops, β-cell failure is also a factor (Sinha et al, 2002). Thus, type 2 diabetes in youth appears to follow a progressive pattern similar to type 2 diabetes in adults.

Successful lifestyle treatment of type 2 diabetes in children and adolescents involves cessation of excessive weight gain, promotion of normal growth and development, and the achievement of blood glucose and A1C goals (ADA, 2000). Nutrition guidelines should also address comorbidities, such as hypertension and dyslipidemia. Behavior modification strategies to decrease intake of high-caloric, high-fat food while encouraging healthy eating habits and regular physical activity for the entire family should be considered. Unfortunately, successful lifestyle treatment regimens for youth with type 2 diabetes have not been defined (ADA, 2002b). Metformin is often used when lifestyle strategies alone have not achieved target glucose goals and has been shown to be safe and effective for the treatment of pediatric type 2 diabetes (Jones et al, 2002). Some youth may also require insulin therapy to achieve adequate glycemic control.

Pregnancy

Normalization of blood glucose levels during pregnancy is very important for women who have preexisting diabetes or who develop GDM. MNT goals are to assist in achieving and maintaining optimal blood glucose control, to provide adequate maternal and fetal nutrition, to supply energy intake for appropriate maternal weight gain, and to provide necessary vitamin and mineral supplements (ADA, 2002b).

Preexisting Diabetes and Pregnancy

Preconception counseling and the ability to achieve near-normal blood glucose levels before pregnancy have been shown to be effective in reducing the incidence of anomalies in infants born to women with preexisting diabetes to nearly that of the general population (Kitzmiller et al, 1996). Normal blood glucose levels are lower during pregnancy. Table 33-9 outlines blood glucose goals during pregnancy for preexisting diabetes and for GDM (ADA, 2002e; Jovanovic, 2000).

As a result of hormonal changes during the first trimester, blood glucose levels are often erratic. Although caloric needs do not differ from those preceding pregnancy, the meal plan may need to be adjusted to accommodate the metabolic changes. Women should be educated about the increased risk of hypoglycemia during pregnancy and cautioned against overtreatment.

The need for insulin increases during the second and third trimesters of pregnancy. This is the reason why screening for GDM is done between weeks 24 and 28 of pregnancy. At 38 to 40 weeks' postconception, insulin needs and levels peak at two to three times prepregnancy levels. Pregnancy-associated hormones that are antagonistic to the action of insulin lead to an elevation of blood glucose levels. For women with preexisting diabetes, this increased insulin need must be met with increased exogenous insulin.

Meal plan adjustments are necessary to provide the additional calories required to support fetal growth. Weight gain should be monitored, and guidelines for appropriate weight gain that apply to women without diabetes also apply to women with diabetes. Regular follow-up visits are needed to also monitor caloric and nutrient intake, blood glucose control, and whether there is starvation ketosis. Urine or blood ketones during pregnancy may signal starvation ketosis that can be caused by inadequate energy or carbohydrate intake, omission of meals or snacks, or prolonged intervals between meals (e.g., more than 10 hours between the bedtime snack and breakfast). Ketonemia during pregnancy has been associated with reduced IQ scores in children (Rizzo et al, 1991). Women should be instructed to test for ketones periodically before breakfast.

Nutrition therapy is individualized according to the food and nutrition history, prepregnancy weight, and physical activity levels. Generally, an additional 100 to 300 kcal daily is added to the meal plan at the beginning of the second trimester. The increased calorie requirement can be met easily by the addition of one or two cups of reduced-fat or skim milk and 1 to 2 oz of meat or meat substitute. This also provides adequately for the increased protein need. Smaller meals and more frequent snacks are often needed to prevent hypoglycemia. A late-evening snack is especially important to decrease the likelihood of overnight starvation ketosis. Records of food intake and blood glucose values are essential for determining whether glycemic goals are being met and for preventing and correcting ketosis.

TABLE 33-9 Plasma Glucose Goals During Pregnancy

TEST	PREEXISTING DIABETES (mg/dl)	GESTATIONAL DIABETES (mg/dl)
Fasting plasma glucose	65-100	80-110
Premeal	65-110	
1 hr postprandial	<145	<155
2 hr postprandial	<135	<130
2 to 6 hr postprandial	65-135	
Normal values during pregnancy		
Fasting plasma glucose:	70-105	
1-2 hr postprandial:	≤140	

Modified from Jovanovic L, editor: *Medical management of pregnancy complicated by diabetes,* ed 3, Alexandria, Va, 2000, American Diabetes Association, and American Diabetes Association: Gestational diabetes mellitus [Position Statement], *Diabetes Care* 25(suppl 1):S94, 2002.

Gestational Diabetes Mellitus

About 7% of all pregnancies are complicated by GDM, resulting in more than 200,000 cases annually (ADA, 2002e). After delivery, about 90% of all women with GDM become normoglycemic but are at increased risk of developing GDM earlier in subsequent pregnancies and are at increased risk for developing type 2 diabetes. Although estimates vary, within 4 years after pregnancy, about 30% to 40% of women with GDM who are obese will develop type 2 diabetes (ADA, 2001). Avoidance of obesity in women before and after pregnancy reduces the risk of subsequent type 2 diabetes.

Because fetal morbidity may be increased, a risk assessment for GDM should be done at the first prenatal visit and for women at high risk (those with marked obesity, previous history of GDM, glycosuria, or a strong family history of diabetes) as soon as possible. An FPG of 126 mg/dl or higher or a casual PG of 200 mg/dl meets the threshold for the diagnosis of diabetes and, if confirmed on a second day, requires no further testing (ADA, 2002a). High-risk women not found to have GDM at the initial screening and average risk women (a few women can be classified as low-risk) should be tested between 24 to 28 weeks' gestation. An oral glucose challenge (which does not have to be preceded by fasting) with a 50-g glucose load is performed, and an elevated plasma glucose level (≥140 mg/dl) 1 hour later is considered an indication of the need for diagnostic testing. The criteria for the diagnosis of GDM based on a 100-g oral glucose tolerance test (OGTT) are listed in Table 33-10. Low-risk women who do not need to be screened must meet all the following criteria: younger than 25 years of age; normal body weight; no family history of diabetes; no history of abnormal glucose tolerance; and not a member of an ethnic or racial group with a high prevalence of diabetes (ADA, 2002a).

Limited research has been done to determine the ideal diet for GDM. In general, the overall nutrition recommendations for preexisting diabetes also apply to GDM, although the diagnosis is generally not made before the second or third trimester. The goal of nutrition therapy is to provide adequate energy levels for appropriate gestational weight gain, achievement and maintenance of normoglycemia, and absence of ketones. Individualization of the meal plan

TABLE 33-10 Diagnosis of Gestational Diabetes Mellitus (GDM)

TYPE OF TEST	RESULTS
Screening during pregnancy—a 50-g oral glucose challenge (does not have to be fasting) at 24 to 28 wk gestation	A plasma glucose level ≥140 mg/dl (≥7.8 mmol/L) 1 hr later indicates the need for further diagnostic testing.
Oral glucose tolerance test with an abnormal screen	After a 100-g oral glucose load, GDM may be diagnosed if two plasma glucose values equal or exceed: **Fasting:** ≥95 mg/dl **1 hr:** ≥180 mg/dl **2 hr:** ≥155 mg/dl **3 hr:** ≥140 mg/dl

Modified from American Diabetes Association: Standards of medical care for patients with diabetes mellitus [Position Statement], *Diabetes Care* 25(suppl 1):S33, 2002.

is recommended, as the ideal percentage and type of carbohydrate is controversial. Monitoring blood glucose, urine and blood ketones, appetite, and weight gain can aid in developing an appropriate, individualized meal plan and in adjusting the meal plan throughout pregnancy (ADA, 2002b).

Nutrition practice guidelines for gestational diabetes have been developed and field-tested (Reader and Sipe, 2001). With input from patients, the dietitian designs a food and meal plan; however, without blood glucose monitoring data, it is impossible to assess its effectiveness. Food and blood glucose records guide nutrition therapy, and alterations to food plans are used to assess outcomes of therapy and, along with weight changes, determine whether insulin therapy is needed. Insulin therapy is added if glucose goals exceed target range (see Table 33-9) on two or more occasions in a 1- to 2-week period without some obvious explanation from food records or if glucose levels are consistently elevated because of patients' dietary indiscretions after MNT intervention. Weight gain or lack of weight gain and ketone testing can be useful in determining whether patients are undereating to keep glucose levels within target range to avoid insulin therapy.

Medical nutrition therapy involves developing a carbohydrate-controlled, consistent food and meal plan. Generally, 40% to 45% of total energy intake will be from carbohydrate, which is distributed throughout the day in three small to moderate-sized meals and two to four snacks. An evening snack is usually needed to prevent accelerated ketosis overnight. Carbohydrate is not as well tolerated at breakfast as it is at other meals because of increased levels of cortisol and growth hormones. To compensate for this, the initial food plan may have 30 to 45 g of carbohydrate at breakfast. To satisfy hunger, protein foods, because they do not affect blood glucose levels, can be added.

Although caloric restriction must be viewed with caution, in obese women with GDM, a 30% caloric restriction (an intake of about 1700 to 1800 kcal daily) can reduce hyperglycemia with no increase in ketonuria (Knopp et al, 1991). Intake below these levels is not advised. The pattern of weight gain during pregnancy for women with GDM should be similar to that of women without diabetes.

Exercise can also assist in overcoming peripheral resistance to insulin and in controlling postprandial hyperglycemia. It may be used as an adjunct to nutrition therapy to improve maternal glycemia. The ideal form of exercise is unknown, but a brisk walk after meals is often recommended.

Older Adults

The prevalence of diabetes and IGT increases dramatically as people age. Many factors predispose older adults to diabetes: age-related decreases in insulin production and increases in insulin resistance, adiposity, decreased physical activity, multiple prescription medications, genetics, and coexisting illnesses. A major factor appears to be insulin resistance. Controversy persists as to whether the insulin resistance is itself a primary change or whether it is attributable to reduced physical activity, decreased lean body mass, and increased adipose tissue, which are all frequently seen in older adults. Abdominal obesity also correlates with insulin resistance in older adults (Kohrt et al, 1993). Furthermore, medications used to treat coexisting diseases may complicate diabetes therapy in older persons.

Despite the increase in glucose intolerance with age, aging per se should not be a reason for suboptimal control of blood glucose. Even if it is incorrectly assumed that preventing long-term diabetic complications is not relevant to the care of older adults, persistent hyperglycemia has deleterious effects on the body's defense mechanisms against infection. It also increases the pain threshold by exacerbating neuropathic pain, and it has a detrimental effect on the outcome of cerebrovascular accidents.

Exercise training can significantly reduce the decline in aerobic capacity that occurs with age, improve risk factors for atherosclerosis, slow the decline in age-related lean body mass, decrease central adiposity, and improve insulin sensitivity.

A daily multivitamin supplement may be appropriate for older adults, especially those with reduced energy intake. All older adults should have a calcium intake of at least 1200 mg daily and a vitamin D intake of 15 μg or 600 IU per day.

Malnutrition, not obesity, is often the more prevalent nutrition-related problem of older adults. It often remains subclinical or unrecognized because the result of malnutrition—excessive loss of lean body mass—resembles the signs and symptoms of the aging process. Until a primary disease develops or chronic problems are exacerbated by illness or some other stress, malnutrition may remain unrecognized. Both malnutrition and diabetes adversely affect wound healing and defense against infection, and malnutrition is associated with depression and cognitive deficits. The most reliable indicator of poor nutritional status in older adults is probably a change in body weight. In general, involuntary weight gain or loss of more than 10 pounds or 10% of body weight in less than 6 months indicates a need to evaluate whether the reason is nutrition related (ADA, 2002b).

Because of concern over malnutrition, it is essential that older adults, especially those in long-term care settings, be provided a diet that meets their nutritional needs, enables them to attain or maintain a reasonable body weight, helps control blood glucose, and is palatable. The imposition of dietary restriction on older residents in long-term health facilities is not warranted. Residents should be served the regular (unrestricted) menu with consistency in the amount and timing of carbohydrate (ADA, 2002f).

In older adults, acute hyperglycemia and dehydration can lead to a serious complication of diabetes: the hyperglycemic hyperosmolar state (HHS). Patients with HHS have a very high blood glucose level (ranging from 400 to 2800 mg/dl, with an average of 1000 mg/dl) without ketones. Patients are markedly dehydrated, and mental status often ranges from mild confusion to hallucinations or coma. Treatment includes provision of adequate fluids as well as blood glucose control.

Box 33-4. Food/Nutrition Assessment

- *Minimum referral data:* age, diagnosis of diabetes and other pertinent medical history, diabetes and other pertinent medications, laboratory data (A1C, cholesterol fractionation, albumin-to-creatinine ratio, and blood pressure), and clearance for exercise
- *Diabetes history:* previous diabetes education, use of blood glucose monitoring, diabetes problems/concerns (hypoglycemia, hyperglycemia, fear of insulin)
- *Food/nutrition history:* current eating habits with beginning modifications
- *Social history:* occupation, hours worked/away from home, living situation, financial issues
- *Medications/supplements:* medications taken, vitamin/mineral/supplement use, herbal supplements

Modified from Franz MJ, Reader D, Monk A: *Implementing group and individual medical nutrition therapy for diabetes,* Alexandria, Va, 2002, American Diabetes Association.

IMPLEMENTING NUTRITION SELF-MANAGEMENT

Medical nutrition therapy begins with developing rapport with the patient, and whether provided individually or in groups, MNT involves a common process—assessment (evaluation at follow-up visits), intervention including self-management education, goal setting, and communication (documentation) (see Chapter 21). If MNT is to be implemented individually, the intervention is then individualized based on the needs of the patient and whether the intervention is for initial, continuing, or intensive care.

Providing MNT in groups is becoming increasingly more important, since reimbursement criteria for diabetes self-management education and for MNT recommend that when possible group sessions are preferable. It is helpful if the group participants are similar in their stage of diabetes management and if they all speak and understand the same language. Group education shifts more responsibility to the patient to provide the needed initial assessment information, to evaluate outcomes, and to decide about therapy changes (Franz, Reader, and Monk, 2002). Group interventions for diabetes self-management education, when compared with individual interventions, have produced similar positive outcomes (Rickheim et al, 2002). Implementation of group MNT is covered in *Implementing Group and Individual Medical Nutrition Therapy for Diabetes* (Franz, Reader, and Monk, 2002).

Assessment

To develop an individualized nutrition care plan, the following parameters are assessed: anthropometric measures (height, weight, BMI), laboratory data, food and nutrition history, learning style, cultural heritage, and socioeconomic status. Box 33-4 provides a summary of such assessment data. Food and eating histories can be done several ways, with the objective being to determine a schedule and pattern of eating that will be the least disruptive to the lifestyle of the individual with diabetes and, at the same time, will facilitate improved metabolic control. With this objective in mind, asking the individual either to record or report what, how much, and when he or she typically eats during a 24-hour period may be the most useful.

Another approach is to ask the patient to keep and bring with him or her a 3-day or 1-week food intake record. This request can be made when an appointment with the dietitian is scheduled. Assessment of the most typical daily pattern can then be made. The history can also reveal other useful information, including (1) usual caloric intake; (2) quality of the usual diet; (3) times, sizes, and contents of meals and snacks; (4) food idiosyncrasies; (5) frequency with which meals are eaten in restaurants; (6) who usually prepares food;

(7) eating problems (e.g., as related to dental, gastrointestinal or other problems); (8) alcoholic beverage intake; and (9) supplements used (see Chapter 17).

It is also essential to learn about the patient's daily routine and schedule. The following information is needed: (1) time of waking; (2) usual meal and eating times; (3) work schedule or school hours; (4) type, amount, and timing of exercise; and (5) usual sleep habits.

Using the assessment data and food and nutrition history information, a preliminary food and meal plan can then be designed and, if the patient desires, sample menus provided. Developing a food and meal plan does not begin with a set calorie or macronutrient prescription; instead, it is determined by modifying the usual food intake as necessary. The worksheet in Figure 33-6 can be used to record the usual foods eaten and to modify the usual diet as necessary. The macronutrient and caloric values for the exchange lists are listed on the form and in Table 33-11. See Appendix 53 for portion sizes of the foods on the exchange lists. These tools are useful in evaluating nutrition assessments. Using the form in Figure 33-6, the dietitian begins by totaling the number of exchanges from each list and multiplying this number by the grams of carbohydrate, protein, and fat contributed by each. Next the grams of carbohydrate, protein, and fat are totaled from each column; the grams of carbohydrate and protein are then multiplied by 4 (4 kcal/g of carbohydrate and protein), and the grams of fat are multiplied by 9 (9 kcal/g of fat). Total calories and percentage of calories from each macronutrient can then be determined. Numbers derived from these calculations are then rounded off. Figure 33-7 provides an example of a preliminary food and meal plan. In this example, the nutrition prescription would be the following:

1900-2000 calories
230 g of carbohydrate (50%)
90 g of protein (20%)
65 g of fat (30%)

The number of carbohydrate choices for each meal and snack is the total of the starch, fruit, and milk servings. Vegetables, unless starchy or eaten in very large amounts (three or more servings per meal), are generally considered "free foods." The carbohydrate choices are circled under each meal and snack column. Table 33-12 is an example of a sample meal plan and menu based on Figure 33-7.

The next step is to evaluate the preliminary meal plan. First and foremost, does the patient with diabetes think it is feasible to implement the meal plan

	Meal/Snack/Time										
Food Group	Breakfast	Snack	Lunch	Snack	Dinner	Snack	Total servings/day	CHO (g)	Protein (g)	Fat (g)	Calories
Starches								15	3	1	80
Fruit								15			60
Milk								12	8	1	90
Vegetables								5	2		25
Meats/ Substitutes									7	5(3)	75(55)
Fats										5	45
CHO Choices							Total grams				
							Calories/ gram	X4=	X4=	X9=	Total calories
							Percent calories				

Calculations are based on medium-fat meats and skim/very low-fat milk. If diet consists predominantly of low-fat meats, use the factor 3 g instead of 5 g fat; if predominantly high-fat meats, use 8 g fat. If low-fat (2%) milk is used, use 5 g fat; if whole milk is used, use 8 g fat.

FIGURE 33-6 • Worksheet for assessment and design of a meal or food plan. *CHO*, Carbohydrate.

into his or her lifestyle? Second, is it appropriate for diabetes management? Third, are the calories appropriate? Fourth, does it encourage healthful eating?

To answer the first question concerning the feasibility of the food plan, the food and meal plan is reviewed with the patient in terms of general food intake. Timing of meals and snacks and approximate portion sizes and types of foods are discussed. Later, a meal-planning approach can be selected that will assist the patient in making his or her own food

TABLE 33-11 Macronutrient and Caloric Values for Exchange Lists*

GROUPS/LISTS	CARBOHYDRATE (g)	PROTEIN (g)	FAT (g)	CALORIES
Carbohydrate Group				
Starch	15	3	0-1	80
Fruit	15	—	—	60
Milk				
Skim	12	8	0-3	90
Reduced-fat	12	8	5	120
Whole	12	8	8	150
Other carbohydrates	15	Varies	Varies	Varies
Vegetables	5	2	—	25
Meat and Meat Substitute Group				
Very lean	—	7	0-1	35
Lean	—	7	3	55
Medium-fat	—	7	5	75
High-fat	—	7	8	100
Fat Group	—	—	5	45

From American Diabetes Association and American Dietetic Association: *Exchange lists for meal planning,* Alexandria, Va, 1995, American Diabetes Association.
*See Appendix 53.

Food Group	Breakfast 7:30 AM	Snack 10:00	Lunch 12:00	Snack 3:00	Dinner 6:30	Snack 10:00	Total servings/day	CHO (g)	Protein (g)	Fat (g)	Calories
Starches	2	1	2–3	1	2–3	1–2	10	15 150	3 30	1 10	80
Fruit	1		1		1	0–1	3	15 45			60
Milk	1				1		2	12 24	8 16	1 2	90
Vegetables			✓		✓			5 10	2 4		25
Meats/ Substitutes			2–3		3–4		6		7 42	5(3) 30	75(55)
Fats	1	0–1	1–2	0–1	1–2	0–1	5			5 25	45
CHO Choices	3–4 CHO	1 CHO	3–4 CHO	1 CHO	4–5 CHO	1–2 CHO	Total grams	229	92	67	
							Calories/ gram	X4= 916	X4= 368	X9= 603	Total calories
							Percent calories	50	19	30	1900–2000

1900–2000 calories
230 g CHO-50%
90 g protein-20%
65 g fat-30%

Calculations are based on medium-fat meats and skim/very low-fat milk. If diet consists predominantly of low-fat meats, use the factor 3 g, instead of 5 g fat; if predominantly high-fat meats, use 8 g fat. If low-fat (2%) milk is used, use 5 g fat; if whole milk is used, use 8 g fat.

FIGURE 33-7 • An example of a completed worksheet from the assessment, the nutrition prescription, and a sample 1900- to 2000-calorie meal plan. *CHO,* Carbohydrate.

TABLE 33-12 Sample Menu for 1900-2000 Kilocalorie Meal Plan

MEAL/TIMING	FOOD SELECTIONS
Breakfast—7:30 AM	
3-4 Carbohydrate choices (i.e., 2 starch, 1 fruit, 1 milk)	Raisin bran cereal, ½ c Bagel, ¼ (1 oz) Cantaloupe (5-inch), ⅓ Skim milk, 1 c
1 Fat	Reduced-fat cream cheese, 1 tbsp
Snack—10:00 AM	
1 Carbohydrate choice (i.e., 1 starch or fruit)	Bagel, ¼ (1 oz)
0-1 Fat	Reduced-fat cream cheese, 1 tbsp
Lunch—Noon	
3-4 Carbohydrate choices (i.e., 2-3 starches, 1 fruit)	Whole-wheat bread, 2 slices Vegetable-beef soup, 1 c Apple, 1 small
Vegetable	Lettuce and tomato slices
2-3 Meats	Turkey, 2 oz
1-2 Fats	Reduced-fat mayonnaise, 1 tbsp
Snack—3:00 PM	
1 Carbohydrate choice (i.e., 1 starch or fruit)	Pretzels, ¾ oz
0-1 Fat	
Dinner—6:30 PM	
4-5 Carbohydrate choices (i.e., 2-3 starch, 1 fruit, 1 milk)	Baked potato, 1 medium Dinner roll, 1 Mandarin oranges, ¾ c Skim milk, 1 c
Vegetables	Broccoli spears, ½ c Dinner salad, 1 small
3-4 Meats	Chicken breast, baked, 3 oz
1-2 Fats	Sour cream, regular, 2 tbsp Reduced-fat salad dressing, 2 tbsp
Snack—10:00 PM	
1-2 Carbohydrate choices (i.e., 1-2 starches, 0-1 fruit)	Ice cream, light, ½ c Strawberries, 1¼ c
0-1 Fat	

Box 33-5. Estimating Approximate Energy Requirements for Adults

• Obese or very inactive persons and chronic dieters	10-12 kcal/lb (20 kcal/kg)
• Persons >55 yr, active women, sedentary men	13 kcal/lb (25 kcal/kg)
• Active men, very active women	15 kcal/lb (30 kcal/kg)
• Thin or very active men	20 kcal/lb (40 kcal/kg)

Data from Franz MJ, Reader D, Monk A: *Implementing group and individual medical nutrition therapy for diabetes,* Alexandria, Va, 2002, American Diabetes Association.

choices. At this point, it needs to be determined whether this meal plan is reasonable for the patient with diabetes. To determine the appropriateness of the meal plan for diabetes management involves assessing both distribution of the meals (and snacks, if desired) and the macronutrient percentages. Appropriateness is based on the types of medications prescribed as well as treatment goals.

For patients receiving MNT alone, often the food and meal plan begins with three or four carbohydrate servings per meal for women and four or five for men, and, if desired, one or two for a snack. Blood glucose monitoring before the meal and 2 hours after the meal is recommended, with the plasma glucose goal being premeal values below 130 mg/dl and 2-hour postprandial values below 160 to 180 mg/dl.

Patients on oral glucose-lowering medications often do better with smaller meals and snacks, especially if they are taking an insulin secretagogue. Persons with type 2 diabetes, however, generally have fewer problems with hypoglycemia and do not need snacks unless this is their choice. If they choose to have snacks, this cannot be in addition to the usual meals. A portion of the meal should be saved to be eaten as a snack between meals.

For patients who require insulin, the timing of eating is extremely important. Food consumption must be synchronized with the time actions of insulin (see previous section on medications). If the eating pattern is determined first, an insulin regimen can be selected that will fit with it. To prevent overnight hypoglycemia, many patients require a bedtime snack. Often individuals who use morning intermediate-acting insulins (NPH or lente) also require an afternoon snack. Individuals using rapid-acting insulin (lispro or aspart) do not need a snack.

The next step is to determine whether the number of calories is appropriate or realistic for the individual patient. Energy requirements depend on several factors, such as age, gender, height, weight, and activity level. Box 33-5 outlines a simple method for determining approximate caloric requirements based on actual weight. Many dietitians use handheld calculators to determine caloric requirements, and the Harris Benedict equation, with modifications, is generally used in their calculations. The determination of a caloric level for a child or adolescent is also based on the nutrition assessment. Table 33-18 can be used to confirm that the child is receiving the minimum necessary calories.

Methods for determining caloric requirements are only approximate. On a practical basis, they do provide a starting point for evaluating the caloric adequacy of the meal plan. Adjustments in calories can be made during follow-up visits. Parameters that should be taken into consideration are weight changes, feelings of satiety and hunger, and concerns about palatability.

The best way to ensure that the meal plan encourages healthful eating is to encourage patients to eat a variety of foods from all the food groups. The Food Guide Pyramid, with its suggested number of servings from each food group, can be used to compare the patient's meal plan with the nutrition recommendations for all Americans (see Chapter 15).

Intervention and Self-Management Education

This step involves selecting an appropriate meal-planning approach and identifying strategies for behavioral change that enhance motivation and adherence to necessary lifestyle changes. A number of meal-planning approaches are available, ranging from simple guidelines or menus to more complex counting methods (Table 33-13). No single meal-planning approach has been shown to be more effective than any other, and the meal-planning approach selected should allow individuals with diabetes to select appropriate foods for meals and snacks.

A popular approach to meal planning is carbohydrate counting. It can be used as a basic meal-planning approach or for more intensive management. Carbohydrate-counting educational tools are based on the concept that after eating, it is the carbohydrate in foods that is the major predictor of postprandial blood glucose levels. One carbohydrate serving contributes 15 g of carbohydrate.

Facilitating Behavioral Changes

The transtheoretic model was proposed by Prochaska as a general model of intentional behavior change (Prochaska et al, 1994). It includes a sequence of stages along a continuum of behavioral change. Different intervention strategies may be needed for individuals at different stages of the change process. Motivational interventions may work best with patients in the earlier contemplative stages, whereas specific skill-training interventions may be most appropriate for persons who have decided to change. Relapse and recycling through the stages occur quite frequently as patients attempt to modify behaviors (see Chapter 22).

Goal Setting

Short-term goals (days or weeks) are often behavioral goals and relate to lifestyle changes. Common self-management behavioral goals are consistent and include appropriate carbohydrate servings, regular physical activity, correct medication dosage (if needed), and blood glucose monitoring as determined to be needed. Goals should be specific, written in behavioral language, and realistic for the patient.

Before the patient leaves the initial session, plans and an appointment for a follow-up session should be identified. In making plans for follow-up, the patient is asked to keep a 3-day or weekly food record with blood glucose–monitoring data.

Evaluation and Documentation

Outcomes must be identified, and the effectiveness of nutrition interventions must be documented. Monitoring of medical and clinical outcomes should be done after the second or third visit to determine whether the patient is making progress toward established goals. If no progress is evident, the individual and dietitian need to reassess and perhaps revise the nutritional care plan. If altering food intake alone is not achieving metabolic target ranges, the dietitian should recommend that medications be added or adjusted.

Finally, documentation is essential for communication and reimbursement. Box 33-6 lists the areas of the nutrition intervention that require documentation.

Follow-Up and Continuing Medical Nutrition Therapy

Successful nutrition therapy involves a process of assessment, problem solving, adjustment, and readjustment. Food records can be compared with the meal plan, which will help to determine whether the initial meal plan needs changing and can be integrated with the blood glucose–monitoring records to determine changes that can lead to improved glycemic control. For patients receiving oral medications or insulin, it can then be determined whether blood glucose values that are outside target ranges can be corrected with adjustments in the meal plan or whether adjustments in medications are needed.

After the basic food and nutrition strategies have been mastered, other aspects of nutrition education should be presented to increase flexibility in food choices and lifestyle while still maintaining glucose control. Of particular importance is information about eating out and the use of information from food labels. Persons using insulin also need information about how to make adjustments in food intake or insulin when schedules are disrupted.

Nutritional follow-up visits should provide encouragement and ensure realistic expectations for the patient. A change in eating habits is not easy for most people, and they become discouraged without appropriate recognition of their efforts. Patients should be encouraged to speak freely about problems they are having with food and eating patterns. Furthermore, there may be major life changes that require changes in the meal plan. Job and schedule changes, travel, illness, and other factors all have an impact on the meal plan.

TABLE 33-13 Food-Planning Approaches for Diabetes

APPROACH	PUBLICATION	DESCRIPTION
Diabetes nutrition guidelines	*The First Step in Diabetes Meal Planning* (American Diabetes Association and American Dietetic Association)	A pamphlet that provides general guidelines for meal planning based on the Food Guide Pyramid. Designed to be given to patients to use until an individualized meal plan can be implemented; however, for some individuals there may be no need to advance to more complex meal-planning approaches.
	Healthy Food Choices (American Diabetes Association and American Dietetic Association)	A pamphlet that promotes healthy eating. It is divided into two sections: (1) guidelines for making healthy food choices and (2) simplified exchanges lists.
	Healthy Eating for People With Diabetes (International Diabetes Center, Minneapolis, Minn.)	Based on the *plate method*, which visualizes kinds and amounts of food and is used to illustrate portions of common foods in relation to plate size. General guidelines for choosing healthy foods, lowering fat intake, and timing of meals and snacks are included.
	Eating Healthy With Diabetes Easy Reading Guide (American Diabetes Association and American Dietetic Association)	A booklet designed specifically for persons with minimal reading skills. The amount of text is limited, symbols and color codes are used, and concepts and foods are presented visually.
Menu approaches	*Month of Meals: Classic Cooking, Old-Time Favorites, Meals in Minutes, Vegetarian Pleasures,* and *Ethnic Delights* (American Diabetes Association)	Separate books with each book containing 28 days of complete menus for breakfast, lunch, dinner, and snacks. Designed to help patients who need help in planning basic menus for their diabetes.
Carbohydrate counting	*Basic Carbohydrate Counting* (American Diabetes Association and American Dietetic Association)	A pamphlet that outlines what foods are carbohydrates, and average portions sizes. It can be used as a basic meal-planning approach for anyone with diabetes and is based on the concept that after eating, carbohydrate in foods has the major impact on blood glucose levels. One carbohydrate serving = 15 g of carbohydrate.
	Advanced Carbohydrate Counting (American Diabetes Association and American Dietetic Association)	A booklet for individuals who have chosen flexible insulin regimens or an insulin pump. The relationship between carbohydrate eaten and insulin injected can be shown as an insulin-to-carbohydrate ratio. This ratio gives the individual a good guide to how much bolus rapid-acting insulin is needed when eating more or less carbohydrate than usual; however, before insulin ratios can be established, blood glucose levels must be under good control and the usual dose of both the basal and rapid-acting (bolus) insulin determined. The grams of carbohydrate consumed at a meal are divided by the number of units of insulin needed to maintain target glucose goals. This is called an *insulin-to-carbohydrate ratio.* For example, 75 g of carbohydrate may require 8 units of rapid-acting insulin and the insulin-to-carbohydrate ratio would be 1:10. Therefore, for each anticipated addition of 10 g of carbohydrate an additional 1 unit of rapid-acting insulin is needed (or for 10 g less of carbohydrate, 1 less unit of rapid-acting insulin is needed).
	My Food Plan (International Diabetes Center, Minneapolis, Minn.)	A pamphlet that combines both carbohydrate counting and calorie control in a simplified approach. It groups carbohydrate, meat, and fat choices by approximate portion sizes. A form for filling in an individualized meal plan is included.
Exchange list approaches	*Exchange Lists for Meal Planning* (American Diabetes Association and American Dietetic Association) (See Appendix 53.)	A booklet that contains lists that group foods in measures that contribute approximately the same number of calories, carbohydrate, protein, and fat. Foods are divided into three basic lists: carbohydrates, meat and meat substitutes, and fat. An individualized food plan that outlines the number of servings from each list for each meal and for snacks is included.

Modified from Franz MJ, Reader D, Monk A: *Implementing group and individual medical nutrition therapy for diabetes,* Alexandria, Va, 2002, American Diabetes Association.

Box 33-6. Nutrition Care Documentation

Documentation of each MNT visit must include:
- Patient name and identification information
- Date of MNT visit and amount of time spent with patient
- Reason for visit
- Patient's current diagnosis (and relevant past diagnoses)
- Pertinent test results and current medications (name, dose)
- Names of others present during MNT
- Physician's referral for MNT (if billing Medicare)

Summaries of:
- Histories: nutrition, medical, social and family
- Nutrition risk factor assessment
- Nutrition problem list
- MNT intervention provided
  - Food and meal plan
  - Short- and long-term goals
  - Educational topics covered
- Short- and long-term goals
- RD's impressions, patient progress
  - Patient acceptance and understanding
  - Anticipated compliance
  - Successful behavior changes
- Plan of care
  - Additional needed skills or information
  - Additional recommendations
  - Plans for ongoing care

From Franz MJ, Reader D, Monk A: *Implementing group and individual medical nutrition therapy for diabetes,* Alexandria, Va, 2002, American Diabetes Association.
MNT, Medical nutrition therapy; *RD,* registered dietitian.

Box 33-7. Common Causes of Hypoglycemia

Medication errors
Excessive insulin or oral medications
Inadvertent or deliberate errors in insulin doses
Improper timing of insulin in relation to food intake
Intensive insulin therapy
Inadequate food intake
Omitted or inadequate meals or snacks
Delayed meals or snacks
Increased exercise or activity
Unplanned activities
Prolonged duration or increased intensity of exercise
Alcohol intake without food

Modified from Skyler JS, editor: *Medical management of type 1 diabetes,* ed 3, Alexandria, Va, 1998, American Diabetes Association.

ACUTE COMPLICATIONS

Hypoglycemia, diabetic ketoacidosis, and hyperglycemic hyperosmolar state (HHS) are acute complications related to diabetes.

Hypoglycemia

Hypoglycemia (or insulin reaction) is a common side effect of insulin therapy, although patients taking insulin secretagogues can also be affected. Autonomic symptoms are often the first signs of mild hypoglycemia and include shakiness, sweating, palpitations, and hunger. Neuroglycopenic symptoms can also occur at similar glucose levels as autonomic symptoms but with different manifestations. The earliest signs of neuroglycopenia include a slowing down in performance and difficulty concentrating and reading. As blood glucose levels drop further, the following symptoms occur: frank mental confusion and disorientation, slurred or rambling speech, irrational or unusual behaviors, extreme fatigue and lethargy, seizures, and unconsciousness.

Several common causes of hypoglycemia are listed in Box 33-7. In general, a glucose of 70 mg/dl or lower should be treated immediately (Cryer et al, 1994). Even a level of 60 to 80 mg/dl may require a management decision (e.g., carbohydrate ingestion, deferral of exercise, change in insulin dosage). Treatment of hypoglycemia requires ingestion of glucose or carbohydrate-containing food. Although any carbohydrate will raise glucose levels, glucose is the preferred treatment. Commercially available glucose tablets have the advantage of being premeasured to help prevent overtreatment. Ingestion of 15 to 20 g of glucose is an effective but temporary treatment. Initial response to treatment should be seen in about 10 to 20 minutes; however, blood glucose should be evaluated again in about 60 minutes because additional treatment may be necessary (Box 33-8). The form of carbohydrate—liquid or solid—used to treat does not make a difference. Furthermore, adding protein to the carbohydrate does not assist in treatment or prevent subsequent hypoglycemia (Gray et al, 1996). If patients are unable to swallow, administration of subcutaneous or intramuscular glucagon may be needed. Parents, roommates, and spouses should be taught how to mix, draw up, and administer glucagon so that they are properly prepared for emergency situations. Kits that include a syringe prefilled with diluting fluid are available.

Self-monitoring of blood glucose is essential for prevention and treatment of hypoglycemia. Changes in insulin injections, eating, exercise schedules, and travel routines warrant increased frequency of monitoring (Cryer et al, 2003). Some patients experience hypoglycemia unawareness, which means that they

Box 33-8. Treatment of Hypoglycemia

- Immediate treatment with carbohydrate is essential.
  - If the blood glucose level falls below 70 mg/dl (3.9 mmol/L), treat with 15 g of carbohydrate, which is equivalent to:
    - 3 glucose tablets
    - Fruit juice or regular soft drinks, ½ c
    - Saltine crackers, 6
    - Sugar or honey, 1 tbsp
- Wait 15 minutes and retest. If the blood glucose level remains ≤70 mg/dl (≤3.9 mmol/L), treat with another 15 g of carbohydrate.
- Repeat testing and treatment until the blood glucose level returns to within normal range.
- Evaluate the time to the next meal or snack to determine the need for additional food. If it is more than an hour to the next meal, add an additional 15 g of carbohydrate.

Modified from Skyler JS, editor: *Medical management of type 1 diabetes*, ed 3, Alexandria, Va, 1998, American Diabetes Association.

do not experience the usual symptoms. Patients need to be reminded of the need to treat hypoglycemia, even in the absence of symptoms. Patients with recurrent hypoglycemia may not be good candidates for intensive insulin therapy.

Hyperglycemia and Diabetic Ketoacidosis

Hyperglycemia can lead to diabetic ketoacidosis (DKA), a life-threatening but reversible complication characterized by severe disturbances in carbohydrate, protein, and fat metabolism. DKA is always the result of inadequate insulin for glucose utilization. As a result, the body depends on fat for energy, and ketones are formed. Acidosis results from increased production and decreased utilization of acetoacetic acid and 3-β-hydroxybutyric acid from fatty acids. These ketones spill into the urine, hence the reliance on testing for ketones.

Diabetic ketoacidosis is characterized by elevated blood glucose levels (≥250 mg/dl but generally <600 mg/dl) and the presence of ketones in the blood and urine. Symptoms include polyuria, polydipsia, hyperventilation, dehydration, the fruity odor of ketones, and fatigue. SMBG, testing for ketones, and medical intervention can all help prevent DKA. If left untreated, DKA can lead to coma and death. Treatment includes supplemental insulin, fluid and electrolyte replacement, and medical monitoring. Acute illnesses, such as flu, colds, vomiting, and diarrhea, if not managed appropriately, can lead to the development of DKA. Patients need to know the steps to take during acute illness to prevent DKA (Box 33-9). During acute illness, oral ingestion of about 150 to 200 g of carbohydrate per day should be sufficient, along with medication adjustments, to keep glucose in the goal range and to prevent starvation ketosis (ADA, 2002b).

Box 33-9. Sick-Day Guidelines for Persons With Diabetes

1. During acute illnesses, take usual doses of insulin. The need for insulin continues, or may even increase, during periods of illness. Fever, dehydration, infection, or the stress of illness can trigger the release of counterregulatory or "stress" hormones, causing blood glucose levels to become elevated.
2. Monitoring of blood glucose levels and urine or blood testing for ketones should be done at least four times daily (before each meal and at bedtime). Blood glucose readings exceeding 240 mg/dl and ketones are danger signals indicating that additional insulin is needed.
3. If regular foods are not tolerated, liquid or soft carbohydrate-containing foods (such as regular soft drinks, soup, juices, and ice cream) should be eaten. At least 50 g of carbohydrate (3 to 4 carbohydrate choices) should be consumed every 3 to 4 hr in small, frequent feedings.
4. Ample amounts of liquid should be consumed every hour. If nausea or vomiting occurs, small sips—1 or 2 tbsp every 15 to 30 min—should be consumed. If vomiting continues, the health care team should be notified.
5. The health care team should be called if illness continues for more than 1 day.

Modified from Franz MJ, Joynes JO: *Diabetes and brief illness*, Minneapolis, 1993, International Diabetes Center.

Fasting Hyperglycemia

The possible reasons for fasting hyperglycemia include waning of insulin action, the dawn phenomenon, and the Somogyi (rebound) effect (phenomenon). The first situation is due to an inadequate insulin dose overnight and requires an adjustment in insulin doses.

The amount of insulin required to normalize blood glucose levels during the night is less in the predawn period (from 1:00 to 3:00 AM) than at dawn (4:00 to 8:00 AM). This rise in fasting blood glucose levels is referred to as the dawn phenomenon and may result if insulin levels decline between predawn and dawn or if overnight hepatic glucose output becomes excessive as is common in type 2 diabetes. Blood glucose level is monitored at bedtime and at 2:00 to 3:00 AM to identify the dawn phenomenon. With the dawn phenomenon, predawn blood glucose levels will be in the low range of normal but not in the hypoglycemic range. For patients with type 2 diabetes, metformin is often used because of its effect on hepatic glucose output. For persons with type 1 diabetes, administering insulin that does not peak at 1:00 to 3:00 AM should be considered. Taking intermediate-acting insulin at bedtime or substituting a peakless, long-acting insulin, such as glargine, is often effective.

Hypoglycemia followed by "rebound" hyperglycemia is called the Somogyi effect. This phenomenon originates during hypoglycemia with the secretion of counterregulatory hormones (glucagon, epinephrine, growth hormone, and cortisol) and is usually caused by excessive exogenous insulin doses. Hepatic glucose production is stimulated, thus raising blood glucose levels. If rebound hyperglycemia goes unrecognized and insulin doses are increased, a cycle of overinsulinization may result. Decreasing evening insulin doses or, as for the dawn phenomenon, taking intermediate-acting insulin at bedtime or substituting a long-acting insulin should be considered.

Hyperosmolar Hyperglycemic State

Hyperosmolar hyperglycemic state is defined as an extremely high blood glucose level, the absence of or the presence of only small amounts of ketones, and profound dehydration. Glucose levels generally range from greater than 600 to 2000 mg/dl. Patients who have HHS have sufficient insulin to prevent lipolysis and ketosis. This condition occurs rarely, usually in older patients with type 2 diabetes. Treatment consists of hydration and small doses of insulin to correct the hyperglycemia.

LONG-TERM COMPLICATIONS

Long-term complications of diabetes include macrovascular diseases, microvascular diseases, and neuropathy. Macrovascular diseases involve diseases of large blood vessels; microvascular diseases associated with diabetes involve the small blood vessels and include nephropathy and retinopathy. In contrast, diabetic neuropathy is a condition characterized by damage to the nerves.

Medical nutrition therapy is important in managing several long-term complications of diabetes. Nutrition therapy is also a major component in reducing risk factors for chronic complications, especially those related to macrovascular disease. The DCCT and the UKPDS provided convincing evidence for the relationship between improved control of blood glucose and decreased risk of microvascular complications (DCCT Research Group, 1993; UKPDSG, 1998a). Although improved glycemic control has not been absolutely proven to reduce macrovascular complications, accumulating evidence is quite suggestive of such a benefit. Blood pressure control is definitely of benefit.

Macrovascular Diseases

Insulin resistance, which may precede the development of type 2 diabetes and macrovascular disease by many years, induces numerous metabolic changes, known as the *metabolic syndrome* or the *insulin resistance syndrome.* It is characterized by intraabdominal obesity or the android distribution of adipose tissue (waist circumference greater than 102 cm [>40 in] in men and greater than 88 cm [>35 inches] in women) and is associated with dyslipidemia, hypertension, glucose intolerance, and increased prevalence of macrovascular complications. Other risk factors include genetics, smoking, sedentary lifestyle, high-fat diet, renal failure, and microalbuminuria.

Macrovascular diseases—including coronary heart disease (CHD), peripheral vascular disease (PVD), and cerebrovascular disease (CVD)—are more common, tend to occur at an earlier age, and are more extensive and severe in people with diabetes. Furthermore, in women with diabetes, the increased risk of mortality from heart disease is greater than in men, in contrast to the nondiabetic population, in which heart disease mortality is greater in men than in women (ADA, 2001).

Dyslipidemia

Lipid abnormalities occur in 11% to 44% of adults in the United States with diabetes. In type 2 diabetes, the prevalence of an elevated cholesterol level is about 28% to 34%, and about 5% to 14% have high triglyceride levels; also, lower HDL cholesterol levels are common. Furthermore, patients with type 2 diabetes typically have smaller, denser LDL particles, which increases atherogenicity even if the total LDL cholesterol level is not significantly elevated. Primary therapy is directed first at lowering LDL cholesterol levels with the goal being to reduce LDL cholesterol concentrations to 100 mg/dl or lower. Lifestyle interventions should be intensified at LDL cholesterol concentrations greater than 100 mg/dl, and pharmacologic therapy with a statin (HMG-CoA reductase inhibitors) should be initiated at LDL cholesterol concentrations of 130 mg/dl or greater. In addition, if the HDL cholesterol is less than 40 mg/dl, a fibric acid such as fenofibrate can be used (ADA, 2002g). Aspirin therapy should be used in all adult patients with diabetes and macrovascular disease and for primary prevention in patients 40 years of age or older with diabetes and one or more cardiovascular risk factors (ADA, 2002a).

Medical Nutrition Therapy for Dyslipidemia

For individuals with elevated LDL cholesterol, saturated fatty acids and trans fatty acids should be limited to less than 10% of energy and perhaps to less than 7% of energy and, if replaced, can be substituted with carbohydrates or monounsaturated fats (ADA, 2002b).

For patients with the metabolic syndrome, improved glycemic control, modest weight loss, restricted intake of saturated fats, increased physical activity, and if weight is not an issue incorporation of monounsaturated fats may be beneficial (ADA, 2002b). In addition, triglyceride lowering can be achieved with very-high-dose statins (for subjects with both high LDL cholesterol and triglyceride levels) or fibric acid derivatives (gemfibrozil or fenofibrate).

Individuals with triglyceride measurements of 1000 mg/dl should restrict all types of dietary fat (except omega-3 fatty acids) and be treated with medication to reduce triglycerides. Supplementation with fish oils may benefit those with resistant hypertriglyceridemia (ADA, 2002b).

Hypertension

Hypertension is a common comorbidity of diabetes, affecting 20% to 60% of persons with diabetes, depending on the person's age, obesity, and ethnicity. Treatment of hypertension in persons with diabetes should also be vigorous to reduce the risk of macrovascular and microvascular disease. Blood pressure should be measured at every routine visit with a goal for blood pressure control of less than 130/80 mm Hg. Patients with a systolic blood pressure of 130 to 139 mm Hg or a diastolic pressure of 80 to 89 mm Hg should be treated with MNT alone for a maximum of 3 months. Patients with a systolic blood pressure of 140 mm Hg or greater or a diastolic pressure of 90 mm Hg or greater should receive drug therapy in addition to MNT. Initial drug therapy may be with angiotensin-converting enzyme (ACE) inhibition, angiotensin receptor blockers (ARBs), β-blockers, or diuretics. Additional drugs may be chosen from these classes or another drug class if necessary to achieve target goals (ADA, 2002a).

Medical Nutrition Therapy for Hypertension

Although blood pressure response varies widely, the lower the sodium intake, the greater the lowering of blood pressure (Sacks et al, 2001). Responses to sodium may be greater in subjects who are "sodium sensitive," a characteristic of many individuals with diabetes. Therefore, in normotensive and hypertensive persons, the goal should be to reduce sodium intake to 2400 mg of sodium or 6000 mg of sodium chloride (salt) per day. A modest amount of weight loss and a low-fat diet that includes fruits and vegetables (five to nine servings per day) and low-fat dairy products (two to four servings per day) will be rich in potassium, magnesium, and calcium and will beneficially affect blood pressure. Drinking small to moderate amounts of alcohol will not adversely affect blood pressure; however, large alcohol intakes (more than three drinks per day) are related to an elevation in blood pressure (ADA, 2002b).

Microvascular Diseases

Nephropathy

In the United States, diabetic nephropathy accounts for about 40% of new cases of end-stage renal disease (ESRD). About 20% to 30% of patients with type 1 or type 2 diabetes develop evidence of nephropathy, but in type 2 diabetes, a considerably smaller number will progress to ESRD; however, because of the greater prevalence of type 2 diabetes, such patients constitute more than half of the patients with diabetes currently starting on dialysis (ADA, 2002h).

The earliest clinical evidence of nephropathy is the appearance of low but abnormal urine albumin levels (>30 mg daily or 20 μg per minute), referred to as *microalbuminuria* or *incipient nephropathy*. Without specific interventions, progression to overt nephropathy or clinical albuminuria (≥300 mg daily or 200 μg per minute) with hypertension and a gradual decline in glomerular filtration rate (GFR) can occur, leading to the development of ESRD in both patients with type 1 diabetes and type 2 diabetes. An annual test for microalbuminuria should be performed in patients who have had type 1 diabetes for more than 5 years and in all patients with type 2 diabetes starting at diagnosis (ADA, 2002h).

Although diabetic nephropathy cannot be cured, persuasive data indicate that the clinical course of the disease can be modified. To reduce the risk or slow the progression of nephropathy, glucose and blood pressure control should be optimized. In hypertensive and nonhypertensive patients with type 1 diabetes, ACE inhibitors are the initial agents of choice. In hypertensive patients with type 2 diabetes, angiotensin receptor blockers (ARBs) are the initial agents of choice. If one class is not tolerated, the other should be substituted and their combination will decrease albuminuria more than use of either agent alone (ADA, 2002h).

Medical Nutrition Therapy for Nephropathy

With the onset of nephropathy, restricted-protein diets may modify the underlying glomerular injury and, along with control of hypertension and hyperglycemia, delay the progression of renal failure (Pedrini et al, 1996; Zeller et al, 1991). Several studies that attempted to reduce protein intake in persons with type 1 or type 2 diabetes and microalbuminuria achieved a protein reduction to about 1.0 g per kilogram of body weight. In a dose-response analysis (Pijls et al, 1999), a 0.1 g per kilogram of body weight per day decrease in the intake of protein was related to an improvement of 11.1% in albuminuria. In studies conducted in subjects with type 1 diabetes and macroalbuminuria (overt nephropathy), the achieved protein restriction was for about 0.8 g per kilogram of body weight daily, which slowed the rate of decline in the GFR significantly over 32 to 35 months (Walker et al, 1989; Zeller et al, 1991). In patients with microalbuminuria, a limit of protein to 0.8 to 1.0 g per kilogram of body weight daily and for patients with overt nephropathy, limiting protein to 0.8 g per kilogram of body weight daily is recommended (ADA, 2002b).

A few studies have explored the potential benefit of plant protein rather than animal protein (Kontesis et al, 1995). In general, the subjects have been normoalbuminuric, normotensive, and not hyperfiltering so that benefits may not have been expected. Furthermore, when plant protein is substituted for animal protein, the amount of protein consumed was also reduced and the beneficial effect may have been from a reduction in protein content or from the change in protein source. Long-term clinical trials are needed to determine whether reductions in animal protein or changes in plant or animal protein will have a beneficial effect on diabetic nephropathy (ADA, 2002b).

Retinopathy

Diabetic retinopathy is estimated to be the most frequent cause of new cases of blindness among adults 20 to 74 years of age. After 20 years of diabetes, nearly all patients with type 1 diabetes and more than 60% of patients with type 2 diabetes have some degree of retinopathy. Laser photocoagulation surgery can reduce the risk of further vision loss but generally is not beneficial in reversing already diminished acuity—thus the importance for a screening program to detect diabetic retinopathy. An initial dilated and comprehensive eye examination should be done in patients 10 years of age and older with type 1 diabetes and in patients with type 2 diabetes shortly after the diagnosis of diabetes. Subsequent examinations for both groups should be done annually (ADA, 2002i).

There are three stages of diabetic retinopathy. The early stages of nonproliferative diabetic retinopathy (NPDR) are characterized by microaneurysms; a pouchlike dilation of a terminal capillary; lesions that include cotton-wool spots (also referred to as *soft exudates*); and the formation of new blood vessels as a result of the retina's great metabolic need for oxygen and other nutrients supplied by the bloodstream. As the disease progresses to the middle stages of moderate, severe, and very severe NPDR, gradual loss of the retinal microvasculature occurs, resulting in retinal ischemia. Extensive intraretinal hemorrhages and microaneurysms are common reflections of increasing retinal nonperfusion.

The most advanced stage—termed *proliferative diabetic retinopathy (PDR)*—is the final and most vision-threatening stage of diabetic retinopathy. It is characterized by the onset of ischemia-induced new vessel proliferation at the optic disk or elsewhere in the retina. The new vessels are fragile and prone to bleeding, resulting in vitreous hemorrhage. With time, the neovascularization tends to undergo fibrosis and contraction, resulting in retinal traction, retinal tears, vitreous hemorrhage, and retinal detachment. *Diabetic macular edema,* which involves thickening of the central (macular) portion of the retina, and glaucoma, in which fibrous scar tissue increases intraocular pressure, are other clinical findings in retinopathy (Aiello et al, 1998).

Neuropathy

Chronic high levels of blood glucose are also associated with nerve damage and affects 60% to 70% of patients with both type 1 and type 2 diabetes (ADA, 2001). Peripheral neuropathy usually affects the nerves that control sensation in the feet and hands. Autonomic neuropathy affects nerve function controlling various organ systems. Cardiovascular effects include postural hypotension and decreased responsiveness to cardiac nerve impulses, leading to painless or silent ischemic heart disease. Sexual function may be affected, with impotence the most common manifestation. Damage to nerves innervating the gastrointestinal tract can cause a variety of problems. Neuropathy can be manifested in the esophagus as nausea and esophagitis, in the stomach as unpredictable emptying, in the small bowel as loss of nutrients, and in the large bowel as diarrhea or constipation. Intensive treatment of hyperglycemia reduces the risk of developing diabetic neuropathy.

Gastroparesis

Gastroparesis (impaired gastric motility) affects about 25% of this population and is perhaps the most frustrating condition that patients and dietitians experience. It results in delayed or irregular contractions of the stomach, leading to various gastrointestinal symptoms, such as feelings of fullness, bloating, nausea, vomiting, diarrhea, or constipation. It can cause detrimental effects on blood glucose control.

Medical Nutrition Therapy for Gastroparesis

Treatment involves minimizing abdominal stress. Small, frequent meals may be better tolerated than three full meals a day, and these meals should be low in fiber and fat. If solid foods are not well tolerated, liquid meals may need to be recommended. As much as possible, the timing of insulin administration should be adjusted to match the usually delayed nutrient absorption. This may even require insulin injections after eating. Frequent blood glucose monitoring is important to determine appropriate insulin therapy.

PREVENTING DIABETES

The development of type 2 diabetes is strongly related to lifestyle factors, thus suggesting to researchers that it might be a preventable disease. Supporting evidence comes from both observational and intervention studies. Observational studies addressing physical activity, weight loss, and dietary intake, including whole grains and fiber and dietary fat, provided evidence for factors that might delay or prevent type 2 diabetes (Wing, 1999). Early intervention trials also provided support for the benefits of lifestyle interventions, but all had methodologic limitations. Based on these observational and intervention studies, the Finnish Diabetes Prevention Study (Tuomilehto et al, 2001) and the Diabetes Prevention Program (Diabetes Prevention Program Research Group, 2002) were designed to investigate the effects of lifestyle interventions on prevention of diabetes in those at high risk (IGT).

In the Finnish study, 522 middle-aged, overweight subjects with IGT were randomized to receive either brief diet and exercise counseling (control group) or intensive individualized instruction on how to reduce weight (goal of 5% weight reduction), total intake of fat (goal of <30% of energy intake), and saturated fat (goal of <10% of energy intake) and how to increase fiber intake (goal of ≥15 g/1000 kcal) and physical activity (goal of >150 minutes weekly). After an average follow-up of 3.2 years, there was a 58% reduction in the incidence of type 2 diabetes in the intervention group compared with the control group. The reduction in the incidence of diabetes was directly associated with the ability of the subjects to achieve one or more of the lifestyle strategies.

The Diabetes Prevention Program (DPP) randomized 3234 persons (45% from minority groups) with IGT to placebo, metformin, or a lifestyle intervention. Subjects in the placebo and medication arms received standard lifestyle recommendations that included written information and an annual 20- to 30-minute individual session. Subjects in the lifestyle arm were expected to achieve and maintain a weight loss of at least 7% and to perform 150 minutes of physical activity per week. Subjects were seen weekly for the first 24 weeks, followed by monthly sessions. After an average follow-up of 2.8 years, a 58% decrease in the progression to diabetes was observed in the lifestyle group and a 31% relative reduction was observed in the metformin group. On average, 59% of the lifestyle group achieved the goal of 7% or greater weight reduction and 74% maintained at least 150 minutes per week of moderately intense activity.

The greater benefit of weight loss and physical activity over medication strongly suggests that lifestyle modification should be the first choices to prevent or delay diabetes. Modest weight loss (5%-10% of body weight) and modest physical activity (30 minutes daily) are the recommended goals (ADA, 2002j). Structured programs that emphasize lifestyle changes are necessary to accomplish these objectives.

No nutritional recommendations can be made for the prevention of type 1 diabetes. Breast-feeding may be of benefit. Although increased obesity in youth may be related to an increased prevalence of type 2 diabetes, research supporting lifestyle interventions is not available. Increased physical activity, reduced energy and fat intake, and resultant weight management may be beneficial.

HYPOGLYCEMIA OF NONDIABETIC ORIGIN

Hypoglycemia of nondiabetic origin has been defined as a clinical syndrome with diverse causes in which low levels of plasma glucose eventually lead to neuroglycopenia (Service, 1995). Hypoglycemia literally means low (hypo) blood glucose (glycemia). Normally, the body is remarkably adept at maintaining fairly steady blood glucose levels—usually between 60 and 100 mg/dl (3.3 to 5.6 mmol/L), despite the intermittent ingestion of food. Maintaining normal levels of glucose is important because body cells, especially the brain and central nervous system, must have a steady and consistent supply of glucose to function properly. Under physiologic conditions, the brain depends almost exclusively on glucose for its energy needs. Even with hunger, either because it is many hours since food was eaten or because the last meal was small, blood glucose levels remain fairly consistent.

Pathophysiology

In a small number of people, however, blood glucose levels become too low. If the brain and nervous system are deprived of the glucose they need to function, symptoms, such as sweating, shaking, weakness, hunger, headaches, and irritability, can develop. Hypoglycemia can be difficult to diagnose because these typical symptoms can be caused by many different health problems besides hypoglycemia. For example, adrenaline (epinephrine), released as a result of anxiety and stress, can trigger the symptoms of hypoglycemia. The only way to determine whether hypoglycemia is causing these symptoms is to measure blood glucose levels while an individual is experiencing the symptoms (Brun, Fedou, and Mercier, 2000). Hypoglycemia, therefore, can best be defined by the presence of three features known as Whipple's triad: (1) a low plasma or blood glucose level; (2) symptoms of hypoglycemia at the same time as the low blood glucose values; and (3) amelioration of the symptoms by correction of the hypoglycemia (Prince, 1997). A fairly steady blood glucose level is maintained by the interaction of several mechanisms. After eating, food is broken down into glucose and enters the bloodstream. As blood glucose levels rise, the pancreas responds by releasing the hormone insulin, which allows glucose to leave the bloodstream and enter various body cells where it fuels the body's activities. Glucose is also taken up by the liver and stored as glycogen for later use. When glucose concentrations from the last meal decline, the body goes from a "fed" to a "fasting" state. Insulin levels decrease, which keeps the blood glucose levels from falling too low. In addition, stored glucose is released from the liver back into the bloodstream with the help of *glucagon*, a hormone that is also released from the pancreas. Normally, the body's ability to balance glucose, insulin, and glucagon (and other counterregulatory hormones) keeps glucose levels within the normal range. Glucagon provides the primary defense against hypoglycemia; without it full recovery does not occur. Epinephrine is not necessary for counterregulation when glucagon is present. In the absence of glucagon, however, epinephrine has an important role (Cryer, 1993).

Symptoms of hypoglycemia have been recognized at plasma glucose levels of about 60 mg/dl, and impaired brain function has occurred at levels of about 50 mg/dl (Mitrakou et al, 1991). Symptoms are classified into two major groups: those that arise from the action of the autonomic nervous system (adrenergic symptoms) and those related to an insufficient supply of glucose to the brain (neuroglycopenic symptoms). Adrenergic symptoms include sweating, trembling, feelings of warmth, anxiety, and nausea. Symptoms of neuroglycopenia include dizziness, confusion, tiredness, difficulty speaking, headaches, and inability to concentrate. Hunger, blurred vision, drowsiness, and weakness are other symptoms some people experience. Symptoms differ for different people but are consistent from episode to episode for any one person. Furthermore, there is not a consistent chronologic order to the evolution of symptoms; autonomic symptoms do not always precede neuroglycopenic ones. In many persons, neuroglycopenic symptoms are the only ones observed. Hypoglycemia is the cause for any of these symptoms only if blood glucose levels are determined to be below normal at the time the symptoms occur.

Types of Hypoglycemia

If blood glucose levels fall below normal limits within 2 to 5 hours after eating, this is often referred to as reactive hypoglycemia (named because the body is reacting to food) or postprandial (reactive) hypoglycemia. Postprandial hypoglycemia can be caused by an exaggerated insulin response caused by either insulin resistance or elevated glucagon-like-peptide-1 (GLP-1), alimentary hyperinsulinism, renal glycosuria, defects in glucagon response, high insulin sensitivity, or rare syndromes, such as hereditary fructose intolerance, galactosemia, leucine sensitivity, or a rare β-cell pancreatic tumor (insulinoma) (Brun, Fedou, and Mercier, 2000).

Alimentary hyperinsulinism is the most common type of documented postprandial hypoglycemia and is seen in patients who have undergone gastric surgery or some other type of gastric surgery (Gebhard et al, 2001) (see Chapter 29). These procedures are associated with rapid delivery of food to the small intestine, rapid absorption of glucose, and exaggerated insulin response. These patients respond best to multiple, frequent feedings (Prince, 1997). α-Glucosidase inhibitors such as acarbose may also be helpful because they decrease the absorption of carbohydrates (Hasler, 2002).

The ingestion of alcohol after a prolonged fast, or the ingestion of large amounts of alcohol and carbohydrate on an empty stomach ("gin-and-tonic" syndrome) may also cause hypoglycemia within 3 to 4 hours in some healthy persons.

Idiopathic reactive hypoglycemia is characterized by normal insulin secretion but increased insulin sensitivity and, to some extent, reduced response of glucagon to acute hypoglycemia symptoms (Brun, Fedou, and Mercier, 2000). The increase in insulin sensitivity associated with a deficiency of glucagon secretion leads to hypoglycemia late postprandially (Leonetti et al, 1996). Idiopathic reactive hypoglycemia has been inappropriately overdiagnosed by both physicians and patients, to the point that some physicians doubt its existence. Although rare, it does exist but can be documented only in persons with hypoglycemia that occurs spontaneously and who meet the criteria of Whipple's triad.

Fasting (food-deprived) hypoglycemia may occur in response to having gone without food for 8 hours or longer; however, generally, fasting hypoglycemia is the result of a serious underlying medical condition. Causes of fasting hypoglycemia include hormone deficiency states (e.g., hypopituitarism, adrenal insufficiency, catecholamine or glucagon deficiency), acquired liver disease, renal disease, certain drugs (e.g., alcohol, propranolol, salicylate), insulinoma (of which most are benign, but 6% to 10% can be malignant), and other nonpancreatic tumors. Factitious hypoglycemia, or self-administration of insulin or sulfonylurea in persons who do not have diabetes, is a common cause as well (Prince, 1997). Symptoms related to fasting hypoglycemia tend to be particularly severe and can include a loss of mental acuity, seizures, and unconsciousness. If the underlying problem can be resolved, hypoglycemia is no longer a problem.

Diagnostic Criteria

One of the criteria used to confirm the presence of hypoglycemia is a blood glucose level of less than 50 mg/dl (<2.8 mmol/L). Previously, the oral glucose tolerance test was the standard test for this condition; however, this test is not helpful because it involves a nonphysiologic stimulus and because results show little correlation with persons who later are documented to have hypoglycemia. Recording fingerstick blood glucose measurements during spontaneously occurring symptomatic episodes at home is a method that is often used to establish the diagnosis. An alternative method is to perform a glucose test in a medical office setting, in which case the patient is given a typical meal that has been documented in the past to lead to symptomatic episodes; Whipple's triad can be confirmed if symptoms occur (Prince, 1997). If blood glucose levels are low during the symptomatic period, and if the symptoms disappear upon eating, hypoglycemia is probably responsible. It is essential to make a correct diagnosis in patients with fasting hypoglycemia because the implications for therapy are serious.

Management of Hypoglycemia

The management of hypoglycemic disorders involves two distinct components: (1) relief of neuroglycopenic symptoms by the restoration of blood glucose concentrations to the normal range and (2) correction of the underlying cause. The immediate treatment is to eat foods or beverages containing carbohydrate. As the glucose from the breakdown of carbohydrate is absorbed into the bloodstream, it will increase the level of glucose in the blood and relieve the symptoms. If an underlying problem is causing hypoglycemia, appropriate treatment of this disease or disorder is essential.

Almost no research has been done to determine what type of food-related treatment is best for the prevention of hypoglycemia. Traditional advice has been to avoid foods containing sugars and to eat protein- and fat-containing foods. Recent research on the glycemic index and sugars has raised questions about the appropriateness of restricting only sugars because these foods have been reported to have a lower glycemic index than many of the starches that were encouraged in the past. Restriction of sugars may contribute to a decreased intake in total carbohydrate, which may be more important than the source of the carbohydrate.

Using the following information, guidelines for the prevention of hypoglycemia have been published (International Diabetes Center, 1998). It is helpful to review metabolism of carbohydrates, protein, and fat; their effects on blood glucose levels and their relationship to insulin secretion. It should be remembered that this research has been conducted using normal subjects, not subjects who have been diagnosed with hypoglycemia.

After digestion, the major macronutrients absorbed are glucose, fructose, galactose, amino acids, and fatty acids that are reconstituted into triglycerides in chylomicrons. Glucose, fructose, and galactose are the major absorbed products of carbohydrate-containing foods, with about 75% being glucose, 22% being fructose and 3% as galactose. The effect of these absorbed sugars on plasma glucose levels and insulin response is different for each (Nuttall and Gannon, 1991a). Fructose ingestion in normal subjects results in little increase in glucose concentrations and little or no change in insulin concentrations. Ingestion of galactose (initially lactose) results in only a modest increase in peripheral glucose concentrations and a modest rise in insulin, which is attributable to the rise in glucose. Fructose and galactose appear to be used primarily for glycogen synthesis in the liver (Gannon et al, 2001). Blood glucose levels generally return to premeal levels after about 4 hours; with smaller amounts of carbohydrate, this time span is shortened.

The amount of insulin secreted after glucose ingestion depends more on the amount of glucose ingested than on the magnitude of the glucose increase (Castro et al, 1970). Quantitatively, the increase in insulin concentration greatly exceeds the increase in glucose concentration. For example, the maximal glucose concentration typically does not exceed 50% of the premeal value, whereas the increase in insulin concentration is commonly 800% to 900%.

Overall, the system is designed to maintain the circulating glucose concentration in the nonfed state within narrowly defined limits. It is also designed to allow only a modest rise in glucose after carbohydrate-containing meals and to return glucose concentrations rapidly to the nonfed state. Most of the insulin secreted during a 24-hour period is secreted during times of the day when ingested food is not being assimilated, that is, as basal insulin secretion (Nuttall and Gannon, 1991a).

Ingested protein does not raise the plasma glucose concentrations in normal subjects, even when ingested in large amounts, although 50% to 70% of the ingested protein can be accounted for by deaminated amino acids and urea synthesis in the liver. Presumably, most deaminated amino acids are converted to glucose (Nuttall and Gannon, 1991b).

Although fat does not independently stimulate insulin secretion, it also does not affect the circulating glucose concentration. However, when fat is ingested with carbohydrate, the plasma glucose and insulin responses are modified. This is an area that requires additional research. Preliminary evidence also suggests that a high fat intake may contribute to insulin resistance.

The goal of treatment is to adopt eating habits that will keep blood glucose levels as static as possible. Recommended guidelines are listed in Box 33-10. Patients with hypoglycemia may also benefit from learning carbohydrate counting and limiting carbohydrate servings (15 g of carbohydrate per serving) to two to four at a meal and one to two for snacks (see Appendix 53). Foods containing protein that are also low in fat can be eaten at meals or with snacks. These foods would be expected to have minimal effect on blood glucose levels and can add extra food for satiety and calories. Because protein as well as carbohydrate stimulates insulin release, however, a moderate intake may be advisable.

Box 33-10. Guidelines for Avoiding Hypoglycemic Symptoms

1. Eat small meals, with snacks interspersed between meals and at bedtime. This means eating five to six small meals rather than two to three large meals to steady the release of glucose into the bloodstream.
2. Spread the intake of carbohydrate foods throughout the day. Eating large amounts of carbohydrate at one time produces increased amounts of glucose and stimulates the release of increased amounts of insulin, which can cause blood glucose levels to drop. Most individuals can eat two to four servings of carbohydrate foods at each meal and one to two servings at each snack. Furthermore, if carbohydrate is removed from the diet, the body loses its ability to handle carbohydrate properly. Carbohydrate foods include starches, fruits and fruit juices, milk and yogurt, and foods containing sugar.
3. Avoid foods that contain large amounts of carbohydrate. Examples of these foods are regular soft drinks, syrups, candy, regular fruited yogurts, pies, and cakes.
4. Avoid beverages and foods containing caffeine. Caffeine can cause the same symptoms as hypoglycemia and make the individual feel worse (Kerr et al, 1993).
5. Limit or avoid alcoholic beverages. Drinking alcohol on an empty stomach and without food can lower blood glucose levels by interfering with the liver's ability to release stored glucose (gluconeogenesis) (Franz, 1999). If an individual chooses to drink alcohol, it should be done in moderation (one or two drinks no more than twice a week), and food should always be eaten along with the alcoholic beverage.
6. Decrease fat intake. A high-fat diet, especially saturated fat, has been shown to affect the body's ability to use insulin (insulin resistance). Decreasing fat intake can also help with weight loss, if weight is a problem. Excess weight also interferes with the body's ability to use insulin.

Modified from International Diabetes Center: *Reactive and fasting hypoglycemia,* Minneapolis, 1998, International Diabetes Center.

SUMMARY

In summary, nutrition is a challenging aspect of the management of diabetes and hypoglycemia of nondiabetic origin. Attention to nutrition and meal-planning principles is essential for glycemic control and overall good health. A registered dietitian who is knowledgeable and skilled in implementing current nutrition principles and making recommendations for diabetes or hypoglycemia of nondiabetic origin is the medical team member who should plan, implement, and evaluate MNT. Outcomes must be identified, and the effectiveness of nutrition interventions continually documented.

Clinical Scenario 1: Type 1 Diabetes

Ellen is a 15-year-old girl with newly diagnosed type 1 diabetes. She is 5 ft 2 in. tall, weighs 115 lb, and is active in cheerleading and basketball in high school. Her physician will be regulating the dosage and timing of her insulin regimen.

Her grandmother has diabetes and is supportive of Ellen's need for education. Ellen's parents are divorced, and she now lives with her grandmother. What steps should you, as her nutrition counselor, take?

1. What food and meal-planning information needs to be shared with the health care team as insulin therapy is integrated into Ellen's normal eating and exercise habits?
2. What guidance should you offer regarding Ellen's sports activities?
3. Ellen is worried about keeping up with her peers. How will you help her adapt to the possible need for snacks during exercise and during a busy school day or during activities with her friends?
4. When Ellen travels on field trips or vacations, what types of food can she pack to take along?
5. What signs and symptoms of lack of diabetes control must Ellen understand to manage her disease? Which problem is she more likely to experience—hyperglycemia or hypoglycemia?

Clinical Scenario 2: Type 2 Diabetes

Debra is a 45-year-old woman with a known diagnosis of type 2 diabetes for 3 years. She has not had a medical check-up for 2 years. She returns at this time with a primary complaint of chronic fatigue. Her laboratory test results show the following: HbA1c 8.3%; serum cholesterol 214 mg/dl; triglycerides 275 mg/dl. Her current weight is 175 lb., and her height is 64 in. (BMI = 30). She states she hasn't returned for any follow-up visits because the only advice she gets is to lose weight and not to eat sugar, neither of which she is able to do.

1. What advice will you offer to improve Debra's metabolic parameters and, in particular, to improve her blood glucose control?
2. What guidelines for carbohydrate intake can help Debra improve her glycemia?
3. What suggestions will you have about fat intake?
4. What information will you share about exercise?
5. What meal-planning method do you suggest for her?
6. What will you recommend regarding her sugar intake?

Clinical Scenario 3: Type 2 Diabetes

John is a moderately obese (BMI = 29) 49-year-old man who complains of increased thirst, polyuria, and fatigue. His family history includes his mother and an older brother with type 2 diabetes. A random (casual) plasma glucose test shows a level of 480 mg/dl. His serum electrolyte level and anion gap are normal.

He reports finding it difficult to control his eating during the evening and because of his long working hours finds it difficult to work in an hour for exercise most days. When asked what he is interested in learning about, he replies that he would like to learn how to control his eating because he is always hungry.

1. What type of diabetes does John likely have? Is it likely to be controlled by nutrition therapy alone?
2. Given the symptoms of hyperglycemia, is it more likely that an oral agent or insulin therapy will be recommended?
3. If John is started on medication, are lifestyle strategies still important?
4. What advice can you give to John to help him with his eating problems?
5. What other lifestyle strategies will be helpful?

Relevant Web Sites

American Association of Diabetes Educators
www.aadenet.org
American Diabetes Association
www.diabetes.org
American Dietetic Association, Diabetes Care and Education Practice Group
www.dce.org
Children With Diabetes
www.childrenwithdiabetes.com
Coverage for Medical Nutrition Therapy
www.eatright.org/gov/reimbursement.html
Healthy Weight Network
www.healthyweight.net
International Diabetes Center, Minneapolis, Minnesota
www.idcdiabetes.org
Lifestyle Manuals Used in the Diabetes Prevention Program
www.bsc.gwu.edu/dpp
National Institute of Diabetes and Digestive Kidney Diseases
www.niddk.nih.gov

Cited References

Aiello LP et al: Diabetic retinopathy [Technical Review], *Diabetes Care* 21:143, 1998.

Albright A et al: American College of Sports Medicine position stand: exercise and type 2 diabetes, *Med Sci Sports Exerc* 32:1345, 2000.

American Diabetes Association: Type 2 diabetes in children and adolescents [Consensus Statement], *Diabetes Care* 23:381, 2000.

American Diabetes Association: *Diabetes 2001 vital statistics,* Alexandria, Va, 2001, American Diabetes Association.

American Diabetes Association: Standards of medical care for patients with diabetes mellitus [Position Statement], *Diabetes Care* 25(suppl 1):S33, 2002a.

American Diabetes Association: Evidence-based nutrition principles and recommendations for the treatment and prevention of diabetes and related complications [Position Statement], *Diabetes Care* 25:202, 2002b.

American Diabetes Association: Diabetes mellitus and exercise [Position Statement], *Diabetes Care* 25(suppl 1):S64, 2002c.

American Diabetes Association: Tests of glycemia in diabetes [Position Statement], *Diabetes Care* 25(suppl 1):S97, 2002d.

American Diabetes Association: Gestational diabetes mellitus [Position Statement], *Diabetes Care* 25(suppl 1):S94, 2002e.

American Diabetes Association: Translation of the diabetes nutrition recommendations for health care institutions, *Diabetes Care* 25(suppl 1):S61, 2002f.

American Diabetes Association: Management of dyslipidemia in adults [Position Statement], *Diabetes Care* 25(suppl 1):S74, 2002g.

American Diabetes Association: Diabetic nephropathy [Position Statement], *Diabetes Care* 25(suppl 1):S90, 2002h.

American Diabetes Association: Diabetic retinopathy [Position Statement], *Diabetes Care* 25(suppl 1):S90, 2002i.

American Diabetes Association: The prevention or delay of type 2 diabetes [Position Statement], *Diabetes Care* 25:2002j.

American Dietetic Association: *Medical nutrition therapy evidence-based guides for practice: nutrition practice guidelines for type 1 and type 2 diabetes,* CD-Rom, Chicago, 2001, American Dietetic Association.

American Diabetes Association and American Dietetic Association: *Exchange lists for meal planning,* Alexandria, Va, 2003, American Diabetes Association.

American Diabetes Association: Economic costs of diabetes in the U.S. in 2002, *Diabetes Care* 26:917, 2003a.

American Diabetes Association: Management of dyslipidemia in children and adolescents with diabetes [Consensus Statement], *Diabetes Care,* 26:2194, 2003b.

Anderson RA et al: Beneficial effects of chromium for people with diabetes, *Diabetes* 46:1786, 1997.

Bantle JP et al: Metabolic effects of dietary fructose in diabetic subjects, *Diabetes Care* 15:1468, 1992.

Bantle JP et al: Metabolic effects of dietary sucrose in type II diabetic subjects, *Diabetes* Care 16:1301, 1993.

Bantle JP et al: Effects of dietary fructose on plasma lipids in healthy subjects, *Am J Clin Nutr* 72:1128, 2000.

Bergman RN, Adler M: Free fatty acids and pathogenesis of type 2 diabetes mellitus, *Trends Endocr Metab* 11:351, 2000.

Bode BW, Strange P: Efficacy, safety, and pump compatibility of insulin aspart use in continuous subcutaneous insulin infusion therapy in patients with type 1 diabetes, *Diabetes Care* 24:69, 2001.

Brodsky IG, Devlin JT: Effects of dietary protein restriction on regional amino acid metabolism in insulin-dependent diabetes mellitus, *Am J Physiol* 270:E148, 1996.

Brown L et al: Cholesterol-lowering effects of dietary fiber: a meta-analysis, *Am J Clin Nutr* 69:30, 1999.

Brun JF, Fedou C, Mercier J: Postprandial reactive hypoglycemia, *Diabetes Metab* 26:337, 2000.

Burge MR, Schade DS: Insulins, *Endocrinol Metab Clin North Am* 26:575, 1997.

Butchko HH, Stargel WW: Aspartame: scientific evaluation in the postmarketing period, *Regul Toxicol Pharmacol* 34:221, 2001.

Carmichael HE et al: Lower fat intake as a predictor of initial and sustained weight loss in obese subjects consuming an otherwise ad libitum diet, *J Am Diet Assoc* 98:35, 1998.

Castro A et al: Plasma insulin and glucose responses of healthy subjects to varying glucose loads during three-hour oral glucose tolerance tests, *Diabetes* 19:842, 1970.

Chandalia M et al: Beneficial effects of a high dietary fiber intake in patients with type 2 diabetes, *N Engl J Med* 342:1392, 2000.

Chaturvedi N, Fuller JH: The WHO Multinational Study of vascular disease in diabetes: mortality risk in body weight and weight change in people with NIDDM, *Diabetes Care* 18:766, 1995.

Chaturvedi N et al: The WHO Multinational Study of vascular disease in diabetes: mortality and morbidity associated with body weight in people with IDDM, *Diabetes Care* 18:761, 1995.

Cheng N et al: Follow-up survey of people in China with type 2 diabetes mellitus consuming supplemental chromium, *J Trace Elem Exp Med* 12:55, 1999.

Coniff RF et al: Reduction of glycosylated hemoglobin and postprandial hyperglycemia by acarbose in patients with NIDDM, *Diabetes Care* 18:817, 1995.

Cowie CC, Harris MI: Physical and metabolic characteristics of persons with diabetes. In National Diabetes Data Group, editors: *Diabetes in America,* ed 2, Bethesda Md, National Institutes of Health, NIDDK, 1995 (NIH publ No. 95-1468).

Cryer PE: Glucose counterregulation: the physiological mechanisms that prevent or correct hypoglycemia. In Frier BM, Fisher BS, editors: *Hypoglycemia and diabetes: clinical and physiological aspects,* London, 1993, Edward Arnold.

Cryer PE et al: Hypoglycemia in diabetes [Technical review], *Diabetes Care* 26:1902, 2003.

Davis SN et al: Effects of antecedent hypoglycemia on subsequent counterregulatory responses to exercise, *Diabetes* 49:73, 2000.

Delahanty LM, Halford BN: The role of diet behaviors in achieving improved glycemic control in intensively treated patients in the Diabetes Control and Complications Trial, *Diabetes Care* 16: 1453, 1993.

Diabetes Control and Complications Trial Research Group: The effect of intensive treatment of diabetes on the development and progression of long-term complications in insulin-dependent diabetes mellitus, *N Engl J Med* 339:977, 1993.

Diabetes Control and Complications Trial Research Group: Implementation of treatment protocols in the Diabetes Control and Complications Trial, *Diabetes Care* 18:36, 1995.

Diabetes Prevention Program Research Group: Reduction in the incidence of type 2 diabetes with lifestyle intervention or metformin, *N Engl J Med* 346:393, 2002.

Drash A: The child, the adolescent and the Diabetes Control and Complications Trial, *Diabetes Care* 16:1515, 1993.

Expert Committee on the Diagnosis and Classification of Diabetes Mellitus: Report of the Expert Committee on the Diagnosis and Classification of Diabetes Mellitus, *Diabetes Care* 20:1183, 1997.

Ferrannini E: Insulin resistance versus insulin deficiency in noninsulin-dependent diabetes mellitus: problems and prospects, *Endocr Rev* 19:477, 1998.

Franz MJ: Alcohol and diabetes. In Franz MJ, Bantle JP, editors: *American Diabetes Association guide to medical nutrition therapy for diabetes,* Alexandria, Va, 1999, American Diabetes Association.

Franz MJ: Protein controversies in diabetes, *Diabetes Spect* 13:132, 2000.

Franz MJ: Carbohydrate and diabetes: is the source or the amount of more importance *Curr Diabetes Rep* 1:177, 2001.

Franz MJ: Nutrition, physical activity, and diabetes. In Ruderman N, editor: *Handbook of exercise in diabetes,* Alexandria, Va 2002, American Diabetes Association.

Franz MJ, Joynes JO: *Diabetes and brief illness,* Minneapolis, 1993, International Diabetes Center.

Franz MJ, Reader D, Monk A: *Implementing group and individual medical nutrition therapy for diabetes,* Alexandria, Va, 2002, American Diabetes Association.

Franz MJ et al: Nutrition principles for the management of diabetes and related complications [Technical Review], *Diabetes Care* 17:490, 1994.

Franz MJ et al: Nutrition practice guidelines and basic care by dietitians for persons with non-insulin-dependent diabetes mellitus: medical and clinical outcomes, *J Am Diet Assoc* 95:1009, 1995.

Franz MJ et al: Evidence-based nutrition principles and recommendations for treatment and prevention of diabetes and related complications [Technical Review], *Diabetes Care* 25:148, 2002.

Gannon MC et al: Effect of protein ingestion on the glucose appearance rate in people with type 2 diabetes, *J Clin Endocrinol Metab* 86:1040, 2001a.

Gannon MC et al: Glucose appearance rate after the ingestion of galactose, *Metabolism* 50:93, 2001b.

Garg A et al: Effects of varying carbohydrate content of diet in patients with non–insulin-dependent diabetes mellitus, *JAMA* 271:1421, 1994.

Gebhard B et al: Postprandial GLP-1, norepinephrine, and reactive hypoglycemia in dumping syndrome, *Dig Dis Sci* 46:1915, 2001.

Giacco R et al: Long-term dietary treatment with increased amounts of fiber-rich low-glycemic index natural food improves blood glucose control and reduces the number of hypoglycemic events in patients with type 1 diabetes, *Diabetes Care* 23:1451, 2000.

Gougeon R et al: Effect of NIDDM on the kinetics of whole-body protein metabolism, *Diabetes* 43:318, 1994.

Gougeon R et al: Effects of oral hypoglycemic agents and diet on protein metabolism in type 2 diabetes, *Diabetes Care* 232:1, 2000.

Gray RO et al: Comparison of the ability of bread versus bread plus meat to treat and prevent subsequent hypoglycemia in patients with insulin-dependent diabetes, *J Clin Endocrinol Metab* 81:1508, 1996.

Hallikainen MA et al: Effects of 2 low-fat stanols ester-containing margarines on serum cholesterol concentrations as part of a low-fat diet in hypercholesterolemic subjects, *Am J Clin Nutr* 69:403, 1999.

Hasler WL: Dumping syndrome, *Curr Treat Options Gastroenterol* 5 (2):139, 2002.

Heilbronn L et al: Effect of energy restriction, weight loss, and diet composition on plasma lipids and glucose in patients with type 2 diabetes, *Diabetes Care* 22:889, 1999.

Henry RR: Protein content of the diabetic diet [Technical Review], *Diabetes Care* 17:1502, 1994.

Hollenbeck CG et al: To what extent does increased dietary fiber improve glucose and lipid metabolism in patients with noninsulin-dependent diabetes mellitus (NIDDM)? *Am J Clin Nutr* 43:16, 1986.

International Diabetes Center: *Reactive and fasting hypoglycemia,* Minneapolis, 1998, International Diabetes Center.

Inzucchi SE: Oral antihyperglycemic therapy for type 2 diabetes [Scientific Review], *JAMA* 287:360, 2002.

Joint National Committee on Prevention, Detection, Evaluation and Treatment of Hypertension: The sixth report of the Joint National Committee on Prevention, Detection, Evaluation and Treatment of High Blood Pressure, *Arch Intern Med* 157:2413, 1997.

Jones KL et al: Effect of metformin in pediatric patients with type 2 diabetes: a randomized controlled trial, *Diabetes Care* 25:89-94, 2002.

Jovanovic L, editor: *Medical management of pregnancy complicated by diabetes,* ed 3, Alexandria, Va, 2000, American Diabetes Association.

Kelley DE et al: Relative effects of caloric restriction and weight loss in non–insulin-dependent diabetes mellitus, *J Clin Endocrinol Metab* 77:1287, 1993.

Kendall A et al: Weight loss on a low-fat diet: consequence of the imprecision of the control of food intake in humans, *Am J Clin Nutr* 53:1124, 1991.

Kerr D et al: Effect of caffeine on the recognition of and responses to hypoglycemia in humans, *Ann Intern Med* 119:799, 1993.

Kitzmiller JL et al: Preconception care of diabetes, congenital malformations, and spontaneous abortions [Technical Review], *Diabetes Care* 19:514, 1996.

Klein R et al: Is obesity related to microvascular complications of diabetes? *Arch Int Med* 157:650, 1997.

Knopp RH et al: Metabolic effects of hypocaloric diets in management of gestational diets, *Diabetes* 40(suppl 2):165, 1991.

Kohrt WM et al: Insulin resistance in aging is related to abdominal obesity, *Diabetes* 42:273, 1993.

Koivisto VA et al: Alcohol with a meal has no adverse effects on postprandial glucose homeostasis in diabetic patients, *Diabetes Care* 16:1612, 1993.

Kontessis PS et al: Renal, metabolic, and hormonal responses to protein of different origin in normotensive, nonproteinuric type 1 diabetic subjects, *Diabetes Care* 18:1233, 1995.

Kulkarni K et al: Nutrition practice guidelines for type 1 diabetes positively affect dietitian practices and patient outcomes, *J Am Diet Assoc* 98:62, 1998.

Kuusisto JL et al: NIDDM and its metabolic control predict coronary heart disease in elderly subjects, *Diabetes* 43:960, 1994.

Lafrance L et al: The effects of different glycaemic index food and dietary fibre intakes on glycaemic control in type 1 patients with diabetes on intensive insulin therapy, *Diabet Med* 15:972, 1998.

Lariviere FJ et al: Effects of dietary protein restriction on glucose and insulin metabolism in normal and diabetic humans, *Metabolism* 43:462, 1994.

Lee DC et al: Cardiorespiratory fitness, body composition, and all-cause and cardiovascular disease mortality in men, *Am J Clin Nutr* 69:373, 1999.

Leonetti F et al: Increased nonoxidative glucose metabolism in idiopathic reactive hypoglycemia, *Metabolism* 45:606, 1996.

Lovejoy JG, DiGirolamo M: Habitual dietary intake and insulin sensitivity in lean and obese adults, *Am J Clin Nutr* 55:1174, 1992.

MacDonald MJ: Postexercise late-onset hypoglycemia in insulin-dependent diabetic patients, *Diabetes Care* 10:584, 1987.

Markovic TP et al: The determinants of glycemic responses to diet restriction and weight loss in obesity and NIDDM, *Diabetes Care* 21:687, 1998a.

Markovic TP et al: Beneficial effect on average lipid levels from energy restriction and fat loss in obese individuals with or without type 2 diabetes, *Diabetes Care* 21:695, 1998b.

Mitchell TH et al: Hyperglycemia after intense exercise in IDDM subjects during continuous subcutaneous insulin infusion, *Diabetes Care* 11:311, 1988.

Mitrakou A et al: Hierarchy of glycemic thresholds for counterregulatory hormone secretion, symptoms, and cerebral dysfunction, *Am J Physiol* 260:E67, 1991.

Mokdad AH et al: The continuing epidemics of obesity and diabetes in the United States, *JAMA* 286:1195, 2001.

Monk A et al: Practice guidelines for medical nutrition therapy for dietitians for persons with non-insulin-dependent diabetes mellitus, *J Am Diet Assoc* 95:999, 1995.

Montori VM et al: Fish oil supplementation in type 2 diabetes: a quantitative systematic review, *Diabetes Care* 23:1407, 2000.

Mooradian AD et al: Selected vitamins and minerals in diabetes mellitus [Technical Review], *Diabetes Care* 17:464, 1994.

Nordt TK et al: Influences of breakfasts with different nutrient contents on glucose, C peptide, insulin, glucagon, triglycerides, and GIP in non-insulin-dependent diabetics, *Am J Clin Nutr* 53:155, 1991.

Nuttall FQ, Gannon MC: Plasma glucose and insulin responses to macronutrients in nondiabetic and NIDDM subjects, *Diabetes Care* 14:824, 1991a.

Nuttall FQ, Gannon MC: Metabolic responses to dietary protein in persons with and without diabetes mellitus, *Diabetes Nutr Metab Clin Exp* 4:71, 1991b.

Nuttall FQ et al: Effect of protein ingestion on the glucose and insulin response to a standardized oral glucose load, *Diabetes Care* 7:465, 1984.

Nuttall FQ et al: The metabolic responses to various doses of fructose in type II diabetic subjects, *Metabolism* 41:510, 1992.

Ohkubbo Y et al: Intensive therapy prevents the progression of diabetic complications in Japanese patients with non-insulin diabetes mellitus: a randomized prospective 6-year study, *Diabetes Res Clin Pract* 28:103, 1995.

Omenn GS et al: Risk factors for lung cancer and for intervention effects in CARET: the Beta Carotene and Retinol Efficacy Trial, *J Natl Cancer Inst* 88:1350, 1995.

Parillo M et al: A high-monounsaturated fat/low carbohydrate diet improves peripheral insulin sensitivity in non-insulin-dependent diabetic patients, *Metabolism* 41:1373, 1992.

Pate RR et al: Physical activity and public health: a recommendation from the Centers for Disease Control and Prevention and the American College of Sports Medicine, *JAMA* 273:402, 1995.

Patti L et al: Long-term effects of fish oil on lipoprotein subfractions and low density lipoprotein size in non-insulin-dependent diabetic patients with hypertriglyceridemia, *Atherosclerosis* 146:361, 1999.

Pedrini MT et al: The effect of protein restriction on the progression of diabetic and nondiabetic renal diseases: a meta-analysis, *Ann Intern Med* 124:627, 1996.

Peters AL, Davidson MB: Protein and fat effects on glucose response and insulin requirements in subjects with insulin-dependent diabetes mellitus, *Am J Clin Nutr* 58:555, 1993.

Peterson DB et al: Sucrose in the diet of patients with diabetes—just another carbohydrate? *Diabetologia* 29:216, 1986.

Pijls LTJ et al: The effect of protein restriction on albuminuria in patients with type 2 diabetes mellitus: a randomized trial, *Nephrol Dial Transplant* 14:1445, 1999.

Prince MJ: Hypoglycemia of nondiabetic origin, *Curr Ther Endocrinol Metab* 6:454, 1997.

Prochaska JO et al: *Changing for good,* New York, 1994, Morrow Press.

Purdon C et al: The roles of insulin and catecholamines in the glucoregulatory response during intense exercise and early recovery in insulin-dependent diabetic and control subjects, *J Clin Endocrinol Metab* 76:566, 1993.

Rabasa-Lhoret R et al: The effects of meal carbohydrate content on insulin requirements in type 1 diabetic patients treated intensively with the basal bolus (ultralenter-regular) insulin regimen, *Diabetes Care* 22:667, 1999.

Rabasa-Lhoret R et al: Guidelines for premeal insulin dose reduction for postprandial exercise of different intensities and durations in type 1 diabetic subjects treated intensively with a basal-bolus insulin regimen (ultralente-lispro), *Diabetes Care* 24:625, 2001.

Ravussin E et al: Effects of a traditional lifestyle on obesity in Pima Indians, *Diabetes Care* 17:1067, 1994.

Reader D, Sipe M: Key components of care for women with gestational diabetes, *Diabetes Spectrum* 14:188, 2001.

Report of a Joint FAO/WHO Expert Consultation: *Carbohydrates in human nutrition,* Rome, Italy, 1998, Food and Agriculture Organization of the United Nations and World Health Organization.

Rickard KA et al: Lower glycemic response to sucrose in the diets of children with type 1 diabetes, *J Pediatr* 133:429, 1998.

Rickheim P et al: Assessment of group versus individual diabetes education: a randomized study, *Diabetes Care* 25:269, 2002.

Rizzo T et al: Correlations between antepartum maternal metabolism and intelligence of offspring, *N Engl J Med* 335:911, 1991.

Sacks FM et al: Effects on blood pressure of reduced dietary sodium and the dietary approaches to stop hypertension (DASH) diet, *N Engl J Med* 344:3, 2001.

Service FJ: Hypoglycemic disorders, *N Engl J Med* 17:1144, 1995.

Sinha R et al: Prevalence of impaired glucose tolerance among children and adolescents with marked obesity, *N Engl J Med* 346:802, 2002.

Skyler JS editor: *Medical management of type 1 diabetes,* ed 3, Alexandria, Va, 1998, American Diabetes Association.

Toeller M et al: Protein intake and urinary albumin excretion rates in the EURODIAB IDDM Complications Study, *Diabetologia* 40:1219, 1997.

Tuomilehto J et al: Prevention of type 2 diabetes mellitus by changes in lifestyle among subjects with impaired glucose tolerance, *N Engl J Med* 344:1390, 2001.

United Kingdom Prospective Diabetes Study Group: UK Prospective Diabetes Study 7: Response of fasting plasma glucose to diet therapy in newly presenting type II diabetic patients, *Metabolism* 39:905, 1990.

United Kingdom Prospective Diabetes Study Group: Intensive blood-glucose control with sulphonylureas or insulin compared with conventional treatment and risk of complications in patients with type 2 diabetes (UKPDS 34), *Lancet* 352:854, 1998a.

United Kingdom Prospective Diabetes Study Group: Tight blood pressure control and risk of macrovascular and microvascular complications in type 2 diabetes (UKPDS 38), *BMJ* 317:703, 1998b.

Vajo Z et al: Recombinant DNA technology in the treatment of diabetes: insulin analogs, *Endocr Rev* 22:706, 2001.

Walker JD et al. Restriction of dietary protein and progression of renal failure in diabetic nephropathy, *Lancet* 2:1411, 1989.

Wasserman DH, Zinman B: Exercise in individuals with IDDM (Technical Review], *Diabetes Care* 17:924, 1994.

Watts NB et al: Prediction of glucose response to weight loss in patients with non–insulin-dependent diabetes mellitus, *Arch Intern Med* 150:803, 1990.

Wing RR: Lifestyle and the prevention of diabetes. In Franz MJ, Bantle JP, editors: *American Diabetes Association guide to medical nutrition therapy for diabetes,* Alexandria, Va, 1999, American Diabetes Association.

Wing RR et al: Long-term effects of modest weight loss in type II diabetic patients, *Arch Intern Med* 147:1749, 1987.

Wing RR et al: Caloric restriction per se is a significant factor in improvements in glycemic control and insulin sensitivity during weight loss in obese NIDDM patients, *Diabetes Care* 17:30, 1994.

Wolever TMS et al: Day-to-day consistency in amount and source of carbohydrate intake associated with improved glucose control in type 1 diabetes, *J Am Coll Nutr* 18:242, 1999.

Yki-Jarvinen H: Acute and chronic effects of hyperglycaemia on glucose metabolism, implications for the development of new therapies, *Diabet Med* 14(suppl 3):S32, 1997.

Yki-Jarvinen H et al: Comparison of insulin regimens in patients with non-insulin-dependent diabetes mellitus, *N Engl J Med* 337:1426, 1992.

Yusuf S et al: Vitamin E supplementation and cardiovascular events in high-risk patients: the Heart Outcomes Prevention Evaluation Study Investigators, *N Engl J Med* 342:154, 2000.

Zeller K et al: Effect of restricting dietary protein and progression of renal failure in patients with insulin-dependent diabetes mellitus, *N Engl J Med* 324:778, 1991.

Additional References

American Diabetes Association: Consensus development conference on insulin resistance [Consensus Report], *Diabetes Care* 21:310, 1998.

American Diabetes Association: The prevention or delay of type 2 diabetes [Position Statement], *Diabetes Care* 26:(suppl 1):S62, 2003.

American Dietetic Association: *Nutrition practice guidelines for type 1 and type 2 diabetes,* CD-Rom, Chicago, 2001, American Dietetic Association.

American Dietetic Association: *Nutrition practice guidelines for gestational diabetes,* CD-Rom, Chicago, 2001, American Dietetic Association.

Anderson BJ, Rubin RR, editors: *Practical psychology for diabetes clinicians,* Alexandria, Va, 1996, American Diabetes Association.

Franz MJ, section editor: Nutritional treatment of type 2 diabetes mellitus and obesity, *Curr Diabetes Rep* 1:159, 2001.

Franz MJ, Bantle JP, editors: *American Diabetes Association guide to medical nutrition therapy for diabetes,* Alexandria, Va, 1999, American Diabetes Association.

Franz MJ et al, editors: *A core curriculum for diabetes educators,* ed 4, Chicago, 2001, American Association of Diabetes Educators.

Franz MJ et al: *Implementing group and individual medical nutrition therapy for diabetes,* Alexandria, Va, 2002, American Diabetes Association.

Rickheim P et al: Type 2 diabetes BASICS. In *A complete curriculum for diabetes education,* Minneapolis, 2000, International Diabetes Center.

Ruderman N et al, editors: *Handbook of exercise in diabetes,* Alexandria, Va, 2002, American Diabetes Association.

Schafer RG et al: Translation of the diabetes nutrition recommendations for health care institutions [Technical Review], *Diabetes Care* 20:96, 1997.

Virally ML, Guillausseau PJ: Hypoglycemia in adults, *Diabetes Metab* 25:477, 1999.

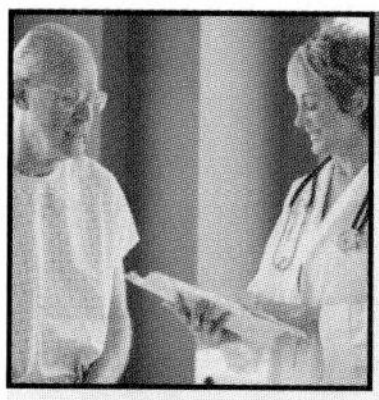

CHAPTER 34

Medical Nutrition Therapy for Anemia

TRACY STOPLER, MS, RD

CHAPTER OUTLINE

- Iron-Related Blood Disorders
- Megaloblastic Anemias
- Other Nutritional Anemias
- Nonnutritional Anemias

KEY TERMS

anemia–a deficiency in the size or number of red blood cells or the amount of hemoglobin they contain that limits the exchange of oxygen and carbon dioxide between the blood and the tissue cells

aplastic anemia–a normochromic-normocytic anemia accompanied by a deficiency of all the formed elements in the blood; can be caused by exposure to toxic chemicals, ionizing radiation, or medications, although the cause is often unknown

ferritin–an iron apoferritin complex; one of the chief storage forms of iron

hematocrit–the volume percentage of erythrocytes in the blood

heme–the nonprotein, iron protoporphyrin constituent of hemoglobin

heme iron–the organic form in which iron occurs in meat, fish, and poultry

hemochromatosis–a genetically determined form of iron overload that results in progressive hepatic, pancreatic, cardiac, and other organ damage

hemoglobin–a conjugated protein containing four heme groups and globin; the oxygen-carrying pigment of the erythrocytes

hemolytic anemia–anemia caused by shortened survival of mature red blood cells

holotranscobalamin II (holo TC II)–vitamin B_{12} attached to the B-globulin, the major circulating vitamin B_{12} delivery protein

hypochromic–characterized by deficient hemoglobin content of red blood cells

intrinsic factor (IF)–a glycoprotein, secreted by the gastric glands, that is necessary for the absorption of exogenous vitamin B_{12} by ileal cell surface receptors for IF-B_{12} complexes

iron deficiency anemia–characterized by the production of small (microcytic) erythrocytes and a diminished level of circulating hemoglobin; the last stage of iron deficiency, which represents the end point of a long period of iron deprivation.

macrocytic anemia–a form of anemia characterized by larger-than-normal red blood cells and increased mean corpuscular volume and mean corpuscular hemoglobin

megaloblastic anemia–a form of anemia characterized by the presence of large, immature, abnormal, red blood cell progenitors in the bone marrow; 95% of cases are attributable to folic acid or vitamin B_{12} deficiency

microcytic anemia–characterized by smaller-than-normal erythrocytes and less circulating hemoglobin; characteristic of iron deficiency and thalassemia

negative vitamin B_{12} balance–a vitamin B_{12} predeficiency stage

nonheme iron–iron that is not a part of the heme complex and that is present in foods, such as eggs, grains, vegetables, and fruits; also present in small amounts in meat, fish, and poultry

pernicious anemia–a macrocytic, megaloblastic anemia caused by a deficiency of vitamin B_{12}, secondary to lack of intrinsic factor

plasma–liquid portion of whole blood that includes coagulation factors

protoporphyrin–an iron-containing portion of the respiratory pigments that, when combined with protein, forms hemoglobin or myoglobin

serum–liquid portion of whole blood without coagulation factors

sickle cell anemia–a chronic hemolytic anemia, occurring most commonly in blacks, that is due to homozygous inheritance of HbS, resulting in a defective hemoglobin synthesis that causes the red blood cells to become sickle shaped

sideroblastic anemia–a microcytic, hypochromic anemia characterized by a derangement in the final pathway of heme synthesis leading to a buildup of iron-containing immature red blood cells; responsive to pharmacologic doses of vitamin B_6

soluble serum transferrin receptors (STFR)–molecules generated on the surface of red blood cells in response to the need for iron

thalassemia–anemia secondary to defective synthesis of the globin part of the hemoglobin

total iron-binding capacity (TIBC)–the capacity of transferrin to take on or become saturated with iron

transferrin–globulin that binds and transports iron from the gut wall to the tissue cells

transferrin receptor–molecule on the surface of the red blood cell that binds transferrin, the transport form of iron

transferrin saturation–a measure of the amount of iron bound to transferrin; a gauge of iron supply to the tissues

Anemia is a condition in which a deficiency in the size or number of erythrocytes, or the amount of hemoglobin they contain, limits the exchange of oxygen and carbon dioxide between the blood and the tissue cells. Classification is based on cell size—*macrocytic* (large), *normocytic* (normal), and *microcytic* (small)—and on hemoglobin content—*hypochromic* (pale color) and *normochromic* (normal color) (Table 34-1). Most anemias are caused by a lack of nutrients required for normal erythrocyte synthesis, principally iron, vitamin B_{12}, and folic acid. Others result from a variety of conditions, such as hemorrhage, genetic abnormalities, chronic disease states, or drug toxicity.

The anemias that result from an inadequate intake of iron, protein, certain vitamins (B_{12}, folic acid, pyridoxine, and ascorbic acid), copper, and other heavy metals are frequently called *nutritional anemias*. The most common nutritional anemias in the United States result from iron or folic acid deficiency.

IRON-RELATED BLOOD DISORDERS

Iron Deficiency Anemia

Iron deficiency anemia is characterized by the production of small (microcytic) erythrocytes and a diminished level of circulating hemoglobin. This microcytic anemia is actually the last stage of iron deficiency, and it represents the end point of a long period of iron deprivation.

Pathophysiology

There are many possible causes of iron-deficiency anemia (Figure 34-1). The condition can arise from (1) inadequate iron intake secondary to a poor diet (such as a vegetarian lifestyle with insufficient heme iron); (2) inadequate absorption resulting from diarrhea, achlorhydria, intestinal disease, atrophic gastritis, partial or total gastrectomy, or drug interference (antacids, cholestyramine, cimetidine [Tagamet], pancreatin, ranitidine [Zantac], and tetracycline); (3) inadequate utilization secondary to chronic gastrointestinal disturbances; (4) increased iron requirement for growth of blood volume, which occurs during infancy, adolescence, pregnancy, and lactation; (5) increased excretion because of excessive menstrual blood (in females); hemorrhage from injury; or chronic blood loss from a bleeding ulcer, bleeding hemorrhoids, esophageal varices, regional enteritis, ulcerative colitis, parasites (hookworm disease), or malignant disease; or (6) defective release of iron from iron stores into the plasma and defective iron utilization owing to a chronic inflammation or other chronic disorder.

With few exceptions, iron deficiency anemia in male adults is the result of blood loss. Large losses of menstrual blood can cause iron deficiency in women, many of whom are unaware that their menses are unusually heavy.

Stages of Deficiency

As shown in Figure 34-2, one's iron status can range from iron overload to iron deficiency anemia. Routine measurement of iron status is necessary because about 6% of Americans have a negative iron balance, about 10% have a gene for positive balance, and about 1% have iron overload.

Deviations from normal iron status have been summarized by Herbert (1992) as follows:

Stages I and II negative iron balance (i.e., iron depletion)—In these stages, iron stores are low and there is no dysfunction. In stage I negative iron balance, reduced iron absorption produces moderately depleted iron stores. Stage II nega-

TABLE 34-1 Morphologic Classification of Anemia

MORPHOLOGIC TYPE OF ANEMIA	UNDERLYING ABNORMALITY	CLINICAL SYNDROMES/CAUSES	TREATMENT
Macrocytic (MCV >94; MCHC >31)			
Megaloblastic	Vitamin B_{12} deficiency	Pernicious anemia	Vitamin B_{12}
	Folic acid deficiency	Nutritional megaloblastic anemias, sprue, and other malabsorption syndromes	Folic acid
	Inherited disorders of DNA synthesis	Orotic aciduria	Treatment based on the nature of the disorder
	Drug-induced disorders of DNA synthesis	Chemotherapeutic agents, anticonvulsants, oral contraceptives	Discontinue offending drug and administer folic acid
Nonmegaloblastic	Accelerated erythropoiesis	Hemolytic anemia	Treatment of underlying disease
	Increased membrane surface area		
Hypochromic Microcytic (MCV <80; MCHC <31)			
	Iron deficiency	Chronic loss of blood, inadequate diet, impaired absorption, increased demands	Ferrous sulfate and correction of underlying cause
	Disorders of globin synthesis	Thalassemia	Nonspecific
	Disorders of porphyrin and heme synthesis	Pyridoxine-responsive anemia	Pyridoxine
	Other disorders of iron metabolism		
Normochromic Normocytic (MCV 82-92; MCHC >30)			
	Recent blood loss	Various	Transfusion, iron Correction of underlying condition
	Overexpansion of plasma volume	Pregnancy	Restore homeostasis
	Hemolytic diseases	Overhydration	Treatment based on the nature of the disorder
	Hypoplastic bone marrow	Aplastic anemia	Transfusions
		Pure red blood cell aplasia	Androgens
	Infiltrated bone marrow	Leukemia, multiple myeloma, myelofibrosis	Chemotherapy
	Endocrine abnormality	Hypothyroidism, adrenal insufficiency	Treatment of underlying disease
	Chronic disorders		Treatment of underlying disease
	Renal disease	Renal disease	Treatment of underlying disease
	Liver disease	Cirrhosis	Treatment of underlying disease

Modified from Wintrobe MM et al: *Clinical hematology*, ed 8, Philadelphia, 1981, Lea & Febiger.
MCV, Mean corpuscular volume = volume of one red blood cell expressed in femtoliters (fl); *MCHC*, mean corpuscular hemoglobin concentration – concentration of hemoglobin expressed in g/dl.

tive iron balance is characterized by severely depleted iron stores. More than 50% of all cases of negative iron balance fall into these two stages. When persons in these two stages are treated with iron, they never develop dysfunction or disease.

Stages III and IV negative iron balance (i.e., iron deficiency)—Iron deficiency is characterized by inadequate body iron, causing dysfunction and disease. In stage III negative iron balance, dysfunction is not accompanied by anemia; however, anemia does occur in stage IV negative iron balance.

Stages I and II positive iron balance—Stage I positive iron balance usually lasts for several years with no accompanying dysfunction. Supplements of iron or vitamin C promote progression to dysfunction or disease, whereas iron removal prevents progression to disease. Iron overload disease develops in persons with stage II positive balance after years of iron overload have caused progressive damage to tissues and organs. Again, iron removal stops disease progression.

Iron status has a variety of indicators. Serum ferritin levels are in equilibrium with body iron stores. Very early (stage I) positive iron balance may best be recognized by measuring total iron-binding capacity (TIBC) (transferrin IBC). Conversely, measurement of serum (plasma) ferritin levels may best reveal early (stages I and II) negative iron balance, although serum total iron-binding capacity may be as good an indicator.

Clinical Findings

Because anemia is the last manifestation of chronic, long-term iron deficiency, the symptoms reflect a malfunction of a variety of body systems. Inadequate muscle function is reflected in decreased work performance and exercise tolerance. Neurologic involvement is manifested by behavioral changes, such as fatigue, anorexia, and pica, especially pagophagia (ice eating) (see Chapter 7). Nokes and colleagues, in their Report of the International Nutritional Anemia Consultative Group (1998) support earlier work by Pollitt and colleagues (1986) that abnormal cognitive devel-

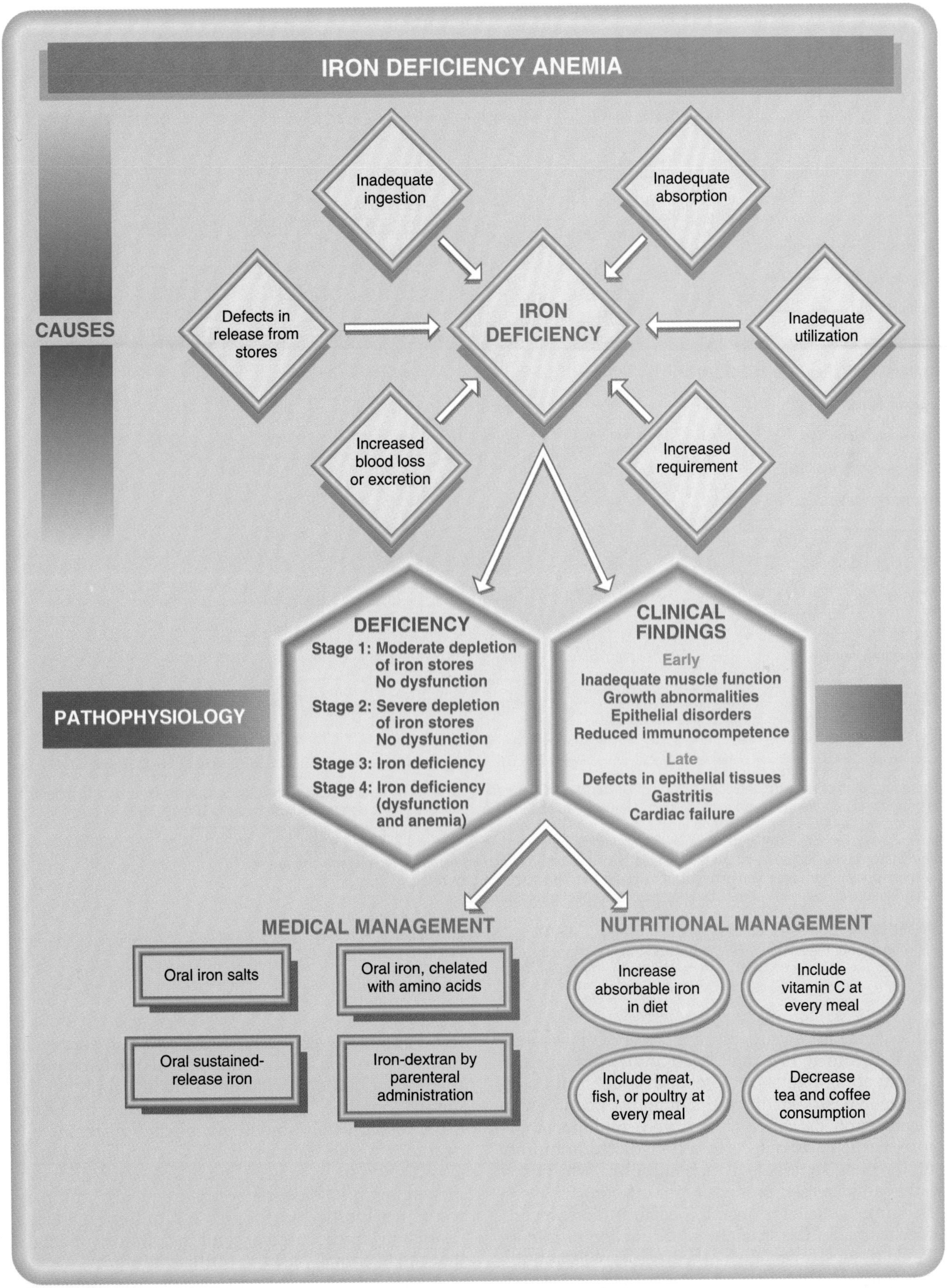

FIGURE 34-1 • Pathophysiology algorithm: iron deficiency anemia. (Algorithm content developed by John Anderson, PhD, and Sanford C. Garner, PhD, 2000. Updated by Tracy Stopler, MS, RD, 2002.)

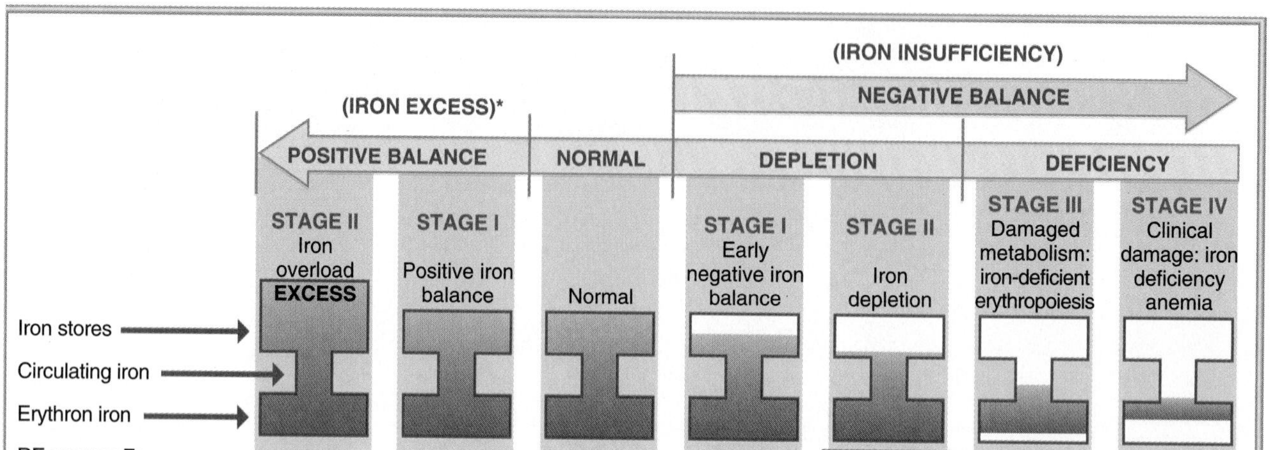

	STAGE II Iron overload EXCESS	STAGE I Positive iron balance	Normal	STAGE I Early negative iron balance	STAGE II Iron depletion	STAGE III Damaged metabolism: iron-deficient erythropoiesis	STAGE IV Clinical damage: iron deficiency anemia
RE marrow Fe	4+	3+	2–3+	1+	0–1+	0	0
Transferrin IBC (μg/100ml)†	<300	<300	330 ± 30	300–360	360	390	410
Plasma ferritin (μg/L)‡	>300	>150	100 ± 60	<25	20	10	<10
Iron absorption (%)	>15	10–15	5–10	10–15	10–15	10–20	10–20
Plasma iron (μg/100ml)†	>175	>150	115 ± 50	<120	115	<60	<40
Transferrin saturation (%)†	>60	>45	35 ± 15	30	30	<15	<15
Sideroblasts (%)	40–60	40–60	40–60	40–60	40–60	<10	<10
RBC protoporphyrin	30	30	30	30	30	100	200
Erythrocytes	Normal	Normal	Normal	Normal	Normal	Normal	Microcytic/ hypochromic
Serum transferrin receptors	Normal	Normal	Normal	Normal-High	High	Very high	Very high
Ferritin-iron (haloferritin) (ng/ml)§	Very high	High	Normal	Normal-Low	Low	Very low	Very low

*Randall Lauffer of Harvard and Joe McCord of University of Colorado–Denver hold that *any* storage iron is excessive because of its potential to promote excessive free radical generation. (Herbert V et al: Most free radical injury is iron related, *Stem Cells* 12:289, 1994.)
†Inflammation reduces transferrin (and the plasma iron on it), because transferrin is a reverse acute-phase reactant.
‡Inflammation produces elevated ferritin, because ferritin protein is an acute-phase reactant.
§Ferritin-iron is unaffected by inflammation, so it is reliable when ferritin, transferrin, and plasma iron are not.
Dallman (pediatrician) definition of negative balance: less absorbed than *excreted.*
Herbert (internist) definition of negative balance: less absorbed than *needed.*

FIGURE 34-2 • Sequential stages of iron status. *RE,* Reticuloendothelial cells; *TIBC,* total iron-binding capacity; *RBC,* red blood cell; *RE,* reticuloendothelial cells; *TIBC,* total iron-binding capacity (Copyright Victor Herbert, 1995).

opment in children suggests the presence of iron deficiency before it has developed into overt anemia. Growth abnormalities, epithelial disorders, and a reduction in gastric acidity are common. A possible sign of early iron deficiency is reduced immunocompetence, particularly defects in cell-mediated immunity and the phagocytic activity of neutrophils, which may lead to an increased propensity for infection.

As iron deficiency anemia becomes more severe, defects arise in the structure and function of the epithelial tissues, especially of the tongue, nails, mouth, and stomach. The skin may appear pale, and the inside of the lower eyelid may be light pink instead of red. Fingernails can become thin and flat, and eventually *koilonychia* (spoon-shaped nails) may be noted (Figure 34-3). Mouth changes include atrophy of the lingual papillae, burning, redness, and, in severe cases, a completely smooth, waxy, and glistening appearance to the tongue *(glossitis). Angular stomatitis* may also occur, as may a form of *dysphagia* (difficulty in swallowing). Gastritis occurs frequently and may result in achlorhydria. Progressive, untreated anemia results in cardiovascular and respiratory changes that can eventually lead to cardiac failure.

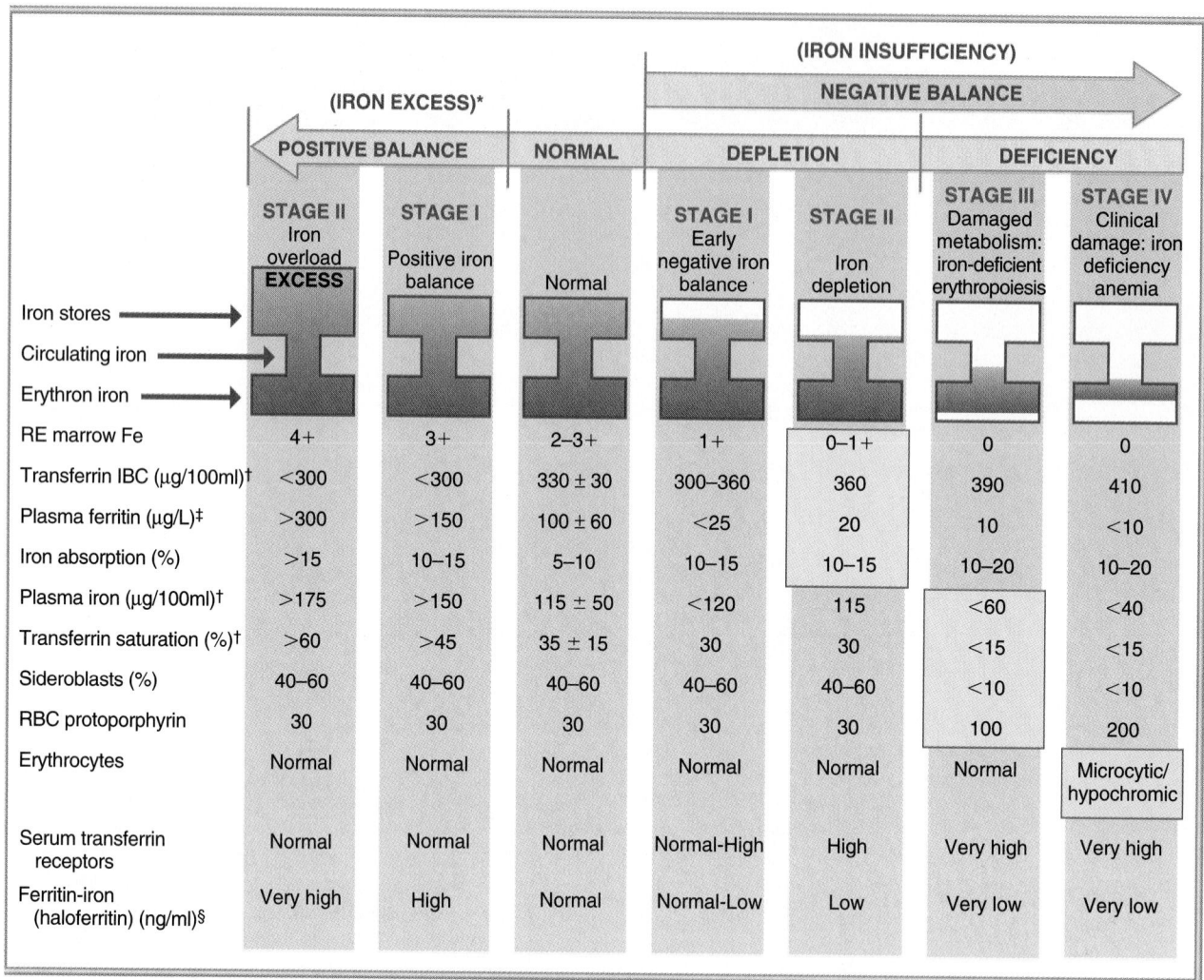

Some behavioral symptoms of iron deficiency seem to respond to iron therapy before the anemia is cured, suggesting they may be the result of tissue depletion of iron-containing enzymes rather than the result of a decreased level of hemoglobin (see Chapters 5 and 18).

Diagnosis

Progressive stages of iron deficiency can be evaluated by six different measurements:

1. Quantity of serum or plasma ferritin.
2. Quantity of serum or plasma iron.
3. Quantity of total circulating transferrin.
4. Percent saturation of circulating transferrin, which measures the iron supply to the tissues. It is calculated by dividing serum iron by the TIBC; levels less than 16% are considered inadequate for erythropoiesis.
5. Percent saturation of ferritin with iron.
6. Quantity of soluble serum transferrin receptor (STFR): Transferrin molecules are generated on the surface of red blood cells in response to the need for iron. With iron deficiency, so many transferrin receptors are on the cell surface looking for iron that some of them break off and float in the blood serum (plasma). Their presence is an early measurement of developing iron deficiency, with a higher quantity meaning greater deficiency of iron.

A definitive diagnosis of iron deficiency anemia requires more than one method of iron evaluation and preferably includes the first three of the measurements just listed. The evaluation should also include an assessment of cell morphology. The serum or plasma ferritin level is the most sensitive parameter of negative iron balance because it decreases only in the presence of true iron deficiency, as with transferrin saturation.

Protoporphyrin, the iron-containing portion of the respiratory pigments that combine with protein to form hemoglobin or myoglobin, can be used to assess iron deficiency. The zinc protoporphyrin (ZnPP)/heme ratio is measured as discussed in Chapter 18. However, this ZnPP/heme ratio and hemoglobin levels are affected by chronic infection and other factors that can produce a condition that mimics iron deficiency anemia when, in fact, iron is adequate (Herbert et al, 1997).

The TIBC declines and serum ferritin levels rise in chronic disease unrelated to iron metabolism (see Table 34-1). By itself, hemoglobin concentration is unsuitable as a diagnostic tool in cases of suspected iron deficiency anemia for three reasons: (1) it is affected only late in the disease; (2) it cannot distinguish iron deficiency from other anemias; (3) hemoglobin values in normal individuals vary widely.

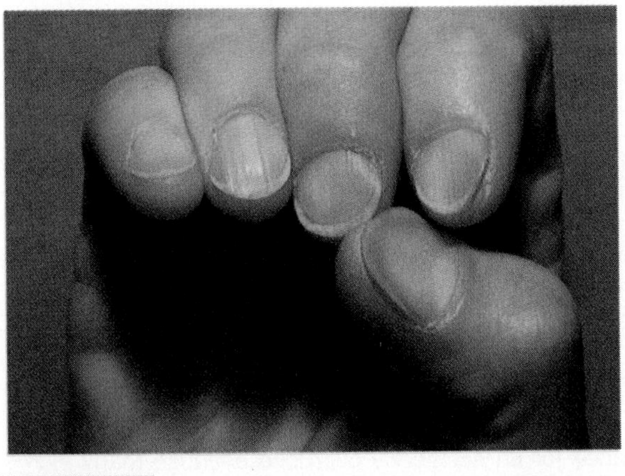

FIGURE 34-3 • Fingernails with cuplike depressions (koilonchia) are a sign of iron deficiency in adults. (From Callen JP et al: *Color atlas of dermatology,* Philadelphia, 1993, WB Saunders.)

Medical Management

Treatment should focus primarily on the underlying disease or situation leading to the anemia, although this is often difficult to determine. Repletion of iron stores, not merely alleviation of the anemia, should be the goal.

Supplementation

The chief treatment for iron deficiency anemia involves oral administration of inorganic iron in the ferrous form. At a dose of 30 mg, absorption of ferrous iron is three times greater than if the same amount were given in the ferric form. At larger doses, the difference is even more marked. The most widely used preparation is ferrous sulfate, and the dose is calculated in terms of the amount of elemental iron provided. Other salts absorbed to about the same degree are the ferrous forms of lactate, fumarate, glycine sulfate, glutamate, and gluconate.

Iron is best absorbed when the stomach is empty; however, under these conditions, it tends to cause gastric irritation. Gastrointestinal side effects can include nausea, epigastric discomfort and distention, heartburn, diarrhea, or constipation. If these side effects occur, the patient is told to take the iron with meals (breakfast, lunch, and dinner) instead of on an empty stomach; however, this sharply reduces the absorbability of the iron. Gastric irritation is a direct result of the quantity of free ferrous iron in the stomach; unfortunately, it is a high quantity of free ferrous iron in the stomach that irritates the gastric mucosa. Health professionals generally prescribe oral iron for iron deficiency for 3 months (three times daily). If it has to be given with meals, treatment should be for 4 to 5 months (see *New Directions:* Getting the Iron—A New Way to Supplement).

Depending on the severity of the anemia and the patient's tolerance of iron supplementation, the daily dose of elemental iron should be 50 to 200 mg for adults and 6 mg per kilogram of body weight for children. Ascorbic acid greatly increases both iron absorption and iron gastric irritation through its capacity to maintain iron in the reduced state.

Absorption of 10 to 20 mg of iron per day permits red blood cell production to increase to about three times the normal rate and, in the absence of blood loss, hemoglobin concentration to rise at a rate of 0.2 g/dl daily. Increased reticulocytosis (an increase in the number of young red blood cells) is seen within 2 to 3 days after iron administration, but affected persons may report subjective improvements in mood and appetite even sooner. The hemoglobin level will begin to increase by day 4 of treatment. Iron therapy should be continued for several months, even after restoration of normal hemoglobin levels, to allow for repletion of body iron reserves.

If iron supplementation fails to correct the anemia, one should consider the following possibilities: (1) the patient may not be taking the medication as prescribed, most likely because of unpleasant side effects; (2) bleeding may be continuing at a rate faster than the erythroid marrow can replace blood cells; or (3) the supplemental iron is not being absorbed, possibly as a result of malabsorption secondary to steatorrhea, celiac sprue, or hemodialysis. In these circumstances, parenteral administration of iron, in the form of iron-dextran, may be necessary (see Figure 34-1). Although replenishment of iron stores by this route is faster, it is more expensive and not as safe as oral administration.

Medical Nutrition Therapy

In addition to iron supplementation, attention should be given to the amount of absorbable dietary iron consumed. Liver, kidney, beef, egg yolk, dried fruits, dried peas and beans, nuts, green leafy vegetables, molasses, whole-grain breads and cereals, and fortified cereals are among the foods that rank highest in iron content (Table 34-2).

It is estimated that 1.8 mg of iron must be absorbed daily to meet the needs of 80% to 90% of adult women and adolescent males and females. Because typical Western diets generally contain 6 mg/1000 kcal of iron, the bioavailability of iron in the diet is clearly more important in correcting or preventing iron deficiency than the total amount of dietary iron consumed.

Bioavailability of Dietary Iron

Several factors influence the bioavailability of dietary iron. The rate of absorption depends on the iron status of the individual, as reflected in the level of iron stores. The lower the iron stores, the greater will be the rate of iron absorption. Individuals with iron deficiency anemia absorb about 20% to 30% of dietary iron compared with the 5% to 10% absorbed by those without iron deficiency.

The form of iron in the diet also influences absorption. Heme iron (about 15% absorbable), present in meat, fish, and poultry (MFP), is much better absorbed than nonheme iron, which can also be found in MFP, as well as in eggs, grains, vegetables, and fruits. The absorption rate of nonheme iron varies between 3% and 8%, depending on the presence of dietary enhancing factors, specifically, ascorbic acid and MFP. Ascorbic acid is not only a powerful reducing agent, but it also binds iron to form a readily absorbed complex. The mechanism by which MFP po-

NEW DIRECTIONS

Getting the Iron—A New Way to Supplement

Treatment of iron deficiency anemia has always been frustrating for clinicians and their patients. Clinically, such large doses of iron are required for a therapeutic amount of elemental iron to be absorbed that patients complain about gastrointestinal upset, gastritis, and constipation. Mothers can be reluctant to give their infants iron-fortified formula because they may remember their own experience with iron supplements during pregnancy and may imagine that their infants have gastrointestinal upset or, in fact, because the infants can really become constipated. For these reasons, compliance with iron therapy is less than optimal, and clinicians and supplement companies are continually looking for new forms in which to give iron supplementation.

Commercial food fortifiction works well to provide iron on a preventive basis, but large amounts of iron (enough to have a therapeutic effect) cannot be provided in this way because the iron causes changes in the taste and color of the food. These problems are even more difficult in developing countries where as many as one third to one half of the population is anemic (World Health Organization, 2000).

To overcome this problem, iron as ferrous fumarate powder along with ascorbic acid is being encapsulated with a soya-based hydrogenated lipid into microencapsulations. Little packets of these microencapsulations can then be sprinkled onto the food that the person is eating and consumed along with the food. The result is the consumption of a large amount of iron without a change in the taste or color of the food. Compared with the use of ferrous sulfate drops in an anemic population in Ghana, the sprinkles were just as effective in treating anemia, and they are less expensive to manufacture and to distribute than the drops. In addition, there is less chance for an accidental overdose because many individual packets would have to be opened and consumed for this to occur (Zlotkin et al, 2001).

TABLE 34-2 Iron Content of Some Common Foods

FOOD	PORTION SIZE	IRON (mg)*
Protein Group		
Chicken, light meat	3 oz	0.9
Chicken, dark meat	3 oz	1.2
Turkey, dark meat	3 oz	2.0
Pork chop	3 oz	0.7
Tenderloin steak	3 oz	1.3
Venison, roasted	3 oz	3.0
Liver, beef	3 oz	5.8
Liver, chicken	3 oz	7.2
Liver, pork	3 oz	15.2
Tuna fish	3 oz	0.6
Swordfish	3 oz	1.1
Oysters, raw	3 oz	5.5
Tofu, raw	½ c	4.0
Black beans	½ c	1.8
Chickpeas	½ c	2.4
Kidney beans	½ c	2.6
Lentil beans	½ c	3.3
Egg	1 whole	0.6
Cashew nuts	1 oz	1.7
Pistachio nuts	1 oz	1.9
Sunflower seeds	1 tbsp	1.9
Dairy Group		
Milk	1 c	0.1
Ricotta, part-skim	½ c	0.6
Soy milk	1 c	1.8
Fruit Group		
Apricots	3 raw	0.6
Apple, dried	10 rings	0.9
Figs, dried	1	0.4
Peaches, dried	5 halves	2.6
Raisins	½ c	1.5
Strawberries	1 c, frozen	1.2
Vegetable Group		
Artichoke, cooked	1 c	5.1
Baked potato	1 medium	2.7
Broccoli	1 medium stalk	2.1
Green pepper	1 medium	0.9
Lima beans	½ c	2.1
Spinach	1 c	1.5
Grain Group		
Pasta (enriched)	1 c	2.0
Rice (enriched)	1 c	1.8
Whole-wheat bread	1 slice	1.0
Bagel	1	1.8
Cereals		
Grapenuts	½ c	18.0
Product 19	¾ c	18.0
Total	1 c	18.0
Wheat germ	1 oz (¼ c)	2.6
Cream of Wheat, instant	¾ c	8.2
Oatmeal, plain, instant	1 packet	6.7
Energy or Sports Bars		
Balance	1 bar, 1.76 oz	4.5
Clif	1 bar, 2.4 oz	4.5
Genisoy	1 bar, 1.76 oz	1.8
Kashi Go Lean	1 bar, 2.75 oz	<1.0
Luna	1 bar, 1.69 oz	6.3
Met Rx (Big 100)	1 bar, 3.5 oz	8.1
Power	1 bar, 2.29 oz	6.3
Pria	1 bar, .98 oz	3.6
Promax	1 bar, 2.7 oz	4.5
Zone	1 bar, 1.76 oz	1.44

*Absorbability of iron from animal foods averages 15%; from plant foods, it averages only 3%.

Box 34-1. Incidence of Hemochromatosis and Iron Deficiency Anemia in Adult Males

1 in 8 have one gene (heterozygous)
1 in 100-200 (approximately ½%-1%) of adult American men have two genes (homozygous) expressing iron overload
1 in 500 have iron deficiency anemia

Stopler T, Herbert V: Nutrition E.T.C. for the millenium, Plainview, NY, 1999, Nutrition ETC.

tentiates the absorption of nonheme iron in other foodstuffs is unknown. MFP digestion may lead to the release of amino acids (particularly cysteine) and polypeptides in the upper small bowel, which then chelate with nonheme iron to form soluble, absorbable complexes (Mulvihill et al, 1998).

Iron absorption can be inhibited to varying degrees by a number of factors that chelate iron, including carbonates, oxalates, phosphates, and phytates (unleavened bread, unrefined cereals, and soybeans). Factors in vegetable fiber may inhibit nonheme iron. Taken with meals, tea and coffee can reduce iron absorption by 50% through the formation of insoluble iron compounds with tannin. Iron in egg yolk is poorly absorbed because of the presence of phosvitin.

In summary, then, to maximize iron absorption and prevent iron deficiency anemia, one should (1) improve food choices to increase total dietary iron intake; (2) include a source of vitamin C at every meal; (3) include MFP at every meal, if possible; and (4) avoid drinking large amounts of tea or coffee with meals.

Hemochromatosis

Hemochromatosis is a genetically predisposed form of iron overload that is present, in heterozygous (one gene) form, in about 12% of nonblacks and about 30% of blacks (www.niddk.nih.gov/health/hematol). About 1 in 200 nonblacks and about 1 in 100 blacks are homozygous (Box 34-1). Homozygotes (two genes) will die of iron overload unless they donate blood frequently. These persons absorb three times more iron from their food than those without hemochromatosis. In women, monthly menses slow the associated organ damage until after menopause.

Pathophysiology

Men are particularly susceptible to hemochromatosis because they have no physiologic mechanisms, such as menstruation, pregnancy, or lactation, for losing iron. The excessive iron intake usually stems from accidental incorporation of iron into the diet from environmental sources. In developing countries, the iron overload can result from eating foods cooked in cast-iron cooking vessels or contaminated by iron-containing soils.

After absorption, iron is transported by plasma transferrin, a β1-globulin (protein) that binds iron derived from the gastrointestinal tract, iron storage sites, or hemoglobin breakdown and transports it to the bone marrow (hemoglobin synthesis), endothelial cells (storage), or placenta (fetal needs). The protein hereditary iron (Fe) (HFE) is the product of the gene responsible for hemochromatosis. It is this protein that interacts with the transferrin receptors on the surface of cells, thus regulating the cells' ability to take up the transferrin-bound iron from the circulation (Cohen, 1998).

Excess iron is stored as ferritin and hemosiderin in the macrophages of the liver, spleen, and bone marrow. The body has a limited capacity to excrete iron. About 1 mg of iron is excreted daily through the gastrointestinal tract, urinary tract, and skin. To maintain a normal iron balance, the daily obligatory loss must be replaced by the absorption of heme and nonheme food iron. Persons with iron overload excrete increased amounts of iron, especially in the feces, to compensate partially for the increased absorption and higher stores (Fairbanks, 1999).

Clinical Findings

In hemochromatosis, iron absorption is enhanced, resulting in a gradual, progressive accumulation of iron. This disease, associated in whites with an abnormal human leukocyte antigen A (HLA-A) gene located on the short arm of chromosome 6, is often underdiagnosed. Most affected persons do not know they have the disease. In its early stages, iron overload may result in symptoms similar to iron deficiency, such as fatigue and weakness; later, it can cause chronic abdominal pain, aching joints, impotence, and menstrual irregularities. A progressive positive iron balance may result in a variety of serious problems, including hepatomegaly, skin pigmentation, diabetes mellitus, arthritis, cancer, heart disease, and hypogonadism. Mortality from hemochromatosis is preventable if excess body iron is removed by phlebotomy therapy before hepatic cirrhosis develops.

Diagnosis

If an iron overload is suspected, the following screening tests should be performed: serum ferritin level (storage iron), serum iron concentration, total iron binding capacity (TIBC), and percent transferrin saturation ([serum iron/TIBC] × 100). Iron overload may be present if the percent of transferrin saturation is greater than 50 in women and 60 in men and if the serum iron level is greater than 180 mg/dl. DNA testing, using blood or cheek cell samples, is also available for early detection of hemochromatosis. Liver biopsy is the "gold standard" for the diagnosis of iron overload.

The patient with iron overload may simultaneously be anemic as a result of damage to the bone marrow or an inflammatory disorder (i.e., arthritis), cancer, internal bleeding, or chronic infection. Iron supplements should not be taken until the cause of the anemia is known.

Medical Management

For patients with significant iron overload, weekly phlebotomy for 2 to 3 years may be required to eliminate all excess iron. Treatment for iron overload may also involve iron depletion with intravenous desferrioxamine-B, a chelating agent that is excreted by the kidneys. Calcium disodium EDTA can also be used. Patients diagnosed as having hemochromatosis should inform all blood relatives so that they too can be evaluated.

Medical Nutrition Therapy

Individuals with iron overload should ingest less heme iron (i.e., from MFP) compared with nonheme iron (plant groups). Persons with iron overload should also avoid alcohol and vitamin C supplements because both enhance iron absorption. Some evidence, however, shows that even though vitamin C enhances iron absorption at a meal, when it is given daily in increased amounts from food or supplements as part of the complete diet, over the long-term, the facilitating effect on iron absorption is far less (Cook and Reddy, 2001). In addition, vitamin C supplements may cause release of harmful free radical–generating excess iron from body stores. Affected persons should also avoid foods that are highly fortified with iron, foods such as many breakfast cereals, many "energy" or sports bars, and many meal-replacement drinks or shakes that are fortified with vitamins and minerals. They should also avoid iron supplements or multiple vitamin-mineral supplements that contain iron. The recommended dietary allowance (RDA) for iron should not be exceeded, and perhaps the intake of iron should be less in some persons. The new RDAs for iron are summarized in Table 5-6 and Table 15-1. The RDA for women in their childbearing years is 18 mg, and the RDA for adult men and women 51 years of age and older is 8 mg (Institute of Medicine, 2001).

Iron Toxicity

Other disorders associated with iron overload include thalassemias, sideroblastic anemia, chronic hemolytic anemia, aplastic anemia, ineffective erythropoiesis, transfusional iron overload (secondary to multiple blood transfusions), porphyria cutanea tarda, and alcoholic cirrhosis. Excess dietary iron intake (as occurs in South African [Bantu] blacks who absorb excess dietary iron from alcoholic beverages fermented in iron stills and food cooked in iron pots) or an overdose of iron medication (as may occasionally occur in children who mistake iron tablets for candy) can be fatal in doses of 3 to 10 g. Excessive iron can cause irritation of the mucosa as well as ulceration and bleeding, hypoxia, metabolic acidosis, alveolar and hepatic damage, and renal failure. Death can occur in 12 to 48 hours.

MEGALOBLASTIC ANEMIAS

Megaloblastic anemia reflects a disturbed synthesis of DNA, which results in morphologic and functional changes in erythrocytes, leukocytes, platelets, and their precursors in the blood and bone marrow. Megaloblastic anemia is usually caused by a deficiency of vitamin B_{12} or folic acid, both of which are essential to the synthesis of nucleoproteins. Hematologic changes are the same for both; however, the folic acid deficiency is the first to appear. Normal body folate stores are depleted within 2 to 4 months in individuals consuming folate-deficient diets; by contrast, vitamin B_{12} stores are depleted only after several years of a vitamin B_{12}–deficient diet. In persons with vitamin B_{12} deficiency, folic acid supplementation can mask B_{12} deficiency (Markle, 1997). In correcting the anemia, the vitamin B_{12} deficiency may remain undetected, leading to the irreversible neuropsychiatric damage that is only prevented with B_{12} supplementation (see Chapter 4).

Pernicious and Other Vitamin B_{12} Deficiency Anemias

Pathophysiology

Pernicious anemia is a megaloblastic macrocytic anemia caused by a deficiency of vitamin B_{12}. Most commonly, the vitamin deficiency is secondary to a lack of intrinsic factor (IF), a glycoprotein in the gastric juice that is necessary for the absorption of dietary vitamin B_{12}. Rarely, vitamin B_{12} deficiency anemia occurs in strict vegetarians whose diet contains no vitamin B_{12} except for traces found in plants contaminated by microorganisms capable of synthesizing vitamin B_{12}. Other causes are shown in Box 34-2.

Ingested vitamin B_{12} is freed from protein by gastric acid and gastric and intestinal enzymes. The free vitamin B_{12} attaches to salivary R-binder, which, at an acid pH (2.3) such as that found in the stomach, has a higher affinity for the vitamin than does IF. Secreted by parietal cells of the gastric mucosa, IF is necessary for the absorption of exogenous vitamin B_{12}. The release of pancreatic trypsin into the proximal small intestine destroys R-binder and releases vitamin B_{12} from its complex with R-protein. At an alkaline pH (6.8), as may be found in the intestine, IF then binds the vitamin B_{12}.

The vitamin B_{12}–IF complex is then carried to the ileum, where in the presence of ionic calcium (Ca^{2+}) and a pH of greater than 6, it attaches to the surface vitamin B_{12}–IF receptors on the ileal cell brush border.

At the brush border, the vitamin B_{12}–IF complex enters the ileal cell, where the vitamin B_{12} is released, attaching to holotranscobalamin II (Holo TC II). Like IF, holo TC II plays an active role in binding and transporting vitamin B_{12}. The TC II–vitamin B_{12} complex then enters the portal venous blood. Other binding proteins in the blood include haptocorrin, also known as transcobalamin I, and transcobalamin III (TC I and TC III). These are α-globulins—larger, macromolecular-weight glycoproteins—that make up the R-binder component of the blood. Unlike IF, the R-proteins are capable of binding not only vitamin B_{12} itself but also many of its biologically inactive analogs.

Although about 75% of the vitamin B_{12} in human serum is bound to haptocorrin, and roughly 25% is bound to TC II, only TC II is important in delivering vitamin B_{12} to all the cells that need it. After transport through the bloodstream, TC II is recognized by receptors on cell surfaces. Patients with haptocorrin abnormalities have no symptoms of vitamin B_{12} deficiency. Those lacking TC II rapidly develop megaloblastic anemia (Herbert, 2001b.)

As a result of normal enterohepatic circulation—that is, excretion of vitamin B_{12} and analogs in bile and reabsorption of mainly vitamin B_{12} in the ileum—it generally takes decades for strict vegetarians who are not receiving vitamin B_{12} supplementation to develop a vitamin B_{12} deficiency. Vitamin B_{12} is also excreted in urine.

Stages of Deficiency

Figure 34-4 shows the sequential biochemical and hematologic stages of vitamin B_{12} deficiency. The sequence of events involves four stages of depletion.

Stage 1—early negative vitamin B_{12} balance—begins when vitamin B_{12} intake is low or absorption is poor, depleting TC II, the primary delivery protein, resulting in a low TC II level (Herzlich and Herbert, 1988). A low TC II (<40 pg/ml) may be the earliest detectable sign of a vitamin B_{12} deficiency (Herbert et al, 1990).

In *stage 2 (vitamin B_{12} depletion)*, besides the low B_{12} on TC II, there is also a gradual lowering of B_{12} on haptocorrin (holohap <150 pg/ml), the storage protein.

Stage 3—damaged metabolism or vitamin B_{12}–deficient erythropoiesis—includes an abnormal deoxyuridine (dU) suppression, hypersegmentation, a decreased TIBC and holohap percent saturation, and a low red blood cell folate level (<140 ng/ml), and subtle neuropsychiatric damage (impaired short-term and recent memory) (Herbert, 2001a).

Stage 4—clinical damage, including vitamin B_{12} deficiency anemia—includes all preceding stages, including macroovalocytic erythrocytes, elevated mean corpuscular volume (MCV), elevated TC II levels, increased homocysteine and methylmalonate levels, and myelin damage.

Box 34-2. Causes of Vitamin B_{12} Deficiency

I. Inadequate ingestion
  A. Poor diet (lacking microorganisms and animal foods, which are the sole sources of vitamin B_{12})
    1. Strict vegetarianism (eating no meat, fowl, seafood, eggs, milk, or any products thereof)
    2. Chronic alcoholism (no vitamin B_{12} or folate in hard liquor; folate deficiency occurs first and is more common, partly because body stores of vitamin B_{12} last much longer than those of folate)
    3. Poverty, religious tenets (Hinduism, Seventh Day Adventism, certain Catholic orders), dietary faddism

II. Inadequate absorption
  A. Gastric disorder producing inadequate or absent secretion by gastric acid and enzymes, reducing ability to split B_{12} from food, followed in several years by loss of intrinsic factor secretion
    1. Addisonian pernicious anemia (PA): that form of vitamin B_{12} deficiency disease that is attributable to inadequate intrinsic factor secretion of uncertain cause
      a) Hereditary absence of normal intrinsic factor secretion: Absent secretion at birth (circulating antibody to intrinsic factor never present) supports the theory that antibody occurs only when antigenic stimulus is produced by intrinsic factor, which enters blood from damaged parietal cells and is recognized as foreign by the immunologic surveillance system; rare
      b) Congenital production of defective intrinsic factor molecule (three published cases)
      c) Autoimmunity-associated gastric atrophy: Affected patients usually have nondiagnostic-for-PA circulating parietal cell antibody, which is an index only of past or present gastric damage and not of the amount of intrinsic factor secretion (circulating diagnostic-for-PA antibody to intrinsic factor is always present in individuals younger than 21 years of age; there is a gradual decrease in measurable antibody, however, so that, by the age of 65 years, only two thirds of patients present with measurable circulating antibody to intrinsic factor)
        (1) Juvenile pernicious anemia (usually presents between the ages of 3 and 14 years)
        (2) Hereditarily determined degenerative gastric atrophy (gradually progresses with increasing age; almost 50% of all adult PA cases fall into this category)
        (3) Acquired gastric atrophy as the end result of superficial inflammatory gastritis such as that produced by *Heliobacter pylori;* superficial gastritis with atrophy (almost 50% of all adult PA cases fall into this category, which includes acquired gastric damage related to iron deficiency or alcohol)
        (4) Endocrine disorders (hypothyroidism, polyendocrinopathy) associated with gastric damage
    2. Gastrectomy
      a) Total
      b) Subtotal (approximately 20% develop PA within 10 years after surgery; associated with atrophy of remaining parietal cells)
        (1) Proximal
        (2) Distal
        (3) Lesions that destroy the gastric mucosa (ingested corrosives, linitis plastica)
        (4) Intrinsic factor inhibitor in gastric section
    3. Antibody to intrinsic factor (in saliva or gastric juice)
      a) "Blocking" antibody (attaches to intrinsic factor to block ability of intrinsic factor to take up vitamin B_{12})
      b) "Binding" antibody (attaches to intrinsic factor at a site distal to the site of vitamin B_{12} attachment)
  B. Small intestinal disorder (affecting ileum, which is the main site of vitamin B_{12} absorption)
    1. Gluten-induced enteropathy (childhood and adult celiac disease); idiopathic steatorrhea; nontropical sprue
    2. Tropical sprue (vitamin B_{12} is often the first nutrient to be subnormally absorbed and the last to return to normal absorption)
    3. Regional enteritis
    4. Strictures or anastomoses of the small bowel; other "stagnant bowel" syndromes
    5. Intestinal resection
    6. Cancers and granulomatous lesions involving the small intestine
    7. Other conditions characterized by chronically disturbed intestinal function
    8. Drugs inhibiting or preventing vitamin B_{12} absorption
      a) Para-aminosalicylic (PAS) acid
      b) Colchicine
      c) Neomycin
      d) Ethanol
      e) Metformin (and possibly other biguanide agents)

Modified from Herbert V, Das KC: Folic acid and vitamin B_{12}. In Shils ME, Olson JA, Shike M, editors: *Modern nutrition in health and disease,* ed 8, vol 1, Philadelphia, 1994, Lea & Febiger.

Box 34-2. Causes of Vitamin B_{12} Deficiency—cont'd

9. Specific malabsorption for vitamin B_{12}
   a) Long-term ingestion of calcium-chelating agents
10. Inadequately alkaline pH in ileum (Zollinger-Ellison syndrome, pancreatic disease)
11. Unknown causes (Lack of intestinal receptors for vitamin B_{12}–intrinsic factor complex? Absence of "releasing factor"?)
    a) Congenital disorder (Imerslund-Graesbeck syndrome; receptors probably functional)
    b) Acquired disorder (forme fruste of sprue; receptors possibly absent or nonfunctional)

C. Competition for vitamin B_{12} by intestinal parasites or bacteria
   1. Fish tapeworm *(Diphyllobothrium latum)*
   2. Bacteria: the blind loop syndrome
   3. *Helicobacter pylori (H. pylori)*

D. Pancreatic disease (normal pancreatic exocrine secretion of trypsin and bicarbonate required for normal vitamin B_{12} absorption)

E. Human immunodeficiency virus (HIV) infection (acquired immunodeficiency syndrome [AIDS]) leading to gastrointestinal dysfunction and malabsorption

III. Inadequate utilization
   A. Vitamin B_{12} antagonists
      1. Substituted vitamin B_{12} amides and anilides (experimental agents)
      2. Cobaloximes (experimental agents)
      3. Anti–vitamin B_{12} analogs?
   B. Congenital or acquired enzyme deficiency or deletion
      1. Methylmalonyl-CoA mutase
      2. Methyltetrahydrofolate-homocysteine methyltransferase
      3. Vitamin B_{12a} reductase
      4. Vitamin B_{12r} reductase
      5. Deoxyadenoxyltransferase
      6. Other enzyme reduction or deletion
   C. Abnormal vitamin B_{12}–binding protein in serum that irreversibly binds vitamin B_{12}, making it unavailable to tissues
      1. Increased TC I or TC III glycoprotein (myeloproliferative disorders; "granulocyte-related" vitamin B_{12} binders)
      2. Increased TC II protein (liver disease; "liver-related" vitamin B_{12} binders)
      3. Other abnormal vitamin B_{12} binding (a glycoprotein in some cases of hepatoma)
   D. Inadequate serum vitamin B_{12}–binding protein (congenital or acquired)
      1. TC II protein (the lack of which produces megaloblastic anemia; it delivers vitamin B_{12} to blood cells as transferrin delivers iron)
      2. TC I glycoprotein (the lack of which is not known to produce megaloblastic anemia; it is mainly a storage protein for vitamin B_{12}, somewhat akin to ceruloplasmin for copper)
      3. TC III (increasing amounts produced in vitro by granulocytes)

IV. Increased requirement (normal adult daily requirement for exogenous sources is 0.1 μg (0.073 nmol)
   A. Hyperthyroidism
   B. Increased hematopoiesis?
   C. Infancy
   D. Parasitization
      1. By fetus
      2. By malignant tissue?

V. Increased excretion
   A. Inadequate vitamin B_{12}–binding protein in serum
   B. Liver disease (inadequate storage capacity for vitamin B_{12})
   C. Renal disease?

VI. Increased destruction by antioxidants
   A. Pharmacologic doses of ascorbic acid

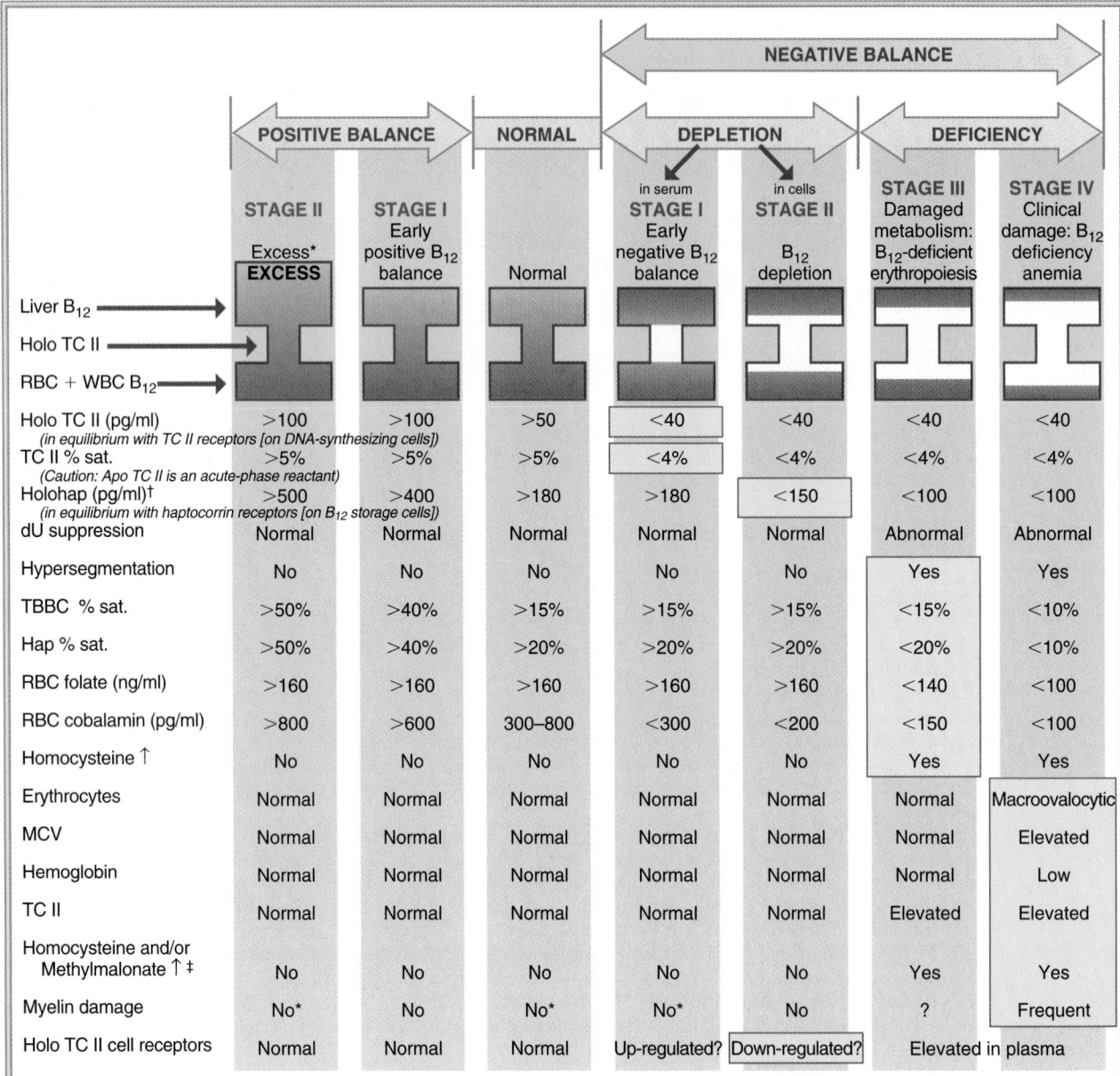

	POSITIVE BALANCE		NORMAL	NEGATIVE BALANCE: DEPLETION		NEGATIVE BALANCE: DEFICIENCY	
				in serum	in cells		
	STAGE II Excess* EXCESS	STAGE I Early positive B_{12} balance	Normal	STAGE I Early negative B_{12} balance	STAGE II B_{12} depletion	STAGE III Damaged metabolism: B_{12}-deficient erythropoiesis	STAGE IV Clinical damage: B_{12} deficiency anemia
Holo TC II (pg/ml)	>100	>100	>50	<40	<40	<40	<40
(in equilibrium with TC II receptors [on DNA-synthesizing cells])							
TC II % sat.	>5%	>5%	>5%	<4%	<4%	<4%	<4%
(Caution: Apo TC II is an acute-phase reactant)							
Holohap (pg/ml)†	>500	>400	>180	>180	<150	<100	<100
(in equilibrium with haptocorrin receptors [on B_{12} storage cells])							
dU suppression	Normal	Normal	Normal	Normal	Normal	Abnormal	Abnormal
Hypersegmentation	No	No	No	No	No	Yes	Yes
TBBC % sat.	>50%	>40%	>15%	>15%	>15%	<15%	<10%
Hap % sat.	>50%	>40%	>20%	>20%	>20%	<20%	<10%
RBC folate (ng/ml)	>160	>160	>160	>160	>160	<140	<100
RBC cobalamin (pg/ml)	>800	>600	300–800	<300	<200	<150	<100
Homocysteine ↑	No	No	No	No	No	Yes	Yes
Erythrocytes	Normal	Normal	Normal	Normal	Normal	Normal	Macroovalocytic
MCV	Normal	Normal	Normal	Normal	Normal	Normal	Elevated
Hemoglobin	Normal	Normal	Normal	Normal	Normal	Normal	Low
TC II	Normal	Normal	Normal	Normal	Normal	Elevated	Elevated
Homocysteine and/or Methylmalonate ↑ ‡	No	No	No	No	No	Yes	Yes
Myelin damage	No*	No	No*	No*	No	?	Frequent
Holo TC II cell receptors	Normal	Normal	Normal	Up-regulated?	Down-regulated?	Elevated in plasma	

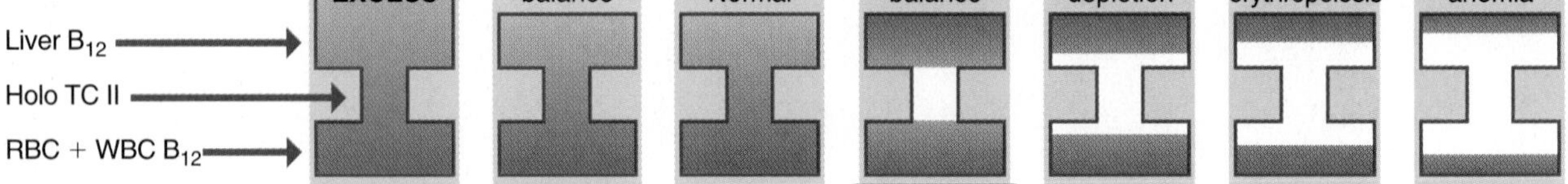

Holo TC II, Holotranscobalamin II; *TBBC,* total B_{12} binding capacity; *% sat.,* percent saturation; *RBC,* red blood cell; *MCV,* mean corpuscular volume.

* Cyanocobalamin excesses (injected or intranasal) produce transient increases in B_{12} delivery protein (TC II); the significance of such increases is unknown. Cyanocobalamin acts as an anti–B_{12} agent in a rare congenital defect in B_{12} metabolism.

† In serum and urine.

‡ Low holohaptocorrin correlates with **liver cell** B_{12} depletion, except in liver disease and myeloproliferative disorders, in which serum B_{12} and binding proteins are artificially elevated.

There may be hematopoietic cell and glial cell B_{12} depletion **prior to** liver cell depletion, and those cells may be in stage III or IV negative B_{12} balance, whereas liver cells are still in stage II.

FIGURE 34-4 • Sequential stages of vitamin B_{12} status. (From Herbert V: Staging vitamin B_{12}. In Ziegler EE, Filer LJ, editors: *Present knowledge in nutrition,* ed 7, Washington, DC, 1996, International Life Sciences Institute Press.)

Clinical Findings

Pernicious anemia affects not only the blood but also the gastrointestinal tract and the peripheral and central nervous systems. This distinguishes it from folic acid deficiency anemia. The overt symptoms, which are caused by inadequate myelinization of the nerves, include paresthesia (especially numbness and tingling in the hands and feet), diminution of the senses of vibration and position, poor muscular coordination, poor memory, and hallucinations. If the deficiency is prolonged, the nervous system damage may be irreversible, even with initiation of vitamin B_{12} treatment.

A link between vitamin B_{12} deficiency (which affects about 10% to 15% of men and women over 60 years of age) and *Helicobacter pylori* bacterium has been found. Researchers at the Turkish Military Medical Academy studied 138 patients with vitamin B_{12} deficiency anemia and found that 77 (58%) had *H. pylori* infection. Treating the infection corrected the anemia and normalized the serum B_{12} levels in 31 (40%) of the 77 infected patients. The researchers concluded that *H. pylori* infection can cause a vitamin B_{12} deficiency, which can be reversed by eradicating the infection (Kaptan et al, 2000; Stopeck, 2000).

Diagnosis

Vitamin B_{12} stores are depleted after several years without vitamin B_{12} intake. The time-consuming microbiologic assays have largely been replaced by the less time-consuming, though still precise, simultaneous radioassays. Radioassays measure more than one component within the same biologic medium (e.g., the Becton-Dickinson SimulTRAC Radioassay Kit measures the levels of serum vitamin B_{12} and serum folate simultaneously in a single test tube). Other laboratory tests that may be helpful in diagnosing a vitamin B_{12} deficiency and determining its cause include measurements of unsaturated B_{12} binding capacity (UBBC), intrinsic factor antibody (IFAB), the Schilling test, the deoxyuridine (dU) suppression test, and tests to determine serum homocysteine and serum methionine levels.

The IFAB and Schilling urinary excretion tests can determine whether the deficiency is caused by a lack of IF. The IFAB assay is performed on a patient's serum, whereas the Schilling test requires that the patient first swallow radioactive B_{12} alone and then a second time with IF.

The vitamin B_{12} assay is performed on the patient's urine after both steps of the Schilling test are completed. Patients with pernicious anemia excrete very little vitamin B_{12} during the first step because little or no vitamin B_{12} is absorbed; during the second step, however, the urinary excretion becomes almost normal because more vitamin B_{12} is absorbed with the addition of the IF. Vitamin B_{12} deficiency secondary to malabsorption syndrome is manifested by a decrease in urinary excretion of B_{12} that remains unchanged with IF administration. A low holo-TC II value (<40 pg/ml) is a sign of early B_{12} deficiency.

Medical Management

Before 1926 pernicious anemia was incurable, and the diagnosis invariably meant death in a relatively short time. In 1926, Minot and Murphy reported on the effectiveness of liver therapy, and active concentrates of liver suitable for oral use were soon developed (Minot and Murphy, 1926). By 1936 relatively purified extracts of liver were available for intramuscular injection. In 1948 vitamin B_{12} was determined to be the active agent in liver, and it is now available for either oral or parenteral administration.

Treatment usually consists of an intramuscular or subcutaneous injection of 100 μg or more of vitamin B_{12} once per week. After an initial response is elicited, the frequency of administration is reduced until remission can be maintained indefinitely with monthly injections of 100 μg. Very large oral doses of vitamin B_{12} (1000 μg daily) are also effective, even in the absence of IF, because about 1% of vitamin B_{12} will be absorbed by diffusion. A nasal gel and sublingual tablets are available and are well absorbed. Initial doses should be increased when vitamin B_{12} deficiency is complicated by debilitating illness, such as infection, hepatic disease, uremia, coma, severe disorientation, or marked neurologic damage.

A response to treatment is evidenced by improved appetite, alertness, and cooperation, followed by improved hematologic results, as manifested by marked reticulocytosis within hours of an injection.

Medical Nutrition Therapy

A high-protein diet (1.5 g/kg of body weight) is desirable both for liver function and for blood regeneration. Because green leafy vegetables contain both iron and folic acid, the diet should contain increased amounts of these foods. Liver should be included frequently because it carries a good supply of iron, vitamin B_{12}, folic acid, and other important nutrients. Meats (especially beef and pork), eggs, milk, and milk products are particularly rich in vitamin B_{12} (Table 34-3). The dietary reference intakes (DRIs) for B_{12} are recommended dietary allowances (RDAs) and are summarized in Table 4-22 and Table 15-1. The RDA for adult men and women is 2.4 μg daily (IOM, 1998).

Folic Acid Deficiency Anemia

Pathophysiology

Folic acid deficiency anemia is associated with tropical sprue, can affect pregnant women, and occurs in infants born to mothers with folic acid deficiency. Folic acid deficiency in early pregnancy can also result in an infant with a neural tube defect (see Chapter 7). Prolonged inadequate diets, faulty absorption and utilization of folic acid, and increased requirements resulting from growth are believed to be the most frequent causes (Box 34-3). Because alcohol interferes with the folate enterohepatic cycle, most alcoholics have a negative folate balance, and most are folate deficient. Alcoholics constitute the only group that generally has all six causes of folic acid deficiency simultaneously—inadequate ingestion, absorption, and utilization and increased excretion, requirement, and destruction of folic acid.

Folate absorption takes place in the small intestine. Enzyme conjugases (pteroylpolyglutamate hydrolase, commonly called folate conjugase), found in the brush border of the small intestine, hydrolyze the polyglutamates to monoglutamates and reduce them to dihydrofolate and tetrahydrofolate (THFA) in the small intestine epithelial cells (enterocytes). From the enterocytes, these forms are transported to the circulation, where they are bound to protein and transported as methyltetrahydrofolate into the cells of the body.

In the absence of vitamin B_{12}, 5-methyltetrahydrofolate (5-methyl THFA), the major circulating and storage form of folic acid, is metabolically inactive. To be activated, the 5-methyl group is removed and THFA is cycled back into the folate pool, where it functions as the main 1-carbon-unit acceptor in mammalian biochemical reactions. THFA may then be converted to the coenzyme form of folate required to convert deoxyuridylate to thymidylate, which is necessary for DNA synthesis.

Methylfolate Trap

Vitamin B_{12} deficiency can result in a folic acid deficiency by causing folate entrapment in the metabolically useless form of 5-methyl THFA (Figure 34-5). The lack of vitamin B_{12} to remove the 5-methyl unit means that metabolically inactive methyl THFA is trapped. It cannot release its 1-carbon methyl group to become THFA, the basic 1-carbon carrier that picks up 1-carbon units from one molecule and delivers them to another. Hence a functional folic acid deficiency results.

TABLE 34-3 Vitamin B_{12} Content of Some Common Foods*

FOOD	PORTION SIZE	VITAMIN B_{12} (μg)
Protein Group		
Chicken/turkey	3 oz	0.3
Hamburger	3 oz	8.0
Pork chop	3 oz	0.9
Tenderloin steak	3 oz	0.5
Liver, chicken	3 oz	16.5
Liver, pork	3 oz	15.8
Kidney, pork	3 oz	6.6
Swordfish	3 oz	1.7
Sardines (tomato sauce)	3 oz	7.7
Salmon	3 oz	5.8
Egg	1 whole	0.5
Dairy Group		
Milk (all varieties)	1 c	0.9
Yogurt	1 c	1.4
Cottage cheese	½ c	0.6
Cheese	1 oz	
Mozzarella/American		0.2
Ricotta/provolone		0.4
Swiss		0.5

*Essentially, vitamin B_{12} is in everything that walks, swims, and flies, and is not in anything that grows in the ground.

Stages of Deficiency

Folate deficiency develops in four stages: two that involve depletion, followed by two marked by deficiency (Figure 34-6) (Herbert, 1999).

Stage 1—Early negative folate balance (serum depletion)—This stage is characterized by a reduction in serum folate levels to less than 3 ng/ml.
Stage 2—Negative folate balance (cell depletion)—Folate depletion is characterized by a decrease in erythrocyte folate levels to less than 160 ng/ml.
Stage 3—Damaged folate metabolism, with folate-deficient erythropoiesis—This stage is characterized by slowed DNA synthesis, manifested by an abnormal diagnostic dU suppression test correctable in vitro by folates, granulocyte nuclear hypersegmentation, and macroovalocytic red cells.
Stage 4—Clinical folate deficiency anemia—This stage is manifested by an elevated mean corpuscular volume (MCV) and anemia.

Clinical Findings

Because of their interrelated roles in the synthesis of thymidylate in DNA formation, a deficiency of either vitamin B_{12} or folic acid will result in the same clinical sign—that is, a megaloblastic anemia. The immature nuclei do not mature properly in the deficient state, and large (macrocytic), immature (megaloblastic) red blood cells are the result.

The common clinical signs of folic acid deficiency include fatigue, dyspnea, sore tongue, diarrhea, irritability, forgetfulness, anorexia, glossitis, and weight loss.

Diagnosis

Normal body folate stores are depleted within 2 to 4 months on a folate-deficient diet, resulting in a macrocytic, megaloblastic anemia. This state is also characterized by a decreased number of erythrocytes, leukocytes, and platelets. Folate deficiency anemia is manifested by very low serum folate (<3 ng/ml) and red cell folate (RCF) levels (<140 ng/ml). Whereas a low serum folate level merely diagnoses a negative balance at the time the blood is drawn, an RCF level measures actual body folate stores and so is the superior measurement for determining folate nutriture. To differentiate folate deficiency from vitamin B_{12} deficiency, levels of serum folate, RCF, serum vitamin B_{12}, and vitamin B_{12} bound to TC II can be measured simultaneously using a radioassay kit. Also diagnostic for folate deficiency is an elevated level of formiminoglutamic acid (FIGLU) in the urine as well

Box 34-3. Causes of Folate Deficiency

I. Inadequate ingestion
   A. Poor diet (lack of unprocessed, fresh, uncooked, or slightly cooked food or fruit juices [folates are heat labile])
      1. Nutritional megaloblastic anemia
         a) Tropical
         b) Nontropical
         c) Scurvy (diets low in vitamin C are also low in folate)
      2. Chronic alcoholism, with or without cirrhosis

II. Inadequate absorption (affecting the upper third of the small intestine, which is the main site of folate absorption. Because most food folates are in polyglutamate forms, biliary and intestinal g-glutamyl conjugases are necessary to split off excess glutamates to make folates absorbable)
   A. Malabsorption syndromes
      1. Gluten-induced enteropathy (childhood and adult celiac disease; idiopathic steatorrhea; nontropical sprue; coincident vitamin B_{12} malabsorption only in rare cases)
      2. Any other chronic functional or structural disorder involving the upper small intestine
         a) Tropical sprue (coincident vitamin B_{12} malabsorption almost invariably present)
         b) Associated with herpetic and other skin disorders
      3. Drugs
         a) Anticonvulsants (e.g., phenytoin, primidone)
         b) Barbiturates
         c) Cycloserine
         d) Ethanol
         e) Metformin
         f) Amino acid excess (glycine or methionine)
         g) Nitrofurantoin? (antimicrobial)
         h) Glutethimide? (sedative)
         i) Cholestyramine
         j) Sulfasalazine (Azulfidine)
   B. Specific malabsorption for folate
      1. Congenital nonconjugase defects (four cases published)
      2. Acquired nonconjugase defects
      3. Inadequate biliary or intestinal conjugases
      4. Conjugase inhibitors (such as those contained in some beans)
   C. Blind loop syndrome (More commonly, bacteria make folate and actually raise the serum folate level of host.)

III. Inadequate utilization (metabolic block)
   A. Folic acid antagonists (dihydrofolate reductase inhibitors)
      1. 4-Amino-4-deoxyfolates, i.e., methotrexate (chemotherapy, immunosuppression, psoriasis)
      2. 2-4-Diaminopyrimidine, e.g., pyrimethiamine, trimethoprin (malaria, toxoplasmosis, antibacterial)
      3. Triamterene (diuretic)
      4. Diamidine compounds, i.e., pentamidine, isothionate (*Pneumocystis carinii*, protozocidal)
   B. Diphenylhydantoin and possibly other anticonvulsants (which may block cell uptake or use folate)
   C. Enzyme deficiency
      1. Congenital
         a) Formiminotransferase
         b) Dihydrofolate reductase
         c) Methyltetrahydrofolate transmethylase
         d) Other enzymes (some of which affect folate secondarily)
      2. Acquired
         a) Liver disease
            (1) Formiminotransferase
            (2) Other enzymes
   D. Vitamin B_{12} deficiency (reduced folate uptake and retention)
   E. Alcohol (both specific and nonspecific damage)
   F. Ascorbic acid deficiency
   G. Dietary amino acid excess (glycine, methionine)

IV. Increased requirement
   A. Extra tissue demand
      1. By fetus
      2. By malignant tissue (especially in lymphoproliferative disorders)
      3. By breast-fed infant
   B. Infancy
   C. Increased hematopoiesis
   D. Increased metabolic activity
   E. Lesch-Nyhan syndrome
   F. Drugs (L-dopa?)

V. Increased excretion
   A. Vitamin B_{12} deficiency (possible obligatory excretion of folate in urine and bile)
   B. Liver disease?
   C. Kidney dialysis
   D. Chronic exfoliative dermatitis

VI. Increased destruction
   A. Oxidant in diet?

Modified from Herbert V, Das KC: Folic acid and vitamin B_{12}. In Shils ME, Olson JA, Shike M, editors: *Modern nutrition in health and disease,* ed 8, vol 1, Philadelphia, 1994, Lea & Febiger.

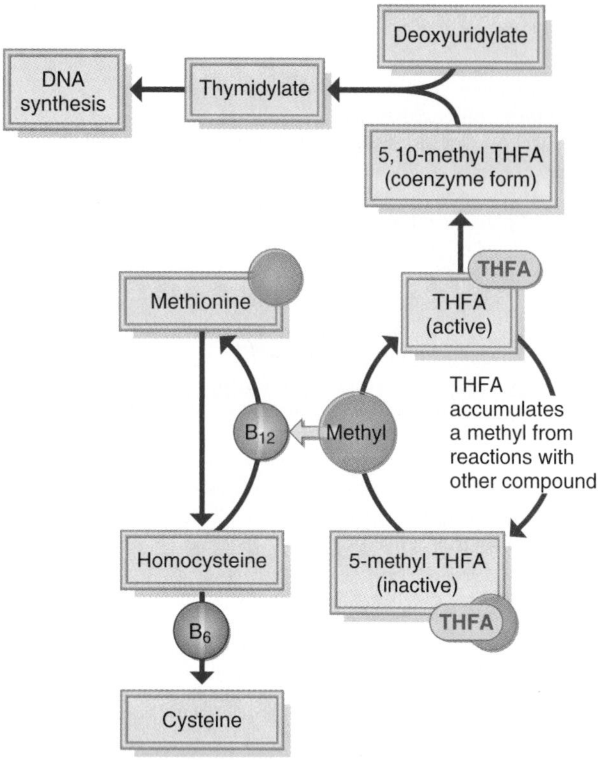

FIGURE 34-5 • Methylfolate trap. A deficiency of vitamin B_{12} can result in a deficiency of folic acid because folate is trapped in the form of 5-methyltetrahydrofolate (5-methyl THFA), which cannot be converted to tetrahydrofolate (THFA) by the vitamin B_{12}–dependent pathway.

as the dU suppression test in bone marrow cells or peripheral blood lymphocytes.

Medical Management

Before treatment is initiated, it is important to diagnose the cause of the megaloblastosis correctly. Administration of folate will correct megaloblastosis from either folate or vitamin B_{12} deficiency, but it can mask the neurologic damage of vitamin B_{12} deficiency, allowing the nerve damage to progress to the point of irreversibility.

A dosage of 1 mg of folate, taken orally every day for 2 to 3 weeks, will replenish folate stores. Maintaining repleted stores requires an absolute minimum oral intake of 50 to 100 μg of folic acid daily. When folate deficiency is complicated by alcoholism or other conditions that suppress hematopoiesis, increase folate requirements, or reduce folate absorption, therapy should begin at a dosage of 500 to 1000 μg daily.

Symptomatic improvement, as evidenced by increased alertness, cooperation, and appetite, may be apparent within 24 to 48 hours, long before hematologic values revert to normal, a gradual process that takes about a month.

Medical Nutrition Therapy

After the anemia is corrected, the patient should be instructed to eat at least one fresh, uncooked fruit or vegetable or to drink a glass of fruit juice daily. One cup of orange juice supplies about 135 μg of folic acid (see Table 34-4 for a list of foods). Fresh, uncooked fruits and vegetables are good sources of folate because folate can easily be destroyed by heat. The DRIs for folate are RDAs and are summarized in Tables 4-20 and 15-1. The RDA for adults is 400 μg daily (IOM, 1998).

OTHER NUTRITIONAL ANEMIAS

Copper-Deficiency Anemia

Copper and other heavy metals are essential for the proper formation of hemoglobin. Ceruloplasmin, a copper-containing protein, is required for normal mobilization of iron from its storage sites to the plasma. In a copper-deficient state, iron cannot be released, leading to low serum iron and hemoglobin levels, even in the presence of normal iron stores. Other consequences of copper deficiency suggest that copper proteins are needed for utilization of iron by the developing erythrocyte and for optimal functions of the erythrocyte membrane (see Chapter 5).

The amounts of copper needed for normal hemoglobin synthesis are so minute that they are usually amply supplied by an adequate diet; however, copper deficiency may occur in infants who are fed cow's milk or a copper-deficient infant formula. It may also be seen in children or adults who have a malabsorption syndrome or who are receiving long-term total parenteral nutrition that does not supply copper.

Anemia of Protein-Energy Malnutrition

Protein is essential for the proper production of hemoglobin and red blood cells. Because of the reduction in cell mass and, thus, oxygen requirements in protein-energy malnutrition (PEM), fewer red blood cells are required to oxygenate the tissue. Because blood volume remains the same, this reduced number of red blood cells with a low hemoglobin level (hypochromic, normocytic anemia), which can mimic an iron deficiency anemia, is actually a physiologic (nonharmful) rather than pharmacologic (harmful) anemia. In acute PEM, the loss of active tissue mass may be greater than the reduction in the number of red blood cells, leading to polycythemia. The body responds to this red blood cell production, which is not a reflection of protein and amino acid deficiency, but of an oversupply of red blood cells. Iron released from normal red blood cell destruction is not reused in red blood cell production but is stored, so that iron

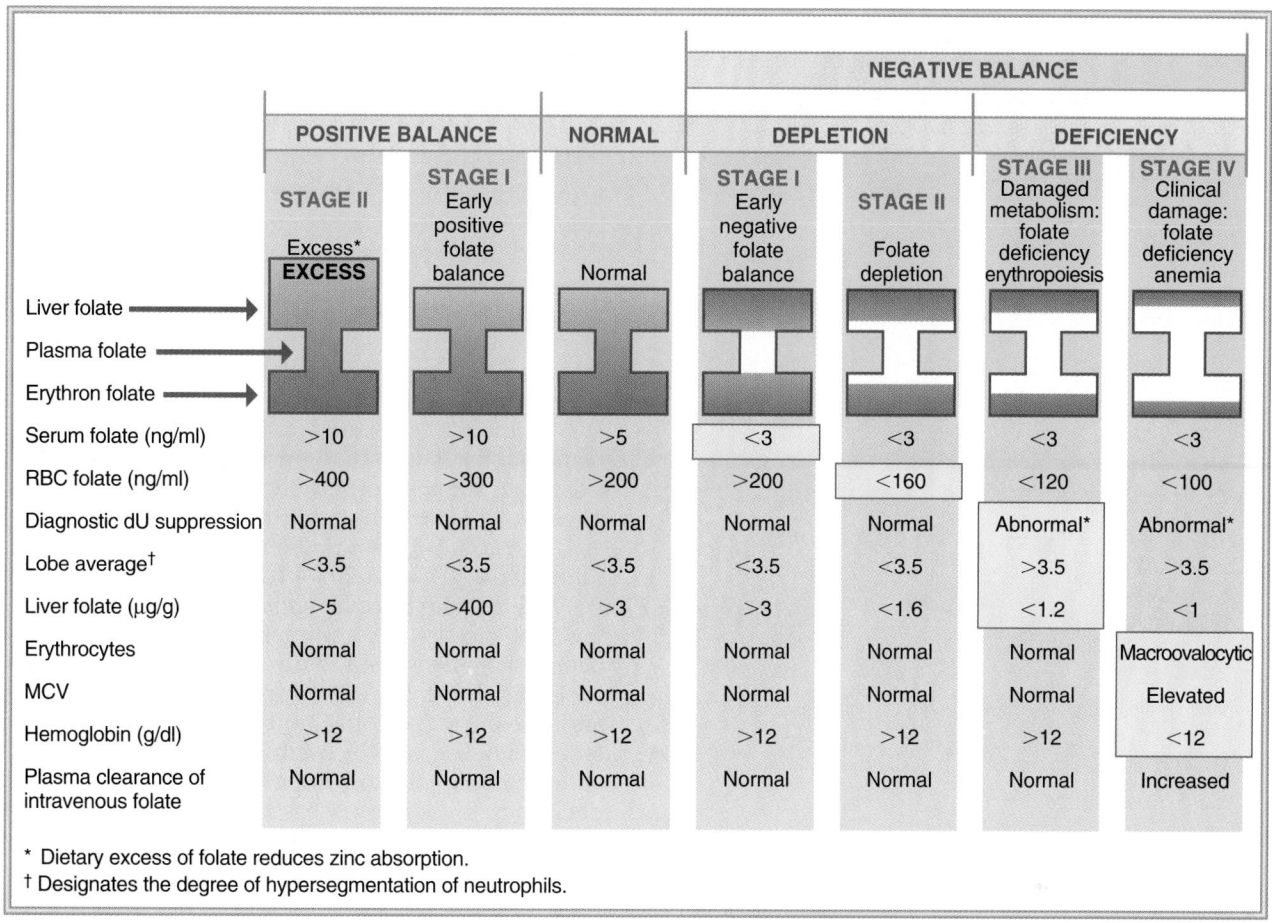

	NEGATIVE BALANCE						
	POSITIVE BALANCE		NORMAL	DEPLETION		DEFICIENCY	
	STAGE II Excess* EXCESS	STAGE I Early positive folate balance	Normal	STAGE I Early negative folate balance	STAGE II Folate depletion	STAGE III Damaged metabolism: folate deficiency erythropoiesis	STAGE IV Clinical damage: folate deficiency anemia
Liver folate / Plasma folate / Erythron folate							
Serum folate (ng/ml)	>10	>10	>5	<3	<3	<3	<3
RBC folate (ng/ml)	>400	>300	>200	>200	<160	<120	<100
Diagnostic dU suppression	Normal	Normal	Normal	Normal	Normal	Abnormal*	Abnormal*
Lobe average†	<3.5	<3.5	<3.5	<3.5	<3.5	>3.5	>3.5
Liver folate (μg/g)	>5	>400	>3	>3	<1.6	<1.2	<1
Erythrocytes	Normal	Normal	Normal	Normal	Normal	Normal	Macroovalocytic
MCV	Normal	Normal	Normal	Normal	Normal	Normal	Elevated
Hemoglobin (g/dl)	>12	>12	>12	>12	>12	>12	<12
Plasma clearance of intravenous folate	Normal	Normal	Normal	Normal	Normal	Normal	Increased

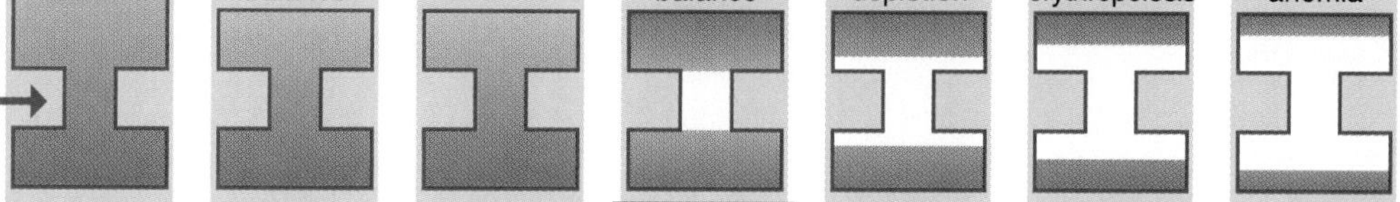

* Dietary excess of folate reduces zinc absorption.
† Designates the degree of hypersegmentation of neutrophils.

FIGURE 34-6 • Sequential stages of folate status. *DU,* Deoxyuridine; *MCV,* mean corpuscular volume; *RBC,* red blood cell. (From Herbert V: Folic acid. In Shils ME, Olson JA, Shike M, editors: *Modern nutrition in health and disease,* ed 9, Philadelphia 1998, Lea & Febiger.)

stores are often adequate. Iron deficiency anemia can reappear with rehabilitation when red blood cell mass expands rapidly.

The anemia of PEM may be complicated by deficiencies of iron and other nutrients and by associated infections, parasitic infestation, and malabsorption. A diet lacking in protein is usually deficient in iron, folic acid, and, less frequently, vitamin B_{12}. The nutrition counselor plays an important role in assessing recent and typical dietary intake of these nutrients.

Sideroblastic (Pyridoxine–Responsive) Anemia

Sideroblastic anemia has four primary characteristics: (1) microcytic and hypochromic red blood cells; (2) high serum and tissue iron levels (causing increased transferrin saturation); (3) the presence of an inherited defect in the formation of δ-aminolevulinic acid synthetase, an enzyme involved in heme synthesis (pyridoxal-5-phosphate is necessary in this reaction); and (4) a buildup of iron-containing immature red blood cells (sideroblasts, for which the anemia is named). The iron that cannot be used for heme synthesis is stored in the mitochondria of immature red blood cells. These iron-laden mitochondria do not function normally, and the development and production of red blood cells become ineffective. The symptoms are those of both anemia and iron overload. The neurologic and cutaneous manifestations of vitamin B_6 deficiency are not observed. The anemia responds to the administration of pharmacologic doses of pyridoxine and thus is referred to as vitamin B_6 (pyridoxine)–responsive anemia, to distinguish it from anemia caused by a dietary vitamin B_6 deficiency.

Treatment consists of a therapeutic trial dose of 50 to 200 mg daily of pyridoxine or pyridoxal phosphate, which is 25 to 100 times the RDA. If the anemia responds to one or the other, pyridoxine therapy is continued for life; however, the anemia is only partially corrected; a normal hematocrit value is never regained. Patients respond to this treatment to varying degrees, and some may achieve near-normal hemoglobin levels.

Unlike the familial sideroblastic anemia just mentioned, acquired sideroblastic anemias, such as those

TABLE 34-4 Folic Acid Content of Some Common Foods

FOOD	PORTION SIZE	FOLATE (μg)
Protein Group		
Chicken, light meat	3 oz	3.0
Chicken, dark meat	3 oz	7.2
Turkey, dark meat	3 oz	7.9
Pork chop	3 oz	5.2
Tenderloin steak	3 oz	5.0
Liver, chicken	3 oz	654.0
Liver, pork	3 oz	139.0
Tuna fish	3 oz	3.5
Sardines (tomato sauce)	3 oz	21.0
Salmon	3 oz	13.0
Tofu, raw	½ c	37.0
Egg	1	23.0
Black beans	½ c	128.0
Kidney beans	½ c	18.0
Lentil beans	½ c	36.0
Soybean nuts	½ c	122.0
Cashew nuts	1 oz	19.6
Dairy Group		
Milk (all varieties)	1 c	13.0
Yogurt	1 c	28.0
Cottage cheese	½ c	10.5
Fruit Group		
Apricots	3 raw	9.1
Orange	1	40.0
Orange juice	1 c	136.0
Strawberries, frozen	1 c	9.7
Banana	1	22.0
Vegetable Group		
Baked potato	1 medium	22.0
Sweet potato	1 medium	26.0
Broccoli	1 c	62.0
Brussels sprouts	½ c	47.0
Endive	½ c	36.0
Spinach	½ c	108.0
Grain Group		
Barley	½ c	13.0
Whole-wheat bread	1 slice	14.0
Wheat germ	¼ c	99.0
Grapenuts cereal	¼ c	101.0

attributable to drug therapy (isoniazid, chloramphenicol), copper deficiency, hypothermia, and alcoholism, are not vitamin B_6 (pyridoxine)–responsive.

Vitamin E–Responsive Anemia

Hemolytic anemia occurs when defects in red blood cell membranes lead to oxidative damage and, eventually, to cell lysis. Vitamin E, an antioxidant, is involved in protecting the membrane against oxidative damage, and one of the few signs noted in vitamin E deficiency is early hemolysis of red blood cells (see Chapter 4). Vitamin E–responsive hemolytic anemia in neonates is discussed in Chapters 8 and 9.

NONNUTRITIONAL ANEMIAS

Sports Anemia (Hypochromic Microcytic Transient Anemia)

Increased red blood cell destruction, along with decreased hemoglobin, serum iron, and ferritin concentrations, may occur at the initiation and early stages of a vigorous training program. Once called *march hemoglobinuria,* this anemia was believed to arise in soldiers as a result of mechanical trauma incurred by erythrocytes (red blood cells) during long marches. The red blood cells in the capillaries are compressed every time the foot lands, until they burst, releasing hemoglobin. It was thought that a similar situation existed in runners, especially long-distance runners; however, it is now thought that it is a *physiologic anemia,* that is, a transient problem of blood volume and dilution (see Chapter 26 for further discussion).

Athletes who have hemoglobin concentrations below that needed for optimal oxygen delivery may benefit from consuming nutrient and iron-rich foods, ensuring that their diets contain adequate protein, and avoiding tea, coffee, antacids, H_2-blockers, and tetracycline, all of which inhibit iron absorption. No athlete should take iron supplements unless true iron deficiency is diagnosed based on a complete blood cell count with differential, serum ferritin level, serum iron level, TIBC, and percent saturation of iron-binding capacity. Athletes who are female, vegetarian, involved in endurance sports, or entering a growth spurt are also at risk for iron deficiency anemia and should therefore undergo periodic monitoring.

Anemia of Pregnancy

Another physiologic anemia is the anemia of pregnancy, which is related to increased blood volume and usually resolves with the end of the pregnancy; however, demands for iron during pregnancy are also increased so that inadequate iron intake may also play a role (see Chapter 7 for further discussion).

Anemia of Inflammation, Infection, or Malignancy (Anemia of Chronic Disease)

Anemia of inflammation, infection, and malignancy occurs because there is decreased red blood cell production, possibly as a result of disordered iron metabolism. Why this happens is unclear, but it may be due to the presence of inflammatory cytokines such as interleukin-1 and tumor necrosis factor, which decrease iron absorption and erythroblast activity (Spivak, 2002). Ferritin levels are normal or increased, but serum iron levels and TIBC are low (see Chapter 18 for further discussion). It is important that this form of anemia, which is mild and normocytic, not be mistaken for iron deficiency anemia and iron supplements be given inappropriately. Recombinant erythropoietin therapy usually corrects this anemia (see Chapter 39).

Sickle Cell Anemia

Pathophysiology

Sickle cell anemia, a chronic hemolytic anemia also known as *hemoglobin S disease,* affects 1 of 600 blacks in the United States as a result of homozygous inheritance of hemoglobin S. This results in defective hemoglobin synthesis, which produces sickle-shaped red blood cells that get caught in capillaries and do not carry oxygen well. The disease is usually diagnosed toward the end of the first year of life.

Clinical Findings

In addition to the usual symptoms of anemia, sickle cell anemia is characterized by episodes of pain resulting from the occlusion of small blood vessels by the abnormally shaped erythrocytes. The occlusions frequently occur in the abdomen, causing acute, severe, abdominal pain. The hemolytic anemia and vasoocclusive disease result in impaired liver function, jaundice, gallstones, and deteriorating renal function. The constant hemolysis of erythrocytes increases iron stores in the liver; however, iron deficiency anemia and sickle cell anemia can coexist. Iron overload is less common and is usually a problem only in those who have received multiple blood transfusions.

Medical Management

No specific treatment exists for sickle cell anemia other than relieving pain during a crisis, keeping the body oxygenated, and, possibly, administering an exchange transfusion. It is important that sickle cell anemia not be mistaken for iron deficiency anemia, which can be treated with iron supplements, because iron stores in the patient with sickle cell anemia secondary to transfusions are frequently excessive.

Zinc can increase the oxygen affinity of both normal and sickle-shaped erythrocytes. Thus, zinc supplements may be beneficial in managing sickle cell disease, especially because decreased plasma zinc is common in children with the SS genotype sickle cell disease and is associated with decreased linear growth and skeletal growth, muscle mass, and sexual maturation (Leonard et al, 1998). Zinc supplementation (as little as 10 mg daily) may also prevent the deficit in growth that also appears in these children (Zemel et al, 2002). Curiously, this growth and development retardation are more apparent in males than in females (Modebe and Ifenu, 1993). Because zinc competes with copper for binding sites on proteins, the use of high doses of zinc may precipitate copper deficiency.

Medical Nutrition Therapy

Children with sickle cell anemia and their families should receive instruction about how they can develop a well-balanced food plan providing enough calories and protein for growth and development. Their dietary intake can be low because of the abdominal pain characteristic of the disease. They may also have increased metabolic rates leading to a need for a higher caloric intake (Singhal et al, 2002). Therefore their diets must be high enough in calories to meet these needs and must promote foods high in the vitamin folate (see Table 34-4) and the trace minerals zinc and copper (see Chapter 5 for sources of these minerals). In addition, they may have intakes low in vitamins A, C, and E, and this needs to be addressed in food choices (Williams et al, 1997).

When assessing the nutritional status of patients with sickle cell anemia, the questions related to the use of vitamin and mineral supplements, the consumption of alcohol (which increases iron absorption), and sources of protein (animal sources being high in both zinc and iron) in the diet must be given special attention. A multivitamin/mineral supplement containing 50% to 150% of the RDA for folate, zinc, and copper (not iron) is recommended; 2 to 3 quarts of water daily is also important. Finally, it is important to remember that patients with sickle cell disease may require higher than RDA amounts of protein.

If it is necessary for the diet to be low in absorbable iron, the diet should emphasize vegetable proteins. Iron-rich foods, such as liver, iron-fortified formula, and iron-fortified cereals, are excluded. Substances such as alcohol and ascorbic acid supplements, both of which enhance iron absorption and free-radical release from iron, should be avoided. It is important to remember, however, that iron deficiency may be present in some patients with sickle cell anemia owing to repeated phlebotomies, excessive transfusions, or hematuria secondary to renal papillary necrosis. This should be assessed and the diet adjusted appropriately. The diet should be high in folate (400 to 600 μg daily) because the increased production of erythrocytes needed to replace the cells being continuously destroyed also increases folic acid requirements (see Table 34-4 for a list of common foods containing folate).

Thalassemias

Thalassemias (α and β) are severe inherited anemias characterized as microcytic, hypochromic, and short-lived red blood cells resulting from defective hemoglobin synthesis, which affects mostly persons in the Mediterranean region. The ineffective erythropoiesis leads to an increase in plasma volume, progressive splenomegaly, and bone marrow expansion with the result of facial deformities, osteomalacia, and bone changes. Ultimately there is increased iron absorption and progressive iron deposition in tissues, resulting in oxidative damage. The accumulation of iron causes dysfunction of the heart, liver, and endocrine glands. Because these patients require transfusions to stay alive, they must also have regular chelation therapy to prevent the damaging buildup of iron that can occur. Malnutrition is common and is an important factor in the stunted growth in these children (Fuchs et al, 1996).

SUMMARY

Anemia is a worldwide problem in persons of all ages. It is not a diagnosis but rather a sign or symptom of an underlying disorder. The goal is to investigate and understand the different stages of anemia and its pathophysiologic mechanism so that proper treatment can begin. Assessment is important, and determination of the underlying cause in nonnutritional anemias such as anemia of inflammation leads to appropriate medical treatment and eventually resolution of the anemia. Identification of a nutritional anemia as the result of inadequate intake, absorption, utilization, or increased requirement is essential to allow for the appropriate medical nutrition therapy. The nutrition practitioner is most effective with a complete understanding of the types of anemia and the ability to translate this understanding into practical advice for the patient.

Dedicated to the memory of Victor Herbert, MD, a pioneer in the area of macrocytic anemia and folic acid and vitamin B_{12} deficiencies.

Clinical Scenario 1

Mary Jo is a 20-year-old black woman who was recently diagnosed as having sickle cell disease. She is a runner and complains about frequent periods of dizziness and weakness. Her hemoglobin level is normal, but recent laboratory studies indicate a low serum folate and vitamin B_{12} level. Her mother has suggested that she take an over-the-counter multiple vitamin/mineral supplement. Mary Jo has called you for guidance. What would you recommend to her?

1. What are the risks of taking a multiple vitamin/mineral supplement when one has sickle cell anemia?
2. What other laboratory data should you obtain before discussing her case with her physician?
3. What foods could be included in her diet that would be beneficial and yet would not contain too much of any single vitamin or mineral?
4. Are there any problems with her usual daily intake of one or two citrus fruits and a quart of juice?
5. What other suggestions would you offer Mary Jo?

Relevant Web Sites

Anemia Institute for Research and Education
www.anemiainstitute.org/
Anemia Lifeline
www.anemia.com/
Iron Disorders Institute
www.irondisorders.org/disorders/aio/
Iron Overload Disease Association
www.ironoverload.org/
National Institutes of Health site
www.niddk.nih.gov/ health/hematol

Cited References

Cohen L: Iron overload gene, *Proc Natl Acad Sci USA* 95:1472, 1998.
Cook JD, Reddy MB: Effect of ascorbic acid intake on nonheme-iron absorption from a complete diet, *Am J Clin Nutr* 73:93, 2001.
Fairbanks VF: Iron in medicine and nutrition. In Shils ME, Olson JA, Shike M, editors: *Modern nutrition in health and disease*, ed 9, vol 1, Philadelphia, 1999, Lea & Febiger.
Fuchs GJ et al: Nutritional factors and thalassaemia major, *Arch Dis Child* 74:224, 1996.
Herbert V: Everyone should be tested for iron disorders, *J Am Diet Assoc* 92:1502, 1992.
Herbert V: Folic acid. In Shils ME, Olson JA, Shike M, editors: *Modern nutrition in health and disease*, ed 9, vol 1, Philadelphia, 1999, Lea & Febiger.

Clinical Scenario 2

Sara is a 22-year-old recent college graduate who has joined the Peace Corp. On arrival in southern Africa, Sarah began feeling fatigued and weak. The site's nurse suggested that her symptoms were indicative of anemia and asked Sarah whether she was taking any multivitamin/mineral supplements. Sarah said she was taking a multivitamin (without iron) and also taking 1000 mg of vitamin C daily. The nurse gave Sarah a 15-mg iron supplement to be taken daily. Sarah's symptoms never subsided, and now, 10 months later, Sarah has begun experiencing abdominal pain, aching joints, and irregular menses. Sarah, now back in the United States, has made an appointment with you.

1. What questions are most relevant for you to ask during her initial evaluation?
2. What potential problems does Sarah face if her condition progresses?
3. What nutrition recommendations would you give to Sarah?
4. Do you think a vegetarian lifestyle would be more or less helpful? Why?
5. Discuss the genetic possibilities (i.e., hemochromatosis/thalassemia) as well as the environmental concerns you have regarding her case.
6. It is clear to you that Sarah needs to make an appointment with her physician. Write a letter to her physician discussing your thoughts and concerns. Also include your care plan and recommendations for laboratory tests that Sarah should have done.

Herbert V: Loss of recent memory (where in the parking lot is my car? etc.) in persons age > 50 is often unrecognized subtle B_{12} deficiency, producing inadequate synthesis of new brain cells, but no anemia, *FASEB J* 15(2, Part I):A59, 2001a.

Herbert V: Vitamin B_{12}. In Bowman BA, Russell RM, editors: *Present knowledge in nutrition,* ed 8, Washington, DC, 2001b, International Life Sciences Institute Press.

Herbert V et al: Low holotranscobalamin is the earliest serum marker for subnormal vitamin B_{12} (cobalamin) absorption in patient with AIDS, *Am J Hematol* 34:132, 1990.

Herbert V et al: Serum ferritin iron, a new test, measures human body iron stores unconfounded by inflammation, *Stem Cells* 15:291, 1997.

Herzlich B, Herbert V: Depletion of serum holotrans cobalamin II: an early sign of negative B_{12} balance, *Lab Invest* 58:3,342, 1988.

Institute of Medicine, Food and Nutrition Board: *Dietary reference intakes for thiamin, riboflavin, niacin, vitamin B_6, folate, vitamin B_{12}, pantothenic acid, biotin and choline,* Washington DC, 1998, National Academy Press.

Institute of Medicine, Food and Nutrition Board: *Dietary reference intakes for vitamin A, vitamin K, arsenic, boron, chromium, copper, iodine, iron, molybdenum, nickel, silicon, vanadium and zinc,* Washington DC, 2001, National Academy Press.

Kaptan K et al: *Helicobacter pylori*—is it a novel causative agent in vitamin B_{12} deficiency? *Arch Intern Med* 160:1349, 2000.

Leonard MB et al: Plasma zinc status, growth, and maturation in children with sickle cell disease, *J Pediatr* 132:467, 1998.

Markle HV: Unmetabolized folic acid and masking of cobalamin deficiency, *Am J Clin Nutr* 66:1480, 1997.

Minot GR, Murphy WP: Treatment of pernicious anemia by special diet, *JAMA* 87:470, 1926.

Modebe O, Ifenu SA: Growth retardation in homozygous sickle cell disease: role of calorie intake and possible gender-related differences, *Am J Hematol* 44:149, 1993.

Mulvihill B et al: Effect of myofibrillar proteins in vitro on bioavailability of non-heme iron, *Int J Food Sci Nutr* 49:187, 1998.

Nokes C, van den Bosch C, Bundy D: The effects of iron deficiency and anemia on mental and motor performance, educational achievement, and behavior in children: an annotated bibliography. A report of the International Nutritional Anemia Consultative Group, September 16-17, 1996, England, University of Oxford, 1998.

Pollitt E et al: Iron deficiency and behavioral development in infants and preschool children, *Am J Clin Nutr* 43:555, 1986.

Singhal A et al: Energy intake and resting metabolic rate in preschool Jamaican children with homozygous sickle cell disease, *Am J Clin Nutr* 75:1093, 2002.

Spivak JL: Iron and the anemia of chronic disease, *Oncology* 16(9 suppl 10):25, 2002.

Stopeck A: Links between *Helicobacter pylori* infection, cobalamin deficiency and pernicious anemia, [Editorial] *Arch Intern Med* 160:1229, 2000.

World Health Organization (WHO): *The global picture,* Geneva, Switzerland, World Health Organization, 2000.

Williams R et al: Nutrition assessment in children with sickle cell disease, *J Assoc Minn Phys* 8:44, 1997.

Zemel BS et al: Effect of zinc supplementation on growth and body composition in children with sickle cell disease, *Am J Clin Nutr* 75:300, 2002.

Zlotkin S et al: Treatment of anemia with microencapsulated ferrous fumarate plus ascorbic acid supplied as sprinkles to complementary (weaning) foods, *Am J Clin Nutr* 74:791, 2001.

■ Additional References

Andrews NC: Disorders of iron metabolism, *N Engl J Med* 341:1986, 1999.

Flynn MA et al: Atherogenesis and the homocysteine-folate-cobalamin triad: do we need standardized analyses? *J Am Coll Nutr* 16:258, 1997.

Hallberg L et al: Iron absorption in man: ascorbic acid and dose-dependent inhibition by phytate, *Am J Clin Nutr* 49:140, 1989.

Herbert V: Vitamin B_{12} and folic acid supplementation, *Am J Clin Nutr* 66:1479, 1997.

Herbert V, Bigaoutte J: Call for endorsement of a petition to the Food and Drug Administration to always add vitamin B_{12} to any folate fortification or supplement, *Am J Clin Nutr* 65:572, 1997.

Herbert V et al: Vitamin C–driven free radical generation from iron, *J Nutr* 126(suppl 4):121, 1996.

Monsen ER: Iron nutrition and absorption: dietary factors [that] impact iron bioavailability, *J Am Diet Assoc* 88:786, 1988.

Olynyk JK et al: A population-based study of the clinical expression of the hemochromatosis gene, *N Engl J Med* 341:718, 1999.

Oski F: Iron deficiency in infancy and childhood, *N Engl J Med* 329:190, 1993.

Pan W, Habicht J: The non-iron deficiency-related differences in hemoglobin concentration between men and women, *Am J Epidemiol* 134:1410, 1991.

Pellegrini B et al: Zinc, copper and iron and their interrelations in the growth of sickle cell patients, *Arch Latinoam Nutr* 45:198, 1995.

Soliman AT et al: Growth and pubertal development in transfusion-dependent children and adolescents with thalassaemia major and sickle cell disease: a comparative study, *J Trop Pediatr* 45 (1):23, 1999.

Steinberg MH: Management of sickle cell disease, *N Engl J Med* 340:1021, 1999.

Stopler T, Herbert V: *Nutrition E.T.C. for the millennium,* 1999, Plainview, NY, Nutrition ETC.

Suitor CW, Bailey LB: Dietary folate equivalents: interpretation and application, *J Am Diet Assoc* 100:88, 2000.

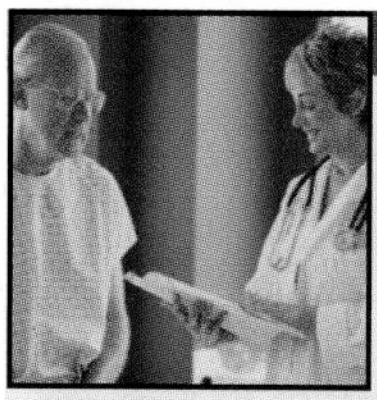

CHAPTER 35

Medical Nutrition Therapy in Cardiovascular Disease

DEBRA A. KRUMMEL, PhD, RD, LD

CHAPTER OUTLINE

- Prevalence and Incidence
- Mortality
- Pathophysiology and Etiology
- Prevention of Coronary Heart Disease
- Lipoprotein Assessment
- Genetic Hyperlipidemias: Classification and Diagnosis
- Dietary Factors
- Treatment

KEY TERMS

apolipoprotein–protein component of lipoproteins that provides structure and controls the metabolic fate of lipoproteins

atheroma–any of the lesions of atherosclerosis; another name for plaque

atherosclerosis–a form of arteriosclerosis; a complex process of thickening and narrowing of the arterial walls caused by the accumulation of lipids, primarily oxidized cholesterol, in the intimal or inner layer in combination with connective tissue and calcification

bile acid sequestrants–drugs that adsorb bile acids and, by preventing their absorption back into the bloodstream, lower blood cholesterol levels

chylomicrons–lipoproteins that transport dietary fat from the gut into the circulation

coronary heart disease (CHD) or coronary artery disease (CAD)–disease involving the network of blood vessels surrounding and serving the heart; manifested in clinical end points of myocardial infarction and sudden death

endothelial dysfunction–abnormalities in vasomotor control, fibrinoloysis and thrombosis, inflammatory response, and growth of vascular smooth muscle

familial combined hyperlipidemia (FCHL)–a common lipid disorder characterized by elevated plasma low-density lipoprotein cholesterol or a triglyceride level above the 90th percentile in at least two family members; the result of overproduction of lipoproteins by the liver

familial dysbetalipoproteinemia–a rare lipoproteinemia characterized by elevated serum total cholesterol and triglycerides and apo E-2 allele

familial dyslipidemia–a common lipid disorder in which at least two family members have fasting triglyceride levels above the 90th percentile

familial hypercholesterolemia (FH)–a genetic defect in the ability to metabolize low-density lipoprotein cholesterol; characterized by hypercholesterolemia (>300 mg/dl), xanthomas, advanced atherosclerosis, and premature death

fatty streaks–earliest lesions in atherosclerosis; characterized by lipid-rich macrophages and smooth-muscle cells

high-density lipoprotein (HDL)–a plasma lipoprotein containing mostly protein and less cholesterol and triglyceride, high levels of which are associated with a decreased risk of coronary heart disease

homocysteine–an amino acid identified as a risk factor for cardiovascular disease

HMG CoA reductase inhibitors–cholesterol-lowering drugs that inhibit the rate-limiting enzyme (HMG CoA reductase) in cholesterol synthesis

hypercholesterolemia–elevated cholesterol level in the blood

hypertriglyceridemia–elevated blood triglyceride level

intermediate-density lipoproteins (IDLs)–lipoproteins that are formed during catabolism; precursors of low-density lipoproteins

ischemia–insufficient blood flow in a tissue resulting from functional constriction or actual obstruction of a blood vessel

lipoproteins–a diverse class of particles containing varying amounts of triglyceride, cholesterol, phospholipids, and protein that solubilize lipids for blood transport

low-density lipoproteins (LDLs)–lipoproteins that are the major cholesterol carriers in the blood; high levels are associated with increased risk of coronary heart disease; main target for interventions

metabolic syndrome–a constellation of risk factors including hypertension, obesity, and hypercholesterolemia associated with insulin resistance

myocardial infarction (MI)–ischemia in the coronary arteries resulting in necrosis, tissue damage, and sometimes sudden death

nitric oxide–key vasodilator produced by endothelial cells; also inhibits platelet aggregation and smooth-muscle cell proliferation and reduces monocyte adherence.

plaque–part of the lesions seen in atherosclerosis; composed of lipids, cholesterol, calcium, and fibrin

risk factors–characteristics found in healthy individuals that increase the likelihood of a person developing a disease; for coronary heart disease, major risk factors are hypercholesterolemia, hypertension, and cigarette smoking

thrombus–an aggregation of blood factors, primarily platelets and fibrin, which, if small, can contribute to the growth of plaque and, if large, can obstruct a blood vessel, resulting in angina, myocardial infarction, or sudden death

very-low-density lipoproteins (VLDLs)–lipoproteins that contain more triglyceride than cholesterol; they transport lipid from the liver to the peripheral circulation

xanthoma–cholesterol deposits (from low-density lipoproteins) seen on tendons and elbows

Since 1900, cardiovascular disease (CVD) has been the leading cause of death in the United States for every year except 1908 (American Heart Association [AHA], 2001). In total, CVD kills almost as many people yearly as the next seven causes of death combined. Of the CVDs, coronary heart disease (CHD) is the most prevalent cause of death, followed by stroke. The morbidity and mortality associated with CVD make it a major public health problem, with costs exceeding $327 billion a year in 2000.

Although most CVD deaths occur in persons 65 years of age and older, one third of deaths occur prematurely. This fact led to extensive research into prevention. Epidemiologic studies (observational studies, such as cohort and cross-sectional studies) and experimental studies (clinical or community trials) have delineated the risk factors associated with CVD development, which has been a major breakthrough for prevention and treatment. One of the greatest public health successes in the twentieth century has been the decline in age-adjusted mortality rates from CVD (CDC, 1999).

PREVALENCE AND INCIDENCE

The United States ranks fourteenth and sixteenth among industrialized nations for the prevalence of CVD in women and men, respectively (Figure 35-1). More than 61 million Americans have at least one form of CVD (i.e., hypertension, CHD, stroke, rheumatic heart disease, or congestive heart failure [CHF]). Most CHD and strokes are the result of ischemia, which is discussed under the topic atherosclerosis (Rosamond, 1999). In adults, the prevalence of CVD is highest in non-Hispanic blacks (~40% for men and women), followed by non-Hispanic whites (30% men, 24% women) and Mexican Americans (29% men, 27% women). As adults age, the prevalence of CVD increases, with a doubling of rates between ages 35 to 44 years of age and 45 to 54 years of age and a continual increase thereafter (Figure 35-2). Of the 61 million Americans with CVD, 13 million have some form of CHD (AHA, 2001).

The incidence of CHD is high; an American experiences a coronary event almost every 29 seconds. In follow-up data of Framingham participants and their offspring (see *Focus on:* Framingham Heart Study), the incidence of a first CVD event is 7 per 1000 in men ages 35 to 44, which steadily rises to 68 per 1000 in men 85 to 94 years of age. Women have comparable rates about 10 to 15 years later than men, but with aging, the gap diminishes (AHA, 2001). Eighty-two percent of coronary events in women are attributable to lack of a healthy lifestyle: unhealthful diet, lack of activity, cigarette use, and overweight (Stampfer et al, 2000).

MORTALITY

Diseases of the heart and stroke cause most deaths in both sexes of all ethnic groups (Figure 35-3). CHD, expressed as myocardial infarction (MI), is the main form of heart disease responsible for these deaths (AHA, 2001). Mortality from all heart diseases increases with age in all races. Until the age of 65 years, black men have the highest rates of CHD deaths; thereafter, white men have the highest rates. Black women have higher rates than white females at all ages. Overall, more men die of CHD than women

Men Ages 35–74

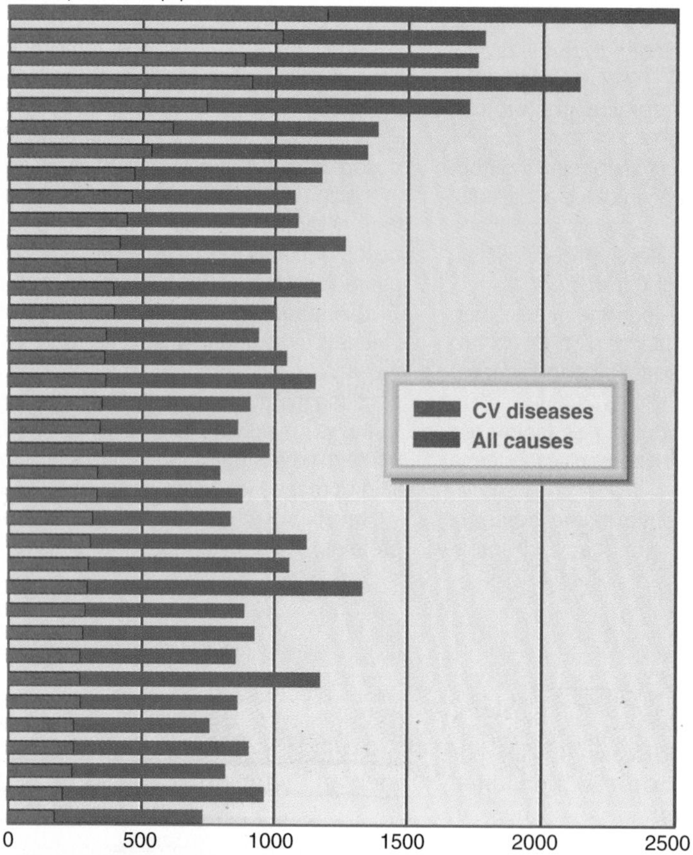

Men Ages 35–74	CVD Deaths	CHD Deaths	Stroke Deaths	Total Deaths
Russsian Federation (98)	1167	639	361	2502
Bulgaria (98)	1008	335	280	1775
Romania (99)+	867	355	282	1751
Hungary (99)+	842	420	207	2131
Poland (96)	735	267	111	1722
Czech Republic (99)+	598	318	120	1377
Argentina (96)	531	140	116	1344
Scotland (99)	460	321	69	1172
Ireland (97)	457	307	61	1072
Finland (98)+	438	288	72	1085
China—Rural (99)	413	64	243	1260
Northern Ireland (99)	406	293	62	983
Colombia (94)	397	190	90	1166
China—Urban (99)	389	106	217	1003
Austria (99)	369	205	59	938
United States (99)+	360	230	41	1024
Denmark (96)+	360	204	66	1144
England/Wales (99)	357	241	52	908
Greece (98)	353	170	82	864
Germany (99)+	347	190	53	973
Sweden (96)	335	216	51	799
Norway (97)+	332	213	51	879
New Zealand (98)	318	222	40	841
Portugal (99)	311	114	130	1116
Belgium (95)	307	153	51	1049
Korea (97)+	304	44	182	1325
Netherlands (99)+	299	151	46	890
Italy (95)	293	140	58	919
Canada (97)	280	184	36	849
Mexico (95)	273	137	61	1172
Israel (97)	270	127	53	868
Australia (98)+	253	172	38	767
Spain (98)	252	121	51	908
Switzerland (96)+	245	137	30	806
France (98)	213	85	41	966
Japan (97)+	186	57	79	743

Women Ages 35–74

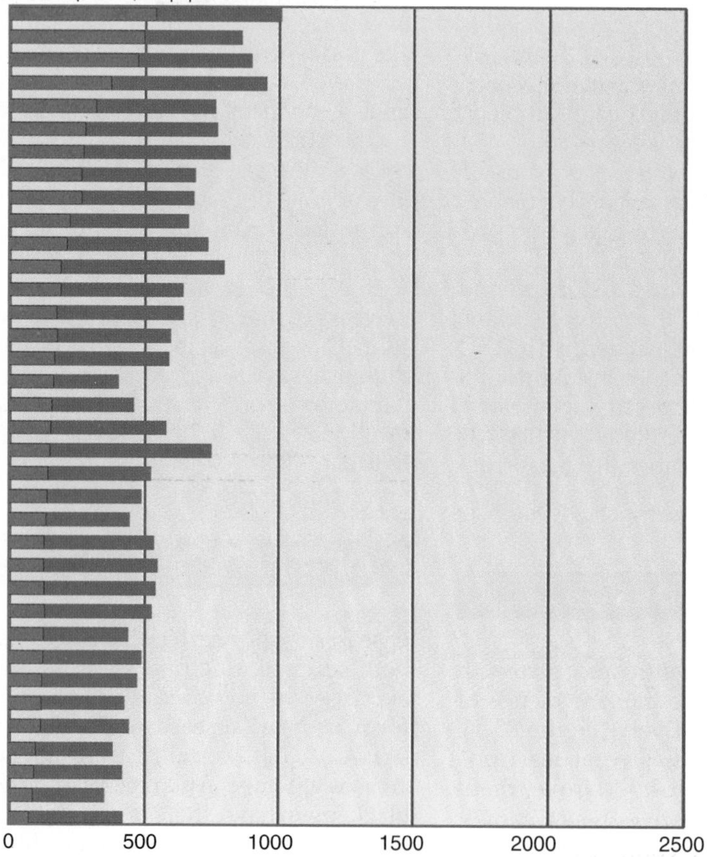

Women Ages 35–74	CVD Deaths	CHD Deaths	Stroke Deaths	Total Deaths
Russian Federation (98)	540	230	229	1001
Bulgaria (98)	504	128	173	839
Romania (99)+	480	167	186	877
Hungary (99)+	380	161	111	928
Poland (96)	325	79	72	742
Colombia (94)	286	110	84	748
China—Rural (99)	279	41	152	799
China—Urban (99)	273	71	147	663
Czech Republic (99)+	273	115	71	659
Argentina (96)	227	39	63	642
Scotland (99)	220	122	54	711
Mexico (95)	197	73	52	773
Ireland (97)	196	109	41	624
United States (99)+	183	95	33	627
Northern Ireland (99)	183	104	47	581
Korea (97)+	177	18	114	561
Greece (98)	170	50	60	429
Austria (99)	168	70	38	469
England/Wales (99)	165	85	41	564
Denmark (96)+	159	76	41	728
Portugal (99)	154	39	77	511
Germany (99)+	149	64	32	490
Finland (98)+	148	81	40	466
Belgium (95)	138	51	34	522
Israel (97)	139	64	33	535
New Zealand (98)	139	71	35	526
Netherlands (99)+	132	51	35	515
Sweden (96)	132	68	34	461
Canada (97)	122	65	25	489
Norway (97)+	119	60	33	485
Italy (97)	116	37	33	418
Australia (98)+	113	61	27	432
Spain (98)	99	32	28	373
Switzerland (96)+	95	40	20	408
Japan (97)+	85	20	41	341
France (98)	78	21	22	409

Rates adjusted to the European Standard population.

* ICD/9 codes are 390–459 for cardiovascular disease; 410–414 for coronary heart disease; and 430–438 for stroke. Exceptions are noted with +.

+ ICD/10 codes are 100–199 for cardiovascular disease; 120–125 for coronary heart disease; and 160–169 for stroke.

FIGURE 35-1 • Death rates for cardiovascular disease, coronary heart disease, stroke, and total deaths in selected countries. (From World Health Organization Web site, www.who.int/whosis/, and National Center for Health Statistics.)

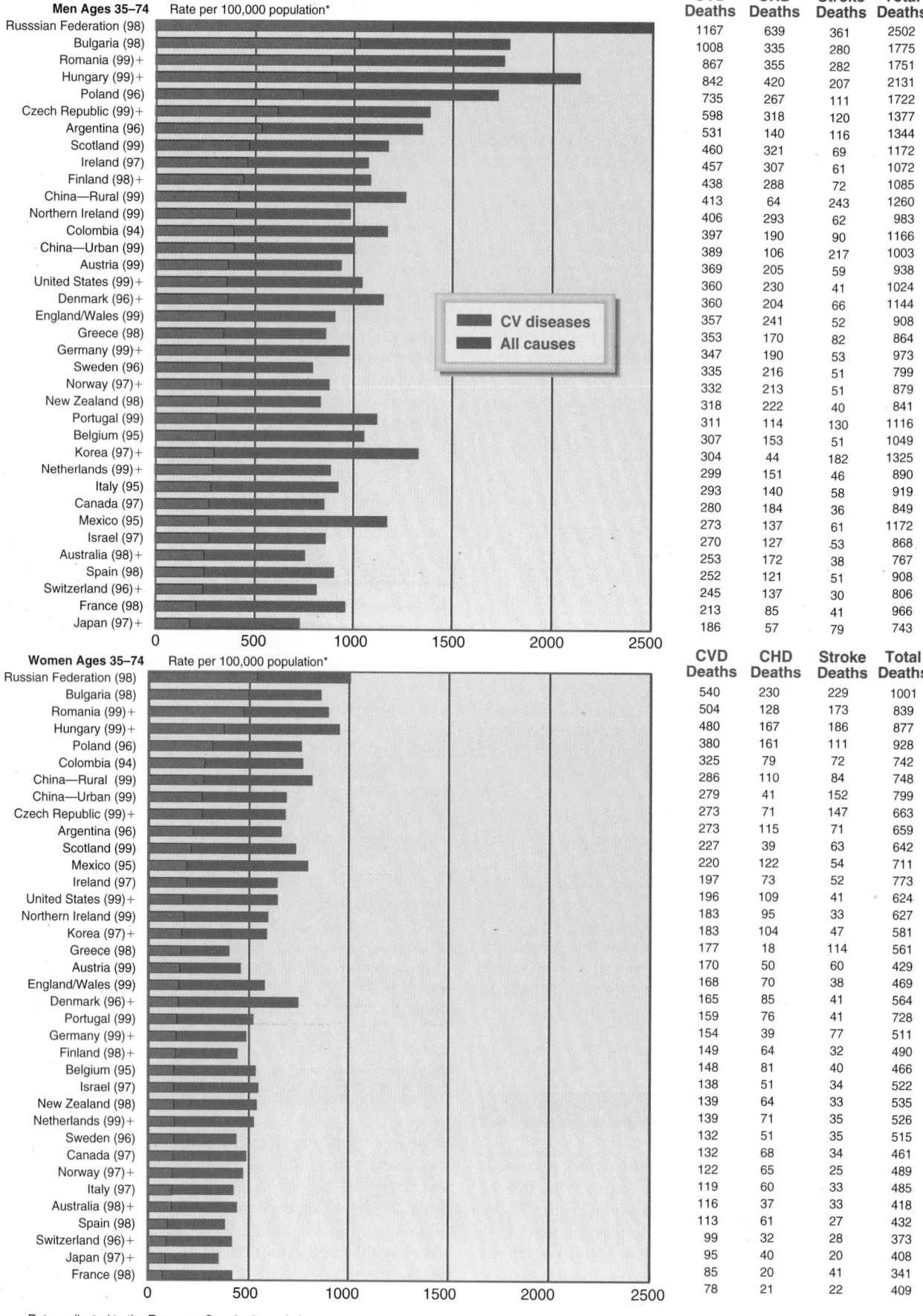

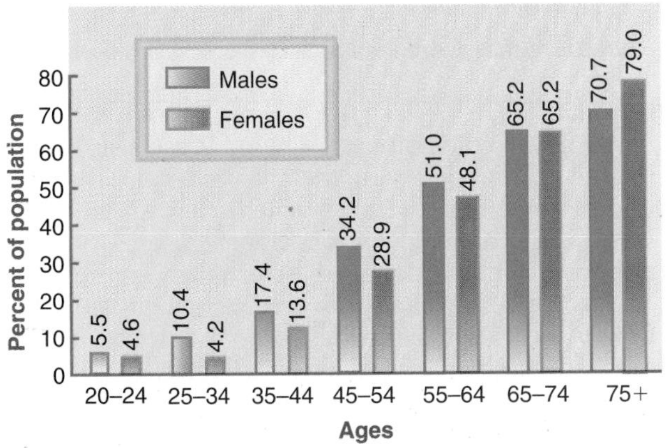

FIGURE 35-2 • Prevalence of cardiovascular disease in Americans 20 years of age and older by age and sex, United States: 1988-1994. (From National Health and Nutrition Examination Survey [1988-1994], Centers for Disease Control and Prevention, National Center for Health Statistics.)

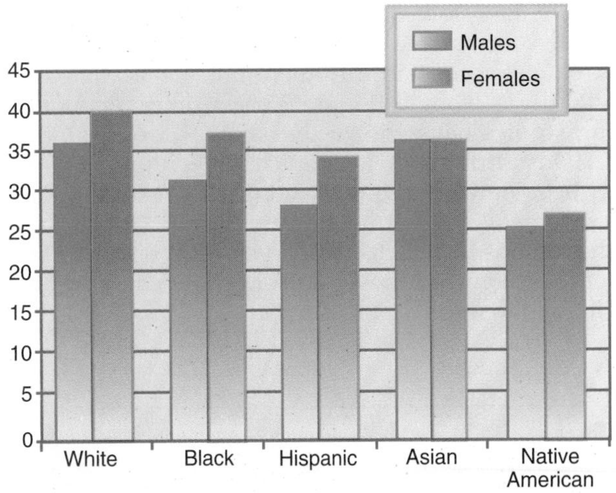

FIGURE 35-3 • Cardiovascular disease for males and females by ethnic group. (From American Heart Association: *2002 Heart and stroke statistical update,* Dallas, 2001, The Association.)

FOCUS ON

Framingham Heart Study

Since 1948 scientists, led by Dr. William Castelli, have been studying the population of Framingham, Massachusetts, to determine the prevalence and incidence of cardiovascular disease and factors related to its development. Study participants (n = 5209) were healthy adults between 30 and 62 years of age. Through this cohort study, the concept of risk factors, and thus prevention, was born. Modifiable risk factors not only predict disease in healthy adults but also contribute to the disease process in those who have atherosclerotic disease.

Highlights of the Framingham Study: Most Significant Milestones

1960 Cigarette smoking found to increase the risk of heart disease

1961 Cholesterol level, blood pressure, and electrocardiogram abnormalities found to increase the risk of heart disease

1967 Physical activity found to reduce the risk of heart disease, and obesity found to increase the risk of heart disease

1970 High blood pressure found to increase the risk of stroke

1976 Menopause found to increase the risk of heart disease

1978 Psychosocial factors found to affect heart disease

1988 High levels of HDL cholesterol found to reduce risk of death

1994 Enlarged left ventricle (one of two lower chambers of the heart) found to increase the risk of stroke

1996 Progression from hypertension to heart failure described

In 1972, a companion study was initiated to measure the influence of heredity and environment on the offspring of the original participants (Wilson et al, 1989). Dietary practices, which were not followed in the initial study, were included along with more sophisticated measurements of physical status. The younger group appears to be more health conscious than the older generation because they have lower smoking rates, lower blood pressure, and lower cholesterol levels than their parents at the same age.

Wilson PF et al: Impact of national guidelines for cholesterol risk factor lowering: the Framingham Offspring Study, *JAMA* 262:41, 1989; and www.nhlbi.nih.gov/about/framingham/timeline.htm.

(Eberhardt MS, Ingram DD, Makuc DM et al, 2001). Among immigrants who migrate from countries with low rates of death from CHD, the death rate is more similar to that of their adoptive country after acculturation than it is to that of their native country.

Of the CVDs, stroke is the third leading cause of death, behind CHD and cancer. From 1989 to 1999, the number of stroke deaths increased by 8.6% (AHA, 2001). More blacks than whites die of strokes.

Epidemic levels of CVD began around 1920, when CHD became the major cause of death in the United States. The age-adjusted death rates for CHD and stroke have declined by 60% and 66%, respectively, between 1963 and 1998 (NHLBI, 2000). The rate of decline has slowed in the last decade for CHD and leveled for stroke. Between the genders, CVD rates have held constant in men but have increased slightly in women (Figure 35-4). Computer modeling studies have shown that 25% of the decline in CHD is attributable to primary prevention and 70% to behavioral changes affecting risk factors or improvements in treatment (Hunink et al, 1997). Thus, the reasons for the decrease in mortality include better treatment and prevention efforts, such as lifestyle changes to modify risk factors.

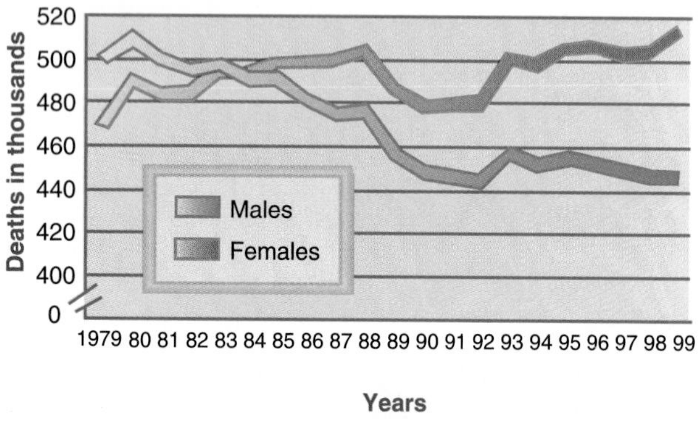

FIGURE 35-4 • Cardiovascular disease mortality trends in men and women, United States, 1979-1999. (From Centers for Disease Control and Prevention, National Center for Health Statistics and the American Heart Association.)

PATHOPHYSIOLOGY AND ETIOLOGY

Coronary heart disease (CHD) results from impeded blood flow to the network of blood vessels surrounding the heart and serving the myocardium. The major underlying cause of CHD is atherosclerosis, which involves structural and compositional changes in the innermost or intimal layer of the arteries (Figure 35-5). These changes produce impaired or inadequate blood flow. Atherosclerosis in the coronary arteries causes MI and angina; in the cerebral arteries it causes strokes; and in the peripheral circulation it causes intermittent claudication and gangrene. Kidneys also can be affected by atherosclerosis (see Chapter 39).

Atherosclerosis

The atherosclerotic process begins in childhood and takes decades to advance. It is now known that the pathogenesis of atherosclerosis is multifactorial. The lesions that develop are the result of (1) proliferation of smooth-muscle cells, macrophages, and lymphocytes (cells involved in the inflammatory response); (2) formation of smooth-muscle cells into a connective tissue matrix; and (3) accumulation of lipid and cholesterol in the matrix around the cells. The lipid deposits and other materials (cellular waste products, calcium, fibrin) that build up in the intimal layer are called plaque or atheroma.

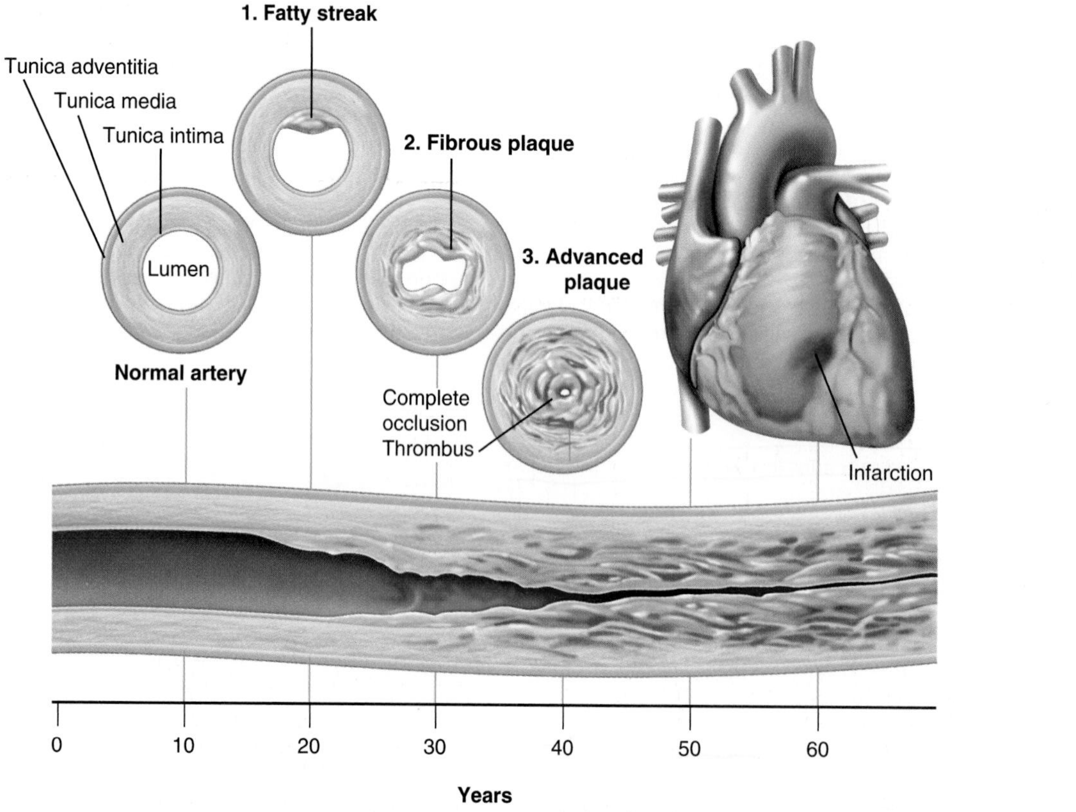

FIGURE 35-5 • Natural progression of atherosclerosis. (From Harkreader H: *Fundamentals,* Philadelphia, 2000, WB Saunders.)

Plaque forms in response to injuries to the endothelium wall. Endothelial dysfunction occurs early in atherogenesis and allows lipoproteins to accumulate in the intima. Some of the factors that cause endothelial injury are hypercholesterolemia, oxidized low-density lipoprotein (LDL), hypertension, cigarette smoking, diabetes, obesity, homocysteine, and diets high in saturated fat and cholesterol. After injury, platelets adhere to the arterial wall and release growth factors that promote lesion development. Thus, atherosclerosis is an inflammatory and proliferative response to arterial wall injuries.

Pathophysiology

There are five phases of atherogenesis, with characteristic lesions and symptoms at each phase (Fuster, 1999; Fuster, Badimon, and Chsebro, 1998). Phase 1, an asymptomatic phase, consists of small fatty streaks, commonly seen in people younger than 30 years of age. Fatty streaks are nonobstructive, lipid-filled cells (macrophages and smooth muscle cells) that form at bends in the artery in response to chronic injury to the arterial endothelium. Not all fatty streaks progress to advanced lesions.

Phase 2 is characterized by plaque with a high lipid content that may be prone to rupture. The lipid is derived from plasma LDL that enters the injured endothelial wall. Because of the instability of the intermediate lesions in phase 2, these lesions can progress to phase 3 (acute, complicated lesions with rupture and nonocclusive thrombus) or phase 4 (acute, complicated lesions with occlusive thrombus). The phase 4 lesions are associated with angina or MI and sudden death. Any complicated lesion can progress to phase 5 (fibrotic or occlusive) lesions with similar clinical outcomes.

Risk factors strongly influence and accelerate progression to more complicated lesions. Oxidized LDL converts macrophages into foam cells. High-density lipoprotein (HDL) can decrease the number and activity of macrophages, which prevents plaque disruption and thrombus formation (Fuster, 1999). Most sudden deaths after MI result from ruptures in the fibrous cap of complicated lesions, leading to hemorrhage in the plaque, thrombosis, and blockage of the artery. Small thrombi help plaque grow, and large thrombi can cause acute clinical events.

The progression of atherosclerotic lesions is not linear or predictable. Lesions can appear in arteries that were judged to be "normal" on angiography months earlier (Fuster et al, 1996) (see Figure 35-6). With prevention, the goal is to regress coronary stenosis, reduce the incidence of plaque rupture, and improve coronary vasomotor function (Paterick and Fletcher, 2001).

Endothelial Dysfunction

An active area of preventive research is the role of endothelial dysfunction in the pathophysiology of clinical ischemia and acute coronary syndromes. Endothelial dysfunction includes abnormalities in vasomotor control (constriction versus dilation), fibrinoloysis and thrombosis, inflammatory response (leukocyte and platelet adhesion), and growth of vascular smooth muscle (Paterick and Fletcher, 2001). Nitric oxide is a key vasodilator produced by endothelial cells. Other key roles of nitric oxide are to inhibit platelet aggregation and smooth-muscle cell proliferation and reduce monocyte adherence. Without nitric oxide–mediated vasodilation, the vasoconstriction increases shear stress, which can increase the likelihood of plaque rupture.

Reduced nitric oxide levels are seen in diabetes, hypertension, or CHD, and people who smoke cigarettes. Thus, restoring nitric oxide levels could have great benefit on endothelial function and cardiovascular health. Nitric oxide is synthesized from the amino acid L-arginine. Dietary supplementation of L-arginine in hypercholesterolemic animals has shown beneficial effects, but data in humans are inconsistent. More long-term trials are needed to determine whether L-arginine supplementation can help restore endothelial function (Preli et al, 2002). The high arginine content of nuts may explain some of the positive associations seen between nut intake and reduced prevalence of CVD (Sabate, 1999). Other nutrients

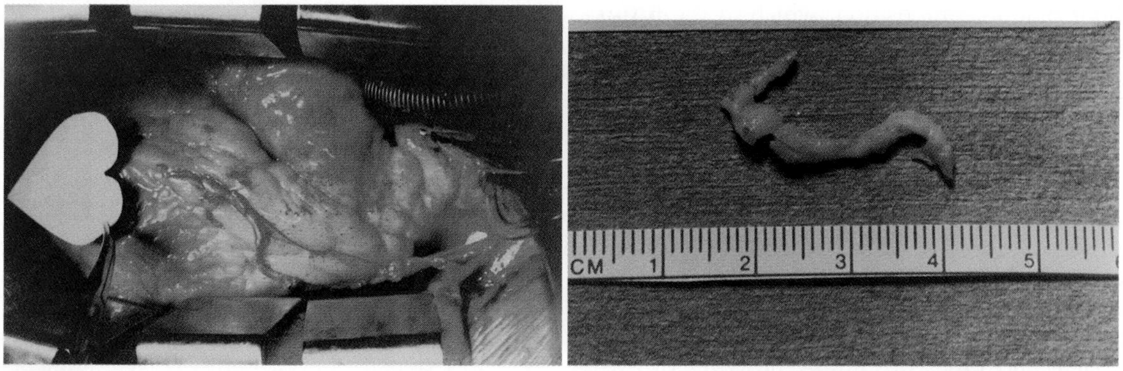

FIGURE 35-6 • Plaque that can be surgically removed from the coronary artery. (Photographs courtesy Ronald D. Gregory and John Riley, MD.)

under investigation for effects on the endothelium are omega-3 fatty acids, vitamins E and C, and folic acid (Brown and Hu, 2001).

Thrombosis

Thrombosis usually is the result of a rupture of the fibrous plaque cap. Thrombus formation and platelet activation are critical to plaque progression and the manifestations of acute angina or MI. Plaque composition, not the severity of stenosis, is a major determinant of which lesions rupture and result in thrombosis (Fuster et al, 1998). Thrombogenic risk factors include local factors, such as the degree of plaque disruption, the degree of stenosis, tissue substrate (lipids), surface of recurring thrombus, and vasoconstriction (platelets, thrombin), as well as systemic factors, such as cigarette smoking; stress; cocaine use; elevated cholesterol, fibrinogen, and lipoprotein(a) levels; impaired fibrinolysis; and infection (*Chlamydia pneumoniae*, cytomegalovirus, *Helicobacter pylori*) (Fuster et al, 1998).

Aspirin, which is commonly used for prevention, blocks only one of three pathways of platelet activation and does not affect the coagulation system. This has led to many antithrombotic drugs being developed and tested. The role of diet in thrombosis and hemostasis is controversial and needs further research (Grundy et al, 2002; Knapp, 1997).

Clinical Determination

Noninvasive tests, such as electrocardiograms, treadmill exercise tests, thallium scans, and echocardiography, are used initially to establish a diagnosis of CHD. A more definitive, invasive test is angiography (cardiac catheterization), in which a dye is injected into the arteries and radiographic images of the heart are obtained. Narrowing and blockages from atherosclerosis are readily apparent on angiograms; however, smaller phase 2 lesions are often not visible on angiography but can cause acute ischemic events. Thus, angiography cannot determine which lesions will rupture or where future occlusion will occur (Fuster et al, 1996).

Intravascular ultrasound detects plaque more frequently than angiography and can provide information about plaque composition, which in the future may affect treatment modalities (Hausmann et al, 1996). Mild coronary lesions have been associated with significant progression to severe stenosis or total occlusion in as many as two thirds of patients with unstable angina or acute coronary syndromes. Thus, early detection is critical.

New techniques, such as subselective coronary artery infusion, intracoronary Doppler velocimetry, and refined quantitative angiography, are being developed to study endothelial function and myocardial ischemia (Paterick and Fletcher, 2001). These methods are invasive and time consuming, however (Brown and Hu, 2001). A noninvasive ultrasound of the brachial artery after infusing acetylcholine or in response to increased flow is closely related to the coronary vasodilation response. This brachial artery method is being used in many studies of endothelial dysfunction.

End Points

About two thirds of the cases of acute coronary syndromes, unstable angina, acute MI, and ischemic sudden death happen in arteries that are minimally or mildly obstructed. The combination of obstruction and thrombosis leads to most acute coronary syndromes (Shah, 2000). In the ischemia of an infarction, the myocardium (or other tissue) is deprived of oxygen and nourishment. Whether the heart is able to continue beating depends on the extent of the musculature involved, the presence of collateral circulation, and the oxygen requirement. Stabilizing plaque (versus reducing plaque) to prevent rupture is an active area of research with much promise (Shah, 2000). Inflammation in the plaque, which can lead to instability, can occur as a result of modified lipids and oxidant and hemodynamic stresses.

PREVENTION OF CORONARY HEART DISEASE

A landmark achievement of epidemiologic research has been the identification of risk factors for CHD. These risk factors were found to be more prevalent in persons who later developed CHD. The primary prevention of CHD involves the assessment and management of these risk factors in asymptomatic person. Persons with multiple risk factors are the target population for primary prevention (National Cholesterol Education Program [NCEP], 2001). Risk factor reduction has been shown to reduce CHD even in older adults (Kannel, 2002; NCEP, 2001) and thus is warranted for all ages.

Blood Lipids and Lipoproteins

Cross-population, within-population, and clinical studies have consistently shown that a high serum cholesterol level causes CHD and mortality. In the last 30 years, the carriers of blood lipids and their carrier proteins, lipoproteins, have come to the forefront as predictors of risk.

Definitions

Blood lipids (cholesterol, triglycerides, and phospholipids) are transported in the blood bound to proteins. These complex particles, called *lipoproteins*, vary in composition, size, and density (Table 35-1). The five classes of lipoproteins—chylomicron, very-low-density lipoprotein (VLDL), intermediate-density lipoprotein (IDL), low-density lipoprotein (LDL), and high-density lipoprotein (HDL)—consist

TABLE 35-1 Characteristics and Functions of the Plasma Lipoproteins

	CLASSES OF LIPOPROTEINS				
CHARACTERISTICS	**CHYLOMICRON**	**VLDL**	**IDL**	**LDL**	**HDL**
Density, g/ml	<0.95	0.95-1.006	1.006-1.019	1.019-1.063	1.063-1.210
Electrophoretic mobility		Pre-β	Pre-β to β	β	α
Origin	Intestine	Liver and intestine	In circulation secondary to catabolism of other lipoproteins Liver	Liver	Liver and intestine
Physiologic role	Transport of dietary triglyceride	Transport of endogenous triglyceride	LDL precursor	Major cholesterol transport lipoprotein	Reverse cholesterol transport
Relative atherogenicity	0	+	+++	++++	Negatively correlated with atherosclerosis
Composition (%)					
Triglyceride	90	60	40	10	5
Cholesterol	5	10	30	50	20
Phospholipid	3	18	20	15	25
Protein	2	10	10	25	50
Major apolipoproteins	A-1 A-IV B-48 CI CII CIII	B-100 CI CII CIII E	B-100 E	B-100	A-I A-II

From Kris-Etherton PM et al: The effect of diet on plasma lipids, lipoproteins, and coronary heart disease, *J Am Diet Assoc* 88:1373, 1988. Copyright the American Dietitic Association.
VLDL, Very-low-density lipoprotein; *IDL,* intermediate-density lipoprotein; *LDL,* low-density lipoprotein, *HDL,* high-density lipoprotein.

of varying amounts of triglyceride, cholesterol, phospholipid, and protein.

Each class of lipoproteins actually represents a continuum of particles. The ratio of protein to fat determines the density; thus, particles with more protein are denser (e.g., HDLs have more protein than LDLs). The physiologic role of lipoproteins includes transporting lipid to cells for energy or storage and serving as a substrate for prostaglandins, thromboxanes, and leukotrienes (see Chapters 3 and 44). Because of different metabolic roles, the lipoproteins also vary in atherogenicity.

Total Cholesterol

A total cholesterol measurement captures cholesterol contained in all lipoprotein fractions: 60% to 70% is carried on LDL, 20% to 30% on HDL, and 10% to 15% on VLDL. There is a direct, positive relationship between total serum cholesterol and CHD. Populations that consume diets high in saturated fatty acids (SFAs) have increased blood cholesterol levels (hypercholesterolemia) and CHD incidence and mortality. Within populations, the blood cholesterol level is a positive, strong predictor of CHD mortality (Figure 35-7). The Third Report of the Expert Panel on Detection, Evaluation, and Treatment of High Blood Cholesterol in Adults (Adult Treatment Panel III [ATP-III]) reaffirms that "lowering total cholesterol and LDL-C reduces CHD risk" (NCEP, 2001). A 10% reduction in total cholesterol would decrease CHD incidence by about 30% (CDC, 2001). Whereas total cholesterol was previously recommended as a screening tool, ATP III now recommends a complete lipoprotein profile for screening.

Numerous factors affect serum cholesterol levels, including age; diets high in fat, saturated fat, and cholesterol and other factors discussed later; genetics; endogenous sex hormones (absence in postmenopausal women or presence during menstrual cycle); exogenous steroids (anabolic or sex hormones); drugs (β-blockers, thiazide diuretics); body weight; glucose tolerance; physical activity level; diseases (diabetes, thyroid, liver); and season of the year. Elevated serum cholesterol, measured in persons in their twenties, is strongly associated later with incidence of CHD (follow-up after 40 years) (Klag et al, 1993).

Serum cholesterol levels in the U.S. population have been declining since 1960, and more than half of that decline occurred between 1976 and 1991, after national preventive education efforts were begun (Johnson, 1993). The proportion of adults with high blood cholesterol (>240 mg/dl) fell from 27% to 19%, which is below the *Healthy People 2000* goal of 20% (NCHS, 2001). Because HDL cholesterol and VLDL cholesterol did not change during this period, the decline in total cholesterol levels is due to decreased LDL cholesterol. CHD mortality rates also fell.

Total Triglycerides

The triglyceride-rich lipoproteins include chylomicrons, VLDL, and any remnants or intermediary products formed in catabolism. Of these triglyceride-rich

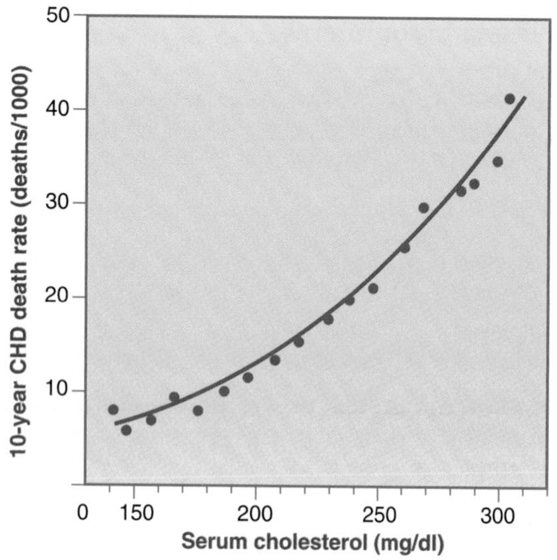

FIGURE 35-7 • Relationship between serum cholesterol level and coronary heart disease (CHD) rate. (From National Cholesterol Education Program: *Report of the Expert Panel on Population Strategies,* Public Health Service, National Institutes of Health, Publication No. 90-3046, Bethesda, Md, 1990, National Heart, Lung, and Blood Institute.)

lipoproteins, IDL and chylomicrons and VLDL remnants are known to be atherogenic. Some research has suggested that postprandial triglyceride measurements may be more predictive of CHD risk than fasting levels (Ginsberg, 1994), with endothelial dysfunction seen after consumption of a high-fat meal as one possible explanation (Plotnick et al, 1997). New data indicate that although patients with CHD have higher fasting and postprandiol levels of triglycerides than controls, the response (percent increase) to a fat-rich meal is comparable in both groups (Schaefer et al, 2001).

Triglyceride levels are classified as *normal* (<150 mg/dl), *borderline high* (150 to 199 mg/dl), *high* (200 to 499 mg/dl), and *very high* (>500 mg/dl) (NCEP, 2001). Patients with familial dyslipidemias will have triglyceride levels in the borderline high or high range (hypertriglyceridemia). Triglycerides in the very high range place the patient at risk for pancreatitis. These patients usually have hyperchylomicronemia and require diets very low in fat (i.e., ≤15% of calories derived from fat). Patients with a deficiency of lipoprotein lipase (LPL) will also have very high triglyceride levels and will require 10% fat diets. Drugs are often necessary to lower triglyceride levels in these patients. Triglyceride measurements are now considered in relationship to other risk factors that can be part of the metabolic syndrome, described in Chapter 12.

Lipoproteins and Metabolism

Chylomicrons

The largest particles, the chylomicrons, transport dietary fat and cholesterol from the small intestine to the liver and periphery (see Chapter 1). Once in the bloodstream, the triglycerides in the chylomicrons are hydrolyzed by lipoprotein lipase (LPL), located on the endothelial cell surface in muscle and adipose tissue. Apo C-II, one of the apolipoproteins in chylomicrons, is a cofactor for LPL. When about 90% of the triglyceride is hydrolyzed, the particle is released back into the blood as a remnant. The liver metabolizes these chylomicron remnants, but some deliver cholesterol to the arterial wall and thus are considered atherogenic. Consumption of high-fat meals produces more chylomicrons and remnants. When fasting plasma studies are done, chylomicrons are normally absent.

Very-Low-Density Lipoprotein

Very-low-density lipoprotein (VLDL) particles are synthesized in the liver to transport endogenous triglyceride and cholesterol. Sixty percent of the VLDL particle is triglyceride (see Table 35-1). VLDL particles are very heterogeneous. The large, buoyant VLDL particle is believed to be nonatherogenic (NIH Consensus Conference, 1993). Vegetarian diets and estrogen increase the formation of large VLDL particles. Smaller VLDL particles (i.e., remnants) are formed from triglyceride hydrolysis by LPL. Normally, these remnants, called *VLDL remnants* or IDL, are taken up by receptors on the liver or converted to LDL.

About 50% of the remnants lose apo E and apo C and become LDL. Some of the smaller LDL particles stay in the blood and become atherogenic when oxidized. These intermediary particles are formed at high rates with excessive cholesterol feeding in animals and in dysbetalipoproteinemia in humans. At present, concentrations of remnants can be determined only by methods (e.g., analytical ultracentrifuge) that are not commonly available in most clinical laboratories. Clinically, a total triglyceride level is a measurement of the triglyceride in VLDL, remnants, and IDL.

Intermediate-Density Lipoprotein

Intermediate-density lipoprotein (IDL) particles are formed with the catabolism of VLDL and are a precursor of LDL. They are rich in cholesterol and apo E (see Table 35-1). High concentrations of IDL and VLDL remnants have been directly related to lesion progression and subsequent coronary events in men and women (NCEP, 2001). As with VLDL remnants, IDL can be measured only by using density-gradient ultracentrifugation, which is not widely available or routinely performed.

Low-Density Lipoprotein

Low-density lipoprotein (LDL) is the primary cholesterol carrier in blood (see Table 35-1); consequently, total cholesterol levels and LDL cholesterol levels are highly correlated. Ninety-five percent of the apolipoproteins in LDL are apo B-100, known, as *apo B.* Apo

B is also present in smaller amounts in VLDL and IDL of hepatic origin.

After LDL is formed in VLDL catabolism, 60% is taken up by LDL receptors on the liver, adrenals, and other tissues. The remainder is catabolized via nonreceptor pathways. Both the number and activity of these LDL receptors are major determinants of LDL cholesterol levels in the blood.

Both LDL cholesterol and apo B are risk factors for atherogenesis and CHD. The atherogenic effect of LDL cholesterol is readily apparent in the genetic disease familial hypercholesterolemia (FH), which is characterized by few or no LDL receptors, resulting in defective LDL metabolism, elevated levels in plasma, and severe premature atherosclerosis and CHD. Without LDL receptors, LDL is metabolized via alternative pathways.

Some LDL can be oxidized and taken up by endothelial cells and macrophages in the arterial wall, leading to the first stages of atherosclerosis. Because of this oxidation, antioxidants are being investigated in clinical trials exploring prevention and treatment of CHD. To date, they have not been shown to be effective.

The effects of other dietary changes, such as replacement of monounsaturates, which would be less susceptible to oxidation than polyunsaturates, are also being investigated. Estrogen has been shown to inhibit LDL oxidation, which may help to explain the lower rates of CHD seen in premenopausal women (Rifici and Khachadurian, 1992).

Like other lipoproteins, LDL particles are heterogeneous in size, density, and lipid components. With the use of sophisticated methods, two LDL subclasses, with different risks, have been identified. Phenotype A is indicated by very large LDL particles, which are not associated with risk of disease. By contrast, phenotype B is typified by small, dense LDL particles that are triglyceride rich and cholesterol depleted and that are predictive of CHD risk in both men and women. Phenotype B, seen in 30% of the general population, tends to occur with low HDL cholesterol and high levels of triglyceride, VLDL, and IDL. Postmenopausal women, who are at increased risk for CHD, have a greater prevalence of smaller LDL than premenopausal women of the same age (Campos et al, 1988).

High-Density Lipoprotein

High-density lipoprotein (HDL) particles contain more protein than any of the other lipoproteins, which accounts for their theoretical metabolic role as a reservoir of the apolipoproteins that direct lipid metabolism. Apo A-I, the main apolipoprotein in HDL, is involved in tissue cholesterol removal. Both apo C and E on HDL are transferred to chylomicrons. Apo E helps receptors recognize and metabolize chylomicron remnants. High HDL levels are therefore associated with low levels of chylomicrons, VLDL remnants, and small, dense LDL. Of the several classes of HDL, HDL-2, which is relatively large and lipid rich, and HDL-3, which is small and relatively dense, predominates in human plasma. The use of these subfractions as predictors of risk has been debated, but total HDL cholesterol remains the best predictor.

LIPOPROTEIN ASSESSMENT

Lipoprotein Profile

A standard lipoprotein profile includes measurement of total cholesterol, LDL cholesterol, HDL cholesterol, and triglyceride levels after fasting. Most clinical laboratories cannot quantify LDL cholesterol directly; the Friedewald formula is used for the calculation. Consequently, a lipid profile must be taken in the fasting state (8 to 12 hours after eating) to allow time for chylomicrons to clear. The Friedewald formula for calculating LDL-C is as follows (NCEP, 2001):

$$\text{LDL-C} = (\text{TC}) - (\text{HDL-C}) - (\text{TG}/5)$$

where LDL-C is low-density lipoprotein cholesterol, TC is total cholesterol, HDL-C is high-density lipoprotein cholesterol, and TG is triglyceride. Calculating the LDL cholesterol level by difference can be done only when triglyceride levels are less than 400 mg/dl.

Adult reference percentiles for total cholesterol, LDL cholesterol, and HDL cholesterol are shown in Tables 35-2 through 35-4. Corresponding levels of lipids, expressed in mmol/L, are given. Total cholesterol and LDL cholesterol increase with aging. Over the 45-year period from age 20 to 65, total cholesterol levels in men increase by 13%. In women, over the same period, the increase is 21%.

A desirable lipoprotein profile is a total cholesterol level of less than 200 mg/dl, LDL cholesterol less than 130 mg/dl, HDL cholesterol greater than 40 mg/dl, and triglyceride level less than 150 mg/dl (NCEP, 2001). Because women have higher HDL cholesterol than men, an HDL cholesterol level of ≥45 mg/dl is recommended to properly assess risk in women (Mosca et al, 1999).

Reference plasma lipid levels for children and adolescents are presented in *Clinical Insight:* NCEP Recommendations for Detection and Management of Hypercholesterolemia in Children and Adolescents. Children of both sexes have similar levels of HDL cholesterol until puberty, after which the levels in females consistently run about 10 mg/dl higher than those in males throughout life. Black men have slightly higher levels of HDL than white men.

Adults older than 20 years of age should have a fasting lipoprotein profile once every 5 years (NCEP, 2001). If nonfasting values are obtained, then only total cholesterol and HDL cholesterol are usable. In this case, a total cholesterol ≥200 mg/dl or HDL choles-

TABLE 35-2 Total Serum Cholesterol Levels (mg/dl) for Persons 20 Years of Age and Older by Race/Ethnicity, Sex, and Age: United States, 1988-1991

RACE/ETHNICITY, SEX, AND AGE (yr)	NO. OF EXAMINED PERSONS	MEAN	SELECTED PERCENTILE								
			5TH	10TH	15TH	25TH	50TH	75TH	85TH	90TH	95TH
Men 20 and Older	3953	205	143	153	162	176	201	231	247	260	276
20-34	1186	189	134	145	151	162	186	211	225	236	260
35-44	653	207	144	155	167	182	205	231	245	258	269
45-54	508	218	152	170	180	191	215	242	257	268	283
55-64	535	221	154	169	180	195	221	245	264	274	285
65-74	557	218	157	173	179	190	214	241	256	270	286
75 and older	514	205	145	156	164	175	202	232	248	257	275
Women 20 and Older	3885	207	143	154	162	175	202	233	252	269	287
20-34	1177	185	134	143	150	160	182	204	218	229	254
35-44	709	195	142	152	159	170	193	215	232	242	254
45-54	464	217	158	165	171	187	212	240	264	279	297
55-64	503	237	168	184	191	204	228	264	280	291	323
65-74	493	234	168	180	186	205	232	261	278	290	308
75 and older	539	230	163	175	184	198	227	263	279	287	316
Mexican American											
Men	1092	202	140	151	159	172	199	225	245	257	277
Women	1046	200	139	149	158	169	195	224	241	258	279
Non-Hispanic Black											
Men	922	199	136	149	156	170	195	224	242	252	276
Women	985	203	137	150	159	172	200	227	248	262	286
Non-Hispanic White											
Men	1816	206	144	154	163	177	203	232	247	260	276
Women	1734	208	144	155	163	176	202	234	254	271	288

Data from National Cholesterol Education Program (NCEP): *Second report of the Expert Panel on Detection, Evaluation, and Treatment of High Blood Cholesterol in Adults (Adult Treatment Panel II)*, NIH Publication No. 93-3095, Bethesda, Md, 1993, National Institutes of Health, National Heart, Lung, and Blood Institute.

TABLE 35-3 Low-Density Lipoprotein Cholesterol Levels (mg/dl) for Persons 20 Years of Age and Older by Race/Ethnicity, Sex, and Age: United States, 1988-1991

RACE/ETHNICITY, SEX, AND AGE (yr)	NO. OF EXAMINED PERSONS	MEAN	SELECTED PERCENTILE								
			5TH	10TH	15TH	25TH	50TH	75TH	85TH	90TH	95TH
Men 20 and Older	1669	131	75	87	95	106	129	154	167	179	194
20-34	487	120	67	78	86	97	121	139	152	165	186
35-44	274	134	85	92	98	111	131	156	166	176	192
45-54	224	138	78	91	100	118	136	163	174	187	195
55-64	228	142	78	90	104	117	143	165	175	194	205
65-74	259	141	93	104	109	119	134	163	177	185	199
75 and older	197	132	83	88	93	106	130	154	170	186	196
Women 20 and Older	1673	126	69	81	88	99	122	150	165	175	191
20-34	525	110	59	70	75	88	108	129	142	155	173
35-44	316	117	67	85	88	97	116	138	146	155	165
45-54	214	132	70	87	93	107	130	157	173	182	198
55-64	213	145	79	90	101	122	145	170	184	189	209
65-74	202	147	92	97	109	119	148	169	185	192	206
75 and older	203	147	90	102	109	121	143	168	189	197	209
Mexican American											
Men	448	124	70	77	85	96	120	148	161	172	188
Women	471	122	67	80	86	95	118	144	158	166	189
Non-Hispanic Black											
Men	393	126	69	76	82	96	123	146	168	186	206
Women	422	126	67	76	86	100	124	147	162	174	192
Non-Hispanic White											
Men	773	132	76	88	97	108	129	154	168	179	194
Women	729	126	69	82	89	99	122	151	166	176	192

Data from National Cholesterol Education Program (NCEP): *Second report of the Expert Panel on Detection, Evaluation, and Treatment of High Blood Cholesterol in Adults (Adult Treatment Panel II)*, NIH Publication No. 93-3095, Bethesda, Md, 1993, National Institutes of Health, National Heart, Lung, and Blood Institute.

TABLE 35-4 High-Density Lipoprotein Cholesterol Levels (mg/dl) for Persons 20 Years of Age and Older by Race/Ethnicity, Sex, and Age: United States, 1988-1991

RACE/ETHNICITY, SEX, AND AGE (yr)	NO. OF EXAMINED PERSONS	MEAN	SELECTED PERCENTILE								
			5TH	10TH	15TH	25TH	50TH	75TH	85TH	90TH	95TH
Men 20 and Older	3920	46.5	28.0	31.0	34.0	37.0	44.1	53.1	59.1	64.0	73.0
20-34	1178	47.1	30.0	34.0	35.1	38.0	46.0	54.0	60.1	64.0	71.0
35-44	642	46.3	28.0	30.0	33.0	37.0	44.0	53.0	58.1	63.0	73.0
45-54	502	46.6	28.0	30.0	33.0	36.0	43.1	53.0	61.0	66.1	77.1
55-64	533	45.6	29.0	31.0	33.0	36.1	43.0	53.0	59.0	62.0	72.0
65-74	553	45.3	28.0	31.0	32.0	36.0	43.0	53.0	58.0	62.1	71.0
75 and older	512	47.2	28.0	32.0	34.0	38.0	45.0	54.0	62.0	67.0	75.1
Women 20 and Older	3855	55.7	34.0	38.0	41.0	44.1	54.0	65.0	71.0	76.1	83.0
20-34	1167	55.7	34.0	38.0	41.0	44.1	54.0	64.1	70.1	75.1	83.1
35-44	701	54.3	33.0	37.0	40.0	44.0	53.0	64.1	69.1	72.1	79.0
45-54	459	56.7	37.0	38.1	41.0	46.0	56.0	65.0	72.1	77.1	84.1
55-64	500	56.1	33.0	37.0	40.0	44.0	53.0	66.0	73.0	79.0	87.1
65-74	492	55.7	34.0	37.0	40.0	44.1	54.0	65.1	73.0	78.0	83.1
75 and older	536	57.1	33.0	39.0	41.0	44.1	56.0	66.1	73.1	78.1	87.0
Mexican American											
Men	1077	46.9	30.0	33.0	34.1	38.0	45.0	54.0	59.0	64.0	69.0
Women	1040	53.3	34.0	37.0	40.0	44.0	52.0	61.0	68.0	72.1	78.0
Non-Hispanic Black											
Men	918	53.3	30.0	35.0	38.0	42.0	51.0	62.0	69.1	75.1	86.1
Women	978	57.8	37.0	40.0	43.0	47.0	55.1	67.1	74.0	78.1	86.0
Non-Hispanic White											
Men	1803	45.5	28.0	30.0	33.1	36.1	44.0	52.1	58.0	62.0	71.1
Women	1717	55.7	33.1	37.0	40.0	44.0	54.0	65.1	71.1	77.0	83.1

Data from National Cholesterol Education Program (NCEP): *Second report of the Expert Panel on Detection, Evaluation, and Treatment of High Blood Cholesterol in Adults (Adult Treatment Panel II)*, NIH Publication No. 93-3095, Bethesda, Md, 1993, National Institutes of Health, National Heart, Lung, and Blood Institute.

CLINICAL INSIGHT

NCEP Recommendations for Detection and Management of Hypercholesterolemia in Children and Adolescents

In 1991 the National Cholesterol Education Program (NCEP) made recommendations for the management of hypercholesterolemia to be applied to adolescents and children older than 2 years of age (National Heart, Lung, and Blood Institute, 1991). This is the first time there has been consensus among pediatric experts, lipid researchers, and nutrition and health care communities on this subject.

For the general population of children and adolescents in the United States, NCEP recommended adoption of eating patterns to meet the following criteria:

- Nutritionally adequate, varied diet
- Adequate energy intake to support growth and development and maintain appropriate body weight
- Saturated fat—less than 10% of total calories
- Total fat—an average of no more than 30% of total calories
- Dietary cholesterol—less than 300 mg/day

Implementation of these dietary patterns requires involvement of the entire community—parents, in selecting and preparing foods; schools, in modifying school food service; health care clinics, in health education; government, in improvement of food labeling; and the food industry, in developing low saturated fat, low-fat foods that are appealing to children.

NCEP also aims to identify and treat individual children and adolescents who have hypercholesterolemia and a family history of premature cardiovascular disease, or whose parents have hypercholesterolemia. For this group, the NCEP recommends:

1. Blood cholesterol screening of children and adolescents whose parents or grandparents, at 55 years or younger, were found to have coronary atherosclerosis; suffered myocardial infarction, peripheral vascular disease, cerebrovascular disease, or sudden death; or underwent invasive cardiac therapy (balloon angioplasty or coronary artery bypass surgery).
2. Blood cholesterol screening of offspring of a parent with a blood cholesterol of 240 mg/dl or greater.

For children with an elevated blood cholesterol level, the Step I Diet is used for 3 months, after which the blood cholesterol level is reassessed. If the desired cholesterol level has not been reached, the Step II Diet is implemented for at least another 6 months. If after 6 months to 1 year of dietary therapy blood lipids lowering is insufficient, drug therapy can be considered in children older than 10 years of age.

Visit the website http://rover.nhlbi.nih.gov/chd for more information.

Levels of Blood Total and LDL Cholesterol in Children and Adolescents

CATEGORY	TOTAL CHOLESTEROL mg/dl	LDL CHOLESTEROL mg/dl
Acceptable	<170	<110
Borderline	170-199	110-129
High	≥200	≥130

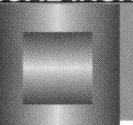

terol <40 mg/dl necessitates a fasting analysis for appropriate LDL management. The ATP-III classification for prevention and treatment is shown in Table 35-5.

Assessing Risk

The American College of Cardiology has categorized risk factors into four categories that match the intensity of risk factor management with the evidence for an association with CVD, clinical usefulness, and response to therapy (Pasternak et al, 1996) (Table 35-6). Category I risk factors are those for which interventions have been proven to lower CVD risk. Category II risk factors are those for which interventions are likely to lower CVD risk. Category III risk factors are those for which additional evidence is needed to determine whether interventions can lower risk. Category IV risk factors are those that cannot be modified.

It is known that diet is the predominant environmental cause of coronary atherosclerosis and that diet modification unequivocally can reduce risk of CHD. Thus, if diet were listed as a separate risk factor, it would be a category I risk factor.

Category I Risk Factors

Cigarette Smoking

The increased risk of CVD from smoking has been recognized for more than 30 years, with definitive evidence presented in several Surgeon General reports. Smoking is the number one cause of preventable death in the United States; one in five CVD deaths are attributable to smoking (AHA, 2001). The economic loss from tobacco use from 1995 through 1999 has been estimated at $157 billion (Fellows and Trosclair, 2002). Since the 1960s, the prevalence of smoking in the United States has fallen by 44% to the current level of 26% in men and 22% in women (Eberhardt, Ingram, Makuc et al, 2001). Among ethnic groups, American Indians/Alaska Natives have the highest prevalence of smoking (41% for both genders). Smoking prevalence is higher in persons with less than a high school education (35%) compared with those with a college education (12%).

Smoking is synergistic with other risk factors (i.e., the risk of CHD is much higher with multiple risk factors) and directly influences acute coronary events, including thrombus formation, plaque instability, and arrhythmias. Over time, smoking increases the risk for carotid stenosis in older patients, who also have high levels of cholesterol and high systolic blood pressure (Wilson et al, 1997). Women who smoke and use oral contraceptives have 10 times the risk of developing CHD than women who do not smoke and who do not use contraceptives. Risk also increases with the number of cigarettes smoked each day; low-tar brands do not reduce the risk. Nicotine and by-products of smoking are involved in the initiation and progression of atherosclerosis. Consequently, any exposure, including passive smoking, increases the risk (Howard and Thun, 1999).

About 37,000 nonsmokers die of CVD yearly from exposure to tobacco smoke (AHA, 2001). Clinically, smoking decreases HDL cholesterol (by an average of 6 to 8 mg/dl) and increases VLDL cholesterol and blood glucose levels. With new therapies, smoking cessation has been attainable for some smokers; 50% of the smoking population from 1965 to 1991 was able to quit. After quitting, CHD risk decreases by 50% and within 15 years the relative risk of CHD mortality approaches that of a lifetime nonsmoker (AHA, 2001).

Low-Density Lipoprotein Cholesterol

As discussed, LDL cholesterol is conclusively linked to CHD development and acute events. Consequently, LDL cholesterol is the primary target for intervention efforts. A decrease of 1 mg/dl in LDL cholesterol results in about a 1% to 2% decrease in the relative risk for CHD. Factors that increase LDL cholesterol include aging, genetics, diet, reduced estrogen levels (as occurs in postmenopausal women), progestins, diabetes, hypothyroidism, nephrotic syndrome, obstructive liver disease, obesity, and some steroid and antihypertensive drugs.

Of these factors, an imprudent diet and obesity are the most prevalent. Diets high in saturated fat and cholesterol elevate LDL by downregulating the LDL receptors in the liver (Woollett et al, 1992). With suppression of LDL receptor activity, less LDL is cleared from the plasma; hence, levels rise. Obesity increases production of apo B–containing lipoproteins: VLDL and, consequently, LDL. For persons who are without disease, LDL levels are classified as near optimal (≤129 mg/dl), borderline high risk (130 to 159 mg/dl), high risk (160 to 189 mg/dl), and very high risk (≥190 mg/dl).

TABLE 35-5 ATP III Classification of LDL, Total, and HDL Cholesterol (mg/dl)

LDL CHOLESTEROL—PRIMARY TARGET OF THERAPY	
<100	Optimal
100-129	Near optimal/above optimal
130-159	Borderline high
160-189	High
≥190	Very high
Total cholesterol	
<200	Desirable
200-239	Borderline high
≥240	High
HDL cholesterol	
<40	Low
≥60	High

From ATP III materials (www.nhlbi.nih.gov/guidelines/cholesterol/atp3_rpt.htm).
LDL, Low-density lipoprotein; *HDL,* high-density lipoprotein.

Lowering LDL cholesterol has been shown to regress lesions; delay progression of atherogenesis; and reduce events, morbidity, and mortality in both primary and secondary prevention trials (Pasternak et al, 1996). The target LDL cholesterol level for persons with disease is less than 100 mg/dl (see Table 35-6). Dietary factors that lower LDL-C include monounsaturated and polyunsaturated fatty acids (when substituted for SFAs), soluble fiber, soy protein, stanols or sterols, and weight reduction.

Hypertension

Hypertension is a risk factor for CHD, stroke, and congestive heart failure. The prevalence of hypertension has been declining and the number of patients being treated increasing with the result of lower CHD mortality rates (NCHS, 2002). About 25% of all adult Americans have hypertension, defined as an average blood pressure of 140/90 mmHg, or use antihypertensive medication (AHA, 2001). The prevalence increases with age, and it is seen more often in blacks than in non-Hispanic whites. Hypertension contributes to disease development by causing vascular injury and stresses to the myocardium. About 50% of first MI patients and 66% of stroke patients have blood pressures higher than 160/90 mm Hg (AHA, 2001). Hypertension is frequently present with other risk factors, such as hypercholesterolemia and obesity, and is one of the risk factors used to determine the presence of metabolic syndrome (see later discussion). Treating hypertension decreases the incidence of stroke, CHD, and CHF (see Chapter 36).

Left Ventricular Hypertrophy

The left ventricle increases in size in response to high blood pressure and increased workload secondary to obesity. In the Framingham Study, left ventricular hypertrophy (LVH) was found to be a strong risk factor for CVD, CHF, and sudden death (Levy et al, 1994). LVH is a risk factor in all age, gender, and ethnic

TABLE 35-6 Cardiovascular Risk Factors: Evidence to Support Interventions

RISK FACTOR	EVIDENCE FOR ASSOCIATION WITH CVD: EPIDEMIOLOGIC	EVIDENCE FOR ASSOCIATION WITH CVD: CLINICAL TRIALS	CLINICAL MEASUREMENT: USEFULNESS	RESPONSE TO: NONPHARMACOLOGIC THERAPY	RESPONSE TO: PHARMACOLOGIC THERAPY
Category I (Risk Factors for Which Interventions Have Been Proven to Lower CVD Risk)					
Cigarette smoking	+++	++	+++	+++	++
LDL cholesterol	+++	+++	+++	++	+++
High-fat/cholesterol diet	+++	++	++	++	−
Hypertension	+++	+++ (stroke)	+++	+	+++
Left ventricular hypertrophy	+++	+	++	−	++
Thrombogenic factors	+++ (fibrinogen)	+++ (aspirin, warfarin)	+ (fibrinogen)	+	+++ (aspirin, warfarin)
Category II (Risk Factors for Which Interventions Are Likely to Lower CVD Risk)					
Diabetes mellitus	+++	+	+++	++	+++
Physical inactivity	+++	++	++	++	−
HDL cholesterol	+++	+	+++	++	+
Triglycerides; small, dense LDL	++	++	+++	++	+++
Obesity	+++	−	+++	++	+
Postmenopausal status (women)	+++	−	+++	−	+++
Category III (Risk Factors Associated With Increased CVD Risk That, if Modified, Might Lower Risk)					
Psychosocial factors	++	+	+++	+	−
Lipoprotein (a)	+	−	+	−	+
Homocysteine	++	−	+	++	++
Oxidative stress	+	−	−	+	++
No alcohol consumption	+++	−	++	++	−
Category IV (Risk Factors Associated With Increased CVD Risk That Cannot Be Modified)					
Age	+++	−	+++	−	−
Male gender	+++	−	+++	−	−
Low socioeconomic status	+++	−	+++	−	−
Family history of early-onset CVD	+++	−	+++	−	−

From Davidson MH, Maki KC: Cardiovascular risk factors: evaluation and treatment goals. In Kris-Etherton PM, Burns JH, editors: Cardiovascular nutrition: strategies and tools for disease management and prevention, Chicago, 1998, American Dietetic Association; and Califf RM et al: Task force 5, *J Am Coll Cardiol* 27:1007, 1996. Copyright American College of Cardiology Foundation.

CVD, Cardiovascular disease; *HDL,* high-density lipoprotein; +, weak, somewhat consistent evidence; ++, moderately strong, rather consistent evidence, +++, very strong, consistent evidence; −, evidence poor or nonexistent.

groups. Intervention trials are being conducted to determine whether regressing LVH will improve the clinical course. In the meantime, the presence of LVH necessitates more intensive risk factor management (see Chapter 37).

Thrombogenic Factors

Most MIs are the result of an intracoronary thrombosis. Prospective studies have shown that plasma fibrinogen is an independent predictor of CHD risk (Ernst and Koenig, 1997). Factors associated with an elevated fibrinogen are smoking, sedentary lifestyle, elevated triglycerides, and genetic factors (Wood, 2001). Genes explain 30% to 50% of the variability in fibrinogen levels (de Maat, 2001). Other thrombogenic factors (factor VII, plasminogen activator inhibitor-1) have inconsistently been related to MI or coronary disease. Platelet aggregation is associated with increased risk of CHD, but measurement inconsistencies make it difficult to include in risk stratification (Wood, 2001). To date, the most widely studied preventive factor for thrombogenesis is the use of aspirin. Daily use of 80 to 325 mg of aspirin is recommended for patients with CHD. Depending on the risk factor profile, aspirin may be recommended for primary prevention also.

Category II Risk Factors likely

Diabetes

Diabetes, like hypertension, is both a disease and a risk factor. It is less prevalent than hypertension, affecting 5% compared with 20% of the population. Both type 1 (insulin-dependent) and type 2 (non-insulin-dependent) diabetes increase the risk for CHD, with occurrence at younger ages. Eighty percent of deaths in persons with diabetes are attributable to atherosclerosis (Pasternak et al, 1996).

Rates of CVD occur four times more often in women 18 to 44 years of age with diabetes compared with women without the disease (CDC, 2001; Hu et al, 2001). The age-adjusted prevalence of CVD in women with diabetes is twice that in women without diabetes. Some of the increased risk for CHD seen in diabetic patients is attributable to the concurrent presence of other risk factors, such as dyslipidemia, hypertension, and obesity (see Chapter 33). Because of this, diabetes is now considered a CHD risk factor. Thus, the LDL cholesterol treatment goal for persons with diabetes is 100 mg/dl. Strict blood glucose control lessens microvascular complications in patients with type 1 and type 2 diabetes.

Physical Inactivity

Physical inactivity, or a low level of fitness, is an independent risk factor for CHD. Twelve percent of all mortality in the United States is related to a sedentary lifestyle, and sedentary people have twice the risk of developing CHD as do active people (Powell et al, 1987). This magnitude of risk is similar to that associated with high blood cholesterol or smoking. Despite public health recommendations to increase activity levels, 29% to 38% of adults in national surveys reported no leisure-time physical activity (Schoenborn and Barnes, 2002).

The least active groups are women, blacks, Hispanics, older adults, and the less affluent (AHA, 2001). Physical inactivity is the most prevalent modifiable risk factor. Thirty minutes of daily activity of moderate intensity is recommended (Pate et al, 1995). Moderate-intensity activities include walking at 3 to 4 mph, climbing stairs, gardening, and housecleaning. Fortunately, the number of Americans engaging in moderate activities five or more time per week increased over the last decade and achieved the goal of 30% of the population (NCHS, 2002).

Physical activity lessens CHD risk by retarding atherogenesis, increasing the vascularity of the myocardium, increasing fibrinolysis, and modifying other risk factors, such as increasing HDL cholesterol, improving glucose tolerance and insulin sensitivity, aiding in weight management, and reducing blood pressure.

High-Density Lipoprotein Cholesterol

Many population studies have shown that HDL cholesterol is a strong, negative, independent predictor of CHD incidence and mortality in men and women. HDL cholesterol is a more powerful predictor of asymptomatic disease observed by intravascular ultrasound than other lipoproteins (Hausmann et al, 1996). In patients with CHD, HDL cholesterol is also inversely related to coronary artery stenosis in both genders. This protective effect of HDL has been confirmed by intervention studies in which HDL cholesterol level was raised.

In the Helsinki Heart Study, simultaneous increases in HDL cholesterol and decreases in LDL cholesterol during drug therapy were accompanied by a 34% reduction in CHD events in middle-age men (Huttunen et al, 1991). After controlling for other risk factors, an increase of 1 mg/dl in HDL cholesterol was shown to reduce CHD risk by 2% to 3% (NIH Consensus Conference, 1993). Because of the inverse relationship between HDL and CHD risk, a high HDL cholesterol level (>60 mg/dl) is now considered protective, and a low HDL cholesterol level (<40 mg/dl) is considered to be a risk factor (NCEP, 2001).

The exact mechanism of HDL's antiatherogenic effect is unknown. Recently, it was shown that artificially raising HDL positively changes the endothelium. Other roles for HDL include transporting excess cholesterol from membranes to triglyceride-rich lipoproteins, which are then removed by receptors on the liver (Patsch, 1994). This process, known as *reverse cholesterol transport*, helps rid the body of cholesterol and prevents lipid accumulation in the arterial wall. A high HDL cholesterol level would mean the system is operating at a high capacity.

It has also been suggested that HDL cholesterol may just be a marker for efficient metabolism of triglyceride-rich lipoproteins with fewer atherogenic remnants being formed (Patsch, 1994). Although the cholesterol involved in lipoprotein metabolism is popularly referred to as "good" (HDL cholesterol) or "bad" (LDL cholesterol), it is, of course, the lipoprotein form, rather than the cholesterol being transported, that is associated with CHD.

Major factors that increase HDL cholesterol level are exogenous estrogen, exercise, loss of excess body fat, and moderate consumption of alcohol. Epidemiologic evidence indicates that consumption of alcoholic beverages, in particular red wine, results in a reduction in cardiovascular risk factors and decreases mortality; but the mechanisms of this cardiovascular protection are unclear. Some evidence suggests that nitric oxide plays a critical role in cardiovascular protection and that nitric oxide synthase is the responsible cardioprotective protein (Parks and Booyse, 2002.)

Obesity, inactivity, cigarette smoking, androgenic and related steroids (anabolic steroids, progesterone-dominant oral contraceptives), β-adrenergic blocking agents, hypertriglyceridemia, and genetic factors lower HDL cholesterol. Dietary factors, discussed in the section on diet and serum lipids, also affect HDL cholesterol levels.

Obesity

Body mass index (BMI) and CHD are positively related; as BMI goes up, the risk of CHD also increases. An estimated 300,000 adults die each year of factors related to obesity. The prevalence of overweight and obesity increased between the National Health and Nutrition Examination Surveys II and III (NHANES II and NHANES III), and preliminary analysis of 1999 indicate the prevalence is still on the rise (NCHS, 2002). Thus, overweight and obesity have reached epidemic proportions in the United States. Mexican Americans have the highest prevalence of obesity, followed by American Indians, non-Hispanic blacks, and non-Hispanic whites. The incidence of diabetes has also increased (Mokdad et al, 2001). A 1-kg increase in weight increases the risk of diabetes by 9% (Mokdad, 2000). The epidemic of obesity and diabetes could reverse the downward trends in CHD mortality if not controlled in the near future.

How obesity affects atherogenesis is not clear, but it is probably related to the coexisting risk factors seen in obese individuals—specifically, glucose intolerance and diabetes, hypertension, dyslipidemia, and increased fibrinogen. Dyslipidemia is directly related to BMI. In women, higher BMIs are associated with triglyceride levels that are 35 to 48 mg/dl higher than average and HDL cholesterol levels that are 5 to 9 mg/dl lower than average (Denke et al, 1994). Weight loss has been correlated with lower fibrinogen (Ditschuneit 1995) and C-reactive protein levels (Tchernof, 2002), both of which are indicative of atherosclerosis.

Weight distribution (upper-body or abdominal versus lower-body distribution) is also predictive of CHD risk and affects glucose tolerance and serum lipid levels. A waist circumference of less than 35 inches for women and 40 inches for men is recommended (NIH, 1998). Small weight losses (10 to 20 lb) can improve risk factors, such as LDL-C, HDL-C, triglycerides, high blood pressure, glucose tolerance, and C-reactive protein levels, even if an ideal BMI is not achieved. Although few studies have explored whether weight loss has any effect on coronary events (Pasternak et al, 1996), predictions indicate that compliance with current NIH recommendations to lower calorie intakes and to increase exercise can help obese persons to achieve and sustain weight loss goals (Carmichael et al, 1998) (see Chapter 24 for managing overweight and Chapter 33 for managing diabetes).

Menopausal Status

Endogenous estrogen confers protection against CVD in premenopausal women, probably by preventing vascular injury. Loss of estrogen following natural or surgical menopause is associated with increased CVD risk. Rates of CHD in premenopausal women are low except in women with multiple risk factors. During the menopausal period, total cholesterol, LDL cholesterol, and triglyceride levels increase and HDL cholesterol level decreases, especially in women who gain weight (Krummel, 1996). In a longitudinal study of women going through menopause, average serum cholesterol levels increased by 19% in the perimenopausal period (van Beresteijn et al, 1993). Hormone replacement therapy (HRT) has been used to correct these negative changes in lipid levels; but HRT should not be used for prevention, because fewer numbers of women had increased risk of CHD in the short term (Grady et al, 2002; Mosca, 2001; Writing Group for the Women's Health Initiative Investigators, 2002). The noncoronary benefits of HRT must be considered, along with the coronary benefits and risks (Nelson et al, 2002).

Category III Risk Factors

Need Evidence

Psychosocial Factors

Psychosocial factors, such as type A personality (time-urgent, impatient, and compulsive), stress, depression, and education level (less than high school) are all associated with increased CVD risk. Interventions for factors that may be amenable to intervention (i.e., stress), however, have not demonstrated a decrease in risk, and more research is needed.

Triglycerides

In ATP III, elevated triglyceride levels are now recognized as an independent risk factor for CHD. Hypertriglyceridemia is most common in metabolic syndrome. Because of their roles in metabolism, triglyceride and HDL cholesterol levels are inversely related; that is, when a patient has high triglyceride levels, the HDL cholesterol levels are usually low. Because of large biologic variability (<20%) in triglyceride measurements, a single sample analyzed for blood triglyceride may not reflect true levels. The 1993 NIH Consensus Conference recommended taking at least two fasting samples 1 week apart before treatment decisions are made (NIH Consensus Conference, 1993).

Factors that increase triglyceride levels are diet (vegetarian, low-fat, refined carbohydrate), estrogens, alcohol, obesity, untreated diabetes, untreated hypothyroidism, chronic renal disease, and liver disease. Treatment of hypertriglyceridemia includes (1) weight loss for overweight patients, (2) consumption of a low saturated fat–low cholesterol diet, (3) decreased intake of refined carbohydrate, (4) increased physical activity, (5) smoking cessation, (6) management of diabetes if present, and (7) restricted alcohol use. Drug therapy is indicated for hypertriglyceridemia when it coexists with established CHD, a positive family history, or concurrent high cholesterol and low HDL cholesterol levels, and when the genetic form is present.

Lipoprotein(a)

Lipoprotein(a) (Lp[a]) is a unique lipoprotein that has been a controversial analyte for more than 30 years. In addition to apo B, Lp(a) has the protein apo (a), which is very similar to plasminogen, a proenzyme involved in the breakdown of fibrin. Many early studies showed that Lp(a) was a strong, independent risk factor for premature CHD; however, large prospective studies have yielded mixed results. The incongruity is due to methodologic differences and the heterogeneity of this particle.

Until further data are available, routine screening of Lp(a) is not recommended. Lp(a) levels are skewed to lower values, and within a given population, the levels can vary by 1000-fold (Pasternak et al, 1996). The 75th and 90th percentiles for Lp(a) are 25 mg/dl and 40 mg/dl, respectively. Lp(a) is a category III risk factor because data are lacking on intervention trials. Estrogens, anabolic steroids, and niacin are known to lower Lp(a).

Homocysteine

Homocysteine was proposed as a risk factor when it was observed that children who were deficient in cystathionine B synthase, the essential catabolic enzyme for homocysteine, were found to have premature atherosclerosis, albeit in veins and not arteries, and mortality. Subsequently, in prospective and case-control studies, moderate hyperhomocysteinemia has been associated with occlusive vascular disease in the coronary, cerebral, and peripheral arteries (Ueland, 2000). Reduced enzyme activity occurs in 5% to 7% of the population; severe deficiency is rare (Welch and Loscalzo, 1998).

Homocysteine as a risk factor is now controversial for several reasons (Braattstrom, 2000). First, elevated plasma homocysteine is strongly and positively related to the other major risk factors for CVD (i.e., age, smoking, blood pressure, high blood cholesterol, and lack of exercise) (Bots, 1997). Second, serum creatinine as an indicator of renal function is a strong predictor of plasma homocysteine levels. Thus, poor renal function due to atherosclerosis raises homocysteine levels, not vice versa. Third, whereas low serum or red cell folate or vitamin B_{12} cause elevations in plasma homocysteine levels, deficiency of either of these vitamins does not produce vascular disease. Elevated homocysteine levels have been most predictive in patients with advanced renal failure or atherosclerosis. Atherogenic mechanics for homocysteine in these patients include procoagulant activity or endothelial injury (Woo et al, 1997).

Genetic factors such as a variant in methylenetetrahydrofolate reductase or inadequate dietary intake of folate, riboflavin, and vitamins B_{12} and B_6 increase plasma homocysteine levels. Thus, ensuring appropriate dietary intake of these B vitamins will reduce plasma homocysteine. Folate fortification lowered homocysteine levels in the Framingham Offspring Study cohort (Jacques et al, 1999), but it is unknown whether increased folic acid intake will lower the prevalence of CVD. Evidently, more research in this area is warranted (Krauss, 2002).

Oxidative Stress

Oxidation of LDL in the vessel wall hastens the atherogenic process by recruiting macrophages, stimulating autoantibodies, increasing LDL uptake, and increasing vascular tone and coagulability (Pasternak et al, 1996). Dietary factors that can decrease LDL oxidation include vitamin C, vitamin E, β-carotene, selenium, flavonoids, magnesium, and monounsaturated fat. Of these, vitamins C and E, and β-carotene have been studied. Recent clinical trials employing vitamin E have provided mixed results indicating either benefit, no effect, or an adverse impact on patients with CVD, but consideration of the design and outcome of these studies suggests approaches for new studies (Blumberg, 2002; Krauss et al, 2000).

Alcohol Consumption

Moderate alcohol consumption (i.e., one or two drinks a day) is associated with a significant reduction in CHD risk (Parks and Booyse, 2002), but the use of alcohol is not recommended as an intervention strategy (see Dietary Factors). The limits on alcohol to no more than two drinks per day for men and one drink per day for women are made because alcohol also raises blood pressure (Krauss et al, 2000).

Category IV Risk Factors

Non-modifiable

Age

Age is a nonmodifiable risk factor for CHD. With increasing age, higher mortality rates from CHD are seen in both genders (see Figure 35-2). Gender, however, is a factor for the assessment of risk. The incidence of premature disease in men 35 to 44 years of age is three times as high as the incidence in women of the same age. Therefore, being older than 45 years of age is considered a risk factor for men (NCEP, 2001). For women, the increased risk comes after the age of 55 years, which is after menopause for most women. Overall, the risk of CHD increases markedly as one ages.

Family History

A family history of premature disease is a strong risk factor, even when other risk factors are considered. A family history is considered to be positive when MI or sudden death occurs before the age of 55 years in a male first-degree relative or the age of 65 in a female first-degree relative (parents, siblings, offspring). Numerous hyperlipidemias are inheritable and lead to premature atherosclerosis and CHD. The presence of a positive family history, although not modifiable, will influence the intensity of risk factor management.

Emerging Risk Factors

Markers of Inflammation

Because atherogenesis is an inflammatory process, markers of inflammation, such as C-reactive protein, have been measured and in epidemiologic studies found to be associated with angina, risk of coronary events, stroke, and peripheral vascular disease, independent of other risk factors (Wood, 2001). Recently, it was demonstrated that weight loss lowers C-reactive protein (Tchernof et al, 2002), which provides another physiologic benefit for weight management as a preventive strategy for CHD reduction.

GENETIC HYPERLIPIDEMIAS: CLASSIFICATION AND DIAGNOSIS

Several relatively rare forms of hyperlipidemia have strong genetic components. Originally, hyperlipidemias were classified according to the predominant aberrant lipoprotein (Table 35-7). For example, type I was defined by the presence of chylomicrons after an individual had fasted; type IIa was evidenced by an abnormal LDL level and a normal VLDL level. Although this system does describe the lipoprotein alteration, it does not provide information about the etiology of the disorder; nor is HDL considered in any of the types. Consequently, this method of classification is being used less often. The heritability of defects in LDL-C metabolism is about 50% and is not an aberration in a single gene.

Familial Hypercholesterolemia

Familial hypercholesterolemia (FH, type IIa; or high LDL cholesterol, normal triglyceride) is one of the LDL defects that are monogenic. A person is heterozygous if only one defective gene is inherited and homozygous if both defective genes are inherited. The heterozygous form (affecting 1 in 500 people in the United States) is much more prevalent than the homozygous form (affecting 1 in 1 million people). In these patients, the LDL receptors are either absent or nonfunctional, resulting in hypercholesterolemia (usually >300 mg/dl), which is present at birth. Early detection with aggressive therapy can prevent or delay CHD. FH accounts for about 2% of CHD occurring before the age of 60 in industrialized countries (Wood, 2001).

Homozygotes have more severe hypercholesterolemia and atherosclerosis, expressed as MI or death in the first or second decade of life. In heterozygotes, the average age of CHD onset is 45 years in men and 55 years in women (Schaefer, 1994a). Clinically, tendon xanthomas (cholesterol deposits from LDLs) seen on tendons and elbows, corneal arcus, premature CHD, and a strong family history of hypercholesterolemia are common. Diagnosis is based on LDL cholesterol levels that lie above the 90th percentile in two or more family members and the presence of tendon xanthomas in members within the family tree.

Treatment for homozygotes involves extreme measures, such as biweekly plasmaphoresis to remove LDL. Liver transplant, gene therapy, and portacaval shunts are experimental modes of treatment. For heterozygotes, therapeutic lifestyle changes with combination drug therapy are usually needed to achieve the goals for LDL levels.

TABLE 35-7 Phenotype Classification of Hyperlipidemias

PHENOTYPE	LIPOPROTEIN ABNORMALITY	BLOOD LIPIDS
Type I	↑↑ Chylomicrons	↑↑↑ Triglycerides ↑ Cholesterol
Type IIa	↑↑ LDL	↑↑ Cholesterol
Type IIb	↑↑ LDL, ↑ IDL, ↑↑ VLDL	↑↑ Cholesterol ↑↑ Triglycerides
Type III	↑ IDL, ↑ VLDL, ↑ remnants	↑↑ Cholesterol ↑↑ Triglycerides
Type IV	↑ VLDL	↑ Cholesterol ↑↑ Triglycerides
Type V	↑↑ Chylomicrons, ↑ VLDL	↑↑ Triglycerides ↑ Cholesterol

Data from Naito HK: The clinical significance of apolipoprotein measurements, *J Clin Immunoassay* 9:11, 1986; and Schonfeld G: The genetic dyslipoproteinemias—nosology update 1990, *Atherosclerosis* 81:81, 1990.
LDL, Low-density lipoproteins; *IDL,* intermediate-density lipoproteins; *VLDL,* very-low-density lipoproteins.

Polygenic Familial Hypercholesterolemia

Polygenic familial hypercholesterolemia is the result of multiple gene defects that have yet to be identified. The diagnosis is based on LDL cholesterol levels above the 90th percentile and the absence of tendon xanthomas in two or more family members. Usually, these patients have lower LDL cholesterol levels than patients with the nonpolygenic form, but they remain at high risk for premature disease. The apo E-4 allele is common in polygenic familial hypercholesterolemia. The treatment is similar to that for heterozygous familial hypercholesterolemia—that is, therapeutic lifestyle changes in conjunction with cholesterol-lowering drugs.

Familial Combined Hyperlipidemia

Familial combined hyperlipidemia (FCHL) is a disorder characterized by serum LDL cholesterol or triglyceride levels above the 90th percentile in at least two family members, with both abnormalities seen in the kindred. Several lipoprotein patterns may be seen in patients with FCHL. These patients can have (1) elevated LDL levels with normal triglyceride levels (type IIa), (2) elevated LDL levels with elevated triglyceride levels (type IIb), or (3) elevated VLDL levels (type IV). Often, these patients have the small, dense LDL associated with CHD. Consequently, all forms of FCHL cause premature disease; about 15% of patients who have an MI before the age of 60 have FCHL. The defect in FCHL is hepatic overproduction of apo B-100 and, thus, VLDL.

Patients with FCHL usually have a constellation of other risk factors—namely, obesity, hypertension, diabetes, and gout. Treatment includes therapeutic lifestyle changes, weight reduction, diabetes control, increased physical activity, and medication if lifestyle measures are ineffective. Patients with elevated triglyceride levels also need to avoid alcohol.

Familial Dyslipidemia

Familial dyslipidemia is a combination of familial hypertriglyceridemia, defined as at least two persons in a family having a triglyceride level above the 90th percentile and a low HDL cholesterol level, defined as less than the 10th percentile (Schaefer, 1994a). Fifteen percent of patients with CHD have familial dyslipidemia. Other risk factors common in these patients are android obesity, insulin resistance, type 2 diabetes, and hypertension. No specific treatment exists except for lifestyle interventions to modify all risk factors.

Familial Dysbetalipoproteinemia

Familial dysbetalipoproteinemia (type III hyperlipoproteinemia) is relatively uncommon (affecting 1 in 5000 persons in the United States). Catabolism of VLDL remnants, IDL, and chylomicron remnants is delayed owing to a basic abnormality in the structure of apolipoprotein E (apo E-2 is present instead of apo E-3 and E-4). For dysbetalipoproteinemia to be seen, other risk factors, such as age, hypothyroidism, obesity, or diabetes, or other dyslipidemias, such as FCHL, must be present. Total cholesterol levels range from 300 to 600 mg/dl, and triglyceride levels range from 400 to 800 mg/dl.

This condition creates increased risk of premature CHD and peripheral vascular disease. Diagnosis is based on determining isoforms of apo E. Treatment involves weight reduction, control of hyperglycemia and diabetes, and dietary restriction of cholesterol and saturated fat. If the dietary regimen is not effective, drug therapy is recommended.

DIETARY FACTORS

For more than 40 years, epidemiologic studies, experimental studies, and clinical trials have shown that numerous dietary risk factors affect serum lipids, atherogenesis, and CHD. The classic Seven Countries Study (Keys, 1970) was the first to show that a population's intake of SFAs was strongly correlated with serum cholesterol levels in the population. Countries with the highest SFA intake (>15% of total kilocalories) and the highest serum cholesterol levels had the highest CHD mortality.

Fat quantity, fat quality, cholesterol, and numerous other dietary substances have been investigated to see how they affect serum lipids and lipoproteins. When studying the effects of fatty acids on serum lipids, two points of comparison are made. First, how do the fatty acids compare with the carbohydrate substitution, which is considered neutral? Second, how do they compare when they replace SFAs?

Saturated Fatty Acids

In general, SFAs tend to elevate blood cholesterol in all lipoprotein fractions (i.e., both LDL and HDL cholesterol) when substituted for carbohydrate or other fatty acids. There is a dose-response relationship between SFA and LDL-C (Van Horn and Ernst, 2001). The most hypercholesterolemic or atherogenic SFAs are lauric (C12:0), myristic (C14:0), and palmitic (C16:0) acids (see Chapter 3). Myristic acid is the most potent, followed by palmitic, and then lauric acid. Although an SFA, stearic acid (C18:0) has no effect on blood lipoproteins and is considered neutral, like carbohydrate (Kris-Etherton and Yu, 1997). Palmitic acid is the most prevalent hypercholesterolemic SFA in the American diet, constituting 60% of total SFA intake. Although palmitate is present in plant sources, most dietary palmitate comes from animal foods. Myristic acid is found mostly in butterfat and coconut and palm kernel oils. It is less prevalent in the American diet than palmitic acid. Lauric acid, the only medium-chain SFA, is found in palm kernel and coconut oils. Of all the added fats in the diet, the most hypercholesterolemic are palm kernel, coconut and palm oils, lard, and butter. In the NHANES III, the mean consumption of SFA was 12% of kilocalories, and this figure did not vary by ethnic group (McDowell et al, 1994). Although progress has been made on reducing SFA consumption, the *Healthy People 2000* goal was not met (NCHS, 2001).

In their classic metabolic ward studies, Keys and colleagues developed equations to predict the blood cholesterol response for changes in SFA, polyunsaturated fatty acid (PUFA), and cholesterol intake. For every 1% increase in total energy intake from SFAs, a 2.7 mg/dl increase in plasma cholesterol level is predicted. For example, raising consumption of SFA (as a percentage of kilocalories) from 7% to 17% increases plasma cholesterol levels by 27 mg/dl. Although SFAs are extremely hypercholesterolemic, not all people respond the same way. People with the apo E-4 phenotype have the greatest blood cholesterol responses to SFA (Grundy, 1994). SFAs raise LDL cholesterol by decreasing LDL receptor synthesis and activity. Regardless of which form, all fatty acids will lower fasting triglycerides if they replace carbohydrate in the diet (Katan, 1994).

Dietary fatty acids have also been associated with the progression of coronary artery disease in men. After controlling for other risk factors, atherosclerosis progressed most in men consuming more stearic acid over a 39-month period (Watts et al, 1996). Palmitic and palmitoleic acids were also associated with disease progression, but not when other risk factors were controlled. The food sources of these fatty acids are milk, cheese, butter, and lamb; bakery goods, fast foods, and snack items provide an additional source in many diets (Elias and Innis, 2002) (see Chapter 3 for more details about *trans*-fatty acids).

In secondary prevention trials, replacement of SFA with MUFA and α-linolenic acid and increased fruits and vegetables prevented fatal and nonfatal CVD events in persons with established disease (de Lorgeril, 1999). Thus, fatty acids affect disease progression through lipids and other mechanisms, possibly thrombosis.

Polyunsaturated Fatty Acids

Omega-6 Polyunsaturated Fatty Acids

If carbohydrate is replaced by linoleic acid (C18:2), the predominant dietary omega-6 polyunsaturated fatty acid (PUFA), LDL cholesterol is lowered and HDL cholesterol is raised. When SFAs are replaced with PUFA in a low-fat diet, LDL and HDL cholesterol levels will be lowered (Nydahl et al, 1994). Overall, eliminating SFA is twice as effective in lowering serum cholesterol levels as is increasing PUFA (Grande et al, 1972; Kris-Etherton et al, 1988). A 1% increase in omega-6 PUFA would lower total cholesterol by 1.4 mg/dl; however, PUFAs have been shown to decrease VLDL, apo B, and HDL synthesis. In the past, a polyunsaturated:saturated ratio (P:S ratio) was used to assess fatty acid composition of foods and diets; however, this ratio is not recommended now because it does not separate the cholesterol-raising SFAs from the neutral SFAs (Denke et al, 1994).

Omega-6 (n-6) PUFAs are widespread in foods, but their major source is vegetable oils, salad dressings, and margarine made with the oils. The U.S. population's intake is at 7% of total kilocalories (McDowell et al, 1994). Because linoleic acid is not consumed in large amounts by any population and experimental feeding of large amounts increases LDL oxidation (Abbey et al, 1993), an increase in linoleic acid is not recommended above current intakes.

Omega-3 Polyunsaturated Fatty Acids

The main omega-3 fatty acids—eicosapentaenoic acid (EPA) and docosahexaenoic acid (DHA)—are high in fish oils, fish oil capsules, and ocean fish. Most studies have shown that omega-3 fatty acids do not affect total cholesterol; however, they do increase LDL cholesterol (5% to 10%) and decrease triglycerides (25% to 30%) (Harris, 1997). LDL cholesterol tends to be raised in patients with hypertriglyceridemia and lowered or unchanged in normal subjects fed concentrated sources of omega-3 fatty acids. Omega-3 fatty acids lower triglyceride levels by inhibiting VLDL and apo B-100 synthesis and by decreasing postprandial lipemia.

The effects of omega-3 fatty acids on triglyceride levels are dose dependent; that is, higher doses produce greater effects. Their greatest clinical utility, therefore, is with hyperlipoproteinemias in which the triglyceride level is also elevated (types II-b, III, IV, and V) (Connor, 1991). Omega-3 fatty acids affect many other steps in atherogenesis; most notably, they are precursors of the prostaglandins that interfere with blood clotting. Therefore, high intakes prolong bleeding times, a condition that is common in Eskimo populations with high dietary intakes and low incidence of CHD. It is now postulated that consumption of fish and fish oils rich in EPA and DHA will lower cholesterol, LDL, and triglyceride levels with a subsequent reduction in sudden cardiac death rates (Albert et al, 1998; Daviglus et al, 1997) (see Chapter 3). Consumption of as little as one fatty fish meal per week (5.5 g of omega-3 PUFAs per month) resulted in a 50% decrease in the risk of cardiac arrest after adjustment for all other risk factors (Siscovick et al, 2000). Dietary supplementation with 1 g of omega-3 PUFA daily reduced the relative risk of CVD death, nonfatal MI, and nonfatal stroke in patients who had recently survived an MI (GISSSI-Prevenzione Investigators, 1999). Thus, omega-3 PUFA has cardioprotective effects in primary and secondary prevention (Kris-Etherton et al, 2001a).

Monounsaturated Fatty Acids

cis-Monounsaturated Fatty Acids

Oleic acid (C18:1) is the most prevalent *cis*-monounsaturated fatty acid (MUFA) in the American diet. Substituting oleic acid for carbohydrate has almost no appreciable effect on blood lipids; however, replacing SFA with MUFA lowers serum cholesterol levels, LDL cholesterol levels, and triglyceride levels to about the same extent as PUFA. The effects of MUFA on HDL cholesterol depend on the total fat content of the diet. When intake of both MUFA (>15% of total kilocalories) and total fat (>35% of kilocalories) is high, HDL cholesterol does not change or increases slightly compared with levels with a lower-fat diet.

In epidemiologic studies, high-fat diets of people in Mediterranean countries have been associated with low blood cholesterol levels and CHD incidence (Trichopoulou et al, 2003). Among other factors, the main fat source is olive oil, which is high in MUFA. This observation led to many studies on the benefits of high-fat and high-MUFA diets. A step I diet (30% total fat, 10% SFAs, 10% MUFAs) and a high-MUFA diet (38% total fat, 10% SFAs, 18% MUFAs) were equally effective in lowering total cholesterol and LDL cholesterol without changing the HDL cholesterol level (Ginsberg et al, 1990). More recently, a Mediterranean-type step I diet was shown to reduce recurrent CVD by 50% to 70% (de Lorgeril, 1999). This modified step I diet emphasizes fruits, root vegetables (carrots, turnips, potatoes, onions, radishes), leafy green vegetables, breads and cereals, fish, foods high in α-linolenic acids (flax, canola oil), vegetable oil products (salad dressing and other products made with nonhydrogenated oils high in α-linolenic acid), and nuts and seeds (walnuts and flaxseed) (Kris-Etherton, 2001b). Although higher-fat diets (low in SFA, with MUFA as the predominant fat) can lower blood cholesterol, they should be used with caution owing to the caloric density of high-fat diets and the results of clinical trials, which have shown new atherosclerotic lesions in men who consume higher-fat diets (Blankenhorn et al, 1990), similar to lesions seen with diets high in SFA in animal studies (Kris-Etherton, 2001).

The negative association between the Mediterranean diet and CHD could be due to factors other than MUFA intake. For example, these populations consume more fruits and vegetables, bread, cereals, fish, and nuts, and less red meat than many populations. Olive oil is the primary source of fat, and eggs are consumed zero to four times per week.

Trans-Fatty Acids

Stereoisomers (*trans* form) of the naturally occurring *cis*-linoleic acid are produced in the hydrogenation process and are widely used in the food industry to harden unsaturated oils (see Chapter 3) and soft margarines. Fifty percent of *trans*-fatty acid intake comes from animal foods (beef, butter, and milk fats), and the other 50% comes from hydrogenated vegetable oils. The major food sources of *trans*-fatty acids in the U.S. diet are stick margarines, shortening, commercial frying fats, and high-fat baked goods (Food and Nutrition Science Alliance, 1994).

Elaidic acid, the *trans*-isomer of oleic acid, raises blood cholesterol if you compare it with PUFA; however, it has less of a cholesterol-raising effect than the saturated myristic and lauric acids (Kris-Etherton and Yu, 1997). Therefore, consuming *trans*-fatty acids at levels typical of American diets (3% of kilocalories) will raise LDL cholesterol levels but to a lesser extent than SFAs such as butter (Judd et al, 1994, 1998). Increased *trans*-fatty acid intakes (6% of energy) also lower HDL cholesterol. Press releases from these and other studies (Willett et al, 1993) led some consumers to switch from margarine to butter; however, margarine contains only 11% of cholesterol-raising saturates plus 1% *trans*, whereas butter contains 40% saturates plus 5% *trans* (Katan, 1994; Katan et al, 1994); hence, soft or spray or liquid margarine is the preferred spread. The average intake of *trans*-fatty acids is estimated to be 7% to 8% of total fat intake (Emken, 1995). Consuming appropriately homemade low-fat desserts, low-fat dairy products, and low-fat meats will lower *trans*-fatty acid intakes.

Amount of Dietary Fat

Total fat intakes are related to obesity, which affects many of the major risk factors for atherosclerosis. Also, high-fat diets increase postprandial lipemia and chylomicron remnants, both of which are associated with increased risk of CHD. When fat is reduced in the diet, and carbohydrate is the replacement source of kilocalories, triglycerides and HDL levels are affected. Low-fat diets (<25% of total kilocalories from fat) raise triglyceride levels (30 to 100 mg/dl) and lower HDL cholesterol levels (3 to 8 mg/dl) (Denke et al, 1994). Although these changes appear to be negative, they are not associated with CHD risk because (1) LDL cholesterol levels are low in persons consuming low-fat diets; and (2) the VLDL that are produced are large, triglyceride-rich VLDL, which are not associated with risk.

Lower-fat diets (<30% of total kilocalories from fat) that are high in SFAs (14% of kilocalories) will not lower LDL cholesterol compared with higher-fat diets (37% of kilocalories from fat) (Barr et al, 1992). Low-fat diets, therefore, lower LDL cholesterol levels only when accompanied by a decrease in SFA. The AHA continues to recommend total fat intakes at less than 30% of calories; the ATP III has broadened the fat recommendation to 25% to 35% of energy, with less than 7% coming from saturated fat (NCEP, 2001).

Dietary Cholesterol

Dietary cholesterol raises total cholesterol and LDL cholesterol, but to a lesser extent than SFAs. A 25-mg increase in dietary cholesterol would raise serum cholesterol by 1 mg/dl (Denke et al, 1994). When cholesterol intakes reach 500 mg per day, even smaller increments in blood cholesterol occur. Thus, there appears to be a threshold for a plasma cholesterol response to dietary cholesterol, which is why experiments that involve feeding eggs to subjects already on the typical American diet fail to affect serum cholesterol levels.

Cholesterol responsiveness also varies widely among individuals. Some people are hyporesponders (i.e., their plasma cholesterol level does not increase after dietary cholesterol challenge), whereas others are hyperresponders (i.e., their plasma cholesterol level responds more strongly than expected to a cholesterol challenge). It has been suggested that hyperresponders may have the apo E-4 allele and poor rates of conversion of cholesterol to bile acids, which causes elevated LDL cholesterol. Feeding cholesterol to animals enriches lipoproteins, which are atherogenic beyond just the rise in serum cholesterol.

Dietary cholesterol intakes in the United States have been declining since the 1960s. Between 1988 and 1991, the average cholesterol intake for the total population was 270 mg (McDowell et al, 1994). Non-Hispanic blacks and Mexican Americans had higher intakes of 301 and 324 mg daily, respectively.

In addition to the effects of dietary cholesterol alone on serum lipids, dietary SFAs and cholesterol have a synergistic effect on LDL cholesterol level. Together they decrease LDL receptor synthesis and activity, increase VLDL enriched with apo E, increase all lipoproteins, and decrease chylomicron size (which is associated with CHD risk) (Kris-Etherton et al, 1988). The intake of cholesterol has generally been positively related to the risk of CHD after adjusting for other risk factors, such as age, blood pressure, serum cholesterol level, and cigarette smoking.

Other Dietary Factors

Fiber

Soluble fibers—pectins, gums, mucilages, algal polysaccharides, and some hemicelluloses—in legumes, oats, fruits, and psyllium lower serum cholesterol and LDL cholesterol. The quantity of fiber needed to produce the lipid-lowering effect varies by food source; higher quantities of legumes are needed than of pectin or gums (Table 35-8).

The average decline in LDL cholesterol is 14% for hypercholesterolemics and 10% for normocholesterolemics when soluble fiber is added to a low-fat diet (Glore et al, 1994). Proposed mechanisms for the hypocholesterolemic effect of soluble fiber include the following: (1) the fiber binds bile acids, which lowers serum cholesterol to replete the bile acid pool; and (2) bacteria in the colon ferment the fiber to produce acetate, propionate, and butyrate, which inhibit cholesterol synthesis.

Insoluble fibers, such as cellulose and lignin, have no effect on serum cholesterol levels. Of the total recommended fiber intake (25 to 30 g daily for adults), about 6 to 10 g should be from soluble fiber. This level is easy to achieve with the recommended five or more servings of fruits or vegetables per day and six or more servings of grains (if whole grains and high-fiber cereals are chosen). The AHA does not recommend fiber supplements for prevention of CVD (Krauss et al, 2000), even though many people use them.

Alcohol

Alcohol affects both total triglyceride and HDL cholesterol levels. The effects of alcohol on triglyceride levels are dose dependent and are greater in persons with triglyceride levels exceeding 150 mg/dl. In population studies, moderate levels of alcohol consumption have been associated with decreased risk of MI and CHD mortality (in white men only) (Coate, 1993). Alcohol raises both the HDL2 and HDL3 cholesterol subfractions of HDL cholesterol. Current alcohol intake among the U.S. population is 2% of total kilocalories (McDowell et al, 1994), and no increase is recommended to decrease CHD risk.

Wine contains resveratrol, an antifungal compound in grape skins that increases HDL cholesterol and inhibits LDL oxidation (Wu et al, 2001.) The French may experience lower rates of CVD, despite a high-fat diet, because of their consumption of red wine: "the French paradox" (Sun et al, 2002.)

Coffee

Mixed results have been shown in studies investigating the effects of coffee on serum lipids. Heavy consumption of regular coffee (720 ml daily) causes minor increases in total cholesterol (9 mg/dl), LDL cholesterol (6 mg/dl), and HDL cholesterol (4 mg/dl) (Fried et al, 1992). Boiled coffee (European method) produces even greater elevations in plasma lipids than filtered coffee (American method) (Hammar et al, 2003; Johansson et al, 1996).

Most large population studies have failed to find associations between coffee consumption and CHD incidence or mortality. Any associations found are related to a constellation of risk factors seen in coffee drinkers. The coffee drinkers consumed more saturated fat and cholesterol, smoked more cigarettes,

TABLE 35-8 Quantity of Soluble Fiber Needed Daily to Produce Lipid-Lowering Effect

SOURCE	QUANTITY (g)
Pectin	6-40
Gums	8-36
Dried beans or legumes	100-150
Dry oat bran	25-100
Oatmeal	57-140
Psyllium	10-30

Data from Glore SR et al: Soluble fiber and serum lipids: a literature review, *J Am Diet Assoc* 94:425, 1994.

and were less likely to exercise than non–coffee drinkers (Puccio et al, 1990).

Antioxidants

Two dietary components that affect the oxidation potential of LDL cholesterol are the level of linoleic acid in the particle and the availability of antioxidants. Vitamins C, E, and β-carotene, at physiologic levels, have antioxidant roles in the body. At supplement levels, they can be either prooxidant or antioxidant, depending on concentrations of other metal ions (Herbert, 1994). Vitamin E is the most concentrated antioxidant carried on LDL, the amount being 20 to 300 times greater than any other antioxidant (Kwiterovich, 1997). A major function of vitamin E is to prevent oxidation of PUFA in the cell membrane. In vitro, vitamin E inhibits LDL oxidation, and it is superior to combined supplementation with vitamins C, E, and β-carotene (Jialal and Grundy, 1993; Witzum et al, 1993). Epidemiologic studies suggest that vitamin E and carotenoids are inversely related to CVD, but randomized trials have not supported these observations (Jha et al, 1995).

For vitamin E, there are no primary prevention trials showing an effect of vitamin E on CVD events. Moreover, in secondary prevention trials, vitamin E, 300 to 400 mg daily, had no benefit (Brown and Hu, 2001; Yusuf, 2000; GISSI-Prevenzione Investigators, 1999). Because data are lacking, the AHA does not recommend vitamin E supplementation for CVD prevention (Krauss et al, 2000). Natural dietary sources of vitamin E are being tested at this time.

β-carotene supplementation has no benefit on CVD events (ATBC, 1994). Consequently, supplementation is not recommended, and consumption of antioxidant-rich, whole foods is recommended instead (Liu et al, 2001).

Calcium

Calcium supplementation produces small decreases in LDL cholesterol in hypercholesterolemic men. In a double-blind, placebo-controlled trial, 1200 mg of calcium carbonate was reported to lower LDL cholesterol by 4.4% and increase HDL cholesterol by 4.1% in men on a step I diet (Bell et al, 1992). Along with current recommendations to increase calcium intakes to prevent osteoporosis, there may be an additional positive lipid-lowering benefit. Part of the rationale includes the possibility that calcium forms insoluble soaps with the available fatty acids; research in this area is ongoing.

Soy Protein

A metaanalysis of 38 studies concluded that substituting soy protein lowers total cholesterol (9%) and LDL cholesterol (13%) and triglycerides (11%) and has no effect on HDL cholesterol (Anderson et al, 1995). The effects on blood lipids are in addition to a NCEP step I diet and appear to occur only in persons with hypercholesterolemia. There is a dose-response relationship between soy protein and blood lipid levels, with lower levels of soy having less effect on blood lipids (Teixeira et al, 2000). At lower doses (25 g daily), soy protein lowered LDL cholesterol by 6% (Crouse, 1999). The effects of soy protein are independent of other risk factors (Wong et al, 1998). Overall, a daily intake of 25 g of soy, with isoflavones intact, will lower LDL cholesterol by 4% to 8% in hypercholesterolemic persons (Erdman, 2000). In 1999, a food claim that 25 g of soy protein daily reduces the risk of CHD was allowed on the food label. Supplements must contain soy protein to confer the phytoestrogenic effect (Jenkins et al, 2002).

Stanols/Sterols

Since the early 1950s plant stanols and sterols, isolated from soybean oils or pine tree oil, have been known to lower blood cholesterol (Lichtenstein et al, 2001). Recently, they have been esterified and made into margarines. Consuming between 2 to 3 g per day lowers cholesterol by 9% to 20% (Lichtenstein, 2001). The mechanism for cholesterol lowering is by inhibiting absorption of dietary cholesterol. ATP III includes stanols as part of dietary recommendations for lowering LDL cholesterol in adults. Because these esters can lower β-carotene, α-tocopherol, and lycopene, further safety studies are needed for use in normocholesterolemic individuals, children, and pregnant women.

TREATMENT

Background

The public health approach to primary prevention of CHD consists of four major dietary guidelines (Table 35-9) that consist of diet and physical activity behavioral changes (AHA, 2000). These guidelines for primary prevention are recommended for the general population over the age of 2 years and must be a way of life for optimal cardiovascular health. A second strategy in primary prevention is reduction of risk factors in persons not yet diagnosed with disease. Hypercholesterolemia has been the target risk factor of the NCEP since its inception in 1985. Five reports have been issued from NCEP, the most recent being the Third Report on Detection, Evaluation, and Treatment of High Blood Cholesterol in Adults, known as ATP III (NCEP, 2001).

Like previous reports, ATP III focuses on LDL cholesterol as the target lipoprotein. New features of ATP III include (1) raising diabetes as an important risk factor for CHD; (2) using Framingham projections of 10-year absolute risk to identify patients for more in-

TABLE 35-9 American Heart Association Dietary Guidelines

POPULATION GOALS			
OVERALL HEALTHY EATING PATTERN	APPROPRIATE BODY WEIGHT	DESIRABLE CHOLESTEROL PROFILE	DESIRABLE BLOOD PRESSURE
Include a variety of fruits, vegetables, grains, low-fat or nonfat dairy products, fish, legumes, poultry, lean meats.	Match energy intake to energy needs, with appropriate changes to achieve weight loss when indicated.	Limit foods high in saturated fat and cholesterol; substitute unsaturated fat from vegetables, fish legumes, nuts.	Limit salt and alcohol; maintain a healthy body weight and a diet with emphasis on vegetables, fruits, and low-fat or nonfat dairy products.

From Krause RM et al: AHA dietary guidelines, revision 2000: a statement for healthcare professionals from the Nutrition Committee of the American Heart Association, *Circulation* 102:2284, 2000.

Box 35-1. Major Risk Factors (Exclusive of LDL Cholesterol) That Modify LDL Goals

- Cigarette smoking
- Hypertension (BP ≥140/90 mm Hg or with antihypertensive medication)
- Low HDL cholesterol (<40 mg/dl)*
- Family history of premature CHD (CHD in male first-degree relative <55 yr; CHD in female first-degree relative <65 yr)
- Age (men ≥45 yr; women ≥55 yr)

From ATPO-III materials (www.nhlbi.nih.gov/guidlines/cholesterol/atp3_rpt.htm).
*HDL cholesterol ≥60 mg/dl counts as a "negative" risk factor; its presence removes one risk factor from the total count.
LDL, Low-density lipoprotein; *BP,* blood pressure; *CHD,* coronary heart disease.

tensive treatment; and (3) identifying persons with multiple metabolic risk factors as candidates for intensified therapeutic lifestyle changes.

Based on animal studies, laboratory investigations, epidemiology, and genetic aberrations in lipid metabolism, LDL cholesterol unequivocally causes CHD and lowering LDL cholesterol reduces the risk of CHD. Thus, the primary goal of therapy and levels for initiating therapy are based on LDL levels. Two calculations are made to assess risk in persons without established disease. First, risk factors are counted (Box 35-1). Second, an algorithm from the Framingham Study is used to determine 10-year risk (Figures 35-8 and 35-9). This system categorizes a patient into one of three categories: (1) highest risk (i.e., 20% of individuals will develop CHD or have a recurrent event within 10 years); (2) moderate risk (i.e., a 10% to 20% risk of new CHD within 10 years); or (3) low risk (less than a 10% risk). With each additional risk factor, the estimated 10-year risk for CHD (Figure 35-10) or stroke (Figure 35-11) increases markedly. LDL and non-HDL goals for therapy are shown in Table 35-10. Persons with CHD or CHD equivalents are in the highest risk category and thus have the lowest LDL cholesterol goal.

The ATP III differentiates other CHD risk factors into lifestyle factors (obesity, physical inactivity, atherogenic diet) and emerging risk factors (lipoprotein(a), homocysteine, prothrombotic and proinflammatory factors, and impaired fasting glucose. The lifestyle factors constitute the intervention areas, and the emerging risk factors guide decisions regarding the intensity of risk reduction therapy.

After the LDL goal is addressed, a second area of intervention is warranted in persons with the metabolic syndrome. This syndrome is a constellation of risk factors associated with insulin resistance. Three of the five risk factors must be present for diagnosis of metabolic syndrome (Table 35-11) (see Chapter 12). In NHANES III, the age-adjusted prevalence of metabolic syndrome was 24% (Ford, 2002). Therapeutic lifestyle changes are the cornerstone of treatment for both elevated LDL and metabolic syndrome.

Therapeutic Lifestyle Changes

Medical nutrition therapy, which includes physical activity, is the primary intervention for patients with elevated LDL cholesterol. The LDL cholesterol levels at which to initiate therapy are shown in Table 35-12. With diet, exercise, and weight reduction, patients can often reach serum lipid goals. Consequently, these interventions are tried before drug therapy. In previous ATP reports, dietary changes were divided into two levels: step I and step II diets. The *step I* diet was more liberal in SFA (up to 10% of energy) and dietary cholesterol (up to 300 mg daily) than the *step II* diet (<8 % of energy as SFA) and cholesterol (up to 200 mg). The ATP III dietary recommendations, known as the *therapeutic lifestyle change (TLC)* diet, are an enhanced step II diet (Table 35-13). SFA recommendations are lowered to less than 7% of calories, and total fat content is changed from less than 30% of energy to a range of 25% to 35% of calories. Consuming 30% to 35% of calories from fat while maintaining a low SFA and *trans*-fatty acid intake is recommended for individu-

Estimate of 10-Year Risk for Women (Framingham Point Scores)

Age	Points
20–34	−7
35–39	−3
40–44	0
45–49	3
50–54	6
55–59	8
60–64	10
65–69	12
70–74	14
75–79	16

HDL	Points
≥60	−1
50–59	0
40–49	1
<40	2

Total cholesterol	Points at age 20–39	Points at age 40–49	Points at age 50–59	Points at age 60–69	Points at age 70–79
<160	0	0	0	0	0
160–199	4	3	2	1	1
200–239	8	6	4	2	1
240–279	11	8	5	3	2
≥280	13	10	7	4	2

	Points at age 20–39	Points at age 40–49	Points at age 50–59	Points at age 60–69	Points at age 70–79
Nonsmoker	0	0	0	0	0
Smoker	9	7	4	2	1

Systolic BP	If untreated	If treated
<120	0	0
120–129	1	3
130–139	2	4
140–159	3	5
≥160	4	6

Point total	10-year risk (%)	Point total	10-year risk (%)
<9	<1	20	11
9	1	21	14
10	1	22	17
11	1	23	22
12	1	24	27
13	2	≥25	≥30
14	2		
15	3		
16	4		
17	5		
18	6		
19	8		

FIGURE 35-8 • Estimate of 10-year coronary heart disease risk: Framingham point scores. (Wilson PWF et al: Prediction of coronary heart disease using risk factor categories, *Circulation* 97:1837, 1998.)

als with metabolic syndrome. This higher fat intake, emphasizing PUFA and MUFA, can be beneficial in lowering triglycerides and raising HDL cholesterol in persons with metabolic syndrome. Also, with a more liberal fat intake, LDL-C can be lowered without exacerbating blood glucose levels.

The time course for medical nutrition therapy is a 3- to 6-month process (Figure 35-12). Lowering SFA and cholesterol is the first level of behavior change. The TLC diet is followed for 6 weeks. At visit 2, the LDL response is evaluated and therapy is intensified as warranted. Adjuncts such as plant sterols/stanols,

Estimate of 10-Year Risk for Men (Framingham Point Scores)

Age	Points
20–34	−9
35–39	−4
40–44	0
45–49	3
50–54	6
55–59	8
60–64	10
65–69	11
70–74	12
75–79	13

HDL	Points
≥60	−1
50–59	0
40–49	1
<40	2

Total cholesterol	Points at age 20–39	Points at age 40–49	Points at age 50–59	Points at age 60–69	Points at age 70–79
<160	0	0	0	0	0
160–199	4	3	2	1	0
200–239	7	5	3	1	0
240–279	9	6	4	2	1
≥280	11	8	5	3	1

	Points at age 20–39	Points at age 40–49	Points at age 50–59	Points at age 60–69	Points at age 70–79
Nonsmoker	0	0	0	0	0
Smoker	8	5	3	1	1

Systolic BP	If untreated	If treated
<120	0	0
120–129	0	1
130–139	1	2
140–159	1	2
≥160	2	3

Point total	10-year risk (%)	Point total	10-year risk (%)
<0	<1	11	8
0	1	12	10
1	1	13	12
2	1	14	16
3	1	15	20
4	1	16	25
5	2	≥17	≥30
6	2		
7	3		
8	4		
9	5		
10	6		

FIGURE 35-9 • Estimate of 10-year stroke risk for men: Framingham point scores. (Wolf PA et al: Probability of stroke: a risk profile from the Framingham Study, *Stroke* 22:312, 1991.)

fiber, and soy are incorporated into education at the second visit. Dietary compliance must be monitored during this period. At visit 3, metabolic syndrome treatment begins if target LDL is reached. Once the maximum LDL reduction has occurred, then management of metabolic syndrome becomes the target for medical nutrition therapy. Increasing physical activity and decreasing energy intake to facilitate weight loss are critical to normalizing risk factor components of the metabolic syndrome. The recommended approaches for weight management can be found in the National Institutes of Health (NIH) Clin-

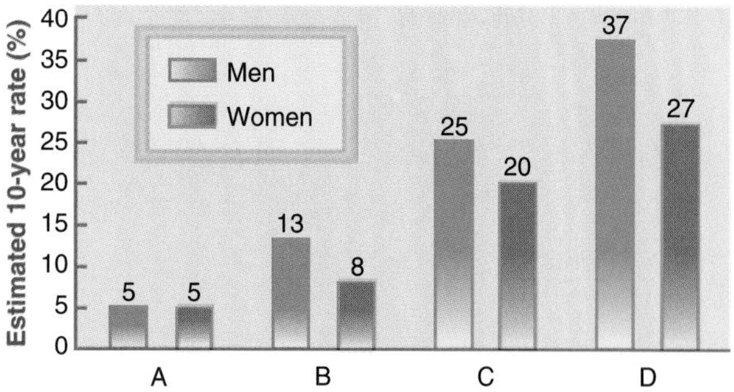

	A	B	C	D
Blood pressure (mm Hg)	120/80	140/90	140/90	140/90
Total cholesterol (mg/dl)	200	240	240	240
HDL cholesterol (mg/dl)	50	50	40	40
Diabetes	No	No	Yes	Yes
Cigarettes	No	No	No	Yes

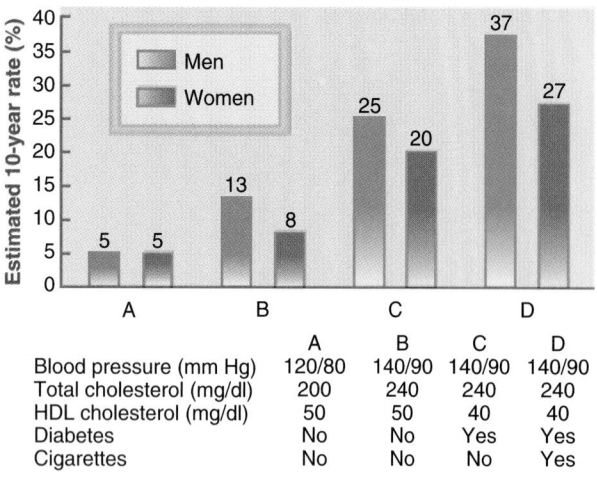

mm Hg, Millimeters of mercury
mg/dl, Milligrams of cholesterol per deciliter of blood

FIGURE 35-10 • Estimated 10-year coronary heart disease risk in 55-year-old adults according to levels of various risk factors: Framingham Heart Study, United States. (From Wilson PWF et al: Prediction of coronary heart disease using risk factor categories, *Circulation* 97:1837-1847, 1998.)

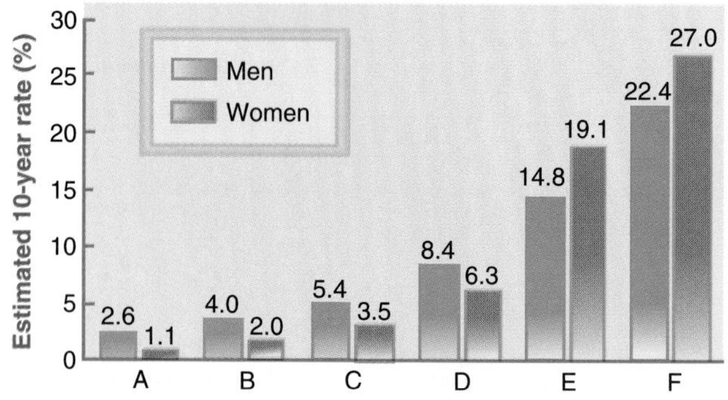

	A	B	C	D	E	F
Systolic BP*	95–105	138–148	130–148	130–148	130–148	130–148
Diabetes	No	No	Yes	Yes	Yes	Yes
Cigarettes	No	No	No	Yes	Yes	Yes
Prior atrial fibrillation	No	No	No	No	Yes	Yes
Prior CVD	No	No	No	No	No	Yes

*Blood pressures are in millimeters of mercury (mm Hg).

FIGURE 35-11 • Estimated 10-year stroke risk in 55-year-old adults according to levels of various risk factors: Framingham Heart Study, United States. (From Wolf PA et al: Probability of stroke: a risk profile from the Framingham Study, *Stroke* 22:312-318, 1991.)

TABLE 35-10 Comparison of LDL Cholesterol and Non-HDL Cholesterol Goals for Three Risk Categories

RISK CATEGORY	LDL GOAL (mg/dl)	NON-HDL-C GOAL (mg/dl)
CHD and CHD risk equivalent (10-yr risk for CHD >20%)	<100	<130
Multiple (2+) risk factors and 10-yr risk ≤20%	<130	<160
0-1 Risk factor	<160	<190

From ATP III materials (www.nhlbi.nih.gov/guidelines/cholesterol/atp3_rpt.htm).
LDL, Low-density lipoprotein; *HDL,* high-density lipoprotein; *CHD,* coronary heart disease.

TABLE 35-11 Clinical Identification of the Metabolic Syndrome

RISK FACTOR	DEFINING LEVEL
Abdominal obesity	Waist circumference
Men	>102 cm (>40 in)
Women	>88 cm (>35 in)
Triglycerides	≥150 mg/dl
HDL cholesterol	
Men	<40 mg/dl
Women	<50 mg/dl
Blood pressure	≥130/≥85 mm Hg
Fasting glucose	≥110 mg/dl

From ATP III materials (www.nhlbi.nih.gov/guidelines/cholesterol/atp3_rpt.htm).

TABLE 35-12 Low-Density Lipoprotein (LDL) Cholesterol Goals and Cutpoints for Therapeutic Lifestyle Changes and Drug Therapy in Different Risk Categories

RISK CATEGORY	LDL-C GOAL	LDL LEVEL AT WHICH TO INITIATE THERAPEUTIC LIFESTYLE CHANGES	LDL LEVEL AT WHICH TO CONSIDER DRUG THERAPY
CHD or CHD risk equivalents (10-yr risk >20%)	<100 mg/dl	≥100 mg/dl	≥130 mg/dl (100-129 mg/dl: drug optional)*
2+ Risk factors (10-yr risk ≤20%)	<130 mg/dl	≥130 mg/dl	10-yr risk 10%-20%: ≥130 mg/dl 10-yr risk <10%: ≥160 mg/dl
0-1 Risk factor†	<160 mg/dl	≥160 mg/dl	≥190 mg/dl (160-189 mg/dl: LDL-lowering drug optional)

From ATP III materials (www.nhlbi.nih.gov/guidelines/cholesterol/atp3_rpt.htm).
*Some authorities recommend use of LDL-lowering drugs in this category if an LDL cholesterol <100 mg/dl cannot be achieved by therapeutic lifestyle changes. Others prefer use of drugs that primarily modify triglycerides and HDL (e.g., nicotinic acid or fibrate). Clinical judgment also may call for deferring drug therapy in this subcategory.
†Almost all people with 0-1 risk factor have a 10-yr risk <10%; thus 10-yr risk assessment in people with 0-1 risk factor is not necessary.
CHD, Congestive heart failure.

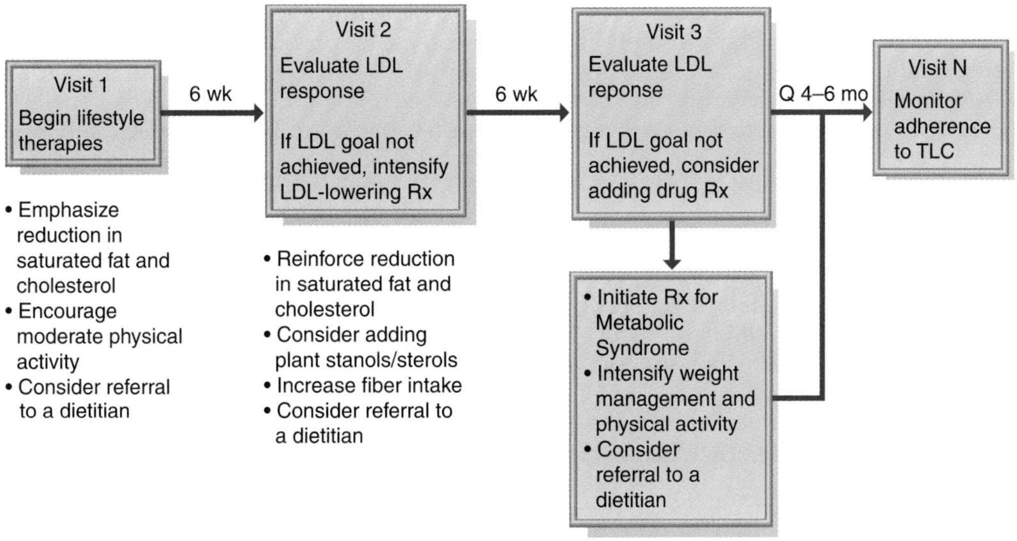

FIGURE 35-12 • Steps in therapeutic lifestyle changes (TLC). (From ATP III materials [www.nhlbi.nih.gov/guidelines/cholesterol/atp3_rpt.htm.])

TABLE 35-13 Nutrient Composition of the Therapeutic Lifestyle Change (TLC) Diet

NUTRIENT	RECOMMENDED INTAKE
Saturated fat*	Less than 7% of total calories
Polyunsaturated fat	Up to 10% of total calories
Monounsaturated fat	Up to 20% of total calories
Total fat	25%-35% of total calories
Carbohydrate†	50% to 60% of total calories
Fiber	20-30 g/day
Protein	Approximately 15% of total calories
Cholesterol	Less than 200 mg/day
Total calories (energy)‡	Balance energy intake and expenditure to maintain desirable body weight/prevent weight gain

From ATP III materials (www.nhlbi.nih.gov/guidelines/cholesterol/atp3_rpt.htm).
**Trans*-fatty acids are another LDL-raising fat that should be kept at a low intake.
†Carbohydrate should be derived predominantly from foods rich in complex carbohydrates, including grains, especially whole grains, fruits, and vegetables.
‡Daily energy expenditure should include at least moderate physical activity (contributing approximately 200 kcal per day).

ical Guidelines (NIH, 1998) and in Chapter 24. Individuals with baseline high-fat diets who lose weight may reduce total cholesterol by 25% or more with good adherence.

Throughout all steps of the TLC, physicians are encouraged to refer patients to registered dietitians for medical nutrition therapy (NCEP, 2001). Medical nutrition therapy, with three to four visits of 50 minutes' duration with a dietitian over several months, has been associated with a significant reduction in serum cholesterol levels and with a savings in health care costs (Sikand et al, 1998). Behavior modification and goal setting are key strategies used by the dietitian to help patients adopt lifestyle changes. Self-efficacy is a strong predictor of fat intake (Humphries and Krummel, 1999). Dietitians can empower patients to increase their confidence and thus make more healthful choices. Behavioral outcomes include appropriate meal planning, food-label reading, knowledge of the soluble fiber content of foods, recipe modification, food preparation, dining out, and food-drug interactions (ADA, 1996). Behavior modification and weight-management programs are discussed in Chapter 24.

For women, adopting a lifestyle that incorporates a healthful diet (highest 40th percentile for cereal fiber, omega-3 fatty acids, and folate; high PUFA-to-SFA ratio and low in *trans* fat and glycemic load), normal BMI (<25), less than half an alcoholic beverage per day, moderate physical activity (30 minutes per day), and smoking avoidance had a very low risk of developing CHD (Stampfer et al, 2000).

Secondary Prevention

Patients with established CHD have a fivefold to sevenfold higher risk of subsequent MI. Secondary prevention includes (1) complete smoking cessation; (2) reducing blood pressure to less than 140/90 or 130/85 if CHF, renal insufficiency, or diabetes is present; (3) reducing LDL cholesterol to less than 100 mg/dl and non-HDL levels less than 130 mg/dl; (4) moderate physical activity for 30 minutes daily three to four days each week; (5) weight management to attain BMI below 25; (6) hemoglobin A1C below 7%; (7) indefinite use of 75 to 325 mg of aspirin daily if not contraindicated; and (8) indefinite use of two antihypertensive drugs (angiotensin-converting enzyme inhibitor [ACE] and β-blockers) following MI, unless contraindicated (Smith, 2001).

Medical nutrition therapy is critical for secondary prevention because SFA levels are related to disease progression in men (Watts et al, 1996). Usually, to attain these lower LDL cholesterol levels, aggressive diet therapy is needed (see the following sections). Major lifestyle interventions can slow lesion development, promote regression of existing lesions, and lessen endothelial dysfunction.

In the Lifestyle Trial, the intervention was a very-low-fat, nearly vegetarian diet (egg whites and nonfat milk allowed; total fat constituting 10% of kilocalories), coupled with exercise, weight reduction, smoking cessation, and stress reduction (Ornish and Brown, 1993). After 1 year, these patients had a 37% reduction in LDL cholesterol, and 82% had overall regression of coronary atherosclerosis. These patients were able to meet the LDL goals without drugs. (The average final LDL cholesterol level was 95 mg/dl.) In a follow-up study, more regression occurred after 5 years than after the 1 year (Ornish et al 1998). Because of the very small sample (n = 35 patients) and lack of women, these data need to be replicated in a larger, more diverse population. Adherence to these lifestyle changes requires a high level of motivation.

In a second study, the intervention involved a less rigorous diet (<20% of kilocalories derived from fat) and exercise. The latter intervention slowed progression of disease and promoted regression more in the intervention patients than in the usual care group (Schuler et al, 1992).

Therapeutic Lifestyle Change Diet

The TLC diet emphasizes grains, cereals, legumes, vegetables, fruits, lean meats, poultry, fish, and nonfat dairy products (Table 35-14). Some different strategies to reduce SFA and *trans*-fatty acids are (1) avoiding hydrogenated fats as spreads or for flavoring, (2) avoiding or reducing the consumption of meat, (3) using specially manufactured low-fat foods (e.g., fat-free salad dressings), (4) using margarines with sterol esters, (5) modifying common foods to be lower in fat (e.g., removing skin from chicken), and (6) replacing high-fat foods with low-fat foods (e.g., substituting skim milk for whole milk).

Because animal fats provide about two thirds of the SFA in the American diet, these foods are limited. High-fat choices are omitted, but low-fat choices can be included. Meat is limited to five or six oz per day and eggs to two or fewer per week. The fat, SFA, and cholesterol content of meat, fish, and poultry are listed in Table 35-15. Lean meats are high in protein, zinc, and iron; hence, if patients wish to consume meat, a 6-oz portion or less is allowed per day. Similarly, with dairy products, nonfat choices are recommended. Neither food group has to be omitted; it is a matter of choice. For lower-fat diets, meats are further restricted.

Some patients, particularly those who need to reduce weight, like to use the exchange system for their dietary modifications (Table 35-16). These plans should be individualized to facilitate long-term compliance. Although some patients prefer the exchange method, others prefer counting grams of fat or SFA (Table 35-17).

The nutrition labels on foods will help patients who want to count fat grams. Labeling terms that relate to diet modifications for CHD are shown in Table 35-18. The limitation of this method is that only fat, SFA, or cholesterol is counted, without attention to calories or to including adequate levels of other nutrients. Many new low-fat products are lacking in essential nutrients, and a diet based on these products without basic foods may be nutritionally incomplete. The TLC diets can be designed using foods from many cultures. Tables 35-19 through 35-21 illustrate menus for the NCEP diets that feature different ethnic cuisines.

With the TLC diet, soluble fiber and use of sterol/stanol esters are encouraged. Soluble fiber intake can be increased by frequent use of legumes, oatmeal or oat bran, fresh fruits, and fibrous vegetables. For women in a low-fat diet trial (intensive intervention with a 20% fat diet), increasing the consumption of grains, fruits, and vegetables was the most difficult change to make (Burrows et al, 1993). Nutrition education efforts are needed in this area. Currently, stanol/sterol esters are widely available only in margarine. More food products are likely to be developed in the future.

Meeting sodium guidelines (2400 mg daily) can be a challenge because lower-fat processed foods often contain salt to increase palatability. Patients may need to limit convenience and processed foods.

Aggressive Diets

For highly motivated patients who want to avoid drug therapy, sometimes very-low-fat diets are effective for reaching blood lipid goals. These diets can also be used as an adjunct to drug therapy for secondary prevention and possible regression of lesions. Such diets contain minimal amounts of animal products; hence, SFA (<3%), cholesterol (<5 mg), and total fat (<10%) intakes are very low. The emphasis is on low-fat grains, legumes, fruits, vegetables, and nonfat dairy foods. Because egg whites are allowed, the plan is a lacto-ovovegetarian regimen. To ensure nutritional adequacy, a food plan, such as that shown in Table 35-22, should be followed. Quick tips are summarized in Box 35-2.

TABLE 35-14 Food Choices for TLC Diets

FOOD GROUP	CHOOSE	DECREASE
Lean meat, poultry, and fish ≤5 oz per day	Beef, pork, lamb—lean cuts, well trimmed before cooking	Beef, pork, lamb—regular ground beef, fatty cuts, spare ribs, organ meats
	Poultry without skin	Poultry with skin, fried chicken
	Fish, shellfish	Fried fish, fried shellfish
	Processed meat—prepared from lean meat (e.g., lean ham, lean frankfurters, lean meat with soy protein or carrageenan)	Regular luncheon meat (e.g., bologna, salami, sausage, frankfurters)
Eggs ≤2 yolks per week, step III	Egg whites (two whites can be substituted for one whole egg in recipes), cholesterol-free egg substitute	Egg yolks (if more than 4 per week on Step I or if more than 2 per week on Step II); includes eggs used in cooking and baking
Low-fat dairy products 2-3 servings per day	Milk—skim, ½%, or 1% fat (fluid, powdered, evaporated), buttermilk	Whole milk (fluid, evaporated, condensed), 2% fat milk (low-fat milk), imitation milk
	Yogurt—nonfat or low-fat yogurt or yogurt beverages	Whole-milk yogurt, whole-milk yogurt beverages
	Cheese—low-fat natural or processed cheese	Regular cheeses (American, blue, Brie, cheddar, Colby, Edam, Monterey Jack, whole-milk mozzarella, Parmesan, Swiss), cream cheese, Neufchatel cheese
	Low-fat or nonfat varieties, such as cottage cheese—low-fat, nonfat, or dry curd (0 to 2% fat)	Cottage cheese (4% fat)
	Frozen dairy dessert—ice milk, frozen yogurt (low-fat or nonfat)	Ice cream
	Low-fat coffee creamer	Cream, half & half, whipping cream, nondairy creamer, whipped topping, sour cream
	Low-fat or nonfat sour cream	
Fats and oils ≤6-8 tsp per day	Unsaturated oils—safflower, sunflower, corn, soybean, cottonseed, canola, olive, peanut	Coconut oil, palm kernel oil, palm oil
	Margarine—made from unsaturated oils listed above; light or diet margarine, especially soft or liquid forms	Butter, lard, shortening, bacon fat, hard margarine
	Salad dressings—made with unsaturated oils listed above; low-fat or fat free	Dressings made with egg yolk, cheese, sour cream, whole milk
	Seeds and nuts—peanut butter, other nut butters	Coconut
	Cocoa powder	Milk chocolate
Breads and cereals ≥6 servings per day	Breads—whole-grain bread, English muffins, bagels, buns, corn or flour tortilla	Bread in which eggs, fat, and butter are a major ingredient; croissants
	Cereals—oat, wheat, corn, multigrain	Most granolas
	Pasta	
	Rice	
	Dried beans and peas	
	Crackers, low-fat—animal type, graham, soda crackers, breadsticks, melba toast	High-fat crackers
	Homemade baked goods using unsaturated oil, skim or 1% milk, and egg substitute—quick breads, biscuits, cornbread muffins, bran muffins, pancakes, waffles	Commercial baked pastries, muffins, biscuits
Soups	Reduced- or low-fat and reduced-sodium varieties (e.g., chicken or beef noodle, minestrone, tomato, vegetable, potato), reduced-fat soups made with skim milk	Soups containing whole milk, cream, meat fat, poultry fat, or poultry skin
Vegetables 3-5 servings per day	Fresh, frozen, or canned, without added fat or sauce	Vegetables fried or prepared with butter, cheese, or cream sauce
Fruits 2-4 servings per day	Fruits—fresh, frozen, canned, or dried	Fried fruit or fruit served with butter or cream sauce
	Fruit juice—fresh, frozen, or canned	
Sweets and modified-fat desserts	Beverages—fruit-flavored drinks, lemonade, fruit punch	
	Sweets—sugar, syrup, honey, jam, preserves, candy made without fat (candy corn, gumdrops, hard candy), fruit-flavored gelatin	Candy made with milk chocolate, coconut oil, palm kernel oil, palm oil
	Frozen desserts—low-fat and nonfat yogurt, ice milk, sherbet, sorbet, fruit ice, popsicles	Ice cream and frozen treats made with ice cream
	Cookies, cake, pie, pudding—prepared with egg whites, egg substitute, skim milk or 1% milk, and unsaturated oil or margarine; ginger snaps; fig and other fruit bar cookies, fat-free cookies; angel food cake	Commercial baked pies, cakes, doughnuts, high-fat cookies, cream pies

Data from National Cholesterol Education Program (NCEP): *Second report of the Expert Panel on Detection, Evaluation, and Treatment of High Blood Cholesterol in Adults* (Adult Treatment Panel II), NIH Publication No. 93-3095, Bethesda, Md, 1993, National Institutes of Health, National Heart, Lung, and Blood Institute.

TABLE 35-15 Fat, SFA, Cholesterol, and Iron Content of Meat, Poultry, and Fish (3-oz Portions) Cooked Without Added Fat

SOURCE	TOTAL FAT (g/3 oz)	SATURATED FAT (g/3 oz)	CHOLESTEROL (mg/3 oz)	IRON (mg/3 oz)
Lean red meats				
Beef (rump roast, shank, bottom round, sirloin)	4.2	1.4	71	2.5
Lamb (shank roast, sirloin roast, shoulder roast, loin chops, sirloin chops, center leg chop)	7.8	2.8	78	1.9
Pork (sirloin cutlet, loin roast, sirloin roast, center roast, butterfly chops, loin chops)	11.8	4.1	77	1.0
Veal (blade roast, sirloin chops, shoulder roast, loin chops, rump roast, shank)	4.9	2.0	93	1.0
Organ meats				
Liver				
Beef	4.2	1.6	331	5.8
Calf	5.9	2.2	477	2.2
Chicken	4.6	1.6	537	7.2
Sweetbread	21.3	7.3	250	1.3
Kidney	2.9	0.9	329	6.2
Brains	10.7	2.5	1747	1.9
Heart	4.8	1.4	164	6.4
Poultry				
Chicken (without skin)				
Light (roasted)	3.8	1.1	72	0.9
Dark (roasted)	8.3	2.3	79	1.1
Turkey (without skin)				
Light (roasted)	2.7	0.9	59	1.1
Dark (roasted)	6.1	2.0	72	2.0
Fish				
Haddock	0.8	0.1	63	1.1
Flounder	1.3	0.3	58	0.3
Salmon	7.0	1.7	54	0.3
Tuna, light, canned in water	0.7	0.2	25	1.3
Shellfish				
Crustaceans				
Lobster	0.5	0.1	61	0.3
Crab meat				
Alaskan King Crab	1.3	0.1	45	0.6
Blue Crab	1.5	0.2	85	0.8
Shrimp	0.9	0.2	166	2.6
Mollusks				
Abalone	1.3	0.3	144	5.4
Clams	1.7	0.2	57	23.8
Mussels	3.8	0.7	48	5.7
Oysters	4.2	1.3	93	10.2
Scallops	1.2	0.1	27	2.6
Squid	2.4	0.6	400	1.2

Data from National Cholesterol Education Program (NCEP): *Second report of the Expert Panel on Detection, Evaluation, and Treatment of High Blood Cholesterol in Adults* (Adult Treatment Panel II), NIH Publication No. 93-3095, Bethesda, Md, 1993, National Institutes of Health, National Heart, Lung, and Blood Institute.
SFA, Saturated fatty acid.

TABLE 35-16 Eating Plans

FOOD GROUP	STEP I DIET 1200 kcal	STEP I DIET 2500 kcal	STEP II OR TLC DIET 1200 kcal	STEP II OR TLC DIET 1600 kcal	STEP II OR TLC DIET 2000 kcal	STEP II OR TLC DIET 2500 kcal
Fats and oils	3	8	3	5	7	8
Fish, poultry, meat	6 oz	6 oz	6 oz	6 oz	6 oz	6 oz
Egg yolks	3/wk	3/wk	1/wk	1/wk	1/wk	1/wk
Dairy foods	2	4	2	2	2	3
Bread, beans, grains, and starches	3	10	4	5	8	10
Fruit	3	5	3	3	4	7
Vegetables	4	4	4	4	4	5
Sugars, sweets, alcohol	0	2	0	2	2	2

Data updated from National Cholesterol Education Program (NCEP): *Second report of the Expert Panel on Detection, Evaluation, and Treatment of High Blood Cholesterol in Adults* (Adult Treatment Panel II), NIH Publication No. 93-3095, Bethesda, Md, 1993, National Institutes of Health, National Heart, Lung, and Blood Institute.
The average daily intake for women is about 1800 kcal; for men, it is about 2500 kcal.
TLC, Therapeutic lifestyle changes.

TABLE 35-17 Maximal Fat and SFA in TLC (Step II Diets)*

	TOTAL CALORIE LEVEL (kcal)							
	1600	1800	2000	2200	2400	2600	2800	3000
Total fat (g)† for 30%	53	60	67	73	80	87	93	100
Saturated fat (g)—step II‡	12	14	16	17	19	20	22	23

Data from National Cholesterol Education Program (NCEP): *Second report of the Expert Panel on Detection, Evaluation, and Treatment of High Blood Cholesterol in Adults* (Adult Treatment Panel II), NIH Publication No. 93-3095, Bethesda, Md, 1993, National Institutes of Health, National Heart, Lung, and Blood Institute.
SFA, Saturated fatty acid; *TLC,* therapeutic lifestyle changes.
*The average daily intake for women is about 1800 kcal; for men, it is about 2500 kcal.
†Total fat content of both diets is 30% of total calories consumed (estimated by multiplying the caloric level of the diet by 0.3 and dividing the product by 9 kcal/g).
‡The recommended intake of saturated fat on the step I diet is 8% to 10% of total calories; saturated fat content is less than 7% for the step II diet.

TABLE 35-18 Nutrition Labeling Terms Related to Modified Diets for Coronary Heart Disease

NUTRIENT	FREE	LOW	REDUCED/LESS/FEWER	OTHER
All	Synonyms for "free": "free of," "no," "zero," "without," "trivial source of," "negligible source of," "dietary insignificant source of"	Synonyms for "low": "contains a small amount of," "low source of," "low in"	Synonyms for "reduced/less/fewer": "reduced in," "lower," "low"	
Kilocalories	<5 kcal/reference serving	<40 kcal/reference serving	Reduced by at least 25%	
Total fat	<0.5 g/reference serving	≤3 g/reference serving Meal and main dish products: ≤3 g/100 g and 30% or less calories from fat	Reduced by at least 25%	"__% fat free," "__% lean," must meet requirements for "low fat"
Saturated fat	<0.5 g/reference serving; levels of *trans*-fatty acids must be 1% or less of total fat	≤1 g/reference serving and 15% or less of calories from saturated fatty acids Meal and main dish products: ≤1 g/100 g and less than 10% of calories from saturated fat	Reduced by at least 25%	
Cholesterol	<2 mg/reference serving; saturated fat content must be 2 g or less	≤20 mg/reference serving; saturated fat content must be 2 g or less per serving Meal and main dish products: ≤20 mg/100 g, with saturated fat content less than 2 g/100 g	Reduced by at least 25% Contains 2 g or less of saturated fat per reference serving	
Sodium	<5 mg/reference serving	≤140 mg/reference serving Meal and main dish products: ≤140 mg/100 g of food	Reduced by at least 25%	"Very low sodium," "Very low in sodium": ≤35 mg/reference serving

Data from National Cholesterol Education Program (NCEP): *Second report of the Expert Panel on Detection, Evaluation, and Treatment of High Blood Cholesterol in Adults* (Adult Treatment Panel II), NIH Publication No. 93-3095, Bethesda, Md, 1993, National Institutes of Health, National Heart, Lung, and Blood Institute.

Medical Intervention

Coronary Angioplasty

Percutaneous transluminal coronary angioplasty (PTCA) is a procedure that uses a balloon to break up plaque deposits in an occluded artery. Because the procedure is performed with the patient under local anesthesia in a cardiac catheterization laboratory, recovery is quicker than with bypass surgery. PTCA is being done more and more frequently every year; 601,000 angioplasty surgeries were performed in 1999. From 1987 to 1999, the number of PTCA procedures increased by 285% (AHA, 2001). PTCA is often possible because of earlier detection of blockages. Cardiac catheterization procedures have been increasing steadily since 1979. Usually, patients with no more than two occluded arteries are candidates for PTCA. The most common problem with PTCA is restenosis of the artery. Therapeutic lifestyle changes, including a more intensive dietary management, should be recommended for these patients.

TABLE 35-19 Sample American Menus for Step I and Step II (TLC) Diets

STEP I: SAMPLE MENUS—TRADITIONAL AMERICAN CUISINE FEMALES 25-49 YEARS*	STEP II: SAMPLE MENUS—TRADITIONAL AMERICAN CUISINE FEMALES 25-49 YEARS*
Breakfast	**Breakfast**
Bagel, plain (½ medium)	Bagel, plain (½ medium)
Cream cheese, low-fat (1 tsp)†	**Margarine** (1 tsp)
Cereal, shredded wheat (1 c)	**Jelly** (1 tsp)
Banana (1 small)	Cereal, shredded wheat (1 c)
Milk, **1%** (1 c)	Banana (1 small)
Orange juice (¾ c)	Milk, **skim** (1 c)
Coffee (1 c)	Orange juice **(1 c)**
Milk, **1%** (1 oz)	Coffee (1 c)
	Milk, **skim** (1 oz)
Lunch	**Lunch**
Minestrone soup, canned, low sodium (½ c)	Minestrone soup, canned, low sodium (½ c)
Roast beef sandwich	Roast beef sandwich
Whole-wheat bread (2 slices)	Whole-wheat bread (2 slices)
Lean roast beef, unseasoned **(3 oz)**‡	Lean roast beef, unseasoned **(2 oz)**‡
American cheese, low-fat and low-sodium (¾ oz)	American cheese, low-fat and low-sodium (¾ oz)
Lettuce (1 leaf)	Lettuce (1 leaf)
Tomato (3 slices)	Tomato (3 slices)
Mayonnaise, low-fat and low-sodium (2 tsp)	**Margarine,** (2 tsp)
Apple (1 medium)	Apple (1 medium)
Water (1 c)	Water (1 c)
Dinner	**Dinner**
Salmon (3 oz)‡	**Flounder** (3 oz)‡
Vegetable oil (1 tsp)	Vegetable oil (1 tsp)
Baked potato (½ medium)‡	Baked potato (½ medium)‡
Margarine (1 tsp)	Margarine (1 tsp)
Green beans (½ c), seasoned with margarine (½ tsp)‡	Green beans (½ c), seasoned with margarine (½ tsp)‡
Carrots (½ c), seasoned with margarine (½ tsp)‡	Carrots (½ c), seasoned with margarine (½ tsp)‡
White dinner roll (1 medium)	White dinner roll (1 medium)
Margarine (1 tsp)	Margarine (1 tsp)
Ice milk (½ c)	**Frozen yogurt** (½ c)
Iced tea, unsweetened (1 c)	Iced tea, unsweetened (1 c)
Snack	**Snack**
Popcorn (2 c)‡	Popcorn (3 c)‡
Margarine **(1 tsp)**	Margarine **(2 tsp)**

TOTALS

Step I				Step II			
Calories:	1831.0	Total carb, % kcal:	52	Calories:	1867.0	Total carb, % kcal:	55
Total fat, % kcal:	30.0	Simple carb, % carb:	37	Total fat, % kcal:	29.0	Simple carb, % carb:	38
SFA, % kcal:	8.7	Complex carb, % carb:	63	SFA, % kcal:	6.8	Complex carb, % carb:	62
Cholesterol, mg:	156.0	Sodium, mg:‡	1415	Cholesterol, mg:	134.0	Sodium, mg:‡	1417
Protein, % kcal:	18.0			Protein, % kcal:	16.0		

Data from National Cholesterol Education Program (NCEP): *Second report of the Expert Panel on Detection, Evaluation, and Treatment of High Blood Cholesterol in Adults* (Adult Treatment Panel II), NIH Publication No. 93-3095, Bethesda, Md, 1993, National Institutes of Health, National Heart, Lung, and Blood Institute.

SFA, Saturated fatty acid; *carb,* carbohydrates.

*100% RDA met for all nutrients except zinc (90%).

† Boldface food items represent differences between the step I and step II diets.

‡No salt is added in recipe preparation or as seasoning. All margarine is low-sodium.

Coronary Bypass Surgery

In *coronary artery bypass graft (CABG)* or *off-bypass coronary artery graft (OBCAG)* surgery, an artery from the chest is used to redirect blood flow around a diseased vessel. Candidates for CABG usually have more than two occluded arteries. CABG surgeries have decreased since 1995 because of more PTCA procedures being done. Still, 571,000 operations were performed in 1999 (AHA, 2001). These surgeries improve survival time, relieve symptoms, and markedly improve the quality of life for patients with CHD. However, CABG does not cure atherosclerosis; the new grafts are also susceptible to atherogenesis. Consequently, restenosis is common within 10 years of surgery. Risk factor modification, including, at a minimum, therapeutic lifestyle changes and probably more aggressive dietary changes are needed to stop progression.

In the postoperative period, post-CABG patients, like others undergoing major surgery, are in a cata-

TABLE 35-20 Sample Mexican American Menus for Step II (TLC) Diets

STEP II: SAMPLE MENUS—MEXICAN AMERICAN CUISINE MALES 25-49 YEARS*

Breakfast
Cantaloupe (½ c)
Farina, prepared with **skim†** milk (1 c)‡
White bread (2 slices)
  Margarine (2 tsp)
  Jelly (2 tsp)
Orange juice (¾ c)
Hot cocoa, prepared with **skim** milk (1 c)

Lunch
Beef enchilada
  Tortilla, corn (2 tortillas)
  Lean roast beef **(2 oz)**‡
  Vegetable oil **(½ tsp)**
  Cheddar cheese, low-fat and low-sodium (1 oz)
  Onion (⅛ c)
  Tomato (⅛ c)
  Lettuce (¼ c)
  Chili peppers (2 tsp)
Refried beans (¾ c), prepared with vegetable oil‡
Carrots (6 sticks), celery (6 sticks)
Milk, **skim** (½ c)

Dinner
Chicken taco
  Tortilla, corn flour (2 tortillas)
  Chicken breast, without skin (3 oz)‡
  Vegetable oil **(½ tsp)**
  Cheddar cheese, low-fat and low-sodium (1 oz)
  Guacamole (2 tbsp)
Corn **(1 c)**, seasoned with margarine **(1 tsp)**‡
Spanish rice (1 c), prepared with margarine‡
Banana (1 medium)
Coffee (1 c)
  Milk, **skim** (1 oz)

Snack
Popcorn (3 c)
  Margarine (1 tbsp)

TOTALS

Calories:	2574.0	Total carb, % kcal:	55
Total fat, % kcal:	28.0	Simple carb, % carb:	36
SFA, % kcal:	6.2	Complex carb, % carb:	64
Cholesterol, mg:	136.0	Sodium, mg:‡	1921
Protein, % kcal:	17.0		

Data from National Cholesterol Education Program (NCEP): *Second report of the Expert Panel on Detection, Evaluation, and Treatment of High Blood Cholesterol in Adults* (Adult Treatment Panel II), NIH Publication No. 93-3095, Bethesda, Md, 1993, National Institutes of Health, National Heart, Lung, and Blood Institute.
SFA, Saturated fatty acid; *carb,* carbohydrates.
*100% RDA met for all nutrients except zinc (90%).
† Boldface food items represent differences between the step I and step II diets.
‡No salt is added in recipe preparation or as seasoning. All margarine is low-sodium.

bolic state; adequate nutritional intake via oral routes is therefore essential. Patients with complications may be at risk for developing cardiac cachexia, which is often associated with heart failure (see Chapter 37). If oral intake is inadequate, tube feeding is indicated to meet increased energy, protein, and nutrient needs (see Chapter 23).

In some facilities, after either cardiac surgery or an acute MI, the dietary regimen starts with a "cardiac liquid" diet (i.e., full liquids with no added salt with the omission of caffeine and restriction of cholesterol). For example, eggnog, high-fat cream soups, caffeinated soda, coffee, and chocolate are excluded.

Once the patient is stabilized and ready to progress to a more complex diet, he or she may choose selections from the appropriate menu. A weight-loss regimen may be recommended in addition to the cardiac restrictions. Patients are discharged on one of the NCEP diets.

Box 35-2. Quick Tips for Aggressive Lipid-Lowering Diets

ABCs of the Reversal Eating Plan

A. Fat intake of 12-14 g/day
B. Vegetarian eating—no meat, poultry, fish
C. No added fats—fat or oil is not added to any food
D. Higher-fat foods are not used—e.g., nuts, seeds, avocado, olives
E. No "fat-free" foods with fat in the ingredient list (e.g., whipped topping mix, dairy creamers, etc.)

Use These Foods Daily

A. Nonfat dairy foods
B. Nonfat egg substitutes and egg whites
C. Nonfat meat substitutes, such as preformed fat-free soy burgers, textured soy nuggets, and wheat gluten
D. Fat-reduced tofu
E. Dried beans and peas
F. Breads, cereals, pasta, starches, rice, and grains
G. Vegetables and fruits

To Make Foods Taste Good: Use for Sauces, Gravies, and Seasonings

A. Nonfat vegetable broth
B. Fat-free, meat-based broth
C. Herbs and seasonings
D. Nonfat butter-flavored sprinkles and liquids

Also use but sparingly: vegetable cooking spray

From Reversal Eating Plan, © 1996 Gerry Krag, MA, RD, Grosse Pte. Park, Mich.

Pharmacologic Management

Determination of drug therapy is dependent on risk category and attainment of the LDL cholesterol goal (see Table 35-12). Many drugs are available for LDL

TABLE 35-21 Sample Asian American Menus for Step I and Step II (TLC) Diets

STEP I: SAMPLE MENUS—ASIAN AMERICAN CUISINE MALES 25-49 YEARS*

Breakfast
Banana (1 medium)
Whole-wheat bread (2 slices)
  Margarine (2 tsp)
Orange juice (¾ c)
Milk, **1%†** (1 c)

Lunch
Beef noodle soup, canned, low-sodium (1 c)
Chinese noodle and beef salad
  Lean roast beef (3 oz)‡
  Peanut oil **(2 tsp)**
  Soy sauce, low-sodium (1 tsp)
  Peanuts, unsalted **(1 T)**
  Carrots (½ c)
  Squash (½ c)
  Onion (½ c)
  Chinese noodles, soft type (¼ c)
Steamed white rice (½ c)‡
Apple (1 medium)
Tea, unsweetened (1 c)

Dinner
Pork stirfry with vegetables
  Pork cutlet **(3 oz)**
  Peanut oil **(2 tsp)**
  Soy sauce, low-sodium (1 tsp)
  Peanuts, unsalted **(1 tbsp)**
  Broccoli (½ c)
  Carrots (½ c)
  Mushrooms (¼ c)
Steamed white rice (1 c)‡
Wonton soup, prepared with low-sodium broth (½ c)‡
Milk, **1%** (1 c)
Tea, unsweetened (1 c)

Snack
Egg roll, vegetarian, baked with peanut oil and low-sodium soy sauce (1 medium)
  Chinese mustard (1 tsp)
  Sweet and sour sauce (1 tsp)
Tea, unsweetened (1 c)

TOTALS

Calories:	2494.0	Total carb, % kcal:	53
Total fat, % kcal:	30.0	Simple carb, % carb:	30
SFA, % kcal:	8.1	Complex carb, % carb:	70
Cholesterol, mg:	238.0	Sodium, mg:‡	1663
Protein, % kcal:	17.0		

STEP II: SAMPLE MENUS—ASIAN AMERICAN CUISINE FEMALES 25-49 YEARS*

Breakfast
Banana **(½ medium)**
Whole-wheat bread (2 slices)
  Margarine (2 tsp)
Orange juice (¾ c)
Milk, **skim** (1 c)

Lunch
Beef noodle soup, canned, low-sodium (½ c)
Chinese noodle and beef salad‡
  Sirloin steak (3 oz)
  Peanut oil **(1 tsp)**
  Soy sauce, low-sodium (1 tsp)
  Carrots (½ c)
  Squash (½ c)
  Onion (¼ c)
  Chinese noodles, soft type (¼ c)
Steamed white rice (½ c)‡
Apple (1 medium)
Tea, unsweetened (1 c)

Dinner
Pork stirfry with vegetables
  Pork cutlet **(2 oz)**
  Peanut oil **(1 tsp)**
  Soy sauce, low-sodium (1 tsp)
  Broccoli (½ c)
  Carrots (½ c)
  Mushrooms (¼ c)
Steamed white rice (½ c)‡
Milk, **skim** (¾ c)
Tea, unsweetened (1 c)

Snack
Wonton soup, prepared with low-sodium broth (½ c)‡
Tea, unsweetened (1 c)

TOTALS

Calories:	1815.0	Total carb, % kcal:	52
Total fat, % kcal:	39.0	Simple carb, % carb:	33
SFA, % kcal:	6.8	Complex carb, % carb:	67
Cholesterol, mg:	176.0	Sodium, mg:‡	1300
Protein, % kcal:	19.0		

Data from National Cholesterol Education Program (NCEP): *Second report of the Expert Panel on Detection, Evaluation, and Treatment of High Blood Cholesterol in Adults* (Adult Treatment Panel II), NIH Publication No. 93-3095, Bethesda, Md, 1993, National Institutes of Health, National Heart, Lung, and Blood Institute.
SFA, Saturated fatty acid; *carb,* carbohydrates.
*100% RDA met for all nutrients except zinc (90%).
† Boldface food items represent differences between the step I and step II (TLC) diets.
‡No salt is added in recipe preparation or as seasoning. All margarine is low-sodium.

lowering (Table 35-23). Regardless of the drug used or category of risk, the therapeutic lifestyle changes underpin all treatment. A regimen combining diet and drugs enables more patients to achieve blood lipid goals than a drug-only regimen (Cobb et al, 1992). A TLC diet with drugs can reduce serum cholesterol levels by up to 40%. More restrictive diets with drugs have not been investigated. The classes of drugs include (1) bile acid sequestrants (cholestyramine), (2) nicotinic acid, (3) HMG CoA reductase inhibitors (lovastatin, pravastatin), (4) fibric acid derivatives (clofibrate, gemfibrozil), and (5) probucol. Classes 1, 2, and 3 are the first choices for treatment (NCEP, 2001).

Most patients can reach lipid goals with diet and a bile acid sequestrant. All these drugs affect nutritional status, which needs to be monitored. Lipid-lowering drugs, once initiated, are required for life. Although most patients will achieve lipid goals with one drug, some require double- or triple-combination therapy. With multiple drugs, a 60% reduction in LDL cholesterol can be achieved (see Chapter 19 for drug-nutrient interactions).

TABLE 35-22 Food Plan for an Aggressive Low-fat Diet (<10% kcal From Fat)

SERVING SIZE	RECOMMENDED DAILY INTAKE	SERVING SIZE	RECOMMENDED DAILY INTAKE
Nonfat Dairy 1 c skim milk 1 c nonfat yogurt 1 oz nonfat cheese* ½ c nonfat cottage cheese* ½ c nonfat ricotta 2 tbsp nonfat cream cheese*	2 servings	**Fruits** 1 medium raw fruit ½ large fruit 1 c fresh fruit ½ c fruit sauce or juice ¼ c dried fruit	≥ 2 (limit of 2/day with elevated triglyceride level)
Protein Dried beans, cooked (4 oz) 4 egg whites (4 oz) ½ c nonfat egg substitute (4 oz) Fat-free gluten meat substitute (4 oz) Reduced-fat tofu or soy protein (4 oz)	4-8 oz	**Breads/Cereals/Starches** 1 slice bread 1 medium potato 1 c pasta, rice, or cereal 6 crackers ½ bagel or English muffin	≥6
Vegetables 1 c raw ½ c cooked ½ c vegetable juice*	≥5 servings	**Nonfat Sweets and Treats**	Rarely

From Reversal Eating Plan, Copyright 1996 Gerry Krag, MA, RD, Grosse Pte. Park, Mich.
*Higher-sodium food.

TABLE 35-23 Drugs Affecting Lipoprotein Metabolism

DRUG CLASS AND AGENTS	LIPID/LIPOPROTEIN EFFECTS	SIDE EFFECTS	CONTRAINDICATIONS	CLINICAL TRIAL RESULTS
HMG CoA reductase inhibitors (statins)*	LDL ↓ 18%-55% HDL ↑ 5%-15% TG ↓ 7%-30%	Myopathy Increased liver enzymes	Absolute: • Active or chronic liver disease Relative: • Concomitant use of certain drugs†	Reduced major coronary events, CHD deaths, need for coronary procedures, stroke, and total mortality
Bile acid sequestrants‡	LDL ↓ 15%-30% HDL ↑ 3%-5% TG No change or increase	Gastrointestinal distress Constipation Decreased absorption of other drugs	Absolute: • Dysbeta-lipoproteinemia • TG >400 mg/dl Relative: • TG >200 mg/dl	Reduced major coronary events and CHD deaths
Nicotinic acid§	LDL ↓ 5%-25% HDL ↑ 15%-35% TG ↓ 20%-50%	Flushing Hyperglycemia Hyperuricemia (or gout) Upper GI distress Hepatotoxicity	Absolute: • Chronic liver disease • Severe gout Relative: • Diabetes • Hyperuricemia • Peptic ulcer disease	Reduced major coronary events, and possibly total mortality
Fibric acids¶	LDL ↓ 5%-20% (may be increased in patients with high TG) HDL ↑ 10%-20% TG ↓ 20%-50%	Dyspepsia Gallstones Myopathy Unexplained non-CHD deaths in WHO study	Absolute: • Severe renal disease • Severe hepatic disease	Reduced major coronary events

*Lovastatin (20-80 mg), pravastatin (20-40 mg), simvastatin (20-80 mg), fluvastatin (20-80 mg), atorvastatin (10-80 mg), cerivastatin (0.4-0.8 mg).
†Cyclosporine, macrolide antibiotics, various antifungal agents and cytochrome P-450 inhibitors (fibrates and niacin should be used with appropriate caution).
‡Cholestyramine (4-16 g), colestipol (5-20 g), colesevelam (2.6-3.8 g).
§Immediate-release (crystalline) nicotinic acid (1.5-3 g), extended release nicotinic acid (Niaspan) (1-2 g), sustained-release nicotinic acid (1-2 g).
¶Gemfibrozil (600 mg bid), fenofibrate (200 mg), clofibrate (1000 mg bid).
CHD, Coronary heart disease; *GI,* gastrointestinal; *HDL,* high-density lipoprotein; *HMG CoA,* hydroxymethylglutaryl enzyme; *LDL,* low-density lipoprotein; *TG,* triglycerides; WHO, World Health Organization.

SUMMARY

Lifestyle changes, with diet at the cornerstone, are pivotal to maintaining cardiovascular health. Because of high hospital costs, efforts to standardize patient care have led to the use of clinical pathways or care maps, which indicate the timing, activities, and services that are provided for the patient. In cardiac units, the clinical pathway designates when patient education will be offered by all disciplines. In many facilities, special group classes are offered to patients after their cardiac event or surgical procedure to encourage them to make permanent lifestyle changes. Diet plays an important role in this process.

Clinical Scenario 1

Lenora is a 60-year-old black woman with type 2 diabetes mellitus, hypertension, and obesity. She lives with her husband of 40 years and maintains a moderate amount of activity. Because their children are grown, many meals are consumed at restaurants. In the past, she has been unsuccessful in maintaining any weight losses. Her family history for CHD is positive. Her height is 5 ft 4 in. and her weight is 250 lb. Her medications are Diabinese, Diazide, Enalapril, and Premarin. At her last checkup, the laboratory tests revealed the following:

TG: 400 mg/dl	Total cholesterol: 253 mg/dl
HDL cholesterol: 37 mg/dl	LDL cholesterol: 185 mg/dl
Fasting blood glucose: 178 mg/dl	

1. What are Lenora's risk factors for CHD?
2. What type of diet would you recommend for Lenora? What additional information needs to be obtained before teaching her about a new eating plan?
3. What suggestions for restaurant eating will help Lenora adhere to the new eating plan?
4. What dietary factors could optimize Lenora's lipid profile?

TG, Triglyceride; *HDL*, high-density lipoprotein; *LDL*, low-density lipoprotein.

Clinical Scenario 2

Jeremiah is a single 30-year-old Hispanic male who has elevated serum cholesterol, serum homocysteine, and blood pressure. He is a migrant worker and has recently emigrated from Mexico to the United States and has become a citizen. He has been referred to your ambulatory nutrition clinic for follow-up. His diet history reveals that he skips meals frequently and cannot predict his income for meal planning. He does not drink milk, but he does like to eat fruits and vegetables when he can afford them. He seldom eats fish but is willing to eat lean poultry.

1. What information do you need to provide further guidance for him?
2. What community resources may be available to assist him with obtaining food on a more regular basis?
3. What type of simple menus can you give Jeremiah that will include foods from the DASH diet plan that he may be willing to consume (see Chapter 36)?

Relevant Web Sites

American Association of Cardiovascular and Pulmonary Rehabilitation
www.aacvpr.org/
American Heart Association
www.americanheart.org/
Heart-Healthy Cookbooks
www.vh.org/Patients/IHB/Dietary/HeartCookBooks.html
Heart Information Network
www.heartinfo.org/
NCEP Adult Treatment Panel Guidelines
www.nhlbi.nih.gov/guidelines/cholesterol/atp_iii.htm
University of California Heart Disease Prevention Program
www.heart.uci.edu/

Cited References

Abbey M et al: Oxidation of low-density lipoproteins: intraindividual variability and the effect of dietary linoleate supplementation, *Am J Clin Nutr* 57:391, 1993.

Albert C et al: Fish consumption and risk of sudden cardiac death, *JAMA* 279:23, 1998.

Allison et al: Annual deaths attributable to obesity in the United States, *JAMA* 282:1530, 1999.

Alpha-Tocopherol, Beta Carotene Cancer Prevention Study Group: The effect of vitamin E and B-carotene on the incidence of lung cancer and other cancers in male smokers, *N Engl J Med* 330:1029, 1994.

American Dietetic Association: *Medical nutrition therapy across the continuum of care,* Chicago, 1996, The Association.

American Heart Association: *2002 Heart and stroke statistical update,* Dallas, 2001, The Association.

Anderson JW et al: Meta-analysis of the effects of soy protein intake on serum lipids, *N Engl J Med* 333:276, 1995.

Barr SL et al: Reducing total dietary fat without reducing saturated fatty acids does not significantly lower total plasma cholesterol concentrations in normal males, *Am J Clin Nutr* 55:675, 1992.

Bass KM et al: Plasma lipoprotein levels as predictors of cardiovascular death in women, *Arch Intern Med* 153:2209, 1993.

Bell L et al: Cholesterol-lowering effects of calcium carbonate in patients with mild to moderate hypercholesterolemia, *Arch Intern Med* 152:2441, 1992.

Blankenhorn DH et al: The influence of diet on the appearance of new lesions in human coronary arteries, *JAMA* 263:1646, 1990.

Blumberg JB: An update: vitamin E supplementation and heart disease, *Nutr Clin Care* 5:50, 2002.

Bots ML et al: Homocysteine, atherosclerosis and prevalent cardiovascular disease in the elderly: the Rotterdam Study, *J Intern Med* 242:339, 1997.

Brattstrom L, Wilcken DE: Homocysteine and cardiovascular disease: cause or effect? *Am J Clin Nutr* 72:315, 2000.

Brown A, Hu F: Dietary modulation of endothelial function: implications for cardiovascular disease, *Am J Clin Nutr* 73:673, 2001.

Brown BG et al: Simvastatin and niacin, antioxidant vitamins, or the combination for the prevention of coronary disease, *N Engl J Med* 345:1583, 2001.

Burrows ER et al: Nutritional applications of a clinical low fat dietary intervention to public health change, *J Nutr Educ* 25:167, 1993.

Bush TL et al: Cardiovascular mortality and noncontraceptive use of estrogen in women: results from the Lipid Research Clinics Program Follow-Up Study, *Circulation* 75:1102, 1987.

Campos H et al: Differences in low density lipoprotein subfractions and apolipoproteins in premenopausal and postmenopausal women, *J Clin Endocrinol Metab* 67:30, 1988.

Carmichael H et al: Lower fat intake as a predictor of initial and sustained weight loss in obese subjects consuming an otherwise ad libitum diet, *J Am Diet Assoc* 98:35, 1998.

Castelli WP: Epidemiology of triglycerides: a view from Framingham, *Am J Cardiol* 70:3H, 1992.

Centers for Disease Control and Prevention (CDC): Declines in death from heart disease and stroke— United States, 1990-1999, *MMWR Morb Mortal Wkly Rep* 48 (3):649, 1999.

Centers for Disease Control and Prevention (CDC): Major cardiovascular disease (CVD) during 1997-1999 and major CVD hospital discharge rates in 1997 among women with diabetes, *MMWR Morb Mortal Wkly Rep* 50:948, 2001.

Coate D: Moderate drinking and coronary artery heart disease mortality: evidence from NHANES I and NHANES I follow-up, *Am J Public Health* 83:888, 1993.

Cobb MM et al: Lovastatin efficacy in reducing low-density lipoprotein cholesterol levels on high- vs. low-fat diets, *JAMA* 265:997, 1992.

Connor WE: *Evaluation of publicly available scientific evidence regarding certain nutrient-disease relationships: omega-3 fatty acids and heart disease,* Washington, DC, 1991, Life Sciences Review Office.

Crouse JR et al: A randomized trial comparing the effect of casein with that of soy protein containing varying amounts of isoflavones on plasma concentrations of lipids and lipoproteins, *Arch Intern Med* 159:2070, 1999.

Daviglus M et al: Fish consumption and the 30-year risk of fatal myocardial infarction, *N Engl J Med* 336:1046, 1997.

de Lorgeril M et al: Mediterranean diet, traditional risk factors, and the rate of cardiovascular complications after myocardial infarction, *Circulation* 99:779, 1999.

de Maat MP: Effect of diet, drugs, and genes on plasma fibrinogen levels, *Ann NY Acad Sci* 936:509, 2001.

Denke MA et al: Excess body weight: an under-recognized contributor to dyslipidemia in white American women, *Arch Intern Med* 154:401, 1994.

Ditschuneit H et al: Fibrinogen in obesity before and after weight reduction, *Obes Res* 3:43, 1995.

Eberhardt MS, Ingram DD, Makuc DM et al: *Urban and rural health chartbook: health, United States, 2001,* Hyattsville, Maryland, 2001, National Center for Health Statistics.

Elias SL, Innis SM: Bakery foods are the major dietary source of trans-fatty acids among pregnant women with diets providing 30 percent energy from fat, *J Am Diet Assoc* 102:46, 2002.

Emken EA: Physiochemical properties, intake, and metabolism of trans fatty acids, *Am J Clin Nutr* 62(suppl):659S, 1995.

Erdman JW et al: Soy protein and cardiovascular disease, *Circulation* 102:2555, 2000.

Ernst E, Koenig W: Fibrinogen and cardiovascular risk, *Vasc Med* 2:115, 1997.

Fellows JL, Trosclair A: Annual smoking—attributable mortality, years of potential life lost, and economic costs—United States, 1995-1999, *MMWR Morb Mortal Wkly Rep* 51:300, 2002.

Food and Nutrition Science Alliance: Statement on trans fatty acids, *J Am Diet Assoc* 94:1098, 1994.

Ford ES et al: Prevalence of the metabolic syndrome among U.S. adults, *JAMA* 287:356, 2002.

Fried RE et al: The effect of filtered-coffee consumption on plasma lipid levels, *JAMA* 267:811, 1992.

Fuentes F et al: Mediterranean and low-fat diets improve endothelial function in hypercholesterolemic men, *Ann Intern Med* 134:1115, 2001.

Fuster V: Understanding the coronary disease process and the potential for prevention: a summary, *Prev Med* 29:S9, 1999.

Fuster V, Badimon J, Chsebro JH: Atherothrombosis: mechanisms and clinical therapeutic approaches, *Vasc Med* 3:231, 1998.

Fuster V et al: Task Force 1: pathogenesis of coronary disease: the biologic role of risk factors, *J Am Coll Cardiol* 27:964, 1996.

Ginsberg HN: Lipoprotein metabolism and its relationship to atherosclerosis, *Med Clin North Am* 78:1, 1994.

Ginsberg HN et al: Reduction of plasma cholesterol levels in normal men on an American Heart Association Step I Diet or a Step I Diet with added monounsaturated fat, *N Engl J Med* 322:574, 1990.

GISSI-Prevenzione Investigators: Dietary supplementation with omega-3 polyunsaturated fatty acids and vitamin E after myocardial infarction: results of the GISSI-Prevenzione Trial, *Lancet* 354:447, 1999.

Glantz SA, Parmley WW: Passive smoking and heart disease: mechanisms and risk, *JAMA* 273:1047, 1995.

Glore SR et al: Soluble fiber and serum lipids: a literature review, *J Am Diet Assoc* 94:425, 1994.

Grady D et al: Cardiovascular disease outcomes during 6.8 years of hormone therapy: Heart and Estrogen/Progestin Replacement Study follow-up (HERS II), *JAMA* 288:49, 2002.

Grande F et al: Diets of different fatty acid composition producing identical serum cholesterol levels in man, *Am J Clin Nutr* 25:53, 1972.

Grundy SM: Influence of stearic acid on cholesterol metabolism relative to other long-chain fatty acids, *Am J Clin Nutr* 60:986S, 1994.

Grundy SM et al: Prevention Conference VI: Diabetes and Cardiovascular Disease: Writing Group IV: lifestyle and medical management of risk factors, *Circulation* 105:153e, 2002.

Hammar N et al: Association of boiled and filtered coffee with incidence of first nonfatal myocardial infarction: the SHEEP and the VHEEP study, *J Intern Med* 253:653, 2003.

Harris WS: OMEGA-3 fatty acids and serum lipoproteins: human studies, *Am J Clin Nutr* 65:1645S, 1997.

Hausmann D et al: Angiographically silent atherosclerosis detected by intravascular ultrasound in patients with familial hypercholesterolemia and familial combined hyperlipidemia: correlation with high density lipoprotein, *J Am Coll Cardiol* 27:1562, 1996.

Herbert V: Antioxidants, pro-oxidants, and their effects, *JAMA* 272:1659, 1994.

Howard G, Thun MJ: Why is environmental tobacco smoke more strongly associated with coronary heart disease than expected? A review of potential biases and experimental data, *Environ Health Perspect* 107:853(S)6, 1999.

Hu FB et al: The impact of diabetes mellitus on mortality from all causes and coronary heart disease in women: 20 years of follow-up, *Arch Intern Med* 161:1717, 2001.

Humphries D, Krummel D: Perceived susceptibility to cardiovascular disease and dietary intake in women, *Am J Health Behav* 23:250, 1999.

Hunink MG et al: The recent decline in mortality from coronary heart disease, 1980–1990: the effect of secular trends in risk factors and treatment, *JAMA* 277:535, 1997.

Huttunen JK et al: The Helsinki Heart Study: central findings and clinical implications, *Ann Intern Med* 23:155, 1991.

Jacques P et al: The effect of folic acid fortification on plasma folate and total homocysteine concentrations, *N Engl J Med* 340:1449, 1999.

Jenkins DJ et al: Effects of high- and low-isoflavone (phytoestrogen) soy foods on inflammatory biomarkers and proinflammatory cytokines in middle-aged men and women, *Metabolism* 51:919, 2002.

Jialal I, Grundy S: Effect of combined supplementation with a-tocopherol, ascorbate, and β-carotene on low-density lipoprotein oxidation, *Circulation* 88:2780, 1993.

Johansson L et al: The Norwegian diet during the last hundred years in relation to coronary heart disease, *Eur J Clin Nutr* 50:277, 1996.

Johnson CL et al: Declining serum total cholesterol levels among U.S. adults: the National Health and Nutrition Examination Surveys, *JAMA* 269:3002, 1993.

Judd JT et al: Dietary trans fatty acids: effects on plasma lipids and lipoproteins of healthy men and women, *Am J Clin Nutr* 59:861, 1994.

Judd JT et al: Effects of margarine compared with those of butter on blood lipid profiles related to cardiovascular disease risk factors in normolipemic adults fed controlled diets, *Am J Clin Nutr* 68:768, 1998.

Kannel WB: Coronary heart disease risk factors in the elderly, *Am J Geriatr Cardiol* 11:101, 2002.

Katan MB: European researcher calls for reconsideration of trans fatty acids [Letter to Editor], *J Am Diet Assoc* 94:1097, 1994.

Katan MB et al: Effects of fats and fatty acids on blood lipids in humans: an overview, *Am J Clin Nutr* 60(suppl):1017S, 1994.

Keys A: Coronary heart disease in seven countries, *Circulation* 41: I-1, 1970.

Kinosian B et al: Cholesterol and coronary heart disease: predicting risk by levels and ratios, *Ann Intern Med* 121:641, 1994.

Klag MJ et al: Serum cholesterol in young men and subsequent cardiovascular disease, *N Engl J Med* 328:313, 1993.

Knapp HR: Dietary fatty acids in human thrombosis and hemostasis, *Am J Clin Nutr* 65:1687S, 1997.

Krauss RM et al: AHA dietary guidelines, revision 2000: a statement for healthcare professionals from the Nutrition Committee of the American Heart Association, *Circulation* 102:2284, 2000.

Kris-Etherton PM, Krummel DA: Role of nutrition in the prevention and treatment of coronary heart disease in women, *J Am Diet Assoc* 93:987, 1993.

Kris-Etherton PM, Yu S: Individual fatty acid effects on plasma lipids and lipoproteins: human studies, *Am J Clin Nutr* 65:1628S, 1997.

Kris-Etherton PM et al: The effect of diet on plasma lipids, lipoproteins, and coronary heart disease, *J Am Diet Assoc* 88:1373, 1988.

Kris-Etherton PM at al: Summary of the Scientific Conference on dietary fatty acids and cardiovascular health, *Circulation* 103: 1034, 2001a.

Kris-Etherton PM et al: Lyon Diet Heart Study. Benefits of a Mediterranean-Style, National Cholesterol Education Program/ American Heart Association Step I dietary pattern on cardiovascular disease, *Circulation* 103:1823, 2001b.

Kritchevsky S et al: Provitamin A carotenoid intake and carotid artery plaques: the Atherosclerosis Risk in Communities Study, *Am J Clin Nutr* 68:726, 1998.

Krummel DA: Cardiovascular disease. In Krummel DA, Kris-Etherton PM, editors: *Nutrition and women's health*, Gaithersburg, Md, 1996, Aspen Publishers.

Kwiterovich PO: The effect of dietary fat, antioxidants, and pro-oxidants on blood lipids, lipoproteins, and atherosclerosis, *J Am Diet Assoc* 97:31S, 1997.

Larsen ML, Illingworth R: Drug treatment of dyslipoproteinemia, *Med Clin North Am* 78:255, 1994.

Levy D et al: Prognostic implications of baseline electrocardiographic features and their serial changes in subjects with left ventricular hypertrophy, *Circulation* 90:1786, 1994.

Lichenstein A et al: Stanol/sterol ester-containing foods and blood cholesterol levels, *Circulation* 103:1177, 2001.

Liu S et al: Intake of vegetables rich in carotenoids and risk of coronary heart disease in men: the Physicians' Health Study, *Int J Epidemiol* 30:130, 2001.

McDowell MA, et al: Energy and macronutrient intakes of persons ages 2 months and over in the United States: *Third National Health and Nutrition Examination Survey, Phase 1, 1988-1991*. Advance data from Vital and Health Statistics, No. 225, Hyattsville, Md, 1994, National Center for Health Statistics.

Meydani S et al: Vitamin E supplementation and in vivo immune response in healthy elderly subjects: a randomized, controlled trial, *JAMA* 277:1380, 1997.

Mokdad A et al: The continuing obesity epidemic in the United States, *JAMA* 284:1650, 2000.

Mokdad A et al: The continuing epidemics of obesity and diabetes in the United States, *JAMA* 286:1195, 2001.

Mosca L et al: Guide to preventive cardiology for women, *J Am Coll Cardiol* 33:1751, 1999.

Mosca L et al: Hormone replacement therapy and cardiovascular disease: a statement for healthcare professionals from the American Heart Association, *Circulation* 104:499, 2001.

National Center for Health Statistics: *Health, United States, 2001*. Hyattsville, Md, 2002, Public Health Service.

National Cholesterol Education Program (NCEP): *Second report of the Expert Panel on Detection, Evaluation, and Treatment of High Blood Cholesterol in Adults* (Adult Treatment Panel II), NIH Publication No. 93–3095, Bethesda, Md, 1993, National Institutes of Health, National Heart, Lung, and Blood Institute.

National Cholesterol Education Program (NCEP): Executive summary of the third report of the National Cholesterol Education Program (NCEP) Expert Panel on Detection, Evaluation, and Treatment of High Blood Cholesterol in Adults (Adult Treatment Panel III), *JAMA* 285:2486, 2001.

National Heart Lung Blood Institute (NHLBI): *Report of the Expert Panel on Blood Cholesterol Levels in Children and Adolescents*, U.S. Department of Health and Human Services, Publication No. 91-2732, Bethesda, Md, September 1991.

National Heart, Lung and Blood Institute (NHLBI): *Fact book fiscal year 1999*. Bethesda, Md, 2000, National Institutes of Health, Public Health Service.

National Institutes of Health (NIH): *NHLBI Obesity Education Initiative Expert Panel on the Identification, Evaluation, and Treatment of Overweight and Obesity in Adults*, Bethesda, MD, The Evidence Report, 1998.

Nelson HD et al: Postmenopausal hormone replacement therapy: scientific review, *JAMA* 288:872, 2002.

NIH Consensus Conference: Triglyceride, high-density lipoprotein, and coronary heart disease, *JAMA* 269:505, 1993.

Nydahl MC et al: Lipid-lowering diets enriched with monounsaturated or polyunsaturated fatty acids but low in saturated fatty acids have similar effects on serum lipid concentrations in hyperlipidemic patients, *Am J Clin Nutr* 59:115, 1994.

Ornish D, Brown SE: Treatment of screening for hyperlipidemia [Letter to Editor], *N Engl J Med* 329:1124, 1993.

Ornish D et al: Intensive lifestyle changes for reversal of coronary heart disease, *JAMA* 280:2001, 1998.

Parks DA, Booyse FM: Cardiovascular protection by alcohol and polyphenols: role of nitric oxide, *Ann NY Acad Sci* 957:115, 2002.

Pasternak RC et al: Task Force 3: spectrum of risk factors for coronary heart disease, *J Am Coll Cardiol* 27:978, 1996.

Pate R et al: Physical activity and public health: a recommendation from the Centers for Disease Control and Prevention with the American College of Medicine, *JAMA* 273:402, 1995.

Paterick TE, Fletcher GF: Endothelial function and cardiovascular prevention: role of blood lipids, exercise, and other risk factors, *Cardiol Rev* 9:282, 2001.

Patsch JR: Triglyceride-rich lipoproteins and atherosclerosis, *Atherosclerosis* 110:S23, 1994.

Plotnick G et al: Effect of antioxidant vitamins on the transient impairment of endothelium-dependent brachial artery vasoactivity following a single high-fat meal, *JAMA* 278:1682, 1997.

Powell KE et al: Physical activity and the incidence of coronary heart disease, *Ann Rev Public Health* 8:243, 1987.

Preli R et al: Vascular effects of dietary L-arginine supplementation, *Atherosclerosis* 162:1, 2002.

Public Health Service: *Healthy People 2000: National health promotion and disease prevention objectives*. Full report with commentary, USDHHS publication No. (PHS) 91-50212, Washington, DC, 1991, U.S. Department of Health and Human Services.

Puccio EM et al: Clustering of atherogenic behaviors in coffee drinkers. *Am J Public Health* 80:1310, 1990.

Rifici VA, Khachadurian AK: The inhibition of low-density lipoprotein oxidation by 17-b estradiol, *Metabolism* 41:1110, 1992.

Rosamond WD et al: Stroke incidence and survival among middle-aged adults: 9-year follow-up of the Atherosclerosis Risk in Communities (ARIC) cohort, *Stroke* 7:736, 1999.

Sabate J: Nut consumption, vegetarian diets, ischemic heart disease risk, and all-cause mortality: evidence from epidemiologic studies, *Am J Clin Nutr* 70:500S, 1999.

Schaefer EJ: Familial lipoprotein disorders and premature coronary artery disease, *Med Clin North Am* 78:21, 1994a.

Schaefer EJ et al: Lipoprotein (a) levels and risk of coronary heart disease in men: the Lipid Research Clinics Coronary Primary Prevention Trial, *JAMA* 271:999, 1994b.

Schaefer EJ et al: Comparison of fasting and postprandial plasma lipoproteins in subjects with and without coronary heart disease, *Am J Cardiol* 88:1129, 2001.

Schoenborn CA, Barnes PM: Leisure-time physical activity among adults: United States, 1997-98. *In advance data from vital and health statistics,* No. 325, Hyattsville, Md, 2002, National Center for Health Statistics.

Schuler G et al: Regular physical exercise and low-fat diet. Effects of progression on coronary artery disease, *Circulation* 86:1, 1992.

Shah P: Plaque disruption and thrombosis, *Cardiol Rev* 8:31, 2000.

Sikand G et al: Medical nutrition therapy lowers serum cholesterol and saves medication costs in men with hypercholesterolemia, *J Am Diet Assoc* 98:889, 1998.

Siscovick DS et al: Dietary intake of long-chain omega-3 polyunsaturated fatty acids and the risk of primary cardiac arrest, *Am J Clin Nutr* 71:208S, 2000.

Smith SC et al: AHA/ACC Guidelines for preventing heart attack and death in patients with atherosclerotic cardiovascular disease: 2001 update, *Circulation* 104:1577, 2001.

Stampfer MJ et al: Primary prevention of coronary heart disease in women through diet and lifestyle, *N Engl J Med* 343:16, 2000.

Sun AY et al: The "French paradox" and beyond: neuroprotective effects of polyphenols(1,2), *Free Radic Biol Med* 32:314, 2002.

Tchernof A et al: Weight loss reduces C-reactive protein levels in obese postmenopausal women, *Circulation* 105:564, 2002.

Teixeira S et al: Effects of feeding 4 levels of soy protein for 3 and 6 weeks on blood lipids and apolipoproteins in moderately hypercholesterolemic men, *Am J Clin Nutr* 71:1077, 2001.

Trichopoulou et al: Adherence to a Mediterranean diet and survival in a Greek population, *N Engl J Med* 348:2599, 2003.

Ueland P et al: The controversy over homocysteine and cardiovascular risk, *Am J Clin Nutr* 72:324, 2000.

U.S. Department of Health and Human Services: *Physical activity and health: a report of the Surgeon General,* Bethesda, Md, 1996, The Department.

van Beresteijn ECH et al: Perimenopausal increase in serum cholesterol: a 10-year longitudinal study, *Am J Epidemiol* 137:383, 1993.

Van Horn L, Ernst N: A summary of the science supporting the new National Cholesterol Education Program dietary recommendations: what dietitians should know, *J Am Diet Assoc* 101:1148, 2001.

Watts GF et al: Dietary fatty acids and progression of coronary artery disease in men, *Am J Clin Nutr* 64:202, 1996.

Welch G, Loscalzo J: Homocysteine and atherosclerosis, *N Engl J Med* 338:1042, 1998.

Willett WC et al: Intake of trans fatty acids and risk of coronary heart disease among women, *Lancet* 341:581, 1993.

Wilson PF et al: Impact of national guidelines for cholesterol risk factor lowering: the Framingham Offspring Study, *JAMA* 262:41, 1989.

Wilson P et al: Cumulative effects of high cholesterol levels, high blood pressure, and cigarette smoking on carotid stenosis, *N Engl J Med* 337:516, 1997.

Witzum JL et al: Studies on the ability of dietary supplementation with β-carotene to protect low-density lipoprotein from oxidative modification, *Ann NY Acad Sci* 691:200, 1993.

Woo KS, et al: Hyperhomocysteinemia is a risk factor for arterial endothelial dysfunction in humans, *Circulation* 96:2542, 1997.

Wood D: Established and emerging cardiovascular risk factors, *Am Heart J* 141:49S, 2001.

Woollett LA et al: Saturated and unsaturated fatty acids independently regulate low density lipoprotein receptor activity and production rate, *J Lipid Res* 33:77, 1992.

Wong W et al: Cholesterol-lowering effect of soy protein in normocholesterolemic men, *Am J Clin Nutr* 68:1385S, 1998.

Writing Group for the Women's Health Initiative Investigators: Risks and benefits of estrogen plus progestin in healthy postmenopausal women: principal results From the Women's Health Initiative randomized controlled trial, *JAMA* 288:321, 2002.

Wu JM et al: Mechanism of cardioprotection by resveratrol, a phenolic antioxidant present in red wine [Review], *Int J Mol Med* 8:3, 2001.

Yusuf S et al: Vitamin E supplementation and cardiovascular events in high-risk patients: Heart Outcomes Prevention Evaluation Study Investigators, *N Engl J Med* 342:164, 2000.

Additional References

Brousseau ME, Schaefer EJ: New targets for medical treatment of lipid disorders, *Curr Atheroscler Rep* 4:343, 2002.

Brynes AE et al: Men at increased risk of coronary heart disease are not different from age- and weight-matched healthy controls in their postprandial triglyceride, nonesterified fatty acid, or incretin responses to sucrose, *Metabolism* 51:195, 2002.

Jha P et al: The antioxidant vitamins and cardiovascular disease: a critical review of epidemiologic and clinical trial data, *Ann Intern Med* 23:860, 1995.

Linton MF, Fazio S: A practical approach to risk assessment to prevent coronary artery disease and its complications, *Am J Cardiol* 92:19i, 2003.

Lotufo PA et al: Diabetes and all-cause and coronary heart disease mortality among US male physicians, *Arch Intern Med* 161:242, 2001.

Mahoney LT et al: Usefulness of the Framingham risk score and body mass index to predict early coronary artery calcium in young adults (Muscatine Study), *Am J Cardiol* 88:467, 2001.

Ostlund RE Jr., et al: Phytosterols that are naturally present in commercial corn oil significantly reduce cholesterol absorption in humans, *Am J Clin Nutr* 75:1000, 2002.

Sharrett AR et al: Coronary heart disease prediction from lipoprotein cholesterol levels, triglycerides, lipoprotein(a), apolipoproteins A-I and B, and HDL density subfractions: The Atherosclerosis Risk in Communities (ARIC) Study, *Circulation* 104:1108, 2001.

Sprecher DL, Pearce GL: Fiber-multivitamin combination therapy: a beneficial influence on low-density lipoprotein and homocysteine, *Metabolism* 51:1166, 2002.

Vapaatalo H, Mervaala E. Clinically important factors influencing endothelial function, *Med Sci Monit* 7:1075, 2001.

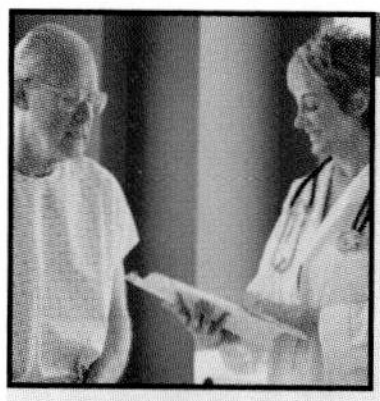

CHAPTER 36

Medical Nutrition Therapy in Hypertension

DEBRA A. KRUMMEL, PhD, RD, LD

CHAPTER OUTLINE

- Definition and Classification
- Prevalence and Incidence
- Morbidity and Mortality
- Pathophysiology
- Primary Prevention
- Medical Management

KEY TERMS

DASH (Dietary Approaches to Stop Hypertension) diet–low-fat eating plan that is high in fruits, vegetables, and low-fat dairy foods; shown to reduce blood pressure

diastolic blood pressure (DBP)–blood pressure during the relaxation phase of the cardiac cycle; 80 mm Hg is optimal

essential hypertension–hypertension of unknown etiology; also known as primary hypertension

hypertension–persistently high arterial blood pressure, defined as systolic blood pressure above 140 mm Hg or diastolic blood pressure above 90 mm Hg

normotensive–relating to a normal blood pressure, which is a systolic blood pressure of 130 mm Hg and a diastolic blood pressure of 85 mm Hg; read as a blood pressure of 130/85

salt-resistant hypertension–elevated blood pressure that is not affected by salt intake

salt-sensitive hypertension–elevated blood pressure that rises or falls with corresponding changes in salt intake

secondary hypertension–elevated blood pressure secondary to another disease

systolic blood pressure (SBP)–blood pressure during the contraction phase of the cardiac cycle; 120 mm Hg is optimal

Hypertension is a common public health problem in developed countries. Untreated hypertension leads to many degenerative diseases, including congestive heart failure, end-stage renal disease, and peripheral vascular disease. It is often called a "silent killer" because people with hypertension can be asymptomatic for years and then have a fatal stroke or heart attack. Although no cure is available, prevention and management decrease the incidence of hypertension and disease sequelae. Some of the decline in cardiovascular disease (CVD) mortality over the last two decades has been attributed to the increased detection and control of hypertension. The emphasis on lifestyle modifications has given diet a prominent role for both the primary prevention and management of hypertension.

Of those with high blood pressure, 90% to 95% have essential or primary hypertension, for which the cause cannot be determined. Most likely there are many causes, including renal dysfunction (Cowley and Roman, 1996). In the remaining 5%, hypertension arises as the result of another disease, usually endocrine, and thus is referred to as secondary hypertension. Depending on the extent of the underlying disease, secondary hypertension can be cured.

DEFINITION AND CLASSIFICATION

A general definition of hypertension is a systolic blood pressure (SBP) of 140 mm Hg or higher or a diastolic blood pressure (DBP) of 90 mm Hg or higher or both. In the Sixth Report of the Joint National Committee on Detection, Evaluation, and Treatment of High Blood Pressure (JNC VI) (Joint National Committee, 1997), hypertension is classified in stages based on the risk of developing CVD (Table 36-1).

A high-normal category is included because these people are at high risk for developing essential hypertension and CVD. Stage 1 hypertension (140 to 159/90 to 99 mm Hg) is the most prevalent level seen in adults. In other words, this is the group most likely to have a myocardial infarction or stroke. The defining point for hypertension is arbitrary because any level of elevated blood pressure is associated with increased incidence of CVD and renal disease. Therefore, normalization of blood pressure is important for all stages of hypertension.

PREVALENCE AND INCIDENCE

About 50 million Americans over 6 years of age have hypertension or are taking antihypertensive medication (American Heart Association [AHA], 2001). Overall, 28% of American adults have high blood pressure *(Healthy People 2010)*. African Americans have a higher prevalence of hypertension (37% of men; 37% of women) than non-Hispanic whites (25% of men; 21% of women) or Mexican Americans (24% of men; 22% of women). The prevalence of high blood pressure in African Americans is among the highest rates seen anywhere in the world. Because African Americans develop hypertension earlier in life and sustain higher blood pressure levels, their risk of fatal stroke (1.8 times higher), heart disease death (1.5 times higher), or end-stage kidney disease (4.2 times higher) is higher than whites.

Blood pressure elevations are seen across the life span. About seven million children have high blood pressure (AHA, 1997). In children, hypertension is defined as blood pressure readings greater than the 95th percentile for age, gender, height on at least three separate occasions (National Heart, Lung, and Blood Institute, 1997). With aging, the prevalence of high blood pressure increases (Figure 36-1). Before the age of 55, more men than women have high blood pressure. After age 65, the rates of high blood pressure in women in each racial group surpass those of the men in their group. Because the prevalence of hypertension rises with increasing age, more than half the older adult population (65 years of age and older) in any racial group has hypertension. The age-related risk for high blood pressure is a function of lifestyle variables, rather than just aging, and is believed to be preventable (Stamler et al, 1993).

TABLE 36-1 Classification of Blood Pressure in Adults Age 18 Years and Older*

	BLOOD PRESSURE (mm Hg)		
CATEGORY	SYSTOLIC		DIASTOLIC
Optimal†	<120	and	<80
Normal	<130	and	<85
High-normal	130-139	or	85-89
Hypertension‡			
Stage 1	140-159	or	90-99
Stage 2	160-179	or	100-109
Stage 3	≥180	or	N≥110

From the Joint National Committee on Prevention, Detection, Evaluation, and Treatment of High Blood Pressure: Sixth Report (JNC VI), *Arch Intern Med* 157:2413, 1997.

*Not taking antihypertensive drugs and not acutely ill. When systolic and diastolic blood pressures fall into different categories, the higher category should be selected to classify the individual's blood pressure status. For example, 160/92 mm Hg should be classified as stage 2 hypertension, and 174/120 mm Hg should be classified as stage 3 hypertension. Isolated systolic hypertension is defined as systolic blood pressure 140 mm Hg or greater and diastolic blood pressure less than 90 mm Hg and staged appropriately (e.g., 170/82 mm Hg is defined as stage 2 isolated systolic hypertension). In addition to classifying stages of hypertension on the basis of average blood pressure levels, clinicians should specify presence or absence of target organ disease and additional risk factors. This specificity is important for risk classification and treatment.

†Optimal blood pressure with respect to cardiovascular risk is less than 120/80 mm Hg. However, unusually low readings should be evaluated for clinical significance.

‡Based on the average of two or more readings taken at each of two or more visits after an initial screening.

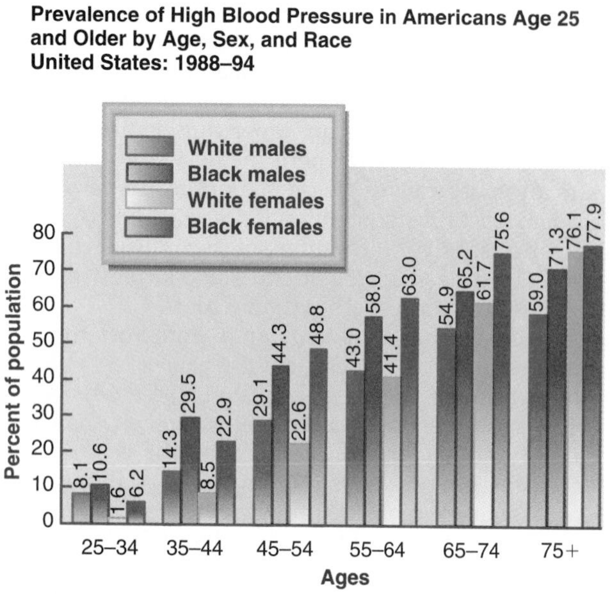

FIGURE 36-1 • Prevalence of hypertension by age. (Data from Wolz M et al: Statement from the National High Blood Pressure Education Program: prevalence of hypertension, *Am J Hypertens* 13:103-104, 2000.) Copyright American Journal of Hypertension Ltd.

Awareness of hypertension, treatment, and control improved over the last three decades and has leveled off since 1993 (JNC, 1997). In the third National Health and Nutrition Examination Survey (NHANES III, 1992-1994), 32% of persons with hypertension were not aware that they had it, 15% were aware and untreated, and 26% received treatment but did not reach recommended blood pressure goals (Hyman and Plavik, 2001). Thus, only 27% of Americans were adequately controlling their blood pressure. Predictors of lack of awareness of high blood pressure included male gender, non-Hispanic black race, age at least 65 years, and not having seen a physician in the past 12 months.

All these variables except race were also associated with poor control of hypertension in adults who knew they had high blood pressure. Younger persons (25 to 44 years of age) were more likely to be adequately treated and controlled (65%) than middle-aged (45 to 64 years) (52%) or older persons (65 of age and older) (34%). Having health insurance and a regular physician were not predictors of blood pressure being diagnosed or controlled. The *Healthy People 2010* goal is for at least 50% of people with hypertension to normalize their blood pressure through lifestyle or pharmacologic treatment (www.health.gov.healthypeople/).

Despite improvements in detection, the prevalence of hypertension has not declined (Kannel, 1996). Efforts at lowering blood pressure work well with committed participants (Wright et al, 2002). Physician treatment practices are partly responsible. Many physicians do not begin treatment until higher levels of blood pressure than recommended are reached, especially in older patients (Hyman and Plavik, 2000). To decrease this public health burden of hypertension, changes in physician practice must occur. In NHANES III, 36% had high normal blood pressure or were taking antihypertensive medication; of these, 5% had no other CVD risk factors; 66% had one major risk factor; and 29% had CVD, diabetes, or target organ disease (Munter et al, 2002). Clearly, a high normal blood pressure is not without risk and should be treated as recommended in the JNC VI (JNC VI, 1997).

In the Framingham Heart Study (see Chapter 35), the incidence of hypertension increased in a stepwise fashion in persons who were normotensive at baseline. For these participants who had an optimal blood pressure at baseline, the incidence over a 4-year period was 5%; for those whose blood pressure was normal, the incidence was 18%; and for those whose blood pressure was high normal, the rate was 37% (Vasan et al, 2001). For persons over 65 years of age, the incidence was 16% for persons with optimal blood pressure at baseline, 26% for persons with normal blood pressure, and 50% for those with high normal blood pressures. Obesity and weight gain were predictive of progression to hypertension; gaining 5% of body weight was associated with a 20% to 30% increase in hypertension.

MORBIDITY AND MORTALITY

Although hypertensive patients are often asymptomatic, hypertension is not a benign disease. Cardiac, cerebrovascular, and renal systems are affected by chronically elevated blood pressure (Table 36-2).

High blood pressure was the primary or a contributory cause in 227,000 of the two million deaths in 1999 (AHA, 2001). Between 1989 and 1999, the age-adjusted death rate from hypertension increased by 21%; overall deaths from hypertension increased by 46%. Death rates from hypertension are about four times higher in blacks than in whites. Atherosclerosis, the underlying cause of much CVD, is a direct result of hypertension-induced end-organ damage (Schwartz et al, 1994). In middle-aged men, a 20 mm Hg increase in SBP results in 60% higher mortality from CVD (Poulter and Sever, 1992). Consequently, 50% of patients with hypertension die of coronary heart disease (CHD) or congestive heart failure, 33% from stroke, and 10% to 15% from renal failure (Kaplan, 1992). Stroke and myocardial infarction also are major contributors to morbidity; between 500,000 and a million people have nonfatal events each year. The factors associ-

TABLE 36-2 Manifestations of Target Organ Disease From Hypertension

ORGAN SYSTEM	MANIFESTATIONS
Cardiac	Clinical, electrocardiographic, or radiologic evidence of coronary artery disease; left ventricular hypertrophy; left ventricular malfunction or cardiac failure
Cerebrovascular	Transient ischemic attack or stroke
Peripheral	Absence of one or more pulses in extremities (except for dorsalis pedis) with or without intermittent claudication; aneurysm
Renal	Serum creatinine >130 μmol/L (1.5 mg/dl); proteinuria (1 + or greater); microalbuminuria
Retinopathy	Hemorrhages or exudates, with or without papilledema

From the Joint National Committee on Prevention, Detection, Evaluation, and Treatment of High Blood Pressure: Fifth report (JNC V), *Arch Intern Med* 153:149, 1993.

Box 36-1. Factors Indicating Poor Prognosis in Hypertension

Black race
Youth
Male
Persistent diastolic pressure >115 mm Hg
Smoking
Diabetes mellitus
Hypercholesterolemia
Obesity
Excessive alcohol intake
Evidence of target organ disease

From Williams GH: Hypertensive vascular disease. In Issilbacher K et al, editors: *Harrison's principles of internal medicine,* ed 13, New York, 1994, McGraw-Hill.

ated with a poor prognosis in hypertension are shown in Box 36-1.

PATHOPHYSIOLOGY

Blood pressure is a function of cardiac output multiplied by the peripheral resistance (the resistance in the blood vessels to the flow of blood). The diameter of the blood vessel markedly affects blood flow. When the diameter is decreased (as in atherosclerosis), resistance and blood pressure increase. Conversely, when the diameter is increased (as with vasodilator drug therapy), resistance decreases and blood pressure is lowered.

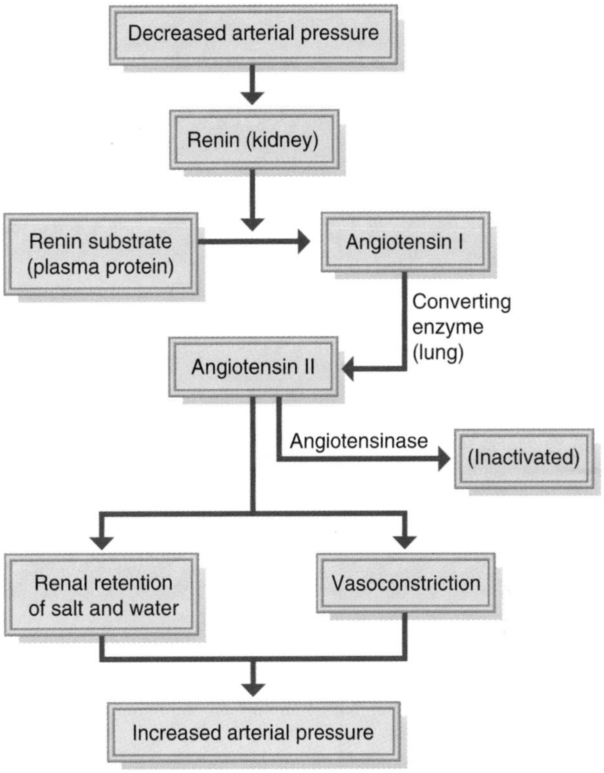

FIGURE 36-2 • Renin-angiotensin cascade.

Many systems maintain homeostatic control of blood pressure. The major regulators are the sympathetic nervous system (for short-term control) and the kidney (for long-term control). In response to a fall in blood pressure, the sympathetic nervous system secretes norepinephrine, a vasoconstrictor, which acts on small arteries and arterioles to increase peripheral resistance and raise blood pressure. The kidney regulates blood pressure by controlling the extracellular fluid volume and secreting renin, which activates the renin–angiotensin system (Figure 36-2).

When the regulatory mechanisms falter, hypertension develops. Plausible causes of hypertension are a hyperactive sympathetic nervous system, a stimulated renin-angiotensin system, a low-potassium diet, and use of the drug cyclosporine (Figure 36-3). All these cause vasoconstriction, which results in ischemia or arterial changes. There are probably many neurohormonal and intrarenal causes of abnormal blood pressure. In most cases of hypertension, peripheral resistance increases. This resistance forces the left ventricle of the heart to increase its effort in pumping blood through the system. With time, left ventricular hypertrophy and eventually congestive heart failure can develop (see Chapter 37).

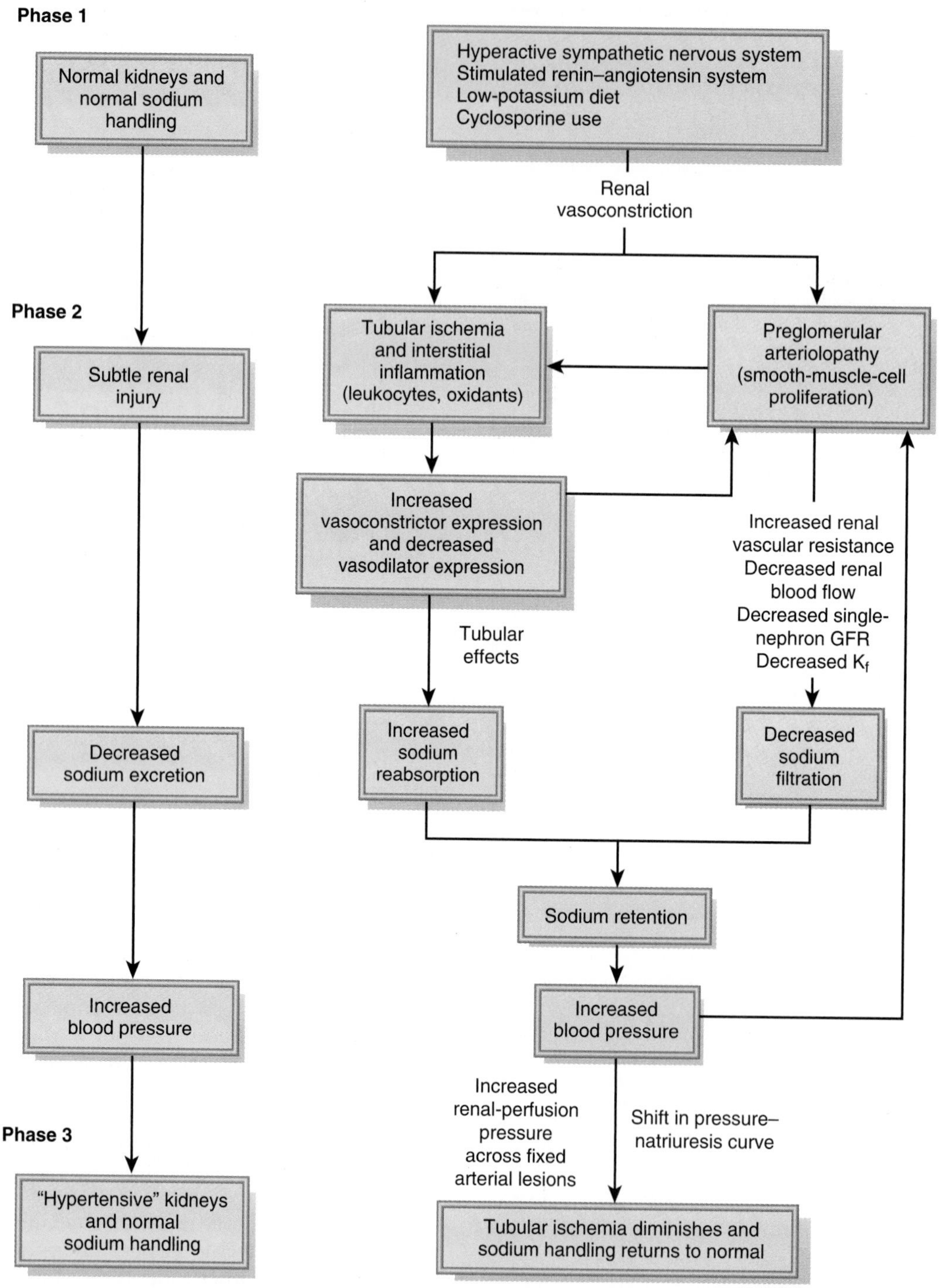

FIGURE 36-3 • Physiology of the development of hypertension. (From Johnson R et al: Subtle acquired renal injury as a mechanism of salt-sensitive hypertension, *N Engl J Med* 346(12):913, 2002. Copyright 2002, Massachusetts Medical Society.)

PRIMARY PREVENTION

The National High Blood Pressure Education Program (NHBPEP) is one of the most successful prevention programs in the twentieth century (Moser, 2002). Through educational efforts, detection, awareness, and treatment have improved over the 30 years since its inception. These changes have contributed to the decline in cardiovascular mortality seen during the same time period.

Primary prevention of hypertension can improve quality of life and costs associated with medical management of hypertension and its complications. A strategy for the population would be to reduce blood pressure in those with higher than optimal levels

Box 36-2. Risk Factors for Developing Hypertension

High-normal blood pressure
Family history of hypertension
African American ancestry
Overweight
Excessive salt consumption
Physical inactivity
Alcohol consumption

Modified from National High Blood Pressure Education Program (NHBPEP) Working Group: report on primary prevention of hypertension, *Arch Intern Med* 153:186, 1993. Copyright 1993, American Medical Association.

(above 120/80) but below the cut points for diagnosis. It was recently shown that these higher than normal blood pressures were associated with an increased risk of cardiovascular disease in the Framingham cohort (Vasan et al, 2001). A downward shift of 3 mm Hg in SBP would decrease the mortality from stroke by 8% and from CHD by 5% (JNC, 1993). Persons at highest risk (Box 36-2) should be strongly encouraged to adopt healthier lifestyles. Several lifestyle changes are essential for both prevention and management of hypertension (Box 36-3).

Box 36-3. Lifestyle Modifications for Hypertension Prevention and Management

Lose weight if overweight
Limit alcohol intake to no more than 1 oz (30 ml) of ethanol (e.g., 24 oz [720 ml] of beer, 10 oz [300 ml] of wine, or 2 oz [60 ml] of 100-proof whiskey) per day for men or 0.5 oz (15 ml) of ethanol per day for women and lighter-weight people
Increase aerobic physical activity to 30-45 min most days of the week
Reduce sodium intake to no more than 100 mmol/day (2.4 g sodium or 6 g sodium chloride)
Maintain adequate intake of dietary potassium (approximately 90 mmol/day)
Maintain adequate intake of dietary calcium and magnesium for general health
Stop smoking
Reduce intake of dietary saturated fat and cholesterol for overall cardiovascular health

From the Joint National Committee on Prevention, Detection, Evaluation, and Treatment of High Blood Pressure: Sixth report (JNC VI), *Arch Intern Med* 157:2413, 1997.

Dietary Factors

Changing four modifiable factors has documented efficacy in the primary prevention and control of hypertension. These four factors are overweight, high salt intake, alcohol consumption, and physical inactivity (JNC, 1997). A 5-year intervention trial in normotensive men and women demonstrated that lifestyle changes could lessen the incidence of hypertension. Intervention goals were to (1) lose 4.5 kg or 5% of body weight (whichever was greater), (2) follow an AHA fat-modified diet (see Chapter 35), (3) reduce sodium intake to 1800 mg daily (78 mEq) or less (see Chapter 37), (4) limit alcohol to no more than two drinks per day, and (5) increase physical activity to 30 minutes three times per week. The incidence of hypertension was 8% in the intervention group and 19% in the control group (Stamler et al, 1989b). Other trials have shown that the incidence of hypertension is significantly lowered by reduction of dietary sodium by 30 to 44 mEq daily (Kaplan, 2000).

Several nutrition intervention studies, the Trials of Hypertension Prevention (TOHP) (Trials, 1997), and Dietary Approaches to Stop Hypertension (DASH) studies (Appel et al, 1997) demonstrated the efficacy of dietary change in preventing hypertension or lowering blood pressure in persons with high-normal pressures. In the TOHP, weight loss (goal 4.5 kg loss) alone or in combination with sodium restriction (daily goal 80 mmol, or 80 mEq) lowered the incidence of hypertension; however, behavior changes were not sustained over time, thus diminishing the positive effects on blood pressure. The DASH study showed that a diet high in fruits, vegetables, and nonfat dairy foods and low in saturated fat and total fat (Table 36-3) decreased SBP an average of 6 to 11 mm Hg (Appel et al, 1997). The total diet was more effective than just adding fruits and vegetables.

The DASH diet is used for both preventing and controlling high blood pressure. Successful adoption of this diet requires many behavioral changes: twice the average number of daily servings of fruits, vegetables, and dairy products; one third the usual intake of beef, pork, and ham; one half the typical use of fats, oils, and salad dressings; and one quarter the number of snacks and sweets (Blackburn, 2001). Lactose-intolerant persons need to incorporate lactase enzyme or other strategies (Chapter 30). Assessing patient readiness to change and engaging patients in problem solving, decision making, and goal setting are behavioral strategies that may improve adherence (Windhauser, 1999) (see Chapter 22).

The high number of fruits and vegetables consumed on the DASH diet is a marked change from typical American patterns. To achieve the 8 to 10 servings, two to three fruits and vegetables are consumed at each meal (Table 36-4). The DASH pattern has been incorporated into the current AHA nutrition guidelines (Krauss, 2000). Servings for different calorie levels are shown in (Table 36-5). A quick assessment tool can help dietitians and patients to monitor progress (Table 36-6).

Excess Body Weight

Body weight is a determinant of blood pressure in most ethnic groups at all ages. The prevalence of high blood pressure in persons with a body mass index (BMI) greater than 30 is 38% for men and 32% for women compared with 18% for men and 17% for women with a normal BMI (<25) (National Institutes of Health [NIH], 1998). The risk of developing elevated blood pressure is two to six times higher in overweight than in normal-weight persons (JNC, 1993). Twenty to 30% of the hypertension seen in this country is attributable to the high prevalence of overweight. Weight gain during adult life is responsible for much of the rise in blood pressure seen with aging. In the Framingham Study, an increase in relative weight of 10% was predictive of a rise in blood pressure of 7 mm Hg.

Some of the physiologic changes proposed to explain the relationship between excess body weight and blood pressure are insulin resistance and hyperinsulinemia (see Chapter 12), activation of the sympathetic nervous and renin-angiotensin systems, and physical changes in the kidney (Hall, 1994). Increased energy intake is also associated with elevated plasma insulin, which is a potent natriuretic factor causing increased renal sodium reabsorption and consequent blood pressure elevation. Weight loss lowers vascular

TABLE 36-3 The DASH Diet*

FOOD GROUP	DAILY SERVINGS (except as noted)	SERVING SIZES	EXAMPLES AND NOTES	SIGNIFICANCE OF EACH FOOD GROUP TO THE DASH EATING PLAN
Grains and grain products	7-8	1 slice bread 1 c dry cereal† ½ c cooked rice, pasta, or cereal	Whole-wheat bread, English muffin, pita bread, bagel, cereals, grits, oatmeal, crackers, unsalted pretzels and popcorn	Major sources of energy and fiber
Vegetables	4-5	1 c raw leafy vegetable ½ c cooked vegetable 6 oz vegetable juice	Tomatoes, potatoes, carrots, green peas, squash, broccoli, turnip greens, collards, kale, spinach, artichokes, green beans, lima beans, sweet potatoes	Rich sources of potassium, magnesium, and fiber
Fruits	4-5	6 oz fruit juice 1 medium fruit ¼ c dried fruit ½ c fresh, frozen, or canned fruit	Apricots, bananas, dates, grapes, oranges, orange juice, grapefruit, grapefruit juice, mangoes, melons, peaches, pineapples, prunes, raisins, strawberries, tangerines	Important sources of potassium, magnesium, and fiber
Low-fat or fat-free dairy foods	2-3	8 oz milk 1 c yogurt 1½ oz cheese	Fat-free (skim) or low-fat (1%) milk, fat-free or low-fat buttermilk, fat free or low-fat regular or frozen yogurt, low-fat and fat-free cheese	Major sources of calcium and protein
Meats, poultry, and fish	2 or less	3 oz cooked meats, poultry, or fish	Select only lean; trim away visible fats; broil, roast, or boil, instead of frying; remove skin from poultry	Rich sources of protein and magnesium
Nuts, seeds, and dry beans	4-5/wk	⅓ c or 1½ oz nuts 2 tbsp or ½ oz seeds ½ c cooked dry beans	Almonds, filberts, mixed nuts, peanuts, walnuts, sunflower seeds, kidney beans, lentils and peas	Rich sources of energy, magnesium, potassium, protein, and fiber
Fats and oils‡	2-3	1 tsp soft margarine 1 tbsp low-fat mayonnaise 2 tbsp light salad dressing 1 tsp vegetable oil	Soft margarine, low-fat mayonnaise, light salad dressing, vegetable oil (such as olive, corn, canola, or safflower)	Besides fats added to foods, remember to choose foods that contain less fat
Sweets	5/wk	1 tbsp sugar 1 tbsp jelly or jam ½ oz jelly beans 8 oz lemonade	Maple syrup, sugar, jelly, jam, fruit-flavored gelatin, jelly beans, hard candy, fruit punch, sorbet, ices	Sweets should be low in fat

From National Institutes of Health (NIH), National Heart, Lung, and Blood Institute (NHLBI): *The DASH diet*, U.S. Department of Health and Human Services, Public Health Services, NIH Publication No. 99-4082, 1999.

*The DASH eating plan shown here is based on 2000 calories a day. The number of daily servings in a food group may vary from those listed depending on your caloric needs. Use this chart to help you plan your menus or take it with you when you go to the store.

†Serving sizes vary between ½ and 1¼ c. Check the product's nutrition label.

‡Fat content changes serving counts for fats and oils: For example, 1 tbsp of regular salad dressing equals 1 serving; 1 tbsp of a low-fat dressing equals ½ serving; 1 tbsp of a fat-free dressing equals 0 servings.

resistance, total blood volume, cardiac output, and sympathetic nervous system activity; suppresses the renin-angiotensin system; and improves insulin resistance (NIH, 1998).

As evidenced by the increasing prevalence of overweight in this country, weight management is a major effort for many persons, especially women. Interventions to prevent weight gain should target groups before they reach midlife. In black women, adolescence is the critical period for intervention (Melnyk and Weinstein, 1994). BMI is recommended as a screening tool for all adolescents (Gardin et al, 2002; Himes and Dietz, 1994). A BMI above 30 is the cutoff for obesity, and referral to a dietitian is warranted. With a large percentage of the population obese and hypertensive, better strategies are needed to prevent excess weight gain and improve compliance with treatment (St. Jeor et al, 1993) (see Chapter 24).

Early identification of children as potential hypertensives has been recommended, and a flowchart for identifying hypertensive children is shown in Figure 36-4 (Strong et al, 1992). Body fatness above 25% in boys and 30% in girls increases the risk of elevated blood pressure (Williams et al, 1992). The goal in children is to prevent the adoption of lifestyle factors (overweight, high salt intake, and sedentary patterns) that are related to the development of hypertension. Strategies for the prevention of obesity and hypertension in children are shown in Chapter 24.

TABLE 36-4 Sample Menu for the DASH Diet

FOOD	AMOUNT	SERVINGS PROVIDED
Breakfast		
Orange juice	6 oz	1 fruit
1% low-fat milk	8 oz (1 c)	1 dairy
Corn flakes (with 1 tsp sugar)	1 c	2 grains
Banana	1 medium	1 fruit
Whole-wheat bread (with 1 tbsp jelly)	1 slice	1 grain
Soft margarine	1 tsp	1 fat
Lunch		
Chicken salad	¾ c	1 poultry
Pita bread	½ slice, large	1 grain
Raw vegetable medley:		
Carrot and celery sticks	3-4 sticks each	1 vegetable
Radishes	2	
Loose-leaf lettuce	2 leaves	
Part-skim mozzarella cheese	1.5 slice (1.5 oz)	1 dairy
1% low-fat milk	8 oz	1 dairy
Fruit cocktail in light syrup	½ c	1 fruit
Dinner		
Herbed baked cod	3 oz	1 fish
Scallion rice	1 c	2 grains
Steamed broccoli	½ c	1 vegetable
Stewed tomatoes	½ c	1 vegetable
Spinach salad:		
Raw spinach	½ c	1 vegetable
Cherry tomatoes	2	
Cucumber	2 slices	
Light Italian salad dressing	1 tbsp	½ fat
Whole-wheat dinner roll	1 small	1 grain
Soft margarine	1 tsp	1 fat
Melon balls	½ c	1 fruit
Snacks		
Dried apricots	1 oz (¼ c)	1 fruit
Mini pretzels	1 oz (¾ c)	1 grain
Mixed nuts	1.5 oz (⅓ c)	1 nuts
Diet ginger ale	12 oz	0

From Appel LJ et al: A clinical trial of the effects of dietary patterns on blood pressure, *N Engl J Med* 336:1117, 1997.

Excessive Consumption of Sodium Chloride

Epidemiologic studies of populations support an etiologic role for salt in hypertension development. Primitive societies in which the intake of sodium is low (70 mEq/day) experience very little hypertension, and the blood pressure increase with age, common in industrialized societies, does not occur (Stamler, 1992). Hypertension is prevalent and stroke is the leading cause of death in countries with very high salt consumption (9 to 12 g daily or 150 to 200 mEq sodium daily). The strength of the relationship between salt consumption and blood pressure is stronger in older people, in those with a family history of hypertension, and in those with higher blood pressures at baseline (Kotchen and McCarron, 1998).

The INTERSALT study, a cross-sectional study involving 52 centers worldwide and more than 10,000 subjects, showed SBP was significantly related to dietary sodium intake (salt-sensitive hypertension) (Elliot et al, 1996). Excreting a 100 mEq difference in sodium in the urine (170 mEq sodium versus 70 mEq) was associated with an increase of 3 to 6 mm Hg in SBP (see *Focus On:* Sodium Equivalents).

In another population study of 24 communities, a difference in sodium intake of 100 mEq/24 hours was associated with a 10 mm Hg fall in SBP in 60- to 69-year-old adults (Stamler et al, 1989a). The rise in SBP seen with aging over a 30-year period would be

TABLE 36-5 DASH Diet Serving Sizes for Different Calorie Levels

CALORIES	GRAINS	VEGETABLES	FRUIT	DAIRY	MEAT, POULTRY, FISH	NUTS, SEEDS, LEGUMES	FATS AND OILS
1600	6	4	4	2	1	0.5	1
2000	8	5	5	3	2	1	2
2600	10	5	5	3	2	1	2
3100	13	6	6	4	2	1	3

TABLE 36-6 What's on Your Plate?

FOOD	AMOUNT (SERVING SIZE)	NO. OF SERVINGS BY DASH FOOD GROUP							
		GRAINS	VEGETABLES	FRUITS	DAIRY FOODS	MEAT, POULTRY, AND FISH	NUTS, SEEDS, AND DRY BEANS	FATS AND OILS	SWEETS
Breakfast *Example: whole-wheat bread and soft margarine*	*2 slices* *2 tsp*	2						2	
Lunch									
Dinner									
Snacks									
DAY'S TOTAL									
Compare yours with the DASH plan		7-8	4-5	4-5	2-3	2 or less	4-5 a week	2-3	5 a week

From the National Institutes of Health (NIH), National Heart, Lung, and Blood Institute (NALBI): *The DASH diet,* U.S. Department of Health and Human Services, Public Health Services, NIH Publication No. 99-4082, 1999.

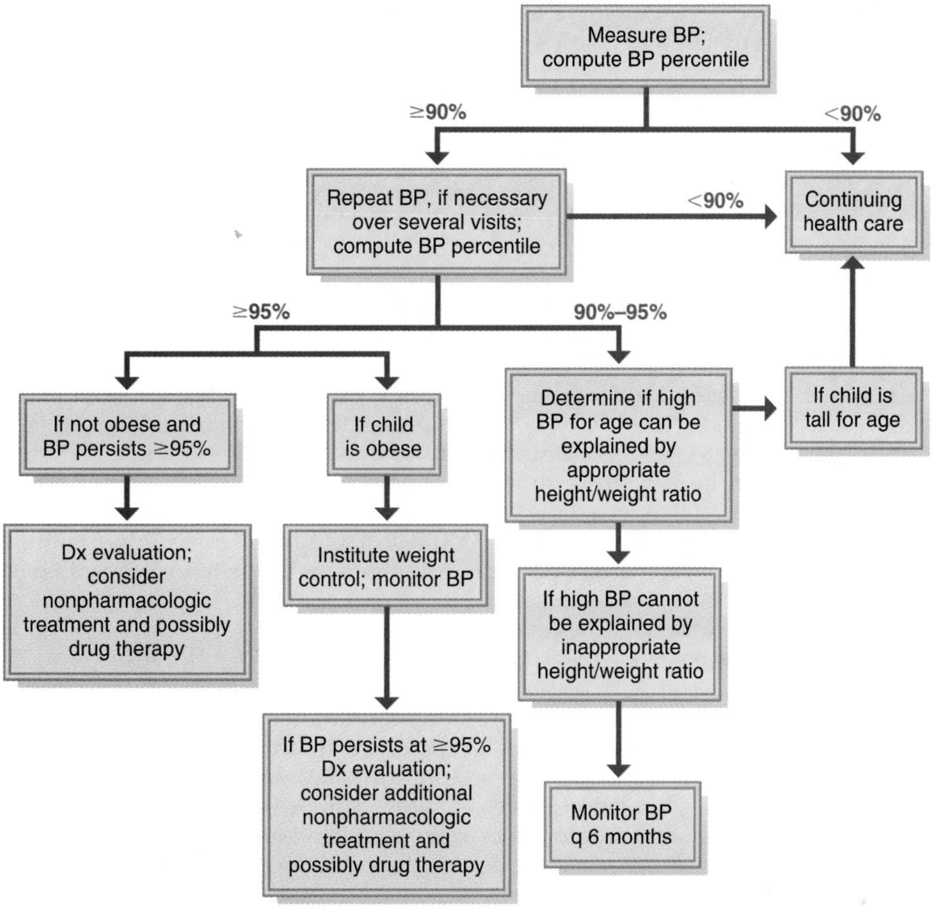

FIGURE 36-4 • Flowchart for identifying children with high blood pressure (BP). (From Strong WB et al: Integrated cardiovascular health promotion in childhood: a statement for health professionals from the Subcommittee on Atherosclerosis and Hypertension in Childhood for the Council on Cardiovascular Disease in the Young, *Circulation* 85:1638, 1992.)

FOCUS ON

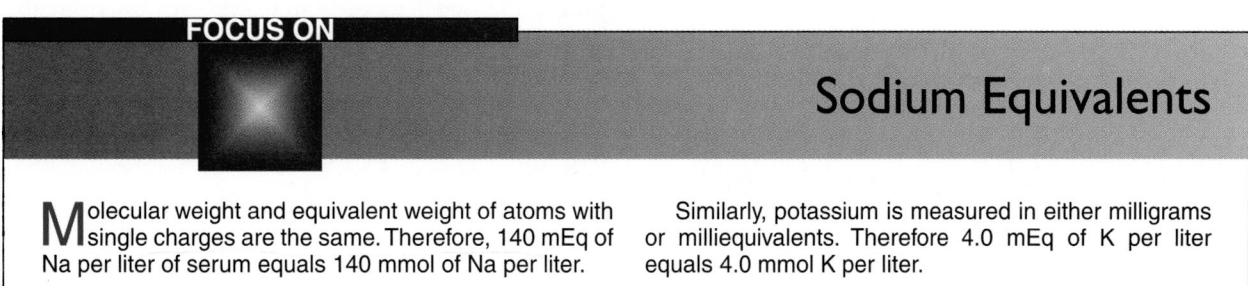

Sodium Equivalents

Molecular weight and equivalent weight of atoms with single charges are the same. Therefore, 140 mEq of Na per liter of serum equals 140 mmol of Na per liter.

Similarly, potassium is measured in either milligrams or milliequivalents. Therefore 4.0 mEq of K per liter equals 4.0 mmol K per liter.

9 mm Hg less and the rise in DBP 4.5 mm Hg less if the average sodium intake were lowered by 100 mEq daily.

Along with the epidemiologic data, clinical trial data also support the positive relationship between sodium and blood pressure. The DASH diet at different levels of sodium intake was tested in the randomized clinical trial. The DASH diet with a low sodium intake (65 mEq daily) produced the lowest blood pressures; that is, SBP was lowered by 12 mm Hg in hypertensives and 7 mm Hg in normotensives (Sacks, 2001). The additive effects of a DASH low sodium diet compared with a DASH high-sodium diet (3.5 g) was a lowering of SBP 3 mm Hg and DBP of 2 mm Hg. A reduction of 2 mm Hg in blood pressure is associated with a 17% reduction in the prevalence of hypertension, 6% reduction in CHD, and 15% reduction in stroke and transient ischemic attacks.

Some persons with hypertension do not increase blood pressure with higher salt intakes (salt-resistant hypertension). About 30% to 50% of hypertensives and 15% to 25% of normotensives are salt sensitive. Features of salt-sensitive hypertension are black race, obesity, advanced age, diabetes, renal dysfunction, and use of the drug cyclosporine (Johnson et al, 2002). Salt-sensitive people experience a decrease of

10 mm Hg in blood pressure when following a low-salt diet after salt loading or a more than 5% increase in blood pressure during salt repletion after restriction (Kotchen, 1991). Currently, methods are lacking for identifying these "salt-sensitive" individuals (see *New Directions:* Method for Determining Salt Sensitivity).

A high salt intake has also been implicated in hypertensive target organ disease (Messerli et al, 1997). Nine studies showed that 24-hour urinary sodium excretion was an independent determinant of left ventricular mass, and other studies have found that salt intake affects hypertensive renal disease and CVD, especially in salt-sensitive individuals. Because one cannot readily determine salt sensitivity, and Americans consume salt in great excess of physiologic requirements, a reduction in salt intake to no more than 6 g daily (100 mEq or 2400 mg Na daily) is recommended to prevent hypertension. This level can be achieved by cooking with as little salt as possible, refraining from adding salt at the table, and avoiding highly salted, processed foods or eating at restaurants where sodium is not controlled (see 2-g sodium diet in Chapter 37).

Alcohol Consumption

Five to 7% of the hypertension in the population is due to alcohol consumption (Joint National Committee, 1997). Three drinks per day (a total of 3 oz of alcohol) is the threshold for raising blood pressure and is associated with a 3 mm Hg rise. For preventing high blood pressure, alcohol intake should be less than two drinks per day (24 oz beer, 10 oz wine, or 2 oz 100-proof whiskey) in men. In women and lighter-weight persons, no more than one drink a day is recommended.

Physical Activity

Less active persons are 30% to 50% more likely to develop hypertension than their active counterparts. In the Framingham Study, medium to high levels of physical activity were protective against developing stroke (Kiely et al, 1994). Despite the benefits of activity and exercise in reducing disease, many Americans remain inactive. Hispanics (50% men, 57% women), blacks (46% men, 57% women), and whites (33% men, 39% women) all have a high prevalence of sedentary lifestyles (AHA, 2001).

Two metaanalyses have demonstrated the beneficial effects of exercise on blood pressure. The first analysis showed that walking reduced blood pressure in adults by an average of 2% (Kelley, 2001). Second, in 54 randomized clinical trials, aerobic exercise reduced blood pressure an average of 4 mm Hg for systolic and 2 mm Hg for diastolic pressure in patients with and without high blood pressure, irrespective of body weight change (Whelton et al, 2002). Thus, increasing the amount of physical activity of low to moderate intensity to 30 to 45 minutes most days of the week is an important adjunct to other strategies for the primary prevention of hypertension.

Other Dietary Factors

Potassium

In population studies, dietary potassium and blood pressure are inversely related; that is, higher potassium intakes are associated with lower blood pressures. More often, the sodium/potassium ratio of the diet is related to blood pressure. With a dietary sodium intake of 100 mmol less than normal and a potassium consumption of up to 70 mmol daily for a sodium/potassium ratio of about 1.0, a 3.4 mm Hg decrease in SBP is predicted. Effects of potassium intake on blood pressure include reduced peripheral vascular resistance by direct arteriolar dilatation, increased loss of water and sodium from the body, suppression of renin and angiotensin secretion, decrease of adrenergic tone, and stimulation of the sodium-potassium pump activity. A metaanalysis found that high dietary potassium may help prevent and control hypertension (Whelton et al, 1997).

NEW DIRECTIONS

Method for Determining Salt Sensitivity

The Salt Step Test was developed to help determine which hypertensive patients are sensitive to salt. The three phases include the following:

Phase 1: Consume a normal diet to establish baseline salt intake. Measure blood pressure. Determine urinary salt excretion.

Phase 2: Consume a 2-g (34 mmol daily equivalent to 745 mg Na daily) salt-restricted diet for 2 weeks. Measure blood pressure. If DBP $<$90 mm Hg, the patient is salt-sensitive and needs a 24-hour urine collection. After 1 month, if DBP is $>$90 mm Hg, with a urinary NaCl of $<$34 mmol/24 hours, then the patient is salt-resistant.

Phase 3: Consume a 2-g salt diet, but add 1 g of salt/day. Each 1-g increase in salt is consumed for 3 days. Blood pressure is measured at each step. When DBP is $>$90 mm Hg, then 24-hour urine is collected. A threshold for salt intake is established.

Data from Espinel C: The salt step test: its usage in the diagnosis of salt hypertension threshold, *J Am Coll Nutr* 11:526, 1992.

Potassium intake has also been related to stroke mortality. In a large population-based cohort, a 10 mEq daily (10 mmol daily) increase in potassium intake—the equivalent of one or two extra servings of fruit, citrus juice, vegetable, or potato—was related to a 40% decrease in the incidence of stroke-related deaths, unrelated to any change in blood pressure (Khaw and Barrett-Connor, 1988). More recently, data from the NHANES survey suggest that low dietary potassium intake is associated with an increased risk of stroke (Bazzano et al, 2001).

The large number of fruits and vegetables recommended in the DASH diet makes it easy to meet the recommendations of the JNC and AHA—that is, a potassium intake of approximately 90 mmol daily (90 mEq daily) (JNC, 1997; Kotchen and McCarron, 1998).

Calcium

Most population studies have found no significant relationship between dietary calcium and the prevalence of hypertension. Where a relationship existed, it appeared more often in African Americans and women. Increasing dairy product consumption (for a total calcium intake of 1500 mg daily) had no effect on blood pressure in hypertensive men (Kynast-Gales and Massey, 1992). Thus, the role of calcium supplementation in preventing hypertension is yet unproved.

The JNC VI includes recommendations for prevention and management of hypertension, including increasing potassium, calcium, and magnesium intake along with aggressive control of blood pressure (Davis and Jones, 2002). An intake of dietary calcium to meet the goal of 1000 to 2000 mg daily is recommended (Kotchen and McCarron, 1998).

Magnesium

Magnesium is a potent inhibitor of vascular smooth-muscle contraction and may play a role in blood pressure regulation as a vasodilator. An inverse relationship has been reported between dietary magnesium and blood pressure (JNC, 1997). In most clinical studies, however, magnesium supplementation has been ineffective in altering blood pressure, possibly because of the confounding effects of antihypertensive medications and the short duration of the studies. Overall, adequate data are lacking to recommend routine supplementation with magnesium to prevent hypertension.

Lipids

Fewer vegans have hypertension than omnivores, even though their salt intake is not significantly different. The vegan diet tends to be higher in polyunsaturated fatty acids (PUFAs), among other nutrients, and lower in total fat, saturated fatty acids, and cholesterol. PUFAs are precursors of prostaglandins, whose actions affect renal sodium excretion and relax vascular musculature. Thus, an effect on blood pressure is plausible.

Both the amount and type of fat have been studied with respect to blood pressure. In a large cohort study of male health professionals (Ascherio et al, 1992), neither total fat nor specific fatty acids were related to baseline blood pressure or incidence of hypertension over a 4-year period. Most other studies have found no hypotensive effect of PUFAs, which led the National High Blood Pressure Education Program Working Group (1994) to conclude that "macronutrient alteration has limited or unproven efficacy in the primary prevention of hypertension." More recently, studies have shown that supplementation with large doses of fish oil (median dose of 3.7 g/day) can give a modest reduction in SBP and DBP, especially in older hypertensive persons (Geleijnse et al, 2002).

Other Factors

Factors other than dietary fat, such as increased potassium levels, appear to lower blood pressure in vegans. Although dietary lipids do not seem to affect blood pressure, they strongly affect CVD risk; thus, the step I diet is recommended for preventing complications from hypertension and CVD (see Chapter 35). Although fatty acids may not directly affect blood pressure, an olive oil–enriched diet has been shown to decrease antihypertensive drug usage by 48% (Ferrara, 2000). Soy protein is another factor that may contribute to the lowering of blood pressure (Hecker, 2001).

Combination of Risk Factors for Cardiovascular Disease

Hypertension often occurs with other risk factors for CVD. In the NHANES III survey (National Education Programs, 1991) 40% of persons with hypertension had high blood cholesterol levels (>240 mg/dl). Fifty-five percent of overweight men have hypertension compared with 27% of normal-weight men. Having a combination of risk factors markedly increases the risk for CVD. A nonsmoker with normal blood cholesterol and blood pressure has one tenth the risk of developing CVD of a person with hypertension and hypercholesterolemia.

Researchers have noted a larger than normal clustering of abdominal obesity, high triglyceride levels, low high-density lipoprotein (HDL) cholesterol, high blood pressure, and high fasting glucose. The most recent recommendations of the National Cholesterol Education Program are calling this metabolic syndrome (NCEP, 2001). For metabolic syndrome to be diagnosed, three of the five risk factors must be present (see Chapter 35). In a large New England sample, the prevalence of dyslipidemic hypertension was 15%, or 1.5 times the expected number if the diseases were independent (Eaton et al, 1993). Lifestyle modifications

Box 36-4. Components of Cardiovascular Risk Stratification in Patients With Hypertension

Major Risk Factors

Smoking
Dyslipidemia
Diabetes mellitus
Age >60 yr
Sex (men and postmenopausal women)
Family history of cardiovascular disease: women <65 yr or men <55 yr

Target Organ Damage/Clinical Cardiovascular Disease

Heart diseases
- Left ventricular hypertrophy
- Angina or prior myocardial infarction
- Prior coronary revascularization
- Heart failure

Stroke or transient ischemic attack
Nephropathy
Peripheral arterial disease
Retinopathy

From the Joint National Committee on Prevention, Detection, Evaluation, and Treatment of High Blood Pressure: Sixth report (JNC VI), *Arch Intern Med* 157:2413, 1997.

can prevent metabolic syndrome from developing (see Chapters 12 and 24). Box 36-4 indicates components of risk stratification related to hypertension.

Medications

A number of medications either raise blood pressure or interfere with the effectiveness of antihypertensive drugs. These include oral contraceptives, steroids, nonsteroidal antiinflammatory drugs (NSAIDs), nasal decongestants and other cold remedies, appetite suppressants, cyclosporin tricyclic antidepressants, and monoamine-oxidase inhibitors (see Chapter 19).

MEDICAL MANAGEMENT

The goal of hypertension management is to reduce morbidity and mortality from stroke, hypertension-associated heart disease, and renal disease. Three objectives for evaluating patients with hypertension are (1) to identify the possible causes, (2) to assess the presence or absence of target organ disease and clinical CVD, and (3) to identify other CVD risk factors that will help guide treatment (JNC, 1997). Weight history, leisure-time physical activity, and dietary assessment of sodium, alcohol, saturated fat, and caffeine are components of the medical history (Figure 36-5). The presence of risk factors and target organ damage determines treatment aggressiveness. As shown in Table 36-7, lifestyle changes are primary therapy in four of the nine risk groups and adjunctive therapy in all other groups.

Lifestyle Modifications

Lifestyle modifications are definitive therapy for some and adjunctive therapy for all persons with hypertension (JNC, 1997). Depending on the risk group, 6 to 12 months of compliant lifestyle modifications should be tried before drug therapy is begun. Even if lifestyle modifications cannot completely correct the blood pressure, they will help increase the efficacy of pharmacologic agents and improve other CVD risk factors. Management of hypertension requires a lifelong commitment.

Weight Management

The effectiveness of weight reduction has been well documented in both mild and severe hypertensives. Hypertensive patients who weigh more than 115% of ideal body weight should be placed on an individualized weight-reduction program that focuses on both hypocaloric dietary intake and exercise. Themes for a weight-reduction program are shown in Box 36-5 (also see Chapter 24).

In the Trial of Antihypertensive Intervention and Management, the goal for energy intake to facilitate weight loss was 25 kcal/kg minus 500 to 1000 kcal daily to produce a 0.5- to 1-kg/week deficit that would reach a total weight loss of 4.5 kg (Wylie-Rosett et al, 1993). This modest loss will not only lower blood pressure but often will normalize blood lipids and glucose. The greater the weight loss, the greater the blood pressure reduction (Stevens et al, 1993). Some stage 1 hypertensives achieve normal blood pressure by weight loss alone.

Another benefit of weight loss on blood pressure is the synergistic effect with drug therapy. In subjects who lost weight and were taking one antihypertensive drug, lowering of blood pressure was greater than in those taking the drug alone (Wylie-Rosett et al, 1993). Therefore, weight loss should be an adjunct to drug therapy because it may decrease the dose or number of drugs necessary to control blood pressure. Furthermore, weight loss lowers blood pressure significantly more than a low-sodium/high-potassium diet. Because weight loss and exercise increase insulin sensitivity, lower levels of triglycerides, and raise HDL cholesterol, this combined intervention is also recommended for treating dyslipidemic hypertension (Eaton et al, 1993).

Once weight is lost, maintenance is critical. Unfortunately, relapse and weight gains are common fol-

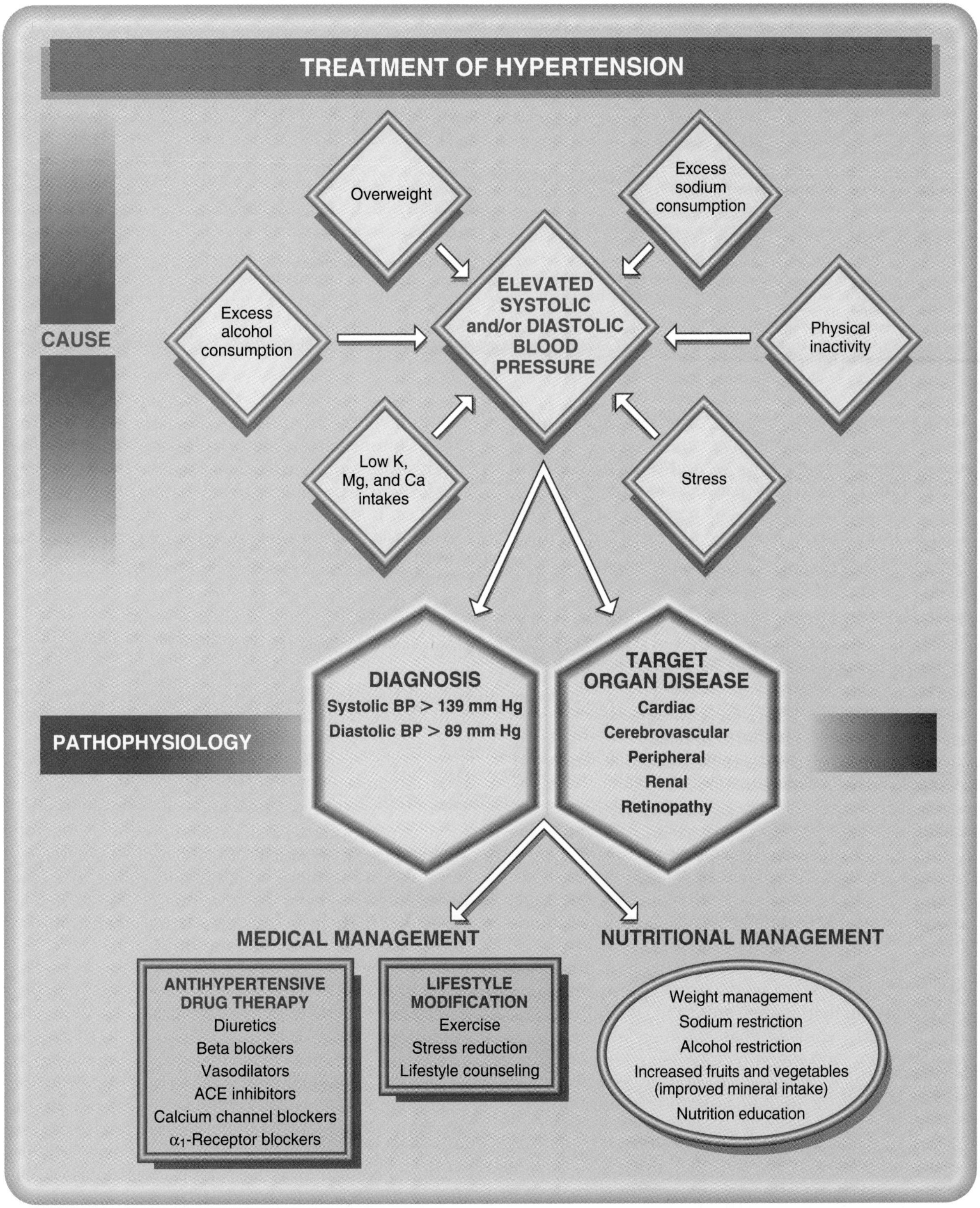

FIGURE 36-5 • Pathophysiology algorithm: treatment of hypertension. *ACE,* Angiotensin-converting enzyme; *BP,* blood pressure. (Algorithm content developed by John Anderson, PhD, and Sanford C. Garner, PhD, 2000.)

TABLE 36-7 Risk Stratification and Treatment

BLOOD PRESSURE STAGES (mm Hg)*	LOW-RISK GROUP (NO RISK FACTORS; NO TOD/CCD†)	MEDIUM-RISK GROUP (AT LEAST 1 RISK FACTOR, NOT INCLUDING DIABETES; NO TOD/CCD)	HIGH-RISK GROUP (TOD/CCD AND/OR DIABETES, WITH OR WITHOUT OTHER RISK FACTORS)
High-normal (130-139/85-89)	Lifestyle modification	Lifestyle modification	Drug therapy§
Stage 1 (140-159/90-99)	Lifestyle modification (up to 12 mo)	Lifestyle modification‡ (up to 6 mo)	Drug therapy
Stages 2 and 3 (≥160/≥100)	Drug therapy	Drug therapy	Drug therapy

Modified from the Joint National Committee on Prevention, Detection, Evaluation, and Treatment of High Blood Pressure: Sixth report (JNC VI), *Arch Intern Med* 157:2413, 1997.
**Note:* For example, a patient with diabetes and a blood pressure of 142/94 mm Hg plus left ventricular hypertrophy should be classified as having stage 1 hypertension with target organ disease (left ventricular hypertrophy) and with another major risk factor (diabetes). This patient would be categorized as "Stage 1, Risk Group C," and recommended for immediate initiation of pharmacologic treatment. Lifestyle modification should be adjunctive therapy for all patients recommended for pharmacologic therapy.
†*TOD/CCD* indicates target organ disease/clinical cardiovascular disease.
‡For patients with multiple risk factors, clinicians should consider drugs as initial therapy plus lifestyle modifications.
§For those with heart failure, renal insufficiency, or diabetes.

lowing weight loss. Some factors associated with effective weight maintenance are exercise, positive self-statements related to weight-reduction efforts, self-monitoring activities (use of a food diary, goal setting, early attention to weight regain), and problem-solving skills in lieu of eating during stressful times (see Chapter 24).

Salt Restriction

Moderate salt restriction (6 g salt, 100 mEq or 2400 mg Na daily) is recommended for treatment of hypertension. The restriction is for salt because the chloride ion with sodium raises blood pressure. In stage 1 hypertension, this level of salt restriction may be sufficient to normalize blood pressure. Patients who require drug therapy also need salt restriction for enhanced drug efficacy. Adherence is better for less restrictive salt reductions. Therefore, more severe salt restrictions are not necessary unless congestive heart failure is present, and 3 g of sodium is what is recommended (see Chapter 37). To assess dietary salt intake, 3 days of diet records and three overnight urine collections provide the best estimate (Dubbert et al, 1992).

Because most dietary salt comes from processed foods and eating out, changes in food preparation and processing can help patients reach the sodium goal. A sensory study showed that commercial processing could develop and revise recipes using lower sodium concentrations (0.15% to 0.30% sodium concentration as the baseline for initial acceptance testing) and reduce added sodium by 30% to 50% without affecting consumer acceptance (Adams et al, 1994).

Other Dietary Modifications

Minerals

Although some data suggest a benefit with increased intakes of potassium, calcium, and magnesium, the information available at this time is insufficient to support a specific recommendation for increased levels of intake, including the use of supplements, except to meet the adequate intake (AI) for calcium and the recommended dietary allowances (RDAs) for magnesium and to increase intakes of fruits and vegetables when possible. Sodium and potassium goals based on body weight are shown in Table 36-8. The DASH diet includes an increase in key minerals as part of the plan.

Lipids

Current recommendations for lipid composition of the diet are those recommended for the National Cholesterol Education Program (NCEP) (see Chapter 35) to help control weight and decrease the risk of CVD.

Alcohol

The diet history should contain information about alcohol consumption. As discussed previously, alcohol intake should be limited to not more than 1 oz of ethanol daily in men, which is equivalent to 2 oz of 100-proof whiskey, 8 oz of wine, or 24 oz of beer. Women or lighter-weight men should consume half this amount (0.5 oz of ethanol/day).

Exercise

Moderate physical activity, defined as 30 to 45 minutes of brisk walking on most days of the week, is recommended as an adjunct therapy in hypertension. Overweight or obese hypertensive patients should strive for 300 to 500 kcal expended in exercise per day or 1000 to 2000 kcal per week to promote weight loss or weight control. Because exercise is strongly associated with success in weight-reduction and weight-maintenance programs, any increase in activity level should be encouraged.

Pharmacologic Treatment

If blood pressure remains elevated after 6 to 12 months of lifestyle changes, antihypertensive medications are

Box 36-5. Programs for Intensive Interventions for Hypertension Management

Weight Control Intervention	Low-Sodium/High-Potassium Intervention
Session 1 • Introduction to program, process, and monitoring • Establishing weight and energy intake goals	**Session 1** • Introduction to program, process, and monitoring • Rationale for low-sodium/high-potassium modification
Session 2 • Assessing lifestyle factors that influence eating • Reading labels focusing on ingredients, kilocalorie information, and serving size (introduction to the concept of caloric density)	**Session 2** • Establishing goals for sodium and potassium intake • Reading labels and identifying foods low in sodium and high in potassium
Session 3 • Identifying and changing eating cues	**Session 3** • Identifying sources of sodium and potassium from diaries
Session 4 • Food shopping, preparation, and restaurant eating	**Session 4** • Changing shopping habits (e.g., reducing number of processed foods) • Selecting low-sodium/high-potassium items from restaurant menus
Session 5 • Assessing social supports and self-reinforcement and establishing control over situations that involve eating	**Session 5** • Examining problem foods that are high in sodium (cue and response analysis)
Session 6 • Identifying low-calorie snack foods, fast foods, and beverages • Establishing routine physical activities	**Session 6** • Preparing foods to maintain maximal potassium content (e.g., steaming, using a minimum amount of water, or consuming raw)
Session 7 • Setting realistic goals • Coping with feelings and behavioral lapses • Evaluating the Trial of Antihypertensive Intervention and Management cookbook	**Session 7** • Learning to use spices and herbs as alternatives to high-sodium seasonings • Evaluating the Trial of Antihypertensive Intervention and Management cookbook
Session 8 • Evaluating and promoting personal motivation and commitment • Evaluating changes in preparation and food selection	**Session 8** • Modifying recipes to lower sodium content • Reviewing low-sodium cookbooks • Preparing low-sodium, high-potassium snacks and desserts
Session 9 • Planning food for a party and for special occasions • Modifying favorite recipes	**Session 9** • Sharing low-sodium and high-potassium recipes • Planning food for special party occasions
Session 10 • Learning how to maintain weight loss and behavioral changes • Reviewing accomplishments (knowledge and skill acquired) • Assessing long-term commitment to new behavior and to follow-up program	**Session 10** • Learning how to maintain changes (e.g., in shopping and food preparation) • Reviewing accomplishments • Assessing long-term commitment and follow-up

Themes presented above are for the 10 group sessions during intensive intervention. The first 15 to 30 minutes of each session are devoted to reviewing (by use of diaries) progress on goals established the previous week. Each session ends with behavioral goal setting.

From Wylie-Rosett J et al: Trial of antihypertensive intervention and management: greater efficacy with weight reduction than with a sodium-potassium intervention, *J Am Diet Assoc* 93:408, 1993.

TABLE 36-8 Goals for Sodium and Potassium Intakes Based on Body Weight

WEIGHT (kg)	SODIUM (mEq)	POTASSIUM (mEq)
≤50.0	52.2	61.5
50.5-60.0	60.1	71.8
60.5-70.0	70.0	82.1
70.5-80.0	78.3	92.3
80.5-90.0	87.5	102.6
≥90.5	100.0	115.4

From Wylie-Rosett J et al: Trial of antihypertensive intervention and management: greater efficacy with weight reduction than with a sodium-potassium intervention, *J Am Diet Assoc* 93:408, 1993.

started. Most patients with hypertension more severe than stage 1 hypertension require drug treatment; however, lifestyle modifications are still a part of therapy even when drugs are used. The standard treatment for hypertension includes diuretics and β-blockers, although other drugs (angiotensin-converting enzyme inhibitors, α1-receptor blockers, and calcium antagonists) are equally effective. All these drugs can affect nutritional status (see Chapter 19 and Appendix 34).

Diuretics lower blood pressure in some patients by promoting volume depletion and sodium loss; however, thiazide diuretics increase urinary potassium excretion, especially in the presence of a high salt intake, thus leading to potassium loss and possibly hypokalemia. Except in the case of a potassium-sparing diuretic, such as spironolactone or triamterene, additional potassium is usually required.

Treatment of Blood Pressure in Older Adults

More than half of the older population has hypertension; this is not a normal consequence of aging, but CVD risk in older adults is two to three times higher than in the middle-age population. The lifestyle modifications discussed previously are the first step in treatment of older adults, as with younger populations. The Trial of Nonpharmacologic Interventions in the Elderly (TONE) study found that losing weight (8 to 10 lb) and reducing salt intake (1800 mg Na daily) can lessen or eliminate the need for drugs in obese, hypertensive older adults (60 to 80 years of age) (Whelton et al, 1998). At the end of the 30-month study, 31% of the sodium-reduction-alone group, 36% of the weight-reduction-alone group, and 53% of the combination group were off medications.

Although this study showed that losing weight and decreasing sodium in older adults were very effective in lowering blood pressure, knowing how to facilitate these changes and promote adherence remains an obstacle for health professionals. Only 38% in the TONE study were able to reach the sodium intake goals. Looking at dose-response analyses, those with greater sodium reduction had fewer occurrences of average SBP over 150 or DBP over 90 (Appel et al, 2001). Severe sodium restrictions are not adopted because these could lead to volume depletion in older patients with renal damage (National High Blood Pressure Education Program, 1994).

Drug treatment in the older adult is supported by very strong data from the Systolic Hypertension in the Elderly Program (Staessen, 1999), which investigated thiazide-based therapy in hypertensives (SBP over 160 mm Hg; normal DBP) over the age of 60 years. After 5 years of treatment with antihypertensive drugs, blood pressures were lowered by 14 mm Hg more than with placebo, which translated into 27% reduction in myocardial infarction, 55% reduction in congestive heart failure, and 37% reduction in stroke. Based on these and other similar data, NHLBI recommends that blood pressures be controlled regardless of age, initial blood pressure level, or duration of hypertension (NHLBI, 1999).

SUMMARY

Several lifestyle changes can lower blood pressure and prevent or control hypertension. Weight control, physical activity, and a low-fat diet rich in fruits and vegetables, with nonfat dairy foods and nuts incorporated have all been shown to lower blood pressure. A major reason for inadequate control of high blood pressure is poor adherence to therapy. The *Healthy People 2000* objective was to increase to at least 90% the number of people with hypertension who were trying to normalize their blood pressure. This goal was not achieved. Thirty-one percent of subjects in NHANES III with high blood pressure were not even aware they had hypertension. Barriers to adherence need to be investigated and remedied.

Clinical Scenario 1

Bob is a 56-year-old white man who works as a truck driver. He is on the road every week and recently saw his physician about headaches, dizziness, and insomnia. He was diagnosed as having hypertension, with three blood pressure tests of 160/90, 175/95, and 177/92. His physician gave him a diuretic, Lasix, and a β-blocker (Inderal). Bob was also given a diet sheet with a brief overview of a no-added-salt diet. Bob has contacted you for assistance in planning menus he can follow.

1. Write a week's set of menus for Bob to follow, starting with a meal at home for breakfast, at a restaurant for lunch, and from a carryout deli late at night.
2. Bob generally consumes one or two beers before bedtime and is willing to give up that habit. What healthy snack habits might Bob have in the evening?
3. Because Bob is on the road so much, food safety might be a problem. What tips would you suggest for meals and snacks that he can keep in his truck?

Clinical Scenario 2

Nell is a 27-year-old white woman who follows traditional Judaism. In her meal planning, she uses many foods that have been prepared in a kosher manner (added salt being part of this process). Nell's blood pressure has been identified as being high, with readings between 150/95 and 160/100. Nell works in an office and does not participate in any physical activity. She will drink milk but does not commonly include milk in her daily diet. She buys her lunch at work, which consists of noodle soup, deli sandwich with large pickle, bottled club soda, and packaged cookies. Nell cooks her own breakfast, consisting typically of eggs, toast, and coffee with real cream. Her dinner is usually a roast, such as brisket, with potatoes and vegetables, and a traditional dessert. She entertains guests frequently and loves to cook. Nell is 5 ft 2 in. tall and weighs 170 lbs.

1. What advice will you give Nell about her meal planning?
2. What resources are there to help her prepare meals that are higher in potassium, calcium, and magnesium?
3. What tips about activity will you share with Nell?
4. If Nell begins a weight-loss program, how much weight should she lose, and how quickly?

■ Relevant Web Sites

DASH Diet
www.nhlbi.nih.gov/hbp/prevent/h_eating/h_eating.htm
National High Blood Pressure Education Program
www.nhlbi.nih.gov
World Hypertension League
www.mco.edu/org/whl

■ Cited References

Adams SO et al: Sodium and potassium mixtures can reduce sodium levels, *J Am Diet Assoc* 94:1313, 1994.

American Heart Association: *1998 Heart and stroke statistical update*, Dallas, 1997, American Heart Association.

American Heart Association: *2001 Heart and stroke statistical update*, Dallas, 2001, American Heart Association.

Appel LJ et al: A clinical trial of the effects of dietary patterns on blood pressure, *N Engl J Med* 336:1117, 1997.

Appel LJ et al: Effects of reduced sodium intake on hypertension control in older individuals, *Arch Intern Med* 161:685, 2001.

Ascherio A et al: A prospective study of nutritional factors and hypertension among US men, *Circulation* 86:1475, 1992.

Bazzano LA et al: Dietary potassium intake and risk of stroke in US men and women: National Health and Nutrition Examination Survey I epidemiologic follow-up study, *Stroke* 32:1473, 2001.

Blackburn GL: The public health implications of the dietary approaches to stop hypertension trial, *Am J Clin Nutr* 74:1, 2001.

Cowley AW, Roman RJ: The role of the kidney in hypertension, *JAMA* 275:1581, 1996.

Davis MM, Jones DW: The role of lifestyle management in the overall treatment plan for prevention and management of hypertension, *Semin Nephrol* 2:35, 2002.

Dubbert P et al: Estimation of sodium intake by analyzing food records with augmented nutrition software and by overnight urine collections, *J Am Diet Assoc* 92:87, 1992.

Eaton CB et al: Prevalence of hypertension, dyslipidemia and dyslipidemic hypertension, *J Fam Pract* 36:17, 1993.

Elliott P et al: INTERSALT revisited: further analyses of 24 hour sodium excretion and blood pressure within and across populations, *BMJ* 312:1249, 1996.

Espinel C: The salt step test: its usage in the diagnosis of salt sensitive hypertension and in the detection of the salt hypertension threshold, *J Am Coll Nutr* 11:526, 1992.

Ferrara LA et al: Olive oil and reduced need for antihypertensive medications, *Arch Intern Med* 160:837, 2000.

Gardin JM et al: Demographics and correlates of five-year change in echocardiographic left ventricular mass in young black and white adult men and women: the Coronary Artery Risk Development in Young Adults (CARDIA) study, *J Am Coll Cardiol* 40:529, 2002.

Geleijnse JM et al: Blood pressure response to fish oil supplementation: meta-regression analysis of randomized trials, *J Hypertens* 20:1493, 2002.

Hall JE: Renal and cardiovascular mechanisms of hypertension in obesity, *Hypertension* 23:381, 1994.

Hecker KD: Effects of dietary animal and soy protein on cardiovascular disease risk factors, *Curr Atheroscler Rep* 3:471, 2001.

Himes JH, Dietz WH: Guidelines for overweight in adolescent preventive services: recommendations from an expert committee, *Am J Clin Nutr* 59:307, 1994.

Hyman DJ, Pavlik VN: Characteristics of patients with uncontrolled hypertension in the United States, *N Engl J Med* 345:479, 2001.

Johnson R et al: Subtle acquired renal injury as a mechanism of salt-sensitive hypertension, *N Engl J Med* 346:913, 2002.

Joint National Committee on the Prevention, Detection, Evaluation and Treatment of High Blood Pressure: Fifth report (JNC V), *Arch Intern Med* 153:149, 1993.

Joint National Committee on the Prevention, Detection, Evaluation and Treatment of High Blood Pressure: Sixth report (JNC VI), *Arch Intern Med* 157:2413, 1997.

Kannel WB: Blood pressure as a cardiovascular risk factor, *JAMA* 275:1571, 1996.

Kaplan NM: Systemic hypertension: mechanisms and diagnosis. In Braunwald E, editor: *Heart disease*, Philadelphia, 1992, WB Saunders.

Kaplan NM: The dietary guideline for sodium: should we shake it up? *No. Am J Clin Nutr* 71:1020, 2000.

Kelley GA et al: Walking and resting blood pressure in adults: a meta-analysis, *Preventive Med* 33:120, 2001.

Khaw K-T, Barrett-Connor E: The association between blood pressure, age, and dietary sodium and potassium: a population study, *Circulation* 77:53, 1988.

Kiely DK et al: Physical activity and stroke risk: the Framingham study, *Am J Epidemiol* 140:608, 1994.

Kotchen TA: *Evaluation of publicly available scientific evidence regarding certain nutrient-disease relationships: sodium and hypertension*, Bethesda, Md, 1991, Life Sciences Research Office, Federation of American Societies for Experimental Biology.

Kotchen TA, McCarron DA: Dietary electrolytes and blood pressure: a statement for healthcare professionals from the American Heart Association Nutrition Commmittee, *Circulation* 98:613, 1998.

Krauss RM et al: Dietary guidelines revision 2000: a statement for healthcare professionals from the Nutrition Committee of the American Heart Association, *Circulation* 102:2284, 2000.

Kynast-Gales SA, Massey LK: Effects of dietary calcium from dairy products on ambulatory blood pressure in hypertensive men, *J Am Diet Assoc* 92:1497, 1992.

Melnyk MG, Weinstein E: Prevention of obesity in black women by targeting adolescents: a literature review, *J Am Diet Assoc* 94:536, 1994.

Messerli F et al: Salt: a perpetrator of hypertensive target organ disease, *Arch Intern Med* 157:2449, 1997.

Moser M: Update on the management of hypertension: do recent clinical trial results indicate a change in national recommmendations for therapy? *J Clin Hypertens* 4:(suppl 2)20, 2002.

Munter P et al: The impact of JNC-VI guidelines on treatment recommendations in the US population, *Hypertension* 39:897, 2002.

National Cholesterol Education Program (NCEP): Summary of the third report of the National Cholesterol Education Program Expert Panel on Detection, Evaluation, and Treatment of High Blood Cholesterol in Adults (Adult Treatment Panel III), *JAMA* 285:2486, 2001.

National Education Programs Working Group: Report on the Management of Patients with Hypertension and High Blood Cholesterol, *Ann Intern Med* 114:224, 1991.

National Heart, Lung, and Blood Institute, National Institutes of Health: *Update on the task force report* (1987) *on high blood pressure in children and adolescents: a working group report from the National High Blood Pressure Program,* NIH Publication No. 97-3790, 1997.

National High Blood Pressure Education Program (NHBPEP) Working Group: report on primary prevention of hypertension, *Arch Intern Med* 153:186, 1993.

National High Blood Pressure Education Program (NHBPEP) Working Group: report on hypertension in the elderly, *Hypertension* 23:275, 1994.

National Institutes of Health (NIH), National Heart, Lung, and Blood Institute (NHLBI): The DASH diet, U.S. Department of Health and Human Services, Public Health Services, NIH Publication No. 99-4082, 1999.

Poulter NR, Sever PS: Intervention in high risk groups: blood pressure. In Marmot M, Elliot P, editors: *Coronary heart disease epidemiology,* New York, 1992, Oxford Medical Publications.

Report of the American Institute of Nutrition (AIN) Steering Committee on Healthy Weight, *J Nutr* 124:2240, 1994.

Sacks F et al: Effects of blood pressure of reduced dietary sodium and the dietary approaches to stop hypertension (DASH) diet, *N Engl J Med* 344:3, 2001.

Schwartz CJ et al: Prevention of atherosclerosis and end-organ damage: a basis for antihypertensive interventional strategies, *J Hypertens* 12(suppl):S3, 1994.

Second Report of the Expert Panel on Detection, Evaluation, and Treatment of High Blood Cholesterol in Adults, NIH Publication No. 93-3095, U.S. Government Printing Office, Bethesda, Md, 1993.

Special Focus: Behavioral Risk Factor Surveillance—United States, 1991, *MMWR Morb Mortal Wkly Rep* 42:1, 1993.

Staessen JA: Overview of the outcome trials in older patients with isolated systolic hypertension, *J Hum Hypertens* 13:859, 1999.

Stamler J et al: Blood pressure, systolic and diastolic, and cardiovascular risks, *Arch Intern Med* 153:598, 1993.

Stamler J et al: INTERSALT study findings: public health and medical care implications, *Hypertension* 14:570, 1989a.

Stamler R: The primary prevention of hypertension. In Marmot M, Elliot P, editors: *Coronary heart disease epidemiology,* New York, 1992, Oxford Medical Publications.

Stamler R et al: Primary prevention of hypertension by nutritional-hygienic means, *JAMA* 262:1801, 1989.

Stevens V et al: Weight loss intervention in phase I of the Trials of Hypertension Prevention, *Arch Intern Med* 153:849, 1993.

St. Jeor ST et al: Obesity, *Circulation* 88:1391, 1993.

Strong WB et al: Integrated cardiovascular health promotion in childhood: a statement of health professionals from the Subcommittee on Atherosclerosis and Hypertension in Childhood of the Council on Cardiovascular Disease in the Young, *Circulation* 85:1638, 1992.

Trials of Hypertension Prevention Collaborative Research Group (TOHP): Effects of weight loss and sodium reduction intervention on blood pressure and hypertension incidence in overweight people with high-normal blood pressure, *Arch Intern Med* 157:657, 1997.

Vasan R et al: Impact of high normal blood pressure on the risk of cardiovascular disease, *N Engl J Med* 345:1291, 2001.

Whelton PK et al: Effects of oral potassium on blood pressure: meta-analysis of randomized controlled clinical trials, *JAMA* 277:1624, 1997.

Whelton PK et al: Sodium reduction and weight loss in the treatment of hypertension in older persons: a randomized controlled Trial of Nonpharmacologic Interventions in the Elderly (TONE), *JAMA* 279:839, 1998.

Whelton PK et al: Effect of aerobic exercise on blood pressure: a meta-analysis of randomized controlled trials, *Ann Intern Med* 136:493, 2002.

Williams DP et al: Body fatness and risk for elevated blood pressure, total cholesterol, and serum lipoprotein ratios in children and adolescents, *Am J Public Health* 82:358, 1992.

Windhauser MM et al: Dietary adherence in the dietary approaches to stop hypertension trial, *J Am Diet Assoc* 99(supp):S76, 1999.

Wright JT Jr et al: Successful blood pressure control in the African American Study of Kidney Diseases and Hypertension, *Arch Intern Med* 162:1636, 2002.

Wylie-Rosett J et al: Trial of antihypertensive intervention and management: greater efficiency with weight reduction than with a sodium-potassium intervention, *J Am Diet Assoc* 93:408, 1993.

■ Additional References

Diez Roux AV et al: Socioeconomic disadvantage and change in blood pressure associated with aging, *Circulation* 106:703, 2002.

Jarvis JK, Miller GD: Overcoming the barrier of lactose intolerance to reduce health disparities, *J Natl Med Assoc* 94:55, 2002.

Lea JP, Nicholas SB: Diabetes mellitus and hypertension: key risk factors for kidney disease, *J Natl Med Assoc* 94:7S, 2002.

Somes GW et al: Body mass index, weight change, and death in older adults: the systolic hypertension in the elderly program, *Am J Epidemiol* 156:132, 2002.

Sorof JM et al: Isolated systolic hypertension, obesity, and hyperkinetic hemodynamic states in children, *J Pediatr* 140:660, 2002.

Wylie-Rosett J et al: Recent dietary guidelines to prevent and treat cardiovascular disease, diabetes, and obesity, *Heart Dis* 4:220, 2002.

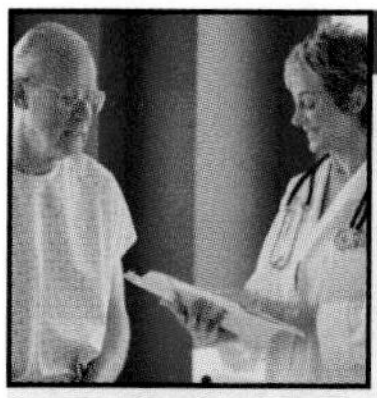

CHAPTER 37

Medical Nutrition Therapy for Heart Failure and Transplant

DEBRA A. KRUMMEL, PhD, RD, LD

CHAPTER OUTLINE

- Heart Failure
- Cardiac Transplantation

KEY TERMS

cachectic heart–a soft, flabby heart characterized by loss of myocardial mass as the result of extreme malnutrition

congestive heart failure (CHF)–a clinical syndrome characterized by progressive deterioration of left ventricular function, inadequate tissue perfusion, fatigue, shortness of breath, and congestion

dyspnea–uncomfortable and distressful breathing caused by heart problems, anxiety, or exercise

edema–abnormal accumulation of fluid in body tissues such as lungs, ankles, feet

heart failure–same as congestive heart failure

left ventricular hypertrophy–enlargement of the left ventricle of the heart, a major risk factor for heart failure

low-salt syndrome–a syndrome characterized by hyponatremia, hypochloremia, and eventually azotemia that occurs when glomerular filtration rate decreases as the result of salt depletion

mild sodium restriction–restriction of dietary sodium to 2 g (87 mEq) per day

moderate sodium restriction–restriction of dietary sodium to 1 g (43 mEq) per day

no-added-salt diet–a diet containing 3 g (130 mEq) of sodium per day

orthopnea–respiratory distress while in a recumbent position

severe sodium restriction–restriction of dietary sodium to 250 mg (11 mEq) per day

strict sodium restriction–restriction of dietary sodium to 500 mg (22 mEq) per day

syncope–lack of oxygen to the brain causing a brief loss of consciousness

Some categories of heart disease, such as chronic heart failure and cardiac cachexia, occur when the heart deteriorates and can no longer adequately pump blood. Nutritional care in these conditions is concerned primarily with the consequences of poor circulation throughout the body. In end-stage heart disease, cardiac transplantation becomes necessary for survival.

HEART FAILURE

Normally, the heart pumps adequate blood to perfuse tissues and meet metabolic needs (Figure 37-1). Heart failure, also known as congestive heart failure (CHF), is a progressive disorder characterized by a complex of symptoms (fatigue, shortness of breath, edema and congestion) that occurs when an impaired left ventricle cannot provide adequate blood flow to the rest of the body. Most people with CHF have left ventricular systolic dysfunction (Box 37-1). Specifically, diseases of the heart (valves, muscle, vessels, arteries) and vasculature (hypertension) can lead to CHF (Figure 37-2). Once the disease is established, conditions such as myocardial infarction (MI), dietary sodium excess, medication noncompliance, arrhythmias, pulmonary embolism, infection, and anemia, can precipitate complete CHF (Rich, 1997). Many cardiovascular diseases end up in this common pathway to CHF.

The prognosis for CHF depends on the causative factors and the individual's response to treatment.

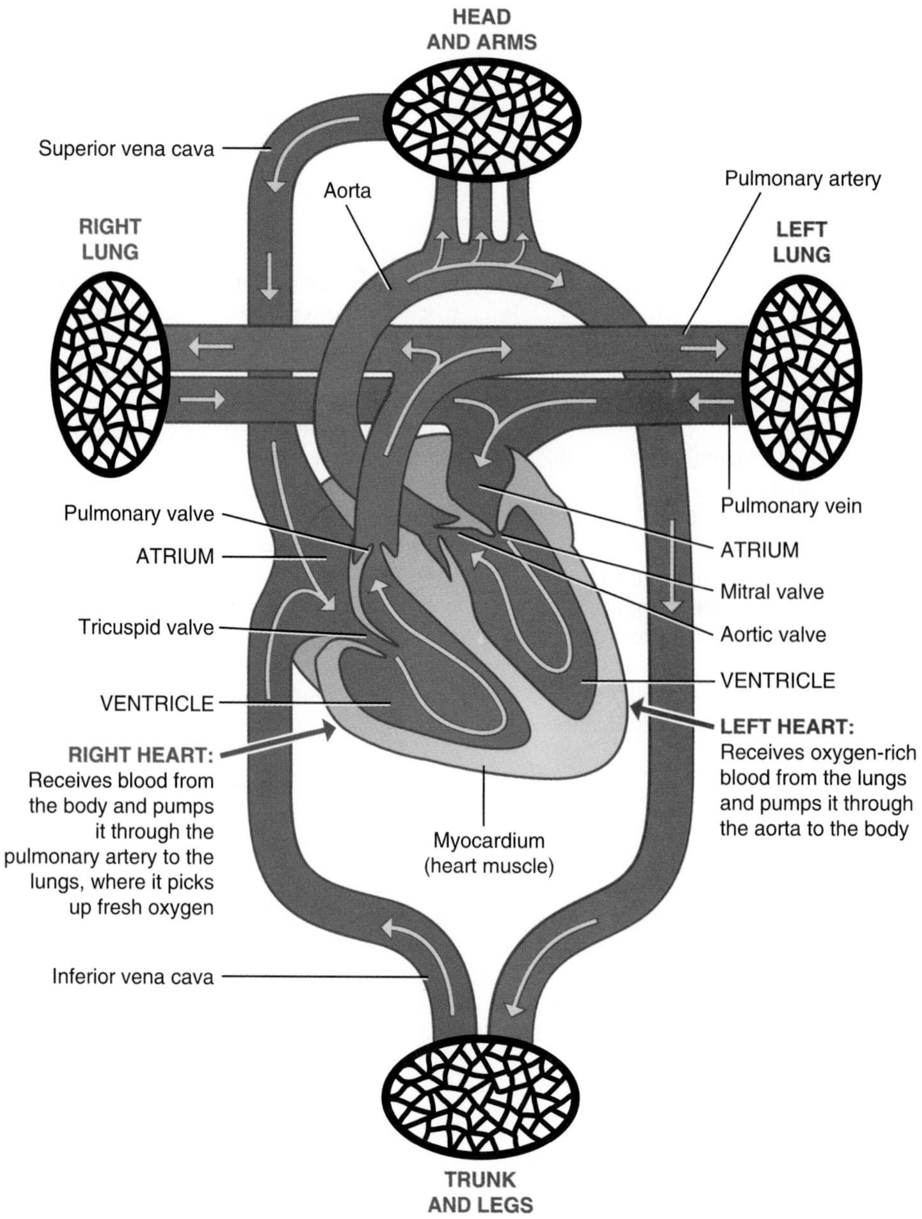

FIGURE 37-1 • Structure of the heart pump.

Overall, the prognosis is poor, with the 5-year mortality rates for advanced CHF approaching 50% and the risk of sudden death sixfold to ninefold higher than that for the general population (Deedwania, 1997).

Prevalence and Incidence

Congestive heart failure has become a major public health problem in the United States over the last 15 years. Unlike other cardiovascular diseases, the number of people being discharged with CHF diagnosis has continued to increase since 1979 (Nohria et al, 2002) (Figure 37-3). About 4.8 million Americans have CHF, with an overall prevalence of 2% to 6% (Miller and Missov, 2001). Between 1979 and 1999, the death rate associated with this disease increased by 145% (American Heart Association [AHA], 2001). The prevalence of CHF increases with age, especially after age 55 years (Figure 37-4). Black men have the highest rates of CHF, followed by Latino women, black women, white men, white women, and Latino men (Miller, 2001).

Box 37-1. Less Common Causes of Left Ventricular Systolic Dysfunction

Infectious agents: viral, bacterial, fungal
Acute rheumatic fever
Infiltrative disorders: amyloid, hemochromatosis, sarcoid
Toxic: heroin, cocaine, alcohol, amphetamines, adriamycin, cyclophosphamide, sulfonamides, lead, arsenic, cobalt, phosphorus, ethylene glycol
Nutritional deficiencies: protein, thiamin, selenium
Electrolyte disorders: hypocalcemia, hypophosphatemia, hyponatremia, hypokalemia
Collagen vascular disorders: lupus erythematosus, rheumatoid arthritis, systemic sclerosis, polyarteritis nodosa, hypersensitivity vasculitis, Takayasu's syndrome, polymyositis, Reiter's syndrome
Endocrine and metabolic diseases: diabetes, thyroid disease (both hypo- and hyper-), hypoparathyroidism with hypocalcemia, pheochromocytoma, acromegaly
Tachycardia-induced: incessant supraventricular tachyarrhythmias or atrial fibrillation with rapid ventricular rates
Miscellaneous: hypereosinophilic syndrome, peripartum cardiomyopathy, sleep apnea syndrome, Whipple's disease, L-carnitine deficiency

From American College of Cardiology, American Heart Association Task Force on Practice Guidelines: Guidelines for evaluation and management of heart failure, *J Am Coll Cardiol* 26:1384, 1995. Copyright American College of Cardiology Foundation.

Most deaths from CHF occur in persons 65 years of age and older. For this Medicare population, CHF is the most common diagnosis, second only to hypertension as the precipitating cause for physician office visits (Rich, 1997). Consequently, more Medicare dollars are spent on CHF than on any other diagnosis; annual costs were approximately $38 billion dollars, or 5% of the U.S. health care budget (Hunt et al, 2001).

The incidence (new cases) of heart failure has risen over the last 20 years because of an aging population and the increased number of people being saved from premature death secondary to MI (Figure 37-5). About 550,000 new cases are diagnosed each year. In persons 65 years of age and older, the incidence of CHF approaches 10 per 1000 people (AHA, 2001). Median survival of men and women is 1.7 years and 3.1 years, respectively (Miller and Missov, 2001). One in five persons with CHF will die within a year of diagnosis.

Risk Factors

The Framingham Study is a 50-year epidemiologic study of the incidence, prevalence, and risk factors for cardiovascular diseases (see *Focus On:* Framingham Heart Study in Chapter 35). In the Framingham population, the risk factors for CHF are hypertension, left ventricular hypertrophy, coronary heart disease, and diabetes. The mean age of onset is 70 years, and 91% of the Framingham cohort had hypertension before CHF (Ho et al, 1993; Levy et al, 1996). Over the last 15 years, at least 60% to 65% of CHF cases were attributable to coronary heart disease (Massie and Shah, 1997).

Prevention

Even with improved therapy for patients with CHF, prognosis remains poor, with annual mortality rates of 5% in stable patients whose symptoms are mild and 30% to 50% in patients in advanced stages (Massie and Amidon, 2002). Because long-term survival rates for persons with CHF are low (24% of men and 31% of women after a 5-year period), prevention is critical. CHF has now been categorized into four stages; the first two of which reflect persons at risk of developing CHF (Table 37-1). For these stages, the primary prevention strategy is the treatment of underlying diseases, such as hypertension, hyperlipidemia, and diabetes, to prevent left ventricular dysfunction and the appearance of CHF symptoms.

Treatment with a cholesterol-lowering drug (simvastatin) in one trial or antihypertensive drugs in another trial decreased the risk of developing heart failure by 20% or 49%, respectively (Kjekshus et al, 1997; Kostis et al, 1997). In previous MI patients, antihypertensive therapy reduced the risk of CHF by 81% (Kostis et al, 1997). Appropriate changes in lifestyle would include a diet low in saturated fat, cholesterol, and sodium; weight management; increased physical activity; smoking cessation; and pharmacologic

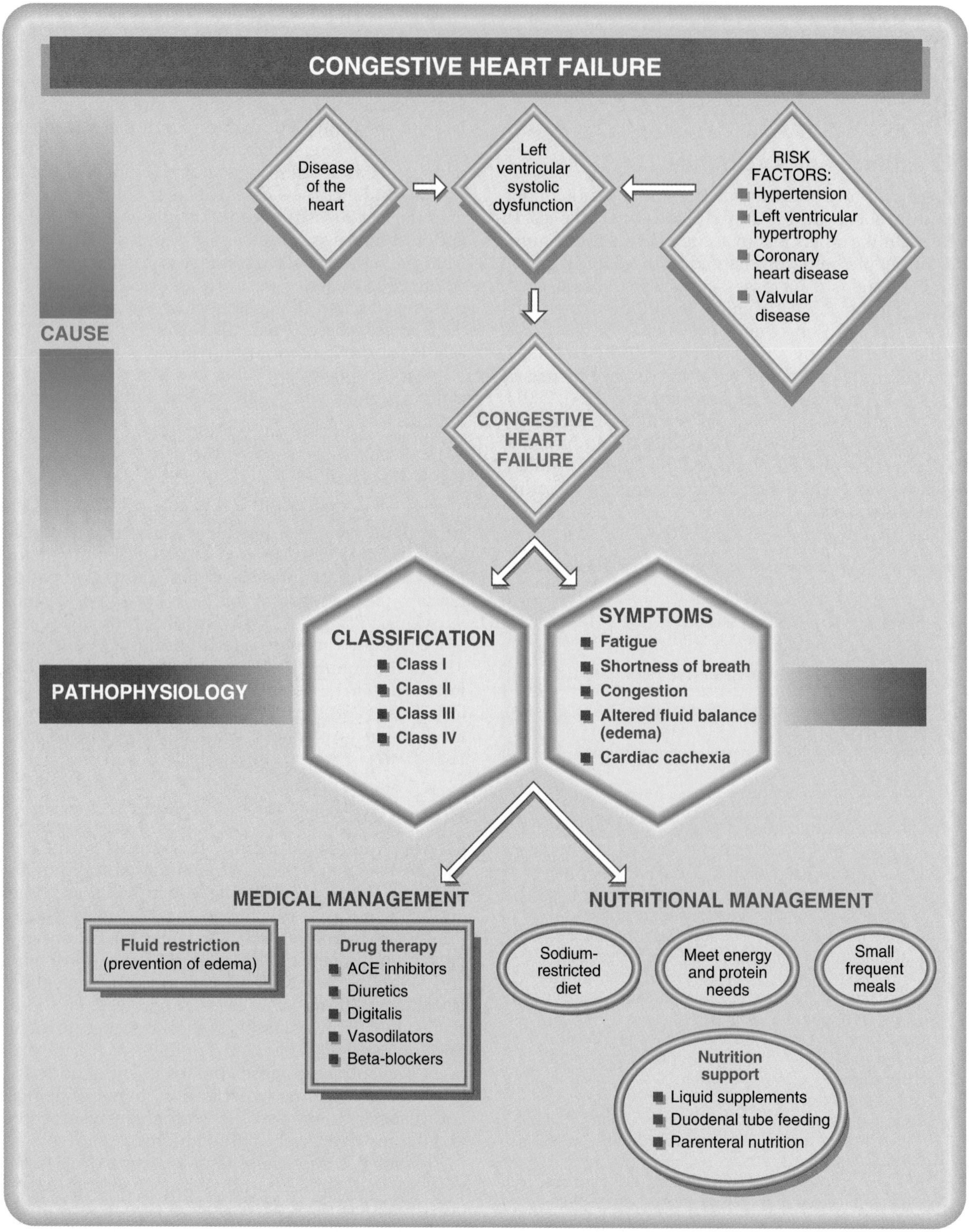

FIGURE 37-2 • Pathophysiology algorithm: congestive heart failure. *ACE,* Angiotensin-converting enzyme. (Algorithm content developed by John Anderson, PhD, and Sanford C. Garner, PhD, 2000. Updated by Debra A. Krummel, PhD, RD, 2002.)

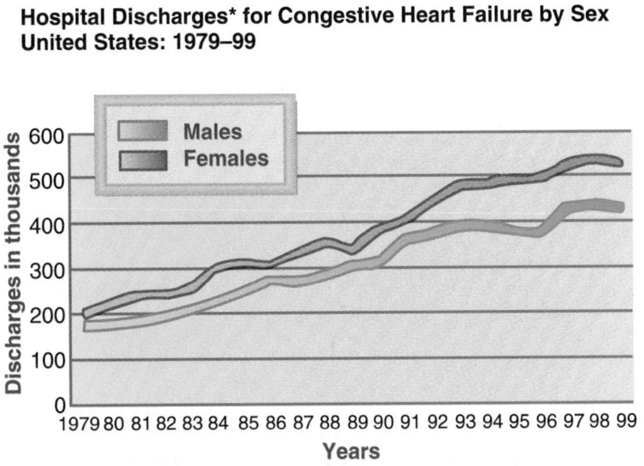

*Hospital discharges include people both living and dead.

FIGURE 37-3 • Hospital discharges with congestive heart failure. (Source: Centers for Disease Control and Prevention/National Center for Health Statistics and American Heart Association.)

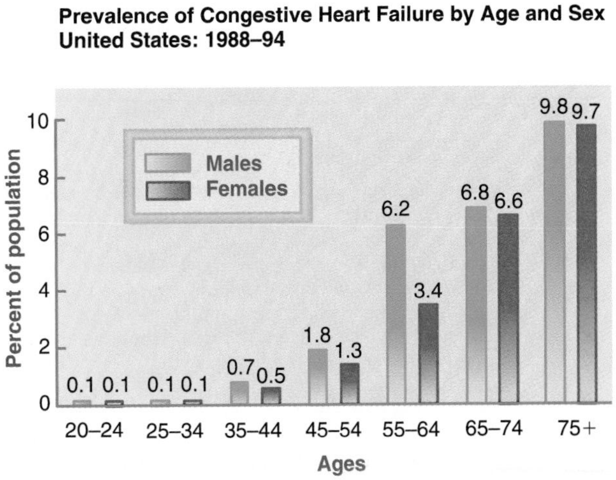

FIGURE 37-4 • Prevalence of congestive heart failure. (Source: National Health and Nutrition Examination Survey III (NHANES III), 1988-1994, Centers for Disease Control and Prevention/National Center for Health Statistics and American Heart Association.)

therapy for those who are not compliant with or responsive to lifestyle change strategies.

For stages C and D, secondary prevention strategies to prevent further cardiac dysfunction are warranted. These strategies include the use of angiotensin-converting enzyme (ACE) inhibitors, β-blockers, aldosterone agonists, antihyperlipidemia therapy, anticoagulation therapy, and coronary revascularization. Use of neurohormonal antagonists (ACE inhibitors and β-blockers) has been shown to reduce CHF mortality (Packer et al, 1999). Early detection, correction of presymptomatic left ventricular dysfunction, and aggressive management of risk factors are needed to lower the incidence and mortality of CHF.

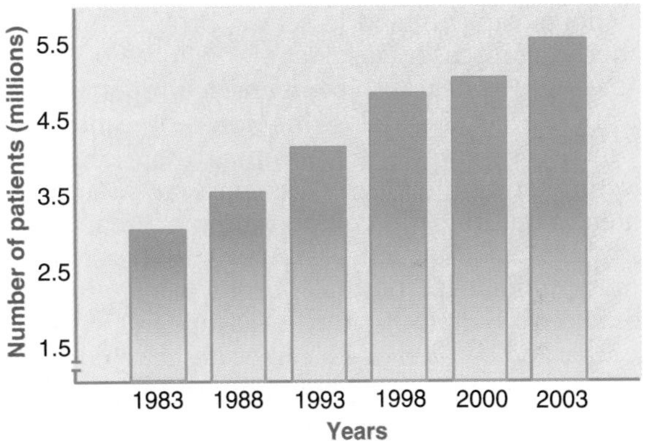

FIGURE 37-5 • Incidence of congestive heart failure. (From American Heart Association: 2001 *Heart and stroke statistical update,* Dallas, 2003, American Heart Association.)

Pathophysiology

The progression of CHF is similar to that of atherosclerosis because there is an asymptomatic phase when damage is silently occurring (stage A) (Figure 37-6). A multitude of factors—nonhemodynamic, genetic, energetic, and neurohormonal—contribute to the progression of heart failure (McMurray and Pfeffer, 2002). CHF is initiated by damage to the heart muscle either of acute (MI) or insidious (hemodynamic pressure or volume overloading) onset (Mann et al, 2002). After damage, compensatory mechanisms such as the adrenergic nervous system, renin–angiotensin system, and cytokine system are activated to restore homeostatic function. Patients are asymptomatic during this phase.

Eventually, overuse of these systems leads to ventricle damage and remodeling, where the heart attempts to decrease wall stress through increases in wall thickness. Remodeling occurs before symptoms are observed and then afterward contribute to worsening symptoms. CHF patients have elevated levels of norepinephrine, angiotensin II, aldosterone, endothelin, and vasopressin, all of which are neurohormonal factors that increase the hemodynamic stress on the ventricle by causing sodium retention and periperheral vasoconstriction. These neurohormones contribute to disease progression; hence, current therapies are trying to inhibit these undesirable pathways and increase desirable ones.

For the final stages of CHF, there is another subjective scale used to classify symptoms based on the degree of limitation in daily activities (Table 37-2). An estimated 33% of CHF patients are in class I, 33% are in class II, 10% to 15% are in class III, and 20% are in class IV (Miller and Missov, 2001). The severity of symptoms in this classification system is weakly related to the severity of left ventricular dysfunction; therefore, treatment encompasses both improving

TABLE 37-1 Stages of Heart Failure

STAGE	DESCRIPTION	EXAMPLES
A	Patients at high risk of developing HF because of the presence of conditions that are strongly associated with the development of HF. Such patients have no identified structural or functional abnormalities of the pericardium, myocardium, or cardiac valves and have never shown signs or symptoms of HF.	Systemic hypertension; coronary artery disease; diabetes mellitus; history of cardiotoxic drug therapy or alcohol abuse; personal history of rheumatic fever; family history of cardiomyopathy.
B	Patients who have developed structural heart disease that is strongly associated with the development of HF but who have never shown signs or symptoms of HF.	Left ventricular hypertrophy or fibrosis; left ventricular dilatation or hypocontractility; asymptomatic valvular heart disease; previous myocardial infarction.
C	Patients who have current or prior symptoms of HF associated with underlying structural heart disease.	Dyspnea or fatigue due to left ventricular systolic dysfunction; asymptomatic patients who are undergoing treatment for prior symptoms of HF.
D	Patients with advanced structural heart disease and marked symptoms of HF at rest despite maximal medical therapy and who require specialized interventions.	Patients who are frequently hospitalized for HF or who cannot be safely discharged from the hospital; patients in the hospital awaiting heart transplantation; patients at home receiving continuous intravenous support for symptom relief or being supported with a mechanical circulatory assist device; patients in a hospice setting for the management of HF.

From Hunt S et al: ACC/AHA: Guidelines for the evaluation and management of chronic heart failure in the adult: executive summary, *Circulation* 104:2996, 2001.
HF, Heart failure.

functional capacity and lessening progression of the underlying disease (Packer et al, 1999).

In CHF, the heart can compensate for poor cardiac output by (1) increasing the force of contraction, (2) increasing in size, (3) pumping more often, and (4) stimulating the kidneys to conserve sodium and water. For a time, this compensation maintains near-normal circulation, but eventually the heart can no longer maintain a normal output *(decompensation)*. Advanced symptoms can develop in weeks or months, and sudden death can occur at any time.

Three symptoms—fatigue, shortness of breath, and fluid retention—are the hallmarks of CHF. Shortness of breath (dyspnea) on exertion is the earliest symptom. The shortness of breath gets worse and occurs at rest (orthopnea) or at night (paroxysmal nocturnal dyspnea). Fluid retention can manifest as pulmonary (congestion) or peripheral edema. Evidence for hypoperfusion includes cool forearms and legs, sleepy feeling, declining serum sodium level, worsening renal function, and narrow pulse pressure (Nohria et al, 2002).

Other symptoms that reflect inadequate blood supply to the abdominal organs include anorexia, nausea, a feeling of fullness, constipation, abdominal pain, malabsorption, an enlarged liver, and liver tenderness. Decreased cranial blood supply can lead to mental confusion, memory loss, anxiety, insomnia, syncope, and headache. The latter symptoms are more common in older patients and often are the only symptoms; this can lead to a delay in diagnosis. Often the first symptom in older adults is a dry cough with generalized weakness and anorexia.

Cardiac Cachexia

Of patients with moderate to severe heart failure, 35% to 53% have malnutrition, known as cardiac cachexia (Carr et al, 1989). Because no standardized criteria for cachexia have been established, indicators of body fat stores, protein nutriture, and immunity have all been used. Unlike normal starvation, which is characterized by adipose tissue loss, cachexia is characterized by a predominant loss of lean body mass greater than 10% of the body total (Anker et al, 1997b; Freeman and Roubenoff, 1994). This loss of lean body mass further exacerbates CHF because of the loss of cardiac muscle and the development of a cachectic heart (Zhao and Zeng, 1997).

Although it is unclear why some patients become cachectic, a variety of factors may play a role (Box 37-2). Impaired fat absorption occurs with severe CHF and contributes to cachexia (King et al, 1996). Other metabolic changes include decreased plasma sodium values and increased catabolic catecholamines (norepinephrine, epinephrine, cortisol) and tumor necrosis factor levels. Tumor necrosis factor causes weight loss in animals and is elevated moderately in CHF patients and markedly in cachectic patients and in patients with other wasting disorders (Zhao and Zeng, 1997). Increased levels of tumor necrosis factor are associated with lowered BMI and plasma total protein levels and decreased skin folds, which indicate a catabolic state.

It appears that CHF progresses to cardiac cachexia when the balance between catabolism and anabolism is impaired (Anker et al, 1997a). Cardiac cachexia can also occur in any case of extreme malnutrition (see Chapter 25). Caloric supplements can help to increase energy intake but rarely reverse malnutrition unless the underlying cause is corrected (Nohria et al, 2002).

The cachectic patient who must undergo cardiac surgery is at increased risk for delayed wound healing, increased time for weaning from ventilator support, postoperative acute renal failure, and

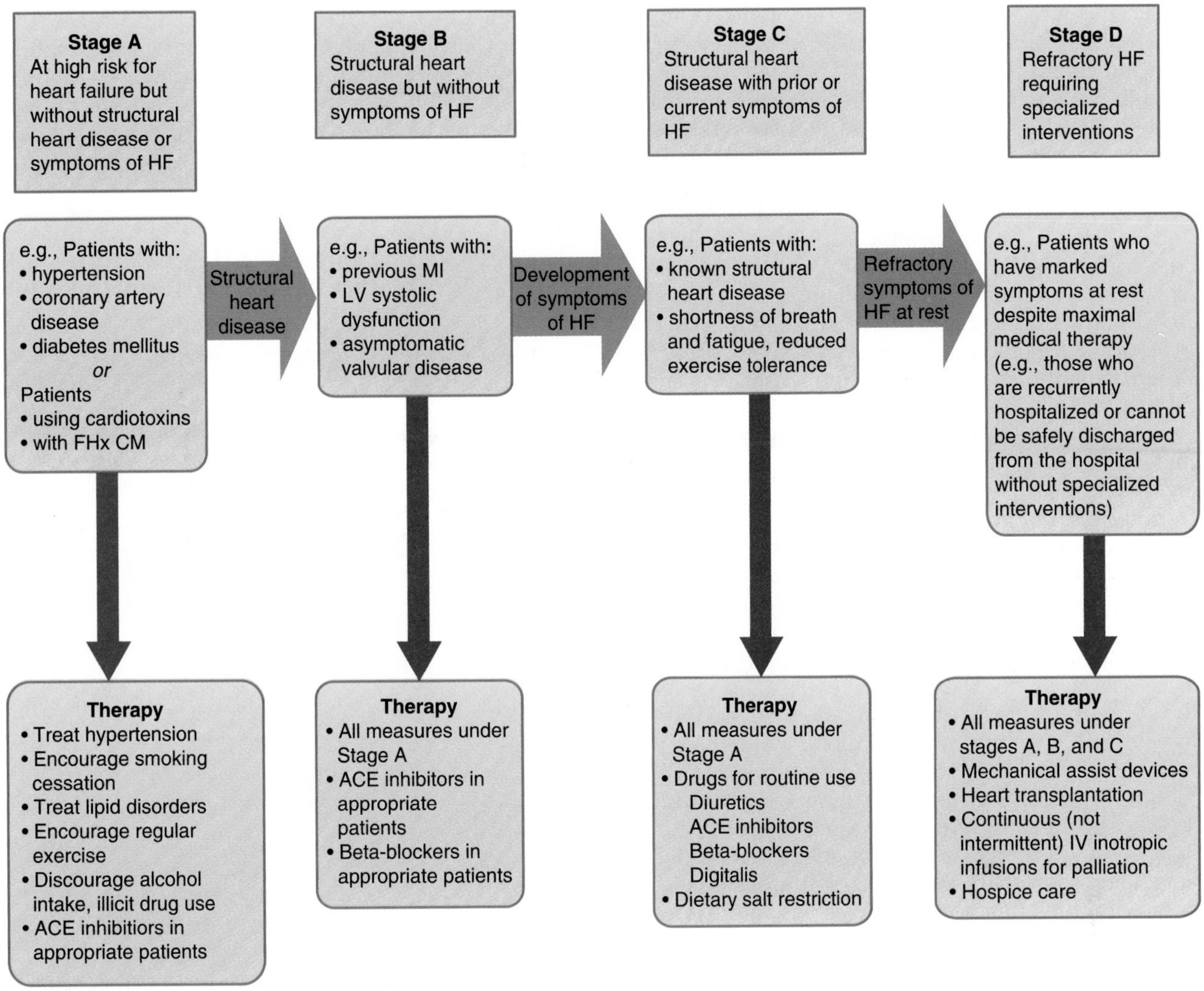

FIGURE 37-6 • Stages in the evolution of heart failure (HF) and recommended therapy by stage. *ACE*, Angiotensin-converting enzyme; *FHx*, family history; *CM*, cardiomyopathy; *MI*, myocardial infarction; *LV*, left ventricular; *IV*, intravenous. (From Hunt S et al: ACC/AHA guidelines for the evaluation and management of chronic heart failure in the adult: executive summary, *Circulation* 104:2996, 2001.)

TABLE 37-2 Classifications of Heart Failure

Class I	No undue symptoms associated with ordinary activity and no limitation of physical activity
Class II	Slight limitation of physical activity; patient comfortable at rest
Class III	Marked limitation of physical activity; patient comfortable at rest
Class IV	Inability to carry out physical activity without discomfort; symptoms of cardiac insufficiency or chest pain at rest

From Bender JR: Heart valve disease. In Zaret BL, Moser M, and Cohen LS, editors: *Yale University School of Medicine heart book,* New York, 1992, Hearst Books.

death. In general, cachectic patients have poorer outcomes and incur higher hospitalization costs than other cardiac patients. Therefore, nutritional support and rehabilitation should begin before surgery and continue after surgery as well.

Medical Management

Therapy recommendations correspond to the stage of CHF (see Figure 37-6). For patients at high risk of developing CHF (stage A), treatment of the underlying conditions (hypertension, hyperlipidemia, thyroid disorders, arrhythmias), avoidance of high-risk behaviors (tobacco, alcohol, illicit drug use), and lifestyle changes (exercise, reduction of sodium intake, nutritional supplements) are recommended. All these recommendations are carried through the other stages. In addition, drugs are added with progressive stages. The last stage also includes medical assistive devices, heart transplantation, continual intravenous therapy, and hospice care at the end of life.

The short-term goals for the treatment of CHF are to relieve symptoms and to improve the quality of life. The degree to which these goals are met by treatment can be assessed by a patient interview. The long-term goal of treatment is to prolong life by lessening, stopping, or reversing left ventricular dysfunction.

Medical management should be tailored to clinical and hemodynamic profiles (evidence of hypoperfusion and congestion) (Nohria et al, 2002).

Initial management of CHF includes a restricted sodium diet (2 to 3 g daily) and regular activity (as symptoms permit). Bed rest is no longer recommended except for those with acute failure. The heart becomes deconditioned with less exercise, whereas with exercise, peak exercise capacity can be increased. Fluids are restricted if hyponatremia develops (serum sodium level <130 mEq/L) (Aronow, 1997). Standard fluid restrictions are to limit total fluids to 2 L (2000 ml daily) (Lutton and Anzlovar, 2001). When patients are severely decompensated, a more restrictive fluid intake (1000 to 1500 ml daily) may be warranted for adequate diuresis. A sodium-restricted diet should be maintained despite low-sodium blood levels because in this case the sodium has shifted from the blood to the tissues.

A combination of four drugs is used initially to treat CHF: a diuretic, an ACE inhibitor, a β-adrenergic blocker, and digoxin. Selected patients may also take aldosterone agonists and vasodilators (e.g., hydralazine) (Weber, 2001). Basically, these drugs reduce excess fluid, dilate blood vessels, and increase the strength of the heart's contraction. Several drugs have neurohormonal benefits along with their primary mechanism of action. For example, ACE inhibitors (e.g., captopril, enalapril) not only inhibit the renin–angiotensin system (see Chapter 36) but also improve symptoms, quality of life, exercise tolerance, and survival. Similarly, spironolactone has both diuretic functions as well as aldosterone-blocking functions that result in reduced morbidity and mortality in patients already taking combination therapy of ACE inhibitor, loop diuretic, or digoxin (Pitt et al, 1999). Most of these drugs can affect nutritional status, as shown in Table 37-3. For a discussion

Box 37-2. Factors Associated With the Development of Cardiac Cachexia

Generalized cellular hypoxia
Decreased energy intake
Anorexia secondary to ascites or drug therapy
Unpalatable diet and fluid restriction
Breathlessness and exhaustion from eating
Altered taste and smell
Depression
Nausea and vomiting
Elevated blood tumor necrosis factor level
Decreased energy assimilation
Increased myocardial oxygen consumption
Increased work of breathing
Elevated basal metabolic rate
Fat malabsorption
Fever
Nutrient losses
Certain diuretics (Zn, Mg, K losses)
Renal protein loss
Poor absorption due to congestion of intestinal veins

TABLE 37-3 Drugs Used to Treat Congestive Heart Failure that Affect Nutritional Status

DRUG CLASS/ GENERIC NAME*	NUTRITIONAL CONSIDERATIONS†
Diuretics	
Furosemide	Avoid taking with natural licorice. Limit alcohol. GI side effects: anorexia, increased thirst, stomach cramps, nausea, vomiting, constipation Monitor Mg, Ca, K, thiamin.
Hydrochlorothiazide	Avoid taking with natural licorice. Use with caution if taken with calcium and/or vitamin D supplements. GI side effects: anorexia, increased thirst, dry mouth, nausea, vomiting, GI irritation, diarrhea, constipation Monitor Mg, Ca, K.
ACE inhibitor	
Enalapril	Avoid taking with salt substitutes, potassium substitutes, or natural licorice.‡ GI side effects: anorexia, taste loss, dry mouth, glossitis, stomatitis, nausea/vomiting, abdominal pain, diarrhea, constipation
Aldosterone agonist	
Spironolactone	Avoid natural licorice. Avoid potassium supplements and salt substitutes. GI side effects: dry mouth, gastritis, nausea, vomiting, cramps, diarrhea, rare gastric bleeding
β-blocker	
Metoprolol	Avoid taking with natural licorice. GI side effects: dry mouth, nausea, dyspepsia, GI upset, flatulence, diarrhea, constipation
Digitalis	
Digoxin	Avoid taking with foods containing high bran fiber, foods with high pectin content, and natural licorice. Use caution if taken with calcium, vitamin D, or magnesium supplements. GI side effects: anorexia, nausea, vomiting, diarrhea
Vasodilator	
Hydralazine HCl	Avoid taking with natural licorice. GI side effects: anorexia, increased thirst, dry mouth, unpleasant taste, nausea, vomiting, GI distress, diarrhea, constipation

*Drugs are those recommended in Armstrong and Moe, 1994.
†Data from Pronsky ZM: *Powers and Moore's food medication interactions*, ed 11, Pottstown, Pa, 2000, Food Medication Interactions.
‡Natural extract of glycyrrhiza root used in some licorice candies (amount in two twists—100 g) can increase sodium and water retention, promote potassium loss, diarrhea, and increased blood pressure.
GI, Gastrointestinal.

of the interrelationships between these drugs and other risk factors for heart disease, refer to Chapters 19 and 35.

Medical Nutrition Therapy

Altered fluid balance complicates assessment and treatment of the patient with CHF, and achievement of a dry weight is a clinical goal. Patients should record daily weights and advise their care providers if weight gain exceeds 2 to 3 lb a day, or 5 lb in a week (Clinical Practice Guidelines, 1994). Restricting sodium and fluids (decreasing by 1 to 1.5 cups) along with diuretic therapy may restore fluid balance and prevent full-blown CHF.

In malnourished patients with CHF, body weight can be either normal or increased as a result of fluid retention. Patients with cardiac cachexia may lose 10% to 15% of their body weight. Other markers of malnutrition (i.e., serum prealbumin and transferrin) may be disproportionately low because of the dilutional effect of excess extracellular fluid. To assess lean body mass, therefore, anthropometrics and diet history must be used. Measurement of calf and thigh circumferences, along with measurement of the mid–upper arm circumference, is the most sensitive indicator of lean body mass in cardiac patients retaining fluid (Poindexter et al, 1989) (see Chapter 17). All patients with CHF should be assessed for cardiac cachexia, especially if they are awaiting surgery.

Energy

Along with the usual factors, the energy needs of patients with CHF depend on their current weight, activity restrictions, and the severity of the heart failure. Overweight patients with limited activity must achieve and maintain an appropriate weight that will not stress the myocardium. For the obese patient, hypocaloric diets (1000 to 1200 kcal daily) will reduce the stress on the heart and facilitate weight reduction. In the undernourished patient with severe CHF, energy needs are increased by 30% to 50% above basal level as a result of the increased energy expenditure of the heart and lungs; 35 kcal/kg of body weight is often used. Patients with cardiac cachexia may require further increases in energy 1.6 to 1.8 times the resting energy expenditure (REE) for nutritional repletion.

Sodium

Edema in patients with decompensated CHF results from impaired cardiac function. Inadequate blood flow to the kidneys leads to aldosterone and antidiuretic hormone secretion. Both these hormones act to conserve fluid. Aldosterone promotes sodium resorption, and antidiuretic hormone promotes water conservation in the distal tubules of the nephron. Sodium and fluid thus accumulate in the tissues. Even asymptomatic patients with mild heart failure (class I to II) and no congestion can retain sodium and water if consuming a high-salt diet (6 g or 250 mEq/day of sodium) (Volpe et al, 1993).

The degree to which sodium and, possibly, fluids are restricted depends on the individual. The most recent consensus recommends a 3-g sodium diet for chronic heart failure (American College of Cardiology, 1995). This level is close to the AHA guideline (2400 mg daily) for optimal cardiovascular health (Krauss et al, 2000). Patients with moderate or severe cardiac failure may require sodium to be restricted to 1 to 2 g daily. It is unknown what sodium level is best for most patients (Dracup et al, 1994). In the rare patient whose sodium intake must be restricted to only 500 mg daily, the period of restriction should be limited, as such a diet is unpalatable and nutritionally inadequate. Indeed, it would be more appropriate to maintain a higher intake of sodium and to increase the use of diuretics. Low-sodium diets enhance the sodium-depleting effects of diuretics. Thus, the diet in conjunction with diuretics yields the best results.

A recent study assessed the ability of CHF patients to adhere to recommended sodium restrictions. Following a dietitian intervention, sodium knowledge scores significantly increased, as did the number of patients who could read the nutrition label (Neily et al, 2002) (see *Clinical Insight:* Sodium and Salt Measurement Equivalents).

CLINICAL INSIGHT

Sodium and Salt Measurement Equivalents

Sodium chloride is approximately 40% (39.3%) sodium and 60% chloride. To convert a specified weight of sodium chloride to its sodium equivalent, multiply the weight by 0.393. Sodium is also measured in milliequivalents (mEq). To convert milligrams of sodium to mEq, divide by the atomic weight of 23.

To convert sodium to sodium chloride (salt), multiply by 2.54.

Millimoles (mmol) and milliequivalents (mEq) of sodium are the same. For example:

1 tsp of salt = approximately 6 g NaCl
= 6096 mg NaCl
6096 mg NaCl × 0.393 = 2396 mg Na (about 2400 mg)
2396 mg Na/23 = 104 mEq Na
1 g Na = 1000 mg/23 = 43 mEq or mmol
1 tsp of salt = ≃ 2400 mg or 104 mEq Na

Sodium-Restricted Diets

The four most common forms of sodium-restricted diets are described as follows:

3 g (131 mEq) of sodium per day/no-added-salt diet: High-sodium foods are limited. An intake of no more than ½ tsp of table salt is allowed daily.

2 g (87 mEq) of sodium per day/mild sodium restriction: High-sodium foods are eliminated; moderate-sodium foods are limited. An intake of no more than ¼ tsp of table salt is allowed daily.

1 g (43 mEq) of sodium per day/moderate sodium restriction: High-sodium and moderate-sodium foods are eliminated. Table salt is not allowed. Canned or processed foods containing salt are omitted. Frozen peas, lima beans, mixed vegetables, and corn are omitted because brine is used during processing. Regular bread and baked goods are limited. This diet may be difficult to maintain at home.

500 mg (22 mEq) of sodium per day/strict sodium restriction: High-sodium and moderate-sodium foods are eliminated. Table salt is not allowed. Canned or processed foods containing salt are omitted.

The frozen vegetables mentioned in the 1-g sodium diet are omitted, as are the following vegetables, which are naturally high in sodium: beets, beet greens, carrots, kale, spinach, celery, white turnips, rutabagas, mustard greens, chard, and dandelion greens. Low-sodium bread replaces regular bread. Meat is restricted to 6 oz daily. This diet is unpalatable and should be used only for short periods. It can be nutritionally deficient if not planned carefully.

The type of sodium restriction prescribed should be the least restrictive diet that will still achieve the desired results. The first step is to minimize or eliminate the use of table salt and high-sodium foods. Box 37-3 lists serving sizes for some common high-sodium foods that should only be used sparingly in the sodium-restricted diet. Other foods that should be limited are shown in Box 37-4. As the restriction becomes more severe, attention is directed toward foods prepared with salt or sodium-containing compounds (Table 37-4). Finally, the intake of foods that naturally contain sodium—milk, meat, and vegetables—must be considered. Table 37-5 lists the sodium content of food groups and the number of servings from each

Box 37-3. Equivalent High-Sodium Foods, Each of Which Contains 400 mg of Sodium

Meats

1 small hot dog or 1 slice of lunchmeat
4 slices bacon
1½ oz cooked pork sausage
1½ oz ham or corned beef
1½ oz regular canned tuna
1½ oz regular canned crab
3 oz regular canned salmon
¾ c cottage cheese
2 oz cheese

Grains

20 small pretzels
¼ of 12 in. thin-crust cheese pizza

Vegetables

2 servings (½ c each) regular canned vegetables
⅓ c canned regular sauerkraut
½ large dill pickle
1 oz (approximately 20) potato chips

Soups

(All soups listed are canned soups diluted with equal amounts of water.)
⅔ c beef broth or vegetarian vegetable
½ c tomato, chicken gumbo, cream of celery
⅓ c cream of mushroom

Miscellaneous

¼ tsp salt, scant
1 tsp soy sauce
4 tsp Worcestershire sauce
2⅓ tbsp catsup
2 tbsp mustard, chili sauce, or barbecue sauce
4⅔ tbsp tartar sauce
2 tbsp French dressing
4 medium olives
4 tbsp sweet pickle relish

Modified from American Dietetic Association: *Manual of clinical dietetics*, ed 5, Chicago, 1996, American Dietetic Association.

Box 37-4. High-Sodium Foods

1. Smoked, processed, or cured meats and fish (e.g., ham, bacon, corned beef, cold cuts, frankfurters, sausage, tongue, salt pork, chipped beef, pickled herring, anchovies, tuna, sardines)
2. Meat extracts, bouillon cubes, meat sauces
3. Salted snacks (potato chips, tortilla chips, corn chips, pretzels, salted nuts, popcorn, and crackers)
4. Prepared salad dressings, condiments, relishes, Worcestershire sauce, barbecue sauce, soy sauce, commercial salad dressings, salsa, catsup, pickles, mustard, olives, sauerkraut
5. Prepackaged frozen foods (although plain vegetables not soaked in brine are excluded): packaged mixes for sauces, gravies, casseroles, and noodle, rice, or potato dishes; Oriental foods; spaghetti; pot pies
6. Canned soup, unless made without salt
7. Cheeses (processed and cheese spreads)

group that can be included at each level of sodium restriction. Table 37-6 presents a plan for a 2-g sodium diet. The National Heart Lung and Blood Institute has helpful tips for consumers trying to reduce sodium intake.

It is important to keep in mind the variety of ways in which dietary goals can be attained. For example, a patient may prefer to follow a 1-g sodium plan, in which regular bread is limited and canned vegetables are omitted, to be allowed to use ½ tsp of salt (1150 mg of sodium) on food throughout the day. This would bring the total sodium intake to 2 g daily.

Experience has shown that patients eating a diet of low-sodium foods do not make up the sodium difference when allowed use of a salt shaker ad libitum. This supports the hypothesis that a substantial reduction in dietary sodium is possible if low-sodium foods are consumed in conjunction with ad libitum use of table salt and that acceptable dietary saltiness can be achieved with less salt (Beauchamp et al, 1987).

TABLE 37-4 Sodium-Containing Additives

NAME	FOODS LIKELY TO CONTAIN
Disodium phosphate	Cereals, cheeses, ice cream, bottled drinks
Monosodium glutamate	Accent (a flavor enhancer), meats, condiments, pickles, soups, candy, baked goods
Sodium alginate	Ice cream, chocolate milk
Sodium benzoate	Fruit juices
Sodium hydroxide	Pretzels, sour cream, cocoa products, canned peas
Sodium propionate	Breads
Sodium sulfite	Dried fruits, cut salad greens
Sodium pectinate	Syrups and toppings, ice cream, sherbet, salad dressings, jams and jellies
Sodium caseinate	Ice cream and other frozen products
Sodium bicarbonate	Baking powder, tomato soup, self-rising flour, sherbets, confections

Dietary Sources of Sodium

Dietary sources of sodium include (1) salt used at the table, (2) salt or sodium compounds added during preparation or processing of foods (see Table 37-4), (3) inherent sodium in foods, and (4) chemically softened water. The average American consumes approximately 4 to 6 g of sodium daily, much more than the minimum 250 mg (9 mEq) required by the human to maintain life. Up to 20% comes from salt added to food during preparation or at the table. Between 35% and 80% of dietary sodium comes from processed foods (Mattes and Donnelly, 1991).

TABLE 37-5 Food Servings for Sodium-Controlled Diets

FOOD GROUP	SERVING SIZE	SODIUM CONTENT		SUGGESTED NUMBER OF SERVINGS FOR VARIOUS RESTRICTED DIETS			
		mg Na^+	mEq Na^+	3 g	2 g	1 g	500 mg
Milk, low sodium	8 oz	7	—				1
Milk, regular	8 oz	120	5	2	2	2	1
Buttermilk, salted	8 oz	280	13	—	—	—	—
Cottage cheese, regular	¼ c	130	6	1	1	1	—
Cheese, regular	1 oz	200	9	1	—	—	—
Meat, fish, poultry, unsalted cheese, tofu (½ c)	1 oz	25	1	6	6	6	5
Fresh shellfish	1 oz	50	2	1	1	—	—
Peanut butter, regular	1 tbsp	80	3	1	1	—	—
Egg	1	70	3	Not restricted		1	1
Vegetables, cooked, fresh, frozen	½ c	10	—			Not restricted	
Vegetables, naturally higher in sodium	½ c	40	2		Not restricted		1
Vegetables, canned, regular	½ c	230	10	—	—	—	—
Vegetable juices, canned	½ c	200	9	—	—	—	—
Fruits	½ c	2	—			Not restricted	
Bread, regular	1 slice	150	7	4	4	1	—
Bread, low sodium	1 slice	5	—			Not restricted	
Quick bread, muffin	1 serving	300	14	1	—	—	—
Cereal, ready-to-eat, salted	1 c	300	14	1	—	—	—
Cereal, unsalted	½ c	5	—			Not restricted	
Butter or margarine, salted	1 tsp	50	2	3	3	2	—
Butter or margarine, unsalted	1 tsp	1	—			Not restricted	
Mayonnaise, regular	1½ tsp	50	2	1	1	1	1
Salad dressing, regular	1 tbsp	350	16	1	—	—	—
Soup, regular	1 c	900	42	—	—	—	—
Soup, low sodium	1 c	25	1			Not restricted	
Desserts, regular	1 serving	300	14	1	—	—	—
Desserts, low sodium	1 serving	15	—			Not restricted	
Salt	1 tsp	2300	10	½ tsp	¼ tsp	—	—

TABLE 37-6 Two-Gram Sodium Diet

FOOD CATEGORY	FOOD RECOMMENDED	FOOD EXCLUDED
Beverages	Milk (limit to 16 oz or 480 ml daily), buttermilk (limit to 1 c/wk or 240 ml/wk); eggnog; all fruit juices; low-sodium, salt-free vegetable juices; low-sodium, carbonated beverages	Malted milk, milkshake, chocolate milk; regular vegetable or tomato juices; commercially softened water used for drinking or cooking
Breads and cereals	Enriched white, wheat, rye, and pumpernickel bread, hard rolls and dinner rolls; muffins, cornbread, and waffles; most dry cereals, cooked cereal without added salt; unsalted crackers and breadsticks; low-sodium or homemade bread crumbs	Breads, rolls, and crackers with salted tops; quick breads; instant hot cereals; pancakes; commercial bread stuffing; self-rising flour and biscuit mixes; commercial bread crumbs or cracker crumbs
Desserts and sweets	All; desserts and sweets made with milk should be within allowance	Instant pudding mixes and cake mixes
Fats	Butter or margarine; vegetable oils; unsalted salad dressings, regular salad dressings limited to 1 tbsp (15 ml); light, sour, and heavy cream	Regular salad dressings containing bacon fat, bacon bits, and salt pork; snack dips made with instant soup mixes or processed cheese
Fruits	Most fresh, frozen, and canned fruits	Fruits processed with salt or sodium-containing compounds (i.e., some dried fruits)
Meats and meat substitutes	Any fresh or frozen beef, lamb, pork, poultry, fish, and shrimp; canned tuna or salmon, rinsed; eggs and egg substitutes; low-sodium cheese, including low-sodium ricotta and cream cheese; low-sodium cottage cheese; regular yogurt; low-sodium peanut butter; dried peas and beans; frozen dinners (<500 mg or 22 mmol sodium/serving)	Any smoked, cured, salted, koshered, or canned meat, fish, or poultry including bacon, chipped beef, cold cuts, ham, hot dogs, sausage, sardines, anchovies, crab, lobster, imitation seafood, marinated herring, and pickled meats; frozen breaded meats; pickled eggs; regular hard and processed cheese, cheese spreads and sauces; salted nuts
Potatoes and potato substitutes	White or sweet potatoes; squash; enriched rice, barley, noodles, spaghetti, macaroni and other pastas cooked without salt; homemade bread stuffing	Commercially prepared potato, rice, or pasta mixes; commercial bread stuffing
Soups	Low-sodium commercially canned and dehydrated soups, broths, and bouillons; homemade broth and soups without added salt and made with allowed vegetables; cream soups within milk allowance	Regular canned or dehydrated soups, broths, or bouillon
Vegetables	Fresh, frozen vegetables and low-sodium canned vegetables	Regular canned vegetables, sauerkraut, pickled vegetables, and others prepared in brine; frozen vegetables in sauces; vegetables seasoned with ham, bacon, or salt pork
Miscellaneous	Salt substitute with physician's approval; pepper, herbs, spices; vinegar, lemon, or lime juice; hot pepper sauce; low-sodium soy sauce (1 tsp or 5 ml); low-sodium condiments (catsup, chili sauce, mustard); fresh ground horseradish; unsalted tortilla chips, pretzels, potato chips, popcorn, salsa (2 tbsp or 30 ml)	Any seasoning made with salt, including garlic salt, celery salt, onion salt, and, seasoned salt; sea salt, rock salt, kosher salt; meat tenderizers; monosodium glutamate; regular soy sauce, barbecue sauce, teriyaki sauce, steak sauce, Worcestershire sauce, and most flavored vinegars; canned gravy and mixes; regular condiments; salted snack foods, olives

From The American Dietetic Association: *Manual of clinical dietetics,* ed 6, Chicago, 2000, American Dietetic Association.

Animal protein foods, such as milk, cheese, eggs, meat, poultry, and fish, have relatively high sodium content. This is because, like human muscle cells, animal tissue cells are surrounded by sodium chloride. Thus, these foods must be limited in strict to severe-sodium-restriction diets. These foods are also restricted because of their saturated fat content to prevent further heart disease. Because Kosher meats and poultry are soaked in salt water for 1 hour after slaughter to remove the blood, even though the meat is washed thoroughly before cooking, the sodium content of such foods may still be increased as much as four times, to a level of 90 to 115 mg per ounce. Acceptable alternatives are to boil the meat and discard the broth before eating or to use low-sodium kosher meats that are available.

Between 4% and 27% of dietary sodium comes from ingested water. The amount of sodium in drinking water is an issue for the person restricted to a 500-mg sodium diet if the sodium concentration in the water is greater than 40 ppm (40 mg or 2 mEq/L). Typical water softeners exchange sodium ions for calcium and other ions that cause water hardness. Use of distilled water may be necessary; alternatively, only the hot water can be chemically softened.

Sodium Labeling

With enactment of the Nutrition Labeling and Education Act (NLEA) of 1990, the Food and Drug Administration (FDA) revised regulations to require labeling of sodium content on foods and provided legal definitions for the terms *low sodium, moderately low sodium,* and *reduced sodium* (Table 37-7). The daily value for sodium was set at 2400 mg. Patients can use the percent daily value to determine whether a certain food would fit into a diet that contains 2400 mg of sodium. The expression of sodium content in milligrams can also help patients determine whether the food is appropriate for their restriction level (Table 37-8).

TABLE 37-7 Food-Labeling Guide for Sodium

Sodium-free	Less than 5 mg per standard serving; cannot contain any sodium chloride
Very low sodium	35 mg or less per standard serving
Low sodium	140 mg or less per standard serving
Reduced sodium	At least 25% less sodium per standard serving than in the regular food
Light in sodium	50% less sodium per standard serving than in the regular food
Unsalted, without added salt, or no salt added	No salt added during processing; the product it resembles is normally processed with salt
Lightly salted	50% less added sodium than is normally added; product must state "not a low-sodium food" if that criterion is not met

Data from U.S. Food and Drug Administration: Scouting for sodium and other nutrients important to blood pressure, FDA Consumer, Publication No. 95-2284, 1995.

Nonnutrient Sources of Sodium

Low-sodium salt substitutes, which contain one third to one half as much sodium as regular table salt, can be calculated into a mildly restricted diet. Vegetized salts, which use powdered dehydrated vegetables, may contain considerable quantities of sodium and should therefore be used only when their sodium content is counted as part of the total intake. Most commercial salt substitutes are mineral bases consisting of potassium chloride, calcium chloride, or ammonium chloride and thus do not contain sodium chloride.

Spices, herbs, and other seasonings (horseradish, tabasco, lemon juice, and vinegar) can be used to improve the flavor of low-sodium foods. Most spices contain less than 0.05% sodium, and almost all contain less than 0.1%. Herb or spice salts, such as garlic salt, should be avoided.

Nondietary Sources of Added Sodium

In addition to the sodium in food and water, incidental amounts may be ingested in the form of medicines and toothpastes. Barbiturates, sulfonamides, antibiotics, and other drugs, as well as cough medications, stomach alkalizers, laxatives, and mouthwashes, may contain large amounts of sodium. For example, some over-the-counter chewable antacid tablets can add 1200 to 7000 mg of sodium daily when used as therapy for ulcer or gastric distress. Aspirin supplies about 50 mg of sodium per tablet. Most medicine contains less than 5 mg of sodium per dose; only those containing 80 to 120 mg per dose contribute substantially to sodium intake.

Low-Sodium or Low-Salt Syndrome

Severe sodium restriction is generally reserved for the hospitalized patient whose sodium tolerance is unusually low. Care should be taken to avoid hyponatremia, hypochloremia, and, eventually, azotemia as the glomerular filtration rate decreases. This low-salt syndrome can also result from adrenal insufficiency, severe and prolonged vomiting, diarrhea, and burns. Symptoms of potential low-sodium syndrome or salt depletion are weakness, lassitude, anorexia, vomiting, abdominal cramps, aching skeletal muscles, and mental confusion.

TABLE 37-8 Sodium and Salt in Gram and Milliequivalent Measures

mEq Na^+ (APPROXIMATE)	mg Na^+	g NaCl (APPROXIMATE)
11	250	0.6
22	500	1.3
43	1000	2.5
65	1500	3.8
87	2000	5.0
130	3000	7.6
174	4000	10.2
217	5000	12.7

Potassium

Some diuretics (e.g., hydrochlorothiazide) increase potassium excretion. Potassium depletion may lead to *digitalis toxicity,* which is characterized by anorexia, nausea and vomiting, abdominal discomfort, hallucinations, depression, drowsiness, and cardiac arrhythmias. For some patients, the inclusion of high-potassium foods in the diet is enough. Other patients require the use of potassium supplements. Another source of potassium is salt substitutes, which can provide between 500 and 2000 mg (13 to 72 mEq) of potassium per teaspoon; however, salt substitutes are contraindicated in patients with renal failure and in those receiving certain medications used to treat CHF (see Table 37-3). Consequently, the approval of a physician should always be sought prior to their use.

Fluids

During hospitalization, fluids are commonly restricted for CHF patients. Intake may be limited to 500 to 2000 ml daily. Occasionally, foods having a high fluid content also must be limited. Foods that are liquid at room temperature such as ice cream, yogurt, gelatin, or popsicles would count toward the total fluid allotment. Freezing pieces of fruit or sucking on sugar-free hard candy can abate the thirst mechanism for patients on fluid restrictions (Lutton and Anzlovar, 2001). Fluid status should be monitored by measuring urine specific gravity and serum electrolyte values and by observing for clinical signs of edema. Restrictions are often discontinued upon the patient's discharge from the hospital.

Calcium and Vitamin D

About half of patients with severe heart failure have osteopenia or osteoporosis (Shane et al, 1997).

Cachectic CHF patients have lower bone mineral density and lower calcium levels than CHF patients without cachexia or normal subjects (Anker, 1999b). Caution must be used with calcium supplements because they may aggravate cardiac arrhythmias.

Magnesium

As with potassium, the diuretics used to treat CHF increase magnesium excretion (Witte et al, 2001). Magnesium deficiency aggravates changes in electrolyte concentration by causing a positive sodium and negative potassium balance. The incidence of magnesium deficiency is not well studied but in one report was estimated at 30% of patients (Wester and Dyckner, 1986). Because deficient magnesium status is associated with poorer prognosis, blood magnesium levels should be measured in CHF patients and treated accordingly (Eichorn et al, 1993; Gottlieb et al, 1990).

Thiamin

Loop diuretics can deplete body thiamin (Brady et al, 1995; Seligmann et al, 1991). Thiamin supplementation for patients taking 80 mg of lasix improved left ventricular ejection fraction and symptoms (Shimon et al, 1995). Thiamin status should be assessed in CHF patients on loop diuretics, and appropriate dietary intake ensured via food intake or supplement.

Feeding Strategies

Patients with CHF often tolerate small, frequent feedings better than larger, infrequent meals because the latter are more tiring to consume, can contribute to abdominal distention, and markedly increase oxygen consumption. All these factors tax the already stressed heart.

Supplements

Many supplements (coenzyme Q10, carnitine, inositol, vitamins) or hormonal therapies (growth hormone) are commonly prescribed for CHF patients (Packer et al, 1999). Coenzyme Q10 is lowered in CHF patients, and it was postulated that repletion could prevent oxidative stress and further myocardial damage. Studies showing a benefit from Q10 supplementation were severely flawed by small sample size, lack of blinding, and lack of randomization of subjects. In two randomized control trials in patients with class III and IV symptoms, coenzyme Q10 had no benefit on ejection fraction, peak oxygen consumption, exercise duration, or quality of life in CHF patients receiving standard therapy (Khatta et al, 2000; Watson et al, 1999).

All guidelines currently avoid recommendation of coenzyme Q10 or any other supplements at this time (American College of Cardiology, 1995; Packer, 1999) and caution against use because of possible interference with the actions of drugs known to be beneficial in CHF patients. More double-blind placebo, randomized control trials are needed to investigate efficacy of dietary supplements in CHF patients (Witte et al, 2001).

CARDIAC TRANSPLANTATION

Cardiac transplant is the only cure for refractory CHF. In 2000, in the United States, 2198 transplants were performed (AHA, 2001), with the highest number in white men 50 to 64 years of age. The survival rates following transplants done between 1994 and 2000 were at 1 year, 84%; at 3 years, 77%; and at 5 years, 69%. Other surgical options are being tested for refractory CHF.

Nutritional care of the heart transplant patient can be divided into three phases: pretransplant, immediate posttransplant, and long-term posttransplant (Table 37-9).

TABLE 37-9 Nutrient Care for Cardiac Transplant Patients

PHASE	MAJOR NUTRITIONAL CONCERNS	ACTIONS
Pretransplant	Cardiac cachexia Sodium and fluid restriction	Evaluate diet, weight history, and functional status. Apply strategies to boost intake. Consider maximally concentrated nutrition support.
Immediate posttransplant	Sufficient calories and protein to promote healing and to help withstand rejection episodes Metabolic and nutritional effects of immunosuppressive regimen	Monitor pertinent assessment data.* Apply strategies to encourage adequate intake. Ensure appropriate calcium intake.
Long-term posttransplant	Hypercholesterolemia and accelerated graft atherosclerosis Long-term metabolic and nutritional effects of immunosuppressive regimen (weight gain, glucose intolerance)	Monitor pertinent assessment data.* Encourage lipid-lowering diet. Apply strategies for weight control. Promote diabetes management.

Data from Rock CL, Leonard LB: Nutrition care of cardiac transplant patients, *Top Clin Nutr* 5(1):1, 1990.

*Body weight, height (in children), dietary intake; serum albumin, prealbumin, glucose, potassium, sodium, magnesium, calcium, and phosphorus levels; hemoglobin, hematocrit values; total blood cholesterol, total fasting triglyceride values; high-density, low-density, and very-low-density lipoprotein cholesterol levels.

Pretransplant Medical Nutrition Therapy

Pretransplant nutritional goals for transplant candidates with adequate nutriture are (1) a body weight that is within 90% to 110% of ideal body weight, (2) a positive nitrogen balance of 3 to 4 g daily, (3) a sodium intake of 2 g daily, (4) a protein intake of 1.0 to 1.2 g per kilogram of body weight, and (5) a caloric intake of 30 kcal per kilogram of body weight (Poindexter et al, 1992). Patients with poor nutritional status would require additional protein (1.5 to 2.0 g/kg) and calories (35 to 40 kcal/kg) for anabolism.

TABLE 37-10 Tube-Feeding Formulas for Posttransplant Patients

CONDITION	SUGGESTED TUBE-FEEDING FORMULA
Normal digestion, immediately posttransplant	Polymeric, high-nitrogen formula
Fluid overload	Concentrated polymeric formula
Hyperglycemia	Diabetic formula
Elevated CO_2 levels in blood	High-fat formula
Fat malabsorption	Low-fat formula or formula containing medium-chain triglycerides
Diarrhea or constipation	High-fiber formula (provide adequate fluid)
Renal failure	Renal formula (concentrated formula with limited potassium, sodium, and phosphorus)
Impaired digestion or immediately after intestinal transplant	Semielemental or glutamine-enhanced formula

From Hasse J: Recovery after organ transplantation in adults: the role of postoperative nutrition therapy, *Top Clin Nutr* 13(2):15, 1998.

Patients awaiting cardiac transplant also need to be evaluated for osteopenic bone disease secondary to prolonged periods of inactivity, malnutrition, and use of loop diuretics (Francisco-Ziller and DiCecco, 1998). Nutritional treatment for osteopenia includes calcium supplementation (1 to 1.5 g daily) and water-miscible vitamin D supplements (see Chapter 27). If oral intake is inadequate, a standard, isotonic enteral feeding is indicated. Patients with comorbid conditions require other tube-feeding formulas (Table 37-10).

Posttransplant Medical Nutrition Therapy

The four goals of medical nutritional therapy for posttransplant patients are (1) to promote healing, (2) to fight infection, (3) to provide energy for ambulation and physical therapy, and (4) to replenish nutrient stores (Hasse, 1998). In the immediate posttransplant period, nutrient needs are increased, as is the case after any major surgery. High caloric and protein intakes (1.3 to 1.5 times basal energy expenditure and 1.2 to 2.0 g/kg of body weight, respectively) are initial goals. Protein intakes are increased because of steroid-induced catabolism, surgical stress, anabolism, and wound healing.

Particular attention should be paid to protein intakes when corticosteroid doses are high because the rate of protein catabolism is proportional to the dose. Patients progress from clear liquids to a soft diet given in small, frequent feedings. Electrolyte disorders secondary to drug therapy and other posttransplant consequences often require nutritional treatment (Table 37-11). Nutritional monitoring in the immediate posttransplant phase is extensive (Table 37-12). Nutrient intake is often maintained by using liquid supplements and foods of high caloric content. In patients with poor appetite, persistence by the

TABLE 37-11 Electrolyte Disturbances in Posttransplant Patients

ELECTROLYTE ABNORMALITY	POSSIBLE CAUSE(S)	SUGGESTED TREATMENT
Hypernatremia	Dehydration; excess sodium intake	Increase fluid intake; decrease sodium intake.
Hyponatremia	Overhydration; total body sodium deficit	Restrict fluid intake; increase sodium intake if there is a total body sodium deficit.
Hyperkalemia	Drugs such as tacrolimus, cyclosporine, potassium-sparing diuretics; renal insufficiency; metabolic acidosis	Restrict potassium intake; administer potassium binder.
Hypokalemia	Potassium-wasting diuretics; refeeding syndrome; diarrhea; fistula; inadequate potassium intake	Increase dietary potassium intake; administer supplements.
Hyperphosphatemia	Renal insufficiency	Restrict phosphorus intake; administer phosphate binders.
Hypophosphatemia	Refeeding syndrome; glucocorticoids	Increase intake of high-phosphorus foods; administer phosphorus supplements.
Hypermagnesemia	Renal insufficiency	Limit magnesium intake.
Hypomagnesemia	Cyclosporine; refeeding syndrome; diabetic ketoacidosis; diuretics; diarrhea	Increase intake of high-magnesium foods; administer magnesium supplements.
Decreased bicarbonate	Increased exocrine drainage (pancreas transplant); intestinal drainage (intestinal transplant)	Administer bicarbonate supplements; if patient is receiving total parenteral nutrition, provide acetate.

From Hasse J: Recovery after organ transplantation in adults: the role of postoperative nutrition therapy, *Top Clin Nutr* 13(2):15, 1998.

medical team and family is the key to achievement of nutritional goals.

Because of longer survival, many transplant patients experience complications such as hyperlipidemia, hypertension, obesity, diabetes, and osteopenia (Weseman and McCashland, 1998). Immunosuppressive drugs have a marked impact on nutritional status and thus influence long-term posttransplant nutrition goals (see Table 37-13). Weight gain and hyperlipidemia are two main sequelae of immunosuppressive drug therapy. Factors found to pose a significant risk for the development of hypercholesterolemia after transplantation are prednisone dose, baseline cholesterol level, blood glucose levels, and weight gain (Kubo et al, 1992). Because graft atherosclerosis is the leading cause of death in long-term survivors, a step II diet (30% of calories derived from fat, less than 7% from saturated fatty acids, and an intake of less than 200 mg of cholesterol daily), along with restriction of sodium to 2 to 4 g per day, is recommended (see Chapter 35). Stricter diets and the use of pharmacologic agents may be necessary to normalize blood lipid levels. Ideal body weight should be achieved and maintained; increasing activity level is important for weight maintenance and the attainment of lipid goals.

TABLE 37-12 Nutritional Monitoring After Transplantation

MONITORING TOOL	INDICATIONS
Indirect calorimetry	When it is difficult to estimate caloric needs and when a patient is receiving adequate nutrition, according to estimates, but is not thriving
Body weight	Daily
Fluid intake and output	Every 8 to 12 hr
Nutrient intake	Daily until adequate
Serum glucose concentration	Every 6 hr initially; less frequently when level normalizes
Serum potassium concentration	Daily
Serum phosphorus level	At least twice per week
Serum bicarbonate level	Daily for small-intestine and pancreas transplant recipients
Serum magnesium level	Once or twice per week

From Hasse JM, DiCecco SR: Solid organ transplantation. In Skipper A, editor: *The dietitian's handbook of enteral and parenteral nutrition,* ed 2, Gaithersburg, Md, 1998, Aspen Publishers.

SUMMARY

Congestive heart failure is most often the end point for other cardiovascular diseases, particularly hypertension and coronary heart disease. Whereas previous therapy focused on alleviation of symptoms,

TABLE 37-13 Common Nutritional Side Effects of Immunosuppressive Medications

DRUG	MECHANISM OF ACTION	SIDE EFFECTS
Cyclosporine A (Sandimmune, Neoral)	Inhibits the response of cytotoxic T cells to interleukin-2 (IL-2) and prevents helper T lymphocytes from producing IL-2	Nephrotoxicity, neurotoxicity (e.g., headache, tremor, seizure); hypertension; hyperglycemia; hyperlipidemia; hyperkalemia; hypomagnesemia; gingival hyperplasia
Tacrolimus (Prograf, FK506)	Inhibits the proliferation of cytotoxic T cells and the synthesis of IL-2	Nephrotoxicity; neurotoxicity; hypertension; hyperglycemia (diabetogenic effects); hyperkalemia; nausea and vomiting; gastrointestinal symptoms (diarrhea)
Corticosteroids (Prednisone, Prednisolone, Solumedrol, Solucortef)	Antiinflammatory response at the arterial site; inhibits IL-1 and decreases IL-2, which suppresses lymphocyte proliferation and decreases circulating lymphocytes	Altered fluid and electrolyte balance; hypertension; adrenal-axis suppression; mood swings (depression, euphoria); peptic ulcer disease; hyperphagia; hyperlipidemia; poor wound healing; cataracts
Azathioprine (Imuran)	Inhibits RNA and DNA synthesis to prevent cytotoxic T-cell and B-cell proliferation and antibody production	Bone marrow suppression (leukopenia, thrombocytopenia, pancytopenia, macrocytic anemia); nausea and vomiting; diarrhea; hepatotoxicity
Mycophenolate mofetil (Cellcept, RS-61443)	Decreases lymphocyte activation and replication by suppressing enzymes in the purine salvage pathway, thereby creating a purine deficiency and inhibiting T- and B-cell proliferation; also suppresses antibody formation	Gastrointestinal symptoms (nausea, vomiting, diarrhea); leukopenia
Antithymocyte globulin (ATGam)	Decreases circulating lymphocytes	Anaphylactic reaction; fever and chills; nausea and vomiting; leukopenia
Muromonab CD3 (OKT3)	Binds to mature T cells to decrease their effector function	Anaphylactic reaction; pulmonary edema (usually first dose only); severe flulike symptoms; headache; increased incidence of lymphoproliferative disorders
Sirolimus (Rapamycin)	Inhibits T- and B-cell proliferation while not affecting IL-2 production	Possible hyperglycemia; possible gastrointestinal symptoms; hyperlipidemia
15-Deoxysperagualin	Inhibits T and B lymphocytes	Leukopenia; thrombocytopenia; gastrointestinal symptoms

From Hasse JM, DiCecco SR: Solid organ transplantation. In Skipper A, editor: *The dietitian's handbook of enteral and parenteral nutrition,* ed 2, Gaithersburg, Md, 1998, Aspen Publishers.

newer treatments include trying to prevent the progressive deterioration in heart function. Through prevention and treatment, medical nutrition therapy for underlying causes (hypertension, coronary heart disease, diabetes) or symptomatic relief (sodium restriction) is pivotal.

Clinical Scenario 1

Evelyn is a 76-year-old white woman with a 25-year history of mild hypertension, controlled by diet and a diuretic. Recently, she has been complaining of a dry cough, headache, dizziness, and shortness or breath while doing yard work. She was admitted to your hospital with the diagnosis of CHF. During her 3-week stay, she has been given oxygen because her Po_2 level was 48 on admission and is now only 60. Lasix, Inderal, and Zaroxolyn have been prescribed. She lives alone, and her two grown daughters live out of state.

1. What are the effects of Evelyn's medications on her nutritional status?
2. She is currently following a 2-g sodium diet but will be following a no-added-salt diet at home. Her favorite foods are ethnic German foods, including sauerkraut, cabbage dishes, pork, and sausage. What dietary adaptations do you suggest?
3. Because shopping is difficult for Evelyn, what types of agency referrals should you seek? What advice will you offer to her daughters, who have called to talk about dietary changes?
4. If Evelyn is discharged to a nursing home, write a draft discharge nutrition summary to send to the dietitian there. What key pieces of information are relevant?
5. What types of instructions should you consider?

Clinical Scenario 2

Leon is a 27-year-old black man who has just seen his physician with complaints of severe chest pain, shortness of breath, and long-term history of hypertension. After extensive testing, he was diagnosed with refractory CHF and is awaiting a heart transplant. He is taking diuretics, follows a 2-g sodium diet but consumes a diet closer to 4 g, and is 30% above his ideal body weight. He is seeing you in your nutrition clinic for the first time tomorrow and will be bringing you some favorite recipes to adapt.

1. What other factors do you need to know to provide Leon with adequate medical nutrition therapy guidance?
2. What tips can you offer him to make his low-sodium diet more palatable?
3. Is this a good time to promote a weight-loss regimen? Why or why not?
4. What are some useful resources for Leon to help him with meal planning before his surgery?

Relevent Web Sites

American Heart Association
www.americanheart.org
National Heart, Lung, and Blood Institute
www.nhlbi.nih.gov/hbp/prevent/sodium/tips.htm
National Institutes of Health Web Site on Heart Failure
www.nhlbi.nih.gov/health/public/heart/other/hrtfail.htm

Cited References

American College of Cardiology/American Heart Association Task Force on Practice Guidelines: Guidelines for evaluation and management of heart failure, *J Am Coll Cardiol* 26:1376, 1995.

American Heart Association (AHA): 2001 Heart and stroke statistical update, Dallas, 2001, American Heart Association.

Anker SD et al: Hormonal changes and catabolic/anabolic imbalance in chronic heart failure and their importance for cardiac cachexia, *Circulation* 96:526, 1997a.

Anker SD et al: Loss of bone mineral in patients with cachexia due to chronic heart failure, *Am J Med* 103:197, 1997b.

Armstrong PW, Moe GW: Medical advances in the treatment of congestive heart failure, *Circulation* 88:2941, 1994.

Aronow WS: Treatment of congestive heart failure in older patients, *J Am Geriatr Soc* 45:1252, 1997.

Beauchamp GK et al: Modification of salt taste, *Ann Intern Med* 98:763, 1987.

Brady JA et al: Thiamine status, diuretic medications and the management of congestive heart failure, *J Am Diet Assoc* 95:541, 1995.

Carr JG et al: Prevalence and hemodynamic correlates of malnutrition in severe congestive heart failure secondary to ischemic or idiopathic dilated cardiomyopathy, *Am J Cardiol* 63:709, 1989.

Clinical Practice Guidelines: Heart failure: management of patients with left ventricular systolic dysfunction, *Am Fam Physician* 50:603, 1994.

Deedwania PC: Underutilization of evidence-based therapy in heart failure, *Arch Intern Med* 157:2409, 1997.

Dracup K et al: Management of heart failure. II. Counseling, education, and lifestyle modifications, *JAMA* 272:1442, 1994.

Eichorn EJ et al: Clinical and prognostic significance of serum magnesium concentration in patients with severe CHF: the PROMISE study, *J Am Coll Cardiol* 21:634, 1993.

Francisco-Ziller N, DiCecco S: Nutritional care of the pretransplant patient, *Top Clin Nutr* 13(2):1, 1998.

Freeman LM, Roubenoff R: The nutrition implications of cardiac cachexia, *Nutr Rev* 52:340, 1994.

Gottlieb S et al: Prognostic importance of the serum magnesium concentration in patients with congestive heart failure, *J Am Coll Cardiol* 16:827, 1990.

Hasse JM: Recovery after organ transplantation in adults: the role of postoperative nutrition therapy, *Top Clin Nutr* 13(2):15, 1998.

Ho KL et al: The epidemiology of heart failure: the Framingham Study, *J Am Coll Cardiol* 22(suppl A):6A, 1993.

Hunt S et al: ACC/AHA guidelines for the evaluation and management of chronic heart failure in the adult: executive summary, *Circulation* 104:2996, 2001.

Khatta M et al: The effect of coenzyme Q10 in patients with congestive heart failure, *Ann Intern Med* 132:636, 2000.

Kjekshus J et al: The effects of simvastatin on the incidence of heart failure in patients with coronary heart disease, *J Card Fail* 3:249, 1997.

King D et al: Fat malabsorption in elderly patients with cardiac cachexia, *Age Ageing* 25(2):144, 1996.

Kostis J et al for the SHEP Cooperative Research Group: Prevention of heart failure by antihypertensive drug treatment in older persons with isolated systolic hypertension, *JAMA* 278:212, 1997.

Krauss RM et al: AHA dietary guidelines, revision 2000: a statement for health care professionals from the Nutrition Committee of the American Heart Association, *Circulation* 102:2284, 2000.

Kubo SH et al: Factors influencing the development of hypercholesterolemia after cardiac transplantation, *Am J Cardiol* 70:520, 1992.

Levy D et al: The progression from hypertension to congestive heart failure, *JAMA* 275:1557, 1996.

Lutton S, Anzlovar N: Nutrition and congestive heart failure. In Coulston AM, Rock CL, Monsen ER, editors: *Nutrition in the prevention and treatment of disease,* San Diego, 2001, Academic Press.

Mann DL et al: New therapeutics for chronic heart failure, *Annu Rev Med* 53:59, 2002.

Massie BM, Amidon TM: Heart. In Tierney LM, McPhee SJ, Papadakis MA, editors: *2002 Current medical diagnosis and treatment,* ed 41, New York, 2002, Lange Medical Books/McGraw Hill.

Massie BM, Shah NB: Evolving trends in the epidemiologic factors of heart failure: rationale for preventive strategies and comprehensive disease management, *Am Heart J* 133:703, 1997.

Mattes RD, Donnelly D: Relative contributions of dietary sodium sources, *J Am Coll Nutr* 10:83, 1991.

McMurray J, Pfeffer MA: New therapeutic options in congestive heart failure, *Circulation* 105:2099, 2002.

Miller LW, Missov ED: Epidemiology of heart failure, *Cardiol Clin* 19:547, 2001.

Neily JB et al: Potential contributing factors to noncompliance with dietary sodium restriction in patients with heart failure, *Am Heart J* 143:29, 2002.

Nohria A et al: Medical management of advanced heart failure, *JAMA* 287:628, 2002.

Packer M et al: Consensus recommendations for the management of chronic heart failure, *Am J Cardiol* 83:1A, 1999.

Pitt B et al: Randomized Aldactone Evaluation Study Investigators: The effect of spironolactone on morbidity and mortality in patients with severe heart failure, *N Engl J Med* 341:709, 1999.

Poindexter SM et al: Potential parameters of nutritional assessment in the congestive heart failure and cardiac transplant patient: circumference measures of waist, lower thigh, and calf, *J Am Diet Assoc* 89:A65, 1989.

Poindexter SM et al: Nutrition support in cardiac transplantation, *Top Clin Nutr* 7(3):12, 1992.

Pronsky Z: *Food medication and interactions,* ed 11, Birchrunville, Pa, 2000, Food Medication Interactions.

Rich MW: Epidemiology, pathophysiology, and etiology of congestive heart failure in older adults, *J Am Geriatr Soc* 45:968, 1997.

Seligmann H et al: Thiamine deficiency in patients with congestive heart failure receiving long-term furosemide therapy: a pilot study, *Am Med J* 91:151, 1991.

Shane E at al: Bone mass, vitamin D deficiency and hypoparathyroidism in congestive heart failure, *Am J Med* 103:197, 1997.

Shimon I et al: Improved left ventricular function after thiamine supplementation in patients with congestive heart failure receiving long-term furosemide therapy, *Am Med J* 98:485, 1995.

Volpe M et al: Abnormalities of sodium handling and cardiovascular adaptations during a high salt diet in patients with mild heart failure, *Circulation* 88:1620, 1993.

Watson PS et al: Lack of effect of coenzyme Q10 on left ventricular function in patients with congestive heart failure, *J Am Coll Cardiol* 33:1549, 1999.

Weber KT: Aldosterone in congestive heart failure, *N Engl J Med* 345:1689, 2001.

Weseman RA, McCashland TM: Nutritional care of the chronic posttransplant patient, *Top Clin Nutr* 13(2):27, 1998.

Wester PO, Dyckner T: Intracelluafar electrolytes in cardiac failure, *Acta Med Scand Suppl* 707:33, 1986.

Witte KK et al: Chronic heart failure and micronutrients, *J Am Coll Cardiol* 37:1765, 2001.

Zhao S-P, Zeng L-H: Elevated plasma levels of tumor necrosis factor in chronic heart failure with cachexia, *Int J Cardiol* 58:257, 1997.

Additional References

Cooper HA et al: Light-to-moderate alcohol consumption and prognosis in patients with left ventricular systolic dysfunction, *J Am Coll Cardiol* 35:1753, 2000.

Horwich TB et al: Anemia is associated with worse symptoms, greater impairment in functional capacity and a significant increase in mortality in patients with advanced heart failure, *J Am Coll Cardiol* 39:1780, 2002.

Masoudi FA et al: The burden of chronic congestive heart failure in older persons: magnitude and implications for policy and research, *Heart Fail Rev* 27:9, 2002.

Neily JB et al: Potential contributing factors to noncompliance with dietary sodium restriction in patients with heart failure, *Am Heart J* 143:29, 2002.

Tresch DD: The clinical diagnosis of heart failure in older patients, *J Am Geriatr Soc* 45:1128, 1997.

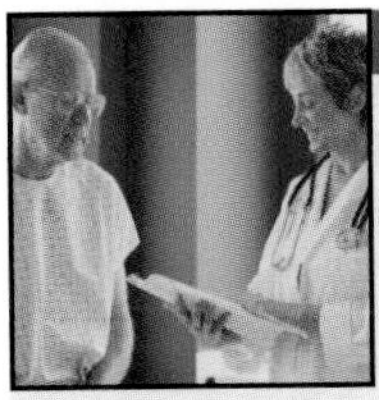

CHAPTER 38

Medical Nutrition Therapy for Pulmonary Disease

DONNA H. MUELLER, PhD, RD, FADA

CHAPTER OUTLINE

- Relationships Between Nutrition and the Pulmonary System
- Overview of Medical Nutrition Therapy in Pulmonary Disease
- Aspiration
- Asthma
- Bronchopulmonary Dysplasia
- Chronic Obstructive Pulmonary Disease
- Cystic Fibrosis
- Lung Cancer
- Pneumonia
- Respiratory Failure
- Tuberculosis

KEY TERMS

acute respiratory distress syndrome (ARDS)–a life-threatening condition characterized by severe hypoxia, bilateral pulmonary fluid infiltration, and decreased lung compliance; usually occurring without prior lung disease but secondary to catastrophic illness

asthma–a condition of hypersensitive airways from allergic and nonallergic causes, generated by immunologic responses

bronchopulmonary dysplasia (BPD)–a chronic lung disease of infancy that commonly arises following respiratory distress syndrome (RDS) and treatment with oxygen; characterized by broncheolar metaplasia and interstitial fibrosis

chronic bronchitis–a chronic, productive cough with inflammation of one or more of the bronchi and secondary changes in lung tissue

chronic obstructive pulmonary disease (COPD)–a process characterized by the presence of chronic bronchitis, emphysema, or both, leading to the development of airway obstruction

coefficient of fat absorption (CFA)–the amount of fat absorbed, based on a 72-hour record of fat intake and a fecal fat collection; calculated by the following equation: CFA = fat intake − fecal fat/fat intake

cor pulmonale–a heart condition characterized by right ventricular enlargement and failure that results from resistance to the passage of blood through the lungs

cystic fibrosis (CF)–an autosomal recessive disorder characterized by dysfunction of the exocrine glands and production of abnormally thick secretions that obstruct airways and pancreatic and other ducts

distal intestinal obstruction syndrome (DIOS)–recurrent distal intestinal impaction; formerly termed *meconium ileus equivalent*

dyspnea–shortness of breath

emphysema–a condition of the lung characterized by abnormal, permanent enlargement of alveoli, accompanied by destruction of their walls without obvious fibrosis

pancreatic enzyme replacement therapy–use of exogenous pancreatic enzymes to produce more normal digestion in persons with pancreatic insufficiency

KEY TERMS—Continued

pulmonary aspiration–the drawing of foreign bodies, such as food or liquid, into the lungs during inspiration

pulmonary function tests–a group of procedures designed to measure the ability of the respiratory system to exchange oxygen and carbon dioxide

respiratory distress syndrome (RDS)–a condition affecting newborn infants, particularly premature neonates and those of low birth weight, that is marked by dyspnea with cyanosis

respiratory quotient (RQ)–the ratio of the volume of carbon dioxide expired to the volume of oxygen inspired (CO_2/O_2)

surfactant–a substance composed of phospholipids (especially dipalmitophosphatidylcholine) and protein that is produced by type II cells of the alveolar epithelium; it lowers surface tension so as to permit gas exchange at the gas-liquid interface

sweat test–a test performed using pilocarpine iontophoreses to determine levels of sodium and chloride in sweat; elevated levels are diagnostic of cystic fibrosis

tachypnea–abnormal rapidity of respiration that, if prolonged, can lead to excess loss of CO_2 and respiratory alkalosis

Respiratory alterations can occur anytime throughout the life cycle: from the premature infant with insufficient surfactant production, to the emaciated teenager with anorexia nervosa, to the young adult with street-drug overdose, to the older adult with severe osteoporosis. Management of the pulmonary problems from these situations along with primary pulmonary system disorders such as asthma, cystic fibrosis, and emphysema, requires attention to the nutritional status and the nutritional intake during the disease and its treatment for best possible outcome.

RELATIONSHIPS BETWEEN NUTRITION AND THE PULMONARY SYSTEM

Optimal Nutrition and the Pulmonary System

Optimal nutrition throughout life promotes anatomic development and physiologic function of the pulmonary system. The respiratory structures include the nose, pharynx, larynx, trachea, bronchi, bronchioles, alveolar ducts, and alveoli. Supporting structures include the skeleton and the muscles (e.g., the intercostal, abdominal, and diaphragm muscles). Nerves, blood, and lymph supply all tissues (Figure 38-1). Within a month after conception, pulmonary system structures are recognizable. The pulmonary system grows and matures during gestation and childhood. Aging results in diminished lung integrity (Rossi et al, 1996).

Gas exchange is the major function of the pulmonary system (Figure 38-2). The lungs enable the body to obtain the oxygen needed to meet its cellular metabolic demands and to remove the carbon dioxide produced by these processes. The lungs also function to filter, warm, and humidify inspired air; synthesize surfactant; regulate body acid–base balance; synthesize arachidonic acid; and convert angiotensin I to angiotensin II.

The relationship between nutrition and lung immune defense mechanisms needs special highlight (Figure 38-3). First, inspired air is laden with particles and microorganisms. Some cells in the airway linings secrete mucus. This mucus keeps the airways moist and traps the particles and microorganisms from inspired air. Most cells that line the trachea, bronchi, and bronchioles have cilia. These constantly beating cilia sweep the particles upward toward the pharynx. Each time a person swallows, the particle- and microorganism-containing mucus passes into the digestive tract. Second, the epithelial surface of the alveoli contains macrophages (Figure 38-4). By the process of phagocytosis, these alveolar macrophages engulf inhaled inert materials and microorganisms and digest them. Third, although the molecular mechanism of action is unknown, the antioxidant nutrients may protect lung tissues from oxidative injury. Thus, overall optimal nutritional status as well as specific nutrients themselves are essential for the formation, development, growth, and protection of healthy lungs and other body structures and processes throughout life.

Impact of Malnutrition on the Pulmonary System

The relationship between malnutrition and respiratory disease has long been recognized (Pingleton, 1998). Malnutrition adversely affects lung structure, elasticity, and function; respiratory muscle mass, strength, and endurance; lung immune defense mechanisms; and control of breathing. For example, protein and iron deficiencies result in low hemoglobin levels, resulting in diminished oxygen-carrying capacity of the blood. Low levels of other minerals, such as calcium, magnesium, phosphorus, and potassium, compromise respiratory muscle function at the cellular level. Hypoproteinemia contributes to the development of pulmonary edema by decreasing colloid osmotic pressure, which allows body fluids to move into the interstitial space. Decreased levels of surfactant, a compound synthesized from proteins and phospholipids, contribute to the collapse of alveoli and thus increase the work of breathing. The sup-

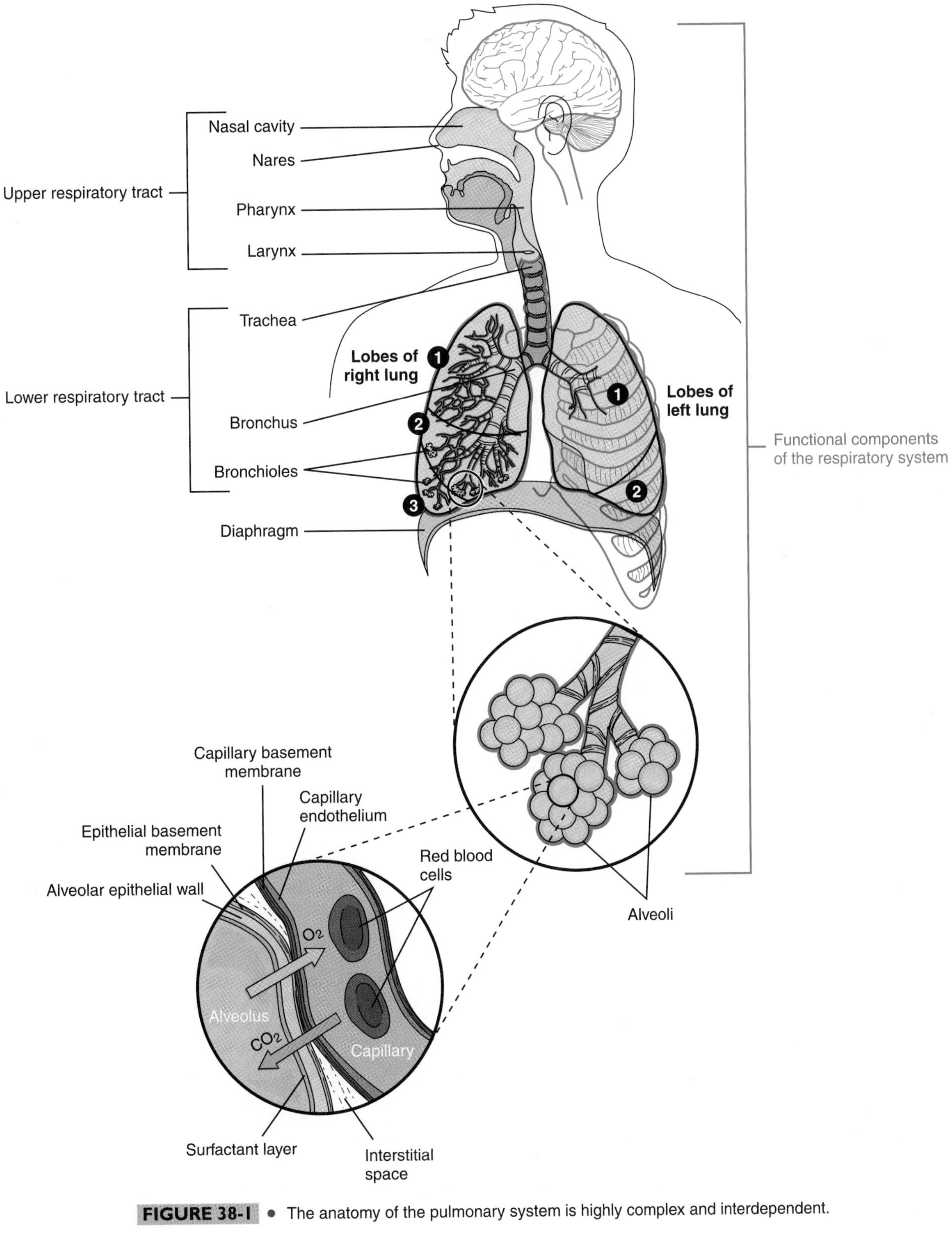

FIGURE 38-1 • The anatomy of the pulmonary system is highly complex and interdependent.

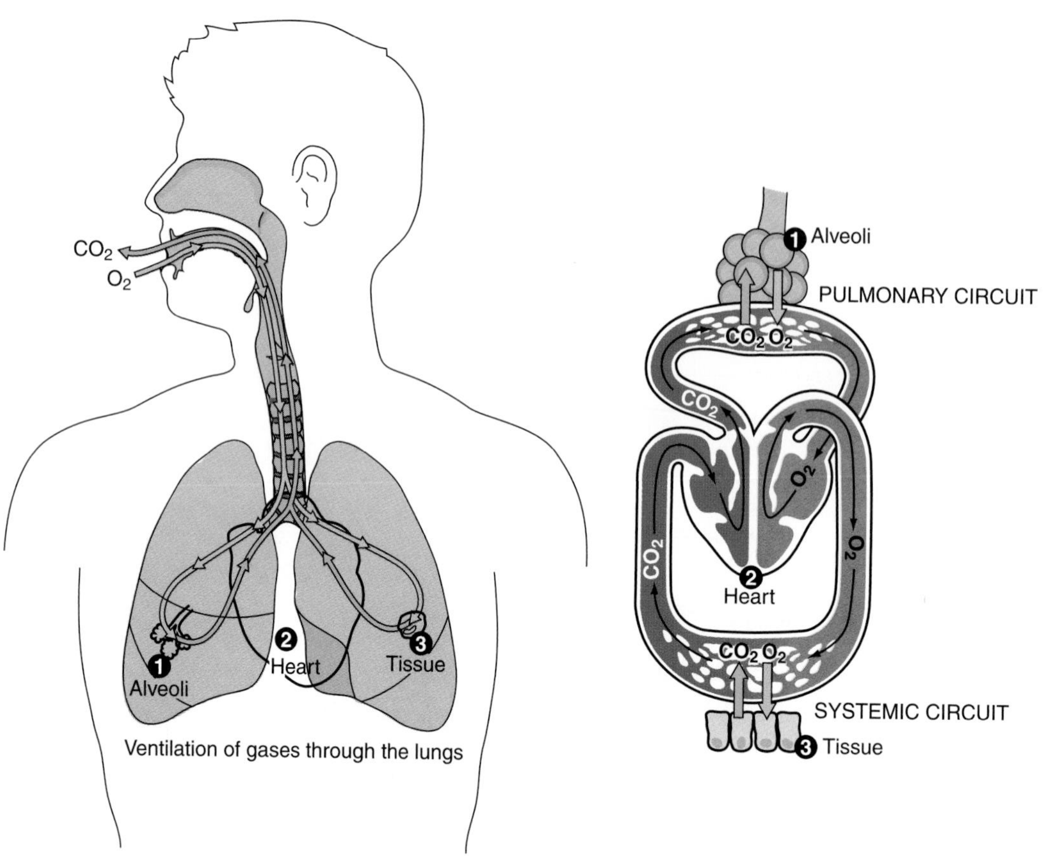

FIGURE 38-2 • The major function of the respiratory tract is to provide the oxygen for cellular metabolism and to remove the carbon dioxide that is produced but not needed.

porting connective tissue of the lungs is composed of collagen, which requires vitamin C for its synthesis. Normal airway mucus is a substance consisting of water, glycoproteins, and electrolytes.

Weight loss from inadequate energy intake is significantly correlated with a poor prognosis in persons with pulmonary diseases. Malnutrition leading to impaired immunity places any patient at high risk for developing respiratory infections. Patients with pulmonary disease who are hospitalized and who are also malnourished are likely to have lengthy hospital stays and are susceptible to increased morbidity and mortality.

Impact of Pulmonary System Disease on Nutritional Status

Pulmonary disease substantially increases energy requirements. This factor explains the rationale for including body composition and weight parameters in nearly all medical, surgical, pharmacologic, and nutritional research studies of people with respiratory diseases. The complications of pulmonary diseases or their treatments can make adequate intake and digestion difficult and absorption, circulation, cellular utilization, storage, and excretion of most nutrients problematic. Some adverse effects of lung disease on nutritional status are listed in Box 38-1.

Drug-nutrient interactions of medications commonly used in pulmonary disease, such as bronchodilators, antibiotics, steroids, and diuretics, are described in Chapter 19 and in Appendix 34. With the burgeoning interest in natural remedies rather than reliance on manufactured pharmaceuticals, people are using botanicals to treat respiratory ailments (Blumenthal et al, 1998; Tyler, 1994). For example, to treat symptomatically the cough from the common cold or flu, herbal remedies fall into two groups: cough suppressants and expectorants. Cough suppressants include the volatile oils of eucalyptus or peppermint. These oils are added to lozenges to increase the production of saliva, thereby increasing the frequency of swallowing to suppress the cough reflex. Teas brewed from herbs are consumed for the mucilages they contain, which may form a protective layer over the mucous membranes of the pharynx, larynx, and trachea. Expectorant herbs include anise, fennel, and thyme (see Chapter 20). This means that the clinician needs to ask about these therapies during the assessment of the patient (see Appendix 35).

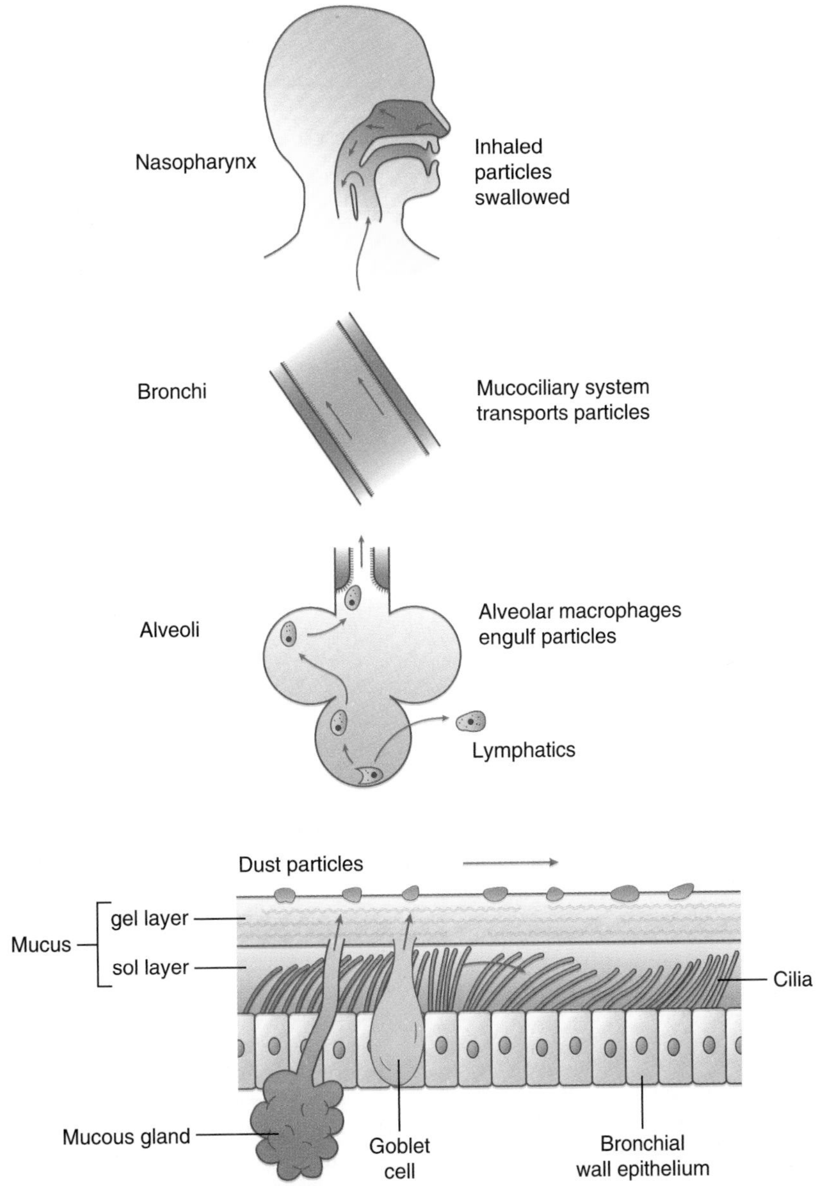

FIGURE 38-3 • The respiratory tract is a protective physical barrier against inhaled particles and microorganisms to prevent them from gaining entrance into the body. (Modified from West JB: *Pulmonary pathophysiology: the essentials,* Baltimore, Md, Williams & Wilkins.)

OVERVIEW OF MEDICAL NUTRITION THERAPY IN PULMONARY DISEASE

Individualized nutrition assessment, intervention, and counseling are integral components of care for each patient with pulmonary system disease. Pulmonary system disorders may be categorized as primary, such as tuberculosis (TB), bronchial asthma, and cancer of the lung, or secondary, such as those associated with cardiovascular disease, obesity, acquired immunodeficiency syndrome (AIDS), sickle cell disease, and scoliosis. Examples of acute conditions include aspiration of enteral feeding liquids, airway obstruction from foods like peanuts, and anaphylaxis from consumption of shellfish. Examples of chronic conditions include cystic fibrosis (CF) and emphysema. Table 38-1 presents a summary of some pulmonary diseases with their nutritional implications.

To determine pulmonary status, the clinician uses the results of numerous diagnostic and monitoring tests, such as imaging procedures, pulmonary function tests, arterial blood gas determinations, sputum cultures, and biopsies. Assessment of the cardiovascular, renal, neurologic, and hematologic systems also is important because diseases involving these systems often produce complications affecting pulmonary anatomy, physiology, and biochemistry.

Nutritionally relevant, common presenting signs and symptoms of pulmonary disease include cough,

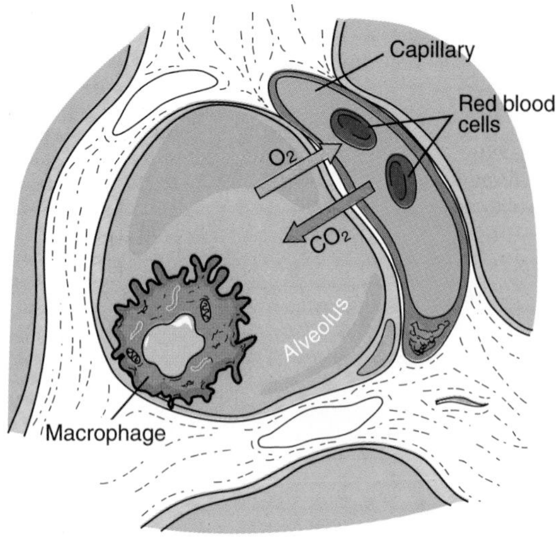

FIGURE 38-4 • Alveolar macrophages are part of the body's systemic immune response. Macrophages are a main defense of the body against harmful cellular debris and microorganisms.

Box 38-1. Adverse Effects of Lung Disease on Nutritional Status

Increased energy expenditure
- Increased work of breathing
- Chronic infection
- Medical treatments (e.g., bronchodilators, chest physical therapy)

Reduced intake
- Fluid restriction
- Shortness of breath
- Decreased oxygen saturation when eating
- Anorexia due to chronic disease
- Gastrointestinal distress and vomiting

Additional limitations
- Difficulty preparing food due to fatigue
- Lack of financial resources
- Impaired feeding skills (for infants and children)
- Altered metabolism

early satiety, anorexia, weight loss, dyspnea (shortness of breath) during preparing food and eating, and fatigue. As pulmonary disease progresses, other related conditions may interfere with food intake or overall nutritional status, especially abnormal production of sputum, vomiting, tachypnea (rapid breathing), hemoptysis, thoracic pain, nasal polyps, anemia, depression, and altered taste secondary to medications.

Assessment of nutritional status is important and should precede any nutritional care or medical treatment unless the treatment is emergent (see Chapters 17 and 18).

TABLE 38-1 Selected Pulmonary Conditions Having Nutritional Implications

CATEGORY	EXAMPLES
Neonate	Bronchopulmonary dysplasia (BPD)
Obstruction	Cystic fibrosis (CF)
	Chronic obstructive pulmonary disease (COPD)
	• Emphysema
	• Chronic bronchitis
	Asthma
	Aspiration (foreign body, food, fluid)
Tumor	Lung cancer
Infection	Pneumonia
	Tuberculosis (TB)
Respiratory failure	Acute respiratory failure (ARF)
	Lung transplantation
Other system abnormalities	
Neuromuscular	Muscular dystrophy
Skeletal	Paralysis
	Osteoporosis
	Scoliosis
Cardiovascular	Pulmonary edema
Endocrine	Severe obesity
	Prader-Willi syndrome

ASPIRATION

Pulmonary aspiration, or the movement of food or fluid into the lungs, can result in pneumonia or even death. Proper body positioning when eating is essential for everyone. At increased risk are infants, toddlers, older adults, and persons with oral, upper gastrointestinal, neurologic, or muscular abnormalities (see Chapter 43). Besides liquids, foods that are most easily aspirated include those that have a round shape, such as nuts, popcorn, hot dog pieces, or chunks of inadequately chewed foods, like meat or raw vegetables. Close attention must be given to people receiving enteral tube feedings (see Chapter 23).

ASTHMA

Pathophysiology

Asthma is a disease of bronchial hyperresponsiveness and airway inflammation, leading to airflow obstruction. The syndrome appears to result from complex interactions among genetic, immunologic, and environmental factors. Continued inadequate management can lead to a life-threatening situation known as *status asthmaticus*. The underlying pathophysiology of primary pulmonary asthma is unclear (Busse and Lemanske, 2001).

Nutritional factors, such as maternal diet during pregnancy, diet during infancy and toddlerhood, and obesity in adolescents and adults have been hypothesized to be implicated in asthma. Asthmatic symptoms may be aggravated by allergen exposure, including foods like shrimp (see Chapter 32); food additives like sulfites (see Chapter 32); and botanicals like citronella in insect repellents, rusty-leafed rhododendron in natural honeys, and strawberry leaf in herbal teas (see Chapter 20).

A common sign of asthma is persistent mouth breathing. In young children, this can result in permanent oral structure malformation lasting into adulthood. The resulting open bite can make biting into nourishing foods, such as sandwiches or fresh fruits and vegetables, difficult.

Medical Nutrition Therapy

Worldwide research results remain controversial but encouraging, and food and individual nutrients are being studied for possible roles in asthma's etiology or treatment. Examples include omega-3 and omega-6 fatty acids (role in decreasing the production of bronchoconstrictive leukotrienes), antioxidant nutrients (role in protecting the airway tissues from oxidative stress), the cation magnesium (role as a smooth-muscle relaxant and antiinflammatory agent), and methylxanthines such as caffeine (role as a bronchodilator). The dilemma for the nutrition care provider is the paucity of evidence-based research to support practice procedures. For example, food and nutrient intakes are based on retrospective food frequency questionnaires (Gilliland et al, 2002; Schwartz, 2000) rather than intervention trials (Mihrshahi et al, 2001). Sufficient measurement of baseline and sequential levels of biochemical parameters, route of nutrient administration (supplement or food), and length of study vary (Nagakura et al, 2000; Okamoto et al, 2000). Laboratory testing methods vary (Dacey, 2001; Mircetic et al, 2001; Saris et al, 2000). Experimental inclusion and exclusion criteria such as severity of disease, status of disease, age, and gender are important confounding variables, thus yielding conflicting results (Hashimoto et al, 2000; Kakish, 2001; Picado et al, 2001; Schenk et al, 2001; Silverman, 2000; Vural et al, 2000). Health care provider and patient participation in scientific nutrition studies aimed at producing evidence-based results are necessary (Baker and Ayres, 2000; Rowe et al, 2001; Smit, 2001).

Nutrition assessment and therapy also must take into account the routinely prescribed medications. These include bronchodilators (to relax the airway smooth muscle) and antiinflammatory agents (to suppress airway inflammation). Patients may experience numerous nutritionally relevant side effects. These include dry mouth and throat, nausea, vomiting, diarrhea, increased serum glucose levels, sodium retention, and hypokalemia, as well as hand tremors, headache, and dizziness (see Chapter 19). Another possible nutritionally related side effect of medications or chronic coughing is gastroesophageal reflux (see Chapter 29). The availability of dual-energy x-ray absorptiometry (DXA) as a nutrition monitoring test is enabling the study of the effect of the chronic use of prescribed corticosteroids on bone mineral density (see Chapters 19 and 27).

Until the etiology of asthma is discovered, general agreement appears to be that nutrition assessment and therapy recommendations include individual evaluation for environmental triggers; a diet of wholesome foods to provide optimal energy, balance of nutrients, and phytonutrients; correction of diagnosed energy and nutrient deficiencies or excesses; careful attention to medication-food-nutrient interactions; frequent monitoring to maintain healthy pulmonary status; and education of the patient, family, and community (American Academy of Allergy, Asthma, and Immunology, 1999; Miller, 2001; National Asthma Education and Prevention Program, 1997).

BRONCHOPULMONARY DYSPLASIA

Pathophysiology

Bronchopulmonary dysplasia (BPD) is a chronic lung condition of infancy in newborns whose lungs appear unable to respond to adverse situations. A major risk factor is the inability of immature lungs to synthesize surfactant that permits inflation for gas exchange. BPD occurs most frequently in infants who are premature or are low birth weight (see Chapter 9). BPD can be a complication in the neonatal period of treating respiratory distress syndrome (RDS) with positive pressure ventilation and oxygen administration. The resulting hyperoxia damages the lung's endothelial cells, perhaps from the free radicals of oxygen. Other risk factors for BPD include meconium aspiration, tracheoesophageal fistula, and infections. Signs and symptoms of BPD include hypercapnia, tachypnea, wheezing, dyspnea, recurrent respiratory infections, cor pulmonale, and a characteristic radiographic appearance of the lungs.

The best nutritional means of prevention is the optimal nutrition status of pregnant women so that infants are born full term and well nourished (see Chapter 7). Infants with severe disease often require prolonged intensive medical care. Therapies such as tube feedings, mechanical ventilation, supplemental oxygen, and medications may be required long after the infant's discharge from the hospital. Because the pathophysiology of BPD is incompletely understood, medical treatment and nutritional intervention are empirically based and often have limited scientific rationale (Hazinski, 1998; Kennedy, 1999).

Medical Nutrition Therapy

Assessment

Because of the fragile nature of affected infants, careful and consistent nutrition assessment is imperative (Mueller, 1998). Growth of infants with BPD is followed closely because it is a major outcome indicator of medical and nutritional status (Farrell and Fiascone, 1997). Because lung size is stature dependent, linear growth is important for the growth of healthy lung tissue and for the resolution of the condition. Observations of growth patterns of infants with BPD suggest that these infants grow more slowly, thereby requiring careful assessment of both respiratory and nutritional status (de Meer et al, 1997; Giacoia et al, 1997; Gregoire et al, 1998).

Reasons for growth failure among infants with BPD include increased energy needs combined with inadequate dietary intake, gastroesophageal reflux, emotional deprivation, and chronic hypoxia (Johnson et al, 1998). Brief episodes of decreased oxygen saturation are thought to occur frequently in infants with BPD, especially during feeding. Thus, whenever growth languishes, low oxygen saturation should be evaluated as a contributing factor. Growth should be evaluated and compared with that of other infants of the same postconceptional age (see Chapter 9). Factors to include in a nutrition assessment are listed in Box 38-2.

Infants with BPD have special short- and long-term nutritional requirements and care considerations related to both their prematurity (see Chapter 9) and their pulmonary status. The general goal of nutritional care is to supply adequate nutrient intakes, promote linear growth, maintain fluid balance, and develop age-appropriate feeding skills (Newkirk et al, 1999). Meeting energy and nutrient needs is a major challenge in the care of infants and toddlers with BPD (Brunton et al, 1998).

Energy

Increased energy needs are well recognized in infants with BPD. Resting energy expenditure for infants with BPD has been documented to be 25% to 50% greater than that in age-matched controls. Infants with BPD who have growth failure may have energy needs that are 50% higher than those who are growing well (Kurzner et al, 1988). Energy needs also vary over the course of the disease. In the acute phase, when infants are kept in controlled temperature environments, are fed parenterally, remain relatively inactive, and are not growing or are growing slowly, energy requirements may be 50 to 85 kcal/kg daily. In contrast, during the convalescent phase, when infants are growing rapidly, being fed orally, and using additional energy for temperature regulation, activity, and the work of breathing, they may require 120 to 130 kcal/kg or more daily (Oh, 1986).

Macronutrients

Protein intake should be within the advised range for infants of comparable postconceptional age. As the caloric density of the diet is increased by the addition of fat and carbohydrate, protein should continue to provide 7% or more of total calories. Lesser amounts may be inadequate for growth.

Additions of fat or carbohydrate should be made to formula only after it has been concentrated to 24 kcal/oz to keep protein at an acceptable level. Fat provides essential fatty acids (EFAs) and helps meet energy demands when tolerance for fluid and carbon dioxide load is limited (see p. 952). Excess sources of carbohydrate may abnormally increase the respiratory quotient (RQ) and the output of CO_2. Continuous calculations of the proportions of the macronutrients related to respiratory status are major considerations in any nutritional evaluation.

Box 38-2. Components of Nutritional Assessment for Infants With Bronchopulmonary Dysplasia

Historical	Medical	Nutritional	Feeding History	Environmental
Birth weight	Respiratory status	Weight	Volume of intake	Parent–child interaction
Gestational age	Oxygen saturation	Length	Frequency of feedings	Home facilities
Medical history	Use of medications	Head circumference	Behavior during feedings	Community resources
Nutritional history	Emesis	Hemoglobin and hematocrit values	Formula composition	Economic resources
Previous growth pattern	Stool pattern	Serum electrolytes	Use of solids	
	Urine output	Other biochemical tests as needed (e.g., serum albumin, alkaline phosphatase, phosphorus levels)	Feeding milestones	
	Urine specific gravity			

Modified from Sirois LW: Nutritional assessment and management of the infant with bronchopulmonary dysplasia, *Nutr Support Serv* 4:62, 1984.

To maintain fluid balance, infants with BPD may require fluid restriction, sodium restriction, and long-term treatment with diuretics, all of which have nutritional implications. When fluid intake is restricted, the use of parenteral lipids or calorically dense enteral feedings may help the infant meet energy needs.

Vitamins and Minerals

Adequate supplies of all vitamins and minerals are essential. Special attention is focused on those related to prematurity, infections, oxygen therapy, and drug-nutrient interactions. Adequate vitamin K is essential for bone development and should be monitored, especially when colon microflora are insufficient for the synthesis of the vitamin.

Because of their role in cell membrane integrity and as antioxidants, vitamins A, C, E and inositol, as well as free fatty acids or the mineral selenium, have been theorized to be implicated in the prevention or treatment of BDP. Of special interest is vitamin A because of its role in the proper development and maintenance of the epithelial cells of the respiratory tract (Verma et al, 1996). Sufficient intake of these nutrients, based on the dietary reference intake (DRI), including total energy, is crucial for the infant's catch-up growth and high metabolic needs (see Chapters 4, 5, and 9). Except for vitamin A, however, evidence-based research for the antioxidant nutrients remains inconclusive. Indeed, vitamin A supplementation (oral supplements; enriched oral or enteral formulas or parenteral solutions; or intramuscular injections) has been reported to be beneficial (Atkinson, 2001; Nolt, 2001; Tyson et al, 1999).

Mineral intake and retention should be monitored regularly and supplemented as needed to maintain normal levels. Determination of mineral requirements is complicated by lack of adequate stores as a result of prematurity (for example, iron, zinc, and calcium), growth delay, and the multiple medications prescribed for infants and toddlers with BPD. Medications include diuretics, bronchodilators, antibiotics, cardiac antiarrhythmics, and corticosteroids. Collectively, these medications are associated with increased urinary loss of minerals, especially chloride, potassium, and calcium (see Chapter 19).

Additional chloride losses may occur in infants with chronic CO_2 retention and respiratory acidosis because of metabolic correction for the acidosis. Deficiencies of chloride or potassium are associated with muscle weakness and impaired growth.

Infants with BPD are at risk for osteopenia (inadequate bone mineralization). Besides limited nutrient intake, other risk factors include inadequate stores of calcium and phosphorus related to prematurity, intermittent respiratory acidosis, chronic use of certain medications, and insufficient physical activity.

For infants sensitive to sodium loads, formulas with lower sodium content can be selected (see Appendix 38 and Table 8-3). Also, the sodium content of medications, water, and foods must be considered.

Feeding Strategies

Barriers to adequate intake include anorexia, fatigue, poor coordination of breathing and swallowing, and weakness of suck. To meet energy needs, calorically dense formulas; small, frequent feedings; use of a soft nipple; and nasogastric or gastrostomy tube feedings may be needed. When calorically dense formulas are used (>24 kcal/oz), the adequacy of fluid intake and urinary output must be monitored closely.

If gastroesophageal reflux is evident, lung disease may worsen owing to aspiration. Associated vomiting with expulsion of feedings leads to inadequate nutritional intake. Treatment includes thickened feedings; upright positioning; medications like antacids or histamine H_2-receptor antagonists; and, in severe cases, surgical fundoplication. To thicken formula, ½ to 1 tbsp of infant cereal is added per ounce of formula, with adjustments made as necessary.

Feeding difficulties frequently occur among infants with BPD. Risk factors include a history of unpleasant oral experiences (e.g., intubation, frequent suctioning, or recurrent vomiting), a history of nonoral feedings, delayed introduction of solids, or discomfort or choking associated with eating solids. Infants may tire easily while breast-feeding or bottle-feeding. Useful approaches that may facilitate feeding acceptance include providing a pleasant and calm mealtime environment, providing oral stimulation during tube feedings, using consistent and appropriate feeding techniques, and gradually introducing progressive texture and flavor changes. An interdisciplinary approach involving all caregivers is recommended.

CHRONIC OBSTRUCTIVE PULMONARY DISEASE

Pathophysiology

Chronic obstructive pulmonary disease (COPD) is characterized by slowly progressive obstruction of the airways. COPD may be subdivided into two categories: emphysema (type I) and chronic bronchitis (type II). Tobacco smoking overwhelmingly is the most important causative factor, although environmental air pollution (including cooking in confined unventilated space) and genetic susceptibility are other etiologic possibilities (Barnes, 2000). Nutritionally, patients with emphysema are thin, often cachectic. They are generally older and have mild hypoxemia but normal hematocrit values. Cor pulmonale develops late in the course of the disease. Conversely, patients with chronic bronchitis are of normal weight and, indeed, are often overweight. Hypoxemia is prominent in these patients, hematocrit values are increased, and cor pulmonale develops early.

Medical Nutrition Therapy

Assessment

Each person with COPD must be individually assessed on a continuous basis. It is important that the age and gender, other acute or chronic medical conditions, medications and other treatments, anthropometric and bone mineral density measurements, past and present state of nutrition, and whether the patient currently is hospitalized or living at home take priority in determining the person's nutritional needs and feeding strategies. Box 38-3 lists major components of nutrition assessment in COPD.

After assessing fluid balance and requirements, energy is the next requirement to determine. Because maintaining energy balance is crucial for combating this progressive disorder, accurate evaluation of both energy intake and energy expenditure is essential.

Decreased food intake is common. Morning headache and confusion from hypercapnia (excessive carbon dioxide in the blood) must be identified because these symptoms may interfere with food preparation or intake. Other pertinent assessments focus on blood oxygen saturation, fatigue, anorexia, difficulty chewing and swallowing from dyspnea, constipation from low-fiber food selections, or diarrhea from impaired peristalsis secondary to lack of oxygen to the gastrointestinal tract.

On the other side of the equation, energy expenditure usually is elevated. This situation appears related to pulmonary complications, such as the degree of airflow obstruction (thus increasing the energy needs due to the increased work of breathing), gas diffusing capacity, CO_2 retention, and respiratory inflammation, or to biochemical mediators like hormones and cytokines (Schols and Wouters, 2000).

Common outcomes are reduced respiratory and limb muscle strength and endurance, increased muscle fatigability, altered pulmonary accessory muscle function, and increased susceptibility to infections. Malnourished patients with COPD have a worse prognosis than those who are well nourished (Thorsdottir et al, 2001).

Nutritional depletion may be evidenced clinically by low body weight for height and reduced triceps fat-fold measurements. However, decreased lean body mass may be occurring, although actual weight may appear stable. Calculation of the body mass index (BMI) may be insufficient to detect alterations. Instead, determination of body composition helps to differentiate lean muscle mass from adipose tissue, and overhydration from dehydration (see Chapter 17). In patients with cor pulmonale resulting in fluid retention, weight maintenance or gain may camouflage actual wasting of lean body mass. Thus, for patients retaining fluids, careful interpretation of both anthropometric measurements and biochemical indicators of nutritional status is necessary, especially because the latter are depressed by hemodilution.

The medication profile should be assessed for food and nutrient interactions. Examples of drugs with potential nutritional implications are bronchodilators, expectorants, and corticosteroids (see Chapter 19). The primary goals of nutritional care for patients with COPD are to facilitate nutritional well-being, maintain an appropriate ratio of lean body mass to adipose tissue, correct fluid imbalance, manage drug-nutrient interactions, and prevent osteoporosis (Berry and Baum, 2001; Harik-Khan et al, 2002).

Energy

Box 38-1 lists factors that can make meeting energy needs difficult. For patients participating in pulmonary inpatient or outpatient rehabilitation programs, adjusted energy requirements depend on the intensity and frequency of exercise therapy (Finnerty et al, 2001; Mador and Bozkanat, 2001). It is crucial to

Box 38-3. Components of Nutritional Assessment for Adults With Chronic Obstructive Pulmonary Disease

Historical	Medical	Nutritional	Diet History	Environmental
Medical history	Respiratory status	Weight	Usual home diet	Home facilities
Nutritional history	Oxygen saturation	Height	Use of supplements	Physical abilities
Usual weight	Dental status	Skin-fold measurements	Where meals are eaten	Financial resources
	Senses of smell and taste	Hemoglobin and hematocrit values	Social companionship with meals	
	Gastrointestinal function	Serum electrolytes		
		Serum proteins		
		Additional biochemical tests as needed (e.g., immunologic testing, creatinine height index, nitrogen balance)		

remember that energy balance and nitrogen balance are intertwined. Consequently, maintaining optimal energy balance is essential to preserving visceral proteins (e.g., albumin, transferrin, retinol-binding protein, and immunoglobulins) and somatic protein mass (e.g., pulmonary tissues and muscles) (see Chapters 2, 3, 17, and 18). Preferably, indirect calorimetry is used to determine energy need predictions, and thus to prescribe and monitor the provision of sufficient, but not excessive, kilocalories. When energy equations are used for predictions, increases for physiologic stress must be included. Caloric needs ranging from 94% to 146% of predicted have been observed (Thorsdottir and Gunnarsdottir, 2002) (see Chapter 2).

Macronutrients

In the person with stable COPD, requirements for water, protein, fat, and carbohydrate are determined by the underlying lung disease, oxygen therapy, medications, weight status, and any acute fluid fluctuations. Sufficient protein, 1.2 to 1.7 g per kilogram of dry body weight, is necessary to maintain or restore lung and muscle strength as well as to promote immune function. A balanced ratio of protein (15% to 20% of calories) with fat (30% to 45% of calories) and carbohydrate (40% to 55% of calories) is important to preserve a satisfactory respiratory quotient (RQ) from substrate utilization (see Chapter 2). Repletion, but not overfeeding, is the long-standing hallmark of nutritional care (Ryan et al, 1993). Often other concurrent disease processes exist, such as cardiovascular or renal disease, cancer, or diabetes mellitus. These underlying conditions affect the total amounts, ratios, and kinds of protein, fat, and carbohydrate prescribed.

Vitamins and Minerals

As with macronutrients, vitamin and mineral requirements for individuals with stable COPD depend on the underlying lung pathology, other concurrent diseases, medical treatments, weight status, and bone mineral density. For people continuing to smoke tobacco, additional vitamin C may be necessary. Research indicates that people who smoke about one pack of cigarettes per day appear to require about 16 mg more ascorbate per day, whereas those who smoke two packs need about 32 mg as replacement (Cross and Halliwell, 1993).

The role of minerals, such as magnesium and calcium, in muscle contraction and relaxation may be important for people with COPD. Intakes at least equivalent to the DRI should be provided (see Table 15-1). Patients who are receiving aggressive nutritional support should undergo routine monitoring of magnesium and phosphorus levels because of their cofactor roles in adenosine triphosphate (ATP) generation. Reduced bone mineral density, measured by DXA, has been demonstrated in patients with COPD, thus providing evidence for the nutritional and exercise concerns related to osteoporosis in this population (Biskobing, 2002; Incalzi et al, 2000). Depending on bone mineral density test results, coupled with food intake history and glucocorticoid medications use, additional vitamins D and K also may be necessary (see Chapter 27).

Some patients with cor pulmonale and fluid retention require sodium and fluid restriction. Depending on the diuretics prescribed, increased dietary intake of potassium may be required (see Chapter 19).

Feeding Strategies

Interdisciplinary team involvement in direct care and education is paramount (Figure 38-5). A modified oral diet usually is preferred. Adequate exercise, fluids, and easily chewed dietary fiber enhance gastrointestinal motility. When abdominal bloating is a problem, limitation of foods associated with gas formation may be helpful (see Chapters 29 and 30). Patients and their families benefit from specific suggestions for enhancing appetite, promoting oral intake, and lessening fatigue when cooking or eating (Figure 38-6). Some suggestions are resting before meals, eating small portions of nutrient-dense foods, and planning expectorant medication use apart from mealtimes. For many patients, using oxygen at mealtimes, eating slowly, chewing foods well, and engaging in social interaction all can enhance food intake, nutrient metabolism, and enjoyment of the experience. To prevent aspiration, special caution must be given to proper sequencing of breathing with swallowing as well as to proper sitting posture during eating (Martin-Harris, 2000). Patients with disease-related physical limitations may be helped by assistance with food shopping and meal preparation. Linkage with community resources, such as congregate meal programs or the Meals on Wheels program, may also be helpful (see Chapter 14).

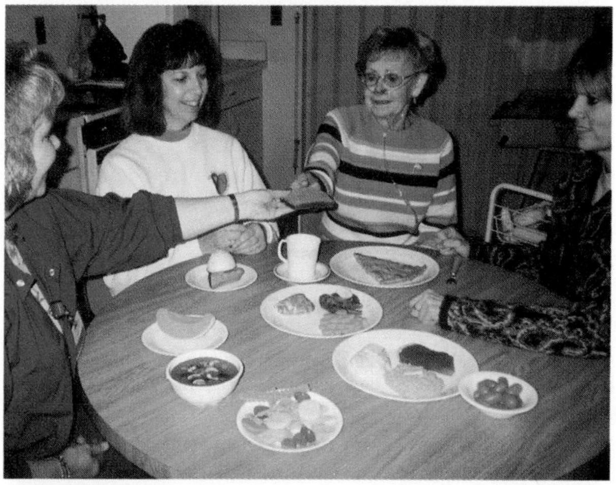

FIGURE 38-5 • During a nutrition education session, a client with chronic obstructive pulmonary disease (COPD) interacts with a dietitian, nurse, and respiratory therapist so that she will achieve optimal nutrition status. (Courtesy Ginny DiNunzio, CRT, Coordinator, Pulmonary Rehabilitation Program, Doylestown Hospital, Doylestown, Pa.)

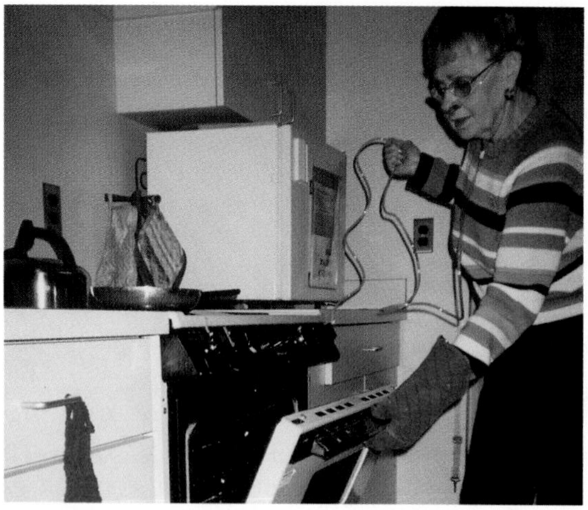

FIGURE 38-6 • While cooking, a client with chronic obstructive pulmonary disease (COPD) must consider the proper care and safety of oxygen and nasal tubing. (Courtesy Ginny DiNunzio, CRT, Pulmonary Rehabilitation Program, Doylestown Hospital, Doylestown, Pa.)

Enteral nutritional supplementation by mouth or by feeding tube can increase total caloric and nutrient intake for some patients with COPD. Decisions to implement this method of nutrition support must take into consideration patient anxiety, labor to perform, and cost. It must be understood that the patient's nutritional status may be improved as long as enteral nutrition is continued but will revert if and when supplementation is discontinued. Besides the potential for aspiration, other negative consequences of nocturnal tube feedings must be considered. Even in healthy adults, oxygen consumption decreases by 15% to 25% during sleep (Schwab, 1995).

CYSTIC FIBROSIS

Pathophysiology and Diagnostic Criteria

Cystic fibrosis (CF) is a complex multisystem disorder that is inherited in an autosomal recessive fashion (Figure 38-7). The first comprehensive description of CF in the United States was published in 1938 (Andersen, 1938). In 1989, the disease's underlying genetic basis was presented (Kerem et al, 1989; Riordan et al, 1989). The CF gene, located on chromosome 7q (the long arm), encodes a membrane-associated protein termed the *cystic fibrosis transmembrane regulator (CFTR)* (see Chapter 16). This protein product appears to be part of a cAMP-regulated chloride channel and appears to regulate chloride and sodium transport across apical membranes of epithelial cells. Nearly a thousand mutations have been identified (Orenstein et al, 2002; Sharer et al, 1998).

Although CF remains one of the most common lethal genetic disorders prevalent in white persons, it is expressed in other population groups as well. About 2% to 5% of white populations are heterozygotes, with a CF incidence of 1:2500 live births. Survival has dramatically improved owing to scientific advancements and improvements in diagnostic and treatment procedures, including nutrition. Of the approximately 30,000 people treated at CF centers in the United States, the median age of patients has surpassed 30 years. Women with CF have delivered healthy infants, and some have chosen to breast-feed their unaffected infants (Michel and Mueller, 1994).

Expression of the CF gene is largely restricted to epithelial cells. Almost all exocrine glands are affected by secretion of abnormally thick, tenacious mucus that obstructs glands and ducts in various organs. The clinical features are dominated by involvement of the respiratory tract, sweat and salivary glands, intestine, pancreas, liver, and reproductive tract. Pulmonary complications include acute and chronic bronchitis, bronchiectasis, pneumonia, atelectasis, and peribronchial and parenchymal scarring. Infection with *Pseudomonas aeruginosa* is typical. Pneumothorax and hemoptysis are common. In advanced stages, cor pulmonale or infection with *Burkholdteria cepacia* may be present, signifying a poor prognosis (Aitken and Fiel, 1993).

Several methods are available for diagnosing CF. For families with previously identified CF, prenatal analysis may be possible. Several countries and some states in the United States conduct routine neonatal screening for the disease (Farrell et al, 2001). The most reliable clinical diagnostic test, known as the sweat test, is performed by pilocarpine iontophoresis. Elevated levels of sodium and chloride (>60 mEq/L) in collected sweat samples are indicative of CF. Criteria for the diagnosis of CF include a positive result on a sweat test and the presence of chronic lung disease, failure to thrive and malabsorption, or a family history of CF.

Cystic fibrosis can have a profound impact on the digestive system. Infants born with meconium ileus have the diagnosis of probable CF until ruled out from other causes. About 85% of persons with CF have pancreatic insufficiency. Plugs of thick mucus reduce the quantity of digestive enzymes released from the pancreas into the small intestine. The resultant enzyme insufficiency causes maldigestion of food and malabsorption of nutrients. Decreased bicarbonate secretion can further reduce digestive enzyme activity. Decreased bile acid reabsorption contributes further to fat malabsorption. The presence of excessive mucus lining the small intestinal tract may interfere with nutrient absorption by the microvilli. Gastrointestinal complications include bulky, foul-smelling stools; cramping and intestinal obstruction; rectal prolapse; and liver involvement. As the disease progresses, damage to the endocrine portion of the pancreas can cause impaired glucose tolerance and development of

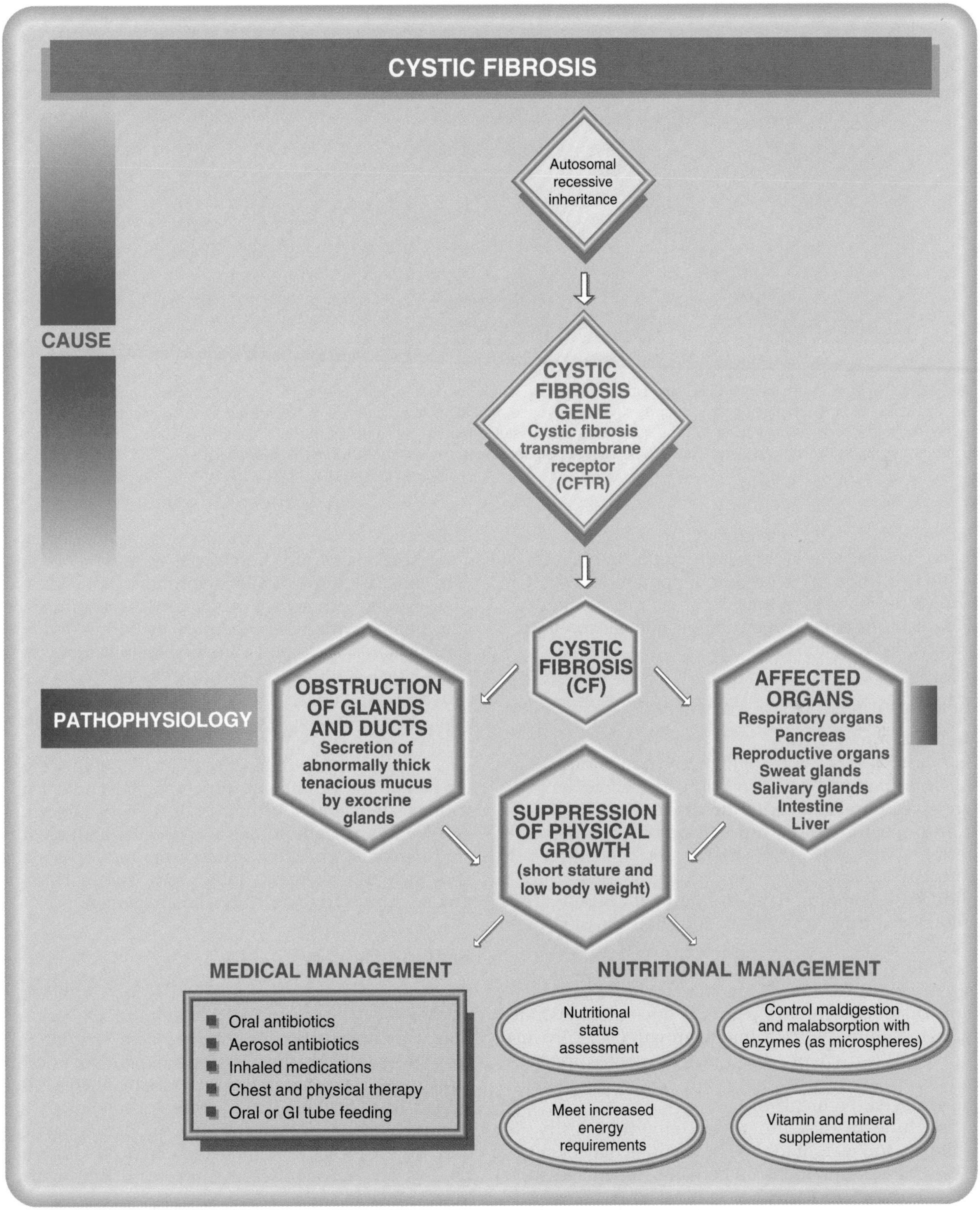

FIGURE 38-7 • Pathophysiology algorithm: cystic fibrosis. (Algorithm content developed by John Anderson, PhD, and Sanford C. Garner, PhD. Updated by Donna H. Mueller, PhD, RD, FADA, 2002.)

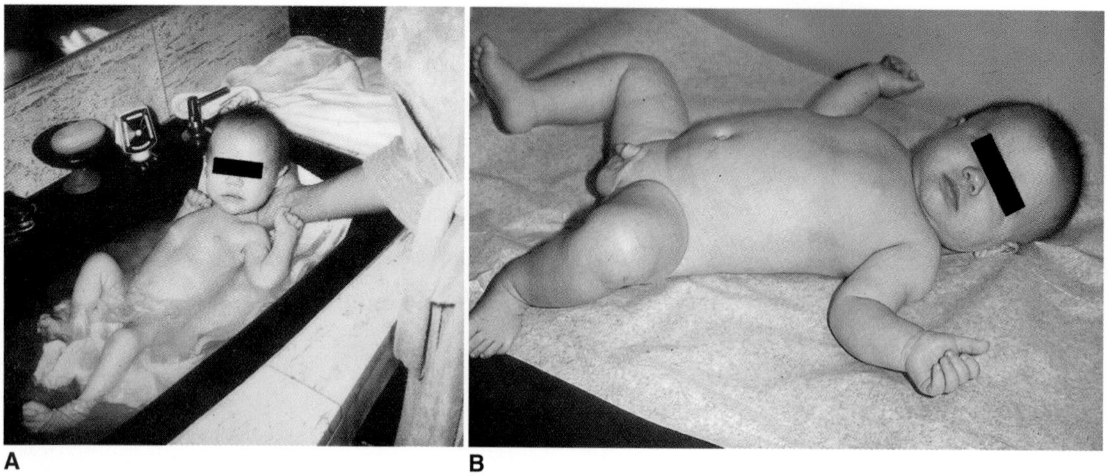

A B

FIGURE 38-8 • **A,** An infant was admitted to the hospital in respiratory failure, with a history of cough, tachypnea, and failure to thrive since 4 weeks of age. Diagnosis of cystic fibrosis (CF) was made on finding sweat chloride of 105 mEq/L and undetectable digestive enzyme levels in duodenal secretions. **B,** The infant was successfully treated with medical and nutritional therapies. (Courtesy Daniel V. Schidlow, MD, Pediatric Pulmonary and Cystic Fibrosis Center, St. Christopher's Hospital for Children, Philadelphia, Pa.)

CF-related diabetes mellitus (CFRD) (Moran et al, 1999). The prevalence of insulin-requiring diabetes is estimated to be 7% in the entire population with CF and up to 15% in the adult CF population. As many as 50% of adults with CF may demonstrate glucose intolerance (see Chapter 33).

Medical Nutrition Therapy

Assessment

Individuals with CF are at high risk for malnutrition. Maldigestion and malabsorption, as well as the progressive complications of the disease, make it difficult to meet increased nutrient needs. Factors interfering with adequate intake and retention of nutrients include dyspnea, coughing and cough-induced vomiting, gastrointestinal discomfort, anorexia during episodes of infection, possible impaired sense of smell and taste, and glucosuria. Growth retardation and difficulty maintaining desired weight for height are common problems. Before diagnosis, infants with CF often demonstrate growth failure. With treatment, growth generally improves. When energy and nutrient intakes are adequate, growth nearly appropriate for age can usually be achieved (Figure 38-8).

As lung disease progresses, growth velocity in children and weight for height in adults may decline. The long-term relationship between nutritional support, growth, and survival is not known; however, improved nutritional status on a long-term basis continues to be suggested as a contributing factor to increased survival. Comprehensive nutrition assessment in individuals with CF was first codified by the Cystic Fibrosis Foundation in 1992 (Ramsey et al, 1992) and updated for children and adolescents in 2002 (Borowitz et al, 2002). Table 38-2 highlights some of the components of nutritional assessment.

Because of all the intricate manifestations and complications of CF, nutritional requirements and care must be individually determined for each patient. Moreover, medical nutrition therapy must be coordinated with other therapies, including oral and aerosol antibiotics, other inhaled medications, and chest physical therapy (Creveling et al, 1997).

Based on clinical research and experience, the goals of nutritional care in CF are to control maldigestion and malabsorption; provide adequate nutrients to promote optimal growth or maintain weight for height and pulmonary function; and prevent nutritional deficiencies (Bruno et al, 1995; Salamoni et al, 1996). Those individuals at especially high risk include infants, children, adolescents, and pregnant and lactating women. Table 38-3 summarizes a graded approach to nutritional management.

Enzyme Therapy

Pancreatic enzyme replacement therapy is the first step taken to correct maldigestion and malabsorption. The introduction of enteric-coated enzyme microspheres in the early 1980s was a major advance in nutritional management. The microspheres, designed to withstand the acidic environment of the stomach, release enzymes in the duodenum, where they digest protein, fat, and carbohydrate. Pharmaceutical advancements have improved the medications available.

The quantity of enzymes to be taken with food depends on the degree of pancreatic insufficiency; the quantity of food eaten; the fat, protein, and carbohydrate content of food consumed; and the type of enzymes used (Borowitz et al, 1995). Enzyme dosage limited to 2500 lipase units per kilogram of body weight per meal is adjusted empirically to control gastrointestinal symptoms, including steatorrhea,

TABLE 38-2 Nutritional Assessment in Cystic Fibrosis

INDEX	MINIMUM FREQUENCY	INDICATION
Anthropometry		
Weight	Every 3 mo	Routine care
Height (children ≥2 yr old), length (children <2 yr old)	Every 3 mo	Routine care
Head circumference	Every 3 months until age 2 yr	Routine care
Mid-arm circumference	Yearly	Routine care, diagnosis
Triceps skin-fold thickness	Yearly	Routine care, diagnosis
Nutritional assessment		
Dietary intake*	Yearly	Routine care, diagnosis
3-d fat balance†	As indicated	Weight loss, growth failure, clinical deterioration, diagnosis
Anticipatory dietary and feeding behavior guidance	Every 3 mo; yearly	Routine care, diagnosis
Laboratory studies		
Complete blood count‡	Yearly	Routine care, diagnosis
Serum or plasma retinol value	Yearly	Routine care, diagnosis
Serum or plasma α-tocopherol value	Yearly	Routine care, diagnosis
Albumin level	Yearly	Weight loss, growth failure, clinical deterioration, diagnosis
Electrolytes and acid-base status	As indicated	Prolonged fever, summer heat, infancy, breast-feeding, diagnosis

Data from Cystic Fibrosis Foundation: *Appendix C: determination of energy requirements.* Consensus Conferences, Concepts in CF Care, *Pediatric nutrition for patients with cystic fibrosis,* X:(1)38, March 28-29, 2001.
*Usually consists of a 24-hr recall with assessment of dietary pattern; should be obtained by a dietitian.
†Includes a diet record to determine energy and fat intake as well as a determination of stool fat excretion. This permits calculation of the coefficient of fat absorption (CFA) and assessment of the degree of malabsorption in malnourished patients.
‡If there is any evidence of iron deficiency, iron status must be measured (i.e., serum iron, iron-binding capacity, and serum ferritin levels).

TABLE 38-3 Categories for Nutritional Management of Patients With Cystic Fibrosis (CF)

CATEGORY	TARGET GROUP	GOALS
Routine management	All patients with CF	Nutritional education, dietary counseling, pancreatic enzyme replacement (for patients with pancreatic insufficiency), vitamin supplementation (for patients with pancreatic insufficiency)
Anticipatory guidance	Patients with CF who are at risk of developing energy imbalance (i.e., severe pulmonary insufficiency, frequent pulmonary infections, periods of rapid growth), but who are maintaining a weight–height index ≥90% of ideal weight	Further education to prepare patients for increased energy needs, increased monitoring of dietary intake, increased caloric density of diet as needed; behavioral assessment and counseling
Supportive intervention	Patients with decreased weight gain velocity and/or a weight–height index 85%-90% of ideal weight	All the above, plus oral supplements as needed
Rehabilitative care	Patients with a weight–height index consistently <85% of ideal weight	All the above, plus enteral supplementation via nasogastric tube or enterostomy, as indicated
Resuscitative and palliative care	Patients with a weight–height index <75% of ideal weight, or progressive nutritional failure	All the above, plus continuous enteral feeds or total parenteral nutrition

From Ramsey BW et al: Nutritional assessment and management in cystic fibrosis: a consensus report, *Am J Clin Nutr* 55:108, 1992.

and to promote growth appropriate for age. If gastrointestinal symptoms cannot be controlled, enzyme dosage, patient adherence, and enzyme type should be reevaluated. Fecal fat or nitrogen balance studies may help to evaluate the adequacy of enzyme supplementation.

For infants or children unable to swallow capsules, the capsules can be opened and the microspheres mixed with a soft food, such as applesauce. Microspheres should not be mixed with foods that have a pH greater than 6.0, such as dairy products (e.g., milk, custard, and ice cream) because the enteric coating will dissolve and the enzymes exposed to the gastric acidity will be inactivated. For the same reason, to retain benefits of the enteric coating, microspheres should not be chewed or crushed.

Distal intestinal obstruction syndrome (DIOS), also known as *recurrent intestinal impaction,* sometimes occurs in children and adults. Prevention of DIOS involves adequate enzymes, fluids, dietary fiber, and regular exercise; treatment includes adding stool softeners, laxatives, hyperosmolar enemas, or intestinal lavage (Gavin et al, 1997).

Energy

Energy needs vary widely from individual to individual and even in the same individual throughout the course of life (Duggan and Gilbert, 1996; Murphy et al, 1995). Factors to consider are gender, age, basal metabolic rate, physical activity, respiratory infection, severity of lung disease, and severity of malabsorption. When indirect calorimetry measurement of energy requirements is unavailable, initial equations for calculating caloric recommendations are convenient to use (see *Clinical Insight:* Estimation of Daily Energy Requirement in Cystic Fibrosis). Patients with CF should not be encouraged to decrease their activity levels but to increase their energy intake instead (Boas, 1997; Michel and Mueller, 1995). Relatively healthy children with CF are able to maintain normal growth and energy stores when fed a high-energy, moderate-fat diet complemented with sufficient pancreatic enzyme supplementation (Kawchak et al, 1996; Tomezsko et al, 1992).

Macronutrients

Dietary protein levels are increased in CF as a result of malabsorption; however, when energy needs are adequately met, individuals with CF generally can meet their protein needs by following a typical North American diet. At least 15% to 20% of the total calories consumed as proteins, or the appropriate RDA for protein for the individual's gender, age, and height, is suggested.

Fat intake should provide 35% to 40% or more of total kilocalories as tolerated. Dietary fat helps to provide the required energy, essential fatty acids (EFAs), and fat-soluble vitamins. Moreover, fat limits the volume of food required to meet energy demands and improves the palatability of the diet.

Indications of fat intolerance include an increase in the number of stools, greasy stools, or abdominal cramping. Essential fatty acid deficiencies may be present, even among patients who are treated adequately with pancreatic enzymes to control malabsorption (Levy et al, 1993). Although clinical signs of EFA deficiency are rare, blood and tissue lipid levels may be abnormal. Even if the visible signs of EFA deficiency (e.g., the typical skin lesions) are not noticeable, the clinician should consider routinely testing for abnormal blood lipid profiles. In addition, patients need to be encouraged to include sources of EFAs (e.g., canola, flaxseed, soybean, or corn oil) as part of their daily fat intake (Benabdeslam et al, 1998; Winklhofer-Roob, 1998).

As the disease progresses, changes in carbohydrate intake may be necessary. Lactose intolerance may become evident, and pancreatic endocrine involvement may require carbohydrate adjustments (see Chapters 30 and 33).

Vitamins and Minerals

With pancreatic enzyme supplementation, the water-soluble vitamins appear to be adequately absorbed in patients with CF, and requirements under normal conditions can usually be met by diet plus a standard age-appropriate multivitamin/mineral supplement; however, monitoring individual variations is important.

Even with pancreatic enzyme supplementation, fat-soluble vitamins usually remain inadequately absorbed (Sokol et al, 1991). Low serum concentrations of vitamin A despite increased hepatic stores have been documented in CF, suggesting impaired mobilization and transport of the vitamin from the liver (Farrell and Hubbard, 1983). Decreased levels of vitamin D metabolites have been observed. This is one of several factors that may be related to the decreased bone mineral content that has been described in populations with CF (Mischler et al, 1979; Reiter et al, 1985). Low vitamin E levels have been associated with hemolytic anemia and abnormal neurologic findings (Cynamon et al, 1988; Peters and Kelly, 1996). Individuals with CF may be at risk for vitamin K deficiency secondary to long-term use of antibiotics or liver disease as well as malabsorption. Although most patients maintain normal prothrombin times without supplementation, decreased biologic activity of vitamin K has been reported (Beker et al, 1997). For all these reasons, vitamin K supplementation is recommended. Table 38-4 summarizes the recommendations for vitamin supplementation in CF during childhood and adolescence. This regimen should be adjusted on an individual basis over time.

Mineral intake should meet the gender and age recommendations according to the DRI or other country-specific recommendations for the general population (see Table 15-1). Special attention must be given to some of the minerals, however. Sodium requirements for infants, children, and adults are increased in CF owing to increased losses in sweat. When sodium intake is inadequate, lethargy, vomiting, and dehydration may occur. Adequate salt is consumed by most children and adults following a typical North American diet with processed foods; however, supplemental salt is required under some conditions. Infants require extra salt owing to the low-sodium content of breast milk, formula, and infant foods; ⅛ to ¼ tsp daily is usually adequate in this situation. Children and adults need additional salt during periods of fever, hot weather, or physical exertion. Table salt or proprietary electrolyte replacement solutions are used.

Other minerals are not routinely supplemented, although mineral status should be evaluated on an individual basis. Decreased bone mineralization, low iron stores, and low magnesium levels have all been described in CF (Green et al, 1985; Pond et al, 1996; Reed et al, 2002). Plasma zinc levels may be low in

CLINICAL INSIGHT

Estimation of Daily Energy Requirement in Cystic Fibrosis

To estimate a caloric prescription, you need the following data:

1. Gender
2. Age
3. Weight
4. Basal metabolic rate
5. Physical activity coefficient
6. Lung disease coefficient
7. Coefficient of fat absorption

If the child is growing adequately or the adult is maintaining weight, and if the pulmonary status and steatorrhea are under good control, the total energy requirement (TEE) is reflective of the person's typical energy use and intake. Compare the typical intake with the recommended dietary allowance (RDA) for gender and age. To enable the child or adult to achieve and maintain healthy growth and body composition, the caloric prescription may approximate the RDA (see Chapter 2).

If the child is not growing adequately or the adult is not maintaining weight or body composition, use the following steps to estimate the TEE.

Step 1

Calculate the basal metabolic rate (BMR) using the World Health Organization (WHO) equations for predicting BMR from body weight (wt).

Equations for Predicting BMR (Kcal) From Body Weight (Kg)

AGE RANGE (yr)	FEMALES	MALES
0-3	61.0 wt − 51	60.9 wt − 54
3-10	22.5 wt + 499	22.7 wt + 495
10-18	12.2 wt + 746	17.5 wt + 651
18-30	14.7 wt + 496	15.3 wt + 679
30-60	8.7 wt + 829	11.6 wt + 879

Step 2

Calculate daily energy expenditure (TEE) by multiplying the BMR by the activity coefficient (AC) and adding the disease coefficient (DC).

$$TEE = BMR \times (AC + DC)$$

Activity Coefficient (AC)

- Confined to bed = 1.3
- Sedentary = 1.5
- Active = 1.7

Disease Coefficient (DC)

- Normal lung function = 0.0
  (forced expiratory volume in 1 second (FEV_1) ≥80% of that predicted)
- Moderate lung disease = 0.2
  (FEV_1 40%-79% of that predicted)
- Severe lung disease = 0.3
  (FEV_1 <40% of that predicted)
- Very severe lung disease = 0.4-0.5
  (FEV_1 <40% of that predicted)
- If pulmonary function tests (PFTs) are unavailable, severity of lung disease is assessed clinically.

Sample Calculation

Data: Male patient; 22 years old; weight = 54 kg; FEV_1 60% of that predicted; attends college; relatively sedentary

Calculation: $TEE = BMR \times (1.5 + 0.2)$
$= [15.3 (54) + 679] \times 1.7$
$= [826.2 + 679] \times 1.7 = 1505.2 \times 1.7$
TEE = 2559 kcal

Step 3

Calculate the total daily energy requirement (DER)* from the total energy expenditure (TEE), taking into account the degree of steatorrhea.

- Pancreatic sufficiency: DER = TEE
  (coefficient of fat absorption [CFA] ≥93% of intake, including patients taking enzymes)
- Pancreatic insufficiency: DER = TEE (0.93/CFA)
  (CFA must be determined as a fraction of fat intake)
- Stool fat collection unavailable: DER = TEE (0.93/0.85)
  (approximate value of 0.85 may be used in the calculation; if possible, obtain fecal fat collection)

Sample Calculation

Assuming the patient had pancreatic insufficiency and is taking enzymes, the daily energy requirement would be computed as follows:

Data: Laboratory analysis of 72-hour fecal fat collection reveals that CFA = 78% of intake.

Calculation: $DER = TEE \times (0.93/CFA)$
$= 2559 \times (0.93/0.78) = 2559 \times 1.19$
DER = 3045 kcal/day

***NOTE:** The DER may be further modified due to infection, fever, or other systemic conditions, such as body composition, cystic fibrosis–related diabetes mellitus, or pregnancy. Careful and frequent reassessment must be accomplished on an anticipatory basis.

Data from Ramsey BW et al: Nutritional assessment and management in cystic fibrosis: a consensus report, *Am J Clin Nutr* 55:108, 1992; and Cystic Fibrosis Foundation: *Appendix C: determination of energy requirements.* Consensus Conferences, Concepts in CF Care, *Pediatric nutrition for patients with cystic fibrosis,* X:(1)38, March 28-29, 2001.

cases of moderate to severe malnutrition (Durie and Pencharz, 1989).

Feeding Strategies

Diet modification focuses on meeting the increased nutritional requirements of CF (Bentur et al, 1996; Collins et al, 1997; Michel and Mueller, 1989). Along with adequate dietary modification, positive eating behaviors must be established (Stark et al, 2000). For infants with CF and their families, the immunologic and psychosocial benefits of breast-feeding are well established, and breast-feeding should not be discouraged (Cannella et al, 1993; Marcus et al, 1991). For the infant with pancreatic insufficiency, enzyme microspheres can be added to a small amount of baby food or placed directly in the infant's mouth. Supplementation with high-calorie formula may be necessary to meet growth goals. For formula-fed infants, standard formulas (20 to 27 kcal/oz), given with supplemental enzymes, are usually adequate. Protein hydrolysate formulas with medium-chain triglycerides may also be used (see Appendixes 39 and 40).

For children and adults, intake can be enhanced by regular and enjoyable mealtimes, larger food portions at meals, extra snacks, and foods selected for high-nutrient density. Table 38-5 shows how energy intake can be boosted. Homemade or proprietary nutritional supplements, such as fortified beverages and puddings, also can help the individual with CF attain nutritional goals.

Supplementation by feeding tube is an alternative for those unable to meet nutritional needs by the oral route. Formulas are provided by continuous infusion through a nasogastric, gastrostomy, or jejunostomy tube, often while the person sleeps (see Chapter 23). Elemental and nonelemental formulas with enzymes have both been used effectively. Enzyme powder can be added directly to the formula. If the nocturnal method is chosen, capsules can be taken by mouth when the feeding is started and again once or twice during the night. Factors to consider in the decision to proceed with nighttime supplementation include nutritional status, medical status (e.g., factors such as the presence of nasal polyps and the degree of oxygenation during sleep), risks associated with tube feeding (e.g., aspiration), and the psychosocial and financial impact (Bowser, 1990). Intensive supplementation has been associated with improved weight gain, slowed decline in pulmonary function, decreased incidence of respiratory infection, and improved sense of well-being (Dalzell et al, 1992).

Although the short-term benefits of supplementation have been well documented, nutritional status is likely to regress when supplementation is discontinued. The long-term impact of intensive supplementation on the disease course has not been determined. Parenteral nutrition is best used for short-term support in patients with clearly evident needs, such as those recuperating from gastrointestinal surgery.

TABLE 38-4 Vitamin Supplementation for Children and Adolescents With Cystic Fibrosis

	INDIVIDUAL VITAMIN DAILY SUPPLEMENTATION*			
	VITAMIN A (IU)	VITAMIN E (IU)	VITAMIN D (IU)	VITAMIN K (mg)
0-12 mo	1500	40-50	400	
1-3 yr	5000	80-150	400-800	0.3-0.5
4-8 yr	5,000-10,000	100-200	400-800	
>8 yr	10,000	200-400	400-800	

Data from Cystic Fibrosis Foundation: *Appendix C: determination of energy requirements.* Consensus Conferences, Concepts in CF Care, *Pediatric nutrition for patients with cystic fibrosis,* X:(1)38, March 28-29, 2001.
*These fat-soluble vitamins are in addition to a standard, age-appropriate dose of non–fat-soluble multivitamins.

TABLE 38-5 Sample Menu: Typical Lunch with Increased Nourishment

TYPICAL LUNCH	CALORIES	BOOSTED LUNCH	CALORIES
Soup		**Soup**	
Tomato (½ c) made with water	50	Tomato, made with ½ c fortified milk*	162
		and 1 tsp margarine	36
Sandwich		**Sandwich**	
Bologna (1 oz)	88	Bologna (2 oz)	176
Cheese (1 oz)	107	Cheese (2 oz)	214
Mustard (1 tsp)	4	Mayonnaise (1 tsp)	34
Bread (2 slices)	124	Bread (2 slices)	124
Salad		**Salad**	
Lettuce and tomato with French dressing	70	Carrot-raisin with mayonnaise	153
Dessert		**Dessert**	
Applesauce (⅓ c)	91	Baked apple (with sugar and margarine)	188
Beverage		**Beverage**	
Whole milk (½ c)	80	Fortified milk* (½ c)	112
TOTAL KILOCALORIES	**614**	TOTAL KILOCALORIES	**1199**

Modified from Michel SH, Mueller DH: Practical approaches to nutrition care of patients with cystic fibrosis, *Top Clin Nutr* 4:46, 1989.
*Fortified milk = 1 c Whole milk plus 4 tbsp powdered nonfat milk.

LUNG CANCER

Lung cancer almost always is the result of persistent tobacco smoking for many years. Smoking cessation sessions are part of most wellness programs and offer ideal settings for nutrition education (Anderson et al, 2002; Young and Wilson, 2002). Since the pulmonary system is exposed to the environment, however, other inhaled pollutants may initiate the malignant condition. The primary sites are usually the bronchi, with subsequent metastasis to other organs, such as the bone, brain, liver, or skin.

In cigarette smokers, food components and specific nutrients have been investigated as either preventive or therapeutic modalities for lung cancer. Findings indicate that high-dose β-carotene supplements may have a negative impact, but that increased consumption of fruits and vegetables may be beneficial (Arora et al, 2001; Cotugna, 2000; Handelman, 1997; Ziegler et al, 1996). Because neither successful prevention nor successful management of lung cancer has been elucidated, the possible role of whole foods or their various components, or botanicals, in lung cancer initiation, promotion, or treatment receives worldwide attention (Sadava et al, 2002; Schwartsmann et al, 2001; Seow et al, 2002).

Currently, the medical treatment of lung cancer involves radiation therapy, chemotherapy, and surgery, which are accompanied by various nutritional side effects (see Chapters 19 and 40 for further discussion.). Patients with lung cancer experience the added stress of respiratory fatigue and diminished residual capacity. Weight loss, along with an associated decline in other anthropometric and laboratory indicators of cancer-related malnutrition, portends a changing prognosis (Chlebowski et al, 1996).

Because of the pulmonary constraints in people with lung cancer, purchasing and preparing foods may be overwhelming tasks. Eating may become an unenjoyable activity owing to severe pain, dyspnea, and dyspepsia. Thus, providing foods, beverages, and nutritional supplements in the forms and at the times best tolerated by the patient is essential. Administering oral medications with calorically dense nutritional supplements is another means of supplying needed nutrients (see Chapter 23).

PNEUMONIA

Among the pulmonary infections with nutritional implications is pneumonia (Nardell and Kent, 1998). Pneumonia usually occurs as a nosocomial infection or as a consequence of aspiration of food, fluid, or secretion (like saliva). Optimal nutritional status and proper feeding techniques aid in preventing this pulmonary infection (Riquelme et al, 1997) (see Chapters 42 and 43). Aspiration is common in infants, children, and adults who are frail, have frequent coughing spasms, are unable to effectively chew or swallow their foods and beverages, or have inadequate head and neck control during eating. Suggestions for preventing aspiration of secretions or food and fluids are located in Appendix 55.

RESPIRATORY FAILURE

Pathophysiology

Respiratory failure (RF) occurs when the pulmonary system is unable to perform its functions. The causes may be traumatic, surgical, or medical. *Multiple organ dysfunction syndrome (MODS)* (see Chapter 42) is the term used to denote abnormal interaction among the organ systems, culminating in relentless dysfunction of all organ systems. The acute respiratory distress syndrome (ARDS) is a common complication of critical illness (Ware and Matthay, 2000). Ultimately, in respiratory failure from any cause, the patient requires oxygen, provided through nasal cannula or by mechanical ventilator support, for varying lengths of time and at various levels of oxygen. Central factors in failure to wean from oxygen support or mechanical ventilation are respiratory muscle weakness and retention of carbon dioxide. The prognosis is precarious for patients with underlying chronic pulmonary disease, such as CF or emphysema, or for those who are otherwise medically compromised, malnourished, or older. Lung transplantation may be a viable option for some patients, especially for those with CF (Pingleton, 1998).

Medical Nutrition Therapy

Nutritional needs vary widely within this group of patients, depending on the underlying disease process, prior nutritional status, and the patient's age. Hypercatabolism or hypermetabolism may be present.

As with most pulmonary diseases, body composition fluctuation is the hallmark nutrition assessment indicator for persons with RF. Most patients become severely underweight. Thus, a series of accurate anthropometric measurements is crucial over the entire course of treatment, sometimes spanning the patient's lifetime (see Chapter 17). Accurate interpretation of laboratory results may be confounded by fluid imbalances, medications, and ventilator support. Other nutritionally relevant factors to assess include immunocompetence, chronic mouth breathing, aerophagia, dyspnea, exercise tolerance, and depression.

The goals of nutritional care in patients with RF are to meet basic nutritional requirements, preserve lean body mass, restore respiratory muscle mass and strength, maintain fluid balance, improve resistance to infection, and facilitate weaning from oxygen support and mechanical ventilation by providing energy substrates without exceeding the respiratory system's capacity to clear carbon dioxide. Methods to provide nutritional support depend on the underlying disease, whether the patient is acutely or chronically ill, and whether ventilator support is necessary (Donahoe, 1997; Thomsen, 1997) (see Chapter 23).

Energy

Because of hypercatabolism and hypermetabolism, energy needs are elevated in RF, and sufficient energy must be supplied to prevent the use of the body's own reserves of protein and fat. Energy requirements fluctuate and so are best determined by continuous individual assessment. To estimate initial caloric requirements, the Harris-Benedict equation, modified for stress and activity as well as the underlying disease, can be used or the new DRI equations (see Chapter 2). Thereafter, indirect calorimetry is most useful, except for some patients who are mechanically ventilated, because their ventilation procedures may negate the results. Overfeeding should be avoided (Barton et al, 1997).

Macronutrients

Because the patient with RF may be in negative nitrogen balance, protein should be supplied to restore balance; however, enterally supplied protein or parenterally supplied amino acids do affect the respiratory quotient. The basic requirements for carbohydrate and fat as actual nutrients for nourishment are influenced by the underlying organ system decompensation, the patient's respiratory status, and the ventilation methods used. Controversy persists concerning the optimal ratio of protein, fat, and carbohydrate supplied to patients with RF (Cook et al, 2001). By general agreement, the most important factor is to provide adequate, but not excessive, kilocalories (Pingleton, 1996.) For example, for the energy prescription, some clinicians start with 1.2 to 1.4 × REE. Protein is calculated as 1.5 to 2.0 g per kilogram of dry body weight. Nonprotein calories are evenly divided between fat and carbohydrate. Daily monitoring of each patient's intake is crucial.

Water requirements must be individualized based on the method of oxygen delivery and environmental factors, coupled with knowledge of underlying disease processes and prescribed medications.

Vitamins and Minerals

Exact requirements for specific vitamins and minerals in RF are unknown. It is assumed that vitamins and minerals need to be supplied at least at the levels of the DRI, plus repletion, based on the gender and age of the patient. The intake of vitamins and minerals necessary for anabolism, wound healing, and immunity, as well as of those with antioxidant functions, may need to be increased. For example, during anabolism, mineral balance must be monitored in an anticipatory manner to prevent the refeeding syndrome (see Chapter 23). Minerals that function as electrolytes need to be monitored closely, especially because of fluid imbalances and the occurrence of respiratory acidosis or alkalosis. As a side effect of medications, potassium, calcium, and magnesium may be lost in the urine.

Feeding Strategies

Diet composition and food selections should be planned to accommodate the nutritional requirements, individual preferences, and living arrangements of the patient. Some people participate in pulmonary rehabilitation programs. Most patients who are not intubated or who have tracheostomies will be able to meet all or most of their nutritional needs by mouth. Small portions and favorite foods enhance oral food intake. Consumption must be monitored to maintain appropriate caloric levels and a suitable ratio of protein, fat, and carbohydrate.

Provision of adequate oxygen is crucial for proper digestion and absorption of food. Patients receiving inadequate oxygen may complain of anorexia, early satiety, malaise, bloating, and constipation or diarrhea. Intubated patients usually require enteral tube feedings or parenteral feedings.

The gastrointestinal route is preferred, although aspiration and bacterial overgrowth are concerns. Feeding procedures that minimize aspiration include the use of a continuous method of feeding rather than large bolus feedings, tube placement in the duodenum rather than the stomach, the use of small-bore nasogastric feeding tubes, chest elevation to at least 45 degrees, frequent evaluation for gastric residuals, and endotracheal tube cuff inflation (Ibanez et al, 2000).

TUBERCULOSIS

Pathophysiology

Tuberculosis (TB) is a bacterial disease caused by mycobacteria, specifically *Mycobacterium tuberculosis, M. bovis, or M. africanum.* The disease traditionally was diagnosed among economically disadvantaged population groups (e.g., immigrants, homeless persons, and children) or those living in close quarters (e.g., prisoners, refugees, and armed forces). The disease is spread from inhalation of organisms dispersed as droplets from the sputum of infected persons (the bacteria-laden droplets can float in the air for several hours). At high risk are health care workers; residents in assisted-living facilities, skilled nursing homes, or hospitals; and people who are immunocompromised, such as those with cancer, chronic renal disease, or human immunodeficiency virus (HIV)/AIDS (Madebo et al, 1997; Schwenk and Macallan, 2000; Taskapan et al, 2000) (see Chapters

39, 40, and 41). Tubercle bacilli increasingly are becoming resistant to drug therapy; strains with increased virulence have emerged. Signs and symptoms of TB with nutritional relevance include undernutrition, weight loss, night sweats, fatigue, dyspnea, and hemoptysis.

Medical Nutrition Therapy

Nutritional assessment and intervention focus on the abnormalities created by the underlying disease or social condition. Unless otherwise contraindicated, people with TB routinely require increased kilocalories and fluids. Pharmacologically, this pulmonary infection is treated with multiple medications, especially antibiotics. First-line drugs are isoniazid (INH), rifampicin, ethambutol, and pyrazinamide. Each has drug–food–nutrient interactions (see Chapter 19). Take isoniazid, for example. Food decreases its absorption; thus, this antibiotic should be administered 1 hour before or 2 hours after mealtimes. It depletes pyridoxine (vitamin B_6). It interferes with vitamin D metabolism, which in turn can decrease absorption of calcium and phosphorus. Patients thus require increased vitamin and mineral intake from food as well as supplements.

SUMMARY

Tremendous advancements have been made in the understanding of pulmonary system physiology, biochemistry, molecular biology, and pharmacology as well as in medical, surgical, and nutritional technology. Discovering the mechanisms of energy generation at the cellular level in respiratory diseases, the methods to promote and maintain body composition of patients, and the specific roles of nutrients and phytonutrients in the etiology or treatment of pulmonary conditions offers promise for the future.

Research findings provide the evidence for a balanced approach to nutrition therapy. Close individualized nutrition assessment, intervention, and monitoring of all patients must be coupled with their pulmonary status over the course of their lifespan. Coordinated, competent, and compassionate interdisciplinary nutrition care is essential for all infants, children, and adults to prevent or treat pulmonary diseases.

Clinical Scenario 1: Cystic Fibrosis

Vanessa is a 30-month-old child who was diagnosed with CF shortly after birth. Her parents report that she now is experiencing food jags and other typical toddler behavior at mealtimes. She presents with recent weight loss (she is at the 5th percentile for weight and at the 25th percentile for height), chronic sinusitis and ear infections, and wheezing. The parents bring you a 3-day food record that includes the time and dosage of the prescribed pancreatic enzymes and vitamin/mineral supplements.

1. What other nutritional assessment information do you need before you see the family?
2. What foods and nutrients will you highlight in Vanessa's diet?
3. What is the goal for weight gain? How long should it take, provided that Vanessa's medicines are effective?
4. The family reads about gene therapy on the Internet and asks you about it. How would you respond?
5. Vanessa is enrolled in a child-care center during the week. What kinds of lunches could her parents pack for her? What kinds of helpful information could her parents provide for the child-care staff? How might you assist?

Clinical Scenario 2: Chronic Obstructive Pulmonary Disease

Rick is a 63-year-old widower who is a retired commercial carpet installer. He started smoking when he was 15, and he smoked two packs per day until 7 years ago. You have an appointment with Rick during his next session at the Outpatient Pulmonary Rehabilitation Program. Significant findings are weight 124 lb, height 5 ft 4 in., blood pressure 127/65, heart rate 82, respiratory rate 18, temperature 98.6° F, Sao_2 95, CO_2 54, FVC 1.04 (28% predicted), FEV_1 0.37 (12% predicted), FEV_1/FVC ratio 36, and $FeF_{25\%-76\%}$ 0.19 (67% predicted). History and physical examination reveal severe dyspnea on exertion (DOE), including showering, carrying packages, making bed, and pushing a vacuum cleaner; orthopnea (two or three pillows); and decreased breath sounds. Prescribed medications include theophylline (300 mg twice daily), prednisone (20 mg one daily in the morning), Flovent (220 mg, four puffs twice daily), albuterol and Atrovent (two puffs as needed), Bactrim DS (1 tablet every 12 hours), and Lasix (as needed). Over-the-counter medications include vitamin C (250 mg twice daily), vitamin E (400 IU daily), and calcium (500 mg daily).

1. What other nutritional assessment information do you need before you see Rick?
2. What are the interrelationships between COPD, food intake, and nutrient metabolism?
3. Are there any food-drug interactions that are a concern for Rick?
4. What are the principles of medical nutrition therapy for Rick? Explain the scientific rationale for each.
5. Write out a day's schedule to include mealtimes, medication administration times, and activities of daily living. Include the foods you might suggest for fulfilling the nutrition prescription. Verify by performing a computerized nutrient analysis.
6. What do you think of Rick's nutrient supplementation program? Would you have Rick change it?
7. You are planning a session on nutrition for the clients and their families who participate in the Outpatient Pulmonary Rehabilitation Program. What topics would you cover? What educational techniques would you use?

Relevant Web Sites

American Institute of Cancer Research
www.aicr.org
American Lung Association
www.lungusa.org
American Thoracic Society
www.thoracic.org/statements
Cystic Fibrosis Foundation
www.cff.org
Cystic Fibrosis Genetic Analysis Consortium
www.genet.sickkids.on.ca/cftr.
***Healthy People 2010* (Office of Disease Prevention and Health Promotion, U.S. Department of Health and Human Services)**
www.health.gov/healthypeople
National Asthma Education and Prevention Program (National Heart, Lung, and Blood Institute; National Institutes of Health)
www.nhlbi.nih.gov/guidelines/asthma

Cited References

Aitken ML, Fiel SB: Cystic fibrosis, *Dis Mon* 39:1, 1993.

American Academy of Allergy, Asthma, and Immunology: *Pediatric asthma: promoting best practice: guide for managing asthma in children,* 1999, www.aaaai.org. Accessed April 21, 2002.

American Cancer Society: Cancer reference information, www.cancer.org. Accessed April 21, 2002.

American Institute for Cancer Research: Research programs, www.aicr.org. Accessed April 21, 2002.

American Lung Association: Lungs. www.lungusa.org/lungs. Accessed April 21, 2002.

American Thoracic Society: Pulmonary rehabilitation. Available at: www.thoracic.org/statements. Accessed April 21, 2002.

Andersen DH: Cystic fibrosis of the pancreas and its relation to celiac disease: a clinical and pathologic study, *Am J Dis Child* 56:344, 1938.

Anderson JE et al: Treating tobacco use and dependence: an evidence-based clinical practice guideline for tobacco cessation, *Chest* 121:932, 2002.

Arora A et al: Interactions of beta-carotene and cigarette smoke in human bronchial epithelial cells, *Carcinogenesis* 22:1173, 2001.

Atkinson SA: Special nutritional needs of infants for prevention of and recovery from bronchopulmonary dysplasia, *J Nutr* 131:942S, 2001.

Baker JC, Ayres JG: Diet and asthma, *Respir Med* 94:925, 2000.

Barnes PJ: Chronic obstructive pulmonary disease, *N Engl J Med* 343:269, 2000.

Barton RG et al: Chemical paralysis reduces energy expenditure in patients with burns and severe respiratory failure treated with mechanical ventilation, *J Burn Care Rehabil* 18:461, 1997.

Beker LT et al: Effect of vitamin K1 supplementation on vitamin K status in cystic fibrosis patients, *J Pediatr Gastroenterol Nutr* 24:512, 1997.

Benabdeslam H et al: Biochemical assessment of the nutritional status of cystic fibrosis patients treated with pancreatic enzyme extracts, *Am J Clin Nutr* 67:912, 1998.

Bentur L et al: Dietary intakes of young children with cystic fibrosis: is there a difference? *J Pediatr Gastroenterol Nutr* 22:254, 1996.

Berry JK, Baum CL: Malnutrition in chronic obstructive pulmonary disease: adding insult to injury, *AACN Clin Issues* 12:210, 2001.

Biskobing DM: COPD and osteoporosis, *Chest* 121:609, 2002.

Blumenthal M et al: *The Complete German Commission E Monographs: therapeutic guide to herbal medicines,* Austin, Tex, 1998, American Botanical Council.

Boas SR: Exercise recommendations for individuals with cystic fibrosis, *Sports Med* 24:17, 1997.

Borowitz DS et al: Consensus report of nutrition for pediatric patients with CF, *J Pediatr Gastroenterol Nutr* 38:246, 2002.

Borowitz DS et al: Use of pancreatic enzyme supplements for patients with cystic fibrosis in the context of fibrosing colonopathy: Consensus Committee, *J Pediatr* 127:681, 1995.

Bowser EK: Evaluating enteral nutrition support in cystic fibrosis, *Top Clin Nutr* 5:55, 1990.

Bruno MJ et al: Maldigestion associated with exocrine pancreatic insufficiency: implications of gastrointestinal physiology and properties of enzyme preparations for a cause-related and patient-tailored treatment, *Am J Gastroenterol* 90:1383, 1995.

Brunton JA et al: Growth and body composition in infants with bronchopulmonary dysplasia up to 3 months corrected age: a randomized trial of a high energy nutrient enriched formula fed after hospital discharge, *J Pediatr* 133:340, 1998.

Busse WW, Lemanske RF: Asthma, *N Engl J Med* 344:350, 2001.

Cannella PC et al: Feeding practices and nutrition recommendations for infants with cystic fibrosis, *J Am Diet Assoc* 93:297, 1993.

Chlebowski RT et al: Recent implications of weight loss in lung cancer management, *Nutrition* 12(suppl):S43, 1996.

Collins CE et al: Fat gram target to achieve high energy intake in cystic fibrosis, *J Paediatr Child Health* 33:142, 1997.

Cook D et al: Trials of miscellaneous interventions to wean from mechanical ventilation, *Chest* 120(6 suppl):438S, 2001.

Cotugna N: Dietary factors and cancer risk, *Semin Oncol Nurs* 16:99, 2000.

Creveling S et al: Cystic fibrosis, nutrition, and the health care team, *J Am Diet Assoc* 97(suppl 2):S186, 1997.

Cross C, Halliwell B: Nutrition and human disease: how much extra vitamin C might smokers need? *Lancet* 341:1091, 1993.

Cynamon HA et al: Effect of vitamin E deficiency on neurologic function in patients with cystic fibrosis, *J Pediatr* 113:638, 1988.

Cystic Fibrosis Foundation: Consensus conferences, *Concepts in CF Care* X(1):1, 2001.

Cystic Fibrosis Foundation: Facts about cystic fibrosis, www.cff.org/facts. Accessed April 21, 2002.

Cystic Fibrosis Genetic Analysis Consortium: Cystic fibrosis mutation data base, www.genet.sickkids.on.ca/cftr. Accessed April 21, 2002.

Dacey MJ: Hypomagnesemic disorders, *Crit Care Clin* 17:155, 2001.

Dalzell AM et al: Nutritional rehabilitation in cystic fibrosis: a 5-year follow-up study, *J Pediatr Gastroenterol Nutr* 15:141, 1992.

de Meer K et al: Total energy expenditure in infants with bronchopulmonary dysplasia is associated with respiratory status, *Eur J Pediatr* 156:299, 1997.

Department of Health and Human Services: Action against asthma: a strategic plan for the Department of Health and Human Services, www.aspe.hhs.gov/sp/asthma. Accessed April 21, 2002.

Donahoe M: Nutritional support in advanced lung disease: the pulmonary cachexia syndrome, *Clin Chest Med* 18:547, 1997.

Duggan MB, Gilbert K: An experimental estimate of the maintenance energy requirement in children with cystic fibrosis, *Eur J Clin Nutr* 50:251, 1996.

Durie PR, Pencharz PB: A rational approach to the nutritional care of patients with cystic fibrosis, *J R Soc Med* 82:11, 1989.

Farrell PA, Fiascone JM: Bronchopulmonary dysplasia in the 1990s: a review for the pediatrician, *Curr Probl Pediatr* 27:129, 1997.

Farrell PM, Hubbard VS: Nutrition in cystic fibrosis: vitamins, fatty acids and minerals. In Lloyd-Still JD, editor: *Textbook of cystic fibrosis,* Boston, 1983, John Wright-PSG.

Farrell PM et al: Wisconsin Cystic Fibrosis Neonatal Screening Study Group: early diagnosis of cystic fibrosis through neonatal screening prevents severe malnutrition and improves long-term growth, *Pediatrics* 107:1, 2001.

Finnerty JP et al: The effectiveness of outpatient pulmonary rehabilitation in chronic lung disease: a randomized controlled trial, *Chest* 119:1705, 2001.

Gavin J et al: Dietary fibre and the occurrence of gut symptoms in cystic fibrosis, *Arch Dis Child* 76:35, 1997.

Giacoia GP et al: Follow-up of school-age children with bronchopulmonary dysplasia, *J Pediatr* 130:400, 1997.

Gilliland FD et al: Dietary magnesium, potassium, sodium, and children's lung function, *Am J Epidemiol* 155:125, 2002.

Green GG et al: Symptomatic hypomagnesemia in cystic fibrosis, *J Pediatr* 107:425, 1985.

Gregoire MC et al: Health and developmental outcomes at 18 months in very preterm infants with bronchopulmonary dysplasia, *Pediatrics* 101:856, 1998.

Handelman GJ: High-dose vitamin supplements for cigarette smokers: caution is indicated, *Nutr Rev* 55:369, 1997.

Harik-Khan RI et al: Body mass index and the risk of COPD, *Chest* 121:370, 2002.

Hashimoto Y et al: Assessment of magnesium status in patients with bronchial asthma, *J Asthma* 37:489, 2000.

Hazinski TA: Bronchopulmonary dysplasia. In Chernick V, Boat TF, editors: *Kendig's disorders of the respiratory tract in children*, ed 6, Philadelphia, 1998, WB Saunders.

Healthy People, 2010: Focus Area 24: Respiratory diseases, www.health.gov/healthypeople/healthfinder. Accessed April 21, 2002.

Ibanez J et al: Incidence of gastroesophageal reflux and aspiration in mechanically ventilated patients using small-bore nasogastric tubes, *JPEN J Parenter Enteral Nutr* 24:103, 2000.

Incalzi RA et al: Correlates of osteoporosis in chronic obstructive pulmonary disease, *Respir Med* 94:1079, 2000.

Johnson DB et al: Nutrition and feeding in infants with bronchopulmonary dysplasia after initial hospital discharge: risk factors for growth failure, *J Am Diet Assoc* 98:649, 1998.

Kakish KS: Serum magnesium levels in asthmatic children during and between exacerbations, *Arch Pediatr Adolesc Med* 155:181, 2001.

Kawchak DA et al: Longitudinal, prospective analysis of dietary intake in children with cystic fibrosis, *J Pediatr* 129:119, 1996.

Kennedy JD: Lung function outcome in children of premature birth, *J Paediatr Child Health* 35:516, 1999.

Kerem BS et al: Identification of the cystic fibrosis gene: genetic analysis, *Science* 245:1073, 1989.

Kurzner SI et al: Growth failure in infants with bronchopulmonary dysplasia: nutrition and elevated resting metabolic expenditure, *Pediatrics* 81:389, 1988.

Levy E et al: Lipoprotein abnormalities associated with cholesteryl ester transfer activity in cystic fibrosis patients: the role of essential fatty acid deficiency, *Am J Clin Nutr* 57:573, 1993.

Madebo T et al: HIV infection and malnutrition change the clinical and radiological features of pulmonary tuberculosis, *Scand J Infect Dis* 29:355, 1997.

Mador MJ, Bozkanat E: Skeletal muscle dysfunction in chronic obstructive pulmonary disease, *Respir Res* 2:216, 2001.

Marcus MS et al: Nutritional status of infants with cystic fibrosis associated with early diagnosis and intervention, *Am J Clin Nutr* 54:578, 1991.

Martin-Harris B: Optimal patterns of care in patients with chronic obstructive pulmonary disease, *Semin Speech Lang* 21:311, 2000.

Michel SH, Mueller DH: Practical approaches to nutrition care of patients with cystic fibrosis, *Top Clin Nutr* 4:46, 1989.

Michel SH, Mueller DH: Impact of lactation on women with cystic fibrosis and their infants: a review of five cases, *J Am Diet Assoc* 94:159, 1994.

Michel SH, Mueller DH: Nutrition and cystic fibrosis, *J Respir Care Pract/RT*, p 27, April/May, 1995.

Mihrshahi S et al: The childhood asthma prevention study (CAPS): design and research protocol of a randomized trial for the primary prevention of asthma, *Control Clin Trials* 22:333, 2001.

Miller AL: The etiologies, pathophysiology, and alternative/complementary treatment of asthma, *Altern Med Rev* 6:20, 2001.

Mircetic RN et al: Magnesium concentration in plasma, leukocytes and urine of children with intermittent asthma, *Clin Chim Acta* 312:197, 2001.

Mischler EH et al: Demineralization in cystic fibrosis, *Am J Dis Child* 133:632, 1979.

Moran A et al: Diagnosis, screening and management of cystic fibrosis related diabetes mellitus: a consensus report, *Diabetes Res Clin Pract* 45: 61, 1999.

Mueller DH: Timeliness of codifying nutrition ABCDEs for BPD, *J Pediatr* 133:315, 1998.

Murphy MD et al: Resting energy expenditures measured by indirect calorimetry are higher in preadolescent children with cystic fibrosis than expenditures calculated from prediction equations, *J Am Diet Assoc* 95:30, 1995.

Nagakura T et al: Dietary supplementation with fish oil rich in omega-3 polyunsaturated fatty acids in children with bronchial asthma, *Eur Respir J* 16:861, 2000.

Nardell EA, Kent D: Respiratory infections in the economically disadvantaged. In Fishman AP, et al, editors: *Fishman's pulmonary diseases and disorders*, ed 3, vol. 2, New York, 1998, McGraw-Hill.

National Asthma Education and Prevention Program (NAEPP), Expert Panel Report 2: Guidelines for the Diagnosis and Management of Asthma, Bethesda, Md, 1997, National Institutes of Health. National Heart, Lung, and Blood Institute, NIH Publication No. 97-4051.

National Cancer Institute: Lung Cancer Home Page, www.nci.nih.gov. Accessed April 21, 2002.

National Institute of Diabetes and Digestive & Kidney Diseases: Cystic Fibrosis Research Directions, www.niddk.nih.gov. Accessed April 21, 2002.

National Institutes of Health: Institutes, Centers & Offices, www.nih.gov/icd. Accessed April 21, 2002.

Newkirk M et al: Nutrition management of bronchopulmonary dysplasia (BPD), *Building Block for Life*. Publication of the Pediatric Nutrition Practice Group of The American Dietetic Association, 22:1, Summer 1999.

Nolt JKB: Does vitamin A supplementation decrease lung disease severity in very low-birthweight infants? *Support Line*. Publication of the Dietitians in Nutrition Support Practice Group of The American Dietetic Association, 23:9, December 2001.

Oh W: Nutritional management of infants with bronchopulmonary dysplasia: bronchopulmonary dysplasia and related chronic respiratory disorders. In *Report of the Ninetieth Ross Conference on Pediatric Research*, Columbus, Ohio, 1986, Ross Laboratories.

Okamoto M et al: Effects of perilla seed oil supplementation on leukotriene generation by leucocytes in patients with asthma associated with lipometabolism, *Int Arch Allergy Immunol* 122:137, 2000.

Orenstein DM et al: Cystic fibrosis: a 2002 update, *J Pediatr* 140:156, 2002.

Peters SA, Kelly FJ: Vitamin E supplementation in cystic fibrosis, *J Pediatr Gastroenterol Nutr* 22:341, 1996.

Picado C et al: Dietary micronutrients/antioxidants and their relationship with bronchial asthma severity, *Allergy* 56:43, 2001.

Pingleton SK. Enteral nutrition in patients with respiratory disease, *Eur Respir J* 9:364, 1996.

Pingleton SK: Nutrition in acute respiratory failure. In Fishman AP et al, editors: *Fishman's pulmonary diseases and disorders*, ed 3., vol 2. New York, 1998, McGraw-Hill.

Pond MN et al: Functional iron deficiency in adults with cystic fibrosis, *Respir Med* 90:409, 1996.

Ramsey BW et al: Nutrition assessment and management in cystic fibrosis: a consensus report, *Am J Clin Nutr* 55:108, 1992.

Reed DW et al: Iron deficiency in cystic fibrosis, *Chest* 121:48, 2002.

Reiter EO et al: Vitamin D metabolites in adolescents and young adults with cystic fibrosis: effects of sun and season, *J Pediatr* 106:21, 1985.

Riordan J et al: Identification of the cystic fibrosis gene: cloning and characterization of the complementary DNA, *Science* 245:1066, 1989.

Riquelme R et al: Community-acquired pneumonia in the elderly: clinical and nutritional aspects, *Am J Respir Crit Care Med* 156:1908, 1997.

Rossi A et al: Aging and the respiratory system, *Aging* 8:143, 1996.

Rowe BH et al: Evidence-based treatments for acute asthma, *Respir Care* 46:1380, 2001.

Ryan CF et al: Energy balance in stable malnourished patients with chronic obstructive pulmonary disease, *Chest* 103:1038, 1993.

Sadava D et al: Effects of four Chinese herbal extracts on drug-sensitive and multidrug-resistant small-cell lung carcinoma cells, *Cancer Chemother Pharmacol* 49:261, 2002.

Salamoni F et al: Bone mineral content in cystic fibrosis patients: correlation with fat-free mass, *Arch Dis Child* 74:314, 1996.

Saris NE et al: Magnesium: an update on physiological, clinical and analytical aspects, *Clin Chim Acta* 294:1, 2000.

Schenk P et al: Intravenous magnesium sulfate for bronchial hyperreactivity: a randomized, controlled, double-blind study, *Clin Pharmacol Ther* 69:365, 2001.

Schols AM, Wouters EF: Nutritional abnormalities and supplementation in chronic obstructive pulmonary disease, *Clin Chest Med* 21:753, 2000.

Schwab RJ: Control of respiration during sleep. In Grippi MA, editor: *Pulmonary pathophysiology,* Philadelphia, 1995, JB Lippincott.

Schwartz J: Role of polyunsaturated fatty acids in lung disease, *Am J Clin Nutr* 71(1 suppl):393S, 2000.

Schwartsmann G et al: Marine organisms as a source of new anticancer agents, *Lancet Oncol* 2:221, 2001.

Schwenk A, Macallan DC: Tuberculosis, malnutrition and wasting, *Curr Opin Clin Nutr Metab Care* 3:285, 2000.

Seow A et al: Diet, reproductive factors and lung cancer risk among Chinese women in Singapore: evidence for a protective effect of soy in nonsmokers, *Int J Cancer* 97:365, 2002.

Sharer N et al: Mutations of the cystic fibrosis gene in patients with chronic pancreatitis, *N Engl J Med* 339:645, 1998.

Silverman R: Treatment of acute asthma: a new look at the old and at the new, *Clin Chest Med* 21:361, 2000.

Smit HA: Chronic obstructive pulmonary disease, asthma and protective effects of food intake: from hypothesis to evidence? *Respir Res* 2:261, 2001.

Sokol RJ et al: Fat-soluble vitamins in infants identified by cystic fibrosis newborn screening, *Pediatr Pulmonol* 7(suppl):52, 1991.

Stark LJ et al: Parent and child mealtime behavior in families of children with cystic fibrosis, *J Pediatr* 136:195, 2000.

Taskapan H et al: The outcome of tuberculosis in patients on chronic hemodialysis, *Clin Nephrol* 54:134, 2000.

Thomsen C: Nutritional support in advanced pulmonary disease, *Respir Med* 91:249, 1997.

Thorsdottir I, Gunnarsdottir I: Energy intake must be increased among recently hospitalized patients with chronic obstructive pulmonary disease to improve nutritional status, *J Am Diet Assoc* 102:247, 2002.

Thorsdottir I et al: Screening method evaluated by nutritional status measurements can be used to detect malnourishment in chronic obstructive pulmonary disease, *J Am Diet Assoc* 101:648, 2001.

Tomezsko JL et al: Dietary intake of healthy children with cystic fibrosis compared with normal control children, *Pediatrics* 90:547, 1992.

Tyler VE: *Herbs of choice: the therapeutic use of phytomedicinals,* New York, 1994, Pharmaceutical Products Press.

Tyson JE et al: Vitamin A supplementation in extremely low birthweight infants, *N Engl J Med* 340:1962, 1999.

U.S. Department of Agriculture: Dietary Guidelines for Americans, www.nutrition.gov. Accessed April 21, 2002.

Verma RP et al: Vitamin A deficiency and severe bronchopulmonary dysplasia in very low birthweight infants, *Am J Perinatol* 13:389, 1996.

Vural H et al: Concentrations of copper, zinc and various elements in serum of patients with bronchial asthma, *J Trace Elem Med Biol* 14:88, 2000.

Ware LB, Matthay MA: The acute respiratory distress syndrome, *N Engl J Med* 342:1334, 2000.

Winklhofer-Roob B: Nutritional status in cystic fibrosis: where to go from here? *Am J Clin Nutr* 67:817, 1998.

Young RC, Wilson CM: Cancer prevention: past, present, and future, *Clin Cancer Res* 8:11, 2002.

Ziegler RG et al: Nutrition and lung cancer, *Cancer Causes Control* 7:157, 1996.

■ Additional References

Andreoli TE et al: *Cecil essentials of medicine,* ed 4, Philadelphia, 1997, WB Saunders, 1997.

Chicago Dietetic Association et al: *Manual of clinical dietetics,* ed 6, Chicago, 2000, American Dietetic Association.

Collins FS: Cystic fibrosis: molecular biology and therapeutic implications, *Science* 256:774, 1992.

Dodge JA: Nutrition in cystic fibrosis: a historical overview, *Proc Nutr Soc* 51:225, 1992.

Escott-Stump S: *Nutrition and diagnosis-related care,* ed 5, Baltimore, 1998, Williams & Wilkins.

Matarese LE: *Contemporary nutrition support practice: a clinical guide,* Philadelphia, 1998, WB Saunders.

West JB: *Pulmonary pathophysiology: the essentials,* Baltimore, Md, 1998, Williams & Wilkins.

Williams CP, editor: *Pediatric manual of clinical dietetics,* Chicago, 1998, American Dietetic Association.

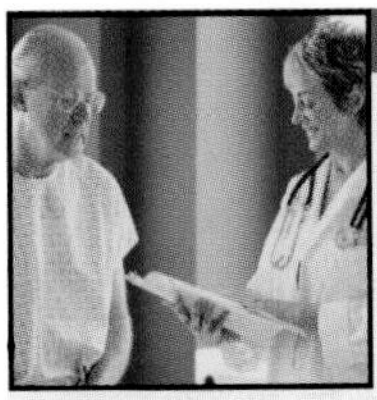

CHAPTER 39

Medical Nutrition Therapy for Renal Disorders

KATY G. WILKENS, MS, RD

CHAPTER OUTLINE

- Physiology and Function of the Kidneys
- Renal Disease
- Glomerular Diseases
- Diseases of the Tubules and Interstitium
- Progressive Nature of Renal Disease
- End-Stage Renal Disease
- Nephrolithiasis (Kidney Stones)*

KEY TERMS

acute glomerulonephritides–a group of diseases characterized by inflammation of the capillary loops of the glomerulus

azotemia–the accumulation in the blood of abnormal quantities of urea, uric acid, creatinine, and other nitrogenous wastes

calciphylaxis–disease characterized by calcium phosphate deposition in soft tissues; occurs when there has been too high a calcium intake for a long time; also called *metastatic calcification*

L-carnitine–an amino acid synthesized in the kidney; required for mitochondrial oxidation of long-chain fatty acids; usually low in dialysis patients; supplementation may be associated with improved muscle function and less leg cramping

continuous arteriovenous hemofiltration (CAVH)–a method of acute renal failure management in which an ultrafiltration membrane, powered by the patient's own blood, produces an ultrafiltrate that can then be replaced by parenteral nutrition fluids

continuous venovenous hemofiltration (CVVH)–a method similar to CAVH that uses the venous system.

dialysate–the solution used in dialysis to remove waste products from the blood; electrolyte content similar to plasma

end-stage renal disease (ESRD)–a disease characterized by the kidney's inability to excrete waste products, maintain fluid and electrolyte balance, and produce hormones

erythropoietin (EPO)–a hormone secreted chiefly by the kidney in the adult and by the liver in the fetus, which acts on stem cells of the bone marrow to stimulate red blood cell production

glomerular filtration rate (GFR)–the quantity of glomerular filtrate formed per unit in all nephrons of both kidneys

hemodialysis–a method of clearing waste products from the blood in which blood passes by the semipermeable membrane of the artificial kidney and waste products are removed by diffusion and fluids by ultrafiltration

hypercalciuria–a urine calcium concentration of 4 mg (0.1 mmol)/kg/day for a random urine collection from a patient on an unrestricted diet.

hyperoxaluria–a urine oxalate concentration of greater than 40 mg per 24-hour urine collection

ischemic acute tubular necrosis–extensive kidney tissue destruction resulting from a prolonged episode of blood deprivation

KT/V–a measurement of the removal of urea from the patient's blood over time; *K* is the urea clearance of the dialyzer, *T* is the length of time of dialysis, and *V* is the patient's total body water volume; also called *kinetic modeling*

*Content for this section was developed by Veena Juneja, MSc, RD.

KEY TERMS—Continued

nephritic syndrome–the syndrome of hematuria, hypertension, and mild loss of renal function that results from acute inflammation of the capillary loops of the glomerulus

nephrolithiasis–a condition marked by the presence of renal calculi (stones)

nephrotic syndrome–a condition resulting from loss of the glomerular barrier to protein; characterized by massive edema, proteinuria, hypoalbuminemia, hypercholesterolemia, hypercoagulability, and abnormal bone metabolism

oliguria–the condition of having urinary volumes of less than 500 ml/day

osteitis fibrosa cystica–inflammation of the bone with fibrous degeneration and formation of cysts secondary to parathyroid gland hyperfunction

peritoneal dialysis–a method of removing waste products from the blood in which diffusion carries them from the blood through the semipermeable peritoneal membrane and into the dialysate; can be either continuous ambulatory or continuous cyclical

pre–end stage renal disease–a decreased level of kidney function for 3 months or more; often called chronic renal failure

pyelonephritis–bacterial infection of the kidneys

renal failure–the inability of a kidney to excrete the daily load of wastes

renal osteodystrophy–metabolic bone disease as a complication of end-stage renal disease

renal tubular acidosis (RTA)–a defect in tubular handling of bicarbonate, treated by different, cause-specific methods

renin-angiotensin mechanism–a major control of blood pressure that involves kidney-secreted renin that acts on angiotensinogen in the plasma to form angiotensin I, which is converted to angiotensin II, a powerful vasoconstrictor and potent stimulus of aldosterone secretion by the adrenal gland

solute load–the end waste products of metabolism

ultrafiltrate–the fluid produced after filtering the blood through the glomerulus; similar in composition to blood until modified by the other segments of the nephron to produce urine

urea reduction rate (URR)–the reduction of urea from before to after dialysis; a form of kinetic modeling

uremia–a clinical syndrome of malaise, weakness, nausea and vomiting, muscle cramps, itching, metallic mouth taste, and often neurologic impairment, which is brought about by an unacceptable level of nitrogenous wastes in the blood

PHYSIOLOGY AND FUNCTION OF THE KIDNEYS

The main function of the kidney is to maintain homeostatic balance with respect to fluids, electrolytes, and organic solutes. The normal kidney can perform this function over a wide range of dietary fluctuations in sodium, water, and various solutes. This task is accomplished by the continuous filtration of blood and by alterations (secretion and reabsorption) in this filtered fluid. The kidney receives 20% of cardiac output, which allows the filtering of approximately 1600 L/day of blood. Approximately 180 L of fluid (ultrafiltrate) is produced in filtering this blood, and through active processes of reabsorbing certain components and secreting others, the composition of this fluid is changed into the 1.5 L of urine excreted in an average day.

Each kidney consists of approximately 1 million functioning units called *nephrons* (Figure 39-1). The nephron consists of a *glomerulus* connected to a series of tubules, which can be broken into functionally different segments: the proximal convoluted tubule, loop of Henle, distal tubule, and collecting duct. Each nephron functions independently in producing a contribution to the final urine, although all are under similar control and are thus coordinated. Nevertheless, when one segment of a nephron is destroyed, that complete nephron is no longer functional.

The glomerulus is a spherical mass of capillaries surrounded by a membrane, *Bowman's capsule.* The function of the glomerulus is production of the large amount of ultrafiltrate, which the following segments of the nephron then modify. The ultrafiltrate produced in the glomerulus is very similar in composition to blood. Because of its barrier function, the glomerulus blocks blood cells as well as molecules of molecular weight greater than 6500 daltons, such as protein. The production of ultrafiltrate is mainly passive and relies on the perfusion pressure generated by the heart and supplied by the renal artery.

The tubules reabsorb the vast majority of components that compose the ultrafiltrate. Much of this process is active and requires a large expenditure of energy in the form of adenosine triphosphate (ATP). A unique structure, differences in permeability between the various segments, and the response to hormonal control allow the tubule to produce a final urine that can vary widely in concentration of sodium, potassium, and other electrolytes; osmolality; pH; and volume.

Ultimately, the final urine produced is funneled into common *collecting tubules* and into the *renal pelvis.* The renal pelvis narrows into a single ureter per kidney, and each ureter carries urine into the bladder, where it accumulates before elimination.

Although the homeostatic mechanisms are interrelated to a large extent, occasional demands are placed on the kidney to regulate one substance while sacrificing tight control of others. In this regard, the control of circulating blood volume predominates over the control of all other parameters. Thus sodium, the most important molecule in determining the body's circulating volume, is regulated at the expense of all other substances. A gain or loss of 1% of circulating volume is reflected in marked changes in urine as well as in serum composition of potassium, bicarbonate, and water.

The kidney has almost unlimited ability to regulate water homeostasis. Its ability to form a large concentration gradient between its inner medulla and outer cortex allows the kidney to excrete urine as dilute as 50 mOsm or as concentrated as 1200 mOsm. Given a daily fixed solute load of about 600 mOsm (the solute load representing the end waste products of normal metabolism), the kidney can get rid of as little as 500 ml of concentrated urine or as much as 12 L. Control of water excretion is regulated by vasopressin, formerly known as *antidiuretic hormone (ADH)*, a small peptide hormone secreted by the posterior pituitary. An excess of relative body water, indicated by a fall in osmolality, leads to prompt shutoff of all vasopressin secretion. Likewise, a small rise in osmolality brings about marked vasopressin secretion and retention of water. However, the need to conserve sodium sometimes leads to a sacrifice of the homeostatic control of water for the sake of volume.

The minimum urinary volume capable of eliminating a relatively fixed 600 mOsm of solute is 500 ml, assuming that the kidney is capable of maximum concentration. Urinary volume of less than 500 ml/day is called oliguria; it is impossible for such a small urine volume to eliminate all of the daily waste.

The majority of the solute load consists of nitrogenous wastes, largely the end products of protein metabolism. Urea predominates in amounts depending on the protein content of the diet. Uric acid, creatinine, and ammonia are present in small amounts. If these normal waste products are not eliminated appropriately, they collect in abnormal quantities in the blood, a condition known as azotemia. The ability of the kidney to adequately eliminate nitrogenous waste products is known as renal function; renal failure is the consequence of inability to excrete the daily load of these wastes.

The kidney also performs functions unrelated to excretion. One of these involves the renin-angiotensin mechanism, a major control of blood pressure. Decreased blood volume causes cells of the glomerulus (the juxtaglomerular apparatus) to react by secreting renin, a proteolytic enzyme. Renin acts on angiotensinogen in the plasma to form angiotensin I, which is converted to angiotensin II, a powerful vasoconstrictor and a potent stimulus of aldosterone secretion by the adrenal gland. As a consequence, sodium is reabsorbed, and blood pressure is returned to normal.

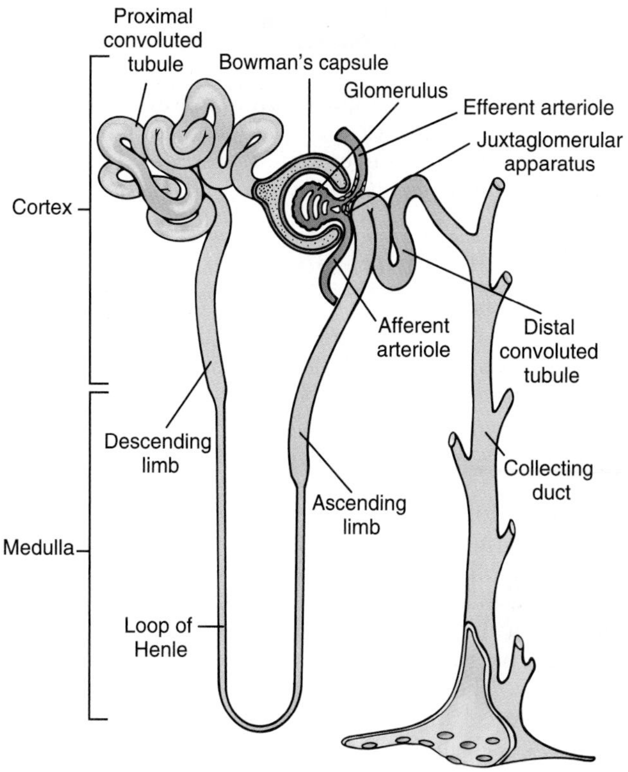

FIGURE 39-1 • The nephron. (From Lewis SM, Heitkemper MM, Dirksen SR: *Medical-surgical nursing: assessment and management of clinical problems*, ed 5, St. Louis, 2000, Mosby.)

The kidney also produces the hormone erythropoietin, a critical determinant of erythroid activity in the bone marrow. Deficiency of erythropoietin is a factor in the severe anemia present in chronic renal disease.

Maintenance of *calcium-phosphorus homeostasis* involves the complex interactions of parathyroid hormone (PTH); calcitonin; vitamin D; and three effector organs, the gut, kidney, and bone. The role of the kidney includes production of the active form of vitamin D—1,25-$(OH)_2D_3$—as well as elimination of both calcium and phosphorus. Active vitamin D promotes efficient absorption of calcium by the gut and is one of the substances necessary for bone remodeling and maintenance (see Chapter 27).

RENAL DISEASE

The manifestations of renal disease are direct consequences of the portions of the urinary tract system most affected. These manifestations include (1) glomerular diseases; (2) acute renal failure (ARF); (3) tubular defects; (4) end-stage renal disease (ESRD); and (5) renal stones. Objectives of nutritional care depend on the abnormality being treated.

GLOMERULAR DISEASES

The functions of the glomerulus that are important with respect to disease are production of an adequate ultrafiltrate and prevention of certain substances from entering this ultrafiltrate.

Nephritic Syndrome

Pathophysiology

Nephritic syndrome incorporates the clinical manifestations of a group of diseases characterized by inflammation of the capillary loops of the glomerulus. These diseases, also called acute glomerulonephritides, are sudden in onset; last a short time; and proceed to either complete recovery, development of chronic nephrotic syndrome (see below), or ESRD.

The primary manifestation of these diseases is hematuria (blood in the urine), a consequence of the capillary inflammation that damages the glomerular barrier to blood cells. The syndrome is also characterized by hypertension and by mild loss of renal function. The most common presentation follows a streptococcal infection and is usually—although not always—self-limiting. Other causes include primary kidney diseases—such as IgA nephropathy and hereditary nephritis—as well as secondary diseases—such as systemic lupus erythematosus (SLE), vasculitis, and glomerulonephritis associated with endocarditis, abscesses, or infected ventriculoperitoneal shunts.

Medical Nutrition Therapy

The treatment of acute glomerulonephritis attempts to maintain good nutritional status while allowing time for the disease to resolve spontaneously. In patients in whom an underlying disease is responsible, treatment of that disease predominates and largely determines outcome. Restricting protein or potassium intake is of no benefit unless significant uremia or hyperkalemia develops. When hypertension is present, it is related mainly to extracellular volume excess and should be treated with sodium restriction (see Chapter 36).

Nephrotic Syndrome

Pathophysiology

Nephrotic syndrome comprises a heterogeneous group of diseases whose common manifestations derive from a loss of the glomerular barrier to protein. Large protein losses in the urine lead to hypoalbuminemia with consequent edema, hypercholesterolemia, hypercoagulability, and abnormal bone metabolism.

More than 95% of the cases of nephrotic syndrome stem from three systemic diseases (diabetes mellitus, systemic lupus erythematosus [SLE], and amyloidosis) and four diseases that are primarily of the kidney (minimal change disease [disease seen only with electron microscopy], membranous nephropathy, focal glomerulosclerosis, and membranoproliferative glomerulonephritis). Although renal function can deteriorate during the course of these diseases, it is not a consistent feature (Hricik et al, 1998).

Medical Nutrition Therapy

The primary objectives of medical nutrition therapy are to manage the symptoms associated with the syndrome (edema, hypoalbuminemia, and hyperlipidemia), decrease the risk of progression to renal failure, and maintain nutritional stores. Patients with an established severe protein deficiency who continue to lose protein may require an extended time of carefully supervised nutritional care.

The diet should attempt to provide sufficient protein and energy to maintain a positive nitrogen balance and to produce an increase in plasma albumin concentration and disappearance of edema. An increase in albumin and positive nitrogen balance are not always achievable, as a high protein diet often leads to increased urinary losses (Mitch, 1996).

Protein

The dietary protein level for patients has changed over time. Historically, these patients received diets high in protein (up to 1.5 g/kg/day) in an attempt to increase serum albumin and prevent protein malnutrition. However, studies have shown that a reduction of protein intake to as low as 0.8 mg/kg/day can decrease proteinuria without adversely affecting serum albumin. To allow for optimal protein use, three fourths of the protein should be from sources of high biologic value (HBV), and energy intake should be about 35 kcal/kg/day for adults and 100 to 150 kcal/kg/day for children (Kaysen, 1997).

Sodium

Edema, the most clinically apparent manifestation of this group of diseases, indicates a state of total body sodium overload. However, because of the low oncotic pressure in the circulating blood volume that results from hypoalbuminemia, the volume of circulating blood may be reduced. Attempts to limit sodium intake more than modestly or to eliminate large amounts of extra sodium with diuretics can cause marked hypotension, exacerbation of the coagulopathy, and deterioration of renal function. Control of edema in this group of diseases should therefore not be complete, should rely to some extent on elastic full-length support hose, and should entail only modest sodium restriction—approximately 3 g of sodium daily (see Chapter 36).

Lipids

The important consequence of hypercholesterolemia lies in the potential for inducing cardiovascular disease. Although a satisfactory answer is not apparent, patients with long-standing nephrotic syndrome are believed to face increased risk (Toto, 1996). Many pediatric patients with frequently relapsing or resistant nephrotic syndrome are at particular risk for premature atherosclerosis. Certain lipid-lowering agents, in combination with a cholesterol-lowering diet, can reduce total cholesterol, low-density lipoprotein (LDL) cholesterol, and triglycerides in patients with nephrotic syndrome (see Chapter 35).

DISEASES OF THE TUBULES AND INTERSTITIUM

To a great extent, the functions of the kidney tubules make them susceptible to injury. The enormous energy requirements and expenditures of the tubules in performing the work of active secretion and reabsorption leave this part of the kidney particularly vulnerable to ischemic injuries. High local concentrations of many toxic drugs can destroy or damage various segments of the tubules. Finally, the high-solute concentration generated in the medullary interstitium exposes it to damage from oxidants and precipitation of calcium-phosphate product (extraosseous calcification) and favors the sickling of red blood cells in sickle cell anemia.

Acute Renal Failure

Pathophysiology

Acute renal failure (ARF) is characterized by a sudden reduction in glomerular filtration rate (GFR) and an alteration in the ability of the kidney to excrete the daily production of metabolic waste (Figure 39-2). It can occur in association with either a reduction in urine output (oliguria, strictly defined as production of less than 500 ml in 24 hours) or normal urine flow. ARF typically occurs in previously healthy kidneys. Its duration varies from a few days to several weeks. The causes of ARF are numerous, and often several occur simultaneously (Box 39-1). These causes are generally classified into three categories: (1) inadequate renal perfusion *(prerenal),* (2) diseases within the renal parenchyma *(intrinsic),* and (3) obstruction *(postrenal).* Generally, if careful attention is directed at diagnosing and correcting the prerenal and obstructive causes, ARF is short-lived and requires no particular nutritional intervention.

Intrinsic ARF can result from toxic drug exposure, a local allergic reaction to drugs, rapidly progressive glomerulonephritis, or a prolonged episode of ischemia leading to ischemic acute tubular necrosis. Of these causes, the latter is the most devastating. Typically, patients develop this illness as a complication of sustained shock caused by an overwhelming infection, severe trauma, surgical accident, or cardiogenic shock.

The clinical course and outcome depend mainly on the underlying cause. Patients with ARF caused by drug toxicity generally recover fully after they stop taking the drug. On the other hand, the mortality rate associated with ischemic acute tubular necrosis caused by shock is approximately 70%. Typically, these patients are highly catabolic, and extensive tissue destruction occurs in the early stages. Hemodialysis is used to reduce the acidosis, correct the uremia, and control hyperkalemia.

If recovery is to occur, it generally takes place within 2 to 3 weeks of the time when the underlying insults have been corrected. The recovery (diuretic) phase is characterized first by an increase in urine output and later by a return of waste elimination. During this period, dialysis may still be required, and careful attention must be paid to fluid and electrolyte balance and appropriate replacement.

Medical Nutrition Therapy

Nutritional care in ARF is particularly important because the patient not only has uremia, metabolic acidosis, and fluid and electrolyte imbalance but also usually also suffers from physiologic stress (e.g., infection or tissue destruction) that increases protein needs. The problem of balancing protein and energy needs with treatment of acidosis and excessive nitrogenous waste is complicated and delicate (see Chapter 42).

In the early stages of ARF, the patient is often moribund and unable to eat. Early attention to nutritional status—often in the form of total parenteral nutrition (TPN) and early dialysis—has been clearly shown to positively affect patient survival (Molina, 1995).

Replacement of renal function during ARF can be carried out as standard hemodialysis, peritoneal dialysis, or continuous arteriovenous hemofiltration (CAVH) or continuous venovenous hemofiltration (CVVH), which use a small ultrafiltration membrane powered by the patient's own blood to produce an ultrafiltrate that can be replaced by parenteral nutrition fluids. This allows parenteral feeding without fluid overload.

Protein

At the onset of ARF, when few patients can tolerate oral feedings because of vomiting and diarrhea, intravenous (IV) preparations can be used to reduce protein catabolism. Some patients can be managed with enteral feedings, depending on the degree of severity of symptoms, but in most ARF patients, IV feeding must be used. Giving carbohydrate alone (e.g., 100 g over a 24-hour period) only reduces protein breakdown by 50%. The preferred treatment is parenteral administration of glucose, lipids, and a mixture of essential and nonessential amino acids. This reduces the protein catabolism and urea production to a minimum until the patient can tolerate oral feeding.

Considerations regarding the amount of protein that should be given to the patient with ARF must

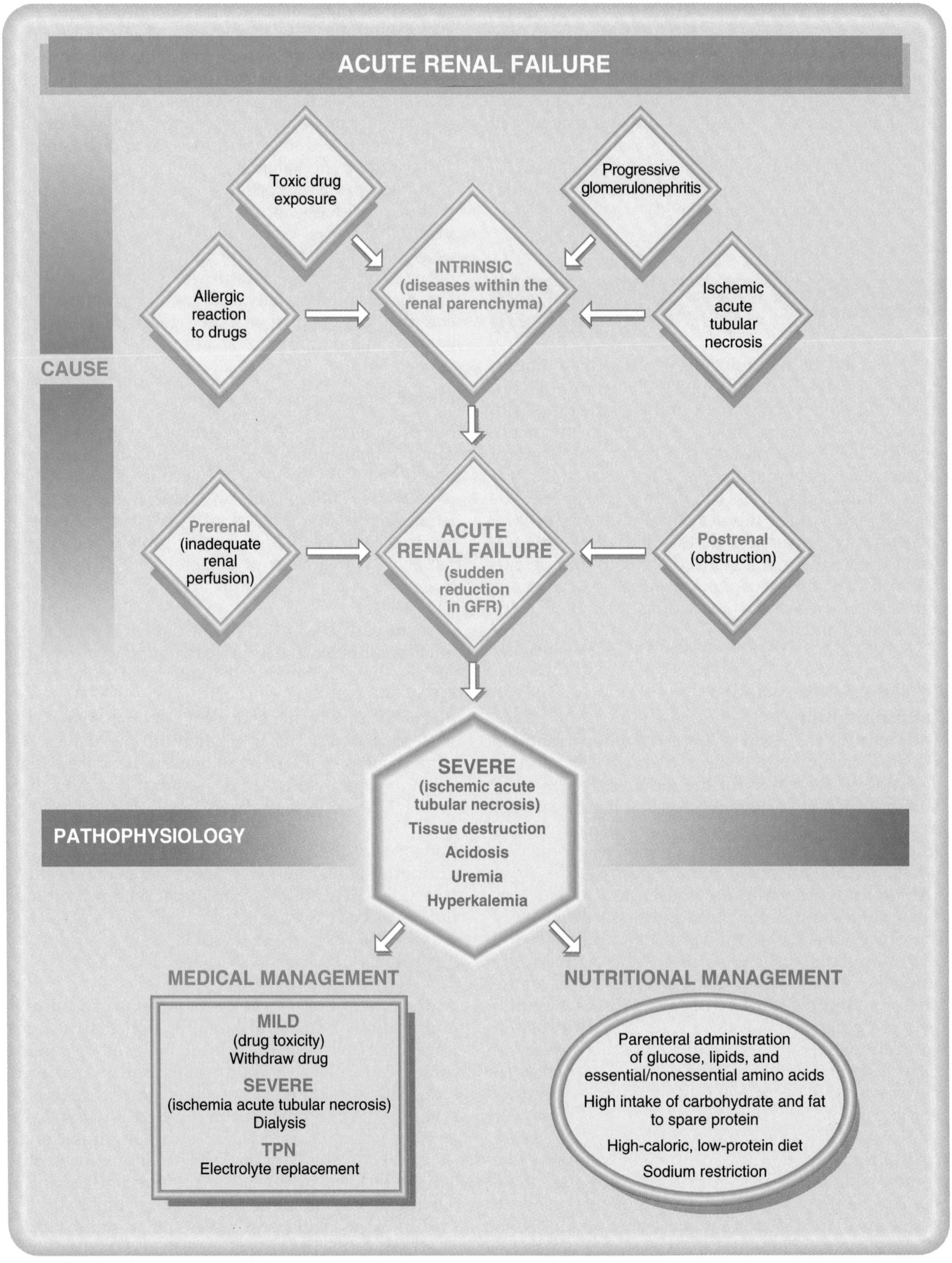

FIGURE 39-2 • Pathophysiology algorithm: acute renal failure. *TPN,* Total parenteral nutrition. (Algorithm content developed by John Anderson, PhD, and Sanford C. Garner, PhD, 2000.)

Box 39-1. Some Causes of Acute Renal Failure

Prerenal

Severe dehydration
Circulatory collapse

Intrinsic

Acute tubular necrosis
- Trauma, surgery
- Septicemia

Nephrotoxicity
- Antibiotics, contrast agents, and other drugs

Vascular disorders
- Bilateral renal infarction

Acute glomerulonephritis of any cause
- Poststreptococcal infection
- Systemic lupus erythematosus

Postrenal Obstruction

Benign prostatic hypertrophy with urinary retention
Carcinoma of the bladder or prostate
Retroperitoneal or pelvic cancer
Bilateral ureteral stones and obstruction

TABLE 39-1 Sample Calculation of Fluid Requirements in Acute Renal Failure

Losses	
Measured urine output of previous 24 hr	−200 ml
Insensible water loss in 24 hr (varies with room temperature, room humidity, and body temperature)	−500 ml
Total water loss in 24 hr	−700 ml
Input	
Water produced by metabolism in 24 hr (provided catabolism and weight loss are not occurring)	500 ml
Water to allow for fluid gain	1000 ml
Water in usual diet in 24 hr	500 ml
Additional fluid intake needed in 24 hr to replace losses in urine	200 ml
Total fluid gain in 24 hr	1700 ml
Total fluid gain minus total fluid loss = fluid gain for 24 hr	1700 ml − 700 ml = 1000 ml
24-hr fluid gain times 2 days between dialyses	1000 × 2 = 2 L fluid gain between dialysis treatments

balance the extraordinary catabolic needs of a patient in intensive care with the inability to excrete the fluid, electrolytes, and solute that this treatment requires. These patients often can receive continuous renal replacement therapies, such as CAVH or CVVH, which are ongoing treatments, rather than periodic dialysis.

A large protein load may otherwise necessitate more frequent dialysis, often in a patient who is not hemodynamically stable, and the patient is at high risk for dialysis complications. This issue is therefore quite controversial. The amount of protein recommended is influenced by the underlying cause of ARF and the presence of other conditions. A range of recommended levels can be found in the literature, from 0.5 to 0.8 g/kg for nondialysis patients, to 1.0 to 2.0 g/kg for dialyzed patients. As the patient's overall medical status stabilizes and improves, metabolic requirements decrease, and dialysis becomes less hazardous. During this stable period before renal function returns, it is generally agreed that a minimum protein intake of 0.8 to 1.0 g/kg of body weight should be given.

Energy

Energy requirements are determined by the underlying cause of ARF and comorbidity. Energy needs can be measured at the bedside by indirect calorimetry in most intensive care settings. If this equipment is not available, calorie needs should be estimated at 30 to 40 kcal/kg dry weight/day. Excessive calorie intake can lead to excess CO_2 production. If peritoneal dialysis or *continuous renal replacement therapy (CRRT)* is used, the amount of glucose absorbed can add significantly to the daily energy intake and should be calculated. Large intakes of carbohydrate and fat will prevent the use of protein for energy production. For patients who receive TPN, high concentrations of both carbohydrate and lipid can be administered to fulfill these needs as long as respiratory status is monitored.

A high-calorie, low-protein diet may be used in cases in which dialysis or hemofiltration is unavailable. In addition to the usual dietary sources of refined sweets and fats, special high-calorie, low-protein, and low-electrolyte formulas have been developed to augment the diet (see Appendix 38). Care must be taken with these products, however, because hyperglycemia is not uncommon as a result of glucose intolerance. Insulin is often needed.

Fluid and Sodium

During the early (often oliguric) phase of ARF, meticulous attention to fluid status is essential. Ideally, fluid and electrolyte intake should balance the net output. With negligible urine output, significant contributions to total body water output include emesis and diarrhea, body cavity drains, and skin and respiratory losses. If fever is present, skin losses can be excessive; whereas if the patient is on humidified air, almost no respiratory losses occur. Table 39-1 provides an example of fluid requirements calculation. Because of the numerous IV drugs as well as blood and blood products necessitated by the underlying disease, the challenge in managing patients at this point becomes how to cut fluid intake as much as possible while providing adequate protein and energy.

Sodium is restricted, depending on the level of urinary excretion. In the oliguric phase when the sodium output is very low, an attempt is made to keep intake low as well, perhaps as low as 20 to 40 mEq/day. However, limiting sodium is often impossible because of the requirement for many IV solutions (including IV antibiotics, medications for blood pressure, and TPN). The administration of these solutions in electrolyte-free water, in the face of oliguria, quickly leads to water intoxication (hyponatremia). For this reason, all fluid above the daily calculated water loss should be presented in a balanced salt solution.

Potassium

Most of the excretion of potassium and the control of potassium balance are normal functions of the kidney. When renal function is impaired, potassium balance should be scrutinized carefully. In addition to dietary sources, all body tissues contain large amounts of potassium; thus tissue destruction can lead to tremendous overload. Potassium levels can shift abruptly and need to be monitored frequently. Potassium intake needs to be individualized according to serum levels.

The primary mechanism of potassium removal during ARF is dialysis. Control of serum potassium levels between dialysis administrations relies mainly on IV infusions of glucose, insulin, and bicarbonate, all of which serve to drive potassium into cells.

Exchange resins such as Kayexalate, which exchange K^+ for Na^+ in the gastrointestinal tract, can be used to treat high K^+ concentrations, but for many reasons these resins are less than ideal. The treatment is unpleasant, regardless of whether it is given orally or by retention enema. In addition, because it can gel in the gastrointestinal tract, thus causing obstruction, it must be given with sorbitol, a nonabsorbable sugar that induces diarrhea. Administration requires a functioning gastrointestinal tract with respect to both absorption and motility, which the critically ill patient often does not have. Finally, the exchanged sodium leads to volume overload, which must also be controlled mainly by dialysis during renal failure. Table 39-2 summarizes medical nutrition therapy for ARF.

Other Tubular or Interstitial Diseases

A wide variety of diseases or disorders of the tubules and interstitium exists. They share common manifestations and can be considered together with respect to dietary management.

Chronic interstitial nephritis can occur as a result of analgesic abuse, sickle cell disease, diabetes mellitus, or vesicoureteral reflux and manifests primarily as an inability to concentrate the urine and as mild renal insufficiency. A hereditary disorder of the interstitium, medullary cystic disease, also presents this picture. Dietary management consists of adequate fluid intake, which can require several liters of extra fluid. This is generally quite well tolerated by the patient, except when intercurrent illness occurs.

Fanconi's syndrome is characterized by an inability to reabsorb the proper amount of glucose, amino acids, phosphate, and bicarbonate in the proximal tubule, thus causing excretion of these substances in the urine. Adults with this syndrome present with acidosis, hypokalemia, polyuria, or osteomalacia, whereas children present with polyuria, growth retardation, rickets, or vomiting. No specific medical treatment is usually available; therefore dietary treatment is the main form of management. Replacement therapy usually consists of large volumes of water as well as dietary supplements of bicarbonate, potassium, phosphate, calcium, and vitamin D.

Other tubular defects, generally affecting reabsorption of only a single solute, are treated with replacement of that particular solute. Renal tubular acidosis (RTA), a defect in tubular handling of bicarbonate, can be caused by either a proximal tubular defect (type 2) or a defect in the distal tubule (type 1). The proximal lesion can be associated with other proximal defects, such as in Fanconi's syndrome, and has very little clinical significance by itself, whereas distal RTA leads to severe osteomalacia, kidney stones, and often nephrocalcinosis (calcification of the kidney). Distal RTA is treated with small amounts of bicarbonate, 70 to 100 mEq/day, with complete resolution of disease manifestations. Isolated proximal RTA in the adult is a benign disease,

TABLE 39-2 Summary of Medical Nutrition Therapy for Acute Renal Failure

NUTRIENT	AMOUNT
Protein	0.8-1.0 g/kg IBW increasing as GFR returns to normal; 60% should be HBV protein
Energy	30-40 kcal/kg body weight
Potassium	30-50 mEq/day in oliguric phase (depending on urinary output, dialysis, and serum K^+ level); replace losses in diuretic phase
Sodium	20-40 mEq/day in oliguric phase (depending on urinary output, edema, dialysis, and serum Na^+ level); replace losses in diuretic phase
Fluid	Replace output from the previous day (vomitus, diarrhea, urine) plus 500 ml
Phosphorus	Limit as needed

GFR, Glomerular filtration rate; *HBV,* high biologic value; *IBW,* ideal body weight.

which is often made worse with bicarbonate treatment and should therefore not be treated.

Pyelonephritis

Pyelonephritis, a bacterial infection of the kidney, does not require extensive dietary management. In chronic cases, however, the use of cranberry juice to reduce bacteriuria has been verified in a double-blind study (Avorn et al, 1994). Concentrated tannins or proanthocyanidins in cranberry juice and apparently blueberry juice seem to inhibit the adherence of *Escherichia coli* bacteria to the epithelial cells of the urinary tract (Howell et al, 1998). The factor does not appear to be hippuric acid acting to make the urine more acidic.

PROGRESSIVE NATURE OF RENAL DISEASE

A wide range of kidney lesions are characterized by a slow, steady decline in renal function. A number of the diseases discussed earlier lead to renal failure in some patients, whereas other patients have a benign course without loss of renal function. The factors involved in producing a benign disease in one patient and renal failure in another patient are not clear. What makes one patient remain with pre–end-stage renal disease for several months to years while others progress rapidly to end-stage renal disease and renal failure and dialysis is unclear. However, it has been recognized in all kidney diseases that once approximately half to two thirds of kidney function has been lost, regardless of the underlying disease, progressive further loss of kidney function ensues. This is true even in diseases in which the underlying cause has been eliminated completely, such as in vesicoureteral reflux, cortical necrosis of pregnancy, or analgesic abuse. The nature of this progressive loss of function has been the subject of an enormous amount of basic and clinical research during the past several decades and the subject of several excellent reviews (Hricik et al, 1998; Pennell, 2001; Remuzzi and Bertani, 1998).

Pathophysiology

It is currently believed that in response to a decreasing GFR, the kidney undergoes a series of adaptations to prevent this decrease. Although in the short term this leads to improvement in filtration rate, in the long term it leads to an accelerated loss of nephrons and progressive renal insufficiency (Table 39-3). The nature of these adaptations involves a change in the hemodynamic characteristics of the remaining glomeruli, specifically leading to increased glomerular pressure. Factors that increase glomerular pressure tend to accelerate this process, whereas factors that decrease glomerular pressure tend to alleviate it.

Medical Nutrition Therapy

The role of dietary protein has been championed as a factor that increases glomerular pressure and thus leads to accelerated loss of renal function (Brenner and Lazarus, 1988). Numerous studies in experimental models of moderate renal insufficiency demonstrate a significant decline in this process with protein restriction. Clinical studies appear to corroborate the experimental models and demonstrate a role for protein restriction in the management of patients with mild to moderate renal insufficiency, for the purpose of preserving renal function (Giordano, 1981; Remuzzi and Bertani, 1998). Although these clinical studies are small, often retrospective, and uncontrolled, the bulk of scientific evidence favors such a role.

A large multicenter trial, Modification of Diet in Renal Disease (MDRD), attempted to determine the role of protein, phosphorus restriction, and blood pressure control in the progression of renal disease. In patients with early renal insufficiency, the projected mean decline in the glomerular filtration rate at 3 years did not differ significantly between the diet groups. In patients with more progressed renal deterioration, those on a very-low-protein diet using ketoanalogs had a somewhat lower rate of decline than those on a low-protein diet only. "In both groups there was no delay in the time to the occurrence of ESRD or death" (Klahr, 1994). Since then, post hoc analysis has indicated that low-protein diets probably do delay the progression of renal failure (Pedrini, 1996).

As a result of this and other related studies, the National Institute of Diabetes and Digestive and Kidney Diseases (NIDDKD) of the National Institutes of Health convened a conference to develop recommendations for the management of patients with progressive renal disease or pre–end-stage renal disease. Recommendations for dietary protein intake in progressive renal failure are 0.8 g/kg/day 60% HBV for patients whose GFR is greater than 55 ml/min, and 0.6 g/kg/day 60% HBV for patients whose GFR is 25 to 55 ml/min (Beto, 1994). More recently, the National Kidney Foundation, Kidney Dialysis Outcome Quality Initiative (KDOQI) panel suggested that patients whose GFR is less than 25 ml/min and who have not yet begun dialysis should be maintained on 0.60 g/

TABLE 39-3 Stages of Chronic Kidney Disease

STAGE	CREATININE	THERAPY
1. Early	<1.5 Female <2.0 Male	Reverse progression
2. Latent	1.5-2.5	Stop progression
3. Emergent	2.5-3.5	Slow progression
4. Imminent	3.5-5.0	Prepare for ESRD
5. ESRD	>5.0	Dialysis/transplant

Modified from National Kidney Foundation: Chronic kidney disease, *Am J Kidney Dis* 39:2(suppl 1), S17-S31, 2002.

kg/day of protein and 35 kcal/kg/day. If patients cannot maintain an adequate caloric intake on this protein recommendation, then their protein intake should be increased to 0.75 g/kg/day. In both cases, about 50% of the protein should be of high biologic value (National Kidney Foundation [NKF], 2000).

Most studies point out that systemic hypertension, another factor that mitigates the progressive loss of renal function, must be well controlled to produce benefits from protein restriction. Also important in the control of the progression of renal failure in people with diabetes is good blood glucose control. In a national multicenter trial, the Diabetes Control and Complications Trial (DCCT) showed that blood glucose control was more important than protein restriction in delaying the onset of renal failure in diabetics (see Chapter 33).

The potential benefits of protein restriction in the patient with moderate renal insufficiency must be weighed against the potential hazards of such treatment—namely, protein malnutrition. Much controversy remains. If protein is restricted, careful monitoring and anthropomorphic studies should be carried out periodically The KDOQI guidelines list these specifically (NKF, 2000; Wiggins, 2002) (see Chapters 17 and 18).

END-STAGE RENAL DISEASE

Pathophysiology

End-stage renal disease (ESRD) can result from a wide variety of different kidney diseases. Currently, 90% of patients reaching ESRD have chronic (1) diabetes mellitus; (2) glomerulonephritis; or (3) hypertension. With ESRD comes a myriad of problems related to the kidney's inability to excrete waste products, maintain fluid and electrolyte balance, and produce hormones. As renal failure slowly progresses, the level of circulating waste products eventually leads to symptoms of uremia (Figure 39-3).

Uremia is defined as the clinical syndrome of malaise, weakness, nausea and vomiting, muscle cramps and itching, metallic taste in the mouth, and—often—neurologic impairment that is brought about by an unacceptable level of nitrogenous wastes in the body. The manifestations are somewhat nonspecific and vary by patient. No reliable laboratory parameter corresponds directly with the beginning of symptoms. However, as a rule of thumb, a blood urea nitrogen (BUN) above 100 mg/dl and a creatinine of 10 to 12 mg/dl are usually quite close to this threshold.

Medical Treatment

Treatment of ESRD requires either transplantation or dialysis. If transplantation is anticipated, it is important to maintain optimal nutritional status so that the patient will be a good candidate for the transplant.

Transplantation

Transplantation involves the surgical implantation of a kidney from a living related donor, a living nonrelated donor, or a cadaver (Figure 39-4). Rejection of the foreign tissue is a major complication. Currently, patients awaiting transplantation far outnumber the donated kidneys available. Registration as an organ donor may be done easily at a local driver's licensing bureau.

Medical Nutrition Therapy

The nutritional care of the adult patient who has received a transplanted kidney is based mainly on the metabolic effects of the required immunosuppressive therapy. Medications typically used for the long term include glucocorticol steroids, cyclosporine, azathioprine, and mycophenolate mofetil. FK506 and OKT3, Thymoglobulin, and Atagam are all used short-term (initially or with acute rejection).

Corticosteroids are associated with accelerated protein catabolism, hyperlipidemia, sodium retention, weight gain, glucose intolerance, and inhibition of normal calcium, phosphorus, and vitamin D metabolism. Cyclosporine therapy is associated with hyperkalemia, hypertension, and hyperlipidemia (see Chapter 19). The doses of these medications used after transplantation are decreased over time until a "maintenance level" is reached.

During the first month after transplantation, a high-protein diet (1.3 to 1.5 g/kg body weight) with an energy intake of 30 to 35 kcal/kg is recommended to prevent negative nitrogen balance (Wiggins, 2002). Higher amounts of protein, 1.6 to 2.0 g/kg, are required in cases of increased needs, such as fever, infection, and increased surgical or traumatic stresses. A moderate sodium restriction (80 to 100 mEq/day) during this period minimizes fluid retention and helps to control blood pressure. After this time, protein intake can be decreased to 1 g/kg, and calorie intake should be at a level sufficient to achieve and maintain an appropriate weight for height. Sodium intakes are individualized, based on fluid retention and blood pressure.

Hyperkalemia, commonly associated with cyclosporine therapy, warrants dietary potassium restriction, although this is usually only temporary. Following transplantation, many patients exhibit hypophosphatemia and mild hypercalcemia caused by bone resorption associated with persistent hyperparathyroidism and the effects of steroids on calcium, phosphorus, and vitamin D metabolism. The diet should contain adequate amounts of calcium and phosphorus (1200 mg of each daily), and serum levels should be monitored periodically. Supplemental phosphorus may be necessary to correct hypophosphatemia.

The majority of transplant recipients have elevated serum triglycerides or cholesterol, or both. The etiology of this hyperlipidemia is multifactorial. In-

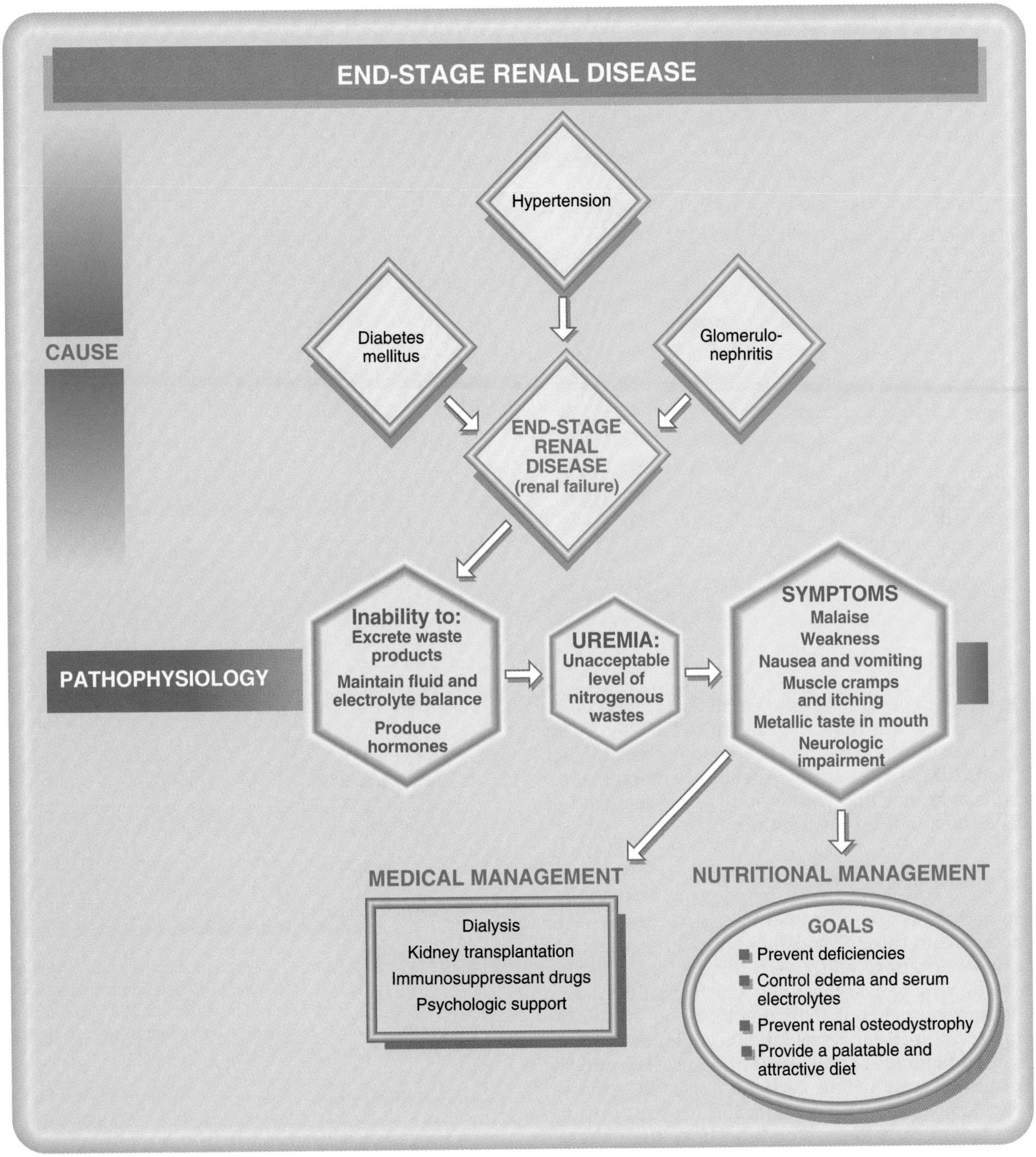

FIGURE 39-3 • Pathophysiology algorithm: end-stage renal disease. (Algorithm content developed by John Anderson, PhD, and Sanford C. Garner, PhD, 2000. Updated by Katy G. Wilkens, MS, RD, 2002.)

tervention consists of calorie restriction for those who are overweight, cholesterol intake limited to less than 300 mg/day, and limited total fat (see Chapter 35). In patients with glucose intolerance, limiting carbohydrates and maintaining a regular moderate exercise regimen are appropriate (Perez, 1993).

In one study of patients who were receiving cyclosporine during their first year posttransplant, the use of 6 g of fish oil, providing omega-3 fatty acids, had a beneficial effect on renal hemodynamics and blood pressure. The 1-year graft survival was also better for those taking the fish oils. The authors speculate that the effect of fish oils on eicosanoid production is probably important and may enhance the immunosuppressive effects of cyclosporine (van der Heide et al, 1993).

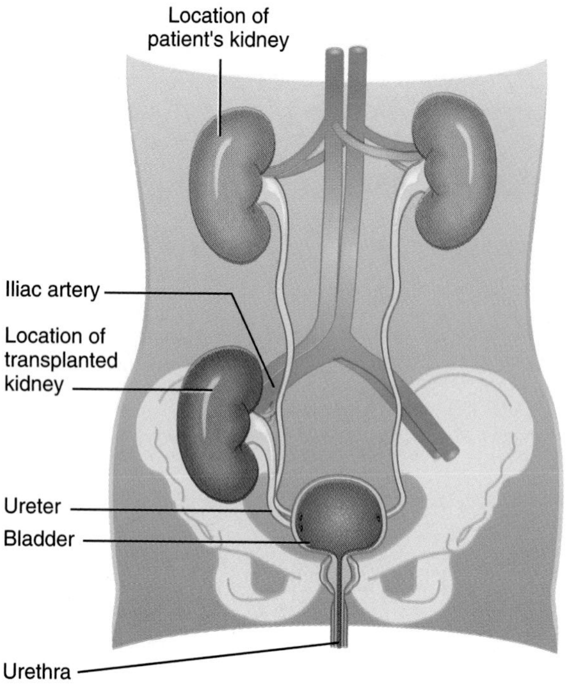

FIGURE 39-4 • Location of a transplanted kidney.

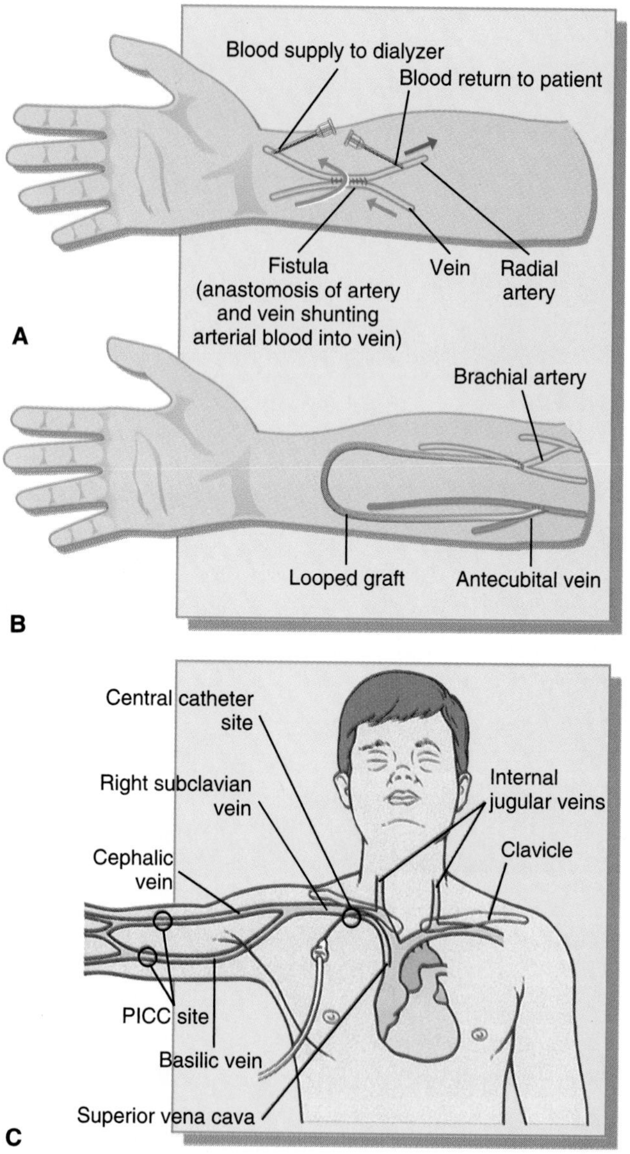

FIGURE 39-5 • Types of access for hemodialysis. **A,** Arteriovenous fistula. **B,** Artificial loop graft. **C,** Subclavian catheter (usually temporary). (**C,** From Lewis SM, Heitkemper MM, Dirksen SR: *Medical-surgical nursing: assessment and management of clinical problems,* ed 5, St. Louis, 2000, Mosby.)

Dialysis

Dialysis can be accomplished either by hemodialysis or by peritoneal dialysis (Pastan and Bailey, 1998). The most common method is hemodialysis, in which blood passes by the semipermeable membrane of the artificial kidney and waste products are removed by diffusion and fluids by ultrafiltration.

Hemodialysis

Hemodialysis requires permanent access to the bloodstream through a fistula created by surgery to connect an artery and a vein (Figure 39-5). Fistulas are often made near the wrist, which greatly enlarges the forearm veins. If the patient's blood vessels are fragile, an artificial vessel called a *graft* may be surgically implanted. Large needles are inserted into the fistula or graft before each dialysis and removed when dialysis is complete. Temporary access through subclavian catheters is common until the patient's permanent access can be created or can mature; however, infection problems make these catheters much less desirable.

The dialysis fluid electrolyte content is similar to that of normal plasma. Waste products and electrolytes move by diffusion, ultrafiltration, and osmosis from the blood into the dialysate and are removed (Figure 39-6). Hemodialysis usually requires treatment of 3 to 5 hours three times per week (Figure 39-7). Dietary protein needs are about 1.2 g/kg, about 50% high biologic value protein, to make up for some losses through the dialysate (Table 39-4).

Peritoneal Dialysis

Peritoneal dialysis makes use of the semipermeable membrane of the peritoneum. A catheter is surgically implanted in the abdomen and into the peritoneal cavity (Figure 39-8). Dialysate containing a high-dextrose concentration is instilled into the peritoneum, where diffusion carries waste products from the blood through the peritoneal membrane and into the dialysate; water moves by osmosis. This fluid is then withdrawn and discarded, and new solution is added. Several types of peritoneal dialysis exist.

Standard peritoneal dialysis is a less efficient method of removing waste products from the blood. Treatments usually last longer than hemodialysis,

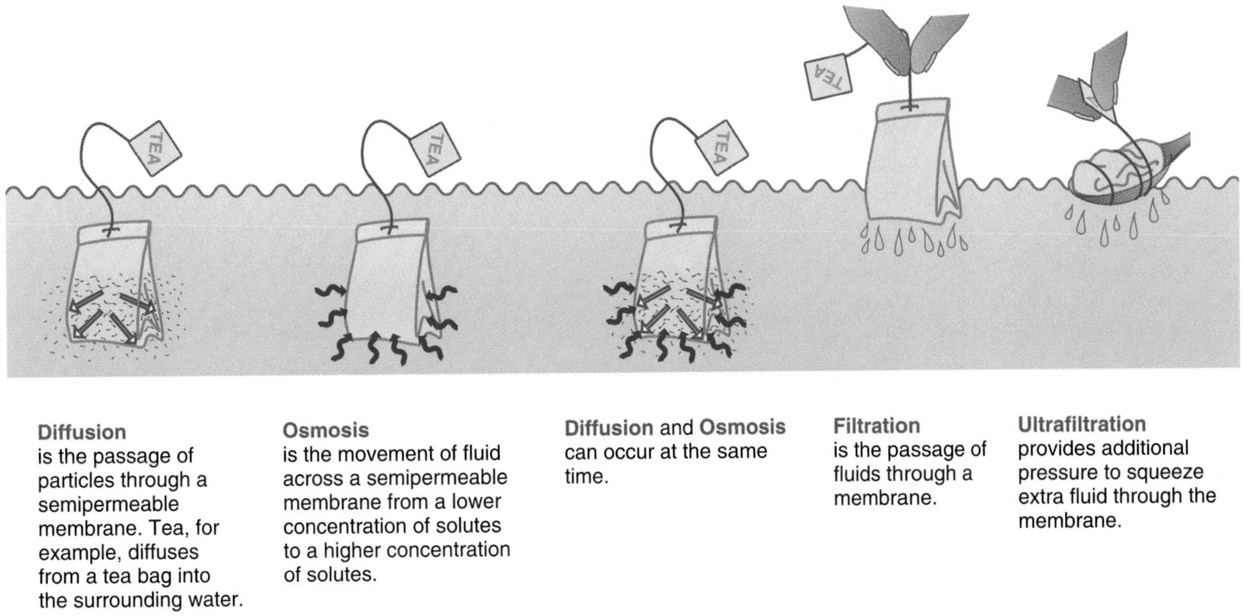
TEA
TEA
TEA
TEA
TEA
Diffusion
is the passage of particles through a semipermeable membrane. Tea, for example, diffuses from a tea bag into the surrounding water.
Osmosis
is the movement of fluid across a semipermeable membrane from a lower concentration of solutes to a higher concentration of solutes.
Diffusion and **Osmosis**
can occur at the same time.
Filtration
is the passage of fluids through a membrane.
Ultrafiltration
provides additional pressure to squeeze extra fluid through the membrane.

FIGURE 39-6 • Dialysis: how it works. (Modified from *Core curriculum for the dialysis technician: a comprehensive review of hemodialysis,* AMGEN, Inc.)

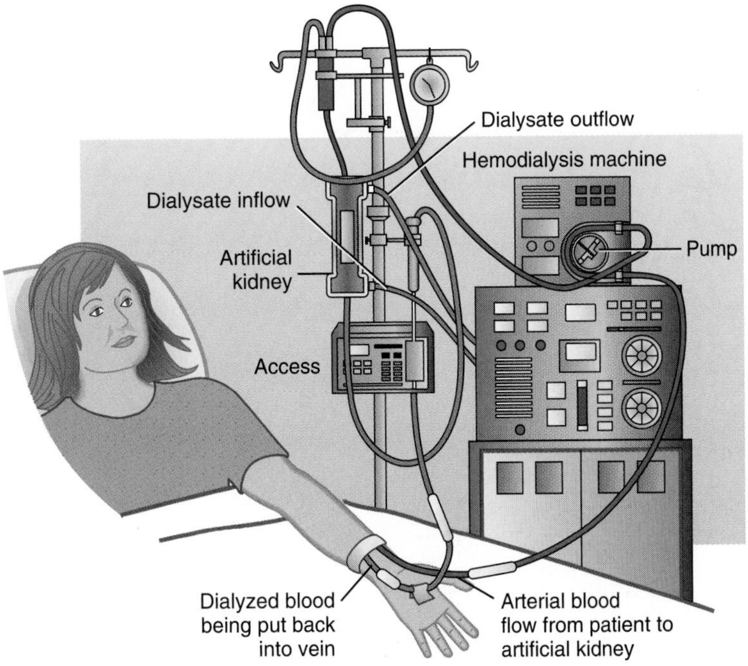
Dialysate outflow
Hemodialysis machine
Dialysate inflow
Artificial kidney
Pump
Access
Dialyzed blood being put back into vein
Arterial blood flow from patient to artificial kidney

FIGURE 39-7 • Hemodialysis. Treatment is usually for 3 to 5 hours, three times per week.

about 10 to 12 hours/day, three times per week. This type of treatment is rarely done anymore. Patients with peritoneal dialysis have higher protein needs (about 1.2 to 1.5 g protein/kg) because of greater protein losses.

Continuous ambulatory peritoneal dialysis (CAPD) is similar to standard peritoneal dialysis, except that the dialysate is left in the peritoneum and exchanged manually so that no machine is required. Exchanges of dialysis fluid are done four to five times daily, making it a 24-hour treatment. Protein losses are somewhat higher than those from regular peritoneal dialysis. Advantages of this form of treatment are avoidance of large fluctuations in blood chemistry and the ability of the patient to achieve a more normal lifestyle.

TABLE 39-4 Nutrient Requirements for Adults With Renal Disease Based on Type of Therapy

THERAPY	ENERGY	PROTEIN	FLUID	SODIUM	POTASSIUM	PHOSPHORUS
Impaired renal function	30-35 kcal/kg IBW	0.6-1.0 g/kg IBW	*Ad libitum*	Variable, 2-3 g/day	Variable, usually ad libitum or increased to cover losses with diuretics	0.8-1.2 g/day or 8-12 mg/kg IBW
Hemodialysis	35 kcal/kg IBW	1.2 g/kg IBW	750-1000 ml/day + urine output	2-3 g/day	2-3 g/day or 40 mg/kg IBW	0.8-1.2 g/day or <17 mg/kg IBW
Peritoneal dialysis (CAPD) (CCPD)	30-35 kcal/kg IBW	1.2-1.3 g/kg BW	*Ad libitum* (minimum of 2000 ml/day + urine output)	2-4 g/day	3-4 g/day	0.8-1.2 g/day
Transplant, 4-6 weeks after transplant	30-35 kcal/kg IBW	1.5-2 g/kg BW	*Ad libitum*	Variable	Variable; may require restriction with cyclosporine-induced hyperkalemia	1.2 g/day Calcium 1.2 g/day
6 weeks or longer after transplant	To achieve/maintain IBW: • Limit simple carbohydrate • Fat <35% of calories • No more than 400 mg/day cholesterol • PUF/SF ratio > 1.0	1 g/kg BW	*Ad libitum*	Variable	Variable	Calcium 1.2 g/day

Modified from National Kidney Foundation: DOQI clinical practice guidelines for nutrition in chronic renal failure, *Am J Kidney Dis* 35(suppl 2), 2000; Wiggins K: *Guidelines for nutrition care of renal patients,* ed 3, Chicago, 2002, American Dietetic Association.

IBW, Ideal body weight; *CAPD,* continuous ambulatory peritoneal dialysis; *CCPD,* continuous cyclical peritoneal dialysis; *PUF,* polyunsaturated fat; *SF,* saturated fat.

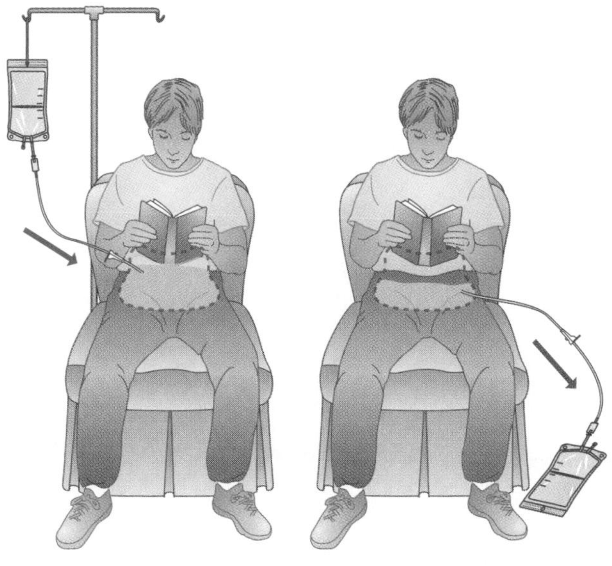

The peritoneal cavity is filled with dialysate, using gravity.

At the end of the exchange, the dialysate is drained into the bag, again using gravity.

FIGURE 39-8 • Continuous ambulatory peritoneal dialysis; 20-minute exchanges are given four to five times daily, every day.

Patients with CAPD have more liberal fluid, sodium, and potassium allowances because the therapy is continuous and more of these products are removed. The loss of sodium can be as much as 6 g/day; thus these patients may need higher sodium intakes, as shown in Table 39-4. Complications associated with CAPD include peritonitis, hypotension that requires additional fluid and sodium replacement, and weight gain. The weight gain is experienced by most patients with CAPD as a result of absorbing 600 to 800 calories/day from the glucose in the dialysate. This may be desirable in patients who are underweight, but eventually dietary intake will have to be modified to account for the energy absorbed from dialysate. Another type of peritoneal dialysis is *continuous cyclical peritoneal dialysis (CCPD)*. In this therapy, which is somewhat the opposite of CAPD, patients' treatments are done at night by a machine that does the exchanges. During the day these patients may keep a single dialysate exchange in the peritoneal cavity for extended periods of time (long dwell), perhaps the entire day. Several combinations of CAPD and CCPD are possible.

Psychological Support

Patients with renal failure must deal not only with conflicting feelings about depending on artificial means of elimination but also with changes in the quality of their lives and the necessity for adapting to a chronic, progressive illness. Control becomes a central issue because they must devote large quantities of time to dialysis, follow fairly strict dietary regimens, and often take several medications. Those who work with renal dialysis patients must be especially empathic to their feelings of thirst, anorexia when faced with eating, and taste changes due to uremia.

Medical Nutrition Therapy

Goals of medical nutrition therapy in the management of ESRD are the following:

1. To prevent deficiency and maintain good nutritional status (and, in the case of children, growth) through adequate protein, energy, vitamin, and mineral intake
2. To control edema and electrolyte imbalance by controlling sodium, potassium, and fluid intake
3. To prevent or retard the development of renal osteodystrophy by controlling calcium, phosphorus, and vitamin D intake
4. To enable the patient to eat a palatable, attractive diet that fits his or her lifestyle as much as possible

Even with the development of dialysis methods and transplantation techniques, nutritional care remains essential to enhance dialysis, maintain optimal nutritional status, and prevent complications.

Because treatment is outpatient or dialysis is done at home, patients with ESRD assume responsibility for their diets. Most long-term patients know their diets very well (Figure 39-9), having been instructed many times by dietitians at their dialysis units. Patients who are relatively new to dialysis may require much more intensive education. Regardless of length of time on dialysis, periodic professional counseling helps all patients who face long-term compliance with difficult diet regimens. Monitoring the patient's long-term nutritional status is an important role of the dietitian. Table 39-5 presents a guide for teaching patients about their blood values and control of their disease.

Fluid and Sodium Balance

The kidney's ability to handle sodium and water in ESRD must be assessed frequently through measurement of blood pressure, presence of edema, serum sodium level, and dietary intake. The diet and fluid intake are then modified accordingly.

Although most patients with ESRD retain sodium, others may lose it. Examples of conditions with a salt-losing tendency are polycystic disease of the kidney, medullary kidney disease, chronic obstructive uropathy, chronic pyelonephritis, and analgesic nephropathy. To prevent hypotension, hypovolemia, cramps, and further deterioration of renal function, extra sodium may be required in these patients. The diet usually contains 130 mEq (3 g) or more of sodium per day, which is the amount in a normal diet without added salt. Adding salt or salty foods can satisfy the need for extra sodium. The number of pa-

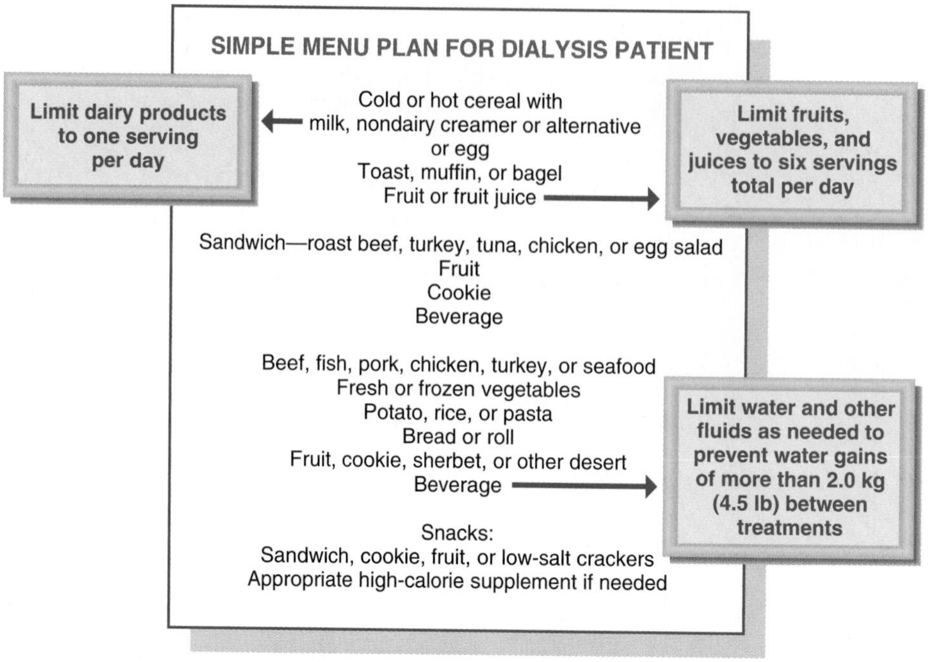

FIGURE 39-9 • A simple menu plan for a patient on dialysis. The diet should allow for no more than 5% weight gain between dialyses.

tients who require this higher sodium intake is few, but these patients exemplify the need for individual consideration of the diet prescription.

Dialysis patients with hypertension and edema may need to restrict intakes of sodium and fluids (see Chapter 36). Even those who do not experience these symptoms, but who put out minimal urine, will benefit from a reduced sodium intake to limit their thirst and prevent large intradialytic fluid gains. The recommended intake of sodium for the vast majority of patients is 2 to 3 g/day. Because solid foods in the average diet contribute approximately 500 to 800 ml of fluid, these foods will replace the 500 ml of net insensible water loss, as shown in Table 39-1. Additional fluid is given to replace urinary and vomitus losses.

Fluid and sodium requirements can increase in the presence of perspiration, vomiting, or fever. Hypotension and the possibility of clotting at the shunt site from overrestriction of fluid and sodium intake must be avoided, although this rarely occurs. Patients who have severe gastropathy or other fluid and electrolyte losses, such as illeostomy, are much more at risk for these problems.

In the patient who is maintained with dialysis, sodium intake and fluid intake are regulated to allow for a weight gain of 4 to 5 lb (2 to 3 kg) from increased fluid in the vasculature between dialyses (Oldenburg, 1988). Other studies support a fluid gain of 2% to 5% of body weight (Sherman et al, 1995). This means a sodium intake of 130 mEq (3 g) daily and a more liberal fluid intake, usually about 1000 ml/day plus the amount equal to the urine output. The dietitian and nursing staff must take care to avoid overrestriction of the patient's intake and resulting malnutrition while they meet the clinical needs for a stable fluid balance. In these situations, interaction between the dietitian and nursing staff is invaluable.

A 130-mEq sodium diet allows for light salting of foods during cooking but no additional salt at the table and no salted, smoked, or cured meat or fish; salted snack foods; canned soups; or high-sodium convenience foods. It is important to remember that the easiest way to reduce the patient's thirst and fluid intake is to decrease the sodium intake. Chapter 37 gives the details of a low-sodium meal plan.

When educating about fluid balance, the health care provider must teach the patient how to deal with thirst without drinking. Sucking on a few ice chips, cold sliced fruit, or sour candies; using artificial saliva; or chewing "sports gum" that contains citric acid may help to alleviate the dryness.

Patients must be taught to measure their fluid intake and urine output, examine their ankles for edema, weigh themselves regularly each morning, and record their weight. Occasionally (in about 15% to 20% of patients), hypertension is not alleviated even after meticulous attention to fluid and water balance. In these patients, hypertension is usually perpetuated by a high level of renin secretion and requires medication for control.

Potassium

Potassium (K^+) usually requires restriction, depending on the individual's body size, the serum K^+ level, urine output, and the frequency of dialysis. High intakes are not tolerated with less frequent dialysis. The daily intake of potassium for most Americans is

TABLE 39-5 Guide to Blood Values

This guide is to help in understanding laboratory reports. In the following table, the normal values are for people with good kidney function. Acceptable values for dialysis patients are given in the next column.

Many things affect blood values. Diet is only one of these. Underlying disease, adequacy of treatment, medications, and complications all may affect laboratory values.

SUBSTANCE	NORMAL VALUES	NORMAL FOR PEOPLE ON DIALYSIS	FUNCTION	DIET CHANGES
Sodium	135-145 mEq/L	Same	Found in salt and many preserved foods. A diet high in sodium will make the patient thirsty. When patients drink too much fluid, it may actuactually dilute their sodium; and serum levels will be low. If patients eat too much sodium and do not drink water, sodium may be high. Too much sodium and water raise blood pressure and can cause fluid overload, pulmonary edema, and CHF.	High: Check fluid status. If high fluid gains, tell patient to eat fewer salty foods (give sodium brochure). If low fluid gains, make sure they are gaining about 1.5 kg between runs (or <4% body weight) and are not dehydrated (this is rare). Low: If high fluid gains, tell patient to eat less salt and fluid. Check fluid status—patient is probably drinking too much fluid. Limit weight gains to under 4% of body weight between runs, and ask them to eat fewer salty foods (give sodium brochure) and to limit fluid to 3 c plus urine output (give fluid brochure).
Potassium	3.5-5.5 mEq/L	3.5-5.5 mEq/L	Found in most high-protein foods, fruits, and vegetables. It affects muscle action, especially the heart. High levels can cause the heart to stop. Low levels can cause symptoms such as muscle weakness and atrial fibrillation.	High: Ascertain that no other causes, such as GI bleeding, trauma, or medications, are are creating high potassium values. Tell patient to avoid foods with over 250 mg/serving and limit daily intake to 2000 mg. Consider lowering potassium in dialysate bath. Recheck blood level next treatment. Low: Add one high-potassium food/day, and recheck blood level (give potassium brochure). Consider raising potassium in dialysate bath if diet changes are not working.
Urea nitrogen (blood urea nitrogen [BUN])	7-23 mg/dl	50-100 mg/dl	Waste product of protein breakdown. Unlike creatinine, this is affected by the amount of protein in the diet. Dialysis removes urea nitrogen.	High: Patient is probably underdialyzed. Check eKT/V. Check nPNA. Low: Underdialysis is also a cause. BUN may decrease if patient is not eating because of uremic symptoms. May also decrease with loss of muscle.
Creatinine	0.6-1.5 mg/dl	Less than 15 mg/dl	A normal waste product of muscle breakdown. This value is controlled by dialysis. Patients have a higher amount because the patient is not dialyzing 24 hours a day, 7 days a week, like the normal kidney does.	Dialysis normally controls creatinine. Low creatinine may indicate good dialysis or low body muscle. Check the KT/V to assess dialysis adequacy. If the patient is losing weight, he or she breaks down more muscle, so creatinine may be higher. The patient may need to eat more protein and calories to stop weight loss.

Developed by Katy G. Wilkens, MS, RD, Northwest Kidney Centers, Seattle, Wash.
ALK phos, Alkaline phosphatase; *HCT,* hematocrit; *LDH,* lactic dehydrogenase; *SGOT,* serum glutamic oxaloacetic transaminase; *CHF,* congestive heart failure.

Continued

TABLE 39-5 Guide to Blood Values—cont'd

SUBSTANCE	NORMAL VALUES	NORMAL FOR PEOPLE ON DIALYSIS	FUNCTION	DIET CHANGES
URR (urea reduction ratio)	n/a	Above 65% (or 0.65)	A measure of reduction of urea that occurs during a dialysis treatment. Postdialysis BUN is subtracted from predialysis BUN.	No diet changes, but catabolism or anabolism will affect values, as with KT/V and eKT/V.
eKT/V (equilibrated clearance of urea during dialysis)	n/a	Above 1.2	A mathematic formula that attempts to quantify how well a patient is dialyzed. Represents the clearance of urea by the dialyzer, multiplied by the minutes of treatment, and divided by the volume of water the patient's body carries.	No diet changes. Low: Values below 1.2 are associated with increased morbidity and mortality. High: Higher values are associated with better outcomes.
KT/V (see p. 980)		Above 1.4-hemodialysis Above 2.0-peritoneal dialysis	Not adjusted for urea equilibration.	No diet changes.
nPNA (normalized protein nitrogen appearance)	n/a	Above 1.2	A calculation used to look at the rate of protein turnover in the body. Assumes the patient is not catabolic because of infection, fever, surgery, or trauma. Can be a good indicator of stable patient's protein intake, when combined with dietary history and albumin. The term *normalized* means that values have been adjusted to the patient's "normal" or ideal weight.	High: Patient may need to decrease protein intake. Have patient consult with nutritionist. Patient may be catabolic. Patient may be eating large amounts of protein. Low: Patient may need to increase protein intake. If patient is putting out urine, a small urine volume can make a big difference in PCR results. Have patient keep a 48-hour urine collection (give patient protein brochure).
Albumin	3.5-5.0 g/dl (bromcresol green) 3.0-4.5 g/dl (bromcresol purple)	Same Above 3.4 g/dl	Albumin is a protein made in the liver. It is a good measure of health. Protein is lost with all dialysis. If albumin is below 2.9, fluid will "leak" from blood vessels into the tissue, thus causing edema. When fluid is in the tissue, it is more difficult to remove with dialysis. Low albumin is closely associated with increased risk of death in dialysis patients.	Low: Increase intake of protein-rich foods: meat, fish, chicken, eggs (give patient protein brochure). A protein supplement may be needed. IV albumin will correct short-term problems with oncotic pressure but will not change serum albumin levels.
Calcium	8.5-10.5 mg/dl	8.5-10.5 mg/dl	Found in dairy products and in some green vegetables. Dialysis patients' intakes are usually low. The body uses it to help muscle movement and build bones. Active vitamin D is needed for absorption. The calcium value multiplied by the phosphorus value should not exceed 60, or patient will get calcium deposits in soft tissue. Because it is bound to albumin, calcium can be falsely lower if albumin is low. Ionized calcium is a more accurate test in this case.	High: Check with doctor if patient is taking calcium supplement or active vitamin D (DHT, Rocaltrol, Hectorol, Calcijex, Zemplar). These should be temporarily stopped. Low: If albumin is low, suggest an ionized calcium be drawn. Patient may need a calcium supplement between meals and/or active vitamin D. Check with physician.

Developed by Katy G. Wilkens, MS, RD, Northwest Kidney Centers, Seattle, Wash.

TABLE 39-5 Guide to Blood Values—cont'd

SUBSTANCE	NORMAL VALUES	NORMAL FOR PEOPLE ON DIALYSIS	FUNCTION	DIET CHANGES
Phosphorus	2.5-4.8 mg/dl	3.0-6.0 mg/dl	Found in milk products, dried beans, nuts, and meats. It is used to build bones and helps the body produce energy. Acceptable levels depend on a variety of factors, including calcium, parathyroid hormone levels, and the level of phosphorus in the diet. If calcium and parathyroid hormone levels are normal, a slightly higher than normal level of phosphorus is acceptable.	High: Limit milk and milk products to 1 serving per day. Remind patient to take phosphate binders as ordered with meals and snacks. Noncompliance with binders is the most common cause of high phosphorus. Low: Add 1 serving milk product or other high-phosphorus food per day, or decrease phosphate binders.
I—PTH (parathyroid hormone intact)	10-65 pg/ml	200-300 pg/ml	A high level of parathyroid hormone indicates calcium is being pulled out of bone to maintain serum calcium levels. This syndrome is called secondary hyperparathyroidism and can lead to osteodystrophy. Pulsed doses of oral or IV vitamin D will usually lower PTH.	High: Check whether patient is taking oral or IV active vitamin D. Contact patient's physician regarding therapy. If patient has no symptoms (high phosphorus, bone pain, fractures), treat less aggressively. Low: No treatment available.
Aluminum	0-10 mcg/L	Less than 40 μg/L	Patients taking aluminum hydroxide phosphate binders may develop aluminum toxicity, which can cause bone disease and dementia. Value should be checked every 6 months.	High: Discontinue aluminum hydroxide treatment. Some patients benefit from deferoxamine treatment, but this also has complications.
Magnesium	1.5-2.4 mg/dl	Same	Magnesium is normally excreted in the urine and can become toxic to dialysis patient. High levels may be caused by antacids or laxatives that contain magnesium like Milk of Magnesia, Maalox, etc.	No dietary changes, except to use nontoxic methods such as fiber to aid in constipation. Magnesium can also be used as a phosphate binder; if so, levels will need to be checked more often.
Ferritin	Male: 20-350 μg/L Female: 6-350 μg/L	>300 μg/L with erythropoietin (EPO); 50 μg/L without EPO	This is the way iron is stored in the liver. If iron stores are low, red blood cell production is decreased.	Low: Iron in food is not well absorbed. Most patients need an oral and/or IV iron supplement. Patients should not take iron at same time as phosphate binders.
CO_2 (carbon dioxide)		22-25 mEq/L	Dialysis patients are often acidotic because they do not excrete metabolic acids in their urine. Acidosis may increase the rate of muscle and bone catabolism.	Low: Review eKT/V, BUN, nPNA. Oral sodium bicarbonate may be given to raise CO_2, but it presents a significant sodium load to patient.
Glucose	65-114 mg/dl	Same for nondiabetic patients Less than 300 mg/dl (diabetic patients)	This sugar in the blood is made from starches and sugar in the diet. The body uses glucose for energy. Because the kidney metabolizes insulin, low blood sugar levels caused by a longer half-life of insulin are possible. For diabetic patients: A high blood sugar may increase thirst.	Most people need 6 to 11 servings of breads/starches or cereals per day and 2 to 4 servings of fruit per day to provide energy. Patients with diabetes should avoid concentrated sweets, unless blood sugar level is low.

75 to 100 mEq (3 to 4 g). This is usually reduced in ESRD to 60 to 80 mEq (2.3 to 3.1 g) per day and is reduced for the anuric patient on dialysis to 51 mEq (2 g) per day. Some patients—those on high-flux dialysis or with increased dialysis times or frequencies—may be able to tolerate higher intakes. Again, a close monitoring of the patient's laboratory values, K^+ content of the dialysate bath, and dietary intake is invaluable.

The potassium content of foods is listed in Box 6-1. When counseling patients on a low-potassium diet, one should take care to point out that many low-sodium foods contain KCl, as a salt substitute, rather than NaCl. Salt substitutes, "lite salt," and low-sodium herb mixtures must all be carefully checked to be sure they do not contain dangerous levels of potassium. Low-sodium soy sauces, sauerkraut, and other special dietary products may need particular review by a trained professional. Reviewing such practices not only with the patient but with other people who may be cooking for the patient—such as a church group or neighbors, who may use salt substitutes in the mistaken belief they are helping the patient avoid salt—is also advisable.

Protein

Dialysis is a drain on body protein, and the daily intake should be increased to compensate for this. Protein losses of 20 to 30 g can occur during a 24-hour peritoneal dialysis, with an average of 1 g/hr. Hourly losses in hemodialysis are similar. Patients who receive hemodialysis three times per week require a daily protein intake of 1.2 g/kg body weight. Patients receiving peritoneal dialysis need 1.2 to 1.3 g/kg body weight. At least 50% should be high biologic value protein. Studies of patients on dialysis indicate that those with low albumin levels have a much higher mortality rate; consequently, more emphasis is placed on adequate protein intake. (Jones, 2002). Protein requirements for patients on different types of dialysis are summarized in Table 39-4. Serum BUN and serum creatinine levels, uremic symptoms, and weight should be monitored, and the diet should be adjusted accordingly (see *Clinical Insight:* When Protein Supplements Are Not "Healthful").

Although serum albumin is a fair indicator of protein status, it may not correlate with other nutritional parameters, because acute or chronic inflammation limits its specificity. In addition, when interpreting albumin values, it is important to know the laboratory's methodology for measuring serum albumin. The bromocresol purple (BCP) test yields lower results than the bromocresol green (BCG) test (see Table 39-5) (Blagg et al, 1993).

Kinetic Modeling

A recent trend in evaluating the efficacy of dialysis relies on measuring the removal of urea from the patient's blood over a given period of time. This method, often called KT/V (where *K* is the urea clearance of the dialyzer, *T* is the length of time of dialysis, and *V* is the patient's total body water volume), should ideally produce a result higher than 1.2. The method for calculating the efficacy of peritoneal dialysis is somewhat different, but a weekly KT/V of 2.0 is the goal. The KT/V can be altered by several patient- and dialysis-associated variables. The calculations for KT/V can also be used to determine the patient's protein nitrogen appearance rate (PNA), which is a simplified nitrogen balance test in the dialysis patient. The PNA values should be above 1.2 g/kg.

A similar method, the urea reduction ratio (URR), looks at the reduction in urea before and after dialysis. The patient is well dialyzed when a 65% or greater reduction in the serum urea occurs. Patients who are poorly dialyzed tend to have lower albumin levels and a higher risk of death (Owen et al, 1993). Serum albumin must be closely monitored. A decreased serum albumin level predicts poor survival in end-stage renal failure. Hypoalbuminemia is multifactorial and related to poor nutrition, inflammation, and comorbid disease (Jones et al, 2002.)

CLINICAL INSIGHT

When Protein Supplements Are Not "Healthful"

The use of protein supplements, especially amino acid supplements, commonly called *aminos*, has become popular lately. They seem harmless, because they "are naturally" from protein—and for most people they probably are. But for those with pre–end-stage or end-stage renal failure, these supplements can be toxic. Because the kidney metabolizes and excretes amino acids, the amino acid profile in renal failure is quite different from that of people who produce good-quality urine. Supplements such as glucosamine, arginase and arginine, lysine, creatine, glutamine, and others may act as toxins in the bodies of patients who cannot metabolize and excrete them. No studies have evaluated these products in patients on dialysis, and use of them should also be discouraged in patients with pre–end-stage or chronic kidney disease because they could be harmful.

Most patients find it challenging to consume adequate protein and still have a palatable diet. In addition, the uremia itself causes some taste aberrations, notably to red meats, sometimes making it difficult to achieve the high (HBV)/low biologic value (LBV) protein ratio (Klahr, 1994).

Exchange lists are no longer used in educating the patient about a renal diet. Rather, a booklet, *The National Renal Diet* (Schiro-Harvey, 2002), available from the American Dietetic Association (see Relevant Web Sites), provides information about food sources of nutrients, adaptation of patients' usual intakes to meet requirements based on their laboratory values, and the decreasing of certain foods when values rise (Wiggins and Schiro-Harvey, 2002). Another resource for patient education is "The Art of Good Eating" (see Relevant Web Sites).

Energy

Energy intake must be adequate to spare protein for tissue protein synthesis and to prevent its metabolism for energy. Depending on the patient's nutritional status and degree of stress, between 25 and 40 kcal/kg body weight should be provided, with the lower amount for transplant and peritoneal dialysis patients. The higher level would be appropriate for the nutritionally depleted patient.

Calcium, Phosphorus, and Vitamin D

A major complication of ESRD is metabolic bone disease, or renal osteodystrophy. The disease is essentially of three types: *osteomalacia*, or bone demineralization; osteitis fibrosa cystica, caused by hyperparathyroidism; and metastatic calcification of joints and soft tissues.

As the GFR decreases, phosphorus, the level of which is controlled by renal excretion, is retained in the plasma. The serum calcium level declines for several reasons. Decreased 1,25-$(OH)_2D_3$, brought about by decreased ability of the kidney to convert the inactive form, appears to be most important. In addition, the calcium-phosphate product, which increases as phosphate increases, leads to extraosseus calcifications throughout the body and brings about a decreased calcium level. The low calcium level triggers several mechanisms by which the healthy body increases calcium to normal. These include the release of PTH from the parathyroid glands as well as increased synthesis of the active form of vitamin D by the kidney. This in turn acts on the gut to increase absorption of both calcium and phosphate and, in concert with PTH, acts to increase bone resorption, thus liberating both calcium and phosphate.

Parathormone also acts on the kidney to increase secretion of phosphate while retaining extra calcium. With decreased ability to produce 1,25-$(OH)_2D_3$, the patient with failing kidneys cannot increase gut absorption of calcium and must therefore rely on the effects of PTH to keep calcium levels up and phosphate down through bone resorption and to increase renal elimination of phosphate. The dependence of calcium-phosphate control on increasing levels of PTH thus leads to a characteristic hyperplastic demineralized bone disease, osteitis fibrosa cystica. The disease is characterized by dull aching bone pain.

Even though the serum calcium level is elevated in response to PTH, the serum phosphate concentration remains high as the GFR falls lower. If the product of the serum calcium level (mg/100 ml) multiplied by the serum phosphate level (mg/100 ml) is greater than 70, metastatic calcification is imminent. Clinical management aims to keep the product below 60 by preventing transient elevations in serum phosphate concentration.

In essence, calcium and phosphorus intake must be controlled to as great a degree as possible to avoid aggravation of the delicate situation posed by hyperparathyroidism, phosphate retention, and hypocalcemia in renal failure. *In practical terms, calcium intake is kept high, and phosphorus intake is kept low.* This is a problem as far as food is concerned because most of the high-calcium foods (milk and milk products) are also high in phosphorus. Consequently, patients must rely on methods in addition to dietary manipulation.

Calcium intake is increased with calcium supplements in the form of calcium carbonate (e.g., Tums), calcium acetate, (PhosLo) lactate, malate, or gluconate, along with the 300 to 500 mg calcium provided in the diet. These supplements are given between meals to increase calcium absorption. Starting calcium supplementation early is more likely to prevent hyperparathyroidism.

Calcium is present in the dialysate bath, and the amount can be somewhat adjusted to help stabilize low calcium values or to decrease serum calcium in patients who have developed hypercalcemia from active vitamin D administration. Patients who receive too large a calcium load may develop calciphylaxis, which occurs when calcium phosphate is deposited in soft tissues. The challenge becomes balancing the patient's need for phosphate binders, with the desire to limit calcium to what is needed, without causing deposition in soft tissues.

Phosphate intake is lowered by restricting dietary sources to 1200 mg or less. A better way to estimate phosphorus restriction is to allow about 17 mg/kg body weight/day. The following regression equation exists for estimating phosphorus intake based on protein intake:

$$128 + 14\ (\text{Grams of protein in diet}) = \text{Milligrams phosphorus per day in the diet}$$

Dietary restrictions alone are not adequate to control serum phosphorus, and nearly all patients who undergo dialysis will require phosphate-binding medication. In the past, aluminum hydroxide products such as Basaljel and Amphojel were used, but the resulting aluminum toxicity in many ESRD patients caused this treatment to be largely abandoned (Andress, 1986; Coburn and Norris, 1986). Current treatment relies on the use of calcium agents to bind phosphorus in the gut. Calcium carbonate, acetate, lactate, or gluconate are routinely used with each meal or snack (Schiller et al, 1989). Calcium citrate is avoided because of its ability to increase aluminum absorption. A complication of use of these calcium-based binders with concomitant use of active vitamin D is hypercalcemia. Because of this, some clinicians have returned to limited use of aluminum binders, in combination with calcium-based binders and sometimes even magnesium-based binders. Obviously, serum levels of aluminum and magnesium need to be watched closely in these patients. A different type of binder, sevelamer hydrochloride, (Renagel) a phosphate-binding resin, is able to reduce serum phosphorus without raising serum calcium because of its composition. Research continues to seek acceptable phosphate-binding medications (Table 39-6).

Severe constipation, leading to intestinal impaction, is a potential risk of excessive consumption of some types of phosphate binders. Occasionally, this may lead to perforation of the intestine, thus resulting in peritonitis and death. Constipation is often the reason why patients do not take the prescribed phosphate binders. Suggestions for using bran or other high-fiber foods and regular light exercise may contribute to patient compliance. Bulking agents such as Citrucel and Metamucil are low in phosphorus and potassium and are often used; however, they require extra fluid to be mixed with them, which needs to be considered with their use.

As with calcium supplementation, the early initiation of phosphate reduction therapies is advantageous for delaying hyperparathyroidism and bone disease. Unfortunately, most patients are asymptomatic during the early phase of hyperparathyroidism and hyperphosphatemia and are not attentive about following a modified diet and taking the calcium supplements and phosphate binders with meals. However, they should be encouraged to do so.

Because of potential *hypermagnesemia,* which can exacerbate the already existent bone disease, magnesium-containing antacids such as Maalox, Gelusil, Milk of Magnesia, or Mylanta should not be used.

Many patients on dialysis suffer from hypocalcemia, despite calcium supplementation. Because of this, the routine drug of choice is 1,25-$(OH)_2D_3$, which is available as calcitriol (Rocaltrol [Roche Labs] and Calcijex [Abbott Labs]). Analogs such as 1-$\alpha(OH)D_3$ (Hectorol) and 19 nor 1-α,25-$(OH)D_3$ (Zemplar) are also all effective in lowering PTH and raising calcium levels to various degrees. Both the oral and IV types are effective.

Hemodialysis, or peritoneal dialysis, does not alleviate osteodystrophy. However, it can reduce the progression of the disease because the infused calcium

TABLE 39-6 Common Medications for Patients With ESRD

1. Phosphate Binders
- Taken with meals and snacks to prevent dietary phosphorous absorption.

Calcium carbonate	**TUMS, Os-Cal, Calci-Chew, Calci-Mix**
Calcium acetate	**PhosLo**
Mg/Ca^{++} carbonate	**MagneBind**
Sevelamer hydrochloride	**Renagel**
Aluminum carbonate	
Aluminum hydroxide	**Alucap, Amphojel**

2. Vitamins
- Increased need for water-soluble vitamins because of losses during dialysis.
- Fat-soluble vitamins A, D, and K are not supplemented.
- Vitamin E may be supplemented.

Dialysis Recommendations:

Vitamin C	60 mg (not to exceed 200 mg daily)
Folic acid	1 mg
Thiamin	1.5 mg
Riboflavin	1.7 mg
Niacin	20 mg
Vitamin B_6	10 mg
Vitamin B_{12}	6 μg
Pantothenic acid	10 mg
Biotin	0.3 mg

- Brand names include **Nephrocap, Neph-ron FA, Nephplex, Renal Caps,** and **Tabron.**

3. Intradialytic Parenteral Nutrition (IDPN)
- Glucose, amino acid, and lipid solution infused during hemodialysis. Solution may include:

CHO	70% dextrose
Protein	15% amino acids
Lipid	20% lipid
Multivitamin	10 ml MVI-12 Infusion

- Fluid volume is removed during the run.
- Insulin often is given for hyperglycemia.

4. Iron
- Iron needs are increased because of EPO therapy.

Oral iron	Ferrous gluconate, ferrous sulphate, **Niferex 150** (polysaccharide iron complex)
IV iron	**Infed** (iron dextran), **Ferrlecit** (iron gluconate) **Venofer** (iron sucrose)

5. Erythropoietin
- Stimulates bone marrow to produce red blood cells.

IV or IM **Epogen** or **EPO** (epoetin)

6. Activated Vitamin D
- Used for the management of hyperparathyroidism.

Oral	**Rocaltrol** (calcitriol), **Hectorol** (doxercalciferol)
IV	**Calcijex** (calcitriol), **Zemplar** (paricalcitriol)

7. Bisphosphonates
- Inhibit bone resorption by blocking osteoclasts.

Oral	**Fosamax** (alendronate)
IV	**Aredia** (pamidronate)

8. Calcium Supplements
TUMS, Os-Cal, Calci-Chew

9. Phosphorous Supplements
KPhos, NutraPhos, NutraPhos K

10. Heavy Metal Chelator
- Binds aluminum and iron and is dialyzed off.

IV **Desferal** (deferoxamine or DFO)

11. Cation Exchange Resin
- For the treatment of hyperkalemia.

Oral or rectal **Kayexalate** (sodium polystyrene sulfonate or SPS)

Developed by Fiona Wolf, RD, and Thomas Montemayor, RPh, Northwest Kidney Centers, Seattle, Wash, 2003.
ESRD, End-stage renal disease.

results in decreased PTH secretion. Patients must still be responsible for following a low-phosphorus diet and for taking calcium to bind the phosphate.

Iron

The hypoproliferative, normochromic, normocytic anemia of chronic renal failure usually stabilizes with dialysis; however, it manifests itself in complaints of fatigue. It is caused by both an inability of the kidney to produce erythropoietin (EPO), a hormone that stimulates the bone marrow to produce red blood cells, and an increased destruction of red blood cells secondary to the circulating uremic waste products.

A synthetic form of EPO, *recombinant human erythropoietin (rHuEPO),* is used to treat the anemia of ESRD. Clinical trials have demonstrated a dramatic effect in the correction of anemia as well as in the restoration of a general sense of well-being (Eschbach et al, 1987). EPO occasionally causes a rise in serum K^+. Whether this is caused by increased blood viscosity impairing dialysis, increased breakdown of erythrocytes causing increased K^+, or an increase in the patient's appetite resulting from the increased sense of well-being is unclear.

Patients should be monitored closely while the EPO dose is adjusted, and they may need increased dialysis or a lower level of K^+ in the dialysate bath. Almost always accompanying the rise in hematocrit is an increased need for iron that requires supplementation intravenously. Oral iron alone is not effective in maintaining adequate iron stores in patients who take EPO. Unless a documented allergic reaction exists, almost all patients taking EPO will require periodic IV or intramuscular iron. For patients who are allergic to IV iron, several much–better-tolerated forms are now available. Iron dextran (Infed), iron gluconate (Ferrlecit), and iron sucrose (Venofer) are examples. For a small minority of patients, oral iron is the only alternative and is usually given in three divided doses. Because of its ability to bind with phosphate binders, oral iron should be taken between meals and not with calcium phosphate binders.

Blood transfusion is not recommended for most patients with ESRD because of (1) its depression of erythropoiesis in the bone marrow; (2) the possibility of overexpansion of the blood volume; (3) the risk of hepatitis; and (4) hemochromatosis and hemosiderosis caused by increased iron stores and the administration of parenteral iron (see Chapter 34).

Serum ferritin is an accurate indicator of iron overload. Patients who have received several transfusions and who are storing extra iron may have serum ferritin levels of 800 to 5000 ng/ml (a normal level is 68 ng/ml for women and 150 ng/ml for men; see Chapter 34). In patients who are receiving EPO, ferritin is kept above 300 ng/dl. When ferritin values fall below 100 ng/ml, IV iron is usually given. The percent of iron saturation (TSAT) is another useful indicator of iron status in these patients. The percent saturation should be greater than 20%.

Vitamins

One of the several causes of vitamin deficiency in uremia is the decreased dietary intake caused by the restriction of dietary phosphorus and potassium. Water-soluble vitamins are usually abundant in high-potassium foods, such as citrus fruits and vegetables, and high-phosphorus foods, such as milk. Diets for patients on dialysis tend to be low in folacin, niacin, riboflavin, and vitamin B_6. Ascorbic acid is marginal. With frequent episodes of anorexia or illness, the vitamin intake is decreased even further.

Altered metabolism and excretory function as well as drug administration also may alter vitamin levels. Little is known about gastrointestinal absorption in uremia, but it may be significantly decreased. Uremic toxins may interfere with the activity of some vitamins; for example, the phosphorylation of pyridoxine (vitamin B_6) and its analogs may be inhibited.

Water-soluble vitamins are also lost during dialysis. In general, ascorbic acid and most of the B-complex vitamins are dialyzable. Because vitamin B_{12} is protein-bound, losses of this B vitamin during dialysis are minimal.

Levels of the fat-soluble vitamins do not usually change as much as levels of the water-soluble vitamins in renal disease. Circulating levels of retinol-binding protein are often high in patients with renal failure, which normally indicates vitamin A toxicity. Whether this indicates toxicity in these patients is unclear. They may have an increased capacity to tolerate vitamin A because of the extra carrying capacity. Because little is known about this, supplementation of vitamin A is not usually recommended. Vitamin D, of course, should only be given in the active D_3 form by prescription, because ESRD patients do not activate this vitamin in its normal dietary or usual supplemental form. Little is known about vitamin E supplementation in chronic renal failure, although some evidence suggests that it does help protect against red blood cell fragility in the uremic patient. However, supplementation is not routinely recommended. Vitamin K supplements are usually avoided because of the large number of patients who take anticoagulants such as Coumadin.

Several vitamin supplements that fit the needs of the uremic patient or the dialysis patient are now available (Nephrocaps [Fleming and Co.], Tabron [Parke-Davis], Neph-plex [Nephro-Tech Inc.], and Renal Caps [Cypress Pharmaceuticals Inc.]). A supplement of vitamin B complex and vitamin C is often used. Additional supplements of folic acid and pyridoxine may also be given. Folic acid supplementation is recommended at 1 mg/day. This level is above that allowed in over-the-counter vitamin preparations and requires a prescription.

Dialysis patients routinely use some form of oral nutritional supplement—the majority of which contain complete vitamin supplementation to the level of the newly defined DRIs in 3 to 4 cans (see Table 15-1). Patients may be getting a significant amount of their vitamin nutriture from these supplements and may not require oral vitamin preparations in addition to their diets. A thorough analysis of the patient's nutrient intake is needed.

Carbohydrate

Glucose intolerance with both hyperglycemia and hypoglycemia commonly is observed in patients with ESRD. It seems to reflect a delayed and erratic action of insulin caused by tissue resistance to insulin action or by an insulin antagonism by the products of uremia. In any case, this glucose intolerance rarely requires administration of insulin but might require control of the carbohydrate in the diet (see Chapter 33). If hypoglycemia becomes a problem, the addition of dextrose to the dialysate usually alleviates the problem.

Lipid

Atherosclerotic cardiovascular disease is the most common cause of death among patients maintained on long-term hemodialysis. This appears to be a function of both underlying disease (e.g., diabetes mellitus, hypertension, nephrotic syndrome) and a lipid abnormality common among patients with ESRD. The patient with ESRD typically has an elevated triglyceride level with or without an increase in cholesterol. The lipid abnormality likely represents both increased synthesis of very-low-density lipoprotein and decreased clearance.

Treatment of hyperlipidemia with diet or pharmacologic agents remains controversial. Epidemiologic evidence demonstrating increased incidence of atherosclerotic coronary disease is balanced by studies that demonstrate that patients with clearly defined clinical evidence of atherosclerosis at the initiation of dialysis are at no increased risk for a cardiovascular event over age-matched cohorts (Ma et al, 1992). Although routine treatment appears unwarranted, a good case can be made for dietary and pharmacologic treatment of patients with ESRD with underlying lipid disorders and evidence of accelerated atherosclerosis. The new generation of lipid-lowering drugs, including lovastatin, may have a significant impact on future management (see Chapter 35).

Improvement of the plasma lipid profile in ESRD may result from supplementation with the amino acid L-carnitine. Because the kidney is a major site of carnitine synthesis, dialysis patients typically have abnormal carnitine metabolism and low plasma-free carnitine levels. However, research has not consistently shown the effectiveness of carnitine supplementation in increasing free and *acyl*-carnitine levels in these patients. Some studies have shown carnitine supplementation associated with improved muscle function and less cramping, fewer hypotensive episodes, and less protein catabolism, but the KDOQI guidelines do not support its routine use (NKF, 2000).

Enteral Tube Feeding

Patients with ESRD who require enteral tube feeding often do quite well on standard formulas used for most tube-fed patients. Patients should receive standard formulas before they try a "specialty" formula, because the former are usually less expensive and typically have lower osmolality than the specific renal products. If electrolyte or fluid concerns arise, patients can switch to one of the formulas now available specifically designed for renal patients: Nepro (Ross Labs), Magnacal Renal (Mead Johnson), Travasorb Renal (Travenol), Novasource Renal (Novartis), and ReNeph (Ross Labs), to name a few (see Appendix 38). If patients are receiving these "renal" products only, they may develop problems with a low phosphorus level if they are experiencing "refeeding syndrome," or if they are taking phosphate binders. The dosage of the phosphate binders may need to be adjusted or eliminated. In some cases patients may need a phosphorus supplement or the addition of milk to their feeding to maintain an acceptable serum phosphorus level.

Some enteral feeding products contain only essential amino acids. These products are designed for use just as the low-protein diet is used in predialysis patients, as a way to lower exogenous protein waste products. One such product is Amin-Aid (McGaw), which contains only the essential amino acids plus histidine in the amount required and which, when mixed with water, provides amino acids, carbohydrate, and a few electrolytes (see Appendix 39). A side effect of this formulation may be diarrhea caused by the high osmolality.

Electrodialyzed whey (lactalbumin treated to remove the electrolytes) combined with glucose and water provides HBV protein with adequate calories and few electrolytes. However, unless the patient is experiencing severe shifts in electrolytes or requires a very large volume, most standard house tube feedings can be tailored to meet the requirements.

Parenteral Nutrition

When a patient with ESRD becomes too ill to maintain an adequate oral intake and when tube feeding is not advisable because of gastrointestinal complications, parenteral nutrition should be considered (see Chapter 23).

Parenteral nutrition in ESRD is similar to parenteral nutrition used for other malnourished patients. The use of essential amino acid solutions, such as Nephramine, formerly were recommended in cases of ARF or when a patient was not receiving dialysis treatment, but this practice has been discontinued because these patients seem to tolerate regular amino acid infusions well. Patients who receive dialysis therapy tolerate routine amino acid solutions, such as Freeamine (McGaw), Travasol 8.5 (Clintec), and Aminosyn (Abbott Labs).

Vitamins and Minerals

Most researchers agree that vitamin needs for ESRD are different from normal requirements during parenteral nutrition but do not agree on their recommendations for individual nutrients. It is generally accepted that folate, pyridoxine, and biotin should be supplemented and that vitamin A should not be provided parenterally unless retinol-binding protein is monitored, because it is elevated in patients with renal failure. Table 39-7 presents vitamin supplementation guidelines.

Little information relating to trace mineral supplementation in renal failure is available. Because most trace minerals, including zinc, chromium, and magnesium, are excreted in the urine, a close monitoring of these minerals in the serum seems to be appropriate.

Hypophosphatemia is a potential complication of parenteral nutrition in ESRD. When the patient is consuming some food and is receiving phosphate binders, this may be of even greater concern. If adequate protein and calories are provided and the patient becomes anabolic, the phosphate-binder regimen may need to be altered to prevent hypophosphatemia and potential respiratory arrest.

TABLE 39-7 Guidelines for Daily Parenteral Vitamin Supplementation in Total Parenteral Nutrition for Patients With Renal Failure*

VITAMIN	SILBERMAN	KOPPLE
A, as retinol (IU)	3300.0	0.0
E, tocopherol (IU)	10.0	10.0
K (mg)		7.5
Niacin (mg)	40.0	20.0
Thiamin HCl (mg)	3.0	2.0
Riboflavin (mg)	3.6	2.0
Pantothenic acid (mg)	15.0	10.0
Pyridoxine (mg)	5.0	10.0
Ascorbic acid (mg)	100.0	100.0
Biotin (mg)	60.0	200.0
Folic acid (mg)	1.0	2.0
B_{12} (mg)	5.0	3.0

From Kouba J: Vitamin and electrolytes in patients with renal failure requiring total parenteral nutrition. In *Dietitians in critical care,* Chicago, 1985, American Dietetic Association.

*These are general guidelines and may need more specific evaluation and adjustment in patients with severe stress or with gastrointestinal losses from diarrhea, ostomies, fistula drainage, etc.

Intradialytic Parenteral Nutrition

Malnourished patients with chronic renal failure who are on hemodialysis have easy access to parenteral nutrition because of the requirements of the dialysis therapy itself. Because direct access to the blood must be made at every treatment, parenteral nutrition can be administered if necessary without additional invasive procedures or surgery.

Intradialytic parenteral nutrition (IDPN) typically is administered through a connection to the venous side of the extracorporeal circuit during dialysis (Olsham et al, 1987). Because of the high blood flow rate achieved through use of the surgically created fistula and the high blood pump speeds that are attained, hypertonic glucose and protein can be administered without danger of phlebitis. Lipids may also be administered (Tables 39-8 and 39-9). Reimbursement issues surrounding this therapy are complex.

Complications

Complications are similar to those encountered in TPN, with the exception of postdialysis hypoglycemia caused the abrupt ending of the glucose supply. To avoid this problem, glucose administration typically is tapered up and down during the first and last half hour of the 3- to 4-hour treatment. Insulin is given often, usually in the bag of dextrose–amino acid solution, so that the patient does not become hypoglycemic if the infusion must be stopped. Blood sugar levels are typically monitored during the therapy. In addition, some patients may benefit from a snack of complex carbohydrate toward the end of the treatment.

Amino acid losses through the dialysate average about 10%. Vitamins and trace minerals are typically not administered with these solutions because patients are able to tolerate oral vitamin preparations and also have some oral dietary intake.

Other potential methods of nutritional support are the use of a hemodialysis dialysate solution that con-

TABLE 39-8 Regimen for Intermittent Parenteral Nutrition Administered During Hemodialysis Therapy

INFUSION	QUANTITY	CALORIES (kcal)	VOLUME (ml)
70% dextrose	350.0 g dextrose	1190	500
15% amino acids	37.5 g protein	Protein should not be counted on to provide calories.	250
20% lipid emulsion	50.0 g fat	450	250
TOTALS		1640	1000*
Monitor serum glucose, sodium, potassium, bicarbonate, phosphate, triglycerides.			

Developed by Katy G. Wilkens, MS, RD, Northwest Kidney Centers, Seattle, Wash.

*Additional volume may include insulin and vitamins.

TABLE 39-9 Regimen for Total Parenteral Nutrition by Subclavian Vein for Dialysis Patients

INFUSION	QUANTITY	CALORIES (kcal)	VOLUME (ml)
70% glucose	700 g glucose	2380	1000
15% amino acids	75 g protein	Protein should not be counted on to provide calories.	500
20% lipid emulsion	100 g fat	900	500
TOTALS		3280	2000*
Monitor serum glucose, sodium, potassium, bicarbonate, phosphate, triglycerides.			

Developed by Katy G. Wilkens, MS, RD, Northwest Kidney Centers, Seattle, Wash.
*Additional volume may include insulin and vitamins.

tains amino acids and a peritoneal dialysate solution that contains amino acids as well as dextrose. These methods are currently in limited usage.

ESRD in Patients With Diabetes

Because renal failure is a complication of diabetes, approximately 40% of all new patients starting dialysis have diabetes. Because of the need to control blood sugar, these patients require even more specialized diet therapy. The diet for diabetes management (see Chapter 33) can be modified for the patient on dialysis. In addition, the diabetic patient on dialysis often has other complications, such as retinopathy, neuropathy, gastroparesis, and amputation, all of which can place this patient at high nutritional risk.

In the presence of hyperglycemia, most patients with diabetes experience thirst, and fluid overload may become a serious problem. Increased osmolarity caused by high serum levels of glucose may cause water and potassium to be pulled out of cells, with resultant hyperkalemia.

ESRD in Children

Renal failure may occur in children at any age, from the newborn infant through the adolescent. As with all children, the major concern is to promote normal growth and development. Without aggressive monitoring and encouragement, the child rarely meets his or her nutritional requirements. If the renal disease is present from birth, nutritional support needs to begin immediately to avoid losing the growth potential of the first few months of life.

Growth in children with ESRD is usually retarded. Although no specific therapy ensures normal growth, factors capable of responding to therapy include metabolic acidosis, electrolyte depletion, osteodystrophy, chronic infection, and protein-calorie malnutrition. Energy and protein needs for children with chronic renal disease are at least equivalent to the DRI for normal children of the same height and age (see Box 10-1 and Table 15-2). If nutritional status is poor, energy needs may be even higher to promote weight gain and linear growth. Feeding by tube is required in the presence of poor intake, particularly in the critical growth period of the first 2 years of life. Gastrostomy tubes are almost always placed in these children to enhance nutritional intake and facilitate growth. TPN is rarely initiated, unless the GI tract is nonfunctional. Table 39-10 presents the nutritional requirements of children with renal failure.

Control of calcium and phosphorus balance is especially important for maintaining good growth. The goal is to restrict phosphorus intake while promoting calcium absorption with the aid of 1,25-$(OH)_2D_3$. This helps prevent renal osteodystrophy, which can cause severe growth retardation during childhood. Use of calcium carbonate formulations to supplement the dietary intake enhances calcium intake while binding excess phosphorus. Aluminum-containing preparations are used only in patients with extreme hyperphosphatemia and only on a short-term basis. Aluminum binders should never be used routinely in children under the age of 10 years.

Persistent metabolic acidosis is often associated with growth failure in infancy. In chronic acidosis, the titration of acid by the bone causes calcium loss and contributes to bone demineralization. Bicarbonate may be added to the formula to counteract this effect.

Restriction of protein in pediatric diets is controversial. The so-called "protective" effect on kidney function must be weighed against the clearly negative effect of possible protein malnutrition on growth. The RDA for protein for age is usually the minimum amount to be given (see Box 10-1).

Each child's diet should be adjusted to his or her food preferences, family eating patterns, and biochemical needs. This is often not an easy task. In addition, care must be taken not to place too much emphasis on the diet to avoid its becoming a manipulative tool and an attention-getting device.

Special encouragement, creativity, and attention are required to help the child with ESRD consume the necessary energy. When possible, *continuous cyclical peritoneal dialysis (CCPD)*, which is intermittent during the day and continuous at night, is a viable therapy of choice for children because it allows liberalization of the diet. The child is more likely to meet nutritional requirements with fewer dietary restrictions and therefore experience better growth.

New developments that may help with treatment of renal disease in children include the use of rHuEPO

TABLE 39-10 Nutrient Requirements Based on Type of Therapy for Children With Renal Disease

THERAPY	ENERGY	PROTEIN: CREATININE CLEARANCE	PROTEIN: PROTEIN REQUIREMENT	FLUID	SODIUM	POTASSIUM	PHOSPHORUS
Impaired renal function (predialysis)	Infant (under 1 yr): 120-150 kcal/kg Child: First 10 kg = 100 kcal/kg Second 10 kg = 50 kcal/kg Every kg thereafter = 20 kcal/kg	10-50	1.5 g/kg	35 ml/100 kcal + urine output	23-69 mg/kg/day (1-3 mEq/kg/day)	29-87 mg/kg/day (1-3 mEq/kg/day)	0.5-1.0 g/day
		<10	1.0 g/kg				
		<5	0.3-0.5 g/kg				
		WEIGHT OF CHILD					
Hemodialysis	Same as above	10-20 kg	2.0 g/kg	Same as above, plus losses from dialysis Child's fluid gains should be about 5% of body weight	57 mg/kg/day (2.5 mEq/kg/day)	Same as above	0.5-1.0 g/day
		20-30 kg	1.5 g/kg				
		30-40 kg	1.0-1.5 g/kg				
		40+ kg	1.0 g/kg				
Intermittent peritoneal dialysis (IPD)	Same as above	10-20 kg	2.0 g/kg	Same as above	Same as above		
Continuous ambulatory peritoneal dialysis (CAPD)	100-120 kcal/kg	20-40 kg 40+ kg 10-20 kg	1.5 g/kg 1.0-1.5 g/kg 2.0-3.0 g/kg	100-160 ml/kg/day + urine output	Same as above	Same as above	0.5-1.0 g/day
Transplant	Normal energy requirement for age; tendency toward obesity because of steroids; not more than 35% of total calories from fat; low saturated fat	20-40 kg 40+ kg	1.5-2.0 g/kg 1.0-1.5 g/kg 2.0-3.0 g/kg	*Ad libitum*	Variable	Variable, usually *ad libitum*	*Ad libitum.* Supplement if necessary Calcium *ad libitum*, supplement if necessary; vitamin D as necessary

Developed by Anne Hetrick, RD, Shands Teaching Hospital, University of Florida, Gainesville, Fla.

and *rDNA-produced growth hormone (rHGH).* Correction of anemia with the use of rHuEPO may increase appetite, intake, and feeling of well-being, but it has not been found to affect growth, even with seemingly adequate nutritional support. Daily rHGH has been shown to increase growth in children with chronic renal failure and ESRD, even when these children have normal endogenous production of growth hormone (Fine et al, 1994).

NEPHROLITHIASIS (KIDNEY STONES)*

Nephrolithiasis, or the presence of kidney stones, is a significant health problem in our population. It is characterized by frequent occurrences between the ages of 30 and 50, predominance in males (three times more often), and a high recurrence rate. The risk doubles in those with a family history of kidney stones.

Pathophysiology

Kidney stone formation is a complex process that consists of saturation, supersaturation, nucleation, crystal growth or aggregation, crystal retention, and stone formation in the presence of promoters, inhibitors, and complexors in urine. Calcium stones are the most common, with calcium oxalate (60%), calcium oxalate and calcium phosphate (10%), calcium phosphate (10%), uric acid (5% to 10%), struvite (5% to 10%), and cystine (1%) (Box 39-2). Low urine volume is the single most important risk factor for urolithiasis.

Medical Management

Uric acid stones are the only type amenable to dissolution therapy. Shockwave lithotripsy and endourologic techniques have almost replaced the open surgical procedures of stone removal of 20 years ago. Management strategies are now aimed at kidney stone prevention and should include a patient evaluation and metabolic workup to identify causes (Goldfarb and Coe, 1999b; Pearl, 2001) (Tables 39-11 and 39-12).

Medical Nutrition Therapy

After corrective treatment for medical disorders, patients should receive nutrition counseling for diet and fluid modification to reduce urinary risk factors for stone disease (Morton et al, 2002). An efficacy of a specific dietary regimen based on comprehensive metabolic evaluation, repeated dietary counseling, and metabolic monitoring was found to be more effective in reducing stone recurrence (7%) than nonspecific measures and limited screening (23%) (Kocvara et al, 1999).

Fluid and Urine Volume

A high fluid intake is the one strategy that can be applied to all types of kidney stones. The objective is to maintain urinary solutes in the undersaturated zone by both an increase in urine volume and a reduction of solute load to inhibit nucleation. High urine flow rate will tend to wash out any formed crystals. A high fluid intake and elimination of dietary excesses controlled stone formation in 60% of patients with idiopathic calcium urolithiasis in a kidney stone clinic (Borghi et al, 1999). A randomized 5-year clinical trial demonstrated decreased recurrence (12% vs. 27%) and a longer time to recurrence (39 months vs. 25 months) in patients who maintained a 2.6-L/day urine volume in comparison to 1.2 L/day (Borghi et al, 1996).

To achieve dilution, the goal for a urine volume should be 2.0 to 2.5 L/day; 250 ml of fluid at each meal, between meals, at bedtime, and when arising to void at night are recommended. Hydration during sleep hours is important to break the cycle of a "most-concentrated" morning urine. Half of the fluid should be taken as water. Higher fluid intake should compensate for gastrointestinal fluid loss, excessive sweating from strenuous exercise, or an excessively

*This section contributed by Veena Juneja, MSc, RD.

Box 39-2. Urinary Risk Factors for Stone Development

Increased Risk	Decreased Risk
Low urine volume	High urine volume and flow
Oxalate	Citrate
Uric acid	Glycoproteins
Sodium	Magnesium
Acid pH	
Stasis	
Calcium	

TABLE 39-11 Causes and Composition of Renal Stones

PATHOGENETIC CAUSES	COMPOSITION OF STONE
Hypercalciuria Hyperoxaluria Hyperuricosuria Hypocitraturia Primary hyperparathyroidism	→ Calcium oxalate
Cystinuria	→ Cystine
Infection	→ Struvite
Acid urine pH Hyperuricosuria	→ Uric acid
Renal tubular acidosis Alkaline urine pH	→ Calcium phosphate

Data from Martini LA, Wood RJ: Should dietary calcium and protein be restricted in patients with nephrolithiasis? *Nutr Rev* 58:111, 2000.

dry environment (such as a commercial airplane cabin). Patients who form idiopathic calcium stones with low urine volume and who are unable to increase urine volume may have altered thirst sensitivity and vasopressin release.

In two large cohort studies, consumption of tea, coffee, beer, and wine was associated with reduced risk of stone formation, but grapefruit juice was not (Goldfarb and Coe, 1999a). However, in a separate study, grapefruit juice ingestion caused no changes in lithogenicity and no net change in calculated supersaturation. Thus, the basis of the observations of epidemiologic studies remains unexplained (Goldfarb and Asplin, 2001). At this point, it is good clinical practice to recommend avoidance of grapefruit juice and also soft drinks that contain phosphoric acid.

Bioavailability and observational studies do not demonstrate brewed tea with added milk as a risk factor, despite tea's high oxalate content. The recommendation for tea drinkers is to drink only a moderate amount of tea (about 2 cups per day), diluted, and with milk.

TABLE 39-12 Baseline Information and Metabolic Evaluation of Urolithiasis

INFORMATION	DESCRIPTION/DATA
History of urolithiasis	History of onset, frequency Family history Spontaneous passage or removal Retrieval, analysis-type of stone Current status with radiologic examination
Medical history, investigations	Hyperparathyroidism Renal tubular acidosis Urinary tract infection Sarcoidosis Hypertension Osteoporosis Inflammatory bowel disease, malabsorption syndrome, intestinal bypass surgery for obesity
Blood tests	Serum—calcium, phosphorus, creatinine, uric acid, CO_2, albumin, parathyroid hormone
Urinalysis	Urine analysis with pH Urine culture
24-hr urine collection	Volume, calcium, oxalate, uric acid, sodium Citrate, magnesium, phosphorus Urea Creatinine Qualitative cystine
Medications and vitamins	Thiazide, allopurinol, vitamin C, vitamin B_6, vitamin D, cod liver oil, calcium carbonate, glucocorticoid therapy
Occupation history and strenuous exercise	Dermal losses, dehydration, low urine volume Type of job and activity level
Environment	Hard water area
Dietary evaluation	Intake of calcium, oxalate, animal protein, salt, purines, herbal products Inadequate fluid intake Type of fluids

Calcium Stones

Calcium

Hypercalciuria is defined as a mean value of calcium in excess of 300 mg (7.5 mmol)/day in men or 250 mg (6.25 mmol)/day in women, or 4 mg (0.1 mmol)/kg/day for either in random urine collections of outpatients on unrestricted diets. Thirty to 40% of patients with calcium stones are hypercalciuric. Hypercalciuria is idiopathic when serum calcium is normal and the usual causes can be excluded. Idiopathic hypercalciuria can result from an exaggerated dietary calcium intake, increased intestinal absorption of calcium that may or may not be vitamin D–mediated, decreased renal tubular reabsorption of calcium, or prolonged bed rest. It can also result from low serum phosphorus levels caused by a renal phosphate leak that stimulates 1,25-dihydroxy vitamin D_3 production and consequently increases intestinal calcium absorption (Morton, Iliescu, and Wilson, 2002). Calcium-loading studies show that urinary calcium rises with an increase in dietary calcium of up to 800 mg (20 mmol)/day. Beyond that point, animal protein may be responsible for the rise in urine calcium (Box 39-3).

For decades, low-calcium diets have been recommended to reduce the high incidence of hypercalciuria in patients who form stones. However, a low-calcium diet was postulated to result in less calcium available to bind oxalate in the gastrointestinal tract and thus to increased passive absorption of free oxalate and eventually to increased urinary oxalate excretion. If low-calcium diets enhance urinary oxalate excretion and thus the risk for an oxalate-containing stone, it was suggested that calcium and oxalate should be restricted simultaneously to prevent a rise in urinary oxalate. However, studies failed to demonstrate a beneficial effect of simultaneous restriction of calcium and oxalate (Massey, Roman-Smith, and Sutton, 1993).

Chronic prolonged calcium restriction may damage the bones of calcium-stone patients because of deficient calcium to meet requirements and increased losses of calcium in the urine. Vertebral mineral density is decreased in calcium-stone formers with idiopathic hypercalciuria. Vertebral fracture risk is in-

Box 39-3. Dietary Factors Associated With Risk of Calcium Stones

Increased Risk	Decreased Risk
Animal protein	Calcium
Oxalate	Potassium
Sodium	Magnesium
	Fluid intake
	Fiber
	Vitamin B_6

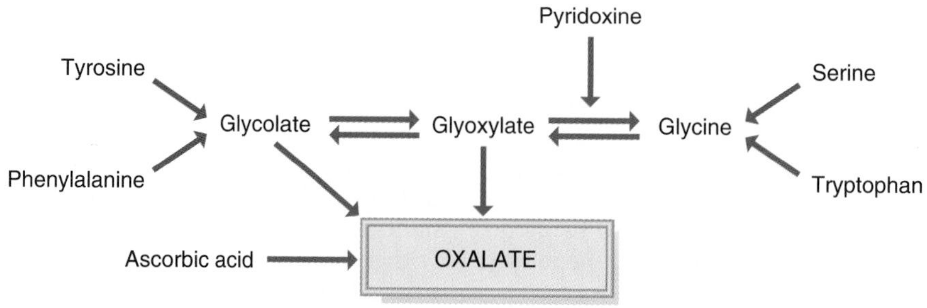

FIGURE 39-10 • Endogenous oxalate formation.

creased by nearly fourfold among urolithiasis patients in comparison with the expected incidence in the general population (Melton et al, 1998). Bone resorption may also be enhanced by a high protein intake of nondairy origin (Bataille et al, 1991).

The relationship between dietary calcium and the incidence of symptomatic kidney stones was examined in two separate long-term prospective studies in men (Curhan et al, 1993) and women (Curhan et al, 1997). Dietary calcium intake was inversely associated with risk of kidney stones, thus conferring a protective effect. Calcium supplements did not have the same protective effect as dietary calcium had and were associated with an increased risk because they may not have been taken with meals to reduce oxalate absorption. Thus far, recommendations for calcium have been made upon observational studies. In a recent randomized trial, a calcium intake of 1200 mg, coupled with restriction of both animal protein and salt intake, was found to be more effective than calcium restriction (400 mg/day) and low oxalate intake in preventing recurrent calcium oxalate stones. After 5 years, only 20% of the men on the normal calcium, reduced-salt, and reduced-protein diet had at least one episode of stone recurrence, whereas 38% of men on the low-calcium diet had at least one stone episode (Borghi et al, 2002). Clearly, calcium restriction does not prevent stone formation and may cause or worsen osteoporosis (Martini, 2002). Current DRIs recommend 1000 mg/day of calcium for men and women age 50 years or younger and 1200 mg/day of calcium for those older than 50 years, which aligns well with calcium recommendations for kidney stone formers (Martini and Wood, 2002).

Oxalate

Dietary oxalate intake affects urinary oxalate (Holmes, Goodman, and Assimos, 2001). Hyperoxaluria plays an important role in calcium stone formation and is observed in up to 20% of recurrent stone formers. The oxalate content of a normal diet is in the range of 80 to 100 mg/day, and absorption does not usually exceed 10% to 20% of the amount in food.

Oxalate cannot be metabolized in the body, and the renal route is the only mode of excretion. Oxalate in urine originates from the absorption of dietary oxalate and endogenous synthesis. Glyoxylic acid accounts for 50% to 70% of urinary oxalate, and ascorbic acid accounts for 35% to 55%. Several amino acids are precursors of oxalate via glyoxylate or glycolate. Pyridoxine acts as a cofactor in the conversion of glyoxylate to glycine, and its deficiency could increase endogenous oxalate production (Figure 39-10).

Normal healthy adults daily excrete 15 to 40 mg of oxalate in urine; this can be increased by 50% by large intakes of oxalate-rich foods. Seasonal variations in oxalate intake are common. Because much less oxalate than calcium exists in urine—the ratio is 1:5—changes in oxalate concentration have a greater impact than changes in calcium concentration on the relative supersaturation of calcium-oxalate crystals.

Patients with inflammatory bowel diseases or gastric bypass develop hyperoxaluria from fat malabsorption. The bile acids produced during the digestive process normally are reabsorbed in the proximal gastrointestinal tract. When this fails to occur, the bile acids bind calcium to form soaps, thus making less calcium in soluble form available to bind oxalate and allowing for increased oxalate absorption from the gut (see Chapter 30). Bile salts and fatty acids also increase colonic permeability to oxalate. Urinary oxalate excretion increases up to two to three times normal in enteric hyperoxaluria.

Primary hyperoxaluria is a feature of an autosomal recessive genetic defect of a hepatic enzyme that results in overproduction of oxalate and a urinary oxalate concentration three to eight times the normal rate. Multiple stones occur in these children and cause renal failure and early death.

Limited data on the oxalate content of foods are available because of inconsistent values from different methodologies used for analysis. Only a few foods have been tested for oxalate bioavailability. High-oxalate foods should not be avoided based on their oxalate content alone when only a limited amount is bioavailable. Foods with a low oxalate content and higher bioavailability may noticeably increase urinary oxalate (Box 39-4; see Appendix 45).

Animal Protein

Epidemiologic studies find a correlation between improved standard of living, high animal protein intake, and a rising incidence of kidney stones. Excessive animal protein intake modulates several urinary

Box 39-4. Foods That Raise Urinary Oxalate Excretion

Rhubarb
Spinach
Strawberries
Chocolate
Wheat bran
Nuts (almonds, peanuts, or pecans)
Beets
Tea (green, black, iced, or instant)

Data from Brinkley LJ et al: A further study of oxalate bioavailability in foods, *J Urol* 144:94, 1990; French AM et al: Urine compositions in normal subjects after oral ingestion of oxalate-rich foods, *Clin Sci* 60:411, 1981; and Massey LK et al: Effect of dietary oxalate and calcium on urinary oxalate and risk of formulation of calcium oxalate kidney stones, *J Am Diet Assoc* 93:901, 1993.

risk factors such as hypercalciuria, hyperuricosuria, hyperoxaluria, low urine pH, and hypocitraturia, all of which increase the risk of kidney stones (Martini and Wood, 2000). Urinary urate acts as a promoter of heterogeneous nucleation of calcium oxalate via epitaxial growth by decreasing its threshold of precipitation. Approximately a third of calcium stone formers are sensitive to meat protein in terms of oxalate excretion. The mechanism does not seem to involve vitamin B_6 deficiency. Prevalence of stone formation in vegetarians is 1.2%, in comparison with 3.8% in the general population (Nguyen et al, 2001; Smith et al, 1981). The male Health Professionals' Observational Study demonstrated a 33% increased risk of kidney stones with a 77-g versus 50-g animal-protein diet (Curhan et al, 1993). A 5-year randomized trial of men on a diet of normal calcium, low salt, and reduced animal protein (52 g with 21 g from meat or fish and 31 g from milk and derivatives) reduced stone incidence by 51%. The diet decreased urine calcium, oxalate, and calcium-oxalate saturation (Borghi et al, 2002). Stone formers with hypercalciuria benefit from decreased intake of animal protein because they may be metabolically more sensitive to a reduction in animal protein intake (Rotily et al, 2000). Moderate protein restriction at 0.8 g/kg and normal calcium intake ameliorates the lithogenic profile and decreases bone resorption (Giannini et al, 1999).

Citrate

Citrate is a urinary stone inhibitor. It forms a complex calcium in urine; thus less calcium is available to bind urinary oxalate, which helps prevent the formation of calcium oxalate or calcium phosphate stones. Distal renal tubular acidosis, acidosis accompanied by hypokalemia, malabsorption syndrome with enteric hyperoxaluria, and excessive meat intake (acid ash) are associated with decreased urinary citrate levels (Morton, Iliescu, and Wilson, 2002). Normal daily urinary citrate level should be more than 640 mg. Lemonade made with lemon juice (4 oz.) diluted to 2 L with water should be encouraged in patients with low urinary citrate (Seltzer et al, 1996). The use of potassium or magnesium citrate to reduce the incidence of kidney stones is currently under investigation.

Sodium

Twenty-four–hour urine sodium and hypercalciuria are directly correlated. A linear increase in urinary calcium occurs as urinary sodium increases from 40 to 200 mmol (920-4600 mg)/day. For every 60-mmol (1380 mg) increase in urine sodium, the relative risk of hypercalciuria increases by 1.63 times. Sodium and calcium are reabsorbed at common sites in the renal tubule. The recommended sodium chloride intake in a recent randomized trial was found to be 50 mmol (1150 mg)/day. However, yearly measurements of urinary sodium were 110 to 130 mmol (2530-2990 mg)/day, which shows the subjects' lack of compliance (Borghi et al, 2002). Salt intake should be lowered in patients with hypercalciuria to less than 100 mmol (2300 mg) per day (Morton, Iliescu, and Wilson, 2002) (see Chapter 36 for sodium content of foods).

Potassium

Stone formers have a low to normal potassium intake (mean 2262 mg (58 mmol)) and high sodium intake (Martini et al, 1998). Potassium intake is inversely related to the risk of kidney stones. Ingestion of potassium at 4042 mg (104 mmol)/day in comparison with 2895 mg (74 mmol)/day caused a 50% reduction in the incidence of kidney stones (Curhan et al, 1993). The level of potassium used in a recent study that reduced stone incidence by 50% was 120 mmol (4680 mg)/day (Borghi et al, 2002). Stone formers should increase potassium in their diets by choosing low-oxalate fruit and vegetables.

Vitamins

Use of vitamin C supplements has been controversial. Improper storage and processing of urine samples led to a conversion of ascorbic acid to oxalate and became the basis for recommendations against vitamin C supplementations (Gerster, 1997). The Health Professionals' study demonstrated no difference in relative risk of kidney stones between those with vitamin C intakes of less than 250 mg/day and with those with intakes equal to or greater than 1500 mg/day, thus suggesting that routine restriction of vitamin C is not warranted (Curhan et al, 1999). A controlled metabolic diet supplemented with 1 g ascorbic acid twice daily was tested in calcium oxalate stone formers and in normal controls, with urine collection under ideal conditions to avoid oxidation. It demonstrated a statistically significant increase in oxalate in both groups. Taking into account the lack of association between vitamin C intake and stone risk in the observational study, Traxer and colleagues (2000) recommended limiting vitamin C to less than 2.0 g/day. Vitamin B_6 intake of greater than or equal to 40 mg/day in comparison with an intake of less than 3 mg/day led to a relative risk reduction of 0.66, thus confirming the role of vitamin B_6 in reducing the incidence of kidney stones (Curhan et al, 1999; Curhan et al, 1996) (see Figure 39-10).

Fiber

Oxalate content of various types of bran varies. The bioavailability of oxalate in wheat bran is high, but oxalate in wheat bran does not seem to be a risk factor for hyperoxaluria. No change in urinary calcium or oxalate is observed when fiber intake from fruit, vegetable and cereal sources is increased up to 25 g/day. Studies of rice bran have shown a reduction in new stone formation (Rotily et al, 2000).

Herbal Products

A study of the lithogenic properties of cranberry concentrate pills in healthy volunteers demonstrated a 43% increase in urinary oxalate, sodium, and calcium (Terris et al, 2001). Patients at risk of nephrolithiasis should be educated to avoid ingestion of cranberry concentrate pills. Long-term use of several products—such as wild yam, flaxseed, zinc, copper, vitamin A, evening primrose oil, and goldenrod, which are promoted to reduce the risk of kidney stones—is not supported by scientific evidence.

Uric Acid Stones

Uric acid is an end product of purine metabolism. The source of purine is food, *de novo* synthesis, and tissue catabolism. About half of the purine load is from endogenous sources and is constant. Exogenous dietary sources provide the other half and account for the variation in uric acid presence in the urine.

Solubility of uric acid depends upon urine volume, the amount excreted, and urine pH (Table 39-13). Uric acid stones form when urine is supersaturated with undissociated uric acid, which occurs at urinary pH less than 5.5. Therefore conditions such as inflammatory bowel disease, which results in chronically acidic urine from dehydration and gastrointestinal bicarbonate loss from diarrhea, predispose patients to uric acid stones. Uric acid stones are also associated with lymphoproliferative and myeloproliferative disorders with increased cellular breakdown that releases purines and thus increases uric acid load.

TABLE 39-13 Effect of Urine pH on Stone Formation

pH	STATE OF URATE	LIKELY STONE DEVELOPMENT
pH <5.5	Undissociated urate	Uric acid stones
5.5-7.5	Dissociated urate	Calcium oxalate stones
>7.5	Dissociated urate	Calcium phosphate stones

Dietary purines should be restricted in patients with uric acid lithiasis and hyperuricosuric calcium oxalate stones. Animal flesh proteins, meat, fish, and poultry are rich in purines and acid ash and should be used in moderation to meet protein requirements (see *Clinical Insight:* "Acid Ash" and "Alkaline Ash" Diets). Foods specifically high in purines should be avoided. These are organ meats, anchovies, herrings, sardines, meat-based broth, and gravy (see Table 44-3). Noncompliance with dietary measures or persistence of hyperuricosuria will warrant use of medication such as allopurinol.

Uric acid stones are the only stones amenable to dissolution therapy by urine alkalinization to a pH of 6.0 to 6.5. Potassium citrate has been used as the therapy of choice. Sodium bicarbonate will increase urinary monosodium urate and calcium and should not be used.

Struvite Stones

Struvite stones comprise magnesium ammonium phosphate and carbonate apatite. They are also known as *triple-phosphate* or *infection stones.* Unlike most urinary stones, they occur more commonly in women than in men, at a ratio of 2:1. They form only in the presence of bacteria such as *Pseudomonas, Klebsiella, Proteus mirablis,* and *Urealyticum* that carry urease, a urea-splitting enzyme. Urea breakdown results in ammonia and CO_2 production, thus raising urine pH and the level of carbonate. Struvite stones grow rapidly to large staghorn calculi in the renal pelvic area. The mainstay of treatment is the surgical removal of calculi alone or with extracorporeal shock-wave lithotripsy with adjunctive culture-specific antimicrobial therapy that uses urease inhibitors. The goal is to eliminate or prevent UTIs by regular screening and monitoring of urine cultures.

Cystine Stones

Cystine stones represent 1% to 2% of urinary calculi and are caused by homozygous cystinuria. Cystine stones affect about one in 15,000 persons in the United States. Most patients with cystinuria will suffer recurrent stone disease during their lifetimes. Whereas normal individuals daily excrete 20 mg or less of cystine in their urine, stone-forming cystinuric patients excrete more than 250 mg/day. Cystine solubility increases when urine pH exceeds 7.0; therefore, an alkaline urine pH must be maintained 24 hours per day, even while the patient sleeps. This is almost always achieved with the use of medication; however, in the past dietary changes have been recommended to change urine pH (see *Clinical Insight:* "Acid Ash" and "Alkaline Ash" Diets). Fluid intake of more than 4 L daily is recommended to prevent cystine crystallization. Lower sodium intake may be useful in reducing cystine in urine.

Methionine is the metabolic precursor of cystine. Severe protein restriction to avoid methionine is impractical, but avoidance of excess may be beneficial. D-Pencillamine is commonly used as a cystine-binding agent to treat cystinuria. The cysteine-pencillamine product is 50 times more soluble than cystine itself.

Diet and fluid modification should be advocated as a first step for the prophylaxis of kidney stone disease to improve the urinary risk profile and reduce recurrence. These modifications, summarized in Table 39-14, are simple, economical, and without side effects.

CLINICAL INSIGHT

"Acid Ash" and "Alkaline Ash" Diets

Dietary intake can influence the acidity or alkalinity of the urine (Sherman and Gettler, 1912). The acid-forming potential is contributed by chloride, phosphorus, and sulfur (anions) and the base-forming potential by sodium, potassium, calcium, and magnesium (cations). Before the use of medication to acidify or alkalinize the urine, dietary changes were commonly used.

In general, fruits and vegetables contribute alkaline "ash" to the urine, except in the case of prunes, plums, and cranberries. These fruits contain benzoic and quinic acids that are excreted in the urine as hippuric acid.

High-protein foods (meat, fish, poultry, eggs, and cheese) and breads and cereals are the primary contributors of acid "ash." Milk contributes to both categories. However, because factors of digestion, absorption, use of salt or medications, hormonal status, and homeostatic mechanisms all affect renal excretion and urine production, urine pH cannot be predicted by calculation of intake. Such information can be obtained only by direct measurement of the urine (Dwyer et al, 1985).

The following food lists serve as a guide to influencing urine pH.

Potentially Acid or Acid-Ash Foods

Meat:	Meat, fish, fowl, shellfish, eggs, all types of cheese, peanut butter, peanuts
Fat:	Bacon, nuts (Brazil nuts, filberts, walnuts)
Starch:	All types of bread (especially whole-wheat), cereal, crackers, macaroni, spaghetti, noodles, rice
Vegetables:	Corn, lentils
Fruits:	Cranberries, plums, prunes
Desserts:	Plain cakes, cookies

Potentially Basic or Alkaline-Ash Foods

Milk:	Milk and milk products, cream, buttermilk
Fat:	Nuts (almonds, chestnuts, coconut)
Vegetables:	All types (except corn, lentils), especially beets, beet greens, Swiss chard, dandelion greens, kale, mustard greens, spinach, turnip greens
Fruit:	All types (except cranberries, prunes, plums)
Sweets:	Molasses

Neutral Foods

Fats:	Butter, margarine, cooking fats, oils
Sweets:	Plain candies, sugar, syrup, honey
Starches:	Arrowroot, corn, tapioca
Beverages:	Coffee, tea

Modified from Pemberton CM et al: *Mayo Clinic diet manual*, ed 6, Toronto, 1988, BC Decker.

TABLE 39-14 Recommendations—Diet, 24-Hour Urine Monitoring

DIET COMPONENT	INTAKE RECOMMENDATION	24-HOUR URINE
Protein	Normal intake: avoid excess	Monitor urinary urea
Calcium	Normal intake: 1000 mg age ≤age 50 years 1200 mg age >age 50 years	Urinary calcium <150 mg/L (<3.75 mmol/L)
Oxalate	Avoid moderate- to high-oxalate foods initially; further restrict if necessary	Urinary oxalate <20 mg/L (<220 umol/L)
Fluids	2.5 L or more; assess type of fluids consumed; provide guidelines	Urine volume >2 L/day
Purines	Avoid excessive protein intake; avoid specific high-purine foods	Uric acid <2 mmol/L (<336 mg/L)
Vitamin C	<2 g/day	Monitor urinary oxalate
Vitamin D; cod liver oil	Supplements not recommended	
Vitamin B_6	40 mg or more/day reduces risk No recommendation made	
Sodium	<100 mmol/day	Monitor urinary sodium

Clinical Scenario 1: Hemodialysis

Mark is a 36-year-old man with a history of drug abuse and cocaine addiction. Recently, he was admitted to the local hospital with acute renal failure and has been started on hemodialysis. He has no prior medical problems or hypertension. His laboratory values include BUN, 90; creatinine, 7; potassium, 6.1; all other laboratory values are currently normal. He is 6 ft 2 in. and weighs 190 lb.

1. What would you suggest for the dialysis nutrition prescription?
2. His physician suggests daily use of a multivitamin supplement containing B-complex vitamins but not the fat-soluble vitamins. Why?
3. What level of protein would you suggest for Mark during dialysis? How much should Mark receive in the way of protein foods?
4. If he goes home without dialysis but has chronic renal failure, what might his doctor suggest for a protein level?
5. What foods will be monitored, according to the National Renal Diet?

SUMMARY

Renal diseases are very complex and often silent in origin. With the increasing incidence of type 2 diabetes and its association with chronic and end-stage renal disease, the incidence of renal disease is also expected to increase.

Early detection of renal deterioration or risk factors for renal stone disease should result in appropriate referrals to specialists. These specialist teams will include nutrition professionals who are familiar with the complex nature of therapy for renal disease and who will play important roles in the management of these patients.

Relevant Web Sites

American Dietetic Association (source of the National Renal Diet)
www.eatright.org
Life Options
www.lifeoptions.org
National Institute of Diabetes and Digestive and Kidney Diseases (NIDDKD)
www.niddk.nih.gov/health/kidney/kidney.htm
National Kidney Foundation
www.kidney.org
Nationwide End-Stage Renal Network
www.esrdnetwork.org
Northwest Kidney Center (source of "The Art of Good Eating," a free workbook for people on dialysis)
www.nwkidney.org
Renal Network
www.renalnet.org

Clinical Scenario 2: Peritoneal Dialysis

Kelsey is a 33-year-old woman with glomerulonephritis who has been on dialysis 8 years. Current laboratory values are the following:

Na: 135	K: 5.9	CO_2: 16
Creat: 9	Ca: 8.7	PO4: 6.9
Alb: 3.4	Ferritin: 82	Wt: 57.2 kg
Ht: 172	Fluid gains: 2.9-3.7 kg	BUN: 70
AMA: <50%	AFA: >8%	

1. Explain why you would expect to see each of the laboratory value discrepancies and what could be done nutritionally to affect each value. Also assess the patient's weight and anthropometric values to determine appropriate nutritional therapy.
2. Kelsey takes the following medications: erythropoietin (EPO), Benadryl, folic acid, prednisone, Nephrocaps, Basaljel, and Tums. The patient dialyzes against the following dialysate fluid: 3 mEq K, 3.5 mg calcium, 35 mEq bicarbonate, 200 g dextrose. Comment on the appropriateness of each. For what are they used? Would you suggest any changes or additional medications?
3. The patient is currently awaiting a cadaveric transplant. She asks you how her diet will change with the transplant. If the transplant does not happen soon, she is considering peritoneal dialysis to give her more freedom from the machine. What would be the nutritional concerns if this were to happen?

Cited References

Andress DL: Aluminum-associated bone disease in chronic renal failure: high prevalance in the long-term dialysis population, *J Bone Miner Res* 1:391, 1986.

Avorn J et al: Reduction of bacteriuria and pyuria after ingestion of cranberry juice, *JAMA* 271:751, 1994.

Bataille P et al: Diet, vitamin D, and vertebral mineral density in hypercalciuric calcium stone formers, *Kidney Int* 39:1193, 1991.

Beto J: Highlights of the consensus conference on prevention of progression in chronic renal disease: implications for dietetic practice, *J Renal Nutr* 4:122, 1994.

Blagg C et al: Serum albumin concentration: HCFA quality assurance criterion is method-dependent, *Am J Kidney Dis* 21:139, 1993.

Borghi L et al: Urinary volume, water, and recurrence in idiopathic calcium nephrolithiasis: a 5-year randomized prospective study, *J Urol* 155:839, 1996.

Borghi L et al: Urine volume: stone risk factor and preventive measure, *Nephron* 81(suppl):31, 1999.

Borghi L et al: Comparison of two diets for the prevention of recurrent stones in idiopathic hypercalciuria, *N Engl J Med* 346:77, 2002.

Brenner BM, Lazarus JM, editors: *Acute renal failure,* ed 2, New York, 1988, Churchill-Livingstone.

Coburn JW, Norris KC: Diagnosis of aluminum-related bone disease and treatment of aluminum toxicity with desferoxamine, *Semin Nephrol* 4:12, 1986.

Curhan GC et al: A prospective study of dietary calcium and other nutrients and the risk of symptomatic kidney stones, *N Engl J Med* 328:833, 1993.

Curhan GC et al: Comparison of dietary calcium with supplemental calcium and other nutrients as factors affecting the risk for kidney stones in women, *Ann Int Med* 126:497, 1997.

Curhan GC et al: Intake of vitamins B6 and C and the risk of kidney stones in women, *J Am Soc Nephol* 10:840, 1999.

Curhan GC, Willet WC, Rim EB: A prospective study of the intake of vitamins C and B_6 in men, *J Urol* 155:1847, 1996.

Eschbach J et al: Correction of the anemia of end-stage renal disease with recombinant human erythropoietin, *N Engl J Med* 316:73, 1987.

Fine RN et al: Growth after recombinant human growth hormone treatment in children with chronic renal failure: report of a multicenter randomized double-blind placebo-controlled study, *J Pediatr* 124:324, 1994.

Gerster H: No contribution of ascorbic acid to renal calcium oxalate stones, *Ann Nutr Metab* 41:269, 1997.

Giannini S et al: Acute effects of moderate dietary protein restriction in patients with idiopathic hypercalcuiria and calcium nephrolithiasis, *Am J Clin Nutr* 69:267, 1999.

Giordano C: Early diet to slow the course of chronic renal failure. In Zurukzoglu W, Papadimetrious M, editors: *Eighth International Congress of Nephrology, June 1981,* Basel, 1981, S Karger.

Goldfarb DS, Asplin JR: Effect of grapefruit juice in urinary litnogenicity, *J Urol* 166:263, 2001.

Goldfarb DS, Coe FL: Beverages, diet and prevention of kidney stones, *Am J Kidney Dis* 33:398, 1999a.

Goldfarb DS, Coe FL: Prevention of recurrent urolithiasis, *Am Fam Physician* 60:2269, 1999b.

Hricik DE et al: Glomerulonephritis, *N Engl J Med* 339:888, 1998.

Holmes RP, Goodman HO, Assimos DG: Contribution of dietary oxalate to urinary oxalate excretion, *Kidney Int* 59:270, 2001.

Howell A et al: Inhibition of the adherence of P-fimbriated Escherichia coli to uroepithelial-cell surface by proanthocyanidin extracts from cranberries *[Letter], N Engl J Med* 339:1085, 1998.

Jones CH et al: The relationship between serum albumin and hydration status in hemodialysis patients, *J Ren Nutr* 12:209, 2002.

Kaysen G: Nutritional management of nephrotic syndrome. In Kopple JD, Massery SG, editors: *Nutritional management of renal disease,* Baltimore, 1997, Williams & Wilkins.

Klahr S: The effects of dietary protein restriction and blood pressure control on the progression of chronic renal disease, *N Engl J Med* 330:877, 1994.

Kocvara R et al: A prospective study of nonmedical prophylaxis after a first kidney stone, *BJU Int* 84:393, 1999.

Ma KW et al: Cardiovascular risk factors in chronic renal failure and hemodialysis populations, *Am J Kid Dis* 19:505, 1992.

Martini LA: Stop dietary calcium restriction in kidney stone-forming patients, *Nutr Rev* 60:212, 2002.

Martini LA, Wood RJ: Should dietary calcium and protein be restricted in patients with nephrolithiasis? *Nutr Rev* 58:111, 2000.

Massey LK, Roman-Smith H, Sutton RAL: Modification of dietary oxalate and calcium reduces urinary oxalate in hyperoxaluric patients with kidney stones, *J Am Diet Assoc* 93:1305, 1993.

Melton LS et al: Fracture risk among patients with urolithiasis: a population-based cohort study, *Kid Int* 53:459, 1998.

Molina M: Nutrition support in the patient with renal failure, *Crit Care Clin* 11:685, 1995.

Mitch WE: Nutritional therapy for the nephrotic syndrome. In Brenner BM, editor: *The kidney,* ed 5, vol 2, Philadelphia, 1996, WB Saunders.

Morton AR, Iliescu EA, Wilson JW: Nephrology. 1. Investigation and treatment of recurrent kidney stones, *Can Med Assoc J* 166:213, 2002.

National Kidney Foundation (NKF): DOQI clinical practice guidelines for nutrition in chronic renal failure, *Am J Kidney Dis* 35(suppl 2), 2000.

Nguyen QY et al: Sensitivity to meat protein intake and hyperoxaluria in idiopathic calcium stone formers, *Kidney Int* 59:2273, 2001.

Oldenburg B: Factors influencing excessive thirst and fluid intakes in dialysis patients, *Dialys Transplant* 17:21, 1988.

Olsham AR et al: Intradialytic parenteral nutrition administration during outpatient hemodialysis, *Dialysis Transplantation* 16:495, 1987.

Owen W et al: The urea reduction ratio and serum albumin concentration as predictors of mortality in patients undergoing hemodialysis, *N Engl J Med* 329:1001, 1993.

Pastan S, Bailey J: Dialysis therapy, *N Engl J Med* 339:1428, 1998.

Pedrini, MT: The effect of dietary protein restriction on the progression of diabetic and nondiabetic renal diseases: a meta-analysis, *Ann Intern Med* 124:627, 1996.

Pennell JP: Optimizing medical management of patients with pre–end-stage renal disease, *Am J Med* 111:559, 2001.

Perez N: Managing nutrition problems in transplant patients, *Nutr Clin Pract* 8(1):28, 1993.

Remuzzi G, Bertani T: Pathophysiology of progressive nephropathies, *N Engl J Med* 339:1448, 1998.

Rotily M et al: Effects of protein or high-fibre diets on urine composition in calcium nephrolithiasis, *Kidney Int* 57:1115, 2000.

Schiller LR et al: Effect of the time of administration of calcium acetate on phosphorous binding, *N Engl J Med* 320:1110, 1989.

Schiro-Harvey K: *The national renal diet,* ed 2, Chicago, 2002, American Dietetic Association.

Seltzer MA et al: Dietary manipulation with lemonade to treat hypocitraturic calcium nephrolithiasis, *J Urol* 156:907, 1996.

Sherman HC, Gettler AO: The balance of acid forming and base forming elements in food and its relation to ammonia metabolism, *J Biol Chem* 11:323, 1912.

Sherman RA et al: Interdialytic weight gain and nutrition parameters in chronic hemodialysis patients, *Am J Kidney Dis* 25:579, 1995.

Smith LH, Robertson WG, Finlayson B, editors: *Urolithiasis: clinical and basic research,* New York, 1981, Plenum Press.

Terris MK, Issa MM, Tacker JR: Dietary supplementation with cranberry concentrate tablets may increase the risk of nephrolithiasis, *Urology* 57:26, 2001.

Toto RD: Treatment of dyslipipedemia in chronic renal failure, lipid abnormalities in patients with renal failure, *Blood Purif* 14:75, 1996.

Traxer O et al: Stone forming risk of ascorbic acid, *J Endourol* 14(suppl 1):A9, 2000.

van der Heide JJH et al: Effect of dietary fish oil on renal function and rejection in cyclosporine-treated recipients of renal transplants, *N Engl J Med* 329:769, 1993.

Wiggins K: *Guidelines for nutritional care of renal patients,* ed 3, Chicago, 2002, American Dietetic Association.

Wiggins KL, Schiro-Harvey K: A review of guidelines for nutrition care of renal patients, *Ren Nutr* 12:190, 2002.

■ Additional References

Brinkley LJ, Gregory J, Pak CYC: A further study of oxalate bioavailability in foods, *J Urol* 144:94, 1990.

Curhan GC et al: Beverage use and risk for kidney stones in women, *Ann Int Med* 128: 534, 1998.

Ebisuno S et al: Results of long term rice bran treatment on stone recurrence in hypercalciuric patients, *Br J Urol* 67:237, 1991.

Evanoff GV et al: Effect of dietary protein restriction on the progression of diabetic nephropathy, *Arch Intern Med* 147:492, 1987.

Hruska KA, Teitelbaum SL: Renal osteodystrophy, *N Engl J Med* 333:166, 1995.

Jones, CA: Low-calcium diet not supported for treatment of renal calculi, *The Integrative Medicine Consult* 4:25, 2002.

Kopple JD: History of dietary protein therapy for the treatment of chronic renal disease from the mid 1800s until the 1950s, *Am J Nephrol* 22:278, 2002.

Kopple JD and National Kidney Foundation K/DOQI Work Group: The National Kidney Foundation K/DOQI clinical practice guidelines for dietary protein intake for chronic dialysis patients, *Am J Kidney Dis* 4(suppl 1):S68, 2001.

Krieger JN et al: Dietary and behavioural risk factors for urolithiasis: potential implications for prevention, *Am J Kidney Dis* 28:195, 1996.

Martini LA et al: Potassium and sodium intake and excretion in calcium stone forming patients, *J Renal Nutr* 8(3):127, 1998.

Mitch W: *Nutrition and the kidney,* ed 3, Baltimore, 1998, Lippincott Williams & Wilkins.

Patel C: *Cultural foods and renal diets for the clinical dietitian,* 2002. Available from Council on Renal Nutrition of Northern California and Northern Nevada, 2002, 1542 Queenstown Court, Sunnyvale, Calif 94087.

Pearle MS: Prevention of nephrolithiasis, *Curr Opin Nephrol Hypertens* 10:203, 2001.

Renal nutrition education materials: an annotated bibliography. Available free from National Kidney and Urologic Diseases Advisory Board, Box NKUDIC, 9000 Rockville Pike, Bethesda, Md 20892; (301) 468-6345.

Rutchik SD, Resnich MI: Cystine calculi: diagnosis and management, *Urol Clin North Am* 24:163, 1997.

Scott P et al: Suggestive evidence for a susceptibility gene near the vitamin D receptor locus in idiopathic calcium stone formation, *J Am Soc Nephrol* 10:1007, 1991.

Sowers MRF et al: Prevalence of renal stones in a population-based study with dietary calcium, oxalates, and medication exposures, *Am J Epidemiol* 147:914, 1998.

Wiggins K, Wilkens K, editors: *Suggested guidelines for nutrition care of renal patients,* ed 3, Chicago, 2002, American Dietetic Association.

■ Resources

The following resources can be ordered by contacting the American Dietetic Association, 216 W Jackson Boulevard, Suite 800, Chicago, IL 60606:

Schiro-Harvey K: *National renal diet,* Chicago, 2002, American Dietetic Association.

Stover J: *A clinical guide to nutrition care in end stage renal disease,* ed 2, Chicago, 1994, American Dietetic Association.

The following resources can be obtained from the National Kidney Foundation, 30 East 33rd Street, New York, NY, 10016:

Educational Resource Directory: *A directory of patient, public and professional educational materials,* New York, 2001, National Kidney Foundation. Also available from NKF Affiliates, National and Local Professional Councils.

McCann L: *The pocket guide to nutritional assessment of renal patients,* ed 3, New York, 2002, National Kidney Foundation.

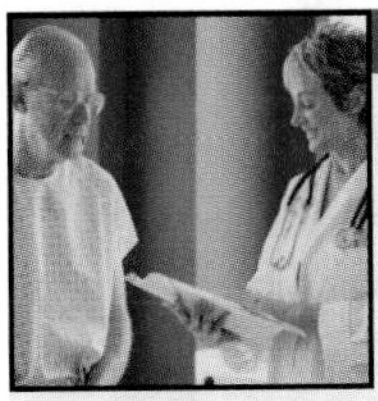

CHAPTER 40

Medical Nutrition Therapy for Cancer Prevention, Treatment, and Recovery

BARBARA ELDRIDGE, MS, RD, LD

CHAPTER OUTLINE

- Diagnosis and Medical Treatment
- Nutrition in the Etiology of Cancer
- Nutritional Implications of Cancer
- Nutritional Implications of Cancer Therapy
- Nutritional Care of Adults Diagnosed With Cancer
- Nutritional Care of Children Diagnosed With Cancer
- Complementary and Alternative Therapies

KEY TERMS

ageusia–loss or absence of the sense of taste

allogeneic marrow transplantation–transfer of marrow from a donor to another person (often a relative, such as a sibling) who is not genetically identical

antineoplastic agents–chemical agents (cytotoxics, immunologic preparations, hormones) or medications used to prevent the development, maturation, or spread of neoplastic cells

antioxidants–molecules, such as some vitamins, that block action of activated oxygen molecules (free radicals) that can damage cells

autologous marrow transplantation–transfer of marrow from the patient's own tissue (from hematopoietic stem cells)

cancer–abnormal division and reproduction of cells that can spread throughout the body, crowding out normal cells and tissues

cancer cachexia–weight loss and lessening of the body's fat and muscle stores that accompanies advanced cancer, even with adequate nutrition

carcinogen–an agent (physical, chemical or viral) that induces cancer in humans and animals

carcinogenesis–the origin or development of cancer; a multistage, biologic process that proceeds on a continuum but is often described in stages of initiation, promotion, and progression

case-control studies–studies in which the diets of individuals with cancer are compared with those of cancer-free controls matched for age, sex, and other key factors

cohort studies–studies in which diets of different groups of subjects are determined before cancer onset and the incidences of developing cancers in each group are compared

cross-sectional studies–studies in which the diets of different groups of subjects are compared, using the same measures at a single point in time

cytokines–protein mediators produced by inflammatory cells in response to exogenous stimuli

dysgeusia–impaired taste

graft-versus-host disease (GVHD)–a disease caused by the immune response of histoincompatible, immunocompetent donor cells against the tissues of an immunoincompetent host; an immunologic reaction of allogeneic donor cells (graft) reacting against the patient (host) tissues

hypogeusia–decreased taste acuity

Revision of chapter previously written by Carol B. Frankmann, MS, RD, LD, CNSD.

KEY TERMS—Continued

initiation–the initial stage of tumorigenesis, involving transformation of cellular DNA

malignant neoplasm–mass of cancer cells that invades surrounding tissues or spreads to distant areas of the body

metastasis–growth of malignant tissue that spreads to surrounding tissues or organs

myelosuppression–suppression of bone marrow cell production

neoplasm–a new and abnormal formation of tissue that serves no useful function

neutropenia–a reduction in white blood cell count (neutrophils) that can be caused by chemotherapy or radiation therapy and that, in turn, results in increased susceptibility to potentially life-threatening infections

pancytopenia–a reduction in all cellular elements of the blood

phytochemicals–nonnutritive compounds in plants thought to influence the process of tumorigenesis

progression–the phase in which tumor cells aggregate, grow autonomously, and form benign tumors that eventually lead to a malignant phenotype with the capacity for tissue invasion and metastasis

promotion–the stage of tumorigenesis in which initiated cells are activated by a promoting agent to multiply and form a discrete tumor

radiation-induced enteritis–a condition of inflammation that can occur after radiation to the intestinal tract and that leads to diarrhea and malabsorption

staging–a classification system known as *TNM* that is used to identify the "extent" of the tumor: its size, the degree of growth and spread; *T* stands for the size of the tumor, *N* for the degree of spread to lymph nodes, and *M* for the presence of metastasis

tumor necrosis factor (cachectin)–a hormone-like protein that releases fat from fat stores, reduces the concentration of enzymes required for the production and storage of fat, and induces a state of anorexia

veno-occlusive disease (VOD)–a symptomatic occlusion of the small hepatic venules caused by hepatotoxins and radiation therapy; may resolve after removal of the offending agent or may progress to portal hypertension and liver failure

xerostomia–mouth dryness

Cancer can be regarded as a disease of the body's cells. Its development involves damage to the DNA of cells; this damage accumulates over time. When these damaged cells escape the mechanisms in place to protect the organism from the growth and spread of such cells, a neoplasm is established. Classification of tumors is based on their tissue of origin, their growth properties, and their invasion of other tissues. The growth of a malignant neoplasm usually destroys surrounding tissue and may eventually spread to distant tissues and organs, a process known as metastasis.

Because cancer occurs in cells that are replicating, the patterns of cancer are quite different in children and adults. In early life, the brain, nervous system, bones, muscles, and connective tissue are still growing. Thus in children, these tissues are more commonly involved with cancerous lesions than they are in adults. Conversely, the common adult tumors involve epithelial linings and are rare in children. Leukemias and lymphomas, which are tumors of the immune system, occur in both children and adults, but the natural history of the disease differs depending on whether they occur early or late (*Food, Nutrition, and the Prevention of Cancer,* 1997).

The study of diet and nutrition as it relates to cancer addresses the causes and the consequences of cancer and its treatment. Carcinogenesis is thought to be a multistage process that proceeds on a continuum but is often described in three progressive phases: initiation, promotion, and tumor progression. Initiation involves a transformation of the cell produced by the interaction of chemicals, radiation, or viruses with cellular DNA. The transformation occurs rapidly, but the resultant cell remains dormant for a variable period until it is activated by a promoting agent. During promotion, initiated cells multiply to form a discrete tumor. From there, progression proceeds, leading eventually to a fully malignant neoplasm with the capacity for tissue invasion and metastasis (Figure 40-1).

DIAGNOSIS AND MEDICAL TREATMENT

Cancer diagnosis can be determined by several methods, including physical examination, blood tests (nonspecific tests and specific markers such as CA-125 or PSA levels), cytology studies and tumor biopsy, imaging (x-rays, CT, MRI, PET scans), and staging (radiographic, pathologic, surgical, or TNM staging for tumor size, nodes, metastasis). Intent of treatment may include cure, control, palliation, or adjuvant therapy. Treatment response is documented as complete, partial, stable, or progressive.

Although the exact mechanisms are unknown, nutrition may modify the carcinogenic process at any stage, including carcinogen metabolism, cellular and host defense, cell differentiation, and tumor growth. Nutrition itself is also adversely affected, both by the

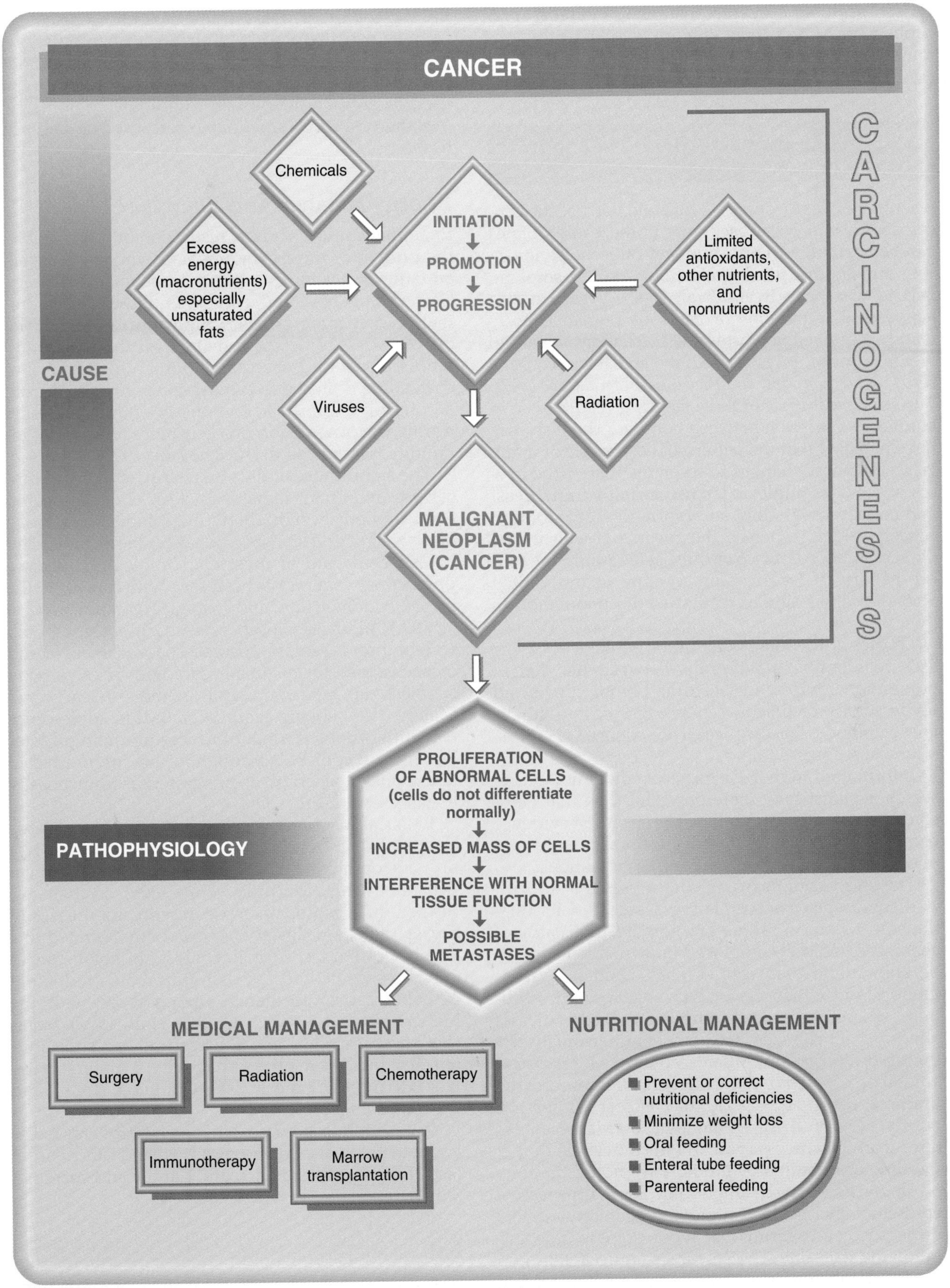

FIGURE 40-1 • Pathophysiology algorithm: carcinogenesis. (Algorithm content developed by John Anderson, PhD, and Sanford C. Gardner, PhD, 2000.)

cancer itself and by the treatment modality prescribed (including chemotherapy, radiation therapy, and surgery).

NUTRITION IN THE ETIOLOGY OF CANCER

Scientific evidence suggests that one third of the cancer deaths that occur each year in the United States can be attributed to nutrition and other lifestyle factors, and another third is related to cigarette smoking and tobacco use (Byers et al, 2002). Evidence also suggests that millions of cases of human cancers could be prevented worldwide by changes in eating, weight control, physical activity, and tobacco usage (*Food, Nutrition, and the Prevention of Cancer,* 1997). The strong influence of these factors is readily seen in studies of migration between cultures. These studies have revealed that the pattern of occurrence of many types of cancer changes to resemble that of the new country. For example, in Japan, mortality from breast and colon cancer is low, and mortality from stomach cancer is high, whereas the reverse is true in the United States. After two or three generations, the cancer pattern of Japanese immigrants to the United States becomes similar to that of the population in their new country.

Studies of the role of diet in the etiology of cancer seek to identify relationships between the diet of population groups and categories of individuals and the incidence of specific cancers. Sets of individuals are compared in case control, cohort, or cross-sectional studies.

Information from these forms of epidemiologic research is statistically more powerful than that gathered from population studies. The strongest evidence comes from consistent findings from different types of epidemiologic studies in diverse populations.

The sheer complexity of diet presents a difficult challenge when contemplating a study of its relationship to cancer. There are literally thousands of chemicals in a diet, some well known; others are little known and unmeasured. Diets contain both inhibitors and enhancers of carcinogenesis. In addition, when one major component of the diet is altered, other changes take place simultaneously. For example, decreasing animal protein also decreases animal fat. This makes the interpretation of research findings difficult because the effects cannot be clearly associated with a single factor. Many cancers have a long latency period, in which case the diet at the time of initiation or promotion—not at the time of diagnosis—may be important. Some prospective epidemiologic studies attempt to circumvent this difficulty by measuring diet at one point in time and following the same subjects for several years.

Studies done with laboratory animals are used to test the effect of food and nutrition on cancer. Since the early part of this century, laboratory scientists have shown that various nutritional manipulations influence the occurrence of tumors in animals. In concert with epidemiologic work, animal studies can be used to provide hypotheses to guide epidemiologic research and reveal modifiable pathways to cancer in humans.

Energy Balance and Exercise

In animal studies, chronic restriction of food inhibits the growth of most experimentally induced cancers and the occurrence of many spontaneous cancers. This effect is observed even when the underfed animals ingest more fat than the controls ingest. The degree of effect depends mainly on the extent and timing of caloric restriction and the tumor type. Underfeeding is most effective when maintained during all phases; if limited to one phase, caloric restriction during the progression phase is more effective in inhibiting tumor growth (Kritchevsky, 1997).

The significance of data on energy intake and cancer risk in humans remains unclear. The relationship between body weight, body mass index, or relative body weight and site-specific cancer has been widely investigated, and in most epidemiologic studies, a positive association has been seen with cancers of the breast, endometrium, and kidney (Trentham-Dietz et al, 1997). In breast cancer, a positive association with weight gain is seen in postmenopausal women, and increased risk for disease occurs with relative body leanness in premenopausal women (Cleary and Maihle, 1997; Huang et al, 1997). BMI in adolescence has implications for risk of cancer mortality in later life; measures of BMI throughout life are needed to determine the period of greatest risk from obesity (Okasha et al, 2002.)

Physical inactivity, high energy intake, and large body mass are associated with an increased risk of developing colon cancer in men and women (Kushner, 2002; Martinez et al, 1997). Conversely, the benefit of regular exercise in reducing the risk of breast and colon cancer has been demonstrated in a number of studies. A metaanalysis of colon cancer and physical activity levels found a 50% reduction in colon cancer incidence among those with the highest level of activity (Colditz et al, 1997). Comprehensive reviews of the literature also substantiate that increased physical activity is inversely related to breast cancer risk (Gammon, John, and Britton, 1998).

In addition to exercise, ongoing controversy exists about the type of calories consumed and cancer onset (see *New Directions:* Pancreatic Cancer and Intake of Starchy Foods).

Fat

Some experimental and epidemiologic data also show a link between some cancers and the amount of fat in the diet. Geographic variations in the incidence and mortality of cancers of the breast, colon, lung, and prostate suggest that high fat intake of both total fat and saturated or animal fat may be related to an increased risk of these cancers (*Food, Nutrition, and the Prevention of Cancer,* 1997). Diets high in fat also tend to be high in calories and contribute to obesity, which in turn is associated with increased risk of cancers at several sites, including the colon and rectum, esophagus, gall bladder, breast (among postmenopausal women), endometrium, pancreas, and kidney (renal cell) (Byers et al, 2002; *Food, Nutrition, and the Prevention of Cancer,* 1997). Because dietary fat intake is correlated with intake of other nutrients and dietary components, it is difficult to distinguish between the effects of dietary fats and protein, total calories, and fiber. A complex interaction of fat with these or other factors may account for inconsistent results of epidemiologic and experimental investigations. For example, several studies have shown that a high consumption of red meats and dairy products is associated with increased risk of prostate cancer (Byers et al, 2002).

Protein

Understanding the role of protein in cancer development is complicated by the fact that most diets high in protein are also high in meat and fat and low in fiber. The effect of protein on experimental carcinogenesis depends on the tissue of origin and the type of tumor as well as on the type of protein and the caloric adequacy of the diet. In general, tumor development is suppressed by diets that contain levels of protein below that required for optimal growth, whereas it is enhanced by protein levels two to three times the amount that is required. The effects may be attributable to specific amino acids, a general effect of protein, or, in the case of low-protein diets, depressed food intake. Epidemiologic data are limited and conflicting. However, increased meat intake has been found to be associated with an increased risk of colon cancer (Potter, 1996) and with advanced prostate cancer (Michaud et al, 2001.)

Because animal studies demonstrate that certain amino acid deficiencies inhibit some tumors, the feeding of amino acid–deficient diets or amino acid antagonists has been proposed as an adjunct to cancer therapy. Although this hypothesis has theoretical appeal, no active clinical research in this area exists currently.

Fiber

Early studies focused much attention on the possible protective role of fiber in preventing cancer of the colon, rectum, breast, and ovaries. Most studies of the relationship between fiber and cancer have measured fiber-rich foods or total dietary crude fiber rather than fiber components. The intake of dietary fiber influences the intake of meat, fat, and refined carbohydrates as well as a number of nutrients and nonnutrients with identified impact on cancer risk.

A number of observational and case-control studies indicate that fiber-rich diets are associated with a protective effect in colon cancer; however, the role of genetics must also be considered. Higher intakes of vegetables were associated inversely with colon cancer risk in one case control study; however, the association with dietary fiber was limited to proximal tumors in older subjects (Slattery et al, 1997). Although the association between fiber and cancer risk remains inconclusive (Fuchs et al, 1999; Schatzkin et al, 2000), consumption of high-fiber foods should still be recommended because of their overall health benefit (lowering heart disease risk) and because they contain other substances that contribute to cancer risk reduction (Byers et al, 2002).

Fruits and Vegetables

A comprehensive review of epidemiologic studies examined the relationship between fruit and vegetable intake and the incidence of cancer and found a

NEW DIRECTIONS

Pancreatic Cancer and Intake of Starchy Foods

Evidence from both animal and human studies suggests that abnormal glucose metabolism plays an important role in pancreatic carcinogenesis. In a cohort of U.S. women (88,802) in the Nurses' Health Study, 180 case subjects with pancreatic cancer were diagnosed during 18 years of follow-up (Michaud et al, 2002.) A food-frequency questionnaire was used to calculate sucrose, fructose, and carbohydrate intakes; glycemic index (postprandial blood glucose response as compared with a reference food); and glycemic load (glycemic index multiplied by carbohydrate content). Carbohydrate and sucrose intake were not associated with overall pancreatic cancer risk. Associations of glycemic load and fructose intakes with pancreatic cancer risk were apparent among women with elevated body mass index (25 kg/m^2) or with low physical activity; impaired glucose metabolism may play a role in pancreatic cancer etiology. A diet high in glycemic load may increase the risk of pancreatic cancer in women who already have an underlying degree of insulin resistance.

statistically significant protective effect in 128 of 156 dietary studies (Block et al, 1992). Increased consumption of fruits and vegetables has been shown to be associated with a lower risk of cancers of the oral cavity, esophagus, stomach, colon, rectum, and bladder (Byers et al, 2002; *Food, Nutrition, and the Prevention of Cancer,* 1997). Evidence is less strong for hormone-related cancers such as breast and prostate cancer (Byers et al, 2002).

Epidemiologic investigators report that consumption of the following groups and types of vegetables and fruits is comparatively low in those who subsequently develop cancer: raw and fresh vegetables, leafy green vegetables, cruciferous vegetables (i.e., broccoli and cabbage), lettuce, carrots, and raw and fresh fruit. Other data suggest that foods high in phytoestrogens—particularly soy—or high in precursor compounds that can be metabolized by gut bacteria into active agents, such as grains and vegetables with woody stems that contain lignans, may be associated with a lower risk of sex hormone–related cancers (Potter and Steinmetz, 1996). Consumption of flavonoids, including soybeans, is thought to contribute to the low incidence of hormone-dependent cancers in Asian countries (Le Marchand, 2002.)

Generally, fruits and vegetables are low in energy and are good sources of fiber, vitamins, minerals, and biologically active substances. Examples of these substances (anticarcinogenic agents) that are found in fruits and vegetables include antioxidants such as vitamins C and E, selenium, and phytochemicals, such as carotenoids, flavonoids, plant sterols, allium compounds, indoles, phenols, and terpenes (see Chapter 12). At this time, which specific substances of fruits and vegetables that are protective against cancer is unclear (Byers et al, 2002). To most effectively reduce cancer risk, the American Cancer Society states that the best advice at present is to consume these substances through food sources rather than supplements (Byers et al, 2002).

Most of the data for the anticarcinogenic potential of all of these substances has been derived from animal and in vitro studies (Craig, 1997; Potter and Steinmetz, 1996). These agents have both complementary and overlapping mechanisms of action, including the induction of detoxification enzymes, inhibition of nitrosamine formation, provision of substrate for formation of antineoplastic agents, dilution and binding of carcinogens in the digestive tract, alteration of hormone metabolism, and antioxidant effects. It appears extremely unlikely that any one substance is responsible for all of the observed associations.

Chemoprevention

Cancer chemoprevention seeks to reverse carcinogenesis in the premalignant phase. Recent experimental evidence indicates that vitamin and mineral deficiencies can lead to DNA damage (Ames and Wakimoto, 2002). Studies have been directed at reversing precancerous lesions, preventing disease in populations at high risk for recurrent or new disease, and reducing the incidence of specific tumors in the general population. Several large-scale, randomized, intervention trials have examined the effects of vitamin and mineral supplementation, with mixed results.

A study in Finland of male smokers who received either α-tocopherol, β-carotene, both, or placebo revealed a 16% higher incidence of lung cancer associated with β-carotene supplementation (ATBC Cancer Prevention Study Group, 1994). A second large study (CARET) of β-carotene and lung cancer also revealed negative effects (Omenn et al, 1996). In both of these studies, heavy alcohol intake appeared to increase the negative effects. The Physician's Health Study found neither increased risk nor benefit from β-carotene supplementation after 12 years of follow-up studies in patients with lung cancer; however, only 11% of the group studied were current smokers (Hennekens et al, 1996). Overall, findings from these β-carotene supplementation trials have been unexpected, and other carotenoids have been studied as a result. Lower risks of lung cancer are observed for the highest versus the lowest quintiles of lycopene (28%), lutein/zeaxanthin (17%), β-cryptoxanthin (15%), total carotenoids (16%), serum β-carotene (19%), and serum retinol (27%), thus suggesting that high fruit and vegetable consumption, particularly a diet rich in carotenoids, tomatoes, and tomato-based products, may reduce the risk of lung cancer (Holick et al, 2002.)

Two large studies were conducted in Linxian, China, to test the effects of vitamin and mineral supplements on cancer incidence in an area that has one of the highest esophageal and gastric cancer mortality rates in the world and a diet low in micronutrients. After 5 years, the group that received two to three times the RDA for β-carotene, vitamin E, and selenium showed significant reduction in mortality due to cancer, especially stomach cancer. No significant effect on mortality was observed for other supplement regimens (Blot, 1994; Blot et al, 1993). A recent investigation found that calcium supplementation is associated with a moderate reduction in the risk of recurrent colorectal adenomas (Baron et al, 1999).

Chemoprevention is also an active area of clinical research that holds promise for patients with cancers commonly associated with recurrence, such as head and neck cancers, as well as for identified high-risk populations, such as former smokers with bronchial metaplasia. The development of second primary tumors is a major cause of treatment failure in patients with head and neck cancers treated in an early stage. Early clinical trials with isotretinoin, a retinoid, decreased the incidence of recurrence; however, significant side effects prevented one third of the patients from completing the treatment (Hong et al, 1990).

Subsequent studies have identified doses that reduce toxicity and show mixed results in reducing recurrence of disease. Trials with precursor lesions are more promising. Antioxidant compounds have been shown to be effective in reversing oral leukoplakia, precursor lesions with a high rate of transformation to malignant disease.

In 2001, the National Cancer Institute began the Selenium and Vitamin E Cancer Prevention (SELECT) Trial to determine whether selenium and vitamin E can prevent prostate cancer. SELECT, which plans to randomize 32,000 men and to follow them for 7 to 10 years, was undertaken in part because of the findings of two studies on the prevention of other cancers. The results of these studies suggested that selenium and vitamin E supplementation might prevent prostate cancer (Clark, 1996; Eichholzer et al, 1996). Another study, the Alpha Tocopheral Beta Carotene (ATBC) Cancer Prevention Study, also suggested the beneficial effect of vitamin E supplementation in prostate cancer risk reduction (Heinonen et al, 1998). To date, chemoprevention studies are in a developmental stage, with no agent showing clear efficacy in reducing incidence or improving survival. However, examples of new studies under development include the following agents: peigallacatechin gallate (green tea) and curcumin, folic acid (Berwick and Schantz, 1997), as well as genistein (soy) and lycopene (tomatoes).

Alcohol

Epidemiologic studies indicate that alcohol has a causal role in carcinogenesis, especially for cancers of the mouth, pharynx, larynx, esophagus, lung, colon, rectum, liver, and breast (*Food, Nutrition, and the Prevention of Cancer,* 1997; U.S. DHHS, 2000). Alcohol appears to have an increased effect on those tissues directly exposed to it during its consumption and tends to act synergistically with tobacco (Marshall and Boyle, 1996). The malnutrition associated with alcoholism is also likely to be important in the increased risk for certain cancers in the alcoholic individual.

Alcohol, especially beer consumption, has been associated with an increased risk for colorectal cancer in a number of studies. The positive relationship between alcohol intake and breast cancer risk has been documented repeatedly, and this correlation may be caused by alcohol-induced increases of endogenous estrogen levels, reduction of folic acid levels, or the direct effect of alcohol or its metabolites on breast tissue (Hunter and Willett, 1996; Smith-Warner et al, 1998).

Coffee and Tea

Coffee intake has been investigated as a possible risk factor for a variety of cancers. Regular consumption of coffee or tea has no significant relationship with the risk of cancer at any site. In fact, studies indicate that regular drinking of green tea and other sources of polyphenols may reduce the risk of stomach cancer (Owuor and Kong, 2002).

Consumption of very hot drinks has been associated with an increased risk of esophageal cancer (Cheng and Day, 1996; Sharp et al, 2001). An association between coffee consumption and pancreatic cancer has been widely publicized, but its carcinogenic effect has not been confirmed by other studies (Byers et al, 2002).

Artificial Sweeteners

Artificial sweeteners have been investigated primarily in relation to bladder cancer. In 1970, cyclamate was banned from use as a food additive in the United States based on the results of a study that demonstrated a significant increase in bladder tumors in rats fed a mixture of cyclamate and saccharin at doses up to 2500 mg/kg/day (Renwick, 1990). During the next 15 years, several intensive reviews were completed. To date, the manufacturer's petition to resume use is pending (FDA, 2002).

The weight of evidence from metabolic studies, short-term tests, animal bioassays, and epidemiologic studies indicates that cyclamate itself is not carcinogenic; however, evidence from in vitro and in vivo studies in animals implies that it may have cancer-promoting or co-carcinogenic activities. Epidemiologic studies indicate that no measurable overall increase in the risk of bladder cancer has been noted in individuals who have used the nonnutritive sweeteners cyclamate and saccharin.

Current evidence does not support a link between aspartame use and increased risk of cancer (Byers et al, 2002), and clinical studies have shown no ill effect in humans who consume large doses (Newberne and Conner, 1986). Epidemiologic data are not available because approval for use is relatively recent.

Nitrates, Nitrites, and Nitrosamines

Nitrates and nitrites have received attention because of their relationship with nitrosamines, which are potent carcinogens in various species. Nitrate can be readily reduced to nitrite, which in turn can interact with dietary substrates, such as amines and amides, to produce N-nitroso compounds, or nitrosamines and nitrosamides. This conversion, known as *N-nitrosation,* has been demonstrated to occur in saliva, as well as in the stomach, colon, and bladder. Diets with high amounts of fruits and vegetables contain vitamin C and phytochemicals that can retard the conversion of nitrites to nitrosamines (Byers et al, 2002).

Nitrates are present in a variety of foods, but the main dietary sources are vegetables and drinking water. Sodium and potassium nitrates are used in the processes of salting, pickling, and curing foods; they also give hot dogs and luncheon meat their pink color. Nitrosamines are present in tobacco and tobacco smoke. Some epidemiologic studies have linked high consumption of processed meat to an increased risk of cancers of the colon, rectum, and stomach (Byers et al, 2002).

Method of Food Preparation

Studies have shown a possible increased cancer risk posed by the formation of polycyclic aromatic hydrocarbons and hetrocyclic amines when high-heat cooking methods such as grilling, broiling, barbecuing, and smoking of meats are used (Wu et al, 2001; *Food, Nutrition, and the Prevention of Cancer,* 1997). These toxic substances are formed during combustion of carbon fuel and pyrolysis of protein. Several investigators have found mutagenic activity in foods after frying and charcoal broiling. Healthier cooking alternatives for meats include boiling, poaching, steaming, stewing, braising, baking, microwaving, and roasting.

Case-control and limited cohort studies suggested that a high salt intake is associated with an increased risk for stomach cancer (Kono and Hirohata, 1996). However, more recent studies question that relationship (Nakaji et al, 2001). Consumption of fruits and vegetables appears to provide a protective effect (Hirohata and Kono, 1997).

Dietary Recommendations for Cancer Prevention

The National Cancer Institute and the Committee on Diet and Health, the Food and Nutrition Board of the National Research Council, and the American Institute for Cancer Research have recommended diet and lifestyle practices that may contribute to cancer prevention. In addition, the recently updated guidelines of the American Cancer Society consist of four recommendations for individual choices (Byers et al, 2002). These recommendations include (1) eating a variety of healthful foods, with an emphasis on plant sources (eating five or more servings of a variety of vegetables and fruits, choosing whole grains, and limiting consumption of red meats); (2) adopting a physically active lifestyle; (3) achieving and maintaining a healthy body weight throughout life; and (4) limiting consumption of alcoholic beverages. In addition, the American Cancer Society presents one key recommendation—community action—which underscores the importance of community measures to support healthy behaviors by increasing access to healthful food choices and opportunities to be physically active (Byers et al, 2002).

Studies indicate that adults who strongly believe in a diet-cancer connection decrease the percentage of energy derived from fat and increase their fiber intake. Perceived ease of eating a healthful diet is a strong predictor of intake (Harnack et al, 1997). Despite recommendations from numerous health agencies for Americans to consume at least five servings of fruits and vegetables daily, consumption remains low.

These findings challenge dietetic professionals to design diet and health promotion programs that address the barriers to dietary change and educate people about the relationship of diet to health. The importance of diet and lifestyle changes is evident in recommendations from the American Institute for Cancer Research (AICR), as well. Box 40-1 summarizes recommendations for cancer prevention; Table 40-1 summarizes the benefit versus harm of existing scientific evidence regarding nutrition and physical activity for cancer prevention.

Box 40-1. American Institute for Cancer Research Diet and Health Guidelines for Cancer Prevention

1. Choose a diet rich in a variety of plant-based foods.
2. Eat plenty of vegetables and fruits.
3. Maintain a healthy weight and be physically active.
4. Drink alcohol only in moderation, if at all.
4. Select foods low in fat and salt.
6. Prepare and store food safely.

And always remember . . . Do not use tobacco in any form.

From American Institute for Cancer Research: Simple steps to prevent cancer, Washington, DC, 2000, AJCR.

NUTRITIONAL IMPLICATIONS OF CANCER

The adverse nutritional effects of cancer can be severe and may be compounded by the effects of the treatment regimens and the psychological impact of cancer. The result is often a profound depletion of nutrient stores. Significant weight loss and poor nutritional status were documented in more than 50% of patients at the time of diagnosis (McMahon, Decker, and Ottery, 1998) and are associated with lower scores on quality-of-life measures (O'Gorman et al, 1998). In early studies, even small amounts of weight loss (less than 5% of body weight) before therapy were associated with a poor prognosis, thus reinforcing the importance of early nutritional assessment and intervention as a preventive measure. Data imply a relationship between nutritional status and the outcome of malignant disease (Figure 40-2).

TABLE 40-1 The American Cancer Society Workgroup Grades for Benefit vs. Harm—Nutrition and Physical Activity for Cancer Prevention

American Cancer Society Guidelines Committee Grades for Benefit vs. Harm

To review the strength of the scientific evidence, a guidelines subcommittee used a method of summarizing the evidence similar to the methods used by other expert panels. For example, the U.S. Preventive Services Task Force judged the scientific evidence related to clinical preventive services with a system that considered both the source and strength of the evidence: from at least one controlled clinical trial, from good uncontrolled trials, from multiple good observation studies, expert opinion, and case reports. They then characterized those guidelines on a five-point grading scheme as to the strength of the guideline: "good for recommending, fair for recommending, insufficient to recommend for or against, fair for not recommending, good for not recommending." The AICR-World Cancer Research Fund project summarized the nature of the scientific evidence for nutritional factors in cancer prevention as being either "Convincing, Probable, Possible, or Insufficient." The American Cancer Society subcommittee employed a method similar to that of both groups. For each issue, the committee judged the likelihood of benefit to the general public as follows:

A1 Convincing evidence for a benefit
A2 Probable benefit
A3 Possible benefit
B Insufficient evidence to conclude benefit or risk
C Evidence of lack of benefit
D Evidence of harm

NUTRITIONAL FACTOR	COLORECTAL CANCER	BREAST CANCER	PROSTATE CANCER	LUNG CANCER	ORAL, ESOPHAGEAL CANCER	STOMACH CANCER	PANCREATIC CANCER	BLADDER CANCER	ENDOMETRIAL CANCER
Increasing vegetable and fruit intake	A2	A3	A3	A2	A2	A2	A3	A3	A3
Limiting intake of red meats	A2	B	A3	B	B	C	A3	C	B
Increasing physical activity	A1	A1	B	B	B	B	B	B	A2
Avoiding overweight	A1	A1	C	B	A2	C	A3	C	A1
Limiting alcohol intake	A3	A2	C	B	A1	C	A3	C	B
Consuming soy foods	B	B	B	B	B	B	B	B	B
Taking β-carotene supplements	B	B	C	D	B	B	B	B	B
Taking vitamin E supplements	B	B	A3	C	B	B	B	B	B
Taking vitamin C supplements	B	B	B	B	B	B	B	B	B
Taking folic acid supplements	A3	A3	B	B	B	B	B	B	B
Taking selenium supplements	A3	B	A3	A3	B	B	B	B	B

From Byers T et al: American Cancer Society's Guidelines on nutrition and physical activity for cancer prevention: reducing the risk of cancer with healthy food choices and physical activity, *CA Cancer J Clin* 52:92, 2002.

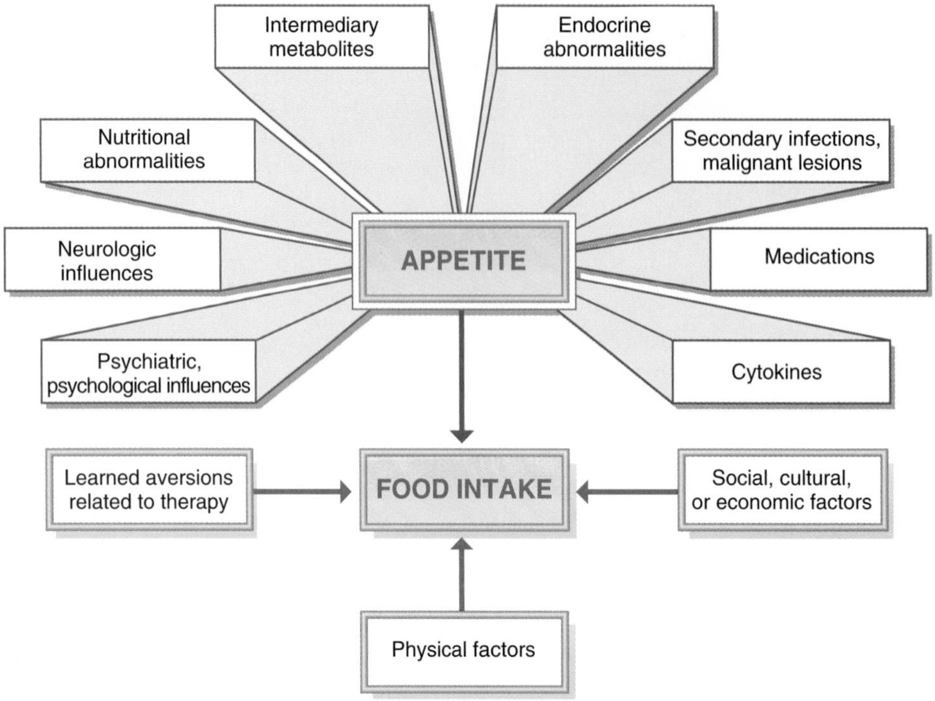

FIGURE 40-2 • Factors that affect appetite, an especially important consideration in cancer patients. (Reference: American Institute for Cancer Research: *Food, nutrition, and prevention of cancer: a global perspective,* Washington, DC, 1997, AICR.)

Cancer Cachexia

A common secondary diagnosis in patients with advanced neoplastic disease is a variant of protein-energy malnutrition. This syndrome is termed cancer cachexia and is characterized by progressive weight loss, anorexia, generalized wasting, immunosuppression, altered basal metabolic rate, and abnormalities in fluid and energy metabolism. The etiology of this complex metabolic derangement is not entirely understood and can manifest in patients with metastatic disease as well as in patients with localized disease. Recent work has focused on the role of cytokines, which, through broad physiologic actions, produce metabolic changes and wasting in the tumor-bearing host that are similar but not identical to those seen in sepsis and inflammation.

Cytokines that are thought to play a role in cancer cachexia include tumor necrosis factor (TNFα and TNTβ (cachectin), interleukin-1, interleukin-6, and interferon-γ. These cytokines have overlapping physiologic activities, which makes it likely that no single substance is the sole cause of cancer cachexia (Matthys and Billiau, 1997; Tisdale, 1997). A pool of anticytokine antibodies or other cytokine inhibitors might be considered as a potential intervention for the treatment of cachectic patients. Trials with single agents and metabolic inhibitors (pentoxyfylline and hydrazine sulfate) have failed to show benefit (Ottery et al, 1998). Administration of thalidomide, an inhibitor of tumor necrosis factor–α, has resulted in weight gain in patients with human immunodeficiency virus (HIV) (Haslett, 1998), but when administered at therapeutic doses, it may cause significant and incapacitating drowsiness.

Pharmaceutical Management of Anorexia-Cachexia Syndrome

A number of pharmacologic agents are under investigation in the management of the anorexia-cachexia syndrome and cancer-related weight loss, including the use of appetite stimulants, metabolic agents and cytokine blockers, prokinetic agents, and anabolic agents (Murphy and Von Roenn, 2000; Von Roenn, 2002) (Box 40-2).

A number of well-designed trials have shown improved appetite and increased energy intake and body weight in cancer patients treated with megestrol acetate, a progestational agent (Ottery et al, 1998). The benefits of megesterol acetate on appetite and weight have been shown to be dose-dependent with greater benefit at higher doses (Murphy and Von Roenn, 2000). Numerous uncontrolled trials indicate that corticosteroids require escalating doses to maintain increased appetite and that improvement in appetite is short-lived and does not translate into weight gain.

Prolonged use of corticosteroids is also associated with negative side effects such as osteoporosis, fluid retention, adrenal suppression, glucose intolerance, electrolyte imbalance, or even arm and leg muscle wasting. Growth hormones have been studied in patients with wasting associated with HIV, but few data are available regarding their use with cancer cachexia and anorexia. In summary, the pharmacologic management of cachexia and anorexia requires careful

Box 40-2. Pharmacologic Agents for Anorexia-Cachexia Syndrome and Weight-Loss Management

Appetite Stimulants

- Megesterol acetate
- Dronabinol
- Corticosteroids

Metabolic Agents and Cytokine Blockers

- Melatonin
- Pentoxifyline
- Hydrazine sulfate
- Eicospentaenoic acid (EPA)

Prokinetic Drugs

- Metaclopramide

Anabolic Agents

- Growth hormone
- Oxandralone
- Nandrolone

Data from Von Roenn JH: Pharmacologic interventions for cancer-related weight loss, *Oncology Issues* 17(suppl):20, 2002; and Murphy S and Von Roenn JH: Pharmacological management of anorexia and cachexia. In McCallum PD, Polisena CG, editors: *The clinical guide to oncology nutrition,* Chicago, 2000, American Dietetic Association.

evaluation based upon the patient's treatment goals and prognosis and upon close monitoring of symptoms and prescribed medications that may interfere with adequate intake (Murphy and Von Roenn, 2000). Ideally, these agents are prescribed in combination with nutritional counseling and physical activity assessment and evaluation.

Energy Metabolism

In chronic starvation, the metabolic rate is reduced as the body adapts to conserve energy and preserve body tissue. However, in comparison with control groups, cancer patients have been reported to have reduced, normal, or increased energy expenditure. The difference in findings is most likely a result of the stages of illness and of nutritional status among the subjects, differing because of methods used in accurately measuring acutely ill individuals. Studies that used indirect calorimetry have shown increased resting energy expenditure (REE) in individuals with some—but not all—tumor types (Dickerson et al, 1995; Gadduci et al, 2001; Jatoi et al, 2001).

In a study of patients with lung cancer, hypermetabolism and weight loss were associated with enhanced levels of inflammatory mediators and acute-phase proteins (Staal van den Brekel et al, 1995). One study of the impact of malignant disease on REE revealed that REE returned to normal levels in patients with lung cancer after curative surgery (Fredrix et al, 1991).

Substrate Metabolism

Energy metabolism is intimately related to carbohydrate, protein, and lipid metabolism, all of which are altered by tumor growth. Tumors exert a consistent demand for glucose. Neoplastic cells exhibit a characteristically high rate of anaerobic metabolism and yield lactate as the end product. This expanded lactic acid pool requires an increased rate of host gluconeogenesis via Cori cycle activity, which is increased in some patients with cancer but not in others. Both protein breakdown and lipolysis take place at increasing rates to maintain high rates of glucose synthesis. A relative state of insulin resistance, characterized by excess fatty acid oxidation and decreased uptake and use of glucose, especially in muscle, may develop (Puccio and Nathanson, 1997).

Alterations in protein metabolism appear to be directed toward providing adequate amino acids for tumor growth. Most notable is the loss of skeletal muscle protein; however, visceral organ atrophy and hypoalbuminemia also occur. Abnormalities of protein metabolism include inappropriate elevations in whole-body protein turnover and increases in skeletal muscle protein synthesis, catabolism, and liver protein synthesis. These changes occur in the presence of reduced nitrogen intake, thus suggesting inability to adapt to diminished protein intake by reducing protein turnover.

Albumin synthesis rates appear to be similar to those in healthy individuals (Fearon et al, 1998); hypoalbuminemia occurs because of increased total body water associated with cancer cachexia, which is more pronounced than the increase in albumin synthesis (Langstein and Norton, 1991).

Lipid metabolism is altered, as evidenced by inappropriate mobilization of free fatty acids from adipose tissues and subsequent depletion of total body fat. Disorders may also be seen in the form of decreased lipid clearance from serum and elevated plasma free fatty acid levels. Supporting evidence suggests that tumors produce lipolytic substances that are directly responsible for increased fat mobilization (Langstein and Norton, 1991).

Other Metabolic Abnormalities

Fluid and electrolyte imbalances are seen in patients with advanced cancer. Hypercalcemia may be seen in bone-metastasizing tumors of the breast, lung, and pancreas as well as in nonmetastatic tumors that induce parathyroid hormone–like peptides. Health care professionals concur that dietary calcium should not be restricted in hypercalcemic patients.

Severe imbalances in fluid and electrolyte status may be present in patients with cancers that promote excessive diarrhea or vomiting. Severe diarrhea can result from tumors that secrete serotonin (carcinoid syndrome), calcitonin, or gastrin (Zollinger-Ellison syndrome). Persistent vomiting is associated with intestinal obstruction or intracranial tumors.

The activities of several enzyme systems can be affected, as can certain endocrine functions. The nature of the alterations varies by tumor type. The patient's immunologic function can be impaired, apparently as the result of both the neoplasm and progressive malnutrition. In addition to the cancer-induced metabolic effects, the mass of the tumor may anatomically alter the normal physiology of specific organ systems.

Sensory Changes

Alterations in taste and smell are common, and they can contribute to the anorexia commonly seen in patients with cancer. Studies of taste sensitivity in malignant disease have shown variable results. Taste alterations are associated with the disease, certain antineoplastic agents, and irradiation or surgery of the head and neck. Chemotherapy-induced, learned taste aversions have been reported in both adults and children.

Patients may also experience a heightened sense of smell that results in sensitivity to food preparation odors and aversions to nonfood items such as soaps or perfumes. Dietary interventions that decrease the aroma of foods, such as serving foods cold instead of hot, may be helpful (Ottery, 1996; Paserot et al, 1997). These sensation abnormalities do not consistently correlate with the tumor site, extent of tumor involvement, tumor response to therapy, or food preferences and intake.

NUTRITIONAL IMPLICATIONS OF CANCER THERAPY

Goals of Nutritional Care

Whether the patient is newly diagnosed, undergoing active therapy, recovering from treatment, or in remission and trying to prevent cancer recurrence, nutrition is an important component of the care and management. The goals of nutrition intervention in cancer are to prevent or reverse nutrient deficiencies, to preserve lean body mass, to minimize nutrition-related side effects, and to maximize the quality of life (Eldridge et al, 2001).

Conventional modalities of cancer treatment include chemotherapy, immunotherapy, radiation therapy, and surgery used alone or in combination. In addition, solid tumors and hematologic malignant diseases such as leukemias, lymphomas, multiple myelomas can be treated by bone marrow or peripheral blood stem cell transplantation. Cancer and its treatment can impact nutritional needs significantly and can affect digestion, absorption, and metabolism. Symptoms with a nutritional impact include nausea and vomiting, changes in taste and smell, bowel changes, dysphagia, anorexia, pain, and fatigue. Table 40-2 describes symptoms that have a nutritional impact.

TABLE 40-2A Nutrition Impact of Cancer Therapies: Chemotherapy

CHEMOTHERAPEUTIC AGENTS	COMMON NUTRITION IMPACT SYMPTOMS
Cytotoxic	
Alkylating agents (cisplatin, ifosfamide, cyclophosphamide, busulfan)	Myelosuppression, anorexia, nausea, vomiting, fatigue, renal toxicities
Antibiotics (doxorubicin, mitomycin, bleomycin)	Myelosuppression, anorexia, nausea, vomiting, fatigue, diarrhea, mucositis
Antimetabolites (5-Fluorouracil, methotrexate, fludarabine)	Myelosuppression, anorexia, nausea, vomiting, fatigue, diarrhea, mucositis
Antimitotic agents (vincristine, vinorelbine, paclitaxel, docetaxel)	Myelosuppression, anorexia, nausea, vomiting, diarrhea, mucositis; fatigue, peripheral neuropathy
Hormonal	
Glucocorticoids (prednisone, dexamethasone)	Sodium and fluid retention, GI upset, glucose intolerance, potassium wasting, osteoporosis
Antiandrogens (flutamide)	Nausea, diarrhea, hot flashes
Antiestrogens (tamoxifen citrate)	Nausea, bone pain, fluid retention, hot flashes, hypercalcemia
Progestins (megesterol acetate)	Increased appetite, weight gain, fluid retention, hypercalcemia
Gonadotropin-releasing hormone analog (leuprolide)	Nausea, bone pain
Immunologic—Biologic Response Modifers	
Interferon alfa	Myelosuppression, anorexia, nausea, vomiting, flulike symptoms
Interleukin	Myelosuppression, nausea, vomiting, hypotension, chills, fatigue, capillary leak syndrome
Monoclonal antibodies (rituximab, trastuzumab)	Myelosuppression, nausea, vomiting, fever, chills, rash
Immunologic—Hematopoietic	
Epoetin alpha (erthropoietin, EPO)	Fever; iron supplementation may be necessary
Filgastim (granulocytic colony-stimulating factor, G-CSF)	Fever, bone pain, flulike symptoms
Sargramostin (granulocytic macrophage-stimulating factor, GM-CSF)	Fever, bone pain, flulike symptoms

Data in Tables 40-2 A-C from Eldridge B: Chemotherapy and nutritional implications. In McCallum PD, Polisena CG, editors: *The clinical guide to oncology nutrition,* Chicago, 2000, The American Dietetic Association; Eldridge B et al: Nutrition and the patient with cancer. In Coulston AM, Rock CL, Monsen ER, editors: *Nutrition in the prevention and treatment of disease,* San Diego, 2001, Academic Press; Polisena CG: Nutrition concerns with the radiation therapy patient. In McCallum RD, Polisena CG, editors: *The clinical guide to oncology nutrition,* Chicago, 2000, American Dietetic Association; Common Toxicity Criteria: Version 2.0 (Publish Date: April 30, 1999). www.ctep.info.nih.gov/2002; Allison G et al: Nutrition implications of surgical oncology. In McCallum PD, Polisena CG, editors: *The clinical guide to oncology nutrition,* Chicago, 2000, American Dietetic Association; and reviewed by James Byron, RPh, BCOP.

TABLE 40-2B Nutrition Impact of Cancer Therapies: Radiation

SITE OF RADIATION THERAPY	COMMON NUTRITION IMPACT SYMPTOMS
Central nervous system (brain and spinal cord)	Acute effects: Nausea, vomiting Elevated blood glucose caused by steroid administration Fatigue Loss of appetite Late effects (>90 days after treatment): Headache, lethargy
Head and neck area (tongue, larynx, pharynx, oropharynx, nasopharynx, tonsils, salivary glands)	Acute effects: Xerostomia Sore mouth and throat Dysphagia, odynophagia Mucositis Alterations in taste and smell Fatigue Loss of appetite Late effects (>90 days after treatment): Mucosal—atrophy and dryness, ulceration Salivary glands—xerostomia, fibrosis Osteoradionecrosis Trismus Alterations in taste and smell
Thorax (esophagus, lung, breast)	Acute effects: Dysphagia, odynophagia Heartburn Fatigue Loss of appetite Late effects (>90 days after treatment): Esophageal—fibrosis, stenosis, necrosis Cardiac—angina on effort, pericarditis, cardiac enlargement Pulmonary—dry cough, fibrosis, pneumonitis
Abdomen and pelvis	Acute effects: Nausea, vomiting Changes in bowel function—diarrhea, cramping, bloating, gas Changes in urinary function—increased frequency, burning sensation with urination Acute colitis or enteritis Lactose intolerance Fatigue Loss of appetite Late effects (>90 days after treatment): Diarrhea, malabsorption, maldigestion Chronic colitis or enteritis Intestinal—stricture, ulceration, obstruction, perforation, fistula Urinary—hematuria, cystitis

TABLE 40-2C Nutrition Impact of Cancer Therapies: Surgery

ANATOMIC SITE	COMMON NUTRITION IMPACT SYMPTOMS
Oral cavity	Difficulty with chewing and/or swallowing Aspiration potential Sore mouth Xerostomia Alterations in taste and smell
Larynx	Alterations in normal swallowing, dysphagia Aspiration potential
Esophagus	Gastroparesis Indigestion and/or acid reflux Alterations in normal swallowing, decreased motility Anastomotic leak
Lung	Shortness of breath Early satiety
Stomach	Dumping syndrome Dehydration Early satiety Gastroparesis Fat malabsorption Vitamin and mineral malabsorption (vitamins B_{12} and D; calcium, iron)
Gallbladder and bile duct	Gastroparesis Hyperglycemia Fluid and electrolyte Fat malabsorption Vitamin and mineral malabsorption (vitamins B_{12}, A, D, E, and K; magnesium, zinc, calcium, iron)
Hepatocellular	Hyperglycemia Hypertriglyceridemia Fluid and electrolyte imbalance Vitamin and mineral malabsorption (vitamins A, D, E, K, and B_{12}; folic acid, magnesium, zinc)
Pancreas	Gastroparesis Fluid and electrolyte imbalance Hyperglycemia Fat malabsorption Vitamin and mineral malabsorption (vitamins A, D, E, K, and B_{12}; calcium, zinc, iron) Chyle leak
Small bowel	Lactose intolerance Bile acid depletion Diarrhea Fluid and electrolyte imbalance Vitamin and mineral malabsorption (vitamins B_{12}, A, D, E, and K; calcium, iron, zinc)
Colorectal	Increased transit time Diarrhea Dehydration Bloating, cramping, and/or gas Fluid and electrolyte imbalance Vitamin and mineral malabsorption (vitamin B_{12}; sodium, potassium, magnesium, calcium)
Gynecologic	Early satiety Bloating, cramping, and/or gas
Brain	Nausea and vomiting If taking corticosteroids, possible hyperglycemia

Common Nutrition Impact Symptoms of Cancer Therapies

Chemotherapy

Chemotherapy is the use of chemical agents or medications to treat cancer. Whereas surgery and radiation therapy are used to treat localized tumors, chemotherapy is a systemic therapy that affects the whole body. The target of action of chemotherapeutic agents is not limited to malignant tissue; it affects normal cells as well. Cells of the body with a rapid turnover such as bone marrow, hair follicles, and the mucosa of the alimentary tract are typically the most affected. Commonly experienced nutrition impact symptoms include myelosuppression, fatigue, nausea and vomiting, loss of appetite, mucositis, changes in taste and smell, xerostomia, dysphagia, and changes in bowel function (see Table 40-2, *A*). As a result, dietary intake and nutritional status can be adversely affected.

The severity of the side effects depends on the specific agent, dosage, duration of treatment, accompanying drugs, individual response, and current health status. The timely and appropriate use of supportive therapies such as antiemetics, antidiarrheals, hematopoietic agents, and antibiotics, as well as dietary changes, are important to the effective management of treatment-related side effects. The reality is that despite the supportive care, many patients still experience significant side effects, especially in "dose-intensive" chemotherapy regimens, and neutropenia and myelosuppression are the primary limiting factors for their administration.

Taste abnormalities lead to anorexia and oligophagy (eating few foods). Diarrhea, constipation, or adynamic ileus (inhibition of bowel motility) may occur. Symptoms of gastrointestinal toxicity are usually not long-lasting; however, some multiagent chemotherapy regimens have severe and prolonged gastrointestinal effects.

Some agents, especially corticosteroids, can cause tissue breakdown and promote excessive urinary loss of protein, potassium, and calcium. The intestinal mucosa and digestive processes are affected, thus altering digestion and absorption to some degree. Protein, energy, and vitamin metabolism may be impaired, although the consequences of this are not known. Total lymphocyte count is depressed and does not accurately reflect nutritional status after antineoplastic agent administration.

Radiation Therapy

Radiation therapy can be delivered externally into the body from a linear accelerator or a cobalt unit or internally by placing a radioactive source (implant) directly inside the body or next to the tumor to deliver a highly localized dose. Whereas chemotherapy is a systemic therapy, radiation therapy affects only the tumor and the surrounding area. The side effects of radiation therapy are usually limited to the specific site being irradiated. Chemotherapy agents may also be given in combination with radiation therapy to produce a radiation-enhancing effect. Patients receiving multimodality therapy often experience more toxic side effects sooner.

When used alone, acute side effects of radiation therapy generally begin around the second or third week of treatment and usually resolve within 2 to 4 weeks after the radiation therapy has been completed. Late effects of radiation therapy may occur several weeks, months, or even years after treatment. Regardless of the area being irradiated, commonly experienced nutrition impact symptoms include fatigue, loss of appetite, skin changes, and hair loss in the area being treated (see Table 40-2, *B*).

Radiation to the head and neck can cause a variety of acute nutrition impact symptoms, including sore mouth, altered taste and smell, dysphagia and odynophagia, mucositis, and xerostomia. Anorexia, fatigue, and weight loss are common in these patients (Hunter, 1996). Current multimodality protocols for treatment of head and neck cancer that utilize chemotherapy and surgery, as well as radiation therapy, should not be used without aggressive supportive care, including enteral nutrition (Mekhail et al, 2001). Late effects of therapy may include dental caries, permanent xerostomia, trismus (lockjaw), and osteoradionecrosis.

Nutrition impact symptoms of radiation therapy to the thorax can include heartburn and acute esophagitis characterized by dysphagia and odynophagia. Late effects include possible esophageal fibrosis and stenosis. When this occurs, patients are generally only able to swallow liquids; esophageal dilations and other means of nutrition support (enteral nutrition) may be necessary to meet nutritional needs.

Radiation therapy to the abdomen may produce acute gastritis or enteritis accompanied by nausea, vomiting, diarrhea, and anorexia. Late effects can include severe gastrointestinal damage that is manifested by malabsorption of disaccharides, fats, and electrolytes. Radiation-induced enteritis can develop into a chronic form of the condition, with symptoms of ulceration or obstruction intensifying the risk of malnutrition. Chronic radiation enteritis combined with massive bowel resection, which results in extensive bowel dysfunction, is called *short bowel syndrome.* The severity of this condition depends on the length and location of the nonfunctional or resected bowel; it is generally diagnosed when the individual has less than 150 cm of remaining small intestine. The sequelae include maldigestion, malabsorption, malnutrition, dehydration, and potentially lethal metabolic aberrations.

Initially, total parenteral nutrition (TPN) is required, and frequent monitoring of fluids and electrolytes may be required for weeks or months. The diet may need to be restricted to defined formula tube feedings or to frequent small meals that are high in complex carbohydrate and protein, low in fat and oxalate, and lactose-free. Medications can be given to decrease intestinal motility. Multivitamin supplements that include vitamin B_{12}; folic acid; and vitamins A, E, and K should be given to prevent deficiencies. Serum concentrations of various minerals should be monitored and adjusted as needed.

Total-body radiation used in bone marrow transplantation protocols may cause all of the aforementioned acute symptoms to some extent.

Surgery

The surgical resection or removal of any part of the alimentary tract—as well as the malignant disease process itself—can impair digestion and absorption significantly. Surgery may be used as the only mode of cancer treatment, or it may be combined with preoperative or postoperative adjuvant chemotherapy or radiation therapy. After surgery, additional energy and protein are required for wound healing and recovery. Commonly experienced nutrition impact symptoms include some degree of fatigue, pain, loss of appetite, and changes in normal eating. Most side effects are temporary and dissipate after a few days following the surgery. However, some surgical interventions have long-lasting nutritional implications. See Table 40-2, *C*, for common nutrition impact symptoms associated with specific surgical interventions for the treatment of cancer.

Patients with head and neck cancer often have impaired mastication and swallowing caused by the tumor mass or the specific surgical intervention required. These patients also present additional problems because of their frequent history of smoking, chronic alcohol use, and poor oral intake. Surgery often necessitates temporary or permanent reliance on enteral nutrition, including percutaneous endoscopic gastrostomy or nasogastric tube feedings. Patients who resume oral intake often have prolonged dysphagia and require modifications of food consistency and extensive training in chewing and swallowing (Meikhail et al, 2001). Referrals to a speech therapist can yield dramatic positive results through evaluation and individualized instruction in swallowing and positioning techniques.

Surgical treatment of esophageal tumors may require partial or total removal of the esophagus. The stomach is commonly used for esophageal reconstruction. A feeding nasojejunostomy or jejunostomy tube can be placed at the time of surgery, permitting early postoperative tube feedings. Usually, the patient is able to progress to oral intake with specific dietary recommendations to minimize nutrition impact symptoms, which include dumping syndrome, gastroparesis, early satiety, and fluid and electrolyte imbalances. Postsurgical dietary recommendations include the intake of a low-fat diet with small, frequent feedings of nutrient-dense foods and avoidance of large amounts of fluids at any time (Grant et al, 1996). New research studies support the use of glutamine-enriched tube-feeding formulas or glutamine supplementation to aid in healing after gastrointestinal surgery (see Chapters 23 and 29).

Total gastrectomy commonly leads to malnutrition secondary to reduced dietary intake and malabsorption. Placement of a jejunostomy feeding tube at surgery is advisable, and enteral nutrition support is generally feasible within a few days after surgery. Fat intolerance may be experienced, especially if the vagus nerves are severed. Administration of pancreatic enzymes with meals may be beneficial for patients for whom the mixing of food and pancreatic juices is inadequate.

When partial gastrectomy is the lower segment of the stomach, dumping syndrome is possible as a result of the rapid transit of foods or liquids (especially those high in simple carbohydrate content) and the dilutional response of the small remaining stomach to highly osmotic bolus feedings. The most common nutrition impact symptom is anemia secondary to malabsorption of iron, folate, and—less commonly—vitamin B_{12} (Grant et al, 1996). Patients may benefit from consumption of six to eight small meals per day, with fluids taken between meals.

Pancreatic cancer, with its attendant surgical resection, has significant nutritional consequences. When more than 70% of the pancreas is removed, insulin is required to regulate glucose metabolism, and a carbohydrate-controlled diet may be warranted. Up to 90% of the pancreas must be removed before clinical symptoms of malabsorption result. Pancreatic enzyme replacement may be used to aid digestion and absorption, and a fat-restricted diet may be indicated (Grant et al, 1996).

Partial or total colectomies may induce profound losses of fluid and electrolytes, the severity of which is related to the length and site of the resection. Resections of as little as 15 cm of the terminal ileum can result in bile salt losses that exceed the liver's capacity for resynthesis, and vitamin B_{12} absorption is affected. With depletion of the bile salt pool, steatorrhea develops. Calcium carbonate should be administered orally to minimize oxalate absorption (Grant et al, 1996). Nutritional support consists of a diet low in fat, osmolality, lactose, and oxalate (see Chapter 30).

Most studies estimate energy requirements to be 1.3 to 1.5 times the basal energy expenditure (BEE) and protein needs to be 1.5 g/kg/day. Increased needs may be observed in children and patients with severe stress, fever, or intestinal losses. Some investigators report that the use of supplemental glutamine in patients who are receiving TPN improves clinical outcome, as evidenced by fewer infections and shortened hospital stays; its use promots lymphocyte recovery (Ziegler et al, 1998).

Immunotherapy

Biologic response modifiers are natural products that are made in quantities through cloning and genetic engineering. Used directly as cytotoxic agents or indirectly as stimulators of the patient's own natural defenses, biologic agents can kill tumor cells. Alpha-interferon is used to treat hairy-cell leukemia. Interleukin-2 is used in the treatment of patients with melanoma and renal cell carcinoma.

Immunotherapy also includes supportive care agents (hematopoietics) such as colony-stimulating factors—cytokines that stimulate the marrow to develop faster—that are used to shorten periods of neutropenia for patients and to enrich the graft for myeloid precursors before harvest of marrow from donors (Isola et al, 1997). Patients in whom these agents are used may experience fatigue, chills, fever, flulike symptoms, and decreased food intake (see Table 40-2, *A*).

Bone Marrow Transplantation

Bone marrow transplantation is performed for the treatment of certain hematologic malignant diseases, such as leukemia and lymphoma, and for solid tumors. The preparative regimen includes cytotoxic chemotherapy, with or without total-body irradiation, to suppress immunological reactivity and eradicate malignant cells. This treatment regimen is followed by intravenous infusion of bone marrow or peripheral stem cells from the patient (autologous) or from a histocompatible related or unrelated donor (allogeneic). With improved tissue typing—resulting from DNA techniques and several million donors worldwide—allogeneic marrow transplantation from an unrelated donor has become a clinical option for many patients who would not previously have been candidates for marrow transplantation (Ringden, 1997) (Figure 40-3).

Bone marrow and stem cell transplant procedures can significantly affect nutrition status. A thorough nutrition assessment—including a comprehensive evaluation of nutrition history, anthropometric biochemical indices, and current medications and health status—should be undertaken before the surgery and then reassessed and monitored throughout the entire transplant course (Charuhas, 2000). The acute toxicities of immunosuppression, which last for 2 to 4 weeks after the transplant, include nausea, vomiting, anorexia, dysgeusia, stomatitis, oral and esophageal mucositis, fatigue and diarrhea. In addition, immunosuppressive medications can also adversely affect nutrition status.

Patients typically have little or no oral intake during the first few weeks posttransplant; therefore alternate routes of nutrition support, including enteral or parenteral nutrition support, are usually considered and have become a standardized component of care. Because the function of the gastrointestinal tract is compromised, TPN is often used. Some investigators who have compared TPN with enteral nutrition support in marrow transplantation cases have established the feasibility of enteral feeding in some—but not all—patients (Miller, 1997; Papdopoulou et al, 1997). Roberts and Miller (1998) report the successful use of gastrostomy tubes for long-term nutritional support in marrow transplant recipients.

TPN should be reserved for patients who cannot tolerate enteral feeding. The administration of optimal levels of TPN is complicated, however, by the frequent need to interrupt it for the infusion of antibiotics, blood products, and medications. This, in turn, necessitates the use of more concentrated nutrient solutions, increased flow rates, and, occasionally, double- and triple-lumen catheters.

Autologous marrow transplantation involves the use of the patient's own marrow to reestablish hematopoietic cell function after the administration of high-dose chemotherapy. The use of mobilized stem cell progenitors has, in some cases, replaced autologous bone marrow as the source of hematopoietic progenitors for transplantation. Their use has shortened the period of pancytopenia, when patients are at risk for bleeding and serious infections that may lead to sepsis. These advances, along with improved prophylactic antibiotic regimens that are relatively easy to administer, have allowed patients to receive autologous marrow transplantation in the outpatient setting. This change has substantially reduced the cost of transplantation and hence has made it available to an increased number of patients (Meisenberg et al, 1997). However, because a majority of these patients receive much of their care outside the hospital, nutritional assessment and monitoring is of critical importance.

The marrow transplantation procedure is associated with severe nutritional consequences and requires prompt, aggressive, nutritional intervention. Nausea, vomiting, and diarrhea are caused by the cytotoxic conditioning regimen and may later accompany antibiotic administration. Antiemetics may be helpful. Complications of delayed onset include varying degrees of mucositis, xerostomia, and dysgeusia. Mucositis, which is often severe and extremely painful, develops in more than 75% of transplant patients (Figure 40-4).

Bland liquids and soft solids are usually better tolerated in patients with treatment-related mucositis. Strong-flavored, acidic, or spicy foods should also be avoided. Herpes simplex virus and *Candida albicans* account for most oral infections (Eisen et al, 1997). Salivary stimulants and substitutes are beneficial for temporary relief of dry mouth; in addition, liquids and foods with sauces and gravies are usually well tolerated.

Severe Oral Mucositis

Because patients become immunocompromised, supportive therapy, including medications and dietary changes, is essential to prevent infection. Patients should be instructed on food safety practices, including the following: avoidance of foods that contain unsafe levels of bacteria (raw meats, spoiled or moldy foods, and unpasteurized beverages); thor-

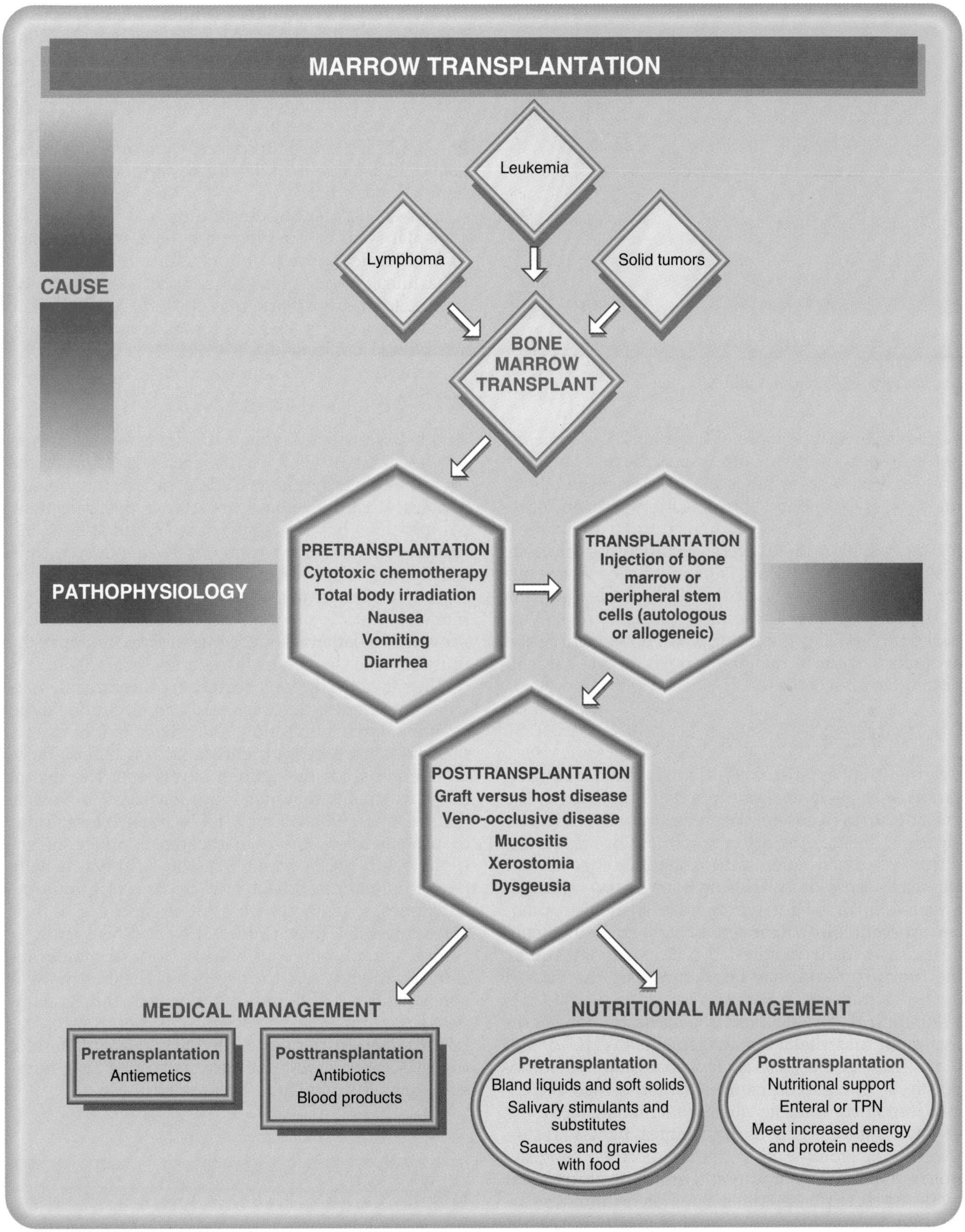

FIGURE 40-3 • Pathophysiology algorithm: marrow transplantation. *TPN,* Total parenteral nutrition. (Algorithm content developed by John Anderson, PhD, and Sanford C. Gardner, PhD, 2000.)

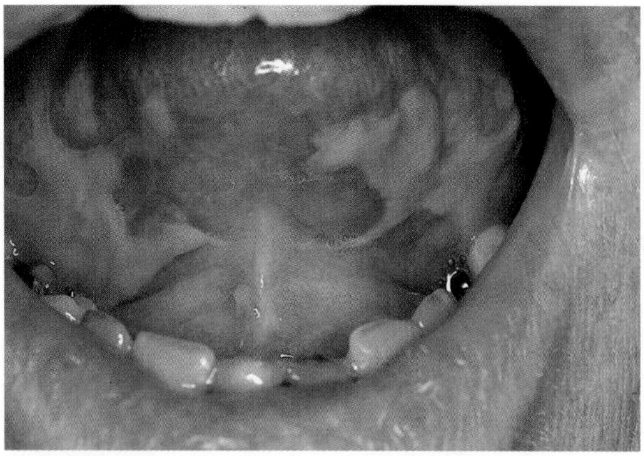

FIGURE 40-4 • Severe oral mucositis after marrow transplantation. This patient also received a course of high-dose cyclophosphamide and whole-body radiation.

ough hand-washing; special handling of raw meats, poultry eggs, utensils, cutting boards, and countertops; and storage of foods at appropriate temperatures (below 40° F and above 140° F) (Eldridge et al, 2001; Charuhas, 2000). Many institutions prescribe a low-microbial or low-bacteria diet (neutropenic diet) for these patients. Its use is chiefly based upon empiric knowledge of the existence of microorganisms in the food supply. These diets consist primarily of cooked foods, and the major restrictions include the avoidance of fresh, raw or uncooked foods and unpasteurized beverages.

Graft-Versus-Host Disease (GVHD)

Graft-versus-host disease (GVHD) is a major complication after allogeneic transplantation, in which the donor marrow cells react against the tissues of the "foreign" host. Although rare, GVHD has also been documented in patients receiving autologous and stem cell transplants. The functions of several target organs (skin, liver, gut, lymphoid cells) are disrupted, and susceptibility to infection is increased. Acute GVHD is usually manifested within 3 months after the transplant and may be seen as early as 7 to 10 days posttransplant. It may resolve, or it may develop into a chronic form that requires long-term treatment and dietary management. GVHD of the liver, evidenced by icterus and abnormal liver function tests, often accompanies gastrointestinal GVHD and further complicates nutritional management.

The symptoms of acute gastrointestinal GVHD are severe. The volume of secretory diarrhea suggests mucosal damage. In addition to immunosuppressive medications, a phased dietary regimen should be instituted (Charuhas, 2000). The first phase consists of total bowel rest until the diarrhea is reduced. Nitrogen losses associated with diarrhea can be severe and are compounded by the high-dose corticosteroids used to treat GVHD. The second phase reintroduces oral feedings of beverages that are isomotic, low-residue, and lactose-free so as to compensate for the loss of intestinal enzymes secondary to alterations in the intestinal villi and mucosa. If these beverages are tolerated, phase three includes the reintroduction of solids that contain low levels of lactose, fiber, fat, and total acidity, and no gastric irritants. In phase four, dietary restrictions are progressively reduced as foods are gradually introduced and tolerance is established. Phase five includes the resumption of the patient's regular diet.

Chronic GVHD can develop up to 3 months posttransplant and is observed with increased frequency in nonidentical related donors and unrelated donors (Charuhas, 2000). Nutrition impact symptoms reported after transplant may include weight gain, weight loss, anorexia, xerostomia, stomatitis, reflux symptoms, and diarrhea.

Veno-Occlusive Disease (VOD)

Another transplant-related complication is veno-occlusive disease (VOD) of the liver; it is characterized by chemotherapy-induced damage to the hepatic venules. It can develop 1 to 3 weeks posttransplant. Symptoms of hepatomegaly, concomitant ascites, and jaundice occur, and in severe cases patients may experience progressive hepatic failure leading to encephalopathy and multiple–organ system failure. Artificial nutrition, total parenteral nutrition in particular, is provided to patients undergoing BMT to minimize the nutritional consequences (Muscaritoli et al, 2002).

Nutritional support requires concentrated parenteral nutrients, judicious fluid and electrolyte management, close monitoring, and adjustment of macronutrients and micronutrients based on the tolerance and response of the individual patient. The use of branched-chain amino acid formulas is controversial. Serum ammonia level may not be a reliable indicator of protein tolerance or of the development of encephalopathy (see Chapter 31). These patients usually have minimal oral intake and are receiving multiple antibiotics, so ammonia may not be generated in their gastrointestinal tract (Miller, 1997). Other acute or chronic complications of marrow transplantation include pulmonary disease, rejection of the graft, growth abnormalities in children, and infection. Nutrition impact symptoms associated with marrow transplantation may persist; patients receiving outpatient marrow transplantation require frequent assessment and intervention by the dietitian.

NUTRITIONAL CARE OF ADULTS DIAGNOSED WITH CANCER

Regardless of the phase of treatment or recovery, individuals diagnosed with cancer should be instructed to consume a nutritionally adequate diet. Ideally, a diet that contains the recommended amounts of essential nutrients, including protein, carbohydrate, fat, vitamins and minerals, and water consumed through a variety of foods each day should be encouraged. As previously discussed, the impact of cancer and its treatment increases nutritional needs, and patients can benefit from individualized nutrition intervention to ensure adequate nutrition intake and weight maintenance.

Body Weight, Energy, and Protein Needs

Patients who are able to maintain their body weight and nutrient stores may be better able to tolerate treatment impact symptoms and recover more quickly from therapy. They also experience improved quality of life. Thus, patients should be advised to consume sufficient energy and protein to maintain their nutrition stores and to achieve and maintain appropriate weight for height. Weight lost during cancer therapy is often more likely caused by the loss of muscle (lean body mass) rather than fat stores. Therefore even if patients are overweight, the maintenance of lean body mass should be encouraged throughout treatment and recovery (Brown et al, 2001). A widely used tool to estimate body weight for height is the body mass index (BMI) that is described in Chapter 17 and Appendix 17. Based on current available evidence, keeping a BMI between 18.5 and 25 throughout life is associated with best overall health (*Food, Nutrition, and the Prevention of Cancer*, 1997).

A patient's need for protein is increased during times of illness and stress. The additional protein is required by the body to repair and rebuild tissues affected by cancer therapy and to maintain a healthy immune system. For the body to most effectively use the protein, adequate energy (calories) should be provided, or the body will use its protein reserves (lean body mass) as a fuel source.

Nutrient Supplementation

Patients diagnosed with cancer often take large amounts of vitamin and mineral supplements because they believe that these products can enhance their immune system or their body's ability to destroy cancer cells (Roberts, 1998). According to a recent epidemiologic review, 50% of all Americans take some kind of nutrient supplementation (Patterson et al, 1997). Many patients may have existing nutritional deficiencies when they are diagnosed with cancer because of poor diet and lifestyle choices and the metabolic effects of the cancer itself, and these deficiencies may worsen as a result of cancer treatment and recovery (Kucuk and Ottery, 2002). Therefore if patients are experiencing difficulty with eating and treatment-related side effects, the use of a multivitamin and mineral supplement that provides no more than 100% of the recommended daily allowances is generally considered safe (Brown et al, 2001; Kogut, 2001).

Controversy about whether the use of antioxidants, such as vitamins A, C, E, β-carotene, and selenium, actually inhibits or enhances the antitumor effects of radiation therapy and chemotherapy continues (Conklin, 2000; Lamson and Brignall, 2000; Miller, 1999; Prasad et al, 2001). Until evidence from well-designed randomized clinical trials of the effects of antioxidants on the potency of anticancer therapies is available, patients should be cautioned against the concurrent use of antioxidant dietary supplements with chemotherapy and radiation therapy (Kucuk and Ottery, 2002).

Nutrition Screening and Assessment

Early intervention is essential. Nutrition screening and assessment for the risk of nutritional problems should be interdisciplinary and instituted at the time of diagnosis and reevaluated and monitored throughout treatment and recovery. With the recent shift of care from the hospital setting to outpatient settings, nutrition screening and assessment throughout the continuum of cancer care are essential. Basic concepts of dietary and clinical assessment as well as nutrition intervention and diet modification are outlined in Chapters 17 and 18.

An example of a tool for nutrition screening and assessment (Detsky et al, 1987) is the Patient Generated–Subjective Global Assessment (PG-SGA), adapted for use with oncology patients (McCallum, 2000; McMahon, Decker, and Ottery, 1998). This tool incorporates sections completed by the patient or caregiver on weight history, food intake, symptoms and functioning. Sections completed by a healthcare member (e.g., physician, nurse, dietitian, social worker) evaluate weight loss, disease, metabolic stress, and a nutrition-related physical examination. Nutrition risk and intervention are then determined by a scoring system (see Chapter 17).

Determining Routes of Nutritional Care

Regardless of which routes of providing nutritional care and support are used, nutritional goals should be specific, achievable, and individualized in scope to encourage patient cooperation. Goals need to be directed toward a visible means of feedback, such as body weight or some other meaningful index. Another goal is to minimize the effects of nutrition impact symptoms and to maximize the patient's nutritional parameters (Wojtaszek, Kochis, and Cunningham, 2002). Consultation with the patient and family members regarding expected problems and their possible solutions should be initiated early in the course of cancer therapy and should continue in conjunction with follow-up nutritional assessment and care.

Oral Nutritional Management Strategies

Ideally, the preferred route of feeding is oral, although patients who experience nutritional impact symptoms such as nausea, anorexia, early satiety, and dysphagia may resist it. Strategies for modifying nutrient intake depend on the specific feeding problem and the extent of depletion. Oral intake may be encouraged with modifications of food and its presentation. Liquid nutritional supplements may be considered for patients unable to consume sufficient energy and protein to maintain their weight and optimal nutritional status (see Chapter 23).

Patients with altered taste acuity (dysgeusia, hypogeusia, ageusia) may benefit from increased use of flavorings and seasonings during food preparation. Meat aversions may require the elimination of red meats, which tend to be strong in flavor, or the substitution of alternative protein sources. Dysphagia secondary to lesions involving the oral and esophageal tissues can be lessened with the intake of foods that are soft or liquefied and served at moderate or room temperature (see Chapter 43).

Artificial saliva preparations and saliva stimulants are often useful in cases of diminished salivation, as are foods with high moisture content and plenty of fluids throughout the day and with meals. Patients with intestinal symptoms may require dietary modifications of lactose, fat, and fiber content as well as alterations in texture. Commercial nutritional supplements can be included in many dietary plans. Management of diarrhea and steatorrhea is discussed in Chapter 30. Guidelines for oral feedings are presented in Table 40-3.

TABLE 40-3 Guidelines for Oral Feeding During Anticancer Therapy

PROBLEM	DIET	SUPPLEMENTS AND AIDS	FOODS TO AVOID
Acute gastrointestinal toxicity; nausea and emesis	Clear, cold nonacidic liquids Light, low-fat foods	None	Milk products, cream soups, fried foods, sandwiches, sweet desserts
Stomatitis, esophagitis	Liquid and soft diet (broth-based soups, fruit ades, carbonated beverages, melons) Alterations in texture and temperature	Mild-flavored supplements, frequent oral hygiene, frequent saline rinses	Juices, especially citrus; bananas; crisp or raw foods; meats; spicy entrees; textured or granular foods; coarse bread products; extremely hot or cold foods
Production of viscous mucus, xerostomia (mouth dryness)	Soft, nonirritating diet; tea with lemon; fruit ades; juices; popsicles; carbonated beverages; broth-based soups; thinned hot cereal	Artificial saliva, frequent saline rinses, and oral hygiene	Thick nectars and liquids, thick cream soups, thick hot cereals, bread products, gelatin, oily foods
Decreased salivation	Regular diet with high-moisture foods (gravies, sauces, casseroles, chicken, fish, beverages with foods, citric acid–containing foods, sherbet, melons, vegetables with sauces)	Artificial saliva; saliva stimulants, such as sugarless lemon drops and gum; frequent saline rinses	Dry foods, bread products, meats, crackers, bananas, excessively hot foods, alcohol
Mouth blindness (hypogeusia)	Regular diet with strongly flavored (spicy) foods Emphasis on aroma and texture	Flavored supplements, frequent saline rinses	Bland foods, plain meats, unsalted foods
Taste alterations (dysgeusia)	Regular diet with many cold foods; milk products Emphasis on experimentation with foods	Fruit-flavored supplements	Red meats, chocolate, coffee, tea
Early satiety	High-calorie diet with calorically dense foods Meat, fish, poultry, eggs, whole milk, cheese, cream soups, ice cream, whole-milk yogurt, creamed vegetables, rich desserts Small, frequent feedings	Calorically dense supplements	Low-fat or nonfat milk products; broth-based soups; green salads; steamed, plain vegetables; low-calorie beverages
Constipation	Regular diet with fiber added; extra fluids	Fiber-enriched supplements, bulking agents	Gas-forming foods and beverages
Myelosuppression (neutropenia)	Safe food diet; well-cooked foods; eliminate foods that could potentially be contaminated with pathogenic organisms	Hand-washing; safe food-handling practices	Raw fish, meats; mold-containing, unpasteurized cheeses, tempe, all miso products, raw fruit and vegetables, dried fruit and raw or fresh roasted nuts, Brewer's yeast, unpasteurized honey, commercial cream-filled pastries that require refrigeration, dry/fresh spices added after cooking, herbal supplements

Guidelines for Oral Feeding During Anticancer Therapy

Chemotherapy-induced nausea and vomiting are commonly classified as anticipatory, acute, or delayed, each of which is manifested by distinct pathophysiologic events and requires different therapeutic interventions. Currently, the most effective agents for treating acute nausea and vomiting are the serotonin antagonists (i.e., ondansetron, granisetron, and dolasetron). Although costly, they are used in conjunction with highly and moderately emetogenic chemotherapeutic regimens. However, these agents are generally thought to be ineffective in the management of delayed nausea and vomiting, and other antiemetic agents—including corticosteroids and dopamine antagonists such as phenothiazines (prochlorperazine) and benzamides (metoclopramide)—may be used (Kennedy, 2000).

Other alternatives include cannabinoids (dronabinol) and benzodiazepines (lorazepam and diazepam). The anticipatory form of nausea and vomiting is a conditioned response that develops by the third or fourth cycle of treatment in about one third of patients. It is primarily a psychological issue and so responds best to behavioral interventions, such as relaxation training or systematic desensitization (Fessele, 1996).

The timing of food presentation also deserves consideration. Patients with cancer often complain of a decreased ability to eat as the day progresses, which means that the morning is often the best time for eating. This phenomenon may be attributable to sluggish digestion and gastric emptying as a result of decreased production of digestive secretions, gastrointestinal mucosal atrophy, and gastric muscle atrophy. It may also be experienced as a result of treatment-related fatigue. Fatigue is one of the most common symptoms reported by patients with cancer and is often characterized as physical tiredness, mental slowness, and lack of emotional resilience (Nail, 2001). Patients should be encouraged to consume more frequent, small feedings, with particular emphasis on morning feedings, and easy-to-eat foods that require less preparation and are easier to consume. Pain can also adversely affect patients' appetite and ability to eat. Pain can be a result of the tumor itself or a consequence of treatment, or it can have a psychological component; appropriate pain management medications, such as topical anesthetics, antiinflammatory agents, and opioid analgesics should be used (Wojtaszek, Kochis, and Cunningham, 2002).

The timing of meals or snacks relative to the gastrointestinal side effects of cancer treatment may have a bearing on subsequent learned food aversions. These aversions develop when specific foods are associated with unpleasant symptoms, such as nausea and vomiting, and psychological stimuli, such as anxiety. The effect may not be limited to new food items but may also involve foods that were included in the patient's usual diet before treatment. Exposure of patients to a "scapegoat" food or beverage just before chemotherapy and (probably) radiotherapy can markedly reduce the incidence of treatment-related aversions to foods in the patient's usual diet (Puccio and Nathanson, 1997).

The dilemma regarding nutrition support in cancer is discussed in *Focus On:* Controversy—Use of Nutrition Support in Patients with Cancer.

FOCUS ON

Controversy—Use of Nutrition Support in Patients With Cancer

Although the detrimental effect of malnutrition on survival is evident, the favorable influence of nutritional intervention is not always as clear. Nutrition support improves nutritional indices and may improve overall patient performance status in cancer patients with malnutrition secondary to gastrointestinal obstruction or treatment toxicity. Moreover, TPN may not benefit patients with advanced cancer whose malignant disease is unresponsive to chemotherapy or radiation therapy (ASPEN, 2002.)

Parenteral nutrition support may, however, benefit some severely malnourished patients with cancer who are undergoing therapy, the intent of which is cancer cure or control. It may also benefit those in whom gastrointestinal toxicities are likely to prevent oral nutritional intake for more than 1 week. Nutritional intervention, when possible, should be provided in conjunction with oncologic therapy to improve quality of life. Specialized nutritional support is not routinely indicated for well-nourished or mildly malnourished patients in whom adequate oral intake is anticipated. The use of TPN requires close monitoring in patients who receive multiple therapies via their catheter access (double- or triple-lumen). The risk of fluid overload, electrolyte imbalance, hyperglycemia, and infection in the immunocompromised patient is of concern.

The controversy persists regarding the merits of nutritional support for patients with cancer. Nevertheless, the adverse effects of malnutrition are clear. Nutrition support is a means of both preventing and treating malnutrition and, as such, plays an important role in the care of the patient with cancer.

Enteral Nutrition

When patients are unable to meet their nutritional needs because of prolonged anorexia, treatment-related toxicities (i.e., dysphagia, odynophagia, mucositis), or mechanical obstruction, other, more aggressive routes of nutrition support need to be considered. If the gut is functional, enteral nutrition is indicated. As described in Chapter 23, enteral nutrition, rather than parenteral nutrition, helps to reduce infectious complications such as bacterial translocation by preserving immune and gut barrier function. Nasogastric or nasojejunal tubes are used most commonly for the short-term administration of enteral nutrition formulas. A percutaneous endoscopic gastrostomy (PEG) or a jejunostomy is used when longer-term enteral nutrition support (for greater than 3 to 4 weeks) is indicated, and patients generally find these routes of nutrition support more acceptable than nasogastric tubes (Mercadante, 1998).

The selection of the enteral nutrition formula is determined by several factors, including the functional capacity of the gut, the physical characteristics of the formula (i.e., osmolality, fiber and protein content, energy density, nutrient content), the patient's metabolic status, and considerations of cost and convenience (Piazza-Barnett and Matarese, 2000). Appendixes 36 to 41 describe available enteral preparations.

General-purpose commercially prepared formulas serve most needs. However, patients with preexisting medical conditions or treatment-related side effects (i.e., radiation enteritis, malabsorption) may benefit from elemental or peptide-based formulas. Beneficial effects have been reported with the use of specialized nutritional formulas supplemented with glutamine (Ziegler et al, 1998) or with arginine, ribonucleic acids, and omega-3 fatty acids (Daly et al, 1995).

Parenteral Nutrition

The use of parenteral nutrition support may be appropriate for some patients with cancer for whom oral intake or enteral nutrition is not an option and who are otherwise expected to survive (Mercadante, 1998). If the gastrointestinal tract is not functioning or enteral nutrition support is not adequate, parenteral nutrition should be considered. This route of nutrition support involves the administration of concentrated nutrient solutions intravenously (see Chapter 23).

The type of parenteral nutrition support is determined by the clinical and nutritional status of the patient and by the type of intravenous (IV) access (DeChicco and Steiger, 2000). Patients diagnosed with cancer often have central IV access to accommodate multiple IV therapies (i.e., chemotherapy, blood products, hydration, and IV medications). Parenteral nutrition support can be delivered via central IV access or via peripheral catheter. Peripheral parenteral nutrition (PPN) mixtures are administered via peripheral catheters and usually are lower in osmolarity and are lipid-based formulas. PPN mixtures are also moderate in protein and usually contain a final dextrose concentration of 10% or less. Total parenteral nutrition (TPN) mixtures are either lipid-based or dextrose-based and are administered via central IV accesses (see Chapter 23). TPN mixtures are not limited by osmolarity because they are infused into larger veins. Energy and protein are usually administered as glucose and a mixture of amino acids (ASPEN, 2002).

Potential complications associated with parenteral nutrition support include potential for fluid overload in patients who receive multiple IV therapies, hyperglycemia resulting from the high concentration of dextrose present in parenteral mixtures, insulin resistance associated with illness and stress, electrolyte imbalance, and increased infection rate (DeChicco and Steiger, 2000). Intense monitoring and specialized care are required for patients who receive TPN. Successful outpatient use of TPN can be achieved when the patient and family are cooperative and instructed properly.

Home Enteral and Total Parenteral Nutrition

Cancer is the largest single diagnosis for patients who are starting home enteral nutrition (HEN) or TPN. The mean survival time of patients with cancer is 6 months after starting nutritional support, but 25% live beyond a year, and 20% resume full oral intake. The outcome is better for children and for patients with leukemia, lymphoma, or small bowel or liver neoplasms. Patients who have survived cancer but who have severe radiation enteritis that requires home TPN can benefit from home parenteral nutrition therapy.

Clinical pathways have been developed to provide a clear, concise, standardized method for monitoring home nutritional support. The average variance from the pathway may be more frequent for oncology patients because of complications and unexpected events (Ireton-Jones et al, 1997).

Rehabilitation and Physical Activity

Rehabilitation is an important concept of cancer care in all settings. The effect of cancer and cancer treatment on the patient's quality of life is addressed throughout the treatment period and continues until the patient is able to successfully resume activities of daily living (Body et al, 1997). Recovery from cancer treatment also requires physical activity to rebuild muscle strength.

Fatigue and impairment of physical performance are common and often severe problems of cancer patients. Psychological and physical factors play roles. Poor nutrition contributes to fatigue; conversely, fatigue may hinder eating and nutritional support regimens. Appropriate exercise may be helpful in treating primary fatigue (Dimeo et al, 1998). In addition, physical activity may improve the immune system, which is important in preventing cancer recurrence (Fairey et al, 2002).

Although little data regarding the role of physical activity in cancer patients are available, physical activity is known to be associated with numerous health benefits, such as reduction of anxiety and depression; improvement in mood, quality of life, and self-esteem; and reduction of symptoms (Brown et al, 2001; Courneya and Friedenreich, 1999). Before participating in any type of physical exercise, patients should be advised to undergo evaluation by qualified professionals, who can then design an individualized physical assessment and activity plan.

Individuals With Advanced Cancer Receiving Palliative Care

Nutrition is an important component in the care and management of individuals with advanced cancer (Brown et al, 2001). The goals of nutrition intervention should focus upon managing nutrition impact symptoms such as pain, weakness, loss of appetite, early satiety, constipation, weakness, dry mouth, and dyspnea (Cox and McCallum, 2000). Another important goal is maintaining strength and energy to enhance quality of life, independence, and ability to perform activities of daily living. Nutrition should be provided "as tolerated or as desired" along with emotional support and awareness of and respect for individual needs and wishes. Thus the pleasurable aspects of eating should be emphasized, without concern for quantity or nutrient and energy content.

Cox and McCallum (2000) define palliative care as the active total care of an individual when curative measures are no longer considered an option by either the medical team or the patient. They go on to state that the goals of palliative care are to provide for optimal quality of life for the individual and the family through the use of a multidisciplinary team approach to managing physiological symptoms as well as psychological, social, and spiritual issues.

NUTRITIONAL CARE OF CHILDREN DIAGNOSED WITH CANCER

Like the adult patient diagnosed with cancer, children with cancer can experience nutrition impact symptoms as a result of their neoplastic disease and its treatment. The incidence of malnutrition ranges from 6% to 50% in the pediatric population, depending on the type, stage, and location of the cancer. It usually has greater severity in the presence of more aggressive cancers in the later stages of the disease (Andrassy and Chwals, 1998).

It is not uncommon for families and caregivers to express their fears of dying through an extreme preoccupation with eating and maintaining weight. Psychogenic food refusal in children requires interventions that address underlying psychological issues. Creative efforts are required to minimize the psychological effects of fear, unpleasant hospital routines, unfamiliar foods, learned food aversions, and pain. Nutrition intervention strategies that use oral intake should stress the maximal use of favorite, nutrient-dense foods during times when intake is likely to be best and food aversions are least likely to occur. Oral nutritional supplements can be useful, but their acceptance is often a problem, so children should be offered a selection from which to choose.

Enteral nutrition support by nasogastric tube is indicated for selected children who are able to cooperate and who have functional gastrointestinal tracts. Some children have even been taught to pass their own nasogastric tube for intermittent or nighttime feedings. It should be remembered, though, that aspiration is always a potential risk. TPN is indicated for children who are receiving intense treatment associated with severe gastrointestinal toxicity and for children with favorable prognoses who are malnourished or have a high risk of developing malnutrition. TPN is seldom indicated for children with advanced cancer associated with significant deterioration or with diseases that are unresponsive to therapy (ASPEN, 2002).

The nutritional requirements of pediatric patients with cancer are similar, with an adjustment for activity level, to those of normal growing children. Often, pediatric patients with cancer are not bedridden but are as active as their healthy peers. Factors that may alter nutrient requirements in cancer include the impact of the malignant disease on host metabolism; the catabolic effects of cancer therapy; and physiologic stress, such as surgery, fever, malabsorption, and infection. Fluid requirements are increased during anticancer therapy or in the presence of fever, diarrhea, or renal failure. Micronutrients may require supplementation during periods of poor intake, stress, or malabsorption. The best long-term indicator of adequate nutrient intake is growth.

The long-term nutritional effects of cancer and its treatment in children are not well documented. Deficiencies in energy and protein can be expected to affect growth adversely, although the impact may be temporary, and catch-up growth may occur after successful tumor therapy is discontinued. However, some cancer treatment regimens may have an effect on growth and development that is independent of nutritional deprivation.

Children have increased nutritional requirements for growth and development that must be met despite extended periods of cancer treatment (ASPEN, 2002.) A special vulnerability exists during the adolescent growth spurt. Ewing's sarcoma is frequently associated with malnutrition. Another reason why children with advanced cancer are at a greater risk of severe nutritional depletion than adults is the frequent use of more aggressive, multimodality treatment.

Marrow transplantation is now an accepted and increasingly successful intensive therapy for a wide range of disorders in children. Many supportive therapies may be safely managed in the outpatient arena, thus reducing the period of hospitalization (Fidler and Hibbs, 1997).

COMPLEMENTARY AND ALTERNATIVE THERAPIES

Complementary and alternative therapies have gained in popularity in recent years. The American Cancer Society defines complementary therapies as supportive methods that are used to complement evidence-based treatment, to help control symptoms, and to improve well-being and quality of life, and alternative therapies as treatments that are promoted as cancer cures and are unproven or scientifically disproved methods (American Cancer Society, 1999). In 1992, the Office of Alternative Medicine (OAM) was established at the National Institutes of Health to provide a structure for the study of alternative and complementary therapies. To facilitate the grant review process, the OAM classified alternative therapies into seven major categories: alternative systems of practice, bioelectromagnetic applications, manual healing methods, mind/body control, pharmacologic and biologic treatments, herbal medicine, and diet/nutrition/lifestyle changes (Barrocas, 1997).

Eisenberg (1997) reports that patients explore alternative therapies when (1) health promotion and disease prevention are sought; (2) conventional therapies have been exhausted; (3) conventional therapies are of indeterminate effectiveness or are commonly associated with side effects or significant risks; (4) no conventional therapy is known to relieve the patient's condition; or (5) the conventional approach is perceived to be emotionally or spiritually without benefit.

Studies indicate that those who use alternative or complementary therapies tend to be Caucasian, more affluent, better educated, and older than nonusers (Newman et al, 1998). In a study of patients at risk for recurrence of breast cancer, 80% reported the use of dietary supplements. The use of herbal and vitamin compounds was inversely related to the months since diagnosis; use of miscellaneous supplements, such as shark cartilage, was directly associated with more advanced disease (Newman et al, 1998). When a child has the malignant disease, the use of alternative medicines may be increased by all members of the family (Mottonen and Uhari, 1997).

In general, examples of complementary and alternative therapies commonly used by cancer patients include nutrition (diet) and metabolic therapies, vitamin/mineral supplementation (single- or multi-agent preparations), and herbal and botanical therapies (Table 40-4), which are discussed extensively in Chapter 20.

Metabolic therapy is a term used for a variety of cancer management methods, including unproven and disproved diagnostic methods and treatments. Metabolic practitioners generally claim that diseases, including cancer, are caused by an accumulation of toxic substances in the body. They allege that if these toxins are removed, the body can heal itself naturally. Three basic steps are common to metabolic therapy: detoxification, strengthening of the immune system, and the use of special modalities to attack cancer. These therapy regimens generally include colonic cleansing with coffee, wheat grass, or other substances; special diets; and vitamin and mineral supplementation. Complications of colonic irrigation include electrolyte imbalance, toxic colitis, bowel perforation, and sepsis. Most regimens promote "natural" and "organic" foods and recommend restriction of animal products, refined flours and sugars, and foods that are processed or contain artificial ingredients.

Nutrition and diet therapies generally are based on the "you are what you eat" principle. A number of diet therapies consist of specific foods prepared and consumed in a specified manner. The macrobiotic diet is a quasi-religious, philosophic system popularized in the United States by Michio Kushi. Currently, the diet derives 50% to 60% of its calories from whole grains; 25% to 30% from vegetables; and the remainder from beans, seaweed, and soups. Meat and certain vegetables are avoided, and soybean consumption is promoted. Past research determined that the diet was deficient in calcium and vitamin B_{12}. Recently, the OAM funded a pilot study of the macrobiotic diet, the principal investigator of which is Lawrence Kushi, ScD, son of Michio Kushi (Cassileth and Chapman, 1996).

Megavitamin therapy, another commonly practiced therapy, is characterized by the use of large doses of one or more vitamins. The treatment is based on the belief that the body's ability to destroy the tumor is enhanced by large doses of vitamins, antioxidants, and other substances, including coenzyme Q_{10} and pangamic acid (Roberts, 1998).

Miscellaneous substances that may be used by patients with cancer include enzymes, which are purported to treat cancer by dissolving the coating of cancer cells so as to allow the immune system to destroy the cancer; melatonin, a hormone that promotes sleep and has strong antioxidant properties; and dehydroepiandrosterone (DHEA), a hormone with unknown safety and effectiveness (Roberts, 1998).

A nutritional history and assessment should always address the patient's use of alternative therapies. Patients often do not inform their health providers about their use of alternative therapies either because they are not asked or because they are afraid of the reaction (Roberts, 1998). Communica-

TABLE 40-4 Commonly Used Complementary and Alternative Therapies (CAM)

CAM THERAPY	BRIEF DESCRIPTION
Nutrition (Diet) and Metabolic Therapies	**Overview and *Caution***
Macrobiotic diet	Emphasis on whole foods (grains, cereals, vegetables, sea vegetables, fermented soy, fruits, nuts, seeds, and soups); individualized diet based on whether cancer is "yin," "yang," or "neutral." *May be inadequate in energy and micronutrients; restrictive; requires considerable meal planning and preparation.*
Vegetarian diet	Includes many health-promoting features (low in saturated fat; high in fiber, vitamins, and phytochemicals). Emphasis on "natural" and "organic" foods. *May be inadequate in energy and micronutrients; restrictive; requires thorough meal planning.*
Gerson therapy	Cleansing and detoxifying program; raw fruit and vegetable regimen that includes juice therapy and fresh calf's liver solution daily. *Restrictive; difficult to follow.*
Kelley/Gonzales regimen	Includes the consumption of 25 nutritional supplements and digestive enzymes; detoxifying treatments such as coffee enemas, moderate exercise, fasting, and purging. *Restrictive and difficult to follow.*
Juice therapies	Includes fresh fruit and vegetable juice regimen to cleanse and detoxify the body. *Inadequate in energy and macro/micronutrients; restrictive; difficult to follow.*
Pharmacologic/Biologic Preparations (Including Vitamin and Mineral Supplements)	**Proposed Use and *Caution***
Shark cartilage	Promoted as an anticancer agent. *Clinical trials currently underway; expensive; may contain possible contaminants.*
DHEA	Promoted as an anticancer agent. *May not be appropriate for people with prostate, breast, or ovarian cancers because of its androgenic effect.*
Enzymes	Promoted as an anticancer agent. *No proven effectiveness in cancer prevention or treatment.*
Oxymedicine	Promoted as an anticancer treatment. *No scientific evidence to treat cancer; if administered incorrectly, may be harmful or toxic.*
Coenzyme Q10 (Ubiquinone)	Promoted as an immune-stimulating agent. *No proven clinical evidence to support immune-enhancing effect.*
Herbals and Botanicals	**Proposed Use and *Caution***
Black cohosh *(Caulophyllum thalictroides)*	Management of menopausal symptoms. *Large doses may cause dizziness, nausea, headaches, hypotension.*
Echinacea (Purple cone flower)	Management of colds, flu, fever, respiratory and urinary tract infections; immune stimulant. *Contraindicated in patients with autoimmune diseases and allergies to daisies; not for long-term use; numbing of the tongue.*
Flaxseed	In animal studies has shown a possible anticancer effect. *Contains compounds that are estrogenic; gastrointestional upset with ingestion of large amounts.*
Ginger (Zingiber officinale)	Antiemetic; digestive aid. *Effectiveness in motion-related nausea, effect on chemotherapy-related nausea under investigation.*
Iscador (Viscum album)	An extract of European mistletoe, used in Germany to treat certain malignancies. *Mistletoe leaves contain cytotoxins; therefore should not be used as a home remedy or beverage.*
Milk thistle (Silybum marianum)	Antioxidant; little evidence to support its protective effect on the liver and anticancer activity. *May delay the clearance of chemotherapeutic agents by the liver.*
PC-SPECS	Combination of seven Chinese herbs and saw palmetto; has estrogenic activity; not a proven treatment for prostate cancer. *Potential side effects include elevation of blood pressure, increased estrogen levels, and formation of blood clots in legs and lungs.*
Saw palmetto *(Serenoa repens)*	Relief of urinary symptoms in benign prostate hyperplasia; not a proven treatment for prostate cancer. *Rare headaches; mild abdominal pain, nausea and dizziness; antiestrogen.*
Soy and soy foods	Inconsistent evidence in the use of soy foods in primary and secondary cancer prevention. *May not be appropriate for women with hormone-responsive cancers.*
Teas (green, black, herbal)	Antioxidant; enhances immune system. *Antiplatelet effect (green); caffeinated varieties may cause insomnia, nervousness, and increased heart rate.*

Data from Brown et al: Nutrition during and after cancer treatment: a guide for informed choices by cancer survivors, *CA Cancer J Clin* 51:153, 2001; Eldridge B et al: Nutrition and the patient with cancer. In Coulston AM, Rock CL, Monsen ER, editors: *Nutrition in the prevention and treatment of disease,* San Diego, 2001, Academic Press; Kogut V: Complementary and alternative dietary therapies, *Clin J Oncol Nurs* 5:283, 2001; and Roberts S: Alternative nutrition therapies used by oncology patients, *Support Line* 20:10, 1998.

tion through open-ended questions, listening with empathy, and an unbiased approach is essential to successful intervention. In that context, the dietetic professionals can then provide sound evidenced-based information about complementary and alternative therapies so that the patient can make informed choices and avoid undesired risks (see Chapter 22).

Dietary Recommendations for Cancer Survivors

The American Cancer Society's (ACS) recommendations for nutrition and physical activity, as well as the American Institute for Cancer Research recommendations (see Box 40-1) provide sound diet and nutrition advice for cancer prevention for all individuals,

TABLE 40-5 The American Cancer Society Workgroup Grading System for Benefit vs. Harm—Nutrition During and After Cancer Treatment

To summarize the strength of the scientific evidence, the ACS Workgroup used a method of summarizing the evidence similar to those used by other expert panels. For example, the U.S. Preventive Services Task Force judged the scientific evidence related to clinical preventive services using a system that considered both the source and strength of the evidence and categorized them as follows: From at least one controlled clinical trial, from good uncontrolled trials, from multiple good observation studies, expert opinion, and case reports. They then characterized those recommendations on a five-point grading scheme as to the strength of the recommendation: "Good for recommending, fair for recommending, insufficient to recommend for or against, fair for not recommending, or good for not recommending."

The AICR-World Cancer Research Fund project summarized the nature of the scientific evidence for nutritional factors in cancer prevention as being either "Convincing, Probable, Possible, or Insufficient."

The ACS committee employed a method of summarizing the evidence that was similar to those used by both groups. For each issue, the committee judged the likelihood of benefit to cancer survivors as follows:

A1	Proven benefit
A2	Probable benefit, but unproven
A3	Possible benefit, but unproven
B	Insufficient evidence to conclude benefit or risk
C	Evidence of possible harm as well as possible benefit
D	Evidence of lack of benefit
E	Evidence of harm

The following table presents a summary of ACS assessments regarding the benefit or harm of 25 dietary factors with respect to their impact on cancer survivors throughout the phases of survivorship.

ACS Workgroup Grades for Benefit vs. Harm

DIETARY FACTOR	PROSTATE CANCER	BREAST CANCER	GI CANCER	LUNG CANCER
Food safety	A1	A1	A1	A1
Intentional weight loss during treatment (if overweight)	E	E	E	E
Intentional weight loss after recovery (if overweight)	B	A2	A3	B
Decreased dietary fats	A3	A2	A3	B
Increased fruits and vegetables	B	A3	A2	A2
Increased physical activity	A3	A2	A2	B
Decreased alcohol	B	A3	A3	B
Fasting therapies	D	D	D	D
Juice therapies	B	A3	A3	A3
Macrobiotic therapies	C	C	C	C
Vegetarian diets	A3	A3	A2	A3
Vitamin and mineral supplements	A3	B	B	C
Flaxseed oil	B	B	B	B
Fish oils	B	B	A3	B
Ginger	B	B	B	B
Soy foods	C	C	B	B
Teas	B	B	B	B
Vitamin E supplements	A3	B	B	B
Vitamin C supplements	B	B	B	B
β-carotene supplements	C	C	C	E
Selenium	A3	B	A3	A3

From Brown J et al: Nutrition during and after cancer treatment: a guide for informed choices by cancer survivors, *CA Cancer J Clin* 51:153, 2001.
Note: Information contained in this table represents studies in progress and presents the best data available at this time. This table will be updated periodically.

including cancer survivors. The American Cancer Society's recently released *Nutrition During and After Cancer Treatment: A Guide for Informed Choices by Cancer Survivors* summarizes current knowledge on nutrition and physical activity guidelines for cancer survivors (Brown et al, 2001). To assist health care professionals in evaluating the strength of existing scientific evidence, the American Cancer Society Workgroup that produced this guide created a grading system to consider benefit versus harm regarding dietary factors and specific cancer sites (Table 40-5).

Cancer survivors represent one of the largest groups of people living with a chronic illness in the United States (Stovall, 1996). Recent studies indicate that an increasing number of patients with cancer are able to return to full function and regain their quality of life, in addition to maintaining their earning potential and employment status (Harrison et al, 1997). This trend is expected to continue because of recent awareness in cancer prevention, advances in cancer detection, development of more effective anticancer therapies, and advancements in determin-

Clinical Scenario 1

Janice is a 55-year-old mother of four. Recently she was diagnosed with breast cancer (estrogen-receptor positive) and has been prescribed surgery and tamoxifen for treatment of her disease. In the next 3 weeks, she will undergo lumpectomy, followed by 5 to 6 weeks of external beam radiation therapy. She is 5 ft, 8 in. tall, weighs 185 lbs, and has a history of mild hypertension that has been controlled with dietary measures. She currently does not engage in regular physical activity but is motivated to make changes in her lifestyle to improve her fitness and overall health. She also is attracted to the use of multiple vitamins and supplements and complementary and alternative therapies for reducing her cancer recurrence risk and managing treatment-related side effects and postmenopausal symptoms.

1. What recommendations would you give Janice to prepare for her surgery?
2. After radiation therapy and surgery, what side effects might Janice experience? List some dietary strategies Janice may follow if she experiences the following: fatigue, intermittent queasiness, a slight difficulty in swallowing (esophagus is in the radiation field), and an increased caloric intake (mostly caused by her need to "take care of" herself) that results in weight gain.
3. Is Janice at her ideal body weight? If not, what suggestions would you recommend? Consider her hypertension, planned surgery, and radiation therapy.
4. What dietary recommendations, if any, are appropriate for a regimen of tamoxifen?
5. What guidance should be provided with regard to the appropriate use of vitamin-mineral supplements and ways to evaluate alternative therapies? How does soy affect estrogen-receptor positive forms of breast cancer? How should she manage hot flashes now that she is not advised to take estrogen replacement therapy?

ing the genetic causes of cancer (Leigh and Thaler-Demers, 2001).

SUMMARY

Nutrition plays an important role in the management of cancer patients from diagnosis through treatment and recovery. Patients have different needs and challenges with regard to their nutritional management, and providing individualized nutrition guidance is an essential component of their care. Prompt and appropriate nutritional management may help to improve patients' tolerance of treatment, minimize nutrition impact symptoms, and maximize quality of life. Patients should be encouraged to actively participate in their care and to communicate with their health care professionals. At a time when patients are often inundated with nutrition-related complementary and alternative therapy choices, dietetic professionals can provide sound guidance for informed decision making.

Clinical Scenario 2

Ed is a 68-year-old white man who has been diagnosed with prostate cancer. He has been sent to your nutrition clinic by his oncologist and expects to undergo surgery in the next few months. His BMI is 35, and he works at home as a computer programmer. His hobbies include reading and making model airplanes. Your diet history reveals a usual daily intake of 12 to 14 oz of meat or poultry, 2 to 3 cups of whole milk, fruits on rare occasion, corn and potatoes with the dinner meal, and a lunch that includes a luncheon meat and cheese sandwich on white bread. Currently, he is taking Proscar and saw palmetto, as prescribed by his physician.

1. What dietary factors are involved with prostate cancer?
2. What types of advice will you offer Ed about his diet?
3. What implications are there for the use of saw palmetto? Are there any studies underway regarding its use in this population?

Relevant Web Sites

American Cancer Society
www.cancer.org
American Institute for Cancer Research
www.aicr.org
Cancer Centers
www.cancerlinksusa.com
Cancer Research Foundation
www.preventcancer.org
National Cancer Institute
www.cancer.gov
Oncology Nutrition Practice Group
www.oncologynutrition.org

Cited References

Allison G et al: Nutrition implications of surgical oncology. In McCallum PD, Polisena CG, editors: *The clinical guide to oncology nutrition,* Chicago, 2000, American Dietetic Association.

American Cancer Society: *American Cancer Society's statement on complementary and alternative methods of cancer management.* Atlanta, 1999, American Cancer Society.

Ames BN, Wakimoto P: Are vitamin and mineral deficiencies a major cancer risk? *Nat Rev Cancer* 2:694, 2002.

Andrassy RJ, Chwals WJ: Nutritional support of the pediatric oncology patient, *Nutrition* 14:124, 1998.

ASPEN (American Society for Parenteral and Enteral Nutrition): Guidelines for the use of parenteral and enteral nutrition in adult and pediatric patients, *J Parenter Enteral Nutr* 26:1, January-February, 2002.

ATBC Cancer Prevention Study Group: The effect of vitamin E and β-carotene on the incidence of lung cancer and other cancers in male smokers, *N Engl J Med* 330:1029, 1994.

Baron JA et al: Calcium supplements for the prevention of colorectal adenomas, *N Engl J Med* 340:101, 1999.

Barrocas A: Complementary and alternative medicine: friend, foe, or OWA? *J Am Diet Assoc* 97:1373, 1997.

Berwick M, Schantz S: Chemoprevention for aerodigestive cancer, *Cancer Metast Rev* 16:329, 1997.

Block G et al: Fruit, vegetables, and cancer prevention: a review of the epidemiologic evidence, *Nutr Cancer* 18:1, 1992.

Blot WJ: Prevention of esophageal cancer: the nutrition intervention trials in Linxian, China, Linxian Nutrition Intervention Trials Study Group, *Cancer Res* 54(suppl):2029S, 1994.

Blot WJ et al: Nutrition intervention trials in Linxian, China: supplementation with specific vitamin/mineral combinations, cancer incidence, and disease-specific mortality in the general population, *J Natl Cancer Inst* 85:1483, 1993.

Body JJ et al: The concept of rehabilitation of cancer patients, *Curr Opin Oncol* 9:332, 1997.

Brown J et al: Nutrition during and after cancer treatment: a guide for informed choices by cancer survivors, *CA Cancer J Clin* 51:153, 2001.

Byers et al: American Cancer Society's Guidelines on nutrition and physical activity for cancer prevention: reducing the risk of cancer with healthy food choices and physical activity, *CA Cancer J Clin* 52:92, 2002.

Cassileth BR, Chapman CC: Alternative cancer medicine: a ten-year update, *Cancer Invest* 14:396, 1996.

Charuhas PM: Medical nutrition therapy in bone marrow transplantation. In McCallum PD, Polisena CG, editors: *The clinical guide to oncology nutrition,* Chicago, 2000, American Dietetic Association.

Cheng KK, Day NE: Nutrition and esophageal cancer, *Cancer Causes Control* 7:33, 1996.

Clark, LC et al: Effects of selenium supplementation for cancer prevention in patients with carcinoma of the skin, *JAMA* 276:1957, 1996.

Cleary MP, Maihle NJ: The role of body mass in the relative risk of developing premenopausal versus postmenopausal breast cancer, *Proc Cox Exp Biol Med* 216: 28, 1997.

Colditz GA et al: Physical activity and reduced risk of colon cancer: implications for prevention, *Cancer Causes Control* 8:649, 1997.

Common Toxicity Criteria: Version 2.0 (Publish Date: April 30, 1999). www.ctep.info.nih.gov/, 2002.

Conklin KA: Dietary antioxidants during cancer chemotherapy: impact on chemotherapeutic effectiveness and development of side effects, *Nutr Cancer* 37:1, 2000.

Courneya K, Friedenreich C: Physical exercise and quality of life following cancer diagnosis: a literature review, *Ann Behav Med* 21:1, 1999.

Cox A, McCallum PD: Medical nutrition therapy in palliative care. In McCallum PD, Polisena CG, editors: *The clinical guide to oncology nutrition,* Chicago, 2000, American Dietetic Association.

Craig WJ: Phytochemicals: guardians of our health, *J Am Diet Assoc* 97(suppl 2):S199, 1997.

Daly JM et al: Enteral nutrition during multimodal therapy in upper gastrointestinal cancer patients, *Ann Surg* 221:327, 1995.

DeChicco RS, Steiger E: Parenteral nutrition in medical/surgical oncology. In McCallum PD, Polisena CG, editors: *The clinical guide to oncology nutrition,* Chicago, 2000, American Dietetic Association.

Detsky A et al: What is subjective global assessment of nutrition status? *J Parenter Enteral Nutr* 11:8, 1987.

Dickerson RN et al: Resting energy expenditure of patients with gynecologic malignancies, *J Am Coll Nutr* 14:409, 1995.

Dickson TC: Clinical pathway nutrition management for outpatient bone marrow transplantation, *J Am Diet Assoc* 97:61, 1997.

Dimeo F et al: Aerobic exercise as therapy for cancer fatigue, *Med Sci Sports Exerc* 30:475, 1998.

Eldridge B: Chemotherapy and nutrition implications. In McCallum PD, Polisena CG, editors: *The clinical guide to oncology nutrition,* Chicago, 2000, American Dietetic Association.

Eldridge B et al: Nutrition and the patient with cancer. In Coulston AM, Rock CL, Monsen ER, editors: *Nutrition in the prevention and treatment of disease,* San Diego, 2001, Academic Press.

Eichholzer M et al: Prediction of male cancer mortality by plasma levels of interacting vitamins: 17-year follow-up of the basal study, *Int J Cancer* 66:145, 1996.

Eisen D et al: Oral cavity complications of bone marrow transplantation, *Semin Cutan Med Surg* 16:265, 1997.

Eisenberg DM: Advising patients who seek alternative medical therapies, *Ann Intern Med* 127:61, 1997.

Fairey AS et al: Physical exercise and immune system function in cancer survivors: a comprehensive review and future directions, *Cancer* 94:539, 2002.

Fearon KC et al: Albumin synthesis rates are not decreased in hypoalbuminemic cachectic cancer patients with an ongoing acute-phase protein response, *Ann Surg* 227:249, 1998.

Fessele KS. Managing the multiple causes of nausea and vomiting in the patient with cancer, *Oncol Nurs Forum* 23:1409, 1996.

Fidler PA, Hibbs CJ: Bone marrow transplant today—home tomorrow: ambulatory care issues in pediatric marrow transplantation, *J Pediatr Oncol Nurs* 14:228, 1997.

Food and Drug Adminstration: Cyclamate petition—FAP 2A36772. Online http://vm.cfsan.fda.gov/~dms/opa-abey.html. Accessed 2002.

Food, nutrition, and the prevention of cancer: a global perspective, Washington, DC, 1997, World Cancer Fund/American Institute for Cancer Research.

Fredrix EWHM et al: Effects of different tumor types on resting energy expenditure, *Cancer Res* 51:6138, 1991.

Fuchs CS et al: Dietary fiber and the risk of colorectal cancer and adenoma in women, *N Engl J Med* 340:169, 1999.

Gadducci A et al: Malnutrition and cachexia in ovarian cancer patients: pathophysiology and management, *Anticancer Res* 21: 2941, 2001.

Gammon MD, John EM, Britton JA: Recreational and occupational physical activities and risk of breast cancer, *J Natl Cancer Inst* 90: 100, 1998.

Grant JP et al: Malabsorption associated with surgical procedures and its treatment, *Nutr Clin Pract* 11:43, 1996.

Harnack L et al: Association of cancer prevention: related nutrition knowledge, beliefs, and attitudes to cancer prevention dietary behavior, *J Am Diet Assoc* 97:957, 1997.

Harrison LB et al: Detailed quality of life assessment in patients treated with primary radiotherapy for squamous cell cancer of the base of the tongue, *Head Neck* 19:169, 1997.

Haslett PA: Anticytokine approaches to the treatment of anorexia and cachexia, *Semin Oncol* 25(2 suppl 6):53, 1998.

Heinonen OP et al: Prostate cancer and supplementation with alpha tocopherol and β-carotene: incidence and mortality in a controlled trial, *J Natl Cancer Inst* 90:440, 1998.

Hennekens CH et al: Lack of effect of long-term supplementation with β-carotene on the incidence of malignant neoplasms and cardiovascular disease, *N Engl J Med* 334:1145, 1996.

Hirohata T, Kono S: Diet/nutrition and stomach cancer in Japan, *Int J Cancer* 10:34S, 1997.

Holick CN et al: Dietary carotenoids, serum β-carotene, and retinol and risk of lung cancer in the alpha-tocopherol, β-carotene cohort study, *Am J Epidemiol* 156:536, 2002.

Hong WK et al: Prevention of second primary tumors with isotretinoin in squamous-cell carcinoma of the head and neck, *N Engl J Med* 323:795, 1990.

Huang Z et al: Dual effects of weight and weight gain on breast cancer risk, *JAMA* 278:1407, 1997.

Hunter AMB: Nutrition management of patients with neoplastic disease of the head and neck treated with radiation therapy, *Nutr Clin Pract* 11:157, 1996.

Hunter DJ, Willett WC: Nutrition and breast cancer, *Cancer Causes Control* 7:56, 1996.

Ireton-Jones C et al: Clinical pathways in home nutrition support, *J Am Diet Assoc* 97:1003, 1997.

Isola LM et al: A pilot study of allogeneic bone marrow transplantation using related donors stimulated with G-CSF, *Bone Marrow Transplant* 20:1033, 1997.

Jatoi A et al: Do patients with nonmetastatic non-small cell lung cancer demonstrate altered resting energy expenditure? *Ann Thorac Surg* 72:348, 2001.

Kennedy LD: Common supportive drug therapies used with oncology patients. In McCallum PD, Polisena CG, editors: *The clinical guide to oncology nutrition,* Chicago, 2000, American Dietetic Association.

Kogut V: Complementary and alternative dietary therapies, *Clin J Oncol Nurs* 5:283, 2001.

Kono S, Hirohata T: Nutrition and stomach cancer, *Cancer Causes Control* 7:41, 1996.

Kritchevsky D: Caloric restriction and experimental mammary carcinogenesis, *Breast Cancer Res Treat* 46:161, 1997.

Kucuk O, Ottery FD: Dietary supplements during cancer treatment, *Oncol Issues* 17(suppl):24, 2002.

Kushner RF: Medical management of obesity, *Semin Gastrointest Dis* 13:123, 2002.

Lamson DW, Brignall MS: Antioxidants in cancer therapy II: quick reference guide, *Altern Med Rev* 5:152, 2000.

Langstein HN, Norton JA: Mechanisms of cancer cachexia, *Hematol/Oncol Clin North Am* 5:103, 1991.

Le Marchand L: Cancer preventive effects of flavonoids: a review, *Biomed Pharmacother* 56:296, 2002.

Leigh S, Thaler-DeMers D: Survivorship. In Gates RA, Fink RM, editors: *Oncology nursing secrets,* ed 2, Philadelphia, 2001, Hanley & Belfus.

Marshall JR, Boyle P: Nutrition and oral cancer, *Cancer Causes Control* 7:101, 1996.

Martinez ME et al: Leisure-time physical activity, body size, and colon cancer in women: Nurses' Health Study Research Group, *J Natl Cancer Inst* 89:948, 1997.

Matthys P, Billiau A: Cytokines and cachexia, *Nutrition* 13:763, 1997.

McCallum PD: Patient-generated subjective global assessment. In McCallum PD, Polisena CG, editors: *The clinical guide to oncology nutrition,* Chicago, 2000, American Dietetic Association.

McMahon K, Decker G, Ottery F: Integrating proactive nutritional assessment in clinical practices to prevent complications and cost, *Semin Oncol* 25(2 suppl 6):20, 1998.

Meikhail TM et al: Enteral nutrition during the treatment of head and neck carcinoma: is percutaneous endoscopic gastrostomy tube preferable to a nasogastric tube? *Cancer* 91:1785, 2001.

Meisenberg BR et al: Outpatient high-dose chemotherapy with autologous stem-cell rescue for hematologic and nonhematologic malignancies, *J Clin Oncol* 15:11, 1997.

Mercadante S: Parenteral versus enteral nutrition in cancer patients: indications and practice, *Support Care Cancer* 6:85, 1998.

Michaud D et al: A prospective study on intake of animal products and risk of prostate cancer, *Cancer Causes Control* 12:557, 2001.

Michaud D et al: Dietary sugar, glycemic load, and pancreatic cancer risk in a prospective study, *J Nat Cancer Inst* 94:1293, 2002.

Miller AL: Should antioxidants be used in cancer therapy? *Altern Med Rev* 4:304, 1999.

Miller JE: Hepatic veno-occlusive disease: a challenging complication of bone marrow transplantation, *Support Line* 19:10, 1997.

Mottonen M, Uhari M: Use of micronutrients and alternative drugs by children with acute lymphoblastic leukemia, *Med Pediatr Oncol* 28:5, 1997.

Murphy S, Von Roenn JH: Pharmacological management of anorexia and cachexia. In McCallum PD, Polisena CG, editors: *The clinical guide to oncology nutrition,* Chicago, 2000, American Dietetic Association.

Muscaritoli M et al: Nutritional and metabolic support in patients undergoing bone marrow transplantation, *Am J Clin Nutr* 75:183, 2002.

Nail LM: Fatigue. In Gates RA, Fink RM, editors: *Oncology nursing secrets,* ed 2, Philadelphia, 2001, Hanley & Belfus.

Nakaji S et al: Relationship between mineral and trace element concentrations in drinking water and gastric cancer mortality in Japan, *Nutr Cancer* 40:99, 2001.

Newberne PM, Conner MW: Food additives and contaminants: an update, *Cancer* 58:1851, 1986.

Newman V et al: Dietary supplement use by women at risk for breast cancer recurrence, *J Am Diet Assoc* 98:285, 1998.

O'Gorman P et al: Impact of weight loss, appetite, and the inflammatory response on quality of life in gastrointestinal patients, *Nutr Cancer* 32: 76, 1998.

Okasha M et al: Body mass index in young adulthood and cancer mortality: a retrospective cohort study, *J Epidemiol Community Health* 56:780, 2002.

Omenn GS et al: Effects of a combination of β-carotene and vitamin A on lung cancer and cardiovascular disease, *N Engl J Med* 334:1150, 1996.

Ottery FD: Supportive nutritional therapy in cancer, *Semin Oncol* 22:3S, 1995.

Ottery FD: Supportive nutritional management of the patient with pancreatic cancer, *Oncology* 10:26, 1996.

Ottery FD et al: Pharmacologic management of anorexia/cachexia, *Semin Oncol* 25:35S, 1998.

Owuor ED, Kong AN: Antioxidants and oxidants regulated signal transduction pathways, *Biochem Pharmacol* 64:765, 2002.

Papdopoulou A et al: Enteral nutrition after bone marrow transplantation, *Arch Dis Child* 77:131, 1997.

Paserot D et al: Evaluation of sensitive alterations in cancer patients treated by chemotherapy: first report, *Proc Annu Meeting Am Soc Clin Oncol* 16:A274, 1997.

Patterson RE et al: Vitamin supplements and cancer risk: the epidemiological evidence, *Cancer Causes Control* 8:786, 1997.

Piazza-Barnett R, Matarese LE: Enteral nutrition in adult medical/surgical oncology. In McCallum PD, Polisena CG, editors: *The clinical guide to oncology nutrition,* Chicago, 2000, American Dietetic Association.

Polisena CG: Nutrition concerns with the radiation therapy patient. In McCallum PD, Polisena CG, editors: *The clinical guide to oncology nutrition,* Chicago, 2000, American Dietetic Association.

Potter JD: Nutrition and colorectal cancer, *Cancer Causes Control* 7:127, 1996.

Potter JD, Steinmetz K: Vegetables, fruit, and phytoestrogens as preventive agents, *IARC Sci Publ* 139:61, 1996.

Prasad KN et al: Scientific rationale for using high-dose multiple micronutrients as an adjunct to standard and experimental cancer therapies, *J Am Coll Nutr* 20:450S, 2001.

Puccio M, Nathanson L: The cancer cachexia syndrome, *Semin Oncol* 24:277, 1997.

Renwick AG: Acceptable daily intake and the regulation of intense sweeteners, *Food Addit Contamin* 7:463, 1990.

Ringden O: Bone marrow transplantation using unrelated donors for hematological malignancies, *Med Oncol* 14:11, 1997.

Roberts S: Alternative nutrition therapies used by oncology patients, *Support Line* 20:10, 1998.

Roberts SR, Miller JE: Success using PEG tubes in marrow transplant recipients, *Nutr Clin Pract* 13:74, 1998.

Schatzkin A et al: Lack of effect of a low-fat, high-fat diet on the recurrence of colorectal adenomas, Polyp Prevention Trial Study Group, *N Engl J Med* 342:1149, 2000.

Sharp L et al: Risk factors for squamous cell carcinoma of the oesophagus in women: a case-control study, *Br J Cancer* 85:1667, 2001.

Slattery ML et al: Plant foods and colon cancer: an assessment of specific foods and their related nutrients (United States), *Cancer Causes Control* 8:575, 1997.

Smith-Warner SA et al: Alcohol and breast cancer in women: a pooled analysis of cohort studies, *JAMA* 270:535, 1998.

Staal van den Brekel AJ et al: Increased resting energy expenditure and weight loss are related to a systemic inflammatory response in lung cancer patients, *J Clin Oncol* 13:600, 1995.

Stovall E: Cancer survivorship in the year 2013: a survivor's perspective. In Brown HG, Seffrin JR, editors: *Horizons 2013: longer, better life without cancer,* Atlanta, 1996, American Cancer Society.

Tisdale MJ: Biology of cachexia, *J Natl Cancer Inst* 89:1763, 1997.

Trentham-Dietz A et al: Body size and risk of breast cancer, *Am J Epidemiol* 145:1011, 1997.

U.S. DHSS: Ninth Report on Carcinogens, Research Triangle Park, NC, 2000, Public Health Service, National Toxicology Program.

Von Roenn JH: Pharmacologic interventions for cancer-related weight loss, *Oncol Issues* 17(suppl):20, 2002.

Wojtaszek CA, Kochis LM, Cunningham RS: Nutrition impact symptoms in the oncology patient, *Oncol Issues* 17(suppl):17, 2002.

Wu AH et al: Dietary heterocyclic amines and microsatellite instability in colon adenocarcinomas, *Carcinogenesis* 22:1681, 2001.

Ziegler TR et al: Effects of glutamine supplementation on circulating lymphocytes after bone marrow transplantation: a pilot study, *Am J Med Sci* 315:4, 1998.

Additional References

Etiology

Ballard-Barbash R et al: Dietary fat, serum estrogen levels, and breast cancer risk: a multifaceted story, *J Natl Cancer Inst* 91:492, 1999.

Day R: Future need for more cancer research, *J Am Diet Assoc* 98:523, 1998.

Holt P et al: Modulation of abnormal colonic epithelial cell proliferation and differentiation by low-fat dairy foods, *JAMA* 280:1074, 1998.

Jacobs ET et al: Intake of supplemental and total fiber and risk of colorectal adenoma recurrence in the wheat bran fiber trial, *Cancer Epidemiol Biomarkers Prev* 11:906, 2002.

Laughlin EW: *Coming to terms with cancer: a glossary of cancer-related terms,* Atlanta, 2000, American Cancer Society.

Rock CL, Demark-Wahnefried W: Nutrition and survival after the diagnosis of breast cancer: a review of the evidence, *J Clin Oncol* 20:3302, 2002.

Tiemersma EW et al: Meat consumption, cigarette smoking, and genetic susceptibility in the etiology of colorectal cancer: results from a Dutch prospective study, *Cancer Causes Control* 13:383, 2002.

Medical Nutritional Therapy

Kalman D, Villani LJ: Nutritional aspects of cancer-related fatigue, *J Am Diet Assoc* 97:650, 1997.

Mason JB: Nutritional chemoprevention of colon cancer, *Semin Gastrointest Dis* 13:143, 2002.

Meydani M, Meydani M: Nutrition interventions in aging and age-associated disease, *Proc Nutr Soc* 61:165, 2002.

Spaulding-Albright N: A review of some herbal and related products commonly used in cancer patients, *J Am Diet Assoc* 97(suppl 2):S208, 1997.

Strasser F, Bruera ED: Update on anorexia and cachexia, *Hematol Oncol Clin North Am* 16:589, 2002.

Walker MS et al: *Oncology nutrition patient education materials,* Chicago, 1998, American Dietetic Association.

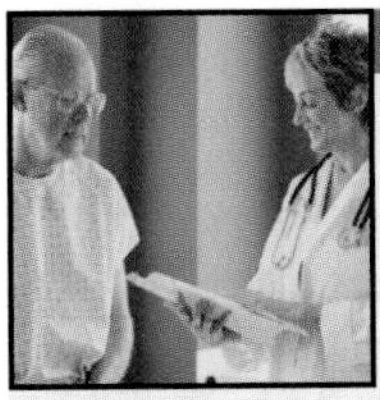

CHAPTER 41

Medical Nutrition Therapy for Human Immunodeficiency Virus (HIV) Disease

MARCY FENTON, MS, RD
ELLYN SILVERMAN, MPH, RD

CHAPTER OUTLINE

- Pathophysiology, Etiology, and Classification
- Epidemiology and Trends
- Manifestations and Stages of HIV Infection
- Opportunistic Infections and Other Complications
- Medical Management
- Women and HIV
- Pediatric Considerations
- Relationship Between Malnutrition and AIDS
- Medical Nutrition Therapy
- Complications With a Nutrition Impact
- Complementary and Alternative Therapies

KEY TERMS

acquired immune deficiency syndrome (AIDS)–HIV infection along with a CD4 cell count of 200 or less (or less than 14%) or dementia, wasting syndrome, malignant diseases such as Kaposi's sarcoma or non-Hodgkin's lymphoma, or one of 26 opportunistic infections

acute human immunodeficiency virus (HIV) infection–the 4- to 7-week period of rapid viral replication immediately after exposure to the virus, characterized by fever, malaise, and other flulike symptoms

AIDS enteropathy–changes in the small and large bowel thought to be attributable to direct HIV infection with no other identifiable pathogen; manifested as chronic diarrhea and possibly malabsorption

asymptomatic–describes a person who tests positive for HIV antibodies but does not exhibit symptoms of the disease

constitutional disease–disease that affects the whole body; common signs include persistent fever, often with night sweats, chronic or intermittent fatigue and malaise, and diarrhea of unknown etiology

cytomegalovirus (CMV)–group of herpes viruses with special affinity for salivary glands; manifesting as mononucleosis-like symptoms

drug resistance–the ability of a disease-causing microorganism, such as HIV, to adapt, grow, and multiply even in the presence of the drugs that are usually effective.

dysesthesia–a painful and persistent sensation induced by gentle touch of the skin

highly active antiretroviral therapy (HAART)–usually a combination of three or more medications used with the goal of suppressing viral replication and progression of HIV disease

HIV-associated nephropathy (HIVAN)–a syndrome of progressive renal failure with HIV infection

HIV encephalopathy (AIDS dementia)–degenerative disease of the brain caused by HIV infection

HIV wasting syndrome–catabolic condition with loss of lean body and muscle mass

KEY TERMS—Continued

human immunodeficiency virus (HIV)–the retrovirus isolated and recognized as the etiologic agent of AIDS

Kaposi's sarcoma–a malignant neoplastic vascular proliferation characterized by the development of bluish-red cutaneous nodules, usually on the surface of the skin or oral cavities

lipodystrophy syndrome–an undefined set of complications that can include disturbed fat metabolism; loss of subcutaneous fat or fat accumulation around the visceral organs and abdomen, breasts, and shoulder blades; metabolic dysregulation of glucose or lipid metabolism and possibly other abnormalities

lymphadenopathy syndrome (LAS)–swollen, firm, and sometimes tender lymph nodes secondary to HIV, influenza, mononucleosis, or lymphoma

myalgia–diffuse muscle pain, usually accompanied by vague feelings of discomfort or weakness

opportunistic infection–infection by an organism that does not ordinarily cause disease but is pathogenic in someone with an impaired immune response

perinatal HIV transmission (PHT)–transmission of HIV infection from mother to infant in utero, during birth, or during breast-feeding

protease inhibitors (PIs)–antiviral drugs that inhibit the viral protease enzyme and prevent viral replication

retrovirus–a virus, such as HIV, that replicates using an enzyme (reverse transcriptase) to copy RNA into DNA when RNA is its natural genetic state; most cells have DNA in their natural state and transcribe to RNA during replication

symptomatic–any perceptible, subjective change in the body or its functions that indicates disease or phases of disease

viral load test–measurement of the quantity of HIV RNA (free virus) in the blood, expressed as copies per milliliter of blood plasma, by PCR or bDNA tests; an optimal result is undetectable with a sensitive testing method

The relationship between immunity and nutrition has been well established. The management of HIV/AIDS draws from established and emerging nutritional science as it is applied and tested in the context of this disease. The nutrition provider must become familiar with HIV disease; its complications and treatment; advances in disease pathophysiology; medications and interactions; and related concerns, such as insulin resistance, lipid dysregulation, hepatitis and kidney diseases, substance abuse, eating disorders, and behavior modification. The medical management of HIV disease has been strengthened by sets of national guidelines, which are updated frequently and are available via the Internet. Numerous nutrition references and protocols exist.

It is considered "necessary for the patient to be entered into a continuum of medical care and services, including social, psychosocial, and nutritional services, with the availability of expert referral and consultation" (Panel on Clinical Practices for the Treatment of HIV, 2001).

After 20 years of AIDS, 22 million have died, and 13.2 million noninfected children have been orphaned. Forty-four million are expected to have died by 2010. Worldwide, people in their communities, corporations, and governments have been challenged, and resources are strained. In June 2001, the United Nations General Assembly held a special session to set a framework for national and international accountability in reaching benchmark targets through a comprehensive response (UNAIDS 2001) (Figure 41-1).

PATHOPHYSIOLOGY, ETIOLOGY, AND CLASSIFICATION

The acquired immunodeficiency syndrome (AIDS) was first described by the Centers for Disease Control (CDC) in 1981 (Gottlieb et al, 1981). Several previously healthy young men were reported to have unusual opportunistic infections—*Pneumocystis carinii* pneumonia, cytomegalovirus, candidiasis, or rare Kaposi's sarcoma associated with severe depression of cellular immunity. These cases presented a previously unknown disorder. In 1983, researchers isolated the etiologic agent, a retrovirus, which was named human immunodeficiency virus (HIV). In 1998, the oldest known original case of human infection by the virus was confirmed using a 1959 blood sample of a man from the Belgian Congo (Zhu et al, 1998).

Primary infection with HIV is the underlying cause of AIDS. HIV invades the genetic core of the CD4+ or T-helper lymphocyte cells, the principal agents involved in protection against infection (Figure 41-2). Although the CD4+ cell count in blood is the common laboratory test used, other distinct compartments contain virus and evolve separately. These compartments are semen, vaginal secretions, the lymph system, and the central nervous system. HIV infection causes a progressive depletion of CD4+ cells, which eventually leads to immunodeficiency, constitutional disease, neurologic complications, opportunistic infections, and neoplasms (Box 41-1).

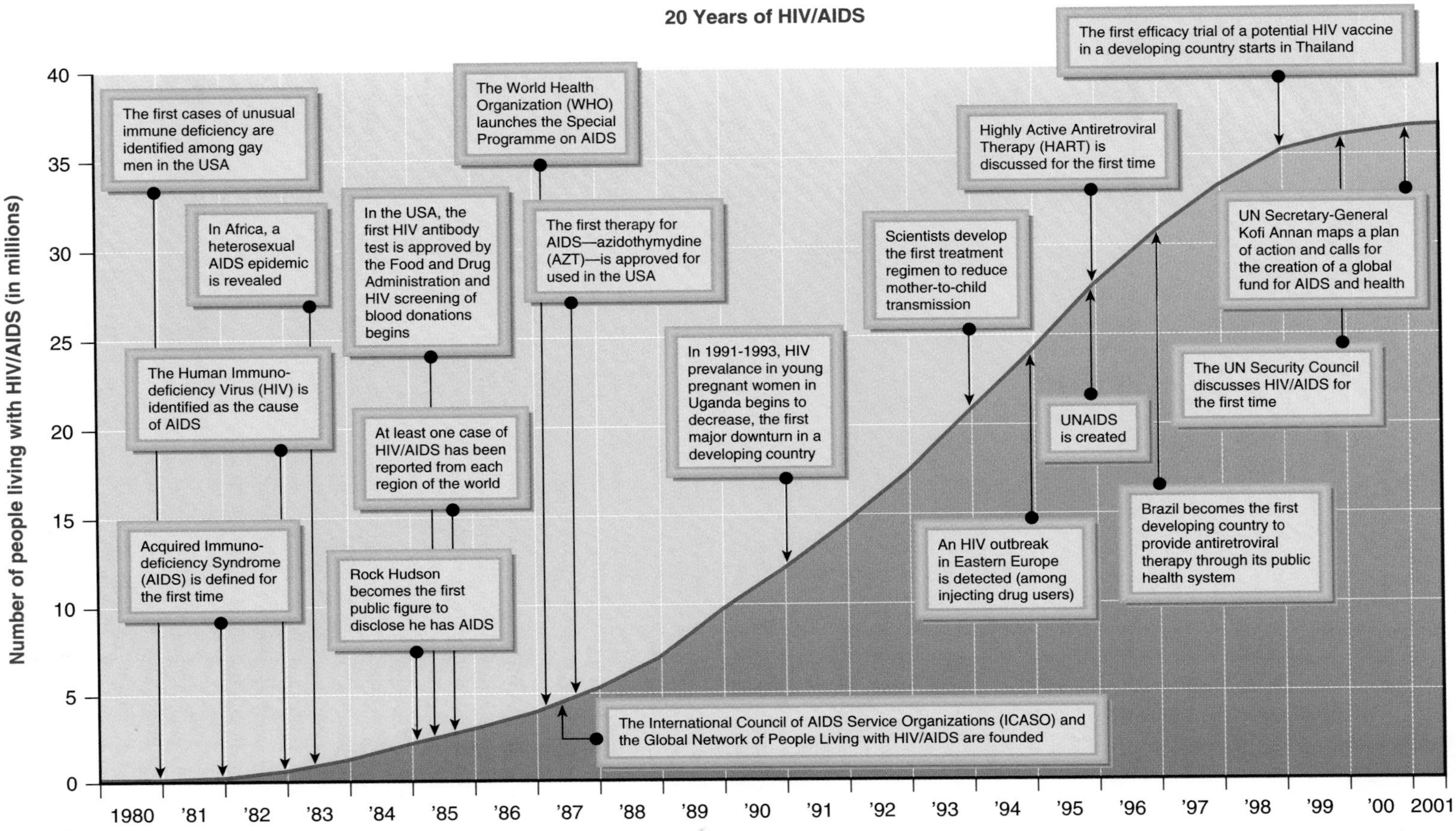

FIGURE 41-1 • Twenty years of HIV/AIDS. (From Joint United Nations Programme on HIV/AIDS: *20 Years of AIDS,* Geneva, Switzerland, 2001, UNAIDS, www.unaids.org/publications/graphics/20 years/Eng/HIV.time.chart.e.jpg.)

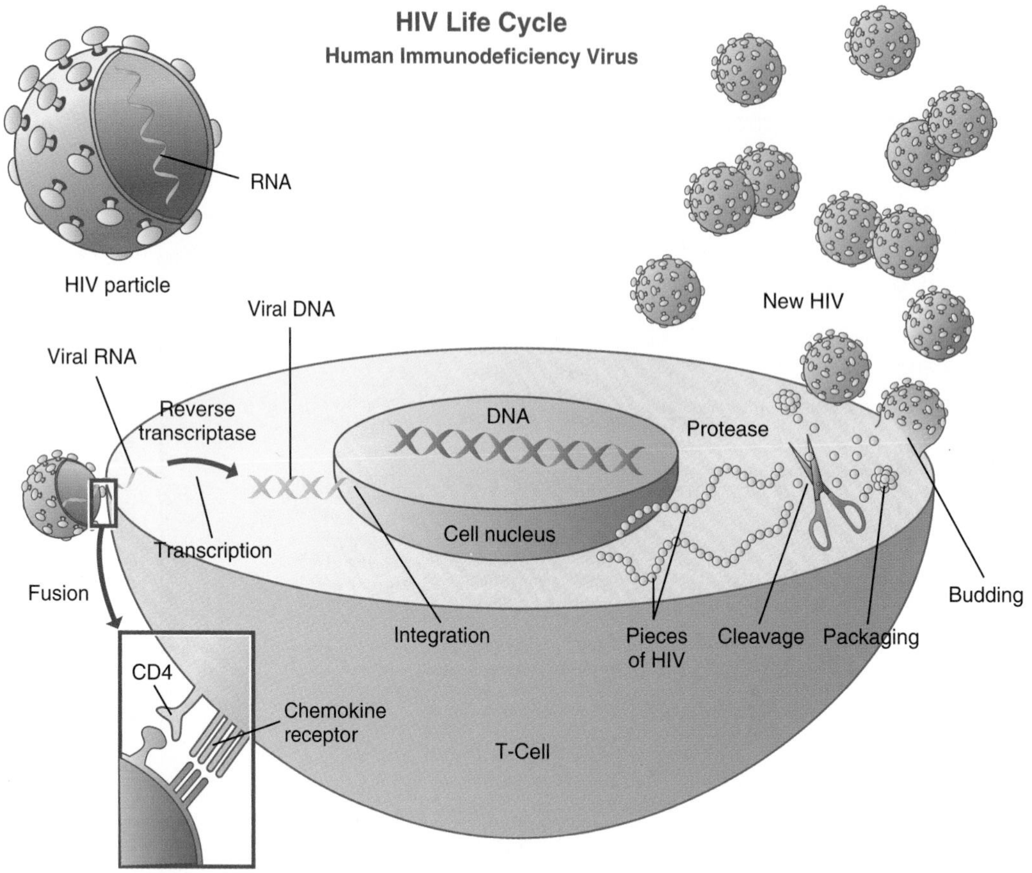

FIGURE 41-2 • HIV life cycle. (Copyright Community Research Initiative on AIDS, Los Angeles, 1998. Courtesy AIDS Community Research Initiative of America [ACRIA], New York.)

HIV progression differs among individuals largely as a result of the complex interaction between viral and genetic host factors. Better understanding of host responses is resulting in new therapeutic approaches for early treatment, immune modulation, structured treatment interruptions, and new chemotherapeutic agents and vaccine development (Hogan, 2001).

HIV can be transmitted via blood, semen, presemenal fluid, vaginal fluid, breast milk, and other body fluids that contain blood. Cerebrospinal fluid surrounding the brain and spinal cord, synovial fluid surrounding bone joints, and amniotic fluid surrounding a fetus are other fluids that can transmit HIV. Saliva, tears, and urine do not contain enough HIV to transmit the virus.

The most common way HIV is transmitted is via blood and semen during unprotected anal or vaginal intercourse with an HIV-infected person. Risk of transmission through oral sex is considered low but not risk-free (CDC, 2001c). Transmission can also occur by sharing of contaminated needles and injection of contaminated blood products and by transfer from an infected mother to her baby before or during birth or through breast-feeding. All persons should use universal precautions to protect both themselves and others when working with body fluids. The virus is not transmitted by casual contact—touching, hugging, or kissing—or through using the same plates, silverware, or drinking glasses.

Two types of HIV—HIV-1 and HIV-2—are transmitted the same way. Most people have HIV-1, and, unless specified, HIV-1 generally is the type to which discussions refer. HIV-2, first isolated in West Africa, is less easily transmitted, and the time between infection and illness is longer than with HIV-1. HIV-1 mutates readily and has different strains, which have many subtypes and groups and are found distributed unevenly throughout the world.

EPIDEMIOLOGY AND TRENDS

The United States

An estimated 850,000 to 950,000 people are currently living with HIV in the United States. Another 40,000 new infections are occurring yearly, of which 70% are in males, 30% are in females, and 1% are in children under the age of 13 years. About 15,000 die each year. Approximately half of those infected are undiagnosed or untreated. The number of infected

Box 41-1. Classification System for HIV Infection and Expanded AIDS Surveillance Case Definition for Adolescents and Adults

Clinical Categories

The clinical categories are defined as follows:

Category A—one or more of the conditions listed here occurring in an adolescent or adult with documented HIV infection. Conditions listed in categories B and C must not have occurred.

- Asymptomatic HIV infection
- Persistent generalized lymphadenopathy (PGL)
- Acute (primary) HIV infection with accompanying illness or a history of acute HIV infection

Category B—symptomatic conditions occurring in an HIV-infected adolescent or adult that are not included among conditions listed in clinical category C and that meet at least one of the following criteria:

1. The conditions are attributed to HIV infection and/or indicate a defect in cell-mediated immunity
2. The conditions are considered by physicians to have a clinical course or management that is complicated by HIV infection

Examples of conditions in clinical category B include but are not limited to the following:

- Bacterial endocarditis,, meningitis, pneumonia, or sepsis
- Candidiasis (vulvovaginal) that is persistent (1 month duration) or is poorly responsive to therapy
- Candidiasis, oropharyngeal (thrush)
- Cervical dysplasia, severe, or carcinoma
- Constitutional symptoms, such as fever (≥38.5° C) or diarrhea lasting >1 month
- Hairy leukoplakia, oral
- Herpes zoster (shingles), involving at least two distinct episodes or more than one dermatome
- Idiopathic thrombocytopenic purpura
- Listeriosis
- *Mycobacterium tuberculosis* infection, pulmonary
- Nocardiosis
- Pelvic inflammatory disease
- Peripheral neuropathy

Category C—any condition listed in the 1987 surveillance case definition for AIDS and affecting an adolescent or adult. The conditions in clinical category C are strongly associated with severe immunodeficiency, occur frequently in HIV-infected individuals, and cause serious morbidity or mortality. Among the conditions listed in the 1993 AIDS surveillance case definition (assuming HIV positivity) are the following:

- Candidiasis of bronchi, trachea, or lungs
- Candidiasis, esophageal
- CD4 lymphocyte counts <200 or a CD4 percent of total lymphocytes <14 if the absolute count is not available
- Cervical cancer, invasive
- Coccidioidomycosis, disseminated or extrapulmonary (Valley fever)
- Cryptococcosis, extrapulmonary
- Cyptosporidiosis, chronic intestinal (>1 month duration)
- Cytomegalovirus disease (other than liver, spleen, or nodes)
- Cytomegalovirus retinitis (with loss of vision)
- HIV encephalopathy
- Herpes simplex: chronic ulcer(s) (>1 month duration) or bronchitis, pneumonitis, or esophagitis
- Histoplasmosis, disseminated or extrapulmonary
- Isosporiasis, chronic intestinal (>1 month duration)
- Kaposi's sarcoma (KS)
- Lymphoma, Burkitt's (or equivalent term)
- Lymphoma, immunoblastic (or equivalent term)
- Lymphoma, primary in brain
- *Mycobacterium avium* complex or *M. kansasii*, disseminated or extrapulmonary
- *M. tuberculosis*, any site, pulmonary or extrapulmonary
- *Mycobacterium*, other species or unidentified species, disseminated or extrapulmonary
- *Pneumocystis carinii* pneumonia (PCP)
- Pneumonia, recurrent
- Progressive multifocal leukoencephalopathy (PML)
- *Salmonella* septicemia, recurrent
- Toxoplasmosis of brain
- Wasting syndrome secondary to HIV

	CLINICAL CATEGORIES		
CD4+ CELL COUNT CATEGORIES (AIDS-INDICATOR CELL COUNT)	A (ASYMPTOMATIC OR PGL)	B (SYMPTOMATIC, NOT A OR C CONDITIONS)	C (AIDS INDICATOR CONDITION)
>500/mm^3	A1	B1	C1
200-499/mm^3	A2	B2	C2
<200/mm^3	A3	B3	C3

From Centers for Disease Control and Prevention: 1993 Revised classification system for HIV infection and expanded surveillance case definition for AIDS among adolescents and adults, *MMWR* 41(No. RR-17), 1992, www.cdc.gov/mmwr/preview/mmwrhtml/00018871.htm.

African Americans and Latinos has been increasing disproportionately. They account for 54% and 19% of the new infections, respectively. Whites account for 26%, and other groups (Asians and Pacific Islanders; American Indians and Alaskan Natives) remain relatively constant at approximately 1% of new cases (CDC, 2001b) (Figure 41-3).

The largest newly infected risk groups in the United States are men who have sex with men (42%), men (9%) and women (24%) infected through heterosexual

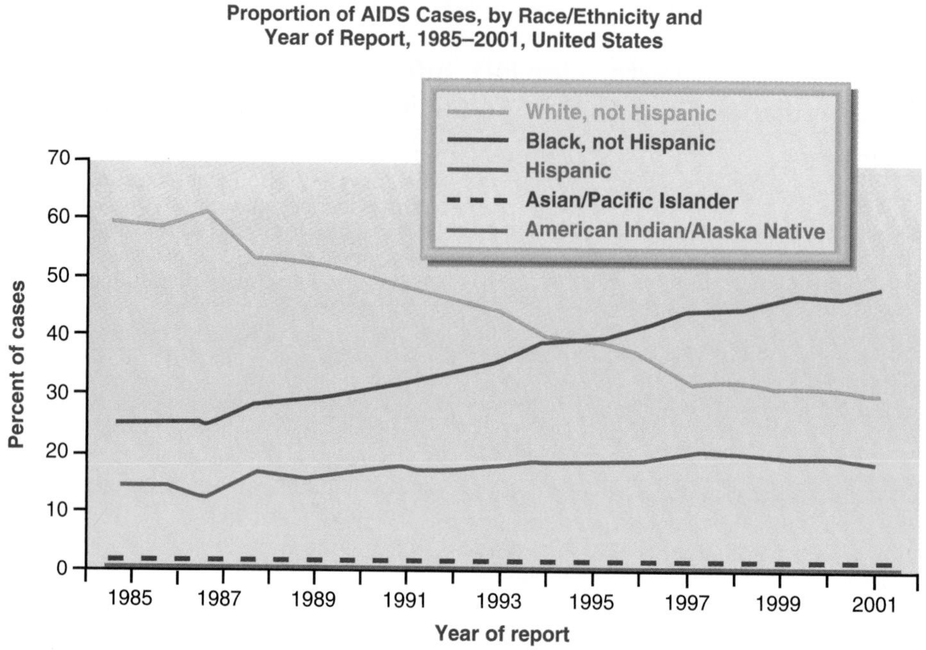

FIGURE 41-3 • Proportion of AIDS cases, by race and ethnicity and year of report, 1985-2000, United States. (From CDC, Division of HIV/AIDS Prevention: *Proportion of AIDS cases, by race/ethnicity and year of report, 1985-2001, United States,* www.cdc.gov/hiv/graphics/images/l238/l238-2.htm, updated February 5, 2003.)

sex, and, in decline, those who use injection drug use (25%) (CDC, 2001b). Improvements in blood-handling management have decreased significantly rates of HIV infection for hemophiliacs and other blood transfusion recipients. There is decreased evidence of HIV in infants born to mothers with HIV-1, thanks to prenatal HIV counseling, voluntary testing, and use of perinatal drug therapy. In 2000, 177 (90%) of the 196 pediatric AIDS cases reported were perinatally acquired, compared with 730 (91%) of the 800 cases in 1995. Representing only 7% of new cases of AIDS in the early part of the epidemic, adult and adolescent females constituted nearly 25% of new cases and 31% of newly diagnosed cases of HIV infection in 2000. Latino and African American women especially have been impacted, and four out of every five new cases of HIV infection are in women of color (CDC, 2001b). Despite new treatments that can extend years and improve quality of life, many women have limited access to quality health care and treatment options.

State and federal correctional facilities have a rate of confirmed AIDS cases five times greater than that of the general U.S. population (Maruschak, 2001). Although 1 in 10 inmates is female, rates of infection are three times higher for women than for men (De Groot, 2000). HIV-infected individuals age 50 years and older represent more than 10% of the total number of AIDS cases reported, and one in every three deaths are in those over 45 years of age (HRSA, 2001). This age group is found to use condoms much less often than 20-year-olds do, is only 20% as likely to get tested for HIV, and is often misdiagnosed and underserved. Postmenopausal women, who are often uninformed of the dangers of HIV transmission, may become increasingly sexually active with more partners who use condoms less often. The physiology of older women increases the risk of transmission, as the vaginal walls are thin, vaginal lubrication decreases, and risk of torn vaginal membranes increases, thus providing easy access for the virus (Engle, 1998).

More than 448,000 deaths from HIV-related causes were reported from the beginning of the epidemic through the end of 2000. Of these deaths, 85% were males, 15% females, 46% whites, 36% African Americans, and 17% Hispanics. With use of HAART and treatment of opportunistic infections, a dramatic decrease in deaths of adults and adolescents with AIDS in the United States occurred; now more people than ever are living with HIV disease (see Table 41-4) (CDC, 2003).

The reporting of AIDS cases is federally mandated but does not reflect an accurate number of people living with HIV, nor does it reflect trends of infection, which makes health and social planning difficult. Thirty-four states, Guam, and the Virgin Islands have now implemented confidential HIV reporting, and gaps are being addressed. The largest source of public health care funding for AIDS care is Medicaid with $7 billion, which covers 55% of adults and 90% of children with AIDS, followed by Medicare and then by Ryan White Comprehensive AIDS Resources Emergency (CARE) Act funding (Bozette et al, 2001;

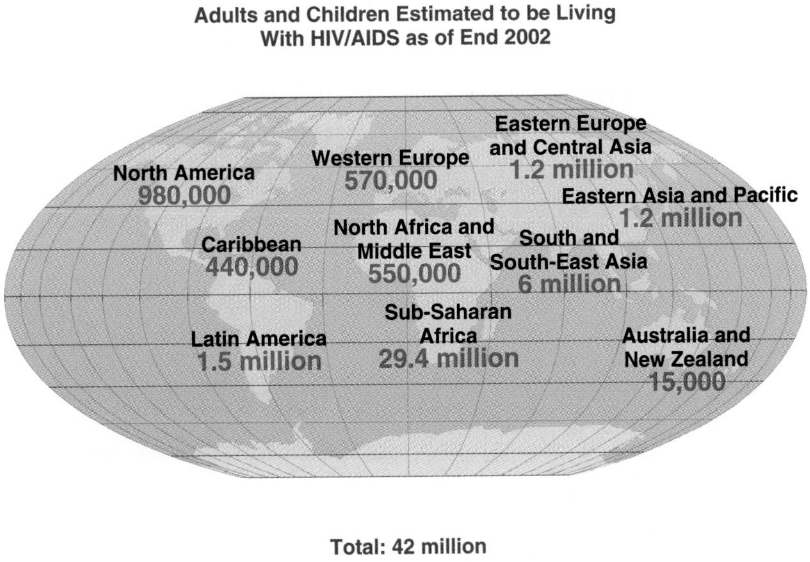

FIGURE 41-4 • Adults and children estimated to be living with HIV/AIDS as of the end of 2002. (From Joint United Nations Programme on HIV/AIDS: *AIDS Epidemic Update*, Geneva, Switzerland, December 2001, UNAIDS, www.unaids.org/worldaidsday/2001/EPIgraphics 2001/EPIcore_en.ppt.)

HRSA, 2002). The U.S. Department of Health and Human Services (DHHS) HIV/AIDS Bureau (HAB) within Health Resources and Services Administration (HRSA, 2002) administers the program.

Primary care programs through Title III CARE Act funding must provide nutrition services on site or at another facility, and the provider has to be a registered or licensed dietitian (HIV/AIDS Bureau, 2001c, 2001d). Funding has been poor, which has left access to adequate HIV nutrition care a goal yet to be achieved.

Worldwide

The Thirteenth World AIDS Conference was held in Durban, South Africa, in 2000. Disparities in access to health care and numbers of HIV infection and related deaths throughout the world became visible. Ninety-five percent of the world's cases of HIV, including those caused by perinatal HIV transmission, are in the developing world (Figure 41-4).

By the end of 2001, 40 million adults and 1.4 million children under 15 years of age were living with HIV disease. Most do not know they are infected. Three million died from AIDS-related causes in 2001. Thirteen million children—10% or more in some countries—have already been orphaned. In the developing world, HIV is primarily spread through sex between men and women; half of the infected are women. In contrast to the education, prevention, health care programs, and access to medications offered in developed nations, less developed countries face a difficult future. The HIV infection rates in some regions have increased by 30% per year; high death rates in many countries cause a decrease in life expectancy. Economically, 15 countries together will experience a reduction of 24 million people from their work force, with a decrease in national incomes, economic growth, and economic potential. In 2000 both the United Nations Security Council and the United States declared HIV/AIDS a security threat (Piot, 2000; Henry J. Kaiser Family Foundation, 2000).

The United Nations urges a comprehensive strategy built on five objectives to fight against HIV/AIDS (Annan, 2001):

1. "Ensure that people everywhere, particularly young people, know what to do to avoid infection.
2. Stop HIV transmission from mother to child.
3. Provide care and treatment for all those infected.
4. Search both for a vaccine and for a cure.
5. Provide care for all people whose lives have been devastated by AIDS, particularly orphans."

Access to food, potable water, and housing and achieving economic stability remain fundamental concerns. The struggle for affordable effective drugs, however, has changed some international pharmaceutical and government agreements.

MANIFESTATIONS AND STAGES OF HIV INFECTION

After exposure and transmission of HIV into the host, HIV spreads throughout the body, and blood CD4+ cell counts fall dramatically. An immune response follows, CD4+ cells can return to almost normal, and virus in the blood falls to an undetectable level. During this period of clinical latency, CD4+ cells decrease to below a level at which increased risks of opportunistic infections occur. Untreated, HIV eventually replicates at 800 billion virus particles per day. Four stages of the disease have been characterized: (1) acute HIV infection; (2) asymptomatic chronic HIV infection; (3) symptomatic HIV infection; and (4) AIDS or advanced HIV (Figure 41-5, Table 41-1; see Box 41-1). Table 41-2 describes the categories as they affect children.

Acute human immunodeficiency virus (HIV) infection is the 4- to 7-week period immediately after infection, when viral replication is rapid. Thirty percent to 60% of newly infected persons develop an acute syndrome with fever, malaise, lymphadenopathy syndrome (LAS), pharyngitis, headache, myalgia, and sometimes rash, which may last for a week to a month. The time period between the initial HIV infection and seroconversion—that is, the development of HIV antibodies—varies from 1 week to several months or more. Once antibodies to HIV appear in the blood, individuals with and without symptoms will test positive for HIV. Viral load is extremely high, and individuals are very infectious at this time.

Asymptomatic HIV is a stage in which few, if any, noticeable symptoms occur, lasting from a few months to as long as 10 years. Subclinical changes have been reported, including a decrease in lean body mass without apparent total body weight change, vitamin B_{12} deficiency, and increased susceptibility to foodborne and waterborne pathogens.

Symptomatic HIV occurs when symptoms appear (see Box 41-1, Category B). These symptoms may include fevers, sweats, skin problems, fatigue, or other symptoms that are not AIDS-defining. A decline in nutrient status or body composition may also occur.

AIDS, or advanced HIV disease, is the diagnostic term reserved for those persons with at least one well-defined, life-threatening clinical condition that is clearly linked to HIV-induced immunosuppression (see AIDS-defining conditions, Category C, in Box 41-1).

A very small number of persons infected with HIV exhibit no signs of disease progression even after 12 or more years. Reasons for long-term nonprogression may include infection by a less virulent strain of the virus, protective genetic mutations, or particular protective characteristics of their immune system or genes. Study of this group will likely assist in the development of protective vaccines.

OPPORTUNISTIC INFECTIONS AND OTHER COMPLICATIONS

Opportunistic infections with bacteria, fungi, protozoa, or viruses are common in this population. They are often the cause of diarrhea, malabsorption, fever, and weight loss as well as many other symptoms.

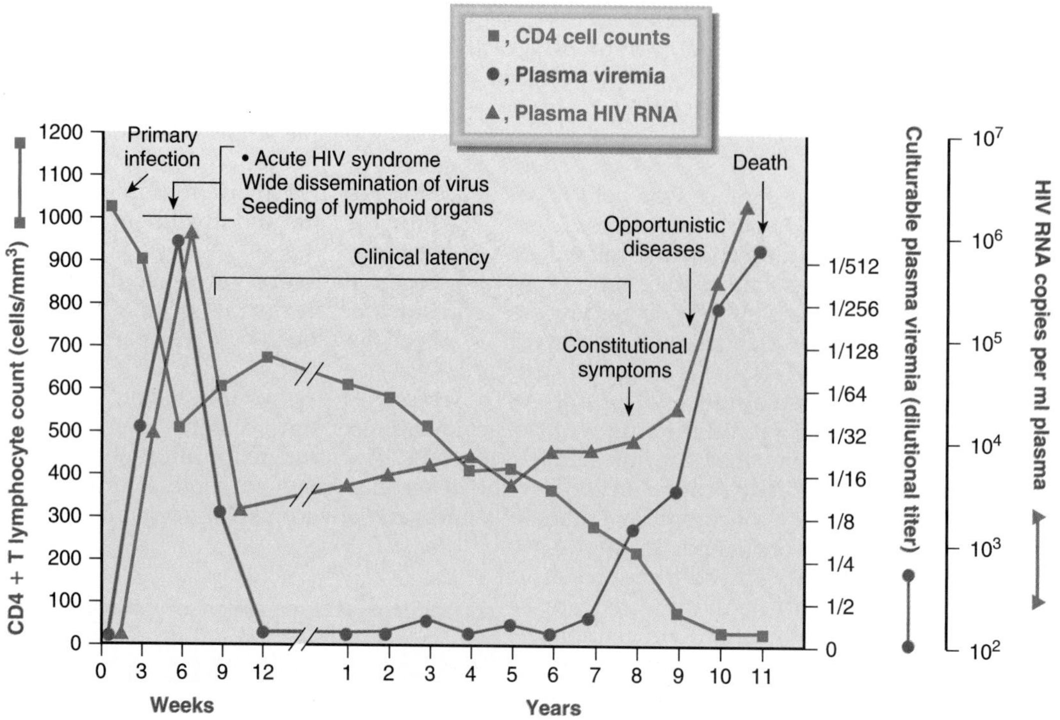

FIGURE 41-5 • Natural history of HIV infection in an average patient without antiretroviral therapy from time of transmission to death at 10 to 11 years. (From Fauci AS et al: Immunopathogenic mechanisms of HIV infections, *Ann Intern Med* 124:654, 1996.)

TABLE 41-1 CD4 Cell Counts and Associated Conditions

CD4 CELL COUNT	CONDITION	COMMON PHYSICAL PROBLEMS AND SYMPTOMS
>550/mm^3	Acute retroviral syndrome	May include fever, adenopathy, pharyngitis, rash, myalgias, diarrhea, headache, nausea and vomiting, hepatosplenomegaly, weight loss, thrush, neurologic symptoms
	Candidial vaginitis	Fungal infection causing itching and swelling of the vulva, thick white-yellow or cheesy discharge, and burning upon urination
	Persistent generalized lymphadenopathy (PGL)	Chronic, diffuse, noncancerous lymph node enlargement
	Guillian-Barré syndrome	The most common form of sudden generalized paralysis
	Myopathy	Progressive muscle weakness
	Aseptic meningitis	An inflammation of the meninges (membranes surrounding the brain or spinal cord), which may be caused by a bacterium, fungus, or virus
200-500 mm^3	Oropharyngeal candidiasis (thrush)	Loss of appetite, white plaques, mouth discomfort, change in taste
	Kaposi's sarcoma	Slightly raised purplish lesions on the skin, mucous membranes, or lymph nodes, usually painless
	Pulmonary tuberculosis reactivation	Cough, blood-stained sputum (hemoptysis), fever, night sweats, weight loss, chest pain, prolonged fatigue, anorexia
	Herpes zoster (shingles) virus	Vesicular skin lesions along dermatomes, pain
	Cryptosporidiosis, self-limited	Watery diarrhea lasting 1 to 4 days or as long as 4 weeks
	Oral hairy leukoplakia	Whitish lesions that appear on the side of the tongue and cheeks with a "hairy" surface
	Pneumococcal and other bacterial pneumonia/ bacterial sinusitis	Inflammation of the nasal cavity and sinuses, congestion, fever, pain, tearing of the eyes and sensitivity to light
	Herpes simplex (virus)	Weeping skin lesions (oral, perirectal), bleeding, rectal discharge, pain
	Cervical intraepithelial neoplasia	Dysplasia of the cervix epithelium, often premalignant, characterized by abnormal keratinization and condylomata
	Cervical cancer	Watery, blood-tinged vaginal discharge more often seen after sexual intercourse
	B-cell lymphoma	The type of lymphoma most commonly associated with HIV in which certain cells of the lymphatic system grow abnormally
	Anemia	A lower than normal number of red cells; fatigue
	Mononeuronal multiplex	A rare type of neuropathy that may be related to the cytomegalovirus (CMV)
	Idiopathic thrombocytopenic purpura	A condition in which the body produces antibodies against the platelets in the blood
	Hodgkin's lymphoma	See B-cell lymphoma
	Lymphocytic interstitial pneumonitis	A type of pneumonia that affects 35%-40% of children with AIDS and causes a hardening of the lung membranes involved in absorbing oxygen
100-200/mm^3	*Pneumocystis carinii* pneumonia (PCP) (fungi)	Fever, chills, night sweats, cough with or without sputum production, shortness of breath, antibiotic side effects, weight loss, weakness
	Disseminated histoplasmosis and coccidioidomycosis	Fever, weight loss, skin lesions, difficulty breathing, anemia, lymphadenopathy, possibly pneumonia
	Miliary/extrapulmonary TB	Refers to the tiny discrete granulomatous lesions in lungs and other organs that result when bloodborne tubercle bacilli seeds many tissues
	Progressive multifocal leukoencephalopathy (PML)	Progressive weakness and dementia, speech problems, forgetfulness, perceptual problems, visual problems, incontinence
	Wasting	Loss of weight and body cell mass
	Peripheral neuropathy	Painful, burning feet or numbness in the feet and/or hands
	HIV-associated dementia	Loss of coordination, mood swings, loss of inhibitions, widespread cognitive dysfunctions
	Cardiomyopathy	Disease of the myocardium associated with ventricular dysfunction
	Vascular myelopathy	Disease of the spinal cord
	Progressive polyradiculopathy	Radiating pain and parathesias that cause mild sensory loss and lower extremity areflexia
	Non-Hodgkin's lymphoma	Depends on location, lumps, fatigue, and/or pain
50-100/mm^3	Microsporidiosis	An intestinal infection from a parasite (microsporidia) that causes diarrhea and wasting in persons with HIV
	Candidial esophagitis	A *Candida* infection of the esophagus that can cause severe problems with swallowing
	Disseminated herpes simplex	A virus that causes cold sores on the mouth and around the eyes or can be transmitted to the genitals
	Cryptoccocus (meningitis)	Headache and fevers, malaise, nausea, fatigue, loss of appetite

Modified from Martin J, Hughes A, Franks P: *AIDS home care and hospice manual,* ed 2, San Francisco, 1990, Visiting Nurses and Hospice of San Francisco; Phair JP, Murphy R: *Contemporary diagnosis and management of HIV/AIDS infections,* Newton, Pa, 1997, Health Care Co.; Bartlett JG, Gallant JE: *Medical management of HIV infection,* 2001-2002 edition, Baltimore, Md, 2002. Johns Hopkins University, Division of Infectious Diseases.

Continued

TABLE 41-1 CD4 Cell Counts and Associated Conditions—cont'd

CD4 CELL COUNT	CONDITION	COMMON PHYSICAL PROBLEMS AND SYMPTOMS
50-100/mm^3—cont'd	Primary tuberculosis	Cough, blood-stained sputum (hemoptysis), fever, night sweats, weight loss, chest pain, prolonged fatigue, anorexia
	Cryptosporidiosis, chronic (protozoa)	Severe chronic, watery diarrhea (up to 15-20/day), severe weight loss, weakness, electrolyte imbalance, abdominal cramping, fever, nausea, vomiting, enlarged lymph nodes
	Toxoplasmosis (protozoa)	Fevers, swollen glands, headaches
0-50/mm^3	Disseminated (CMV)	Blindness or visual loss (retinitis), fever, fatigue and severe malaise, weight loss, facial edema (secondary to adrenalitis), enteritis, colitis
	Disseminated *Mycobacterium avium* complex (MAC)	Fever, severe weight loss/cachexia, abdominal pain, diarrhea, malabsorption, antibiotic side effects
	Central nervous system lymphoma	A lymphoma limited to the cranial-spinal axis without systemic disease

TABLE 41-2 Immunologic Categories for HIV-Infected Children Based on Age-Specific CD4+ T-Lymphocyte Counts and Percentage of Total Lymphocytes

	CELL COUNTS (CELLS/μL [%]*) ACCORDING TO AGE		
IMMUNOLOGIC CATEGORY	<12 MONTHS	1-5 YEARS	6-12 YEARS
No evidence of suppression	≥1500 (≥25)	≥1000 (≥25)	≥500 (≥25)
Evidence of moderate suppression	750-1499 (15-24)	500-999 (15-24)	200-499 (15-24)
Severe suppression	<750 (<15)	<500 (<15)	<200 (<15)

Modified from Centers for Disease Control and Prevention: 1997 USPHS/IDSA guidelines for the prevention of opportunistic infection in persons infected with human immunodeficiency virus, *MMWR* 46(No. RR-12):27, 1997.
*Percentage of total lymphocytes.

Common infections, their relationships to CD4+ counts, and their manifestations are summarized in Table 41-1.

Malignant Disease

Kaposi's sarcoma (KS) is a malignant disease of the peripheral blood mononuclear cells that manifests as purple nodules on the skin, mucous membranes, or lymph nodes or throughout the gastrointestinal tract. Incidence of KS has greatly declined with combination therapy and greater viral control. KS lesions in the oral cavity or esophagus may cause pain and difficulty with chewing and swallowing, and lesions in the intestinal tract have been implicated in diarrhea and intestinal obstruction. Localized KS lesions can be treated with surgery or radiation therapy, and chemotherapy is often used to treat persons with disseminated disease. Disseminated KS is difficult to control because chemotherapy can further suppress immune function in persons with other HIV-related complications.

Lymphomas, including non-Hodgkin's lymphoma and Burkitt's lymphoma that involve the small bowel, can cause malabsorption, diarrhea, or intestinal obstruction. Primary lymphoma in the brain can cause alterations in personality and in motor and cognitive abilities. Lymphomas of these types often respond poorly to multiagent chemotherapies; preexisting immune suppression often limits the amount and frequency of treatment.

Neuromuscular Diseases

Immediately following infection, HIV enters the brain and may result in HIV encephalopathy (AIDS dementia), myelopathy, peripheral neuropathy, and myopathy. Secondary neurologic complications may result from toxoplasma encephalitis, progressive multifocal leukoencephalopathy, cytomegalovirus (CMV) encephalitis, radiculomyelitis, cryptococcal meningitis, primary central nervous system lymphoma, and neurosyphilis.

Before there were medications to control viral replication, dementia affected 25% of those living with HIV; today the rate of HIV-associated dementia is below 10% (Diesing, 2002). Symptoms of AIDS dementia may include deterioration in cognition (concentration, recall, new memory development, language), motor function (coordination, gait, bladder control), and behavior (psychosis, depression, withdrawal). The presence of one or more factors may be necessary for AIDS dementia to be identified: cytokines, calcium-mediated toxicity, excitatory amino acids (glutamate, quinolinic acid), arachidonic acid, oxidative mechanisms, platelet-activating factor, or apoptosis (programmed cell death). Viral load in the brain and the level of neurologic decline are not strongly correlated.

Myelopathy (disease of the spinal cord) may occur in as many as 25% of those with advanced HIV disease and can result in partial paralysis of the lower extremities (paraparesis). Myelopathy affects motor and sensory functions and is manifested by spasticity and, in some, weakness in the legs and bladder. Approximately 20% of patients with AIDS experience peripheral neuropathy, which is characterized by sensory loss, pain, weakness, and wasting of muscle in the hands or legs and feet. The first signs are tingling, burning, or numbness in the toes and fingers. Peripheral neuropathy may be caused by the virus or by drugs (zalcitabine, didanosine, and stavudine).

Myopathy—progressive muscle weakness—is usually a result of HIV infection or toxicity from AZT. If AZT is the underlying cause, creatine kinase levels are usually elevated (Clifford et al, 1999).

HIV-Liver Disease

Hepatitis C (HVC) is now considered an HIV opportunistic infection, and deaths from liver disease have increased significantly. Approximately 170 million persons worldwide are infected with the hepatitis C virus (HVC)—1.8 percent of people in the United States, about 25% of those with HIV infection (Lauer and Walker, 2001). Those with both HIV and HVC have a faster progression to AIDS and death (Piroth et al, 1998), and current HVC treatments do not seem to alter outcome in HIV-infected persons (Murphy, 2003). The FDA has approved α-interferon with ribaviron for treatment. When ribaviron is not tolerated, α-interferon alone is also FDA-approved and used (see Chapter 31).

Liver function may be compromised through the use of highly active antiretroviral therapy and by infection with cytomegalovirus (CMV), cryptosporidia, and hepatitis B or by hepatic malignant diseases, such as KS or lymphoma. Dosing of drugs must be adjusted for those with liver failure.

Tuberculosis and Lung Diseases

There has been a drop in deaths caused by tuberculosis. Although most cases of tuberculosis (TB) caused by *Mycobacterium tuberculosis* affect the lungs, the disease may also occur, especially in HIV-infected persons, in extrapulmonary sites, such as in the larynx, lymph nodes, brain, kidneys, or bones. Medical conditions that increase the risk of TB infection include HIV infection; a body weight that is 10% or more below ideal weight; immunosuppressive therapy; and hematologic disorders, such as leukemia and lymphomas. Other risk factors include underfeeding, alcoholism, intravenous (IV) drug use, and homelessness (see Chapter 38).

It is estimated that 10% of all HIV-infected persons may be tuberculin-positive (Jacobson et al, 1992) and that, although the risk of active TB is 10% over a lifetime in those infected with only *M. tuberculosis,* the risk increases to 7% to 10% per year for persons coinfected with *M. tuberculosis* and HIV (Selwin et al, 1989). *M. tuberculosis* and HIV coinfection causes immune activation and a rapid increase in the rate of HIV replication. Early and aggressive treatment of TB and HIV is critical to controlling the progression of both diseases. Survival rates have increased with use of HAART, possibly by decreasing the risk of other life-threatening opportunistic infections (Girardi et al, 2001). Dietary recommendations include liberal amounts of protein and calories; sufficient—but not excessive—calcium and vitamin D; iron; supplemental vitamin B_6 and vitamin A (as carotene is poorly converted); adequate fluids (unless contraindicated); and adjustments of TB medications because of nutrient-drug interactions (see Chapter 19).

HIV-Associated Nephropathy

A syndrome of progressive renal failure, HIV-associated nephropathy (HIVAN), may occur. Proteinuria may also result from repeated infections, volume depletion, or nephrotoxic drugs. At one time, 20% of hospitalized HIV-infected patients were reported to have acute renal failure (creatinine >2.0 mg/dl) (Valeri and Neusy, 1991), and 30% to 60% have hyponatremia associated with increased morbidity and mortality (Tang et al, 1993). Deaths from kidney disease have increased; the number of dialysis centers serving HIV-infected patients has also increased. Dosing of drugs and nutrition therapy must be adjusted for those with renal failure (see Chapter 39).

Other Affected Organ Systems

Other nutritionally pertinent organs affected by HIV infection or its treatment include the gastrointestinal tract and the pancreas. *Mycobacterium avium* complex (MAC), greatly decreased in incidence since the use of powerful HIV medications, can be seen in the lymph nodes, liver, bone marrow, blood, and urine of patients with AIDS. Cytomegalovirus (CMV) can affect the eye, causing retinitis; and if left untreated, it may progress to blindness (Drew et al, 2002).

Chronic diarrhea may persist in the absence of identifiable enteric pathogens as a result of what is known as AIDS enteropathy. Intestinal injury is related to specific complications rather than to the immunodeficiency caused by HIV (Kotler, 1999). Persons with HIV enteropathy may have villous atrophy and abnormal results on tests of small bowel function, including 72-hour fecal fat, D-xylose, and paraaminobenzoic acid (PABA) absorption (Cello, 1997). Because of the vulnerability of persons with immune suppression to foodborne and waterborne pathogens, food and water safety is a concern (see *Focus On:* Reducing Infections).

MEDICAL MANAGEMENT

Disease progression differs among individuals, and treatment decisions must be individualized. With the advent of viral load testing and highly active antiretroviral therapy (HAART), clinical and therapeutic

FOCUS ON

Reducing Infections

The CDC has emphasized the need to consider blood and other body fluids from all persons to be potentially infective (CDC, 2001a). In the hospital setting, nursing and nutrition service employees should follow their institution's appropriate universal precaution policies and procedures to prevent the transmission of HIV. Hospital personnel need not wear gowns, masks, or gloves while performing general patient care unless respiratory or strict isolation is indicated.

Persons with HIV and their caregivers should be instructed in food and water safety practices at home and for eating out or traveling abroad. Tips from the Centers for Disease Control (CDC, 1987) to reduce the risk of cryptosporidiosis include careful hand-washing; avoiding sex that involves contact with stool; avoiding touching of farm animals or the stool from pets; carefully washing and cooking of foods; exercising caution when swimming in pools, jacuzzis, or lakes; drinking only safe water; and exercising caution with food and water while traveling.

TABLE 41-3 Indications for the Initiation of Antiretroviral Therapy in the Chronically HIV-1-Infected Patient

CLINICAL CATEGORY	CD4+ T CELL COUNT	PLASMA HIV RNA	RECOMMENDATION
Symptomatic (AIDS, severe symptoms)	Any value	Any value	Treat.
Asymptomatic, AIDS	CD4+ T cells $>200/mm^3$	Any value	Treat.
Asymptomatic	CD4+ T cells $\geq 350/mm^3$	Any value	Treatment generally should be offered, although it is controversial.
Asymptomatic	CD4+ T cells $>350/mm^3$	>55,000 (by bDNA or RT-PCR)	Some experienced clinicians would recommend initiating therapy, recognizing that the 3-year risk of developing AIDS in untreated patients is >30%. In the absence of very high levels of plasma HIV RNA, some would defer therapy and monitor the CD4+ T cell count and level of plasma HIV RNA more frequently.
Asymptomatic	CD4+ T cells $>350/mm^3$	<55,000 (by bDNA or RT-PCR)	Many experienced clinicians would defer therapy and observe, recognizing that the 3-year risk of developing AIDS in untreated patients is <15%.

Modified from Guidelines for the use of antiretroviral agents in HIV-infection, *MMWR* 47(No. RR-4), 1998, updated 7/2003, www.aidsinfo.nih.gov.

management of HIV-infected adults is based upon numerous considerations (CDC, 1998). Viral load tests, CD4+ cell counts—along with the patient's clinical condition and readiness and likelihood to comply—guide decisions of when to start or change therapies (Table 41-3). One recent medical development is the use of immune-based therapies, which affect the activity of the immune system. Immune-based therapies may help restore immune responsiveness, suppress viral infections, or even counteract the bone marrow toxicity of some anti-HIV drugs.

The overall goals of medical management of HIV are to prolong life and improve the quality of life for the long term; maximize suppression of viral replication to undetectable levels (currently defined as <50 CD4+ cell copies/ml); optimize and extend the usefulness of currently available therapies; and minimize drug toxicity and manage side effects.

Because medical management evolves continuously, care providers need to stay informed about new developments (Table 41-4). Quickly approved antiretroviral medications expanded the use of viral load measurements, HIV drug resistance, and drug blood tests; and new research and emerging complications are complex and integral to medical monitoring.

HAART usually consists of a combination of at least three antiretroviral agents used with the intent to suppress viral replication and progression of HIV disease. The use of only one antiretroviral drug has been recognized as leading to drug-resistant mutants of the virus; this practice has been discontinued. HAART therapy considers:

1. Viral load levels (HIV-RNA), which predict the risk of HIV disease progression, and when to initiate or change therapy

TABLE 41-4 Additional FDA-Approved Drugs for HIV and AIDS-Related Conditions

GENERIC NAME	BRAND AND OTHER NAMES	PROBLEM TREATED OR PREVENTED
1. Alitretinoin	Panretin	Kaposi's sarcoma
2. Amphotericin B liquid complex	Abelcet, ABLC, Ambisome	Aspergillosis
3. Atovaquone	Mepron, 566C80	*Pneumocystis carinii* pneumonia (PCP)
4. Azithromycin	Zithromax	*Mycobacterium avium* complex
5. Cidofovir	Vistide, HPMPC	Cytomegalovirus retinitis
6. Clarithromycin	Biaxin, Klacid	*Mycobacterium avium*-intracellular complex (MAC)
7. Daunorubicin-liposomal	DaunoXome	Advanced Kaposi's sarcoma
8. Doxorubicin hydrochloride-liposomal	Doxil	Kaposi's sarcoma
9. Dronabinol	Marinol	Anorexia associated with weight loss
10. Erythropoietin	EPO, Epogen, Procrit	Anemia related to AZT therapy
11. Famciclovir	Famvir	Mucocutaneous herpes simplex
12. Fluconazole	Diflucan	Oropharyngeal and esophageal candidiasis; cryptococcal meningitis
13. Fomivirsen sodium injection	Vitravene intravitreal injectable	Cytomegalovirus (CMV)
14. Foscarnet	Foscavir	CMV retinitis; acyclovir-resistant mucocutaneous herpes simplex virus
15. Ganciclovir (IV, oral)	Cytovene, DHPG	CMV retinitis; CMV disease
16. Ganciclovir (implant)	Vitrasert	Cytomegalovirus retinitis
17. Immune globulin (IV)	Gamimune N, Gamma Globulin, IGIV	Bacterial infections (pediatric)
18. Interferon Alfa-2a	Roferon-A	Kaposi's sarcoma
19. Interferon Alfa2b	Intron-A	Kaposi's sarcoma, chronic non-A, non-B hepatitis
20. Itraconazole	Sporanox	Histoplasmosis, blastomycosis, and aspergillosis; pulmonary and extrapulmonary aspergillosis; oropharyngeal and esophageal candidiasis
21. Megestrol acetate	Megace, Ovarian	Anorexia, cachexia, or unexplained, significant weight loss
22. Paclitaxel	Taxol	Kaposi's sarcoma
23. Pentamidine (aerosolized)	NebuPent	*Pneumocystis carinii* pneumonia
24. Rifabutin	Ansamycin, Mycobutin	*Mycobacterium avium* complex
25. Somatropin rDNA	Serostim	AIDS wasting and cachexia
26. Sulfamethoxazole/trimethoprim	Bactrim in combination with trimethoprim; Septra in combination with trimethoprim; SMX	*Pneumocystis carinii* pneumonia (PCP)
27. Trimethoprim/Sulfamethoxazole	Bactrim in combination with sulfamethoxazole; Septra in combination with sulfamethoxazole; SMX	*Pneumocystis carinii* pneumonia (PCP)
28. Trimetrexate glucuronate	Leucovorin (Neutrexin, TMTX)	*Pneumocystis carinii* pneumonia
29. Oral valganciclovir	Valcyte, HCL	CMV retinitis

Modified from U.S. Food and Drug Administration: *Approved drugs for HIV/AIDS and AIDS-related conditions*, Washington, DC, accessed 11/7/2001, www.fda.gov/oashi/aids/stat.

2. Current and lowest CD4+ counts for the extent of HIV-induced immune damage and the risk for opportunistic infections
3. Current and past clinical conditions and symptoms of HIV disease, including history of treatment outcomes
4. Life stage: children, adolescents and pregnant women warrant special considerations.

Between effective treatments for opportunistic infections and the introduction of HAART, deaths and severe illnesses attributable to complications of AIDS have sharply declined. In the United States the number of AIDS deaths dropped dramatically by 44% in the first half of 1997, in comparison with the same period in 1996, when the number of AIDS cases dropped only 12%. The largest decreases have been seen in the incidence of *Pneumocystis carinii* pneumonia, wasting syndrome, Kaposi's sarcoma, *Mycobacterium avium* complex, cytomegalovirus retinitis, and—to a lesser extent—toxoplasmosis, dementia, esophageal candidiasis, cryptococcal meningitis, and cryptosporidiosis (Michaels et al, 1998). However, serious concerns about HAART that need to be considered in developing nutritional plans include the following:

1. Viral resistance can occur. More new HIV infections involve strains resistant to at least one class of medications, leaving fewer treatment options (Kuritzkes et al, 2003). HIV mutates rapidly, and resistance to one medication often results in resistance to others. Genotypic testing helps identify which specific genetic mutations are causing drug resistance and drug failure, and phenotypic testing directly measures the sensitivity of HIV to specific drugs.
2. Patients must adhere to daily—and often very complicated—drug schedules, which may have bothersome meal and food requirements (Table 41-5). With less virus in the body, fewer muta-

TABLE 41-5 HIV Antiretroviral Medications and Nutritional Complications

MEDICATION: BRAND, GENERICS AND OTHER NAMES	A	D	C	N	V	F	H	FOOD EFFECTS AND RECOMMENDATIONS	OTHER CONSIDERATIONS, ADVERSE EFFECTS, AND NOTES (NOT ALL-INCLUSIVE)
Nucleoside Analogue Reverse Transcriptase Inhibitors (NRTIs)									
Combivir-Lamivudine/Zidovudine		x		x		x	x	If possible, take on empty stomach. Low-fat meal can reduce side effects. Avoid alcohol.	See individual drugs (Retrovir and Epivir).
Emtriva-emtricitabine		x		x				Take with or without food.	Monitor patients with renal disease; may cause abnormal dreams, tingling in hands and feet, and lactic acidosis (www.emtriva.com).
Epivir-3TC, Lamivudine	x	x		x	x	x	x	Food may reduce GI side effects. Avoid alcohol.	Malaise
HIVID-ddC-Zalcitabine	x	x	x	x	x	x	x	Taken with food decreases complications by 14% (not clinically significant). Avoid alcohol.	Peripheral neuropathy; oral and esophageal ulcers; pancreatitis; avoid taking with antacids containing magensium or aluminum.
Retrovir-Zidovudine-AZT-Azidothymidine		x		x	x	x	x	If possible, take on empty stomach. Low-fat meal can reduce side effects. Avoid alcohol.	Dysphoria; bone marrow suppression (anemia, neutropenia); rash. Peak plasma with food is decreased.
Trizivir-fixed dose combination of Ziagen, Retrovir, and Epivir								If possible, take on empty stomach. Low-fat meal can reduce side effects. Avoid alcohol.	Rash (may be part of hypersensitivity reaction—*do not rechallenge!*) See individual drugs (Ziagen, Retrovir, and Epivir).
Videx, Videx EC-Didansosine-ddI-Dideoxyinosine		x	x	x	x		x	Take on empty stomach, at least 30-60 minutes before or 2 hours after a meal; take with water. Avoid alcohol.	Peripheral neuropathy; pancreatitis; abnormal liver function tests; avoid antacids that contain magnesium or aluminum; chewable/dispersible, buffered tablets (or pediatric powder for oral formulation) thoroughly chewed, manually crushed, or dispersed in water (stable for 1 hour) before swallowing.
Zerit-Stavudine-d4T	x	x		x	x		x	Food has little effect on absorption. Avoid alcohol.	Peripheral neuropathy; CNS changes (agitation, dysphoria); pancreatitis.
Ziagen-Abacavir		x		x	x	x	x	Avoid alcohol; can be taken with or without food.	Rash (may be part of hypersensitivity reaction—*do not rechallenge!*), alcohol increases ABC AUC by 41%.
Non-Nucleoside Analogue Reverse Transcriptase Inhibitors (NNRTIs)									
Rescriptor-Delavirdine mesylate-DLV	x	x		x	x	x	x	Can be taken without regard to food. Avoid alcohol. Avoid taking with antacids. Do not take St. John's wort.	Rash; antacids that contain aluminum and magnesium and ddI reduce absorption and should be taken at least 1 hour after DLV.
Sustiva-Efavirenz				x		x	x	Low-fat meals improve EFV tolerability; avoid high-fat meal (increases bioavailability and CNS effects). Do not take if pregnant! Do not take St. John's wort. Alcohol may increase CNS side effects.	Rash; CNS changes (vivid dreams, dizziness, euphoria, dysphoria, hallucinations). Take in the evening to minimize CNS effects.
Viramune-Nevirapine				x			x	Can be taken without regard to food. Avoid alcohol. Do not take St. John's wort.	Rash.
Nucleotide Analogue Reverse Transcriptase Inhibitors (NtRTIs)									In general: Lactic acidosis and severe hepatomegaly with steatosis, including fatal cases, have been reported with the use of nucleoside analogues alone or in combination with other antiretrovirals.
Viread-Tenofovir disoproxil fumarate		x		x	x		x	Should be taken with meal to enhance drug bioavailability. Study meal, 700-1000 kcal, 40%-50% fat, increased AUC by 40%.	Asthenia, abdominal pain, flatulence, and—for a few—anorexia. Contains lactose. Drug is not a substrate of the CYP450 enzymes.
Fusion Inhibitor							x		May cause pain at injection site, dizziness, numbness in feet and hands, insomnia, www.rocheusa.com

Protease Inhibitors (PIs)									PIs in general: Lipodystrophy syndrome: fat maldistribution (increased fat in waist, neck, breasts; decrease in extremities, buttocks, face); elevated cholesterol and/or triglycerides, insulin resistance (or frank diabetes mellitus); abnormal liver function tests (increased enzymes: SGOT [ALT] and SGPT [AST], alkaline phosphatase, bilirubin, GGT); bone density, hair and nail changes. Substrates of the CYP450 enzymes in varying degrees.
Agenerase-Amprenavir		x		x	x	x	x	Take with or without food; if taken with food, no more than 67 g of fat, which decreases absorption. Do not take St. John's wort.	Rash; tingling around the mouth (parathesia). Avoid extra vitamin E above a general multiple vitamin; each 150-mg capsule contains 109 IU vitamin E; each milliliter of solution contains 46 IU. High doses of vitamin E may exacerbate blood coagulation defect of vitamin K deficiency caused by anticoagulation therapy or malabsorption; grapefruit juice may be a concern; increase fluid intake. Do not take antacids within 1 hour of taking medication. Oral solution contains a propylene glycol excipient and is contraindicated in infants and children under 4 years, pregnant women, patients with hepatic or renal failure, and patients receiving disulfiram or metronidazole.
Crixivan-Indinivir sulfate	x	x		x	x	x	x	Take on empty stomach at least 1 hour before or 2 hours after a meal. Wait 2 hours after last meal/snack; take drug and wait 1 hour to eat again. May take with light meals that total no more than 2 g of fat, 5.6 g of protein, 65 g of carbohydrate, and fewer than 300 calories. Must drink approximately 48 ounces extra water daily. Avoid grapefruit juice. Do not take St. John's wort.	Must be taken every 8 hours and requires careful meal/snack coordination. In combination with ritonavir, it significantly increases blood levels of indinavir, eliminating the need to fast. Kidney stones; abdominal, back or flank pain; elevated serum bilirubin (jaundice); dizziness; dry skin; rash. Take 1 hour before or after ddI (buffer in ddI impairs absorption.
Kaletra-Lopinavir/Ritonavir								Take with food to increase absorption. Do not take St. John's wort.	Store capsules in the refrigerator.
Viracept-Nelfinavir mesylate, NFV		x		x	x		x	Food increases absorption 2 to 3 times more than fasted state and reduces GI side effects. Bioavailability was better with test meal of 500 kcal, 11.3 g fat, 20.5 g pro, 99.2 g cho, than test meal of 125 kcal, 3.1 g fat, 10.0 g pro, 14.6 g cho (Peterson et al, 2003). Lactase enzyme or lactose free dairy products may reduce diarrhea; avoid acidic food or liquid. Do not take St. John's wort.	Rash; flatulence; abdominal pain; asthenia.
Norvir-Ritonavir-ABT-538	x	x		x	x	x	x	Take with food to increase absorption. Do not take St. John's wort.	Oral and peripheral paresthesia; hyperasthesia; vasodilation. Store capsules in the refrigerator; mix oral solution with chocolate milk or supplements or intensely flavored food to mask taste.
Invirase-Saquinavir mesylate		x		x	x			Take within 5 minutes or up to 2 hours after a full (high-fat) meal to increase absorption. Grapefruit juice increases absorption. Avoid alcohol. Do not take St. John's wort.	Another formulation is under development to be taken with ritonavir.
Fortovase-Saquinavir mesylate		x		x	x	x	x	Take with or up to 2 hours after a full (high-fat) meal to increase AUC 670%. Avoid alcohol. Do not take St. John's wort.	Store capsules in the refrigerator.
Reyataz-atazanavir sulfate E		x		x	x		x	Take with food and 1 hour away from antacids. Do not take St. John's wort.	Can cause high levels of bilirubin and jaundice, which dissipate after stopping medication. Can cause tingling in hands and feet, abdominal pain, and depression, www.reyataz.com

Modified from Fenton M: *HIV antiretroviral medications and nutritional complications,* Los Angeles, 2001, AIDS Project Los Angeles. For more information on these and new medications, refer to most current version of: Panel on Clinical Practices for the Treatment of HIV: guidelines for the use of antiretroviral agents in HIV-infected adults and adolescents, *MMWR* 1998 47(No. RR-5), updated July 2003, www.aidsinfo.nih.gov.
X, Possible complication; *A*, Appetite loss; *D*, diarrhea; *C*, constipation; *N*, nausea; *V*, vomiting; *F*, Fatigue; *H*, Headache.

tions will occur, and nonadherence is associated with increased levels of plasma HIV. One must be more than 95% adherent for medications to work correctly (Horn, 2001). Late, missed, or non–meal-coordinated medications increase risks for suboptimal dosing, viral breakthrough, and the development of drug-resistant strains of HIV. One study found adherence was poor in 28% (<80% antiretrovirals per day), fair for 23% (80% to 99% per day), and excellent in 50% (100% per day). Barriers to adherence are as follows: being busy with other things or forgot (52%), away from home (46%), changed daily routines (45%), depression (27%), drug holiday (20%), ran out (20%), too many medications (19%), worried about becoming immune to medications (19%), drugs too toxic (18%), drug side effects (17%), didn't want others to notice (17%), and taking drugs is a reminder of HIV infection (16%) (Gifford et al, 2000).

3. Not all patients tolerate antiretroviral drugs. Although some side effects diminish after the start of medication treatment, some persist, and bothersome HIV-related side effects continue to be substantial. One multisite national study identified the prevalence of side effects in over 4000 HIV-infected adults: fever/night sweats (51.1%), diarrhea (51%), nausea/anorexia (49.8%), dysesthesias (48.9%), severe headache (39.9%), weight loss, (37.1%), vaginal symptoms (35.6% of women), sinus symptoms (34.8%), eye trouble (32.4%), cough dyspnea (30.4%), thrush (27.3%), rash (24.3%), oral pain (24.1%), and Kaposi's sarcoma (4%). Numbers and severity of symptoms varied and were greatest in women, patients with lower education income levels, and Medicare enrollment, and those who were followed at teaching hospitals (Mathews et al, 2000).
4. New adverse complications have emerged: body fat accumulation and fat atrophy, hyperlipidemia, insulin resistance or glucose intolerance, osteopenia and osteoporosis, avascular necrosis and bone fracture, lactic acidosis, and mitochondrial toxicity. The loosely termed lipodystrophy syndrome stems from one or more of the following causes: (1) drug side effects; (2) extended exposure to the virus or activated immune cells characteristic of HIV infection; or (3) immune system alterations along with suppression of the virus by the drugs.
5. Medication costs can be about $12,000 to $25,000 annually per person, and medications are not available to all patients. Many state-based and private health insurance policies do not cover all FDA-approved HIV-related medications.

WOMEN AND HIV

Prenatal Considerations

Perinatal use of combination therapy and special drug therapy sharply reduces HIV transmission from mother to baby. The AIDS Clinical Trial Group study showed that perinatal HIV transmission could be reduced by two thirds when oral zidovudine was initiated at 14 to 34 weeks of gestation, administered intravenously during labor, and then administered to the neonate for 6 weeks (Connor et al, 1997). An even shorter and less costly course of zidovudine therapy was shown to reduce perinatal HIV transmission by half.

A joint Uganda–United States study, HIVNET 012, demonstrated that one dose of nevirapine given during labor and to the neonate within the first 72 hours decreased transmission of HIV by 47%. Current guidelines call for standard antiretroviral therapy to be offered to HIV-infected pregnant women with zidovudine incorporated into the regimen (Public Health Service Task Force, 2001a). Many short-term and long-term risks and benefits, including birth defects and issues regarding the health of the baby versus the mother, are problematic.

Guidelines also recommend preconceptional counseling for optimal nutritional status because malnutrition increases the risk of postcesarean complications and postpartum morbidity, which are especially prevalent in HIV-infected women (Public Health Service Task Force, 2001a). Other guidelines address the safety and toxicity of antiretrovirals in this population, including reports on placental and breast milk passage of HIV in animal and human studies (Public Health Service Task Force, 2001b). Changes in absolute CD4+ count during pregnancy may reflect the physiologic changes of pregnancy on hemodynamic parameters and blood volume as opposed to a long-term influence of pregnancy on CD4+ count (Colgrove et al, 1998).

Poor nutritional status may also increase the risk of perinatal HIV transmission. Through randomized, placebo-controlled studies, vitamin A and other supplemented vitamins were shown, not to affect transmission at birth (Dreyfuss and Fawzi, 2002; French et al, 2002). Poor prenatal nutrition, apart from HIV status, can result in delayed growth of the fetus and inadequate growth for gestational age, thus contributing to decreased cellular immunity and low T-cell levels, small thymus size, and increased rate of infection (Stiehm, 1995). Nutrient deficiencies can result from the increased nutritional demands for fetal growth and development. HIV further increases these demands especially in developing countries, where deficiencies of vitamin A, folate, iron, and zinc are common.

Breast-Feeding

Breast-feeding recommendations for developed and "resource-poor" settings are different. It is recommended that in developed countries HIV-positive mothers refrain from breast-feeding (Public Health Services Task Force, 2001b). The risk of breast milk transmission is estimated to range from 14% to 22% and is the cause of 5% to 15% of perinatal HIV transmissions. Banked milk may be an option for some mothers.

Infants in South Africa who received early mixed feedings were found to have significantly increased the risk of maternal-to-child transmission of HIV compared with exclusively breast-fed infants at 3 months of age. Potential mechanisms for this may be that earlier introduction of solid foods causes physical damage to the GI tract and increases the likelihood of viral particle penetration of the intestinal lining, or that early addition of solid foods causes an allergic reaction (Coutsoudis et al, 1999). Mortality rates are higher for infants breast-fed by HIV-infected mothers. Formula feeding with adequate education and clean water results in a lower mortality rate for these infants than for those who breast-feed (Mbori-Ngacha et al 2001). However, these and other related concerns are not resolved, and more studies are underway (Papathakis, 2001). Although the policies are still controversial, the World Health Organization recently reconfirmed the following policies on breast-feeding and infant feeding by HIV-infected women (World Health Organization, 2001):

1. Exclusive breastfeeding should be protected, promoted, and supported for 6 months. This applies to women who are known to be free from HIV and for women whose infection status is unknown.
2. When replacement feeding is acceptable, feasible, affordable, sustainable, and safe, avoidance of all breast-feeding by HIV-infected mothers is recommended; otherwise, exclusive breast-feeding is recommended during the first months of life.
3. To minimize HIV transmission risk, breast-feeding should be discontinued as soon as feasible, taking into account local circumstances, the individual woman's situation, and the risks of replacement feeding, which include infections other than HIV and malnutrition.
4. HIV-infected women should have access to information, follow-up clinical care, and support, including family planning services and nutritional support.

WHO recommends that programs to prevent perinatal HIV transmission include the prevention and treatment of opportunistic infections, treatment with antiretroviral drugs where possible, and psychosocial and nutritional support.

Other General Considerations for Women

Women should be counseled on real-life strategies and referrals to improve their health and nutrition status, living situation, access to food, income, and practical solutions to exercise. Some women access a registered dietitian through the Women, Infant, and Children Program (WIC); however, their HIV statuses are often not disclosed, and the opportunity to receive appropriate HIV medical nutrition therapy is lost.

Other barriers for HIV-positive women that prevent access to care include low socioeconomic situations, multiple children for whom they care and whose needs are placed before their own, lack of child care or transportation, isolation, and fear of disclosure. Moreover, women may have been or are currently at subsistence level and may eat a less than nutritionally adequate diet. Women may seek ways to lose weight quickly, such as starvation or fad dieting to decrease weight and fat mass, and may have no regular exercise regimen.

Most research on HIV-related medications and side effects, body composition, and nutritional deficiencies has been done on men, but gender differences are now recognized. Women have lower viral loads than men but lose CD4+ cells and develop AIDS just as quickly (Sterling et al, 2001). Drug metabolism and excretion are different in women than in men; women experience more drug-related gastrointestinal symptoms. Women tend to gain more fat weight and less lean muscle mass than men. Many women have little or no health insurance or access to quality health care providers (Shapiro et al, 1999); they are often diagnosed and seek care later, when they have a greater viral load and disease progression (Anastos et al, 1999). Women are less likely to be taking combination therapy and appropriate prophylaxis medications then men.

PEDIATRIC CONSIDERATIONS

Today, the important role of pediatric nutrition support is well recognized. Children born to mothers with HIV are often born with weight and height below the 50th percentile, and although uninfected children catch up, HIV-infected children do not. An earlier and more pronounced deficit in height for age is noted, especially by 15 months of age (Saavedra et al, 1995). Growth failure and neurodevelopmental deterioration may be manifestations of pediatric HIV disease. Pediatric guidelines recognize that monitoring growth and development is essential and nutritional support is an intervention that affects immune function, quality of life, and bioactivity of antiretroviral drugs. Growth failure, a persistent decline in weight-gain velocity despite adequate nutritional support and without other explanation, is a reason to consider changing antiretroviral therapy. Change in CD4+ percentage, not number, may be a better marker of identifying disease progression in children (Guidelines for the Use of Antiretroviral Agents in Pediatric HIV Infection, 2001). Every child with the infection should be assessed within 3 months of diagnosis and every 1 to 6 months thereafter, relative to age, problems, and nutritional status (Heller 2000).

Current guidelines acknowledge that management of the complex and diverse needs of HIV-infected infants, children, adolescents, and their families requires a multidisciplinary team of physicians, nurses, social workers, psychologists, nutritionists, outreach workers, and pharmacists (Guidelines for the Use of Antiretroviral Agents in Pediatric HIV Infection, 2001). The health care professional's role may be direct or may involve referral to an appropriate agency or individual. When working with the HIV-infected child, one must consider the total family unit and environment, including social and financial issues, cultural issues, and caregiver support in dealing with a chronically ill child. For example, adherence to medication schedules may involve setting meal and medication times or including particular foods and activities in specific sequences.

Clinical trials on antiretroviral drugs have often not included children; as a result, 11 of the 15 antiretroviral drugs approved for adults and adolescents are used for children, although they are not labeled for this population. Current pediatric guidelines detail drug dosing for neonatal, pediatric, and adolescent patients and detail toxicities; interactions; and special instructions, including food and nutrition concerns. Some drugs are in liquid form for dosing according to weight and for easier administration. Tube feeding, more prevalent in this population, is sometimes initiated to administer crucial medications.

RELATIONSHIP BETWEEN MALNUTRITION AND AIDS

Wasting and Metabolic Disorders

Malnutrition is an important and complicated consequence of HIV infection, and deaths from wasting have increased. Problems leading to malnutrition may involve ingestion, absorption, digestion, metabolism, and use of nutrients; these influence immunocompetence, reproductive health and function, physical activity, and work performance and cognition (Raiten, 2001). Without successful antiretroviral therapy, protein-energy malnutrition (PEM) is a frequent complication of AIDS.

HIV wasting syndrome, a constitutional disease, is diagnostic of AIDS in the HIV-positive individual for whom no other cause of weight loss can be identified. It is defined as meeting one of the following criteria (Polsky et al, 2001):

- Unintentional weight loss of 10% over 12 months
- Unintentional loss of 10% of body weight over 6 months
- Loss of 5% of lean body mass within 6 months
- In men: body cell mass (BCM) <35% of total body weight (BW) and body mass index (BMI) <27
- In women: BCM <23% of total BW and BMI <27kg/m^2
- BMI <20 kg/m^2

Involuntary weight loss of 10% to 15% in AIDS is common, and as little as a 5% weight loss has been associated with a significantly increased risk of opportunistic infections and death (Wheeler et al, 1998). Weight loss, lean body mass depletion, decreased skin-fold thickness and midarm circumference, decreased iron-binding capacity, decreased serum in potassium and intracellular water, and hypoalbuminemia are reported commonly.

Before widespread use of potent antiretroviral therapy, HIV wasting syndrome had been the second most commonly reported AIDS-indicator condition for adults, and the fourth for children younger than 13 years of age (CDC, 1996). CDC no longer reports AIDS-indicator conditions that include the incidence of wasting; however, a recent report showed that wasting still occurs. Of 466 patients who received medical care, 18% lost over 10% body weight since their first visit; 21% lost over 5% usual body weight in 6 months; and many sustained that loss over a year. Eight percent had a BMI less than 20 kg/m^2 since the most recent visit (Wanke et al, 2000). Weight loss and wasting are multifactorial. The major contributing factors are lack of adequate intake, malabsorption, metabolic irregularities, uncontrolled opportunistic infection, and lack of physical activity. Decreased oral intake is very common and can result from anorexia secondary to medications; depression; infection; symptoms such as nausea, vomiting, diarrhea, dyspnea, or fatigue; or neurologic disease.

Low oral intake can also be attributable to disorders of the mouth and esophagus, such as candidiasis (thrush), herpes simplex, aphthous ulcers, or CMV. Malabsorption—often suspected in the event of loose stools, diarrhea, or vomiting—can be caused by medications; HIV infection; opportunistic infections, such as CMV, MAC, or cryptosporidiosis; or a developed intolerance to lactose, fat, or—possibly—gluten. At the same time, fevers and infection may increase energy and protein needs. HIV-induced metabolic changes and host responses are poorly understood. Resting energy expenditure (REE) is elevated in asymptomatic HIV-infected persons and relates to viral load (Mulligan et al, 1997). Lipid metabolism and transport may also be affected by infection, thus causing wasting of lean body mass.

Women have been found to lose more body fat than lean body mass during both the early and advanced stages of wasting, whereas men lose greater amounts of lean body mass while sparing body fat. Furthermore, women have less growth hormone resistance as a function of weight loss in comparison with men (Office of AIDS Research, 1998).

The malnutrition associated with HIV infection and AIDS has characteristics similar to other infectious processes and some that are unique to HIV. Nutrition status is a major factor in survival, and in the absence of disease, starvation usually leads to death when the victim reaches 66% of ideal body weight. Body cell mass, the amount of functional protoplasm in lean body mass (muscle and viscera) may be the best predictor of death (Flier and Underhill, 1992). As the wasting of lean body mass nears 55% of normal for age, sex, and height, death is imminent, regardless of the causes of malnutrition (Keusch and Thea, 1993; Kotler, 1992).

Body fat is not a predictable marker of wasting. Persons with AIDS, men more than women, tend to lose body cell mass with less loss of fat, in contrast to uncomplicated starvation, in which fat stores are depleted. As with HIV wasting syndrome, host resistance to infection causes changes in metabolism, as mediated by cytokines. The search for host mediators of metabolic disturbances initially resulted in the cachectin hypothesis, related to tumor necrosis factor (TNF) (see Chapter 40). Other theories have also been evaluated.

Immune changes associated with PEM are similar to those seen in AIDS. Both conditions are marked by multiple opportunistic infections of viral, bacterial, parasitic, and fungal origin. KS and B-cell lymphomas have been reported in individuals in Central and East Africa, where PEM is common. Malnutrition may contribute to the frequency and severity of infection seen in AIDS by compromising immune function. Deficiencies of protein; calories; copper; zinc; selenium; iron; essential fatty acids; pyridoxine; folate; and vitamins A, C, and E all interfere with immune function. Severe weight loss can also result in organ damage, which may increase the risk of death from infections.

Direct and indirect mechanisms are responsible for the impact of nutrition on HIV. Directly, nutritional factors are required for specific immune-cell triggering, interaction, and expression. Clinical trials with supplementation of specific nutrients at different stages of HIV disease are needed. Indirectly, nutritional factors are essential for DNA and protein synthesis and for the physiologic integrity of cell tissues and organ systems, including lymphoid tissues.

Simply, maintaining and restoring weight and lean body mass requires (1) eliminating or mitigating the deleterious effects of the infectious agent; (2) ample caloric and nutrient intake; and (3) sufficient exercise. Nutrition counseling has been recognized as a necessary component in the treatment of HIV-associated wasting (Fisher 2001; New York State Department of Health AIDS Institute, 2001; Polsky et al 2001).

Adequate resistance exercise is important to ensure gain in lean body mass (Roubenoff et al, 2001). Moderate physical exercise three to four times a week has been found to increase CD4+ counts and offer a more protective effect than daily exercise (Mustafa et al, 1999).

Megestrol acetate (Megace), dronabinol (Marinol), and—experimentally—medical marijuana are appetite stimulants considered to combat HIV anorexia. Megace, the more powerful appetite stimulant, reduces testosterone levels and increases body fat. Marinol, a derivative of marijuana, produces undesired central nervous side effects. Weight gains from these agents are primarily—but not all—in the fat compartment (Mulligan et al, 2001). Although exercise may be necessary to increase lean body mass, clinicians want for better appetite stimulants.

Prescriptive drug treatments used to prevent and help restore weight and body cell mass loss have become available. Other drug treatments that may be considered for use in wasting and preservation of lean body mass are anabolic agents to promote positive nitrogen balance and cytokine inhibitors to slow protein breakdown.

Decreases in testosterone levels have been associated with lower libido and loss of bone density (Laboratory Corporation of America, 2001). Testosterone exists in serum both free and bound to albumin and to sex hormone–binding globulin (SHBG). Unbound (free) testosterone, usually less than 2% of the total testosterone concentration, reflects an individual's biologically active circulating testosterone and is considered the true test for judging testosterone production. Amounts vary greatly. HIV-infected men and women should be routinely monitored for serum levels of both free and total testosterone and treated for testosterone deficiency. Testosterone is obtainable in injected, patch, gel, and oral synthetic forms.

Anabolic agents include nandrolone, oxandralone, stanozolol, oxymethalone, nandrolone decanoate, and recombinant human growth hormone. Cytokine inhibitors include thalidomide, cyprohedptadin, ketotifen, pentoxifylline, fish oil, and *N*-acetylcysteine. Anabolic steroids, which are still controversial, require adequate caloric intake and progressive resistance exercise to maintain and maximize increases in lean body mass. Recombinant human growth hormone, a lipolytic agent, promotes lean body mass at the expense of fat stores, and adequate energy intake is necessary. Side effects vary with the individual drug and include mood changes, skin problems, hair

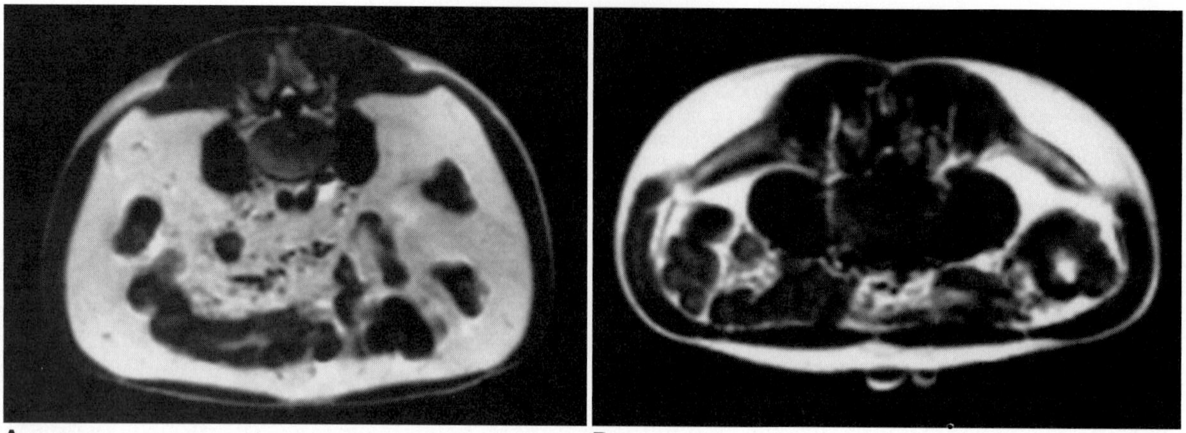

FIGURE 41-6 • **A,** Abdominal magnetic resonance image (MRI) of an HIV-infected man with visceral adiposity syndrome. **B,** Abdominal MRI of a non–HIV-infected man similar in race, age, height, weight, and total adiposity. (From Engelson et al: Fat distribution in HIV-infected patients reporting truncal enlargement quantified by whole-body magnetic resonance imaging, *Am J Clin Nutr* 69[6]:1162-1169, 1999. Reproduced with permission by the *American Journal of Clinical Nutrition.* Copyright *American Journal of Clinical Nutrition,* Society for Clinical Nutrition.)

growth, menstrual irregularities, changes in libido and potency, fluid retention, abnormal liver enzymes, altered blood glucose, and even diabetes.

Lipodystrophy Syndrome

Body shape changes may include depletion of subcutaneous adipose tissue (SAT) with thinning of the arms and legs, buttocks, and face (maxillary, nasolabial, and temporal areas). Changes may also include accumulation of visceral adipose tissue (VAT) (Figure 41-6), as well as a dorsocervical (buffalo hump), mammary adipose tissue, adipose tissue in axillary regions, and lipomas. Prominent veins from loss of subcutaneous fat and ingrown toenails have also been reported.

Metabolic alterations include low serum testosterone concentrations in both women and men and elevations in serum triglyceride, insulin, glucose, and blood pressure (Dubé and Sattler, 1998; Kotler and Muurahainen, 1998). REE may be increased with lipodystrophy and insulin resistance (Kosmiski et al, 2001).

People living with HIV have changes in bone metabolism. Factors for this may include low body mass, wasting, poor nutrition, previous corticosteroid use, or hormonal deficiencies. Potent antiretroviral therapy seems to further increase new bone formation and bone destruction, with greater bone turnover and loss of bone mineral density. Early studies suggest that HIV-positive subjects who take protease inhibitors (PIs), those who take them for longer duration, and those with lipodystrophy syndrome may develop bone loss, osteopenia, and osteoporosis (Duran et al, 2001; Moyle, 2001) Suggestions include use of improved diet; calcium and vitamin D dietary supplements; exercise; and—when indicated—hormone replacements and biphosphonates, such as alendronate or risedronate (Mondy and Tebas, 2003) (see Chapter 27).

Avascular necrosis, also called *asceptic necrosis* or *osteonecrosis,* has been occurring at greater rates in the HIV-infected than in the noninfected populations. Whether HIV is an independent risk factor is unknown. A suggested reason for the increased rate is the occurrence of the following risk factors in this population: hyperlipidemia, alcohol abuse, pancreatitis, corticosteroid use, and hypercoaguability (Scribner et al, 2000).

MEDICAL NUTRITION THERAPY

Nutrient deficiencies may play important roles in the pathogenesis of HIV disease. Medical nutrition therapy with individualized counseling is critical in overall treatment. The goals of nutrition intervention are the following:

1. Maintain and expand nutrition knowledge and empowerment.
2. Maintain or restore healthy body weight and normal morphology.
3. Preserve or restore optimal somatic and visceral protein status.
4. Prevent nutrient deficiencies or excesses known to compromise immune function.
5. Treat or minimize HIV or medication-related complications that interfere with either intake or absorption of nutrients.
6. Correct metabolic abnormalities.
7. Support optimal therapeutic drug levels.
8. Prolong and optimize quality of life.

When adequately provided, timely HIV nutrition therapy should decrease health care costs. In the context of the unique HIV disease complications, the nutrition practitioner should apply basic nutrition fundamentals in assessment and interventions, including nutritional support decisions (see Chapters 21 to 23). Achieving nutritional health and preventing malnutrition are essential in maintaining positive health outcomes for persons with HIV (American Dietetic Association, 2000; LACCHHS, 1999).

Screening

Ideally, all persons with HIV infection should be screened for nutritional problems and concerns at the time of their first contact with a health care professional, and routine monitoring should continue on an ongoing basis. The occurrence of nutrition-related symptoms should trigger automatic referrals for nutrition intervention as identified by any member of the health care team. Box 41-2 lists nutrition referral criteria for adults and adolescents, and Box 41-3 provides referral criteria specific to pediatric patients.

Assessment

Referral information for further nutrition assessment should include the following: consent of client to release medical information (usually necessary when clients are seen outside of their primary medical setting); current diagnosis and medical history; referring health care provider's nutrition prescription or desired outcome; clinical symptoms and feeding route; weight history and body composition; biochemical data; current medications, including prescription and nonprescription drugs, vitamins, minerals, other dietary supplements and use of complementary and alternative therapies; functional status; and lifestyle, including substance use patterns, psychosocial status, and activity and exercise routine.

A comprehensive nutritional assessment should be performed. Factors include HIV infection–associated symptoms, dietary patterns, the use of nontraditional therapies, and the impact of these treatments on the person (see Chapter 17). The diet should be evaluated for nutrient adequacy, especially for nutrients involved with immune function, and for a possible history of erratic and inadequate intakes. Individuals who follow nontraditional diet therapies should be made aware of any potentially harmful effects. Psychosocial conditions (fear, anxiety, depression, and social isolation) all affect appetite and nutrient intake. Illness or ostracism often leads to a lack of employment and subsequent loss of social contacts as well as income and medical insurance.

Evaluating weight in terms of the percentage of usual weight is useful for this population, although percent of goal body weight is an important marker. Monitoring changes in anthropometric measurements over time is feasible because many patients will have multiple clinic visits and hospitalizations. Useful measurements include height, weight, waist or hip or neck circumferences, waist/hip ratio, and measurements of either lean body mass (using triceps skin-fold and midarm muscle circumference) or body cell mass (using bioelectric impedance analysis or other techniques). These calculations can be compared with each other and with published reference data (see Chapter 17).

Laboratory values, such as serum albumin, prealbumin, retinol-binding protein, transferrin, and total iron-binding capacity, can be used to monitor changes in visceral protein status (see Chapter 18). These parameters are especially useful when compared over time. Total lymphocyte count and delayed hypersensitivity skin testing should not be used, as these immune functions are impaired in this population and therefore do not indicate nutritional status (Collins, 1988). Other laboratory values to monitor include fasting lipids, fasting blood sugar and insulin, alkaline phosphatase, and liver function tests. Evaluation of drug therapy is essential, as many side effects complicate nutritional status (see Table 41-5).

Interventions

All persons with HIV infection and AIDS need early, ongoing medical nutrition therapy. The goals should be to educate individuals about the importance of consuming a well-balanced diet, to provide adequate nutrition for maintenance or improvement in nutritional status, and to prevent protein-energy malnutrition and vitamin and mineral deficiencies. Counseling should be individualized, considering barriers to adequate intake, and supported with practical written materials (Box 41-4). Mapping out one's meal and medication schedule is part of medical nutrition therapy and is an important component for supporting adherence to the drug regimen.

Energy and Activity

Energy and protein needs vary depending on the health status of the individual at the time of HIV infection, the progression of the disease, and the development of complications that impair nutrient intake and use. The Harris-Benedict equation or the new DRI equations for energy intake (see Chapter 2) can be used to determine basal energy expenditure (BEE), which can be multiplied by a stress factor to allow for maintenance and anabolism. An adjustment must also be made in the presence of fever. Energy requirements increase by 13% (Grunfeld and Feingold, 1992) and protein requirements by 10% for every degree Celsius of temperature elevation above normal. Keusch and Thea (1993) suggest the following guidelines for determining energy requirements: BEE $\times$ 1.3 for maintenance and BEE $\times$ 1.5 for weight gain.

Activity can also affect energy requirements. Chronic exercise and high-fat diets have often been

Box 41-2. Nutrition Referral Criteria for Adults (18+ Years) With HIV/AIDS

Screen every 6 months or more often if there is a status change. Automatically refer to a registered dietitian for any of the following:

A. Diagnosis and Nutrition Assessment

1. ☐ Newly diagnosed HIV infection
2. ☐ Newly diagnosed with AIDS
3. ☐ Any change in disease or nutritional status
4. ☐ No nutrition assessment by a registered dietitian or not seen by a registered dietitian in 6 months

B. Physical Changes and Weight Concerns

1. ☐ >3% unintentional weight loss from usual body weight in the last 6 months or since last visit (% wt loss formula: usual body wt − current body wt/usual body wt × 100)
2. ☐ Visible wasting, <90% ideal body weight, BMI <20, or decrease in body cell mass (BCM)
3. ☐ Use of anabolic steroids or growth hormone for weight, muscle gain, or metabolic complications
4. ☐ Lipodystrophy: Lipoatrophy, central fat adiposity or fat accumulation on the neck, upper back, breasts, or other areas
5. ☐ Abdominal obesity: Waist circumference >102 cm (40 in) for men and >88 cm (35 in) for women
6. ☐ Client or MD–initiated weight management, or obesity: BMI >30

C. Oral/GI Symptoms

1. ☐ Use of an appetite stimulant or suppressant
2. ☐ Loss of appetite, desire to eat, or poor oral intake of food or fluid for more than 3 days
3. ☐ Missing teeth, severe dental caries, difficulty chewing or swallowing
4. ☐ Mouth sores; thrush; or mouth, tooth, or gum pain
5. ☐ Persistent diarrhea, constipation, or change in stools (color, consistency, frequency, smell)
6. ☐ Persistent nausea or vomiting
7. ☐ Persistent gas, bloating, or heartburn
8. ☐ Changes in perception of taste or smell
9. ☐ Food allergies or food intolerances (e.g., fat, lactose, wheat)
10. ☐ Medication involving food or meal modification
11. ☐ Need for enteral or parenteral nutrition

D. Metabolic Complications and Other Medical Conditions

1. ☐ Diabetes mellitus, impaired glucose tolerance, impaired fasting glucose, insulin resistance, hypoglycemia, or hyperglycemia
2. ☐ Hyperlipidemia: Cholesterol >200 mg/dl, triglycerides ≥150 mg/dl, LDL >130 g/dl, or HDL <40 mg/dl in men and <50 mg/dl in women
3. ☐ Hypertension: Three BP readings ≥135/85 mm Hg or diagnosed with HTN
4. ☐ Hepatic disease: Hepatitis C, hepatitis B, cirrhosis, steatotosis, or other:
5. ☐ Osteopenia/osteoporosis risk: Per elevated alkaline phosphatase, DEXA of the hip and spine, low T-scores
6. ☐ Other conditions: Renal disease, anemia, heart disease, pregnancy, cancer, or other:
7. ☐ Albumin <3.5 mg/dl, prealbumin <19 mg/dl, or cholesterol <120 mg/dl
8. ☐ Scheduled chemotherapy or radiation therapy

E. Barriers to Nutrition, Living Environment, Functional Status

Usually or always needs assistance with:

1. ☐ Eating
2. ☐ Preparing food
3. ☐ Shopping for food and necessities

1. ☐ Homebound
2. ☐ Homeless
3. ☐ Unable to secure food

Patient is:

4. ☐ Has limited or no cooking skills
5. ☐ Lives on income of less than $6,000/yr
6. ☐ Has no stove or refrigerator

F. Behavioral Concerns or Unusual Eating Behaviors

1. ☐ Binges, purges, purposely skips meals, or avoids eating when hungry
2. ☐ Consumes more than two alcoholic beverages per day
3. ☐ Intravenous or recreational drug use
4. ☐ Vegetarianism
5. ☐ Client-initiated vitamin/mineral supplementation >RDA, or complementary or alternative diet-related therapies

From HIV/AIDS Dietetic Practice Group: *Nutrition screen and referral criteria for adults (18+ years) with HIV/AIDS: ADA medical nutrition therapy evidenced-based guides for practice,* American Dietetic Association, 2002, www.hivaidsdpg.org/Data/QM/HIV_Adult_Nutrition_Screen_Referral_Criteria_200207.pdf. With information from Anderson JA, et al: Nutrition referral criteria for adults (+18 years) with HIV/AIDS. In *Guidelines for implementing HIV medical nutrition therapy,* Los Angeles 1999, Los Angeles County Commission on HIV Health Services.

Box 41-3. Nutrition Referral Criteria for Pediatrics (<18 years) With HIV/AIDS

In addition to conditions listed in Box 41-2, referral to a registered dietitian when any one of the following conditions exist:

1. Not seen by a registered dietitian in 3 months
2. Weight for age <10th percentile (National Center for Health Statistics [NCHS])
3. Height for age <10th percentile if weight for age is also <10th percentile for age (NCHS)
4. Weight for height ≥95% of standard or weight for height ≤25th percentile
5. Downward crossing of one major "weight for age" percentile measurement
6. Visible wasting, <95% ideal body weight, BMI ≤25th percentile for age and gender, or any decrease in body cell mass (BCM)
7. Poor appetite, food or fluid refusals
8. Prolonged bottle-feeding or severe dental caries
9. Change in stools (color, consistency, frequency, smell)
10. For children 0-12 months: Low birth weight
11. For children 0-12 months: No weight gain for 1 month
12. For children 0-12 months: Diarrhea or vomiting for 2 days
13. For children 0-12 months: Poor suck
14. For children 1-3 years: No weight gain for several consecutive months
15. For children 1-3 years: Diarrhea or vomiting for 3 days
16. For children 4-16 years: No weight gain for 3 consecutive months
17. For children 4-18 years: Diarrhea or vomiting for 4 days
18. Poor feeding skills
19. Food allergies or intolerances (formula, fat, lactose, wheat, etc.)
20. Inborn error of metabolism
21. Prealbumin: 9-22 mg/dl (0-6 months), 11-29 mg/dl (6 months-6 years), 15-37 mg/dl (6-16 years)
22. Cholesterol <65 mg/dl or >175 mg/dl
23. Triglycerides <40 mg/dl and >160 mg/dl

Modified from Fenton M et al: Nutrition referral criteria for pediatrics (<18 years) with HIV/AIDS. In *Guidelines for implementing HIV medical nutrition therapy,* Los Angeles, 1999, Los Angeles County Commission on HIV Health Services.

associated with immune suppression. However, one study of HIV-infected individuals found that exercise has mixed effects and that a high-fat diet has no adverse effect on runners' immune systems (Venkatraman et al, 1997). CD8 suppressor T-cell levels were higher in men than in women; numbers of killer cells were 2.5 times higher after exercise than at rest and were positively related to dietary fat levels. In men—but not in women—levels of proinflammatory cytokines were lower after exercise than at rest. Activity can be successfully planned for HIV patients.

Protein

High-protein diets might safely promote positive nitrogen balance and lean body mass repletion, but studies to clarify the ability of a high-protein diet to reverse HIV-malnutrition and body composition changes are still needed. HIV-infected persons, like the uninfected, have a normal metabolic response to a high-protein diet; protein supplementation stimulates protein metabolism (Engelson et al, 1998). Protein requirements may be estimated at 1.0 to 1.4 g/kg for maintenance and 1.5 to 2.0 g/kg for repletion. Because of the increased protein requirements, protein restriction is indicated only in persons with severe hepatic or renal disease. Dietary intervention for these further compromised patients is the same as for noninfected persons (see Chapters 29 and 40).

Fat

Fat tolerance varies from person to person. In individuals with malabsorption or diarrhea, use of a low-fat diet may aid in management. Use of the more readily absorbed medium-chain triglyceride (MCT) oil is considered better than long-chain triglyceride–based supplements for decreasing stool fat and stool nitrogen content and in reducing the number of bowel movements and abdominal symptoms.

Fish oil (omega-3 fatty acids), when given with MCT oil, may improve immune function because this combination is less inflammatory than the usual omega-6 fatty acids. However, if triglyceride and cholesterol levels are increased, leading clinicians have speculated that following the guidelines established in the National Cholesterol Education Program could be beneficial (see Chapter 35).

Fluids and Electrolytes

Fluid needs in HIV-infected individuals are similar to those of well individuals and are calculated to be 30 to 35 ml/kg (8 to 12 cups for adults) per day, with additional amounts to compensate for losses from diarrhea, nausea and vomiting, night sweats, and prolonged fever. Replacement of electrolyte losses (sodium, potassium, and chloride) in the presence of vomiting and diarrhea is also recommended.

Box 41-4. Practical Eating Suggestions for Symptom Management

SYMPTOM/PROBLEM	MANAGEMENT
Nausea	Small, frequent meals Avoidance of high-fat, greasy foods Cool or room-temperature foods Avoidance of lying down flat after eating Take medications after meal
Sore mouth or throat	Soft, moist foods Avoidance of spicy or acidic foods Experimentation with temperature of foods (avoidance of very hot or very cold foods; cool or room-temperature foods are best) Use of nutrient- and energy-dense foods to maximize oral intake
Xerostomia (dry mouth)	Use of foods that are moist or served with a sauce or gravy Consumption of liquids at mealtimes and extra fluids between meals Emphasis on good oral hygiene: flossing, brushing, and rinsing; regular dental care Use of fluoride gels or mouthwashes Consideration of prophylactic antifungal therapy Chewing of sugarless gum or sucking of mints
Difficulty with breathing	Use of easy-to-eat foods Use of nutrient- and energy-dense foods
Diarrhea	Fluid and electrolyte replacement Low-insoluble and high-soluble–fiber diet Possible benefits from low-lactose diet Low-fat diet (may be indicated) Avoidance of gas-causing foods and beverages Avoidance of caffeine Take medications after meal
Constipation	Increased fluid intake Increased dietary fiber intake
Inadequate oral intake	Use of nutrient- and energy-dense foods, including nutritional supplements Use of small, frequent meals and snacks Consideration of alternative nutrition support or appetite stimulant such as Megace or Marinol
Fatigue	Adequate sleep, relaxation, exercise Adequate diet, especially foods rich in vitamins B_{12}, A, C, folate, and carotene or zinc; inadequate amounts may cause fatigue (Coodley et al, 1993; Tang et al, 1996) Avoidance of caffeine, alcohol, cigarette smoking, and recreational drug use Avoidance of stress and treatment of anxiety or depression Identification and management of possible causes for anemia: • Medications: AZT, bactrim, dapsone, gancyclovir, interferon, pyrimethamine • Other causes: alcohol abuse, bleeding, *Mycobacterium avium* complex, tuberculosis, fungal infections, cytomegalovirus Check lactic acid levels for indications of mitochondrial toxicity
Body cell mass loss	Adequate diet Resistance exercise Correct for testosterone deficiency Consider anabolic agents (Rx from MD)

Vitamins and Minerals

The importance of nutrition for the immune system has been well established. The research on micronutrients and their effects on the immune system is often contradictory, and randomized control studies are needed to better identify relationships of vitamin and mineral intakes, levels, deficiencies, needs, and supplementation with HIV infection and with opportunistic infections, complications and side effects, disease progression, and medications. Blood or serum micronutrient levels may not reflect actual status; dietary intake measurements may be helpful in determining the nutritional condition (Kupka and Fawzi, 2002).

One dietary study found nutrient intakes for a large percentage of women and minorities to be less than the recommended levels and suggested dietary assessments and counseling (Woods et al, 2002). The need for increased intake of micronutrients has been suggested, and HIV nutrition practitioners commonly recommend that patients take a daily multivitamin-mineral supplement that provides 100% of the RDA and a basic B-complex supplement. In adults, supplements up to 55% of the RDA for riboflavin and thiamin have improved survival rates (Heller, 1997).

Special Micronutrient Concerns in Pediatric Patients

In addition to supporting optimal function of the immune system, nutrition is especially critical in children for normal growth and development (Heller, 1997). Children should be growing consistently, and weight gain and linear growth must be monitored carefully from baseline and at least every 3 months (see Box 41-3). In some studies, failure to thrive and growth stunting have been identified. Changes in adipose and muscle stores may occur as a result of metabolic changes. The goal is to preserve lean body mass. Serum prealbumin, a sensitive predictor of visceral protein stores, is used to measure the effectiveness of nutrition intervention (Heller, 1997).

Each infected child should undergo a baseline nutritional assessment, with follow-up every 4 to 6 months, depending on the child's age, nutritional status, and nutritional symptoms (see Boxes 41-3 and 41-4). As in adults, nutrition changes in children with HIV/AIDS are not always apparent, and poor intake is usually the major reason for weight loss. General nutrition recommendations for children include high-energy, high-protein, nutrient-dense foods, as protein needs may vary from 150% to 200% of the RDA and energy needs from 100% to 200% of the RDA (Bentler and Stanish, 1987). Nutrient and caloric intake must be assessed. Children with severe encephalopathy may be bedfast and require fewer total calories.

Weight loss may be attributable to poor energy intake, malabsorption, and opportunistic infections. Stunting and failure to thrive (FTT) have been identified in nearly all HIV-infected children. Skin-fold measurements should be taken for comparison. The goal is simply to preserve lean body mass.

A multivitamin supplement is needed to provide at least 100% of the RDAs. Poor absorption may be a problem for vitamins A, C, B_6, B_{12}, and folate; and the minerals iron; selenium; and zinc (Heller, 1997). Tube feeding via gastrostomy tube may improve the weight and fat mass of children with HIV. Higher age-adjusted CD4+ cell counts and lower weight-for-height scores at baseline have been significant predictors of a positive response to gastrostomy tube feedings (Miller et al, 1995).

Treatment for children with HIV includes the use of potent antiretroviral medications. These medications, when used in children, are associated with adverse side effects and difficulty with maintaining a rigid dosage schedule. Children and their caregivers need assistance from dietetics professionals in identifying creative ways of adhering to medication schedules and reducing the flavor and smells of medications. Medications can be mixed into foods or beverages, such as shakes, ice cream, or cranberry or apple sauces, so that they are consumed in sufficient quantities to be effective. Table 41-5 presents HIV medications, along with their dietary considerations and side effects. Although reducing fat intake may decrease difficulty with diarrhea and malabsorption, decreasing fat in a child's diet, especially before the age of 2 years, may directly and negatively impact the growth and development of the child (Leung, 1989).

Mild to severe developmental delays are estimated to occur in up to 80% of HIV-infected children, and as a result, feeding skills may also be impaired (Heller, 1997). A child's oral-motor and self-feeding skills, especially during the first 3 years of life, should be monitored closely. Oral and esophageal manifestations, such as *Candida* or herpes simplex infections, can make it painful for the child to eat. In such cases, the family may benefit from guidelines and suggestions as to soft, cold, and nonacidic foods and beverages that can help support the child's nutrition status. Resolving barriers to adequate nutrition intake, ensuring regular access to food, eliminating stress in the environment, and increasing financial resources can help to improve the child's nutrition status.

COMPLICATIONS WITH A NUTRITION IMPACT

If the disease progresses, signs and symptoms of HIV infection and AIDS will be manifested along with increased nutrition complications. Pre-HAART studies show that wasting and diarrhea will occur sooner or later during the course of AIDS. In many persons, death appears to have been determined more by nutritional status than by any particular opportunistic infection (Keusch and Thea, 1993). Other common nutrition-related complications are anorexia, fatigue, fever, dehydration, nausea, and fat and metabolic abnormalities. Successful lowering of the viral load, especially through the use of combination antiretroviral therapies, helps to maintain nutritional status.

Diarrhea and Malabsorption

Persons with the greatest risk of developing diarrhea are those with a CD4+ cell count of less than 200 to 250 cells/mm^3. Fifty percent of all persons with HIV/AIDS will develop diarrhea at sometime during the clinical course of their disease (Cello, 1997). Diarrhea and malabsorption are the major nutritional problems for this population, and they are often the most difficult problems to resolve. Abnormal D-xylose absorption and steatorrhea are common. Malabsorption of fat, monosaccharides, disaccharides, nitrogen, vitamin B_{12}, folate, minerals, and trace elements occurs in patients with intestinal infections of

TABLE 41-6 Possible Causes of HIV-Related Diarrhea

CATEGORY	SPECIFIC AGENTS/CONDITIONS
Bacteria	*Campylobacter* species
	Clostridium difficile
	Enteroadherent *Escherichia coli*
	Mycobacterium avium complex/ *M. tuberculosis*
	Salmonella species
	Shigella
	Vibrio
Parasites	*Cryptosporidium*
	Cyclospora
	Giardia
	Isospora
	Microsporidia
	Entamoeba histolytica
Fungi	*Histoplasma capsulatum*
Viruses	Adenovirus
	Cytomegalovirus
	Herpes simplex
	HIV (possibly)
Nutritional causes	Fat malabsorption
	High-fiber diet
	Hypoalbuminemia
	Lactose intolerance
	Kaposi's sarcoma
	Malnutrition
	Caffeine
	Sorbitol
Drugs	
Antacids	Mg^{++}-containing
Antiretrovirals	Didanosine (Videx, ddI)
	Nelfinavir (Viracept)
	Ritonavir (Norvir)
	Saquinavir (Fortovase)
Antimicrobials	Amphotericin
	Macrolide antibiotics
	Azithromycin
	Clorithromycin
	Pentamidine
Vitamins (high dose)	Vitamin C

Modified from Dieterich DT: *Diarrhea in the HIV/AIDS patient,* 1997, Golden Colo, Medical Education Collaborative and Oestreicher Medical Communications, Inc.

TABLE 41-7 Nutrition Intervention for Diarrhea

TYPE OF DIARRHEA	INTERVENTION
Treatable diarrhea	Maintain adequate nutritional intake for bowel regeneration
	Enhance absorption by using elemental diets
	Control infection and symptoms with antibiotics and antidiarrheals
	Provide fiber-containing supplements; follow general guidelines
Diarrhea resistant to treatment	Promote patient comfort
	Maintain adequate hydration; intravenous hydration may be indicated
	Control symptoms by using antidiarrheals or antispasmodics
	TPN may be indicated
	Calcium carbonate (500 mg bid)
Diarrhea resulting from AIDS enteropathy	Incorporate small frequent meals into daily plan
	Avoid lactose-containing foods and medications or use lactase enzyme
	Reduce high fructose–containing foods (apple and pear juices, grapes, honey, dates, nuts, figs, soft drinks)
	Limit sorbitol, hexitols, and mannitol in "sugar-free" products
	Limit carbonated beverages
	Limit fat if steatorrhea is present; try medium-chain triglyceride(MCT) oil
	Consider a lactobacillus replacement or probiotics if patient is receiving long-term antibiotic therapy
	Consider prescriptive pancreatic enzymes
	Consider L-glutamine (.4 g/kg up to 30 g/day for 5-14 days, followed by 5-10 g/day)
	Recommend a multivitamin/mineral supplement
	Gradually reintroduce suspect foods, one at a time, and check for tolerance
General guidelines for diarrhea	Consume foods at room temperature
	Limit insoluble and bran-type, high-fiber foods
	Avoid foods that cause gas

the small bowel. When the large bowel is infected, malabsorption of fluids and electrolytes is seen. Diarrhea and malabsorption can lead to subtherapeutic blood levels of medications, thereby negatively influencing treatment outcomes (Patel et al, 1995).

The causes of diarrhea can be multifactorial, and its etiology must be pursued. In an early study, 80% to 85% of persons with AIDS-associated diarrhea were found to have one or more identifiable enteric pathogens (Cello et al, 1991). These pathogens and other factors that cause diarrhea are listed in Table 41-6.

Regardless of whether the cause of diarrhea is identified, intervention and treatment must be pursued. Treatment often uses a combination of antidiarrheal agents, including cholestyramine and fiber supplements; antimotility agents, such as codeine phosphate, Lomotil, Imodium, morphine, and paragoric; and hormones, such as octreotide and Sandostatin (Dieterich, 1997). Table 41-7 provides information on the nutritional management of diarrhea.

Disorders of the Oral Cavity and Esophagus

Oral lesions are common and usually are neoplastic, bacterial, viral, or fungal in origin. They often are the first sign of HIV infection that leads to diagnosis and can mark immunodeficiency and disease progression. Symptoms of oral candidiasis (thrush) include soreness of the mouth and tongue, often described as a "burnt" feeling, and pain or difficulty with swallowing (Figure 41-7).

Dysgeusia may also be present secondary to medication, zinc, and other nutrient deficiencies; candidiasis; xerostomia; or excessive mucus production. Conventional as well as necrotizing ulcerative periodontitis (NUP)—formerly called HIV-periodontal—disease is often seen. Frequent dental care and routine hygiene are essential. NUP is associated with severe pain and bleeding as well as bone and soft tissue loss (Greenspan and Greenspan, 1997).

KS or herpes in the oropharyngeal or esophageal area can also inhibit normal chewing and swallowing, thus limiting nutritional intake. Patients with extensive or chronic lesions may require alternative nutritional support, such as enteral or parenteral nutrition.

Use of specially designed formulas may slow the progressive decline toward malnutrition. Box 41-4 lists suggestions for improving the dietary intake of the patient who has a painful mouth. For painful mouth sores, the patient can swish and spit "magic mouthwash," consisting of equal parts 2% viscous lidocaine, Benadryl, and Maalox, that can be prescribed by the physician and formulated by the pharmacist.

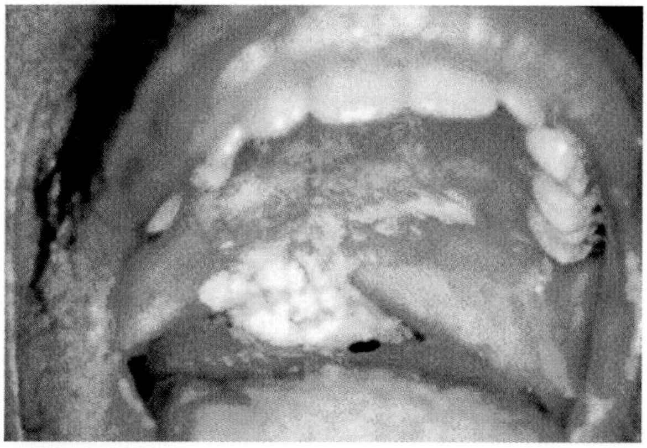

FIGURE 41-7 • Fluconazole-resistant pseudomembranous candidiasis. (Copyright 1996-2000 David Reznik, DDS. All rights reserved. Used with permission by HIVdent and Dr. Reznik.)

Neurologic Disorders

CNS manifestations of AIDS, ranging from psychomotor impairment to severe dementia, can significantly affect the ability of an infected individual to maintain adequate nutrition. Moreover, decreased sensory perception when chewing and swallowing can increase the risk of aspiration. Working closely with occupational and physical therapists, speech pathologists, the nursing staff, and others involved in overall patient care is important in helping the patient maintain adequate nutritional intake.

Alterations in Metabolism and Body Shape

Distinguishing body composition changes that indicate wasting, lipodystrophy, or obesity from a healthy and nonthreatening weight loss is important. Monitoring body composition provides a picture of body shape changes over time. Measuring waist, hip and waist-hip ratio, midarm, breast, and neck circumferences, in addition to weight should be done every 3 to 6 months. Bioelectrical impedance analysis (BIA) is an inexpensive and easy tool for measuring body cell mass, loss of which may indicate wasting. BIA does not indicate regional differences in fat and therefore is not useful in identifying fat redistribution. Expensive tools, such as dual-energy x-ray absorptiometry (DEXA or DXA), computed tomography (CT) scans, and magnetic resonance imaging (MRI), are mostly used for research and provide the most accurate assessment of these body composition changes.

The use of potent anti-HIV therapies, especially protease inhibitors, has increased the incidence of insulin resistance, type 2 diabetes, hypercholesterolemia, pancreatitis, and hypertriglyceridemia in the HIV/AIDS population. Principles developed for diabetes or from the National Cholesterol Education Program are used in an effort to control these conditions (see Chapters 33 and 35). Oral hypoglycemics and insulin are being used, as are lipid-lowering drugs. Supplements often promoted for these conditions include omega-3 fatty acids, α-lipoic acid, and L-carnitine.

Treatment for body-shape changes has been both difficult and confusing. The stigma and psychological discomfort associated with the condition can be devastating. Discontinuing antiretroviral therapy is not a favorable option, and less offending regimens are under active study. Those that can afford them are using cosmetic surgery, such as liposuction or implants, anabolic therapy, or a combination of these options. Aerobic exercise may have a role in reducing truncal adiposity, along with a moderate–fat and carbohydrate and high–fiber diet (Roubenoff et al 1999, 2002).

Growth hormone, approved for AIDS wasting or cachexia based on evidence that it increased lean body mass and decreased fat mass, may have a role in reducing HIV-associated fat accumulation. Transient worsening of both insulin sensitivity and glucose tolerance of most individuals and increased insulin-like growth factor I levels can occur. An oral glucose tolerance test has been recommended to identify those at risk for growth hormone–induced hyperglycemia (Lo et al, 2001).

A pilot study that used low-dose metformin resulted in reductions of insulin resistance and visceral adipose tissue; however, subcutaneous adipose tissue was also reduced, which was undesirable for some (Hadigan et al, 2000). Metformin has been associated with lactic acidosis and must be used cautiously in this population. The use of metformin and of pioglitazone and rosiglitazone, other insulin-sensitizing agents, are being studied actively. Implementing changes in diet and exercise, core components in treating insulin resistance, are prudent while awaiting formal studies in this population (Currier 2000; Grinspoon, 2001).

COMPLEMENTARY AND ALTERNATIVE THERAPIES

People with HIV disease often become frustrated with the lack of definitive medical therapies, and some turn to unconventional nutritional therapies. "Alternative medicine" describes treatments and practices that (1) lack sufficient documentation of safety and effectiveness against specific diseases and conditions; (2) are not readily taught in U.S. medical schools; and (3) are not generally reimbursable by health insurance providers (Stehlin, 1995). The National AIDS Health Fraud Task Force uses the definition of AIDS fraud as "the sale, advertising, or promotion (usually for profit) of products, therapies or services to diagnose, prevent, cure or treat HIV disease or AIDS which are unproven, unscientific or harmful" (California AIDS Fraud Task Force, 1996). Among the major questions to consider in assessing therapies are the following:

- Is the product or treatment harmful?
- Are there harmful drug-drug interactions with prescription or over-the-counter medications or nutrients?
- Are unproven treatments being used while effective conventional treatment(s) are being delayed?
- Does the therapy work?
- Is the financial expense worth the benefit?

One must be wary of products or services when their promotion uses sensationalism, testimonials, or claims that they are based on a secret formula or when promotional literature accuses the government or Western physicians of neglect.

Many herbs that might have been dismissed casually as safe are contraindicated when used with antiretroviral medications. St John's wort, an inducer in the cytochrome P450 pathway, was found to substantially decrease plasma concentrations of the protease inhibitor indinavir, which is metabolized in the cytochrome P450 pathway. Drug resistance and treatment failure could occur because of this pharmacokinetic interaction. Researchers and the FDA have cautioned that other protease inhibitors, nonnucleoside reverse transcriptase inhibitors, and other drugs using the same pathway would be negatively affected as well (Lumpkin and Alpert, 2000; Piscitelli et al 2000). Garlic supplements reduced blood concentrations of saquinavir by about 50% and after a wash-out period of 10 days by 35% (Piscitelli et al, 2001).

Concern has been raised about silymarin, the flavonoid extract from *Silybum marianum* (milk thistle). Although silymarin is promoted and used to protect the liver, one study showed that it reduced the activity of CYP3A4 enzyme in human hepatocyte cultures, which could lessen metabolism of coadministered medications and increase toxicity (Venkataramanan et al, 2000).

Addressing alternative therapies should be a customary part of both the medical and nutrition assessment and intervention. Therapies that people who live with HIV may try include exercise, lifestyle changes, dietary supplements, herbal medications, megavitamins, counseling, and prayer therapy. Nutrition supplements formulated and marketed for this population have yet to be substantiated.

Specific dietary supplements often used by this population include echinacea, St John's wort, cat's claw, protein supplements, creatine, anabolic steroids, and Chinese herbs. Reiki, massage, yoga, and acupunture are also used often (see Chapter 20 and Appendix 35). One study found 56% of patients had informed their physicians about using alternative therapies, but the information was found in the medical charts of only 13% of the patients (Southwell, 2001).

SUMMARY

HIV disease involves multiple systems and has complex psychological, social, and economic ramifications. However, until recently, research, medical care, and education about HIV have been less than ideal throughout the world. These factors must be considered to find the best ways to provide appropriate HIV medical nutrition therapy. Advocacy for improving these inequities will undoubtedly improve outcomes for people with HIV in the United States and in the rest of the world.

Clinical Scenario I

Gary is a 41-year-old male HIV-positive patient who also is diagnosed with hepatitis C and recently had shingles. His current HIV antiretroviral regimen is Viracept, Zerit, and Videx. His last viral load was 250,000; his CD4+ cell count was 14; and his serum triglycerides were at 890 mg/dl. He lives alone and gets one meal per day from a community meal provider. He has chronic diarrhea, with four to five loose stools per day. He has recurrent heartburn and bloating after meals. He is on disability and has no extra money to join a gym. Gary smokes 1 pack of cigarettes per day and is in an outpatient alcohol recovery program. He is 5 ft 10 in., weighs 150 lb, and his dietary intake as shown from a recent 24-hour recall is 1650 kcal with 40 g protein.

1. What energy and protein recommendations would you make? How does this compare with the recommended amount for his age, sex, and size?
2. What recommendations would you make to his meal provider?
3. Would you recommend any other laboratory tests? If so, which ones?
4. What exercise recommendations would you make given his limited funds?

Clinical Scenario 2

Miguel is a 34-year-old man infected with HIV for over 10 years. His current viral load is undetectable at below 50 copies, and his CD4+ count is 563. He is 6 ft 0 in. and weighs 202 lb. He has been on antiretroviral therapy for 8 years and currently takes Kaletra, Epivir, and Rescriptor. Miguel drinks two alcoholic drinks per week and works out at the gym twice a week, where he walks on a treadmill for 30 minutes and weight trains for 1 hour. Over the last year he has noticed that his body composition has changed with an increasing abdominal girth. His last fasting lipid profile was abnormal with a total cholesterol of 280 mg/dl, triglycerides 455 mg/dl, HDL 29 mg/dl, and LDL 148 mg/dl. He has a positive family history for both cardiovascular disease and diabetes.

1. What do you think are the reasons for Miguel's expanding waist?
2. Calculate Miguel's daily energy and protein needs.
3. What risk factors does he have for developing diabetes or heart disease?
4. What are your dietary, exercise, and lifestyle recommendations?

Relevant Web Sites

AIDS Education Global Information System
www.aegis.com
AIDS Treatment Information Service (ATIS)
www.hivatis.org
Association of Nutrition Services Agencies
www.aidsnutrition.org
CDC Division of HIV/AIDS Protection
www.cdc.gov/hiv/dhap.htm
Division of Acquired Immunodeficiency Syndrome (DAIDS), NIH Research
www.niaid.nih.gov/daids/
HIV and Hepatitis.com
www.hivandhepatitis.com
HIV Fitness Guidelines
www.hivfitness.org
HIV Nutrition Education
www.apla.org
HIV Resources
www.hivresources.com
HIV/AIDS Dietetic Practice Group
www.hiavaidsdpg.org
HIVdent
www.hivdent.org
Project Inform
www.proinform.com

Cited References

Adams M et al: Battling HIV on many fronts, *N Engl J Med* 338:198, 1998.

American Dietetic Association: *HIV/AIDS medical nutrition therapy protocol: medical nutrition therapy across the continuum of care,* ed 2, Chicago, 1998, ADA.

American Dietetic Association (ADA): Position of the American Dietetic Association and dietitians of Canada: nutrition intervention in the care of persons with human immunodeficiency virus infection, *J Am Diet Assoc* 100:717, 2000.

Anastos K et al: The relative value of CD4 cell count and quantitative HIV-1 RNA in predicting survival in HIV-1 infected women: results of the Women's Intraagency HIV Study, *AIDS* 13:1717, 1999.

Annan K: Address to the World Health Assembly, Geneva, May 2001, http://www.unaids.org/whatsnew/speeches/eng/SG1705wha.htm.

Bentler M, Stanish M: Nutrition support of the pediatric patient with AIDS, *J Am Diet Assoc* 87:488, 1987.

Bozette S et al: For the HIV Cost and Services Utilization Study Consortium. Expenditures for the care of HIV-infected patients in the era of highly active anti-retroviral therapy, *NEJM* 344:11, 2001.

California AIDS Fraud Task Force: *Stop AIDS health fraud,* Los Angeles, 1996, California AIDS Fraud Task Force.

Cello JP: Gastrointestinal tract manifestations of AIDS. In Sande MA, Voberding PA, editors: *The medical management of AIDS,* Philadelphia, 1997, WB Saunders.

Cello JP et al: Effect of octreotide on refractory AIDS-associated diarrhea, *Ann Intern Med* 115:705, 1991.

Centers for Disease Control: Recommendations for prevention of HIV transmission in health care settings, *MMWR* 36:1, 1987.

Centers for Disease Control and Prevention: *HIV/AIDS Surveillance Report* 8(2):1, 1996, www.cdc.gov/hiv/stats/hivsur82.pdf.

Centers for Disease Control and Prevention: 1997 USPHS/IDSA guidelines for the prevention of opportunistic infection in persons infected with human immunodeficiency virus, *MMWR* 46(No. RR-12):27, 1997. Available at www2.cdc.gov/mmwr.

Centers for Disease Control: CDC report of the NIH Panel to define principles of therapy of HIV infection and guidelines for the use of antiretroviral agents in HIV-infected adults and adolescents, *MMWR* 47(RR-5):1, 1998.

Centers for Disease Control and Prevention: *You can prevent crypto (cryptosporidiosis): a guide for people with HIV infection,* Atlanta, 2001a, CDC, www.cdc.gov/hiv/pubs/brochure/oi_cryp.htm.

Centers for Disease Control and Prevention: *HIV/AIDS surveillance report, year-end edition,* vol 12(12), updated 9/24/2001b, www.cdc.gov/hiv/stats/hasrlink.htm.

Centers for Disease Control and Prevention: *Primary HIV infection associated with oral transmission,* updated 2/2001c, www.cdc.gov/hiv/pubs/facts/oralsexqa.htm.

Centers for Disesae Control and Prevention: *Characteristics of persons living with AIDS and HIV 2001, HIV/AIDS Surveillance Suppl Rep* 9(2):1, 2003, www.cdc.gov/hiv/stats/hasrsupp92/commentary.htm.

Clifford DB et al: HAART improves prognosis in HIV-associated progressive multifocal leukoencephalopathy, *Neurology* 52:623, 1999.

Colgrove RC et al: Selective vertical transmission of HIV-1 antiretroviaral reisistance mutations, *AIDS* 12:2281, 1998.

Collins CL: Nutrition care in AIDS, *Diet Curr* 15:1, 1998.

Community Research Initiative on AIDS: *HIV lifecycle; human immunodeficiency virus,* 1998, AIDS Community Research Initiative of America.

Connor EM et al: Reduction of maternal-infant transmission of human immunodeficiency virus type 1 with zidovudine treatment, *N Engl J Med* 331:1173, 1997.

Coodley GO et al, β-carotene in HIV infection, J AIDS 6:272, 1993.

Coutsoudis A et al: Influence of infant-feeding patterns on early mother-to-child transmission of HIV-1 in Durban, South Africa: a prospective cohort study, *Lancet,* 353:786, 1999.

Currier J: How to manage metabolic complications of HIV therapy: what to do while we wait for answers, *AIDS Reader* 10(3):162, 2000.

De Groot AS: HIV infection among incarcerated women: epidemic behind bars, *AIDS Reader* 10(5):287, 2000.

Diesing TS et al: HIV-1-associated dementia: a basic science and clinical perspective, *AIDS Read* 12(8):358, 2002, 2002 Cliggott Publishing, Division of SCP Communications, 09/20/2002, www.medscape.com/viewarticle/441085.

Dieterich DT: *Diarrhea in the HIV/AIDS patient,* 1997, Medical Education Collaborative and Oestreicher Medical Communications, Inc.

Division of HIV/AIDS Prevention: *Proportion of AIDS cases, by race/ethnicity and year of report, 1985-200, United States,* updated 9/19/01, Centers for Disease Control and Prevention, www.cdc.gov/hiv/graphics/minority.htm.

Drew WL et al: New perspectives on CMV and other viruses in the immunocompromised patient, *Medscape Today,* March 2003, University of Minnesota, www.medscape.com/viewprogram/2255.

Dreyfuss ML and Fawzi WW: Micronutrients and vertical transmission of HIV-1, *Am J Clin Nutr* 75:959, 2002.

Dubé MP, Sattler FR: Metabolic complications of antiretroviral therapies, *AIDS Clin Care* 10:1, 1998.

Duran A et al: Bone loss associated with lipodystrophy syndrome [Abstract]. *Conference on HIV Pathogenesis and Treatment, First IAS Conference in Buenos Aires,* July, 2001, www.aids2001ias.org.

Engelson ES et al: Nutrition and testosterone status of HIV+ women, [Abstract No. Tu. B 2382], *International Conference on AIDS, July 7-12, 1996,* 11:1, 332.

Engelson ES et al: Effect of a high protein diet upon protein metabolism in HIV-infected men and women. *[Abstract No. 32166], Twelfth World AIDS Conference,* Geneva, Switzerland, 1998.

Engelson ES et al: Fat distribution in HIV-infected patients reporting truncal enlargement quantified by whole-body magnetic resonance imaging, *Am J Clin Nutr* 69:1162, 1999.

Engle L: Old AIDS, *Body Positive* XI:11, 1998.

Fisher K: Wasting and lipodystrophy in patients infected with HIV: a practical approach in clinical practice, *The AIDS Reader* 11(3):132, 2001.

Flier J, Underhill L: Metabolic disturbances and wasting in the acquired immunodeficiency syndrome, *N Engl J Med* 327:329, 1992.

French AL et al: Vitamin A deficiency and genital viral burden in women infected with HIV-1, *Lancet* 359:1210, 2002.

Gifford AL et al: Predictors of self-reported adherence and plasma HIV concentrations in patients on multidrug antiretroviral regimens, *J Acquir Immune Defic Syndr* 23:386, 2000.

Girardi E et al: Changing clinical presentation and survival in HIV-associated tuberculosis after highly active antiretroviral therapy, *J Acquir Immun Defic Syndr* 26(4):326, 2001.

Gottlieb MS et al: Pneumocystis pneumonia—Los Angeles, *MMWR* 30:250, 1981.

Greenspan D, Greenspan JS: Oral manifestations of HIV infection, *AIDS Clinical Care* 9:4, 1997.

Grinspoon S: Insulin resistance in HIV disease, *The PRN Notebook* June 2001.

Grunfeld C, Feingold KR: Metabolic disturbances and wasting in the acquired immunodeficiency syndrome, *N Engl J Med* 327:329, 1992.

Guidelines for the use of antiretroviral agents in pediatric HIV infection, *MMWR* 47(No RR-4), 1998, updated 08/08/01, www.hivatis.org.

Hadigan C et al: Metformin in the treatment of HIV lipodystrophy syndrome: a randomized controlled trial, *JAMA* 284:472, 2000.

Hammett TM et al: *1996-1997 Update: HIV/AIDS, STDs, and TB in correctional facilities,* July 1999, National Institute of Justice.

Hayes C, editor: Integrating nutrition therapy into medical management of human immunodeficiency virus, *Clin Infect Dis* 36(suppl 2), April 2003, www.journals.uchicago.edu/CID/journal/contents/v36nS2.html.

Health Resources and Services Administration: *Health care and HIV: nutritional guide for providers and clients,* June 2002, HRSA, HIV/AIDS Bureau, www.aids-etc.org/aidsetc.

Health Resources and Services Administration: HIV disease in individuals ages fifty and above, *HRSA Care ACTION,* February 2001.

Health Resources and Services Administration HIV/AIDS Bureau. Ryan White CARE Act 2001. Data Report for Title I, Title II, AIDS Assistance Program, Health Insurance Program. USDHHS, HRSA, 2002, http://hab.hrsa.gov/reports/saar2001/saar2001report.htm#_Toc40130325.

Heller L: Nutrition support for children with HIV/AIDS, *J Am Diet Assoc,* 97:473, 1997.

Heller L: Nutrition support for children with HIV/AIDS, *AIDS Reader* 10(2):109, 2000, www.medscape.com/viewarticle/410256.

Henry J Kaiser Family Foundation: *Daily Reports, national security: Clinton administration explains AIDS as a security threat,* 6/8/2000, www.kaisernetwork.org.

HIV-AIDS Bureau: *Title III EIS Grant Application Guidance.* DHHS, HRSA, HAB, 2001, http://hab.hrsa.gov/grants/newcompetingguide.doc.

HIV-AIDS Bureau. *Title I Grant Application Guidance.* DHHS, HRSA, HAB, 2001d, http://hab.hrsa.gov/grants/newcompetingguide.doc.

Hogan CM, Hammer SM: Host determinants in HIV infection and disease. Part 1: cellular and humoral immune responses, *Ann Intern Med* 1:134(9 Pt1):761, 2001.

Horn T: HIV drug resistance and drug-resistance testing, just FAQs, *CRIA Update,* Community Research Initiative on AIDS (10)4, Fall 2001.

Jacobson MA et al, editors: *Medical management of AIDS,* ed 3, Philadelphia, 1992, WB Saunders.

Joint United Nations Programme on HIV/AIDS: *20 years of AIDS,* 2001, www.unaids.org/publications/graphics/20years/Eng/HIV.time.chart.e.jpg.

Joint United Nations Programme on HIV/AIDS: Adults and children estimated to be living with HIV/AIDS as of end 2001, *AIDS Epidemic Update,* December 2001, www.unaids.org/worldaidsday/2001/EPIgraphics2001/EPIcore_en.ppt.

Keusch GT, Thea DM: Malnutrition in AIDS, *Med Clin North Am* 77:795, 1993.

Kosmiski LA et al: Fat distribution and metabolic changes are strongly correlated and energy expenditure is increased in the HIV lipodystrophy syndrome, *AIDS* 15:1193, 2001.

Kotler DP: Nutritional effects and support in the patient with acquired immunodeficiency syndrome, *J Nutr* 122:723, 1992.

Kotler DP: Characterization of intestinal disease associated with human immunodeficiency virus infection and response to antiretroviral therapy, *J Infect Dis* 179:4545, 1999.

Kotler DP, Muurahainen N: Nutritional and gastrointestinal syndromes: complications of HIV infection and treatment. In *Clinical Care Options for HIV, Conference Summaries, Fifth Conference on Retroviruses and Opportunistic Infections,* 1998, www.healthcg.com.

Kupka R, Fawzi W: Zinc nutrition and HIV infection, *Nutr Rev* 60(3):69, 2002.

Kuritzkes DR et al: Current management challenges in HIV: antiretroviral resistance, *AIDS Read.* Cliggott Publishing, Division of SCP Communications, 13(3):133, 2003, www.medscape.com/viewarticle/451678.

Laboratory Corporation of America: *Directory of services and interpretive guide,* 2001, Laboratory Corporation of America, Burlington, NC, Holdings and Lexi-Comp Inc.

Leung J: An approach to feeding HIV-infected infants and toddlers, *Top Clin Nutr* 4:27-37, 1989.

Lo JC et al: The effects of recombinant human growth hormone on body composition and glucose metabolism in HIV-infected patients with fat accumulation, *J Clin Endocrinol Metab* 86(8):3480, 2001.

Los Angeles County Commission on HIV Health Services (LACCHHS): *Guidelines for Implementing HIV medical nutrition therapy guidelines,* approved 9/9/1999.

Luaer GM and Walker BD: Hepatitis C virus infection, *N Engl J Med* 345:141, 2001.

Lumpkin MM, Alpert A: Risk of drug interactions with St John's wort and indinavir and other drugs, *FDA Public Health Advisory,* February 2000.

Maruschak L: HIV in prisons and jails, 1999, *Bureau of Justice Statistics Bulletin* NCJ 187456, July 2001.

Mathews WC et al: National estimates of HIV-related symptom prevalence from the HIV Cost and Services Utilization Study, *Med Care* J 38(7):750, 2000.

Mbori-Ngacha D et al: Morbidity and mortality in breastfed and formula-fed infants of HIV-1-infected women, a randomized trial, *JAMA* 286:2413, 2001.

Michaels S et al: Differences in the incidence rates of opportunistic processes before and after the availability of protease inhibitors, *Fifth Conference on Retrovirus and Opportunistic Infections,* Chicago, February 1-5, 1998.

Miller Get al: Gastrostomy tube supplementation for HIV-infected children, *Pediatrics* 96:696, 1995.

Mondy K, Tebas P: *Emerging problems of bone in HIV disease, Clin Infect Dis* 36(S101-S105), April 2003.

Moyle G: Adverse events with antiretrovirals. In *Highlights from the First International AIDS Society (IAS) Conference on HIV Patho-*

genesis and Treatment, July 8-11, 2001, Buenos Aires, Argentina 2001.

Mulligan K et al: Energy expenditure in human immunodeficiency virus, *N Engl J Med* 336:70, 1997.

Mulligan K et al: Body composition changes in HIV-infected men consuming self-selecting diets during a placebo-controlled inpatient study of cannabinoids. In *Eighth Conference on Retroviruses and Opportunistic Infections,* [Abstract No. 647], 2001.

Murphy RL et al: Strategies for Concurrent Treatment of HIV and HCV: A Practical Approach for Managing Coinfected Patients. AdvancMed. Release date: April 28, 2003. http://www.medscape.com/viewprogram/2233.

Mustafa T et al: Association between exercise and HIV disease progression in a cohort of homosexual men, *Ann Epidemiol* 9:127, 1999.

New York State Department of Health AIDS Institute: General nutrition, weight loss and wasting syndrome. In *Adult HIV Guidelines,* March 2001, www.hivguidelines.org/public_html/CENTER/clinicalguidelines/adult_hiv_guidelines/ADULTS.htm.

Office of AIDS Research in Collaboration with the NIH Institutes, Centers, and Divisions: *Report on current NIH-supported research activities on women and HIV/AIDS,* Bethesda, Md, 1998, NIH.

O'Neill JF: *About HIV/AIDS bureau,* http://hab.hrsa.gov/aboutus.htm. 2001.

Panel on Clinical Practices for the Treatment of HIV: Guidelines for the use of antiretroviral agents in HIV-infected adults and adolescents, *MMWR* 47(No.RR-5), 1998, updated 7/14/03, www.aidsinfo.nih.gov.

Papathakis P: Personal communication, November 27, 2001.

Patel KB et al: Drug malabsorption and resistant tuberculosis in HIV-infected patients, *N Engl J Med* 332:336, 1995.

Peterson C et al: Pharmacokinetics of nelfinavir (Virecept 250 mg tablet): effect of food intake on single-dose PK parameters, *Abstracts of the Tenth Conference on Retroviruses and Opportunistic Infections,* Chicago, February 2003.

Piot P: *Update on the development of the global strategy framework and UN system strategic plan 2001-2005,* Ninth Meeting, Geneva, May 25-26, 2000, UNAIDS.

Piroth L et al: Does hepatitis C virus coinfection accelerate clinical and immunological evolution of HIV-infected patients? *AIDS* 12:381, 1998.

Polsky B et al: HIV-associated wasting in the HAART era: guidelines for assessment, diagnosis, and treatment, *AIDS Patient Care and STDs* 15(8):411, 2001.

Piscitelli SC et al: Indinavir concentrations and St John's wort, *Lancet* 355:547-548, 2000.

Piscitelli SC et al: The effect of garlic supplements on the pharmacokinetics of saquinavir, *Clinical Infectious Diseases* electronic edition, 12/3/2001.

Public Health Service Task Force: Safety and Toxicity of Individual Antiretroviral Agents in Pregnancy, *MMWR* 47(No. RR-2), 1998, updated 12/5/01, www.hivatis.org/guidelines/perinatal/Dec_01/perin1205.pdf.

Public Health Service Task Force: Recommendations for Use of Antiretroviral Drugs in Pregnant HIV-1 Infected Women for Maternal Health and Interventions to Reduce Perinatal HIV-1 Transmission in the United States, *MMWR* 47(No. RR-2), 1998, updated as a Living Document on December 5, 2001a, www.aidsinfo.nih.gov.

Public Health Service Task Force: Safety and Toxicity of Individual Antiretroviral Agents in Pregnancy: *MMWR* 47(No. RR-2), 1998, updated as a Living Document on December 5, 2001b, www.aidsinfo.nih.gov.

Raiten DJ: *Nutrition and HIV infection: a review and evaluation of the extant knowledge of the relationship between nutrition and HIV infection* (FDA Contract No. 223-88-2124), 1990.

Roubenoff R, Wilson IB: Effect of resistance training on self-reported physical functioning in HIV infection, *Med Sci Sports Exerc* 33:1811, 2001.

Roubenoff R et al: A pilot study of exercise training to reduce trunk fat in adults with HIV-associated fat redistribution, *AIDS* 13(11):1373, 1999.

Roubenoff R et al: Reduction of abdominal obesity in lipodystrophy associated with human immunodeficiency virus by means of diet and exercise: case report and proof of principle, *Clin Infect Dis* 34:390, 2002.

Saavedra J et al: Longitudinal assessment of growth in children born to mothers with human immunodeficiency virus infection, *Arch Pediatr Adolesc Med* 149:497, 1995.

Scribner AN et al: Osteonecrosis in HIV: a case-control study, *J Acquir Immune Defic Syndr* 25:19, 2000.

Selwin PA et al: A prospective study of the risk of tuberculosis among intravenous drug users with human immunodeficiency virus infection, *N Engl J Med* 320:545, 1989.

Shapiro MF et al: Variation in the care of HIV infected adults in the US: results from the HIV Cost and Services Utilization Study, *JAMA* 2305, 1999.

Southwell H et al: Use of alternative therapy among HIV-infected patients at an urban tertiary center, [Abstract No. 497], *Eighth Conference on Retroviruses and Opportunistic Infections,* 2001.

Stehlin IB: An FDA guide to choosing medical treatments, *FDA Consumer,* June, 1995.

Sterling T et al: Initial plasma HIV-1 RNA levels and progression to AIDS in women and men, *N Engl J Med* 344:720, 2001.

Stiehm RE: Newborn factors in maternal-infant transmission of pediatric HIV infection. In *Nutrition in pediatric HIV infection setting: the research agenda,* Bethesda, Md, 1995, NIH.

Tang W et al: Hyponatremia in hospitalized patients with acquired immunodeficiency syndrome, *Am J Med* 94:164, 1993.

United Nations Programme on HIV/AIDS (UNAIDS) and World Health Organization (WHO): *Joint AIDS Epidemic Update,* 2001, UNAIDS/WHO, www.unaids.org/worldaidsday/2001/Epiupdate2001/EPIupdate2001_en.doc.

Valeri A, Neusy A: Acute and chronic renal disease in hospitalized patients, *Clin Nephrol* 33:110, 1991.

Venkatraman J et al: Influence of the level of dietary lipid intake and maximal exercise on the immune status in runners, *Med Sci Sports Exercise* 29:333, 1997.

Venkataramanan R et al: Milk thistle, an herbal supplement, decreases the activity of CYI and uridine diphosphglucuronosyl transferase in human hepatocyte cultures, *Drug Metab Dispos* 28(11):1270, 2000.

Wanke CA et al: Weight loss and wasting remain common complications in individuals infected with human immunodeficiency virus in the era of highly active antiretroviral therapy, *Clin Infect Dis* 31:803, 2000.

Wheeler D et al: Weight loss as a predictor of survival and disease progression in HIV infection, *J AIDS Hum Retroviral* 18:80, 1998.

World Health Organization: Effect of breastfeeding on mortality among HIV-infected women, WHO Statement, June 7, 2001.

Woods MN et al: Nutrient intake and body weight in a large HIV cohort that includes women and minorities, *J Am Diet Assoc* 102:203, 2002.

Zhu T, Korber B, Nahinias AJ: An African HIV-1 sequence from 1959 and implications for the origin of the epidemic, *Nature* 391:594, 1998.

■ Additional References

Bartlett JG, Gallant JE: *Medical management of HIV infection,* 2001-2002 edition, Baltimore, Md, 2002, Johns Hopkins University, Division of Infectious Diseases.

Fauci AS et al: Immunopathogenic mechanisms of HIV infections, *Ann Intern Med* 124:654, 1996.

Fenton M et al: *HIV/AIDS adults: medical nutrition therapy across the continuum of care,* ed 2, Chicago, 1998, American Dietetic Association.

Fenton M et al: Nutrition referral criteria for pediatrics (<18 years) with HIV/AIDS. In *Guidelines for implementing HIV/AIDS medical nutrition therapy,* Los Angeles, 1999, Los Angeles County Commission on HIV Health Services.

Henderson R et al: Serum and plasma markers of nutritional status in children infected with the human immunodeficiency virus, *J Am Diet Assoc* 97:1377, 1997.

Raiten DJ: *Nutrition and HIV/AIDS: data needs and definitions of endpoints.* 2001, Office of Prevention Research and International Programs, NICHD/NIH.

Kruse LM: Nutrition assessment and management for patients with HIV disease, *AIDS Reader* 8(3):121, 1998.

Wanke CA et al: Clinical evaluation and management of metabolic and morphologic abnormalities associated with human immunodeficiency virus, *Clin Infect Dis* 34:248, 2002.

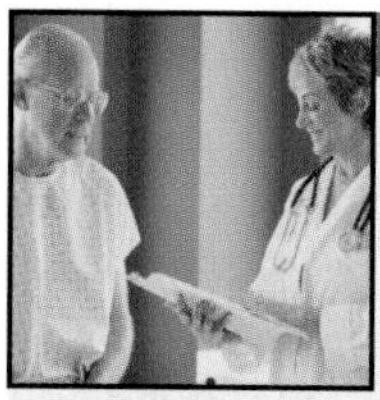

CHAPTER 42

Medical Nutrition Therapy for Metabolic Stress: Sepsis, Trauma, Burns, and Surgery

MARION F. WINKLER, MS, RD, LDN, CNSD
AINSLEY M. MALONE, MS, RD, CNSD

CHAPTER OUTLINE

- Metabolic Response to Stress
- Starvation Versus Stress
- Systemic Inflammatory Response Syndrome and Multiple Organ Dysfunction Syndrome
- Head Injury
- Major Burns
- Surgery

KEY TERMS

acute-phase proteins–secretory proteins in the liver that are altered in response to injury or infection; positive acute-phase proteins, C-reactive protein, α_1-antitrypsin, and fibronectin are increased; negative acute-phase proteins, immunoglobulin G and M, complement, prealbumin, transferrin, ceruloplasmin, and albumin are decreased

adrenocorticotropic hormone (ACTH)–a hormone secreted by the anterior pituitary gland that acts primarily on the adrenal cortex, thus stimulating its growth and secretion of corticosteroids

bacterial translocation–morphologic changes from acute insult to the gastrointestinal tract that may allow entry of bacteria from the gut lumen into the body; associated with a systemic inflammatory response that may contribute to multiple organ dysfunction syndrome

catecholamines–hormones (epinephrine and norepinephrine) released by the adrenal medulla in response to shock and a higher glucagon/insulin ratio; stimulate hepatic glycogenolysis, fat mobilization, and gluconeogenesis

cytokines–proinflammatory proteins released by macrophages that act as mediators of shock, multiple organ dysfunction syndrome, and sepsis; examples include tumor necrosis factor, interleukin-1, and interleukin-6

ebb phase–initial response to bodily insult characterized by lower blood pressure, cardiac output, body temperature, and oxygen consumption; associated with hypovolemia, hypoperfusion, and lactic acidosis

flow phase–a neuroendocrine response to physiologic stress that follows the ebb phase; characterized by hypermetabolism and hypercatabolism

Glascow Coma Scale (GCS)–system for determining the degree of neurologic insult and a patient's level of consciousness by assessing responses to eye opening and motor and verbal response

glutamine–an amino acid that is the preferential fuel for enterocytes in the gut mucosa, especially during stress; it enhances cell mass and the height of the mucosal villi

growth hormone–an anabolic agent mediated by insulin-like growth factor 1 (IGF-1); thought to accelerate

Chapter previously developed with the assistance of Susan Manchester, RD, CNSD.

growth in children and improve protein synthesis in injured patients

gut-associated lymphoid tissue (GALT)–a component of the gut intestinal mucosal barrier that may protect against multiple organ dysfunction syndrome; contains 40% of the immune effector cells in the body

hemodynamics–physiologic processes involving blood flow in circulation; blood pressure and cardiac output are key components in hemodynamic stability

interleukin-1 (IL-1)–a cytokine mediator induced by tumor necrosis factor (TNF) and produced by endothelial cells and monocytes; induces fever by stimulating prostaglandin production

multiple organ dysfunction syndrome (MODS)–organ dysfunction that results from direct injury, trauma, or disease or as a response to inflammation; the response usually is in an organ remote from the original site of infection or injury

sepsis–the systemic response to an identifiable infectious agent

shock–severe sepsis with hypotension, hypoperfusion, lactic acidosis, oliguria, and acute change in mental status

structured lipid–fat composed of rearranged triglycerides that contain both medium- and long-chain fatty acids; may improve hepatic protein synthesis and reduce protein catabolism and energy expenditure

systemic inflammatory response syndrome (SIRS)–sepsis that occurs without evidence of invasive bacterial or fungal infection; can result in multiple organ dysfunction syndrome

tumor necrosis factor (TNF)–a cytokine produced by activated cells, Kupffer cells in the liver, and macrophages that is stimulated by endotoxin or by bacterial, viral, and fungal infection; initiates an inflammatory response and stimulates skeletal muscle catabolism

Trauma from motor vehicle accidents, gunshots, stab wounds, falls, and burns is a major cause of death and disability. Unintentional injuries and motor vehicle accidents are ranked as the fifth leading cause of death—after heart disease, malignant neoplasm, cerebrovascular disease, and chronic respiratory diseases. Injury results in profound metabolic alterations beginning at the time of injury and persisting until wound healing and recovery are complete. Whether the event is sepsis (infection), trauma (including burns), or surgery, once the systemic response is activated, the physiologic and metabolic changes that follow are similar and may lead to shock and other outcomes (Figure 42-1). Variable responses relate in part to the patient's age, previous state of health, preexisting disease, type of infection, and presence of multiple organ dysfunction syndrome (MODS).

METABOLIC RESPONSE TO STRESS

The metabolic response to critical illness, traumatic injury, sepsis, burns, or major surgery is complex and involves most metabolic pathways. This state is characterized by an accelerated catabolism of lean body or skeletal mass that clinically results in negative nitrogen balance and muscle wasting. The response to critical illness, injury, and sepsis characteristically involves both the ebb and flow phases (Cuthbertson, 1979) (Table 42-1; see Chapter 18). The ebb phase, occurring immediately following injury, is associated with hypovolemia, shock, and tissue hypoxia. Typically, decreased cardiac output, oxygen consumption, and body temperature characterize this phase. Insulin levels fall in direct response to the increase in glucagon, most likely as a signal to increase hepatic glucose production (Souba and Wilmore, 1994).

Increased cardiac output, oxygen consumption, body temperature, energy expenditure, and total body protein catabolism characterize the flow phase, which follows fluid resuscitation and restoration of oxygen transport. Physiologically, a marked increase occurs in glucose production, free fatty acid release, circulating levels of insulin, catecholamines, glucagon, and cortisol. The magnitude of hormonal response appears to be associated with the severity of injury.

Hormonal and Cell-Mediated Response

Metabolic stress is associated with an altered hormonal state that results in an increased flow of substrate but poor utilization of carbohydrate, protein, fat, and oxygen (Table 42-2). Counter-regulatory hormones, which are elevated after injury and sepsis, play a role in the accelerated proteolysis that characteristically is seen. Glucagon promotes gluconeogenesis, amino acid uptake, ureagenesis, and protein catabolism. Cortisol, which is released from the adrenal cortex in response to stimulation by adrenocorticotropic hormone (ACTH), enhances skeletal muscle catabolism and promotes hepatic use of amino acids for gluconeogenesis, glycogenolysis, and acute-phase protein synthesis.

After injury or sepsis, energy production becomes increasingly protein-dependent. Branched-chain amino acids (BCAA-leucine, isoleucine, and valine) are oxidized from skeletal muscle as a source

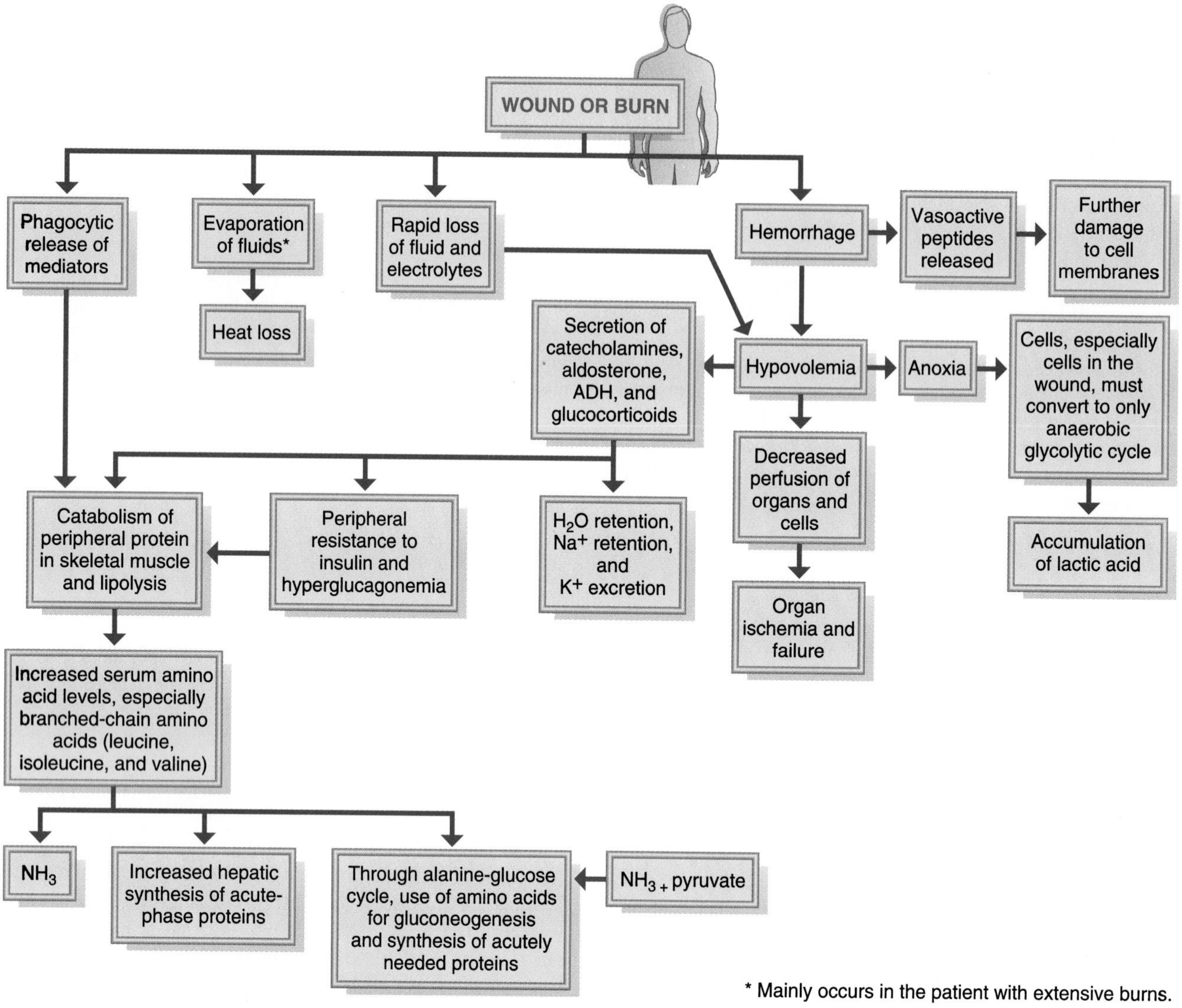

FIGURE 42-1 • Physiologic and metabolic changes immediately after an injury or burn. The extent of these changes depends on the severity of the trauma. *ADH,* Antidiuretic hormone (or vasopressin); *NH_3,* ammonia.

TABLE 42-1 Characteristics of Metabolic Phases Occurring After Severe Injury

EBB-PHASE RESPONSE	FLOW PHASE	
	ACUTE RESPONSE	ADAPTIVE RESPONSE
Hypovolemic Shock ↓ Tissue perfusion ↓ Metabolic rate ↓ Oxygen consumption ↓ Blood pressure ↓ Body temperature	**Catabolism Predominates** ↑ Glucocorticoids ↑ Glucagon ↑ Catecholamines Release of cytokines, lipid mediators Production of acute-phase proteins ↑ Excretion of nitrogen ↑ Metabolic rate ↑ Oxygen consumption Impaired use of fuels	**Anabolism Predominates** Hormonal response gradually diminishes ↓ Hypermetabolic rate Associated with recovery Potential for restoration of body protein Wound healing depends in part on nutrient intake

From *Enteral nutrition support in critical care,* Columbus, Oh, 1994, Ross Products Division, Abbott Laboratories.

TABLE 42-2 Metabolic Responses During Sepsis

ORGAN	RESPONSE
Liver	↑ Glucose production ↑ Amino acid uptake ↑ Acute-phase protein synthesis ↑ Trace metal sequestration
Central nervous system	Anorexia Fever
Circulation	↑ Glucose ↑ Triglycerides ↓ Amino acids ↑ Urea ↓ Iron ↓ Zinc
Skeletal muscle	↑ Amino acid efflux (especially glutamine), leading to loss of muscle mass
Intestine	↓ Amino acid uptake from both luminal and circulating sources, leading to gut mucosal atrophy
Endocrine	↑ ACTH ↑ Cortisol ↑ Growth hormone ↑ Epinephrine ↑ Norepinephrine ↑ Glucagon ↑ Insulin (usually)

From Michie HR: Metabolism of sepsis and multiple organ failure, *World J Surg* 20:461, 1996.

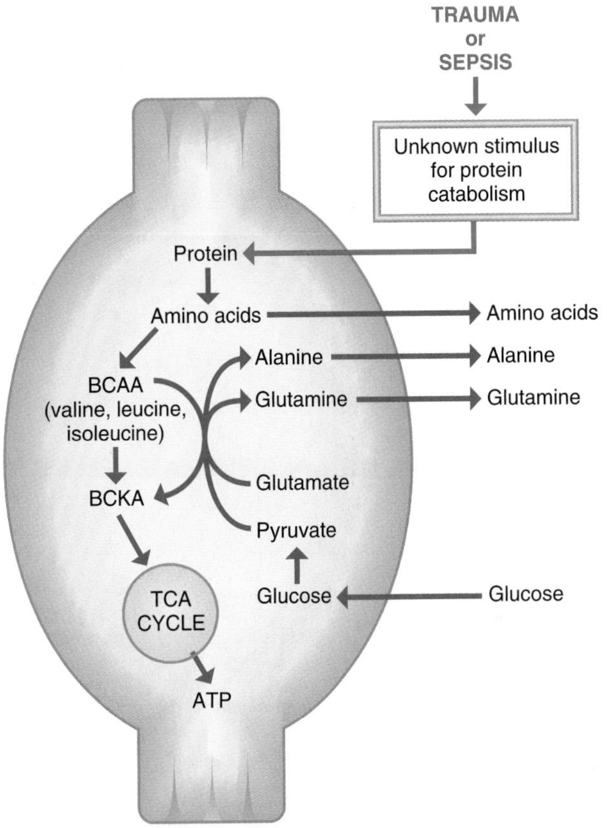

FIGURE 42-2 • Skeletal muscle proteolysis. Breakdown of skeletal muscle protein leads to increases in amino acid levels. Amino acids are transaminated with glutamate or pyruvate to form alanine and glutamine. The muscle preferentially uses branched-chain amino acids (BCAA) for energy through transamination with the formation of branched-chain ketoacids (BCKA), which can enter the tricyclic acid (TCA) cycle for energy production. (From Simmons RL, Steed DL: *Basic science review for surgeons*, Philadelphia, 1992, WB Saunders.)

of nitrogen, energy for the muscle, and carbon skeletons for the glucose-alanine cycle and muscle glutamine synthesis. The fate of amino acid generation from muscle catabolism is shown in Figure 42-2.

The mobilization of acute-phase proteins results in rapid loss of lean body mass and an increased negative nitrogen balance, which continues until the cause of the stress is relieved. Breakdown of protein tissue also causes increased urinary losses of potassium, phosphorus, and magnesium. Lipid metabolism is also altered in stress and sepsis. Increased circulation of free fatty acids is thought to result from increased lipolysis caused by elevated catecholamines and cortisol as well as a marked elevation in the ratio of glucagon to insulin. The free fatty acids can be oxidized and used to form ketones, which provide energy to non–glucose-dependent tissues, or to resynthesize triglyceride.

Most notable is the hyperglycemia observed during stress. This initially results from a marked increase in glucose production and uptake secondary to gluconeogenesis and to elevated levels of hormones, including epinephrine, that diminish insulin release. Stress also initiates the release of aldosterone, a corticosteroid that causes renal sodium retention, and of vasopressin (antidiuretic hormone [ADH]), which stimulates renal tubular water resorption. The action of these hormones results in conservation of water and salt and support of the circulating blood volume.

The response to injury is also regulated by metabolically active cytokines such as interleukin-1 (IL-1), interleukin-6 (IL-6), and tumor necrosis factor (TNF), which are released by phagocytic cells in response to tissue damage, infection, inflammation, and some drugs and chemicals. Cytokines are thought to stimulate hepatic amino acid uptake and protein synthesis, accelerate muscle breakdown, and induce gluconeogenesis. IL-1 appears to have a major role in stimulating the acute-phase response. This includes fever, leukocytosis, skeletal muscle proteolysis, and acute-phase protein synthesis (Bessey, 1993). As part of the acute-phase response, serum iron and zinc levels also decrease, and levels of ceruloplasmin increase primarily because of sequestration and—in the case of zinc—increased urinary zinc excretion. The net effect of the hormonally and cell-mediated response is an increase in oxygen supply and a greater availability of substrates for metabolically active tissues.

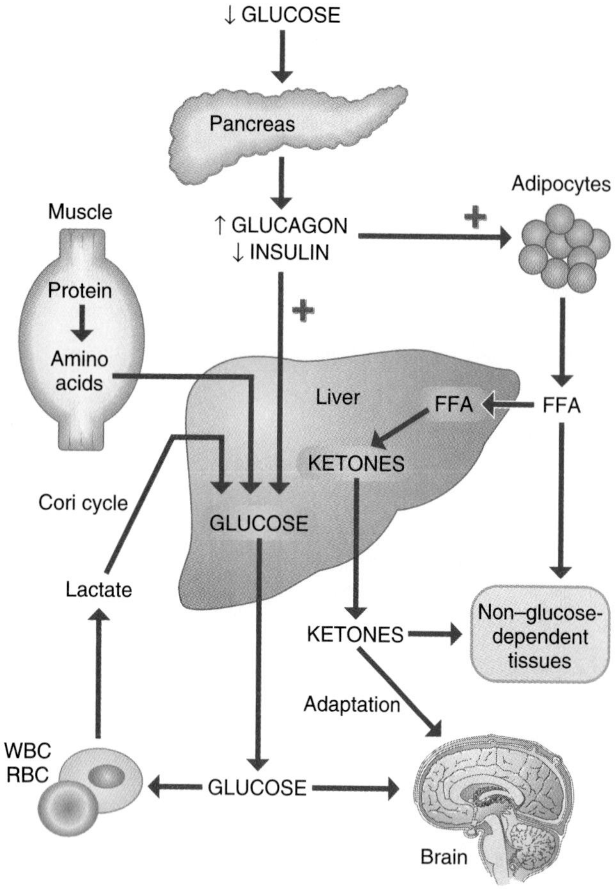

FIGURE 42-3 • Metabolic changes in starvation. *FFA*, Free fatty acids; *RBC*, red blood cells; *WBC*, white blood cells. (From Simmons RL, Steed DL: *Basic science review for surgeons*, Philadelphia, 1992, WB Saunders.)

STARVATION VERSUS STRESS

The metabolic response to critical illness is very different from simple or uncomplicated starvation, in which loss of muscle is much slower in an adaptive response to preserve lean body mass. Stored glycogen, the primary fuel source in early starvation, is depleted in about 24 hours. After the depletion of glycogen, glucose is available from the breakdown of protein to amino acids as depicted in Figure 42-3. The depressed glucose levels lead to decreased insulin secretion and increased glucagon. During the adaptive state of starvation, protein catabolism is reduced and hepatic gluconeogenesis decreases. Lipolytic activity is also different in starvation and in stress. After 1 week of fasting or food deprivation, a state of ketosis—in which ketones supply the bulk of energy needs, thus reducing the need for gluconeogenesis and conserving body protein to the greatest possible extent—develops. In late starvation as in stress, ketone body production is increased, and fatty acids serve as a major energy source for all tissues except the glucose-obligated brain, nervous system, and red blood cells.

TABLE 42-3 Comparison of Starvation and Stress Hypermetabolism*

	STARVATION	STRESS HYPERMETABOLISM
Resting energy expenditure	Decreased	Increased
Respiratory quotient	(0.6-0.7)	(0.8-0.9)
Mediator activation	—	+++
Primary fuels	Fat	Mixed
Proteolysis	+	+++
Branched-chain oxidation	+	+++
Hepatic protein synthesis	+	+++
Ureagenesis	+	+++
Urinary nitrogen loss	+	+++
Gluconeogenesis	+	+++
Ketone body production	++++	+

From Barton RG: Nutrition support in critical illness, *Nutr Clin Pract* 9:127, 1994. Modified from the American Society for Parenteral and Enteral Nutrition (ASPEN).

*Patients fall in a continuum between the extremes of starvation and stress hypermetabolism.

Starvation is characterized by decreased energy expenditure, diminished gluconeogenesis, increased ketone body production, and decreased ureagenesis. Conversely, energy expenditure in stress is markedly increased, as are gluconeogenesis, proteolysis, and ureagenesis. As discussed, the stress response is activated by hormonal and cell mediators—counterregulatory hormones such as catecholamines, cortisol, and growth hormone. This mediator activation does not occur in starvation. Table 42-3 highlights the physiologic differences between starvation and stress.

SYSTEMIC INFLAMMATORY RESPONSE SYNDROME AND MULTIPLE ORGAN DYSFUNCTION SYNDROME

Pathophysiology

Sepsis and the systemic inflammatory response syndrome (SIRS) often complicate the course of a critically ill patient. The term *sepsis* is used when a patient has a documented infection and an identifiable organism. Bacteria and their toxins lead to a stronger inflammatory response. Other microorganisms that lead to an inflammatory response include viruses, fungi, and parasites. *SIRS* is the preferred terminology to describe the widespread inflammation that can occur in infection, pancreatitis, ischemia, burns, multiple trauma, hemorrhagic shock, and immunologically mediated organ injury (Bone, 1992). The inflammation is usually present in areas remote from the primary site of injury and affects otherwise

Box 42-1. Diagnosis for Systemic Inflammatory Response Syndrome

Site of infection established and at least two of the following are present:

- Body temperature above 38° C or less than 36° C
- Heart rate more than 90 beats/min
- Respiratory rate greater than 20 breaths/min (tachypnea)
- $Paco_2$ of less than 32 mm Hg (hyperventilation)
- White blood cell count above 12,000/mm^3 or less than 4000/mm^3
- Bandemia—the presence of more than 10% bands (immature neutrophils) in the absence of chemotherapy-induced neutropenia and leukopenia

Data from Bone et al: ACCP/SCCM Consensus Conference: Definitions for sepsis and organ failure and guidelines for the use of innovative therapies in sepsis, *Chest* 101: 1664, 1992.

healthy tissue. Each condition leads to release of cytokines, proteolytic enzymes, or toxic oxygen species and activation of the complement cascade. SIRS is diagnosed according to criteria shown in Box 42-1.

A common complication of SIRS is the development of multiple organ dysfunction syndrome (MODS). The syndrome generally begins with lung failure and is followed by failure of the liver, intestines, and kidney. Hematologic and myocardial failure usually manifest later; however, central nervous system changes can occur at any time (Deitch, 1992). MODS can be primary and the direct result of injury to an organ from trauma. Examples of primary MODS include pulmonary contusion, renal failure due to rhabdomyolysis, or coagulopathy from multiple blood transfusions (Bone, 1992). Secondary MODS occurs in the presence of inflammation or infection in organs remote from the initial injury. Patients with SIRS and MODS are clinically hypermetabolic and exhibit high cardiac output, low oxygen consumption, high venous oxygen saturation, and lactic acidemia. Patients generally have a strong positive fluid balance associated with massive edema and a decrease in plasma protein concentrations.

Multiple hypotheses have been proposed to explain the development of SIRS or MODS. In some animal models and clinical studies, SIRS leading to MODS appears to be mediated by excessive production of proinflammatory cytokines and other mediators of inflammation. Much of the research has focused on trying to understand what triggers this response. The gut hypothesis suggests that the trigger is injury or disruption of the gut barrier function, with corresponding translocation of enteric bacteria

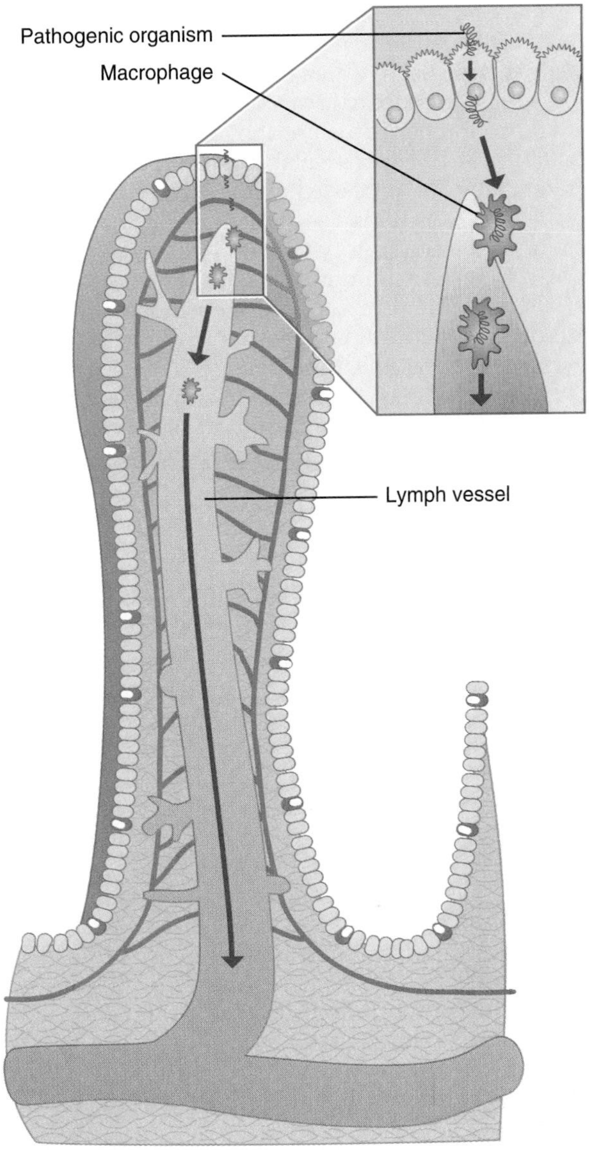

FIGURE 42-4 • Bacterial translocation across microvilli and the way in which it spreads into the bloodstream.

into the mesentary lymph nodes, liver, and other organs (Figure 42-4).

Enteral feeding is thought to restore gut function and influence the clinical course. Enteral nutrition may act at several levels by altering antigen exposure, modulating splanchnic immune responses, enhancing mucosal protection, or influencing oxygenation and blood supply to the mucosa (Reynolds, 1996; Reynolds et al, 1996). Poor gut function, secondary to dependence on parenteral nutrition or the lack of enteral stimulation, might be caused by an exaggerated cytokine response as a result of loss of intestinal barrier function (Swank and Deitch, 1996). Alterations in intestinal gut barrier function associated with malnutrition are thought to occur through weight loss and villous atrophy. Because enteral feeding maintains the villous height and brush border enzymes, feedings may be better tolerated when initiated promptly while this absorptive area remains intact.

Aspects of gut barrier function related to immunity and the route and type of nutrition support are active areas of research. Experimental and clinical data demonstrate that cells processed within the gut-associated lymphoid tissue (GALT) can migrate outside of the intestine to the respiratory tract and other mucosal surfaces and induce immunity (Kudsk, 2002). Lack of enteric stimulation is associated with mucosal atrophy and decreased intestinal absorption; this is thought to negatively affect the host defense against bacterial and toxin products in the intestine in septic patients. This bacterial translocation from the intestinal lumen to the mesenteric lymph nodes is well documented in animals, especially rats, but does not occur to the same extent in humans (Alpers, 2002).

Medical Nutrition Therapy

Nutritional Assessment

The critically ill patient typically enters an intensive care unit (ICU) because of a cardiopulmonary diagnosis, intraoperative or postoperative complication, multiple trauma, burn injury, or sepsis. Figure 42-5 illustrates the scene observed when entering an ICU room: patients often have numerous catheters for intravenous (IV) fluids and invasive hemodynamic monitoring, as well as tubes for drainage of body fluids.

Traditional methods of assessing nutritional status are often of limited value in the critical care setting. The severely injured patient is usually unable to provide a dietary history. Values for weight may be erroneous after fluid resuscitation, and anthropometric measurements are not easily attainable, nor are they sensitive to acute changes. Abnormal serum albumin may result from the effects of both undernutrition and the severity of illness or underlying disease (ASPEN Board of Directors, 2002). Because of the difficulties in conducting a nutritional assessment in a critically ill patient, clinical judgment must play a major role in deciding when to offer nutrition support. The ability to predict the clinical course and when the patient will resume adequate oral food intake is a key component of this process (Pomp et al, 1988).

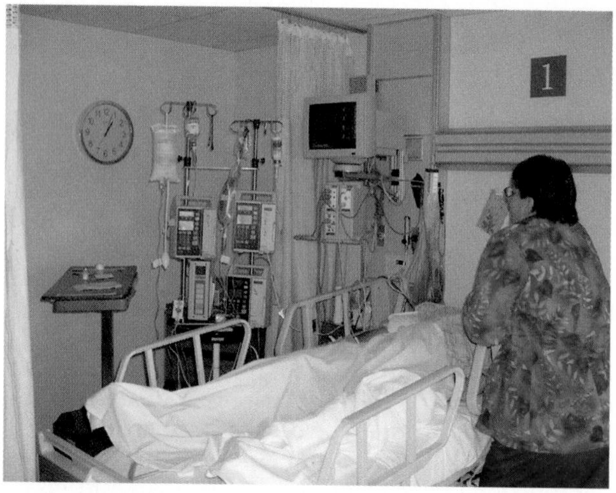

FIGURE 42-5 • View of intensive care unit (ICU) room. (Courtesy Carol Landry, RN, Rhode Island Hospital, 2002.)

In general, assessment focuses on the preadmission, preoperative, or preinjury nutrition status, presence of any organ system dysfunction, the need for early nutrition support, and options that exist for enteral or parenteral access. Care planning should consider the factors in Box 42-2. When monitoring critically ill patients, one must focus on laboratory data, not to define or determine nutritional status, but to design the nutritional prescription (see Chapter 18). Practitioners should review indices of organ system function, blood glucose, and laboratory abnormalities, specifically electrolytes and acid-base balance, that may impact enteral and parenteral formulations or the diet order. Urine urea nitrogen (UUN) excretion in grams per day has been used to evaluate the degree of hypermetabolism. A UUN value of 0 to 5 corresponds with no stress, 5 to 10 with mild hypermetabolism or level 1 stress, 10 to 15 with moderate hypermetabolism or level 2 stress, and greater than 15 with a severe hypermetabolic state or level 3 stress (Blackburn et al, 1977).

Goals of Nutrition Support

The goals of nutrition support during sepsis and after injury include minimization of starvation, prevention or correction of specific nutrient deficiencies, provision of adequate calories to meet energy needs, and fluid and electrolyte management to maintain adequate urine output and normal homeostasis (see Figure 42-6). The first emphasis of care is fluid resuscitation and the removal of the inflicting stress through wound repair, abscess drainage, burn wound debridement and grafting, or treatment of infection. Nutrition support should begin as soon as the patient is hemodynamically stable (stabilized vital functions, fluid and electrolyte and acid-base balance, and adequate tissue perfusion to allow transport of oxygen and fuel).

Recognizing that the provision of nutrition support alone cannot abolish the hypermetabolic response and the subsequent muscle breakdown seen in acute injury or illness is important (Wolfe and Martini, 2000). Critically ill patients who are injured, septic, or bedridden cannot be expected to gain weight, lean body mass, or strength until the source of hypermetabolism is treated or corrected and physical therapy or exercise is begun. The ASPEN practice guidelines for critical care are outlined in Box 42-3.

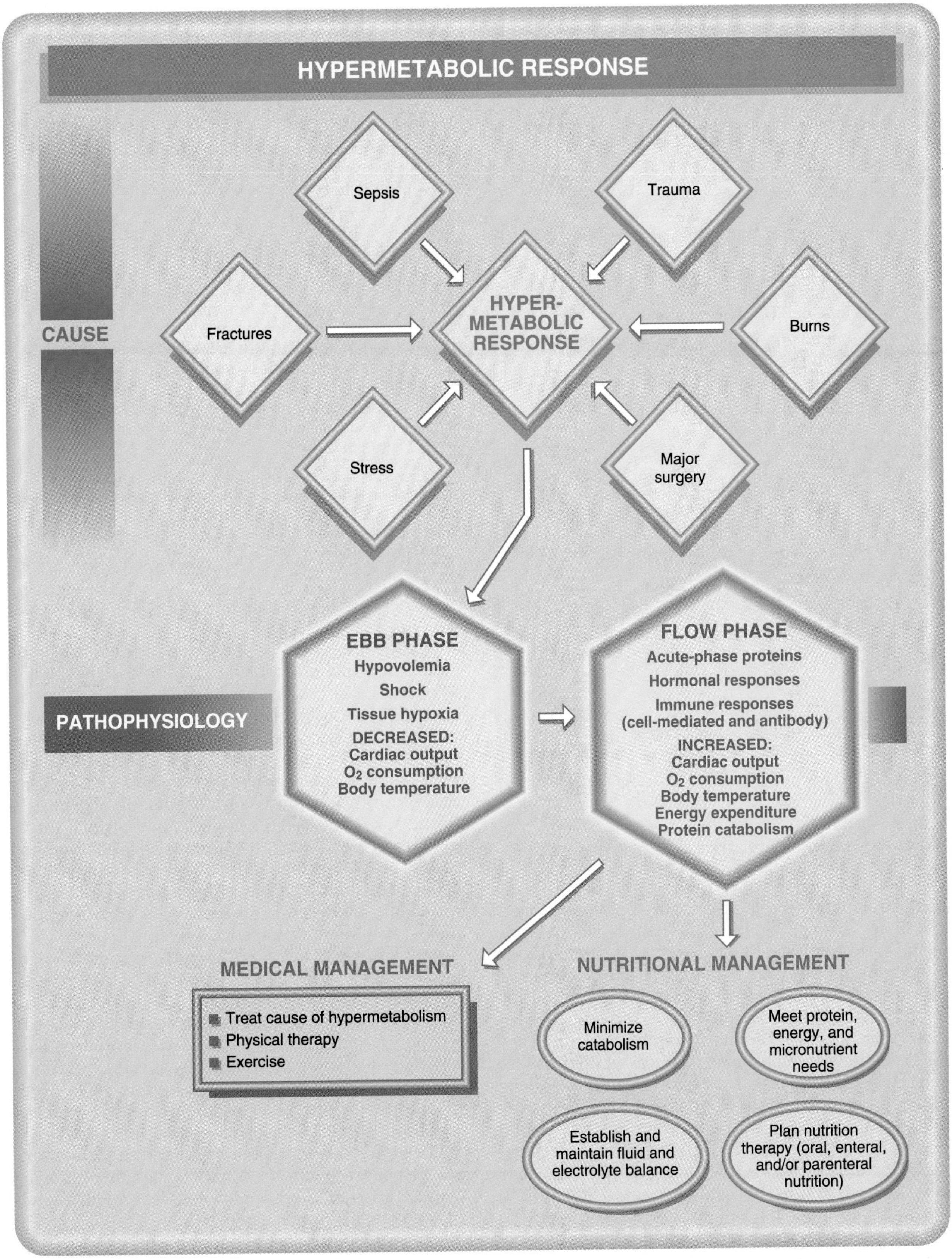

FIGURE 42-6 • Pathophysiology algorithm: hypermetabolic response to stress. (Algorithm content developed by John Anderson, PhD, and Sanford C. Garner, PhD, 2000. Updated by Marion F. Winkler, MS, RD, LDN, CNSD, and Ainsley Malone, MS, RD, CNSD, 2002.)

Box 42-2. Factors to Consider in Screening an ICU Patient

Factors to Consider With ICU Medical Admission

Preadmission nutrition status
Organ function
Use of pharmacologic agents, vasopressors, and other paralytic agents
Ability to predict clinical course (i.e., length of intubation or ventilator dependence)
Need for enteral or parenteral nutrition

Factors to Consider With Postoperative ICU Admission

Intraoperative complications
Preoperative nutrition status
Cardiopulmonary event
Diagnosis
Sepsis or SIRS
Gastrointestinal function
Ability to predict return of GI function
Nutrition support access options

Factors to Consider With Burn or Trauma Admission

Preinjury nutrition status
Type of trauma
Extent of injury
Surgical findings
Gastrointestinal function
Enteral access options

ICU, Intensive care unit; *SIRS,* systemic inflammatory response syndrome; *GI,* gastrointestinal.

Box 42-3. ASPEN Practice Guidelines for Critical Care

- Patients with critical illnesses are at nutrition risk and should undergo nutrition screening to identify those who require formal nutrition assessment with development of a nutrition care plan.
- Specialized nutrition support should be initiated when it is anticipated that critically ill patients will be unable to meet their nutrient needs orally for a period of 5 to 10 days.
- Enteral nutrition is the preferred route of feeding in critically ill patients who require specialized nutrition support.
- Parenteral nutrition should be reserved for those patients who require specialized nutrition support and in whom enteral nutrition is not possible.

Data from ASPEN Board of Directors: Guidelines for the use of parenteral and enteral nutrition in adult and pediatric patients, *J Parenter Enteral Nutr* 26(suppl) 1S, 2002.

Determination of Nutrient Requirements

Energy

Critically ill patients should receive feedings at rates of 25 to 30 kcal/kg (ASPEN Board of Directors, 2002). Although adequate energy is essential to metabolically stressed patients, excess calories can result in complications such as hyperglycemia, hepatic steatosis, and excess carbon dioxide production, which can exacerbate respiratory insufficiency or prolong weaning from mechanical ventilation (see Chapter 38). Persistent hyperglycemia can also lead to hyperosmolar nonketotic coma and glucose-obligated diuresis, which may complicate fluid and electrolyte management. Hyperglycemia associated with insulin resistance in critically ill patients may also lead to complications and increased susceptibility to severe infection. Intensive insulin therapy to maintain blood glucose at or below 110 mg/dl is associated with reduced morbidity and mortality from multiple organ failure with sepsis, episodes of septicemia, the need for prolonged antibiotic therapy, and acute renal failure in surgical ICU patients (Van Den Berghe et al, 2001).

Energy requirements can be estimated with the Harris-Benedict equation or the new DRI equation (see Chapter 2). Because avoiding overfeeding the critically ill, stressed patient is important, adding a factor for stress of 1.3 may be prudent. Once the patient is hemodynamically stable and is ambulating or undergoing rehabilitation, caloric delivery can be in a higher anabolic range. Energy requirements can also be estimated at 25 to 30 kcal/kg (see *Clinical Insight:* Estimating Energy and Protein Requirements). Either method may overestimate the caloric requirements of mechanically ventilated and sedated patients, in whom neuromuscular paralysis may decrease energy requirements, even in septic patients, by as much as 30%.

Indirect calorimetry is the preferred method for measurement of oxygen consumption in severely injured patients (Epstein et al, 2000). Oxygen consumption is an essential component in the determination of energy expenditure (see Figure 2-4). Many investigators have examined the alterations in energy expenditure associated with critical illness and have documented substantial increases, particularly in septic and trauma patients (Moriyama et al, 1999; Uehara et al, 1999). Indirect calorimetry can be performed serially as a patient's clinical status changes, thus allowing a more accurate assessment of energy requirements over a patient's course in the ICU.

Indirect calorimetry is not appropriate for all patients, however, and must be performed and interpreted by experienced clinicians. High oxygen requirements, the presence of a chest tube, acidosis,

CLINICAL INSIGHT

Estimating Energy and Protein Requirements

A 64-year-old man underwent surgery for a ruptured colonic diverticulum. He developed an intraabdominal abscess that drained through the wound, and he had repeated temperature spikes. An ileus was noticed on the x-ray. Physical examination revealed an edematous, toxic-appearing patient with a poorly healing abdominal wound. His preoperative weight was 147 lb (67 kg) and his height was 5 ft 9 in. (180 cm).

1. Using the Harris-Benedict Equation: BEE (male) = 66.47 + 13.75 (W) + 5 (H) − 6.76 (age) = 1455 kcal
2. Using a factor of 1.3 to account for surgical stress and sepsis: 1455 kcal × (1.3) = 1892 kcal
3. Using 25 to 30 kcal/kg = 1675-2010 kcal/day
4. Protein requirement using 1.5-2.0 g/kg = 100 − 134 g/day

and the use of supplemental oxygen are several factors that will produce invalid results. In these situations, measurement of energy expenditure by indirect calorimetry is not recommended (Malone, 2002). Unstable, critically ill patients often need hemodynamic monitoring through a pulmonary artery catheter. The data obtained from these measurements allow calculation of oxygen consumption and hence energy expenditure, using the Fick equation (Liggett et al, 1987).

Glucose is the primary caloric substrate in a parenteral nutrition formulation. The maximum rate of glucose oxidation is approximately 5 to 7 mg/kg/min or 7.2 g/kg/day (Wolfe et al, 1979). Part of this glucose load is provided endogenously via gluconeogenesis. Carbohydrate should constitute approximately 60% to 70% of energy. Parenteral nutrition should be initiated with a low dextrose infusion rate, and blood and urine glucose should be closely monitored in patients with diabetes or risk of glucose intolerance. Insulin should be administered to maintain blood glucose levels at less than 200 mg/dl (ASPEN Board of Directors, 2002). Fat provides the remainder of energy, at about 15% to 40% of the calories. Fat is used not only to prevent essential fatty acid deficiency but also to meet elevated energy requirements, particularly in the presence of glucose intolerance. The use of intravenous fat emulsion in stressed and trauma patients should be carefully monitored because fatty acids modulate the immune response (Grimm et al, 1994).

Protein

Amino acids are supplied to critically ill patients as part of the total nutrition regimen to support the synthesis of proteins required for defense and recovery, to spare lean body mass, and to reduce the amount of endogenous protein catabolism for gluconeogenesis. For the unstressed adult patient with adequate organ function requiring nutrition support, 0.8 g/kg per day may be adequate, but requirements may rise with metabolic demands to levels of about 2 g/kg per day (ASPEN Board of Directors, 2002). Providing exogenous amino acids does not alter the catabolic state, but it does decrease the characteristic negative nitrogen balance by supplying the liver with substrates for protein synthesis and subsequently reducing the need for endogenous proteins from peripheral tissue (Gilder, 1986).

Vitamins, Minerals, and Trace Elements

No specific guidelines exist for the provision of vitamins, minerals, and trace elements in metabolically stressed individuals. Micronutrient needs are elevated during acute illness because of increased urinary and cutaneous losses and diminished gastrointestinal absorption, altered distribution, and altered carrier protein concentrations (Prelack and Sheridan, 2001). With increased caloric intake there may be an increased need for B vitamins, particularly thiamin and niacin. Catabolism and loss of lean body tissue increase the loss of potassium, magnesium, phosphorus, and zinc. Gastrointestinal and urinary losses, organ dysfunction, and acid-base imbalance necessitate that mineral and electrolyte requirements be determined and adjusted individually. Fluid and electrolytes should be provided to maintain adequate urine output and normal serum electrolytes.

Feeding Strategies

The preferred route for nutrient delivery is an oral diet. However, critically ill patients are often unable to eat because of endotracheal intubation and ventilator dependence. Furthermore, oral feeding may be delayed by impairment of chewing, swallowing, or anorexia induced by pain-relieving medications or posttraumatic shock and depression. Patients who are able to eat may not be able to meet the increased energy and nutrient requirements associated with metabolic stress and recovery and often require combinations of oral nutritional supplements, enteral tube nutrition, and parenteral nutrition. When enteral nutrition fails to meet nutritional requirements or when gastrointestinal feeding is contraindicated, parenteral nutrition support should be initiated (Figure 42-7).

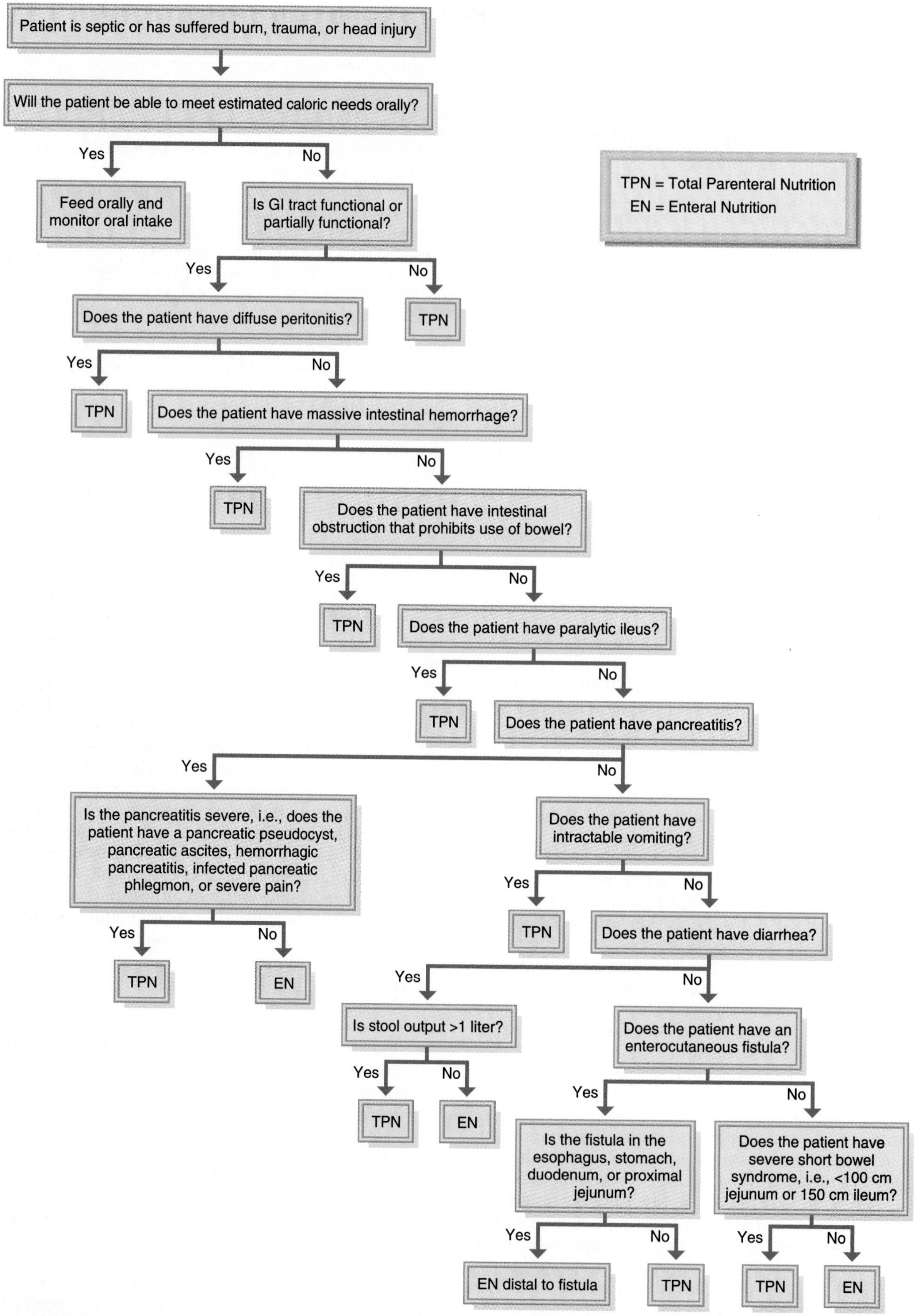

FIGURE 42-7 • Determining the route of nutrition support in the critically ill patient. (ASPEN Nutrition Support Practice Manual: *Determining the route of nutrition support in the critically ill,* Silver Spring, Md, 1998, ASPEN. [ASPEN does not endorse the use of this material in any form other than in its entirety.])

Timing and Route of Feeding

Successful enteral nutrition for surgical or stressed patients may require access to the small bowel. Critically ill patients are presumed to be at a higher risk of aspiration because of conditions such as respiratory insufficiency, gastric dysmotility, or neuromuscular paralysis. Studies in surgical patients, however, have demonstrated that the rate of aspiration when patients are fed into the stomach versus the small bowel is not significantly different (Fox et al, 1995). Gastric motility is usually impaired for 12 to 24 hours after laparotomy, whereas a colonic ileus may last up to 5 days. Generally, small bowel motility returns within 4 to 6 hours postoperatively.

An enteric feeding tube may be placed if the patient is expected to be unable to consume food by mouth for an extended period. Tubes can be placed under x-ray guidance, endoscopically, or intraoperatively into the stomach or small bowel (see Chapter 23). Initially, patients with multiple intestinal injuries, small bowel ileus, high-output intestinal fistulas, severe pancreatitis, or other severe intestinal insults may require TPN. However, because of the demonstrated benefits of early enteral nutrition, tube feedings can often be administered simultaneously with TPN at low rates to maintain gut integrity (Zaloga et al, 1992). This allows adequate nutrient delivery while helping to preserve the intestinal mucosa.

Although early enteral feeding has proven benefits, waiting until the patient is hemodynamically stable before beginning remains important. Anaerobic metabolism during shock and after resuscitation differs, and the aggressive delivery of enteral nutrients in a state of intestinal hypoperfusion may result in increased intestinal ischemia and necrosis (Tappenden et al, 1998).

Formula Selection

Choosing an enteral product should be based on fluid, energy, and nutrient requirements, as well as gastrointestinal function. Most standard polymeric enteral formulas can be used to feed the critically ill patient. Some critically ill patients demonstrate intolerance to standard diets because of the fat content of the formula and temporarily require a lower-fat diet or a product containing a higher ratio of medium-chain triglycerides. Several commercially available products are marketed specifically for trauma and metabolic stress. These products typically have higher protein content and a higher ratio of BCAA or additional glutamine or arginine (see Appendixes 38 and 39).

Specialized enteral formulas designed to enhance the immune system have been investigated for their role in improving patient outcomes. Complex pharmaconutrient formulas that contain arginine, glutamine (GLN), and omega-3 fatty acids have been proven to shorten hospital stay, decrease the incidence of infection, and reduce hospital costs in selected groups of patients (Alexander, 2002). The effects are greatest in those patients with severe trauma, including burn injury; major surgical procedures, especially when malnourished; and critical illness with existing infection and ICU admittance. In the septic population, however, there is concern that the use of specialized enteral formulas may have a detrimental effect (Consensus Recommendations, JPEN, 2001). Before prescribing immune-enhancing formulas, clinicians must evaluate the potential benefit in their specific patient populations.

Alterations in glutamine levels may develop during critical illness and can negatively affect gut health. GLN supplementation has important effects in catabolic surgical patients, but the exact mechanisms to explain these events remain unknown; more research is required to explain the benefits (Wilmore, 2001). Figure 42-8 depicts glutamine metabolism and demonstrates its uptake by the kidney and the intestine as a preferential fuel for enterocytes.

Parenteral nutrition formulations have not traditionally contained glutamine because of instability in the solution, and as a result, TPN has been thought to contribute to this deficiency. Glutamine supplementation of TPN solutions has been shown to partially reverse mucosal atrophy, attenuate the reduction of intestinal immunoglobulin A, and improve upper respiratory immunity to influenza virus in mice (Li et al, 1997).

Dietary fiber is known to maintain colonic integrity. The colonic fermentation of fiber and other nondigestible carbohydrates produces the short-chain fatty acids (SCFA) of proprionate, acetate, and butyrate. These substances are readily absorbed, are trophic to the colonocyte, stimulate water and sodium absorption, and may provide a significant source of energy. Much experimental work has focused on whether SCFA could improve immunocompetence by maintaining the gastrointestinal mucosal barrier in the presence of intestinal atrophy and immunosuppression (Koruda et al, 1986). SCFA from dietary fiber fermentation in the colon or added as a supplement to TPN has been shown in rats to prevent the TPN-associated mucosal atrophy (Tappenden et al, 1997) and to improve nonspecific immunity after small bowel resection (Pratt et al, 1996). Whether the effects of SCFA are through stimulation of gastrointestinal growth factors or direct action on the enterocyte is unknown (Tappenden et al, 1996) (see Chapters 1 and 30).

Anabolic Hormones

Combinations of anabolic hormones, growth factors, and specific nutrients have been used to enhance nutrition support and modify the metabolic response to trauma and critical illness. Growth hormone (GH) stimulates growth, antagonizes the action of insulin, and has lipolytic activity. In trauma patients with low growth hormone levels, the administration of human growth hormone has been shown to improve protein and fat metabolism (Jeevanandam et al, 1992). Hu-

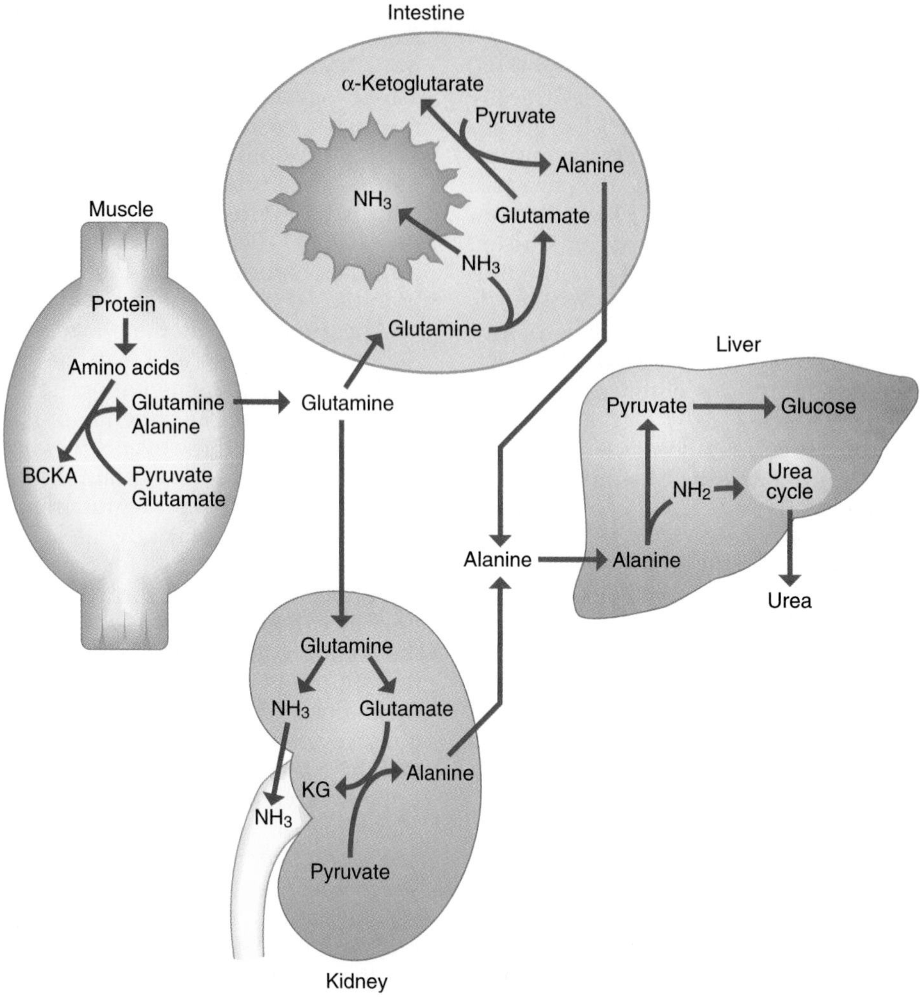

FIGURE 42-8 • Glutamine metabolism. Glutamine is generated by skeletal muscle from glutamate by transamination. Glutamine is taken up by the intestine and kidney, where deamination and ammonia elimination occur. The glutamate formed is transaminated with pyruvate to form alanine, which goes to the liver for gluconeogenesis, and α-ketoglutarate (KD), which can be used for energy production by the muscle or kidney. *NH_2*, Amine; *NH_3*, ammonia. (From Simmons RL, Steed DL: *Basic science review for surgeons,* Philadelphia, 1992, WB Saunders.)

man growth hormone improves nitrogen balance and normalizes plasma free amino acid levels in hypermetabolic and acute trauma patients (Jeevanandam et al, 1995). The administration of growth hormone to mechanically ventilated patients with acute respiratory failure promotes marked nitrogen retention and increased fat-free mass and total body water, yet these results are not accompanied by improved muscle strength or shortened time on the ventilator (Pichard et al, 1996).

Growth hormone administration with nutrition support could have a role in improving protein economy and enhancing recuperation in the face of catabolic illness related to insulin-like growth factor-1 (IGF-1) (Young and Persinger, 1994). Clinical findings associated with growth hormone therapy include hyperglycemia, insulin resistance, and mild sodium and fluid retention. At least one report in a large multicenter European trial suggests that growth hormone therapy may be associated with a twofold higher mortality in intensive care unit patients (Ziegler, 1998). These findings underscore the need to evaluate carefully clinical trials and appropriately apply the results to practice. Caution in the use of growth hormone therapy in critically ill patients in intensive care units is currently warranted.

HEAD INJURY

Pathophysiology

Patients with traumatic brain injury (TBI) are severely hypermetabolic and catabolic. The more severe the head injury, the greater is the release of catecholamines (norepinephrine and epinephrine) and cortisol and the hypermetabolic response. Although most brain-injured patients are well nourished before injury, without aggressive nutrition support, rapid loss in lean body mass and immunosuppression can occur. With evidence that neurons are capable of regenerating, it becomes even more crucial to provide an environment conducive for repair (Ott and Young, 1991). The Glascow Coma Scale (GCS) is a commonly used tool for quantifying a patient's state of consciousness. A score of 14 to 15 indicates minor head injury; 9 to 13 corresponds to moderate injury; and a less than 8 reflects severe injury (Hester, 1993) (see Chapter 43).

Medical Nutrition Therapy

Energy Requirements

Most studies show that the measured energy expenditure in TBI is about 40% greater than predicted by the Harris-Benedict equation (Hadley et al, 1986; Ott and Young, 1991). Patients with a GCS of 4 to 5 often have the highest energy expenditure. Braindead patients or those who receive sedatives, barbiturates, or musculoskeletal blocking agents often have lower than predicted energy expenditure, averaging about 14% less (Hester, 1993; Ott and Young, 1991). The use of indirect calorimetry is helpful in determining the caloric requirements of these patients, because overfeeding or underfeeding can be harmful. A study that compared predictive formulas like the Harris-Benedict equation with measured energy expenditure determined by indirect calorimetry demonstrated significant discrepancies (Sunderland and Heilbrun, 1992). In the absence of indirect calorimetry, energy requirements should be estimated for patients with TBI by using the Harris-Benedict equation and applying a stress factor of 1.4 (Annis et al, 1991) (see Chapter 2).

Protein Requirements

Patients with TBI will probably be in a negative nitrogen balance for 2 to 3 weeks, regardless of the quantity of protein provided (Annis et al, 1991). Steroid administration can further increase urinary nitrogen losses during the first 6 days after the injury (Greenblatt et al, 1989), but then nitrogen losses remain similar regardless of steroid administration (Annis et al, 1991). The administration of branched chain amino acids (BCAAs) may aid in restoring plasma amino acid profiles to normal and improving nitrogen balance (Ott and Young, 1991). Protein requirements are generally estimated at 1.5 to 2.2 g/kg of body weight (Hester, 1993). Provision of more protein results in a heightened nitrogen excretion (Hadley et al, 1986). An adequate amount of nonprotein calories is essential for protein sparing. Because achieving early nitrogen equilibrium is very difficult, minimizing catabolism is paramount.

Vitamins, Minerals, and Fluid

Although the requirements for vitamins and minerals are not well established for brain-injured individuals, studies have shown decreased plasma levels of many B vitamins and vitamin C. Urinary zinc excretion increases significantly during stress, and serum zinc levels are often low. Because salt-wasting occasionally occurs in the brain-injured patient, treatment may consist of restricting fluids, providing additional sodium, or both. In addition, osmotic dehydration may be performed to control cerebral swelling.

Methods of Nutrition Support

Brain-injured individuals are often unable to take oral nutrition. However, patients with a GCS greater than 12 are usually able to consume food (Ott and Young, 1991). Thirty percent or more of brain-injured patients experience dysphagia. The impairment can be physiologic or cognitive. These individuals may have a delayed or absent swallowing reflex, reduced lingual control, prolonged oral transit time, reduced pharyngeal peristalsis, or laryngeal incompetence (see Chapter 43).

Patients may be easily distracted, which greatly prolongs mealtime and results in inadequate intake. Conversely, some brain-injured patients eat rapidly and consume excessive amounts of food—even nonfood items (Wood, 1990). Early nutrition support is essential. In addition to providing adequate nutrition, early enteral feeding may help blunt the stress response by decreasing the intestinal permeability to toxins, which could otherwise stimulate the release of toxic inflammatory mediators (Annis et al, 1991). Furthermore, prompt use of the gut should maintain the intestinal absorptive area. Patients commonly experience impaired gastric emptying, which hinders the ability to feed via a nasogastric or gastrostomy tube. Access to the small bowel has allowed for successful enteral feeding in many instances, and parenteral and enteral nutrition support often is combined.

MAJOR BURNS

Pathophysiology

Major burns result in severe trauma. Energy requirements can increase as much as 100% above resting energy expenditure (REE), depending on the extent and depth of the injury (Figure 42-9). Exaggerated protein catabolism and increased urinary nitrogen excretion accompany this hypermetabolism. Protein is also lost through the burn wound exudate. Burn patients are particularly susceptible to infection, and this markedly increases requirements for both energy and protein. Because patients with major burns may develop an ileus (loss of intestinal peristalsis or lack of effective coordinated peristalsis) and are anorexic, nutrition support can be a real challenge.

Medical Management

Fluid and Electrolyte Repletion

The first 24 to 48 hours of treatment for thermally injured patients are devoted to fluid and electrolyte replacement. A variety of formulas have been developed to calculate the volume of resuscitation fluid needed. Most agree that half of the calculated volume for the first 24 hours should be given during the first 8 hours, because this is the period of greatest intravascular loss.

The volume of fluid needed is based on the age and weight of the patient and the extent of the burn. Variations of a standard known as the Lund and Browder chart (Herndon et al, 1985; Lund and Browder, 1944) can be used to determine the percentage of total body surface area (TBSA) burned. Once resuscitation is complete, ample fluids must be given to cover both maintenance requirements and evaporative losses that continue through open wounds. Evaporative water loss can be estimated at 2.0 to 3.1 ml/kg of body weight per 24 hours per percent TBSA burn. Serum sodium, osmolar concentrations, and body weight are used to monitor fluid status. Providing adequate fluids and electrolytes as early as possible after injury is paramount for maintaining circulatory volume and preventing ischemia (Warden, 1992).

Wound Management

Wound management depends on the depth and extent of the burn. Current surgical management promotes early debridement, excision, and grafting. Energy expenditure may be reduced slightly by the practice of covering wounds as early as possible to reduce evaporative heat and nitrogen losses, and to prevent infection.

Ancillary Measures

Physical therapy helps prevent muscle wasting and atrophy. A warm environment minimizes heat loss and the expenditure of energy to maintain body temperature. Thermal blankets, heat lamps, and individual heat shields are often used to maintain environmental temperature near 30° C (86° F). Minimizing fear and pain with reassurance from the staff and adequate pain medication can also reduce catecholamine stimulation and help to avoid increases in energy expenditure. Finally, antacids are given to patients with major burns to prevent formation of stress-related Curling's ulcers in the gastric or duodenal mucosa.

Medical Nutrition Therapy

Along with early wound coverage and infection control, nutrition support is recognized as one of the most significant aspects of care for the burned pa-

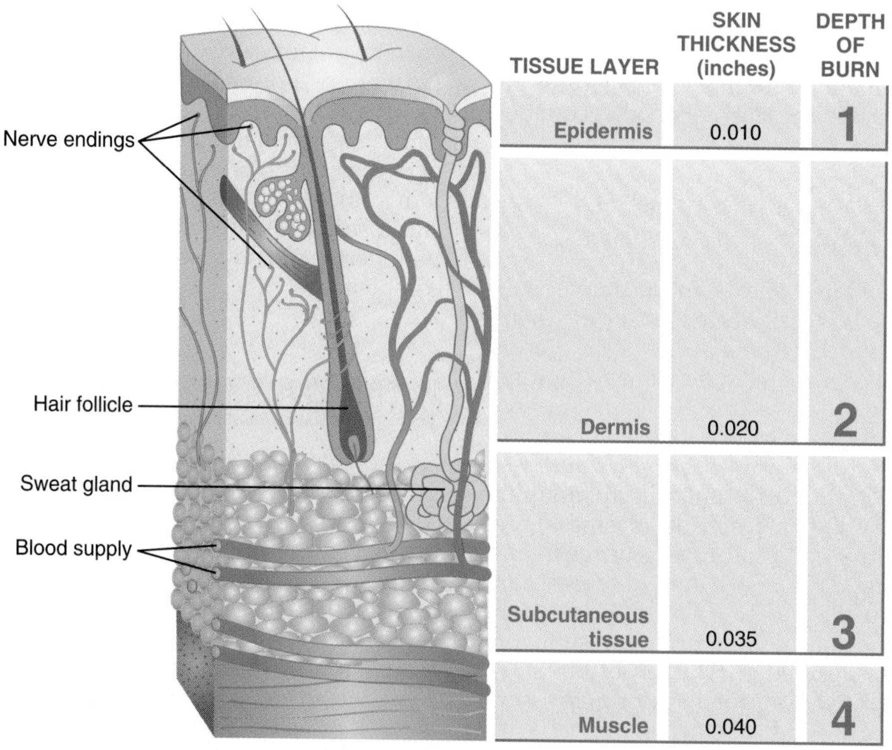

FIGURE 42-9 • Interpretation of burn classification based on damage to the integument.

tient. Wound healing can occur only in an anabolic state. Feeding should be initiated soon after resuscitation is complete. In fact, very early enteral feeding (within 4 to 12 hours of hospitalization) has been shown to be successful in decreasing the hypercatabolic response, thus decreasing the release of catecholamines, decreasing glucagon, reducing weight loss, and shortening the hospital length of stay (Chiarelli et al, 1990; McClave et al, 2002).

Achievement of enteral access and provision of a sufficient volume of enteral nutrients early in the hospital course of a critically ill patient afford an opportunity to improve the outcome of that patient. Enteral feeding provides a conduit for the delivery of immune stimulants and serves as effective prophylaxis against stress-induced gastropathy and gastrointestinal hemorrhage (McClave et al, 2002). Tube placement beyond the stomach into the small bowel in hypermetabolic, severely ill patients prone to ileus and disordered gut motility may aid delivery of enteral nutrients while reducing risk of aspiration.

Placement of enteral tubes during surgery has also been practiced at some burn centers in an effort to minimize the length of time a burn patient is without nutrition support (Jenkins et al, 1994). Nutritional goals for the burned patient are shown in Box 42-4.

Energy Requirements

The increased energy needs of the burned patient vary according to the size of the burn. Various formulas have been developed for estimating energy needs. The Curreri formula is the following (Curreri, 1979):

$$\text{kcal needed per day} = 24 \text{ kcal} \times \text{kg usual body weight} + 40 \text{ kcal} \times \text{\% TBSA burned (using a maximum of 50\% burn)}$$

The measurement of metabolic rate by indirect calorimetry has confirmed that the Curreri formula exceeds actual energy expenditure (Saffle et al, 1990). It is likely that the Curreri formula overestimates energy expenditure because of overall improvements in burn care and management since the formula was developed (Gottschlich and Ireton-Jones, 2001).

Once a burn exceeds 50% to 60% TBSA, minimal increases in energy expenditure occur (Waymack and Herndon, 1992). Some formulas do not establish an upper limit to the number of calories required. When these formulas are used, it should be noted that the maximum caloric load that the body can handle is approximately 100% above resting metabolic expenditure (2 × REE) (Cunningham et al, 1989).

Measuring energy expenditure via indirect calorimetry is the most reliable method for assessing energy expenditure in burn patients. Increasing energy expenditure by 20% to 30% is necessary to account for energy expenditure associated with wound care, physical therapy, etc. An alternate equation for assessing energy expenditure in the burn patient has been developed that accounts for burn injury and ventilatory status. The Ireton-Jones equation, which follows, has been repeatedly validated since its initial development (Gagliardi, Brathwaite, and Ross, 1995; Ireton-Jones, 1992, 1997, 2002; Wall et al, 1995).

$$EEE = 1784 - 11(A) + 5(W) + 244(G) + 239(T) + 804(B)$$

EEE = Estimated energy expenditure (kcal/day)
A = Age
W = Weight (kg)
G = Gender (female = 0, male = 1)
T = Diagnosis of trauma (absent = 0, present = 1)
B = Diagnosis of burn (absent = 0, present = 1)

Additional calories may be required to meet the needs because of fever, sepsis, multiple trauma, or the stress of surgery. Although weight gain may be desirable for the severely underweight patient, this is generally not feasible until after the acute illness. Weight maintenance should be the goal for overweight patients until the healing process is complete. Obese individuals may be at higher risk of wound infection and graft disruption. The energy requirement for the obese burned person is probably more than that calculated when ideal body weight is used but less than that calculated when actual body weight is used. Indirect calorimetry is the most accurate method of determining the energy needs of the obese patient (Gottschlich, 1993).

An accurate formula for calculating the nutritional needs of the pediatric burn patient remains to be developed. Because basic requirements depend on the stage of growth and development, providing a formula to cover all age groups is difficult. The commonly used Galveston formula estimates the caloric requirements as 1800 kcal/m^2 + 2200 kcal/m^2 of

Box 42-4. Nutritional Care Goals for Burned Patients

1. Minimize metabolic response by:
   - Controlling environmental temperature
   - Maintaining fluid and electrolyte balance
   - Controlling pain and anxiety
   - Covering wounds early
2. Meet nutritional needs by:
   - Providing adequate calories to prevent weight loss of greater than 10% of usual body weight
   - Providing adequate protein for positive nitrogen balance and maintenance or repletion of circulating proteins
   - Providing vitamin and mineral supplementation as indicated
3. Prevent Curling's ulcer by:
   - Providing antacids or continuous enteral feedings

burn (Waymack and Herndon, 1992). Mayes and colleagues estimate caloric need for children younger than 3 years of age as 108 + (68 × kg weight) + 3.9 × % body surface area burn (Mayes, et al).

Energy Sources

Carbohydrates are excellent for protein sparing. However, although carbohydrate is recommended as the chief energy source in burn patients, there appears to be a maximum glucose load of 7 mg/kg/min above which glucose is not oxidized but rather is converted to fat (Wolfe et al, 1979). This state of lipogenesis causes increased oxygen consumption and carbon dioxide production (see Chapter 38). Excessive carbohydrate can aggravate hyperglycemia and cause osmotic diuresis, dehydration, and respiratory difficulty.

Although lipids are a concentrated source of calories, high levels of lipids may cause deleterious immunologic responses and increased susceptibility to infections (Gottschlich et al, 1990). The composition of the lipid is important because diets high in omega-3 fatty acids may result in improved immune response and in tube-feeding tolerance (Alexander and Gottschlich, 1990). The omega-3 fatty acids inhibit the production of prostaglandin E2 and leukotrienes, which have immunosuppressive properties.

The administration—both enterally and parenterally—of a low-fat formula results in less pneumonia, improved respiratory function, faster recovery of nutritional status, and a shorter length of care (Garrel et al, 1995). A reasonable approach is to begin by limiting lipid to 12% to 15% of the nonprotein calories, giving attention to indicators of immune function, feeding tolerance, and serum triglycerides before higher amounts are used (Mayes and Gottschlich, 2003).

Both medium-chain triglycerides and structured lipids are currently under investigation. Medium-chain triglycerides are theoretically preferentially oxidized, thus leaving little tendency for deposition in adipose tissue or clogging of the reticuloendothelial system of the mitochondria (Tredget and Yu, 1992). Structured lipids may improve hepatic protein synthesis and reduce protein catabolism and energy expenditure.

Protein

The protein needs of burned patients are elevated because of losses through urine and wounds, increased use in gluconeogenesis, and wound healing. Recent evidence promotes the use of high-protein feeding. Provision of 20% to 25% of total calories as protein of high biologic value is suggested (Mayes and Gottschlich, 2003). Protein need in thermally injured children is generally agreed to be higher than the recommended dietary allowance. Feeding 2.5 to 3.0 g/kg protein has been suggested (Cunningham et al, 1990). The ability of pediatric burn patients to tolerate protein depends on their renal function and fluid balance.

The BCAAs seem to have no beneficial effect in burn patients (Alexander and Gottschlich, 1990). However, the conditionally essential amino acid, arginine, may improve cell-mediated immunity and wound healing (Mayes and Gottschlich, 2003; Tredget and Yu, 1992). Arginine may also affect anabolic hormone production (Gottschlich et al, 1990). A recent study showed that glutamine enhances the ability of neutrophils to kill certain bacteria (Ogle et al, 1994). For all patients who receive high-protein diets, blood urea nitrogen, serum creatinine, and hydration must be monitored.

Assessment of Energy and Protein Adequacy

The adequacy of protein and energy intake is best evaluated by monitoring wound healing, graft take, and basic nutritional assessment parameters. Wound healing or graft take may be delayed if weight loss exceeds 10% of the usual weight. An exact evaluation of weight loss may be difficult to obtain because of fluid shifts or edema or because of differences in the weights of dressings or splints. The coordination of weight measurement with dressing changes or hydrotherapy may allow recording of a weight without dressings and splints (Mayes and Gottschlich, 2003). Generally, the fluid gained during the resuscitation period is lost within 2 weeks. Weight-change trends can then be identified.

Nitrogen balance often is used to evaluate the efficacy of a nutritional regimen, but it cannot be considered accurate without accounting for wound losses. The following formulas have been used to estimate wound nitrogen losses (Mayes and Gottschlich, 2003):

$<$10% open wound = 0.02 g nitrogen/kg/day
11% to 30% open wound = 0.05 g nitrogen/kg/day
$>$31% open wound = 0.12 g nitrogen/kg/day

During the first 4 weeks, nitrogen balance studies may be the most reflective measure in nutritional monitoring (Carlson et al, 1991). Nitrogen excretion should begin to decrease as wounds heal or are grafted or covered; however, serum albumin levels usually remain depressed until major burns are healed. Proteins with shorter half-lives, such as serum prealbumin, retinol-binding protein, and transferrin, help to assess the protein status of burn patients (see Chapter 18).

Vitamins and Minerals

Vitamin needs generally increase for burn patients, but exact requirements have not been established. Supplements may be needed for patients who are eating food; however, most patients who receive tube feeding or TPN receive amounts of vitamins in excess

FOCUS ON

Maximizing Oral Nutrient Intake

A 58-year-old woman suffered third-degree burns over her lower extremities that resulted in a 15% total body surface burn. Because of her small overall burn size, the clinical dietitian recommended providing optimal nutrition via the oral route. The patient's energy and protein requirements were determined to be approximately 2100 kcal/day (measured via indirect calorimetry) and 155 g protein/day. A high-calorie, high-protein diet was provided via three meals and two snacks daily. Examples of meal and snack items are the following:

Breakfast

Orange juice with added Polycose
Cereal with fortified whole milk*
Scrambled eggs
Toast with margarine and jelly

Lunch

Cream-of-potato soup
Ham and cheese sandwich with mayonnaise
Fruited gelatin salad
Chocolate pudding with added protein supplement

Afternoon Snack

Instant Breakfast milkshake with protein powder supplement

Dinner

Tossed salad with Parmesan cheese and Italian dressing
Spaghetti with meat sauce
Cheesecake
Fortified whole milk

Evening Snack

Fruit slush with protein supplement

This meal plan offers approximately 2700 kcal/day and 175 g protein.

*Milk supplemented with protein (via either Carnation instant nonfat dry milk powder or general protein supplement).
Note: Enteral manufacturers offer a wide variety of fortified foods for maximizing oral nutrient intake; please refer to individual manufacturers for specific items (see Appendixes 36 to 41).

of the DRIs because of the high calorie intake. Vitamin C is involved in collagen synthesis and immune function and may be required in increased amounts for wound healing. Doses of 500 mg twice daily are the routine protocol at some burn centers (Mayes and Gottschlich, 2003). Vitamin A is also an important nutrient for immune function and epithelialization. Provision of 5000 IU of vitamin A per 1000 calories of enteral nutrition is often recommended (Mayes and Gottschlich, 2003).

Electrolyte imbalances that involve serum sodium or potassium are usually corrected by adjusting fluid therapy. Hyponatremia may be seen in patients whose evaporative losses are reduced drastically by the application of dressings or grafts; who have had changes in maintenance fluids; or who have been treated with silver nitrate soaks, which tend to draw sodium from the wound. Restricting the oral consumption of free water and sodium-free fluids may help correct hyponatremia. Hypokalemia often occurs after the initial fluid resuscitation and during protein synthesis. A slightly elevated serum potassium may indicate inadequate hydration.

Depression of serum calcium levels may be seen in patients with burns that involve more than 30% TBSA. Hypocalcemia often accompanies hypoalbuminemia. Calcium losses may be exaggerated if the patient is immobile or being treated with silver nitrate soaks. Early ambulation and exercise should help minimize these losses. Administration of calcium supplements may be necessary to treat symptomatic hypocalcemia.

Hypophosphatemia has also been identified in patients with major burns. This occurs most commonly in patients who receive large volumes of resuscitation fluid along with parenteral infusion of glucose solutions and large amounts of antacids for stress ulcer prophylaxis. Serum levels need to be monitored, and appropriate phosphate supplementation provided. Magnesium levels may also require attention because a significant amount of magnesium can be lost from the burn wound. Supplemental phosphorus and magnesium are often given parenterally to prevent gastrointestinal irritation.

A depressed serum zinc level has been reported in burn patients, but whether this is representative of total body zinc nutriture or is an artifact of hypoalbuminemia is unclear, because zinc is bound to serum albumin. Zinc is a cofactor in energy metabolism and protein synthesis. Supplementation with 220 mg zinc sulfate is appropriate (Mayes and Gottschlich, 2003). The anemia initially seen following a burn is usually unrelated to iron deficiency and is treated with packed red blood cells.

Methods of Nutrition Support

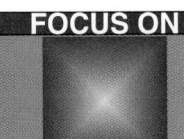

Methods of nutrition support need to be implemented on an individual basis. Most patients with burns of less than 20% TBSA are able to meet their needs with a regular, high-calorie and high-protein diet (see *Focus On:* Maximizing Oral Nutrient Intake). Often the use of concealed nutrients such as adding protein to puddings, milks, and gelatins is helpful because consuming large volumes of foods can be overwhelming to the patient and can lead to overeating after the burns are healed. Patients with major burns, extraordinarily high energy expenditure, or poor appetites usually require tube feeding or TPN.

Enteral feeding is the preferred method of nutrition support for burn patients, but parenteral nutrition may be necessary with early excision and grafting so as to avoid the frequent interruptions in enteral nutrition support required for anesthesia. Because ileus is often present only in the stomach, severely burned patients can be successfully fed into the small bowel. This is a routine practice in many burn centers. IGF-1 and human growth hormone in conjunction with nutrition support have been shown to blunt the stress response and improve nitrogen balance in burn patients (Goodwin, 1993; Waymack and Herndon, 1992). Anabolic steroids such as oxandrolone, when combined with a high-protein diet (2 g/kg/day) have also been shown to significantly increase the rate at which patients restore lost weight after burn injury (Demling and Desanti, 1997).

TPN may be the method of choice for patients with persistent ileus who do not tolerate tube feedings or who have a high risk of aspiration. With careful monitoring, central lines for TPN can be maintained through burn wounds.

SURGERY

Although surgical morbidity correlates best with the extent of the primary disease and the nature of the operation performed, malnutrition may compound the severity of complications (Mullen et al, 1979). A well-nourished patient usually tolerates major surgery better than a severely malnourished patient; malnutrition is associated with a high incidence of operative complications and death (Campos and Mequid, 1992). The National Veterans Affairs Surgical Risk Study evaluated 87,000 noncardiac surgeries in 44 Veterans' Administration medical centers and found preoperative serum albumin to be the strongest predictor of postoperative mortality (Khuri et al, 1997).

Medical Nutrition Therapy

Preoperative Nutritional Care

A chemically defined or elemental liquid diet with minimal residue can be used preoperatively for patients at nutritional risk. A large multicenter study of surgical patients concluded that the use of preoperative TPN should be limited to patients who exhibit signs of severe malnutrition, unless other specific indications exist (Veterans Affairs TPN Cooperative Study Group, 1991). Except for patients who are unable to take food enterally or who are malnourished, no conclusive evidence suggests that perioperative nutritional support (other than in the form of oral intake) is effective in reducing operative complications and death. Preoperative nutrition support should be administered for 7 to 14 days to moderately or severely malnourished patients who are undergoing major gastrointestinal surgery, if the operation can be safely postponed (ASPEN Board of Directors, 2002).

It is important that the stomach be empty of food at the time of the operation to avoid the danger of vomitus aspiration during the induction of anesthesia or on awakening. In elective cases, no food is allowed by mouth for at least 6 hours before surgery. In emergency cases, gastric lavage is advisable to remove stomach contents before anesthesia is started.

Before abdominal surgery, the colon should be free of residue to prevent postoperative infection. Colonic bacteria are reduced when less food residue is present. Low-fiber foods or a liquid diet are commonly given for 2 to 3 days before surgery, and the patient receives an enema a few hours before going to the operating room. Enteral products that are low in residue can be used for colon preparation prior to surgery (see Appendixes 38 and 39).

Postoperative Nutritional Care

In the postoperative period, nutrition support is used to reduce nutritional deficits that ordinarily develop in untreated patients during the period of NPO (nothing by mouth) after surgery. The length of time a patient can tolerate remaining NPO after surgery without complications is unknown, but it is probably influenced by the patient's preexisting nutritional status, the severity of the operative stress, and the nature and severity of the illness. Postoperative nutrition support should be administered to patients when they are anticipated to be unable to meet their nutrient needs orally for a period of 7 to 10 days (ASPEN Board of Directors, 2002).

The introduction of solid food depends on the condition of the gastrointestinal tract. Oral feeding is often delayed for the first 24 to 48 hours after surgery to await the return of bowel sounds or passage of flatus. A general practice has been to progress over a period of several meals from clear liquids to full liquids and finally to solid foods. However, no physiologic reason exists for solid foods not to be introduced as soon as the gastrointestinal tract is functioning and a few liquids are being tolerated. Multiple studies have now demonstrated that after surgery, patients can be fed a regular solid-food diet rather than a clear liquid diet (Bickel et al, 1992; Jeffery et al, 1996; Martindale, 1998).

If oral feeding is not possible, or an extended NPO period is anticipated, an access device for enteral feeding should be inserted at the time of surgery. Combined gastrostomy-jejunostomy tubes offer significant advantages over standard gastrostomies because they allow for simultaneous gastric

Clinical Scenario 1

Michael, a 22-year-old man, was involved in a motor vehicle accident as an unbelted rear-seat passenger and sustained a skull fracture, left subdural hematoma, and right pneumothorax that requires a chest tube. Glasgow Coma Scale was 10. Michael's weight on admission to the surgical intensive care unit was 162 lb, and his height is 6 ft 4 in. He has no previous significant medical or nutrition history.

Michael was stabilized and was given slightly less than his maintenance fluid requirements and a diuretic to prevent brain swelling. He was maintained on a respirator. A nasogastric tube was placed for drainage.

On hospital day 4, TPN was initiated because of continued high nasogastric drainage. Michael began running high fevers. The diuretic was discontinued, and the fluid restriction was liberalized because he was becoming too dehydrated. Using the Harris-Benedict equation with an injury factor of 1.4, the registered dietitian calculated his energy requirements at 2681 calories. Indirect calorimetry indicated that Michael's measured energy expenditure (MEE) was 2990 kcal/day. The nutritional goal was to feed the patient his actual measured energy needs. Protein requirements were calculated to provide approximately 1.5 g/kg, or 110 g, of protein per day. The serum albumin level of 4.3 g/dl on admission, dropped to 2.9 g/dl after rehydration.

A concentrated intact nutrient formula was started at 20 ml/hr via the nasogastric tube on hospital day 6. Feedings were successfully advanced to the goal rate of 85 ml/hr by day 9. This provided 3060 calories and 124 g protein per day. TPN was discontinued as Michael continued to tolerate enteral nutrition. Rapid turnover proteins were low; retinol-binding protein was 1.3 mg/dl (normal 3.0 to 6.0 mg/dl); and prealbumin was 4.8 mg/dl (normal 10 to 40 mg/dl). Zinc was normal at 83 (63 to 147 mg/dl). Total urinary nitrogen excretion was 27 g/day.

On hospital day 11, a nasojejunal tube replaced the nasogastric tube to lessen the risk of aspiration for this unresponsive patient. Michael continued to run a fever and was often treated with a cooling blanket. Because of anticipated continued ventilator dependence and neurologic impairment, gastrostomy (G-tube) and jejunostomy (J-tube) tubes were surgically placed. Since the initiation of nutrition support, Michael has received 90% or more of his measured nutritional requirements. His weight is now 132 lbs. Diarrhea and copious airway secretions began during hospital week 3. An infectious cause of diarrhea was ruled out. A less concentrated tube-feeding formula is provided for hydration and to perhaps lessen stooling.

1. What indications of hypermetabolism are evident in this patient's history?
2. Compare Michael's measured energy expenditure with that calculated by the Harris-Benedict equation. What are the differences? Also compare it in kilocalories per kilogram.
3. What nutritional recommendations would you make for the remainder of his hospital stay?

Clinical Scenario 2

Thomas, a 61-year-old man, was admitted with gastric outlet obstruction secondary to gastric carcinoma. Surgical intervention was planned, but because of his history of a 30-lb weight loss over 2 months, parenteral nutrition was initiated with surgery scheduled for his fifth day of hospitalization. His weight on admission was 135 lb, and his height is 5 ft 10 in. Thomas' usual body weight is 165 lb, which he also reported weighing 3 months ago. According to Thomas, he was easily able to consume liquids when his symptoms initially began, but within the past 2 weeks he has had difficulty consuming liquids without emesis. He has not been able to consume solid foods during the past 3 months.

His initial laboratory work included a BUN of 2 mg/dl, an albumin of 3.5 g/dl, and serum triglycerides of 65 mg/dl. Indirect calorimetry testing revealed a resting energy expenditure (REE) of 1460 kcals/day. His respiratory quotient (RQ) was 0.72. His past medical history was significant for type I diabetes mellitus and chronic bronchitis.

Thomas underwent a total gastrectomy with jejunostomy tube placement on his fifth hospital day. He experienced blood pressure instability in the initial postoperative period and required multiple fluid boluses and large amounts of pharmacologic agents to maintain adequate blood pressure. On postoperative day (POD) one, Thomas' abdomen was firm and distended, and bowel sounds were absent. His laboratory work postoperatively included a blood glucose level of 275 mg/dl, a serum albumin of 1.9 g/dl, and a prealbumin of 5.7 mg/dl. Repeated indirect calorimetry revealed an energy expenditure of 1925 kcal/day and an RQ of 0.85. Urinary urea nitrogen excretion was 21 g/day.

On postoperative day 3, Thomas' abdomen was soft and nondistended, and bowel sounds were hypoactive. An intact nutrient formula with added arginine, omega-3 fatty acids, and nucleotides was initiated at 20 ml/hr via the jejunostomy tube. Thomas tolerated this initial enteral regimen but demonstrated abdominal distention and pain when attempts were made to advance his feeding rate. Consequently, his TPN continued at the goal rate. On postoperative day 7, the tube-feeding rate was increased to 30 ml/hr with subsequent tolerance. Feeding advancement continued and reached the goal rate of 55 ml/hr. TPN infusion remained at the goal rate. On postoperative day 8, Thomas' serum glucose level was 310 mg/dl. and his arterial P_{CO_2} was 52 mg/dl. His TPN was slowly discontinued over 2 hours, and on postoperative day 9, his glucose is now 205 mg/dl, and his arterial P_{CO_2} has decreased to 38 mg/dl.

1. Describe Thomas' nutritional status. What assessment parameters are used for evaluation? Was preoperative TPN indicated?
2. What are the differences in metabolic response between Thomas' initial presentation and his postoperative status?
3. Why may an immune-enhancing enteral formula be beneficial for Thomas?
4. What may have been the explanation for Thomas' increased glucose and P_{CO_2} levels during his combined TPN and tube feeding therapies?

drainage from the gastrostomy tube and enteral feeding via the jejunal tube.

SUMMARY

The combined impact of the metabolic alterations that occur in stress with bed rest can lead to rapid and severe depletion of lean body mass. Nutrition support cannot fully prevent or reverse the metabolic alterations and disruptions in body composition associated with critical illness. However, nutrition support likely ameliorates the rate of net protein catabolism. Initial assessment of the critically ill patient should include an evaluation of the patient's preexisting nutritional status. Clinical judgment is paramount in making decisions about the need to initiate nutrition support. For patients who will require enteral or parenteral nutrition, it should begin as soon as hemodynamic stability is achieved. Critically ill patients who are injured, septic, or bedridden cannot be expected to gain weight, lean body mass, or strength until the hypermetabolism resolves and physical therapy, exercise, and rehabilitation begin.

■ Relevant Web Sites

American College of Surgeons
www.facs.org
American Gastroenterology Association
www.gastro.org
American Society for Clinical Nutrition (ASCN)
www.faseb.org/ASCN
American Society for Parenteral and Enteral Nutrition (ASPEN)
www.clinnutr.org/
Burn Nutrition
www.burnsurgery.org/modules/burnnutrition/
Burn Survivor Resource Center
www.burnsurvivor.com/nutrition.html

■ Cited References

Alexander JW: Nutritional pharmacology in surgical patients, *Am J Surg* 183:349, 2002.

Alexander JW, Gottschlich MM: Nutritional immunomodulation in burn patients, *Crit Care Med* 18:S149, 1990.

Alpers DH: Enteral feeding and gut atrophy, *Curr Opin Clin Nutr Metab Care* 5:679, 2002.

Annis K et al: nutrition support of the severe head-injured patient, *Nutr Clin Pract* 6:245, 1991.

ASPEN Board of Directors: Guidelines for the use of parenteral and enteral nutrition in adult and pediatric patients, *J Parenter Enteral Nutr* 26:1S, 2002.

Bessey PQ: Parenteral nutrition and trauma. In Rombeau J, Caldwell MD, editors: *Parenteral nutrition,* ed 2, Philadelphia, 1993, WB Saunders.

Bickel A et al: Early oral feeding following removal of nasogastric tube in gastrointestinal operations, *Arch Surg* 127:287, 1992.

Blackburn GL et al: Nutritional and metabolic assessment of the hospitalized patient, *J Parenter Enteral Nutr* 1:11, 1977.

Bone RC: Toward an epidemiology and natural history of SIRS (systemic inflammatory response syndrome), *JAMA* 268:3452, 1992.

Bone RC et al: ACCP/SCCM Consensus Conference: definitions for sepsis and organ failure and guidelines for the use of innovative therapies in sepsis, *Chest* 101:1644, 1992.

Campos A, Meguid M: A critical appraisal of the usefulness of perioperative nutrition support, *Am J Clin Nutr* 55:117, 1992.

Carlson DW et al: Evaluation of serum visceral protein levels as indicators of nitrogen balance in thermally injured patients, *J Parenter Enteral Nutr* 15:440, 1991.

Chiarelli A et al: Very early nutrition supplementation in burned patients, *Am J Clin Nutr* 51:1035, 1990.

Consensus recommendations from the U.S. summit on immune-enhancing enteral therapy, *J Parenter Enteral Nutr* 25:S61-S62, 2001.

Cunningham J et al: Measured and predicted calorie requirements of adults during recovery from severe burn trauma, *Am J Clin Nutr* 49:404, 1989.

Cunningham J et al: Calorie and protein provision for recovery from severe burns in infants and young children, *Am J Clin Nutr* 51:553, 1990.

Curreri PW: Nutritional replacement modalities, *J Trauma* 19:904, 1979.

Cuthbertson DP: The metabolic response to injury and its nutritional implications: retrospect and prospect, *J Parenter Enteral Nutr* 3:108, 1979.

Deitch EA: Multiple organ failure, *Ann Surg* 216:117, 1992.

Demling RH, Desanti L: Oxandrolone, an anabolic steroid, significantly increases the rate of weight gain in the recovery phase after major burns, *J Trauma* 43:47, 1997.

Epstein CD et al: Comparison of methods of measurements of oxygen consumption in mechanically ventilated patients with multiple trauma: the Fick method versus indirect calorimetry, *Crit Care Med* 28:1363, 2000.

Fox KA et al: Aspiration pneumonia following surgically placed feeding tubes, *Am J Surg* 170:560, 1995.

Gagliardi E, Brathwaite CE, Ross SE: Predicting energy expenditure in trauma patients: validation of the Ireton-Jones equations, *J Parenter Enteral Nutr* 19(suppl):22S, 1995 (abstract).

Garrel DR et al: Improved clinical status and length of care with low-fat nutrition support in burn patients, *J Parenter Enteral Nutr* 19:482, 1995.

Gilder H: Parenteral nourishment of patients undergoing surgical or traumatic stress, *J Parenter Enteral Nutr* 10:88, 1986.

Goodwin CW: Parenteral nutrition in thermal injuries. In Rombeau J, Caldwell MD, editors: *Clinical nutrition: parenteral nutrition,* ed 2, Philadelphia, 1993, WB Saunders.

Gottschlich MM, Ireton-Jones CS: The Curreri formula: a landmark process for estimating caloric needs of burn patients, *Nutr Clin Pract* 16:172, 2001.

Gottschlich MM et al: Differential effects of three enteral dietary regimens on selected outcome variables in burn patients, *J Parenter Enteral Nutr* 14:225, 1990.

Gottschlich MM et al: Significance of obesity on nutritional, immunologic, hormonal, and clinical outcome parameters in burns, *J Am Diet Assoc* 93:1261, 1993.

Greenblatt SH et al: Catabolic effect of dexamethasone in patients with major head injuries, *J Parenter Enteral Nutr* 13:372, 1989.

Grimm H et al: Immunoregulation by parenteral lipids: impact of the ω-3 to ω-6 fatty acid ratio, *J Parenter Enteral Nutr* 18:417, 1994.

Hadley MN et al: nutrition support and neurotrauma: a critical review of early nutrition in forty-five acute head injury patients, *Neurosurgery* 19:367, 1986.

Herndon DN et al: Treatment of burns in children, *Pediatr Clin North Am* 32:1311, 1985.

Hester DD: Neurologic impairment. In Gottschlich MM et al, editors: *Nutrition support dietetics core curriculum,* ed 2, Silver Spring, Md, 1993, American Society for Parenteral and Enteral Nutrition.

Ireton-Jones CS, Jones JD: Why use predictive equations for energy expenditure assessment? *J Am Diet Assoc* 97 (suppl):A-44, 1997 (abstract).

Ireton-Jones C, Jones JD: Improved equations for predicting energy expenditure in patients: the Ireton-Jones equations, *Nutr Clin Pract* 17:29, 2002.

Ireton-Jones CS et al: Equations for the estimation of energy expenditures in patients with burns with special reference to ventilatory status, *J Burn Care Rehabil* 13:330, 1992.

Jeevanandam M et al: Decreased growth hormone levels in the catabolic phase of severe injury, *Surgery* 111:495, 1992.

Jeevanandam M et al: Adjuvant recombinant human growth hormone normalizes plasma amino acids in parenterally fed trauma patients, *J Parenter Enteral Nutr* 19:137, 1995.

Jeffery KM et al: The clear liquid diet is no longer a necessity in the routine postoperative management of surgical patients, *Am Surg* 62:167, 1996.

Jenkins ME et al: Enteral feeding during operative procedures in thermal injuries, *J Burn Care Rehabil* 15:199, 1994.

Khuri SF et al: Risk adjustment of the postoperative mortality rate for the comparative assessment of the quality of surgical care: results of the National Veterans Affairs Surgical Risk Study, *J Am Coll Surg* 185:315, 1997.

Koruda MJ et al: Effect of parenteral nutrition supplemented with short-chain fatty acids on adaptation to massive small bowel resection, *Gastroenterology 95:*715, 1986.

Kudsk KA: Current aspects of mucosal immunology and its influence by nutrition, *Am J Surg* 183:390, 2002.

Li J et al: Effect of glutamine-enriched total parenteral nutrition on small intestinal gut-associated lymphoid tissue and upper respiratory tract immunity, *Surgery* 121:542, 1997.

Liggett SB et al: Determination of resting energy expenditure utilizing the thermodilution pulmonary artery catheter, *Chest* 91:562, 1987.

Lund CL, Browder NC: The estimation of areas of burns, *Surg Gynecol Obstet* 79:352, 1944.

Malone AM: Methods of assessing energy expenditure in the intensive care unit, *Nutr Clin Pract* 17:21, 2002.

Martindale R: Clear liquid diets: tradition or intuition? *Nutr Clin Pract* 13:186, 1998.

Mayes T, Gottschlich MM: Burns and wound healing. In Matarase LE, Gottschlich MM, editors: *Contemporary nutrition support practice: a clinical guide,* ed 2, Philadelphia, 2003, WB Saunders.

Mayes TM, et al: An evaluation of predicted and measured energy requirements in burn children, *J Am Diet Assoc* 96(1):24, 1996.

McClave SA et al: Enteral access for nutrition support: rationale for utilization, *J Clin Gastroenterol* 35:209, 2002.

Moriyama S et al: Evaluation of oxygen consumption and resting energy expediture in critically ill patients with systemic inflammatory response syndrome, *Crit Care Med* 27:2133, 1999.

Mullen JL et al: Implication of malnutrition in the surgical patient, *Arch Surg* 114:121, 1979.

Ogle CK et al: Effect of glutamine on phagocytosis and bacterial killing by normal and pediatric burn patient neutrophils, *J Parenter Enteral Nutr* 18:128, 1994.

Ott L, Young B: Nutrition in the neurologically injured patient, *Nutr Clin Pract* 6:223, 1991.

Pichard C et al: Lack of effects of recombinant growth hormone on muscle function in patients requiring prolonged mechanical ventilation: a prospective, randomized, controlled study, *Crit Care Med* 24:403, 1996.

Pomp A et al: Specialized nutrition support in surgical patients, *Prob Gen Surg* 5:271, 1988.

Pratt VC et al: Short-chain fatty acid-supplemented TPN improves nonspecific immunity after intestinal resection in rats, *J Parenter Enteral Nutr* 20:264, 1996.

Prelack K, Sheridan RL: Micronutrient supplementation in the critically ill patient: strategies for clinical practice, *J Trauma* 51:601, 2001.

Reynolds JV: Gut barrier function in the surgical patient, *Br J Surg* 83:1668, 1996.

Reynolds JV et al: Impaired gut barrier function in malnourished patients, *Br J Surg* 83:1288, 1996.

Saffle JR et al: A randomized trial of indirect calorimetry-based feedings in thermal injury, *J Trauma* 30:776, 1990.

Souba W, Wilmore D: Diet and nutrition in the case of the patient with surgery, trauma and sepsis. In Shils ME et al, editors: *Modern nutrition in health and disease,* vol 2, ed 8, Philadelphia, 1994, Lea & Febiger.

Sunderland PM, Heilbrun MP: Estimating energy expenditure in traumatic brain injury: comparison of indirect calorimetry with predictive formulas, *Neurosurgery* 31:246, 1992.

Swank GM, Deitch EA. Role of the gut in multiple organ failure: bacterial translocation and permeability changes, *World J Surg* 20:411, 1996.

Tappenden KA, et al: Short-chain fatty acids increase proglucagon and ornithine decarboxylase messenger RNAs after intestinal resection in rats, *J Parenter Enteral Nutr* 20:357, 1996.

Tappenden KA et al: Short-chain fatty acid-supplemented total parenteral nutrition enhances functional adaptation to intestinal resection in rats, *Gastroenterology* 112:792, 1997.

Tappenden KA et al: Early enteral nutrition may have detrimental effects in patients with gastrointestinal hypoperfusion (abstract). Presented at the Twenty-second Clinical Congress, American Society for Parenteral and Enteral Nutrition, January 1998.

Tredget EE, Yu YM: The metabolic effects of thermal injury, *World J Surg* 16:68, 1992.

Uehara M et al: Components of energy expenditure in patients with severe sepsis and major trauma: a basis for clinical care, *Crit Care Med* 27:1295, 1999.

Van Den Berghe G et al: Intensive insulin therapy in critically ill patients, *N Engl J Med* 345:1359, 2001.

Veterans Affairs Total Parenteral Nutrition Cooperative Study Group: Perioperative total parenteral nutrition in surgical patients, *N Engl J Med* 325:525, 1991.

Wall J et al: A validation of equations for predicting the energy expenditures of hospitalized patients, *J Am Diet Assoc* 95(suppl): A-24, 1995 (abstract).

Warden GD: Burn shock resuscitation, *World J Surg* 16:16, 1992.

Waymack JP, Herndon DN: nutrition support of the burned patient, *World J Surg* 16:80, 1992.

Wilmore DW: The effect of glutamine supplementation in patients following elective surgery and accidental injury, *J Nutr* 131: 2543S, 2001.

Wolfe RR, Martini WZ: Changes in intermediary metabolism in severe surgical illness, *World J Surg* 24:639, 2000.

Wolfe R et al: Glucose metabolism in man: responses to intravenous glucose infusion, *Metabolism* 28:210, 1979.

Wood P: Managing dysphagia in patients with traumatic brain injury: news and views, *Mead Johnson Nutritionals Newsletter* (2)1, 1990.

Young LS, Persinger RL: The utility of growth hormone in nutrition support, *Support Line* 16:6, 1994.

Zaloga GP et al: Effect of rate of enteral nutrient supply on gut mass, *J Parenter Enteral Nutr* 16:39, 1992.

Ziegler TR: Anabolic agents in nutrition support. Presented at the Twenty-second Clinical Congress, American Society for Parenteral and Enteral Nutrition, January 1998.

Additional References

Albina JE: Nutrition and wound healing, *J Parenter Enteral Nutr* 18:367, 1994.

Alpers DH: Enteral feeding and gut atrophy, *Curr Opin Clin Nutr Metab Care* 5:679, 2002.

Cahill GF: Starvation in man, *N Engl J Med* 282:668, 1980.

Cioffi WG: What's new in burns and metabolism, *J Am Coll Surg* 192:241, 2001.

Demling RH, Seigne P: Metabolic management of patients with severe burns, *World J Surg* 24:673, 2000.

Field CJ et al: Glutamine and arginine: immunonutrients for improved health, *Med Sci Sports Exerc* 32:S377, 2000.

Kudsk KA et al: A randomized trial of isonitrogenous enteral diets after severe trauma: an immune enhancing diet reduces septic complications, *Ann Surg* 224:531, 1996.

Lewis SJ et al: Early enteral feeding versus "nil by mouth" after gastrointestinal surgery, *BMJ* 323:773, 2001.
Magnuson B et al: Pentobarbital coma in neurosurgical patients: nutritional considerations, *Nutr Clin Pract* 9:146, 1994.
Mayes T, Gottschlich MM. Burns. In Matarese LE, Gottschlich MM, editors: *Contemporary nutrition support practice,* Philadelphia, 1998, WB Saunders.
Moore FA et al: Early enteral feeding, compared with parenteral reduces postoperative septic complications: the results of a meta-analysis, *Ann Surg* 216:172, 1992.
Mueller C: Inflammatory response and sepsis. In Matarese LE, Gottschlich MM, editors: *Contemporary nutrition support practice,* Philadelphia, 1998, WB Saunders.
Ott L et al: Altered gastric emptying in the head injured patient: relationship to feeding intolerance, *J Neurosurg* 74:738, 1991.
Pratt VC et al: Alterations in lymphocyte function and relation to phospholipid composition after burn injury in humans, *Crit Care Med* 30:1753, 2002.
Silk DBA, Gow NM: Postoperative starvation after gastrointestinal surgery: early feeding is beneficial, *BMJ* 323:761, 2001.
Thomas SJM: The effect of prolonged euglycemic hyperinsulinemia on lean body mass after severe burn, *Surgery* 132:341, 2002.
Winkler MF: Nutritional assessment in critical care. In: Simko MD et al, editors: *Nutrition assessment: a comprehensive guide for planning intervention,* Rockville, Md, 1995, Aspen Publishers.
Winkler MF: Surgery and wound healing. In Skipper A, editor: *Dietitian's handbook of enteral and parenteral nutrition,* Gaithersburg, Md, 1998, Aspen Publishers.

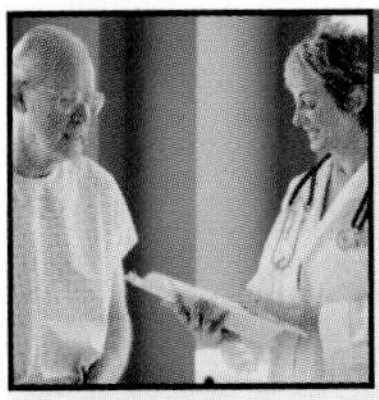

CHAPTER 43

Medical Nutrition Therapy for Neurologic Disorders

VALENTINA M. REMIG, PhD, RD, LD, FADA
CECILIA ROMERO, MD

CHAPTER OUTLINE

- Neurologic Disease Classification
- Nervous System Wiring and Lesions
- Medical Nutrition Therapy
- Problems With Procurement of Food
- Neurologic Diseases Arising From Nutritional Deficiencies or Excesses
- Neurologic Diseases With Nonnutrition Etiologies

KEY TERMS

adrenoleukodystrophy (ALD)–rare congenital enzyme deficiency in young men that affects the metabolism of very-long-chain fatty acids (VLCFAs) in the paroxisomes

agne–distorted perception of the surrounding world and related auditory, visual, or tactile sensations; common in Alzheimer's disease

agnosia–loss of comprehension that occurs as a manifestation of Alzheimer's disease

Alzheimer's disease (AD)–a progressive degenerative brain disease characterized by α-amyloid protein and endoplasmic reticulum–associated binding protein in the brain, that begins gradually, advances, and eventually leads to confusion, personality and behavior changes, and impaired judgment

amyotrophic lateral sclerosis (ALS)–a degenerative disease that causes progressive denervation atrophy and muscle weakness

anomia–inability to remember names of objects; a common manifestation of Alzheimer's disease

anosmia–loss or impairment of smell

aphasia–impaired or absent comprehension or communication because of an acquired lesion of the dominant cerebral hemisphere

apraxia–inability to perform purposeful movements although there is no sensory or motor impairment

aspiration–inhalation of foreign object(s), including contents of gastric reflux, into the lungs; can lead to aspiration pneumonia

ataxia–impaired muscular movement, especially voluntary movement

corpus callosum–the bridge between the two hemispheres of the brain, consisting of white matter

cortical blindness–blindness resulting from a lesion of the visual area of the cerebral cortex

deglutitory dysfunction–swallowing irregularity

dysarthria–impairment of the tongue or other muscles essential to speech, which makes speaking difficult

dysgeusia–impaired taste

dysomia–distortion of normal smell

dysphagia–difficulty swallowing

echolalia–repeating of words spoken by others; manifestation of Alzheimer's disease and psychotic disorders

embolic stroke–occlusion of an artery by cholesterol plaque, which deprives part of the brain of its oxygen supply

epidural hematoma–bleeding between the skull and the dura mater; usually a result of trauma

epilepsy–an intermittent derangement of the nervous system presumably caused by sudden, excessive, disorderly discharge of cerebral neurons

Guillain-Barré syndrome (GBS)–an acute-onset, inflammatory, demyelinating polyneuropathy that affects the proximal motor nerves, including the cranial nerves and the diaphragm

---

Chapter written by LeeAnn R. Shiveley, MPH, RD, and Patrick J. Connolly, MD, for the previous edition of this text.

KEY TERMS—Continued

hemiparesis–weakness that affects only one side of the body

hemianopsia–blindness for half of the visual field; vision in one eye

hemotympanum–fluid or blood behind the eardrum or leaking from the ear; suggests a skull base fracture

hydrocephalus–accumulation of cerebrospinal fluid within ventricles of the brain

hyperosmia—abnormally increased sensitivity to odors

multiple sclerosis (MS)–often debilitating, sometimes fatal disease, featuring autoimmune inflammatory attack against the myelin insulation of neurons

myasthenia gravis (MG)–autoimmune disease of the neuromuscular junction characterized by an immune response to acetylcholine receptors (AChR), which renders them ineffective and causes muscle weakness

myelopathy–any pathologic condition of the spinal cord

nystagmus–constant, involuntary movement of the eyeball

otorrhea–clear fluid running from the ear; suggests a skull base fracture

paresthesia–numbness sensation and heightened sensitivity; experienced in central and peripheral nerve lesions and in locomotor ataxia

Parkinson's disease (PD)–a progressive, disabling, neurodegenerative disease characterized by slow and decreased movement, muscular rigidity, resting tremor, and postural instability

peripheral neuropathy–functional disturbance or pathologic changes in the peripheral nervous system; noninflammatory lesions in the peripheral nervous system

petit mal seizure–one of three former classifications of epilepsy; "absence" seizure

subarachnoid hemorrhage (SAH)–bleeding into the subarachnoid space, often caused by a ruptured aneurysm in the arteries at the base of the brain

subdural hematoma–blood collection between the dura mater and arachnoid membrane

thromboembolic event–obstruction of a blood vessel by a thrombus that has become detached from its site of formation

thrombotic stroke–the rupturing of a cholesterol plaque in an artery with subsequent platelet aggregation to clot an already narrowed artery

tonic-clonic seizure–"grand mal" seizure characterized by generalized involuntary muscular contraction and cessation of respiration; may occur singly or in close succession with a sensory warning or aura preceding each seizure

transient ischemic attack (TIA)–a brief attack that lasts from a few minutes to hours of cerebral dysfunction of vascular origin with no persistent neurologic defect

Diseases of the nervous system pose serious health problems of worldwide magnitude and are seen in epidemic proportions. For example, between 1991 and 1994, when sudden economic and political changes occurred in Cuba, the Cuban Ministry of Public Health reported over 50,000 cases of optic and peripheral neuropathy among its population of 10.8 million. The pathogenesis was associated with an acute nutritional deficiency and the toxic effects of tobacco. A significant number of patients improved after treatment with parenteral administration of vitamin B-complex vitamins (high doses of thiamin, riboflavin, B_6, and B_{12}); oral supplements of vitamins A, E, and folic acid; and consumption of a high-protein diet for 10 days. Prophylactic vitamin supplements were subsequently distributed to the entire population, and after only 2 months, the incidence of disease had plummeted (Ordunez-Garcia et al, 1996). Fortunately, in this situation, nutrition was assessed, and inexpensive vitamin B therapy prevented a major catastrophe. Complaints of even minor symptoms such as headaches, dizziness, insomnia, weakness, pain, and discomfort must be skillfully evaluated for the presence of a nutrition component in their cause and treatment.

NEUROLOGIC DISEASE CLASSIFICATION

The medical or health history is often the most important part of the neurologic evaluation. Numerous symptoms and malnutrition may accompany the various types of neurologic disease. Primary prevention is the cornerstone of management for neurologic diseases that arise from nutritional deficiencies as described in the previous section, or nutritional excesses. Diseases of the nervous system that have a nutrition etiology are often attributed to malabsorption, alcoholism, or malnutrition. For the management of malabsorption refer to Chapter 30.

Not all neurologic diseases have a nutrition etiology, yet nutritional considerations are integral to effective medical and clinical management (Table 43-1). Many neurologic dysfunctions occur secondary to a deficiency of a single or several vitamins; other diseases of the nervous system may be attributed to dietary excess (Table 43-2).

A second category of neurologic disease has a nonnutrition etiology, but nutrition therapies are adjuncts to disease management. Many elements of nutrition

TABLE 43-1 Nutritional Considerations for Neurological Conditions

MEDICAL CONDITION	RELEVANT NUTRITION THERAPY
Adrenoleukodystrophy	Dietary avoidance of very-long-chain fatty acids (VLCFA) has not been proven Lorenzo's oil lowers VLCFA levels
Alzheimer's disease	Assess nutritional status of patient Minimize distractions at mealtime Initiate smell or touch of food Hand guidance to initiate eating Provide nutrient-dense foods and omega-3 fatty acids
Amyotrophic lateral sclerosis	Intervention to prevent malnutrition and dehydration Monitor dysphagia
Epilepsy	Ketogenic diet
Guillain-Barré syndrome	Attain positive energy balance with high-energy, high protein tube feedings Assess dysphagia
Migraine headache	Follow general recommendations about food avoidance Maintain adequate dietary intake Extensive record keeping of symptoms and foods
Myasthenia gravis	Provide nutritionally dense foods at beginning of meal Small, frequent meals recommended Limit physical activity before meals Temporary feeding tube
Multiple sclerosis	Antioxidant supplements Possibly linoleic acid supplement Evaluate health status of patient Nutrition support may be needed in advanced stages Distribute fluids throughout waking hours; limit before bed
Neurotrauma	Enteral or parenteral nutrition support
Parkinson's disease	Focus on drug-nutrient interactions Minimize dietary protein at breakfast and lunch Ensure nutritionally complete diet
Pernicious anemia	Vitamin B_{12} injections Diet liberal in HBV protein Diet supplemented with Fe+, vitamin C, and B complex vitamins
Spinal trauma	Enteral/parenteral nutrition support High-fiber, adequate hydration to minimize constipation Dietary intake to maintain nutrition health and adequate weight
Stroke	Primary prevention to include dietary alterations Maintain good nutritional status Assess possible dysphagia Enteral or parenteral nutrition support may be needed
Wernicke-Korsakoff syndrome	Thiamin Adequate hydration Diet liberal in high-thiamin foods Eliminate alcohol Dietary protein may need to be restricted

care for neurologic disease are similar, regardless of the origin of the disease process.

NERVOUS SYSTEM WIRING AND LESIONS

The central nervous system (CNS) in mammals is differentiated functionally into three dimensions. This implies that lesions of the nervous system can leave a unique "calling card" of localized dysfunction. Localizing the defect (lesion) to muscle, nerve, spinal cord, or brain is part of the diagnosis. This chapter provides an emphasis on conditions with nutritionally significant dysfunction.

Nerve tracts coming to and from the brain cross to opposite sides in the CNS (Figure 43-1). Therefore a lesion in the brain that affects the right arm would be found on the left side of the brain. Signs of weakness are the most quantifiable clinical signs of nervous system disease.

The neurons in the motor strip (upper motor neurons) receive input from all parts of the brain and project their axons all the way to their destinations in the spinal cord. Here they connect to the spinal cord motor neurons (lower motor neurons). These neurons extend from the spinal cord to muscles without interruption. The location of a lesion in the central nervous system can often be deduced clinically by observing stereotypical abnormalities of either upper or lower motor neurons (Table 43-3).

Localizing Signs of Mass Lesions

The frontal lobes in the brain are the source of our most complex activities and therefore commonly offer the most complex presentations. Psychiatric manifestations such as depression, mania, or personality change may herald a tumor or other frontal lobe mass, either right or left. If the tumor is near the base of the skull, one may also lose the sense of smell or experience visual changes because the olfactory and optic nerves track along the bottom of the frontal lobes. Chemosensory losses of smell have been described in stages: anosmia (absence of smell), hyperosmia (increased sensitivity of smell), and dysomia (distortion of normal smell). Compensation for taste and smell losses with flavor-enhanced food recently has been found to improve palatability and intake, increase salivary flow and immunity, reduce chemosensory complaints in both healthy and sick elderly, and lessen the need for table salt (Schiffman and Graham, 2000).

Lesions in the central portion of the frontal lobes may present as motor apraxia. With apraxia, the patient cannot properly execute a complex activity, although he or she is strong and understands a request to perform the activity. The frontal lobes are larger

TABLE 43-2 Neurologic Syndromes Attributed to Nutritional Deficiency or Excess

NUTRITIONAL DEFICIENCY	
SITE OF MAJOR SYNDROME	NAME
Encephalon	Hypocalcemia (lack of vitamin D), tetany, seizures
	Mental retardation (protein-calorie deprivation)
	Cretinism (lack of iodine)
	Wernicke-Korsakoff syndrome (thiamin)
Corpus callosum	Marchiafava-Bignami disease
Optic nerve	Nutritional deficiency optic neuropathy ("tobacco-alcohol amblyopia")
Brain stem	Central pontine myelinolysis
Cerebellum	Alcoholic cerebellar degeneration
	Vitamin E deficiency in bowel disease
Spinal cord	Combined system disease (B_{12} deficiency)
	Tropical spastic paraparesis (some forms?)
Peripheral nerves	Beriberi (thiamin), pellagra (nicotinic acid)
	Hypophosphatemia
	Tetany (vitamin D deficiency)
Muscle	Myopathy of osteomalacia

NUTRITIONAL EXCESS		
SYNDROME	CONDITION	AGENT
Increased intracranial pressure	Self-medication	Vitamin A
Encephalopathy	Phenylketonuria	Phenylalanine
	Water intoxication	Water
	Hepatic encephalopathy	Protein (and NH_3)
	Ketotic or nonketotic coma in diabetes	Glucose
Strokes	Hyperlipidemia	Lipid
Peripheral neuropathy	Hypochondriasis	Pyridoxine
	Insomnia, anxiety	Tryptophan, contaminated
Myopathy	Anorexia nervosa, bulimia	Emetine, ipecac
Myoglobinuria	Constipation	Licorice

than normal, and the posterior portions of the frontal lobes are where the motor strips are located. Lesions here will exhibit upper motor neuron signs in the part of the body governed by this cortex. Temporal lobes control memory and speech functions; thus lesions here may affect these abilities.

Although any lesion of cerebral gray matter may produce seizures, the temporal lobes are particularly prone to seizures. Masses in the right parietal lobe may cause the patient to exhibit chronic inability to focus attention, thus completely ignoring the left side of the body. The speech centers are located near the junction of the left temporal, parietal, and frontal lobes. Pathology in this region may cause speech problems.

The occipital lobes are reserved for vision, and dysfunction here may bring about cortical blindness of varying degrees. In this condition, the patient is unaware that he or she cannot see. Lesions at other points along the visual pathway can cause several different types of visual field deficits.

Lesions of the cerebellum and brain stem may obstruct the ventricular system where it is most narrow. This obstruction may precipitate life-threatening hydrocephalus, a condition of increased intracranial pressure (ICP) that may quickly result in death. Other signs of hydrocephalus include balance, walking, and coordination abnormalities; marked sleepiness; and headache that is worse on awakening. Lesions in the brain stem may infiltrate any of the cranial nerves (Table 43-4) that enervate structures of the face and head, including the eyes, ears, jaw, tongue, pharynx, and the facial muscles. These lesions have consequences for nutrition because the patient is often unable to eat without risking aspiration of food or liquids into the lung. Tumors or other lesions in the medulla may infiltrate respiratory and cardiac centers, and dysregulation of these centers has grim consequences. Providing nutrition through other means is often necessary.

Lesions in the spinal cord are much less common than brain tumors and ordinarily cause lower motor neuron signs at the level(s) of the mass and upper motor signs in segments above the level of the mass (NIH, 2002). Spinal cord injury is the most common cause of pathology in this region. Other examples of spinal cord abnormalities are multiple sclerosis, amyotrophic lateral sclerosis (ALS), tumor, syrinx (fluid-filled neuroglial cavity), chronic meningitis, vascular insufficiency, and mass lesions of the epidural space.

Lesions of the pituitary gland and hypothalamus are often heralded by systemic manifestations that may include electrolyte and metabolic abnormalities secondary to adrenocortical, thyroid, and antidiuretic hormone dysregulation. Because of the proximity to the visual pathways, visual field, acuity, and binocular deficits are also often present. The syndrome of inappropriate secretion of antidiuretic hormone (SIADH)

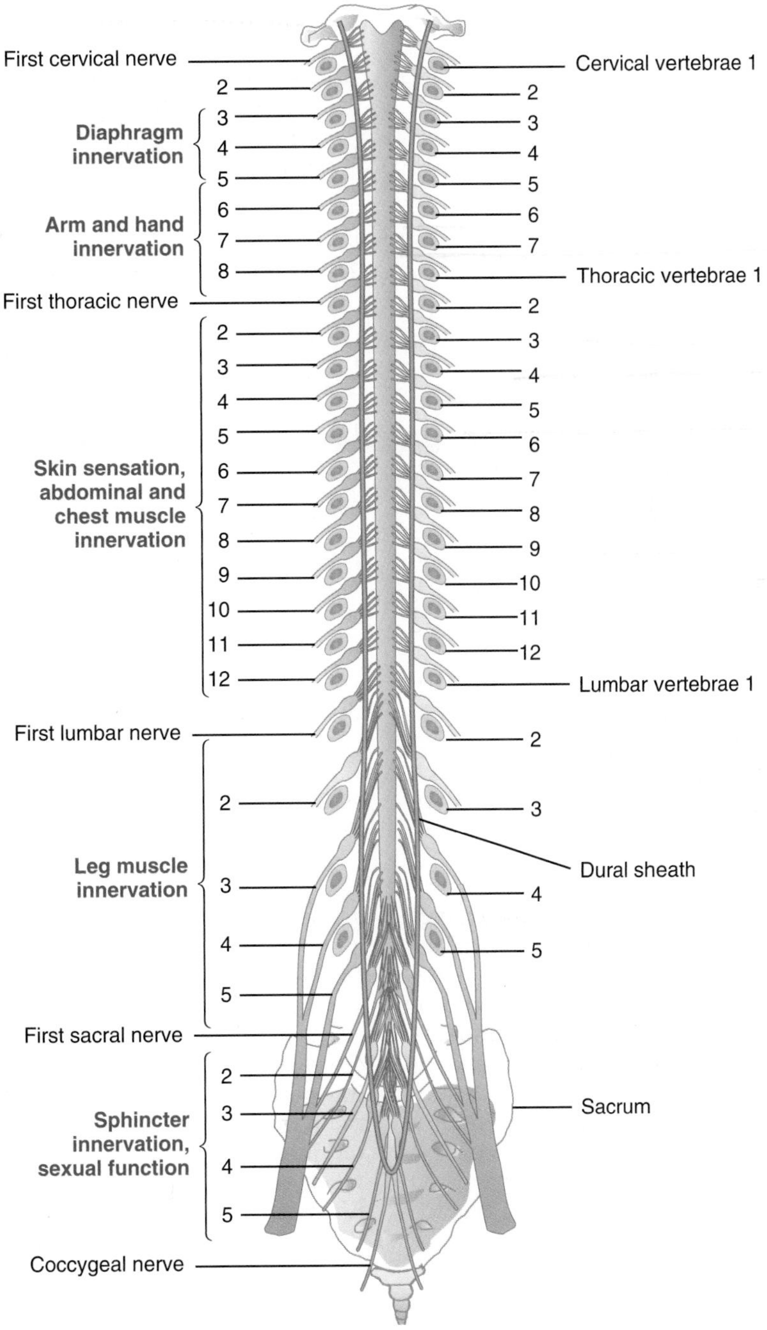

FIGURE 43-1 • Spinal cord lying within the vertebral canal. Spinal nerves are numbered on the left side; vertebrae are numbered on the right side; body areas supplied by various levels are in blue.

is often a complication, and consideration of volume status is important here; hyponatremia is essential to the diagnosis. Because the hypothalamus is the regulatory center for hunger and satiety, lesions here may present as anorexia or as overeating.

Finally, disorders of peripheral nerves and the neuromuscular junction can also affect one's ability to maintain proper nutrition. Disorders such as Guillain-Barré syndrome (GBS) (the most common acquired demyelinating neuropathy) or myasthenia gravis

TABLE 43-3 Clinical Differences Between Upper and Lower Motor Neuron Lesions

UPPER MOTOR NEURON FINDINGS	LOWER MOTOR NEURON FINDINGS
Weakness	Weakness
Stiff limbs	Floppy limbs
Sensory loss less common	Sensory loss more common
Increased reflexes	Decreased reflexes

TABLE 43-4 Basic Functions of Cranial Nerves

CRANIAL NERVE (NUMBER)	MOTOR FUNCTION	SENSORY FUNCTION
Olfactory (I)	None	Smell
Optic (II)	None	Vision
Oculomotor (III)	1. Eye movement 2. Pupil constriction	None
Trochlear (IV)	Eye movement	None
Trigeminal (V)	Mastication	1. Facial heat, cold, and touch 2. Noxious odors 3. Input for corneal reflex
Abducens (VI)	Eye movement	None
Facial (VII)	1. All muscles of facial expression 2. Corneal reflex	1. Facial pain 2. Taste on anterior two thirds of tongue
Vestibulocochlear (VIII)	None	Hearing and head acceleration and input for oculocephalic reflex
Glossopharyngeal (IX)	1. Swallowing 2. Gag reflex	Palatal, glossal, and oral sensation
Vagus (X)	1. Heart rate, GI activity, sexual function 2. Cough reflex	Taste on posterior third of tongue
Spinal accessory (XI)	1. Trapezius 2. Sternocleidomastoid	None
Hypoglossal (XII)	Tongue movement	None

(MG) may aggravate the patient's natural efforts to maintain metabolic balance. Many parts of the nervous system are required to eat and drink effectively; thus a problem at any step along the way can result in an inability to meet the body's metabolic demands.

MEDICAL NUTRITION THERAPY

The nutritional management of patients with neurologic disease is complex. Severe neurologic impairments often compromise the physical and cognitive abilities needed for adequate nourishment. Not only do many of these patients have dysphagia (difficulty swallowing), but the ability to obtain, prepare, and present food to the mouth may also be compromised. As a result, all neurologic patients are at high risk for malnutrition. Early recognition of signs and symptoms, implementation of an appropriate care plan to meet the unique nutritional requirements of the individual, and counseling for the patient and family members on dietary choices are first steps. Regular evaluation of the patient's nutritional status in relation to the disease management is essential, with the ultimate goal of improving outcomes and the patient's quality of life.

Nutrition assessment is the first step in managing the patient. It should include a detailed diet history as well as measurement and history of weight change. The diet history is helpful to assess patterns of normal chewing, swallowing, and rate of ingestion. Weight loss and history establish a baseline weight. A weight loss of 10% or more indicates nutrition risk. Anemias should be noted because the synthesis of the neurotransmitters dopamine and serotonin require adequate iron nutriture (Connor and Beard, 1997). For explicit information on nutrition assessment, refer to Chapters 17 and 18.

PROBLEMS WITH PROCUREMENT OF FOOD

With chronic neurologic diseases, a decline in function may hinder the ability for self-care. Home care services and grocery home-delivery services are being used more commonly and allow persons to remain independent in their homes for a longer period of time (Marino et al, 1998). Fulfilling nutritional needs and malnutrition are concerns, however. The procurement of food and satisfying basic needs may depend on the involvement of family, friends, or professionals. With acute neurologic situations, such as trauma, stroke, or Guillain-Barré syndrome, the entire process of eating can be interrupted abruptly and further, the patient may require enteral nutrition support for a period of time until overall function improves and eating can be resumed.

Meal Preparation

Confusion, dementia, impaired vision, or poor ambulation may also contribute to difficulty with meal preparation, thus hindering even the enjoyment of eating. An increased reliance on comfort or convenience foods such as prepackaged single servings can be encouraged as a way to maintain nourishment obtained independently.

TABLE 43-5 Common Disorders of Neurologic Diseases

SITE IN THE BRAIN	IMPAIRMENT	RESULTS
Cortical lesions of the parietal lobe (perception of sensory stimuli)	Sensory deficits	Fine regulation of muscle activities impossible if the patient is unable to perceive joint position and motion and tension of contracting muscles
Lesions of the nondominant hemisphere	Hemiinattention syndrome (neglect)	Patient neglects that side of the body
Optic tract lesions (usually of the middle cerebral artery or the artery near the internal capsule)	Visual field cuts	Patient reads one half of a page, eats from only half of the plate, and so forth (see Fig. 43-2).
Loss of subcortically stored pattern of motor skills	Apraxia	Inability to perform a previously learned task (e.g., walking, rising from a chair), but paralysis, sensory loss, spasticity, and incoordination are not present
No identification with a particular brain disorder or a specifically located lesion	Language apraxia	Inability to produce meaningful speech, even though oral muscle function is intact and language production has not been affected
Lesion of Broca's area	Nonfluent aphasia	Thought and language formulation are intact, but the patient is unable to connect them into fluent speech production
Lesion of Wernicke's area	Fluent aphasia	Flow of speech and articulation seem normal, but language output makes little or no sense
Extensive brain damage	Global aphasia	Both expression and speech perception are severely impaired
Brain stem lesions, bilateral hemispheric lesions, cerebellar disorders	Dysarthria	Inability to produce intelligible words with proper articulation

From Steinberg FU: Rehabilitating the older stroke patient: what's possible? *Geriatrics* 41:85, 1986.

Feeding Issues: Presentation of Food to the Mouth

The patient with neurologic disease may be unable to feed himself or herself because of limb weakness, poor body positioning, hemianopsia, apraxia, confusion, or neglect. The damaged region of the CNS determines the resulting disability (Table 43-5). Tremors—as with Parkinson's disease—spastic movements, or involuntary motor manifestations as occur with cerebral palsy, Huntington's disease, or tardive dyskinesia may further restrict dietary intake.

If limb weakness or paralysis occurs on the dominant side of the body, poor coordination—resulting from a new reliance on the nondominant side—may make eating difficult and unpleasant. The patient may have to adjust to eating with one hand. Small, frequent feedings can help if fatigue or early satiety is a problem. An occupational therapist may be helpful with recommendations for specific adaptive eating utensils.

Hemiparesis, or weakness that causes the body to slump toward the affected side, may increase a patient's risk of aspiration. It is important to have the patient sit as upright (at a 90 degree angle) as possible. If the patient must be in bed during mealtime, pillows can be used to bank and support the paretic side.

Hemianopsia is blindness in one half of the field of vision. The patient must learn to recognize that he or she no longer has a normal field of vision and to compensate by turning the head. Neglect indicates inattention to a weakened or paralyzed side of the body; this occurs when the nondominant (right) parietal side of the brain is affected. The patient ignores the affected body part, and his or her perception of the body's midline is shifted. Hemianopsia and neglect can occur together and severely impair the patient's function. A patient may eat only half of the contents of a meal as a result because he or she recognizes only half of it; assistance or supervision may be needed (Figure 43-2).

Another potential interference with self-feeding is apraxia, in which the patient has difficulty with perceptual motor planning. Even though the patient knows what needs to be done and has the physical ability to do it, he or she may be unable to carry out an action and follow directions. Demonstration may make it possible to do the action; however, judgment may be affected as well and can result in the performance of dangerous tasks. This makes leaving the patient alone unsafe.

Eating: The Oral Process

Dysphagia, or difficulty in swallowing, may accompany neurologic disease. Symptoms of dysphagia include drooling, choking, or coughing during or following meals; inability to suck from a straw; a gurgly voice quality; holding pockets of food in the buccal recesses (of which the patient may be unaware); absent gag reflex; and chronic upper respiratory infections. Weight loss and anorexia are features of nutritional concern. Dysphagia often leads to malnutrition because of inadequate intake. Environmental distractions and conversations during mealtime increase the risk for aspiration and should be curtailed. See

Appendix 55 for the different stages of the National Dysphagia Diet.

Reports of coughing and unusually long mealtimes are often associated with tongue, facial, and masticator muscle weakness. Observation during meals allows the nurse or dietitian to screen informally for signs of dysphagia problems and bring them to the attention of the health care team. Changing the consistency of foods served may be beneficial. A swallowing evaluation by a speech pathologist is in order. Patients with late- or intermediate-stage Parkinson's disease, multiple sclerosis, amyotrophic lateral sclerosis (ALS), dementia, or stroke are particularly at risk.

Swallowing

Proper position for effective swallowing should be encouraged (i.e., sitting bolt upright with the head in a chin-down position). Concentrating on the swallowing process can also help reduce choking.

Initiation of the swallow begins voluntarily but is completed reflexively. Normal swallowing allows for safe and easy passage of food from the oral cavity through the pharynx and esophagus into the stomach by propulsive muscular force with some benefit from gravity. The process of swallowing can be organized into three phases, as shown in Figure 43-3.

Oral Phase

During the preparatory and oral phases of swallowing, food is placed in the mouth, where it is combined with saliva, chewed if necessary, and formed into a bolus by the tongue. The tongue pushes the food to the rear of the oral cavity by gradually squeezing it backward against the hard and soft palate (see Figure 43-3). Increased intracranial pressure (ICP) or cranial nerve damage may result in weakened or poorly coordinated tongue movements and lead to problems in completing the oral phase of swallowing. Weakened lip muscles result in the inability to completely seal the lips, form a seal around a cup, or suck through a straw. Patients are embarrassed by drooling and may not want to eat in front of others. The patient may have difficulty forming a cohesive bolus and moving it through the oral cavity. Food can become pocketed in the buccal recesses, especially if cheek sensation is lost or facial weakness exists.

Pharyngeal Phase

The pharyngeal phase is initiated when the bolus is propelled past the faucial arches. Four events must occur in rapid succession during this phase. The soft palate elevates to close off the nasopharynx and prevent oropharyngeal regurgitation. The hyoid and larynx elevate, and the vocal cords adduct to protect the airway. The pharynx sequentially contracts while the cricopharyngeal sphincter relaxes to allow the food to pass into the esophagus. Breathing resumes at the end of the pharyngeal phase. Symptoms of poor coordination during this phase include gagging, choking, and nasopharyngeal regurgitation.

Esophageal Phase

The final or esophageal phase, during which the bolus continues through the esophagus into the stomach, is completely involuntary. Difficulties that occur

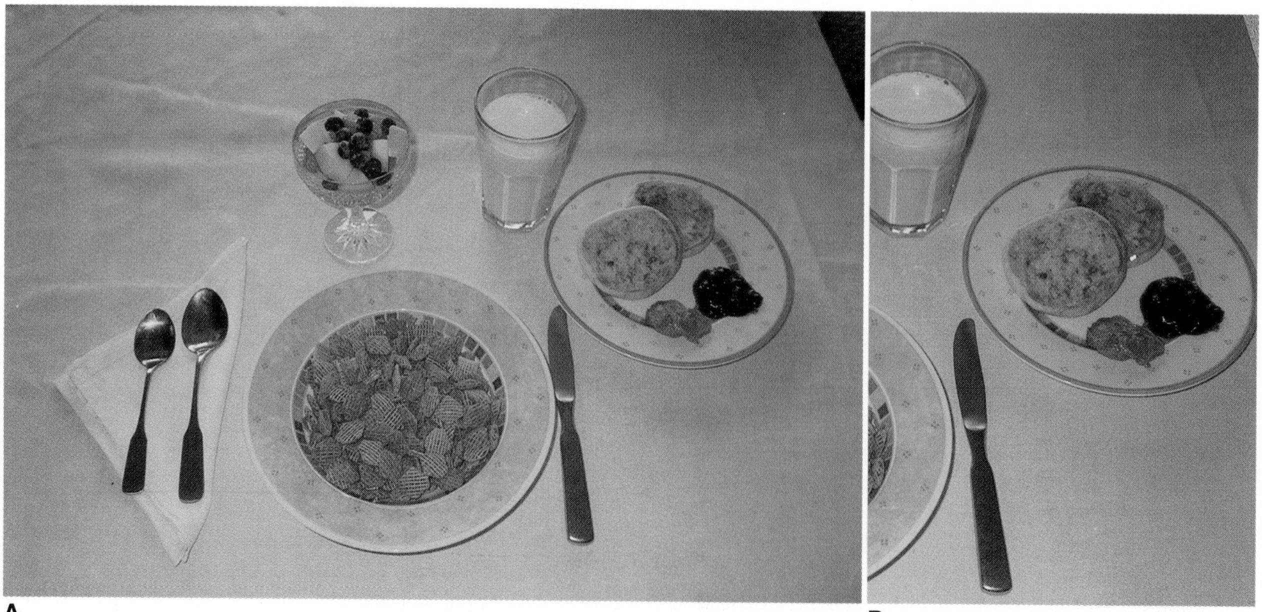

A B

FIGURE 43-2 • **A,** Normal vision. **B,** Vision with hemianopsia.

during this phase are generally the result of a mechanical obstruction, but neurologic disease cannot be ruled out. For example, impaired peristalsis can arise from a brain stem infarct.

Liquids

Swallowing liquids of thin consistency (including water) requires the most coordination and control. Liquids are easily aspirated into the lungs and may pose a life-threatening event because aspiration pneumonia may ensue, even from sterile water in the lungs. Sterile water is no longer sterile once it is introduced to the bacterial load of the oral cavity. If a patient has difficulty consuming thin liquids, fluid requirements may be met by thickening liquids. Liquids of all types can be thickened with nonfat dry milk powder, cornstarch, modular carbohydrate supplements, or commercial thickeners that contain a modified cornstarch thickener, such as Thick-It or Thick-n-Easy.

Thick liquids that contain a high percentage of water need to be emphasized to maintain fluid balance. Fatigue and malaise often are associated with a "mild chronic dehydration" that results from decreased fluid intake. Popsicles, ice, and fresh fruit are additional sources of free water. Encourage use of noncaffeinated beverage sources because caffeine has a diuretic effect that further contributes to dehydration, fatigue, and thickened saliva.

Milk is considered a liquid with unique properties. Some people associate consumption of milk with symptoms of excess mucus production; however, no statistically significant data have proven a link between milk or dairy products and symptoms of mucus production (Arney and Pinnock, 1993). The dysphagic patient, however, often reports increased phlegm after milk consumption, which may actually be a consequence of poor swallowing ability rather than mucus production. Patients are encouraged to "chase" the milk products with appropriately thickened liquids to help flush the throat, rather than to eliminate dairy products.

Neurogenic bladder (the main feature is urinary retention) is a common sign and management issue in patients with a myelopathy, or spinal cord injury. This predisposes the individual to urinary tract infections and miscalculation of fluid balance. Alter-

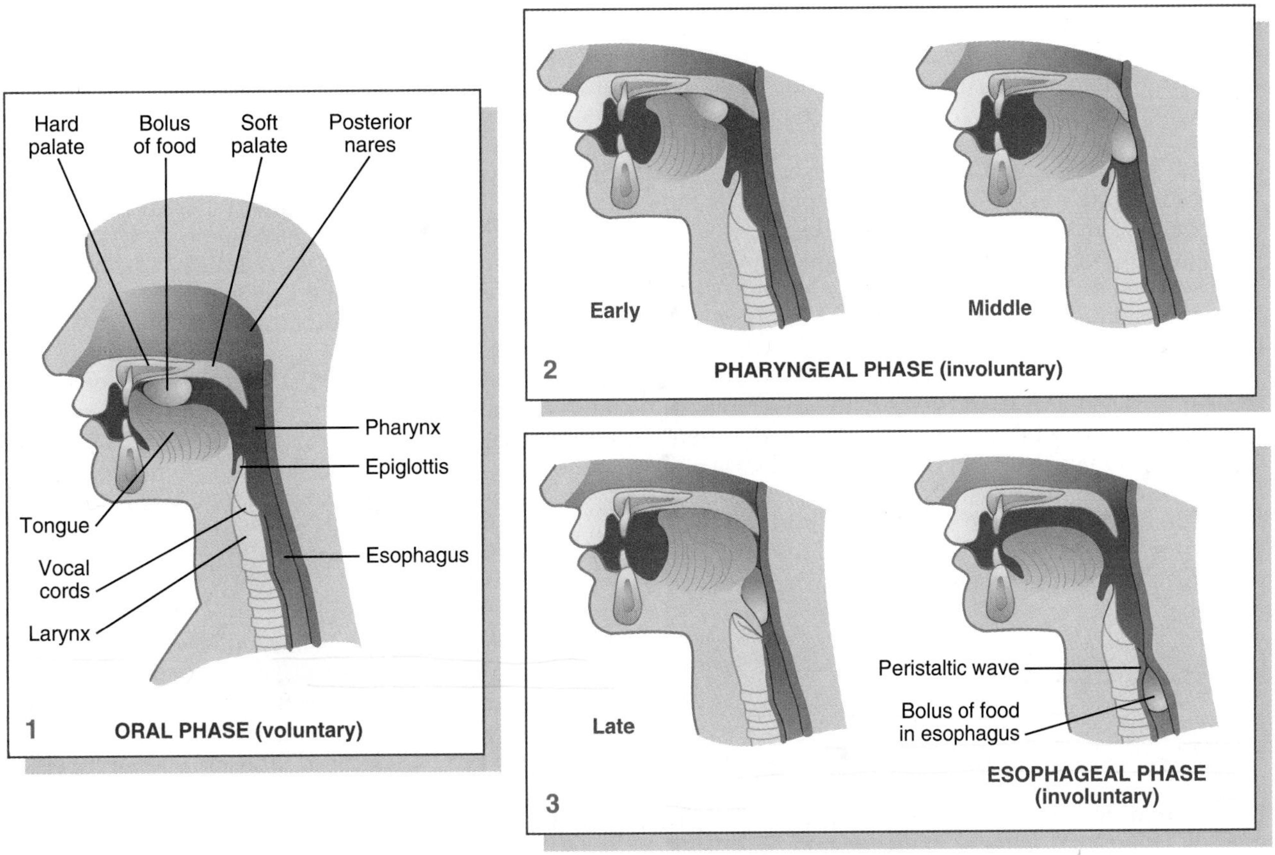

FIGURE 43-3 • Swallowing occurs in three phases: (1) Voluntary or oral phase. Tongue presses food against the hard palate, forcing it toward the pharynx; (2) Involuntary, pharyngeal phase. *Early:* wave of peristalsis forces a bolus between the tonsillar pillars. *Middle:* soft palate draws upward to close posterior nares, and respirations cease momentarily. *Late:* vocal cords approximate, and the larynx pulls upward, covering the airway and stretching the esophagus open; (3) Involuntary, esophageal phase. Relaxation of the upper esophageal (hypopharyngeal) sphincter allows the peristaltic wave to move the bolus down the esophagus.

nately, myelopathy and spinal cord injury may result in urinary urgency, frequency, and incontinence. To minimize these problems, distributing fluids evenly throughout the waking hours and limiting them before bedtime is helpful. Some patients limit fluid intake severely to decrease urgency or frequent urination. This practice increases the risk of urinary tract infection (UTI) and is not recommended. One nontraumatic source of myelopathy and neurogenic bladder is multiple sclerosis (MS), an unpredictable severe, progressive disease of the central nervous system. Individuals with MS (women are affected more often than men) have a higher incidence of UTIs. Increased intake of cranberry juice may reduce the frequency of UTIs (see Chapter 39).

Textures

As chronic disease progresses, cranial nerves become damaged, thus leading to neurologic deficits manifested by dysphagia and possible elimination of entire food groups. Nutrition intervention should be individualized according to the type and extent of dysfunction. Vitamin and mineral supplementation may be necessary. If chewable supplements are not handled safely, liquid forms may be added to acceptable foods. The dietitian can ensure that the diet remains palatable and nutritionally adequate by recommending changes in food consistency to mechanical soft or a pureed consistency to reduce the need for oral manipulation and to conserve energy while eating. Box 43-1 describes key points of the National Dysphagia Diet (see Appendix 55).

Small, frequent meals may also encourage increased intake. Swallowing can also be improved by emphasizing the taste, texture, and temperature of foods. Juices can be substituted for water and will provide taste, nutrients, and calories. A cool temperature facilitates the swallowing mechanism; therefore cold food items may be better tolerated. Carbonation may also be better tolerated because of the beneficial effect of texture. Sauces and gravies lubricate foods for ease in swallowing and can help prevent fragmentation of foods within the oral cavity. Moist pastas, casseroles, and egg dishes are well tolerated.

Nutrition Support

Patients with acute and chronic neurologic diseases may benefit from nutrition support. For acute disease, nutrition support may be required in the early term until a degree of function is regained, whereas chronic neurologic disease may require nutrition support in the late stages of the disease to meet changing metabolic demands. Nutrition support helps to avert complications of aspiration, pneumonia, or sepsis, which can compound the deteriorating effects of these diseases.

Enteral tube feedings may be necessary if the risk of aspiration from eating is high or if the patient cannot eat enough to meet nutritional needs. In the latter case, nocturnal tube feedings can bridge the gap between oral intake and actual nutritional requirements. This should allow the normal sensation of hunger to be generated and provide freedom from tube feeding during the day.

In most instances, the gastrointestinal tract function remains intact, and enteral nutrition is the preferred method of support. One noted exception occurs after spinal cord injury. In this instance, ileus is common for 7 to 10 days after the insult, and parenteral nutrition may be needed.

Although a nasogastric tube can be a short-term option, a percutaneous endoscopic gastrostomy (PEG) tube or gastrostomy-jejunostomy (PEG-J) tube placed with the patient under local anesthesia is preferred for long-term management. These should be considered for patients whose swallowing function is inadequate to ensure nutritional health (see Chapter 23). Malnutrition itself can produce neuromuscular weakness and thereby adversely affect quality of life; it is therefore a prognostic factor for poor survival.

In the acute care setting, when a previously well-nourished individual is unable to resume oral alimentation within 7 days, nutrition support may be required to prevent decline in nutrition health and to aid recovery. For the majority of patients, this intervention is commonly used until oral nourishment can be resumed. Conversely, in the chronic care setting, nutrition support is an issue that each patient eventually must address because it may result in prolonged therapy. However, adequate nutrition can prolong the health of the individual and may be a welcome relief to the patient who has become overburdened with the difficulties of sustenance.

Malnutrition was cited in 16% to 50% of ALS patients (Desport et al, 2000). Although the effect on survival may be controversial, one study of patients with amyotrophic lateral sclerosis (ALS) demonstrated improved survival after 6 months of nutritional support via PEG (Mazzini et al, 1995). A hypermetabolic status for ALS patients was confirmed by using resting energy expenditure measurements, which means that these patients require more calories than usual (Desport et al, 2001).

Some patients may decline, however, with early placement of a feeding tube because of the emotional, economic, or physical impact of this choice. In advanced stages of disease one may refuse tube feedings, choosing not to prolong life. Nutrition support should enhance the quality of life, and the health care team has an important role in alleviating patient and family concerns and fostering informed decisions (Mitsumoto and Del Bene, 2000). The patient needs to be fully informed about the impact of a tube feeding on daily life. Discussion of both the advantages and the disadvantages of nutritional support should be initiated with the patient and family well ahead of need; options

Box 43-1. Guidelines for Feeding the Dysphagic Patient

Part One: The Dysphagia Outcome and Severity Scale

Full PO: Normal Diet

Level 7: Normal in All Situations

- Normal diet
- No strategies or extra time needed

Level 6: Within Functional Limits/Modified Independence

- Normal diet, functional swallow
- Patient may have mild oral or pharyngeal delay, retention, or trace epiglottal undercoating but *independently and spontaneously* compensates and clears
- May need extra time for meal
- No aspiration with different consistencies

Full PO: Modified Diet and Independence

Level 5: Mild Dysphagia: Distant Supervision; May Need One Diet Consistency Restricted

May exhibit one or more of the following:

- Aspiration of thin liquids only but with strong reflexive cough to clear completely
- Airway penetration midway to cords or to cords with one consistency but *clears spontaneously*
- Retention in pharynx that is *cleared spontaneously*
- Mild oral dysphagia with reduced mastication or oral retention that is *cleared spontaneously*

Level 4: Mild-Moderate Dysphagia: Intermittent Supervision/Cueing; One to Two Diet Consistencies Restricted

May exhibit one or more of the following:

- Retention in pharynx that is *cleared with cue*
- Retention in the oral cavity that is *cleared with cue*
- Aspiration with one consistency, airway penetration to the level of the vocal cords *with cough* with two consistencies, or airway penetration to the level of the vocal cords *without cough* with one consistency

Level 3: Moderate Dysphagia: Total Assist, Supervision, or Strategies; Two or More Diet Consistencies Restricted

May exhibit one or more of the following:

- Moderate retention in pharynx that is *cleared with cue*
- Moderate retention on oral cavity that is *cleared with cue*
- Airway penetration to the level of the vocal cords *without cough* with two or more consistencies or aspiration with two consistencies

Nonoral Nutrition Necessary

Level 2: Moderately Severe Dysphagia: Maximum Assistance or Maximum Use of Strategies With Partial PO Only

May exhibit one or more of the following:

- Severe retention on pharynx, *unable to clear or needs multiple cues*
- Severe oral stage bolus loss or retention, *unable to clear or needs multiple cues*
- Aspiration with two or more consistencies, *no reflexive cough, and weak volitional cough;* or aspiration with one or more consistencies, *no cough,* and airway penetration to cords with one or more consistencies, *no cough*

Level 1: Severe Dysphagia: NPO: Unable to Tolerate Any PO Safely

May exhibit one or more of the following:

- Severe retention in pharynx, *unable to clear*
- Severe oral stage bolus loss or retention, *unable to clear*
- Silent aspiration with two or more consistencies, nonfunctional volitional cough or unable to achieve swallow

Part Two: Techniques for Improving Acceptance

Feeding individuals with dysphagia requires extra care and consideration. Food is enjoyed with all of the senses. Pureed meals need to look good, smell good, and taste good. Here are some ideas to improve the sensory experience for those with dysphagia. Start simple and build a puree program to be creative and serve attractive meals.

Aroma

- Good-smelling food and a pleasant atmosphere may increase appetite and improve consumption.
- Serve foods seasoned with aromatic ingredients such as garlic, pepper, onions, and cinnamon.

Seasoning

- Individuals with dysphagia often have a dulled sense of taste.
- Taste all foods and adjust seasoning as needed.
- Serve foods that have stronger flavors such as chili, spaghetti, and apple pie.

Layering/Swirling

- Swirling vegetables together is simple and makes a great plate presentation; peas and carrots are striking together and taste great.
- Use standardized recipes to make attractive layered casseroles such as shepherd's pie, lasagna, or chicken á la king.

Piping

- Place pureed food into a pastry bag and pipe for a lovely plate presentation.
- Simple and fun with pureed pasta.

Molding

- To mold, use a thickener or a shaping or enhancing product.
- For hot foods: prepare per recipe, freeze and heat to temperature before serving.
- For cold foods: prepare per recipe, freeze, set on plate, and serve (will thaw quickly).

Modified from the American Dietetic Association: *National dysphagia diet: standardization for optimal care,* Chicago, 2003, ADA.

Continued

Box 43-1. Guidelines for Feeding the Dysphagic Patient—cont'd

Part Two: Techniques for Improving Acceptance—cont'd

Slurries

- Prepare a slurry with thickener and juice or milk.
- Prepare a slurry with a liquid that goes well with the food being prepared.
- Slurry shortcake with juice and serve with pureed strawberries.
- Slurry sugar cookies with milk.
- Slurries work well with biscuits, cakes, graham crackers, muffins, and brownies.

Garnishing

- Garnishing is often overlooked but makes a big visual impact.
- Only garnish with foods appropriate for the diet consistency.
- Use sauces, gravies, and syrups and try putting in squeeze bottles and decorating plates.
- Pipe garnishes around edges such as piping lettuce around the edge of a pureed sandwich.
- Cut shapes out of cranberry sauce and serve with turkey.

These are a few simple ideas to keep in mind when serving modified-consistency foods. Beautiful plate presentations and good-tasting foods will help maintain good consumption and ultimately good nutritional status. Resident and patient dignity is very important. Good-looking and good-tasting food can help people feel more dignified.

Modified from the American Dietetic Association: *National dysphagia diet: standardization for optimal care,* Chicago, 2003, ADA.

should include a description of feeding schedules, tube placement procedures, and appropriate training.

NEUROLOGIC DISEASES ARISING FROM NUTRITIONAL DEFICIENCIES OR EXCESSES

Primary Prevention Strategies: Beriberi and Pellagra

The major manifestations of thiamin deficiency in humans involve the cardiovascular (wet beriberi) and nervous (dry beriberi, neuropathy, and/or Wernicke-Korsakoff syndrome) systems (Singleton and Martin, 2001). Pellagra is another condition that affects the nervous system; it is less common in the United States today than decades ago because of the variety of foods consumed (see Chapter 4).

Pernicious Anemia

Historically, pernicious anemia and vitamin B_{12} (cobalamin) deficiencies have been the more common neurologic syndromes caused by a single nutrient. The classic triad of anemia, neurologic deficits, and epithelial atrophy of the tongue was well recognized at the turn of the century. Until 1926, when replacement therapy was introduced, the term "pernicious" appropriately described the outcome of events for those afflicted with this disease: "destructive, harmful, and fatal." Consumption of liver was prescribed empirically, and only in 1948 was vitamin B_{12} recognized as the healing agent (Rowland, 1995).

Given the technology for measuring vitamin B_{12} levels in the blood, early detection during the preclinical phase of disease is the rule. As a result, pernicious anemia is rarely seen in medical centers in developed countries. For those who develop pernicious anemia, only 20% are younger than age 50; most are over 60. The effectiveness of diagnosis and treatment has been remarkable. Over 90% of symptomatic patients regain independence in conducting activities of daily living (ADL) (see Chapter 34 on anemias).

Pathophysiology

In the nervous system, lesions occur initially in the myelin sheaths of optic nerves, cerebral white matter, and peripheral nerves. Conceivably, the presence of abnormal fatty acids may explain the structural changes observed in central and peripheral myelin of these patients (Adams et al, 1997).

Medical Treatment

Most neurologic manifestations of vitamin B_{12} deficiency are associated with the typical macrocytic anemia of pernicious anemia. General weakness, especially paresthesia, constitutes the earliest and most common symptoms, with tingling or the feeling of "pins and needles" in hands or feet. This tends to be constant and steadily progressive. If left untreated, the following signs may ensue: dysgeusia (impaired taste), impaired gait, spasticity, and contracture; mental signs of irritability, apathy, somnolence, emotional instability, marked confusion, and depression; and visual impairment. Fortunately, for the majority of patients today, the disease is detected before neurologic symptoms or signs develop.

Early diagnosis of pernicious anemia can be somewhat complicated, however, because hematologic and neurologic signs do not always correlate. A significant component of primary prevention is the determination of serum vitamin B_{12} because it is the best, most readily available test for evaluating vitamin B_{12} status. Serum levels less than 150 pg/ml are considered to represent deficiency (Beers and Berkow, 1999). Chapter 18 offers more information about available tests.

The duration of symptoms before treatment is the factor most likely to influence treatment response; neurologic manifestations that occur in less than 3 months are rapidly and completely reversible. Amelioration of symptoms occurring between 6 to 12 months is variable, and in extreme cases, arrest of disease progression is the most that can be accomplished. Prompt initiation of therapy is imperative. Monthly maintenance doses of cyanocobalamin are administered for life if lack of intrinsic factor is apparent (see Chapter 34).

Medical Nutrition Therapy

For the majority of individuals with pernicious anemia, inadequate dietary intake of vitamin B_{12} is unrelated to this disease; most have inadequate absorption. It is recommended that in addition to the injections of vitamin B_{12}, the diet be liberal in use of high–biologic value proteins and supplemented with iron, vitamin C, and other B vitamins (including folic acid).

Wernicke-Korsakoff Syndrome

Wernicke-Korsakoff syndrome (WKS) is a disease of the cerebellum and brain stem that results from chronic thiamin deficiency with continued carbohydrate ingestion. It most commonly occurs in alcoholics and is one of the gravest consequences of alcoholism (Singleton and Martin, 2001). WKS is actually two separate diseases—Wernicke's encephalopathy and Korsakoff's psychosis; their common association has led to inclusion into one syndrome with characteristic memory defects.

The incidence of WKS may be underreported because it is often undiagnosed. Alcoholism is more prevalent in the homeless populations, in which access to medical care is limited. Because clinical findings are subtle, diagnosis of WKS is often made at autopsy. The rat model has also shown that chronic alcohol intake interferes with retinoid metabolism and signaling (Wang, 1999).

Although the epidemiology of WKS cannot be precisely quantified, the risk factors can be accurately described. In North America and Europe, this nutritional disorder is the most commonly encountered manifestation acquired from thiamin deficiency; it often develops after severe or repeated attacks of postalcoholic delirium tremens. It has also been seen in patients who are nutritionally depleted from anorexia nervosa, gastrointestinal disease, or HIV infection. It also may follow ischemic stroke or subarachnoid or thalamic hemorrhage.

Pathophysiology

Thiamin deficiency is the accepted primary cause of WKS. Depletion of body stores of thiamin can occur rapidly, within 7 to 8 weeks, especially in alcoholics. The pathology in this acute and severe nutritional deficiency is restricted to the CNS, but not all regions of the nervous system are affected equally (Langlais, 1996).

The exact relationship between the lesions induced by thiamin deficiency and their effect on the brain remains unclear. However, one certain thing is the effect of treatment on outcome. Wernicke's encephalopathy is responsive to thiamin, whereas Korsakoff's psychosis is not; unfortunately, the mental derangements precipitated by Korsakoff's psychosis are irreversible.

Medical Treatment

Wernicke's disease is characterized by the "classic triad" of disturbances in mentation (encephalopathy), vision (nystagmus), and gait (ataxia), but they are present simultaneously in only 10% to 33% of cases (Greenberg, 1997). This is one reason why clinical diagnosis is deferred until confirmed at autopsy.

Korsakoff's psychosis presents as an amnesia, a confabulatory mental disorder in which retentive memory is significantly impaired in comparison with other cognitive functions. Memory is diminished; the patient is unable to learn new things; conceptual or perceptual functions decline; and as the disease progresses, confabulation is less apparent.

Treatment with thiamin should be started immediately, and adequate hydration should be provided if WKS is suspected. Thiamin is administered prophylactically to alcoholics to prevent disease progression and even to reverse the brain abnormalities that are not yet permanent changes. From 50 to 100 mg of parenteral thiamin should be administered for several days because of the possibility of coexisting gastrointestinal malabsorption.

Glucose must never be given before thiamin because sudden increases in brain glucose levels may precipitate symptoms of WKS in patients with marginal thiamin reserves. Glucose and metabolic stress also increase requirements for thiamin (Adams et al, 1997).

The response to therapy depends on the conversion of thiamin to its active form in the liver. With concomitant liver disease, response may be delayed. Ophthalmologic symptoms generally respond rapidly to thiamin, whereas ataxia and encephalopathy respond more slowly. Mental deficits of Korsakoff's psychosis do not improve. A decrease in erythrocyte transketolase activity correlates well with improvement in the clinical picture, as a normal value is a sensitive measure of adequate thiamin nutriture.

Medical Nutrition Therapy

First and foremost, the nutritional deficiency should be corrected if possible. With thiamin deficiency, not only should therapeutic supplementation be administered, but nutrient-dense foods containing thiamin, such as whole-grain or enriched breads and cereals, should be incorporated into the diet as well. Alcohol must be eliminated.

Because no singular food item contains large amounts of thiamin, one serving of a nutrient-dense food item contributes about 10% of an individual's daily need. A diet of a variety of food items is required to ensure that the recommended dietary allowance (RDA) for thiamin is met (see Chapter 4). In the presence of concomitant encephalopathy, repletion of dietary protein may be limited or restricted. For a complete discussion of nutritional therapy in liver disease, refer to Chapter 31.

Stroke

Stroke is the most rampant clinical entity of cerebrovascular disease in developed countries. It is defined as an acute onset of focal or global neurologic deficit that lasts more than 24 hours and is attributable to diseases of the intracranial or extracranial neurovasculature. Severe strokes are often preceded by transient ischemic attacks (TIAs).

Stroke is the third most common cause of death in the United States and, after Alzheimer's disease, is the second most common cause of neurologic disability (Beers and Berkow, 1999). Old age is the most significant risk factor. Among modifiable risk factors, hypertension and smoking contribute most to the risk of stroke. Other factors include coronary heart disease; atrial fibrillation; diabetes; and oral contraceptive use, particularly by female smokers.

Stroke is a disease of the twentieth century that in large part has resulted from tobacco use and obesity. Although the incidence of stroke has declined over the last 30 years, it appears now to have leveled off. The National Stroke Association is reported to estimate the cost of stroke for the United States to be about $43 billion a year; direct costs for medical care and therapy average $28 billion a year (NIH, 2002). This high cost may be attributed in part to the high degree of disability imparted by cerebrovascular events.

Pathophysiology

Eighty-five percent of strokes are incited by a thromboembolic event, which may be aggravated by atherosclerosis, hypertension, diabetes, and gout (Figure 43-4).

Embolic stroke occurs when a cholesterol plaque is dislodged from a proximal vessel and travels to the brain and blocks an artery, most commonly the middle cerebral artery (MCA). In patients with dysfunctional cardiac atria, clots may be dislodged from there and embolize. In thrombotic stroke, a cholesterol plaque within an artery ruptures, and platelets subsequently aggregate to clog an already narrowed artery.

Intracranial hemorrhage is less common (15% of strokes) but more often fatal immediately. Both varieties of intracranial hemorrhage occur more commonly in individuals with hypertension. The first is intraparenchymal hemorrhage. Among patients with intraparenchymal hemorrhage, the prevalence of hypertension is 80%. This event occurs when a vessel inside the brain ruptures. A variation of intraparenchymal hemorrhage is a lacunar (from the Latin *lacus,* or *lake* or *deep pool*) infarct. These smaller infarcts occur in the deep structures of the brain, such as the internal capsule, basal ganglia, pons, thalamus, and cerebellum. Even a small lacunar infarct can produce significant disability because the brain tissue in the deep structures is so densely functional.

The second type of intracranial hemorrhage is subarachnoid hemorrhage (SAH). This occurs most commonly as a result of head trauma but almost as often as a result of a ruptured aneurysm of a vessel in the subarachnoid space. Ruptured aneurysms more commonly result in clinically significant SAH than trauma does.

Medical Treatment

The medical history can give some evidence about the mechanism of a new infarct. Hemorrhage is suspected when the patient presents with headache, decreased level of consciousness, and vomiting, all of which evolve over minutes to hours. A thromboembolic stroke is more likely when the patient is fully conscious but onset of motor or sensory findings occurs suddenly (Greenberg, 1997). As with all neurologic disease, the clinical presentation depends on the location of the abnormality. An infarction of a particular cerebrovascular territory can be suspected by seeking out various constellations of neurologic deficits. A middle cerebral artery (MCA) occlusion will betray itself by producing paresis and sensory deficits of limbs on the opposite side of the body because this artery supplies the motor and sensory strips. If the left MCA is occluded, aphasias may also be present.

In the past, treatment for embolic stroke was supportive; it focused on prevention of further brain infarction and rehabilitation. Recently, use of thrombolytic or "clot-busting" drugs has allowed reversal of brain ischemia by lysing thromboembolic clots in selected patients. Evaluation and initiation of therapy needs to occur within 6 hours of the onset of symptoms. Use of aspirin may be of some value in preventing further cerebrovascular events, but its effectiveness has not yet been demonstrated definitively.

Controlling intracranial pressure (ICP) while maintaining sufficient perfusion of the brain is the treatment for intracranial hemorrhage. This may include surgical evacuation of large volumes of intracranial blood, ventricular drainage, or other neurosurgical interventions. Rehabilitation is a key component of therapy. Hemorrhage—particularly SAH—commonly has more severe functional consequences and therefore has a longer period of convalescence than ischemic stroke.

Medical Nutrition Therapy

Primary prevention is the cornerstone for managing stroke. This can be accomplished in part by dietary means as well as by other lifestyle behaviors (Feldman, 2001). These nutrition-related factors have shown a salutory effect on reducing the incidence of stroke and have been compiled from various large population-based prospective studies (Box 43-2).

Given the prevalence of stroke and its associated burden of disease, treatment for those afflicted with this disease cannot be ignored. The average cost per patient for the first 90 days after a stroke is reported to be $15,000 with 10% of patients incurring costs ex-

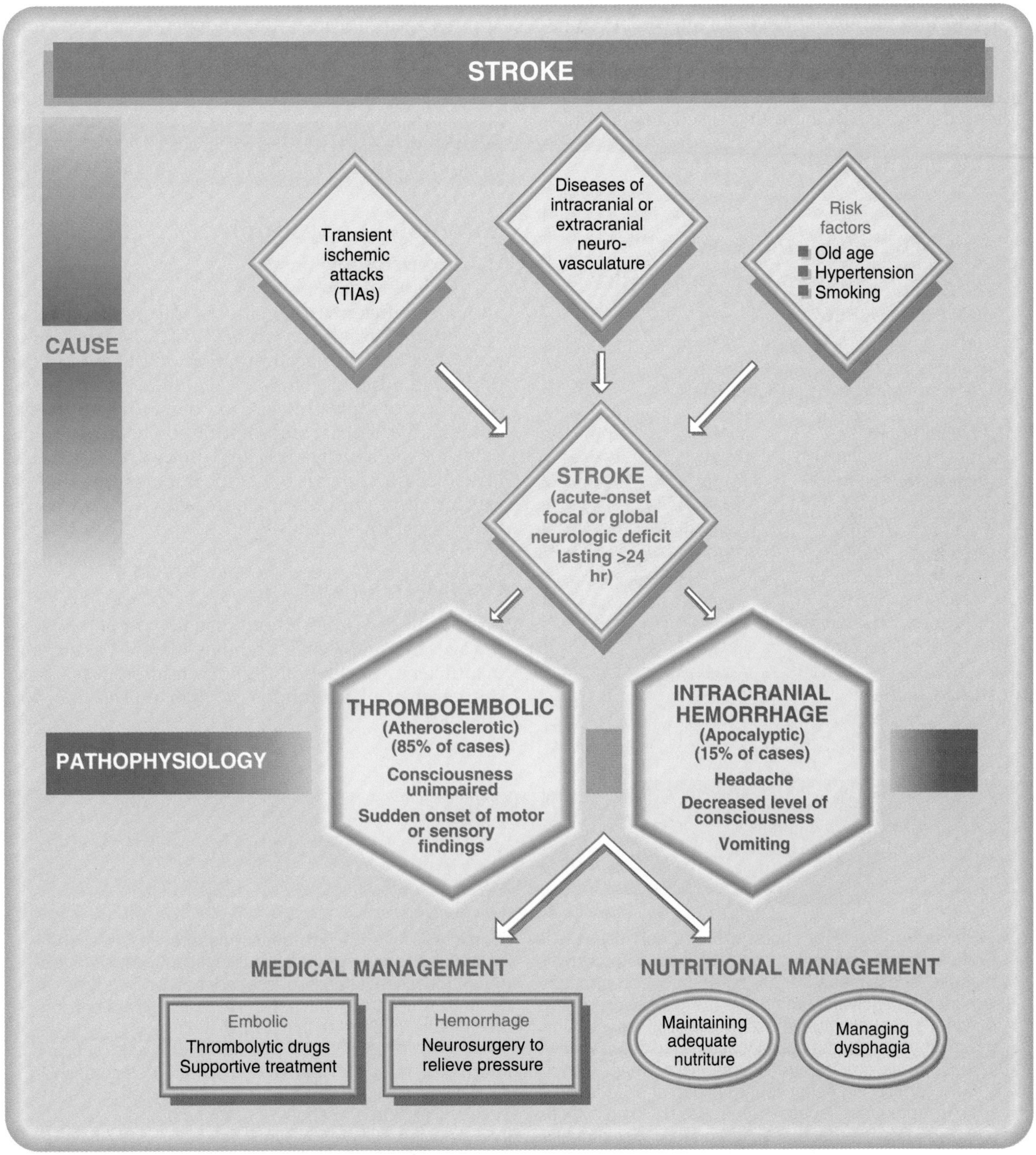

FIGURE 43-4 • Pathophysiology algorithm: stroke. (Algorithm content developed by John Anderson, PhD, and Sanford C. Garner, PhD, 2000.)

ceeding $35,000 (NIH, 2002). Malnutrition predicts a poor outcome. Once stroke does occur, dietary reduction of cholesterol, fat, and salt is of questionable benefit. Efforts should be directed toward maintaining the overall health of the patient. Under ideal circumstances, nutritional status would be maintained; however, even in the presence of adequate intake, nutriture of the patient is not always guaranteed (Davalos et al, 1996) (Box 43-2; see Appendix 55).

Feeding difficulties are determined by the extent of the stroke and the area of the brain affected. Dysphagia, an independent predictor of mortality, commonly accompanies stroke and contributes to complications and poor outcome from increased malnutrition, pulmonary infections, disability, increased length of hospital stay, and institutional care (Mann et al, 1999). Patients admitted to the hospital after stroke who exhibit difficulties chewing or swallowing should be promptly evaluated for dysphagia, and dietary interventions should be implemented accordingly.

In some instances, nutrition support is temporarily required to maintain nutritional health until oral alimentation can be resumed. As motor functions improve, eating and other activities of daily living are fundamental to the patient's rehabilitation process and necessary for resuming independence (see *Focus On:* Cholesterol and Stroke).

Box 43-2. Nutrition-Related Factors and Stroke Risk

Risk Factors for Stroke

BMI >27 kg/m^2 in women
Weight gain >11 kg over 16 years in women
Waist-to-hip ratio >0.92 in men
Diabetes
Hypertension
Cholesterol in hemorrhagic stroke

Protective Factors for Stroke

High intake of total dietary fat
Daily consumption of fresh fruit
Flavonoid consumption >4.7 cups green tea/daily
Fish consumption in white and black women and black men
Cholesterol in ischemic stroke

BMI, Body mass index.

NEUROLOGIC DISEASES WITH NONNUTRITION ETIOLOGIES

Adrenoleukodystrophy

Pathophysiology

Adrenoleukodystrophy (ALD) is a rare congenital enzyme deficiency that affects the metabolism of very-long-chain fatty acids (VLCFAs) in young men. This leads to accumulation of VLCFAs in the brain and adrenal glands. The mental and physical deterioration progresses to dementia, aphasia, apraxia, dysarthria, and blindness. The incidence is 1/20,000 male births. It is an X-linked recessive disorder characterized by skin hyperpigmentation, myelopathy, peripheral neuropathy, and cerebral demyelination.

Medical Treatment

First clinical manifestations usually occur between the ages of 4 and 8 years and may manifest as adrenal insufficiency or cerebral decompensation. Dysarthria (impairment of the tongue or other muscles needed

FOCUS ON

Cholesterol and Stroke

Although the role of cholesterol in heart disease is well known, its role in predisposing some individuals to stroke is less clear. Dietary cholesterol and monounsaturated and polyunsaturated fat are not always related to risk of any stroke subtype. Low intake of saturated fat and animal protein has actually been associated with an increased risk of intraparenchymal hemorrhage, which is more common in Asian countries (Iso et al, 2001).

Data from the Diabetes Control and Complications Trial (DCCT) show that those individuals under intensive treatment for diabetes had nearly one half the number of cerebrovascular events as conventionally treated patients (DCCT, 1995). Low-density lipoproteins, total cholesterol, and triglycerides were significantly lower in the group receiving intensive treatment. This suggests a beneficial effect of intensive diabetes treatment on macrovascular disease in type 2 diabetes.

Current research will continue to delineate cholesterol's role in stroke and will guide future recommendations on cholesterol reduction (Barzilay et al, 2001; Meigs et al, 2002). It should be remembered, however, that reducing elevated serum cholesterol does have a proven role in preventing coronary artery disease.

for speech) or dysphagia may interfere with oral alimentation. Bronzing of the skin is a late clinical sign. In the face of adrenal insufficiency, physiologic replacement of steroids, which may improve neurologic symptoms and prolong life, is indicated. Numerous therapies have been directed at the root of the disorder but have been disappointing. The selective use of bone marrow transplant is one current therapy, and gene therapy holds promise for the future.

Medical Nutrition Therapy

Nutritional therapy by dietary avoidance of VLCFAs is still being studied. It does not lead to biochemical change because of endogenous synthesis. A speciality altered fatty acid product, Lorenzo's oil, lowers the VLCFA level; however, the clinical course is not significantly improved (Suzuki et al, 2001). A slower decline in function may be the more important result.

Alzheimer's Disease

Alzheimer's disease (AD) is the most common form of dementia. It is named after Alois Alzheimer, who in 1907 first described the clinical features and pathologic changes of this complex degenerative brain disease. It begins gradually, advances, and eventually leads to confusion, personality and behavior changes, and impaired judgment. A loss of independence, disordered eating behavior, and weight loss may accompany other symptoms.

Manifestations of AD result in a progressive dementia with increasing loss of memory, intellectual function, and disturbances in speech. Initially, day-to-day events are forgotten—possessions are misplaced, and appointments are forgotten—while memories are retained. Cerebral function declines, but this decline only becomes evident after the loss in memory is pronounced. Speech becomes impaired—names of objects are not remembered (anomia); words spoken by others are repeated (echolalia); and comprehension is lost (agnosia). Over time, motor skills deteriorate, as evidenced by changes in reflexes and a shuffling gate. Clinical findings are consistent when disease progression reaches the terminal stage. Bowel and bladder control is lost; limb weakness and contractures occur; and intellectual activity ceases. The patient becomes completely incapacitated in a vegetative state as death approaches.

The incidence rate of new cases of AD is similar for both sexes and throughout the world, increasing exponentially after age 40. Prevalence of AD among white males at age 100 is 41.5%; heterogeneity in the differences of APo-E genotype for AD causes the incidence rate to level off at about 11.7% per year at age 102 (Ewbank, 2002). The higher prevalence rate seen in women (three times higher than in men) is a result of a lower overall mortality than that of men. Given its prevalence, the personal, familial, financial, and clinical impact of AD is staggering.

Pathophysiology

No single factor has been established as a risk factor for AD. The risk factors commonly believed to be associated with AD are genetic factors, birth order, mother's age at birth, head injury, level of education, free radical action, vascular compromise, and presence of Down syndrome (Maimone et al, 2001) (Figure 43-5). β-Amyloid protein and endoplasmic reticulum–associated binding protein are central to the pathophysiology (Geula et al, 1998; Yan et al, 1997). More recent studies suggest that damage to key mitochondrial components may play a role, and inappropriate response to insulin may also be relevant (Blass et al, 2002).

Several genes have been identified as increasing the susceptibility for developing AD, but only one, the allele apolipoprotein-E4 (Apo-E4), has possible nutritional implications (Igbavboa et al, 2002). Apo-E4, a protein located on chromosome 19, binds β-amyloid, which is involved in the transport of cholesterol.

Medical Treatment

Alzheimer's disease is diagnosed by histopathology. Clinically, the diagnosis is presumptive and one of exclusion. As a result, studies may be subjected to criticism based on the absence of a confirmatory diagnosis.

Treatment directed at the impairment of brain metabolism may improve neuropsychological functions in AD patients (Blass et al, 2002). Hyperhomocysteinemia also has been proposed to play a role in the pathogenesis of AD. Findings from the Boston Veterans' Affairs Normative Aging Study show that plasma homocysteine concentrations correlated negatively with spatial copying skills (Riggs et al, 1996); other studies that implicated homosyteinemia did not find statistically significant relationships between elevated homocysteine levels and cognitive function assessments (Miller, 1999). Vascular disease, however, may contribute to the disorder and needs further exploration.

No definitive treatment currently exists; cerebral vasodilators, stimulants, L-dopa, and megadoses of vitamins C or E, and thiamin remain unproven therapies. Certain drugs may be effective in suppressing aberrant behavior or aiding disturbed sleep. Estrogen administration seemed to be beneficial for some postmenopausal women (Wickelgren, 1997), but this remains controversial. Based on research findings from rat studies, injections of testosterone have also been suggested as an effective treatment; however, widespread safety data are lacking (Guillozet et al, 2003). Neurofibrillary tangles and amyloid plaques are found in AD; studies of various nutrient relationships continue. In particular, omega-3 fatty acids seem to be essential (Igbavboa et al, 2002).

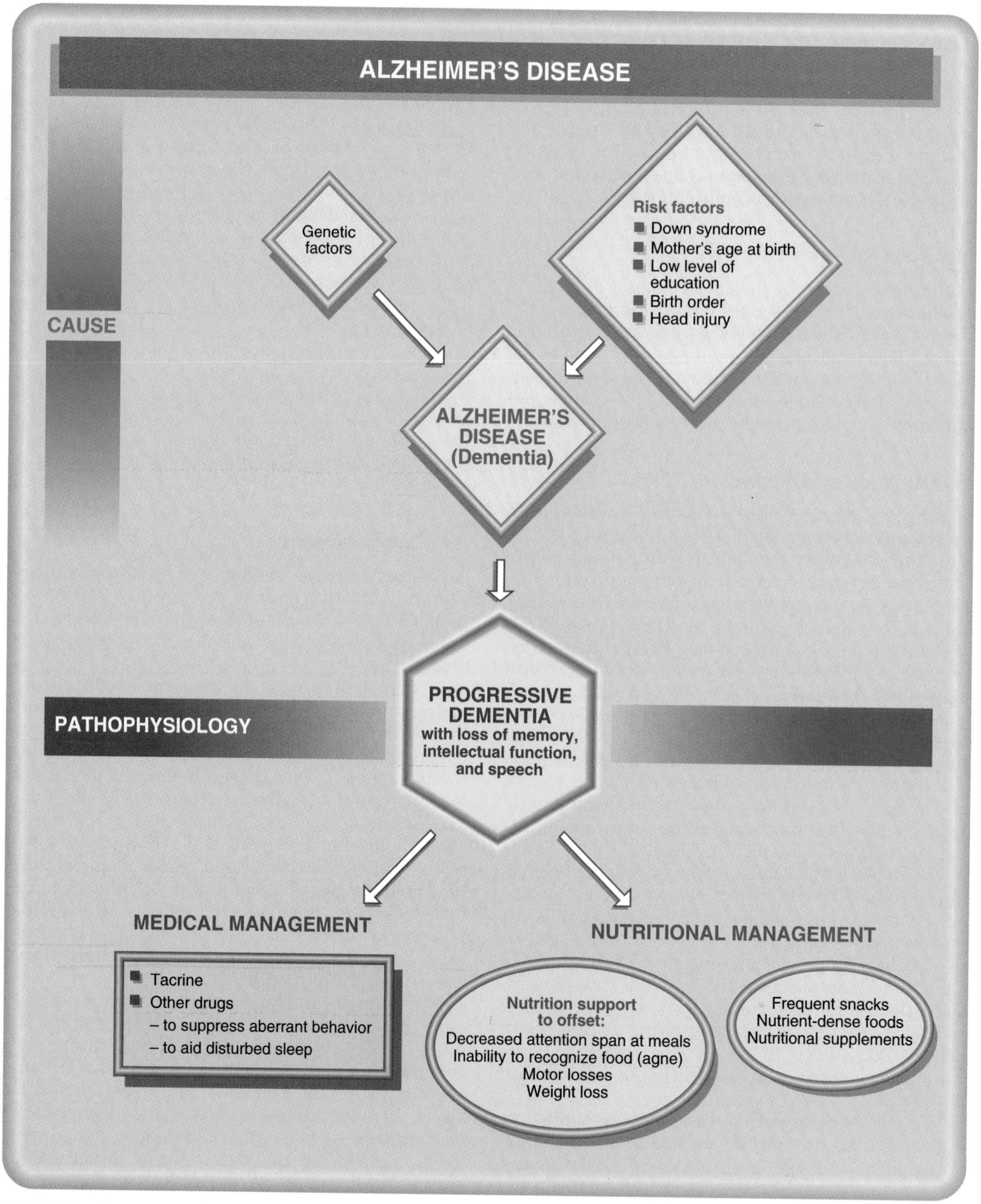

FIGURE 43-5 • Pathophysiology algorithm: Alzheimer's disease. (Algorithm content developed by John Anderson, PhD, and Sanford C. Garner, PhD, 2000.)

Drug treatment remains experimental, and combinations of drugs (e.g., acetylcholine, vitamin E, other antioxidants, and nonsteroidal antiinflammatory drugs in combination) are currently believed to be most effective. Tacrine (the first cholinesterase inhibitor approved by the FDA for use in the treatment of AD) resulted in only modest improvement in both noncognitive function and cognition (Raskind et al, 1997). It requires four doses a day, however, and has been replaced with drugs that have safer side effect profiles and that are taken twice daily (Rivastigmine) or once daily (Donepezil).

Primary care management is the effective treatment. Empathic support is important. Assessment of the following domains is fundamental to maximizing health, function, and quality of life of patients and family members: patient, individual family caregivers, family function, and availability of community services (Cohen, 1994).

Medical Nutrition Therapy

Determination of the nutritional status of the patient is essential because this population is often malnourished, and poor nutrition has untoward consequences (Cohen, 1994). Although a gluttonous appetite may develop in some individuals with AD (with accompanying weight increase), generally the global nutritional finding is weight loss. Whether an increased resting metabolic rate or increased energy expenditure causes weight loss is unclear. The latter is probably true because energy output associated with constant pacing may be increased. For others, eating is neglected, and weight loss is caused by an inadequate food intake that results from decreased independence and impaired self-feeding. In still other cases, weight loss may be secondary to a higher basal energy expenditure as a result of higher rates of infection. Weight loss increases the risk of infections, skin ulcers, and consequently a decreased quality of life (Riviere et al, 1999).

Proper inclusion of specific nutrients, such as antioxidants, may play a role in protecting the AD patient from further decline (Meydani, 2001) (see *Focus On:* Herbs, Nutrients, and Ginkgo in Alzheimer's Disease and Other Neurologic Conditions).

Alzheimer's disease is a disease of cortical neurons. The frontal lobe controls behavior, reasoning, emotion, and cognition; the temporal lobe controls hearing, memory, smell, and language; and the parietal lobe controls sensory perception, hearing, and body image. As a result, a wide range of neurologic functions that interfere with numerous activities involved with eating are impaired.

Cognitive losses impair attention span, reasoning, and judgment. This includes the ability to recognize feelings of hunger, thirst, and satiety. As the disease progresses, the attention span decreases, and meals may be forgotten as soon as they are eaten or may not be eaten at all. Dehydration is also a problem; recognizing thirst and then seeking water is often neglected. Attempts should be made to minimize distractions at mealtimes. Noise can be distracting, and therefore the radio or television should be turned off during mealtime. Food may need to be placed on small plates or bowls and given one at a time so as not to stress the individual by offering too wide a choice of foods. As social inhibitions decrease, the pa-

FOCUS ON

Herbs, Nutrients, and Ginkgo in Alzheimer's Disease and Other Neurologic Conditions

The tight microglial cellular junctions that form the blood-brain barrier (BBB) protect the CNS from large molecules. Diseases such as Alzheimer's disease (AD) and stress can make the BBB more permeable (Friedman et al, 1996). Proper inclusion of specific nutrients, such as antioxidants, may play a role in maintaining this barrier.

Antioxidants, especially vitamin E, have been studied for their role in AD. Alpha-tocopherol and the drug selegiline have been found to be useful in slowing the progression of moderately severe AD (Sano et al, 1997). Antioxidants in foods have been shown to be effective in maintaining memory; folate, vitamin C, and beta-carotene seem to be the best protective agents in fruits and vegetables (Warsama Jama et al, 1996; Tufts University, 1998). Cognitive ability is also supported by adequate intakes of vitamins B_6 and B_{12} in addition to folate.

Ginkgo biloba extract (GBE) has been promoted in Asian countries and was recently approved for use in Germany to treat dementia (LeBars et al, 1997). Studies in the United States have tested the effectiveness of ginkgo in a 1-year double-blind, randomized trial. Results found no improvement in memory or functioning in the treatment group but significant worsening among the placebo group. Although the mechanism is not yet clear, a role for this extract may exist in the dementia population.

Products on the market do not always provide predictable levels of the effective ingredient, and home remedies may not be safe to use because they may have other contaminants. Further study is warranted (see Chapter 20; see Appendix 35).

tient may take another person's food. The patient consuming inedible items, spoiled foods, or hazardous fluids reflects impaired reasoning. These patients should be served first and be closely supervised during meals.

Visual agne, with the inability to recognize food, is manifested by not eating. The touch or smell of food is needed to initiate eating responses. Another sensory loss is the inability to recognize food when it is served in a bowl the same color as the food item. Use of colored bowls and plates that are in contrast to the color of the food may be necessary so that food can be distinguished from the place setting. Patients may also have difficulties using eating utensils, but they can model behaviors if demonstrated by staff or caregivers.

Motor losses occur over the course of the illness. Some clients may need hand guidance to initiate eating. Usually, after the activity has been initiated, the patient can continue the activity as long as verbal cues continue. As motor skills decline, use of eating utensils will become limited; over time the patient may be able to use only a spoon. Eating utensils should not be removed prematurely because this may contribute to agitation, excessive disability, lack of eating, and eventually weight loss.

Assessment of motor skills should be done routinely. Finger foods may be useful when use of utensils becomes difficult—but only if the patient has no difficulty with chewing or swallowing. If the patient is inclined to swallow large boluses of food, finger foods are not appropriate. Although adaptive equipment is useful in certain situations, it may be unfamiliar to the patient with AD and not as helpful. As end-stage disease approaches, swallowing often becomes impossible; dysphagia should be assessed to prevent the risk of aspiration (Finley, 1997). Table 43-6 lists additional interventions for eating-related behavioral problems in individuals with dementia.

Frequent snacks, nutrient-dense foods, and nutritional supplements need to be provided to combat weight loss. Behavior modification, along with altered food items, will improve the quality of life of the individual for as long as possible. Evaluation of nutritional status is needed throughout the stages of AD to ensure that objectives of nutritional therapy continue to be met.

TABLE 43-6 Examples of Practical Intervention for Eating-Related Behavioral Problems Common in Individuals With Dementia

BEHAVIORAL PROBLEM	INTERVENTION
Attention/or concentration deficit	Verbally direct client through each step of eating process Place utensils in hand Make food and fluids available and visible
Combative, throws food	Identify provocative agent, remove Feeder stands or sits on nondominant side Provide nonbreakable dishes with suction holder Give one food at a time Reward appropriate mealtime behavior
Chews constantly	Tell client to stop chewing after each bite Serve soft foods to reduce the need to chew Offer small bites
Eats nonedible things	Remove nonedibles from reach Provide finger foods Provide edible centerpiece or table decorations
Eats too quickly	Set utensils down between bites Offer food items separately Offer bulky foods that require chewing Use a smaller spoon or cup
Eats too slowly	Monitor eating place and provide verbal cues: "chew," "take a bite" Serve first to allow more time Use insulated dishes to maintain proper temperatures
Forgetful or disoriented	Simple routines Constant environment Assigned seating Minimize distractions Limit choices
Forgets to swallow	Tell client to swallow Feel for swallow before offering next bite Stroke upward on larynx
Inappropriate emotional expression	Engage in conversation Ignore emotional display Provide quiet environment
Paces	Sit beside client at table Change dining location Aerobic exercise before meals Finger foods Cups with covers or spouts
Plays in food	Serve one food at a time Fill glass or plate half full at refill Finger food Cups with covers or spouts
Shows paranoia	Provide structured routine Present food in a consistent manner Serve foods in closed containers Do not put medicine in food
Spits	Evaluate chewing and swallowing ability Tell client not to spit Place away from others who would be offended Provide mealtime supervision
Will not go into dining room	Ask why Change dining location Provide a single dining partner versus a group Serve meals in room

Modified from the Nutrition Screening Initiative, a project of the American Academy of Family Physicians, The American Dietetic Association, and the National Council on the Aging, Inc., and funded in part by a grant from Ross Products Division, a division of Abbott Laboratories.

Amyotrophic Lateral Sclerosis

Amyotrophic lateral sclerosis (ALS), also called *Lou Gehrig's disease* after the famous baseball player afflicted with the disease, is the most common type of motor system disease. Incidence is 1 to 2/100,000 (Sathasivam et al, 2001). ALS involves a progressive denervation atrophy and weakness of muscles—hence the term *amyotrophy,* the hallmark sign and symptom. Both upper and lower motor neurons are lost in the spinal cord, brain stem, and motor cortex and thus contribute to the clinical manifestations, which are characterized by generalized skeletal muscular weakness, atrophy, and hyperreflexia. The natural history of disease for ALS is unpleasant; the course is relentless and without remissions, relapses, or plateaus; it usually progresses to death in 2 to 6 years (Adams et al, 1997).

Pathophysiology

Risk factors of occupation, trauma, diet, or socioeconomic status are not consistent. The prevalence is constant throughout the world, and men are affected more than women. The average age of onset is the mid-50s (more often found in the 40- to 70-year age group) but ranges from the late teens to the 80s (Mitsumoto, 1994).

ALS is known as the neurodegenerative disease of the aging nervous system, but its etiology is unknown. The pathologic basis of weakness in ALS is the selective death of motor neurons in the ventral gray matter of the spinal cord and in the motor cortex (Kasarskis and Neville, 1996). Only about 5% to 10% of cases are familial; the remainder are sporadic (90% to 95%). Genetic analysis of patients with familial, chromosome 21–linked ALS has suggested that mutations in the copper-zinc superoxide dismutase (SOD1) gene may be involved in the etiology (Jonsson et al, 2002).

Several different mechanisms have been proposed for the loss of neurons, including increased intracellular calcium, oxidative stress and free radical damage, mitochondrial dysfunction and neurofilament aggregation, and dysfuntion of transport mechanisms (Appel et al, 2001). The possible role of antioxidant status in prevention and therapeutic intervention needs further investigation. Studies involving the use of vitamin C and vitamin E are recommended to further define the role or possible benefits of antioxidant therapy in ALS.

Medical Treatment

Given the classic signs of this disease, ALS can be accurately diagnosed by clinical examination 90% to 95% of the time. The typical presentation is evidenced with both lower motor neuron (weakness, wasting, fasciculation) and upper motor neuron deficits (hyperactive tendon reflexes, Hoffman signs, Babinski signs, or clonus). Muscle weakness commences in the legs and hands and progresses to the proximal arms and oropharynx. As these motor nerves deteriorate, almost all of the voluntary skeletal muscles are at risk for atrophy and complete loss of function. This loss of spinal motor neurons causes the denervation of voluntary skeletal muscles of the neck, trunk, and limbs and results in muscle wasting, flaccid weakness, and fasciculations that lead to loss of mobility. The progressive loss of function in cortical motor neurons can lead to spasticity of jaw muscles resulting in dysarthria (slurred speech) (Kasarskis and Neville, 1996).

The onset of dysphagia is usually insidious, and the functional deficits affect dysphagia and speech similarly; swallowing difficulties usually follow speech difficulties. Despite the presence of impaired speech, patients often do not report difficulties swallowing. Although some weight loss is inevitable, given the muscle atrophy, consistent or dramatic loss may indicate probable chewing difficulties or dysphagia (Strand et al, 1996).

Eye movement and eye blink are spared, as are the sphincter muscles of the bowel and bladder. Incontinence is rare. Sensation remains intact, and, except in rare cases, mental acuity is maintained. Although mechanical ventilation can extend the life of patients, most decline this option because the quality of life is poor in advanced ALS.

No effective therapy can cure or even slow the disease progression. Research has shown no benefit from immunosuppression, immunoenhancement, plasmapheresis, lymph node irradiation, glutamate antagonists, nerve growth factors, or antiviral agents. Therefore only supportive measures can be used to maintain the optimal quality of life. The ALS Severity Scale, developed by Hillel and colleagues (1989), is one guideline used to assess the functional level of swallowing, speech, and upper and lower extremities. Once the severity of deficits has been identified, appropriate interventions can be implemented (Box 43-3).

Medical Nutrition Therapy

The nutritional changes during the different stages of ALS have not been well documented. However, Kasarskis and colleagues (1996) studied the effects of ALS on nutritional status with relation to the proximity of death to characterize the natural history of ALS with regard to nutritional status (Table 43-7). Their results demonstrate decreases in body fat, lean body mass, muscle power, and nitrogen balance and an increase in resting energy expenditure as death approaches.

The relationship of dysphagia and respiratory status in disease progression is important. As ALS progresses, a progressive loss of function in bulbar and respiratory muscles contributes to oral and pharyngeal dysphagia. In late stages, the respiratory status is impaired such that the patient is not a good candidate for PEG placement. Although the PEG is placed with the patient under local anesthesia, the patient may not be able to lie prone for tube placement without respiratory decompensation. This reinforces the need for early versus late education about dysphagia management and initiation of discussion about whether to place a feeding tube. Placing a feeding tube will not lengthen life (Thornton et al, 2002).

The clinician should become familiar with common clinical findings throughout the natural history of disease progression to prevent secondary complications of malnutrition and dehydration. The functional status of each patient should be monitored closely so that timely intervention with the appropriate management techniques can be started. In particular, dysphagia should be monitored closely.

Box 43-3. Amyotrophic Lateral Sclerosis Severity Scale

Swallowing Scale

Rating

NORMAL EATING HABITS

10 Normal Swallowing: Person denies any difficulty chewing or swallowing. Examination demonstrates no abnormality.

9 Nominal Abnormality: Only the individual with ALS notices slight indicators, such as food lodging in the recesses of the mouth or sticking in the throat.

EARLY EATING PROBLEMS

8 Minor Swallowing Problems: Complains of some swallowing difficulties. Maintains essentially a regular diet. Isolated choking episodes.

7 Prolonged Time or Small Bite Size: Mealtime has significantly increased, and smaller bite sizes are necessary. Must concentrate on swallowing liquids.

DIETARY CONSISTENCY CHANGES

6 Soft Diet: Diet is limited primarily to soft foods. Requires some special meal preparation.

5 Liquified Diet: Oral intake adequate. Nutrition limited primarily to liquefied diet. Thin liquid intake usually a problem. May force self to eat.

NEEDS TUBE FEEDING

4 Supplemental Tube Feedings: Oral intake alone is no longer adequate. Person uses or needs a tube to supplement intake. Person continues to take significant nutrition (greater than 50%) by mouth.

3 Tube Feeding With Occasional Oral Nutrition: Primary nutrition and hydration accomplished by tube. Receives less than 59% of nutrition by mouth.

NOTHING BY MOUTH

2 Secretions Managed With Aspirator/Medication: Cannot safely manage any oral intake. Secretions managed by aspirator and/or medications. Swallows reflexively.

1 Aspiration of Secretions: Secretions cannot be managed noninvasively. Rarely swallows.

Speech Scale

Rating

NORMAL SPEECH PROCESSES

10 Normal Speech: Individual denies any difficulty speaking. Examination demonstrates no abnormality.

9 Nominal Speech Abnormality: Only the individual with ALS or spouse notices that speech has changed. Maintains normal rate and volume.

DETECTABLE SPEECH DISTURBANCE

8 Perceived Speech Changes: Speech changes are noted by others, especially during fatigue or stress. Rate of speech remains essentially normal.

7 Obvious Speech Abnormalities: Speech is consistently impaired. Affected are rate, articulation, and resonance. Remains easily understood.

BEHAVIORAL MODIFICATIONS

6 Repeats Messages on Occasion: Rate is much slower. Repeats specific words in adverse listening situations. Does not limit complexity or length of message.

5 Frequent Repeating Required: Speech is slow and labored. Extensive repetition or a "translator" is commonly needed. Person probably limits the complexity or length of message.

USE OF AUGMENTATIVE COMMUNICATION

4 Speech Plus Augmentative Communication: Speech is used in response to questions. Intelligibility problems need to be resolved by writing or a spokesperson.

3 Limits Speech to One-Word Response: Vocalizes one-word response beyond yes/no; otherwise writes or uses a spokesperson. Initiates communication nonvocally.

LOSS OF USEFUL SPEECH

2 Vocalizes for Emotional Expression: Uses vocal inflection to express emotion, affirmation, and negation.

1 Nonvocal: Vocalization is difficult, limited in duration, and rarely attempted. May vocalize for crying or pain.

X Tracheostomy

Upper Extremities Scale Rating

Rating

NORMAL FUNCTION

10 Normal Function: Person denies any weakness or unusual fatigue of upper extremities. Examination demonstrates no abnormality.

9 Suspected Fatigue: Person suspects fatigue in upper extremities during exertion. Cannot sustain work for as long as normal. Atrophy not evident on examination.

INDEPENDENT AND COMPLETE SELF-CARE

8 Slow Self-Care Performance: Dressing and hygiene performed more slowly than usual.

7 Laborious Self-Care Performance: Requires significantly more time (usually double or more) and effort to accomplish self-care. Weakness is apparent on examination.

INTERMITTENT ASSISTANCE

6 Mostly Independent: Handles most aspects of dressing and hygiene alone. Adapts by resting, modifying (electric razor), or avoiding some tasks (e.g., buttons, tie).

5 Partial Independence: Handles some aspects of dressing and hygiene alone. However, routinely requires assistance for many tasks such as makeup, combing, shaving, etc.

NEEDS ATTENDANT FOR SELF-CARE

4 Attendant Assists Person: Attendant must be present for dressing and hygiene. Person performs the majority of each task with the assistance of the attendant.

From Hillel AD et al: ALS Severity Scale, *J Neuroepidemiol* 8:142, 1989. Reproduced with permission of J. Karger AG, Basel, Switzerland.

Box 43-3. Amyotrophic Lateral Sclerosis Severity Scale—cont'd

3 Person Assists Attendant: The attendant assists the person with ALS for most all tasks. The person moves in a purposeful manner to assist the attendant. Does not initiate self-care tasks.

TOTAL DEPENDENCE

2 Minimal Movement: Minimal movement of one or both arms. Cannot reposition arms.

1 Paralysis: Flaccid paralysis. Unable to move upper extremities.

Lower Extremities Scale

Rating

NORMAL

10 Normal Ambulation: Person denies any weakness or fatigue. Examination detects no abnormality.

9 Fatigue Suspected: Person suspects weakness or fatigue in lower extremities during exertion.

EARLY AMBULATION PROBLEM

8 Difficulty With Uneven Terrain: Difficulty and fatigue when walking long distances, climbing stairs, and walking over uneven ground (even thick carpet).

7 Observed Changes in Gait: Noticeable change in gait. Pulls on railing when climbing stairs. May use leg brace.

WALKS WITH ASSISTANCE

6 Walks With Mechanical Device: Needs or uses canes, walker, or assistant to walk. Probably uses wheelchair away from home.

5 Walks With Mechanical Device and Attendant: Does not attempt to walk without an attendant. Ambulation limited to less than 50 feet. Avoids stairs.

FUNCTIONAL MOVEMENT ONLY

4 Able to Support Weight: At best can shuffle a few steps with the help of an attendant for transfers.

3 Purposeful Leg Movements: Unable to take steps but can position legs to assist an attendant in transfers. Moves legs purposefully to maintain mobility in bed.

NO PURPOSEFUL LEG MOVEMENT

2 Minimal Movement: Minimal movement of one or both legs. Cannot reposition legs independently.

1 Paralysis: Placcid paralysis. Cannot move lower extremities.

TABLE 43-7 Nutritional and Metabolic Changes During the Progression of Amyotrophic Lateral Sclerosis

	EARLY PHASE	LATE PHASE
Pathophysiology	Cycles of muscle denervation, muscle catabolism and atrophy, reinnervation, and protein synthesis	Net muscle catabolism and atrophy
Functional status	Mild functional restriction of physical activity Mild impairment of respiration	Progressive limitation of physical activity Increased work of ventilation
Nutritional and metabolic changes	Positive nitrogen balance Normal resting energy expenditure Probable neutral energy balance	Negative nitrogen balance Increased resting energy expenditure Decrease in body fat

From Kasarskis EJ et al: Nutritional status of patients with amyotrophic lateral sclerosis: relation to the proximity of death, *Am J Clin Nutr* 63:130, 1996. Printed in USA. Copyright 1996 *Am J Clin Nutr*, American Society for Clinical Nutrition.

Oropharyngeal weakness affects survival in ALS by placing the patient at continuous risk of aspiration, pneumonia, and sepsis and by curtailing the adequate intake of energy and protein (Kasarskis and Neville, 1996). These problems can compound the deteriorating effects of the disease. Therefore Strand and colleagues (1996) have outlined the timing of dysphagia intervention on a continuum of five stages that correlate to the ALS Severity Scale:

1. *Normal Eating Habits (ALS Severity Scale Rating 10-9).* Early assessment and intervention are critical for maintaining nutritional health in ALS. This is the appropriate time to begin educating the patient, before the development of speech or swallowing symptoms. Hydration and maintenance of nutritional health are critical at this stage. Fluid intake of at least 2 quarts daily from noncaffeinated sources is important because caffeine has a diuretic effect, which contributes to dehydration. Dehydration contributes to fatigue and thickens saliva. For patients with spinal ALS, emphasis on fluids is important because they may intentionally limit fluid intake because of difficulties with toileting. The diet history is helpful to assess patterns of normal chewing, swallowing, and the rate of ingestion; weight loss history establishes a baseline weight. A weight loss of 10% or more indicates increased nutritional risk.

2. *Early Eating Problems (Severity Scale Rating 8-7).* At this point, patients begin to report difficulties eating; reports of coughing and unusually long mealtimes are associated with tongue, facial, and masticator muscle weakness. Dietary intervention begins to focus on modification of consistency, avoidance of thin liquids, and use of foods that are easier to chew and swallow.
3. *Dietary Consistency Changes (Severity Scale Rating 6-5).* As symptoms progress, the oral transport of food becomes difficult as dry crumbly foods will tend to break apart and cause choking. Foods that require more chewing, such as raw vegetables or steak, are typically avoided. As dysphagia progresses, ingestion of thin liquids, especially water, may become more problematic. Often the patient has fatigue and malaise, which may be associated with a mild chronic dehydration due to a decreased fluid intake. Dietary intervention should change food consistency to mechanical soft or pureed (see Appendix 55) to reduce the need for oral manipulation and to conserve energy (Table 43-8). Small, frequent meals may also increase intake. Thick liquids that contain a high percentage of water as well as attempts to increase fluid intake need to be emphasized to maintain fluid balance. Popsicles, gelatins, ice, and fresh fruit are additional sources of free water. Liquids can be thickened with a modified cornstarch thickener.

   Swallowing can be improved by emphasizing taste, texture, and temperature. Juices can be substituted for water to provide taste, nutrients, and calories (see Box 43-1). A cool temperature facilitates the swallowing mechanism and therefore cold food items may be better tolerated. Heat does not provide the same advantage. Carbonation may also be better tolerated because of the beneficial effect of texture.

   Instructions for preventing aspiration should be addressed. Proper position for safe swallowing should be achieved (i.e., sitting bolt upright with the head in a chin-down position). Concentrating on the swallowing process can also help reduce choking. Environmental distractions and conversation during mealtime increase the risk for aspiration; however, families should be encouraged to maintain as normal mealtime behavior as possible. As dysphagia progresses, the limitation of food consistencies may result in the exclusion of entire food groups. Vitamin and mineral supplementation may be necessary. If chewable supplements are not handled safely, liquid forms may be added to acceptable foods. Fiber may also need to be added along with fluids for constipation problems.
4. *Tube Feeding (Severity Scale Rating 4-3).* Dehydration will occur acutely before malnutrition, a more chronic state, is exhibited. This may be an early indication of the need for nutrition support. Weight loss from muscle wasting and dysphagia will eventually lead to placement of a PEG tube for nutrition and protection against aspiration caused by dysphagia. Enteral nutrition support is preferred over parenteral nutrition support because the gastrointestinal tract should be functioning properly. Given the progressive nature of ALS, placing feeding tubes when dysphagia and dehydration are evident is probably better than initiating this therapy later in the course after the patient has become overtly malnourished or after respiratory status is

TABLE 43-8 Diet for Easy Chewing and Swallowing

TYPE OF FOOD	FOODS GENERALLY INCLUDED	FOODS COMMONLY EXCLUDED
Fluids	Thick juices,* sherbet,* sherbet shakes,* popsicles,* gelatin,* thin liquids thickened with Thick-It†	Water, thin juices, milk, coffee, tea
Bread and cereals	Bread, toast, cooked cereal, quick breads without nuts or raisins, pancakes, moist pastas, and casseroles	Crackers, dry rice, dry cereal flakes, crumbly bread, soft white bread
Dairy products	Butter, margarine, creamy or blenderized cottage cheese, soft cheeses, yogurt, thickened milk or dairy substitutes, and ice cream if tolerated	Dry cottage cheese, melted hot cheese
Eggs	Medium-cooked, poached, scrambled, soft omelet, custard	Runny eggs, thin eggnogs
Meat, fish, and poultry	Moist ground meat in casseroles, meatloaf, meatballs, ground meat with sauces and gravies, moist, tender fish without bones	Dry ground meat, chunky meats, dry fish, or fish with bones
Fruits	Soft canned fruits with seeds, pits, and skin removed; ripe bananas; chilled, thick pureed fruits; soft fruits in gelatin	Raw fruits except bananas, thin pureed fruits, stringy pineapple
Vegetables	Soft canned vegetables; baked, mashed, or boiled potatoes with margarine or gravy; whipped squash with margarine; scalloped potatoes; thick pureed vegetables; minced vegetables in gelatin	Raw vegetables, chunky vegetables such as diced beets, stringy vegetables such as spinach, corn, firm peas
Soups	Thick soups (blenderized)	Thin soups or chunky-style soups
Desserts	Fruit whip, gelatin,* apple or peach crisp, moist cookies without nuts or raisins, custard, pudding, sherbet, ice cream if tolerated	Dry cakes and cookies; dessert with raisins, nuts, seeds, or coconut; hard candies and chocolate

*Safety with these foods may depend on oral retention times because they melt in the mouth and become difficult to manage.
†Thick-It is a modified cornstarch used to thicken both hot and cold liquids. Made by Milani, Precision Foods, St. Louis, and available nationwide.

marginal. The decision of whether to place a feeding tube for nutrition support is part of the decision-making process each patient must face. However, it might be added that adequate nutriture can maintain health of the individual longer.

The initiation of nutrition support may be a welcome relief for the patient who has become overburdened with all of the difficulties of sustaining himself or herself. The purpose of nutrition support should be to enhance the quality of life. Long-term access should be considered via a PEG or percutaneous endoscopic jejunostomy (PEJ) tube (see Chapter 23).

5. *Nothing by Mouth (Severity Scale Rating 2-1).* The final level of dysphagia is reached when the patient cannot eat orally. Nor can the patient manage his or her own oral secretions. Although saliva production is not increased, it tends to pool in the front of the mouth because of declining swallow response. Once the swallowing mechanism is absent, mechanical ventilation is required to manage saliva flow. Tube feeding is permanent at this stage.

Epilepsy

Epilepsy is an intermittent derangement of the nervous system presumably caused by a sudden, excessive, disorderly discharge of cerebral neurons. It is estimated that 2.3 million individuals in the United States have epilepsy, and 14% of those are younger than 15 years of age. Direct medical costs for persons with continued seizure activity is reported to be 55% higher than the average costs for all persons with epilepsy (Mandel et al, 2002).

Pathophysiology

Most seizures begin in early life, but a resurgence of epileptic events occurs after age 60. The first occurrence of a seizure in adults should prompt investigation into a cause. A clinical work-up usually reveals no anatomic abnormalities, and the cause of the seizure may remain unknown (idiopathic).

Seizures before age 2 are usually caused by developmental defects, birth injuries, or a metabolic disease (see Chapter 45). The medical history is the key component for suggesting further avenues of diagnostic investigation, especially in children. An electroencephalogram can help to delineate seizure activity and is most helpful in localizing partial complex seizures.

Medical Treatment

The dramatic tonic-clonic (formerly *grand mal*) seizure is the most common image of a seizure (lasting 1-2 minutes), yet numerous classifications of seizures, each with a different and often less dramatic clinical presentation, exist. A generalized seizure is one that involves or appears to involve the entire brain cortex from its beginning phases and is characterized by complete loss of muscle tone and consciousness. The tonic-clonic seizure comes under this heading. After such a seizure the patient will wake up slowly after a time; he or she will be groggy and disoriented for minutes to hours after the event. This is termed the *postictal phase* and is characterized by deep sleep, headache, confusion, and muscle soreness.

The absence seizure (formerly petit mal seizure) is also generalized in nature. A patient with absence seizures may appear to be daydreaming during an episode, but he or she recovers consciousness within a few seconds and has no postictal fatigue or disorientation. Partial seizures occur when there is a discrete focus of epileptogenic brain tissue. A simple partial seizure involves no loss of consciousness, whereas a complex partial seizure is characterized by a change in consciousness. This implies a spread to the brain stem areas that govern consciousness. Partial seizures may also secondarily generalize, where the electrical activity in the seizure focus spreads across the entire brain.

Determining the seizure type is key to implementing effective therapy. Generalized seizures are ordinarily managed with valproate or phenytoin. These drugs are difficult to use because they interact with other drugs metabolized in the liver and have a proclivity to cause liver damage. Liver enzymes and serum drug levels must be monitored periodically. Phenytoin metabolism has unusual kinetics; thus toxic levels may be attained with very small dosage adjustments. Gabapentin has been introduced recently, and it is rapidly gaining popularity because of its safety and ease of use.

Carbamazepine or phenytoin can usually control partial seizures. Failure of partial seizure control may prompt consideration of seizure surgery. A localized focus resected from nonessential brain will render a patient seizure free in 75% of cases. Use of phenobarbital is usually avoided because its use has been associated with decreased intelligence quotient (IQ) in children. It is occasionally considered for use after failure of other antiepileptic drugs.

Medications used in anticonvulsant therapy may alter the nutritional status of the patient. Phenobarbital, phenytoin, and primidone interfere with intestinal absorption of calcium by increasing vitamin D metabolism in the liver. Long-term therapy with these drugs may lead to osteomalacia in adults or rickets in children. Vitamin D supplementation is essential. Folic acid supplementation interferes with phenytoin metabolism, so it contributes to difficulties in achieving therapeutic levels. For this reason, sporadic folic acid supplementation should be avoided (see Chapter 19). Phenytoin and phenobarbital are bound primarily to albumin in the bloodstream. Decreased serum albumin levels in malnutrition or with reduced albumin synthesis secondary to advanced cirrhosis limit the amount of drug that can be bound.

This results in an increased free drug concentration and possible drug toxicity with administration of a standard dose.

New guidelines for treating seizures have been released by the Epilepsy Foundation (see Relevant Web Sites). The guidelines emphasize the special needs of women and older Americans in optimizing treatment strategies and the recommend use of just one antiseizure medication initially and resorting to combination therapies only when needed.

Alcohol consumption results in the loss of the intended effect of phenytoin, possibly inducing seizures. Absorption of phenobarbital is delayed by the consumption of food; therefore administration of the drug must be staggered around mealtimes if it is used.

Continuous enteral feeding slows the absorption of phenytoin, thus necessitating an increase in the dose to achieve a therapeutic level. Decreased serum phenytoin concentrations associated with enteral feeding may increase the risk of seizures; a patient-specific care plan that includes consideration of the enteral feeding formulation and method of administration, as well as the phenytoin dosage form, schedule of administration, and monitoring, is needed (Au Yeung and Ensom, 2000). This is an area in which much more research is needed because significant individual variability exists.

Recommendations to separate phenytoin suspension from tube-feeding formulas are common. Stopping the tube feeding before and after the phenytoin dose is generally suggested, but recommendations vary from 1- to 4-hour intervals. The most common is a two-hour feeding-free interval before and after the dose of phenytoin is administered (Au Yeung and Ensom, 2000). Whenever tube feedings are stopped, the dose of phenytoin needs to be adjusted to avoid toxicity.

Medical Nutrition Therapy

A ketogenic diet previously has been reserved as a last resort for treatment of all types of seizures in children in whom all drug therapies have failed. This treatment, however, is financially beneficial, particularly in comparison to total costs for care (Mandel et al, 2002). A recent report that evaluated medical costs for children (2 to 18 years of age) with drug refractory epilepsies demonstrated cost advantage, reduction in seizures, and a reduced need for drugs (Mandel et al, 2002).

The ketogenic diet has minimal side effects and may be curative. Although it is initially demanding, the diet will completely control epilepsy in one third of the children whose seizures are otherwise uncontrollable. For another one third of children, the diet will either markedly decrease the frequency of seizures or allow medications to be reduced (Freeman et al, 1996). The new guidelines for epilepsy treatment can be found from the Epilepsy Foundation.

The diet is designed to create and maintain a state of ketosis. Although its mechanism of action is not clearly understood, the beneficial effect in epilepsy may be caused by a change in neuronal metabolism, whereby a ketone body behaves as an inhibitory neurotransmitter, thus producing an anticonvulsant effect on the body. Raised levels of free plasma polyunsaturates could contribute to the beneficial effect of the ketogenic diet in refractory epilepsy not only by helping sustain ketosis but also by their own direct yet poorly defined antiseizure effects (Cunnane et al, 2002). Mild dehydration is important with this diet to prevent dilution of the level of ketones circulating at any time (Berryman, 1997).

Two forms of the ketogenic diet are in use: the "traditional" approach, developed in the 1920s, and the medium-chain triglyceride (MCT)-based approach. With either approach, the child fasts in the hospital for 24 to 72 hours until a 4+ ketonuria is produced. For the majority of patients, if the diet is going to work, it will usually work during the initial fasting period. It should also be noted that antiepileptic drugs need to be stopped when administering the ketogenic diet.

In the traditional approach, once ketosis is established, caloric intake is resumed in a 4:1 ratio of fat to protein and carbohydrate kilocalories. For a child, kilocalories are calculated to provide 75% of the calories needed as fat. Protein is calculated to provide appropriate intake for growth (about 1 g/kg/day). Carbohydrates are added to make up the remaining portion of protein and carbohydrate energy needs (usually a minimal to negligible amount). The exchange lists (see Appendix 53) can be used to adjust the carbohydrate amount. Fluids are also carefully controlled—about 65 ml/kg/day but not to exceed 2 L/day is recommended (Kinsman et al, 1992). A multiple vitamin and calcium supplement is recommended to ensure that the diet is nutritionally complete; this should be provided in a sugar-free form.

The MCT-based ketogenic diet replaces the long-chain fats of the traditional diet with MCT. MCT oil is available as an odorless, colorless, tasteless oil and was originally used as a means of improving the palatability of the diet. A greater amount of nonketogenic foods, such as fruits and vegetables and small amounts of bread and other starches, can be allowed because ketosis from MCT can be more readily achieved (Table 43-9). Fluids are not limited in this diet.

Initiating the ketogenic diet is intense. Further, the diet may seem unpalatable as well as complex, thus making compliance difficult to achieve. To be successful, children may benefit from behavioral techniques while parents most often require substantial psychosocial support. Intensity required during the follow-up phase will vary and is affected by the patient's health status, growth, development, and caregiver's level of anticipation. For the child whose epilepsy is controlled on the diet, complying with the diet is much easier than dealing with devastating seizures and associated injuries. Fortunately, the du-

TABLE 43-9 Typical Ketogenic Diet Menu Using MCT Oil

FOOD ITEM	AMOUNT (g)	CARBOHYDRATE (g)	PROTEIN (g)	FAT (g)	ENERGY (kcal)
Breakfast					
White bread	5	2.8	0.4	0.2	13
Egg, scrambled	48		6.1	5.5	74
Cream, heavy whipping	10	0.3	0.3	3.8	36
Margarine	5			5.0	45
MCT oil	12			12.0	108
Fat	11			11.0	99
Koolaid, with nonnutritive sweetner	240				
TOTAL		2.8	6.8	37.5	375
Lunch					
American cheese	12	2.2	2.8	3.6	52
Ham	23	0.7	3.7	3.9	53
MCT oil mayonnaise	11			11.0	99
Fat	19			19.0	171
Koolaid, with nonnutritive sweetner	240				
TOTAL		2.9	6.5	37.5	375
Dinner					
Turkey	19		6.3	0.7	32
Tomato	10	0.5	0.1	0.0	3
Green beans	10	0.6	0.2	0.0	3
Potatoes	12	1.7	0.2	0.0	8
Margarine	15			15.0	135
MCT oil mayonnaise	11			11.0	99
Fat	10			10.0	90
Koolaid, with nonnutritive sweetner	240				
TOTAL		2.8	6.8	36.7	370
DAILY TOTAL:		8.5	20.1	111.7	1120

ration of the diet is limited; it can often be discontinued after 2 to 3 years.

Guillain-Barré Syndrome

Guillain-Barré syndrome (GBS) is an acute-onset, inflammatory, demyelinating polyneuropathy that has a predilection for proximal motor nerves, including the cranial nerves and the diaphragm. The incidence is approximately 2/100,000, and the cause is most likely mediated by the immune system. Guillain-Barré syndrome is the most common paralytic illness of children and adolescents in countries with established immunization programs (Joseph and Tsao, 2002).

Pathophysiology

In 60% of cases, the disorder follows an infection, surgery, or an immunization. Some of the more common organisms are *Campylobacter jejuni* (Fields and Swerdlow, 1999), *Mycoplasma,* and some herpes viruses (Griffin, 1996). Several pathologic varieties exist, and the nature of the distinction is related to the segment of the immune system that is inflicting nerve damage. The clinical course of GBS is similar regardless of subtype, although GBS after a *Campylobacter* infection tends to be more severe. Relatively symmetric weakness with paresthesia usually begins in the legs and progresses to the arms. It is reported that more than 50% of patients with severe disease have weakness of facial and oropharyngeal muscles and 5% to 10% may need intubation because of respiratory failure (Beers and Berkow 1999).

The loss of function in affected nerves occurs because of demyelination. Myelin is the specialized fatty insulation that envelops the conducting part of the nerve, the axon. In GBS the immune system recognizes myelin and mounts an attack against it. Presumably, myelin shares a common characteristic with the pathogen from the antecedent infection, so the immune system cannot differentiate what is foreign (the pathogen) from what is native (myelin). When myelin is removed from a nerve, its ability to conduct signals is severely impaired, and this results in neuropathy.

Medical Treatment

The most common sequence of symptoms is areflexia, followed by proximal limb weakness, followed finally by cranial nerve weakness, and then by respiratory insufficiency. These symptoms may progress for up to 1 month but normally peak by 2 weeks. Diagnosis is ordinarily made on clinical grounds, but nerve conduction studies are revealing.

Before the clinical course is apparent, myelopathic disorders need to be considered. GBS will reveal itself in a matter of days.

Because of the potentially precipitous progression of GBS, hospitalization is in order, if only for observation. Vital capacity and swallowing function may deteriorate rapidly such that intensive care is sometimes necessary. Intubation and respiratory support should be instituted early in the face of respiratory decline to avoid the need for resuscitation. Plasmapheresis, the exchange of the patient's plasma for albumin, is often helpful. This reduces the load of circulating antibodies. Also, intravenous immunoglobulin has been shown to be of benefit. Steroids may be used in conjunction with the above measures (Cecil and Underlie, 1997).

Medical Nutrition Therapy

Guillain-Barré syndrome evolves quickly, and during this acute stage, the metabolic response of GBS is similar to the stress response that occurs in neurotrauma. Researchers studied 21 patients with GBS admitted to an intensive care unit. Energy needs assessed by indirect calorimetry were 40 to 45 nonprotein kcal/kg, and protein needs assessed by 24-hour urine urea nitrogen were 2.0 to 2.5 g/kg. Supportive care by immediate attainment of positive energy balance provided by high-energy and protein tube feedings may help to reestablish a positive nitrogen balance and attenuate muscle wasting (Roubenoff et al, 1992).

For a small percentage of patients, affected oropharyngeal muscles may lead to dysphagia and dysarthria. In this situation, a visit by the dietetics professional at mealtime can be an invaluable way to observe difficulties the patient may have with chewing or swallowing. Such difficulties warrant evaluation by a swallowing specialist. The swallow therapist can evaluate the degree of dysphagia and make appropriate dietary recommendations pertaining to texture, and the patient can be ensured adequate nourishment (Curran, 1997).

Migraine Headache

The syndrome is defined clinically as an episodic intense, throbbing head pain that lasts from 4 to 72 hours. It is usually on one side of the head and becomes worse with exertion. It may be accompanied by nausea and classically is associated with a prodrome of visual disturbances or unusual olfactory and gustatory perception. Most persons report an associated transient visual aura, including flashing lights.

Pathophysiology

Although the cause is unknown, migraine headache is thought to be vascular in origin and follows a family history of migraines or of visual prodromata. The leading theory proposes that dural blood vessels become dilated, and the pulsatile blood flow through these vessels distends and irritates the highly pain-sensitive dura mater. This would explain the throbbing quality of the headache. An inflammatory component to migraine headache has also been proposed.

In two methodologically identical national surveys that were completed 10 years apart, an increase in individuals suffering from migraine was consistent with population growth; 23.6 million people suffered from migraine in 1989 and 27.9 million in 1999. The prevalence and distribution of migraine have remained stable over the last decade. From the most recent survey (29,727 respondents) prevalence of migraine headaches was greater among females (18.2%) than among males (6.5%) and higher in whites than in blacks (Lipton et al, 2001).

Medical Treatment

Treatment depends on the frequency of attacks and the presence of comorbid illness. A thorough history is the key to diagnosis. To qualify for a diagnosis of migraine headache, the headache must be throbbing, episodic, and supremely intense. The excruciating headache must not be prematurely considered to be a migraine. A history of intercurrent nausea, vomiting, photophobia, and visual or olfactory auras is sought. Less commonly, the examiner can identify a neurologic deficit.

Numerous medicines are used to prevent or abort migraine, indicating a less than crystal clear understanding of its pathophysiology. Nonsteroidal antiinflammatory drugs are often the first line, followed by sympathomimetics and serotonin agonists such as sumitriptan. Prophylaxis can include calcium channel antagonists, beta-adrenergic blockers, and serotonin antagonists. The addictive nature of some of the analgesic drugs used with migraine sufferers is noted (Silberstein, 2001).

Medical Nutrition Therapy

Migraine attacks are triggered by a variety of factors, including food, and respond to a variety of treatments (Rapoport and Edmeads, 2001). Foods implicated in one individual may not trigger attacks in another, and food intolerance thresholds vary over time. Therefore general recommendations about food avoidance are ill-advised. The proposed mechanisms that predicate migraine headache on nutritional factors are poorly understood. One recent study suggests that riboflavin may be beneficial because its derivatives participate in mitochondrial dysfunction that plays a part in migraine pathogenesis (Schoenen et al, 1998). Additional research is needed in this area.

Another obstacle to dietary management occurs when dietary restriction of the offending foods contributes to inadequate nutritional intake. Because suspect food items can only be correctly identified if eliminated and then reintroduced into the diet, the dietetics professional should offer alternative food suggestions so that eliminated dietary items are replaced with foods of similar nutritional value, thus ensuring adequate food intake and optimal nutritional status.

Foods that may contribute to migraine attacks include citrus fruits, tea (flavonoids), coffee, pork, chocolate, milk, nuts, vegetables, and cola drinks. Substances that modify vascular tone are tyramine, phenylalanine, phenolic flavonoids, alcohol, food additives (sodium nitrate, aspartame), and caffeine. Foods thought to trigger migraines subsequent to hypoglycemia are chocolate; cheese; citrus fruits; bananas; nuts; cured meats; dairy products; cereals; beans; hot dogs; pizza; food additives; coffee; tea; cola drinks; and alcoholic drinks such as red wine, beer, or whiskey distilled in copper stills (Leira and Rodriguez, 1996). Initiation of therapy will require trial and error and extensive record-keeping of symptoms and food intake on the part of the patient. Chapter 32 offers a Food and Symptom Diary Form.

Myasthenia Gravis

Myasthenia gravis (MG) is not only the most well-known disorder of the neuromuscular junction, but it is also one of the most well-characterized autoimmune diseases, a class of disorders in which the body's immune system raises a response to acetylcholine receptors (AChRs). The incidence of MG is 14 in 100,000 people (www.myasthenia.org/information/summary.htm).

Pathophysiology

The neuromuscular junction is the site on the striated muscle membrane where a spinal motor neuron connects. Here, the signal from the nerve is carried to the muscle via a submicron-sized gap, a synapse. The molecule that carries the signal from the nerve ending to the muscle membrane is acetylcholine (ACh), and AChRs populate the muscle membrane. These receptors translate the chemical signal of ACh into an electrical signal that is required for contraction of muscle fibers.

In MG, the body unwittingly makes antibodies to AChRs. These antibodies are the same that fight off colds and give immunity. The AChR antibodies bind to AChRs and make them unresponsive to ACh. Neither disorder of nerve conduction nor intrinsic disorder of muscle exists. The characteristic weakness in MG occurs because the nervous system signal to the muscle is garbled at the neuromuscular junction. Patients with MG commonly have an overactive thymus gland. This gland resides in the anterior thorax and plays a role in the maturation of B lymphocytes, the cells that are charged with synthesizing antibodies.

Medical Treatment

Relapsing and remitting weakness and fatigability, the period of which varies from minutes to days, characterize MG. The most common presentation is diplopia (double vision) caused by extraocular muscle weakness—followed by dysarthria, facial muscle weakness, and dysphagia. Thirty-three percent of patients with MG are estimated to have significant swallowing disorders caused by fatigue after mastication (Miller, 1997). In 10% of this population, muscular wasting has been encountered, primarily in patients with malnutrition caused by dysphagia (Rowland, 1995). Less commonly, proximal limb weakness (i.e., in hips and shoulders) may be present. In 10% of patients, severe diaphragmatic weakness can result in respiratory difficulty. No involvement of sensory nerves occurs.

Anticholinesterases are medicines that inhibit acetylcholinesterase. They serve to increase the amount of ACh in the neuromuscular junction. Removal of the thymus results in symptomatic improvement in most patients. Corticosteroids are immunosuppressive. In the event that respiratory failure occurs, intubation and temporary cessation of anticholinesterases are the proper course of action until the crisis resolves (Greenberg, 1997).

Medical Nutrition Therapy

Chewing and swallowing are often compromised in MG. Because this occurs with fatigue, it is important to provide nutritionally dense foods at the beginning of meals before the patient tires. Small frequent meals that are easy to chew and swallow are helpful. Difficulties holding a bolus on the tongue have also been observed, which suggests that foods that do not fall apart easily may be better tolerated. For patients treated with anticholinesterase drugs, it is crucial to time medication with feeding to facilitate optimal swallowing.

Physical activity should be limited before mealtime to ensure maximal strength to eat a meal. In certain patients, even nonstrenuous activities such as talking can mean the difference between consuming an oral diet versus requiring enteral nutrition support (Miller, 1997). It is important not to encourage food consumption once the patient begins to tire because this may contribute to aspiration.

If and when respiratory crisis occurs, it is usually temporary. Nutrition support via nasogastrointestinal tube may be implemented in the interim to assist in maintaining the vital function of the patient until the crisis subsides. Once the patient is extubated, a swallow evaluation using cinefluoroscopy is appropriate to assess the degree of deglutitory dysfunction or swallowing irregularity and the risk of aspiration associated with resuming an oral diet.

Multiple Sclerosis

Multiple sclerosis (MS) is a chronic disease that affects the CNS and is characterized by destruction of the myelin sheath, the function of which is transmission of electrical nerve impulses. MS is called "multiple" because multiple areas of optic nerves, spinal cord, and brain undergo "sclerosis," whereby myelin is replaced with sclera or scar tissue. As with other complex conditions and diseases, no single test can ascertain whether a patient has MS; however, new diagnostic criteria have been developed for use by practicing clinicians (Vastag, 2001).

The signs and symptoms of MS are easily distinguished features, despite remitting to a varying extent, and they recur over the natural history of this disease. The prevalence is less than 1/100,000 in equatorial areas; 6 to 14/100,000 in the southern United States and southern Europe; and 30 to 80/100,000 in Canada, northern Europe, and the northern United States (www.mmss.org). In the worst scenario, MS can render a person unable to write, speak or walk, but the vast majority of patients are only mildly affected.

Pathophysiology

The precise cause of MS remains undetermined, and the epidemiology is difficult to establish in view of the uncertainty of the diagnosis and relative rarity of the disease. A number of well-established findings have been incorporated into a hypothesis to explain the etiology of MS. Although a familial predisposition to MS has been noted in a minority of cases, familial tendency is not well established; no consistent pattern of Mendelian inheritance has emerged (Adams et al, 1997). The tendency to consider diseases with an increased familial incidence as inherited exists; however, instances of the same condition in several family members may reflect exposure to a common agent. Hence, environmental factors compete for this distinction, and two of these are geographic latitude and diet.

Epidemiologic studies have linked the incidence of MS to geographic location rather than to a particular ethnic group. This increased incidence from the equator northward has been explained by exposure to the sun. Exogenous 1,25-dihydroxyvitamin D_3 (hormonal form of vitamin D_3) has been associated with preventing experimental autoimmune encephalomyelitis (EAE) in mice, thus focusing attention on the possible relationship of MS to vitamin D. Researchers hypothesize that the degree of sunlight exposure catalyzing the production of vitamin D_3 in skin is an environmental factor and that the hormonal form of vitamin D_3 is a selective immune system regulator inhibiting this autoimmune disease (Hayes et al, 1997). Low sunlight exposure yields insufficient vitamin D_3, which limits 1,25-dihydroxyvitamin D_3 and increases the risk for MS.

Diet is another environmental risk factor associated with the development of MS (Payne, 2001). One ecologic study compared sex-specific mortality rates of MS from the World Health Statistics with the consumption of various saturated fats obtained from the food balance sheets of the United Nations Food and Agriculture Organization (FAO). A higher prevalence of disease was noted in populations that consume diets rich in animal fats containing saturated fatty acids. Ecologic studies are a good starting point in determining whether an association exists. However, the exposure (dietary fat) and outcome (incidence of disease) data for each individual are unknown, and therefore a causal relationship of dietary fat to the incidence of MS cannot be concluded (Gordis, 1996). It appears that both environmental factors are compelling, but circumstantial evidence warrants further studies.

More recent data from two large cohorts (the Nurses Health Study with 92,422 individuals and the Nurses Health Study II with 95,389) were analyzed for associations between intakes of total and specific types of fat and the risk of MS (Zhang et al, 2000). Omega-3 fatty acids from fish were found to be unrelated to risk, and although not statistically significant, a lower risk of MS existed with a higher intake of linolenic acid, a polyunsaturated fatty acid found in vegetable oils—particularly flaxseed oil and nuts such as walnuts (see Chapter 3). Age, smoking, and tier at birth (i.e., geographic region) were the variables found to be risk factors for MS when analyses were completed. Although conclusions about results from previous studies are inconsistent (Polish, New Zealand, Italian, and French investigations), most investigators report that use of dietary fats are unrelated to MS risk or are inconclusive (Payne, 2001; Zhang et al, 2000).

Medical Treatment

Fluctuating symptoms and spontaneous remissions make treatments difficult to evaluate. Currently no proven treatment for changing the course of MS, preventing future attacks, or preventing deterioration exists. Initially, recovery from relapses is nearly complete, but over time, neurologic deficits remain (Figure 43-6). Therefore measures to maximize recovery from initial attacks or exacerbations, prevent fatigue and infection, and use all of the available rehabilita-

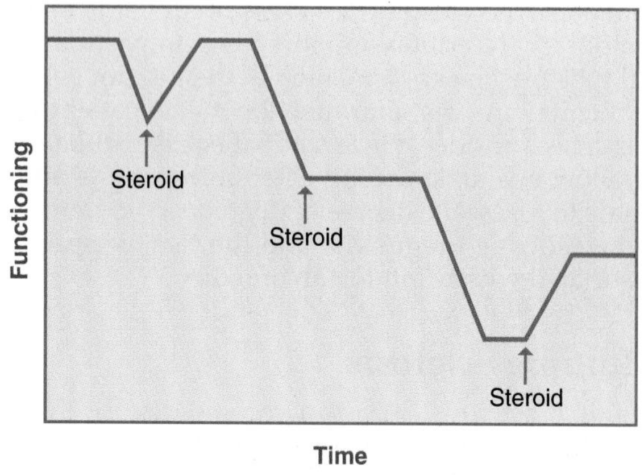

FIGURE 43-6 • The progression of multiple sclerosis.

tive measures to postpone the bedridden stage of disease are imperative. Physical and occupational therapies are standard for weakness, spasticity, tremor, uncoordination, and other symptoms.

Drugs for spasticity can be initiated at a low dose and cautiously increased until the patient responds. Physical therapy for gait training and range-of-motion exercises for weak spastic limbs helps (Beers and Berkow, 1999). Steroid therapy is used in treating exacerbations; adrenocorticotrophic hormone (ACTH) and prednisolone are the drugs of choice. However, treatment is not consistently effective and tends to be more useful in cases of less than 5 years' duration. Side effects of short-term steroid treatment include increased appetite, weight gain, fluid retention, nervousness, and insomnia. Methotrexate may also be used with ACTH, thus causing anorexia and nausea. Drug therapies may therefore be a challenge (see Chapter 19).

Reduced cerebrospinal fluid and serum levels of vitamin B_{12} and folate have been noted in MS patients who receive high-dose steroids. Because a deficiency of these two nutrients has been associated with cerebral demyelination and subacute combined degeneration of the spinal cord, it might be desirable to administer vitamin B_{12} and folate or at least monitor the levels of these nutrients (Frequin et al, 1993). A more recent therapy used by researchers in Dallas identified improvement in T cells in healthy people, but the cells function abnormally for those with MS. Use of α-interferon (Avonex, Betaseron, Copaxone) has been available because it interferes with viral replication. Treatment with α-interferon seems to delay neurologic deterioration, but a drawback is expense.

Medical Nutrition Therapy

With respect to research, environmental factors such as nutrition have dominated over therapeutic trials aimed at treating the disease once it has occurred. Several dietary regimens for managing MS have been studied, including low-fat, gluten-free diets and fatty acid supplements, all of which have yielded equivocal results.

Data suggest that dietary supplementation with linoleic acid (safflower oil, soybean oil) may have some beneficial effects, although this therapy remains investigational. Other trials have used 1.7 g/day of eicosapentanoic acid (EPA) and 1.1 g/day of docosahexaenoic acid (DHA), with the controls receiving 10 g/day of oleic acid (olive oil) for a period of 2 years; evidence is inconclusive as well (Wozniak-Wowk, 1993).

Past trials of various diets—such as allergen-free, gluten-free, pectin-free, and fructose-restricted diets; the raw food Evers diet; the MacDougal diet (no gluten, low sugar, and no refined sugar; a low-fat diet high in polyunsaturated fatty acids, with megadoses of vitamins and minerals); the Cambridge liquid diet (330 kcal/day with 22 g protein); and vitamin/mineral therapies (zinc phosphates, calcium, other combinations) have generally been ruled ineffective (Wozniak-Wowk, 1993).

Although no valid clinical trials have supported the efficacy of nutrition in delaying the progression of MS, the nutrition professional's careful evaluation of nutritional status of the patient, maximizing nutritional status as an adjunct to the medical care plan, is imperative. As the disease progresses, neurologic deficits, dysphagia in particular, may occur as the result of damaged cranial nerves. Hence, diet consistency may need to be modified to prevent aspiration. Additional problems include impaired vision, dysarthria, and poor ambulation, which make eating less enjoyable by turning meal preparation into a difficult task. In this situation, reliance on comfort foods and prepackaged, single-serving, or convenience foods often permits independent preparation of meals. Given the chronic nature of this debilitating disease, patients may require enteral nutrition support.

Neurogenic bladder is common. It causes urinary incontinence, urgency, and frequency. To minimize these problems, distributing fluids evenly throughout the waking hours and limiting them before bed is helpful. Some patients limit fluid intake severely to decrease frequency of urination but thereby increase the risk of urinary tract infection (UTI). UTIs are common in patients with MS, and some patients increase their intake of cranberry juice as a form of self-treatment (see Chapter 39). Neurogenic bowel can cause either constipation or diarrhea, and incidence of fecal impaction is increased in MS. A diet that is high in fiber with additional prunes and adequate fluid can moderate both problems.

Parkinson's Disease

Parkinson's disease (PD) is a progressive, disabling, neurodegenerative disease described by James Parkinson in 1817. It is characterized by slow and decreased movement, muscular rigidity, resting tremor, and postural instability. Although the natural history of this disease can be remarkably benign in some cases, approximately 66% of patients are disabled within 5 years, and 80% are disabled after 10 years (Adams et al, 1997). PD is one of the most common neurologic diseases in North America; it affects approximately 1% of the population over 65 years of age. The incidence is similar across socioeconomic groups, but PD is less common in African Americans and Asians in comparison with whites. It most commonly occurs between the ages of 40 and 70 (Adams et al, 1997).

Pathophysiology

Although the cause of PD remains unclear, the pathogenesis is well described. It involves an interaction of inheritance with environmental factors. There is a marked loss of dopaminergic neurons (pigmented cells) in the substantia nigra as well as tyrosine hydroxylase, the rate-limiting enzyme for dopamine. Three theories are postulated for the etiology of PD: (1) altered dopamine metabolism from neural injury; (2) exposure to environmental neurotoxins; and (3) predisposition (Standaert and Stern, 1993). The genetic and environmental factors have been confirmed more recently (Gwinn-Hardy, 2002).

The role of endogenous toxins from cellular oxidative reactions has emerged because aging has been associated with a loss of neurons that contain dopamine and an increase in monoamine oxidase. When metabolized (enzymatic oxidation and auto-oxidation), dopamine produces endogenous toxins (hydrogen peroxide and free radicals), thus causing peroxidation of membrane lipids and cell death. In the presence of an inherited or acquired predisposition, severe oxidative injury may lead to substantial loss of dopaminergic neurons similar to that observed in PD.

Several other environmental factors have also been implicated in the etiology of PD, and this theory of etiology has been strengthened considerably by the onset of the disease in intravenous drug users who self-administered an opiate substance, 1-methyl-4-phenyl-1,2,3,6-tetrahydropyridine (MPTP). This neurotoxin produces a rapidly progressive Parkinsonian syndrome that selectively destroys dopamine cells in the substantia nigra (Gelinas and Martinoli, 2002).

Dietary lipids and antioxidants are other environmental factors implicated in the etiology of PD. A case-controlled study found evidence that links high-fat intake from animal sources and PD (Logroscino et al, 1996). It has long been recognized that supplementing deficient subjects with vitamin E is an important preventive measure, given the devastating peripheral neuropathy and ataxia that may result from vitamin E deficiency (Traber and Sies, 1996). Although serum levels of vitamin E were not significantly lower in patients with PD than in control subjects, researchers have concluded that a prolonged and severe vitamin E deficiency can result in loss of nigrostriatal nerve endings (Fernandez-Calle et al, 1992). These nutrient-related findings support the hypothesis that oxidative stress may contribute to the pathogenesis of PD; however, data do not support an affect for any single vitamin supplement.

The third environmental factor associated with the incidence of PD is geography. There is a greater incidence of PD in industrialized countries and agrarian areas where toxins are more commonly used. No one chemical toxin or heavy metal has been shown to definitely cause PD (Adams et al, 1997), but an overload of dietary iron and manganese are thought to be related (Powers et al, 2003). More research is needed.

The genetic susceptibility for developing PD remains an area of study. Twin studies are inclusive, and most cases are sporadic, despite a family incidence rate of about 5% (Maher, 2002). Maher (2002) reported that female-female sibling pairs more often had other relatives with PD than did the male siblings who were studied. Women may have a stronger genetic component to their disease.

Medical Treatment

The "classic triad" of signs—tremor, rigidity, and bradykinesia—first described by James Parkinson, remain the accepted clinical criterion for diagnosis. However, it was well over a century before an effective therapy, levodopa (L-dopa) (the current cornerstone of treatment) was introduced for controlling symptoms. Because dopamine does not readily cross the blood-brain barrier, L-dopa, a precursor to dopamine, is administered and subsequently converted to dopamine by dopa decarboxylase, and it crosses the blood-brain barrier (Calne, 1993).

Pharmacotherapy agents as well as surgical interventions and physical therapy are adjunct therapies for treating PD. Deprenyl (a monoamine oxidase inhibitor)—but not vitamin E (2000 IU daily)—was shown to delay the onset of disability associated with early otherwise untreated PD (Parkinson's Study Group, 1993). In older patients, drug-induced PD may occur as a side effect of neuroleptics or metoclopramide (see Chapter 19).

Medical Nutrition Therapy

The primary nutritional intervention in counseling patients with PD, especially with patients having refractory fluctuations of dyskinesias, should be to focus on drug-nutrient interactions; in particular, drug-nutrient interactions between dietary protein and L-dopa should be reviewed. Large neutral amino acids are thought to compete for the transport mechanism in the gastrointestinal tract altering the rate of entry of L-dopa into circulation and uptake into the brain.

For some patients, symptoms may be reduced by eliminating (minimizing) dietary protein at breakfast and lunch and adding it to the evening meal. Several studies have claimed to reduce L-dopa fluctuations by restricting daytime protein to only 10 g and redistributing protein intake to the evening meal to meet the RDA protein requirement. Daytime mobility was improved, whereas rigidity occurred overnight (Karstaedt and Pincus, 1992; Pare et al, 1992). Table 43-10 presents a sample menu for this diet.

Any benefit from this diet should be apparent within 1 week, and a special effort should be made to ensure that the diet is not deficient in other nutrients such as calcium, iron, B vitamins, and fiber. Results of these diet studies are conflicting, but dietary manipulation is harmless if the diet is nutritionally complete, and it may be adjunctive therapy.

Pyridoxine and aspartame have also been studied for their possible interaction with L-dopa. Decarboxylase, the enzyme required to convert L-dopa to dopamine, depends on pyridoxine. If excessive

TABLE 43-10 Protein Redistribution in L-Dopa Therapy

Breakfast	**Amount of Protein (g)**
½ cup oatmeal	2
1 orange	0.5
1 cup Polyrich (nondairy creamer)	0.5
Egg Replacer (unlimited)	0
Low-protein bread, toasted	0
Margarine or butter (unlimited)	0
Jelly or jam (unlimited)	0
Sugar or sugar substitute (unlimited)	0
Coffee or tea (unlimited)	0
Lunch	
½ cup vegetable soup	2
1 cup tossed salad	1
Salad dressing (unlimited)	0
1 banana	1
Low-protein pasta (unlimited)	0
Margarine or butter (unlimited)	0
Low-protein cookies (unlimited)	0
Soda pop, coffee, tea, or water	0
Afternoon Snack	
Gum drops or hard candy (unlimited)	0
Apple or cranberry juice (unlimited)	0
TOTAL	7
Dinner	
4 oz beef, pork, veal, chicken (at least)	28 or more
1 cup stuffing	4
Gravy	0
½ cup peas	2
1 cup pudding	8
1 cup milk	8
Evening Snack	
1 oz cheese	7
4 crackers	2
Soda pop	0
DAILY TOTAL	66 or more

amounts of the vitamin are present, L-dopa may be metabolized in the periphery—not in the CNS, where its therapeutic activity occurs. Therefore vitamin preparations that contain pyridoxine should not be taken with doses of L-dopa.

Side effects of medications for PD include anorexia, nausea, reduced sense of smell, constipation, and dry mouth. To diminish the gastrointestinal side effects of L-dopa, it should be taken with meals. Additional foods, especially broad beans (fava beans), naturally contain L-dopa. A diet that substitutes these legumes for other protein foods may be useful in reducing fluctuations in response to L-dopa medication (Kempster and Wahlqvist, 1994).

As the disease progresses, rigidity of the extremities can interfere with the patient's ability to care for himself or herself, including self-feeding. Rigidity also interferes with the ability to control the position of the head and trunk, necessary for eating. Eating is slowed; mealtimes may take up to 1 hour. Simultaneous movements such as those required to handle both a knife and fork become increasingly difficult. Tremor in the arms and hands increases caloric needs and may make self-feeding of liquids impossible without spilling. Perception, including spatial organization, can become impaired and further impact effective ambulation (Burns and Carr-Davis, 1994).

Dysphagia is a late complication but is not due to dopaminergic degeneration (Nilsson et al, 1996). A large number of patients may be silent aspirators, which affects nutritional status. One study identified a fourfold increase in weight loss greater than 10 lb in patients with PD in comparison with matched control patients (Beyer et al, 1995). Encouragement and support to consume adequate amounts of nourishment are key.

Experimental treatment procedures are being tested and reported with increasing frequency (e.g., progress with deep brain penetration and other surgical interventions), and efforts with stem cell research continue in hopes that the "cure" is not far off.

Neurotrauma

Head trauma refers to any of the following, alone or in combination: brain injury; skull fractures; extraparenchymal hemorrhage—epidural, subdural, subarachnoid—or hemorrhage into the brain tissue itself, including intraparenchymal or intraventricular hemorrhage. In the United States, trauma is the leading cause of death in persons up to 44 years of age, and more than half of these deaths result from head injuries (Adams et al, 1997). The annual incidence is estimated to be 200/100,000 people, with a peak frequency between 15 and 24 years of age.

Even though relatively much is known about different types of head injuries, it is difficult to accurately predict neurologic recovery. Morbidity is also high, as estimated by the 74,000 newly disabled each year, yielding an incidence of 31 to 42/100,000 (Rowland, 1995). Motor vehicle collisions are the major source of injury. Despite intensive intervention, long-term disability occurs in a large portion of the survivors of severe head injury.

Pathophysiology

Brain injury can be subdivided into three types: concussion, contusion, and diffuse axonal injury. A concussion is a brief loss of consciousness (<6 hours) with no evidence of damage found on computed tomography (CT) or magnetic resonance imaging (MRI) scans. Microscopic studies have failed to find any evidence of structural damage in areas of known concussion, although evidence of change in cellular metabolism exists. Contusion is similar to a bruise on the skin. It is characterized by damaged capillaries and swelling, followed by resolution of the damage. Note that large contusions may dramatically increase intracranial pressure (ICP) and may lead to ischemia or herniation. Contusions can be detected by CT or MRI scans. Diffuse axonal injury results from the shearing of axons by a rotational acceleration of the brain inside the skull. Damaged areas are often found in the corpus callosum and the upper outer portion of the brain stem.

Skull fractures of the calvarium and the base are described in the same manner as other fractures. Comminution involves splintering of bone into many fragments. Displacement occurs when bones are displaced from their original apposition to each other. *Open* or *closed* describes whether a fracture is exposed to air. Open fractures dramatically increase the risk of infection (osteomyelitis), and open skull fractures in particular carry an increased risk for meningitis because the dura mater is often violated.

Epidural and subdural hematomas are often corrected by surgical intervention. The volume of these lesions often displaces the brain tissue and may cause diffuse axonal injury and swelling. When the lesion becomes large enough, it may cause herniation of brain contents through various openings of the skull base. Consequent compression and ischemia of vital brain structures may rapidly lead to death.

Medical Treatment

The body's response to stressors such as that seen in neurotrauma results in the production of cytokines such as interleukin-1, interleukin-6, interleukin-8, and tumor necrosis factor. These are elevated in the body after head injury and are associated with the hormonal milieu that negatively affects metabolism and organ function (see Chapters 18 and 42). Some of the metabolic events include fever, neutrophilia, muscle breakdown, altered amino acid metabolism, production of hepatic acute-phase reactants, increased endothelial permeability, and expression of endothelial adhesion molecules. It has also been proposed that specific cytokines cause organ demise. Specific tissue damage has been observed in the gut, liver, lung, and brain.

The molecular basis of functional recovery is poorly understood. Clinical observations and research that use experimental injury models implicate several metabolites in neuronal degeneration (Liu et al, 2002). The levels of intracellular ATP (energy source) and pH are decreased, whereas levels of extracellular glutamate, intracellular calcium ions, and oxidative damage to RNA and DNA, protein, and lipid are increased (Liu et al, 2002).

Clinical findings of brain injury often include a transient decrease in consciousness level. Headache and dizziness are relatively common and are less worrisome unless they become more intense or are accompanied by vomiting. Focal neurologic deficits, progressively decreasing level of consciousness, and penetrating brain injury are more ominous risk factors and demand prompt neurosurgical evaluation (Greenberg, 1997).

Skull fractures are suspected underneath lacerations, can often be felt as a "drop off" or discontinuity on the surface of the skull, and are readily identifiable by CT scan. Basilar skull fractures are manifested by otorrhea, hemotympanum, and rhinorrhea (salty fluid dripping from the nose or down the pharynx). Other signs include raccoon eyes and Battle's sign—blood behind the mastoid process. Basilar skull fractures may precipitate injuries to cranial nerves, which are essential for chewing, swallowing, taste, and smell.

Epidural and subdural hematomas are neurosurgical emergencies because they may rapidly progress to herniation of brain contents through the skull base with subsequent death. These lesions may present similarly, with decreased level of consciousness, contralateral hemiparesis, and pupillary dilation. Classically, epidural hematoma presents with progressively decreasing consciousness after an interval of several hours in which the patient has been awake after a brief loss of consciousness. The subdural hematoma usually features progressively decreasing consciousness from the time of injury. These lesions damage brain tissue by gross displacement and traction. Sequelae most commonly include epilepsy and the postconcussive syndrome and a constellation of headache, vertigo, fatigue, and memory difficulties.

Treatment approaches for these patients can become highly complex, but the two goals of any therapeutic intervention are to maintain cerebral perfusion and to regulate ICP. Of the possible interventions, perfusion and pressure control do have implications for nutritional therapy in the patient with a head injury.

Medical Nutrition Therapy

The goal of nutritional management is to oppose the hypercatabolism and hypermetabolism associated with the inflammation. Hypercatabolism is manifested by protein degradation and is evidenced by profound urinary urea nitrogen excretion. Data in non–head-injured patients show that a 30% weight loss increases mortality rate; further, starved head-injured patients lose sufficient nitrogen to reduce weight by 15% per week (Liebert, 2000). Nitrogen catabolism in a fasting normal human is only 3 to 5 g nitrogen per day, whereas nitrogen excretion is 14 to 25 g nitrogen per day in the fasting patient with severe head injury. In the absence of nutritional intake, this degree of nitrogen loss can result in a 10% decrease in lean mass within 7 days. If sequelae were to continue unabated, within 2 to 3 weeks a weight loss of 30% could impact mortality significantly (Brain Trauma Foundation, 1996) (see Chapter 42).

Hypermetabolism contributes to increased energy expenditure. Correlations between the severity of brain injury as measured by the Glascow Coma Scale and energy requirements have been shown (see Chapter 42). The mean resting metabolic rate in patients with head trauma is approximately 140% to 160% of the expected normal basal metabolic rate. In patients paralyzed with pancuronium bromide or barbiturates, metabolic expenditure may be decreased to 100% to 120% of basal metabolic rate. This decreased metabolic rate in pharmacologically paralyzed patients suggests that maintaining muscle tone is an important part of metabolic expenditure since the energy requirements would be 140% to 160% of BMR in the unparalyzed patient. Nutriture of the neurologically critically ill patient is accomplished by administering either enteral or parenteral nutrition support. Routine intragastric feedings are safe and well tolerated (Klodell et al, 2000). Nutrition support is usually begun within 72 hours after injury and is necessary in order to achieve nutritional replacement by 7 days after injury. Both modes of therapy must be initiated at levels below actual requirements and increased gradually to meet nutritional requirements. For guidelines on estimating nutritional requirements in head trauma, refer to *Clinical Insight:* Estimating Nutrition Requirements in Neurotrauma.

Spine Trauma

The term *spine trauma* encompasses many types of injuries ranging from stable fractures of the spinal column to catastrophic transsection of the spinal cord. Of nutritional significance is neurologic injury. A complete spinal cord injury (SCI) is defined as a lesion without preservation of motor or sensory function more than three segments below the level of the injury (Greenberg, 1997). With an incomplete injury, some degree of residual function, motor or sensory, exists more than three segments below the lesion. Spinal cord injury is somewhat less common than head injury with an annual incidence of 40/1,000,000 people (Greenberg, 1997). SCI, like head injury, is most often seen in the young. Motor vehicle collisions account for one third to one half of SCIs; the balance is caused by athletic injuries and domestic and industrial accidents.

Pathophysiology

The spinal cord responds to insult in a manner similar to that of the brain. Bleeding, contusion, and shorn axons appear first and are followed by a several-year remodeling process that consists of gliosis and fibrosis. Liquefactive necrosis may predispose to the formation of a syrinx, a fluid collection in the center of the spinal cord, whose mass effect may manifest as a slowly progressive neurologic deficit. Although SCI may strike at a single location, the significance of the injury lies more in the disruption of descending axons at that level than in injury to the segment itself.

Traumatic extraparenchymal hematomas in the spine are unusual; however, SCIs are almost invariably associated with spinal column fractures and ligament instability. Such processes may be amenable to either surgical or nonsurgical reduction and stabilization.

CLINICAL INSIGHT

Estimating Nutrition Requirements in Neurotrauma

It is difficult to estimate nutritional requirements precisely, but they can be generalized as follows:

1. Ideally, caloric requirements should be measured by indirect calorimetry but may be estimated from the Harris-Benedict equation if indirect calorimetry is not available: 140% to 160% of basal energy expenditure for severe head injuries; 100% to 120% of basal energy expenditure in pharmacologically paralyzed patients.
2. Protein requirements are accentuated in comparison with calorie requirements. Protein intake should be 15% to 20% of total calories, and requirements should be measured by using urinary urea nitrogen in an attempt to achieve positive nitrogen balance. Initially, attenuation of negative nitrogen balance rather than achievement of positive nitrogen balance may be all that is possible. Other factors that mediate protein requirements are hepatic and renal function. Renal function may be altered, especially in the head-injured patient, because of dehydration therapy.
3. Free water should be given in accordance with the needs of either dehydration (increased ICP or hydrocephalus) or hypervolemic therapy (vasospasm risk). Concentrated enteral formulas that provide 2 kcal/ml can be used to maintain adequate nutritional intake while providing minimal free water; about 2000 kcal can be provided in only 730 ml of free water. Merely reducing the rate of infusion is not advised because this will contribute to nutritional deficits.
4. Nonprotein calories should be provided to prevent deleterious effects of excessive carbohydrate (hyperglycemia, hyperinsulinemia, gluconeogenesis, and hypercarbia) and fat (immunosuppression and hyperlipidemia) intake. Carbohydrate administration should range between 3 and 5 mg/kg/min/day with a minimum of about 150 g carbohydrate/day to prevent gluconeogenesis. Lipids should not exceed 2 g/kg/day and should come from sources of omega-6 fatty acids.
5. Vitamin and mineral supplementation to meet the RDAs is important. Additional supplementation with calcium, phosphorus, and magnesium is often required when patients are on steroids, diuretics, or some other therapy.

Medical Treatment

Spinal cord injuries have numerous clinical manifestations, depending on the level of the injury. Complete transsection results in complete loss of function below the level of the lesion, including the bladder and sphincters. Numerous incomplete cord syndromes have been described (see Table 43-8).

After the patient is stabilized hemodynamically, the next step is to evaluate the degree of neurologic deficit. Patients with suspected SCI are usually immobilized promptly in the field. Complete radiographic evaluation of the spinal column is obligatory in multitrauma and unconscious patients. In the awake patient, clinical evidence of spine compromise is usually sufficient to determine the need for further workup. CT and MRI are used to more accurately delineate bony damage and spinal cord compromise. A dismal 3% of patients with complete spinal cord insults will recover some function after 24 hours. Failure to regain function after 24 hours predicts a 0% chance of reestablishment of function in the future. Incomplete spinal cord syndromes, described in Table 43-11, have variably improved outcomes.

TABLE 43-11 Incomplete Spinal Cord Injury Syndromes*

SYNDROME	RECOVERY (%)
Anterior cord: Paraplegia and heat or temperature sensation loss. Fine sensation preserved.	10-20
Brown-Sequard: Cord hemisection. Ipsilateral hemiparesis, fine sensation impaired. Contralateral pain and temperature sense loss.	90
Central cord: Upper extremities weaker than lower extremities. Bladder ileus. Variable sensory loss.	50
Posterior cord: Dysesthesias in neck, upper arms, and waist. Upper extremity hemiparesis.	Rare

Modified from Greenberg MS: *Handbook of neurosurgery,* ed 4, Lakeland, Fla, 1997, Greenberg Graphics.
*The more common incomplete spinal cord injury syndromes. A course of steroids is strongly indicated for each of these.

Medical Nutrition Therapy

Morbidity and mortality rates associated with SCI have improved dramatically, particularly in the last two decades. Advances in acute-phase care have reduced early mortality and prevented complications

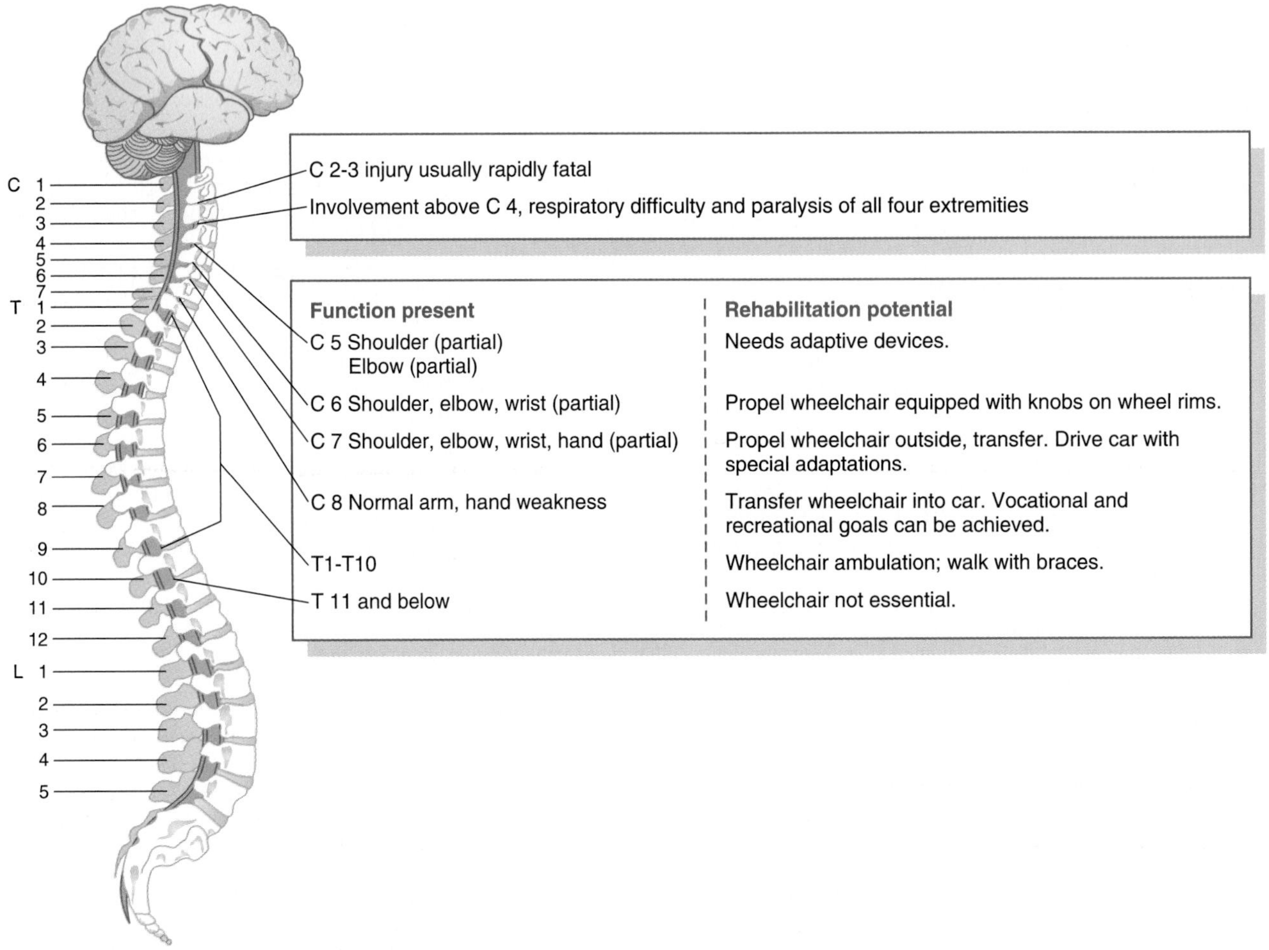

FIGURE 43-7 • Sequelae of spinal cord injury and rehabilitation changes.

frequently associated with early death, such as respiratory failure and pulmonary emboli. Fewer than 10% of patients with SCI die from the acute injury. Technologic advances in enteral and parenteral feeding techniques and formulas have also played a role in maintaining nutritional status of these patients. Although the metabolic response to neurotrauma has been studied extensively, the acute metabolic response to SCI has not, but it is similar to that seen in neurotrauma during the acute phase. Initially, paralytic ileus may occur but may resolve within 72 hours after injury. See section on nutritional management for neurotrauma.

For those who survive the injury but are disabled for life, there are significant alterations in lifestyle as well as the need for prevention of developing secondary complications that follow SCI. In general, the number and frequency of complications, constipation, pressure ulcers, obesity, and pain vary but are interrelated to nutrition. Figure 43-7 describes the rehabilitation potential based on the level of injury.

Constipation is a problem that can adversely affect appetite. Therapeutic diets of high fiber and adequate water intake alone will not suffice for treatment of constipation. More than likely, a routine bowel preparation program is required. The individual with SCI is at risk for developing pressure ulcers, which, if left uncared for, can contribute to morbidity. Maintenance of nutritional health is one factor in preventing the development of pressure ulcers because poor nutrition is an underlying risk factor for infection.

Loss of muscle tone caused by skeletal muscle paralysis below the level of injury contributes to decreased metabolic activity, initial weight loss, and predisposition to osteoporosis. Acutely, the patient experiences some weight loss. Guidelines for accepted weights adjusted for paraplegia and quadriplegia are as follows: the paraplegic should weigh 10 to 15 lb less than ideal body weight (IBW); the quadriplegic should weigh 15 to 20 lb less than IBW (Blissitt, 1990). The ability to maintain adequate weight is important for a number of reasons. Basal metabolic rates may be lower than predicted and significantly correlated with the level of the lesion. The higher the injury, the lower the metabolic rate. Quadriplegic patients have lower metabolic rates than paraplegic patients; it is proportional to the amount of denervated muscle that results in part from the loss of residual motor function.

In the rehabilitation phase, quadraplegics may require approximately 25% to 50% fewer calories than conventional equations would predict. Hence, these patients have the potential to become overweight. Obesity actually has been proposed to influence the eventual rehabilitation process by limiting functional outcome. As a consequence of bone loss because of the loss of mineralization that results from immobilization, SCI is associated with osteopenia and osteoporosis, and the prevalence of long bone fractures is increased.

SUMMARY

A diverse array of physical and psychosocial issues—such as anemia, respiratory paralysis, pneumonia, ileus, pressure ulcers, hemorrhage, neurogenic bowel and bladder, depression, and social support—affect the nutritional status of the neurologic patient. The nutritionist plays an important role in not only the acute care but also the long-term care as these patients adjust to life with differing function levels. Activities related to feeding, exercise, and maintaining optimal health and appropriate nutritional care can help tremendously.

■ Relevant Web Sites

Amyotrophic Lateral Sclerosis Association (ALS)
www.alsa.org/als
www.msif.org.uk
Archives of Neurology
archneur.ama-assn.org/issues/v57n8/ffull
Brain Injury Diseases and Disorders
www.neurosurgery.ucla.edu/diagnoses/braininjury
Epilepsy Foundation
www.efa.org
JAMA and Archives
www.ama-assn.org/special/infohome.htm
Neurological Disorders
www.ninds.nih.gov
Parkinson's Disease
www.pdf.org/index/cfm or www.parkinsons.org

Clinical Scenario 1: Seizures

Clarence, a hospitalized patient who is receiving enteral nutrition support, is having mild seizure activity. Tube feedings have been infused via a PEG over 12 hours. Therapeutic serum level for phenytoin has not been achieved despite the patient's receiving a normal prescribed dose of phenytoin. The physicians would like input regarding the drug-nutrient interaction to achieve therapeutic serum phenytoin levels for control of the seizures.

1. As the clinician managing the nutritional care of this patient, what would you consider to be the most appropriate action based on the current enteral support regimen?
   a. Hold the feedings 2 hours before and after administering the phenytoin.
   b. Change the tube-feeding regimen to gravity drip infusions of 480 ml four times per day.
   c. Change the tube-feeding formula to a blenderized formula.
   d. Suggest dosing phenytoin once per day via sustained-release capsule so that the tube-feeding formula will not bind with the medication.
   e. Continue the present enteral support regimen because answers a and c will not result in therapeutic phenytoin levels without increasing the dose of phenytoin.
2. Clarence's wife has suggested adding bolus feedings so the patient can walk with her more often. How would you design the feeding frequency, and how will this affect the phenytoin administration?

Clinical Scenario 2: Alzheimer's Disease

Carina, an 83-year-old Hispanic woman—height: 5 ft 1 in, weight: 92 lb,—is brought to the physician's office because her family is concerned about her apparent weight loss. They had noticed changes in her behavior and thought that her clothes were fitting more loosely. On questioning they state that most of this has happened over the past 3 months. They report that Carina "paces a great deal of the time, and wanders off more frequently than she used to do," especially when left alone. They have noticed an increase in her forgetfulness.

1. Why is Carina losing weight?
2. What is helpful for Carina? Is it more beneficial to give many different foods, allowing choices, or is it better to give small amounts of one food at a time?
3. The patient does not recognize the food being offered. What might be suggested? Consider her cultural preferences.
4. The patient has difficulty using utensils and seems confused when considering which one to use. Loss of motor function may be gradual; later hand guidance may be needed; assess motor skills routinely. What should be planned?

Cited References

Adams RD et al: *Principles of neurology,* ed 6, New York, 1997, McGraw-Hill, Health Professions Division.

Appel SH et al: Calcium: the Darth Vader of ALS, *Amyotroph Lateral Scler Other Motor Neuron Disord* 2(1):47S, 2001.

Arney WK, Pinnock CB: The milk mucus belief: sensations associated with the belief and characteristics of believers, *Appetite* 20:53, 1993.

Au Yeung SC, Ensom MH: Phenytoin and enteral feedings: does evidence support an interaction? *Ann Pharmacother* 34:896, 2000.

Barzilay JI et al: Baseline characteristics of the diabetic participants in the Antihypertensive and Lipid-Lowering Treatment to Prevent Heart Attack Trial (ALLHAT), *Diabetes Care* 24:654, 2001.

Beers M, Berkow R: *The Merck manual of diagnosis and therapy,* Whitehouse Station , NJ 1999, Merk Research Laboratories.

Berryman MS: The ketogenic diet revisited, *J Am Diet Assoc* 97:S192, 1997.

Beyer PL et al: Weight change and body composition in patients with Parkinson's disease, *J Am Diet Assoc* 95:979, 1995.

Blass JP et al: The role of the metabolic lesion in Alzheimer's disease, *J Alzheimers Dis* 4:225, 2002.

Blissitt PA: Nutrition in acute spinal cord injury, *Crit Care Nurs Clin North Am* 2:375, 1990.

Brain Trauma Foundation: Nutritional support of brain-injured patients, *J Neurotrauma* 13(11):721, 1996.

Burns BL, Carr-Davis EM: Nutritional management of Parkinson's disease. In Weiner WJ, Cohen A, editors: *Interdisciplinary treatment of Parkinson's disease,* New York, 1994, Demos Publication.

Calne DB: Treatment of Parkinson's disease, *N Engl J Med* 329:1021, 1993.

Cecil RL, Underlie TE: *Cecil essentials of medicine,* ed 4, Philadelphia, 1997, WB Saunders.

Cohen D: A primary care checklist for effective family management, *Med Clin North Am* 78(4):795, 1994.

Connor JR, Beard JL: Dietary iron supplements in the elderly: to use or not to use, *Nutr Today* 32(3):102, 1997.

Cunnane S et al: Potential role of polyunsaturates in seizure protection achieved with the ketogenic diet, *Prostaglandins Leukot Essent Fatty Acids* 67:131, 2002.

Curran JE: Nutritional considerations in dysphagia. In Groher ME, editor: *Dysphagia: diagnosis and management,* ed 3, Boston, 1997, Butterworth-Heinemann.

Davalos A et al: Effect of malnutrition after acute stroke on clinical outcome, *Stroke* 27(6):1028, 1996.

Desport JC et al: Nutritional assessment and survival in ALS patients, *Amyotroph Lateral Scler Other Motor Neuron Disor* 1:91, 2000.

Desport JC et al: Factors correlated with hypermetabolism in patients with amyotrophic lateral sclerosis, *Am J Clin Nutr* 74:328, 2001.

Diabetes Control and Complications Trial Research Group: Effect of intensive diabetes management on macrovascular events and risk factors in the Diabetes Control and Complications Trial, *Am J Cardiol* 75:894, 1995.

Ewbank DC: A multistate model of the genetic risk of Alzheimer's disease, *Exp Aging Res* 28:477, 2002.

Feldman EB: Fruits and vegetables and the risk of stroke, *Annu Rev Nutr* 59:24, 2001.

Fernandez-Calle P et al: Serum levels of alpha-tocopherol (vitamin E) in Parkinson's disease, *Neurology* 42:1064, 1992.

Fields PI, Swerdlow DL: Campylobacter jejuni, *Clin Lab Med* 19:489, 1999.

Finley B: Nutritional needs of the person with Alzheimer's disease: practical approaches to quality care, *J Am Diet Assoc* 97(10 suppl 2):S177, 1997.

Freeman JM et al: *The epilepsy diet treatment: an introduction to the ketogenic diet,* ed 2, New York, 1996, Demos.

Frequin STFM et al: Decreased vitamin B_{12} and folate levels in cerebrospinal fluid and serum of multiple sclerosis patients after high-dose intravenous methylprednisolone, *J Neurol* 240:305, 1993.

Friedman A et al: Pyridostigmine brain penetration under stress enhances neural excitability and induces early immediate transcriptional response, *Nat Med* 2:1382, 1996.

Gelinas S, Martinoli MG: Neuroprotective effect of estradiol and phytoestrogens on MPP+-induced cytotoxicity in neuronal PC12 cells, *J Neurosci Res* 70:90, 2002.

Geula C et al: Aging renders the brain vulnerable to amyloid β-protein neurotoxicity, *Nat Med* 4:827, 1998.

Gordis L: *Epidemiology,* Philadelphia, 1996, WB Saunders.

Greenberg MS: *Handbook of neurosurgery,* ed 4, Lakeland, Fla, 1997, Greenberg Graphics.

Griffin JW: Neurological disorders. In Bennett JC, Plum F, editors: *Cecil textbook of medicine,* ed 20, Philadelphia, 1996, WB Saunders.

Guillozet AL et al: Neurofibrillary tangles, amyloid, and memory in aging and mild cognitive impairment, *Arch Neurol* 60:729, 2003.

Gwinn-Hardy K: Genetics of parkinsonism, *Mov Disord* 17:645, 2002.

Hayes CE et al: Vitamin D and multiple sclerosis (review), *Proc Soc Exp Biol Med* 216(1):21, 1997.

Hillel AD et al: ALS Severity Scale, *J Neuroepidemiol* 8:142, 1989.

Igbavboa U et al: A new role for apolipoprotein E: modulating transport of polyunsaturated phospholipid molecular species in synaptic plant membranes, *J Neurochem* 80:255, 2002.

Iso H et al: Prospective study of fat and protein intake and risk of intraparenchymal hemorrhage in women, *Circulation* 103:856, 2001.

Jacob RA, Milne DB: Biochemical assessment of vitamins and trace minerals, *Clin Lab Med* 13(2):371, 1993.

Jonsson P et al: CuZn-superoxide dismutase in D90A heterozygotes from recessive and dominant ALS pedigrees, *Neurobiol Dis* 10:327, 2002.

Joseph SA, Tsao CY: Guillain-Barré syndrome, *Adolesc Med* 13:487, 2002.

Kasarskis EJ et al: Nutritional status of patients with amyotrophic lateral sclerosis: relation to the proximity of death, *Am J Clin Nutr* 63:130, 1996.

Kasarskis EJ, Neville HE: Management of ALS: nutritional care, *Neurology* 47(4 suppl 2):S118, 1996.

Karstaedt PJ, Pincus JH: Protein redistribution diet remains effective in patients with fluctuating Parkinsonism, *Arch Neurol* 49(2):149, 1992.

Kempster PA, Wahlqvist ML: Dietary factors in the management of Parkinson's disease, *Nutr Rev* 52(2 pt 1): 51, 1994.

Kim YI: To feed or not to feed: tube feeding in patients with advanced dementia, *Annu Rev Nutr* 59:86, 2001.

Kinsman SL et al: Efficacy of the ketogenic diet for intractable seizure disorders: review of 58 cases, *Epilepsia* 33:1132, 1992.

Klodell CT et al: Routine intragastric feeding following traumatic brain injury is safe and well tolerated, *Am J Surg* 179: 168, 2000.

Koehler KM: The New Mexico aging process study, *Annu Rev Nutr* 52:34S, 1994.

Langlais PJ: Neuropathology of thiamine deficiency: an update on the comparative analysis of human disorders and experimental models, *Metab Brain Dis* 11(1):19, 1996.

LeBars PI et al: A placebo-controlled, double-blind, randomized trial of an extract of ginkgo biloba for dementia, *JAMA* 278: 1327, 1997.

Leira R, Rodriguez R: Diet and migraine: review, *Revista de Neurologia* 24(129):534, 1996.

Liebert M: Nutrition, *J Neurotrauma* 17:539, 2000.

Lipton RB et al: Prevalence and burden of migraine in the United States: data from the American migraine study II, *Headache* 41:646, 2001.

Liu PK et al: The association between neuronal nitric oxide synthase and neuronal sensitivity in the brain after brain injury, *Ann NY Acad Sci* 962:226, 2002.

Logroscino G et al: Dietary lipids and antioxidants in Parkinson's disease: a population-based, case-control study, *Ann Neurol* 39(1):89, 1996.

Maher NE: Epidemiologic study of 203 sibling pairs with Parkinson's disease, *Neurology* 58:79, 2002.

Maimone D et al: Pharmacogenomics of neurodegenerative diseases, *Eur J Pharmacol* 413:11, 2001.

Mandel A et al: Medical costs are reduced when children with intractable epilepsy are successfully treated with the ketogenic diet, *J Am Diet Assoc* 102:396, 2002.

Mann G et al: Swallowing function after stroke: prognosis and prognostic factors at 6 months, *Stroke* 30(4):744, 1999.

Marino DD et al: Unique grocery home delivery service aids older adults, *Journal of Nutrition for the Elderly*, 1998, The Haworth Press, Inc.

Mazzini L et al: Percutaneous endoscopic gastrostomy and enteral nutrition in amyotrophic lateral sclerosis, *J Neurol* 242:695, 1995.

Meigs JB et al: Fasting and glycemia and cardiovascular disease risk: the Framingham Offspring Study, *Diabetes Care* 25:1845, 2002.

Meydani M: Antioxidants and cognitive function, *Annu Rev Nutr* 59:75S, 2001.

Miller J: Homocysteine and Alzheimer's disease, *Annu Rev Nutr* 57:126, 1999.

Miller RG et al: Practice parameter: the care of the patient with amyotrophic lateral sclerosis (an evidence-based review): report of the Quality Standards Subcommittee of the American Academy of Neurology: ALS practice parameters task force, *Neurology* 52:1311, 1999.

Miller RM: General treatment of neurologic swallowing disorders. In Groher ME, editor: *Dysphagia: diagnosis and management*, ed 3, Boston, 1997, Butterworth-Heinemann.

Mitsumoto H: Classification and clinical features of amyotrophic lateral sclerosis. In Mitsumoto H, Norris FH, editors: *Amyotrophic lateral sclerosis: a comprehensive guide to management*, New York, 1994, Demos.

Mitsumoto H, Del Bene M: Improving the quality of life for people with ALS: the challenge ahead, *Amyotroph Lateral Scler Other Motor Neuron Disord* 1:329, 2000.

NIH: http://www.ninds.nih.gov/health_and_medical/pubs/brain_tumor_hope_through_research.html, 2002.

Nilsson H et al: Quantitative assessment of oral and pharyngeal function in Parkinson's disease, *Dysphagia* 11(4):274, 1996.

Ordunez-Garcia et al: Cuban epidemic neuropathy, 1991 to 1994: history repeats itself a century after the "amblyopia of the blockade," *Am J Public Health* 86(5): 738, 1996.

Pare S et al: Effect of daytime protein restriction on nutrient intakes of free-living Parkinson's disease patients, *Am J Clin Nutr* 55:701, 1992.

Parkinson's Study Group: Effects of tocopherol and deprenyl on the progression of disability in early Parkinson's disease, *N Engl J Med* 328:176, 1993.

Payne A: Nutrition and diet in the clinical management of multiple sclerosis, *J Hum Nutr Diet* 14:349, 2001.

Powers et al: Parkinson's disease risks associated with dietary iron, manganese, and other nutrient intakes, *Neurology* 60:1761, 2003.

Radunovic A et al: Copper and zinc levels in familial amyotrophic lateral sclerosis patients with CuZnSOD gene mutations, *Ann Neurol* 42:130, 1997.

Rapoport A, Edmeads J: Migraine: the evolution of our knowledge, *Arch Neurol* 57(8):1221, 2000.

Raskind MA et al: Effect of tacrine on language, praxis and noncognitive behavioral problems in Alzheimer disease, *Arch Neurol* 54(7):838, 1997.

Riggs KM et al: Relations of vitamin B_{12}, B_6, folate, and homocysteine to cognitive performance in the normative aging study, *Am J Clin Nutr* 63: 306, 1996.

Riviere S et al: Nutrition and Alzheimer's disease, *Annu Rev Nutr* 57:363, 1999.

Roubenoff RA et al: Hypermetabolism and hypercatabolism in Guillain-Barre syndrome, *J Parenter Enteral Nutr* 16(5):464, 1992.

Rowland LP: Merritt's textbook of neurology, ed 9, Baltimore, Md, 1995, Williams & Wilkens.

Sano M et al: A controlled trial of selegitine, alpha-tocopherol or both as treatment for Alzheimer's disease, *N Engl J Med* 336:1216, 1997.

Sathasivam S et al: Apoptosis in amytrophic lateral sclerosis: a review of the evidence, *Neuropathol Appl Neurobiol* 27: 257, 2001.

Schiffman S: Changes in taste and smell: drug interactions and food preferences, *Annu Rev Nutr* 52: S11, 1994.

Schoenen J et al: Effectiveness of high-dose riboflavin in migraine prophylaxis: a randomized controlled trial, *Neurology* 50:466, 1998.

Silberstein SD: Butalbital in the treatment of headache: history, pharmacology, and efficacy, *Headache* 41:953, 2001.

Singleton CK, Martin PR: Molecular mechanisms of thiamine utilization, *Curr Mol Med* 1(2):197, 2001.

Standaert DG, Stern MB: Update on the management of Parkinson's disease, *Med Clin North Am* 77(1):169, 1993.

Strand EA et al: Management of oral-pharyngeal dysphagia symptoms in amyotrophic lateral sclerosis, *Dysphagia* 11:129, 1996.

Suzuki Y et al: The clinical course of childhood and adolescent adrenoleukodystrophy before and after Lorenzo's oil, *Brain Dev* 23:30, 2001.

Thornton FJ et al: Amyotrophic lateral sclerosis: enteral nutrition provision endoscopic or radiologic gastrostomy? *Radiology* 224:713, 2002.

Traber MG, Sies H: Vitamin E in humans: demand and delivery [Review]. *Annu Rev Nutr* 16:321, 1996.

Tufts University: *Health and Nutrition Letter*, p 7, February 1998.

Vastag B: New diagnostic criteria for MS issued, *JAMA* 286:1703, 2001.

Wang X: Chronic alcohol intake interferes with retinoid metabolism and signaling, *Nutr Rev* 57(2):51, 1999.

Warsama Jama J et al: Dietary antioxidants and cognitive function in a population-based sample of older persons: the Rotterdam Study, *Am J Epidemiol* 144:275, 1996.

Wickelgren I: Estrogen stakes claim to cognition, *Science* 276:675, 1997.

Wozniak-Wowk CS: Nutrition intervention in the management of multiple sclerosis, *Nutr Today* 28(6):12, 1993.

Yan SD et al: An intracellular protein that binds amyloid-B peptide and mediates neurotoxicity in Alzheimer's disease, *Nature* 389:689, 1997.

Zhang S et al: Dietary fat in relation to risk of multiple sclerosis among two large cohorts of women, *Am J Epidemiol* 152:1056, 2000.

Additional References

Alpert JE et al: Folinic acid (leucovorin) as an adjunctive treatment for SSRI-refractory depression, *Ann Clin Psychiatry* 14:33, 2002.

Ascherio A et al: Epstein-Barr virus antibodies and risk of multiple sclerosis: a prospective study, *JAMA* 286:3083, 2001.

Daly BJ: Special challenges of withholding artificial nutrition and hydration, *J Gerontol Nurs* 26:25, 2000.

Grap MJ, Munro CL: Ventilator-associated pneumonia: clinical significance and implications for nursing, *Heart Lung* 26(6):419, 1997.

Hansen HS: New biological and clinical roles for the *n*-6 and *n*-3 fatty acids, *Annu Rev Nutr* 52:162, 1994.

Hernandez-Rodriguez J, Manjarrez-Gutierrez G: Macronutrients and neurotransmitter formation during brain development, *Annu Rev Nutr* 59:49S, 2001.

Lang AE, Lozano AM: Parkinson's disease, part I, *N Engl J Med* 339:1044, 1998.

Lecours AR, Mandujano M, Romero G: Ontogeny of brain and cognition: relevance to nutrition research, *Annu Rev Nutr* 59: 7S, 2001.

Lieberman HR: The effects of ginseng, ephedrine, and caffeine on cognitive performance, mood and energy, *Annu Rev Nutr* 59:91, 2001.

Lucas A et al: Nutrition and mental development, *Annu Rev Nutr* 59:24S, 2001.

Pauloski BR et al: Swallow function and perception of dysphagia in patients with head and neck cancer, *Head Neck* 24:555, 2002.

Pina Latorre MA et al: Parkinsonism and Parkinson's disease associated with long-term administration of sertraline, *J Clin Pharm Ther* 26:111, 2001.

Ramulu P et al: Wernicke's encephalopathy, *Neurology* 59:846, 2002.

Rosenberg IH: B vitamins, homocysteine, and neurocognitive function, *Nutr Rev* 59:69S, 2001.

Sano M et al: A controlled trial of selegiline, alpha tocopherol, or both as treatment for Alzheimer's disease, *N Engl J Med* 336:1216, 1997.

Schiffman SS et al: Taste, smell, and neuropsychological performance of individuals at familial risk for Alzheimer's disease, *Neurobiol Aging* 23:397, 2002.

Uauy R et al: Essential fatty acids in visual and brain development, *Lipids* 36:885, 2001.

Uauy R, Mena P: Lipids and neurodevelopment, *Annu Rev Nutr* 59:34S, 2001.

Wauben IPM, Wainwright P: The influence of neonatal nutrition on behavioral development: a critical appraisal, *Annu Rev Nutr* 57:35, 1999.

Youdim M: Deficiency and excess of iron in brain function and dysfunction, *Annu Rev Nutr* 59: S83, 2001.

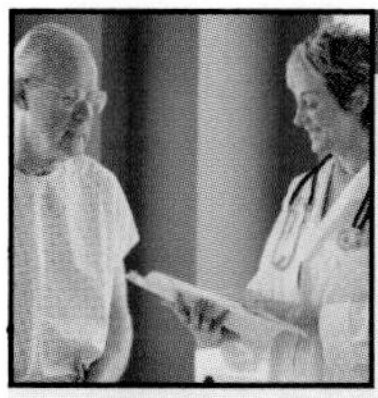

CHAPTER 44

Medical Nutrition Therapy for Rheumatic Disorders

LISA DORFMAN, MS, RD, LMHC

CHAPTER OUTLINE

- Etiology
- Pathophysiology of Inflammation in Rheumatic Diseases
- Drugs Commonly Used to Reduce Inflammation
- Osteoarthritis
- Rheumatoid Arthritis
- Sjögren's Syndrome
- Temporomandibular Joint Syndrome
- Gout
- Scleroderma
- Systemic Lupus Erythematosus
- Chronic Fatigue Disorder Syndrome and Fibromylagia
- Controversies and Unproven Remedies for Rheumatic Disorders

KEY TERMS

arachidonic acid–a polyunsaturated fatty acid with four double bonds on the 5, 8, 11, and 14 carbon positions; a precursor for eicosanoid production

autoimmune–having a specific type of humoral or cell-mediated immune response against constituents of the body's own tissues

cytokines–small proteins, including lymphokines and monokines, that are produced by immunocytes, macrophages, and fibroblasts and that mediate or increase an inflammatory response

fibromyalgia–generalized, widespread, nonarticular pain or inflammation

gout–a group of disorders of purine and pyrimidine metabolism characterized by hyperuricemia and deposition of uric acid crystals

juvenile rheumatoid arthritis–a chronic, autoimmune, multisystem condition occurring in children (mostly girls) that primarily affects the joints, with changes in the synovial membranes and joint structures, atrophy, and osteopenia

osteoarthritis (OA)–a degenerative nonsystemic joint disease, the "wear-and-tear" disease, that occurs mainly in older persons; characterized by degeneration of the joint cartilage, hypertrophy of bone at the margins, and changes in the synovial membrane

prostaglandin (PG)–any of a group of components derived from unsaturated 20-carbon fatty acids that are extremely potent mediators of a diverse group of physiologic processes; the series is designated with a subscript 1, 2, or 3, depending on the number of double bonds in the hydrocarbon skeleton and the fatty acid from which it was synthesized

purines–the nitrogenous bases adenine and guanine, which are constituents of nucleoproteins, the metabolic end product of which is uric acid

rheumatic diseases–manifestations of systemic connective tissue and arthritic disease marked by degener-

Chapter written by Therese Ann Franzese, MS, RD, CD-N, for the previous edition of this text.

KEY TERMS—Continued

ation, inflammation, pain, and swelling of the joints; thought to have an autoimmune component.

rheumatoid arthritis (RA)–chronic inflammatory autoimmune systemic disease primarily of the joints, characterized by changes in the synovial membranes, atrophy of joints, and osteopenia

rheumatoid factor (RF)–abnormal circulating proteins found in the serum of individuals with rheumatoid arthritis; a group of immunoglobins that have been classified as antibodies

scleroderma–progressive, systemic inflammation and hardening of the skin with deposition of fibrous connective tissue in the skin and visceral organs, including the gastrointestinal tract

Sjögren's syndrome–a chronic inflammatory disorder characterized by diminished production of both saliva and tears in the eye

synovial fluid–transparent, alkaline fluid secreted by the synovial membrane and located in joints

systemic lupus erythematosus (SLE)–a chronic, inflammatory, multisystem disorder of connective tissue, primarily affecting women, that involves the skin, joints, kidneys, and serosal membranes; of presumed immune-mediated etiology

xerophthalmia–dryness of the cornea and conjunctiva of the eyes; manifestations include dry, sandy eyes with thick, white mucosa

xerostomia–dryness of the mouth secondary to reduced or absent saliva; leads to increased risk of dental decay, gingivitis, and difficulty chewing and swallowing

Rheumatic diseases and related conditions include more than 100 different manifestations of connective tissue and systemic, arthritic disease marked by degeneration, inflammation, pain, and swelling of the joints. Because no identifiable cause nor cure is known, pharmacotherapy, physical and occupational treatment, and medical nutrition therapy (MNT) play important roles in managing the symptoms.

Recent increases in the frequency of these conditions may be due to the aging of the U.S. population. At least 70% of individuals over 70 years old (1.5 million women) have radiologic evidence of osteoarthritis. Only half will develop symptoms, whereas almost everyone over 75 is affected in at least one joint (www.arthritis.org).

Body changes associated with aging—including decreased body protein, body fluid, and bone density as well as an increased proportion of total body fat—may contribute to the onset and progression of arthritis. The aging body mass causes changes in neuroendocrine regulators, immune regulators, and metabolism that affect the inflammation process (Roubenoff et al, 1997).

Rheumatic diseases affect all population groups. As many as 285,000 children (including those with juvenile rheumatoid arthritis) are diagnosed with arthritis. Osteoarthritis affects 21 million; gout, 2.1 million; and rheumatoid arthritis, 2.1 million Americans (Lawrence et al, 1998). Conditions such as lupus (affecting 300,000 people), fibromyalgia (affecting 100,000), Sjögren's syndrome (affecting 2 to 4 million), and scleroderma have a great impact on the American population.

Arthritis is a generic term that comes from the Greek word *arthro,* which means *joint,* and *itis,* which means *inflammation.* There are two distinct categories of diseases: systemic, autoimmune rheumatic disease and nonsystemic osteoarthritis. The autoimmune arthritis group includes rheumatoid arthritis (RA), juvenile rheumatoid arthritis (JRA), gout, Sjögren's syndrome, fibromyalgia, lupus, and scleroderma. The osteoarthritis group includes osteoarthritis, bursitis, and tendonitis.

Arthritis is one of the most prevalent chronic disease conditions in the United States, currently affecting an estimated 24.3 million persons (Singh et al, 2002), and is projected to affect 60 million (more than 18% of the population) by 2020 (Lawrence et al, 1998). According to the Arthritis Foundation (AF), arthritis is the leading cause of disability; it is associated with total direct costs to the U.S. economy of $65 billion per year in medical care and lost wages.

ETIOLOGY

The etiology of most rheumatic conditions remains unknown. In addition, some forms of rheumatic conditions can affect other organs, like the skin or blood vessels. Rheumatic conditions have no known cure and are usually chronic but may present as acute episodes with short or intermittent duration. Chronic arthritic conditions are associated with alternating periods of remission, absence of symptoms, and flares or worsening of symptoms, which often occur without any identifiable etiology.

Although various alternative diet theories and supplement regimens have been proposed for the management of rheumatic conditions, the scientific data are either limited or based on anecdotal or nonscientific data. In addition, because no identifiable cure for rheumatic conditions is usually available, in-

TABLE 44-1 Overview of Medical Nutrition Therapy for Rheumatic Disorders

DISEASE	MEDICAL NUTRITION THERAPY	COMPLEMENTARY THERAPY	SUPPLEMENTS/HERB	UNPROVEN/ QUESTIONABLE TX
Rheumatoid arthritis	Monitored fast 7-10 days; vegetarian diet; vegan diet; diet rich in folic acid	Exercise	Antioxidants when diet does not reach DRI	Feverfew
Osteoarthritis	Weight management; decrease weight to reach ideal body weight; diet adequate in vitamins B_6, B_{12}, and folate	Exercise, acupuncture, massage	1200 mg Calcium; 400 IU vitamin D	Glucosamine and chondroitin, capsaicin
Gout	Purine-controlled diet, 50%-55% carbohydrates, 30% fat or less, moderate protein; restrict or eliminate alcohol; include tofu as protein source; increase water consumption	Exercise for weight and visceral fat management	—	—
Lupus	Tailor diet to individual needs; calories to promote ideal body weight; restrict fluid and sodium	—	30 g Ground flaxseed daily?: enteral or parenteral nutrition as needed	Restrict calories, fat, and protein?
Scleroderma	High-energy protein supplements to correct weight loss	—	Vitamin and mineral, fatty acid supplements with malabsorption/diarrhea	—
Fibromylagia	Vegan diet	Exercise, acupuncture	—	"Living food diet"
Sjögren's syndrome	Balanced diet rich in vitamin B_{12}, folate, and iron; moist, ready-to-eat foods; diet to relieve symptoms	Lemon drops to increase salivary flow; frequent rinsing and teeth-brushing	—	DHEA?
TMJ	Mechanical soft diet; alter food consistency	Exercise, massage	—	

DRI, Dietary restriction intake; *DHEA*, dehydroepiandrosterone; *TMJ*, temporomandibular joint.

dividuals with arthritis often seek remedies from unorthodox sources. For these reasons, helping individuals with rheumatic disorders is a continuing challenge for nutritionists (Table 44-1).

PATHOPHYSIOLOGY OF INFLAMMATION IN RHEUMATIC DISEASES

Inflammation, which is the predominant cause of pain, is the most debilitating component of all forms of arthritis. Pain reflects a neuroendocrine process associated with levels of corticotrophin-releasing hormone, methyl-D-aspartate, inflammatory mediators, unmyelinated C fibers sensitized to noradrenaline, and biologically active peptides (Harris, 1997). The inflammatory process normally occurs to protect and repair tissue damaged by infections, sports injuries, toxicity, or wounds via accumulation of fluid and cells. Once the cause is resolved, the inflammation usually subsides. Whether inflammation is attributable to stress on the joints (osteoarthritis) or is an autoimmune response (rheumatoid arthritis), in most forms of arthritis, the inflammatory reaction continues out of control, thus causing more damage than repair.

The complex inflammatory process is initiated by the production of histamine, prostaglandins (PGs), plasma proteases, and plasma-activating factors. Many specific prostaglandins and other mediators (i.e., PGE1 and PGE2, thromboxanes and leukotrienes, respectively) potentiate the effects of inflammatory mediators such as histamine. Arachidonic acid, when released from cell membranes, is oxygenated to several classes of eicosanoids, including prostaglandins, thromboxanes, leukotrienes, and prostacyclins, all of which are proinflammation. Glucocorticoid therapy decreases the release of arachidonic acid from cell membrane phospholipids by binding to the receptor in the cell cytoplasm, thus forming a complex that moves into the nucleus as a transcription factor and interferes with expressions for the enzyme phospholipase (Harris, 1997). Thromboxane activates platelet aggregation to initiate clotting and to release growth factors and proteases. Leukotrienes stimulate the attraction of neutrophils, macrophages, and fibroblasts into the circulating joint fluid. Prostacyclin (PGI2) has the opposite effect of PGE1 and PGE2; it relaxes the smooth muscle and inhibits platelet aggregation.

Prostaglandins are produced by neutrophils, macrophages, and synovial fibroblasts in large quantities in synovial tissue as a response to specific cytokines (activating protein hormones such as tumor necrosis factors, interferons, and interleukins) acting on oxygenated arachidonic acid. Prostaglandins play a major role in the depletion of bone in rheumatoid arthritis, and tumor necrosis factor (TNF-α) has assumed particular importance (Firestein and Zvaifler, 1997; Harris, 1997).

DRUGS COMMONLY USED TO REDUCE INFLAMMATION

Many of the drugs used in treating rheumatic diseases affect the synthesis of prostaglandins, usually by diminishing their production. Nonsteroidal anti-inflammatory drugs (NSAIDs), which include Advil,

Nuprin, Motrin, and Aleve, slow down the body's production of prostaglandins by inhibiting cyclooxygenase (COX), an enzyme that leads to the suppression of COX-1–mediated production of gastrointestinal protective prostaglandins (Emery et al, 1999). Although long-term use of NSAIDs is often associated with gastrointestinal problems such as irritation, ulcers, abdominal burning, pain, cramping, nausea, and GI bleeding as well as renal failure (Perneger et al, 1994), they are still the most popular pain-relieving medications used in the management of most rheumatic disorders. New COX-2 inhibitors like Celecoxib, Nimesulide, and Naproxen have been shown to provide comparable relief over other NSAIDs but have potentially less gastrointestinal toxicity (Emery et al, 1999). However, the cost of COX-2 inhibitors may be more expensive—up to $10,000 each year or more (www.rheumatology.org).

OSTEOARTHRITIS

Pathophysiology

Osteoarthritis (OA), formally known as degenerative arthritis or degenerative joint disease (DJD), is the most prevalent form of arthritis. Obesity, aging, gender, and congenital abnormalities appear to be the major risk factors; other factors include obesity, bone density, and genetics (Sowers, 2001). Osteoarthritis is a chronic process characterized by the softening of the articular (joint) cartilage and includes reactive chemically mediated phenomena, such as vascular congestion and osteoblast activity in underlying bone, new growth of cartilage and bone (osteophytes) at the joint margins, and capsular fibrosis (Figure 44-1). It is mechanically driven.

The major difference between osteoarthritis and rheumatoid arthritis is that osteoarthritis is not systemic or autoimmune in origin but involves cartilage destruction with asymmetrical inflammation. It is caused by joint overuse, whereas rheumatoid arthritis is a systemic autoimmune disorder that results in symmetrical joint inflammation.

The joints most often affected in osteoarthritis are the distal interphalangeal joints; the thumb joint; and, in particular, the joints of the knees, hips, ankles, and spine, which bear the bulk of the body's weight. The elbow, wrist, and ankle are less often affected. The early stage of the disease is marked by stiffness, usually upon arising from a chair or after standing; this then progresses to generalized "soreness." One or more joints may be affected, and symptoms are usually confined to the afflicted parts. Diseases of the joints influenced by congenital and mechanical derangements of the joints may contribute to osteoarthritis. Inflammation occurs at times; however, it is not a primary symptom of this condition.

Medical Management

According to the American College of Rheumatology (ARC) Guidelines, the patient's medical history and level of pain should determine the most appropriate treatment (www.rheumatology.org). Nonpharmacologic therapies should always be included in the treatment regimen and should be followed by acetaminophen or NSAIDS for mild to moderate pain and opioids for severe pain (Todd, 2002). Adjunctive treatments, intraarticular corticosteroid injections, and surgery are also viable options for some patients.

Surgery

Surgical reconstruction (total joint replacement) may be considered for patients with osteoarthritis who are not responding to other medical therapies and who are good candidates for surgery (Creamer et al, 1998). Surgical reconstruction has been quite successful but should not be viewed as a replacement for overall good nutrition, maintenance of healthy body weight, and exercise.

Exercise

The disease limits the ability to increase energy expenditure through exercise. It is critical for the exercise to be done in correct form so as not to cause damage or exacerbate an existing problem. Nonloading aerobic (swimming), range-of-motion, and weight-bearing exercise have all been shown to reduce symptoms, increase mobility, and lessen continuing damage from osteoarthritis (Fisher et al, 1997; Fransen et al, 1997; Rejeski et al, 1998). Non–weight-bearing exercise may also serve as an adjunct to NSAID use (Clyman, 2001; Nicolakis et al 2002; Toda, 2001).

Sports or strenuous activities that subject joints to repetitive high impact and loading increase the risk of joint cartilage degeneration (Spector, 1996). Therefore increased muscle tone and strength, correct form, general flexibility, and conditioning will help protect these joints in the habitual exerciser (Buckwalter and Lane, 1997).

Medical Nutrition Therapy

Excess weight puts an added burden on the weight-bearing joints. Epidemiologic studies have shown that obesity and injury are the two greatest risk factors for osteoarthritis (Cooper et al, 1998). The risk for knee osteoarthritis increases as the BMI increases (Coggon et al, 2001). Controlling obesity can reduce the burden of knee osteoporosis. Weight-reduction medications have sometimes been used in problematic cases, but close monitoring of potential side effects is essential, and these medications should not be used when risks are high (see Chapter 24).

A well-balanced diet that is consistent with established dietary guidelines and that promotes attain-

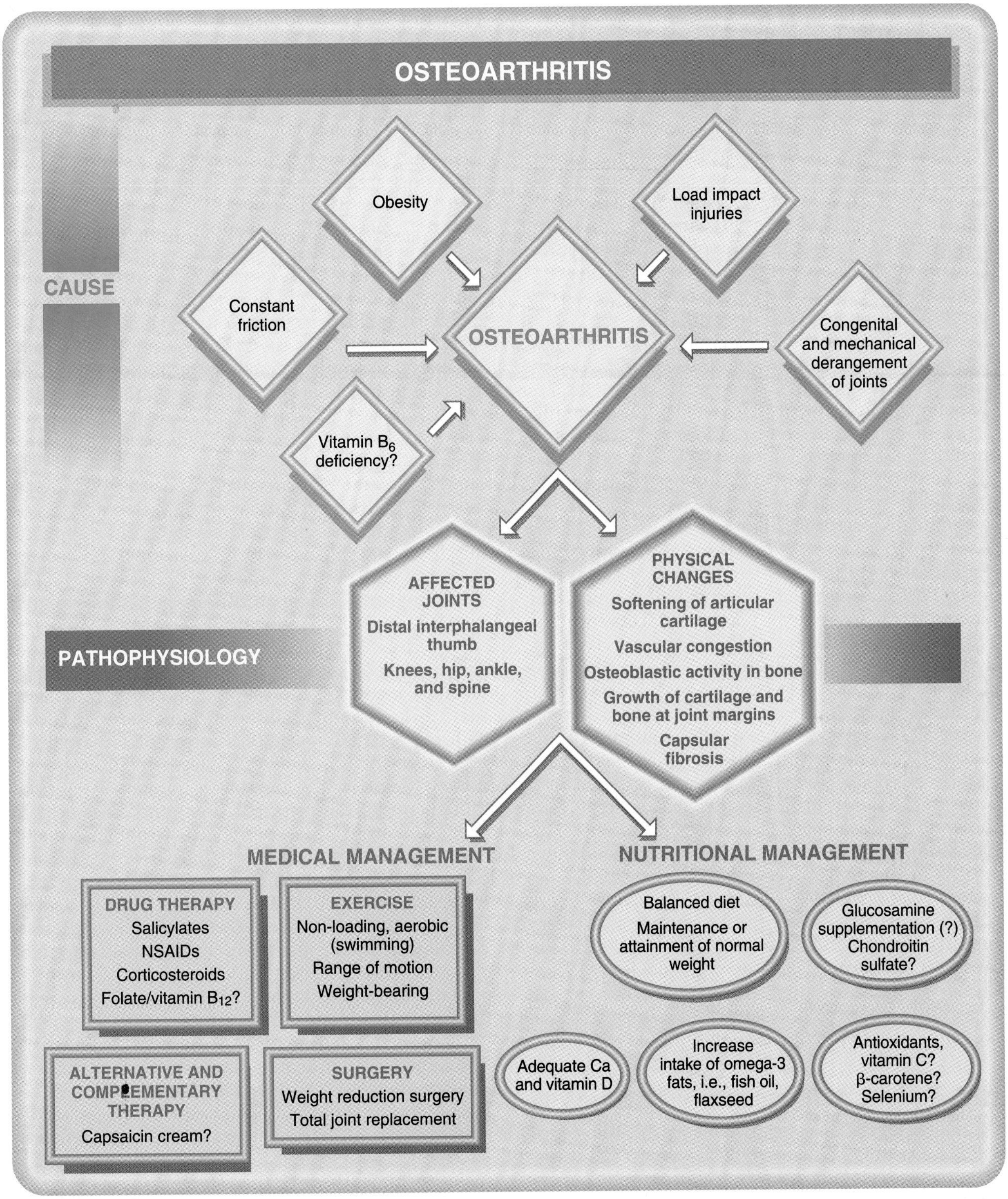

FIGURE 44-1 • Pathophysiology algorithm: osteoarthritis. (Algorithm content developed by John Anderson, PhD, and Sanford C. Garner, PhD, 2000. Updated by Lisa Dorfman, MS, RD, LMHC, 2002.)

ment and maintenance of a desirable body weight is an important part of medical nutrition therapy for osteoarthritis (Johnson and Kennedy, 2000).

Vitamins and Minerals

Experimental data have shown that vitamin B_6 deficiency may be responsible for the development of osteoarthritis-type lesions (Koopman, 1997). Comprehensive nutrition interviewing and counseling should include a determination of acceptable sources of all nutrients for the patient as well as integration of sufficient amounts in the diet to achieve the recommended levels (van Weel, 1997).

A folate and cobalamin (vitamin B_{12}) supplement has been tested as a treatment for osteoarthritis of the hands, with fairly good results, minimal cost, and no side effects. Supplements with 6400 μg of folate plus 20 μg of cobalamin were randomly allocated to a small group of patients who were found to improve grip values; these results have not been duplicated with larger groups (Flynn et al, 1994.)

Cumulative damage to tissues mediated by reactive oxygen species has been implicated as a pathway that leads to many of the degenerative changes seen with aging. Large doses of dietary antioxidants—including vitamin C, the tocopherols (vitamin E), beta-carotene, and selenium—have had a beneficial effect on osteoarthritis (Darlington and Stone, 2001; McAlindon et al, 1996a). One follow-up study showed no benefit for the management of symptomatic OA with supplemental 500 IU vitamin E per day for 6 months (Brand et al, 2001). In another study that examined serum levels of carotenoids, some levels were associated with protecting against knee OA, whereas others were shown to increase knee OA (DeRoos et al, 2001). Further studies are warranted before recommendations for routine dietary supplementation can be made.

Many patients with osteoarthritis have been shown to be deficient in the consumption of dairy products and calcium, and have a low intake of vitamin D. Low serum levels of vitamin D have been shown to be associated with progression of osteoarthritis (McAlindon et al, 1996a). Improving intake to at least DRI levels is suggested.

Herbs and Complementary Therapy

Some alternative "investigative dietary therapies" that are being used to help lessen the need for NSAIDs, aspirin, and acetaminophen are glucosamine, chondroitin sulfate, oils, and herbs. Advocates of these alternative modalities cite reports of progressive and gradual decline of joint pain and tenderness, improved mobility, sustained improvement after drug withdrawal, and a lack of toxicity associated with short-term use of these agents (Brief et al, 2001).

Chondroitin sulfate and glucosamine are both molecules that produce cartilage, but the mechanism for eliminating pain has not been identified. In an analysis of studies between 1975 and 1997, limited data suggest that glucosamine sulfate administered orally, intravenously, intramuscularly, and intraarticularly may produce a gradual and progressive reduction in joint pain and tenderness as well as improved range of motion and walking speed (daCamara and Dowless, 1998). Results of the trials have also shown that glucosamine has produced consistent benefits, including greater than 50% improvement in symptom scores in patients with OA. In some cases glucosamine may be equal or superior to ibuprofen.

However, no reliable scientific evidence that these two substances have structure-modifying actions with respect to prohibiting, healing, or restoring cartilage exists (Hauselmann, 2001). The majority of the relevant clinical trials investigating glucosamine have small sample size; short terms for examining safety, efficacy, and optimal dosage; and serious deficiencies in design (Brief et al, 2001; daCamara and Dowless, 1998). A large trial will be completed in March 2005 (NIH, 2001b).

Although it is not effective for all afflicted individuals, the Arthritis Foundation suggests a safe and suggested dose of glucosamine and chondroitin sulfate to be 500 mg three times each day and 400 mg three times each day, respectively (Horstman, 2001). Those persons with shellfish allergies should avoid glucosamine supplementation.

A variety of complementary therapies have been proposed as a solution to managing pain in osteoarthritis, including topical aids, manipulative therapies, and acupuncture. Capsaicinoids, derived from chili peppers, have a fatty acid receptor that stimulates, then blocks, small-diameter pain fibers by depleting them of the neurotransmitter substance P, thought to be the principal chemomediator of pain impulses from the periphery (Robbins, 2000). A randomized, double-blind study on osteoarthritic patents showed that capsaicin, applied with glyceryl trinitrate to reduce on-site burning, reduces pain in OA patients (McCleane, 2000). Certain pulsed electromagnetic fields can also affect the growth of bone and cartilage with potential use in osteoarthritis, and use of static magnets may provide temporary pain relief under certain circumstances (Trock, 2000).

Herbs and botanicals are also popular. Willow bark has gained a great deal of attention, since it contains salaicin, the chemical from which aspirin is derived. In one double-blind placebo-controlled study, a dose equivalent to 240 mg salaicin per day was shown to have a moderate analgesic effect on osteoarthritic patients (Schmid et al, 2001). However, the Arthritis Foundation suggests that it is safer to take aspirin because willow bark supplements are unregulated.

RHEUMATOID ARTHRITIS

Rheumatoid arthritis (RA) is a debilitating and frequently crippling disease with overwhelming personal, social, and economic effects. Although less common than osteoarthritis, RA may be more severe. The most frequently affected tissues are the interstitial tissues, blood vessels, cartilage, bone, tendons, and ligaments as well as the synovial membranes that line joint surfaces. Rheumatoid arthritis occurs more frequently in women than in men (1.5 million women vs. 600,000 men) (Lawrence et al, 1998). Although the peak onset commonly occurs between 20 and 45 years years of age, it often strikes individuals in their twenties or thirties. Numerous remissions and exacerbations generally follow its onset.

Rheumatoid arthritis is postulated to be caused by a virus or by constant stress (from obesity or inappropriate strenuous exercise) that initiates the inflammatory process. Epidemiologic studies have documented that onset in the northern hemisphere is more common in winter than in summer and that exacerbations of the disease are more common in winter (Kelly et al, 1997). Decaffeinated coffee intake has been independently and positively associated with RA onset in a prospective study of 31,336 women ages 55 to 69 years; further investigations are needed to verify these findings and explore a biologic basis (Mikuls et al, 2002).

Pathophysiology

Rheumatoid arthritis (RA) is a chronic, autoimmune, systemic disorder of unclear etiology. The inflammatory process, which involves cytokines, seems to play a role (Firestein and Zvaifler, 1997; Moreland et al, 1997). Rheumatoid arthritis has articular manifestations that involve chronic inflammation that begins in the synovial membrane and progresses to subsequent damage in the joint cartilage. Although any joint may be affected by rheumatoid arthritis, involvement of the small joints of the extremities—typically the proximal interphalangeal joints of the hands and feet—is most common (Figure 44-2).

Pain, stiffness, and swelling are frequent complaints. The swelling or puffiness is caused by the accumulation of synovial fluid in the membrane lining the joints and inflammation of the surrounding tissues (Figure 44-3). The appearance of rheumatoid factor (RF), an abnormal circulating protein that is an immunoglobulin-classified antibody, may precede symptoms of RA (Kelly et al, 1997). Anemia may also be present.

Medical Management

Pharmacologic therapy to control pain and inflammation is the mainstay of treatment for rheumatoid arthritis. The primary drug classifications used to treat rheumatoid arthritis are salicylates, NSAIDs, antimalarial agents, immunosuppressive agents, remittive agents, and steroids. The choice of drug class and type is based on patient response to the medication, incidence and severity of adverse reactions, and patient compliance. Drug-nutrient side effects can occur with any of the drugs. Side effects of drug use may influence ingestion, digestion, and absorption, and hence nutritional status (Table 44-2; see Chapter 19).

Salicylates are usually the first line of drug therapy. However, chronic aspirin ingestion is associated with gastric mucosal injury and bleeding, increased bleeding time, and increased urinary excretion of vitamin C. Taking aspirin with milk, food, or an antacid often alleviates the gastrointestinal symptoms. Vitamin C supplementation is prescribed when serum and platelet levels of ascorbic acid are abnormally low.

The second line of drug therapy involves the use of nonsteroidal antiinflammatory drugs (NSAIDs). The effectiveness of aspirin and NSAIDs lies in the inhibition of prostaglandin synthesis and immune modulation.

Immunosuppressive agents such as methotrexate (MTX) are the most commonly prescribed drugs for rheumatoid arthritis. Adverse effects of methotrexate include folate antagonism (Endresen and Husby, 2001). Treatment with MTX induces a significant rise in *p*-homocysteine, which is neutralized by folic acid supplementation (Slot, 2001). For many patients, a properly balanced diet is sufficient to avoid folate deficiency (Endresen and Husby, 2001). However, folic acid supplementation is needed to offset the toxicity of this drug, for protection against gastrointestinal disturbances, and for maintenance of red blood cell production (Shahin et al 2001; van Ede et al 2001). Fortunately, folic acid supplementation does not decrease the efficacy of methotrexate therapy (Griffith et al, 2000). Long-term supplementation in patients on MTX is important in order to prevent neutropenia and to avoid discontinuation of treatment because of mouth ulcers, nausea, and vomiting (Griffith et al, 2000). See Chapter 19 for more information about drug therapies.

Low doses of *steroids* such as prednisone will control most of the inflammatory features of early polyarticular RA (Conn, 2001). As the most potent of the antiinflammatory drugs used to treat rheumatoid arthritis, steroids have extensive catabolic impact that can result in negative nitrogen balance. Hypercalciuria and reduced calcium absorption can increase the risk of osteoporosis (see Chapter 27). Concomitant calcium (1 g) and vitamin D (500 IU) and monitoring of bone status can minimize osteopenia (Conn, 2001; Canoso, 1997). Care must be taken to avoid serum calcium levels greater than 11.0 mg/dl (Harris, 1997). Edema often occurs and may require diet modification, including a sodium-restricted diet and fluid restriction. Other side effects of steroid use include Cushingoid changes in the body, gastrointestinal bleeding, and diabetes mellitus.

"Remittive agents," including gold salt therapy, antimalarials, and D-penicillamine, may lead to a remission in RA symptoms. Proteinuria may occur with administration of gold and D-penicillamine. Therefore, toxicity from these drugs must be monitored continually.

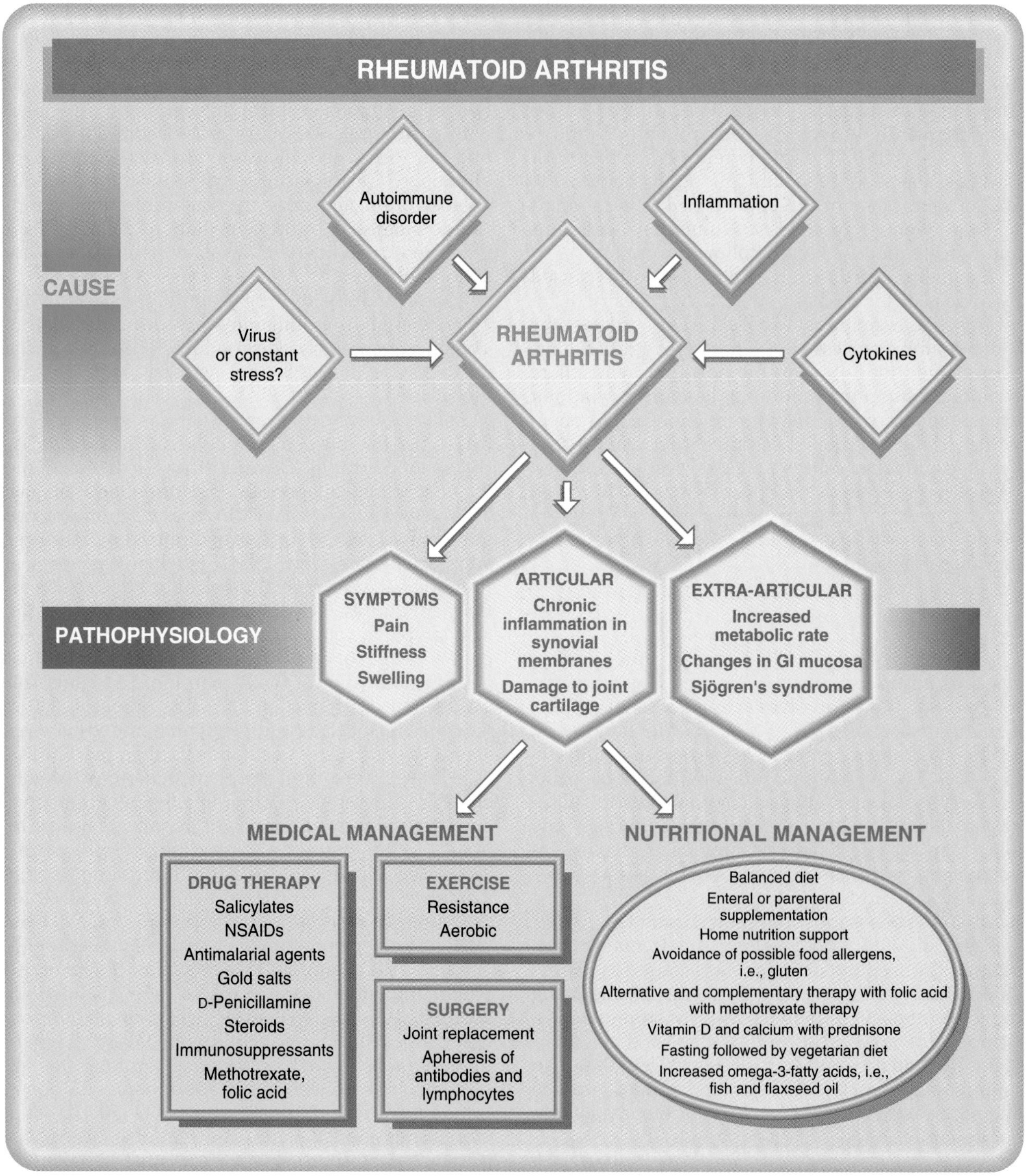

FIGURE 44-2 • Pathophysiology algorithm: rheumatoid arthritis. (Algorithm content developed by John Anderson, PhD, and Sanford C. Garner, PhD, 2000. Updated by Lisa Dorfman, MS, RD, LMHC, 2002.)

Medical Nutrition Therapy

A comprehensive nutritional assessment of individuals with rheumatoid arthritis is essential. The medical history should include a review of systems to determine the systemic impact of the disease process. A physical examination provides diagnostic signs and symptoms of nutrient deficits. Use of a "likelihood of malnutrition index" has been suggested for this population (Alarcon and Morgan, 1997), considering the number of medications often used. A physical and occupational therapy evaluation helps to determine actual range of motion and activities that the individual can do independently.

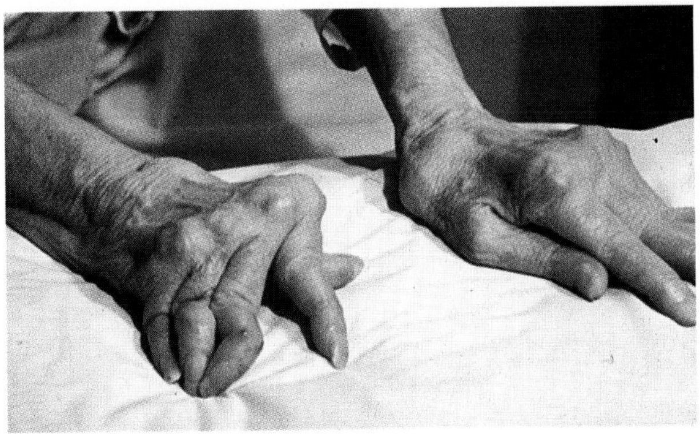

FIGURE 44-3 • A patient with advanced rheumatoid arthritis. The twisted hands and the puffiness of the metacarpal joints are typical of the disease. (From Damjanov I: *Pathology for the health-related professions*, Philadelphia, 1996, WB Saunders.)

Articular and extra-articular manifestations of rheumatoid arthritis affect the nutritional status of individuals in several ways. Articular involvement of the small and large joints may limit the ability to perform activities of daily living (ADL), including shopping for, preparing, and eating food. Involvement of the temporomandibular joint can impact the ability to chew and swallow and may necessitate changes in diet consistency. Extra-articular manifestations include increased metabolic rate secondary to the inflammatory process, Sjögren's syndrome, and changes in the gastrointestinal mucosa.

The increase in metabolic rate secondary to the inflammatory process leads to increased nutrient needs, often in the face of a diminishing nutrient intake. Taste alterations secondary to xerostomia and dryness of the nasal mucosa, dysphagia secondary to pharyngeal and esophageal dryness, anorexia secondary to medications, fatigue, and pain may reduce dietary intake. Changes in the gastrointestinal mucosa affect intake, digestion, and absorption. The impact of RA and of the medications used may be evident throughout the GI tract, from the oral cavity to the small and large intestines (Bossingham and Hawkey, 1993) (see Chapter 19).

Current weight and history of weight change over time are the least expensive, least invasive, and most reliable assessment tools to use with this population. Studies demonstrate that weight change is an important measure in rheumatoid arthritis. Increased cytokine production in rheumatoid arthritis may lead to reduced body cell mass and altered energy intake and metabolism (Roubenoff et al, 1994). Patients with rheumatoid arthritis may also be obese and have abnormal vitamin levels and poor nutrient intakes (Morgan et al, 1997a).

The diet history should review the usual diet; the impact of the handicap; types of food consumed; and changes in food tolerance secondary to oral, esophageal, and intestinal disorders. Impact of the disease on food shopping and preparation; self-feeding ability; appetite; and intake also need to be assessed. The use of elimination or other diets purported to treat or cure arthritis should be evaluated.

The association of foods with disease flares should be discussed because of the possibility of undetected food allergies (see Chapter 32). Whether food intake can modify the course of rheumatoid arthritis is an issue of continued scientific debate and interest. Dietary manipulation either by modifying food composition or by reducing weight may give some clinical benefit in improving RA symptoms (Danao-Camara and Shintani, 1999). Some benefits may be related to a reduction in immunoreactivity to food antigens eliminated by a change in diet (Hafstrom et al, 2001) (see *Clinical Insight:* Fasting and Vegetarian Diets in Rheumatoid Arthritis).

Energy

Objective measures of actual energy needs for this population have not been determined. It is important to remember that the actual impact of the inflammatory response on the metabolic rate is unknown and may vary from individual to individual. In addition, activity levels vary greatly.

Although traditional measures to assess energy requirements can be used, weight should be monitored and energy intake modified as needed to achieve desirable or usual body weight. Methods to determine energy requirements include the Harris-Benedict formula (see Chapter 2) and the DRI equations for resting energy expenditure (REE), with an additional factor for injury. During active disease, a factor of 1.14 to 1.35 times REE may be used to cover the effects of hypermetabolism. An activity factor of 1.2 times REE can be used for patients with limited mobility who are receiving physical therapy, and a factor of 1.3 times REE can be used for those receiving intensive daily physical therapy (Touger-Decker, 1988). For patients who are totally sedentary, calculations should be estimated at the REE and adjusted for weight changes that occur over time. When intakes are poor, enteral or parenteral supplementation may be required, and home nutritional support is beneficial for chronic cases.

Protein

Well-nourished individuals require protein at levels comparable to the recommended dietary allowances (RDAs) for age and sex. One study revealed that patients with rheumatoid arthritis have increased whole-body protein breakdown (regardless of age), which correlates with growth hormone factor, glucagon, and tumor necrosis factor production (Rall et al, 1996b). Rall also concluded that strength training for patients receiving methotrexate yielded normal rates of protein catabolism (Rall et al, 1996a). Requirements of patients who are poorly nourished or are in an inflammatory phase

TABLE 44-2 Nutritional Side Effects of Arthritis Medications

SIDE EFFECTS	SALICYLATES	NSAIDS	ANTI-MALARIALS	D-PENICILLAMINE	CORTICO-STEROIDS	IMMUNOSUPPRESSIVE AGENTS	GOLD
Nutritional							
Anorexia			x	x		x	
Stomatitis		x		x		x	x
Nausea	x	x	x	x	x	x	
Vomiting	x	x	x	x			x
Gastritis	x						
Duodenal ulcer		x			x		
Peptic ulcer	x						
Constipation		x					
Gastrointestinal bleeding	x	x					
Diarrhea		x*	x	x		x	x
Altered taste				x		x	
Metabolic							
Glucose intolerance					x		
Proteinuria				x			x
Negative nitrogen balance					x		x
Altered serum K	x				x		
Edema		†			x		
Depressed total lymphocyte count (TLC)					x	x	
Anergy					x	x	
Increased BUN value		x					
Anemia	x	x		x			
Decreased Vitamin/Mineral							
Ascorbic acid	x						
Folate	x					x‡	
Zinc				x			
Copper				x			
Calcium					x	x	
Iron				x			

Modified from Touger-Decker R: Nutritional considerations in rheumatoid arthritis, *J Am Diet Assoc* 88:329, 1988.
NSAIDs, Nonsteroidal antiinflammatory drugs; *BUN,* blood urea nitrogen.
*Meclomen only.
†May occur with preexisting edema.
‡Methotrexate only.

CLINICAL INSIGHT

Fasting and Vegetarian Diets in Rheumatoid Arthritis

Scientific literature validates the use of fasting in the control of joint inflammation. Fasting followed by a vegetarian diet may produce a sustained positive response measured clinically and by laboratory variables of inflammation (Danao-Camara and Shintani, 1999; Kjeldsen-Kragh, 1999; Muller et al, 2001). Researchers pooled the results of four controlled studies for a duration of 3 months or more from 31 studies and showed a statistically and clinically significant long-term effect of fasting followed by a vegetarian diet (Muller et al, 2001).

A vegan, gluten-free diet causes improvement in some patients, perhaps because of the reduction of immunoreactivity to food antigens eliminated by the change in diet (Hafstrom et al, 2001). Uncooked, lactobacilli-rich, vegan diets have also been suggested to have a positive outcome. Large amounts of living lactobacilli and chlorophyll-rich drinks and increased fiber intake seem to have positive effects on objective measures of RA and decrease the need for medications (Nenonen et al, 1998). Additional research is warranted to confirm the efficacy of these diet modifications.

of the disease increase to approximately 1.5 to 2 g/kg/day (Touger-Decker, 1988).

Lipids

The generation of reactive oxygen species is an important factor in the development and maintenance of rheumatoid arthritis (Darlington and Stone, 2001). Low-fat diets (including use of low-fat substitutes) lead to low serum levels of vitamin A and E and actually stimulate lipid peroxidation and eicosanoid production, thus aggravating rheumatoid arthritis (Adam et al, 1995). Therefore the typical emphasis on low-fat or fat-free dieting that has been the cornerstone of healthy eating in the United States may actually be counterproductive for patients susceptible to or afflicted by rheumatoid arthritis.

Rather than eliminating fat, changing the type of fat in the diet is probably more useful. Omega-3 fatty acids, either in tablet form or as they occur in oils, have increased in popularity in the management of rheumatoid arthritis because of their role in inflammatory pathways (see Box 44-1 and *Focus On:* Omega-3 Fatty Acids and the Inflammatory Process).

Some other oils of marine origin and a range of vegetable oils (olive and evening primrose oil) have indirect antiinflammatory actions probably mediated via prostaglandin E_1 (Belch and Hill, 2000; Darlington and Stone, 2001). Flaxseed oil contains the 18-carbon, omega-3 fatty acid alpha-linolenic acid, which can be converted to EPA after ingestion; it can be just as effective as fish oil in inhibiting arachidonic acid (AA) conversion to eicosanoids (James, Gibson, and Cleland, 2000).

In conclusion, swaying the balance of dietary fats in favor of the omega-3 and omega-6 fatty acids has an antiinflammatory effect but does not appear to correct the basic immunologic processes involved in the development of the arthropathies (Danao-Camara and Shintani, 1999; Sarzi-Puttini et al, 2000).

Box 44-1. Production of Eicosanoids From Omega-3 and Omega-6 Fatty Acids

Omega-6: Linoleic Acid 18:2~6 and Arachidonic Acid 20:4~6

Thromboxane$_2$ (vasoconstrictor)—Platelet aggregation
Prostaglandin$_2$ (vasodilator)—Platelet antiaggregation
Leukotriene$_4$—Elongation
Desaturation—In platelets, blood vessels, leukocytes

Omega-3: Linolenic Acid 18:3~3 and Eicosapentaenoic Acid 20:5~3

Thromboxane$_3$ (vasoconstrictor)
Prostaglandin$_3$ (vasodilator)
Leukotriene$_5$

Minerals, Vitamins, and Antioxidants

Animal studies have shown that vitamin E—in addition to omega-3 and omega-6 fatty acids—may also affect cytokine and eicosanoid production by decreasing proinflammatory cytokines and lipid mediators (Tidow-Kebritchi and Mobahan, 2001). In one human study, several antioxidant enzymes were efficient suppressors of oxygen radical overproduction in RA patients (Ostrakhovitch and Afanas'ev, 2001). Selenium, used in some trials, does not show specific clinical benefits (Peretz et al, 2001).

Earlier studies have shown that juvenile arthritis patients have reduced serum concentrations of an-

FOCUS ON

Omega-3 Fatty Acids and the Inflammatory Process

Two classes of polyunsaturated fatty acids—omega-6 and omega-3—are metabolized competitively, including conversion of their 20-carbon chain by oxygenase enzymes to form eicosanoids (*eicosa* means 20 in Greek). Prostaglandins, thromboxanes, leukotrienes, and prostacyclins are eicosanoids. Eicosapentaenoic acid (EPA) has a 20-carbon chain, and docosahexaenoic acid (DHA) has a 22-carbon chain; these are the omega-3 polyunsaturated fatty acids that are abundant in fish, such as salmon, mackerel, herring, tuna, and some other fish oils. Alpha-linolenic acid (ALA) has an 18-carbon chain with an omega-3 bond and is found in abundance in flaxseed, walnuts, and soy and canola (rapeseed) oils.

EPA, DHA, and ALA have all been shown to reduce the synthesis of aggressive inflammatory response cytokines by interfering with the conversion of arachidonic acid in various pathways, thus suppressing activation of cytokines in the cell membrane. Cytokines are produced by antagonistic omega-6 polyunsaturated acids that are mostly formed from linoleic acid found in safflower and other oils (Grimble and Tappia, 1998). The type of inflammatory mediator that is produced is determined by the composition of cellular membrane lipids, which in turn is influenced by the nature of the fatty acids in the diet. By increasing the amount of omega-3 fatty acids in the diet, the production of mediators with antiinflammatory effects improves the overall effectiveness.

Studies over the past two decades have clearly shown beneficial changes in cytokine and eicosanoid metabolism with fish oil supplementation in patients with rheumatoid arthritis (Tidow-Kebritchi and Mobahan, 2001; James, Gibson, and Cleland, 2000). Although fish oil seems to exert an antiinflammatory effect in short term studies, these effects may vanish during long-term treatment because of decreased numbers of autoreactive T cells via apoptosis. In already existing disease, increased consumption might not be beneficial over a long period (Ergas et al, 2002).

Although most studies (Ariza-Ariza et al, 1998; Hansen et al, 1998) have demonstrated improvement in arthritic conditions and modulation of the inflammatory response with the administration of omega-3, lowered intake of omega-6 fatty acids and increased intake of omega-3 oils should not replace conventional drug therapies. These oils should be used in conjunction with improved eating habits. Research continues to determine whether the source of omega-3 fatty acids (from a variety of whole food sources, like fish and oil-containing plants, rather than from pills) is significant. Counselors should advise their patients that fish oil supplements are not without their own side effects, such as increased bleeding time, gastrointestinal distress, and fishy taste or odor.

tioxidants in comparison to healthy controls and may benefit from dietary supplements when the dietary intake does not reach desired intake levels (Helgeland et al, 2000). European clinical trials have shown significant pain reduction in RA patients treated with vitamin E and other antioxidants (Tidow-Kebritchi and Mobahan, 2001; Ostrakhovitch and Afanas'ev, 2001).

Patients often have nutritional intakes below the RDA for calcium, folic acid, vitamin E, zinc, and selenium (Stone et al, 1997). This confirms earlier research in which more than 50% of patients studied had dietary intakes that provided less than 67% of the RDA for zinc, vitamin E, folic acid, pyridoxine, and magnesium (Morgan et al, 1993).

Independent of drug-induced alterations in specific vitamin or mineral levels, mounting evidence supports supplementation beyond the minimum levels for some nutrients. Vitamin therapy may complement conventional drug therapy, especially in the case of vitamin E (Edmonds et al, 1997; Tidow-Kebritchi and Mobahan, 2001), folic acid (Griffith et al, 2000; Martin, 1998), zinc (Naveh et al, 1997), and vitamin D (Deluca and Cantorna, 2001; DeLuca and Zierold, 1998).

Strong evidence suggests that patients with rheumatoid arthritis are under pathophysiologic oxidative stress (Chiriac et al, 1996; Gambhir et al, 1997). Degradation of collagen and eicosanoid stimulation are associated with oxidative damage; therefore increased intakes of supplemental antioxidants have been linked with beneficial effects in terms of both prevention and therapy for rheumatoid arthritis (Aaseth et al, 1998; Comstock et al, 1997; Hansen et al, 1998).

When metabolic bone disease, such as osteoporosis and osteomalacia, is present, calcium and vitamin D supplementation is indicated (Gough et al, 1998). Results from animal studies have shown that the role of vitamin D as a selective immunosuppressant is illustrated by its ability to either prevent or markedly suppress animal models of rheumatoid arthritis and lupus erythematosus (Deluca and Cantorna, 2001). Although, the action of vitamin D depends on the animal's maintenance of a normal or high-calcium diet in almost every case, these interesting findings warrant further research.

Calcium and vitamin D malabsorbtion and bone demineralization are characteristic of advanced stages of the disease, which may lead to osteoporosis. Supplementation with calcium and vitamin D has been shown to help prevent and reduce these detrimental conditions (Buckley et al, 1996; Oelzner and Hein, 1997) (see Chapter 28).

Use of methotrexate in rheumatoid arthritis may be associated with elevated homocysteine levels caused by low folate levels. Thus in patients with rheumatoid arthritis paying special attention to adequate intakes of folate and vitamins B_6 and B_{12} makes sense (Morgan et al, 1998; Roubenoff et al, 1997) (see Chapter 19).

Elevated levels of copper and ceruloplasmin in serum and joint fluid are seen in rheumatoid arthritis. Plasma copper levels correlate with the degree of joint inflammation, decreasing as the inflammation is diminished. Elevated plasma levels of ceruloplasmin, the carrier protein for copper, may have a protective role because of its antioxidant activity.

Variations in serum ferritin levels are less common in elderly persons than in young adults; this is true in rheumatoid arthritis as well (Lammi-Keefe et al, 1996). Plasma transferrin receptor levels are reliable for assessing iron status in this population. No special requirement for iron supplementation appears to exist in cases of rheumatoid arthritis.

Herbs and Complementary Therapy

The increasing popularity of the use of complementary and alternative treatments appears to be particularly evident with people afflicted with chronic diseases. One therapy that has been identified to have a potential benefit in the treatment of rheumatoid arthritis is herbal therapy (Little and Parsons, 2001; Tao et al, 2001). However, concerns of toxicity must also be addressed because the FDA provides relatively little regulation of herbal therapies (Klepser and Klepser, 1999; Ramgolam et al, 2000).

Gamma-linolenic acid (GLA), which the body uses to produce antiinflammatory prostaglandins, may relieve pain, morning stiffness, and joint tenderness with no serious side effects. Further studies are required to establish optimum dosage and duration (Horstman, 2001; Little and Parsons, 2001).

Thunder god vine (*Tripterygium wilfordii*) has been widely used in China to treat patients with a number of autoimmune diseases (Horstman, 2001; Ramgolam et al, 2000). It has been shown to inhibit mitogen-stimulated lymphoprolifieration and inhibit production of proinflammatory cytokines by monocytes, lymphocytes, and prostaglandin E_2 production via the COX-2 pathway (Lipsky and Tao, 1997). One placebo-controlled double-blind trial has clearly demonstrated its efficacy in rheumatoid arthritis (Lipsky and Tao, 1997). In one study, doses greater than 360 mg/day were associated with a clinical benefit in patients with RA (Tao et al, 2001). It should be explored further in autoimmune disorders like RA (Chen, 2001).

Feverfew is reputed by folklore to be effective in arthritis. The ingredient that is primarily responsible for this effect is parthenolide, a sesquiterpene lactone; however, its concentration varies widely in samples (Miller and Murray, 1998). Formulations that contain curcumin reduce inflammation and disability in double-blind clinical trials in patients with RA (Lodha and Bagga, 2000).

Other Medical Treatments and Exercise

Surgery replaces irreversibly damaged joints, improves the functional capacity of damaged joints, and prevents damage to otherwise healthy joints. Circulating antibodies and lymphocytes are sometimes removed by a process called *aphaeresis*.

Regular resistance and aerobic activity in patients with rheumatoid arthritis increases their range of motion, improves strength and endurance, preserves bone mass, preserves lean body mass, prevents fatigue, decreases depression, and distributes the forces of muscle contraction more evenly over joint surfaces (Hakkinen et al, 2001; Neuberger et al, 1997; Van den Ende et al, 1998).

Research on the use of recombinant human tumor necrosis factor receptor (p75)–Fc protein has shown that it can diminish inflammatory symptoms of rheumatoid arthritis (Moreland et al, 1997).

SJÖGREN'S SYNDROME

Sjögren's syndrome, a chronic inflammatory disorder, is characterized by polyglandular tissue destruction leading to keratoconjunctivitis, diminished production of tears and saliva, xerostomia, and xerophthalmia (Tabbara and Vara-Cristo, 2000). Half of the patients with Sjögren's syndrome also have rheumatoid arthritis (www.rheumatology.org).

The goal of dietary management in individuals with Sjögren's syndrome is relief of symptoms and eating discomfort, which can result in lack of appetite, weight loss, fatigue, difficulty chewing and swallowing, cavities, and anemia. Management of xerostomia should also include strategies for reducing the risk of dental decay (see Chapter 28), including frequent rinsing with water, tooth-brushing, or using topical fluorides.

Because swallowing is a problem, ready-to-eat foods may be useful. Foods should all be moist, and extremes in temperature should be avoided. The tartness of artificially sweetened lemon drops may help stimulate salivary flow. Artificial saliva or products such as lemon glycerine may also be recommended by dental or dietetic professionals. Iron and vitamin deficiencies such as low vitamin B_{12} and folate are possible and should be treated with a well-balanced diet (Lundstom and Lindstrom, 2001).

Dehydroepiandrosterone (DHEA), a hormone made by the adrenal glands whose production declines with aging, has benefited some patients and has been suggested as an adjunct treatment to corticosteroids (Straub et al, 2000). Currently a clinical trial is studying the effectiveness of DHEA with 18- to 75-year-old women (National Institutes of Health, 2001a).

TEMPOROMANDIBULAR JOINT SYNDROME

Severe temporomandibular joint (TMJ) syndrome, which may be associated with rheumatoid arthritis, results in pain with eating. The goal of dietary management is to alter food consistency to reduce chewing pain. Diet consistency should be mechanical soft, and all foods should be cut into bite-size pieces to minimize the individual's need to chew.

To facilitate self-feeding in individuals with rheumatoid arthritis, the dietitian or nurse should work closely with the occupational therapist to design a diet that maximizes independence in preparation and consumption of food and minimizes pain and frustration. Finger foods that do not fall apart easily may be helpful.

GOUT

Pathophysiology

Gout, one of the oldest diseases in recorded medical history, is a disorder of purine metabolism in which abnormally high levels of uric acid accumulate in the blood (hyperuricemia). As a consequence, sodium urates are formed and deposited as tophi in the small joints and surrounding tissues. Renal disease is common, and uric acid nephrolithiasis can occur. In chronic gout, a classic site is the helix of the ear (Figure 44-4); a more common site is the large toe or the elbow (Figure 44-5).

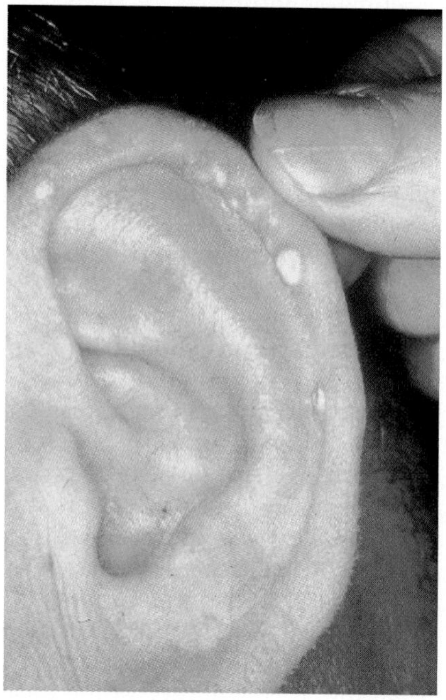

FIGURE 44-4 • Tophi on the ear of a patient who has had gout for many years. (Courtesy American College of Rheumatology, Atlanta.)

The disease, which usually occurs after the age of 35 years and predominantly affects men, is characterized by the sudden and acute onset of localized arthritic pain that usually begins in the big toe and continues up the leg. In one retrospective study, those with familial gout had an onset 7.5 years earlier than environmentally afflicted subjects and had lower serum triglyceride and cholesterol levels and less hypertension than nonfamilial gout sufferers (Chen et al, 2001). These urate deposits can destroy joint tissues, leading to chronic symptoms of arthritis (Figure 44-6).

One comorbidity of gout is obesity (WHO, 2000). Increased visceral adipose tissue (VAT) seems to aggravate the risks of insulin resistance in gout and may leave these patients at an increased risk of atherosclerotic disease (Takahashi et al, 2001). Ketosis associated with fasting or a low-carbohydrate diet can also precipitate an attack; occasionally, the disturbance follows surgery. As the disease advances, symptoms occur more frequently and are more prolonged. Trivial injury or unaccustomed exertion may precipitate the episodes, and attacks have been related to excessive eating, drinking, and exercise.

Medical Management

Gout is treated with drugs that inhibit or eliminate uric acid synthesis. Probenecid and sulfinpyrazone decrease the blood uric acid level by increasing elimination through the kidneys. Allopurinol inhibits uric acid production. Both probenecid and sulfinpyrazone often are used in conjunction with colchicine, a

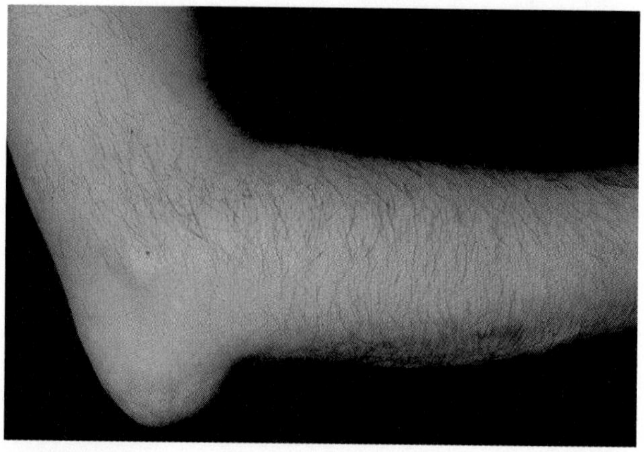

FIGURE 44-5 • Gout. This markedly enlarged olecranon bursa is caused by gout. (From the Clinical Slide Collection on the Rheumatic Diseases, copyright 1991, 1995, 1997. Used by permission of the American College of Rheumatology, Atlanta.)

drug that has no effect on uric acid metabolism but has been shown to relieve the joint pain of gouty arthritis. Colchicine is most valuable during the acute stage but may be needed during symptom-free periods as a preventive measure (for the nutritional effects of colchicine, see Chapter 19). Other antiinflammatory agents, such as indomethacin or phenylbutazone, are sometimes used in the acute stage of gout. NSAIDs are favored unless the side effects are too troublesome (Emmerson, 1996).

Medical Nutrition Therapy

Role of Proteins and Purines

Uric acid, derived from the metabolism of purines, constitutes a part of nucleoproteins. Although gout has traditionally been treated with a low-purine diet, drugs have largely replaced the need for rigid restriction of dietary purines. Endogenous formation of uric acid from simple metabolites—as well as from purine breakdown—accounts for 85% of the urate and is apparently influenced very little by dietary regulation. Even though limiting dietary purines is unlikely to decrease the uric acid pool significantly, individuals with gout should be encouraged to limit or avoid foods high in purines, to reduce metabolic stress (such as ketosis from excessive dieting), and to reduce medication use, if possible.

Intake of fluids (3 L/day) should be encouraged to assist with the excretion of uric acid and to minimize the possibility of renal calculi formation. Because urate excretion tends to be reduced by fats and enhanced by carbohydrates, the diet should be relatively high in carbohydrate (50% to 55% of calories), low in fat (30% of calories), modified in cholesterol (<300 mg/day), and moderate in protein. During an interval stage between attacks, dietary treatment for patients who are receiving maintenance medication for gout involves a normal, adequate diet adjusted to achieve and maintain a desirable body weight and to avoid ketosis.

Traditionally, restriction of foods that contain purines has been recommended in the acute stage of gout to avoid adding exogenous purines to the existing high uric acid load. When purine is restricted, as in severe gout, it should be restricted to 100 to 150 mg/day; the groupings in Box 44-2 can be used, allowing for considerable individualization among patients.

Tofu (bean curd) has been suggested as a preferable source of protein in patients with gout. Tofu ingestion has been shown to alter plasma protein concentration and to increase uric acid clearance and excretion (Yamakita et al, 1998). Ethanol does increase uric acid production but does not always cause an attack of gout. The patient should be advised not to consume an excess of alcohol.

SCLERODERMA

Pathophysiology

Scleroderma is a progressive, systemic sclerosis characterized by deposition of fibrous connective tissue in the skin and visceral organs, including the gastrointestinal tract (Escott-Stump, 2002). Women tend to be afflicted four times more often than men. The five-year survival rate is 80% to 85%. One manifestation of scleroderma is Raynaud's syndrome (ischemia or coldness in the small extremities, such as

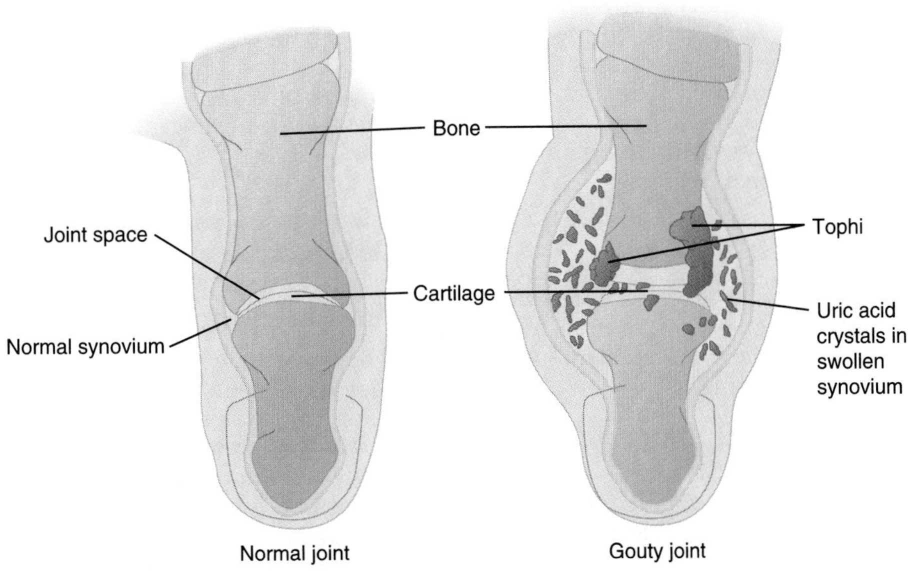

FIGURE 44-6 • Comparison of a gouty joint and a normal joint. (From Black JM et al: *Medical surgical nursing*, ed 5, Philadelphia, 1996, WB Saunders.)

Box 44-2. Foods Grouped According to Purine Content

Group 1: High Purine Content (100 to 1000 mg of Purine Nitrogen per 100 g of Food)

Anchovies	Mackerel
Bouillon	Meat extracts
Brains	Mincemeat
Broth	Mussels
Consommé	Partridge
Goose	Roe
Gravy	Sardines
Heart	Scallops
Herring	Sweetbreads
Kidney	Yeast (baker's and brewer's), taken as supplement

Foods in this list should be omitted from the diet of patients who have gout (acute and remission stages).

Group 2: Moderate Purine Content (9 to 100 mg of Purine Nitrogen per 100 g of Food)

Meat and Fish (except those listed in group 1):	Vegetables
Fish	Asparagus
Poultry	Beans, dried
Meat	Lentils
Shellfish	Mushrooms
	Peas, dried
	Spinach

One serving (2 to 3 oz) of meat, fish, or fowl or 1 serving (½ cup) of vegetables from this group is allowed daily (depending on condition) during remissions.

Group 3: Negligible Purine Content

Bread, white, and crackers	Fruit
Butter or margarine (in moderation)*	Gelatin desserts
Cake and cookies	Herbs
Carbonated beverages	Ice cream
Cereal beverage (e.g., Postum)	Milk
Cereals and cereal products	Macaroni products
Cheese	Noodles
Chocolate	Nuts
Coffee	Oil
Condiments	Olives
Cornbread	Pickles
Cream (in moderation)*	Popcorn
Custard	Puddings
Eggs	Relishes
Fats (in moderation)*	Rennet desserts
Vegetables (except those in group 2)	Rice
	Salt
	Sugar and sweets
	Tea
	Vinegar
	White sauce

Foods included in this group may be used daily.

*Recommended in moderation because of fat content.

the fingers), which causes difficulty in preparation and consumption of meals. Sjögren's syndrome is often also present. Gastrointestinal symptoms include heartburn, nausea and vomiting, dysphagia, diarrhea, constipation, and fecal incontinence (Weston et al, 1998). Weight loss, renal dysfunction, and multiple organ system dysfunctions may result.

Medical Management

The disease is progressive, and no current treatment produces a cure. Side effects of specific drug therapies, as prescribed for specific symptoms and organ involvement, are noted in Chapter 19.

Medical Nutrition Therapy

Dysphagia may be one symptom that requires nutritional interventions (see Chapter 43). Malabsorption of lactose, vitamins, fatty acids, and minerals can cause further nutritional problems; supplementation may be required. A high-energy, high-protein supplement or enteral feeding may be effective in correcting or preventing weight loss, which is a common manifestation. Home enteral or parenteral nutritional support is often required when problems, such as chronic diarrhea, persist (see Chapter 23).

SYSTEMIC LUPUS ERYTHEMATOSUS

Pathophysiology

Systemic lupus erythematosus (SLE) has an unclear etiology. A genetic predisposition (genetic marker HLA, or human leukocyte antigen), the presence of anti-DNA antibodies, and environmental factors, such as a viral infection, are thought to be involved. The condition is most prevalent in women of childbearing age and is more common in African Americans than in Caucasians. In 1954 the survival rate was 50%; today it is 97%. About 25% of persons with SLE also develop Sjögren's syndrome (www.sjögrens.org).

Medical Management

SLE is considered to be an autoimmune disease that affects all organ systems. The disease itself, as well as the medications (e.g., steroids) that are commonly used to treat SLE, affect nutrient metabolism, needs, and excretion. Renal function is deranged, thus causing excessive excretion of protein and, often, renal failure. Corticosteroids alter protein, sodium, fluid, and calcium needs. Plaquenil, an antimalarial drug, appears to be effective in clearing up skin lesions for some individuals but has side effects that include nausea, abdominal cramping, and diarrhea. Immunosupressants, such as azathioprine, may be used in the event of brain or renal involvement, but gastrointestinal side effects may occur.

Medical Nutrition Therapy

At this time, no specific dietary guidelines for managing SLE exist. Rather, the diet needs to be tailored to the individual needs of the patient. Priorities include addressing the sequelae of the disease and the pharmacologic effects on organ function and nutrient metabolism (see Table 44-2). Protein requirements are altered as a result of disordered renal function caused by the disease and steroid-induced side effects. Sodium and fluid intakes are typically restricted for the same reasons. Although a diet low in saturated fats has been recommended, further studies are necessary to document effectiveness.

The effect of dietary modifications has been extensively studied in lupus animal models. Energy needs should be tailored to the individual's dry weight. The goal in determining caloric requirements should be to attain and maintain the usual body weight. Calorie, protein, and especially fat restriction may cause a significant reduction in immune-complex deposition in the kidney and proteinuria and may prolong the life span (Leiba et al, 2001). The addition of polyunsaturated fatty acids such as from 30 g of ground flaxseed daily for 1 year in a small group of subjects is protective of the kidneys, but more large-scale studies are recommended (Clark et al, 2001). Nutrition support may be required in chronic cases.

CHRONIC FATIGUE DISORDER SYNDROME AND FIBROMYALGIA

Disorders such as chronic fatigue disorder syndrome (CFDS) and fibromyalgia have rheumatic symptoms but no proven cure. About 2% of 5 million Americans are afflicted, women seven times more frequently than men—more often during the child-bearing years (www.fmpartnership.org).

In CFDS, chronic fatigue is the major symptom. It lasts 6 months or longer and is accompanied by hypotension, sore throat, multiple joint pains, headaches, postexertion lethargy, muscle pain, and impaired concentration. CFDS mimics autoimmune disorders such as SLE or hypothyroidism. Graduated exercise programs, low-fat diets, antioxidant therapy, massive doses of vitamins, magnesium sulfate use, and costly intravenous immunoglobin therapy have been recommended, but their efficacy is as yet unconfirmed by controlled studies. When hypotension is identified medically, increases in sodium and fluid intakes have been suggested.

In fibromyalgia, nonarticular aches and fatigue cause disabling symptoms that are similar to those of rheumatoid arthritis. Muscle tenderness, sleep disturbances, fatigue, morning stiffness, numbness and tingling, chronic headaches, irritable bowel, and irritable bladder have all been reported to be associated with the "fibromyalgia syndrome." Several hypotheses have been proposed, including central pain derangement; central nervous system dysfunction; nutrient deficiencies of magnesium, malic acid, manganese, or thiamin; and other systemic abnormalities. Pain therapy, use of calcium channel blockers, physical reconditioning, psychological therapy, and alternative approaches have been recommended, but further studies are needed to evaluate their effectiveness.

Medical Nutrition Therapy

A vegan diet has been shown to have beneficial effects on fibromyalgia patients, at least for the short term (Kaartinen et al, 2000). Eighteen patients followed a strict, low-salt, uncooked-vegetable, lactobacteria-rich diet for a 3-month period and were able to reduce their BMI, total cholesterol, and urine sodium. Results revealed significant improvements in pain, joint stiffness, and sleep quality. In another study, the shift to a vegan "living food" diet of berries, fruits, vegetables and roots, nuts, germinated seeds, and sprouts rich in carotenoids and vitamins C and E resulted in a decrease in joint stiffness (Hanninen et al, 2000). Longer studies are needed to confirm these findings.

Complementary Therapy

The treatment options for fibromyalgia appear to be limited and generally unsatisfactory; long-lasting effects have not been evaluated. Nonetheless, the National Institutes of Health (NIH) Consensus Development Statement on Acupuncture states that musculoskeletal conditions such as fibromyalgia and myofascial pain are conditions in which acupuncture may be beneficial (National Institutes of Health, 2000).

Exercise has also been shown to be effective with fibromylagia patients. In one study, three 30-minute classes for 23 weeks appeared to be successful in improving mood and physical function (Gowans et al, 2001).

CONTROVERSIES AND UNPROVEN REMEDIES FOR RHEUMATIC DISORDERS

Because modern medicine cannot promise a cure or even permanent relief of symptoms, many persons with rheumatic disorders understandably turn to folk medicine and even quackery for help. Surveys in the United States and other countries show that 50% to 94% of those affected try at least one self-help remedy—usually more than one (Jarvis, 1990). Favorable effects of self-help treatments are often reported anecdotally, but as a rule, no cause-and-effect relationships are documented. Any amelioration can usually be attributed to the placebo effect or to characteristic cycles of worsening, followed by periods of improvement.

Megavitamin therapy and special foods and diets are among the most popular self-help remedies. Dietary variations are often unusual, as evidenced by the "honey and apple cider vinegar" treatment or use of kombucha tea. According to the Arthritis Foundation, kombucha tea has a high risk of contamination with anthrax and other bacteria (Horstman, 2001). Ground bovine cartilage at best may cause allergic reactions and at worst Mad Cow Disease (Horstman, 2001).

Some seemingly "natural" remedies have their roots in medicine, as in the case of willow bark and copper bracelets. Salicylates, as in aspirin and derived from willow bark, have been around as a medicinal remedy for pain and inflammation since 1763; some have even traced their use back to ancient Egypt (Vane, 2000). Willow bark as such is of little use because it has the same gastrointestinal side effects as aspirin or NSAIDs and can increase the effects of blood-thinning drugs or supplements (Hedner and Everts, 1998; Horstman, 2001). Although the folk remedy of wearing a copper bracelet to relieve arthritis pain has been suggested as a means of promoting copper absorption through the skin, no clinical studies have substantiated this claim.

Rhizoma smilacis glabrae, also known as glabrous green briar rhizome (china root), is an extract used in Chinese herbal medicine that has been shown to act as a therapeutic agent in rheumatoid arthritis, and it is without side effects (Jiang et al, 1997). Initial studies suggest that china root extract acts through selective suppression of the cellular immune response involved in inflammation as well as through a direct antiinflammatory mechanism, including inhibition of PGE2. This is not yet a proven remedy.

Shark cartilage is a popular remedy because it is a cheap source of chondroitin sulfate, but no studies of the effect of shark cartilage on joint disease have occurred. Even with positive-effect evidence for cow trachea chondroitin sulfate and other promising "natural" remedies, some difficulties persist, including the following: (1) lack of regulation of such supplements in terms of dosage, purity, or claims; (2) the fact that using these nonregulated remedies is, in effect, self-medication without monitoring; and (3) lack of understanding of other drug interactions or long-term safety (see Chapter 20 and Appendix 35).

Although much of the dietary experimentation is harmless (except for the cost of special foods or popular diet books), some self-treatment modalities can be harmful. Both comfrey and alfalfa are herbs that have been promoted as potential cures for arthritis, yet both have been deemed toxic by the scientific community. Rattlesnake meat has been touted as a remedy, but the risk of salmonella poisoning is high.

Finally, the use of pulsed electromagnetic fields (PEMF) has been shown to affect the growth of bone and cartilage in vitro with potential application as an arthritis treatment, but the data are limited (Trock, 2000).

SUMMARY

Because no known cure for the arthritic condition exists, pharmacotherapy, physical and occupational treatment, and medical nutrition therapy (MNT) can help to manage the symptoms associated with this group of disorders. Some alternative diet therapies, supplements, and programs currently under investigation appear to be promising in reducing the need for toxic medications and for alleviating some of the symptoms and managing the pain. Medical nutrition therapy appears to play a key role in the treatment of rheumatic disorders and holds promise for managing these patients for the span of their lifetimes.

Clinical Scenario I

Dana is a 49-year-old woman who has been diagnosed with the early stages of knee-and-elbow osteoarthritis. Until diagnosis, she was an avid tennis player who enjoyed a country club lifestyle entertaining with her executive husband. Her weight has reached 150 lb for her 5 ft 5 in. frame. Her physician has prescribed a nonsteroidal antiinflammatory drug for pain and suggested that she speak with a registered dietitian about a weight-loss program to decrease her symptoms and the progression of the disease. She comes to see you and presents a list of supplements and herbs her friends have suggested she take to control her osteoarthritis naturally because the NSAIDs seem to affect her stomach.

1. How would you approach Dana's diet, considering the social constraints she will have?
2. What type of foods and fluids would you recommend she consume more often to help her reduce her weight, control the side effects of the NSAIDs, and prevent her from feeling deprived?
3. What type of exercise and alternative therapy might you recommend as a possibility to help improve her weight and manage the pain?
4. What advice would you give her regarding the use of herbs and supplements? What type of information is available (i.e., research; Web sites; organizations that may be able to provide information on the efficacy, safety, and hazards of consuming specific vitamin/mineral supplements and herbs)?

Clinical Scenario 2

Sam is a 52-year-old white man who lives with his wife in a rural area. He is 5 ft 10 in. and weighs 230 lb. He has recently been diagnosed with osteoarthritis. A nonsteroidal antiinflammatory drug was prescribed for severe flare-ups of the condition. Although the medication is generally effective, Sam now wants you to develop a special diet for him. He has heard that liver extract, bee pollen, and gold tablets will cure his condition. He brought you a bag full of various remedies and has displayed them on your desk.

1. How will you tactfully advise him about these so-called remedies that are not likely to be useful and may actually cause some harm?
2. He has read in the newspaper that vitamin E and other antioxidants are useful in alleviating his condition, but you have no scientific articles to prove this. How will you discuss this topic with Sam?
3. From his diet history, it appears that Sam eats little at breakfast and has a heavy, high–saturated fat lunch. He eats no fish, few fruits and vegetables, and drinks a cocktail before dinner. What dietary changes would you suggest to improve his diet?
4. Sam does not mention his overweight. How would you bring up the subject, and what steps would you recommend for him?

Relevant Web Sites

American College of Rheumatology
www.rheumatology.org/index.asp
Arthritis Foundation
www.arthritis.org
Lupus Foundation of America
www.lupus.org
National Fibromyalgia Partnership
www.fmpartnership.org
National Institute of Arthritis, Musculoskeletal and Skin Diseases
www.nih.gov/niams
Scleroderma Foundation
www.scleroderma.org/
Scleroderma Research Foundation
www.SRFCure/org
Sjögrens Syndrome Foundation
www.sjogrens.org

Cited References

Aaseth J et al: Rheumatoid arthritis and metal compounds: perspectives on the role of oxygen radical detoxification, *Analyst* 123:3, 1998.

Adam O et al: Low-fat diet decreases alpha-tocopherol levels, and stimulates LDL oxidation and eicosanoid biosynthesis in man, *Eur J Med Res* 1:65, 1995.

Alarcon GS, Morgan SL: Guidelines for folate supplementation in rheumatoid arthritis patients treated with methotrexate: comment on the guidelines for monitoring drug therapy, *Arthritis Rheum* 40:391, 1997.

Anderson LS, Hansen TM: Prospectively measured red cell folate levels in methotrexate treated patients with rheumatoid arthritis: relation to withdrawal and side effects, *J Rheumatol* 25:830, 1997.

Ariza-Ariza R et al: Omega-3 fatty acids in rheumatoid arthritis: an overview, *Semin Arthritis* Rheum 27:366, 1998.

Belch JJ, Hill A: Evening primrose oil and borage oil in rheumatologic conditions, *Am J Clin Nutr* 71: 352S, 2000.

Bossingham D, Hawkey CJ: Gastroenterology in the rheumatic diseases, *Gastroenterol Rheum* Dis 1:138, 1993.

Brand C et al: Vitamin E is ineffective for symptomatic relief of knee osteoarthritis: a six-month double blind, randomized, placebo controlled study, *Ann Rheum Dis* 60: 946, 2001.

Brief AA et al: Use of glucosamine and chondroitin sulfate in the management of osteoarthritis, *J Am Acad Orthop Surg* 9: 71, 2001.

Buckley LM et al: Calcium and vitamin D_3 supplementation prevents bone loss in the spine secondary to low-dose corticosteroids in patients with rheumatoid arthritis: a randomized, double-blind, placebo-controlled trial, *Ann Intern Med* 125:961, 1996.

Buckwalter JA, Lane NE: Athletics and osteoarthritis, *Am J Sports Med* 25:873, 1997.

Canoso JJ: *Rheumatology in primary care,* Philadelphia, 1997, WB Saunders.

Chen SY et al: Clinical features of familial gout and effects of probable genetic association between gout and its related disorders, *Metabolism* 50:1203, 2001.

Chiriac R et al: The antioxidant systems in rheumatoid polyarthritis, *Rev Med Chir Soc Med Nat Iasi* 100:79, 1996.

Clark WF et al: Flaxseed in lupus nephritis: a two-year non placebo controlled crossover study, *J Am Coll Nutr* 20:143S, 2001.

Clyman B: The value of aerobic or resistance training supported studies not without statistical and methodological imperfections, *Curr Rheumatol Rep* 3; 520, 2001.

Coggon D et al: Knee osteoarthritis and obesity, *Int J Obes Relat Metab Disord* 25: 622, 2001.

Comstock GW et al: Serum concentrations of alpha-tocopherol, beta-carotene, and retinol preceding the diagnosis of rheumatoid arthritis and systemic lupus erythematosus, *Ann Rheum Dis* 56:323, 1997.

Conn DL: Resolved: low dose prednisone is indicated as a standard treatment in patients with rheumatoid arthritis, *Arthritis Rheum* 45: 462, 2001.

Cooper C et al: Individual risk factors for hip osteoarthritis: obesity, hip injury, and physical activity, *Am J Epidemiol* 147:516, 1998.

Creamer P et al: Management of osteoarthritis in older adults, *Clin Geriatr Med* 14:435, 1998.

DaCamara CC, Dowless GV: Glucosamine for osteoarthritis, *Ann Pharmacother* 32: 58, 1998.

Danao-Camara TC and Shintani TT: The dietary treatment of inflammatory arthritis: case reports and review of the literature, *Hawaii Med J* 58:126, 1999.

Darlington LG, Stone TW: Antioxidants and fatty acids in the amelioration of rheumatoid arthritis and related disorders, *Br J Nutr* 85:251, 2001.

Deluca HF, Cantorna MT: Vitamin D: its role and uses in immunology, *FASEB J* 15:2579, 2001.

DeLuca HF, Zierold C: Mechanisms and functions of vitamin D, *Nutr Rev* 56:S4, 1998.

DeRoos AJ et al: Serum caratenoids and radiologic knee osteoarthritis: the Johnston County Osteoarthritis Project, *Public Health Nutr* 4:935, 2001.

DHEA: Monograph. *Altern Med Rev* 6: 314, 2001.

Emery P et al: Celecoxib verses diclofenac in long-term management of rheumatoid arthritis: randomized, double blind comparison, *Lancet* 354:2106, 1999.

Emmerson B: The management of gout, *N Engl J Med* 334:445, 1996.

Endresen GK, Husby G: Folate supplementation during methotrexate treatment of patient with rheumatoid arthritis: an update and proposals for guidelines, *Scand J Rheumatol* 30:129, 2001.

Ergas D et al: N-3 fatty acids and the immune system in autoimmunity, *Isr Med Assoc J* 4: 34, 2002.

Escott-Stump S: *Nutrition and diagnosis-related care,* ed 5, Baltimore, 2002, Lippincott Williams & Wilkins.

Firestein G, Zvaifler N: Anticytokine therapy in rheumatoid arthritis, *N Engl J Med* 337:195, 1997.

Fisher NM et al: Muscle function and gait in patients with knee osteoarthritis before and after muscle rehabilitation, *Disabil Rehabil* 19:47, 1997.

Flynn M et al: The effect of folate and cobalamin on osteoarthritic hands, *J Am Coll Nutr* 13:351, 1994.

Fransen M et al: A revised group exercise program for osteoarthritis of the knee, *Physiother Res Int* 2:30, 1997.

Gambhir JK et al: Correlation between blood antioxidant levels and lipid peroxidation in rheumatoid arthritis, *Clin Biochem* 30:351, 1997.

Gough A et al: Effect of vitamin D receptor gene alleles on bone loss in early rheumatoid arthritis, *J Rheumatol* 25:864, 1998.

Gowans SE et al: Exercise can improve mood and physical function, *Arthritis Rheum* 45:519, 2001.

Griffith SM et al: Do patients with rheumatoid arthritis established on methotrexate and folic acid 5 mg daily need to continue folic acid supplements long term? *Rheumatology* 39:1102, 2000.

Grimble RF, Tappia PS: Modulation of pro-inflammatory cytokine biology by unsaturated fatty acids, *Z Ernahrungswiss* 37:57, 1998.

Hafstrom I et al: A vegan diet free of gluten improves the signs and symptoms of rheumatoid arthritis: the effects on arthritis correlate with a reduction in antibodies to food antigens, *Rheumatology* 40:1175, 2001.

Hakkinen A et al: A randomized two-year study of the effects of dynamic strength training on muscle strength, disease activity, functional capacity and bone mineral density in early rheumatoid arthritis, *Arthritis Rheum* 44: 515, 2001.

Hanninen O et al: Antioxidants in vegan diet and rheumatic disorders, *Toxicology* 155:45, 2000.

Hansen G et al: Nutritional status of Danish patients with rheumatoid arthritis and effects of a diet adjusted in energy intake, fish content and antioxidants, *Ugeskr Laeger* 160:3074, 1998.

Harris ED: *Rheumatoid arthritis,* Philadelphia, 1997, WB Saunders.

Hauselmann HJ: Nutripharmaceuticals for osteoarthritis, *Best Pract Res Clin Rheumatol* 15:595, 2001.

Hedner T, Everts B: The early clinical history of salicylates in rheumatology and pain, *Clin Rheumatol* 17:17, 1998.

Helgeland M et al: Dietary intake and serum concentrations of antioxidants in children with juvenile arthritis, *Clin Exp Rheumatol* 18:637, 2000.

Horstman J: *2001 supplement guide,* 2001, Arthritis Foundation.

James MJ, Gibson RA, Cleland LG: Dietary polyunsaturated fatty acids and inflammatory mediator production, *Am J Clin Nutr* 71:343S, 2000.

Jarvis WT: Arthritis: folk remedies and quackery, *Nutr Forum* 7(1):1, 1990.

Jiang J et al: Anti-inflammatory activity of the aqueous extract from rhizome smilacis glabrae, *Pharmacol Res* 36:309, 1997.

Johanning GL: Modulation of breast cancer cell adhesion by unsaturated fatty acids, *Nutrition* 12:810, 1996.

Johnson RK, Kennedy E: The 2000 dietary guidelines for Americans: what are the changes and why were they made? The Dietary Guidelines Advisory Committee, *J Am Diet Assoc* 100:769, 2000.

Kaartinen K et al: Vegan diet alleviates fibromylagia symptoms, *Scand J Rheumatol 29*:308, 2000.

Kelly WN et al: *Textbook of rheumatology,* vol 2, Philadelphia, 1997, WB Saunders.

Kjeldsen-Kragh J: Rheumatoid arthritis treated with vegetarian diets, *Am J Clin Nutr* 70:594S, 1999.

Klepser TB, Klepser ME: Unsafe and potentially safe herbal therapies, *Am J Health Syst Pharm* 15:125, 1999.

Koopman WJ: *Arthritis and allied conditions: a textbook of rheumatology,* vol 2, Baltimore, 1997, Williams & Wilkins.

Lammi-Keefe C et al: Day-to-day variation in iron status indexes is similar for most measures in elderly women with and without rheumatoid arthritis, *J Am Diet Assoc* 96:247, 1996.

Lawrence RC et al: Estimates of the prevalence of arthritis and selected musculoskeletal disorders in the United States, *Arthritis Rheum* 41:778, 1998.

Leiba A et al: Diet and lupus, *Lupus* 10:246, 2001.

Lipsky PE, Tao XL: A potential new treatment for rheumatoid arthritis: thunder god vine, *Semin Arthritis Rheum* 26:713, 1997.

Little C, Parsons T: Herbal therapy for treating rheumatoid arthritis, *Cochrane Database Syst Rev* (1):CD002928, 2001.

Lodha R, Bagga A: Traditional Indian systems of medicine, *Ann Acad Med Singapore* 29:37, 2000.

Lundstrom IM, Lindstrom FD: Iron and vitamin deficiencies, endocrine and immune status in patients with primary Sjogren's syndrome, *Oral Dis* 7:144, 2001.

Martin RH: The role of nutrition and diet in rheumatoid arthritis, *Proc Nutr Soc* 57:231, 1998.

McAlindon TE et al: Do antioxidant micronutrients protect against the development and progression of knee osteoarthritis? *Arthritis Rheum* 39:648, 1996a.

McAlindon TE et al: Relation of dietary intake and serum levels of vitamin D to progression of osteoarthritis of the knee among participants in the Framingham Study, *Ann Intern Med* 125:353, 1996b.

McCleane G: The analgesic efficacy of topical capsaicin is enhanced by glyceryl trintrate in painful osteoarthritis: a randomized, double-blind, placebo controlled study, *Eur J Pain* 4:355, 2000.

Mikuls TR et al: Coffee, tea and caffeine consumption and risk of rheumatoid arthritis: results from the Iowa Women's Health Study, *Arthritis Rheum* 46:83, 2002.

Miller L, Murray W: *Herbal medicinals: a clinician's guide,* New York, 1998, Haworth Press.

Moreland L et al: Treatment of rheumatoid arthritis with a recombinant human tumor necrosis factor receptor (p75)-Fc protein, *N Engl J Med* 337:141, 1997.

Morgan S et al: Nutrient intake patterns, body mass index, and vitamin levels in patients with rheumatoid arthritis, *Arthritis Care Res* 10:9, 1997a.

Morgan S et al: Methotrexate in rheumatoid arthritis: folate supplementation should always be given, *BioDrugs* 8:164, 1997b.

Morgan S et al: Folic acid supplementation prevents deficient blood folate levels and hyperhomocysteinemia during long-term, low dose methotrexate therapy for rheumatoid arthritis: implications for cardiovascular disease prevention, *J Rheumatol* 25:441, 1998.

Morgan SL et al: Dietary intake and circulating vitamin levels of rheumatoid arthritis patients treated with methotrexate, *Arthritis Care Res* 6:4, 1993.

Muller H et al: Fasting followed by a vegetarian diet in patients with rheumatoid arthritis: a systemic review, *Scand J Rheumatol* 30:1, 2001.

National Institutes of Health: Acupuncture in fibromylagia, National Center for Complementary and Alternative Medicine (NCCAM), www.clinicaltrials.org, 2000.

National Institutes of Health: DHEA Treatment for Sjogren's syndrome, www.clinicaltrials.gov. April 2001a.

National Institutes of Health: Glucosamine/chondroitin arthritis intervention trail, www.clinicaltrials.org, 2001b.

National Institutes of Health: Cost-effectiveness of and long-term outcomes following acupuncture treatment for osteoarthritis of the knee, www.clinicaltrials.org, 2001c.

Naveh Y et al: Zinc metabolism in rheumatoid arthritis: plasma and urinary zinc and relationship to disease activity, *J Rheumatol* 24:643, 1997.

Nenonen T et al: Uncooked, lactobacilli-rich, vegan food and rheumatoid arthritis, *Br J Rheumatol* 37:274, 1998.

Neuberger GB et al: Effects of exercise on fatigue, aerobic fitness, and disease activity measures in persons with rheumatoid arthritis, *Res Nurs Health* 20:195, 1997.

Nicolakis P et al: Long-term outcome after treatment of temporomandibular joint osteoarthritis with exercise and manual therapy, *Cranio* 20:23, 2002.

Oelzner P, Hein G: Inflammation and bone metabolism in rheumatoid arthritis: pathogenetic viewpoints and therapeutic possibilities, *Med Klin* 92:607, 1997.

Ostrakhovitch EA, Afanas'ev IB: Oxidative stress in rheumatoid arthritis leukocytes: suppression by rutin and other antioxidants and chelators, *Biochem Pharmacol* 62:743, 2001.

Peretz A et al: Selenium supplementation in rheumatoid arthritis investigated in a double blind, placebo controlled trial, *Scand J Rheumatol* 30:208, 2001.

Perneger TV et al: Risk of kidney failure associated with the use of acetaminophen, aspirin, and nonsteroidal anti-inflammatory drug, *N Engl J Med* 331:1675, 1994.

Rall LC et al: Effects of progressive resistance training on immune response in aging and chronic inflammation, *Med Sci Sports Exerc* 28:1356, 1996a.

Rall LC et al: Protein metabolism in rheumatoid arthritis and aging: effects of muscle strength training and tumor necrosis factor cc, *Arthritis Rheum* 39:1115, 1996b.

Ramgolam V et al: Traditional Chinese medicines as immunosuppresive agents, *Ann Acad Med Singapore* 29:11, 2000.

Rejeski WJ et al: Treating disability in knee osteoarthritis with exercise therapy: a central role for self-efficacy and pain, *Arthritis Care Res* 11:94, 1998.

Robbins W: Clinical applications of capsaicinoids, *Clin J Pain* 16: 86S2, 2000.

Roubenoff R et al: Rheumatoid cachexia: cytokine-driven hypermetabolism accompanying reduced body cell mass chronic inflammation, *J Clin Invest* 93:2379, 1994.

Roubenoff R et al: Abnornal homocysteine metabolism in rheumatoid arthritis, *Arthritis Rheum* 40:718, 1997.

Sarzi-Puttini P et al: Diet therapy for rheumatoid arthritis: a controlled double-blind study of two different dietary regimens, *Scand J Rheumatol* 29: 302, 2000.

Schmid B et al: Efficacy and tolerability of a standardized willow bark extract in patients with osteoarthritis: randomized placebo controlled, double blind clinical trial, *Phytother Res* 15: 344, 2001.

Shahin AA et al: Protective effect of folinic acid on low-dose methotrexate genotoxicity, *Z Rheumatol* 60: 63, 2001.

Singh G et al: Prevalence of cardiovascular disease risk factors among US adults with self-reported osteoarthritis: data from the Third National Health and Nutrition Examination Survey, *Am J Manag Care* 8:383S, 2002.

Slot O: Changes in plasma homocysteine in aryhritis patients starting treatment with low-dose methotrexate subsequently supplemented with folic acid, *Scand J Rheumatol*, 30:305, 2001.

Sowers M: Epidemiology of risk factors for osteoarthritis: systemic factors, *Curr Opin Rheumatol* 13:447, 2001.

Spector TD et al: Risk of osteoarthritis associated with long-term weight-bearing sports: a radiologic survey of the hips and knees in female ex-athletes and population controls, *Arthritis Rheum* 39:988, 1996.

Stone J et al: Inadequate calcium, folic acid, vitamin E, zinc, and selenium intake in rheumatoid arthritis patients: results of a dietary survey, *Semin Arthritis Rheum* 27:180, 1997.

Straub RH et al: Replacement therapy with DHEA plus corticosteroids in patients with chronic inflammatory diseases—substitutes of adrenal and sex hormones, *Z Rheumatol* 59,108S2, 2000.

Tabbara KF, Vera-Cristo CL: Sjögren syndrome, *Curr Opin Opthalmol* 11:449, 2000.

Takahashi S et al: Increased visceral fat accumulation further aggravates the risks of insulin resistance in gout, *Metabolism* 50: 393, 2001.

Tao X et al: A phase I study of ethyl acetate extract of the Chinese antirheumatic herb *tripterygium wilfordii* hook f in rheumatoid arthritis, *J Rheumatol* 28:2160, 2001.

Tidow-Kebritchi S, Mobahan S: Effects of diets containing fish oil and vitamin E on rheumatoid arthritis, *Nutr Rev* 59(10):335, 2001.

Toda Y: The effect of energy restriction, walking and exercise on lower extremity lean body mass in obese women with osteoarthritis of the knee, *J Orthop Sci* 6: 148, 2001.

Todd C: Meeting the therapeutic challenge of the patient with osteoarthritis, *J Am Pharm Assoc* 42:74, 2002.

Touger-Decker R: Nutritional considerations in rheumatoid arthritis, *J Am Diet Assoc* 88:327, 1988.

Trock DH: Electromagnetic fields and magnets: investigational treatment for musculoskeletal disorders, *Rheum Dis Clin North Am* 26:51, 2000.

Van den Ende CH et al: Dynamic exercise therapy in rheumatoid arthritis: a systematic review, *Br J Rheumatol* 37:677, 1998.

Van Ede AE et al: Effect of folic or folinic acid supplementation on the toxicity and efficacy of methotrexate in rheumatoid arthritis: a forty-eight week, multicenter, randomized, double-blind, placebo controlled study, *Arthritis Rheum* 44: 1515, 2001.

van Weel C: Morbidity in family medicine: the potential for individual nutritional counseling, an analysis from the Nijmegen continuous morbidity registration, *Am J Clin Nutr* 65:1928S, 1997.

Vane JR: The fight against rheumatism: from willow bark to cox-1 sparing drugs, *J Physiol Pharmacol* 51:573, 2000.

Weston S et al: Clinical and upper gastrointestinal motility features in systemic sclerosis and related disorders, *Am J Gastroenterology* 93:1085, 1998.

World Health Organization: Obesity: preventing and managing the global epidemic: report of a WHO consultation, *World Health Organ Tech Rep Ser* 894:i-xii, 1-253, 2000.

Yamakita J et al: Effect of tofu (bean curd) ingestion on uric acid metabolism in healthy and gouty subjects, *Adv Exp Med Biol* 431:839, 1998.

Additional References

Chinn KS et al: Modulation of adjuvant-induced arthritis by dietary arachidonic acid in essential fatty acid–deficient rats, *Lipids* 32:979, 1997.

Edmonds SE et al: Putative analgesic activity of repeated oral doses of vitamin E in the treatment of rheumatoid arthritis: results of a prospective placebo controlled double blind trial, *Ann Rheum Dis* 56:649, 1997.

Fiechtner JJ and Brodeur RR: Manual and manipulation techniques for rheumatic disease, *Med Clin North Am* 86:91, 2002.

Hunt PG et al: The effects of daily intake of folic acid on the efficacy of methotrexate therapy in children with juvenile rheumatoid arthritis: a controlled study, *J Rheumatol* 24:2230, 1997.

Kriegel W et al: Double blind study comparing the long term efficacy of the COX-2 inhibitor nimesulide and naproxen in patients with osteoarthritis, *Int J Clin Pract* 55:510, 2001.

Martin RH: The role of nutrition and diet in rheumatoid arthritis, *Proc Nutr Soc* 57:231, 1998.

McAlindon TE et al: Glucasomine and chondroitin for treatment of Osteoarthritis: a systematic quality assessment and metaanalysis, *JAMA* 283: 1469, 2000.

Ortiz Z et al: The efficacy of folic acid and folinic acid in reducing methotrexate gastrointestinal toxicity in rheumatoid arthritis: a meta-analysis of randomized controlled trials, *J Rheumatol* 25:36, 1998.

Peltonen R et al: Faecal microbial flora and disease activity in rheumatoid arthritis during a vegan diet, *Br J Rheumatol* 36:64, 1997.

Pettersson T et al: Serum homocysteine and methylmalonic acid in patients with rheumatoid arthritis and cobalaminopenia, *J Rheumatol* 25:859, 1998.
Philbin EF et al: Osteoarthritis as a determinant of an adverse coronary heart disease risk profile, *J Cardiovasc Risk* 3:529, 1996.
Shiroky JB: The use of folates concomitantly with low-dose pulse methotrexate, *Rheum Dis Clin North Am* 23:969, 1997.
White-O'Connor B et al: Dietary habits, weight history, and vitamin supplement use in elderly osteoarthritis patients, *J Am Diet Assoc* 89:378, 1998.
Woolf K, Manore M: Nutrition, exercise, and rheumatoid arthritis, *Top Clin Nutr* 14(3):30, 1999.

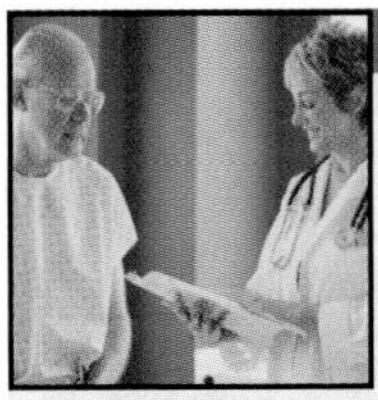

CHAPTER 45

Medical Nutrition Therapy for Metabolic Disorders

CRISTINE M. TRAHMS, MS, RD, CD, FADA

CHAPTER OUTLINE

- Newborn Screening
- Goals of Medical Nutrition Therapy
- Disorders of Amino Acid Metabolism
- Disorders of Organic Acid Metabolism
- Disorders of Urea Cycle Metabolism
- Disorders of Carbohydrate Metabolism
- Disorders of Fatty Acid Oxidation
- Other Disorders
- Role of Nutritionist in Medical Nutrition Therapy for Metabolic Disorders

KEY TERMS

argininosuccinic aciduria (ASA)–the presence of argininosuccinic acid in the blood and urine as a result of argininosuccinate lyase deficiency

autosomal recessive–incapable of expression unless the responsible allele is carried by both members of a pair of homologous chromosomes that are not sex chromosomes

carbamyl-phosphate synthetase (CPS) deficiency–a defect in urea cycle metabolism that causes hyperammonemia and elevated plasma glycine

L-carnitine–a substance that functions as a carrier of fatty acids across the mitochondrial membranes

citrullinemia–elevated citrulline in the blood and urine secondary to a deficiency of argininosuccinic acid synthetase in the metabolism of citrulline to argininosuccinic acid

endocrine disorders–diseases caused by the disorder of any of the glands of internal secretion; newborn screening programs often include screening for congenital adrenal hyperplasia and congenital hypothyroidism

galactosemia–a disturbance in the conversion of galactose to glucose because of the absence of the enzyme galactokinase or galactose-1-phosphate uridyl transferase

gluconeogenesis–the formation of glucose from noncarbohydrate molecules, such as glycerol, and the carbon skeletons of amino acids

glycogen storage diseases–a group of inherited disorders of glycogen metabolism, such as glycogenosis, in which an enzyme deficiency causes glycogen to accumulate in abnormally large amounts in various parts of the body, especially the liver

glycogenolysis–the breakdown of glycogen to glucose

hemoglobinopathies–a group of disorders characterized by the production of abnormal hemoglobin β-chains (e.g., sickle cell disease, β-thalassemia)

ketone utilization disorder–possibly mitochondrial 2-methylacetoacetyl-CoA thiolase deficiency; a disorder of isoleucine and ketone body metabolism

long-chain 3-hydroxyacyl-CoA dehydrogenase deficiency (LCHAD)–a disorder of long-chain fatty acid oxidation

maple syrup urine disease (MSUD) or **branched-chain ketoaciduria**–an autosomal recessive metabolic

KEY TERMS—Continued

defect in decarboxylation that affects the metabolism of branched-chain amino acids

medium-chain acyl-CoA dehydrogenase deficiency (MCAD)–a disorder of medium-chain fatty acid oxidation

methylmalonic acidemia–an excess of methylmalonic acid in the blood and urine because of a defect of methylmalonyl-CoA mutase or other similar enzyme

ornithine transcarbamylase (OTC) deficiency–a sex-linked recessive disorder in the conversion of ornithine and carbamyl-phosphate to citrulline; usually lethal in males

phenylketonuria (PKU)–hyperphenylalaninemia in which phenylalanine is not metabolized to tyrosine because of a deficiency of phenylalanine hydroxylase

propionic acidemia–an excess of propionic acid in the blood secondary to defective propionyl-CoA reductase

Metabolic disorders or inborn errors of metabolism are inherited traits that result in the absence or reduced activity of a specific enzyme or cofactor. Most metabolic disorders are inherited as autosomal recessive traits (see Chapter 16). The treatment for many metabolic disorders is with medical nutrition therapy and medications specific to the disorder. In some instances, in phenylketonuria, for example, when treatment is initiated early in the newborn period and meticulously continued for a lifetime, the affected individual usually is cognitively and physically normal. In other instances, in galactosemia, for example, meticulously applied early and continued treatment does not always prevent cognitive and physical damage.

It is important to remember that biochemical disorders vary from normal variations in enzyme activity that are benign and do not require intervention to severe manifestations that are incompatible with life. For many of the metabolic disorders, significant questions related to diagnosis and treatment still need to be answered.

NEWBORN SCREENING

Most inherited metabolic disorders are associated with severe clinical illness that often appears soon after birth. Mental retardation and severe neurologic involvement may be quickly apparent. Diagnosis of a specific disorder may be difficult, and appropriate treatment measures may be uncertain. Prenatal diagnosis is available for many metabolic disorders, but it usually requires the identification of a family at risk, which can be done only after the birth of an affected child. However, effective newborn screening programs as well as advanced diagnostic techniques and treatment modalities have improved the outcome for many of these infants.

Infants suspected of having a metabolic disorder should be afforded access to care offered by centers with expertise in treating these disorders. Infants who are afebrile but—for no apparent reason—are lethargic, vomiting, in respiratory distress, or having seizures should be evaluated for an undiagnosed metabolic disorder. The initial assessment should include blood gas measurements, electrolyte values, glucose and ammonia testing, and a urine test for ketones.

Advances in newborn screening technology have offered opportunities for earlier diagnosis, prevention of neurologic crisis, and improved intellectual and physical outcomes. When tandem mass spectrometry techniques are used in newborn screening laboratories, infants with a broader range of metabolic disorders can be identified, and identification can be earlier than ever before (see *New Directions:* Newborn Screening).

GOALS OF MEDICAL NUTRITION THERAPY

The goals of medical nutritional therapy for metabolic disorders are to maintain biochemical equilibrium for the affected pathway, provide adequate nutrients to support typical growth and development, and support social and emotional development.

Nutritional treatment is designed to circumvent the missing or inactive enzyme by (1) restricting the amount of substrate available; (2) supplementing the amount of product; (3) supplementing the enzymatic cofactor; or (4) combining any or all of these approaches (Table 45-1).

DISORDERS OF AMINO ACID METABOLISM

Nutritional therapy for amino acid disorders most commonly consists of substrate restriction, which involves limiting one or more essential amino acids to the minimum requirement while providing adequate energy and nutrients to promote typical growth and development—for example, restricting

NEW DIRECTIONS

Newborn Screening

Since the 1960s, many states in the United States have adopted as state law mandatory newborn screening. These programs were developed as a result of the efficacy of the Guthrie bacterial inhibition assay, in which dried blood spots were assayed. This simple, sensitive, and inexpensive screening test became the basis for population-based screening systems for newborns. The hemoglobinopathies, endocrine disorders, metabolic disorders, and some infectious disorders can be effectively identified in this way. Most states screen for 5 to 10 disorders. Tandem mass spectrometry is a new method that offers the opportunity to screen for 30 or more disorders affecting newborns. Many states have evaluated the preliminary studies of this new technology and have implemented newborn screening program changes (Albers et al, 2001).

phenylalanine in phenylketonuria. An inadequate intake of an essential amino acid is often as detrimental as excess. Supplementation of the product of the specific enzymatic reaction is usually required in nutritional therapy for amino acid disorders; for example, tyrosine is supplemented in formulas for treatment of phenylketonuria.

Requirements for individual amino acids are difficult to determine because typical growth and development can be achieved over a wide range of intake. The data of Holt and Snyderman (1967) are often used as the basis for prescribing amino acid intakes (Table 45-2). Careful and frequent monitoring is required to ensure the adequacy of the nutritional prescription (Acosta and Yannicelli, 1993). Although nitrogen studies would be the most precise, weight gain in infants is a sensitive and easily monitored index of well-being and nutritional adequacy.

Phenylketonuria

Of the amino acid disorders listed in Table 45-1, phenylketonuria provides a reasonable model for detailed discussion because PKU (1) occurs relatively frequently, and most neonates are screened for it; (2) has a predictable course, with the greatest available documentation of "natural" and "intervention" history (see *Focus On:* Time Line of Events in the Diagnosis and Treatment of Phylketonuria); and (3) has a successful medical nutrition therapy.

Phenylketonuria (PKU) is the most common of the hyperphenylalaninemias. In this disorder, phenylalanine (Phe) is not metabolized to tyrosine (Tyr) because of a deficiency or inactivity of *phenylalanine hydroxylase,* as shown in Figure 45-1. Nutritional treatment involves restricting the substrate (Phe) and supplementing the product (Tyr) (Figure 45-2). Most affected infants exhibit phenylalanine hydroxylase deficiency; the remainder (less than 3%) have defects in associated pathways. Low-phenylalanine nutritional therapy does not prevent the neurologic deterioration present in the disorders of associated pathways (Pass et al, 2000).

Diagnostic Criteria and Outcome

All states have newborn screening programs for phenylketonuria and other metabolic disorders. The Guthrie bacterial inhibition assay, performed on blood, has been the most commonly used screening test. The American Academy of Pediatrics (AAP) has recommended that neonates with a positive screening result be tested again by both qualitative and quantitative methods (AAP, 1996).

Diagnostic criteria for phenylketonuria include blood concentrations of phenylalanine that consistently exceed 6 to 10 mg/dl (360 to 600 μmol/L) and tyrosine levels of less than 3 mg/dl (165 μmol/L). Outcome, measured in terms of intelligence quotient (IQ) attainment or intellectual function, depends on the age of the infant at diagnosis and start of nutritional therapy, as well as the infant's biochemical control over time. Because infants with PKU do not manifest any clinical signs of abnormality in the immediate postnatal period, the age of the infant at diagnosis and start of nutritional therapy depend on the effectiveness of the screening program and an organized follow-up program. The advantage of rigorous nutritional therapy has been demonstrated by measurements of intellectual function. Individuals who do not receive diet therapy are severely mentally retarded (mean IQ of about 40), whereas individuals who are on therapy from the early neonatal period have IQs in the normal range of intellectual function (Legido et al, 1993; NIH, 2001; Williamson et al, 1981).

Medical Nutrition Therapy for Infants and Children

Formula

Restricted-phenylalanine dietary therapy is planned around the use of a formula/medical food with phenylalanine removed from the protein. The formulas/

TABLE 45-1 Selected Metabolic Disorders That Respond to Dietary Treatment

DISORDER	ENZYME DEFECT	INCIDENCE	CLINICAL/BIOCHEMICAL FEATURES	DIETARY TREATMENT
Urea Cycle Disorders				
Carbamyl-phosphate synthetase deficiency	Carbamyl-phosphate synthetase	Rare	Vomiting; seizures; sometimes, coma → death Survivors usually have MR ↑ Plasma ammonia and glutamine levels	*Long-term treatment:* low-protein diet as tolerated and phenylbutyrate *Acute treatment:* hemodialysis or peritoneal dialysis with energy and fluids
Ornithine transcarbamoylase deficiency	Ornithine transcarbamyolase (X-linked)	Rare	Vomiting; seizures; coma → death as a newborn ↑ Plasma ammonia, glutamine, glutamic acid, and alanine levels	Low-protein diet and phenylbutyrate
Citrullinemia	Argininosuccinic acid synthetase	Rare	*Neonatal:* vomiting; seizures; coma → death *Infantile:* vomiting; seizures; progressive developmental delay ↑ Plasma citrulline, ammonia, and alanine levels	Low-protein diet; arginine supplements; phenylbutyrate
Argininosuccinic aciduria	Argininosuccinic acid lyase	Rare	*Neonatal:* hypotonia, seizures *Subacute:* vomiting, FTT, progressive developmental delay ↑ Plasma argininosuccinic acid, citrulline, and ammonia levels	Low-protein diet; arginine supplements; dialysis for crisis; phenylbutyrate
Argininemia	Arginase	Rare	Periodic vomiting; seizures; coma Progressive spastic diplegia and developmental delay ↑ Arginine and ↑ ammonia levels with protein intake	Low-protein diet
Organic Acidemias				
Methylmalonic acidemia	Methylmalonyl-CoA mutase or similar	Rare	Metabolic acidosis; vomiting; seizures; coma; often death ↑ Organic acid and ammonia levels	*Long-term:* ↑ kcal, ↓ protein diet; ↓ isoleucine, methionine, threonine, valine, vitamin B_{12} supplements *Acute:* IV fluids, bicarbonate
Propionic acidemia	Propionyl-CoA carboxylase or similar	Rare	Metabolic acidosis; ↑ ammonia level; ↑ propionic acid in blood, ↑ methylcitric acid in urine	*Long-term:* ↑ kcal, ↓ protein diet *Acute:* IV fluids, bicarbonate
Isovaleric acidemia	Isovaleryl-CoA dehydrogenase	Rare	Poor feeding, lethargy, seizures, metabolic ketoacidosis, hyperammonemia	↓ Protein, leucine, glycine; supplement with L-carnitine
Ketone-use disorder	2-Methylacetoacetyl-CoA-thiolase or similar	Unknown	Vomiting, dehydration, metabolic ketoacidosis	↓ Protein intake, prevent fasting, provide complex carbohydrates, L-carinitine, and Bicitra (to buffer acid-base balance)
Carbohydrate Disorders				
Galactosemia	Galactose-1-phosphate uridyl transferase	<1:65,000	Vomiting, hepatomegaly, hypoglycemia, FTT, cataracts, MR, and often, early sepsis ↑ Urine/blood galactose levels	Low-galactose and lactose-free diet
Galactokinase deficiency	Galactokinase	1:40,000	Cataracts ↑ Blood/urine galactose levels after lactose feeding	Same as for galactosemia
Hereditary fructose intolerance	Fructose-1-phosphate aldolase	Rare	Vomiting, hepatomegaly, hypoglycemia, FTT, renal tubular defects after fructose introduction ↑ Blood/urine fructose levels after fructose feeding	Fructose-, sucrose, and sorbitol-free diet; prevent fasting

Phe, Phenylalanine; *MR,* mental retardation; *FTT,* failure to thrive; nitisinone, formerly *NTBC,* 2-(2-nitro-4-trifluoro-methyl-benzoyl)-1,3-cyclohexanedione, commercially available as Orfadin; *IV,* intravenous.

TABLE 45-1 Selected Metabolic Disorders That Respond to Dietary Treatment—cont'd

DISORDER	ENZYME DEFECT	INCIDENCE	CLINICAL/BIOCHEMICAL FEATURES	DIETARY TREATMENT
Carbohydrate Disorders—cont'd				
Fructose 1,6-diphosphatase deficiency	Fructose-1,6-diphosphatase	Rare	Hypoglycemia, hepatomegaly, hypotonia, metabolic acidosis upon fructose introduction No ↑ fructose level in blood or urine	Same as for hereditary fructose intolerance
Glycogen storage disease, type Ia	Glucose-1–6-phosphatase	1:60,000	Profound hypoglycemia, hepatomegaly	Exogenous glucose from uncooked cornstarch Avoidance of fructose, lactose ↑ Complex carbohydrate intake, ↓ fat intake
Amino Acid Disorders				
Hyperphenylalaninemias				
Phenylketonuria	Phenylalanine hydroxylase	<1:10,000	Blood Phe >20 mg/dl ↑ Phenylketones in urine Progressive severe MR, which can be prevented by early treatment	↓ Phe, ↑ tyrosine diet to maintain serum Phe at 2-6 mg/dl
Mild phenylketonuria	Phenylalanine hydroxylase	<1:13,000	Blood Phe >6 mg/dl ↑ Phenylketones in urine	↓ Phe, ↑ tyrosine diet to maintain serum Phe at 2-6 mg/dl
Offspring of maternal phenylketonuria	None		Fetal brain damage	None
Dihydropteridine reductase deficiency	Dihydropteridine reductase	Rare	Blood Phe <20 mg/dl Irritability, developmental delay, seizures	None
Tyrosinemias				
Tyrosinemia, type I	Fumaryl-acetoacetate hydroxylase	<1:120,000	Vomiting, acidosis, diarrhea, FTT, hepatomegaly, rickets; ↑ blood/urine tyrosine, methionine; ↑ urine para-hydroxy derivatives of tyrosine; often fatal	Nitisinone; ↓ tyrosine, ↓ Phe diet
Tyrosinemia, type II	Tyrosine aminotransferase	Rare	Keratosis; MR; corneal dystrophy ↑ Blood/urine tyrosine levels; ↑ levels of urine parahydroxy derivatives of tyrosine	↓ Tyrosine, ↓ Phe diet
Maple Syrup Urine Disease (MSUD)				
MSUD	Ketoacid decarboxylase (<2% activity)	1:250,000	Early onset; seizures; acidosis; severe MR; often, death Plasma leucine, isoleucine, and valine levels 10 × normal	↓ Leucine, isoleucine, valine diet
Intermittent MSUD	Ketoacid decarboxylase (<20% activity between episodes)	Rare	Intermittent symptoms can cause death and some MR Plasma leucine, isoleucine, and valine levels 10 × normal during episodes	As for MSUD
Homocystinuria				
	Cystathionine synthase or similar enzyme	1:300,000	Arterial and venous thromboses; bony abnormalities; dislocated lens; fair hair and skin; mild to moderate MR, ↑ methionine; ↑ homocysteine	Trial of 500 mg of vitamin B_6/day for 1 month (if folate levels are normal) Low-protein, low-methionine diet with added L-cystine, betaine

medical foods described in Table 45-3 provide a major portion of the daily protein and energy needs for affected infants, children, and adults. In general, the protein source in the formula/medical food is L-amino acids, with the critical amino acids (i.e., phenylalanine) omitted. Carbohydrate sources are corn syrup solids, modified tapioca starch, sucrose, and hydrolyzed cornstarch. Fat is provided by a variety of oils. Some formulas and medical foods contain no fat or carbohydrate; therefore these components must be provided from other sources. The additional protein, carbohydrate, or fat that must be provided is specific to the formula or medical food chosen for use. Most formulas or medical foods contain calcium, iron, and all other necessary vitamins and minerals, and are a reliable source of these nutrients; others are devoid of these nutrients and require supplementation to ensure nutritional adequacy.

TABLE 45-2 Approximate Daily Requirements for Selected Dietary Components and Amino Acids in Infancy and Childhood

DIETARY COMPONENT/ AMINO ACID	AGE/REQUIREMENT BIRTH TO 12 MO (mg/kg)	1 TO 10 YR (mg/day)
Phenylalanine	1-5 mo: 47-90 6-12 mo: 25-47	200-500*
Histidine	16-34	
Tyrosine†	1-5 mo: 60-80 6-12 mo: 40-60	25-85 (mg/kg)
Leucine	76-150	1000
Isoleucine	1-5 mo: 79-110 6-12 mo: 50-75	1000
Valine	1-5 mo: 65-105 6-12 mo: 50-80	400-600
Methionine‡	20-45	400-800
Cyst(e)ine§	15-50	400-800
Lysine	90-120	1200-1600
Threonine	45-87	800-1000
Tryptophan	13-22	60-120
Energy	1-5 mo: 108 kcal/kg 6-12 mo: 98 kcal/kg	70-102 kcal/kg
Water	100 ml/kg	1000 ml
Carbohydrate	kcal × 0.5 ÷ 4 = g/day	kcal × 0.5 ÷ 4 = g/day
Total protein	1-5 mo: 2.2 g/kg 6-12 mo: 1.6 g/kg	16-18
Fat	kcal × 0.35 ÷ 9 = g/day	kcal × 0.35 ÷ 9 = g/day

Modified from Committee on Nutrition, American Academy of Pediatrics: Special diets for infants with inborn errors of metabolism, *Pediatrics* 57:783, 1976.

Compiled from amino acid data of Holt and Snyderman. Information on amino acid requirements of infants and children at different ages is limited; the figures given here are in excess of minimum requirements. Consequently, this table should be used only as a guide and should not be regarded as an authoritative statement to which individual patients must conform.

*More phenylalanine (>800 mg) is required in the absence of tyrosine.

†Total phenylalanine plus tyrosine should be considered in the prescription, as most phenylalanine is converted to tyrosine.

‡More methionine is required in the absence of cyst(e)ine.

§More cyst(e)ine is required in the presence of a blocked *trans*-sulfuration outflow pathway for methionine metabolism.

Phenylalanine-free formula is supplemented with regular infant formula or breast milk during infancy and cow's milk in early childhood to provide high biologic value (HBV) protein, nonessential amino acids, and sufficient phenylalanine to meet the individualized requirements of the growing child. The phenylalanine-free formula and milk mixture should provide about 90% of the protein and 80% of the energy needed by infants and toddlers. A method for calculating the appropriate quantities of a phenylalanine-free formula is shown in Table 45-4. It must be stressed that formula calculations should provide adequate but not excessive energy intake for infants as well as appropriate fluid to maintain hydration. To support metabolic control effectively, formulas and medical foods must be consumed in three or four nearly equal portions throughout the day.

Low-Phenylalanine Foods

Foods of moderate- or low-phenylalanine content are used as a supplement to the formula or medical food mixture. These foods are offered at the appropriate ages to support developmental readiness and to meet energy needs. Puréed foods from a spoon might be introduced at 5 to 6 months of age, finger foods at 7 to 8 months, and the cup at 8 to 9 months, using the same timing and progression of texture recommended for typical children. Table 45-5 suggests typical low-phenylalanine food patterns for young children.

Low-protein pastas, breads, and baked goods made from wheat starch add variety to the food pattern and allow children to eat some foods "to appetite." Table 45-6 compares low-protein and regular food items. The relative protein and energy values indicate the advantage of the low-protein products in meeting energy needs. Sources for low-protein products are given in *Clinical Insight:* Sources of Low-Protein Foods. In many cases, parents create recipes or adapt family favorites to meet the needs of their children. These recipes offer the children a variety of textures and food choices, allowing them to participate in family meals. Families are also able to meet the energy and phenylalanine needs of their children without resorting to excessive intakes of sugars and concentrated sweets. The availability of aspartame (Nutrasweet), an artificial sweetener that contains phenylalanine, has made food choices more difficult, as it may be an ingredient in otherwise low-phenylalanine foods, for example, sugarless chewing gum.

A formula or medical food that is free of phenylalanine and has a more appropriate amino acid, vitamin, and mineral composition for an older child is generally introduced in the toddler or preschool period. The criterion for introduction of the "next step" formula is that the child accept the food pattern and formula well and reliably consume a wide variety of foods from the low-phenylalanine food list. Successful management with consistently low blood phenylalanine levels is based on habit—that is, the formula/medical food is offered and consumed without negotiation or threat. Children respond favorably to the regularity of the time of ingestion of the formula/medical food and the familiarity of its taste and presentation. Table 45-7 compares a restricted phenylalanine food pattern with a typical food pattern for a child of the same age.

FOCUS ON

Time Line of Events in the Diagnosis and Treatment of Phenylketonuria

1934: A. Folling identifies phenylpyruvic acid in the urine of mentally retarded siblings.

Early 1950s: G. Jervis demonstrates a deficiency of phenylalanine oxidation in the liver tissue of an affected patient.

Early 1950s: H. Bickel demonstrates that dietary phenylalanine restrictions lower the blood concentration of phenylalanine.

Early 1960s: R. Guthrie develops a bacterial inhibition assay for measuring blood phenylalanine levels.

Mid-1960s: Semisynthetic formulas restricted in phenylalanine content become commercially available.

1965-1970: States adopt newborn screening programs to detect phenylketonuria (PKU).

1967-1980: Collaborative Study of Children Treated for Phenylketonuria is conducted. Data from this study form the basis for treatment protocols for PKU clinics in the United States.

Late-1970s: Detrimental effects of maternal phenylketonuria are recognized as a significant public health problem.

1980s: Lifelong restriction of phenylalanine intake becomes the standard of care for PKU clinics in the United States.

1983: The Maternal PKU Collaborative Study begins to study the effects of treatment on the pregnancy outcome of women with phenylketonuria.

1987: Techniques for carrier detection and prenatal diagnosis of phenylketonuria are developed.

Late-1980s: The gene for phenylalanine hydroxylase deficiency (MIM No. 261600) is located on chromosome 12q22-q24.1. DNA mutation analysis can be accomplished with peripheral leukocytes.

1990s: Phenylalanine level of 1-6 mg/dl (60-360 μmol/L), lower than the previous level of less than 10 mg/dl, becomes the new standard of care for treatment of phenylketonuria.

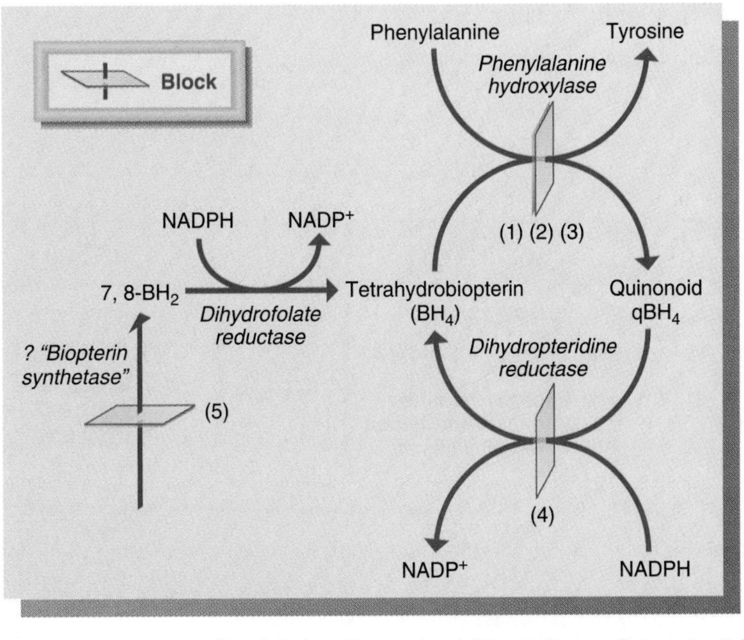

FIGURE 45-1 • Hyperphenylalaninemias. *1,* "Classic" phenylketonuria. *2,* "Atypical" phenylketonuria. *3,* Benign hyperphenylalaninemia. *4,* Dihydropteridine reductase deficiency. *5,* "Bipterin synthetase" deficiency. *NADPH,* Nicotinamide-adenine dinucleotide phosphate (reduced form); *NADP+,* nicotinamide-adenine dinucleotide phosphate (oxidized form).

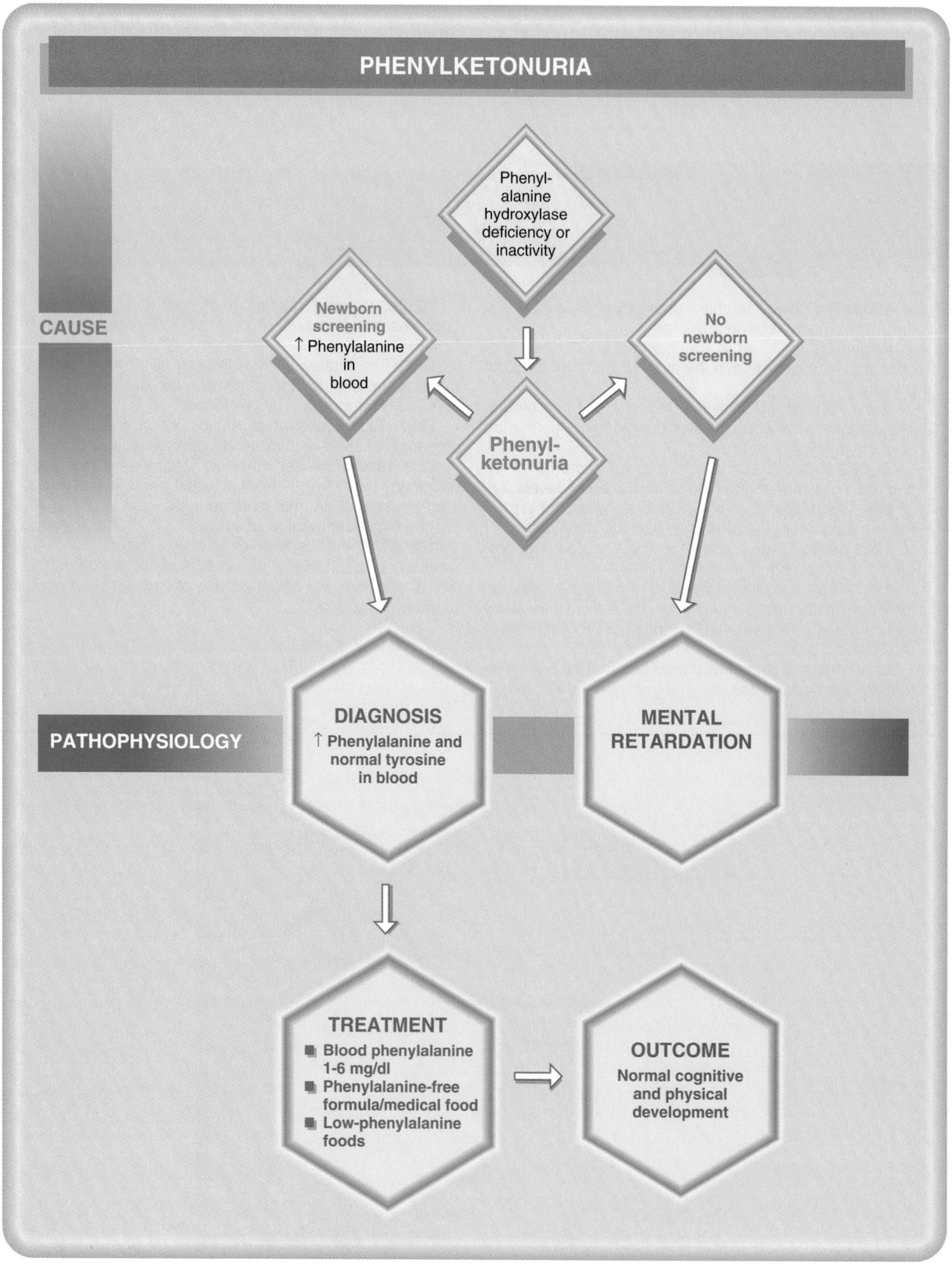

FIGURE 45-2 • Pathophysiology algorithm: phenylketonuria.

TABLE 45-3 Formulas/Medical Foods for the Management of Selected Metabolic Disorders

DISORDER	FORMULAS	COMPOSITION
Phenylketonuria	Phenex-1,2,* Phenyl-Free-1,2#, XP Analog, Periflex+	Protein-L-amino acids (each product has amino acids limited for a specific disorder), carbohydrate, fat, vitamins, and minerals. (There are two versions of many of these products for the treatment of each disorder—[1] infant and [2] child-adult with age-appropriate protein, energy, fat, and vitamin/mineral modifications.)
Maple syrup urine disease	Ketonex-1,2,* MSUD Diet Powder, BCAD-2#, MSUD Analog+	
Isovaleric acidemia	I-Valex-1,2,* XLEU Analog+	
Glutaric aciduria, type 1	Glutarex-1,2,* XLYS,TRY Analog+	
Homocystinuria	Hominex-1,2,* HCY-2#, XMET Analog+	
Propionic acidemia and methylmalonic acidemia	Propimex-1,2,* XMTVI Analog+	
Tyrosinemia	Tyrex-1,2,* 3200AB,Tyros-2#, XPHEN, XTYR Analog+	
Urea cycle disorders	Cyclinex-1,2,* WND-2#	
Phenylketonuria	PKU-1,2#	Protein-L-amino acids (each product has amino acids limited for a specific disorder), carbohydrate, no fat. (There are two versions of products for the treatment of each disorder—[1] infant and [2] child-adult- with age appropriate protein and vitamin/mineral modifications.)
Maple syrup urine disease	MSUD-1,2#	
Homocystinuria	HOM-1,2#	
Propionic acidemia and methylmalonic acidemia	OS-1,2#	
Tyrosinemia	TYR-1,2#	
Urea cycle disorders	UCD-1,2#	
Phenylketonuria	XP Maxamaid, Maxamum+	Protein-L-amino acids (each product has amino acids limited for a specific disorder), carbohydrate, no fat, vitamins and minerals. (Maxamaid is designed for children, Maxamum for adults.)
Maple syrup urine disease	MSUD Maxamaid, Maxamum+	
Isovaleric acidemia	XLEU Maxamaid, Maxamum+	
Glutaric aciduria, type 1	XLYS,TRY Maxamaid, Maxamum+	
Homocystinuria	XMET Maxamaid, Maxamum+	
Propionic acidemia and methylmalonic acidemia	XMTVI Maxamaid, Maxamum+	
Other products	Pro-Phree*, 80056#, PFD-2#	Protein-free, carbohydrate, fat, vitamins, and minerals
	ProViMin*	Carbohydrate and fat-free, protein, vitamins, and minerals
	RCF,* 3232A#	Carbohydrate-free, protein, fat, vitamins, and minerals
Phenylketonuria	Phlexy-10 drink, capsules, bar+	L-amino acids only

Data from *Ross Metabolic Formula System Products, www.ross.com/; Mead Johnson Nutritionals, www.meadjohnson.com, +Scientific Hospital Supplies, www.shsna.com.

Blood Phenylalanine Control

The blood phenylalanine concentration must be checked regularly, depending on the age and health status of the child, to be sure it remains within the range of 2 to 6 mg/dl or 120 to 360 μmol/L (Medical Research Council, 1993a,1993b; NIH, 2001). Phenylalanine-containing foods are offered as tolerated as long as the blood concentration of phenylalanine remains in the range of good biochemical control. The child's rate of growth and mental development must be carefully monitored. Effective management requires a cohesive team in which the child, parents, registered dietitian, pediatrician, psychologist, social worker, and nurse work together to achieve and maintain biochemical control and provide an atmosphere for normal mental and emotional development.

An essential management tool for parents, children, and clinicians is the food diary, an example of which is shown in Figure 45-3. Daily record-keeping supports compliance with treatment and builds self-management skills. An accurate record of food and formula intake for at least the 3 days before a laboratory specimen is obtained is mandatory for accurate interpretation of the results and subsequent adjustment of the phenylalanine prescription.

Elevations in blood phenylalanine concentration are generally caused by either excessive phenylalanine intake or tissue catabolism. Intake of phenylalanine in excess of the amount required for growth accumulates in the blood. Deficient energy intake or the trauma of illness or infection can result in protein breakdown and the release of amino acids, including phenylalanine, into the blood. In general, the anorexia of illness limits energy intake. Preventing tissue catabolism by maintaining the intake of formula/medical food as much as possible is essential. Although it may occasionally be necessary to offer only clear liquids during an illness, the phenylalanine-free formula/medical food should be reintroduced as soon as it is feasible.

The necessity of continuing the restricted-phenylalanine dietary therapy beyond adolescence is a consideration in the management of children with PKU. Progressively decreasing IQs, learning difficulties, poor attention span, and behavioral difficulties have been reported in children who have discontinued the dietary regimen (Koch et al, 1982; Legido et al, 1993; Smith et al, 1978). As the cohort of children

TABLE 45-4 Guidelines for Low-Phenylalanine Food Pattern Calculations

Case Study
Molly is a 6-month-old infant with phenylketonuria.

Baseline Data

Age	6 mo
Sex	Male
Weight (kg)	7.7
Weight percentile	50th
Height (cm)	67.8
Length percentile	50th
Head circumference (cm)	43.3
General health	Good
Activity	Very active

Step 1. Calculate the child's requirement for phenylalanine, protein, and energy (kcal) by using the information in Table 45-2.

A. Phenylalanine
7.7 kg body weight × 60* mg phenylalanine/kg/day = 462 mg phenylalanine/day

B. Protein
7.7 kg body weight × 3.3† g protein/kg/day = 25.4 g protein/day

C. Energy
7.7 kg body weight × 115† kcal/kg/day = 885 kcal/day

Step 2. Determine the amount of phenylalanine-free formula required per day. This information is determined from the infant's protein requirement.
For example: 25.4 g protein/day × 90% of protein from phenylalanine-free formula powder (Phenex I) = 23 g protein = 145 g of formula powder per day.

Step 3. Determine the amount of standard infant formula to be included in the formula.

Step 4. Determine the amounts of phenylalanine, protein, and energy in the phenylalanine-free formula and infant formula as shown in the examples below.

Step 5. Determine the amount of water to mix with the phenylalanine-free formula. The consistency of the formula will vary according to the infant's age and fluid requirements.
For example: To prepare formula for the infant described in the case study, mix 145 g of Phenex I and 120 g Enfamil powder with 4 oz of water to prevent lumps from forming. Then add water to make a total of 32 oz of formula. This provides 4 bottles of 8 oz each.

FORMULA	PHENYLALANINE (mg)	PROTEIN (g)	ENERGY (kcal)
Phenex I powder (145 g)	0	23.0	695
Enfamil powder (120 g)	410	4.8	120
TOTAL	410	27.8	815

Step 6. Determine the amount of phenylalanine, protein, and energy to be obtained from foods other than the formula mixture.

Total phenylalanine	462 mg/day
Phenylalanine in formula	410 mg/day
Phenylalanine from other foods	52 mg/day
Total protein	25.4 g/day
Protein in formula	27.8 g/day
Protein from other foods	1.0-2.0 g/day
Total energy	885 kcal/day
Energy in formula	815 kcal/day
Energy from other foods	70 kcal/day

Step 7. Determine the amount of foods other than formula to be included in the dietary plan.‡

	PHENYLALANINE (mg)	PROTEIN (g)	kcal
Baby rice cereal, 1 Tbsp	9	0.2	9
Green beans, strained, 1 Tbsp	9	0.2	4
Banana, mashed, 50 g	22	0.6	44
Carrots, strained, 3 Tbsp	9	0.3	12
TOTAL	49	1.3	69

Step 8. Determine the actual amounts of phenylalanine, protein, and energy/kg of body weight by dividing the total available nutrients by the body weight (in kg).

Phenylalanine (mg)
460 mg phenylalanine ÷ 7.7 kg body weight = 60 mg phenylalanine/kg/day

Protein
29.1 g protein ÷ 7.7 kg body weight = 3.8 g protein/kg/day

Energy
885 kcal ÷ 7.7 kg body weight = 115 kcal/kg/day

*A phenylalanine intake of 60 mg/kg/day is chosen as a moderate intake level. The prescription for phenylalanine must be adapted to individual needs as judged by growth and blood levels.

†Although these intakes are higher than the RDA, they are the intakes found by the Collaborative Study to promote normal growth with consumption of protein hydrolysate–based formula.

‡Total energy intake must be adjusted to meet individual needs, and an excess must be avoided.

TABLE 45-5 Typical Menus for a 3-Year-Old With Phenylketonuria

Tolerance: 300 mg phenylalanine/day
Formula/medical food for 24 hours: 100 g Phenyl-Free-2, 125 g 2% milk, water to 34 oz
This formula mixture provides 25.8 g protein, 670 kcal energy, 200 mg phenylalanine.

Menu for 100 mg Phenylalanine From Food	Amount Phenylalanine
Breakfast	
Formula mixture, 10 oz	
Kix cereal, 4 g (3 Tbsp.)	15 mg
Peaches, canned, 60 g (¼ c)	9 mg
Lunch	
Formula mixture, 8 oz	
Low protein bread, ½ slice	7 mg
Jelly 1 tsp	0
Carrots, cooked, 40 g (¼ c)	13 mg
Apricots, canned, 25 g (½ c)	6 mg
Snack	
Apple slices, peeled, 4	4 mg
Goldfish crackers, 10	18 mg
Formula mixture, 8 oz	
Dinner	
Formula mixture, 8 oz	
Low-protein pasta, ½ c, cooked	5 mg
Tomato sauce, 2 Tbsp	16 mg
Green beans, cooked, 17 g (2 Tbsp)	9 mg
TOTAL PHENYLALANINE FROM FOOD	102 mg

Tolerance: 400 mg phenylalanine/day
Formula/medical food for 24 hours: 100 g Phenyl-Free-2, 125 g 2% milk, water to 34 oz.
This formula mixture provides 25.8 g protein, 670 kcals energy, 200 mg phenylalanine.

Menu for 200 mg Phenylalanine From Food	Amount Phenylalanine
Breakfast	
Formula mixture, 10 oz	
Rice Krispies, 20 g (¼ c)	22 mg
Nondairy creamer, ¼ c	19 mg
Lunch	
Formula mixture, 8 oz	
Vegetable soup (¼ c soup plus ¼ c water)	52 mg
Grapes, 50 g (10)	9 mg
Low-protein crackers, 5	3 mg
Low-protein cookie, 2	2 mg
Snack	
Rice cakes, 6 g (2 mini)	18 mg
Jelly 1 tsp	0
Formula mixture, 8 oz	
Dinner	
Formula mixture, 8 oz	
Potato, diced, 50 g (5 Tbsp)	50 mg
Dairy-free margarine, 1 tsp	0 mg
Zucchini, sauteed, ¼ c (45 g)	18 mg
TOTAL PHENYLALANINE FROM FOOD	193 mg

TABLE 45-6 Comparison of Protein and Energy Content of Foods Used in Low-Protein Diets

FOOD ITEM	ENERGY (kcal)	PROTEIN (g)
Pasta, ½ c, cooked		
Low-protein	107	0.15
Regular	72	2.4
Bread, 1 slice		
Low-protein	135	0.2
Regular	74	2.4
Cereal, ½ c, cooked		
Low-protein	45	0.0
Regular	80	1.0
Egg, 1		
Low-protein egg replacer	30	0.0
Regular	67	5.6

enrolled in the National Collaborative Study matured, those who maintained well-controlled blood phenylalanine levels demonstrated comparatively higher intellectual achievement (Azen et al, 1991, 1996; Michals et al, 1988). Good dietary control of blood phenylalanine concentrations by nutritional therapy is the best predictor of IQ, whereas "off-diet" blood phenylalanine concentrations of greater than 20 mg/dl (1200 μmol/L) are the best predictors of IQ loss (Waisbren et al, 1987). Subtle deficits in higher-level cognitive function may persist even at blood phenylalanine levels of 6 to 10 mg/dl (360 to 600 μmol/L) (Diamond, 1994); thus most clinics are recommending treatment blood levels of 1 to 6 mg/dl (60 to 1360 μmol/L). The current recommendation is that restricted-phenylalanine therapy should be continued for life to maintain normal cognitive function (NIH, 2001; Ris et al, 1994).

Education About Therapy Management

The energy needs and amino acid requirements of children with PKU do not differ appreciably from those of children in general. With proper management, typical growth can be expected (Figure 45-4). However, parents may tend to offer excessive energy as sweets because they feel the child is being deprived of food experiences. Health care providers and parents need to understand that children with PKU are well children who must make careful food choices for themselves, not chronically ill children who require food indulgences.

Appropriate clinical interaction with the family provides them with the information and skills to differentiate between food behaviors that are typical for the age and developmental level of the child and those related specifically to PKU (Keickhefer and Trahms, 2000; Trahms, 1986). To avoid power struggles and conflicts over food, it is advisable to involve the child in choosing appropriate foods at an early age. Two- and 3-year-old children can master the concept of appropriate choices when foods are categorized as *yes* foods and *no* foods. The concept of an appropriate quantity of a food can be introduced to

CLINICAL INSIGHT

Sources of Low-Protein Foods

Low-protein products add energy, texture, and variety to restricted–amino acid and low-protein food patterns. A variety of low-protein pastas, rice, breads, rusks, crackers, cookies, egg replacers, and gelled dessert mixes is available. Wheat starch and a variety of low-protein baking mixes for breads, cakes, and cookies are also available.

These selected companies provide low-protein baking ingredients, breads, pastas, cereals, cookies, recipes, and low-protein cookbooks.

Company	Telephone	Web address
Dietary Specialties Whippany, NJ 07951	(888) 640-2800	www.dietspec.com
Med-Diet Inc. Plymouth, MN 55447	(800) 633-3438	www.med-diet.com
Ener-G Foods Seattle, WA 98124-5787	(800) 331-5222	www.ener-g.com
Scientific Hospital Supplies Gaithersburg, MD 20884	(877) 482-7845	www.shsna.com
Cambrooke Foods Framingham, MA 01701	(866) 456-9776	www.cambrookfoods.com

TABLE 45-7 Comparison of Menus Appropriate for Children With and Without Phenylketonuria (PKU)

MEAL	MENU FOR PKU	PHENYLALANINE (mg)	REGULAR MENU	PHENYLALANINE (mg)
Breakfast	Phenylalanine-free formula	0	Milk	450
	Rice Krispies		Rice Krispies	
	Orange juice		Orange juice	
Lunch	Jelly sandwich with low-protein bread	18	Jelly sandwich with white bread	260
	Banana		Banana	
	Carrot and celery sticks		Carrot and celery sticks	
	Low-protein chocolate chip cookies	4	Chocolate chip cookies	60
	Juice		Juice	
Snack	Phenylalanine-free formula	0	Milk	450
	Orange		Orange	
	Potato chips (small bag)		Potato chips	
Dinner	Phenylalanine-free formula	0	Milk	450
	Salad		Salad	
	Low-protein spaghetti with tomato sauce	8	Spaghetti	240
			Spaghetti with tomato sauce and meatballs	600
	Baskin-Robbins fruit ice	10	Ice cream	120
ESTIMATED INTAKE		400		2900

a 3- or 4-year-old child in terms of "how many" by counting crackers or raisins and then in terms of "how much" by weighing or measuring foods, such as cereal or fruit. The child then moves to more complex tasks (e.g., formula and food preparation) and planning of meals (e.g., breakfast or a packed lunch). Responsibility for planning a full day's menu by calculating the quantity of phenylalanine in portions of food and compiling the daily total is the ultimate goal. These age-related tasks are shown in Table 45-8.

Psychosocial Development

The necessity of carefully controlling food intake may prompt parents to overprotect their children and perhaps to restrict their social activities. The children, in turn, may react negatively to their parents and to their nutritional therapy. The ability of the family to respond to the stresses of PKU, as reflected by adaptability and cohesion scores, is demonstrated by improved blood phenylalanine concentrations and the positive coping behaviors of older children

MY PKU FOOD RECORD

Name ______________________

Date ______________________

My formula is

_____ g (product)

_____ oz water

My prescription is ________ mg PHE per day

NAME OF FOOD Was it fresh, canned, cooked?	HOW MUCH I ATE Use cups, tablespoons, pieces	PHENYLALANINE IN FOOD (use your list)

Today I drank _____ oz of formula

FIGURE 45-3 • Sample phenylketonuria (PKU) food record. *PHE*, Phenylalanine.

with PKU (Kazak et al, 1988; Nowak-Cooperman et al, 1987; Trahms et al, 1987). Thus, continuing nutritional therapy beyond early childhood requires that children become knowledgeable about and responsible for managing their own food choices (Figure 45-5). The health care team becomes responsible for working with families and children to provide strategies that enable children and adolescents to participate in social and school activities, interact with peers, and progress through the typical developmental stages with self-confidence and self-esteem (Keickhefer and Trahms, 2000; Sullivan, 2001).

Children require parental and professional support as they begin to assume responsibility for their food management. Self-management of food choices avoids the risk of the child using dietary noncompliance as a wedge against parental restrictions. Normal intellectual development is a laudable goal of management of PKU, but to be entirely successful, children with PKU concomitantly need to develop self-assurance and a strong self-image. This can be achieved in part by fostering self-management, independence, and a typical lifestyle for these children.

Nutritional Care in Maternal Phenylketonuria

A pregnant woman with elevated blood phenylalanine concentrations endangers her fetus because of the amplified transport of amino acids across the placenta. The fetus is exposed to about twice the phenylalanine level contained in normal maternal blood. Babies whose mothers have elevated blood phenylalanine concentrations have an increased occurrence of cardiac defects, retarded growth, microcephaly, and mental retardation, as presented in Table 45-9. The fetus appears to be at risk of damage even with minor elevations in maternal blood phenylalanine levels, and the higher the level, the more severe the effect will be (Levy et al, 2001; Platt et al, 2000; Rouse et al, 2000; Waisbren et al, 2000). Strict control of maternal phenylalanine levels before conception and throughout pregnancy offer the

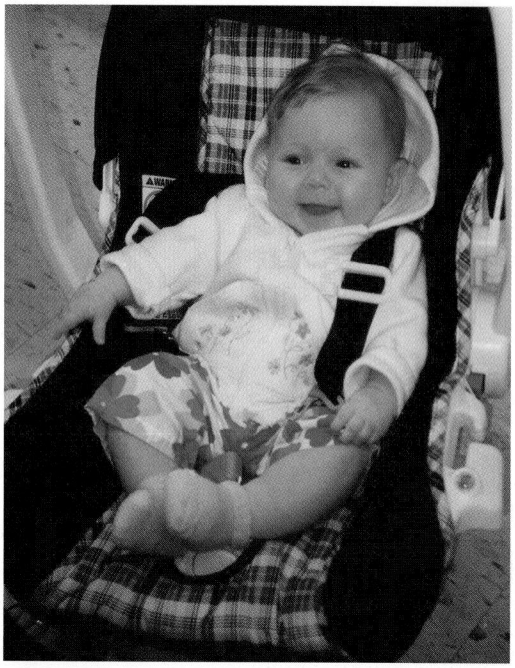

FIGURE 45-4 • Infant with phenylketonuria, who was identified by a newborn screening program and started on treatment by 7 days of age, demonstrates typical growth and development (Courtesy Cristine M. Trahms, Seattle).

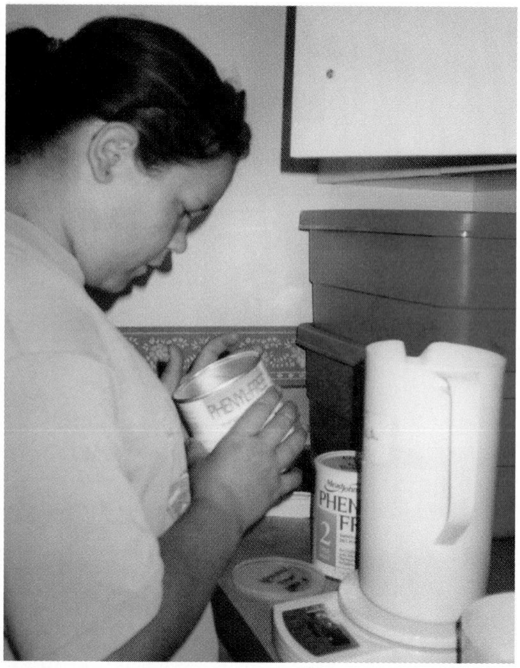

FIGURE 45-5 • A preadolescent girl demonstrates her self-care skills by preparing her own formula/medical food (Courtesy Cristine M. Trahms, Seattle).

TABLE 45-8 Tasks to be Expected of Children With Phenylketonuria (PKU) by Age Level

AGE (yr)	SCHOOL LEVEL	TASK
2-3	Preschool	Distinguishing between yes and no foods
3-4	Preschool	Counting: how many?
4-5	Preschool	Measuring: how much?
5-6	Kindergarten	Preparing own formula; using scale
6-7	Grade 1-2	Writing basic notes in food diary
7-8	Grade 2	Making some decisions on after-school snack
8-9	Grade 3	Preparing breakfast
9-10	Grade 4	Packing lunches
10-14	Middle school	Managing food choices with increasing independence
14-18	High school	Independently managing PKU

TABLE 45-9 Frequency of Abnormalities in Children Born to Mothers With Phenylketonuria (PKU)

COMPLICATION (% OF OFFSPRING)	MATERNAL PHENYLALANINE LEVELS (mg/dl)				
	20	16-19	11-15	3-10	NON-PKU MOTHER
Mental retardation	92	73	22	21	5.0
Microcephaly	73	68	35	24	4.8
Congenital heart disease	12	15	6	0	0.8
Low birth weight	40	52	56	13	9.6

Modified from Lenke RR, Levy HL: Maternal phenylketonuria and hyperphenylalaninemia: an international survey of the outcome of untreated and treated pregnancies, *N Engl J Med* 303:1202, 1980.

best opportunity for normal fetal development (AAP, 2001).

The management of nutritional therapy during pregnancy for a women with hyperphenylalaninemia is complex. The changing physiology of pregnancy and changing nutritional needs are difficult to monitor with the precision required to maintain appropriately low blood-phenylalanine concentrations.

Even with meticulous attention to phenylalanine intake, blood concentrations, and the nutritional requirements of pregnancy, a woman cannot be ensured of a normal infant. The risks of abnormal development of the fetus, even with therapeutic dietary management and maintenance of blood phenylalanine concentrations at 1 to 5 mg/dl (60 to 300 μmol/L), are an important consideration for young women with PKU considering pregnancy (Brenton and Lilburn, 1996; Brenton et al, 1994).

Nutritional management during pregnancy is difficult, even for women who have consistently followed a low-phenylalanine dietary regimen since infancy. Women who have discontinued treatment find that reinstituting medical food consumption and limitation of food choices is difficult, if not overwhelming. Inadequate maternal nourishment (i.e., inadequate intakes of total protein, fat, and energy) may also contribute to poor fetal development (Acosta et al, 2001). Adherence to nutritional therapy during pregnancy for even the well-motivated woman requires family and professional support as well as frequent monitoring of biochemical and nutritional aspects of both pregnancy and phenylketonuria.

Medical Nutrition Therapy for Adults With Phenylketonuria

Many adults with PKU have had the benefits of early diagnosis and treatment and are less likely to be affected by neurologic damage. However, among those who have had some degree of mental retardation, hyperactivity and self-abuse are often major concerns. Not all patients have responded with improved behavioral or intellectual function. For the difficult-to-manage older patient, a trial of a low-phenylalanine food pattern is recommended. If successful, continued phenylalanine restriction therapy may facilitate behavioral management.

The current recommendation of most clinics is effective management of blood phenylalanine concentrations throughout one's lifetime. This recommendation is based on disturbing reports of declining intellectual capabilities (Smith et al, 1990), magnetic resonance imaging (MRI) studies that demonstrate white matter changes in the brain after prolonged, significant elevation of phenylalanine concentrations (Brismar et al, 1990; Shaw et al, 1991), and negative neuropathologic developments (Waisbren and Levy, 1991).

Reinstituting a phenylalanine-restricted food pattern is difficult after the eating pattern has been liberalized (Finkelson, Bailey, and Waisbren, 2001). However, the efficacy of continued treatment throughout adulthood has been documented by reports of improved current intellectual performance, especially in terms of response time (Krause et al, 1985) and improved problem-solving abilities (Ris et al, 1994) when blood phenylalanine concentrations are kept low.

Maple Syrup Urine Disease

Maple syrup urine disease (MSUD), or branched-chain ketoaciduria, results from a defect in decarboxylation that affects the metabolism of the branched-chain amino acids (BCAAs) leucine, isoleucine, and valine (Figure 45-6). MSUD is an autosomal recessive disorder. Infants appear normal at birth, but by 4 or 5 days of age, they demonstrate poor feeding, vomiting, lethargy, and periodic hypertonia. A characteristic sweet, malty odor from the urine and perspiration can be noted toward the end of the first week of life. Failure to treat this condition leads to acidosis, neurologic deterioration, seizures, and coma, proceeding eventually to death. Management of acute disease requires peritoneal dialysis and hydration. BCAAs are introduced gradually into the diet when plasma leucine concentrations are sufficiently decreased (Chuang and Shih, 2001).

The precise mechanism for the complete decarboxylase reaction and the resultant neurologic damage is not known. Neither is the reason why leucine metabolism is significantly more abnormal than that of the other two BCAAs understood. Clinical relapse is most often related to the degree of abnormality of the leucine concentrations, and these relapses often are related to infection. Acute infections represent life-threatening medical emergencies in this group of children. If the plasma leucine concentration increases rapidly during illness, BCAAs should be removed from the diet immediately and intravenous therapy started.

Depending on the severity of the enzyme defect, early intervention and meticulous biochemical control can provide a more hopeful prognosis for infants and children with MSUD. Reasonable growth and intellectual development in the normal to low-normal range have been described (Hilliges et al, 1993). Diagnosis before 7 days of age and long-term metabolic control are critical factors in long-term normalization of intellectual development (Kaplan et al, 1991; Nord et al, 1991). Maintenance of plasma leucine concentrations at between 2 and 5 mg/dl (150 to 380 μmol/L) is recommended. Concentrations above 10 mg/dl (760 μmol/L) are often associated with alpha-ketoacidemia and neurologic symptoms.

Nutritional therapy requires very careful monitoring of blood concentrations (especially leucine, isoleucine, valine, and alloisoleucine), growth, and general nutritional adequacy. Several formulas specifically designed for the treatment of this disorder are now available to provide a reasonable amino acid and vitamin mixture (see Table 45-3). These are generally supplemented with a small quantity of standard infant formula or cow's milk to provide the BCAAs needed to support growth and development. Some infants and children may require additional supplementation with L-valine or L-isoleucine to maintain biochemical balance. Typical leucine-modified menus for young children are presented in Table 45-10.

DISORDERS OF ORGANIC ACID METABOLISM

Pathophysiology

The organic acid disorders are a group of disorders characterized by the accumulation in the blood of non–amino acid organic acids. Most of the organic acids are efficiently excreted in the urine. Diagnosis is based on excretion of compounds not normally present or abnormally high amounts of other compounds in the urine.

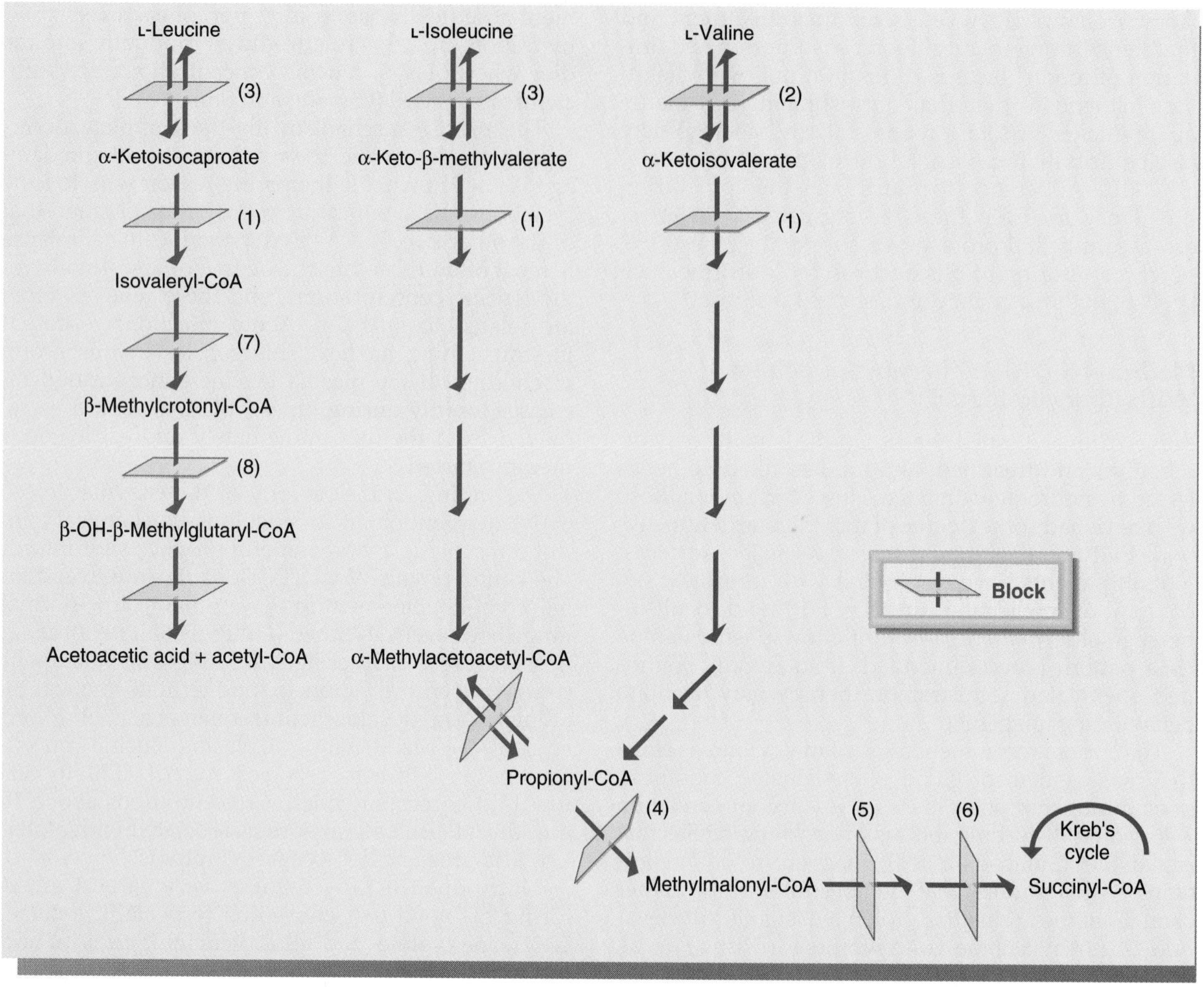

FIGURE 45-6 • Organic acidemias and maple syrup urine disease (MSUD). *1,* Branched-chain ketoacid decarboxylase (MSUD). *2,* Valine aminotransferase. *3,* Leucine-isoleucine aminotransferase. *4,* Propionyl-CoA carboxylase (propionic acidemia). *5,* Methylmalonyl-CoA racemase (methylmalonic aciduria). *6,* Methylmalonyl-CoA mutase (methylmalonic aciduria). *7,* Isovaleryl-CoA dehydrogenase (isovaleric acidemia). *8,* Beta-methylcrotonyl-CoA carboxylase (biotin-responsive multiple carboxylase deficiency).

Propionic acidemia is a defect of propionyl-CoA carboxylase in the pathway of propionyl-CoA to methylmalonyl-CoA, as illustrated in Figure 45-6. The clinical course can vary but is generally marked by vomiting, lethargy, hypotonia, dehydration, seizures, and coma. Survivors often have permanent neurologic damage. Metabolic acidosis with a marked anion gap and hyperammonemia is characteristic. Long-chain ketonuria may also be present. Some patients with propionic acidemia may respond to pharmacologic doses of biotin (Fenton, Gravel, and Rosenblatt, 2001). Long-term outcome in propionic acidemia is variable; hypotonia and cognitive delay may result even in children who are diagnosed early and who receive rigorous treatment (North et al, 1995).

At least five separate enzyme deficiencies have been identified that result in methylmalonic acidemia. The defect of methylmalonyl-CoA mutase apoenzyme is the most frequently identified (see Figure 45-6). The clinical features are similar to those of propionic acidemia. Acidosis is common, and diagnosis is confirmed by the presence of large amounts of methylmalonic acid in blood and urine. Other findings include hypoglycemia, ketonuria, and elevation of plasma ammonia and lactate levels. Some patients may respond to pharmacologic doses of vitamin B_{12} (Fenton, Gravel, and Rosenblatt, 2001). Progressive renal insufficiency is often a long-term outcome of methylmalonic acidemia (Molteni, et al, 1991).

Medical Nutrition Therapy

The goals of managing acute episodes of propionic acidemia and methylmalonic acidemia are to achieve and maintain normal nutrient intake and biochemical balance. Maintenance of energy and fluid intake is important to prevent tissue catabolism and dehydration. IV fluids correct electrolyte imbalances, and abnormal metabolites are removed through urinary excretion, promoted by a high fluid intake. Relapses of

TABLE 45-10 Typical Menus for a 2-Year-Old With Maple Syrup Urine Disease (MSUD)

Tolerance: 450 mg leucine/day
Formula/medical food for 24 hours: 100 g Ketonex-2, 38 g Isomil powder, water to 28 oz
This formula mixture provides 34.2 g protein, 570 kcal energy, 388 mg leucine.

Menu for 50 mg Leucine From Food	Amount Leucine
Breakfast	
Formula mixture, 6 oz	
Kix cereal, 1 g (1 Tbsp)	5 mg
Peaches, canned, 60 g (¼ c)	9 mg
Lunch	
Formula mixture, 6 oz	
Low protein bread, 1 slice	4 mg
Jelly 1 tsp	0
Carrots, cooked, 20 g (2 Tbsp)	9 mg
Apricots, canned, 25 g (½)	9 mg
Snack	
Apple slices, peeled, 4	4 mg
Low-protein crackers, 5	3 mg
Formula mixture, 6 oz	
Dinner	
Formula mixture, 6 oz	
Low protein pasta, ½ c, cooked	5 mg
Dairy-free margarine	0
Green beans, cooked, 9 g (1 Tbsp)	7 mg
TOTAL FROM FOOD	55 mg

Tolerance: 550 mg leucine/day
Formula/medical food for 24 hours: 100 g Ketonex-2, 38 g Isomil powder, water to 28 oz
This formula mixture provides 34.2 g protein, 570 kcal energy, 388 mg leucine.

Menu for 150 mg Leucine From Food	Amount Leucine
Breakfast	
Formula mixture, 6 oz	
Rice Krispies, 6 g (¼ c)	35 mg
Nondairy creamer, 2 Tbsp	7 mg
Lunch	
Formula mixture, 6 oz	
Vegetable soup (2 Tbsp soup plus ¼ c water)	30 mg
Grapes, 50 g (10)	7 mg
Low-protein crackers, 5	3 mg
Low-protein cookie, 3	3 mg
Snack	
Rice cakes, 1 g (1 mini)	7 mg
Jelly 1 tsp	0
Formula mixture, 6 oz	
Dinner	
Formula mixture, 6 oz	
Potato, diced, 30 g (3 Tbsp)	33 mg
Dairy-free margarine, 1 tsp	0
Zucchini, sautéed, ¼ c (45 g)	24 mg
TOTAL FROM FOOD	149 mg

metabolic acidosis may result from excessive protein intake, infection, or unidentified factors. Parents become skilled at identifying early signs of illness. Treatment for these episodes must be rapid because coma and death can occur quickly.

Restricted protein intake is an essential component of the treatment of organic acid disorders. A daily protein intake of 1 to 1.5 g/kg of body weight is often an effective treatment modality for infants who have a mild form of their disorder. This can be supplied by diluting standard infant formula to decrease the protein content and adding a protein-free formula to meet nutrient needs. Specialized formulas (see Table 45-3) that limit threonine and isoleucine and omit methionine and valine are used, as clinically indicated, to support an adequate protein intake and growth.

Requirements for the limited amino acids may vary widely. Growth rate, state of health, residual enzyme activity, and overall protein and energy intakes must be monitored carefully and correlated with plasma amino acid levels. An adequate fluid intake is required to normalize blood ammonia levels. Food refusal and lack of appetite may complicate nutritional therapy, which compromises medical management.

Ketone utilization disorders (mitochondrial 2-methylacetoacetyl-CoA thiolase deficiency or similar enzyme defect) are disorders of isoleucine and ketone body metabolism. Affected individuals are usually older infants or toddlers who present with ketoacidosis, vomiting, and lethargy with secondary dehydration and, sometimes, coma. This event often is preceded by febrile illness or fasting (Slovik, 1993). The treatment is dietary protein restriction (usually 1.5 g of protein per kilogram of body weight per day); 100 to 300 mg of L-carnitine, a substance that functions as a carrier of fatty acids across the mitochondrial membranes, per kilogram of body weight per day; avoidance of fasting by providing small, frequent meals that consist primarily of carbohydrates; and the use of Bicitra to treat ketoacidosis.

DISORDERS OF UREA CYCLE METABOLISM

Pathophysiology

All urea cycle defects result in an accumulation of ammonia in the blood. The clinical signs of elevated ammonia are vomiting and lethargy, which may progress to seizures, coma, and ultimately death. In infants, the adverse effects of elevated ammonia levels are rapid and devastating. In older children, symptoms of elevated ammonia may be preceded by hyperactivity and irritability. Neurologic damage may result from frequent and severe episodes of hyperammonemia. The severity and variation of the clinical courses of all urea cycle defects may be related to the degree of residual enzyme activity. The common urea cycle defects are discussed in a progression that proceeds around the urea cycle, as shown in Figure 45-7. A recent conference summarized the diagnosis and treatment concerns for persons with urea cycle disorders (Proceedings of a Consensus Conference, 2001).

Ornithine transcarbamylase (OTC) deficiency is an X-linked recessive disorder marked by blockage in the conversion of ornithine and carbamyl phosphate to citrulline. OTC deficiency is identified by hyperammonemia and increased urinary orotic acid, with normal levels of citrulline, argininosuccinic acid, and arginine (Brusilow and Horwich, 2001). OTC deficiency is usually lethal in males, whereas heterozygous females with various degrees of enzyme activity may not demonstrate symptoms until they are induced by stress, as from an infection, or a significant increase in protein intake.

Citrullinemia is the result of a deficiency of argininosuccinic acid synthetase in the metabolism of citrulline to argininosuccinic acid. Citrullinemia is identified by markedly elevated citrulline levels in the urine and blood. Symptoms may be present in the neonatal period, or they may develop gradually in early infancy. They may include poor feeding and recurrent vomiting which, without immediate treatment, progress to seizures, neurologic abnormalities, and coma (Brusilow and Horwich, 2001).

Argininosuccinic aciduria (ASA) results from deficiency of argininosuccinate lyase, which is involved in the metabolism of argininosuccinic acid to arginine. ASA is identified by the presence of argininosuccinic acid in urine and blood. L-Arginine must be supplemented to provide an alternative pathway for waste nitrogen excretion (Brusilow and Horwich, 2001).

Carbamyl-phosphate synthetase (CPS) deficiency is the result of deficient activity of carbamylphosphate synthetase. The onset is usually in the early neonatal period, with vomiting, irritability, marked hyperammonemia, respiratory distress, altered muscle tone, lethargy, and often coma. Specific laboratory findings usually include low plasma levels of citrulline and arginine and normal orotic acid levels in urine (Brusilow and Horwich, 2001).

Medical Nutrition Therapy

The aim of therapy for the urea cycle disorders is to prevent or decrease hyperammonemia and the detrimental neurologic consequences associated with it. Treatment is similar for all of the disorders. For mildly affected infants, a standard infant formula can be diluted to 1.0 to 1.5 g of protein per kilogram of body weight per day. The energy, vitamin, and mineral concentrations can be brought up to recommended intake levels with the addition of a protein-free formula. However, specialized formulas are often needed to adjust protein composition in an effort to limit ammonia production.

L-Arginine is supplemented based on individual needs, except in the case of arginase deficiency (Brusilow and Howich, 2001). Phenylbutyrate or other compounds that enhance alternative metabolic pathways are usually required to normalize ammonia levels.

Acute episodes of illness are managed by discontinuing protein intake and administering intravenous fluids and glucose to correct dehydration and provide energy. If hyperammonemia is severe, peritoneal dialysis, hemodialysis, or exchange transfusion may be required. Intravenous sodium benzoate or other alternative pathway compounds have been beneficial in reducing the hyperammonemia.

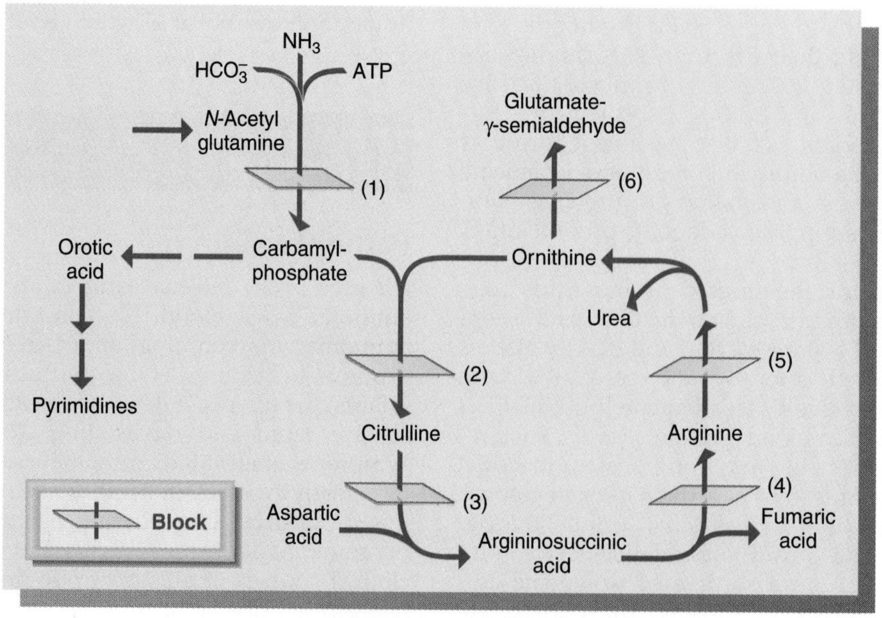

FIGURE 45-7 • Urea cycle disorders. *1,* Carbamyl-phosphate synthetase (CPS) deficiency. *2,* Ornithine carbamyl transferase (OTC) deficiency. *3,* Argininosuccinic acid synthetase (citrullinemia). *4,* Argininosuccinic acid lyase (argininosuccinic aciduria). *5,* Arginase (argine-mia). *ATP,* Adenosine triphosphate.

Long-term therapy consists of restricting dietary protein to 1.0 to 2.0 g/kg/day, depending on individual tolerance. For most infants and children with these disorders, except for arginase deficiency, L-arginine supplements are required to prevent arginine deficiency and assist in waste nitrogen excretion. Phenylbutyrate or other alternative pathway compounds are prescribed to aid in ammonia excretion. Because of the effect of infection and illness on the urea cycle, infections should be treated aggressively.

Neurologic outcome and intellectual development in individuals with urea cycle disorders vary, with a range from normal IQ and motor function to severe mental retardation and cerebral palsy. Although information on long-term follow-up is limited, the use of alternative pathways for waste nitrogen excretion and a protein-restricted food pattern to control ammonia levels may improve the outcome.

Protein-Restricted Diets

Infants and children with metabolic disorders, such as urea cycle defects or organic acidemias, generally require restricted-protein intakes and specialized formulas. The most usual restrictions are for 1.0 g, 1.5 g, and 2.0 g of protein per kilogram of body weight. The appropriate prescription for protein level is based on the individual's tolerance or residual enzyme activity, age, and projected growth rate (Trahms, 1987). The highest protein level tolerated should be given to ensure adequate growth and a margin of nutritional safety. The steps for effective planning of a low-protein food pattern are shown in Box 45-1.

In general, low-protein or restricted-protein food patterns can be formulated from readily available, lower-protein infant, toddler, and table foods. Special low-protein foods (see Table 45-6) can be used to provide energy, texture, and variety in the food pattern without appreciably increasing the protein load. Infant formula can be diluted with a protein-free formula product to meet the prescribed protein level. Supplementing carbohydrate and fat makes up the resultant energy deficit. Specialty formulas are also available (see Table 45-3). The appropriate choice depends on the level of protein restriction, age, and condition of the child. Formulas should contain 20 kcal/oz and should supply at least 100 kcal/kg of energy, depending on age. Osmolality of the formula must be considered; feedings of no more than 400 mOsm/L of solution have been recommended. The usual recommendations for vitamins and minerals are appropriate to support growth for this group of infants and children.

Box 45-1. Steps in Organizing a Low-Protein Food Pattern

1. Determine the protein tolerance of the individual based on (a) diagnosis; (b) age; and (c) growth. Consider the metabolic stability and total protein intake required for the infant's or child's weight.
2. Calculate the protein and energy needs of the individual based on age, activity, and weight.
3. Provide at least 70% of total protein as high-biologic value (HBV) protein—from formula for infants and from milk or dairy foods for older children. Use a specialized formula if the infant or child cannot tolerate all of the protein intake from intact protein.
4. Provide energy and nutrient sources to meet basic needs.
5. Add water to meet fluid requirements and to maintain appropriate concentration of formula mixture.
6. For the older infant and child, provide foods to meet food variety, texture, and energy needs.
7. Provide adequate intake of calcium, iron, and all other vitamins and minerals for age.

DISORDERS OF CARBOHYDRATE METABOLISM

Disorders of carbohydrate metabolism are varied in presentation, clinical course, and clinical outcome. Some of the disorders present in the early newborn period with life-threatening seizures and sepsis (e.g., galactosemia); others may present in midinfancy at the time of introduction of solids that contain offending ingredients (e.g., hereditary fructose intolerance) or at the time of spacing of feedings and subsequent hypoglycemia (e.g., glycogen storage disease). All of these disorders require early and aggressive nutritional therapy.

Galactosemia

Pathophysiology

Galactosemia—a high level of plasma galactose-1-phosphate combined with galactosuria—is found in two autosomal recessive metabolic disorders: galactokinase deficiency and galactose-1-phosphate uridyl transferase deficiency, which is also called *classic galactosemia.*

Galactosemia results from a disturbance in the conversion of galactose to glucose because of the absence of one of the enzyme activities shown in Figure 45-8. The enzyme deficiency causes an accumulation of galactose, or galactose and galactose-1-phosphate, in body tissues. Galactose-1-phosphate in intercellular fluids is believed to cause the cellular disturbances in classic galactosemia.

If an infant has no galactose-1-phosphate uridyl transferase activity, illness generally occurs within the first 2 weeks of life. Symptoms are vomiting, diar-

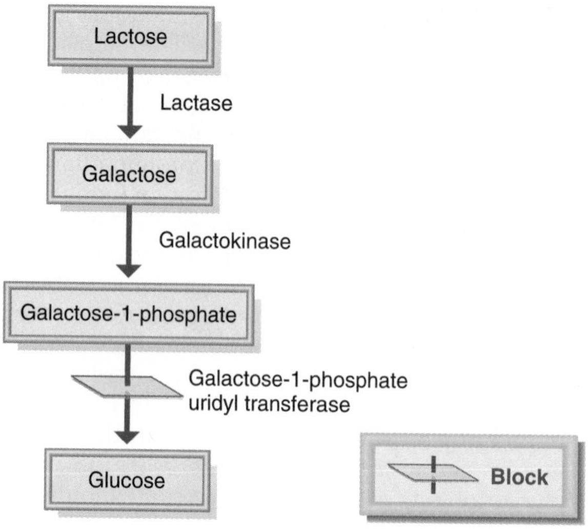

FIGURE 45-8 • Schematic diagram of the metabolism of galactose in galactosemia.

rhea, lethargy, failure to thrive, jaundice, hepatomegaly, and cataracts. Infants with galactosemia may be hypoglycemic and are susceptible to infection from gram-negative organisms. If the condition is not treated, death frequently ensues secondarily to septicemia. If diagnosis and therapy are delayed, mental retardation can result (Holton, Walter, and Tyfield, 2001).

Diagnosis of transferase deficiency is accomplished in a stepwise fashion. Sick neonates are first screened for urinary non–glucose-reducing sugars, which are identified by a positive result from Benedict's test and a negative result from a glucose paper strip test. This is followed by the Beutler test for transferase enzyme activity and confirmation of diagnosis by specific enzyme tests.

With early diagnosis and treatment, physical and motor development should proceed normally. However, intellectual achievement may be depressed; patients often have an IQ of 85 to 100, and visual-perceptual and speech difficulties are common (Kaufman et al, 1995). Ovarian failure is a recognized problem that affects about 95% of women with galactosemia (Kaufman et al, 1995; Liu, Hale, and Hughes, 2000).

Medical Nutrition Therapy

Galactosemia is treated by lifelong galactose restriction. Although galactose is required for the production of galactolipids and cerebrosides, it can be produced by an alternative pathway if galactose is omitted from the diet. Galactose restriction mandates strict avoidance of all milk and milk products and lactose-containing foods because lactose is hydrolyzed into galactose and glucose. Infants are fed soy-based formula. Recent data suggest the restriction of fruits and vegetables that contain significant amounts of galactose is also necessary. Dates, papayas, bell peppers, persimmons, tomatoes, and watermelons all contain more than 10 mg of galactose per 100 g fresh weight of product (Acosta and Gross, 1995; Gropper et al, 2000). Whether these sources of galactose contribute to the pathophysiology of the disorder is unclear. Effective galactose restriction requires careful reading of food product labels. Milk is added to many products, and lactose often appears in the coating of the tablet form of medications (Weese et al, 2003). Table 45-11 presents a low-galactose food pattern.

Galactokinase deficiency requires the same galactose-restricted regimen as galactosemia. Cataracts form, but the other sequelae of galactosemia have not been described.

Glycogen Storage Diseases

Pathophysiology

Glycogen storage diseases, as a group, reflect an inability to metabolize glycogen to glucose in the liver. There are a number of possible enzyme defects along the pathway. The most common of the disorders are types I and III. Their symptoms are poor physical growth, hypoglycemia, hepatomegaly, and abnormal biochemical parameters, especially for cholesterol and triglycerides. Advances in the treatment of glycogen storage diseases have improved the quality of life for affected children.

Glycogen storage disease type Ia (GSD Ia) is a defect in the enzyme glucose-1–6-phosphatase, which impairs gluconeogenesis and glycogenolysis. The affected person is unable to metabolize glycogen stored in the liver. Severe hypoglycemia can result and can causes irreparable damage.

Amylo-1, 6-glucosidase deficiency (GSD III or debrancher enzyme deficiency) prevents glycogen breakdown beyond branch points. This disorder is similar to GSD I in that glycogenolysis is inefficient but glu-

TABLE 45-11 Food Lists for Low-Galactose Food Pattern

ALLOWABLE FOODS	GALACTOSE-CONTAINING FOODS TO BE AVOIDED*
Milk and Milk Substitutes	
Isomil (Ross) Prosobee (Mead Johnson) Alsoy (Carnation) Gerber Soy (Gerber)	Breast milk All forms of animal milk Imitation or filled milk Cream, butter, some margarines Cottage cheese, cream cheese Hard cheeses Yogurt Ice cream, ice milk, sherbet
Fruits	
All fresh, frozen, canned, or dried fruits except those processed with unsafe ingredients†	Dates, papayas, bell peppers, persimmons, tomatoes, and watermelons, which contain >10 mg galactose/100 g fresh weight Intake of fruits and vegetables containing galactose needs to be monitored carefully.
Vegetables	
All fresh, frozen, canned, or dried vegetables except those processed with unsafe ingredients,† seasoned with butter or margarine, breaded, or creamed	
Meat, Poultry, Fish, Eggs, Nuts	
Plain beef, lamb, veal, pork, ham, fish, turkey, chicken, game, fowl, Kosher frankfurters, eggs, nut butters, nuts	
Breads and Cereals	
Cooked and dry cereals, bread or crackers without milk or unsafe ingredients,† macaroni, spaghetti, noodles, rice, tortillas	
Fats	
All vegetable oils; all shortening, lard, margarines, and salad dressings except those made with unsafe ingredients†; mayonnaise; olives	

*NOTE: Lactose is often used as a pharmaceutical bulking agent, filler, or excipient; thus tablets, tinctures, and vitamin and mineral mixtures should be evaluated carefully for galactose content. The *PDR (Physician's Desk Reference)* now lists active and inactive ingredients in medications, as well as manufacturers' telephone numbers.

†Unsafe ingredients include milk, buttermilk, cream, lactose, galactose, casein, caseinate, whey, dry milk solids, or curds. Labels should be checked regularly and carefully, as formulations of products change often.

coneogenesis is amplified to help maintain glucose production. The symptoms of GSD III are usually less severe and range from hepatomegaly to severe hypoglycemia (Chen, 2001).

Medical Nutrition Therapy

The rationale for intervention is to maintain plasma glucose in a safe range and prevent hypoglycemia by providing a constant supply of exogenous glucose. Currently, administration of raw cornstarch at regular intervals and a high-carbohydrate, low-fat dietary pattern are advocated to prevent hypoglycemia. Young infants may require administration of pancreatic enzyme before ingesting uncooked cornstarch, to increase its effectiveness (Goldberg and Slonin, 1993). Some infants and children do very well with oral cornstarch administration, whereas others require glucose polymers administered via continuous-drip gastric feedings, to prevent hypoglycemic episodes during the night (Wolfsdorf and Crigler, 1997). The dose of cornstarch should be individualized; however, doses of 1.75 to 2.5 g/kg at 4- to 6-hour intervals have proved to be effective for young children (Lee, Dixon, and Leonard, 1996). Overnight glucose delivery rates of 4 to 6 mg/kg/min have proved adequate (Goldberg and Slonin, 1993). Adolescents may be able to maintain plasma glucose concentrations with a single dose of cornstarch at bedtime (Wolfsdorf and Crigler, 1997). The glucose vehicle suggested is a lactose-free formula. Iron supplementation is required to maintain adequate hematologic status because cornstarch interferes with iron absorption.

The outcome of treatment has been good. The hazard of severe hypoglycemic episodes is diminished; physical growth is improved; and liver size is decreased. However, the risk of progressive renal dysfunction is not entirely eliminated by current treatment modalities (Lee, Dixon, and Leonard, 1996; Wolfsdorf et al, 1997).

To some extent, treatment protocols for the glycogen storage diseases are still evolving. The protocols include various kinds of carbohydrates at various doses during the day and night. Individual tolerance, body weight, state of health, ambient temperature, and physical activity all play important roles in designing the specific pattern of carbohydrate administration. The goal for all of the protocols remains the same: normalization of blood glucose levels.

DISORDERS OF FATTY ACID OXIDATION

Pathophysiology

Recent laboratory advancements in the identification of disorders involving fatty acid oxidation have enabled the treatment of medium-chain acyl-CoA dehydrogenase deficiency (MCAD) and long-chain 3-hydroxyacyl-CoA dehydrogenase deficiency (LCHAD) (Figure 45-9).

Children affected by LCHAD or MCAD are generally identified during periods of fasting or clinical illness. These children present with symptoms of variable severity, including failure to thrive, episodic vomiting, and hypotonia. Children with LCHAD become hypoglycemic and demonstrate abnormal liver function, reduced or absent ketones in the urine, and often secondary carnitine deficiency. Children with MCAD have mild metabolic acidosis and a similar presentation (Roe and Ding, 2001).

Medical Nutrition Therapy

The concept underlying effective treatment is straightforward: avoidance of fasting. This is accomplished by the regularly spaced intake of foods that provide an adequate energy intake and that are high in carbohydrates. A low-fat diet is advocated because fats are not effectively metabolized. Consumption of 15% to 20% of calories as fat has been recommended. Supplementation with L-carnitine, a substance that functions as a carrier of fatty acids across the mitochondrial membranes, is often required. Children often do very well with three meals and three snacks offered at regular intervals. Some children may require additional carbohydrate feedings during the night.

OTHER DISORDERS

Table 45-1 outlines additional disorders by the enzymatic defects, distinctive clinical and biochemical features, and current approaches to dietary therapy.

ROLE OF NUTRITIONIST IN MEDICAL NUTRITION THERAPY FOR METABOLIC DISORDERS

The role of the nutritionist in the treatment of metabolic disorders is a complex one that requires expertise in medical nutrition therapy for the specific disorder and access to detailed information about the disorders and treatment modalities (see *Clinical Insight:* Resources for Management of Metabolic Disorders). A family-centered counseling approach, feeding skill development, and behavioral modification, as well as the support and counsel of a team of health care providers involved in the care of the patient, is required. Nutritional intervention is often a lifelong consideration. Specific objectives of nutritional care are shown in Box 45-2.

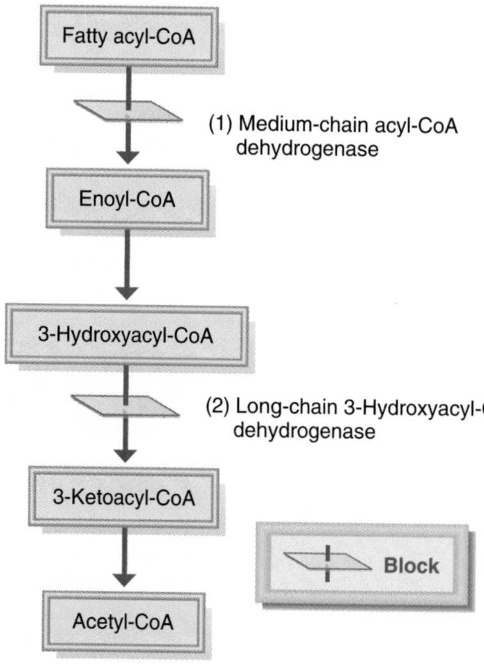

FIGURE 45-9 • Mitochonrial fatty acid oxidation disorders: *1*, Medium-chain acyl-CoA dehydrogenase deficiency (MCAD), the most common fatty acid oxidation disorder. *2*, Long-chain 3-hydroxyacyl-CoA dehydrogenase deficiency (LCHAD).

CLINICAL INSIGHT

Resources for Management of Metabolic Disorders

These selected companies provide infant formulas and medical foods, product descriptions, protocols for treatment and referral information to the nearest genetics center or treatment program for metabolic disorders.

Company	Telephone	Web address
Ross Laboratories Columbus, OH 43216	(800) 551-5838	www.ross.com
Mead Johnson Nutritionals Evansville, IN 47721	(800) 755-4805	www.meadjohnson.com
Scientific Hospital Supplies Gaithersburg, MD 20884	(800) 365-7354	www.shsna.com

Box 45-2. Intervention Objectives for the Nutritionist Involved in the Treatment of Metabolic Disorders

In the clinic, the nutritionist has a major role in ongoing therapy and planning for each child. These responsibilities include gathering of objective food intake data from the family, assessing the adequacy of the child's intake, and working with the family to teach its members appropriate ways to monitor the restricted food intake pattern.

The child with a metabolic disorder often presents a wide range of concerns, which may include unstable biochemical levels, failure to gain weight, excessive weight gain, difficulty adhering to the diet, and behaviors that cause an adverse feeding situation. Thus managing a child with a metabolic disorder requires input from the entire health care team. The nutritionist uses skills and a basic knowledge of foods as sources of nutrients, parent-child relationships, growth, development, and interviewing to obtain the necessary information for assessing and planning for the child with a metabolic disorder.

I. The nutritionist functions as an effective interdisciplinary team member by doing the following:
   A. Becoming familiar with the background and current status of the child through the medical record
   B. Recognizing and accepting the responsibility as the nutritionist by doing the following:
      1. Identifying appropriate intake of nutrients for growth, activity, and biochemical balance
      2. Identifying developmental stages of feeding behavior
      3. Understanding the concept of food as a support of developmental progress
      4. Identifying behavior as it affects nutrient intake
   C. Understanding, respecting, and using the expertise of the team disciplines in providing care for the child with a metabolic disorder

II. The nutritionist provides adequate and supportive patient services by doing the following:
   A. Establishing a positive, cooperative working relationship with the parent and child
   B. Interviewing the parents about dietary intake and the feeding situation in a nonjudgmental manner
   C. Assessing the parent-child relationship as it relates to dietary management and control of the disorder
   D. Developing a plan for appropriate dietary management based on growth, biochemical levels, nutrient needs, and developmental progress
   E. Developing a plan that includes appropriate foods and recognizes the parents' skills in food preparation as well as family routines
   F. Working with the parents to establish a method to deal effectively with negative feeding behaviors, if necessary
   G. Contacting the family after receiving laboratory results and calculating food records to make necessary and appropriate changes in diet prescription
   H. Supporting parents in their efforts at effective dietary and behavior management

III. The nutritionist develops a professional database by doing the following:
   A. Becoming familiar with the current literature on the treatment of metabolic disorders
   B. Understanding the genetic basis of metabolic disorders

IV. The nutritionist works with the team members to develop an understanding of long-term patient care and a written care plan for the patient.

Clinical Scenario 1: Newborn Infant With Phenylketonuria

The 1-day newborn screening test result for phenylalanine (Guthrie method) for a 7-lb, 4-oz male child was 3 mg/dl. The infant was breast-fed with no supplemental formula. A repeat sample was requested to further document the phenylalanine concentration in the infant's blood. The result from this sample, collected on day 5 of life, was 24 mg/dl. To confirm the diagnosis for this child, who was considered to be "presumptive positive," a quantitative sample was obtained, and phenylalanine and tyrosine levels were measured. On day 9 of life, the serum phenylalanine concentration was 25.5 mg/dl, and the tyrosine level was 1.1 mg/dl.

To provide adequate protein and energy intake, and at the same time decrease the serum phenylalanine concentration, a phenylalanine-free formula was introduced at standard dilution without a phenylalanine supplement. Within 24 hours, the infant's serum phenylalanine concentration had decreased to 16.5 mg/dl while the infant was being provided an intake of 16 oz of formula. Within 48 hours, the level was 8.8 mg/dl, with an intake of 18 oz of formula. At this point, standard infant formula was added to bring the calculated phenylalanine intake to about 60 mg/kg and to maintain a generous protein and energy intake for this 3.6-kg infant.

Phenylalanine concentrations were measured on alternate days for 4 days, and the levels were 7.6 mg/dl and 5.6 mg/dl, respectively. In subsequent weeks, growth and serum phenylalanine concentrations continued to be monitored carefully, and energy and phenylalanine intakes were adjusted as necessary to maintain blood phenylalanine concentrations between 1 and 6 mg/dl and to maintain growth in appropriate channels.

1. What is the expected energy requirement for this infant with phenylketonuria?
2. What baseline formula would you use for this infant to provide phenylalanine at 60 mg/kg, formula at 20 kcal/oz, and protein and energy intakes at recommended levels?
3. What are the growth expectations for this infant?
4. What steps would you take if the plasma phenylalanine concentration exceeded 6 mg/dl on subsequent measurements?

Families require support from the expert clinic staff at the tertiary care center, from community providers, and from each other. Support groups have been formed for several disorders. Because of these organizations, families are able to share personal stories, support each other through the emotional turmoil of the daily management of metabolic disorders, share management tips, and develop a community (see Relevant Web Sites).

SUMMARY

Advances in newborn screening technology have improved the early identification of infants with some metabolic disorders. The treatment for these disorders is medical nutrition therapy in conjunction with medications specific to the disorder. With early identification and initiation of treatment many infants have a brighter developmental future. This requires lifetime treatment, for example, with phenylketonuria. Many infants and children with metabolic disorders are "medically fragile" and require intensive medical and nutritional treatment to survive—for example, those with disorders of the urea cycle. All families require the support of an expert team of health care providers accustomed to managing the detailed treatment modalities. Research efforts currently are focused on enzyme and gene therapy to discover whether outcomes and quality of life can be improved for these children.

Clinical Scenario 2: Toddler With Phenylketonuria

Tia is a 3-year-old girl with phenylketonuria. Her diagnosis was established when she was 8 days of age. Her parents have meticulously followed the dietary recommendations made by the PKU clinic staff. Tia consumes 1 L of formula/medical food at a 20-kcal/oz concentration per day. Her phenylalanine tolerance has been established at 350 mg phenylalanine from foods per day. Her growth has been at the 50th percentile for weight and stature for the past year. Tia's blood phenylalanine determinations have ranged between 3 and 6 mg/dl on a monthly basis with a single elevation to 12 mg/dl when she was ill.

Tia's mother has questions for the clinic staff.

1. Tia's mother feels that Tia is not growing rapidly enough. She would like to increase the amount of phenylalanine that Tia ingests each day in an effort to increase her growth rate. Would increasing Tia's phenylalanine intake increase her growth rate?
2. Do you think that Tia has had good biochemical control? What would you expect her intellectual development to be?
3. What additional information would you need from Tia's mother to assess Tia's intake and evaluate her growth?

■ Relevant Web Sites

Families with children with similar disorders have organized groups such as the following to cope with the daily stresses of managing difficult metabolic disorders:

Children's PKU Network
www.pkunetwork.org/PKU.html
Fatty Acid Oxidation Disorder Communication Network
www.fodsupport.org
Maple Syrup Urine Disease Newsletter
www.msud-support.org
National Organization for Rare Disorders (NORD)
www.rarediseases.org/cgi-bin/nord

National PKU News
www.pkunews.org
National Urea Cycle Disorders Foundation
www.NUCDF.org/
Organic Acidemia Association, Inc.
www.oaanews.org
Parents of Galactosemic Children, Inc.
www.galactosemia.org

Cited References

Acosta PB, Gross KC: Hidden sources of galactose in the environment, *Eur J Pediatr* 154:S87, 1995.

Acosta PB, Yannicelli S: Nutrition support of inherited disorders of amino acid metabolism, part I, *Top Clin Nutr* 9(1):65, 1993.

Acosta PB et al: Intake of major nutrients by women in the Maternal Phenylketonuria (MPKU) Study and effects on plasma phenylalanine concentrations, *Am J Clin Nutr* 73:792, 2001.

Albers S et al: New England Consortium: a model for medical evaluation of expanded newborn screening with tandem mass spectrometry, *J Inherit Metab Dis* 24:303, 2001.

American Academy of Pediatrics, Committee on Genetics: Newborn screening fact sheets, *Pediatrics* 98:473, 1996.

American Academy of Pediatrics, Committee on Genetics: Maternal phenylketonuria, *Pediatrics* 107:427, 2001.

Azen CG et al: Intellectual development in 12-year-old children treated for phenylketonuria, *Am J Dis Child* 145:35, 1991.

Azen CG et al: Summary of findings from the United States Collaborative Study of Children Treated for Phenylketonuria, *Eur J Pediatr* 155:S29, 1996.

Brenton DP, Lilburn M: Maternal phenylketonuria: a study from the United Kingdom, *Eur J Pediatr* 155:S177, 1996.

Brenton DP et al: Maternal phenylketonuria: preconception dietary control and outcome, *Int Pediatr* 9(suppl 2):5, 1994.

Brismar J et al: Malignant hyperphenylalaninemia: CT and MRI of the brain, *Am J Neurol Res* 11:135, 1990.

Brusilow SW, Howich AL: Urea cycle enzymes. In Scriver CR et al, editors: *The metabolic and molecular bases of inherited disease*, ed 8, New York, 2001, McGraw Hill.

Chen YT: Glycogen storage diseases. In Scriver CR et al, editors: *The metabolic and molecular bases of inherited disease*, ed 8, New York, 2001, McGraw Hill.

Chuang DT, Shih VE: Maple syrup urine disease (branched-chain ketoaciduria). In Scriver CR et al, editors: *The metabolic and molecular bases of inherited disease*, ed 8, New York, 2001, McGraw Hill.

Diamond A: Phenylalanine levels of 6-10 mg/dL may not be as benign as once thought, *Acta Paediatr* [Suppl] 407:89, 1994.

Diamond A et al: Prefrontal cortex cognitive deficits in children treated early and continuously for phenylketonuria, *Monog Soc Res Child Dev* 62(4):1, 1997.

Fenton WA, Gravel RA, Rosenblatt DS: Disorders of propionate and methylmalonate metabolism. In Scriver CR et al, editors: *The metabolic and molecular bases of inherited disease*, ed 8, New York, 2001, McGraw Hill.

Finkelson L, Bailey L, Waisbren SE: PKU adults and their return to diet: predicting diet continuation and maintenance, *J Inherit Metab Dis* 24:515, 2001.

Goldberg T, Slonin AE: Nutritional therapy for hepatic glycogen storage diseases, *J Am Diet Assoc* 93:1423, 1993.

Gropper SS et al: Free galactose content of fresh fruits and strained fruit and vegetable baby foods: more foods to consider for the galactose-restricted diet, *J Am Diet Assoc* 100:573, 2000.

Hilliges C et al: Intellectual performance of children with maple syrup urine disease, *Eur J Pediatr* 152:145, 1993.

Holt LE, Snyderman SE: The amino acid requirements of children. In Nyhan WL, editor: *Amino acid metabolism and genetic variation*, New York, 1967, McGraw-Hill.

Holton JB, Walter JH, Tyfield LA: Galactosemia. In Scriver CR et al, editors: *The metabolic and molecular bases of inherited disease*, ed 8, New York, 2001, McGraw Hill.

Kaplan P et al: Intellectual outcome in children with maple syrup urine disease, *J Pediatr* 119:46, 1991.

Kaufman FR et al: Cognitive functioning, neurological status, and brain imaging in classical galactosemia, *Eur J Pediatr* 154:52, 1995.

Kazak AE et al: Childhood chronic disease and family functioning: a study of phenylketonuria, *Pediatrics* 81:224, 1988.

Keickhefer G, Trahms CM: Supporting development of children with chronic conditions: from compliance toward shared management, *Pediatr Nurs*, 26(4): 354, 2000.

Koch R et al: Preliminary report on the effects of diet discontinuation on PKU, *J Pediatr* 100:870, 1982.

Krause W et al: Biochemical and neuropsychological effects of elevated plasma phenylalanine in patients with treated phenylketonuria, *J Clin Invest* 75:40, 1985.

Lee PJ, Dixon MA, Leonard JV: Uncooked cornstarch: efficacy I type 1 gluconeogenosis, *Arch Dis Child* 74: 546, 1996.

Legido A et al: Treatment variables and intellectual outcome in children with classic phenylketonuria, *Clin Pediatr* 32:417, 1993.

Levy HL et al: Congenital heart disease in maternal phenylketonuria: report from the Maternal PKU Collaborative Study, *Pediatr Res* 49:636, 2001.

Liu G, Hale GE, Hughes CL: Galactose metabolism and ovarian toxicity, *Reprod Toxic* 14:377, 2000.

Medical Research Council Working Party on Phenylketonuria: Phenylketonuria due to phenylalanine hydroxylase deficiency: an unfolding story, *BMJ* 306:115, 1993a.

Medical Research Council Working Party on Phenylketonuria: Recommendations on the dietary management of phenylketonuria, *Arch Dis Child* 68:426, 1993b.

Michals K et al: Blood phenylalanine levels and intelligence of 10-year-old children with PKU in the National Collaborative Study, *J Am Diet Assoc* 88:1226, 1988.

Molteni KH et al: Progressive renal insufficiency in methylmalonic acidemia, *Pediatr Nephrol* 5:323, 1991.

National Institutes of Health: Report of an NIH Consensus Conference on Phenylketonuria: Screening and Management, 2001, National Institute of Child Health and Human Development, Washington, DC, www.consensus.nih.gov/.

Nord A et al: Developmental profile of patients with maple syrup urine disease, *J Inherited Metab Dis* 14:881, 1991.

North KN et al: Neonatal onset propionic acidemia: neurologic and developmental profiles and implications for management, *J Pediatr* 126:916, 1995.

Nowak-Cooperman KM et al: The impact of assertiveness, self-concept and coping behavior on self-management abilities in adolescents with phenylketonuria [Abstract], *J Adolesc Health Care* 8:305, 1987.

Ohtani Y et al: Secondary carnitine deficiency in hyperammonemic attacks of ornithine transcarbamylase deficiency, *J Pediatr* 112:409, 1988.

Pass KA et al: U.S. newborn screening system guidelines II: follow-up of children, diagnosis, management, and evaluation, *J Pediatr* 137: S1, 2000.

Platt LD et al: The international study of pregnancy outcome in women with phenylketonuria: report of a 12-year study, *Am J Obstet Gynecol* 182: 326, 2000.

Proceedings of a Consensus Conference for the Management of Patients with Urea Cycle Disorders, *J Pediatr* 138: S1, 2001.

Ris MD et al: Early-treated phenylketonuria: adult neuropsychologic outcome, *J Pediatr* 124:388, 1994.

Robertson A, Singh RH: Outcomes analysis of verbal dyspraxia in classic galactosemia, *Genet Med* 2:142, 2000.

Roe CR, Ding J: Mitochondrial fatty acid oxidation disorders. In Scriver CR et al, editors: *The metabolic and molecular bases of inherited disease*, ed 8, New York, 2001, McGraw Hill.

Rouse B et al: Maternal phenylketonuria syndrome: congenital heart defects, microcephaly, and developmental outcomes, *J Pediatr* 136:57, 2000.

Shaw DWW et al: MR imaging of phenylketonuria, *Am J Neurol Res* 12:403, 1991.

Shield JPH et al: The relationship of genotype to cognitive outcome in galactosemia, *Arch Dis Child* 83:248, 2000.

Slovik O: Mitochondrial 2-methylacetoacetyl-CoA thiolase deficiency: an inborn error of isoleucine and ketone body metabolism, *J Inherited Metab Dis* 16:46, 1993.
Smith I et al: Effect of stopping low-phenylalanine diet on intellectual progress of children with phenylketonuria, *BMJ* 2:723, 1978.
Smith I et al: Effect on intelligence of relaxing the low phenylalanine diet in phenylketonuria, *Arch Dis Child* 65:311, 1990.
Sullivan JE: Emotional outcome of adolescents and young adults with early and continuously treated phenylketonuria, *J Pediatr Psychol* 26:477, 2001.
Trahms CM: Long-term nutrition intervention model: the treatment of phenylketonuria, *Top Clin Nutr* 1(1):62, 1986.
Trahms CM: Low protein diets for children: guidelines for treatment of common organic acidemias and urea cycle disorders, *Top Clin Nutr* 2(3):49, 1987.
Trahms CM et al: Impact of patient attitudes and family function on compliance with treatment of phenylketonuria [Abstract], *J Adolesc Health Care* 8:305, 1987.
Waisbren SE, Levy HL: Agoraphobia in phenylketonuria, *J Inherited Metab Dis* 14:755, 1991.
Waisbren SE et al: Predictors of intelligence quotient and intelligence quotient change in persons treated for phenylketonuria early in life, *Pediatrics* 79:351, 1987.
Waisbren SE et al: Outcome at age 4 years in offspring of women with maternal phenylketonuria: the Maternal PKU Collaborative study, *JAMA* 283:756, 2000.
Weese et al: Galactose content of baby food meats: considerations for infants with galactosemia, *J Am Diet Assoc* 103:373, 2003.
Williamson MS et al: Correlates of intelligence tests results in treated phenylketonuric children, *Pediatrics* 68:161, 1981.
Wolf B et al: Propionic acidemia: a clinical update, *J Pediatr* 99:835, 1981.
Wolfsdorf JI, Crigler JF: Cornstarch regimens for nocturnal treatment of young adults with type I glycogen storage disease, *Am J Clin Nutr* 65:507, 1997.
Wolfsdorf JI et al: Metabolic control and renal dysfunction in type I glycogen storage disease, *J Inherited Metab Dis* 20:559, 1997.

Additional References

Clarke JTR: *A clinical guide to inherited metabolic disease,* Cambridge University Press, 2001, London.
DeVivo DC: *Universal Newborn Screening,* Orandell, NJ, 2001, The EP Foundation for Education.
Fernandes J, Saudubray J-M, van den Berghe G, editors: *Inborn metabolic diseases: diagnosis and treatment,* ed 3, Berlin, 2000, Springer.
Nutrition Support Protocols: *The Ross Metabolic Formula System,* ed 4, Columbus, Ohio: Ross Products Division, 2001, Abbott Laboratories.
Schoen EJ: *Cost-benefit analysis of universal tandem mass spectrometry for newborn screening,* Pediatrics 110:781, 2002.
Scriver CR et al, editors: *The metabolic and molecular bases of inherited disease,* ed 8, New York, 2001, McGraw Hill.
Winter SC, Buist NRM: Guidelines: clinical treatment guide to inborn errors of metabolism, *J Rare Dis* 4:18, 1998.

Appendixes

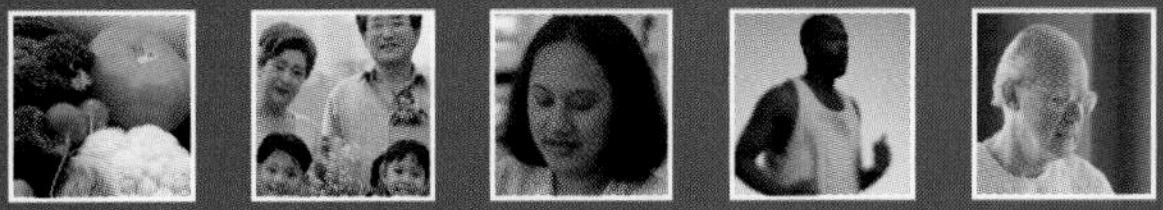

Appendix I General Abbreviations

ABGs arterial blood gases
ACTH adrenocorticotropic hormone
AD Alzheimer's disease
ADH antidiuretic hormone
ADI acceptable daily intake
ADL activities of daily living
AI adequate intake
AIDS acquired immunodeficiency syndrome
ALS amyotrophic lateral sclerosis
AP angina pectoris
ARF acute renal failure
ASHD atherosclerotic heart disease
ATP adenosine triphosphate
BCAA branched-chain amino acid
BEE basal energy expenditure
BHA butylated hydroxyanisole
BHT butylated hydroxytoluene
BMR basal metabolic rate
BMT bone marrow transplantation
BPD bronchopulmonary dysplasia
BSA body surface area
BV biologic value
CA cancer
CAD coronary artery disease
CAPD continuous ambulatory peritoneal dialysis
CAVH continuous arteriovenous hemofiltration
CC cardiac cachexia
CCK cholecystokinin
CCU coronary care unit
CDC Centers for Disease Control and Prevention
CHD coronary heart disease
CHF congestive heart failure
CHI closed head injury
CNS central nervous system
COPD chronic obstructive pulmonary disease
CPN central parenteral nutrition
CSII continuous subcutaneous insulin infusion
CSF cerebrospinal fluid
CVA cerebrovascular accident
DCCT Diabetes Control and Complications Trial
DHA docosahexaenoic acid
DHEW Department of Health, Education,and Welfare
DHHS Department of Health and Human Services
DJD degenerative joint disease
DKA diabetic ketoacidosis
DM diabetes mellitus
DNA deoxyribonucleic acid
DRI dietary reference intake
ECG/EKG electrocardiogram
EDTA ethylenediaminotetraacetate
EFA essential fatty acid
EPA eicosapentaenoic acid
EPO erythropoietin
ERT enzyme replacement therapy
ERT estrogen replacement therapy
ESR erythrocyte sedimentation rate
ESRD end-stage renal disease
FAD flavin adenine dinucleotide
FBG fasting blood glucose
FBS fasting blood sugar
FFA free fatty acids
FIGLU formimino glutamic acid
FMN flavin mononucleotide
FPG fasting plasma glucose
FTT failure to thrive
FX fracture
GB gallbladder
GFR glomerular filtration rate
GI gastrointestinal
GIP gastric inhibitory polypeptide
GTF glucose tolerance factor
GTT glucose tolerance test
GVHD graft-versus-host disease
HA hyperalimentation
HAV hepatitis A virus
Hgb hemoglobin
HBV hepatitis B virus
HBv high biologic value
HCT hematocrit
HDL high-density lipoprotein
HE hepatic encephalopathy
HGB hemoglobin
HIV human immunodeficiency virus
HPN home parenteral nutrition
HSL hormone-sensitive lipase
HTN hypertension
HX history
IBD inflammatory bowel disease
IBS irritable bowel syndrome
IBW ideal body weight
ICU intensive care unit
IDDM insulin-dependent diabetes mellitus
IF intrinsic factor
IgE immunoglobulin E
IGT impaired glucose tolerance
IL-2 interleukin-2
IM intramuscular
INH isonicotinic acid hydrazide
IV intravenous
IVH intravenous hyperalimentation
J joule
kcal (Cal) kilocalorie
kJ kilojoule
KS Kaposi's sarcoma
KUB kidney, ureter, bladder
LBM lean body mass
LCT long-chain triglyceride
LDL low-density lipoprotein
LES lower esophageal sphincter
LFT liver function test
LNA α-linolenic acid
LPL lipoprotein lipase
MAOI monoamine oxidase inhibitor
MCH mean corpuscular hemoglobin
MCT medium-chain triglyceride
MCV mean corpuscular volume
MET metabolic equivalent
MFOS mixed-function oxidase system
MI myocardial infarction
MOM Milk of Magnesia
MSG monosodium glutamate
MSUD maple syrup urine disease
NANB non-A, non-B hepatitis virus
NCEP National Cholesterol Education Program
NCJ needle catheter jejunostomy
NG nasogastric
NI nutritional index
NIDDM non–insulin-dependent diabetes
NPO nothing by mouth
NPU net protein utilization
NSAID nonsteroidal antiinflammatory drug
NSP nonstarch polysaccharide
N & V nausea and vomiting
OC oral contraceptive
OGTT oral glucose tolerance test
OHA oral hypoglycemic agent
PBI protein-bound iodine
PCM protein-caloric malnutrition

Continued

Appendix 1 General Abbreviations—cont'd

PD	Parkinson's disease
PEG	percutaneous endoscopic gastrostomy
PEM	protein energy malnutrition
PER	protein efficiency ratio
PG	prostaglandin
PHE	phenylalanine
PKU	phenylketonuria
PLP	pyridoxal phosphate
PPN	peripheral parenteral nutrition
PT	patient
PTA	prior to admission
PU	peptic ulcer
PUFA	polyunsaturated fatty acid
RAST	radioallergosorbent test
RBC	red blood cell
RDA	recommended dietary allowance
RDS	respiratory distress syndrome
REE	resting energy expenditure
RMR	resting metabolic rate
RNA	ribonucleic acid
R/O	rule out
ROS	review of systems
RQ	respiratory quotient
RS	resistant starches
RTA	renal tubular acidosis
SCA	sickle cell anemia
SCT	short-chain triglyceride
SFA	saturated fatty acid
SLE	systemic lupus erythematosus
SMBG	self-monitoring of blood glucose
SOB	shortness of breath
TBSA	total body surface area
TC	total cholesterol
TEE	total energy expenditure
TEF	thermic effect of food
TG	triglyceride or triacylglycerol
THFA	tetrahydrofolate
TIA	transient ischemic attack
TIBC	total iron-binding capacity
TNF	tumor necrosis factor
TPN	total parenteral nutrition
TS	transferrin saturation
UL	tolerable upper intake level
URI	upper respiratory infection
UTI	urinary tract infection
VLCD	very-low-calorie diet
VLDL	very-low-density lipoprotein
VOD	venous occlusive disease
VS	vital signs
WNL	within normal limits

Appendix 2 Unit Abbreviations

Along with the specialized vocabulary that is used in the medical, dietetic, and nursing fields, there are acceptable forms of abbreviations. The following is a list of abbreviations commonly used.

aa: Gr. *ana;* of each
ac: L. *ante cibum;* before meals
ad, add: L. *adde, addatus,* or *addantur;* add or added
ad lib: L. *ad libitum;* at pleasure, as desired
aq: L. *aqua;* water
aq dest: L. *aqua destillata;* distilled water
bid, bis in d: L. *bis in die;* twice a day
c: L. *cum;* with
c: cup
cc: cubic centimeter
Cent; cent; C: centrigrade, Celsius
cm: centimeter
dilut: L. *dilutus;* dilute
div: L. *divide;* divide
fac: make
g: gram
gr: L. *granum;* grain
gtt: L. *guttae;* drops
hs: L. *hora somni;* at hour of sleep
IU: international unit
kcal: kilocalorie
kg: kilogram
kJ: kilojoule
lb: pound
μg: microgram
mcg: microgram
μU: microunit
mEq: milliequivalent
mg: milligram
mil or ml: milliliter
mM: millimole
mOsm: milliosmole
oz: ounce
prn: L. *pro re nata:* may be repeated according to instructions
pt: pint
pulv: L. *pulvis;* powder
qd: L. *quaque die:* every day
QID, qid: L. *quater in die;* four times daily
q3h: every 3 hours
qs: L. *quantum satis;* a sufficient quantity
qt: quart
RE: retinol equivalent
s: L. *sine;* without
sol: solution
ss: L. *semis;* half
stat: L. *statim;* immediately
t, tsp: teaspoon
T, tbsp: tablespoon
tid. L. *ter in die:* three times a day

Appendix 3 Potential ICD-9-CM Codes for Nutrition Services

Carcinoma (Primary)

195.2	Carcinoma, abdomen
188	Carcinoma, bladder, ADR
170	Carcinoma, bone and articular cartilage, ADR
191	Carcinoma, brain, ADR
174	Carcinoma, breast (female), ADR
154.0	Carcinoma, colon
189.0	Carcinoma, kidney, except pelvis, NOS
155.0	Carcinoma, liver
145	Carcinoma, mouth, ADR
183.0	Carcinoma, ovary
157	Carcinoma, pancreas, ADR
185	Carcinoma, prostate
154.1	Carcinoma, rectum
173	Carcinoma, skin, ADR
151	Carcinoma, stomach, ADR
193	Carcinoma, thyroid
162	Carcinoma, trachea, lung and bronchus, ADR
182	Carcinoma, body of uterus, ADR

Cardiovascular

413.9	Angina pectoris, U, N
411.1	Angina, unstable
424.1	Aortic valve disorders, NOS
427.9	Arrythmia, NOS, U
785.9	Bruit, arterial, N
429.2	Cardiovascular disease, U, N
786.50	Chest pain, U, N
428.0	Congestive heart failure
414.01	Coronary atherosclerosis, of native coronary artery
401.1	Hypertension, essential, benign
401.1	Hypertension, essential, malignant
401.9	Hypertension, U, N
402.90	Hypertensive heart disease, U, w/o CHF
402.91	Hypertensive heart disease, U, w/CHF
403.00	Hypertensive renal disease, malignant, w/o renal failure
403.01	Hypertensive renal disease, malignant, w/renal failure
458.0	Hypotension, orthostatic
410.00	Myocardial infarction, of anterolateral wall, episode of care unspec., N
410.01	Myocardial infarction, acute, of other anterolateral wall, episode of care unspec., N
412	Myocardial infarction, status post
443.9	Peripheral vascular disease, U, N
416.0	Primary pulmonary hypertension
436	Stroke, acute but ill-defined, NOS
785.0	Tachycardia, U, N
435.9	Transient cerebral ischemia, U, N

Endocrine and Metabolic Disorders

790.2	Abnormal glucose tolerance test
255.4	Addison's disease, NOS
255.0	Cushing's syndrome
277.00	Cystic fibrosis, w/o meconium ileus
277.01	Cystic fibrosis, w/meconium ileus
253.5	Diabetes insipidus
250.0	Diabetes mellitus (DM), w/o mention of complications, ADR*
250.1	Diabetes w/ketoacidosis, ADR*
250.2	Diabetes w/hyperosmolar coma, ADR*
250.3	Diabetes w/other coma, ADR*
250.4	Diabetes w/renal manifestations, ADR*
250.5	Diabetes w/ophthalmic manifestations, ADR*
250.6	Diabetes w/neurological manifestations, ADR*
250.7	Diabetes w/peripheral circulatory disorders, ADR*
250.8	Diabetes w/other specified manifestations, ADR*
357.2	Diabetic polyneuropathy, NPD
271.1	Galactosemia
785.4	Gangrene, NOS
240.9	Goiter, U, N
242.00	Grave's disease, w/o thyrotoxic crisis or storm
242.01	Grave's disease, w/thyrotoxic crisis or storm
255.1	Hyperaldosteronism
275.42	Hypercalcemia
272.0	Hypercholesterolemia, pure
272.1	Hyperglyceridemia, pure
272.2	Hyperlipidemia, mixed
252.0	Hyperparathyroidism
242.9	Hyperthyroidism, NOS, N
275.41	Hypocalcemia
251.2	Hypoglycemia, U, N
252.1	Hypoparathyroidism
244.0	Hypothyroidism, postsurgical
244.9	Hypothyroidism, U, N, NOS
758.7	Klinefelter's syndrome
270.3	Maple syrup urine disease
276.2	Metabolic acidosis
278.00	Obesity, U, N, NOS
278.01	Obesity, morbid
270.1	Phenylketonuria

Gastrointestinal

571.2	Alcoholic cirrhosis of liver
571.0	Alcoholic fatty liver
535.30	Alcoholic gastritis, w/o hemorrhage
535.31	Alcoholic gastritis, w/hemorrhage
571.1	Alcoholic hepatitis, acute
571.3	Alcoholic liver damage, U, N
579.2	Blind loop syndrome
574.50	Calculus of bile duct w/o cholecystitis, w/o obstruction
574.51	Calculus of bile duct w/o cholecystitis, w/obstruction
579.0	Celiac disease
575.0	Cholecystitis, acute
575.10	Cholecystitis, chronic, U, N
571.5	Cirrhosis of liver, w/o mention of alcohol
749.10	Cleft lip, U, N
749.20	Cleft palate w/cleft lip, U, N
749.00	Cleft palate, U, N
558.2	Colitis and gastorenteritis, toxic
556.9	Colitis, ulcerative, U, N
564.0	Constipation
555.0	Crohn's disease, small intestine
555.1	Crohn's disease, large intestine
564.5	Diarrhea, functional
562.10	Diverticulosis
562.11	Diverticulitis
564.2	Dumping syndrome
536.8	Dyspepsia, other disorders of stomach, N

Reference: International Classification of Diseases, Clinical Modification, 1997.
(ICD-9-CM), Delaware: American Medical Association, 1996.

Each year, the ICD-9-CM is updated. Check the most recent publication year for accurate information, clarification, and additional digits not listed here.
To obtain an ICD-9-CM book, contact the AMA at (800) 621-8335 or visit their Web site @ http://www.cdc.gov/nchs/about/otheract/icd9/abticd9.htm.
ICD-10 codes are the next generation of codes not yet implemented in the United States.
Reference: The American Dietetic Association, Reimbursement Team, Chicago, 1998, The American Dietetic Association.

*The following fifth digit is for use with category 250:
0 type 2 diabetes
1 type 1 diabetes

ADR, Additional digit required; *N*, Nonspecific code; *NOS*, Not otherwise specified; *NEC*, Not elsewhere classified; *NPD*, Not a primary diagnosis; *U*, Unspecified.

Note: Dietitic professionals are encouraged to use ICD-9-CM codes in conjunction with medical nutrition therapy (MNT) codes for charting or billing purposes. Physicians make the medical diagnoses from which these codes are derived.

Continued

Appendix 3 Potential ICD-9-CM Codes for Nutrition Services—cont'd

787.2	Dysphagia
787.3	Flatulence
575.9	Gallbladder, disorder, U
535.00	Gastritis, acute, w/o hemorrhage
535.01	Gastritis, acute, w/hemorrhage
558.9	Gastroenteritis, NOS, N
523.0	Gingivitis, acute
523.1	Gingivitis, chronic
529.0	Glossitis
787.1	Heartburn
578.0	Hematemesis
578.9	Hemorrhage of GI tract, U, N
573.3	Hepatitis, U, N
789.1	Hepatomegaly
271.2	Hereditary fructose intolerance
553.3	Hiatal hernia
536.2	Hyperemesis (not of pregnancy)
560.1	Ileus, paralytic
560.30	Impaction of colon, N
536.8	Indigestion
569.61	Infection, colostomy or enterostomy
564.1	Irritable colon (irritable bowel syndrome)
579.8	Steatorrhea, chronic, N
271.3	Malabsorption, glucose, lactose, sucrose
579.9	Malabsorption syndrome, NOS
578.1	Melena
787.01	Nausea with vomiting
787.02	Nausea alone
560.9	Obstruction, intestinal, U, N
577.9	Pancreas, unspec. disease of, N
577.0	Pancreatitis, acute
577.1	Pancreatitis, chronic
569.89	Pericolitis, intestine, N
528.9	Sore mouth, denture, N
528.0	Stomatitis
787.7	Stool, abnormal
525.1	Teeth loss
569.82	Ulceration, intestine
533.00	Ulcer, peptic, acute w/hemorrhage, w/obstruction
533.10	Ulcer, peptic, acute w/perforation, w/ obstruction
557.0	Vascular insufficiency of intestine, chronic
560.2	Volvulus
787.03	Vomiting alone
536.2	Vomiting, persistent

Genitourinary

626.0	Amenorrhea
753.10	Cystic kidney disease, U, N
595.9	Cystitis, U, N
276.9	Dialysis disequilibrium syndrome
625.3	Dysmenorrhea
403.9	Hypertensive renal disease, U, ADR
592.0	Kidney stones
627.2	Menopause symptoms
626.9	Menstrual disorders, U, N
626.0	Menstruation, absence
626.4	Menstruation, irregular
583.0	Nephritis, w/proliferative glomerulonephritis
583.9	Nephritis, NOS, N
583.81	Nephritis and nephropathy, NPD
626.1	Oligomenorrhea
625.4	Premenstrual tension syndromes
791.0	Proteinurea
590.80	Pyelonephritis, U, N
584.9	Renal failure, acute, U, N
585	Renal failure, chronic
592.9	Urinary calculus, U, N
599.0	Urinary tract infection, unspec. site, N

Hematology

285.9	Anemia, U, N
281.2	Anemia, folate deficiency
281.3	Anemia, folate and B_{12} deficiency
282.2	Anemia, G-6-PD deficiency
280.9	Anemia, iron deficiency, U, N
281.4	Anemia, protein deficiency
280.1	Anemia, secondary to lack of dietary iron intake
282.60	Anemia, sickle cell, U, N
281.9	Anemia, simple chronic
281.1	Anemia, vitamin B_{12} deficiency, U, N
276.9	Electrolyte and fluid disorders, NEC, N
275.4	Hypocalcemia
251.2	Hypoglycemia, U, N
276.8	Hypokalemia
282.5	Sickle cell trait
282.4	Thalassemias

Infections

006.9	Amoebiasis, U, N
114.9	Coccidioidomycosis, U, N
078.5	Cytomegaloviral disease
008.00	*E. coli* infection, U, N
487.0	Flu w/pneumonia
008.8	Gastroenteritis, viral, N, NEC
007.1	Giardiasis
573.3	Hepatitis, U, N
070.1	Hepatitis A, viral, w/o hepatic coma
070.3	Hepatitis B, viral, w/o hepatic coma, acute, N
054	Herpes simplex, ADR
042	Human immunodeficiency virus (HIV) disease
075	Mononucleosis, infectious
136.3	Pneumocystosis
480.0	Pneumonia, due to adenovirus
481	Pneumonia, pneumococcal
486	Pneumonia, organism unspec., N
031.0	Pulmonary disease, mycobacterium infection
034.0	Streptococcal sore throat
112.0	Thrush, oral
463	Tonsillitis, acute
130.9	Toxoplasmosis, U, N
079.98	Viral and chlamydial infections, U, N

Musculoskeletal

714.0	Arthritis, rheumatoid
274.0	Arthropathy, gouty
724.5	Backache, U, N
727.3	Bursitis, NOS, N
724.2	Lumbago (low back pain)
340	Multiple sclerosis
729.1	Myalgia and myositis, U, N
268.2	Osteomalacia, U, N
730.00	Osteomyelitis, site unspec., N
733.00	Osteoporosis, U, N

Reference: International Classification of Diseases, Clinical Modification, 1997.
(ICD-9-CM), Delaware: American Medical Association, 1996.

Each year, the ICD-9-CM is updated. Check the most recent publication year for accurate information, clarification, and additional digits not listed here. To obtain an ICD-9-CM book, contact the AMA at (800) 621-8335 or visit their Web site @ http://www.cdc.gov/nchs/about/otheract/icd9/abticd9.htm. ICD-10 codes are the next generation of codes not yet implemented in the United States.

Reference: The American Dietetic Association, Reimbursement Team, Chicago, 1998, The American Dietetic Association.

*The following fifth digit is for use with category 250:
0 type 2 diabetes
1 type 1 diabetes

ADR, Additional digit required; *N*, Nonspecific code; *NOS*, Not otherwise specified; *NEC*, Not elsewhere classified; *NPD*, Not a primary diagnosis; *U*, Unspecified.

NOTE: **Dietitic professionals are encouraged to use ICD-9-CM codes in conjunction with medical nutrition therapy (MNT) codes for charting or billing purposes. Physicians make the medical diagnoses from which these codes are derived.**

Appendix 3 Potential ICD-9-CM Codes for Nutrition Services—cont'd

Nervous System

305.00 Alcohol abuse, U, N
331.0 Alzheimer's disease
305.20 Cannabis abuse, U, N
343.9 Cerebral palsy, NOS, U
304.40 Drug dependence—amphetamines, U, N
304.10 Drug dependence—barbiturates, U, N
304.30 Drug dependence—cannabis, U, N
304.20 Drug dependence—cocaine, U, N
304.00 Drug dependence—opioid type, U, N
311 Depression disorder, NEC
300.4 Depression disorder, neurotic
345.0 Epilepsy, nonconvulsive, ADR
345.1 Epilepsy, convulsive, ADR
345.2 Epilepsy, petit mal status
345.3 Epilepsy, grand mal status
742.1 Microcephalus
346.9 Migraine, U, N, ADR
359.0 Muscular dystrophy, congenital hereditary
300.01 Panic disorder
780.50 Sleep disturbances, U, N
300.23 Social phobia, fear of eating in public
780.2 Syncope and collapse

Nutritional

790.6 Abnormal blood level, iron, zinc, N
783.1 Abnormal weight gain
783.2 Abnormal weight loss
783.0 Anorexia, loss of appetite (not nervosa)
307.1 Anorexia nervosa
263.2 Arrested development following protein-calorie malnutrition
265.0 Beriberi
307.51 Bulimia, nonorganic nature
267.0 Deficiency, ascorbic acid (Vit C)
264.7 Deficiency, vitamin A, xeropthalmia, N
266.9 Deficiency, vitamin B, U, N
265.1 Deficiency, vitamin B_1, U, N
266.0 Deficiency, vitamin B_2
266.1 Deficiency, vitamin B_6
266.2 Deficiency, B_{12} or folic acid
269.3 Deficiency, calcium
261 Deficiency, calorie (marasmus)
268.9 Deficiency, vitamin D, U, N
280.9 Deficiency, iron, anemia, U, N
271.3 Deficiency, lactose
265.2 Deficiency, niacin (pellagra)
269.9 Deficiency, nutritional, U
276.5 Dehydration, volume depletion
781.1 Disturbances of sensation of smell and taste
783.4 Failure to thrive
783.3 Feeding problem, elderly or infant
779.3 Feeding problem, newborn
005.9 Food poisoning, U, N
278.3 Hypercarotenemia
278.2 Hypervitaminosis A
278.4 Hypervitaminosis D
264.8 Keratosis, vitamin A deficiency, N
260 Kwashiorkor
579.3 Malnutrition, malabsorption, post–gastro surgery, N
278.01 Obesity, morbid
307.52 Pica
263.9 Protein-calorie malnutrition, U, N
263.0 Protein-calorie malnutrition, moderate
783.6 Polyphagia
268.0 Rickets, active
783.4 Short stature

Perinatal

789.00 Abdominal pain, colic, unspec. site, N
758.0 Down syndrome
676.4 Lactation, failure, U, ADR
675.20 Mastitis, nonpurulent, U, ADR
775.1 Neonatal diabetes mellitus
760.70 Noxious substance, affecting fetus via placenta or breast milk, U, N
656.50 Poor fetal growth, unspec. as to care

Pregnancy

646.3 Aborter, habitual, ADR
648.8 Diabetes mellitus (gestational), U
V23.3 Grand multiparity
643.0 Hyperemesis gravidarum, ADR
646.8 Insufficient weight gain
V61.5 Multiparity
642.7 Pre-eclampsia or eclampsia superimposed on pre-existing hypertension, unspec. as to care
642.4 Pre-eclampsia, U or mild, ADR
643.9 Vomiting of pregnancy, U, N, ADR

Respiratory

786.09 Apnea, N
493.9 Asthma, U, N, ADR
466.0 Bronchitis, acute
491.0 Bronchitis, simple, chronic
491.1 Bronchitis, chronic, recurrent
492.8 Emphysema, NOS, N
780.53 Hypersomnia, w/sleep apnea
474.1 Hypertrophy of tonsils and adenoids
786.01 Hyperventilation
487.1 Influenza w/other respiratory manifestations, N
780.51 Insomnia, w/sleep apnea
482.9 Pneumonia, bacterial, U, N
480.9 Pneumonia, viral, U, N
472.0 Rhinitis, chronic (excludes allergic)
474.0 Tonsillitis, chronic

Signs and Symptoms

995.3 Allergy, excludes hayfever, dermatitis, allergic diarrhea, U, N
796.2 Blood pressure, elevated, w/o hypertension
782.3 Edema
780.7 Fatigue and malaise
783.3 Feeding difficulties and management
780.6 Fever
784.0 Headache
789.1 Hepatomegaly
782.4 Jaundice, not of newborn, U
785.6 Lymph nodes, enlargement
789.2 Splenomegaly

Skin

682.9 Cellulitis and abscess, site unspec., N
707.0 Pressure ulcer
708.9 Hives, NOS, N
696.1 Psoriasis, other, N
782.1 Rash and other nonspecific skin eruption, N
707.1 Ulcer of lower limbs, except decubitus

Appendix 4 Milliequivalents and Milligrams of Electrolytes

TO CONVERT MILLIGRAMS TO MILLIEQUIVALENTS

Divide milligrams by atomic weight and then multiply by the valence:

$$\frac{\text{Milligrams}}{\text{Atomic weight}} \times \text{Valence} = \text{Milliequivalents}$$

MINERAL ELEMENT	CHEMICAL SYMBOL	ATOMIC WEIGHT	VALENCE
Calcium	Ca	40.0	2
Chlorine	Cl	35.4	1
Magnesium	Mg	24.3	2
Phosphorus	P	31.0	2
Potassium	K	39.0	1
Sodium	Na	23.0	1
Sulfate	SO_4	96.0	2
Sulfur	S	32.0	

TO CONVERT SPECIFIC WEIGHT OF SODIUM TO SODIUM CHLORIDE

Multiply by 2.54.
Example:
1000 mg Sodium = 1000 × 2.54 = 2540 mg Sodium chloride (2.5 g)

TO CONVERT SPECIFIC WEIGHT OF SODIUM CHLORIDE TO SODIUM

Multiply by 0.393.
Example:
2.5 g Sodium chloride = 2.5 × 0.393 = 1000 mg sodium

MILLIGRAMS	SODIUM VALUES (MILLIEQUIVALENTS)	GRAMS OF SODIUM CHLORIDE
500	21.8	1.3
1000	43.5	2.5
1500	75.3	3.8
2000	87.0	5.0

Modified from Nelson JK et al: *Mayo clinic diet manual,* ed 7, St Louis, 1994, Mosby.

Appendix 5 Approximate Conversions to and From Metric Measures

APPROXIMATE CONVERSIONS TO METRIC MEASURES

WHEN YOU KNOW	MULTIPLY BY	TO FIND
Length		
Inches	2.5	Centimeters
Feet	30.0	Centimeters
Yards	0.9	Meters
Miles	1.6	Kilometers
Area		
Square inches	6.5	Square centimeters
Square feet	9.09	Square meters
Square yards	0.8	Square meters
Square miles	2.6	Square kilometers
Acres	0.4	Hectares
Mass (weight)		
Ounces	28.0	Grams
Pounds	0.45	Kilograms
Short tons (2,000 lb)	0.9	Tonnes
Volume		
Teaspoons	5.0	Milliliters
Tablespoons	15.0	Milliliters
Fluid ounces	30.0	Milliliters
Cups	0.24	Liters
Pints	0.47	Liters
Quarts	0.95	Liters
Gallons	3.8	Liters
Cubic feet	0.03	Cubic meters
Cubic yards	0.76	Cubic meters
Temperature		
Fahrenheit	$^5/_9$ (after subtracting 32)	Celsius

APPROXIMATE CONVERSIONS FROM METRIC MEASURES

WHEN YOU KNOW	MULTIPLY BY	TO FIND
Length		
Millimeters	0.04	Inches
Centimeters	0.4	Inches
Meters	3.3	Feet
Meters	1.1	Yards
Kilometers	0.6	Miles
Area		
Square centimeters	0.16	Square inches
Square meters	1.2	Square yards
Square kilometers	0.4	Square miles
Hectares (10,000 m^2)	2.5	Acres
Mass (weight)		
Grams	0.035	Ounces
Kilograms	2.2	Pounds
Tonnes (1000 kg)	1.1	Short tons
Volume		
Milliliters	0.03	Fluid ounces
Liters	2.1	Pints
Liters	1.06	Quarts
Liters	0.26	Gallons
Cubic meters	35	Cubic feet
Cubic meters	1.3	Cubic yards
Temperature		
Celsius	$^9/_5$ (then add 32)	Fahrenheit

Modified from Nelson JK, et al: *Mayo clinic diet manual,* ed 7, St Louis, 1994, Mosby; and U.S. Department of Commerce, National Bureau of Standards: *Metric conversion card* (NBS Special Publication 365), Washington, DC, 1972, U.S. Government Printing Office.

Appendix 6 Birth to 36 Months: Boys Length-for-Age and Weight-for-Age Percentiles

NAME ______________________

RECORD# ____________

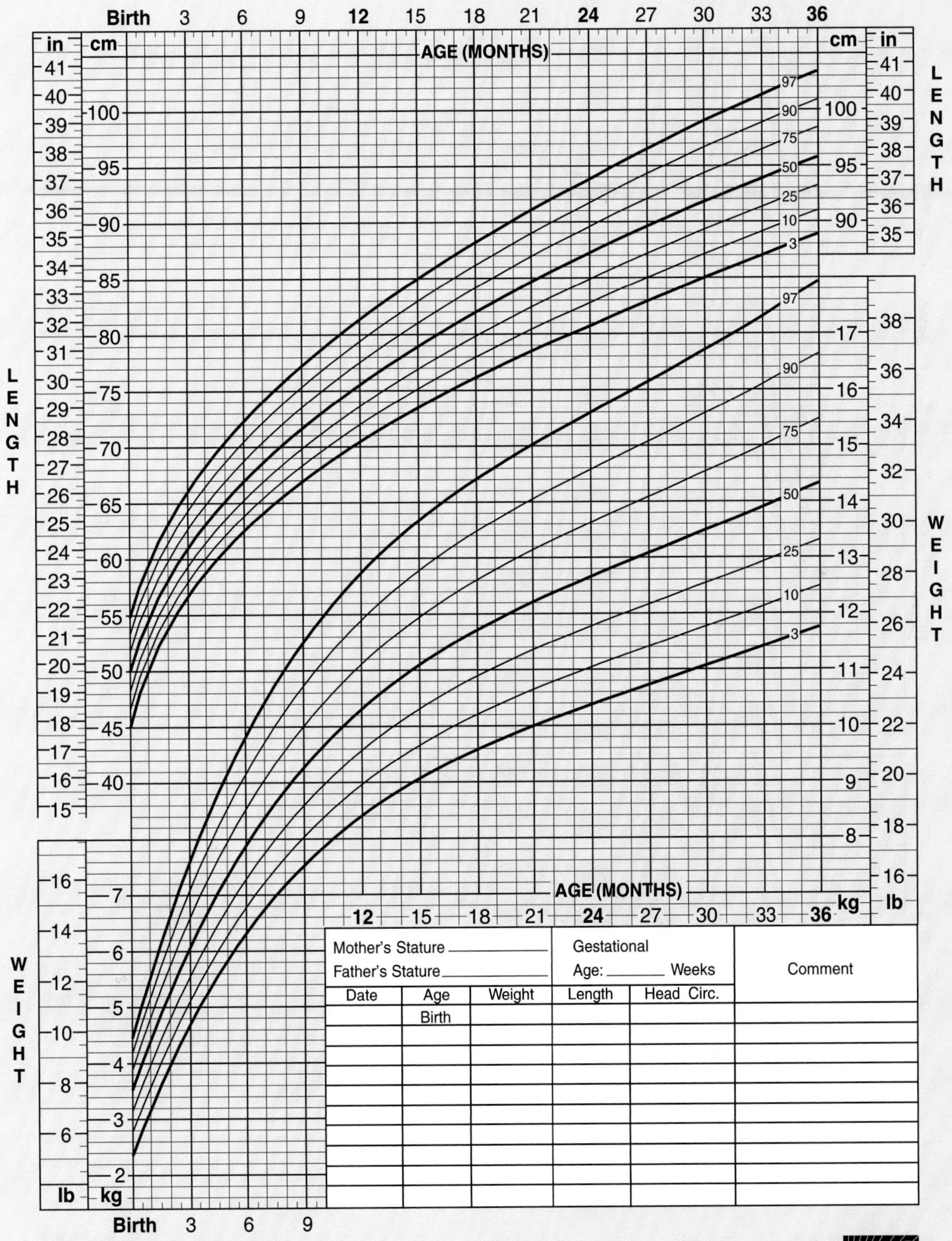

Published May 30, 2000 (modified 4/20/01).
SOURCE: Developed by the National Center for Health Statistics in collaboration with the National Center for Chronic Disease Prevention and Health Promotion (2000).
http://www .cdc.gov/growthcharts

CDC
SAFER•HEALTHIER•PEOPLE

Appendix 7 Birth to 36 Months: Boys Head Circumference-for-Age and Weight-for-Length Percentiles

NAME ______________________

RECORD # ____________

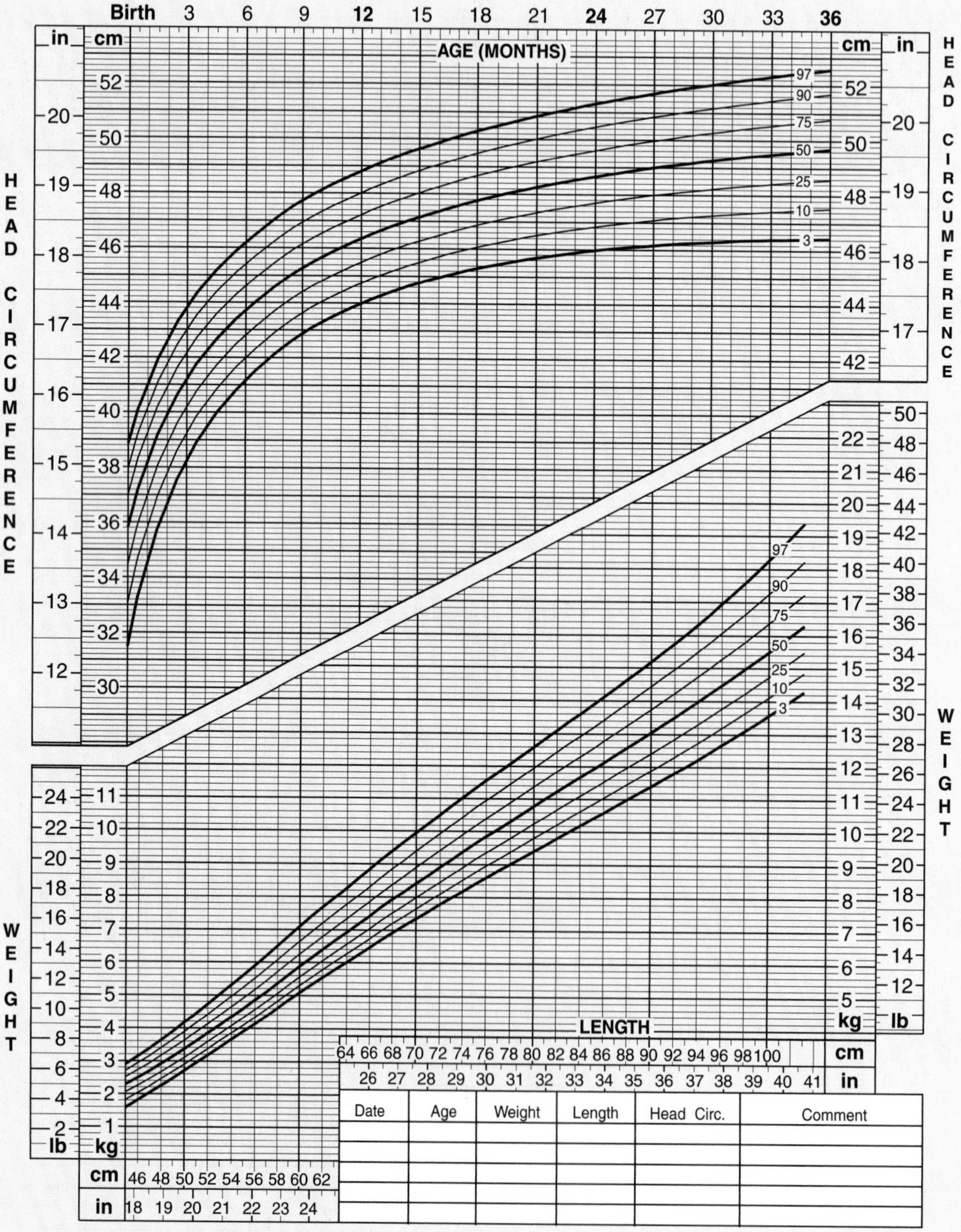

Date	Age	Weight	Length	Head Circ.	Comment

Published May 30, 2000 (modified 10/16/00).
SOURCE: Developed by the National Center for Health Statistics in collaboration with
the National Center for Chronic Disease Prevention and Health Promotion (2000).
http://www.cdc.gov/growthcharts

CDC SAFER•HEALTHIER•PEOPLE

Appendix 8 2 to 20 Years: Boys Stature-for-Age and Weight-for-Age Percentiles

NAME ____________________

RECORD # __________

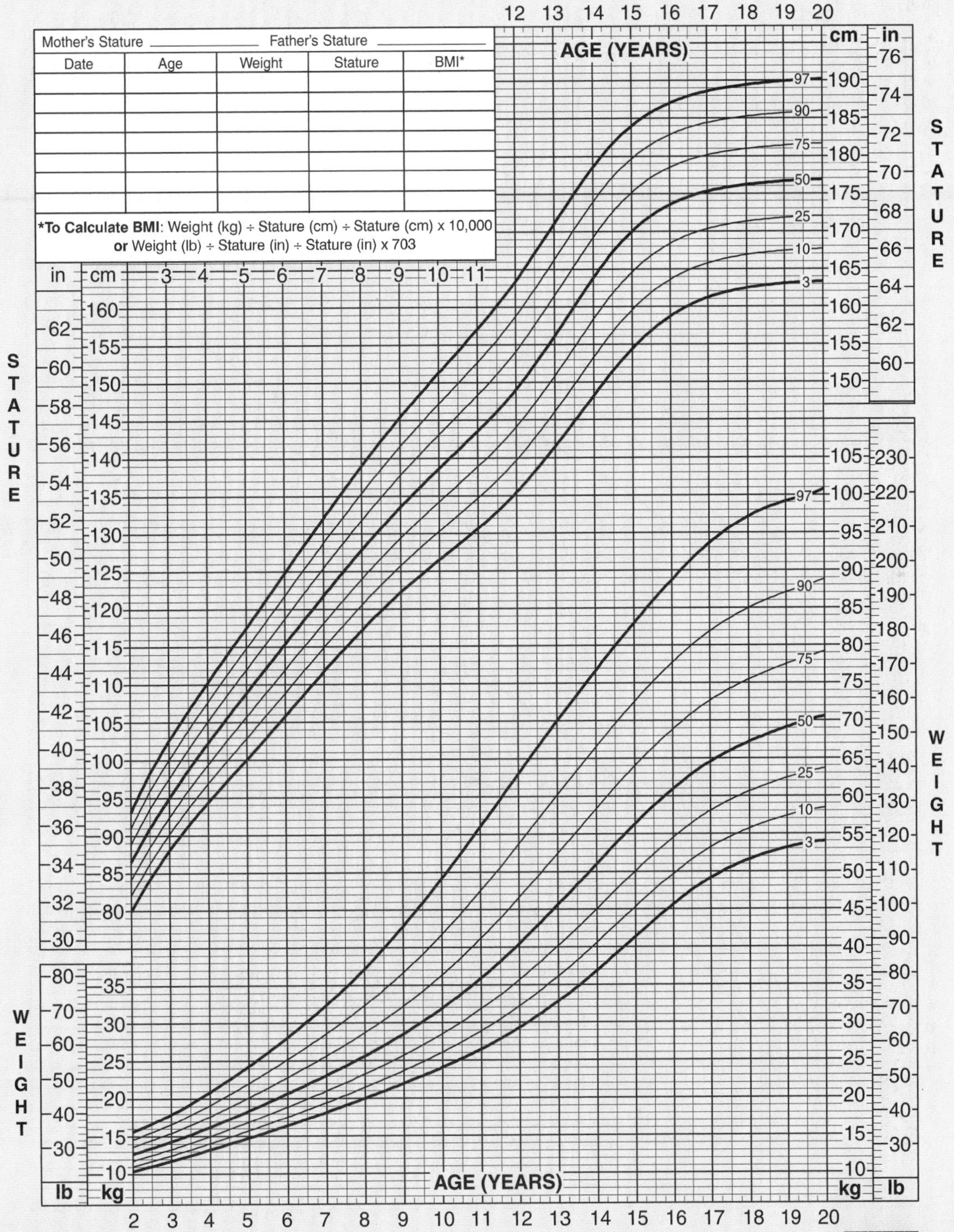

Published May 30, 2000 (modified 11/21/00).
SOURCE: Developed by the National Center for Health Statistics in collaboration with the National Center for Chronic Disease Prevention and Health Promotion (2000). http://www.cdc.gov/growthcharts

CDC
SAFER•HEALTHIER•PEOPLE

Appendix 9 Birth to 36 Months: Girls Length-for-Age and Weight-for-Age Percentiles

NAME ______________________

RECORD # ____________

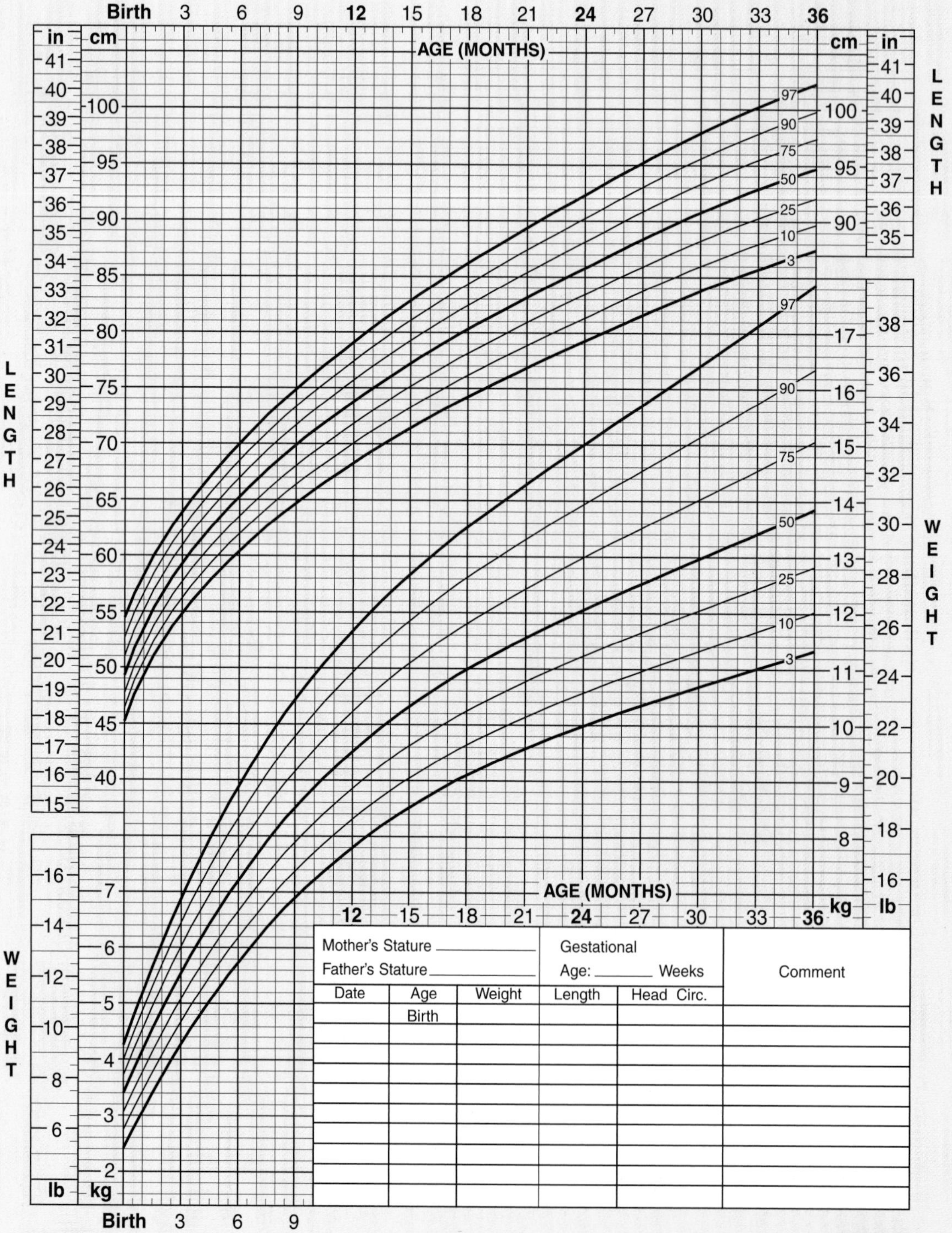

Published May 30, 2000 (modified 4/20/01).
SOURCE: Developed by the National Center for Health Statistics in collaboration with the National Center for Chronic Disease Prevention and Health Promotion (2000).
http://www.cdc.gov/growthcharts

SAFER•HEALTHIER•PEOPLE

Appendix 10 Birth to 36 Months: Girls Head Circumference-for-Age and Weight-for-Length Percentiles

NAME ______________________

RECORD # ____________

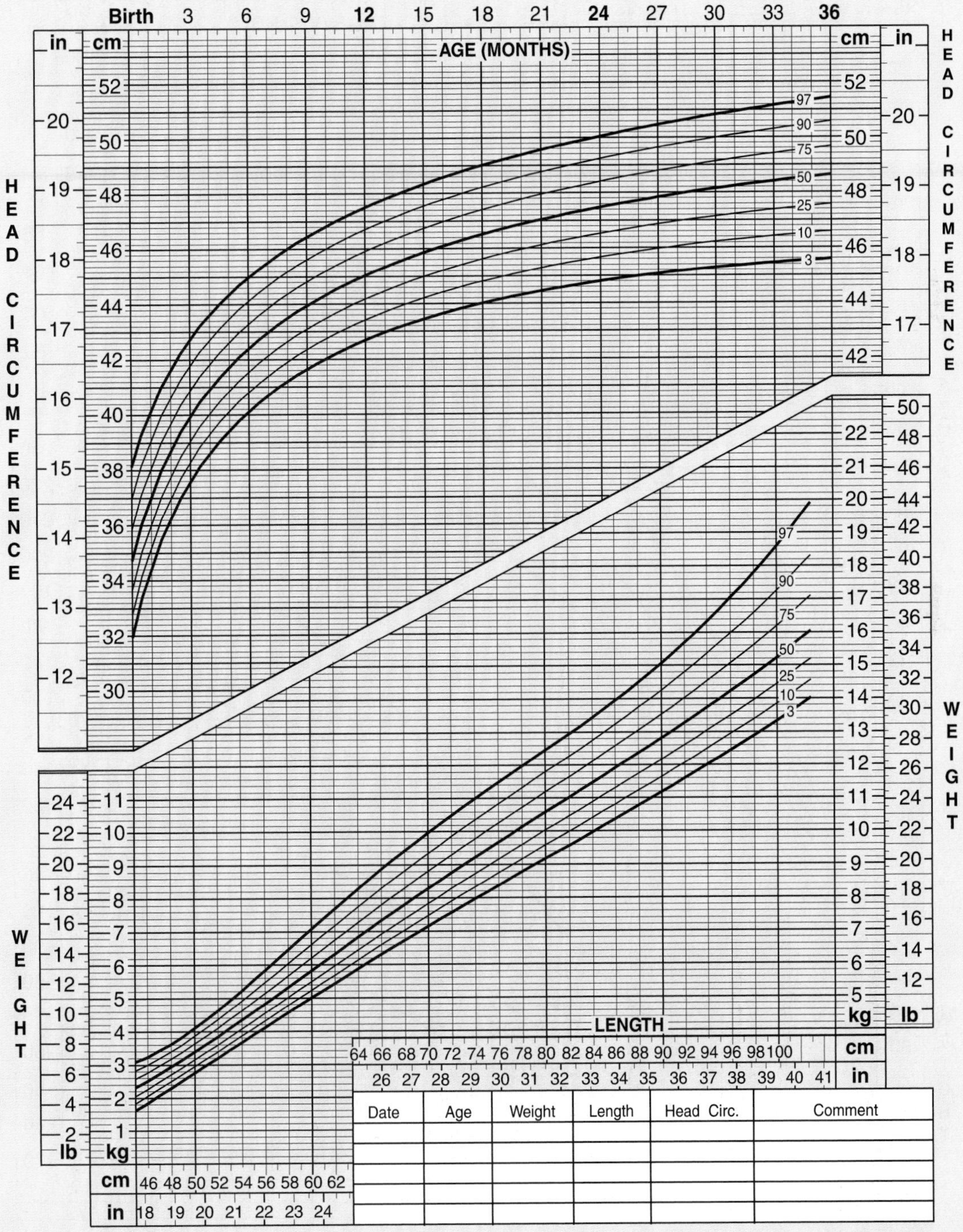

Date	Age	Weight	Length	Head Circ.	Comment

Published May 30, 2000 (modified 10/16/00).
SOURCE: Developed by the National Center for Health Statistics in collaboration with the National Center for Chronic Disease Prevention and Health Promotion (2000).
http://www.cdc.gov/growthcharts

CDC SAFER•HEALTHIER•PEOPLE

Appendix 11 2 to 20 Years: Girls Stature-for-Age and Weight-for-Age Percentiles

NAME ____________________

RECORD # ____________

Mother's Stature ____________ Father's Stature ____________

Date	Age	Weight	Stature	BMI*

***To Calculate BMI**: Weight (kg) ÷ Stature (cm) ÷ Stature (cm) x 10,000
or Weight (lb) ÷ Stature (in) ÷ Stature (in) x 703

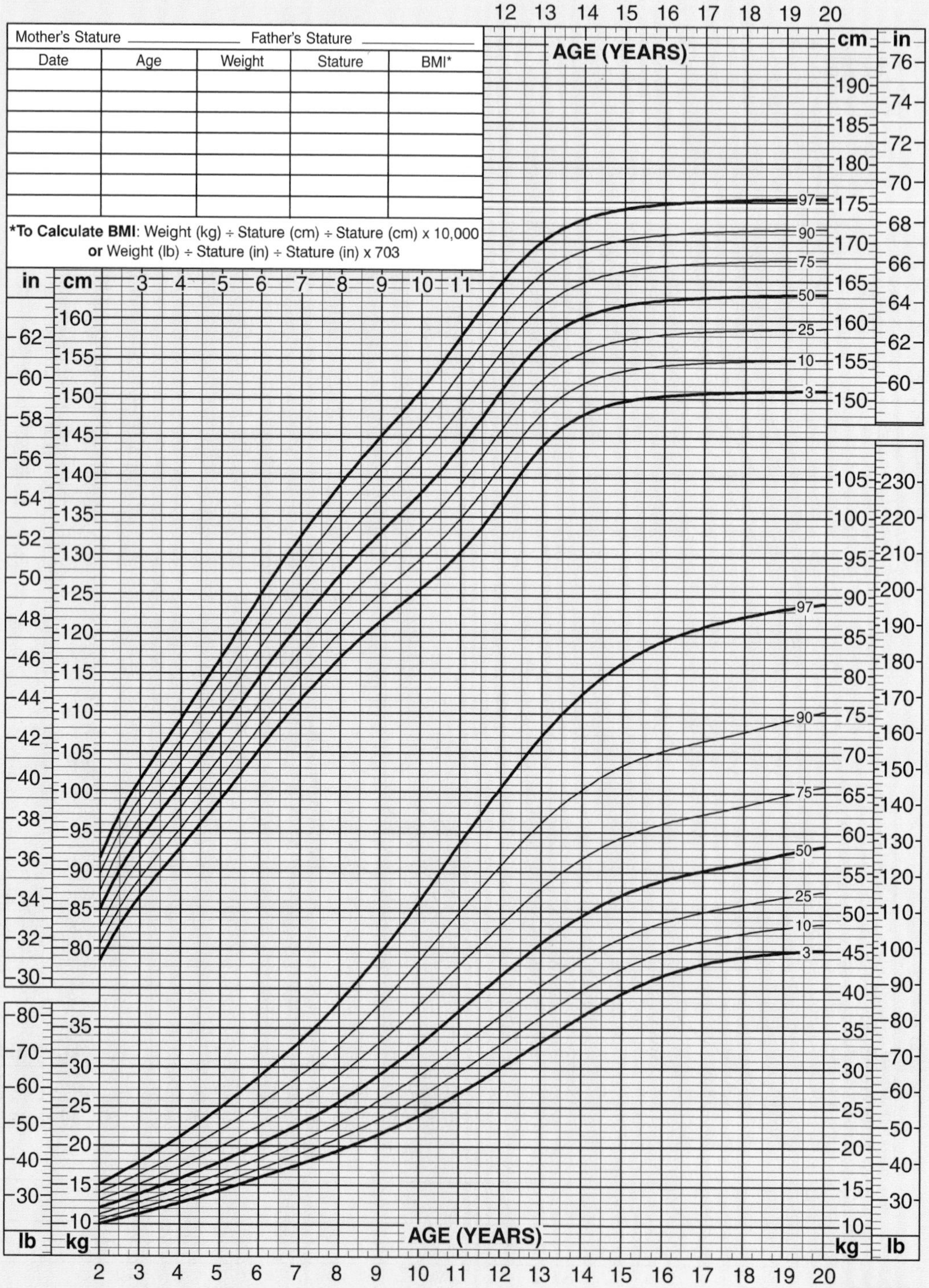

Published May 30, 2000 (modified 11/21/00).
SOURCE: Developed by the National Center for Health Statistics in collaboration with the National Center for Chronic Disease Prevention and Health Promotion (2000).
http://www.cdc.gov/growthcharts

CDC
SAFER•HEALTHIER•PEOPLE

Appendix 12 Tanner Stages of Adolescent Development for Females

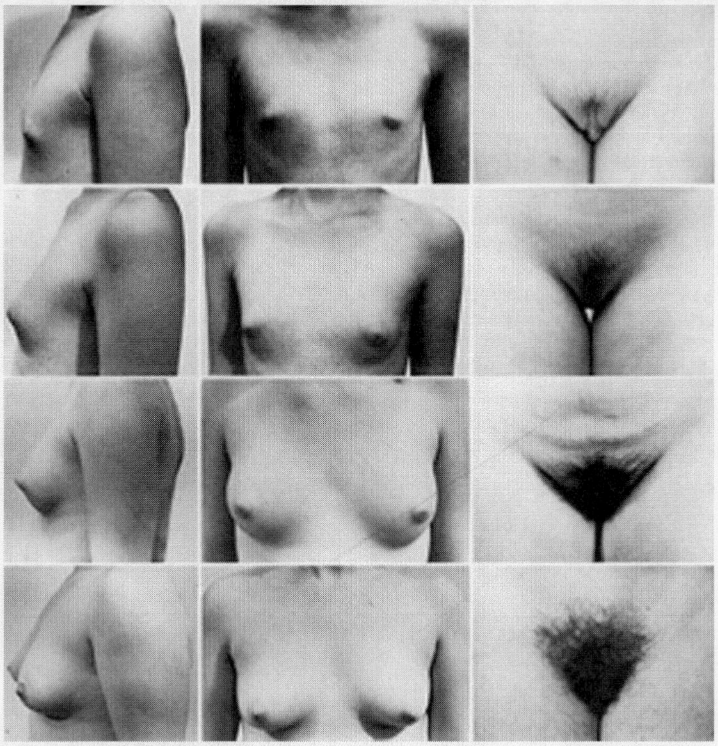

From Mahan LK, Rees JM: *Nutrition in adolescence,* St. Louis, 1984, Mosby.

Appendix 13 Tanner Stages of Adolescent Development for Males

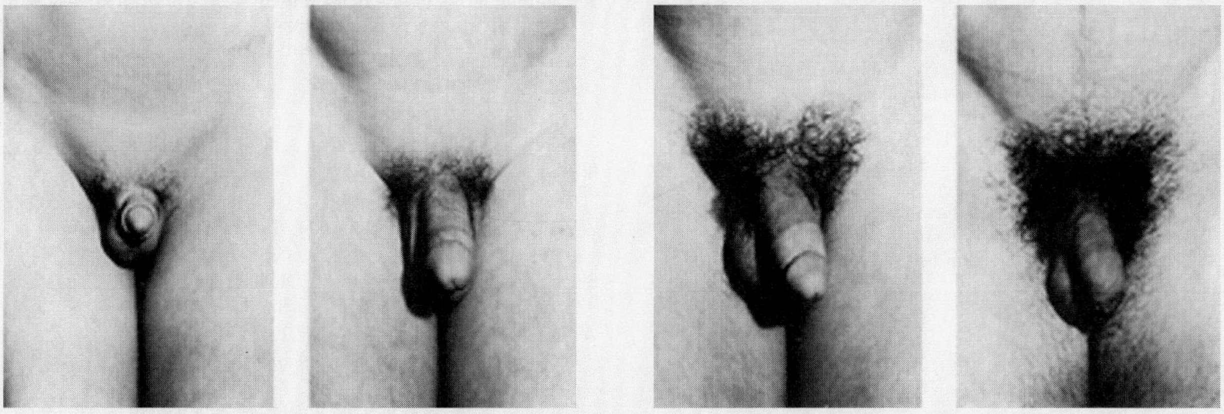

Chronologic age is not always the best way to assess adolescent growth because of individual variations in beginning and completing the growth sequence. A more useful way of describing pubertal development, and thus the varying needs for nutrients throughout adolescence, is to divide growth into stages of breast and pubic hair development in girls (Appendix 12) and pubic hair and penis and testicle development in boys (Appendix 13). These are termed the Tanner Stages of Adolescent Development. Nutritional requirements vary depending on the stage of development.

From Mahan LK, Rees JM: *Nutrition in adolescence,* St. Louis, 1984, Mosby.

Appendix 14 Direct Methods for Measuring Height and Weight

Height

1. Height should be measured without shoes.
2. The individual's feet should be together, with the heels against the wall or measuring board.
3. The individual should stand erect, neither slumped nor stretching, looking straight ahead, without tipping the head up or down. The top of the ear and outer corner of the eye should be in a line parallel to the floor (the "Frankfort plane").
4. A horizontal bar, a rectangular block of wood, or the top of the statiometer should be lowered to rest flat on the top of the head.
5. Height should be read to the nearest ¼ inch or 0.5 cm.

Weight

1. Use a beam balance scale, not a spring scale, whenever possible.
2. Periodically calibrate the scale for accuracy, using known weights.
3. Weigh the subject in light clothing without shoes.
4. Record weight to the nearest ½ lb or 0.2 kg for adults and ¼ lb or 0.1 kg for infants. Measurements above the 90th percentile or below the 10th percentile warrant further evaluation.

Appendix 15 Indirect Methods for Measuring Height

Measuring Arm Span

Steps:

1. The arms are extended straight out to the sides at a 90-degree angle from the body.
2. The distance from the longest fingertip of one hand to the longest finger of the other hand is measured.

Adult Recumbent

Steps:

1. Stand on right side of the body.
2. Align body so that the lower extremities, trunk, shoulders, and head are straight.
3. Place a mark at the top of the sheet in line with the crown of the head and one at the bottom of the sheet in line with the base of the heels.
4. Measure length between marks with measuring tape.

Knee Height*

Knee height measurement is highly correlated with upright height. It is useful in those who cannot stand and in those who may have curvatures of the spine.

Steps:

1. Use the left leg for measurements.
2. Bend the left knee and the left ankle to 90-degree angles. A triangle may be used if available.
3. Using knee height calipers, open the caliper and place the fixed part under the heel. Place the sliding blade down against the thigh (approximately 2 inches behind the patella).
4. Measure from the heel to the anterior surface of thigh using a cloth measuring tape.
5. Obtain the measurement and convert it to centimeters by multiplying by 2.54.
6. Formulas to use to calculate estimated knee height:

Men (ht in cm) = 64.19 − (0.04 × Age) + (2.02 × Knee height in cm)

Women (ht in cm) = 84.8 − (0.24 × Age) + (1.83 × Knee height in cm)

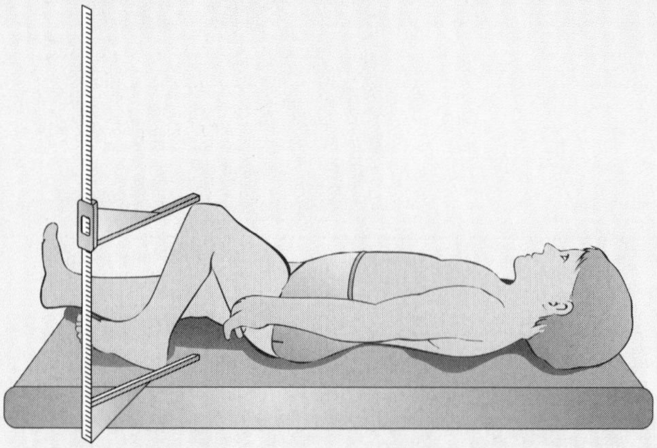

Recommended equations for predicting stature from knee height in adults (18 to 60 years of age) and children (6 to 18 years of age)

GROUP	EQUATION[a]
White men	Stature = 71.85 + (1.88 knee height) R^2 = .65; RMSE[a] = 3.97; SEI[b] = 3.97 cm; CV[c] = 2.28.
Black men	Stature = 73.42 + (1.79 knee height) R^2 = .69; RMSE = 3.60; SEI = 3.60 cm; CV = 2.08.
White women	Stature = 70.25 + (1.87 knee height) − (0.06 age) R^2 = .66; RMSE = 3.60; SEI = 3.60 cm; CV = 2.23.
Black women	Stature = 68.10 + (1.86 knee height) − (0.06 age) R^2 = .69; RMSE = 3.80; SEI = 3.80 cm; CV = 2.36.
White boys	Stature = 40.54 + (2.22 knee height) R^2 = .96; RMSE = 4.16; SEI = 4.21 cm; CV = 2.79.
Black boys	Stature = 39.60 + (2.18 knee height) R^2 = .95; RMSE = 4.44; SEI = 4.58 cm; CV = 2.99.
White girls	Stature = 43.21 + (2.15 knee height) R^2 = .95; RMSE = 3.84; SEI = 3.90 cm; CV = 2.63.
Black girls	Stature = 46.59 + (2.02 knee height) R^2 = .94; RMSE = 4.25; SEI = 4.39 cm; CV = 2.91.

[a]*RMSE,* Root mean square error; [b]*SEI,* standard error for an individual; [c]*CV,* coefficient of variation.

*Data from Chumlea WC et al: *Nutritional assessment of the elderly through anthropometry,* Columbus, Ohio, 1984, Ross Laboratories.

Appendix 16 Determination of Frame Size

Method 1*

Height is recorded without shoes.
Wrist circumference is measured just distal to the styloid process at the wrist crease on the right arm using a tape measure.
The following formula is used:

$$r = \frac{\text{Height (cm)}}{\text{Wrist circumference (cm)}}$$

Frame size can be determined as follows:

MALES	FEMALES
r >10.4 small	r >11.0 small
r = 9.6–10.4 medium	r = 10.1–11.0 medium
r <9.6 large	r <10.1 large

Method 2†

The patient's right arm is extended forward perpendicular to the body, with the arm bent so the angle at the elbow forms 90° with the fingers pointing up and the palm turned away from the body. The greatest breadth across the elbow joint is measured with a sliding caliper along the axis of the upper arm, on the two prominent bones on either side of the elbow. This is recorded as the elbow breadth. The following tables give the elbow breadth measurements for medium-framed men and women of various heights. Measurements lower than those listed indicate a small frame size; higher measurements indicate a large frame size.

MEN		WOMEN	
HEIGHT IN 1″ HEELS	ELBOW BREADTH	HEIGHT IN 1″ HEELS	ELBOW BREADTH
5′2″–5′3″	2½″–2⅞″	4′10″–4′11″	2¼″–2½″
5′4″–5′7″	2⅝″–2⅞″	5′0″–5′3″	2¼″–2½″
5′8″–5′11″	2¾″–3″	5′4″–5′7″	2⅜″–2⅝″
6′0″–6′3″	2¾″–3⅛″	5′8″–5′11″	2⅜″–2⅝″
6′4″	2⅞″–3¼″	6′0″	2½″–2¾″

*From Grant JP: *Handbook of total parenteral nutrition*, Philadelphia, 1980, WB Saunders.
†From Metropolitan Life Insurance Co., 1983.

Appendix 17 Body Mass Index (BMI) Table

BMI	19	20	21	22	23	24	25	26	27	28	29	30	31	32	33	34	35
Height								***Weight (in pounds)***									
4′10″ (58″)	91	96	100	105	110	115	119	124	129	134	138	143	148	153	158	162	167
4′11″ (59″)	94	99	104	109	114	119	124	128	133	138	143	148	153	158	163	168	173
5′ (60″)	97	102	107	112	118	123	128	133	138	143	148	153	158	163	168	174	179
5′1″ (61″)	100	106	111	116	122	127	132	137	143	148	153	158	164	169	174	180	185
5′2″ (62″)	104	109	115	120	126	131	136	142	147	153	158	164	169	175	180	186	191
5′3″ (63″)	107	113	118	124	130	135	141	146	152	158	163	169	175	180	186	191	197
5′4″ (64″)	110	116	122	128	134	140	145	151	157	163	169	174	180	186	192	197	204
5′5″ (65″)	114	120	126	132	138	144	150	156	162	168	174	180	186	192	198	204	210
5′6″ (66″)	118	124	130	136	142	148	155	161	167	173	179	186	192	198	204	210	216
5′7″ (67″)	121	127	134	140	146	153	159	166	172	178	185	191	198	204	211	217	223
5′8″ (68″)	125	131	138	144	151	158	164	171	177	184	190	197	203	210	216	223	230
5′9″ (69″)	128	135	142	149	155	162	169	176	182	189	196	203	209	216	223	230	236
5′10″ (70″)	132	139	146	153	160	167	174	181	188	195	202	209	216	222	229	236	243
5′11″ (71″)	136	143	150	157	165	172	179	186	193	200	208	215	222	229	236	243	250
6′ (72″)	140	147	154	162	169	177	184	191	199	206	213	221	228	235	242	250	258
6′1″ (73″)	144	151	159	166	174	182	189	197	204	212	219	227	235	242	250	257	265
6′2″ (74″)	148	155	163	171	179	186	194	202	210	218	225	233	241	249	256	264	272
6′3″ (75″)	152	160	168	176	184	192	200	208	216	224	232	240	248	256	264	272	279

Data from NIH/National Heart, Lung, and Blood Institute (NHLBI): *Evidence report of clinical guidelines on the identification, evaluation, and treatment of overweight and obesity in adults,* Bethesda, Md, 1998, NIH/NHLBI.

19-24, Minimal health risk; *25-26,* low health risk; *27-29,* moderate health risk; *30-34,* high health risk; *35-39,* very high health risk; *40+,* extremely high health risk.

Appendix 18 Body Mass Index-for-Age Percentiles: Boys, 2 to 20 Years

NAME ____________________

RECORD # ____________

Date	Age	Weight	Stature	BMI*	Comments

***To Calculate BMI**: Weight (kg) ÷ Stature (cm) ÷ Stature (cm) x 10,000
or Weight (lb) ÷ Stature (in) ÷ Stature (in) x 703

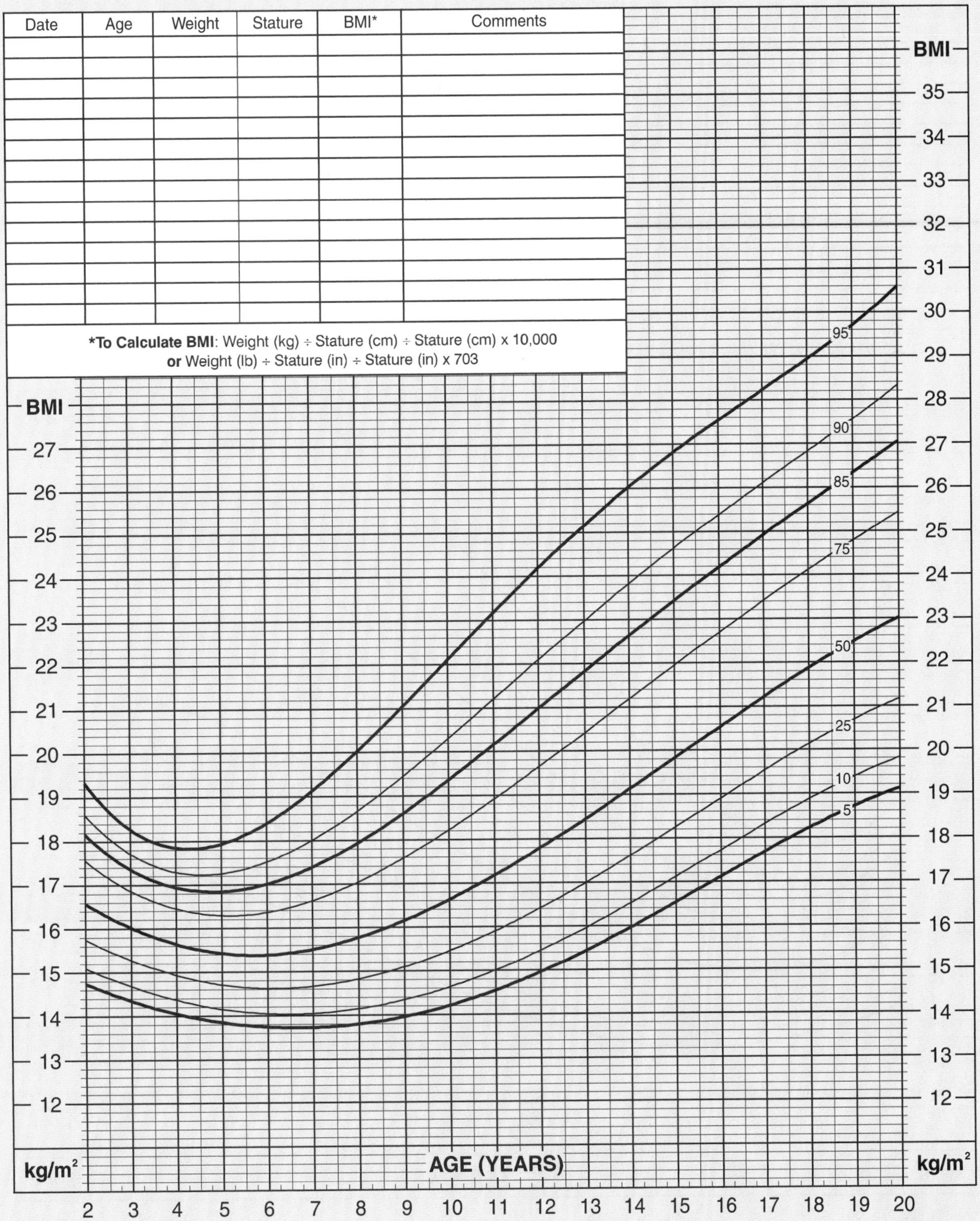

Published May 30, 2000 (modified 10/16/00).
SOURCE: Developed by the National Center for Health Statistics in collaboration with the National Center for Chronic Disease Prevention and Health Promotion (2000).
http://www.cdc.gov/growthcharts

CDC
SAFER•HEALTHIER•PEOPLE

Appendix 19 Body Mass Index-for-Age Percentiles: Girls, 2 to 20 Years

NAME ______________________

RECORD # __________

Date	Age	Weight	Stature	BMI*	Comments

***To Calculate BMI**: Weight (kg) ÷ Stature (cm) ÷ Stature (cm) x 10,000
or Weight (lb) ÷ Stature (in) ÷ Stature (in) x 703

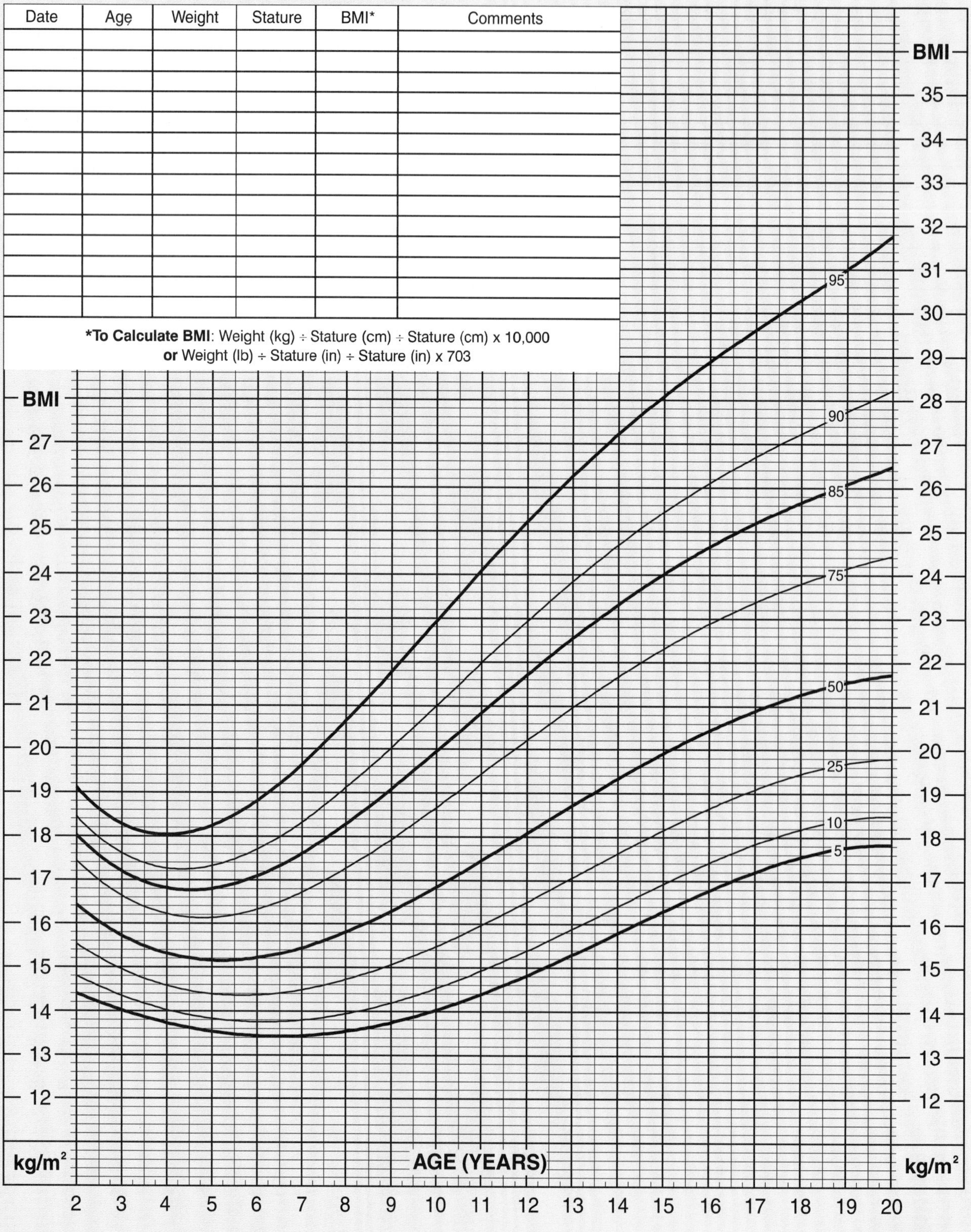

Published May 30, 2000 (modified 10/16/00).
SOURCE: Developed by the National Center for Health Statistics in collaboration with the National Center for Chronic Disease Prevention and Health Promotion (2000).
http://www.cdc.gov/growthcharts

SAFER•HEALTHIER•PEOPLE

Appendix 20A Body Mass Index, Mid-Upper Arm Circumference, Triceps Skinfold Thickness, and Arm Muscle Circumference for Men 50 Years of Age and Older Examined in the Third National Health and Nutrition Examination Survey (1988-1994)

			SELECTED PERCENTILE						
VARIABLE AND AGE GROUP[a]	n	MEAN ± SE[b]	10TH	15TH	25TH	50TH	75TH	85TH	90TH
Body Mass Index[c]									
50-59 yr	855	27.8 ± 0.23	22.6	23.5	24.7	27.2	30.7	32.1	33.5
60-69 yr	1175	27.3 ± 0.18	21.9	23.1	24.4	27.1	30.0	31.7	32.8
70-79 yr	875	26.7 ± 0.21	21.5	22.3	23.8	26.1	29.3	30.7	31.7
80+ yr	699	25.0 ± 0.22	19.8	21.1	22.4	25.0	27.1	28.7	29.5
Mid–Upper Arm Circumference (cm)									
50-59 yr	824	33.7 ± 0.18	29.2	30.0	31.1	33.7	35.6	37.2	37.9
60-69 yr	1126	32.8 ± 0.15	28.4	29.2	30.6	32.7	35.2	36.2	37.0
70-79 yr	832	31.5 ± 0.17	27.5	28.2	29.3	31.3	33.4	35.1	36.1
80+ yr	642	29.5 ± 0.19	25.5	26.2	27.3	29.5	31.5	32.6	33.3
Triceps Skinfold Thickness (mm)									
50-59 yr	813	13.7 ± 0.29	7.5	8.0	9.4	12.6	16.0	18.7	21.8
60-69 yr	1122	14.2 ± 0.25	7.7	8.5	10.1	12.7	17.1	20.2	23.1
70-79 yr	825	13.4 ± 0.28	7.3	7.9	9.0	12.4	16.0	18.8	20.6
80+ yr	641	12.0 ± 0.28	6.6	7.6	8.7	11.2	13.8	16.2	18.0
Arm Muscle Circumference (cm)[d]									
50-59 yr	811	29.2 ± 0.15	25.6	26.2	27.4	29.2	31.1	32.1	33.0
60-69 yr	1119	28.3 ± 0.13	24.9	25.6	26.7	28.4	30.0	30.9	31.4
70-79 yr	824	27.3 ± 0.14	24.4	24.8	25.6	27.2	28.9	30.0	30.5
80+ yr	639	25.7 ± 0.16	22.6	23.2	24.0	25.7	27.5	28.2	28.8

From Kuczmarski MF et al: Descriptive anthropometric reference data for older Americans, *J Am Diet Assoc* 100:59, 2000. Copyright American Dietetic Association.
[a]All racial/ethnic groups included.
[b]SE=Standard error.
[c]Calculated as kg/m^2.
[d]Arm muscle circumference=mid-arm circumference (cm)−π×triceps skinfold thickness (cm).

Appendix 20B Body Mass Index, Mid-Upper Arm Circumference, Triceps Skinfold Thickness, and Arm Muscle Circumference for Women 50 Years of Age and Older Examined in the Third National Health and Nutrition Examination Survey (1988-1994)

VARIABLE AND AGE GROUP[a]	n	MEAN ± SE[b]	SELECTED PERCENTILE 10TH	15TH	25TH	50TH	75TH	85TH	90TH
Body Mass Index[c]									
50-59 yr	1006	28.4 ± 0.31	21.0	22.2	23.6	27.2	32.1	35.1	37.1
60-69 yr	1172	27.6 ± 0.27	20.9	21.8	23.5	26.6	30.8	33.6	35.7
70-79 yr	985	26.9 ± 0.28	20.7	21.4	22.6	25.9	29.9	32.1	34.5
80+ yr	788	25.2 ± 0.26	19.3	20.3	21.7	25.0	28.4	30.0	31.4
Mid–Upper Arm Circumference (cm)									
50-59 yr	970	32.5 ± 0.25	26.6	27.5	28.7	32.0	35.3	37.5	39.2
60-69 yr	1122	31.7 ± 0.21	26.2	26.9	28.3	31.2	34.3	36.5	38.3
70-79 yr	914	30.5 ± 0.23	25.4	26.1	27.4	30.1	33.1	35.1	36.7
80+ yr	712	28.5 ± 0.25	23.0	23.8	25.5	28.4	31.5	33.2	34.0
Triceps Skinfold Thickness (mm)									
50-59 yr	929	26.7 ± 0.40	16.4	18.3	20.6	26.7	32.1	35.2	37.0
60-69 yr	1090	24.2 ± 0.37	14.5	15.9	18.2	24.1	29.7	32.9	34.9
70-79 yr	902	22.3 ± 0.39	12.5	14.0	16.4	21.8	27.7	30.6	32.1
80+ yr	705	18.6 ± 0.42	9.3	11.1	13.1	18.1	23.3	26.4	28.9
Arm Muscle Circumference (cm)[d]									
50-59 yr	927	23.8 ± 0.15	20.4	20.9	21.5	23.3	25.4	26.5	27.8
60-69 yr	1090	23.8 ± 0.12	20.6	21.1	21.9	23.5	25.4	26.6	27.4
70-79 yr	898	23.4 ± 0.14	20.3	20.8	21.6	23.0	24.8	26.3	27.0
80+ yr	703	22.7 ± 0.16	19.3	20.0	20.9	22.6	24.5	25.4	26.0

From Kuczmarski MF et al: Descriptive anthropometric reference data for older Americans, *J Am Diet Assoc* 100:59, 2000. Copyright American Dietetic Association.
[a] All racial/ethnic groups included.
[b] SE=Standard error.
[c] Calculated as kg/m^2.
[d] Arm muscle circumference=mid-arm circumference (cm)−π×triceps skinfold thickness (cm).

Appendix 21 Arm Anthropometry for Children

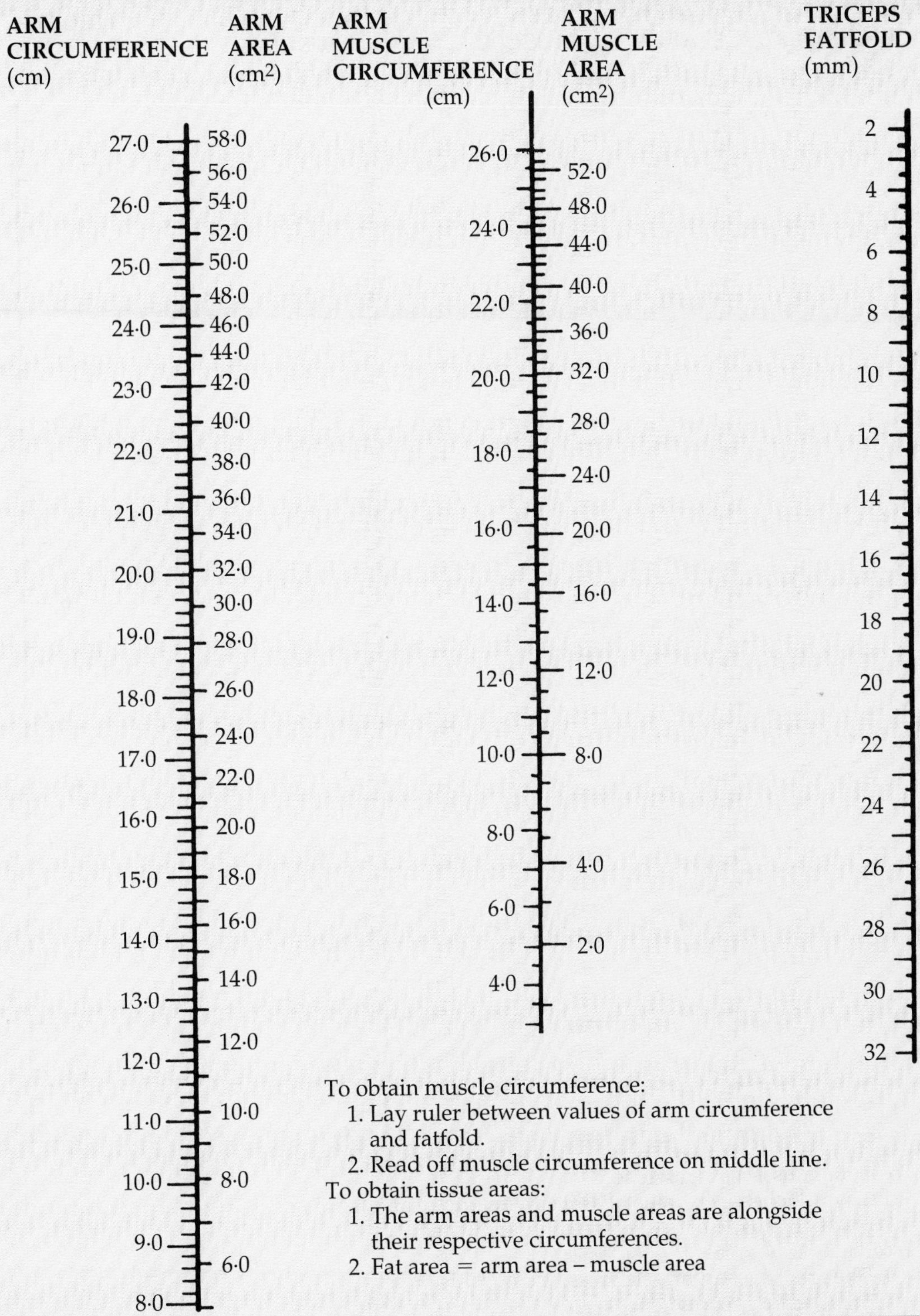

To obtain muscle circumference:

1. Lay ruler between values of arm circumference and fatfold.
2. Read off muscle circumference on middle line.

To obtain tissue areas:

1. The arm areas and muscle areas are alongside their respective circumferences.
2. Fat area = arm area – muscle area

From Gurney JM, Jelliffe DB: Arm anthropometry in nutritional assessment: nomogram for rapid calculation of muscle circumference and cross-sectional muscle fat areas, *Am J Clin Nutr* 26:913, 1973.

Appendix 22 Arm Anthropometry for Adults

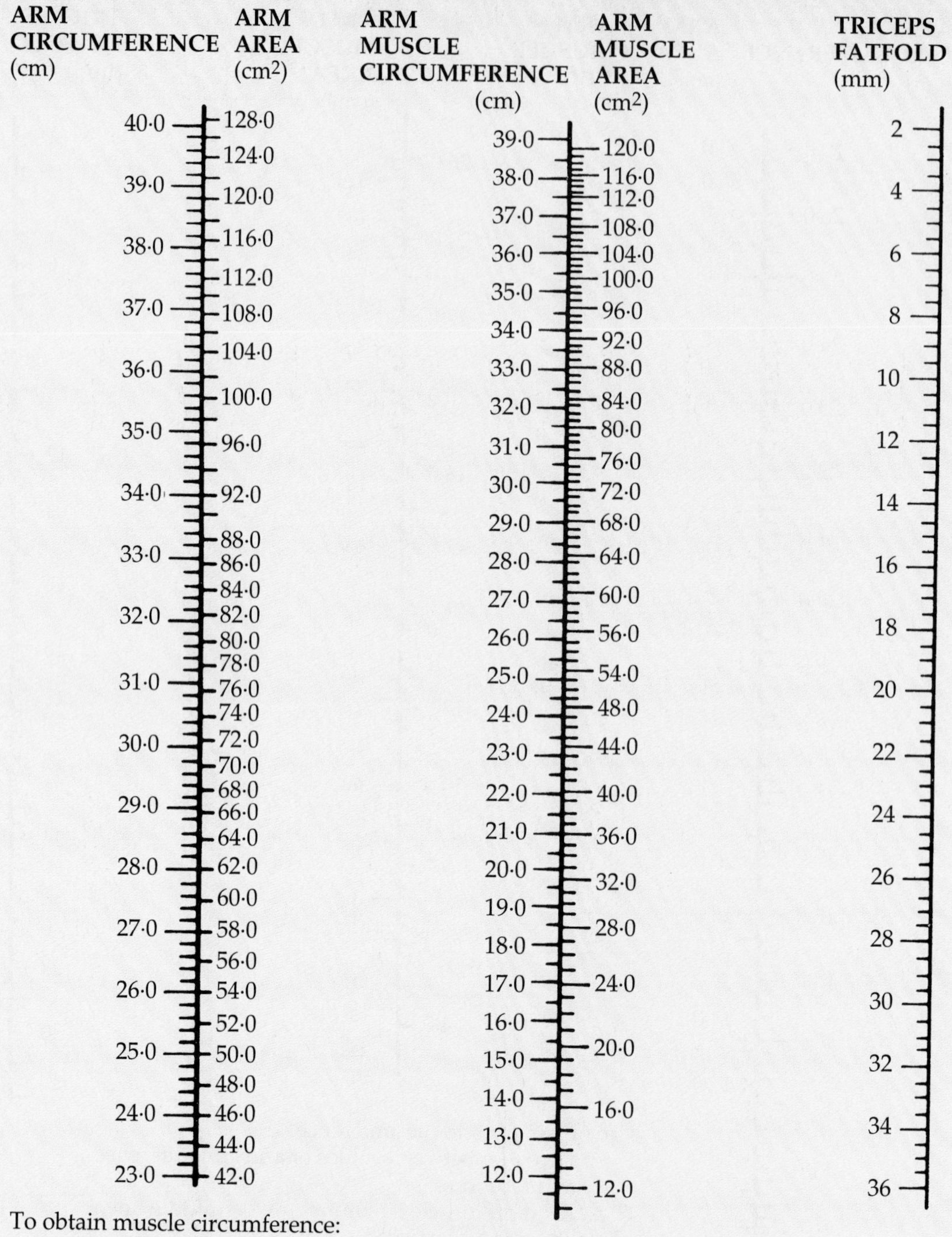

To obtain muscle circumference:

1. Lay ruler between value of arm circumference and fatfold.
2. Read off muscle circumference on middle line.

To obtain tissue areas:

1. The arm area and muscle area are alongside their respective circumferences.
2. Fat area = arm area – muscle area

From Gurney JM, Jelliffe DB: Arm anthropometry in nutritional assessment: nomogram for rapid calculation of muscle circumference and cross-sectional muscle fat areas, *Am J Clin Nutr* 26:913, 1973.

Appendix 23 Means, Standard Deviations, and Percentiles of Weight (kg) by Height (cm) for Males of 2 to 74 Years

				PERCENTILES								
HEIGHT (cm)	N	MEAN	SD	*5*	*10*	*15*	*25*	*50*	*75*	*85*	*90*	*95*
Boys: 2 to 11 Years												
84-86	75	12.1	1.1	10.7	10.9	11.1	11.3	11.9	12.8	13.1	13.5	14.3
87-89	170	12.8	1.1	11.2	11.4	11.7	12.0	12.7	13.4	13.8	14.2	14.6
90-92	207	13.5	1.0	11.9	12.1	12.5	12.8	13.6	14.2	14.6	14.9	15.2
93-95	278	14.4	1.2	12.7	13.0	13.4	13.6	14.3	15.1	15.5	15.8	16.3
96-98	310	15.0	1.3	13.3	13.6	13.8	14.2	15.0	15.6	16.1	16.4	17.0
99-101	300	16.0	1.3	13.9	14.4	14.7	15.1	15.9	16.7	17.2	17.6	18.3
102-104	290	16.9	1.4	15.1	15.4	15.6	15.9	16.8	17.7	18.0	18.5	19.3
105-107	291	17.6	1.6	15.4	15.9	16.2	16.6	17.5	18.4	19.0	19.4	19.8
108-110	298	18.7	1.7	16.7	17.0	17.1	17.6	18.5	19.6	20.1	20.5	21.3
111-113	274	20.0	2.2	17.0	17.8	18.1	18.7	19.6	21.0	21.7	22.4	23.4
114-116	223	20.9	2.2	18.6	19.0	19.2	19.6	20.5	21.7	22.3	22.7	23.6
117-119	199	21.9	2.3	19.0	19.6	20.2	20.5	21.5	23.0	23.8	24.3	26.0
120-122	177	23.3	2.4	19.8	20.8	21.2	21.9	23.1	24.5	25.4	26.0	27.3
123-125	174	25.0	2.8	21.5	22.0	22.7	23.4	24.5	26.2	27.0	28.2	30.0
126-128	185	26.5	3.8	22.6	23.1	23.8	24.3	25.9	27.8	29.4	30.6	32.0
129-131	174	27.6	3.1	23.5	24.4	24.7	25.6	27.3	28.9	30.0	31.0	32.9
132-134	180	29.3	3.5	25.1	25.7	25.8	26.8	28.5	31.0	33.0	34.4	35.4
135-137	175	31.4	4.6	26.2	27.1	27.6	28.5	30.4	33.0	34.9	37.4	41.5
138-140	150	33.5	4.7	28.2	28.9	29.4	30.5	32.3	35.1	37.8	39.9	42.0
141-143	153	36.1	5.0	30.4	31.3	31.8	33.0	34.9	38.2	40.5	43.3	45.4
144-146	114	38.9	6.6	31.6	32.7	33.1	35.1	37.6	41.2	43.9	46.3	50.7
147-149	87	40.9	6.8	33.6	34.3	35.3	35.9	39.2	43.8	47.3	51.5	56.7
Boys: 12 to 17 Years												
144-146	59	38.1	5.5	31.1	32.4	33.6	34.6	36.5	40.3	42.1	46.1	53.0
147-149	77	40.9	7.1	33.6	34.0	34.7	36.5	38.3	43.8	47.4	49.4	59.8
150-152	103	43.4	6.6	36.3	37.2	38.0	38.7	41.4	46.5	51.5	54.7	56.7
153-155	106	45.9	7.9	36.5	38.1	39.1	40.6	43.7	49.7	51.9	55.2	60.9
156-158	113	48.5	9.2	39.9	40.7	41.3	42.5	45.8	50.0	57.9	62.0	67.3
159-161	146	51.1	9.2	40.8	42.9	43.9	45.6	48.6	53.6	60.9	65.4	68.4
162-164	177	54.8	8.9	44.7	45.9	46.9	49.1	53.2	58.4	61.8	64.3	69.1
165-167	197	57.3	9.2	47.1	48.8	49.9	51.3	55.3	61.0	64.8	68.6	73.3
168-170	235	61.4	10.4	49.2	51.4	52.4	55.0	59.9	65.5	69.6	72.5	79.1
171-173	233	62.8	8.8	51.4	53.4	54.8	56.9	61.3	66.1	71.2	73.7	78.2
174-176	202	66.7	10.9	52.3	55.7	57.4	60.0	64.8	71.2	75.5	81.4	89.9
177-179	166	68.8	12.0	55.8	58.7	59.6	61.6	66.3	72.3	75.5	79.6	88.0
180-182	103	71.8	9.7	60.2	60.9	62.1	64.0	70.1	79.5	82.2	85.2	88.7
183-185	64	73.5	9.1	62.4	63.6	65.4	67.8	72.1	77.3	79.4	89.9	91.1
Males: 18 to 74 Years												
153-155	56	64.6	13.0	48.6	51.3	54.5	57.1	62.0	66.8	76.8	80.6	83.5
156-158	140	65.5	11.2	48.3	51.4	54.0	57.4	64.9	72.0	77.3	79.3	86.0
159-161	292	66.2	10.8	49.1	53.8	56.4	59.2	66.0	71.2	76.9	80.2	84.3
162-164	643	68.0	10.5	52.2	55.2	57.0	60.4	67.3	74.5	79.1	81.6	86.9
165-167	1147	70.8	11.6	53.0	56.6	59.6	62.7	70.3	77.6	82.3	85.2	90.1
168-170	1582	73.5	12.0	55.9	58.6	61.3	65.9	72.7	80.2	84.5	87.9	93.4
171-173	2047	76.1	12.5	58.2	61.3	63.6	67.6	75.1	83.2	88.1	92.0	97.8
174-176	2053	78.3	12.7	60.0	63.8	66.1	69.5	77.3	84.9	90.1	93.8	99.7
177-179	1750	80.3	12.8	61.9	65.1	67.5	71.4	79.4	87.3	92.6	96.5	102.6
180-182	1252	82.6	13.6	63.4	67.3	69.6	72.9	81.4	90.1	95.0	99.4	105.7
183-185	833	85.2	13.9	65.1	69.2	71.5	75.3	83.3	93.4	99.1	103.2	110.4
186-188	398	88.0	13.3	68.9	72.3	74.8	79.4	86.6	95.1	100.4	103.5	109.8
189-191	161	92.0	16.0	71.3	75.3	77.8	80.7	89.9	99.4	105.0	110.8	123.7
192-194	66	95.9	15.8	71.8	78.6	80.2	84.8	94.2	105.2	109.1	111.8	123.8

From Frisancho AR: *Anthropometric standards for the assessment of growth and nutritional status,* Ann Arbor, 1990, The University of Michigan Press.

Appendix 24 Means, Standard Deviations, and Percentiles of Weight (kg) by Height (cm) for Females of 2 to 74 Years

HEIGHT (cm)	N	MEAN	SD	PERCENTILES 5	10	15	25	50	75	85	90	95
Girls: 2 to 10 Years												
81-83	36	11.2	.8	10.1	10.2	10.3	10.4	11.0	11.7	12.1	12.6	12.6
84-86	118	11.9	.9	10.5	10.8	11.0	11.3	12.0	12.5	12.7	13.0	13.6
87-89	156	12.5	1.2	11.0	11.3	11.6	11.8	12.4	13.0	13.6	13.8	14.6
90-92	229	13.2	1.2	11.6	11.8	12.0	12.3	13.0	13.8	14.3	14.6	15.2
93-95	259	13.9	1.2	12.0	12.6	12.8	13.1	13.8	14.6	15.1	15.5	16.1
96-98	275	15.0	1.3	13.1	13.5	13.7	14.1	14.9	15.6	16.3	16.7	17.2
99-101	272	15.8	1.6	13.8	14.1	14.3	14.6	15.5	16.6	17.2	17.6	18.4
102-104	278	16.6	2.0	14.2	14.6	15.0	15.5	16.4	17.3	18.0	18.5	19.4
105-107	270	17.6	1.6	15.3	15.8	16.1	16.6	17.3	18.4	19.2	19.4	20.1
108-110	275	18.3	1.6	15.9	16.6	16.8	17.2	18.1	19.2	20.0	20.4	21.1
111-113	251	19.4	1.9	16.6	17.1	17.3	17.9	19.4	20.4	21.2	21.8	22.8
114-116	215	20.7	2.5	17.5	18.3	18.6	19.0	20.2	21.8	22.9	23.9	25.7
117-119	191	21.9	2.6	19.0	19.4	19.5	20.2	21.4	23.0	24.0	24.8	26.6
120-122	181	23.1	2.5	20.1	20.4	20.9	21.5	22.6	24.0	25.3	26.2	27.7
123-125	162	24.5	2.5	21.2	21.8	22.3	22.8	24.0	25.9	26.5	27.2	29.0
126-128	172	26.2	3.1	22.6	23.0	23.4	23.9	25.6	27.7	29.4	30.0	31.5
129-131	157	28.0	3.8	23.6	24.3	24.8	25.6	27.3	29.4	31.1	33.4	36.6
132-134	148	30.3	4.4	25.1	25.8	26.2	27.0	29.4	32.3	34.5	37.2	39.9
135-137	135	32.1	5.4	25.6	27.2	27.7	28.3	30.8	33.9	35.8	41.6	44.1
138-140	124	34.6	7.3	27.6	28.8	29.1	30.6	32.5	35.5	40.9	43.5	47.5
141-143	97	36.0	6.3	28.8	29.8	30.7	32.2	34.8	37.9	41.3	45.6	49.9
144-146	65	39.2	7.0	31.0	31.9	32.9	34.5	37.6	42.9	45.3	48.4	51.8
147-149	45	40.0	7.3	30.7	32.3	34.0	35.0	38.3	44.2	48.0	50.8	54.8
Girls: 11 to 17 Years												
141-143	54	37.1	7.8	28.9	29.8	31.1	32.2	34.9	38.6	42.4	45.7	59.5
144-146	67	38.5	6.8	30.4	30.8	31.6	32.9	38.4	41.4	44.1	46.5	52.4
147-149	127	43.4	10.0	32.7	34.3	35.4	37.0	40.7	46.7	51.3	56.4	61.2
150-152	180	45.8	9.1	34.7	36.3	37.4	39.5	44.1	49.9	54.3	56.1	61.9
153-155	235	48.8	8.9	38.0	39.5	40.6	43.1	46.7	53.6	56.5	60.0	66.3
156-158	352	52.3	10.4	39.7	41.7	43.1	45.1	49.9	57.5	62.5	66.0	72.3
159-161	372	55.1	11.0	42.2	44.3	46.0	48.3	52.8	59.2	62.9	68.4	77.6
162-164	344	56.6	9.9	44.9	46.6	47.5	50.2	54.4	60.6	65.3	68.6	73.8
165-167	243	60.0	12.5	46.3	48.8	50.1	52.8	57.6	62.7	69.4	74.7	84.7
168-170	124	61.2	10.8	48.9	49.2	51.1	53.5	59.0	65.7	73.4	75.1	82.4
171-173	74	67.5	15.0	53.0	54.3	54.9	57.7	62.1	72.3	80.1	89.1	104.2
Females: 18 to 74 Years												
141-143	64	55.9	10.2	39.2	41.3	43.9	49.0	56.5	63.3	64.9	67.7	76.6
144-146	178	57.1	14.2	38.7	42.0	44.3	48.1	54.3	64.4	71.3	74.6	82.0
147-149	430	59.4	13.2	41.5	44.6	46.8	50.1	56.9	66.9	71.9	76.1	84.8
150-152	928	61.1	13.2	43.1	46.5	48.1	51.5	59.0	68.3	74.3	78.4	86.2
153-155	1685	63.0	13.7	45.3	47.5	49.8	53.2	60.7	70.2	77.3	81.6	88.6
156-158	2670	63.8	14.6	46.6	49.1	50.8	53.5	60.7	70.9	77.1	82.3	90.0
159-161	3041	65.3	14.5	47.7	50.2	52.0	55.2	62.3	72.6	79.4	84.6	92.9
162-164	2849	66.9	14.6	49.4	51.5	53.4	56.6	63.5	74.2	81.4	86.0	94.9
165-167	2327	68.2	15.3	50.3	52.8	54.9	57.8	64.5	74.7	82.4	88.6	98.2
168-170	1327	69.5	15.1	52.5	54.7	56.5	59.2	65.4	76.1	83.5	90.1	99.4
171-173	685	71.8	15.8	54.1	55.9	57.9	60.5	67.6	78.9	86.1	93.9	105.0
174-176	334	72.9	17.3	56.1	57.9	59.6	62.3	68.4	77.6	85.7	93.1	106.9
177-179	97	75.3	16.5	57.6	59.9	60.7	64.4	71.2	81.8	89.6	102.1	112.8

From Frisancho AR: *Anthropometric standards for the assessment of growth and nutritional status,* Ann Arbor, 1990, The University of Michigan Press.

Appendix 25 Means, Standard Deviations, and Percentiles of Weight (kg) by Age for Adult Males of Small, Medium, and Large Frames

				PERCENTILES								
AGE (yr)	N	MEAN	SD	5	10	15	25	50	75	85	90	95
Males With Small Frames												
18.0-24.9	444	69.9	11.5	54.5	57.4	59.0	62.3	68.3	76.1	80.5	83.8	89.8
25.0-29.9	318	73.4	12.0	56.7	60.3	61.9	65.1	71.8	79.4	84.7	87.5	97.9
30.0-34.9	239	75.7	12.5	57.9	61.6	63.2	67.0	74.6	83.1	87.8	92.9	98.0
35.0-39.9	212	75.5	12.0	56.0	59.9	62.1	66.6	75.9	83.5	87.8	91.4	96.0
40.0-44.9	210	78.3	12.4	58.8	62.8	65.4	70.3	76.1	86.3	92.3	94.8	101.0
45.0-49.9	220	76.3	11.7	57.7	60.9	63.2	67.6	76.2	83.6	89.0	92.1	95.8
50.0-54.9	225	75.4	11.9	57.3	60.2	64.5	67.1	74.7	82.8	88.2	90.5	99.3
55.0-59.9	204	74.5	12.0	54.7	58.2	61.5	66.7	74.8	81.9	87.2	90.6	94.7
60.0-64.9	318	74.0	12.3	54.2	59.2	62.5	65.9	73.4	80.7	85.7	88.4	93.8
65.0-69.9	446	70.7	12.1	50.8	55.4	57.8	61.9	70.3	79.0	83.3	86.8	92.4
70.0-74.9	315	70.5	12.5	49.9	54.4	57.3	61.9	70.1	78.4	83.0	85.5	92.8
Males With Medium Frames												
18.0-24.9	877	74.0	12.7	57.5	60.6	62.3	65.3	71.5	80.3	86.0	91.6	99.6
25.0-29.9	627	77.0	13.2	58.5	61.8	64.5	68.4	75.9	84.1	88.3	92.4	100.4
30.0-34.9	473	78.5	12.9	59.8	63.0	65.9	69.5	77.8	85.8	91.1	93.8	98.8
35.0-39.9	419	80.5	12.8	58.7	64.8	68.4	72.9	80.4	87.4	91.5	95.9	102.5
40.0-44.9	414	80.1	12.4	60.8	64.2	67.9	71.9	79.3	88.1	92.4	96.8	102.6
45.0-49.9	436	80.7	13.0	60.3	65.1	67.1	71.9	79.8	88.7	93.3	96.7	101.3
50.0-54.9	441	79.0	13.7	58.4	62.5	65.8	70.0	78.3	86.3	91.7	96.6	103.1
55.0-59.9	404	78.8	12.7	59.9	64.5	66.7	70.5	77.9	85.3	91.1	95.4	102.2
60.0-64.9	629	76.7	11.9	58.3	61.5	64.5	68.7	76.3	84.4	88.4	91.6	97.8
65.0-69.9	886	75.0	12.2	56.1	59.5	62.5	66.9	74.5	82.9	86.9	90.8	97.2
70.0-74.9	627	73.6	12.2	54.3	58.3	61.1	65.5	72.6	81.0	86.1	89.8	93.9
Males With Large Frames												
18.0-24.9	433	77.5	15.4	58.2	61.3	62.6	67.4	74.7	85.0	91.2	95.0	104.9
25.0-29.9	310	84.3	17.4	61.2	66.0	68.4	72.6	82.2	91.6	99.8	102.8	115.2
30.0-34.9	233	86.5	16.6	65.5	68.4	70.2	75.2	85.4	94.0	101.6	106.7	116.7
35.0-39.9	206	85.0	15.0	59.6	67.4	71.8	75.4	84.1	93.1	98.9	104.1	113.3
40.0-44.9	205	85.8	16.4	63.7	67.7	68.8	74.3	84.9	94.5	100.3	107.4	113.3
45.0-49.9	215	85.5	16.5	62.7	67.0	69.4	74.0	84.0	94.0	101.3	105.9	119.2
50.0-54.9	216	84.7	14.7	64.4	66.9	68.8	73.3	83.1	94.3	101.7	103.6	108.4
55.0-59.9	199	85.7	15.7	64.5	67.1	70.3	74.8	84.5	93.5	100.5	103.5	121.1
60.0-64.9	313	82.1	14.6	61.5	66.6	69.3	73.1	80.7	89.4	94.5	98.9	107.7
65.0-69.9	440	79.5	13.8	57.0	61.5	64.9	70.4	78.9	87.8	93.0	96.3	104.0
70.0-74.9	310	77.1	13.8	55.3	59.9	63.6	67.9	76.7	84.1	90.5	95.8	101.4

From Frisancho AR: *Anthropometric standards for the assessment of growth and nutritional status,* Ann Arbor, 1990, The University of Michigan Press.

Appendix 26 Means, Standard Deviations, and Percentiles of Weight (kg) by Age for Adult Females of Small, Medium, and Large Frames

				PERCENTILES								
AGE (yr)	N	MEAN	SD	*5*	*10*	*15*	*25*	*50*	*75*	*85*	*90*	*95*
Females With Small Frames												
28.0-24.9	652	56.2	8.7	44.0	46.1	48.0	50.3	55.1	60.9	64.4	66.9	71.5
25.0-29.9	487	56.9	9.5	44.1	47.3	48.6	50.9	55.6	61.1	64.5	67.6	72.6
30.0-34.9	413	59.1	10.0	45.7	48.2	50.0	52.7	57.6	63.4	68.1	71.8	77.7
35.0-39.9	369	61.1	11.4	45.8	48.2	50.8	53.4	59.5	66.7	71.9	76.0	79.5
40.0-44.9	353	60.6	9.4	48.1	50.3	51.8	54.5	59.1	66.1	70.0	73.6	80.3
45.0-49.9	244	61.4	11.1	46.3	47.8	50.8	53.6	60.3	67.3	71.4	75.1	80.8
50.0-54.9	257	61.3	10.8	46.3	49.1	51.7	54.5	60.3	66.9	71.0	73.1	78.4
55.0-59.9	224	61.3	11.1	47.3	49.5	52.2	54.7	59.9	65.3	70.2	73.6	81.5
60.0-64.9	351	61.9	11.0	46.4	48.9	50.6	54.2	60.9	68.5	71.7	74.0	82.2
65.0-69.9	491	61.1	10.7	44.9	48.4	50.7	53.6	60.2	67.4	71.7	74.0	79.3
70.0-74.9	369	60.6	12.1	42.6	45.9	48.5	51.6	60.2	67.0	72.3	75.4	81.0
Females With Medium Frames												
18.0-24.9	1297	59.5	10.4	46.0	48.4	50.0	52.5	58.1	64.4	69.5	72.8	78.4
25.0-29.9	967	60.9	11.5	46.9	49.1	50.6	53.0	58.6	66.3	72.2	76.9	83.0
30.0-34.9	815	63.5	13.4	47.2	50.0	51.7	54.3	60.7	69.3	76.7	80.6	87.2
35.0-39.9	730	64.1	12.1	49.2	51.7	53.0	56.1	61.8	69.8	74.7	79.4	87.9
40.0-44.9	700	65.6	13.3	48.8	51.3	53.6	57.0	62.8	71.8	77.3	82.4	92.1
45.0-49.9	484	65.8	13.4	48.3	51.4	53.3	56.4	63.4	72.2	77.8	83.1	91.6
50.0-54.9	504	66.4	12.2	48.9	52.0	54.4	57.7	64.4	73.1	79.3	82.8	89.7
55.0-59.9	444	68.0	15.3	48.2	51.1	54.3	58.1	66.3	74.8	81.0	86.2	92.1
60.0-64.9	695	66.2	12.4	49.1	52.3	54.0	57.5	64.5	73.5	78.1	82.2	89.0
65.0-69.9	973	66.2	12.7	48.1	51.4	53.6	57.1	64.9	73.1	78.7	82.4	88.8
70.0-74.9	731	64.3	11.9	46.8	50.5	52.5	56.8	62.9	70.8	76.9	80.2	84.7
Females With Large Frames												
18.0-24.9	642	68.0	17.2	48.9	51.3	53.1	56.3	62.9	76.2	83.8	89.0	102.7
25.0-29.9	480	72.6	17.7	49.9	53.4	55.6	59.3	68.7	82.9	90.9	98.8	105.0
30.0-34.9	402	76.4	19.7	51.1	54.9	57.7	61.1	72.7	88.4	97.3	102.8	111.9
35.0-39.9	361	79.1	19.5	52.8	56.1	59.1	64.5	76.7	90.4	98.1	106.0	117.9
40.0-44.9	346	79.7	19.8	53.4	57.3	60.7	65.7	77.1	91.3	99.2	104.9	114.2
45.0-49.9	240	80.1	19.6	54.5	60.1	63.2	66.7	76.8	86.6	97.6	105.0	116.9
50.0-54.9	250	79.4	16.9	55.6	60.0	63.0	67.8	77.7	88.8	97.1	103.3	112.1
55.0-59.9	218	79.8	17.5	56.4	60.2	62.5	67.6	77.6	89.9	97.0	101.6	111.3
60.0-64.9	346	77.8	15.6	56.0	59.4	62.8	66.8	76.8	85.7	92.8	100.0	104.8
65.0-69.9	484	76.6	15.4	55.3	59.4	62.0	65.8	74.5	84.6	91.7	97.8	105.0
70.0-74.9	363	74.9	14.0	53.5	57.9	60.9	65.8	74.5	82.7	87.9	91.3	99.1

From Frisancho AR: *Anthropometric standards for the assessment of growth and nutritional status,* Ann Arbor, 1990, The University of Michigan Press.

Appendix 27 Means, Standard Deviations, and Percentiles of Triceps Skinfold Thickness (mm) by Age for Males and Females of 1 to 50 Years

				PERCENTILES								
AGE (yr)	N	MEAN	SD	*5*	*10*	*15*	*25*	*50*	*75*	*85*	*90*	*95*
Males												
1.0-1.9	681	10.4	2.9	6.5	7.0	7.5	8.0	10.0	12.0	13.0	14.0	15.5
2.0-2.9	677	10.0	2.9	6.0	6.5	7.0	8.0	10.0	12.0	13.0	14.0	15.0
3.0-3.9	717	9.9	2.7	6.0	7.0	7.0	8.0	9.5	11.5	12.5	13.5	15.0
4.0-4.9	708	9.2	2.7	5.5	6.5	7.0	7.5	9.0	11.0	12.0	12.5	14.0
5.0-5.9	677	8.9	3.1	5.0	6.0	6.0	7.0	8.0	10.0	11.5	13.0	14.5
6.0-6.9	298	8.9	3.8	5.0	5.5	6.0	6.5	8.0	10.0	12.0	13.0	16.0
7.0-7.9	312	9.0	4.0	4.5	5.0	6.0	6.0	8.0	10.5	12.5	14.0	16.0
8.0-8.9	296	9.6	4.4	5.0	5.5	6.0	7.0	8.5	11.0	13.0	16.0	19.0
9.0-9.9	322	10.2	5.1	5.0	5.5	6.0	6.5	9.0	12.5	15.5	17.0	20.0
10.0-10.9	334	11.5	5.7	5.0	6.0	6.0	7.5	10.0	14.0	17.0	20.0	24.0
11.0-11.9	324	12.5	7.0	5.0	6.0	6.5	7.5	10.0	16.0	19.5	23.0	27.0
12.0-12.9	348	12.2	6.8	4.5	6.0	6.0	7.5	10.5	14.5	18.0	22.5	27.5
13.0-13.9	350	11.0	6.7	4.5	5.0	5.5	7.0	9.0	13.0	17.0	20.5	25.0
14.0-14.9	358	10.4	6.5	4.0	5.0	5.0	6.0	8.5	12.5	15.0	18.0	23.5
15.0-15.9	356	9.8	6.5	5.0	5.0	5.0	6.0	7.5	11.0	15.0	18.0	23.5
16.0-16.9	350	10.0	5.9	4.0	5.0	5.1	6.0	8.0	12.0	14.0	17.0	23.0
17.0-17.9	337	9.1	5.3	4.0	5.0	5.0	6.0	7.0	11.0	13.5	16.0	19.5
18.0-24.9	1752	11.3	6.4	4.0	5.0	5.5	6.5	10.0	14.5	17.5	20.0	23.5
25.0-29.9	1251	12.2	6.7	4.0	5.0	6.0	7.0	11.0	15.5	19.0	21.5	25.0
30.0-34.9	941	13.1	6.7	4.5	6.0	6.5	8.0	12.0	16.5	20.0	22.0	25.0
35.0-39.9	832	12.9	6.2	4.5	6.0	7.0	8.5	12.0	16.0	18.5	20.5	24.5
40.0-44.9	828	13.0	6.6	5.0	6.0	6.9	8.0	12.0	16.0	19.0	21.5	26.0
45.0-49.9	867	12.9	6.4	5.0	6.0	7.0	8.0	12.0	16.0	19.0	21.0	25.0
Females												
1.0-1.9	622	10.4	3.1	6.0	7.0	7.0	8.0	10.0	12.0	13.0	14.0	16.0
2.0-2.9	614	10.5	2.9	6.0	7.0	7.5	8.5	10.0	12.0	13.5	14.5	16.0
3.0-3.9	652	10.4	2.9	6.0	7.0	7.5	8.5	10.0	12.0	13.0	14.0	16.0
4.0-4.9	681	10.3	3.0	6.0	7.0	7.5	8.0	10.0	12.0	13.0	14.0	15.5
5.0-5.9	673	10.4	3.5	5.5	7.0	7.0	8.0	10.0	12.0	13.5	15.0	17.0
6.0-6.9	296	10.4	3.7	6.0	6.5	7.0	8.0	10.0	12.0	13.0	15.0	17.0
7.0-7.9	330	11.1	4.2	6.0	7.0	7.0	8.0	10.5	12.5	15.0	16.0	19.0
8.0-8.9	276	12.1	5.4	6.0	7.0	7.5	8.5	11.0	14.5	17.0	18.0	22.5
9.0-9.9	322	13.4	5.9	6.5	7.0	8.0	9.0	12.0	16.0	19.0	21.0	25.0
10.0-10.9	329	13.9	6.1	7.0	8.0	8.0	9.0	12.5	17.5	20.0	22.5	27.0
11.0-11.9	302	15.0	6.8	7.0	8.0	8.5	10.0	13.0	18.0	21.5	24.0	29.0
12.0-12.9	323	15.1	6.3	7.0	8.0	9.0	11.0	14.0	18.5	21.5	24.0	27.5
13.0-13.9	360	16.4	7.4	7.0	8.0	9.0	11.0	15.0	20.0	24.0	25.0	30.0
14.0-14.9	370	17.1	7.3	8.0	9.0	10.0	11.5	16.0	21.0	23.5	26.5	32.0
15.0-15.9	309	17.3	7.4	8.0	9.5	10.5	12.0	16.5	20.5	23.0	26.0	32.5
16.0-16.9	343	19.2	7.0	10.5	11.5	12.0	14.0	18.0	23.0	26.0	29.0	32.5
17.0-17.9	291	19.1	8.0	9.0	10.0	12.0	13.0	18.0	24.0	26.5	29.0	34.5
18.0-24.9	2588	20.0	8.2	9.0	11.0	12.0	14.0	18.5	24.5	28.5	31.0	36.0
25.0-29.9	1921	21.7	8.8	10.0	12.0	13.0	15.0	20.0	26.5	31.0	34.0	38.0
30.0-34.9	1619	23.7	9.2	10.5	13.0	15.0	17.0	22.5	29.5	33.0	35.5	41.5
35.0-39.9	1453	24.7	9.3	11.0	13.0	15.5	18.0	23.5	30.0	35.0	37.0	41.0
40.0-44.9	1391	25.1	9.0	12.0	14.0	16.0	19.0	24.5	30.5	35.0	37.0	41.0
45.0-49.9	962	26.1	9.3	12.0	14.5	16.5	19.5	25.5	32.0	35.5	38.0	42.5

From Frisancho AR: *Anthropometric standards for the assessment of growth and nutritional status,* Ann Arbor, 1990, The University of Michigan Press.

Appendix 28 Means, Standard Deviations, and Percentiles of Upper Arm Muscle Area (cm^2) by Height (cm) for Boys and Girls of 2 to 17 Years

				PERCENTILES								
HEIGHT (cm)	N	MEAN	SD	*5*	*10*	*15*	*25*	*50*	*75*	*85*	*90*	*95*
Boys: 2 to 11 Years												
87-092	94	12.9	2.2	9.3	10.4	10.6	11.2	12.9	14.2	15.0	15.8	16.5
93-098	373	13.7	2.4	10.2	10.9	11.2	12.1	13.5	15.3	15.9	16.5	17.0
99-104	587	14.6	3.1	10.9	11.7	12.2	13.0	14.5	15.9	16.5	17.1	18.4
105-110	587	15.7	3.1	12.0	12.8	13.3	14.1	15.4	17.0	17.8	18.6	19.8
111-116	588	16.7	2.9	12.6	13.6	14.3	15.0	16.6	18.1	18.9	19.6	20.7
117-122	496	18.1	3.5	14.1	14.5	15.0	16.1	17.7	19.7	20.7	21.6	23.4
123-128	376	19.5	3.6	15.0	15.9	16.3	17.4	19.2	21.2	22.3	23.2	24.2
129-134	359	21.6	4.3	16.1	17.3	18.4	19.3	21.1	23.2	24.7	25.3	27.9
135-140	354	22.9	4.2	17.2	18.1	18.9	20.4	22.6	24.9	26.1	27.2	30.2
141-146	325	25.1	5.2	19.3	20.1	20.8	21.9	24.0	27.2	29.0	30.5	34.0
147-152	266	27.5	4.8	21.2	22.4	23.2	24.8	27.0	29.8	31.8	32.9	34.4
153-158	150	29.8	7.2	22.3	23.2	24.3	25.4	28.4	32.2	34.8	36.9	40.1
159-164	65	32.5	6.5	23.7	24.5	25.3	27.5	31.9	35.6	39.7	41.4	44.5
Boys: 12 to 17 Years												
141-146	31	26.8	4.7	20.7	21.4	22.7	24.1	25.6	30.3	32.8	33.9	36.3
147-152	90	28.2	4.1	22.4	23.4	24.1	25.6	27.5	30.2	33.1	34.2	36.1
153-158	181	31.4	6.4	22.7	24.9	26.1	27.5	30.4	34.1	36.4	39.1	41.5
159-164	218	35.0	7.7	23.7	26.7	27.8	30.2	34.1	38.6	41.5	44.3	48.4
165-170	323	40.8	9.3	28.1	29.7	31.5	34.2	40.0	45.6	49.0	52.9	58.9
171-176	431	46.6	9.9	32.8	35.2	36.6	39.5	45.8	52.6	56.0	59.1	66.0
177-182	431	50.3	9.3	36.1	38.7	40.8	43.4	49.5	56.4	59.4	62.6	65.9
183-188	269	53.4	11.2	38.3	41.3	42.8	46.1	52.6	57.8	63.0	67.5	74.3
189-194	99	55.4	9.9	41.4	44.2	45.7	48.9	53.9	60.3	65.0	68.5	74.0
Girls: 2 to 10 Years												
87-092	154	12.6	2.1	9.5	10.1	10.5	11.0	12.6	14.2	14.8	15.5	16.2
93-098	384	13.2	2.1	10.1	10.7	11.0	11.8	13.2	14.4	15.3	15.8	16.9
99-104	533	14.1	2.3	10.6	11.2	11.7	12.5	14.0	15.5	16.4	16.9	18.0
105-110	550	14.8	2.4	11.3	11.9	12.4	13.2	14.6	16.3	17.3	17.9	18.9
111-116	543	15.9	2.8	12.3	13.0	13.5	14.2	15.7	17.4	18.4	19.1	20.3
117-122	465	17.0	2.8	13.0	13.9	14.4	15.2	16.7	18.5	19.6	20.3	21.4
123-128	372	18.2	2.8	14.2	15.0	15.5	16.2	17.9	19.6	20.8	21.6	22.9
129-134	333	20.1	4.6	15.3	16.1	16.8	17.6	19.7	21.7	22.9	23.8	25.4
135-140	303	21.6	4.2	16.1	17.4	18.1	19.2	21.1	23.8	24.8	26.3	27.9
141-146	258	23.3	4.0	17.6	18.5	19.5	20.5	23.0	25.8	27.9	28.8	30.6
147-152	161	25.2	5.2	18.5	20.0	20.7	21.7	24.4	27.8	30.0	31.2	32.9
153-158	66	26.7	6.7	19.4	20.1	22.4	23.0	25.4	29.2	31.8	34.0	38.2
Girls: 11 to 17 Years												
141-146	53	23.8	4.4	17.1	19.3	19.5	21.0	23.4	25.5	27.9	28.6	33.4
147-152	119	25.2	4.6	18.5	19.7	20.9	22.0	24.3	28.0	29.8	30.3	34.4
153-158	305	29.1	6.4	20.8	22.0	23.0	24.7	28.3	32.9	35.0	37.5	39.2
159-164	587	32.2	7.1	23.3	24.8	26.0	27.7	31.2	35.7	38.0	40.1	43.5
165-170	715	34.2	7.4	25.0	26.6	27.8	29.5	33.2	37.6	40.2	42.8	46.9
171-176	367	34.9	8.0	25.9	27.1	28.0	29.9	33.7	38.0	41.2	43.5	47.6
177-182	113	37.8	8.4	28.6	29.5	30.5	31.7	35.9	41.1	45.9	47.8	58.2

From Frisancho AR: *Anthropometric standards for the assessment of growth and nutritional status,* Ann Arbor, 1990, The University of Michigan Press.

Appendix 29 Means, Standard Deviations, and Percentiles of Upper Arm Muscle Area (cm^2) by Age for Adult Males of Small, Medium, and Large Frames

AGE (yr)	N	MEAN	SD	PERCENTILES 5	10	15	25	50	75	85	90	95
Males With Small Frames												
18.0-24.9	443	45.6	10.6	30.8	33.8	35.8	38.7	44.6	51.3	55.2	58.1	63.2
25.0-29.9	318	48.2	9.8	33.5	36.8	39.2	41.8	47.6	53.5	57.7	61.2	63.7
30.0-34.9	237	49.6	10.2	35.0	37.5	38.9	42.0	48.8	56.4	60.0	62.7	66.9
35.0-39.9	212	51.2	10.4	34.7	38.7	40.9	44.1	50.7	57.5	61.7	63.8	70.0
40.0-44.9	210	51.5	10.1	34.9	38.1	40.6	44.2	51.6	58.2	61.6	64.5	66.9
45.0-49.9	220	49.7	10.8	32.8	36.5	38.9	42.9	49.1	55.7	59.5	63.3	68.8
50.0-54.9	225	49.1	11.2	33.8	36.0	38.2	41.5	47.6	55.5	60.7	63.8	69.3
55.0-59.9	204	47.9	10.1	31.2	35.4	37.8	41.7	47.8	54.3	58.8	61.4	64.2
60.0-64.9	318	48.7	11.2	32.5	36.3	38.7	41.4	48.0	54.6	59.6	62.2	68.0
65.0-69.9	446	45.1	10.7	26.7	31.5	34.7	37.6	44.7	52.5	56.1	58.5	62.7
70.0-74.9	314	43.5	10.3	27.7	30.8	32.9	36.1	43.4	49.6	53.4	56.6	59.9
Males With Medium Frames												
18.0-24.9	875	50.5	10.5	35.5	38.2	40.8	43.6	49.5	56.5	60.8	63.2	69.3
25.0-29.9	626	54.0	11.3	37.0	40.1	42.9	46.8	53.2	60.9	65.6	67.7	73.0
30.0-34.9	472	55.0	10.4	38.5	42.2	44.8	48.0	54.3	61.8	65.7	68.6	72.7
35.0-39.9	416	56.7	11.7	39.9	43.1	45.2	48.8	55.9	64.0	69.0	71.6	75.6
40.0-44.9	413	56.7	11.0	39.2	42.6	45.8	49.2	56.3	64.0	68.0	71.1	74.4
45.0-49.9	433	56.6	11.2	39.0	42.6	45.6	49.4	55.9	63.7	69.6	72.8	76.2
50.0-54.9	440	55.3	11.7	37.6	41.8	44.5	47.7	54.2	62.5	65.9	69.6	74.1
55.0-59.9	403	55.4	10.8	39.2	42.5	44.4	48.5	54.8	62.2	66.7	69.5	75.0
60.0-64.9	627	52.3	10.8	34.5	38.3	41.6	45.0	52.1	59.2	63.3	66.3	70.4
65.0-69.9	886	49.8	10.5	33.4	37.2	39.6	43.0	49.2	56.7	60.1	62.4	68.1
70.0-74.9	626	47.8	10.8	30.8	34.6	36.9	40.6	47.5	54.4	59.1	62.0	66.8
Males With Large Frames												
18.0-24.9	431	55.7	12.2	37.6	40.8	43.0	47.3	54.6	63.5	67.0	71.6	76.7
25.0-29.9	305	60.3	12.0	42.6	45.7	48.4	52.6	60.4	67.3	72.8	75.8	81.2
30.0-34.9	230	62.8	13.4	44.2	46.9	49.2	53.3	62.6	70.6	75.3	78.8	84.0
35.0-39.9	203	61.6	13.3	43.2	46.0	48.9	51.8	59.9	70.3	76.6	79.4	82.8
40.0-44.9	204	61.8	12.3	44.9	47.4	49.6	53.2	60.0	69.8	74.4	79.4	83.7
45.0-49.9	214	61.1	13.0	42.9	46.3	48.1	52.4	59.6	67.5	71.1	74.9	86.4
50.0-54.9	214	60.5	12.8	41.8	46.0	47.8	51.6	59.4	67.6	72.5	77.6	85.4
55.0-59.9	198	60.2	12.0	42.3	45.0	47.9	52.9	59.8	66.9	71.8	75.3	83.8
60.0-64.9	311	57.9	12.1	38.9	43.9	46.8	50.1	57.5	65.8	69.0	71.8	77.4
65.0-69.9	439	54.5	12.7	35.6	39.4	41.7	46.0	53.7	62.7	66.9	70.7	75.6
70.0-74.9	310	52.0	12.4	33.2	38.3	40.3	43.6	51.6	59.0	63.8	67.2	72.2

From Frisancho AR: *Anthropometric standards for the assessment of growth and nutritional status*, Ann Arbor, 1990, The University of Michigan Press.
Note: Values for males age 18 years and older have been adjusted for bone area by subtracting 10.0 cm^2 from the calculated mid–upper arm muscle area.

Appendix 30 Means, Standard Deviations, and Percentiles of Upper Arm Muscle Area (cm^2) by Age for Adult Females of Small, Medium, and Large Frames

AGE (yr)	N	MEAN	SD	PERCENTILES 5	10	15	25	50	75	85	90	95
Females With Small Frames												
18.0-24.9	651	26.2	6.0	18.2	19.6	20.7	22.5	25.5	29.2	31.2	32.8	36.2
25.0-29.9	486	27.8	7.4	19.5	20.6	21.6	23.2	26.9	30.8	33.3	35.2	38.1
30.0-34.9	413	28.6	7.8	19.1	21.6	22.4	24.5	27.8	31.4	33.7	36.2	38.8
35.0-39.9	368	29.8	10.1	19.7	21.4	22.9	24.4	28.8	32.5	35.4	37.5	42.2
40.0-44.9	350	29.8	6.6	20.9	22.1	23.4	25.7	28.9	33.2	36.0	37.9	41.8
45.0-49.9	241	29.2	7.4	19.1	21.5	22.6	24.3	28.3	33.3	36.1	38.7	41.2
50.0-54.9	256	30.3	7.3	20.8	22.1	23.9	25.5	29.1	33.4	36.7	38.5	41.3
55.0-59.9	223	30.9	7.6	20.4	22.3	23.6	25.8	30.2	34.8	37.6	41.3	45.1
60.0-64.9	351	31.9	8.7	20.9	22.4	23.6	25.8	31.2	36.4	39.1	41.1	46.2
65.0-69.9	491	31.3	8.1	19.4	22.1	23.7	25.7	30.6	35.4	39.8	41.8	45.7
70.0-74.9	367	32.0	9.9	20.3	22.5	24.1	25.9	30.3	36.1	39.8	42.6	47.3
Females With Medium Frames												
18.0-24.9	1296	29.3	7.0	19.8	21.9	23.2	24.9	28.4	32.8	35.2	37.2	40.7
25.0-29.9	964	30.0	7.2	20.7	22.1	23.3	25.0	29.0	33.9	36.8	39.0	43.3
30.0-34.9	814	32.0	9.1	21.4	23.1	24.2	26.3	30.8	36.1	39.4	41.8	46.4
35.0-39.9	728	32.7	8.4	21.4	23.6	24.9	27.3	31.4	37.3	40.8	43.0	47.0
40.0-44.9	696	33.7	12.1	21.2	23.2	25.1	27.2	31.6	37.7	43.1	47.1	52.3
45.0-49.9	484	33.8	8.8	22.2	23.6	25.5	27.9	32.2	37.9	42.5	45.4	49.6
50.0-54.9	502	35.0	9.7	22.8	25.2	26.2	28.5	33.7	40.0	43.5	46.7	51.4
55.0-59.9	442	36.3	11.5	23.7	25.3	26.6	28.7	34.5	41.5	44.9	49.2	53.4
60.0-64.9	695	35.1	9.1	23.0	25.3	26.5	29.2	33.9	39.9	43.7	46.1	49.4
65.0-69.9	971	35.7	10.0	22.4	24.8	26.4	29.1	34.6	40.7	44.5	48.1	51.9
70.0-74.9	731	35.3	9.7	22.2	24.3	26.1	28.9	34.0	40.0	44.4	46.7	51.3
Females With Large Frames												
18.0-24.9	641	34.4	10.7	21.9	23.8	25.3	27.3	31.9	38.7	43.9	47.5	55.8
25.0-29.9	471	36.7	11.5	22.2	25.4	26.8	29.3	34.5	42.0	46.8	50.3	60.1
30.0-34.9	392	38.8	12.3	24.0	25.8	27.3	30.1	36.3	45.1	50.7	55.1	61.2
35.0-39.9	357	41.6	14.4	23.9	27.4	29.1	32.2	39.1	47.2	53.7	61.0	72.1
40.0-44.9	344	43.5	16.6	26.2	28.8	30.5	32.9	40.3	49.5	54.4	58.7	71.6
45.0-49.9	236	43.0	15.8	25.0	28.0	29.4	32.5	39.7	49.0	58.3	62.8	69.9
50.0-54.9	246	42.4	13.1	25.1	28.4	30.1	33.4	39.6	49.5	54.8	59.7	68.4
55.0-59.9	213	45.2	16.9	27.0	30.0	32.4	35.8	42.0	51.0	58.5	62.2	65.7
60.0-64.9	341	43.1	14.2	26.6	29.1	31.2	33.9	40.7	49.8	54.8	57.5	67.6
65.0-69.9	482	42.5	13.4	26.4	28.4	30.6	33.5	40.0	48.7	55.3	58.7	66.5
70.0-74.9	363	41.5	11.6	25.7	28.8	30.2	32.8	40.1	48.7	51.4	54.8	60.3

From Frisancho AR: *Anthropometric standards for the assessment of growth and nutritional status,* Ann Arbor, 1990, The University of Michigan Press.
Note: Values for females age 18 years and older have been adjusted for bone area by subtracting 6.5 cm^2 from the calculated mid–upper arm muscle area.

Appendix 31 Means, Standard Deviations, and Percentiles of Upper Arm Fat Area (cm^2) by Age for Males and Females of 1 to 74 Years

				PERCENTILES								
AGE (yr)	N	MEAN	SD	5	10	15	25	50	75	85	90	95
Males												
1.0-1.9	681	7.5	2.2	4.5	4.9	5.3	5.9	7.4	8.9	9.6	10.3	11.7
2.0-2.9	672	7.4	2.3	4.2	4.8	5.1	5.8	7.3	8.6	9.7	10.6	11.6
3.0-3.9	715	7.6	2.4	4.5	5.0	5.4	5.9	7.2	8.8	9.8	10.6	11.8
4.0-4.9	707	7.3	2.5	4.1	4.7	5.2	5.7	6.9	8.5	9.3	10.0	11.4
5.0-5.9	676	7.4	3.1	4.0	4.5	4.9	5.5	6.7	8.3	9.8	10.9	12.7
6.0-6.9	298	7.7	4.1	3.7	4.3	4.6	5.2	6.7	8.6	10.3	11.2	15.2
7.0-7.9	312	8.1	4.2	3.8	4.3	4.7	5.4	7.1	9.6	11.6	12.8	15.5
8.0-8.9	296	8.9	5.0	4.1	4.8	5.1	5.8	7.6	10.4	12.4	15.6	18.6
9.0-9.9	322	10.1	6.2	4.2	4.8	5.4	6.1	8.3	11.8	15.8	18.2	21.7
10.0-10.9	333	12.0	7.3	4.7	5.3	5.7	6.9	9.8	14.7	18.3	21.5	27.0
11.0-11.9	324	13.6	9.4	4.9	5.5	6.2	7.3	10.4	16.9	22.3	26.0	32.5
12.0-12.9	348	13.9	9.6	4.7	5.6	6.3	7.6	11.3	15.8	21.1	27.3	35.0
13.0-13.9	350	13.0	9.2	4.7	5.7	6.3	7.6	10.1	14.9	21.2	25.4	32.1
14.0-14.9	358	13.3	10.2	4.6	5.6	6.3	7.4	10.1	15.9	19.5	25.5	31.8
15.0-15.9	356	12.8	9.0	5.6	6.1	6.5	7.3	9.6	14.6	20.2	24.5	31.3
16.0-16.9	350	13.9	9.5	5.6	6.1	6.9	8.3	10.5	16.6	20.6	24.8	33.5
17.0-17.9	337	12.9	8.9	5.4	6.1	6.7	7.4	9.9	15.6	19.7	23.7	28.9
18.0-24.9	1752	16.9	10.8	5.5	6.9	7.7	9.2	13.9	21.5	26.8	30.7	37.2
25.0-29.9	1250	18.8	11.6	6.0	7.3	8.4	10.2	16.3	23.9	29.7	33.3	40.4
30.0-34.9	940	20.4	11.4	6.2	8.4	9.7	11.9	18.4	25.6	31.6	34.8	41.9
35.0-39.9	832	20.1	10.5	6.5	8.1	9.6	12.8	18.8	25.2	29.6	33.4	39.4
40.0-44.9	828	20.4	11.2	7.1	8.7	9.9	12.4	18.0	25.3	30.1	35.3	42.1
45.0-49.9	867	20.1	11.0	7.4	9.0	10.2	12.3	18.1	24.9	29.7	33.7	40.4
50.0-54.9	879	19.4	10.3	7.0	8.6	10.1	12.3	17.3	23.9	29.0	32.4	40.0
55.0-59.9	807	19.2	10.2	6.4	8.2	9.7	12.3	17.4	23.8	28.4	33.3	39.1
60.0-64.9	1259	19.1	10.2	6.9	8.7	9.9	12.1	17.0	23.5	28.3	31.8	38.7
65.0-69.9	1773	18.0	9.8	5.8	7.4	8.5	10.9	16.5	22.8	27.2	30.7	36.3
70.0-74.9	1250	17.5	9.4	6.0	7.5	8.9	11.0	15.9	22.0	25.7	29.1	34.9
Females												
1.0-1.9	622	7.3	2.3	4.1	4.6	5.0	5.6	7.1	8.6	9.5	10.4	11.7
2.0-2.9	614	7.7	2.3	4.4	5.0	5.4	6.1	7.5	9.0	10.0	10.8	12.0
3.0-3.9	651	7.8	2.5	4.3	5.0	5.4	6.1	7.6	9.2	10.2	10.8	12.2
4.0-4.9	680	8.0	2.6	4.3	4.9	5.4	6.2	7.7	9.3	10.4	11.3	12.8
5.0-5.9	672	8.5	3.4	4.4	5.0	5.4	6.3	7.8	9.8	11.3	12.5	14.5
6.0-6.9	296	8.7	3.9	4.5	5.0	5.6	6.2	8.1	10.0	11.2	13.3	16.5
7.0-7.9	329	9.8	4.5	4.8	5.5	6.0	7.0	8.8	11.0	13.2	14.7	19.0
8.0-8.9	275	11.3	6.5	5.2	5.7	6.4	7.2	9.8	13.3	15.8	18.0	23.7
9.0-9.9	321	13.1	7.3	5.4	6.2	6.8	8.1	11.5	15.6	18.8	22.0	27.5
10.0-10.9	329	14.1	7.7	6.1	6.9	7.2	8.4	11.9	18.0	21.5	25.3	29.9
11.0-11.9	302	16.3	9.7	6.6	7.5	8.2	9.8	13.1	19.9	24.4	28.2	36.8
12.0-12.9	323	16.9	8.9	6.7	8.0	8.8	10.8	14.8	20.8	24.8	29.4	34.0
13.0-13.9	360	19.1	11.0	6.7	7.7	9.4	11.6	16.5	23.7	28.7	32.7	40.8
14.0-14.9	370	20.4	11.0	8.3	9.6	10.9	12.4	17.7	25.1	29.5	34.6	41.2
15.0-15.9	309	20.7	11.4	8.6	10.0	11.4	12.8	18.2	24.4	29.2	32.9	44.3
16.0-16.9	343	23.5	10.9	11.3	12.8	13.7	15.9	20.5	28.0	32.7	37.0	46.0
17.0-17.9	291	23.9	13.0	9.5	11.7	13.0	14.6	21.0	29.5	33.5	38.0	51.6
18.0-24.9	2588	25.2	13.4	10.0	12.0	13.5	16.1	21.9	30.6	37.2	42.0	51.6
25.0-29.9	1921	28.1	14.7	11.0	13.3	15.1	17.7	24.5	34.8	42.1	47.1	57.5
30.0-34.9	1619	31.6	16.1	12.2	14.8	17.2	20.4	28.2	39.0	46.8	52.3	64.5
35.0-39.9	1453	33.6	16.8	13.0	15.8	18.0	21.8	29.7	41.7	49.2	55.5	64.9
40.0-44.9	1390	34.3	16.2	13.8	16.7	19.2	23.0	31.3	42.6	51.0	56.3	64.5
45.0-49.9	961	36.0	17.2	13.6	17.1	19.8	24.3	33.0	44.4	52.3	58.4	68.8
50.0-54.9	1004	36.7	15.9	14.3	18.3	21.4	25.7	34.1	45.6	53.9	57.7	65.7
55.0-59.9	879	37.6	17.7	13.7	18.2	20.7	26.0	34.5	46.4	53.9	59.1	69.7
60.0-64.9	1389	37.1	16.0	15.3	19.1	21.9	26.0	34.8	45.7	51.7	58.3	68.3
65.0-69.9	1946	34.7	15.1	13.9	17.6	20.0	24.1	32.7	42.7	49.2	53.6	62.4
70.0-74.9	1463	32.9	14.6	13.0	16.2	18.8	22.7	31.2	41.0	46.4	51.4	57.7

From Frisancho AR: *Anthropometric standards for the assessment of growth and nutritional status*, Ann Arbor, 1990, The University of Michigan Press.

Appendix 32 Nutrition-Focused Physical Assessment

SYSTEM	NORMAL FINDINGS	ABNORMAL FINDINGS	POSSIBLE NUTRITION/ METABOLIC ASSOCIATIONS	NONNUTRITIONAL EXAMPLES
general survey	weight for height appropriate, well-nourished, alert, and cooperative	loss of weight, muscle mass and fat stores, growth retardation	protein-calorie deficiency	endocrine disorders, osteogenic disorders, menopausal disorders secondary to estrogen depletion
		excess fat stores	excess calorie intake	
		fatigue, anemia	iron deficiency	
skin	pink, soft, moist, turgor with instant recoil, smooth appearance	poor wound healing, ulcers	protein, vitamin C, or zinc deficiency	diabetes, steroids
		dry with fine lines and shedding, scaly (xerosis)	essential fat, or vitamin A deficiency	environmental or hygiene factors
		spinelike plaques around hair follicles on buttocks, thighs, or knees (follicular hyperkeratosis)	vitamin A or essential fat deficiency	
		pellagrous dermatitis (hyperpigmentation of skin exposed to sunlight)	niacin or tryptophan deficiency	thermal, sun, or chemical burns; Addison's disease
		pallor	iron or folic acid deficiency	skin pigmentation disorders, hemorrhage
		yellow pigmentation	carotene excess	jaundice
		poor skin turgor	fluid loss	
		petechiae, ecchymoses	vitamin K or C deficiency	aspirin overdose, liver disease, or trauma
nails	smooth, translucent, slightly curved nail surface and firmly attached to nail bed; nail beds with brisk capillary refill	spoon-shaped (koilonychia)	iron deficiency	chronic obstructive pulmonary disease, heart disease, aortic stenosis
		dull, lackluster	protein or iron deficiency	chemical effects
		pale, mottled	vitamin A or C deficiency	infection, chemical effects
scalp	pink, no lesions, tenderness; fontanels without softening, bulging	softening or craniotabes	vitamin D deficiency	
		open anterior fontanel (usually closes by ~18 months of age)	vitamin D deficiency	hydrocephalus
hair	natural shine, consistency in color and quantity, fine to coarse texture	lack of shine and luster, thin, sparse	protein, zinc, or linoleic acid deficiency	hypothyroidism, chemotherapy, psoriasis, color treatment
		easily pluckable	protein deficiency	hypothyroidism, chemotherapy, psoriasis, color treatment
		alternating bands of light and dark hair in young children (flag sign)	protein deficiency	chemically processed or bleached hair
face	skin warm, smooth; dry, soft, moist with instant recoil	diffuse depigmentation, swollen	protein deficiency	steroids and other medications
		pallor	iron, folate, or B_{12} deficiency	low perfusion, low volume states
		moon face	protein, calorie	Cushing's disease
		bilateral temporal wasting	protein, calorie	neuromuscular disorders
eyes	evenly distributed brows, lids, lashes; conjunctiva pink without discharge sclerae, without spots; cornea clear; skin without cracks or lesions	pale conjunctiva	iron, folate, or B_{12} deficiency	
		night blindness	vitamin A deficiency	
		dry, grayish, yellow or white foamy spots on whites of eyes (Bitot's spots)	vitamin A deficiency	pterygium, Gaucher's disease

		dull, milky, or opaque cornea (corneal xerosis)	vitamin A deficiency	
		dull, dry, rough appearance to whites of eyes and inner lids (conjunctival xerosis)	vitamin A deficiency	chemical, environmental
		softening of cornea (keratomalacia)	vitamin A deficiency	
		cracked and reddened corners of eyes (angular palpebritis)	riboflavin, niacin deficiency	infection, foreign objects
nose	uniform shape, septum slightly to left of midline, nares patent bilaterally, mucosa pink and moist, able to identify smells	scaly, greasy, with gray or yellowish material around nares (nasolabial seborrhea)	riboflavin, niacin, pyridoxine deficiency	
		inflammation, redness of sinus tract, discharge, obstruction or polyps	irritation of skin membranes	need to reconsider if placing feeding tube; evaluate for non-food allergies
Oral Cavity				
lips/mouth	pink, symmetrical, smooth intact	bilateral cracks, redness of lips (angular stomatitis)	riboflavin, niacin, pyridoxine deficiency	poor-fitting dentures, herpes, syphilis
		vertical cracks of lips (cheilosis)	riboflavin, niacin deficiency	AIDS (Kaposi's sarcoma), environmental exposure
tongue	pink, moist, midline, symmetrical with rough texture	magenta	riboflavin deficiency	
		smooth, slick, loss of papillae (atrophic filiform papillae)	folate, niacin, riboflavin, iron, or B_{12} deficiency	
		beefy red color, atrophied taste buds, and mucosa red and swollen	niacin, folate, riboflavin, iron, B_{12}, or pyridoxine deficiency	Crohn's disease, infection
		decreased taste (hypoguesia)	zinc deficiency	cancer therapy
gums	pink, moist without sponginess	spongy, bleeding, receding	vitamin C deficiency	dilantin and other medication, poor hygiene, lymphoma, polycythemia, thrombocytopenia
teeth	repaired, no loose teeth; color may be various shades of white	missing, poor repair, caries, loose	excess sugar	trauma, syphilis, aging, poor dental hygiene
		white or brownish patches (mottled)	excess flouride	enamel hypoplasia, erosion
cranial nerves	intact	abnormal	influences feeding route	
gag reflex	intact	absent	affects route of feeding	
jaw	proper alignment, movement from side to side	improper alignment and movement	may influence intake by ability to chew properly	
parotid gland	located anterior to earlobe, no enlargement	bilateral enlargement	protein deficiency	bulimia, cysts, tumors, hyperparathyroidism
neck nodules	trachea midline, freely movable without enlargement or nodules	enlarged thyroid	iodine deficiency	cancer, allergy, cold infection
Cardiopulmonary				
chest/lungs	anterior and posterior thorax; adequate muscle and fat stores, respirations even and unlabored, symmetrical rise and fall of chest during inspiration and expiration, lung sounds clear	somatic muscle- and fat-wasting; labored respirations; breath sounds such as crackles, rhonchi, and wheezing: evaluate for fluid status versus tenacious secretions that may labor breathing and increase energy expenditure; also consider increased rate and depth, decreased rate and depth	protein-calorie deficiency metabolic acidosis metabolic alkalosis	respiratory disease: COPD, etc.

Modified from Rindall J: *Physical assessment of the malnourished patient.* Presented at Eighteenth Clinical Congress of the American Society for Parenteral and Enteral Nutrition, San Antonio, Tex, February 1, 1994; with permission; Hammond K: Physical assessment: a nutritional perspective, *Nurs Clin North Am* 32(4):779, 1997.
NOTE: This chart is not intended to be a comprehensive list for all nutritional or metabolic deficiencies or nonnutrition examples.

Continued

Appendix 32 Nutrition-Focused Physical Assessment—cont'd

SYSTEM	NORMAL FINDINGS	ABNORMAL FINDINGS	POSSIBLE NUTRITION/ METABOLIC ASSOCIATIONS	NONNUTRITIONAL EXAMPLES
heart	rhythm regular and rate within normal range; S_1 and S_2 heart sounds	irregular rhythm	potassium deficiency or excess calcium deficiency magnesium deficiency or excess phosphorus deficiency	cardiopulmonary disease states
		pounding pulse	fluid overload (hypervolemia)	cardiopulmonary disease
		small, weak pulse	fluid deficiency (hypovolemia)	
		palpitations	hypoglycemia	
		tachycardia	thiamin deficiency	
		enlarged heart	thiamin deficiency associated with anemia and beri beri	
vascular access devices intact	no swelling, redness, drainage	purulent drainage, swelling, excessive redness	influences nutrition if device has to be removed	
abdomen	soft, nondistended, symmetrical, bilateral without masses, umbilicus in midline, no ascites, bowel sounds present and normoactive; tympanic on percussion; feeding device intact without redness, swelling	generalized symmetrical distention	obesity	enlarged organs, fluid, or gas
		protruding, everted umbilicus, tight glistening appearance (ascites)	influences protein, fluid, sodium concerns of feeding	
		scaphoid appearance	protein-calorie deficiency	
		increased bowel sounds	influences nutrition in gastroenteritis (normal if hunger pains)	
		high-pitched tinkling	influences nutrition if intestinal fluid and air present, indicating early obstruction	
		decreased bowel sounds	influences nutrition if peritonitis or paralytic ileus present	
kidney, ureter, bladder	urine golden yellow (ranges from pale yellow to deep gold), clear without cloudiness, adequate output	decreased output, extremely dark, concentrated	dehydration	
musculoskeletal	full range of motion without joint swelling or pain, adequate muscle strength	inability to flex, extend, and rotate neck adequately	influences nutrition by interfering with ability to feed or make hand-to-mouth contact	
		decreased range of motion, swelling, impaired joint mobility of upper extremities; muscle wasting on arms, legs; skin folding on buttocks	protein-calorie deficiency	
		swollen, painful joints	vitamin C deficiency	connective tissue disease
		enlargement of epiphyses at wrist, ankle, or knees	vitamins D or C deficiency	trauma, deformity, or congenital cause
		bowed legs	vitamin D deficiency, calcium deficiency	

		beading of ribs	vitamin D deficiency, calcium deficiency	renal rickets, malabsorption
		pain in calves, thighs	thiamin deficiency	deep vein thrombosis, other neuropathy
neurologic	alert, oriented, hand-to-mouth coordination; no weakness or tremors	decreased or absent mental alertness; inadequate or absent hand-to-mouth coordination	influences nutrition by the ability to feed or make hand-to-mouth contact	
		psychomotor changes, confusion, peripheral neuropathy	protein deficiency thiamin, pyridoxine, vitamin B_{12} deficiency	trauma, neurologic disease
		tetany	calcium, magnesium deficiency	
	cranial nerves intact: primary nutritionally focused ones include trigeminal, facial, glossopharyngeal, vagus, and hypoglossal			
	reflexes (biceps, brachioradialis patella, and Achilles common in exam), functioning within normal range of 2+ +	hyperactive reflexes	hypocalcemia	tetany, upper motor neuron disease
	hypoactive reflexes	hypokalemia	associated with metabolic diseases such as diabetes mellitus and hypothyroidism	
		hypoactive achilles, patellar reflex	thiamin, vitamin B_{12}	neurologic disorders

Modified from Rindall J: *Physical assessment of the malnourished patient*. Presented at Eighteenth Clinical Congress of the American Society for Parenteral and Enteral Nutrition, San Antonio, Tex, February 1, 1994; with permission; Hammond K: Physical assessment: a nutritional perspective, *Nurs Clin North Am* 32(4):779, 1997.
Note: This chart is not intended to be a comprehensive list for all nutritional or metabolic deficiencies or nonnutrition examples.

Appendix 33 A Guide to the Use of Laboratory Data in Nutritional Assessment and Monitoring

I. Principles of Nutritional Laboratory Testing

A. Purpose

Laboratory-based nutritional testing, used to estimate nutrient availability in biologic fluids and tissues, is critical for assessment of both clinical and subclinical nutrient deficiencies. Laboratory data are the only objective data used in nutritional assessment that are "controlled"—that is, the validity of the method of its measurement is checked each time a specimen is assayed by also assaying a sample with a known value. The known sample is called a control, and if the value obtained for the sample is outside the range of normal analytical variability, both the specimen and control are measured again.

The nutrition professional can use laboratory data to reduce the time required to gather subjective data and to eliminate the inevitable inconsistency associated with subjective judgment. Furthermore, because numeric values do not themselves connote personal judgment, this kind of data can often be passed on to a patient or client without implicit or perceived blame.

B. Specimen Types

Ideally, the specimen to be tested reflects the total body content of the nutrient to be assessed. Often, however, the best specimen is not readily available. The most common specimens for analysis are the following:

Whole blood—Must be collected with an anticoagulant if entire content of the blood is to be evaluated. The two common anticoagulants for whole blood-analyses are ethylenediaminetetraacetic acid (EDTA), a calcium chelator used in hematologic analyses, and heparin (maintains the blood in its most natural state)[1]

Blood cells—Separated from anticoagulated whole blood for measurement of cellular analyte content.

Plasma—The uncoagulated fluid that bathes the formed elements (blood cells).

Serum—The fluid that remains after whole blood or plasma have coagulated. Coagulation proteins and related substances are missing or significantly reduced.

Urine—Contains a concentrate of excreted metabolites.

Feces—Important in nutritional analyses when nutrients are not absorbed and are therefore present in fecal material.

Hair—An easy-to-collect tissue; usually a poor indicator of actual body levels.

Other tissues—*Buccal cells* and *solid organ biopsy* specimens are rarely used in nutritional laboratory assessment.

C. Interpretation of Laboratory Data

As with all data, nutritional data may be quantitative (how much, how often, how fast, etc.), semiquantitative (many, most, few, a lot, usually, majority, several, etc.), or qualitative (color, shape, species, etc.). The advantage of quantitative data is that they are less ambiguous or more objective than other types of observations. Although objective laboratory data are extremely important resources in nutrition assessment, one should be extremely cautious about using a single isolated laboratory test value to make an assessment. One value is often misleading, especially when taken out of the context of an individual's habits, clinical status, and dietary and medical histories. The best data are obtained from analysis of changes in laboratory values.

When monitoring patients for changes in nutrition test values, one must consider how much change is necessary to give confidence that a difference is significant. The change required for statistical significance has been called the *critical difference*. It is calculated from measurement of the variances calculated from repeated measurements of an analyte in (1) specimens that have been obtained, at several different times, from each of several healthy persons (intrasubject variation); and (2) separate samples from a large specimen pool (analytic variation).

The critical differences for some plasma proteins of nutritional significance are the following:[2]

PROTEIN	CRITICAL DIFFERENCE
Albumin	8%
Transthyretin	32%
C-Reactive protein	175%

The statistical probability that two consecutive albumin measurements are statistically different requires that the concentration change by 8% or more. Therefore an albumin increase, for example, from 30.0 g/L to 32.4 g/L indicates that a statistically significant change has occurred. For transthyretin (prealbumin), an increase from 30.0 mg/dl to 39.6 mg/dl would be significant, and for C-reactive protein, an increase from 3.0 mg/L to 8.2 mg/L would be significant. There are two reasons for the large discrepancy in the critical differences for these three proteins. The major reason is that the albumin level is very stable in healthy persons, whereas transthyretin and C-reactive protein concentrations vary considerably. Also contributing to these differences is the fact that the currently available methods measure albumin more precisely than transthyretin or C-reactive protein.

In practice, assessments are not based on the measurement of a single analyte at one point in time. If you monitor, for example, transthyretin and C-reactive protein simultaneously, and both change so as to indicate a clinical improvement (opposite numerical directions), the amount of change required for significance decreases. The changes in laboratory data may precede changes in other nutritional indices, but generally, although not always, the data available should point to the same conclusion.

D. Reference Ranges

To determine whether a particular laboratory value is abnormal, particularly when serial data are not available, the value is generally compared to a reference range. The reference range is constructed from a large number of test values (20 to >1000). The average value and the standard deviation for these data are determined, and the reference range is calculated from the mean ±2 standard deviations.

Appendix created by Timothy H. Carlson, PhD, RD.

[1]Samples obtained for blood coagulation tests are diluted with solutions containing sodium citrate (a calcium chelator). Because of the dilutional effect of the anticoagulant solutions, citrated samples are not suitable for measurement of the concentrations of analytes.

[2]Clark GH, Fraser CG: Biological variation of acute phase proteins, *Ann Clin Biochem* 30:373, 1993.

[3]Monsen ER: The *Journal* adopts SI units for clinical laboratory values, *J Am Diet Assoc* 37:356, 1987.

Appendix 33 A Guide to the Use of Laboratory Data in Nutritional Assessment and Monitoring—cont'd

If the sample group is representative of the reference population, the reference range will include values that reflect those found in approximately 95% of the reference population. About 2.5% of this normal population will have values greater than the upper end of the reference range, and 2.5% will have values less than the lower end. This means that one normal individual in 20 would have a value below or above the reference range.

Reference ranges can be made for different populations. For example, reference ranges based on gender, age, race, and so forth, can be developed. In practice the differences between populations are often ignored because the importance of small differences in a nutrient analyte is not usually significant. However, in the event of borderline values, the possible influence differences between the population of which the patient is a member and the reference population may need to be taken into account. Reference ranges often are determined by obtaining blood from personnel working in or near the clinical laboratory. This population is often skewed toward younger persons, has few minorities, and is overrepresented by women.

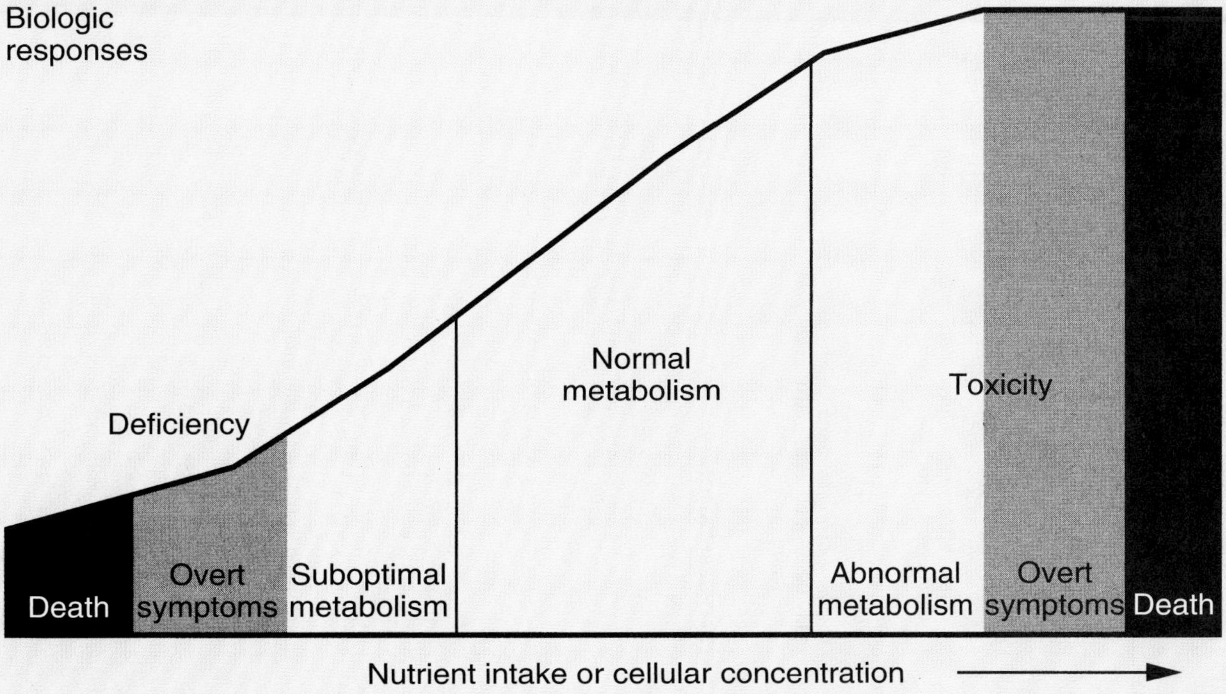

E. Units

Many types of units are used in reporting nutrient-dependent laboratory values. Two basic systems of units are in common use: the conventional system and the SI system (Système Internationale d'Unités).[3] The conventional system sometimes lacks convention, and so different laboratories adopt different units to report the same analyte! For example, the conventional report of an ionized calcium value could be 2.30 mEq/L, 46 mg/L, or 4.6 mg/dl. In the SI system, however, only 1.15 mmol/L is allowed.

F. Nature of Nutritional Testing and Types of Tests

Typically, laboratory tests are *static* assays (i.e., the concentration of an analyte is measured in a biologic fluid [e.g., a fasting blood specimen] at a point in time. Assessment of nutrient status made by this approach is often inaccurate or distorted as explained in Chapter 18.

Some nutrients can be assessed by tests that are based on measurements that reflect the endogenous availability of a nutrient to a measurable biologic function (e.g., biochemical, tissue, or organ). Most often, *functional* assessment of nutrient status may be done by measurement of a biochemical marker (i.e., a normal or abnormal metabolite) of function. The results of this type of testing can be reliably considered to reflect the adequacy of a nutrient pool (see Chapter 18).

As shown in the figure above, the size of a nutrient pool can vary continuously from frankly deficient, to adequate, to toxic. Most of these states can be assessed in the laboratory. This allows nutritional intervention before frank deficiency occurs. Furthermore, the response of the patient's body pool to nutritional intervention or change in patient behavior can be assessed before clinical or anthropometric changes take place.

Continued

Appendix 33 A Guide to the Use of Laboratory Data in Nutritional Assessment and Monitoring—cont'd

II. A. Laboratory Measurement of Body Composition

TEST	PRINCIPLE AND REQUIREMENTS	INTERPRETATION	REFERENCE RANGE	LIMITATIONS
Creatinine-height ratio (CHR) and creatinine-height index (CHI)	Creatinine is a continuously released by-product of energy metabolism in muscle. $CHR = \frac{\text{Urine creatinine/24 hr (mg)}}{\text{Height (cm)}}$ CHI = CHR (subject)/CHR (ideal)	Creatinine excretion related to muscle mass; tables of normal CHI values used to calculate percent deficit; % Deficit = 100 − CHI (%).	% Deficit 5-15 = mild 6-30 = moderate >30 = severe	Diet (creatinine in meat) and stress (infection, exercise, injury) ↑ creatinine excretion; age and renal insufficiency ↓ excretion; variability occurs during menstrual cycle.
3-Methylhistidine (3-MH)	3-MH, an amino acid found only in muscle, is measured by chromatographic analysis of 24-hour urine collections.	3-MH excretion is related to muscle mass of adults; may be useful in monitoring or assessment for research purposes.	155-304 μmol/24 hr (young males; meat-free diet)	3-MH in meat; effects of age and hormone status not known; probably not useful in stressed patients or after intense muscular activity.
Hydroxyproline (HPro) index (HI)	HPro, an amino acid found in the collagen of connective tissue and bone, measured in random urine; HPro excretion related to tissue growth and repair.	$HI = \frac{\text{mg HPro per ml urine}}{\text{mg Creatinine per ml urine}}$ Can assess growth rate in children. May monitor effect of nutrition support on wound healing.	Normal children: 0.7-4.7	HPro found in gelatin and other animal products; affected by age, sex, presence of parasites, sprue, arthritis, and rheumatic fever.

II. B. Tests of Protein-Energy Status

TEST	PRINCIPLE AND REQUIREMENTS	INTERPRETATION	REFERENCE RANGE	LIMITATIONS
Urea urinary N (UUN)	The protein pool (visceral and somatic) N is catabolized to urea; urine urea represents ~80% of N catabolized; requires accurate estimate of protein intake, so usually used only for TPN or tube-feeding patients.	UUN is compared with the actual N intake. $\text{N balance} = \frac{\text{protein (g)}}{6.25^*} - \text{UUN} + 4;$ *Factor = 5.95 for TPN; reflects severity of metabolic stress.	− = Catabolism 0 = Catabolism + = Anabolism (3-6 g/24 hr = optimal use range)	Urine collection must be quantitative (complete); UUN not appropriate in renal insufficiency; does not account for wound leakage, cell losses, or diarrhea; inaccurate in metabolically stressed patients.
Total urinary N (TUN)	Some N is excreted as nonurea N (e.g., ammonia and creatinine); 24-hour TUN reflects total protein catabolism, accounting for all sources of urinary N; as for UUN, requires accurate protein intake.	TUN is compared with the actual N intake; $\text{N balance} = \frac{\text{Protein (g)}}{6.25^*} - \text{TUN} + 2;$ *Factor = 5.95 for TPN; reflects severity of metabolic stress; TUN gives the most accurate estimation of total protein catabolism.	− = Catabolism 0 = Catabolism + = Anabolism (3-6 g/24 hr = optimal use range)	Urine collection must be quantitative (complete); TUN not appropriate in renal insufficiency; not done in many institutions; does not account for wound leakage, cell losses, or diarrhea.
Urea kinetics	Formulas used to estimate protein catabolic rate (PCR) from changes in blood urea nitrogen (BUN) concentration in patients with impaired renal function.	Urinary urea (residual renal urea clearance—KrU) and BUN levels (urea generation rate—GU) are used to determine PCR; 1- to 3-day diet intake compared with PCR.	In protein balance, PRC = protein intake	Urea lost in dialysis must be accounted for in calculating urea nitrogen appearance. Dietary protein intake hard to estimate.
Visceral Proteins				
Total protein (TP)	Protein concentration in serum is easily measured colorimetrically; largely reflects albumin (50%-60% of TP).	TP levels parallel clinical signs of malnutrition; plasma TP is 0.4 g/dl greater than serum TP.	6.4-8.3 g/dl (64-83 g/L)	Does not reflect status during inflammatory (acute-phase) response; conditions that affect individual protein affect TP.
Albumin	Easily and quickly measured colorimetrically; large body pool (3-5 g/kg body weight), ~60% is outside the plasma (in the extravascular pool); long half-life of 3 weeks.	Decreased levels can occur following short-term protein and energy deficiency; often associated with other deficiencies (i.e., zinc, iron, and vitamin A).	3.5-5.0 g/dl (35-50 g/L)	Significance confounded by acute stress reaction, liver disease, protein-losing enteropathy, nephrotic syndrome, pregnancy, oral contraceptive use, strenuous exercise, and hemodilution.

Transferrin	Iron transport protein; smaller extravascular pool than albumin; measured by immunoassay or calculated from TIBC (see p. 1215); half-life ~8 days.	Levels increased during iron deficiency and decreased by protein-energy deficiency. Calculated values give inexact estimates of serum concentration.	200-400 mg/dl (2.0-4.0 g/l)	Significance confounded by acute stress reaction, liver disease, protein-losing enteropathy, nephrotic syndrome, pregnancy or estrogen administration, and hemodilution.
Transthyretin	Transports thyroxin and acts as a carrier for retinol-binding protein; also called prealbumin and thyroxin-binding prealbumin; half-life ≈2 days. Soon will be available for routine laboratory measurement.	More sensitive protein-energy balance indicator than albumin or transferrin; responds rapidly to nutritional intervention; reportedly more sensitive to energy intake than to protein intake.	19-43 mg/dl (190-430 g/l) (Reference range varies considerably depending on methodology)	Very sensitive to stress response; also ↓ in liver disease, protein-losing enteropathy, nephrotic syndrome, and hemodilution.
Retinol-binding protein (RBP)	Transports retinol; because of low molecular weight, RBP is filtered by glomerulus and catabolized by the kidney tubule; half-life ≈0.5 days.	More sensitive protein-energy balance indicator than albumin or transferrin; responds rapidly to nutritional intervention; reportedly more sensitive to protein intake than to energy intake.	2.1-6.4 mg/dl (21-64 mg/l) (Children's values ~½ of adults until puberty)	Very sensitive to stress response; also ↓ in liver disease, protein-losing enteropathy, nephrotic syndrome, vitamin A and zinc deficiencies, and hemodilution; ↑ in chronic renal disease.
Insulin-like growth factor-1 (IGF-1) (Somatomedin C)	The peptide mediator of growth-hormone activity produced by the liver; half-life of a few hours; much less sensitive to stress response than other proteins.	Low in chronic undernutrition; increases rapidly during nutrition support when albumin, transferrin, transthyretin, and RBP are not affected.	95-395 ng/ml (95-395 μg/l)	Reduced levels seen in hypopituitarism, hypothyroidism, liver disease, and with estrogen use. Not generally available clinically.
Metabolic Indicators				
Amino acid ratio	Serum ratio of nonessential to essential amino acids is an index of protein-energy status in kwashiorkor.	NEAA:EAA ratio $= \frac{\text{Gly + Ser + Gln + Tau}}{\text{Ile + Leu + Val + Met}}$ Decreased ratio in kwashiorkor but not marasmus.	*Risk* / *Ratio* Low <2.0 Medium 2.0-3.0 High >3.0	Not usually done because amino acid analysis is too expensive for this application.
Urea/creatinine ratio	Urinary urea/creatinine ratio (U:Cr) in fasting, first-void urine used to compare amino acid catabolism (BUN) with muscle mass (creatinine).	$\text{U:Cr} = \frac{\text{Urine urea (mg/dl)}}{\text{Urine creatinine (mg/dl)}}$ Can be used in uncomplicated protein-energy deficiency to approximate status.	*Risk* / *Ratio* Low >12.0 Medium 6.0-12.0 High <6.0	Affected by recent protein intake, therefore not useful for estimating long-term status; ratio not used for accurate assessment or monitoring.

II. C. Immunologic Tests

TEST	PRINCIPLE AND REQUIREMENTS	INTERPRETATION	REFERENCE RANGE	LIMITATIONS
Total lymphocyte count (TLC)	Calculated from the percentage of lymphocytes reported in the hemogram and the WBC count. Units = cells/μl or cells/mm^3	Decreased in protein-energy malnutrition and immunocompromised state.	Normal >2700 Moderate depletion 900-1500 Severe depletion <900	Decreased by viral infection, chemotherapy, radiation, and drugs (e.g., steroids, penicillin, sulfonamides, Lasix, phenylbutazone); increased by tissue necrosis and other types of infection.
Delayed cutaneous hypersensitivity	Anergy for antigens, such as mumps and *Candida;* occurs in malnutrition; antigens injected intradermally and redness (erythema) and hardness (induration) read 1, 2, or 3 days later.	Response affected by protein-energy status and vitamin A, iron, zinc, and vitamin B_6 deficiencies.	*Induration* 1+ <5 mm 2+ = 6-10 mm 3+ = 11-20 mm 4+ >20 mm Erythema + or −	Usefulness in acute care limited by drugs, effect of aging and disease (metabolic, malignant, and infectious diseases); difficult to administer and interpret results. Semiquantitative.

Appendix created by Timothy H. Carlson, PhD, RD.

Continued

Appendix 33 A Guide to the Use of Laboratory Data in Nutritional Assessment and Monitoring—cont'd

II. D. Prognostic Indices

TEST	PRINCIPLE AND REQUIREMENTS	INTERPRETATION	REFERENCE RANGE	LIMITATIONS
Albumin	↓ Levels associated with increased incidence of medical or nutritional complications (morbidity), length of hospital stay, and mortality.	Levels <3.5 g/dl indicate need for further patient evaluation; <3.0 g/dl can be associated with edema; <2.5 g/dl implies extreme medical and nutritional risk.	See interpretation	Albumin responds slowly to treatment because of long $t_{1/2}$; markedly decreased during the metabolic response to injury.
Cholesterol	Low levels (< 80 mg/dl) are associated with increased incidence of medical or nutritional complications and death.	Levels <150 indicate increased risk; concentration correlates with ↓ albumin, transthyretin, iron, zinc, and vitamins A and E.	See interpretation	Decreasing levels of total cholesterol may be more significant than absolute values.
Prognostic nutritional index (PNI)	PNI uses the following parameters to estimate nutritional risk: albumin (g/dl) transferrin (mg/dl) TSF = triceps skinfold (mm) DH = delayed hypersensitivity (0-nonreactive; 1 = <5 mm; 2 = >5 mm)	PNI (%) = 158 − 16.6 [Alb] − 0.78 (TSF) − 0.2 [Tfn] − 5.8 (DH) Prospectively identifies patients who benefit from nutrition support.	*PNI* Low risk <40% Moderate 40%-50% High risk >50%	Does not predict outcome in acute trauma; does not give specific information on nutritional deficiencies.

III. Tests of Carbohydrate Absorption

TEST	PRINCIPLE AND REQUIREMENTS	INTERPRETATION	REFERENCE RANGE	LIMITATIONS
Lactose Intolerance				
Breath hydrogen	Lactose loading (2 g/kg) in lactase deficiency allows bacterial metabolism of lactose with production of H_2 gas. Breath analyzed for H_2 by gas chromatography.	Breath H_2 measured fasting and 0.5 and 2 hours after dosing with lactose; a significant increase is associated with malabsorption.	Normal increase: <50 parts/million (i.e., <50 ppm)	Bacterial overgrowth can cause false positive results; consumption of soluble fiber or legumes and smoking are associated with H_2 production; false negative results caused by antibiotics.
Lactose tolerance test	Lactose loading (50 g) followed by blood sampling at 5, 10, 30, 60, 90, and 120 min after dose; glucose produced from lactose is assayed.	Lactase deficiency associated with <20 mg/dl increase in glucose.	Normal glucose increase ≥20 mg/dl	Test is not specific (many false positives) or sensitive (many false negatives).

IV. Tests of Lipid Status

TEST	PRINCIPLE AND REQUIREMENTS	INTERPRETATION	REFERENCE RANGE	LIMITATIONS
Fat Malabsorption				
Fecal fat screening	Microscopic inspection of fat-stained (Sudan stain) specimens for the presence of lipid droplets.	Trained observers are able to identify excessive fat in ~80% of persons with fat malabsorption.	Qualitative results	Patient must be consuming sufficient fat for analysis to reveal malabsorption. Semiquantitative.
Prothrombin time (PT)	Absorption of fat-soluble vitamins, including vitamin K, decrease in fat malabsorption; vitamin K impairs coagulation, causing an ↑ in PT.	A prolonged PT is a relatively sensitive but nonspecific indicator of fat malabsorption.	10.4-12.8 sec	Oral anticoagulant and other drugs, ↓ platelet count, acquired and hereditary bleeding diseases and liver disease ↑ PT.
Serum carotene (total serum carotenoids)	Carotenoids, fat-soluble pigments in plant foods, are poorly absorbed in fat malabsorption; extracted by organic solvents for quantification.	A serum carotene level of less than 50 mg/dl is seen in ~85% of patients with fat malabsorption.	90-280 μg/dl (1.6-5.1 μmol/L)	Decreased serum carotenoid levels are also seen in low vegetable/fruit diets (e.g., in TPN or tube feeding), liver failure, and some lipoprotein disorders.

Quantitative fecal fat determination	Patient must consume 100 g fat/day (4 × 8 oz whole milk/day, and 2 tbs vegetable oil/meal) during and for 2 days before collection.	Quantitative 72-hour stool collection required for accurate assessment; average daily discharge used for interpretation.	Normal: <5 g fat/24 hr Malabsorption: ≥10 g/24 hr	Failure to adhere to the diet invalidates the results.
Essential Fatty Acid Deficiency				
Fatty acid analysis	Levels of eicosapentaenoic acid (C20:3n9) and linoleic acid (C18:2n6) reflect essential fatty acid status; fatty acids in plasma or blood cell fractions assayed by gas chromatography.	Endogenous synthesis of C20:3n9 greatly increases during linoleic acid deficiency; plasma phospholipid C20:3n9/C18:2n6 ratio used to assess status.	C20:3n9/C18:2n6 ratio >0.2 confirms deficiency	Test available only from laboratories specializing in nutritional or lipid analyses.
Nonesterified Fatty Acids				
Serum-free fatty acids (FFA or NEFA)	Measured by a simple colorimetric procedure.	↑ When medium-chain fatty acids are administered.	8-25 mg/dl (0.28-0.89 mmol/L)	Many conditions ↑ FFA including hyperthyroidism, alcoholism, diabetes, acute myocardial infarct; also ↑ in fasting and strenuous exercise.

V. Tests for Nutrition-Influenced Risk Factors for Atherosclerotic Diseases

TEST	PRINCIPLE AND REQUIREMENTS	INTERPRETATION	REFERENCE RANGE	LIMITATIONS
High-sensitivity C-reactive protein (hs-CRP)	CRP is an acute-phase protein used to assess inflammatory status. Measured by a variety of immunoassay techniques.	When slightly increased, CRP has been shown to be associated with increased risk for coronary heart disease and other cardiovascular disease.	Low risk: <1.0 mg/l Moderate risk: 1.5-3.0 mg/l High risk: >3mg/l	Is not specific for risk of artherosclerotic disease; relatively minor injuries and other causes of inflammation also increase CRP levels.
Total serum or plasma cholesterol	Cholesterol is enzymatically released from cholesterol esters. Free cholesterol measured in automated enzyme assays.	Total cholesterol correlated with risk for cardiovascular diseases but not as good an indicator as HDL-c and LDL-c. See National Cholesterol Education Program (NCEP) guidelines.	Desirable: <200 mg/dl (<5.2 μmol/L) Borderline: 200-239 mg/dl (5.2-6.2 μmol/L) High risk: ≥240 mg/dl (≥6.2 μmol/L)	Cholesterol measurements have considerable within-subject variability. May partly result from variability in specimen collection or handling.
HDL cholesterol (HDL-c)	LDL-c (and VLDL-c) are precipitated from the serum before measurement of residual HDL-c; direct measurement of HDL-c is now done in some laboratories.	HLD-c is called "good cholesterol" to indicate that it is a negative risk factor.	Desirable: >35 mg/dl (0.9 μmol/L)	Some precipitation methods cause underestimation of HDL. HDL can be divided into classes: HDL_1, HDL_2, and HDL_3; HDL_3 best correlates with risk of CHD.
LDL cholesterol (LDL-c)	LDL-c is estimated by the Friedewald formula, LDL-c = total cholesterol − HDL-c − TG/5, or by new direct assays.	LDL-c is called "bad cholesterol" to indicate that it is a positive risk factor. See NCEP guidelines.	Desirable: <130 mg/dl (<3.4 μmol/L) Borderline: 130-159 mg/dl (3.4-4.1 μmol/L) High risk: ≥160 mg/dl (≥4.1 μmol/L)	Calculation only valid when TG concentration is <400 mg/dl, so cannot be determined in nonfasting serum or plasma.
Triglycerides (TG)	Lipases release glycerol and fatty acids from TG; glycerol measured in automated enzyme assays.	The association of TG and CHD has been shown; may be a more important risk factor in women.[1]	<160 mg/dl (<1.80 mmol/L)	Fasting specimen is essential; alcohol ingestion can increase; some anticoagulants affect.
Lipoprotein (a) Lp(a)	Measured by a variety of immunoassay techniques.	Positive associations exists between CHD risk and serum Lp(a). Influence of diet is uncertain.		Results of different assay methods may not be comparable.

Continued

Appendix created by Timothy H. Carlson, PhD, RD.
[1]See Austin MA, Hokanson JE: Epidemiology of triglycerides, small dense low-density lipoprotein, and lipoprotein(a) as risk factors for coronary heart disease, *Med Clin North Am* 78:99, 1994.

Appendix 33 A Guide to the Use of Laboratory Data in Nutritional Assessment and Monitoring—cont'd

TEST	PRINCIPLE AND REQUIREMENTS	INTERPRETATION	REFERENCE RANGE	LIMITATIONS
LDL subclass pattern and size	LDL particles of different sizes (densities) can be assessed by electrophoresis or other techniques.	Pattern B (small, dense LDL) is associated with ↑ risk of CHD and is responsive to diet. Pattern A (larger, buoyant LDL) is not associated with risk.		Measurements are generally inaccurate and imprecise. Only available from special laboratories.
Homocysteine (Hcy)	Total Hcy (oxidized + reduced forms) are measured by chromatography or by more rapid immunoassays that have recently become available.	Hcy level is an independent risk factor for CHD, venous thrombotic, and other diseases; folic acid and vitamins B_{12} and B_6 reduce plasma Hcy levels.	Normal: 3.8-18.6 μmol/L ♂ 0.2-20.1 μmol/L ♀ In CAD: 4.4-21.7 μmol/L ♂ 0-27.8 μmol/L ♀	Small Hcy differences between CAD and normal subjects; as for LDL cholesterol, risk is increased even at slightly elevated levels.

VI. Tests of Micronutrient Status

TEST	PRINCIPLE AND REQUIREMENTS	INTERPRETATION	REFERENCE RANGE	LIMITATIONS
A. Vitamins				
Thiamin (B_1)[2]	Thiamin status is usually assessed by measuring the amount of thiamin pyrophosphate (TPP) needed to fully activate the RBC enzyme, transketolase.	The TPP needed to fully activate transketolase is inversely related to B_1 status; percent stimulation by TTP.	% Stimulation >20% (index >1.2) indicates deficiency	Amount (and activity) of enzyme affected by drugs, iron, folate, or vitamin B_{12} status, malignant or GI diseases, and diabetes.
Riboflavin (B_2)	Riboflavin status is assessed by measuring the amount of FAD needed to fully activate RBC enzyme, glutathione reductase (GR).	The FAD needed to fully activate GR is inversely related to B_2 status; percent stimulation.	% Stimulation >40% (index >1.4) indicates deficiency	Amount and/or activity of enzyme may change with age, iron status, liver disease, and glucose-6-phosphate dehydrogenase deficiency.
Niacin (B_3)[3]				
Pyridoxyl (PLP) compounds (B_6)[4]	1) RBC enzymes, ALT (GPT) or AST (GOT), are assayed for the presence of PLP as the enzymes' cofactor.[5]	1) Difference between enzyme activities before and after addition of PLP is inversely related to B_6 status.	1) % ALT stimulation of >25% or AST activity of >50% in deficiency	1) Disease and drugs that affect the liver and heart and pregnancy confound interpretation.
	2) Plasma PLP can be directly measured by chromatography.	2) PLP is the major transport form of B_6; therefore serum levels reflect body stores.	2) Normal: 0.50-3.0 μg/dL (20-120 nmol/L)	2) Deficiency may be seen clinically before plasma PLP levels ↓.
	3) Tryptophan (Trp) load test, measures excretion of the PLP-dependent, metabolite xanthurenic acid (XA).	3) In this functional test, the levels of urinary XA should ↑ significantly when 2-5 g of Trp is ingested.	3) Marginal status: >50 mg/24 hr	3) Steroid drugs and estrogen ↑ enzyme activity, some drugs cause analytic errors.
Folate[6]	1) Because of ↓ DNA synthesis large RBCs are produced.	1) Deficiency leads to increase in MCV (mean cell volume).	1) Normal: MCV <100	1) Not sensitive or specific for folate.
	2) Shape of neutrophil nucleus affected by folate deficiency.	2) ↑ Neutrophil lobe count seen in folate deficiency.	2) Normal: ≤4 lobes per neutrophil	2) Lobe count sensitive but not specific.
	3) Folate levels can be directly measured by radio-immunoassay.	3) Both red cell and serum folate are indicators of body stores.	3) 2-10 μg/L serum; 140-960 ng/L RBC (3.2-22 nmol/L)	3) Plasma from nonfasted subjects may reflect recent intake; RBC folate is not measured accurately.
	4) Functional folate status assayed by formimino-glutamic acid (FIGLU) in 24-hour urine or after oral histidine loading.	4) After 2-15 g loading dose, 10-50 mg of FIGLU should be excreted in 8 hours.	4) Normal: <7.4 mg/24 hours (<42.6 μmol/24 hr) without loading	4) FIGLU affected by vitamin B_{12}, drugs, liver disease, cancer, TB, and pregnancy.
Cobalamin (B_{12})	1) Because of ↓ DNA synthesis large RBCs are produced.	1) Deficiency leads to increase in MCV (mean cell volume).	1) Normal: MCV <100	1) Not sensitive or specific for B_{12}

	2) Shape of neutrophil nucleus is affected by B_{12} deficiency.	2) ↑ Neutrophil lobe count in B_{12} deficiency.	2) Normal: ≤4 lobes per neutrophil	2) Lobe count sensitive but not specific
	3) B_{12} can be directly measured by radioimmunoassay.	3) Levels <150 ng/L indicate deficiency (age affects level).	3) 200-1000 ng/L 150-750 pmol/L)	3) Marginal deficiency not correlated with level
	4) Methylmalonic acid excretion reflects B_{12} available for branched-chain AA metabolism.	4) Methylmalonic acid excretion >300 mg/24 hr in B_{12} deficiency.	4) Normal excretion: ≤9.0 mg/24 hr (≤76 μmol/24 hr)	4) Specific for B_{12} but requires normal BCAA levels; done only in specialized laboratories
	5) Schilling test for intrinsic factor and B_{12} absorption assesses radiolabeled B_{12} absorption as reflected by urinary excretion.	5) Abnormal B_{12} absorption indicated by excretion <3% of B_{12} radioactivity per 24 hours.	5) Normal excretion: ≈8% of radioactivity per 24 hours	5) Test must be repeated with oral administration of intrinsic factor (IF) to differentiate IF deficiency and malabsorption.
Ascorbic acid (C)	Plasma or leukocyte C measured by (1) chromatography; (2) ascorbate oxidase; (3) spectrophotometrically by reaction with 2,4-dinitrophenylhydrazine.	Leukocyte C is less affected by recent intake, but well-fasted plasma levels parallel leukocyte levels; plasma preferred for acutely ill patients because leukocyte level is affected by infection, some drugs, and hyperglycemia; <0.2 mg/dl (<10 μg/10^8 WBC).	Plasma: 0.50-1.40 mg/dl (30-80 μmol/L) Leukocyte deficiency: 20-50 μg/10^8 WBC (1.1-3.0 fmol/cell)	Blood samples must by carefully prepared for assay to prevent C breakdown. Oxalate, glucose, and proteins interfere with some assays; recent intake can mask deficiency.
Retinols (A)	Serum retinol and retinol esters extracted by organic solvents and measured by chromatography; functional tests (e.g., dark adaptation) only detect severe deficiency.	Retinol levels <100 g/L indicate severe deficiency; retinol ester >5% of total retinols indicates hypervitaminosis A.	30-80 μg/dl (1.0-2.8 μmol/L)	Exposure of serum to bright light or oxygen destroys vitamin A; low retinol-binding protein level associated with low vitamin A (see protein-energy section).
Tocopherols (E)	Serum tocopherols measured by chromatography; α- and β-tocopherols serve different antioxidant functions.	Lower values found in infants; level associated with deficiency not determined.	0.5-1.8 mg/dl (12-42 μmol/L)	Plasma level dependent on recent intake and level of lipids, especially triglycerides, in blood.
Cholecalciferol (D_3) calcidiol calcitriol	1) Alkaline phosphatase activity reflects level of bone activity and, indirectly, D status.	1) Serum levels >190 units/L D deficiency; 30% is the form from bone.	1) Adult: 25-100 U/L 1-12 yr < 350 U/L	1) Not specific, but a sensitive indicator; serum Ca and PO_4 should also be ↑
Calciferol (D_2) ercalcidiol/ ercalcitriol	2) Calcidiol and ercalcidiol (25-OH-D) are assayed together by chromatography or radioimmunoassay.	2) <3 ng/ml (7.4 nmol/L) indicates deficiency; >200 ng/mL (500 nmol/L) indicates hypervitaminosis D.	2) 15-80 μg/L) summer (37-200 nmol/L) 14-42 μg/L winter (35-105 nmol/L)	2) Best indicator of status (liver stores), but marginal levels hard to interpret
	3) Calcitriol [1,25-(OH)2-D_3] is assayed by chromatographic or immunoassay procedures.	3) Used to show that vitamin D metabolism is occurring normally.	3) 2.5-4.5 ng/dl (60-108 pmol/L) (little seasonal change)	3) Poor indicator of status because of tight control of synthesis independent of body stores.
Phyloquinone (K_1) and menadione (K_2)	Normal coagulation factor synthesis requires K; prothrombin (PT) assesses coagulation status.	In K deficiency, PT increases with increasing production of abnormal coagulation factors.[7]	10.4-12.8 slc (varies significantly with method)	The level of vitamin K available for vitamin K–dependent bone proteins may not be reflected by the PT.

Appendix created by Timothy H. Carlson, PhD, RD.

Continued

[2]Red blood cells are separated from plasma by centrifugation and washed with saline; after hemolyzing the cells the intracellular material is analyzed for vitamin availability.

[3]No biochemical tests have been developed to assess B_3 status; the fraction of whole blood niacin as NAD is a potentially useful test (see Powers HJ: Current knowledge concerning optimum nutritional status of riboflavin, niacin, and pyridoxine. *Proceedings Nutrition Society* 58:435, 1999).

[4]Several tests in addition to the ones described here have been used to assess B_6 status—for example, urinary B_6/creatinine ratios, urinary 4-pyridoxic acid excretion, and the kynurenine load test are tests for B_6, but these are not usually available for clinical use.

[5]ALT (alanine aminotransferase) and GPT (glutamic-pyruvate transaminase) are the same enzyme; AST (aspartate aminotransferase) and GOT (glutamic-oxalacetic transaminase) are the same enzyme.

[6]Microbiologic growth assays, the deoxyuridine suppression test and recently developed research tests for folate and vitamin B_{12} are not generally offered in the contemporary clinical laboratory.

[7]More sensitive procedures for measurement of vitamin K include serum chromatography and determination of the serum level of vitamin K–dependent bone protein called osteocalcin. Deficiency significantly increases the amount of abnormal forms of this protein. These tests are not yet widely available.

Appendix 33 A Guide to the Use of Laboratory Data in Nutritional Assessment and Monitoring—cont'd

TEST	PRINCIPLE AND REQUIREMENTS	INTERPRETATION	REFERENCE RANGE	LIMITATIONS
B. Minerals				
Electrolytes				
Sodium (Na^+)[8,9]	Serum electrolytes, including bicarbonate, are usually measured together by ion-specific electrodes in autoanalyzers; sometimes Na and K are measured by flame emission spectrophotometry.	↑ Serum Na seen in water loss; ↓ Na occurs in many conditions.	135-145 mEq/L (1 mEq/L = mmol/L)	Electrolytes change rapidly in response to changes in physiology (e.g., hormonal stimulus, renal and other organ dysfunction, acid-base balance changes, and drug action); serum electrolytes are minimally affected by diet.
Potassium (K^+)		↑ Serum K seen in renal diseases and ↓ Na; ↓ K usually indicates ↓ intake or ↑ cellular uptake.	3.5-5.1 mEq/L (1 mEq/L = mmol/L)	
Chloride (Cl^-)		Chloride levels change with cation and osmotic changes in the body.	100-110 mEq/L (1 mEq/L = mmol/L)	
Bicarbonate or total CO_2		Bicarbonate levels reflect acid-base balance.	21-30 mEq/L (1 mEq/L = mmol/L)	
Major minerals				
Calcium (Ca^{2+})	1) Total serum Ca^{2+} measured as chromogenic or fluorescent complexes, or by atomic absorption. 2) Ionized (free) Ca^{2+} measured by ion-specific electrodes.	Usually, slightly more than half of the serum Ca^{2+} is bound to albumin, or complexed with other molecules; the remaining Ca^{2+} is called ionized Ca (ICA); ICA is available physiologically.	1) 8.8-10 mg/dl (2.2-2.5 mmol/L) 2) 2.3-2.6 mEq/L (1.15-1.30 mmol/L)	Calcium status is related to many factors, including vitamin D, phosphate, parathyroid function and malignancy, and renal function.
Phosphate (H_2PO_4, PO_4^2, and PO_4^{3-}) (Phosphorous)	Usually measured spectrophotometrically after reaction with ammonium phosphomolybdate.	Abnormal P level is most closely associated with disturbed intake, distribution, or renal function.	2.7-4.5 mg/dl (0.87-1.45 mmol/L) (higher in children)	Reported as phosphorus (P), not phosphate; hemolyzed blood cannot be used because of high RBC phosphate levels.
Magnesium (Mg^{2+})	1) Total serum Mg^{2+} measured after reaction to form chromogenic or fluorescent complexes or by atomic absorption 2) Ionized (free) Mg^{2+} measured by ion-specific electrodes.	Neuromuscular function (hyperirritability, tetany, convulsion, and electrocardiographic changes) affected when levels of total serum Mg^{2+} fall to <1.0 mEq/L.	1) 1.4-2.3 mEq/L (0.70-1.15 mmol/L) 2) 0.7-1.2 mEq/L (0.35-0.60 mmol/L)	Usually, about 45% of the serum Mg^{2+} is complexed with other molecules; the remaining Mg^{2+} is called ionized magnesium; serum levels remain constant until body stores are nearly depleted.
Trace minerals				
Iron				
Complete blood count[10] (CBC) and red cell indices	HCT = % RBC in whole blood Hb = blood Hb concentration MCV = mean red blood cell volume	A CBC with red cell indices is one of the first set of tests that a patient receives; although CBC data are not specific for nutritional status, their universal and repeated presence in the patient's record make them very important.	42-52 (male) 37-47 (female)[11] 14-18 g/dl (male) 12-16 g/dl (female) 80-99 fl all except 96-108 in newborns.	These tests are affected only when iron stores are essentially depleted; HCT and Hb are sensitive to hydration status; low MCV also occurs in thalassemias and lead poisoning.
Serum iron (Fe)	Serum Fe^{3+} reduced to Fe^{2+} and then complexed with chromogen.	Slightly higher in males than in premenopausal females; reflects recent Fe intake.	50-175 μg/dl (9-31 μmol/L)	Very insensitive index of total Fe stores; extremely variable (day-to-day and diurnal).
Total iron binding capacity (TIBC)	TIBC determined by saturating serum transferrin with Fe and then remeasuring serum Fe.	Reflects transferrin concentration.	250-450 μg/dl (45-81 μmol/L)	TIBC does not increase until Fe stores are essentially completely depleted.
Transferrin saturation (Tf-sat)	Tf-sat = serum Fe/TIBC × 100	Used like TIBC in assessment of Fe deficiency; useful in diagnosis of iron toxicity or excess storage (hemochromatosis).	20-50% ♂ 15-50% ♀	↓ When Fe stores essentially depleted; ↑ in ↓ vitamin B_6 aplastic anemia.

Zinc protoprophyrin (ZPP)	1) ZPP/heme ratio measured by hematofluorometry; a single drop of blood required. 2) Free erythrocyte protoporphyrin (FEP) measures total red cell ZPP. These tests reflect substitution of zinc for iron during iron-deficient heme synthesis and erythropoiesis.	1) Because a ratio is measured, ZPP:H is insensitive to hemodilution. 2) Both ZPP:H and FEP also detect lead poisoning and hereditary tyrosinemia.	1) 30-80 μmol/mol 2) 17-77 μg/dl (cells) (0.27-1.23 μmol/L)	ZPP/heme ratio and FEP ↑ as iron availability ↓; both are excellent for screening and monitoring iron stores, but must be interpreted in light of possible lead poisoning and chronic inflammation.
Red cell distribution width (RDW)	Measurement of variation in RBC diameter (anisocytosis); reported to be helpful in distinguishing iron deficiency and anemia associated with chronic inflammation.	Very sensitive indicator of Fe status; normal RDW reportedly rules out anemia caused by chronic inflammatory diseases.[12]	Normal value <16% (varies considerably with instrument used for measurement)	Specificity of RDW for Fe deficiency is relatively low; interpretation confounded by red cell transfusion; measurement usually not reported.
Ferritin	Intracellular Fe-storage protein; serum levels parallel iron stores; measured by immunoassays.	Best biochemical index of uncomplicated iron deficiency or overload (iron toxicity) and excess storage.	Males: 15-200 ng/ml (15-200 μg/L) Females: 12-150 ng/ml (12-150 μg/L)	Increases during metabolic response to injury, even when Fe stores are adequate; not useful in anemia of chronic disease.
Zinc (Zn)[13]	Serum levels measured by atomic absorption spectrophotometry.	Serum levels affected by diet and the inflammatory response. Zinc deficiency associated with many diseases and trauma.	0.7-1.5 mg/L (11-23 mmol/L)	Serum levels detect frank— but not marginal—deficiency; blood must be collected in zinc-free tubes.
Copper (Cu)	1) Serum levels measured by flame emission atomic absorption spectrophotometry. 2) Ceruloplasmin is the major Cu-containing plasma protein; measured by immunoassay (e.g., nephelometry).	1) Cu deficiency is associated with neutropenia, anemia, and scurvylike bone disease. 2) Ceruloplasmin is required for conversion of Fe^{3+} to Fe^{2+} during cellular Fe uptake; anemia can result from ↓ ceruloplasmin.	1) 70-140 μg/dl ♂ (11-22 mmol/L) 80-155 μg/dl ♀ (13-24 μmol/L) 2) 150-600 mg/L	1) Serum levels detect frank but not marginal deficiency; use of oral contraceptives ↑ serum Cu 2) Ceruloplasmin not a useful marker of Cu status but can be used to assess changes in status after supplementation.
Selenium (Se)	1) Serum levels measured by atomic absorption spectrophotometry. 2) Whole blood levels (measured by same methods) better reflect long-term status.	Margin between deficiency and toxicity is narrower for Se than any other trace component of the antioxidant enzyme element; important glutathione peroxidase.	1) 80-320 μg/L (1.0-4.0 μmol/L) 2) 60-340 μg/L (0.75-4.3 μmol/L)	Cutoff points for deficiency or toxicity are not well established.

Appendix created by Timothy H. Carlson, PhD, RD.

[8]These substances are measured by similar techniques when the concentration in urine or other body fluids is determined.

[9]These tests are combined with serum glucose, creatinine, and BUN on a test battery or panel. This set of tests is among the first and most frequently administered laboratory tests.

[10]The CBC includes the red cell count, the red cell indices, hemoglobin concentration (Hb), hematocrit (HCT), mean red blood cell volume (MCV), mean cell hemoglobin (MCH), mean cell hemoglobin concentration (MCHC), and white cell and platelet counts. Only HCT, Hb, and MCV are discussed here (see Savage RA: The red cell indices: yesterday, today, and tomorrow, *Clin Lab Med* 13:773-785, 1993).

[11]Ranges are for adult men and premenopausal women. Pregnant women, infants, and children have different reference ranges.

[12]See van Zeben D et al: Evaluation of microcytosis using serum ferritin and red cell distribution width, *Eur J Haematol* 44:106-109, 1990.

[13]Taste acuity tests can be used to supplement laboratory methods (see, e.g., Gibson RS et al: A growth limiting mild zinc deficiency syndrome in some Southern Ontario boys with low growth percentiles, *Am J Cli Nutr* 49:1266, 1989).

Continued

Appendix 33 A Guide to the Use of Laboratory Data in Nutritional Assessment and Monitoring—cont'd

TEST	PRINCIPLE AND REQUIREMENTS	INTERPRETATION	REFERENCE RANGE	LIMITATIONS
Iodine (I)	Urinary excretion is best indicator of I status, either μg/24 hr or μg/g creatinine; thyroid hormone level related to I status.	Excretion should be ≥RDA for 24-hour urine or >50 μg/g creatinine; thyroid hormone = T_3 or T_4.	No urinary I reference range T_4 reference range: 5.0-12.0 μg/dl (65-155 nmol/L)	Thyroid hormone levels are affected by many factors beside iodine status.
Ultra-trace minerals				
Chromium (Cr)	Urinary excretion usually tested by atomic absorption spectrophotometry.	Excretion should be ≥DRI; deficiency reported in patients on long-term TPN; ↓ levels in diabetes mellitus.	10-200 ng/dl (1.9-38 nmol/L)	Test not available in most clinical laboratories; special handling required to prevent specimen contamination during collection.
Manganese (Mn)	Whole blood or serum assayed by atomic absorption spectrophotometry.	Mn is a cofactor for a variety of enzymes; ↑ in rheumatoid arthritis.	Plasma: 0.7-1.2 μg/L (13-22 nmol/L) Whole blood: 8.0-19 μg/L (150-340 nmol/L)	Test not available in most clinical laboratories; special handling required to prevent specimen contamination during collection.
Fluorine/fluoride (FI)	Serum assayed by gas chromatography.	Levels >10-200 μg/L are usually observed.	10-200 μg/L (0.5-10 μmol/L)	Not available in most clinical laboratories.

VII. Blood Gases and Water Status

TEST	PRINCIPLE AND REQUIREMENTS	INTERPRETATION	REFERENCE RANGE	LIMITATIONS
pH	pH = $-\log [H^+]$; H^+ depends mainly on the CO_2 from respiration: CO_2 + $H_2O \Leftrightarrow H_2CO_3 \Leftrightarrow HCO_3 + H^+$ Measured by ion-selective electrodes (like those found in common pH meters).	In: Acidosis pH <7.35 Alkalosis pH >7.45 pH compatible with life 6.80-7.80.	Whole blood: Arterial 7.35-7.45 Venous 7.32-7.42	Blood must not be exposed to air before or during measurement.
pO_2 or Po_2 and O_2 saturation	Whole blood O_2 measured by oxygen electrode; Po_2 = "pressure" contributed by O_2 to the total "pressure" of all the gases dissolved in blood Saturation = $\frac{\text{Content}}{\text{Capacity}}$ (× 100).	Affected by alveolar gas exchange, ventilation/perfusion inequalities, and generalized alveolar hypoventilation.	Arterial blood: pO_2: 83-108 mm Hg <40 mm Hg = critical value (gravely dangerous) O_2 saturation: 0.95-0.98 (95%-98%)	Blood must not be exposed to air before or during measurement.
pCO_2 or Pco_2	Measured by ion-selective electrode; "pressure" contributed by CO_2 to the total "pressure" of all the gases dissolved in blood.	↑ In respiratory acidosis (↑ CO_2 in inspired air or ↓ in alveolar ventilation) and ↓ in respiratory alkalosis (e.g., in hyperventilation from anxiety, mechanical ventilator, or closed head injury [damaged respiratory center]).	Whole blood: Arterial 35-48 mm Hg ♂ 32-45 mm Hg ♀ Venous 6-7 mm Hg higher	Blood must not be exposed to air before or during measurement.
Bicarbonate (HCO_3^-) and total CO_2 (tCO_2)	For whole blood [HCO_3^-] is calculated from the equation given in pH section.	↑ In compensated respiratory acidosis and in metabolic acidosis; ↓ in metabolic acidosis and in compensated respiratory alkalosis.	Whole blood: Arterial 18-23 mEq/L (18-23 mmol/L)	Blood must not be exposed to air before or during measurement.
Osmolality (Osmol)	Osmol is dependent on amount of particles (solutes) dissolved in a solution; measurement based on relationship between solute concentration and freezing point; serum osmol assesses hydration status and solute load.	Osmolality increases in dehydration, diabetic coma, diabetic ketoacidosis; also estimated from the formula: mOsmol/L = 1.86 [Na^+] + [Glucose]/18 + [BUN]/2.8	282-300 mOsmol/kg (1 Osmol = 1 mol of solute particles; 1 kg serum ≈ 1 L)	Freezing point depression gives a more accurate estimate of osmolality than the calculated value (e.g., in ketoacidosis).

VIII. Tests of Antioxidant Status/Oxidative Stress

TEST	PRINCIPLE AND REQUIREMENTS	INTERPRETATION	REFERENCE RANGE	LIMITATIONS
Water-soluble compounds	See Vitamin C.			
Lipid-soluble compounds: see Vitamin E: Carotenoids Coenzyme Q10	The carotenoids: lutein, xanthein zeaxanthein, α- and β-carotene, and lycopene; carotenoids and coenzyme, Q10 (ubiquinone-10) are measured chromatographically.	Reference ranges for these compounds vary greatly, depending on the method used for their assay.	See reference for carotenoid range under fat malabsorption	Tests for carotenoids and coenzyme Q are not yet available for routine clinical use.
Total antioxidant capacity: e.g., ORAC TEAC FRAP	ORAC: Oxygen radical absorbance capacity TEAC: Trolox-equivalent antioxidant capacity FRAP: Ferric reducing ability of plasma	These assays reflect the presence of all of plasma or serum antioxidants, including vitamins C and E, carotenoids, coenzyme Q10, glutathione, uric acid, bilirubin, superoxide dismutase, catalase, glutathione peroxidase, and albumin.		These assays are now commercially available but are currently performed only in specialized laboratories.
Oxidative stress markers: e.g., *o*-tyrosine, nitrotyrosine, 8-isoprostane, 4-hydroxynonenal, malondialdehyde	Free radical oxidation products of lipids (e.g., malondialdehyde, 8-isoprostane), proteins (e.g., *o*-tyrosine and nitrotyrosine), or secondary oxidation products (e.g., 4-hydroxynonenal) can be measured chromatographically or by immunoassay.	8-Isoprostane (also called 8-epi-prostaglandin $F_{2\alpha}$) increases in plasma or urine of patients with lung disease, hypercholesterolemia, or diabetes mellitus.		8-Isoprostane assays are now commercially available. Markers of oxidative stress are currently assayed only in specialized laboratories.

IX. Tests for Monitoring Nutrition Support

TEST	PRINCIPLE AND REQUIREMENTS	INTERPRETATION	REFERENCE RANGE	LIMITATIONS
C-reactive protein (CRP)	CRP is an acute-phase protein used to assess inflammatory status. Measured by a variety of immunoassay techniques.	Large increases in CRP are associated with development of a catabolic state during the stress response; CRP levels begin to fall when the anabolic phase is entered.	>5 mg/L	Serial values rather than a single value must be used to specify the stage of the stress response.
Chemistry panel with phosphate and Mg^{2+}	Panel includes electrolytes, glucose, creatinine, BUN, and total CO_2 (bicarbonate); see earlier discussion for additional test information.	Used to monitor carbohydrate tolerance, hydration status, and major organ system function.	See earlier discussion	Very frequently ordered test panel.
Osmolality (see earlier discussion)	Can be measured or calculated from chemistry-panel data.	Used to assess hydration status.	See earlier discussion	Measured value accounts for substances in blood not accounted for by calculation.
Protein-Energy Balance				
Serum proteins (see earlier discussion)	Transthyretin, retinol-binding protein, transferrin, albumin most often available.	These visceral proteins aid in assessing protein and energy balance.	See earlier discussion	Stress reaction can markedly affect these and confound their interpretation as protein-energy indicators.
Nitrogen balance: UUN, TUN (see earlier discussion)			Nitrogen balance in hospitalized patients ranges from −20 g to +6 g/day	UUN may greatly underestimate nitrogen excretion.

Appendix created by Timothy H. Carlson, PhD, RD.
DRI, Dietary reference intake.

Continued

Appendix 33 A Guide to the Use of Laboratory Data in Nutritional Assessment and Monitoring—cont'd

TEST	PRINCIPLE AND REQUIREMENTS	INTERPRETATION	REFERENCE RANGE	LIMITATIONS
Minerals: Zn, Cu, Se, Cr (see earlier discussion)			See earlier discussion	Most trace minerals are measured only in long-term nutrition support patients.
Vitamins C and A (see earlier discussion)	Because vitamin C and vitamin A are important in immune function and wound healing, they should be assessed regularly.	Vitamin C levels can ↓ sharply in response to stress.	See earlier discussion	Systematic, regular monitoring protocol should be followed.
Liver function tests (TPN only)	Bilirubin, alanine aminotransferase (ALT), gamma glutamyl transferase (GGT), and alkaline phosphatase (AlkP) assess liver function.	Excessive glucose or lipid administration, EFAD, impaired bile flow, or specific amino acid deficiency can ↑ liver enzymes and affect bilirubin.	ALT: 7-24 U/L GGT: 8-40 U/L AlkP: 20-90 U/L Bilirubin: 0.2-1.0 mg/dl (3.4-17.1 μmol/L)	Values for males generally slightly higher than for females; enzyme values are sensitive but not specific.
Triglycerides (TG) (see earlier discussion)	Sepsis and stress can alter ability to metabolize fat; therefore TG should be regularly measured.	↑ TG indicates fat overload syndrome; measure TG before and after initial lipid infusion and postinfusion, weekly thereafter.	See earlier discussion	Measurement only after lipid infusion may make interpretation impossible.
Vitamin K status (TPN only) (see earlier discussion)	Contribution of the gut flora to vitamin K status is absent during TPN, and basic TPN formulas are devoid of it.	Prothrombin time (PT) is used to assess status.	See earlier discussion	PT is affected by many other factors besides vitamin K status.

X. Tests for Metabolic Disease

TEST	PRINCIPLE AND REQUIREMENTS	INTERPRETATION	REFERENCE RANGE	LIMITATIONS
Amino acidurias	Dietary treatment is the major therapy for many of these genetic diseases: PKU, cystinuria, maple syrup urine disease, tyrosinemia, homocysteinuria, Hartnup disease.	Monitoring amino acid level in urine or serum is necessary to assess adequacy of treatment.	Examples: Phe 1-16 g/L (35-90 μmol/L) Cys 2-22 g/L (10-90 μmol/L) Val 17-37 g/L (145-315 μmol/L) Tyr 4-16 g/L (20-90 μmol/L)	There are several methods used to measure, e.g., phenylalaline; these usually do not have exactly equivalent reference ranges.

Diabetes Mellitus				
Diabetes diagnosis	1) Serum or whole blood glucose: after fasting 8-16 hours, or on a casual blood sample.	1) ≥2 fasting levels >126 mg/dl are diagnostic; casual level ≥200 followed by fasting level >126 are diagnostic. Fasting levels of 110 to 126 indicate impaired glucose tolerance (IGT).	See Chapter 33	1) Elevated glucose levels are normal in physiologic stress; whole blood gives slightly lower values.
	2) Glucose tolerance test (GGT); 75 g glucose (100 g during pregnancy) given after fasting; serum glucose measured by before and five times during the next 3 hours after oral dosing. Glucose measured by automated chemistry procedure.	2) Serum levels of >200 at 2-hour point is diagnostic; 2-hour level <140 and all 0 to 2-hour levels <200 are normal; 140-199 at 2 hours indicates IGT. Gestational diabetes: fasting >105, 1-hour GGT >190, 2-hour GGT >165, and 3-hour GGT >145.		2) Often used for confirmation; ambulatory patients only; bedrest or stress impairs GGT; inadequate carbohydrate consumption before test invalidates results.
Diabetes monitoring	1) Blood glucose—monitoring requires that *the patient* monitor blood glucose level	1) Tight diabetes control of requires frequent monitoring of glucose levels.	1) 70-110 mg/dl (3.9-6.1 mmol/L)	A combination of glucose monitoring (by patient) and laboratory measurement of glycated proteins is needed to effectively monitor glucose control; fructosamine must be interpreted in light of plasma protein half-lives, and HbA_{1c} must be interpreted in light of red cell half-life.
	2) Serum fructosamine—assesses medium-term glucose control by measured glycated serum proteins; currently only tested in the laboratory	2) Allows assessment of average glucose levels for previous 2-3 weeks.	2) Normal levels: 1%-2% of total protein	
	3) Serum glycated hemoglobin or HbA_{1c}—assesses longer-term glucose control; currently only tested in the laboratory.	3) Allows assessment of average glucose levels for previous 2-3 months and verification of patient's serum glucose log.	3) Normal levels: 5.0%-7.5%	

Appendix created by Timothy H. Carlson, PhD, RD.

Appendix 34 Nutritional Implications of Selected Drugs

DRUG	CATEGORY	DRUG EFFECT	NUTRITIONAL IMPLICATIONS/CAUTIONS
Antiinfective Agents			
Penicillins	Antibacterial agents	Long-term use may lead to oral candidiasis, diarrhea, epigastric distress. Some products contain high amounts of potassium and/or sodium. May cause *Clostridium difficile* pseudomembranous colitis.	Caution with low-sodium diet or potassium supplements. Take most oral forms 1 hour before or 2 hours after food to improve absorption. Take amoxicillin/potassium clavulanate with food to decrease GI distress. Focus on fluid and electrolyte replacement for diarrhea.
Azithromycin (Zithromax) Claritromycin (Biaxin) Erythromycin (Ery-Tab)	Macrolide antibacterial agent Macrolide antibacterial agent Macrolide antibacterial agent	May cause GI distress, anorexia, stomatitis, bad taste in the mouth, or diarrhea. May increase sedative effect of alcohol. May cause *Clostridium difficile* pseudomembranous colitis.	Take with food to decrease GI distress. Eat frequent, small, appealing meals to counteract anorexia. Use mouth rinses, sugarless gum, or lemon water for abnormal taste in mouth. Focus on fluid and electrolyte replacement for diarrhea. Avoid alcohol.
Sulfamethoxazole/ trimethoprin (Bactrim, Bactrim DS)	Sulfonamide combination Antibacterial agent	May interfere with folate metabolism, especially with long-term use. May cause stomatitis, anorexia, nausea/vomiting, severe allergic reactions. May cause *Clostridium difficile* pseudomembranous colitis.	Take with food and 8 ounces of fluid to lessen nausea, vomiting, and anorexia. Folate supplement may be necessary. Discontinue drug and consult physician at first sign of allergic reaction. Focus on fluid and electrolyte replacement for diarrhea.
Cephalexin (Keflex) Cefproxil (Cefzil)	Cephalosporin antibacterial agent Cephalosporin antibacterial agent	May cause stomatitis, sore mouth, tongue and interfere with eating. May cause diarrhea. May cause *Clostridium difficile* pseudomembranous colitis.	Focus on fluid and electrolyte replacement for diarrhea. Eat moist, soft, low-salt foods as well as cold foods such as ice chips, sherbet, and yogurt for stomatitis and sore mouth.
Ciprofloxacin (Cipro)	Fluoroquinolone antibacterial agent	Drug may rarely precipitate in renal tubules. Drug will bind to magnesium, calcium, zinc, and iron, forming an insoluble, unabsorbable complex. Ciprofloxacin inhibits the metabolism of caffeine, thereby causing increased CNS stimulation.	Take drug with 8 ounces of fluid; maintain adequate fluid intake. Limit caffeine intake.
Levofloxacin (Levaquin)	Fluoroquinolone antibacterial agent	May cause *Clostridium difficile* pseudomembranous colitis.	Take drug at least 2 hours before or 6 hours after antacids, magnesium, calcium, iron, or zinc supplements or multivitamin with minerals. Focus on fluid and electrolyte replacement for diarrhea.
Tetracycline (Sumycin)	Antibacterial agent	Drug may cause anorexia. Drug will bind to Mg+, Ca++, Zn++, and Fe++, forming an insoluble, unabsorbable complex. May decrease bacterial production of vitamin K in intestinal tract. May cause vitamin B deficiency with long-term use. Drug combined with vitamin A may increase the risk of benign intracranial hypertension. May cause *Clostridium difficile* pseudomembranous colitis.	Take supplements separately by 3 hours. Eat frequent, small, appealing meals to decrease anorexia. Avoid excessive vitamin A while taking drug. Vitamin K and B supplement may be necessary with long-term use. Focus on fluid and electrolyte replacement for diarrhea.
Metronidazole (Flagyl)	Antibacterial agent/ antiprotozoal agent	May cause anorexia, GI distress, stomatitis, and metallic taste in mouth. May cause disulfiram-like reaction when ingested with alcohol.	Take with food to avoid GI distress. Eat frequent, small, appealing meals to decrease anorexia. Avoid all alcohol during use and for 3 days after discontinuation.

Nitrofurantoin (Macrobid)	Nitrofuran antibacterial agent	Drug may cause peripheral neuropathy, muscle weakness, and muscle wasting, especially in individuals with preexisting anemia, vitamin B deficiency, and electrolyte abnormalities. May cause *Clostridium difficile* pseudomembranous colitis.	Drug should be taken with adequate calories, protein, and vitamin B complex. Avoid in G-6-PD deficiency because of increased risk of hemolytic anemia. Focus on fluid and electrolyte replacement for diarrhea.
Gentamicin (Garamycin)	Aminoglycoside antibacterial agent	Drug may be ototoxic and nephrotoxic. Dehydration increases the risk of toxicity.	Adequate fluid intake/hydration necessary to lower risk of toxicity.
Amikacin (Amikin)	Aminoglycoside antibacterial agent		
Isoniazid (Nydrazid)	Antitubercular agent	Drug may cause pyridoxine (vitamin B_6) and niacin (vitamin B_3) deficiency, resulting in peripheral neuropathy and pellagra. Drug may affect vitamin D metabolism and decrease calcium and phosphate absorption. Drug processes MAO inhibitor-like activity.	Avoid use in malnourished individuals and others at increased risk for peripheral neuropathy. Supplement with 25 to 50 mg of pyridoxine and possibly B-complex if skin changes occur. Avoid foods high in tyramine (e.g., aged cheeses). Maintain adequate calcium and vitamin D intake.
Rifampin (Rifadin)	Antitubercular agent	Drug may increase the metabolism of vitamin D. Rare cases of osteomalacia have been reported.	May need vitamin D supplement with long-term use.
Ethambutol (Myambutol)	Antitubercular agent	Drug may decrease body copper and zinc. Drug may decrease the excretion of uric acid, leading to hyperuricemia and gout.	Increase intake of foods high in copper and zinc; take daily multivitamin with minerals when drug is used long-term. Maintain adequate hydration and purine-restricted diet.
Pyrazinamide	Antitubercular agent	Drug may decrease the excretion of uric acid, leading to hyperuricemia and gout.	Maintain adequate hydration and purine-restricted diet.
Amphotericin B (Fungizone)	Antifungal agent	Drug may cause anorexia and weight loss. Drug causes loss of potassium, magnesium, and calcium.	Eat frequent, small, appealing meals high in magnesium, potassium, calcium. Ensure adequate hydration.
Ketoconazole (Nizoral)	Antifungal agent	Drug does not dissolve at pH >5.	Take with food to increase absorption. Take with acidic liquid (e.g., cola) especially individuals with achlorhydria.
Amprenavir (Agenerase)	Antiretroviral agent	Drug provides 1744 IU of vitamin E with daily adult dose.	Avoid vitamin E supplements.
Hematologic Agents			
Warfarin (Coumadin)	Anticoagulant	Prevents the conversion of oxidized vitamin K to the active form. Produces a state of systemic anticoagulation. May inhibit mineralization of newly formed bone.	Dietary and supplemental (i.e., in vitamins) intake must be consistent to achieve desired state of anticoagulation. Monitor bone mineral density in individuals on long-term therapy.
Aspirin (Ecotrin)	Salicylate platelet inhibitor	Drug may cause GI irritation and bleeding. Drug may decrease uptake of vitamin C by leukocytes and increase urinary loss; decreases systemic levels of iron, folic acid, sodium, potassium especially with high dose, long-term use.	Incorporate foods high in vitamin C and folic acid into diet. Monitor electrolytes, hemoglobin for need for potassium, iron supplements. Avoid alcohol consumption.

Appendix created by Sr. Jeanne P. Crowe, PharmD, RPh.

Modified from Pronsky ZM: *Food medication interactions,* ed 13, Birchrunville, Pa, 2004, Waza, Inc, T/A Food Medication Interactions. Used by permission; may not be copied or reprinted without permission from Waza, Inc.

Continued

Appendix 34 Nutritional Implications of Selected Drugs—cont'd

DRUG	CATEGORY	DRUG EFFECT	NUTRITIONAL IMPLICATIONS/CAUTIONS
Hormonal/Metabolic Agents			
Metformin (Glucophage)	Biguanide	Drug may decrease absorption of vitamin B_{12}, folic acid. May cause lactic acidosis.	Maintain prescribed diabetic diet. Increase foods high in vitamin B_{12} and folic acid or supplement if necessary. Avoid alcohol to decrease risk of lactic acidosis.
Prednisone (Deltasone) Methylprednisolone (Medrol)	Corticosteroid Corticosteroid	Drug induces protein catabolism, resulting in muscle wasting, atrophy of bone protein matrix, delayed wound healing. Drug decreases intestinal absorption of calcium; promotes urinary loss of calcium, potassium, zinc, vitamin C, nitrogen; causes sodium retention.	Maintain diet high in calcium, vitamin D, protein, potassium, zinc, and vitamin C and low in sodium. Calcium and vitamin D supplements recommended for prevention of osteoporosis with long-term use of drug.
Alendronate (Fosamax)	Biphosphonate	Drug may induce mild decrease in serum calcium.	Diet high in calcium or calcium and vitamin D supplement.
Estrogen (Premarin) Oral contraceptives	Sex hormone	Drug may decrease absorption and tissue uptake of vitamin C. Drug may increase absorption of vitamin A. May inhibit folate conjugase and decrease serum folic acid levels. Drug may decrease serum levels vitamins B_6 and B_{12}, riboflavin, magnesium, zinc.	Maintain diet with adequate magnesium, folic acid, vitamins B_6 and B_{12}, riboflavin, and zinc. Calcium and vitamin D supplement may be recommended with estrogen as hormone replacement for postmenopausal women.
Cardiovascular Agents			
Digoxin (Lanoxin)	Cardiac glycoside	Drug may increase urinary loss of magnesium and decrease serum levels of potassium.	Hypokalemia, hypomagnesemia, and hypercalcemia increase drug toxicity. Maintain diet high in potassium and magnesium. Caution with calcium supplements and antacids.
Propranolol (Inderal) Metoprolol (Lopressor, Toprol XL) Atenolol (Tenormin)	Beta-adrenergic antagonist Beta-adrenergic antagonist Beta-adrenergic antagonist	Drug may mask sympathetic signs of hypoglycemia. Drug may prolong hypoglycemia. Drug may decrease insulin release in response to hyperglycemia.	Maintain prescribed diabetic diet. Monitor blood glucose for hyperglycemia. Monitor for nonsympathetic signs of hypoglycemia.
Benazepril (Lotensin) Enalapril (Vasotec) Foxinopril (Monopril) Lisinopril (Zestril, Prinivil)	ACE inhibitor ACE inhibitor ACE inhibitor ACE inhibitor	Drug may increase serum potassium levels.	Caution with high-potassium diet or potassium supplements. Avoid salt substitutes. Ensure adequate fluid intake/hydration.
Clonidine (Catapres)	Alpha-adrenergic agonist	Drug commonly causes dizziness, drowsiness, and sedation.	Avoid alcohol/alcohol products. Drug increases sensitivity to alcohol, which may increase sedation caused by drug alone.
Hydralazine (Apresoline)	Peripheral vasodilator	Drug interferes with pyridoxine (vitamin B_6) metabolism. May result in pyridoxine deficiency.	Maintain a diet high in pyridoxine. Supplementation may be necessary.
Quinidine (Quinaglute)	Antiarrhythmic agent	Cardiac toxicity of drug is increased in the presence of hypokalemia, hypomagnesemia, and/or hypocalcemia.	Diet adequate in potassium, magnesium, calcium to maintain normal serum levels. Supplementation may be necessary.

Antihyperlipidemic Agents			
Atorvistatin (Lipitor) Simvastatin (Zocor) Fluvastatin (Lescol) Pravastatin (Pravachol)	HMG Co-A reductase inhibitor HMG Co-A reductase inhibitor HMG Co-A reductase inhibitor HMG Co-A reductase inhibitor	Drug may cause significant reduction in coenzyme Q10. Drug lowers LDL cholesterol; raises HDL cholesterol.	Supplementation with coenzyme Q10 is controversial. Drug is adjunct to diet therapy. Maintain low-fat, low-cholesterol diet for optimal drug effect.
Gemfibrozil (Lopid) Fenofibrate (Tricor)	Fibric acid derivative Fibric acid derivative	Drug decreases serum triglycerides.	Maintain low-fat, low-sucrose diet; avoid alcohol for optimal therapeutic effect.
Cholestyramine (Questran)	Bile acid sequestrant	Drug binds fat-soluble vitamins (A,E,D,K), beta carotene, calcium, magnesium, iron, zinc, and folic acid.	Take fat-soluble vitamins in water-miscible form or take vitamin supplement at least 1 hour before first dose of drug daily. Maintain diet high in folic acid, magnesium, calcium, iron, zinc, or supplements when necessary. Monitor serum nutrient levels with long-term use of drug.
Niacin (Niaspan)	Nicotinic acid	High dose may elevate blood glucose and uric acid.	Maintain diabetic, low-purine diet if necessary.
Diuretics			
Furosemide (Lasix) Bumetanide (Bumex)	Loop diuretic Loop diuretic	Drug increases urinary excretion of sodium, potassium, magnesium, calcium.	Maintain diet high in potassium, magnesium, and calcium. Avoid natural licorice, which may counteract the diuretic effect of the drug. Monitor electrolytes; supplementation may be necessary.
Hydrochlorothiazide (Hydrodiuril)	Thiazide diuretic	Drug increases urinary excretion of sodium, potassium, magnesium. Drug increases renal reabsorption of calcium.	Maintain diet high in potassium and magnesium. Avoid natural licorice, which may counteract the diuretic effect of the drug. Monitor electrolytes; supplementation may be necessary. Caution with calcium supplements.
Triamterene (Dyrenium) Spironolactone (Aldactone)	Potassium-sparing diuretic Potassium-sparing diuretic	Drug increases renal reabsorption of potassium.	Avoid salt substitutes. Caution with potassium supplements. Avoid excessive potassium intake in diet.
Analgesics			
Acetaminophen (Tylenol)	Analgesic	Drug may cause hepatotoxicity at high dose. Chronic alcohol ingestion increases the risk of hepatotoxicity.	Maximum safe adult dose is <4 g/day. Avoid alcohol or limit to <2 drinks/day.
NSAIDs (ibuprofen, naproxen, nabumetone)	Analgesic, anti-arthritic	Drug may cause GI irritation and bleeding, both acute and occult.	Take drug with food or milk to decrease risk of GI toxicity.
Antidepressants			
Fluoxetine (Prozac)	Selective serotonin reuptake inhibitor	Fluoxetine may cause anorexia and weight loss.	Monitor weight and caloric intake if necessary.
Paroxetine (Paxil)	Selective serotonin reuptake inhibitor	Fluoxetine may decrease the absorption of leucine.	Avoid tryptophan, St. John's wort. Additive effects may produce adverse effects/serotonin syndrome.
Sertraline (Zoloft)	Selective serotonin reuptake inhibitor	Some herbal/natural products may increase toxicity.	
Nefazodone (Serzone) Trazodone (Desyrel) Venlafaxine (Effexor XR)	Unclassified antidepressant Unclassified antidepressant Unclassified antidepressant	Some herbal/natural products may increase toxicity.	Avoid tryptophan, St. John's wort. Additive effects may produce adverse effects/serotonin syndrome.
Amitriptyline (Elavil)	Tricyclic antidepressant	Drug may cause increased appetite (especially for carbohydrates and sweets) and weight gain. High fiber may decrease drug absorption.	Monitor caloric intake. Maintain consistent amount of fiber in diet.

Continued

Appendix created by Sr. Jeanne P. Crowe, PharmD, RPh.
Modified from Pronsky ZM: *Food medication interactions,* ed 13, Birchrunville, Pa, 2004, Waza, Inc, T/A Food Medication Interactions. Used by permission; may not be copied or reprinted without permission from Waza, Inc.

Appendix 34 Nutritional Implications of Selected Drugs—cont'd

DRUG	CATEGORY	DRUG EFFECT	NUTRITIONAL IMPLICATIONS/CAUTIONS
Antidepressants—cont'd			
Phenelzine (Nardil)	MAO inhibitor	Drug may cause increased appetite (especially for carbohydrates and sweets) and weight gain. Risk for severe reaction with dietary tyramine.	Avoid foods high in tyramine during drug use and for 2 weeks after discontinuation to prevent hypertensive crisis. Monitor caloric intake to avoid weight gain.
Lithium carbonate (Lithobid)	Antimanic/antidepressant	Sodium intake affects drug levels. Low-sodium diet, dehydration increase drug toxicity. Drug may cause GI irritation.	Drink 2 to 3 L of fluid daily to avoid dehydration. Maintain consistent dietary sodium intake. Take with food to decrease GI irritation.
Antipsychotic Agents			
Clozapine (Clozaril)	Atypical antipsychotic	Drug may cause increased appetite and weight gain. Drug may cause life-threatening toxic agranulocytosis.	Monitor for weight gain/calorie count. Individual must be enrolled in and adhere to requirements of Clozaril program, including a weekly white blood cell count.
Olanzapine (Zyprexa) Risperidone (Risperdal)	Atypical antipsychotic Atypical antipsychotic	Drug may cause increased appetite and weight gain.	Monitor weight and food intake.
Chlorpromazine (Thorazine)	Typical antipsychotic, low potency	Drug may impair glucose tolerance and insulin release. May cause increased appetite and weight gain. Risk for tardive dyskinesia.	Closer monitoring of blood glucose in the diagnosed patient with diabetes. Periodic check of blood glucose in the "at-risk" nondiabetic individual. Monitor weight/calorie count. Tardive dyskinesia may interfere with biting, chewing, swallowing.
Haloperidol (Haldol)	Typical antipsychotic, high potency	May cause increased appetite and weight gain. Risk for tardive dyskinesia.	Monitor weight/calorie count. Tardive dyskinesia may interfere with biting, chewing, swallowing.
Antianxiety and Hypnotic Agents			
Lorazepam (Ativan) Diazepam (Valium) Alprazolam (Xanax) Clonazepam (Klonopin)	Benzodiazepine Benzodiazepine Benzodiazepine Benzodiazepine	Drugs may cause significant sedation.	Avoid concurrent ingestion of alcohol, which will produce CNS depression. Limit or avoid caffeine, which may decrease the therapeutic effect of the drug.
Temazeopam (Restoril)	Benzodiazepine hypnotic		Caution with herbal/natural products that cause CNS stimulation or sedation
Zolpidem (Ambien)	Nonbenzodiazepine hypnotic		
Anticonvulsant Agents			
Carbamazepine (Tegretol)		Drug may decrease biotin, folic acid, and vitamin D levels.	Maintain diet high in folic acid and vitamin D. Calcium and vitamin D supplementation may be necessary for long-term therapy to prevent loss of bone mineral density.
Phenytoin (Dilantin)	Hydantoin	Drug may decrease serum levels of folic acid, calcium, vitamin D, biotin, thiamin.	Folic acid, calcium, and vitamin D supplement may be recommended with long-term use.
Phenobarbital	Barbiturate	Drug may induce rapid metabolism of vitamin D and produce deficiency of vitamin D and calcium. Drug may increase the metabolism of vitamin K, decrease serum folic acid and vitamin B_{12} levels.	Increase dietary intake of calcium, vitamin D, and folic acid. May need calcium, vitamin D, folic acid, and vitamin B_{12} supplementation with long-term use of drug.

Anti-Alzheimer's Agents			
Donepezil (Aricept)	Cholinesterase inhibitor	Drug is highly cholinergic; may cause anorexia, nausea, vomiting, diarrhea, increased gastric acid secretion, GI bleeding.	Take drug with food to prevent GI irritation. Monitor food intake and weight.
Rivastigmine (Exelon)	Cholinesterase inhibitor		
Galantamine (Reminyl)	Cholinesterase inhibitor		
Gastrointestinal Agents			
Famotidine (Pepcid)	H-2 receptor antagonist	Drug may reduce the absorption of vitamin B_{12} and iron.	Monitor iron studies, vitamin B_{12} level while on long-term therapy. Supplement if necessary.
Nizatidine (Axid)	H-2 receptor antagonist		
Ranitidine (Zantac)	H-2 receptor antagonist		
Omeprazole (Prilosec)	Proton pump inhibitor	Inhibition of acid secretion may inhibit the absorption of iron and vitamin B_{12}.	Monitor iron studies and vitamin B_{12} levels with long-term use of drug. Supplement if necessary.
Lansoprasole (Prevacid)	Proton pump inhibitor		
Metoclopramide (Reglan)	Prokinetic agent	Drug increases gastric emptying; may change insulin requirements in people with diabetes; may increase CNS depressant effects of alcohol. Drug may cause tardive dyskinesia with extended use.	Monitor blood glucose in diabetic individuals carefully when drug is initiated. Avoid alcohol. Tardive dyskinesia may interfere with biting, chewing, swallowing.
Antineoplastic Agents			
Methotrexate	Folate antagonist	Drug inhibits dihydrofolate reductase; decreased formation of active folate. Drug may cause GI irritation or injury.	Maintain diet high in folic acid and vitamin B_{12}. Daily folic acid supplement recommended with antirheumatic doses. Leucovorin rescue may be necessary with antineoplastic doses.
Cyclophosphamide (Cytoxan)	Alkylating agent	Drug metabolite causes bladder irritation, acute hemorrhagic cystitis.	Maintain high fluid intake (2-3 L daily) to induce frequent voiding.
Neoplastic agents		All agents are cytotoxic; could damage intestinal mucosal.	Extensive effects discussed in Chapter 40.
Carbidopa/Levodopa (Sinemet)	Dopamine precursor	Carbidopa protects levodopa against pyridoxine-enhanced peripheral decarboxylation to dopamine.	Pyridoxine supplements in excess of 10-25 mg daily may increase carbidopa requirements and increase adverse effects of levodopa.
Bromocriptine (Parlodel)	Dopamine agonist	Drug may cause GI irritation, nausea, vomiting, and GI bleeding.	Take drug with food to prevent GI irritation. Take drug at bedtime to decrease nausea.
Selegiline (Eldepryl)	MAO-B inhibitor	Drug selectively inhibits MAO-B at 10 mg or less per day. Drug loses selectivity at higher doses.	Avoid high-tyramine foods at doses greater than 10 mg per day. May precipitate hypertension.
Entacapone (Comtan)	COMT inhibitor	Drug chelates iron; may decrease serum iron levels.	Take iron supplement separately from drug.
CNS Stimulants			
Methylphenidate (Ritalin, Concerta)	CNS stimulant	Drug may cause anorexia, weight loss, and decreased growth.	Ensure adequate calorie intake. Limit ingestion of caffeine; avoid alcohol and herbal products. Monitor children's weight and growth.
Amphetamine (Adderall, Dexedrine)	CNS stimulant	Drug may cause anorexia, decreased weight loss, and decreased growth.	Ensure adequate calorie intake. Limit ingestion of caffeine; avoid alcohol and herbal products. High-dose vitamin C may decrease drug absorption, increase drug excretion, and decrease half-life of drug. Monitor children's weight and growth.

Appendix created by Sr. Jeanne P. Crowe, PharmD, RPh.
Modified from Pronsky ZM: *Food medication interactions*, ed 13, Birchrunville, Pa, 2004, Waza, Inc, T/A Food Medication Interactions. Used by permission; may not be copied or reprinted without permission from Waza, Inc..

Appendix 35 Counseling Patients on Dietary Supplements

1994 Dietary Supplement Health and Education Act
Gives FDA authority to establish GMPs
Defines dietary supplements and ingredients
Makes manufacturer responsible for ensuring safety
Allows third-party literature at point of sale
Regulates support statements
Establishes label requirements
Requires that new ingredients be submitted to the FDA 75 days before marketing product
Establishes the Office of Dietary Supplements and the Commission on Dietary Supplements

Dietary Supplement Label Requirements
Identity
Contents
Structure-function claims
Directions
Facts panel
Ingredients in descending order
Correspondence address

Safety Issues
Lack of quality control
Misidentification of plants
Contents not verified
Potential allergic reactions
Adulteration with prescription drugs
Lack of regulation
Contamination with heavy metals and pesticides
Raw animal parts; obscure labeling; no restriction on source of animal tissues
Variation in chemical composition of plants
Overharvesting of endangered species
Substitution of herbs
Standardized to only one component
Lack of research supporting use
Effective dosage not established
Misleading labels and advertising

High-Risk Patients
Elderly and children
Those taking prescription or OTC medicines, especially if more than three drugs or high-risk drugs are involved
Pregnant or breast-feeding
Chronically ill
Those with kidney disease and on dialysis; whether herbs can be used is unknown

---

From Herr SM: *Herb-drug interaction handbook,* ed 2, Nassau, NY, 2002, Church Street Books. Used with permission from Sharon M. Herr, RD, CDN.
[1]May contain or be adulterated with aristolochic acid.
GMP, Good manufacturing practices.

Appendix 35 Counseling Patients on Dietary Supplements—cont'd

High-Risk Drugs

Digoxin
Drugs used during transplantation
Rifamycin agents
Theophylline
Antifungals
Chemotherapy agents
Macrolides
Warfarin
Antiepileptics

Pharmacokinetic Interactions

Altered absorption or distribution
Inhibition or induction of metabolism
Additive activity
Alteration in protein-binding sites
Altered renal elimination
Synergistic activity

Herbs That May Have Adverse Health Effects

Chaparral
Ephedra
Lobelia
Slimming/dieter's tea
Wormwood
Bragantia wallichii[1]
Asarum spp[1]
Cocculus spp[1]
Menispernum dauricum[1]
Sinomenium acutum[1]
Vladimiria souliei[1]
Comfrey
Germander
Magnolia-stephania preparations
Willow bark
Aristolochia spp[1]
Akebia spp[1]
Clematis spp[1]
Diploclisia spp[1]
Saussurea lappa[1]
Stephania spp[1]
Triatricol

Herb Safety

Encourage patients to discuss supplements with their physicians.
Do not combine herbs and drugs having similar actions.
Urge caution with patients who are taking drugs with a narrow margin of safety, who are on multiple drugs, or who are scheduled for elective surgery.
Do not exceed dosages on supplement label.
Use nationally known brands or brands tested by independent labs, such as Consumer Labs.
Collect data on supplement use. Compare supplement use against verifiable changes in health status.
Report any suspected interactions to MedWatch at the FDA.
Keep up-to-date information on dietary supplements.

Communicating With Patients

Ask patient about supplement use. Patient may consider herbs natural and safe.
Patient might not acknowledge the need to report use to health care providers. Review ingredients in vitamin/mineral supplements.
Ask about herbal teas and their ingredients. Practitioner should examine how he or she feels about complementary and alternative medicine.
Do not be judgmental. Body language is as important as words.
Assess patient's knowledge about supplements used. Who recommended the supplement? Is scientific research available to support that use?
Provide reliable resources for patients.

Appendixes 36 to 41 provide basic nutritional information and unique product components. The tables were compiled by Ainsley M. Malone, MS, RD, CNSD. Product information was obtained from the following companies:

B. Braun Medical—Bethlehem, Pennsylvania
Baxter Healthcare—Deerfield, Illinois
Corpak MedSystems—Wheeling, Illinois
Mead-Johnson Nutritionals—Evansville, Indiana
Nestle Clinical Nutrition—Deerfield, Illinois
Novartis Nutrition—Minneapolis, Minnesota
Ross Products Division, Abbott Laboratories—Columbus, Ohio
Scandipharm—Birmingham, Alabama

Appendix 36 Milk-Based Formulas or Products Designed to Be Mixed With Milk

PRODUCT	MANUFACTURER	kcal/ml	% CHO kcal	% PRO kcal	% FAT kcal	FLAVORS	COMMENTS
Carnation Instant Breakfast	Nestlé	1.06	63	19	18	Vanilla, chocolate, strawberry, café mocha, chocolate malt	Mixed as directed with 2% milk
Sugar-Free Carnation Instant Breakfast	Nestlé	1.0	51	25	24	Vanilla, chocolate, strawberry, chocolate malt	Mixed as directed with 2% milk
Resource Instant Breakfast	Novartis	1.2	51	21	28	Vanilla, strawberry	Mixed as directed with whole milk
Forta Shake	Ross Products	1.2	50	24	26	Vanilla, chocolate, strawberry, eggnog	Mixed as directed with 2% milk
Meritene Powder	Novartis	1.08	45	26	29	Vanilla, chocolate	Mixed as directed with whole milk
Ultra Slim Fast	Slim Fast Food Company	0.74	66	27	5		Mixed as directed with skim milk

Appendix created by Ainsley M. Malone, MS, RD, CNSD.

Appendix 37A Whole-Protein, Lactose-Free Formulas With 0.5 kcal/ml

PRODUCT	MANUFACTURER	kcal/ml	% CHO kcal	% PRO kcal	% FAT kcal	VOLUME TO MEET 100% RDI (ml)	COMMENTS
Introlite	Ross Products	0.53	53.3	16.7	30	1320	Unflavored

Appendix created by Ainsley M. Malone, MS, RD, CNSD.

Appendix 37B Whole-Protein, Lactose-Free Formulas With 1 to 1.2 kcal/ml

PRODUCT	MANUFACTURER	kcal/ ml	% CHO kcal	% PRO kcal	% FAT kcal	VOLUME TO ACHIEVE 100% RDI (ml)	COMMENTS
Boost	Mead-Johnson	1.01	67.0	17.0	16	—	Six available flavors
Boost High Protein	Mead-Johnson	1.01	55.0	24.0	21	—	Chocolate Strawberry Vanilla
Boost With Fiber	Mead-Johnson	1.01	67.0	17.0	16	—	Chocolate Vanilla 3 gm fiber/8 oz
Compleat	Novartis	1.07	53.0	16.0	31	1500	Unflavored 4.3 gm fiber/L (soluble and insoluble)
Ensure	Ross Products	1.06	63.9	14.1	22	948	Eight available flavors
Ensure High Calcium	Ross Products	0.95	54.7	21.3	24	—	Chocolate Vanilla 400 mg calcium/8 oz
Ensure High Protein	Ross Products	0.95	54.7	21.3	24	—	Four available flavors 12 gm protein/8 oz
Ensure With Fiber	Ross Products	1.06	63.9	14.1	22	948	Contains fructooligosaccharides 2.8 gm fiber/8 oz
Fibersource	Novartis	1.2	57.0	14.0	29	1165	Unflavored 10 gm fiber/L (soluble and insoluble)
Fibersource HN	Novartis	1.2	53.0	18.0	29	1165	Unflavored 10 gm fiber/L (soluble and insoluble)
Isocal	Mead-Johnson	1.06	50.0	13.0	37	1890	Unflavored
Isocal HN	Mead-Johnson	1.06	46.0	17.0	37	1180	Unflavored
Isocal HN Plus	Mead-Johnson	1.2	53.0	18.0	29	1000	Unflavored
Isosource	Novartis	1.2	57.0	14.0	29	1165	Unflavored
Isosource HN	Novartis	1.2	53.0	18.0	29	1165	Unflavored
Isosource VHN	Novartis	1.0	50.0	25.0	25	1250	Unflavored 10 gm fiber/L (soluble and insoluble) High protein
Jevity	Ross Products	1.06	54.3	16.7	29	1321	Mild flavor 14.4 gm fiber/L
Jevity Plus	Ross Products	1.2	52.5	18.5	29	1000	Unflavored 12 gm fiber/L (soluble and insoluble) Contains fructooligosaccharides
Modulen IBD	Nestlé	1.0	44.0	14.0	42	2000	Contains transforming growth factor designed for Crohn's disease
Nubasics	Nestlé	1.0	53.0	14.0	33	—	Chocolate Strawberry Vanilla
Nutren 1.0	Nestlé	1.0	51.0	16.0	33	1500	Unflavored
Nutren 1.0 With Fiber	Nestlé	1.0	51.0	16.0	33	1500	Unflavored 14.0 gm fiber/L
Osmolite	Ross Products	1.06	57.0	14.0	29	1887	Mild flavor
Osmolite HN	Ross Products	1.06	54.3	16.7	29	1321	Mild flavor

Appendix created by Ainsley M. Malone, MS, RD, CNSD.

Continued

Appendix 37B Whole-Protein, Lactose-Free Formulas With 1 to 1.2 kcal/ml —cont'd

PRODUCT	MANUFACTURER	kcal/ml	% CHO kcal	% PRO kcal	% FAT kcal	VOLUME TO ACHIEVE 100% RDI (ml)	COMMENTS
Osmolite HN Plus	Ross Products	1.2	52.5	18.5	29	1000	Mild flavor
Probalance	Nestlé	1.2	52.0	18.0	30	1000	Vanilla 10 gm fiber/L (soluble and insoluble)
Promote	Ross Products	1.0	52.0	25.0	23	1000	Vanilla High-protein
Promote With Fiber	Ross Products	1.0	50.0	25.0	25	1000	Vanilla 14.4 gm fiber/L (soluble and insoluble)
Protain XL	Mead-Johnson	1.0	52.0	22.0	26	1250	Unflavored 9.1 gm fiber/L Fortified with vitamins A, C, zinc, and β-carotene
Replete	Nestlé	1.0	45.0	25.0	30	1000	Vanilla High-protein Fortified with vitamins A, C, zinc, and β-carotene
Replete With Fiber	Nestlé	1.0	45.0	25.0	30	100	Vanilla High-protein, 14.0 gm fiber/L Fortified with vitamins A, C, zinc, and β-carotene
Resource Standard	Novartis	1.06	64.0	14.0	22	1180	Chocolate Strawberry Vanilla
Ultracal	Mead-Johnson	1.06	50.0	17.0	33	1120	Unflavored 14.4 gm fiber/L
Ultracal HN Plus	Mead-Johnson	1.2	53.0	18.0	29	1000	Unflavored 10 gm fiber/L

Appendix created by Ainsley M. Malone, MS, RD, CNSD.

Appendix 37C Whole-Protein, Lactose-Free Formulas With 1.5 and 2.0 kcal/ml

PRODUCT	MANUFACTURER	kcal/ ml	% CHO kcal	% PRO kcal	% FAT kcal	VOLUME TO ACHIEVE 100% RDI (ml)	COMMENTS
Boost Plus	Mead-Johnson	1.52	50.0	16.0	34.0	—	Chocolate Strawberry Vanilla
Comply	Mead-Johnson	1.5	46.0	16.0	36.0	830	Unflavored MCT/LCT 20/80
Ensure Plus	Ross Products	1.5	56.4	14.6	29.0	1185	Six flavors
Ensure Plus HN	Ross Products	1.5	47.3	16.7	30.0	947	Chocolate Vanilla
Ensure Plus HN for tube feeding	Ross Products	1.5	54.3	16.7	29.0	1000	Unflavored
Isosource 1.5	Novartis	1.5	44.0	18.0	38.0	933	Unflavored 8 gm fiber/L (soluble and insoluble)
Nubasics Plus	Nestlé	1.5	47.0	14.0	39.0	—	Chocolate Strawberry Vanilla
Nutren 1.5	Nestlé	1.5	45.0	16.0	39.0	1000	Unflavored MCT/LCT 50/50
Nutrifocus	Ross Products	1.5	53.7	16.7	29.6	—	Chocolate Vanilla 10 gm fiber/500 ml Contains fructooligo-saccharides Fortified with vitamins A, C, and zinc
Resource Plus	Novartis	1.5	58.0	14.0	28.0	946	Chocolate Strawberry Vanilla
2.0 kcal/ml							
Deliver 2.0	Mead-Johnson	2.0	40.0	15.0	45.0	1000	Vanilla MCT/LCT 30/70
Novasource 2.0	Novartis	2.0	43.0	18.0	39.0	948	Orange crème Vanilla
Nutren 2.0	Nestlé	2.0	45.0	16.0	39.0	750	Vanilla MCT/LCT 75/25
Twocal HN	Ross Products	2.0	43.2	16.7	40.1	948	Butter pecan Vanilla Contains fructooligosac-charides
VHC 2.25	Nestlé	2.25	35.0	16.0	49.0	—	Vanilla Designed as a medication pass beverage

Appendix created by Ainsley M. Malone, MS, RD, CNSD.

Appendix 38 Specially Designed Formulas: Clear Liquid, Fat Malabsorption, Glucose Intolerance, Hepatic, Immune-Support, Metabolic Stress, Pulmonary, Renal

PRODUCT	MANUFACTURER	kcal/ml	% CHO kcal	% PRO kcal	% FAT kcal	FLAVORS	COMMENTS
Clear Liquid Formulas							
Forta Drink	Ross Products	0.52	67.5	26.0	6.5	Fruit punch Orange	Powder form
Nubasics Juice Drink	Nestlé	1.0	83.0	16.0	—	Berry Orange	5.5-oz serving size
Resource Arginaid Extra	Novartis	1.06	83.0	17.0	—	Berry Orange	Fortified with arginine, zinc, vitamins C and E
Resource Fruit Beverage	Novartis	1.06	86.0	14.0	—	Berry Orange Peach	
Formulas for Fat Malabsorption							
Lipisorb	Mead-Johnson	1.35	48.0	17.0	35.0	Vanilla	MCT/LCT 85/15

PRODUCT	MANUFACTURER	kcal/ml	% CHO kcal	% PRO kcal	% FAT kcal	VOLUME TO ACHIEVE 100% RDI (ml)	COMMENTS
Formulas for Glucose Intolerance							
Choice DM	Mead-Johnson	1.06	40.0	17.0	43.0	1120	MCT/LCT 10/90 soluble and 14.4 gm fiber/L (soluble and insoluble)
Diabetisource AC	Novartis	1.2	36.0	20.0	44.0	1120	10.0 gm fiber/L (soluble and insoluble) Supplemented with arginine, vitamins C and E, and chromium
Glucerna	Ross Products	1.0	34.3	16.7	49.0	1442	14.1 gm fiber/L 100% insoluble
Glytrol	Nestlé	1.0	40.0	18.0	42.0	1400	15 gm fiber/L (soluble and insoluble)
Hepatic Disease Formulas							
Hepatic-Aid II	B. Braun	1.2	57.3	15.0	27.7	Incomplete	Increased levels of leucine, isoleucine, and valine Minimal phenylalanine, tryptophan, and tyrosine content
Nutri-Hep	Nestlé	1.5	77.0	12.0	11.0	1000	Contains standard amounts of vitamins and minerals; 50% BCAA and 50% AAA 66% of fat is MCT

Appendix created by Ainsley M. Malone, MS, RD, CNSD.

Appendix 38 Specially Designed Formulas: Clear Liquid, Fat Malabsorption, Glucose Intolerance, Hepatic, Immune-Support, Metabolic Stress, Pulmonary, Renal—cont'd

PRODUCT	MANUFACTURER	kcal/ ml	% CHO kcal	% PRO kcal	% FAT kcal	VOLUME TO ACHIEVE 100% RDI (ml)	COMMENTS
Formulas for Immune-Support							
Advera	Ross Products	1.28	65.5	18.7	15.8	1184	Fortified with vitamins C, E, B_6, and folic acid Protein is hydrolyzed
Crucial	Nestlé	1.5	33.7	23.5	39.0	1000	Fortified with arginine, vitamins A, C, zinc, and β-carotene MCT/LCT 50/50
Immune-Aid	B. Braun	1.0	48.0	32.0	25.0	2000	Powder form Fortified with arginine, glutamine, BCAAs, and nucleic acids
Impact	Novartis	1.0	53.0	22.0	25.0	1500	Fortified with arginine and nucleotides Menhaden oil as source of ω-3 fatty acids
Impact 1.5	Novartis	1.5	38.0	22.0	40.0	1250	Fortified with arginine and nucleotides Menhaden oil as source of ω-3 fatty acids
Impact Glutamine	Novartis	1.3	46.0	24.0	30.0	1000	Fortified with arginine, glutamine, and nucleotides Menhaden oil as source of ω-3 fatty acids 10 gm fiber/L
Impact with Fiber	Novartis	1.0	53.0	22.0	25.0	1500	Fortified with arginine and nucleotides Menhaden oil as source of ω-3 fatty acids 10 gm fiber/L
Impact Recover	Novartis	1.0	46.0	24.0	30.0	—	Oral supplement powder Fortified with arginine, glutamine, and nucleotides
Intensical	Mead-Johnson	1.3	46.0	25.0	29.0	1000	Fortified with arginine Menhaden oil as source on ω-3 fatty acids
Formulas for Metabolic Stress							
Perative	Ross Products	1.3	42.0	15.8	8.8	1155	Protein in peptide form Fortified with arginine
Prosure	Ross Products	1.25	64.0	21.3	14.7	—	Banana Vanilla Oral supplement 1 gm eicosapentanoic acid/serving to modulate metabolism
Traumacal	Mead-Johnson	1.5	38.0	22	40.0	2000	Vanilla Fortified with vitamins B complex, C and E

Continued

Appendix 38 Specially Designed Formulas: Clear Liquid, Fat Malabsorption, Glucose Intolerance, Hepatic, Immune-Support, Metabolic Stress, Pulmonary, Renal—cont'd

PRODUCT	MANUFACTURER	kcal/ ml	% CHO kcal	% PRO kcal	% FAT kcal	VOLUME TO ACHIEVE 100% RDI (ml)	COMMENTS
Pulmonary Disease Formulas							
NovaSource Pulmonary	Novartis	1.5	40.0	20.0	40.0	933	8.0 gm fiber/L
NutriVent	Nestlé	1.5	27.0	18.0	55.0	1000	MCT/LCT 40/60
Oxepa	Ross Products	1.5	28.1	16.7	55.2	947	Fortified with vitamins C, E, and β-carotene, eicoaspentanoic acid, and borage oil
Pulmocare	Ross Products	1.5	28.2	16.7	55.1	947	MCT/LCT 25/75 MCT/LCT 20/80
Respalor	Mead-Johnson	1.5	40.0	20.0	40.0	1000	MCT/LCT 30/70 Fortified with vitamins C, E, and β-carotene

PRODUCT	MANUFACTURER	kcal/ ml	PROTEIN (gm)*	POTASSIUM (mEq)*	PHOSPHORUS (mg)*	MAGNESIUM (mg)*	COMMENTS
Renal Disease Formulas							
Magnacal Renal	Mead-Johnson	2.0	37.5	16	400	100	Added carnitine, ↓ vitamins C, D, and K 1000 ml to achieve RDI
Nepro	Ross Products	2.0	35.0	14	343	108	Added carnitine, ↓ vitamins A and D, ↑ calcium 947 ml to achieve RDI
NovaSource Renal	Novartis	2.0	37.0	14	325	100	Added carnitine, ↓ vitamins A, C, D, and E 1000 ml to achieve RDI
Nutrirenal	Nestlé	2.0	14.0	16	350	100	Fortified with vitamins C, B complex, folic acid, zinc, and selenium 750 ml to achieve RDI
Suplena	Ross Products	2.0	15.0	14	365	108	Added carnitine, ↓ vitamins C, D, and K, ↑'d calcium 947 ml to achieve RDI
Renalcal	Nestlé	2.0	17.0	Negligible	Negligible	Negligible	Added carnitine No fat-soluble vitamins

Appendix created by Ainsley M. Malone, MS, RD, CNSD.
*Per 1000 kcal.

Appendix 39 Defined Formulas

PRODUCT	MANUFACTURER	kcal/ml	% CHO kcal	% PRO kcal	% FAT kcal	VOLUME TO ACHIEVE 100% RDI (ml)	COMMENTS
Alitraq	Ross Products	1.0	65.7	21.1	13.2	1500	Vanilla Fortified with arginine and glutamine
Criticare HN	Mead-Johnson	1.06	81.0	14.4	4.5	1890	50% peptides and 50% FAA Increased levels of vitamins C and B complex
FAA	Nestlé	1.0	70.0	20.0	10.0	1000	100% FAA
Optimental	Ross Products	1.0	54.5	20.5	25.0	1422	Vanilla Fortified with arginine Contains fructooligo-saccharides
Peptamen	Nestlé	1.0	51.0	16.0	33.0	1500	MCT/LCT 70/30
Peptamen with FOS	Nestlé	1.0	51.0	16.0	33.0	1500	MCT/LCT 70/30 Contains fructooligo-saccharides
Peptamen 1.5	Nestlé	1.5	49.0	18.0	33.0	1500	MCT/LCT 70/30
Peptamen VHP	Nestlé	1.0	42.0	25.0	33.0	1500	MCT/LCT 70/30 High-protein
Peptinex	Novartis	1.0	65.0	20.0	15.0	1500	Peptides FAA (16%) Vanilla
Peptinex DT	Novartis	1.0	65.0	20.0	15.0	1500	Greater percentages of smaller peptides FAA (40%)
Reabilan*	Nestlé	1.0	52.5	12.5	35.0	2000	Peptides MCT/LCT 50/50
Reabilan HN*	Nestlé	1.33	47.5	17.5	35.0	1500	Peptides
Subdue	Mead-Johnson	1.0	50.0	20.0	30.0	1180	Chocolate Orange Increased levels of vitamins C, E, and β-carotene
Subdue Plus	Mead-Johnson	1.5	50.0	20.0	30.0	946	Chocolate Orange Increased levels of vitamins C, E, and β-carotene
Tolerex	Novartis	1.0	91.0	8.0	1.0	1800	Powder form Protein is 100% FAA
Vivonex Plus	Novartis	1.0	76.0	18.0	6.0	1800	Powder form Protein is 100% FAA
Vivonex RTF	Novartis	1.0	70.0	20.0	10.0	1500	Liquid form Protein is 100% FAA
Vivonex TEN	Novartis	1.0	82.0	15.0	3.0	2000	Powder form Protein is 100% FAA
Vivonex HN	Novartis	1.0	73.8	16.7	9.5	1500	Powder form Protein is 100% FAA

Appendix created by Ainsley M. Malone, MS, RD, CNSD.
*No longer available in some markets.

Appendix 40 Pediatric Specialized Formulas

PRODUCT	MANUFACTURER	kcal/ ml	% CHO kcal	% PRO kcal	% FAT kcal	VOLUME (ml) TO ACHIEVE 100% RDA	COMMENTS
Compleat Pediatric	Novartis	1.0	50.0	15	35.0	900	Unflavored Blenderized feeding 4.4 gm fiber/L
Enfamil Kindercal	Mead-Johnson	1.06	52.0	11	37.0	946	Vanilla
Enfamil Kindercal With Fiber	Mead-Johnson	1.06	52.0	11	37.0	946	Vanilla 6.3 gm fiber/L
Pediasure	Ross Products	1.0	43.9	12	44.1	1000	Four flavors
Pediasure Enteral	Ross Products	1.0	43.9	12	44.1	1000	Vanilla
Pediasure Enteral With Fiber	Ross Products	1.0	43.9	12	44.1	1000	5.0 gm fiber/L
Peptamen Junior	Nestlé	1.0	55.0	12	33.0	1000	Vanilla Whey-based peptides MCT/LCT 60/40
Portagen	Mead-Johnson	0.68	46.0	14	40.0	—	Powder form MCT/LCT 86/14
Resource Just for Kids	Novartis	1.0	44.0	12	44.0	1000	Chocolate Strawberry Vanilla
Resource Just for Kids With Fiber	Novartis	1.0	44.0	12	44.0	1000	Vanilla 6 gm fiber/L
Vivonex Pediatric	Novartis	0.80	63.0	12	25.0	1170	Flavor packets Powder form Protein is 100% FAA

Appendix created by Ainsley M. Malone, MS, RD, CNSD.

Appendix 41 Modular Components for Enteral Feedings

PRODUCT	MANUFACTURER	kcal/ SERVING	CHO (g)/ SERVING	PRO (g)/ SERVING	FAT (g)/ SERVING	SERVING SIZE	COMMENTS
Protein							
Casec	Mead-Johnson	17	—	4.0	0.09	1 tablespoon	Caseinates
Promix	Corpak	82	7.2	15.0	1.0	1 packet	Whey protein Lecithin
Promod	Ross Products	28	0.67	5.0	0.60	1 scoop	Whey protein
Resource Arginaid	Novartis	35	4.0	4.5	—	1 packet	4.5 g arginine
Resource Glutasolve	Novartis	90	7.0	15.0	—	1 packet	L-Glutamine
Resource Protein Powder	Novartis	25	0	6.0	0	1 scoop	Whey protein
Sympt-X Glutamine	Baxter	60	5.0	10.0	—	1 packet	L-Glutamine
Carbohydrate							
Karo Syrup	Best Foods	120	30.0	—	—	30 ml	Corn syrup
Moducal	Mead-Johnson	30	7.5	—	—	1 tablespoon	Glucose polymers
Polycose Liquid	Ross Products	60	15.0	—	—	30 ml	Glucose polymers
Polycose Powder	Ross Products	23	5.6	—	—	1 tablespoon	Glucose polymers
Fat							
MCT oil	Mead-Johnson	115	—	—	14.0	1 tablespoon	
Microlipid	Mead-Johnson	135	—	—	15.2	30 ml	
Vegetable oil		120	—	—	13.3	1 tablespoon	

PRODUCT	MANUFACTURER	kcal/ 100 g	g CHO/ 100 g	g PRO/ 100 g	g FAT/ 100 g	COMMENTS
Mixed						
Scandical	Scandipharm	538	62	—	38	Powder form Maltodextrin Coconut and soy oils

Appendix created by Ainsley M. Malone, MS, RD, CNSD.

Appendix 42 Fiber Content of Selected Foods

FOOD	AMOUNT	GRAMS OF FIBER	CALORIES
Very Good Sources: More than 3.0 Grams per Serving			
Baked beans, canned in sauce	1 cup	16.0	180
Black beans, cooked	1 cup	15.0	227
Bran Buds cereal	⅓ cup	12.0	88
Figs, dried	3	10.5	120
Pinto beans, cooked	½ cup	7.3	117
Lima or butter beans, mature	½ cup	7.0	115
All-Bran cereal	½ cup	6.6	54
Kidney beans (red), cooked	½ cup	6.5	112
Chickpeas, canned	½ cup	5.3	143
Apple, baked	1 large	5.0	100
Grape Nuts cereal	½ cup	5.0	200
Potato, baked with skin	1 medium	4.8	220
Raspberries, fresh or frozen	½ cup	4.6	20
Peanuts, dry roasted	¼ cup	4.6	332
Lentils, cooked	⅔ cup	4.5	160
Artichoke hearts, canned	4 or 5 small	4.5	24
English muffin, whole-wheat	1 whole	4.4	134
Oat bran	¼ cup	4.4	63
Whole-wheat bread	2 slices	4.0	120
Shredded wheat, spoon size	½ cup	4.0	100
Eggplant, baked with tomatoes	2 thick slices	4.0	42
Greens, cooked	1 cup	4.0	42
Pear, with skin	1 medium	4.0	100
Green peas, cooked	½ cup	3.9	58
Blackberries, raw, plain	½ cup	3.8	37
Sauerkraut	⅔ cup	3.8	29
Beets, whole	3 small	3.7	48
Apple, with skin	1 medium	3.7	80
Grape Nuts cereal	½ cup	3.6	208
Squash, winter, baked	¾ cup	3.5	60
Sweet potato with skin, baked	1 medium	3.4	117
Strawberries, raw	1 cup	3.4	45
Good Sources: 2.0 to 3.0 Grams per Serving			
Cheerios	1 cup	3.0	110
Broad beans (Italian)	¾ cup	3.0	30
Sweet potatoes, baked	1 medium	3.0	100
Plums, dried (prunes)	5	3.0	100
Rolled oats	¾ cup cooked	3.0	70
Cabbage, cooked	1 cup	3.0	30
Raisin bran cereal	¾ cup	3.0	200
Orange, Valencia, raw	1 medium	3.0	59
Almonds, sliced	1 oz	2.9	171

Data from: Anderson JW, Bridges SR: Dietary fiber content of selected foods, *Am J Clin Nutr* 47:440, 1988; and Pennington J: *Bowe's and Church's food values of portions commonly used,* ed 17, Baltimore, Md, 1998, Lippincott-Williams & Wilkins.

Appendix 42 Fiber Content of Selected Foods—cont'd

FOOD	AMOUNT	GRAMS OF FIBER	CALORIES
Good Sources: 2.0 to 3.0 Grams per Serving—cont'd			
Raisins, seeded	¼ cup	2.8	111
Banana	1 medium	2.7	105
Shredded wheat	⅔ cup	2.6	102
Green beans, frozen, whole	½ cup	2.5	30
Rhubarb, cooked with sugar	½ cup	2.4	139
Broccoli, cooked	½ cup	2.3	22
Carrots	1 medium	2.2	31
Okra, boiled	½ cup	2.2	30
Corn, whole-kernel, canned	⅔ cup	2.1	44
Bran meal	1 tbsp	2.0	9
Plums	2 small	2.0	40
Pineapple, canned in water	1 cup	2.0	150
Whole-wheat bread	1 slice	2.0	60
Fair Sources: Less Than 2.0 Grams			
Asparagus, small spears	½ cup	1.7	17
Avocado, diced	¼ cup	1.7	97
Peach, raw	1 medium	1.7	37
Watermelon	2 cups	1.6	102
Peppers, green (cooked)	1 cup	1.6	36
Melon, honeydew	3-in slice	1.5	42
Mushrooms, raw	5 small	1.4	4
Tomato	1 medium	1.4	26
Brussels sprouts	¾ cup	1.3	20
Cauliflower	½ cup	1.3	13
Peanut butter, chunky	1 tbsp	1.1	94
Peanut butter, creamy	1 tbsp	1.1	86
Cantaloupe	¼ small, whole	1.0	38
Grapes, white	20	1.0	75
Popcorn, no additives	1 cup	1.0	20
Poor Sources: Less Than 1.0 Gram per Serving			
Celery	2 tbsp	1.0	3
Cucumbers	10 thin slices	0.7	12
Lettuce	1 cup	0.8	5
Onions	½ cup	1.5	22
Grapefruit	½	0.8	30
Fruit and vegetable juice	½ cup	0	Variable
Cornflakes or Rice Krispies	1 cup	0.5 less than 1.0	Variable
Refined white flour products (white bread, rolls, bagels, most pastas, pizza crust, crackers)	Usual portion		

Appendix 43 Caffeine Content of Foods

CAFFEINE CONTENT	SERVING (mg)
Coffee, 6-oz Cup	
Brewed, drip method	103
Brewed, percolator method	75
Instant, 1 rounded tsp	57
Decaffeinated	2
Flavored, regular and sugar-free	25-75
Espresso, 1 ounce	40
Tea	
3-minute brew, 6-oz cup	36
Instant, 1 rounded tsp in 8 oz of water	25-35
Decaffeinated, 5-minute brew, 6-oz cup	1
Cola Beverages, 12 oz	
Regular or diet	35-50
Decaffeinated	Trace
Cherry Colas, Dr. Pepper, Mr. Pibb, 12 oz	
Regular or diet	35-50
Decaffeinated	Trace
Mellow Yellow, 12 oz	
Regular or diet	52
Mountain Dew, 12 oz	
Regular or diet	54
Cocoa and Chocolate	
Cocoa beverage, 6-oz cup	4
Chocolate milk, 8 oz	8
Chocolate, sweet, semisweet, dark, milk, 1 oz	8-20
Chocolate, baking, unsweetened, 1 oz	58
Chocolate-flavored, syrup, 1 oz	5
Chocolate pudding, ½ cup	4-8

Modified from Pennington JA: *Bowe's and Church's food values of portions commonly used,* ed 17, Baltimore, 1998, Lippincott-Williams & Wilkins.

Appendix 44 Nutritive Values for Alcoholic Beverages and Mixes

BEVERAGE	SERVING (oz)	ALCOHOL (g)	CARBOHYDRATE (g)	CALORIES	EXCHANGES FOR CALORIE CONTROL
Beer					
Regular	12.0	13.0	13	150	1 Starch, 2 fat
Light	12.0	11.0	5	100	2 Fat
Near beer	12.0	1.5	12	60	1 Starch
Distilled spirits					
80-proof (gin, rum, vodka, whiskey, scotch)	1.5	14.0	Trace	100	2 Fat
Dry brandy, cognac	1.0	11.0	Trace	75	1.5 Fat
Table wine					
Dry white	4.0	11.0	Trace	80	2 Fat
Red or rosé	4.0	12.0	2	85	2 Fat
Sweet wine	4.0	12.0	5	105	⅓ Starch, 2 fat
Light wine	4.0	6.0	1	50	1 Fat
Wine cooler	12.0	13.0	30	215	2 Fruit, 2 fat
Dealcoholized wines	4.0	Trace	6-7	25-35	0.5 Fruit
Sparkling wines					
Champagne	4.0	12.0	4	100	2 Fat
Sweet kosher wine	4.0	12.0	12	132	1 Starch, 2 fat
Appetizer/dessert wines					
Sherry	2.0	9.0	2	74	1.5 Fat
Sweet sherry, port, muscatel	2.0	9.0	7	90	0.5 Starch, 1.5 fat
Cordials, liqueurs	1.5	13.0	18	160	1 Starch, 2 fat
Vermouth					
Dry	3.0	13.0	4	105	2 Fat
Sweet	3.0	13.0	14	140	1 Starch, 2 fat
Cocktails					
Bloody Mary	5.0	14.0	5	116	1 Vegetable, 2 fat
Daiquiri	2.0	14.0	2	111	2 Fat
Manhattan	2.0	17.0	2	178	2.5 Fat
Martini	2.5	22.0	Trace	156	3.5 Fat
Old-fashioned	4.0	26.0	Trace	180	4 Fat
Tom Collins	7.5	16.0	3	120	2.5 Fat
Mixes					
Mineral water	Any	0.0	0	0	Free
Sugar-free tonic	Any	0.0	0	0	Free
Club soda	Any	0.0	0	0	Free
Diet soda	Any	0.0	0	0	Free
Tomato juice	4.0	0.0	5	25	1 Vegetable
Bloody Mary mix	4.0	0.0	5	25	1 Vegetable
Orange juice	4.0	0.0	15	60	1 Fruit
Grapefruit juice	4.0	0.0	15	60	1 Fruit
Pineapple juice	4.0	0.0	15	60	1 Fruit

From: Franz MJ: Alcohol and diabetes: its metabolism and guidelines for its occasional use, Part II, *Diabetes Spectrum* 3(4):210-216, 1990.

Caloric Value of Alcoholic Beverages

The caloric contribution from alcohol of an alcoholic beverage can be estimated by multiplying the number of ounces by the proof and then again by the factor 0.8. For beers and wines, kilocalories from alcohol can be estimated by multiplying ounces by percentage of alcohol (by volume) and then by the factor 1.6.

Appendix 45A Oxalate Content of Foods*

FOOD	OXLATE (mg)
Cereal and Cereal Products	
Bread, white	4.9
Cake, fruit	11.8
Cake, sponge	7.4
Cornflakes	2.0
Crackers, soybean	207.0
Egg noodle (chow mein)	1.0
Grits (white corn)	41.0
Macaroni, boiled	1.0
Oatmeal, porridge	1.0
Spaghetti, boiled	1.5
Spaghetti in tomato sauce	4.0
Wheat bran	92.0†
Wheat germ	269.0
Milk and Milk Products	
Butter	0.0
Cheese, cheddar	0.0
Margarine	0.0
Milk	0.15
Meats and Eggs	
Bacon, streaky, fried	3.3
Beef, canned corned	0.0
Beef, topside roast	0.0
Chicken, roasted	0.0
Eggs, boiled	0.0
Fish:	
Haddock	0.2
Plaice	0.3
Sardines	4.8
Ham	1.6
Hamburger, grilled	0.0
Lamb, roast	Trace
Liver	7.1
Pork, roast	1.7
Vegetables	
Asparagus	5.2
Beans, green, boiled	15.0
Beans in tomato sauce	19.0
Beetroot, boiled	575.0
Beetroot, pickled	500.0
Broccoli, boiled	Trace
Brussels sprouts, boiled	0.0
Cabbage, boiled	0.0
Carrots, canned	4.0
Cauliflower, boiled	1.0
Celery	20.0
Chard, Swiss	645.0
Chive	1.1
Collards	74.0
Corn, yellow	5.2
Cucumber, raw	1.0
Dandelion greens	24.6
Eggplant	18.0
Escarole	31.0
Kale	13.0
Leek	89.0
Lettuce	3.0
Lima beans	4.3
Mushrooms	2.0
Mustard greens	7.7
Okra	132.0†
Onion, boiled	3.0
Parsley, raw	100.0
Parsnips	10.0
Peas, canned	1.0
Vegetables—cont'd	
Pepper, green	16.0
Pokeweed	476.0
Potatoes, white, boiled	0.0
Potatoes, sweet	56.0
Radishes	0.3
Rice, boiled	0.0
Rutabagas	19.0
Spinach, frozen	618.0†
Squash, summer	22.0
Tomatoes, raw	2.0
Turnip greens	6.0†
Watercress, early fine curled	10.0
Fruits	
Apples, raw	3.0
Apricots	2.8
Avocado	0.0
Banana, raw	Trace
Berries:	
Black	18.0
Blue	15.0
Dew	14.0
Green goose	88.0
Raspberries, black	53.0
Raspberries, red	15.0
Strawberries	18.0
Cherries:	
Bing	0.0
Sour	1.1
Currants:	
Black	4.3
Red	19.0
Fruit salad, canned	12.0
Grapes:	
Concord	25.0
Thompson seedless	0.0
Lemon peel	83.0
Lime peel	110.0
Mangoes	0.0
Melons:	
Cantaloupe	0.0
Casaba	0.0
Honeydew	0.0
Watermelon	0.0
Nectarines	0.0
Orange, raw	4.0
Peaches:	
Alberta	5.0
Canned	1.2
Hiley	0.0
Stokes	1.2
Pears:	3.0
Bartlett, canned	1.7
Pineapple, canned	1.0
Plums:	
Damson	10.0
Golden gage	1.1
Greengage	0.0
Preserves:	
Red plum jam	0.5
Strawberry jam	9.4
Prunes, Italian	5.8
Rhubarb:	
Stewed, no sugar	767.0†
Nuts	
Almonds	131.0†
Peanuts, roasted	116.0†
Pecans	11.2†
Confectionary	
Chocolate, plain	117.0†
Jelly, with allowed fruit	0.0
Marmalade	10.8
Sweets, boiled (plain candies)	0.0
Beverages, Nonalcoholic	
Barley water, bottled	0.0
Coca-Cola	Trace
Coffee (0.5 g Nescafe/100 ml)	3.2
Lemon squash drink (lemonade)	1.0
Orangeade	2.5
Ovaltine drink, 2 g in 100 ml	10.0
Pepsi-Cola	Trace
Ribena, concentrate (black currant drink)	2.0
Tea, Indian:	
2-min infusion	55.0
4-min infusion	72.0
6-min infusion	78.0
Tea, instant (10 g)	66.0
Tea, brewed, 500 ml water	1400.0†
Juices	
Apple juice	Trace
Cranberry juice	6.6†
Grape juice	5.8
Grapefruit juice	0.0
Orange juice	0.5†
Pineapple juice	0.0
Tomato juice	5.0
V-8 Juice	6.5
Beverages, Alcoholic	
Beer:	Trace
Bottled	0.0
Draft	1.0
Lager draft, Tuborg Pilsner	4.0
Stout, Guiness Draft	2.0
Cider	0.0
Sherry, dry	Trace
Wine:	
Port	Trace
Rosé	1.5
White	0.0
Miscellaneous	
Chocolate	139.0†
Cocoa, dry powder	623.0
Coffee powder (Nescafé)	33.0
Chicken noodle soup	1.0
Lemon juice	1.0
Lime juice	0.0
Ovaltine, powder, canned	35.0
Oxtail soup	1.0
Pepper	419.0
Tomato soup	3.0
Vegetable soup	5.0

Modified from Ney DM et al: *The low oxalate diet book for the prevention of oxalate kidney stones*, San Diego, 1981, University of California.
*Per 100 grams of edible portion.
†See Appendix 45B for bioavailability of oxalate from foods.

Appendix 45B Bioavailability of Oxalate

FOOD	QUANTITY	OXALATE CONTENT (mg)	BIOAVAILABILITY (%)
Brewed tea	10 g 500 ml Water	1400 mg	0.08
Tea	10 g 250 ml water 250 ml milk	1402	0.03
Instant tea	10 g	66	6.2
Peanuts	100 g	116	3.8
Almonds	100 g	131	2.8
Pecans	60 g	7	42.9
Spinach	200 g	1236	2.4
Turnip greens	200 g	12	5.8
Okra	200 g	264	0.1
Beets	200 g	1150	
Rhubarb	200 g	1534	
Strawberries	200 g	15-36	
Chocolate	90 g	126	2.6
Wheat bran	24 g	52	
V-8 Juice	500 ml	26	2.3
Orange juice	500 ml	2	20.0
Cranberry juice	500 ml	22	21.8

Data from Brinkley LJ et al: A further study of oxalate bioavailability in foods, *J Urol* 146:1377, 1991.

Appendix 46 Omega-6 and Omega-3 Fatty Acids in Selected Foods*

TYPE OF FOOD	OMEGA-6	OMEGA-3 LNA	OMEGA-3 EPA	OMEGA-3 DHA
Seafood				
Anchovies	0.2	—	0.5	0.9
Bass, freshwater	0.4	Trace	0.1	0.2
Bass, striped	—	Trace	0.2	0.6
Bluefish	0.4	—	0.4	0.8
Burbot	0.1	—	0.1	0.1
Carp	0.8	0.3	0.2	0.1
Catfish, channel	0.7	Trace	0.1	0.2
Cod, Atlantic	Trace	Trace	0.1	0.2
Cod, Pacific	Trace	Trace	0.1	0.1
Eel, European	0.5	0.7	0.1	0.1
Flounder	0.1	Trace	0.1	0.1
Haddock	Trace	Trace	0.1	0.1
Hake, Atlantic	0.1	Trace	Trace	Trace
Hake, Pacific	0.2	Trace	0.2	0.2
Halibut, Greenland	0.5	Trace	0.5	0.4
Halibut, Pacific	0.2	0.1	0.1	0.3
Herring, Atlantic	0.4	0.1	0.7	0.9
Herring, Pacific	0.6	0.1	1.0	0.7
Mackerel, Atlantic	1.1	0.1	0.9	1.6
Mackerel, King	1.0	—	1.0	1.2
Ocean perch	0.3	Trace	0.2	0.1
Pike, northern	0.1	Trace	Trace	0.1
Pike, walleye	0.1	Trace	0.1	0.2
Pollock	Trace	—	0.1	0.4
Rockfish, brown	0.3	Trace	0.3	0.4
Rockfish, canary	0.1	Trace	0.2	0.3
Sablefish	0.5	0.1	0.7	0.7
Salmon, Atlantic	0.7	0.2	0.3	0.9
Salmon, chinook	0.6	0.1	0.8	0.6
Salmon, chum	0.4	0.1	0.4	0.6
Salmon, coho	0.7	0.2	0.3	0.5
Salmon, pink	0.4	Trace	0.4	0.6
Salmon, sockeye	0.6	0.1	0.5	0.7
Sardines, canned	—	0.5	0.4	0.6
Sea bass, Japanese	0.1	Trace	0.1	0.3
Shark, unspecified	—	—	Trace	0.5
Smelt, rainbow	0.1	0.1	0.3	0.4
Snapper, red	0.2	Trace	Trace	0.2
Sole	0.1	Trace	Trace	0.1
Sprat	0.2	—	0.5	0.8
Sturgeon, Atlantic	0.6	Trace	1.0	0.5
Sturgeon, common	0.1	0.1	0.2	0.1
Swordfish	—	—	0.1	0.1
Trout, brook	0.3	0.2	0.2	0.2
Trout, lake	1.4	0.4	0.5	1.1
Trout, rainbow	0.6	0.1	0.1	0.4
Tuna, albacore	0.3	0.2	0.3	1.0
Tuna, bluefin	—	—	0.4	1.2
Tuna, skipjack	—	—	0.4	1.2
Whitefish, lake	0.7	0.2	0.3	1.0
Whiting, European	—	Trace	Trace	0.1
Wolfish, Atlantic	0.2	Trace	0.3	0.3

Data from Simopoulos AP, Kifer RR, Martin RE: *The health effects of polyunsaturated fatty acids in seafoods,* Washington D.C., 1986, Academic Press and Human Nutrition Information Service, USDA: Provisional table on the content of omega-3 fatty acids and other fat components in selected foods, *HNIS/PT-103,* 1988.
*Per 100 grams of edible portion.
LNA, α-Linolenic acid; *EPA,* eicosapentaenoic acid; *DHA,* docosahexaenoic acid.
NOTE: "Trace" signifies trace amounts; "—" signifies lack of reliable data for a nutrient known to be present.

Appendix 46 Omega-6 and Omega-3 Fatty Acids in Selected Foods*—cont'd

TYPE OF FOOD	OMEGA-6	OMEGA-3		
		LNA	EPA	DHA
Crustaceans				
Crab, Alaska king	Trace	Trace	0.2	0.1
Crab, blue	0.1	Trace	0.2	0.2
Crab, Dungeness	Trace	—	0.2	0.1
Crawfish	0.2	Trace	0.1	Trace
Lobster, European	Trace	—	0.1	0.1
Lobster, northern	Trace	—	0.1	0.1
Shrimp, Atlantic brown	0.2	Trace	0.2	0.1
Shrimp, Japanese	0.5	Trace	0.3	0.2
Mollusks				
Abalone	—	Trace	Trace	—
Clam, littleneck	—	Trace	Trace	Trace
Clam, Japanese	—	—	0.1	0.1
Clam, softshell	0.2	Trace	0.2	0.2
Conch	0.1	Trace	0.6	0.4
Mussel, blue	0.1	Trace	0.2	0.3
Mussel, Mediterranean	0.1	—	0.1	0.1
Octopus	0.1	—	0.1	0.1
Oyster, eastern	0.3	Trace	0.2	0.2
Oyster, European	0.1	0.1	0.3	0.2
Oyster, Pacific	0.3	Trace	0.4	0.2
Scallops	0.1	Trace	0.1	0.1
Squid, Atlantic	0.1	Trace	0.1	0.3
Squid, short-finned	0.1	Trace	0.2	0.4
Fats and Oils				
Butter	1.8	1.2	—	—
Canola oil (rape seed oil)	22.2	11.2	—	—
Chicken fat	19.9	1.0	—	—
Duck fat	11.9	1.0		
Flax seed oil (linseed oil)	12.7	53.5	—	—
Margarine, hard, soybean	19.4	1.5	—	—
Rice brain oil	33.4	1.6	—	—
Safflower oil	77.0	1.0	—	—
Mayonnaise, soybean	37.1	4.2	—	—
Soybean oil	51.1	6.8	—	—
Walnut oil	52.9	10.4	—	—
Wheat germ oil	54.8	6.9	—	—
Nuts and Seeds				
Beechnuts, dried	18.4	1.7	—	—
Butternuts, dried	34.0	8.7	—	—
Chia seeds, dried	3.4	3.9	—	—
Hickory nuts, dried	20.9	1.0	—	—
Soybean kernels, roasted	11.2	1.5	—	—
Walnuts, black	34.2	3.3	—	—
Walnuts, English	32.3	6.8	—	—

Appendix 47 Carotenoid Content of Fruits and Vegetables

	β-CAROTENE[a,b]		α-CAROTENE[a,b]		LUTEIN + ZEAXANTHEIN		LYCOPENE	
	MEDIAN	CONF CODE[c]	MEDIAN	CONF CODE	MEDIAN	CONF CODE	MEDIAN	CONF CODE
	⟵ μg/100g ⟶		⟵ μg/100g ⟶		⟵ μg/100g ⟶		⟵ μg/100g ⟶	
Apple, raw	26	C	0[d]	C	45	C	0	C
Apricot, canned, drained	1500[e]	B	0	C	2	C	65	C
Apricot, dried	17,600[e]	C	—	—	0	C	864	C
Apricot, raw	3524	C	0	C	0	C	5	C
Asparagus, raw	449	C	9	C	—	—	—	—
Avocado, raw	34	C	—	—	320	C	—	—
Banana, raw	0	C	0	B	0	C	0	C
Basil, not dried	350	B	—	—	—	—	—	—
Beet greens	2560	B	3	B	—	—	—	—
Beet, canned	1	C	0	C	4	C	0	C
Bitter melon, raw	50	C	—	—	—	—	—	—
Blueberries	—	—	0	C	—	—	—	—
Bottle gourd, raw	4	C	—	—	—	—	—	—
Broccoli, cooked	1300	A	—	—	1800	A	—	—
Broccoli, raw	700	A	1[e]	B	1900	C	0	C
Brussels sprouts	480	A	6	C	1300	A	0	C
Cabbage, Chinese, bok choy, raw	62	C	1	C	40	C	0	C
Cabbage, Chinese, wild	530	B	—	—	—	—	—	—
Cabbage, red, raw	15	C	1	C	26	C	0	C
Cabbage, white	80[e]	A	0	C	150	C	0	C
Cantaloupe, raw	3000[e]	A	35	C	0	C	0	C
Carrot, cooked, canned, frozen	9800	A	3700	A	—	—	0	C
Carrot, raw	7900	A	3600	A	260	C	0	C
Carrot, A+ variety, raw	18,250	C	10,650	C	—	—	0	C
Carrot, A+ variety, cooked	25,650	C	15,000	C	—	—	0	C
Cashew apple, raw	155	C	14	C	—	—	—	—
Cashew apple juice	80	C	—	—	—	—	—	—
Cassava leaf	3000	C	—	—	—	—	—	—
Cauliflower	8[e]	B	0	B	33[e]	B	0	C
Celeriac, raw	0	C	0	C	1	C	0	C
Celery	710	B	0	C	3600	C	0	C
Chicory leaf, raw	3430	C	—	—	—	—	—	—
Coriander, not dried	2000	C	—	—	—	—	—	—
Corn, yellow	51	C	50	C	780	A	0	C
Cranberries, raw	22	C	1	C	28	C	0	C
Cress leaf, raw	4150	C	—	—	—	—	—	—
Cucumber, pickled	180	C	0	C	510	C	0	C
Cucumber, raw	6[e]	C	0	C	240	C	0	C
Currants, raw	62	C	0	C	240	C	0	C
Dill, not dried	4500	C	0	C	6700	C	0	C
Eggplant	35	B	—	—	—	—	—	—
Endive	1300	C	—	—	—	—	—	—
Fennel leaves	4440	C	—	—	—	—	—	—
Grapefruit, pink, raw	1310	C	0	C	0	C	3362	C

Modified from Mangels A et al: Carotenoid content of fruits and vegetables: an evaluation of the analytic data, *J Am Diet Assoc* 93:284, 1993.
[a]Missing values for minimum and maximum (min-max) alone indicate that only one acceptable analytic value was found for that carotenoid in that food.
[b]Missing value for median, minimum, maximum, and confidence code indicate that no acceptable analytic values were found for that carotenoid in that food. Refer below for imputed values.
[c]Conf code = Confidence code; see chart below.
[d]Zeroes represent values reported as not detected at a detection limit specified in the acceptable references.
[e]Mean for acceptable foods more than two times median.
[f]Values based only on data for Finnish catsup that contained carrots.
See also website www.nal.usda.gov/fnic/foodcomp/Data/car98/car98.html.

Appendix 47 Carotenoid Content of Fruits and Vegetables—cont'd

	β-CAROTENE[a,b]		α-CAROTENE[a,b]		LUTEIN + ZEAXANTHEIN		LYCOPENE	
	MEDIAN	CONF CODE[c]	MEDIAN	CONF CODE	MEDIAN	CONF CODE	MEDIAN	CONF CODE
	←— μg/100g —→		←— μg/100g —→		←— μg/100g —→		←— μg/100g —→	
Grapefruit, white, raw	14[e]	B	1e	B	10	C	0	C
Grapes, raw	33	C	1	C	72	C	0	C
Green beans	630	A	44	C	740	B	0	C
Greens, collard	5400	B	—	—	—	—	—	—
Greens, fiddlehead	1950	B	280	B	—	—	—	—
Greens, mustard	2700	B	—	—	9900	C	—	—
Guava juice	270	C	—	—	—	—	3340	C
Guava, raw	812	C	—	—	—	—	5400	C
Jackfruit, raw	23	C	—	—	—	—	—	—
Jellies, jams, preserves	16	C	1	C	6	C	0	C
Kale	4700	A	—	—	21900	B	—	—
Kale, Chinese	140	C	—	—	—	—	—	—
Kiwi fruit, raw	43	C	0	C	180	C	0	C
Leeks, raw	1000	C	0	C	1900	C	0	C
Lemon, raw	3	C	0	C	12	C	0	C
Lettuce, iceberg	480	C	4	C	—	—	—	—
Lettuce, leaf	1200	C	1	C	1800	C	0	C
Lettuce, romaine	1900	B	—	—	—	—	—	—
Lima beans, cooked	—	—	0	C	—	—	—	—
Loofah fruit, raw	47	C	—	—	—	—	—	—
Mango, raw	1300	A	0	C	0	C	0	C
Mint, not dried	730	C	—	—	—	—	—	—
Mushroom	0	C	0	C	0	C	0	C
Mushroom, chanterelle, raw	1300	C	1	C	0	C	0	C
Nectarine, raw	103	C	0	C	—	—	—	—
Okra, raw	170	C	28	C	—	—	—	—
Olive, green	280	C	0	C	510	C	0	C
Onion, yellow, raw	160	C	0	C	16	C	0	C
Orange juice	7	A	6	A	74	A	0	B
Orange, raw	39[e]	B	20[e]	B	14	C	0	C
Papaya, raw	99	C	0	C	—	—	0	C
Parsley, not dried	5300	C	0	C	10,200	C	0	C
Peach, canned, drained	100	B	0	C	28	B	0	C
Peach, dried	9256	C	—	—	188	C	0	C
Peach, raw	99	B	1	C	14	B	0	C
Pear, raw	17	C	0	C	110	C	0	C
Peas, green	350	A	16	C	1700	A	0	C
Pepper, green, raw	230	B	11	B	700	C	0	C
Pepper, red	2200	B	60	C	—	—	—	—
Pepper, yellow, raw	150	C	92	C	770	C	0	C
Pigeon peas	40	C	—	—	—	—	—	—
Pineapple, canned, drained	18	C	1	C	2	C	—	—
Plum, raw	430	C	—	—	240	C	0	C
Potato salad	12	C	2	C	—	—	0	C
Potato, white, cooked	0	C	0	C	0	C	0	C
Potato, white, raw	6	C	0	C	36	C	0	C
Prune, dried	140	C	31	C	120	C	0	C
Pumpkin	3100	A	3800	A	1500	C	0	B

Continued

Appendix 47 Carotenoid Content of Fruits and Vegetables—cont'd

	β-CAROTENE[a,b]		α-CAROTENE[a,b]		LUTEIN + ZEAXANTHEIN		LYCOPENE	
	MEDIAN	CONF CODE[c]	MEDIAN	CONF CODE	MEDIAN	CONF CODE	MEDIAN	CONF CODE
	← μg/100g →		← μg/100g →		← μg/100g →		← μg/100g →	
Radish, raw	9	C	0	C	12	C	0	C
Raisins	0	C	0	C	1	C	0	C
Raspberries, raw	6	C	6	C	76	C	0	C
Rhubarb, raw	61	C	0	C	170	C	0	C
Roquette, raw	3460	C	—	—	—	—	—	—
Rose hip, purée, canned	420	C	0	C	—	—	780	C
Rutabaga, raw	1	C	0	C	0	C	0	C
Scallion, raw	850	C	6	C	2100	C	—	—
Spinach, cooked, drained	5500	A	—	—	12,600	A	—	—
Spinach, raw	4100	A	0	B	10,200	C	0	C
Squash, summer	420	C	12	C	1200	C	—	—
Squash, winter, cooked	2400	A	12e	B	38	C	—	—
Squash, winter, raw	820[e]	A	12[e]	B	38	C	—	—
Strawberries	9	C	2	C	31	C	0	C
Sweet potato, cooked	8800	A	0	C	—	—	0	C
Sweet potato, raw	8900	B	0	C	—	—	0	C
Swiss chard, raw	3647	C	45	C	—	—	—	—
Tangerine, tangelo juice	8e	B	5	B	135	C	—	—
Tangerine, raw	38	C	20	C	20	C	—	—
Tomato catsup	5000[f]	C	0[f]	C	210[f]	C	9900[f]	—
Tomato juice, canned	900	C	—	—	—	—	8580	B
Tomato paste, canned	1700	C	—	C	—	—	6500	B
Tomato sauce, canned	1000	C	—	—	—	—	—	—
Tomato, raw	520	A	—	—	100	C	3100	A
Turnip, raw	72	C	1	C	1	C	0	C
Watermelon, raw	230	C	1	C	14	C	4100	B
Yard-long beans, raw	44	C	—	—	—	—	—	—

Modified from Mangels A et al: Carotenoid content of fruits and vegetables: an evaluation of the analytic data, *J Am Diet Assoc* 93:284, 1993.
[a]Missing values for minimum and maximum (min-max) alone indicate that only one acceptable analytic value was found for that carotenoid in that food.
[b]Missing value for median, minimum, maximum, and confidence code indicate that no acceptable analytic values were found for that carotenoid in that food. Refer below for imputed values.
[c]Conf code = Confidence code; see chart below.
[d]Zeroes represent values reported as not detected at a detection limit specified in the acceptable references.
[e]Mean for acceptable foods more than two times median.
[f]Values based only on data for Finnish catsup that contained carrots.
See also website www.nal.usda.gov/fnic/foodcomp/Data/car98/car98.html.

A. The consensus of experts in carotenoid analysis is that this food does not contain detectable levels of this carotenoid. Impute the carotenoid level as 0.
B. Carotenoid present in similar food. For imputation purposes, cooked broccoli was used to estimate missing values for asparagus; guava for guava juice; white cabbage for iceberg lettuce; raw peach for raw nectarine; cucumber for okra; orange juice for oranges; green pepper for red pepper; tangerine juice for tangerines; tomato for tomato juice, tomato paste, and tomato sauce; and a mixture of greens (mustard greens, kale, parsley, raw spinach, and cooked spinach) for beet greens, chicory, cress leaf, endive, collard greens, romaine lettuce, and Swiss chard. Impute carotenoid using the ratio of the missing carotenoid to β-carotene in similar food multiplied by the β-carotene content of the food with missing carotenoid.
C. Impute using unpublished preliminary data for guava from Nutrient Composition Laboratory, Beltsville Human Nutrition Research Center, Agriculture Research Service, Beltsville, Md.
D. Impute value from similar food with highly similar levels of other carotenoids. For imputation purposes, carotenoid content of cloud berries (29) was used to replace missing values for blueberries, raw broccoli for cooked broccoli, and raw carrots for cooked carrots.
E. Impute based on unpublished preliminary data, 1988, for blueberries from Arthur D. Little, Inc., Cambridge, Mass.

Appendix 48 Vitamin D Content of Foods*

FOOD ITEM	VITAMIN D (µg)	VITAMIN D (IU)
Breakfast Cereals[1]		
All-Bran	3.5	140
Apple Jacks	3.5	140
Cap'n Crunch	†	140
Cheerios	3.5	140
Cinnamon Toast Crunch	3.5	140
Cocoa Pebbles	3.5	140
Corn Chex	†	140
Corn Pops	3.5	
Cracklin' Oat Bran	3.5	140
Crispix	3.5	140
Froot Loops	3.5	140
Frosted Flakes, Kellogg's	3.5	140
Frosted Mini-Wheats	†	
Fruity Pebbles	3.5	140
Golden Grahams	3.5	140
Grape-Nuts Brand Cereal	3.5	140
Honeycomb	3.5	140
Honey Nut Cheerios	3.5	140
Honey Smacks	3.5	140
Just Right With Fruit and Nuts	2.7	108
Kellogg's Bran Flakes	3.5	140
Kellogg's Corn Flakes	3.5	140
Kix	3.5	140
Life	†	
Lucky Charms	3.5	140
Nabisco Shredded Wheat	†	
Nabisco Shredded Wheat'n Bran	†	
Natural Bran Flakes	3.5	140
Natural Raisin Bran	3.8	152
Nut & Honey Crunch	3.5	140
Oatmeal Raisin Crisp	3.5	140
Product 19	3.5	140
Raisin Bran, Kellogg's	2.5	100
Rice Chex	†	
Rice Krispies	3.5	140
Special K	3.5	140
Spoon-Size Shredded Wheat	†	
Super Golden Crisp	3.5	140
Total	3.5	140
Trix	3.5	140
Wheaties	3.5	140
Dairy and Egg Products		
Milk, cow, fortified[2]:		
Whole, 3.3% fat	1.0	40
Low-fat, 2% fat	1.0	40
Low-fat, 2% fat with nonfat milk solids added	1.0	40
Low-fat, 2% fat, protein fortified	1.0	40
Low-fat, 1% fat	1.0	40
Low-fat, 1% fat, with nonfat milk solids added	1.0	40
Low-fat, 1% fat, protein fortified	1.0	40
Skim	1.0	40
Skim, with nonfat milk solids added	1.0	40
Skim, protein fortified	1.0	40
Dairy and Egg Products—cont'd		
Dry, whole	7.8	312
Dry, nonfat, regular	8.3	332
Dry, nonfat, instantized	11.0	440
Evaporated, skim	2.0	80
Chocolate, whole	1.0	40
Chocolate, low-fat, 2% fat	1.0	40
Chocolate, low-fat, 1% fat	1.0	40
Milk, cow, fluid, whole, unfortified[3]:		
Summer	0.08	3
Winter	0.03	1
Season not specified	0.06	2
Milk, goat, whole, fluid	0.3	12
Milk, human, whole, fluid	0.09	4
Cheese:		
Camembert	0.3	12
Cheddar	0.3	12
Edam	0.9	36
Parmesan	0.7	28
Swiss	1.1	44
Cream, heavy whipping, fluid	1.3	52
Egg, chicken:		
Whole, fresh or frozen	1.3	52
Whole, dried	4.7	188
White, fresh	0	0
Yolk, fresh	3.7	148
Fast Foods		
Cheeseburger		
Regular	0.3	12
4-ounce	0.3	12
Eggs, scrambled	1.7	68
English muffin with egg, cheese, and bacon	0.8	32
Fish sandwich, regular, with cheese	0.5	20
Hamburger:		
Regular	0.3	12
Double meat and double-decker roll	0.4	16
4-ounce patty, regular roll	0.4	16
Ice cream cone	0.2	8
Shake:		
Chocolate	0.4	16
Strawberry	0.2	8
Vanilla	0.2	8
Sundae:		
Caramel	0.2	8
Hot Fudge	0.3	12
Strawberry	0.3	12
Fats		
Butter	1.4	56
Margarine, fortified[4]:		
Fleischmann's	1.5	60
Mazola	1.5	60
Promise	1.5	60
Margarine, unfortified	0	0

Continued

Data from USDA Nutrient Data Laboratory, www.nal.usda.gov/fnic/foodcomp.
µg = Microgram.
IU = International Unit (1.0 µg = 40 IU).
*Per 100 grams of edible portion.
†Level in unfortified cereals is negligible.
[1]Values for breakfast cereals are based on label claim information.
[2]Fortified so that 1 quart of milk contains 10 µg, or 400 IU, of vitamin D.
[3]Level of vitamin D varies with season.
[4]Values based on label claim information.

Appendix 48 Vitamin D Content of Foods*—cont'd

FOOD ITEM	VITAMIN D (μg)	VITAMIN D (IU)
Fats—cont'd		
Fish oils:		
Cod liver:		
Medicinal, regular	417.5	16,700
Medicinal, high-potency	1010.0	40,400
Low-potency	125.0	5000
Commercial, refined	250.0	10,000
Dogfish liver	60.5	2420
Halibut liver	9200.0	368,000
Mackerel	3250.0	130,000
Rockfish liver	2445.0	97,800
Sardine, Atlantic or Pacific	8.3	332
Swordfish liver	17,325.0	693,000
Tuna liver	3250.0	130,000
Fish oil, unspecified	5.0	200
Fish and Related Products		
Finfish, fillet, raw:		
Catfish, channel	12.5	500
Cod	1.1	44
Eel, European	5.0	200
Flounder	1.5	60
Garfish	8.5	340
Halibut, Greenland	15.0	600
Herring, Atlantic	40.7	1628
Mackerel, Atlantic	9.0	360
Finfish roe, canned:		
Caviar, sturgeon	5.8	232
Cod	2.1	84
Herring:		
Pickled	17.0	680
Smoked	3.0	120
Mackerel, Atlantic:		
Canned in oil	5.7	228
Canned in tomato sauce	6.0	240
Mackerel, Pacific:		
Canned in oil	6.3	252
Salmon, canned:		
Chinook	8.1	324
Chum	5.6	224
Pink	15.6	624
Sardines:		
Atlantic, canned in oil	6.8	272
Pacific, canned in oil	8.3	332
Unspecified, canned in tomato sauce	12.0	480
Shellfish:		
Clam	0.1	4
Oyster	8.0	320
Shrimp	3.8	152
Sprat, smoked	3.0	120
Tuna, light meat, canned in oil, drained	5.9	236

FOOD ITEM	VITAMIN D (μg)	VITAMIN D (IU)
Meat and Related Products		
Beef:		
Kidney	0.8	32
Lean cuts	0.3	12
Liver	0.4	16
Bologna:		
Beef	0.7	28
Beef and pork	1.1	44
Pork	1.4	56
Bratwurst, pork, smoked	1.1	44
Braunschweiger	1.2	48
Frankfurter:		
Beef	0.9	36
Beef and pork	0.9	36
Loaves:		
Beef, honeyroll	1.0	40
Pork:		
Ham and cheese	1.1	44
Luxury	0.7	28
Mother's loaf	1.0	40
Olive	1.1	44
Pickle and pimiento	1.1	44
Pork and beef:		
Barbecue	0.9	36
Honey	0.9	36
Old-fashioned	1.0	40
Peppered	0.8	32
Picnic	1.2	48
Salami:		
Beef:		
Beer	0.9	36
Cotto	1.2	48
Pork, beer	0.9	36
Sausage:		
Beef, summer	1.1	44
Beef and pork:		
Raw	1.1	44
Cooked	0.7	28
Pork	1.3	52
Vegetables		
Mushrooms:		
Chanterelle	2.1	84
Morel	3.1	124
Shitake, fresh	2.5	100
Shitake, dried	41.5	1660
Yellow Boletus	3.1	124
Unspecified	1.9	76

Data from USDA Nutrient Data Laboratory, www.nal.usda.gov/fnic/foodcomp.
μg = Microgram.
IU = International Unit (1.0 μg = 40 IU).
*Per 100 grams of edible portion.
†Level in unfortified cereals is negligible.
[1]Values for breakfast cereals are based on label claim information.
[2]Fortified so that 1 quart of milk contains 10 μg, or 400 IU, of vitamin D.
[3]Level of vitamin D varies with season.
[4]Values based on label claim information.

Appendix 49 Vitamin E Content of Foods as α-Tocopherol (mg)

Chips and Snacks	
Potato chips—1 oz (28 g)	1.20
Potato sticks—1 oz (28 g)	2.23
Eggs, Chicken	
Whole, fresh/frozen—1 large (50 g)	0.88
Yolk, fresh—yolk of large egg (17 g)	0.87
Entrées, Box Mix	
Pizza, cheese, from Contadina Pizzeria Kit	
Thick crust—¼ pizza (128 g)	0.14
Thin crust—¼ pizza (104 g)	0.14
Fats, Oils, and Shortenings	
Animal Fats	
Beef tallow, raw—1 T (13 g)	0.30
Pork fat (lard), raw—1 T (13 g)	0.20
Vegetable Oils	
Almond oil—1 T (14 g)	5.30
Coconut oil—1 T (14 g)	0.10
Corn oil—1 T (14 g)	1.90
Corn oil, Mazola—1 T (14 g)	3.00
Cottonseed oil—1 T (14 g)	4.80
Olive oil—1 T (14 g)	1.60
Palm oil—1 T (14 g)	2.60
Peanut oil—1 T (14 g)	1.60
Safflower oil—1 T (14 g)	4.60
Sesame oil—1 T (14 g)	0.20
Soybean oil—1 T (14 g)	1.50
Soybean oil, hydrogenated—1 T (14 g)	1.10
Sunflower oil—1 T (14 g)	6.10
Vegetable-oil spray, Mazola No Stick—2.5-sec spray (0.7 g)	0.51*
Wheat-germ oil—1 T (14 g)	20.30
Fruit and Vegetable Juices	
Apple juice, canned/bottled—8 fl oz (248 g)	0.03
Grapefruit juice, canned—8 fl oz (247 g)	0.10
Orange juice, fresh—8 fl oz (248 g)	0.10
Tomato juice—6 fl oz (182 g)	0.40
Fruits	
Apple	
Raw, with skin—1 med (138 g)	0.81
Raw, without skin—1 med (128 g)	0.35
Apricots, cnd, in heavy syrup—4 halves (90 g)	0.80
Banana, raw—1 med (114 g)	0.31
Blackberries, raw—½ cup (72 g)	0.35
Cantaloupe, raw—1 cup pieces (160 g)	0.22
Cherries, sour, raw—½ cup (78 g)	0.10
Currants, European black, raw—½ cup (56 g)	0.56
Currants, red and white, raw—½ cup (56 g)	0.06
Gooseberries, raw—1 cup (150 g)	0.56
Grapefruit, raw, red and white—½ med (123 g)	0.30
Mango, raw—1 med (207 g)	2.32
Mixed fruit, frozen, in syrup, Bird's Eye—½ cup (142 g)	0.06
Orange, navel or valencia, raw—1 fruit (131 g)	0.30
Pear, raw—1 med (166 g)	0.83
Pineapple, raw—1 cup pieces (155 g)	0.16
Raspberries	
Raw—1 cup (123 g)	0.37
Frozen, in lite syrup, Bird's Eye—½ cup (142 g)	0.27
Strawberries	
Raw—1 cup (149 g)	0.18
Frozen, in lite syrup, Bird's Eye—½ cup (142 g)	0.13
Frozen, sweetened or unsweetened—1 cup (149 g)	0.31
Grain Products	
Pasta	
Macaroni, enriched, cooked—1 cup (140 g)	1.03
Spaghetti, enriched, cooked—1 cup (140 g)	1.03
Nuts, Nut Products, and Seeds	
Almonds	
Dried—1 oz (24 nuts) (28 g)	6.72
Oil-roasted—1 oz (22 nuts) (28 g)	1.55
Toasted—1 oz (28 g)	1.41
Whole, Blue Diamond—1 oz (28 g)	1.66
Brazil nuts, dried—1 oz (8 med nuts) (28 g)	2.13
Cashews, dry roasted—1 oz (28 g)	0.16
Coconut, raw—1 piece (2″ × 2″ × ½″) (45 g)	0.33
Filberts (hazelnuts), dried—1 oz (28 g)	6.70
Peanut butter, creamy/smooth, Skippy—1 T (16 g)	3.00
Peanut butter, chunk style/crunchy, Skippy—1 T (16 g)	3.00
Peanuts	
Dried—1 oz (28 g)	2.56
Dry roasted—1 oz (28 g)	2.18
Oil roasted—1 oz (28 g)	2.07
Pecans, dried—1 oz (31 large nuts) (28 g)	0.87
Pistachio nuts, dried—1 oz (47 nuts) (28 g)	1.46
Sesame seeds, whole, dried—1 T (9 oz)	0.20
Walnuts, English/Persian, dried—1 oz (14 halves) (28 g)	0.73
Spreads	
Butter—1 T (15 g)	0.20
Margarine by brand	
Mazola—1 T (14 g)	8.00
Mazola unsalted—1 T (14 g)	8.00
Margarine by form and type of oil	
Liquid, soybean and cottonseed—1 t (5 g)	0.20
Stick, safflower and soybean—1 t (5 g)	0.80
Stick soybean—1 t (5 g)	0.10
Stick, soybean and cottonseed—1 t (5 g)	0.30
Tub, corn—1 t (5 g)	0.50
Tub, safflower—1 t (5 g)	0.60
Tub, soybean—1 t (5 g)	0.10
Tub, soybean and cottonseed—1 t (5 g)	0.30
Margarine, imitation (diet) by brand	
Mazola diet—1 T (14 g)	3.00
Parkay, diet soft—1 T (14 g)	0.40
Margarine, imitation (diet) by form and type of oil	
Tub, soybean and cottonseed—1 t (5 g)	0.40
Mayonnaise	
Best Foods/Hellman's—1 T (14 g)	11.00
Soybean—1 T (14 g)	2.90
Miracle Whip, Kraft—1 T (14 g)	0.50
Miracle Whip, light, Kraft—1 T (14 g)	0.40
Sandwich spread, Best Foods/Hellmann's—1 T (15 g)	5.00
Vegetables	
Asparagus	
Canned—½ cup (121 g)	0.46
Frozen, boiled—4 spears (60 g)	0.81
Raw—4 spears (58 g)	1.15
Avocado, raw, Californian—1 med (173 g)	2.32
Beet greens, raw—1 cup (38 g)	0.57
Beets, canned, Harvard—½ cup slices (123 g)	0.04
Broccoli, raw—½ cup chopped (44 g)	0.20
Brussels sprouts	
Raw—½ cup chopped (44 g)	0.39
Boiled—½ cup (4 sprouts) (78 g)	0.66

From Pennington JA: *Bowe's and Church's food values of portions commonly used*, ed 17, Baltimore, Md, 1998, Lippincott-Williams & Wilkins.
*Specified as tocopherols.

Continued

Appendix 49 Vitamin E Content of Foods as α-Tocopherol (mg)—cont'd

Vegetables—cont'd	
Cabbage, Chinese (bok-choy), raw—½ cup shredded (35 g)	0.05
Cabbage, green, raw—½ cup shredded (35 g)	0.04
Carrots	
Raw—1 med (72 g)	0.32
Boiled—½ cup slices (78 g)	0.33
Cauliflower, raw—½ cup pieces (50 g)	0.02
Celery, raw—1 stalk (7.5″ long) (40 g)	0.14
Corn, sweet, yellow/white, canned—½ cup (128 g)	0.05
Corn, sweet, yellow/white, frozen—½ cup (82 g)	0.02
Cucumber, raw—½ cup slices (⅙ cucumber) (52 g)	0.08
Dandelion greens, raw—½ cup chopped (28 g)	0.70
Eggplant, raw—½ cup pieces (41 g)	0.01
Garden cress, raw—½ cup (25 g)	0.18
Garlic, raw—3 cloves (9 g)	0.001
Green beans (snap beans)	
Raw—½ cup (55 g)	0.01
Canned—½ cup (68 g)	0.03
Frozen—½ cup (62 g)	0.06
Frozen, boiled—½ cup (68 g)	0.09
Leeks, raw—¼ cup chopped (26 g)	0.24
Lettuce, iceberg, raw—¼ head (135 g)	0.54
Mushrooms, raw—½ cup pieces (35 g)	0.03
Mustard greens, raw—½ cup chopped (28 g)	0.56
Onion rings, frozen, heated—7 rings (70 g)	0.48
Onions, raw—½ cup chopped (80 g)	0.25
Parsley, raw—½ cup chopped (30 g)	0.52
Parsnips, raw—½ cup (67 g)	0.67
Peas, green	
Raw—½ cup (78 g)	0.10
Frozen—½ cup (72 g)	0.09
Frozen, boiled—½ cup (80 g)	0.10
Peppers, sweet raw—½ cup chopped (50 g)	0.34
Potato	
Raw without skin—1 potato (112 g)	0.07
Baked without skin—1 potato (156 g)	0.05
Boiled without skin—1 potato (135 g)	0.05
French fried, frozen, heated—10 pieces (50 g)	0.10
Pumpkin, raw—½ cup (58 g)	0.58
Rutabaga, boiled—½ cup cubes (85 g)	0.13
Seaweed, kelp (kombu/tangle), raw—3.5 oz (100 g)	0.87
Spinach	
Raw—½ cup chopped (28 g)	0.53
Canned—½ cup (107 g)	0.02
Squash, winter, all varieties, baked—½ cup cubes (102 g)	0.12
Sweet potato, raw—1 med (130 g)	5.93
Tomato, red, raw—1 tomato (123 g)	0.42
Turnip greens, raw—½ cup chopped (28 g)	0.63
Watercress, raw—½ cup chopped (17 g)	0.17

From Pennington JA: *Bowe's and Church's food values of portions commonly used*, ed 17, Baltimore, Md, 1998, Lippincott-Williams & Wilkins.
*Specified as tocopherols.

Appendix 50 Vitamin K Content of Foods*

FOOD ITEM	VITAMIN K (μg/100 g)
Apples, raw:	
Unpeeled	4.0
Peeled	0.46
Asparagus spears:	
Raw	39.0
Frozen	27.0
Bananas, raw	0.5
Beans, mung:	
Mature seeds, dry	170.0
Mature seeds, sprouted, raw	33.0
Beans, snap:	
Raw	28.0
Frozen	32.0
Beef, raw:	
Ground, regular	4.0
Ground, lean	0.6
Beef heart, raw	0
Beef kidney, raw	0
Beets, raw	5.0
Blueberries, canned	0.5
Broccoli, spears:	
Raw	154.0
Frozen	68.0
Cabbage, raw	149.0
Carrots, raw	13.0
Cauliflower, raw	191.0
Chicken breast, raw	0.01
Chickpeas:	
Mature seeds, dry	264.0
Mature seeds, sprouted, raw	48.0
Cola:	
Regular	0.01
Diet	0
Corn, sweet, yellow, raw	7.0
Cranberry juice	<0.005
Cranberry sauce	1.4
Cucumbers, raw	5.0
Eggs:	
Whole	50.0
Yolk	147.0
White	0.02
Farina, dry	0.15
Fruit juice blend	<0.005
Garlic powder	0.72
Ginger ale, regular	0.01
Grapefruit juice	0.02
Honey	0.02
Kale, raw	275.0
Lentils:	
Mature seeds, dry	264.0
Mature seeds, sprouted, raw	48.0
Lettuce, iceberg, raw	113.0
Lemonade	0.03
Liver, raw:	
Beef	104.0
Chicken	80.0
Lamb	0
Pork	88.0
Rabbit	35.0
Turkey	0
Veal	27.0
Milk, cow:	
Whole	4.0
Skim	4.0
Nonfat dry, regular	10.0
Milk, human	2.0
Mushrooms, raw	8.0
Mustard, dry	0.3
Nettle leaves, raw	372.0
Oats, rolled, dry	63.0
Oils:	
Almond	7.0
Canola	830.0
Coconut	10.0
Corn	5.0
Cottonseed	0
Olive	58.0
Palm	8.0
Peanut	2.0
Safflower	7.0
Sesame	12.0
Sunflower	10.0
Soybean	200.0
Walnut	16.0
Onions, mature, raw	0.52
Oranges, raw	1.35
Orange juice, fresh	0.04
Peaches, canned	3.0
Peanut butter	0.11
Pears, canned	0.46
Peas:	
Mature seeds, dry	81.0
Mature seeds, sprouted, raw	28.0
Pork, lean, raw	0.01
Potatoes, baked:	
Flesh and skin	0.53
Flesh	0.22
Pumpkin, canned	15.0
Rice flour:	
Brown, regular	0.04
White, regular	0.05
White, instant	0.01
Salt	0.01
Seaweed, raw:	
Dulse (*Rhocimeria palmenta*)	255.0
Rockweed (*Ascophyllum nodosum*)	255.0
Seagrass (*Enteromorpha clathrata*)	246.0
Sealettuce (*Ulva lactuca*)	68.0
Soybean, mature seeds, dry	190.0
Spinach:	
Raw	266.0
Frozen	138.0
Strawberries, raw	14.0
Sugar	0.01
Sweet potatoes, raw	4.0
Tea, black, brewed	0.05
Tea, black, decaffeinated, brewed	0.02
Tomatoes, raw:	
Green	47.0
Ripe	23.0
Vinegar	<0.005
Wheat:	
Whole grain	20.0
Bran, crude	83.0
Germ, crude	39.0
Flour, all-purpose	0.5
Flour, whole-wheat	1.1
Starch	0.15
Wine, sherry	<0.005

Data from USDA Nutrient Data Laboratory, www.nal.usda.gov/fnic/foodcomp.
*Per 100 grams of edible portion.

Appendix 51 Selenium Content of Foods*

FOOD ITEM	MEAN (μg)
Baked Products	
Bagels	32.0
Biscuits, refrigerated dough, baked	17.8
Bread:	
Cornbread mix	5.6
Prepared	9.9
Cracked-wheat	25.3
French or Vienna	31.5
Italian	27.2
Pita:	
White	27.1
Whole-wheat	44.0
Raisin	20.0
Rye	30.9
Wheat	30.9
White	28.2
Whole-wheat	36.6
Bread crumbs, dry, grated, plain	37.7
Bread stuffing, mix, dry	48.0
Cake:	
Chocolate, with chocolate frosting	3.3
Yellow:	
Prepared with chocolate frosting	3.4
Dry mix, pudding-type	2.4
Prepared with white frosting	3.3
Coffeecake	17.2
Cookies:	
Animal crackers	7.0
Chocolate chip	6.0
Chocolate sandwich with creme filling	5.0
Fig bars	3.3
Graham crackers	10.2
Oatmeal	9.8
Peanut butter:	
Regular	5.9
Soft	4.4
Refrigerated dough, baked	5.1
Peanut butter sandwich	7.7
Sugar	2.1
Vanilla wafers	11.3
Crackers:	
Cheese	8.6
Melba toast	34.8
Rye wafers	23.8
Saltines	11.7
Standard snack-type:	
Regular	6.6
Sandwich with peanut butter filling	4.8
Wheat	6.3
Whole-wheat	14.7
Danish pastry or sweet rolls	17.0
Doughnuts:	
Cake-type	9.3
Yeast-leavened	19.8
English muffins	20.1
Toasted	27.0
French toast, frozen	16.7
Ice cream cone	4.8
Muffins:	
Plain or blueberry	11.2
Corn	15.2
Baked Products—cont'd	
Pancake mix	12.9
Prepared	9.8
Pie:	
Apple	1.0
Pumpkin	2.6
Rolls:	
Dinner	27.2
Hamburger or hot dog	26.5
Hard	39.1
Toaster pastries, fruit	4.4
Tortillas:	
Corn	5.5
Flour	23.4
Waffles, frozen, toasted	16.0
Beef Products	
Retail cuts:	
Chuck, separable lean:	
Raw	16.6
Cooked, braised	26.7
Cooked, roasted	24.0
Rib, whole, separable lean, raw	17.1
Round, full cut, separable lean, raw	20.8
Round, bottom round, separable lean, cooked, braised	28.1
T-bone, top loin, tenderloin, porterhouse: separable lean, raw	17.8
Top sirloin, separable lean:	
Raw	19.8
Cooked, broiled	32.9
Cooked, pan-cooked	23.6
Ground:	
Extra lean, raw	13.9
Lean:	
Raw	15.7
Cooked, broiled, medium	29.0
Regular:	
Raw	12.7
Cooked, baked	19.4
Variety meats:	
Kidneys, raw	148.8
Liver:	
Raw	41.3
Cooked, pan-fried	57.0
Beverages	
Beer	1.2
Cola, carbonated	0.1
Chocolate-flavor mix, powder	2.6
Cocoa mix, prepared with water	0.4
Coffee, brewed	0.1
Coffee, instant powder	12.6
Fruit punch drink, canned	0
Orange drink, canned	0
Orange-flavor drink, powder, prepared with water	0.1
Shake, fast-food, chocolate	1.7
Tea:	
Brewed	0
Instant, unsweetened, powder	5.3
Thirst-quencher drink, bottled	0.3
Wine, white	0.2

Data from USDA Nutrient Data Laboratory, www.nal.usda.gov/fnic/foodcomp.
*Per 100 grams of edible portion.

Appendix 51 Selenium Content of Foods*—cont'd

FOOD ITEM	MEAN (μg)
Breakfast Cereals	
Cereals, ready-to-eat:	
All-Bran	9.4
Bran Buds	28.9
Bran Flakes, Kellogg's	10.5
Cheerios	37.5
Corn Chex	3.5
Corn Flakes, Kellogg's	5.1
Corn Pops	6.5
Froot Loops	7.3
Frosted Flakes, Kellogg's	4.4
Frosted Mini-Wheats	4.1
Golden Crisp	48.6
Granola, commercial, plain	20.3
Grape-Nuts Brand Cereal	9.6
Honey Nut Cheerios	23.5
Life	23.6
Lucky Charms	19.8
Multi-Bran Chex	9.0
100% Bran, Nabisco	8.0
100% Natural Cereal	17.3
Product 19	12.0
Raisin Bran	7.0
Rice Chex	3.9
Rice Krispies	15.4
Rice, puffed	10.5
Special K	54.9
Wheat germ, toasted	65.0
Wheat, puffed	123.1
Wheat, shredded	5.9
Wheaties	4.7
Cereals, to-be-cooked:	
Corn grits, regular, quick and instant:	
Dry	17.0
Cooked	3.1
Cream of Wheat:	
Regular, dry	20.0
Quick, cooked	12.8
Instant, cooked	11.4
Farina:	
Dry	23.5
Cooked	9.1
Oats, regular, quick, and instant:	
Dry	34.0
Cooked	8.1
Cereal Grains and Pasta	
Cereal grains:	
Bulgur, dry	2.3
Corn	15.5
Corn flour, masa	15.0
Cornmeal, degermed	7.8
Cornstarch	2.8
Oat bran	45.2
Rice, brown:	
Raw	23.4
Cooked	9.8
Rice, white:	
Regular:	
Raw	15.1
Cooked	7.5

FOOD ITEM	MEAN (μg)
Cereal Grains and Pasta—cont'd	
Rice, white (continued):	
Parboiled:	
Dry	23.0
Cooked	8.2
Precooked or instant:	
Dry	46.9
Prepared	4.2
Rice bran	15.6
Rye flour	35.7
Wheat bran	77.6
Wheat germ	79.2
Wheat flour:	
Whole-grain	70.7
White:	
All-purpose	33.9
Bread	39.7
Cake	4.9
Wild rice, raw	2.8
Pasta:	
Macaroni or spaghetti:	
Dry	62.2
Cooked	21.3
Noodles, Chinese, chow mein	43.0
Noodles, egg:	
Dry	59.2
Cooked	21.7
Dairy and Egg Products	
Cheese:	
Cheddar	13.9
Cottage, creamed	9.0
Cream	2.4
Feta	15.0
Mozzarella, low-moisture, part-skim	16.3
Parmesan, grated	26.2
Pasteurized process, American:	
Cheese	14.4
Cheese food	16.1
Cheese spread	11.3
Swiss	12.7
Cream:	
Sour, cultured	2.2
Sweet, fluid:	
Half and half	1.8
Light, coffee, or table	0.6
Cream substitute, powdered	0.6
Milk, cow:	
Fluid:	
Whole (3.3% fat)	2.0
Low fat, 2% fat	2.2
Skim	2.1
Buttermilk, cultured	2.0
Chocolate, low fat	1.9
Dry, nonfat	27.3
Evaporated, whole, canned	2.3
Milk, human, whole, mature, fluid	1.8
Yogurt, lowfat:	
Plain	3.3
Fruit-flavored	2.3

Continued

Appendix 51 Selenium Content of Foods*—cont'd

FOOD ITEM	MEAN (μg)
Dairy and Egg Products—cont'd	
Eggs:	
Raw:	
Whole	30.8
White	17.6
Yolk	45.2
Cooked:	
Fried	26.9
Scrambled	22.5
Fast Food	
Chicken, breaded, fried, boneless pieces	16.3
Hamburger sandwich:	
Regular, single meat patty, with condiments	19.5
Large, single meat patty:	
Plain	19.8
With condiments and vegetables	15.4
Pizza:	
Cheese	21.4
Sausage	20.6
Fats and Oils	
Lard	0.2
Salad dressings:	
Blue cheese	1.0
Mayonnaise	1.7
Thousand Island	2.1
Finfish and Shellfish	
Finfish:	
Catfish, channel, raw	12.6
Cod:	
Raw	33.1
Cooked	37.6
Fish portions and sticks, frozen, reheated	16.6
Flounder:	
Raw	32.7
Cooked	58.2
Haddock:	
Raw	30.2
Cooked	40.5
Mackerel, Atlantic:	
Raw	44.1
Cooked	51.6
Canned	52.8
Ocean perch, raw	43.3
Pollock, walleye, raw	21.9
Salmon, pink:	
Raw	44.6
Canned	33.2
Salmon, sockeye:	
Raw	33.7
Cooked	37.8
Canned, no bones or skin	38.6
Snapper, raw	38.2
Swordfish, raw	48.1
Tuna, canned, drained:	
Light meat:	
In oil	76.0
In water	80.4
White meat:	
In oil	60.1
In water	65.7

FOOD ITEM	MEAN (μg)
Finfish and Shellfish—cont'd	
Finfish—cont'd	
Whiting, raw	32.1
Shellfish:	
Crustaceans:	
Crab, blue:	
Canned	31.8
Cooked, moist heat	40.2
Shrimp:	
Raw	38.0
Breaded and fried	41.7
Canned, frozen or cooked	39.6
Mollusks:	
Clams, canned, drained	48.6
Oysters:	
Raw	63.7
Cooked	71.6
Scallops, mixed species, raw	22.2
Fruits and Fruit Juices	
Apples, raw	0.3
Apple juice, bottled	0.1
Applesauce, canned	0.3
Avocados	0.4
Bananas, raw	1.1
Fruit cocktail, canned, heavy syrup, drained	0.5
Grapes, raw	0.2
Melons, cantaloupe, raw	0.4
Olives, ripe, canned	0.9
Oranges, raw	0.5
Orange juice, frozen concentrate, diluted with 3 parts water by volume	0.1
Peaches, raw	0.4
Peaches, canned, heavy syrup, drained	0.3
Pears, raw	1.0
Pineapple, raw	0.6
Pineapple, canned, drained	0.4
Raisins, seedless	0.7
Raisins, seeded	0.6
Strawberries, frozen, sweetened	0.7
Watermelon, raw	0.1
Lamb and Veal	
Lamb, separable lean:	
Raw	23.4
Cooked	26.1
Lamb, chops, pan-cooked with added fat	22.9
Lamb kidney, raw	126.9
Lamb liver, raw	82.4
Veal, separable lean, cooked	13.0
Veal cutlet, breaded, pan-fried	13.5
Legumes	
Baked beans, canned	4.7
Beans, great northern:	
Raw	12.9
Cooked	4.1
Beans, kidney, cooked or canned	1.2
Beans, lima, large:	
Raw	7.2
Cooked	4.5

Data from USDA Nutrient Data Laboratory, www.nal.usda.gov/fnic/foodcomp.
*Per 100 grams of edible portion.

Appendix 51 Selenium Content of Foods*—cont'd

FOOD ITEM	MEAN (μg)
Legumes—cont'd	
Beans, navy:	
Raw	11.0
Cooked	5.8
Beans, pinto:	
Raw	18.5
Cooked or canned	7.1
Cowpeas:	
Raw	9.0
Cooked	2.5
Canned	2.3
Peas, split, raw	1.6
Peanuts, roasted	7.5
Peanut butter	7.5
Soybeans, roasted	19.1
Soy sauce	0.8
Tofu, raw	8.9
Nuts and Seeds	
Almonds	4.7
Brazil nuts	2960.0
Cashew nuts, roasted	11.4
Coconut, dried, sweetened	16.1
Filberts or hazelnuts	4.0
Pecans	5.2
Sunflower seed kernels:	
Dried	59.5
Roasted	78.2
Walnuts, black	17.0
Walnuts, English	4.6
Pork Products	
Pork, fresh:	
Separable lean (see individual cuts)	
Separable fat:	
Raw	8.0
Cooked	16.3
Loin:	
Whole, separable, lean, roasted	35.1
Backribs, separable lean and fat:	
Raw	24.0
Roasted	39.3
Blade or country-style ribs, separate lean only:	
Raw	32.6
Roasted	42.3
Center loin (loin chops or roast), separable lean only:	
Raw	32.5
Broiled	47.3
Center rib (ribs or roasts), separable lean only:	
Raw	35.4
Roasted, bone-in or boneless	43.2
Broiled (see Center loin, broiled)	
Sirloin, separable lean only:	
Raw	33.2
Broiled	51.6
Roasted	43.1
Tenderloin, separable lean only:	
Raw	28.9
Roasted	48.1
Toploin (loin chops, boneless), separable lean only:	
Raw (see Center loin, raw)	
Broiled (see Center loin, broiled)	
Roasted	48.2
Pork Products—cont'd	
Pork, fresh—cont'd	
Shoulder:	
Blade, Boston, separable lean only:	
Raw	28.9
Broiled	39.3
Ground:	
Raw	24.6
Cooked	35.4
Pork kidney, raw	190.0
Pork products, cured:	
Bacon:	
Raw	25.0
Cooked	24.7
Canadian-style bacon	25.0
Ham, canned	29.8
Ham, center slice, lean only, unheated	21.4
Ham, fully cooked, separable lean only, roasted	25.4
Poultry	
Chicken:	
Flesh and skin, cooked:	
Fried, flour-coated	21.7
Roasted	23.9
Livers:	
Raw	64.1
Cooked, broiled	70.9
Parts:	
Breast, meat only, roasted	27.6
Thigh, meat only, roasted	29.0
Turkey:	
Dark meat, without skin, roasted	40.9
Light meat, without skin, roasted	32.1
Sausages and Luncheon Meats	
Bologna, beef or beef and pork	11.3
Chicken roll	12.5
Frankfurters:	
Beef or beef and pork	13.8
Chicken	18.4
Ham, chopped	17.4
Ham, sliced	16.4
Kielbasa, Polish sausage	17.7
Liverwurst	58.0
Luncheon meat:	
Beef, sliced	28.2
Pork, canned	28.0
Pork sausage, fresh:	
Raw	11.5
Cooked	18.2
Salami, cooked	14.6
Turkey breast meat	30.8
Snacks and Sweets	
Snacks:	
Corn-based, extruded:	
Chips or tortilla chips	6.7
Puffs or twists, cheese-flavor	3.0
Popcorn, oil-popped	7.3
Potato chips	8.1
Pretzels, hard	5.8

Continued

Appendix 51 Selenium Content of Foods*—cont'd

FOOD ITEM	MEAN (μg)
Snacks and Sweets—cont'd	
Sweets:	
Candies:	
Caramels	1.8
Kit Kat Wafer Bar	4.7
Milk chocolate	3.9
Snickers Bar	4.6
Cocoa, dry powder, unsweetened	14.3
Desserts:	
Egg custard, dry mix, prepared	14.1
Gelatins:	
Dry mix	6.7
Prepared with water	0.3
Dry powder, unsweetened	39.5
Pudding, chocolate, dry mix, instant or regular, prepared	1.7
Frozen desserts:	
Ice cream, chocolate	2.5
Ice cream sandwich	3.2
Ice milk, vanilla	2.8
Honey	0.8
Molasses	17.8
Sugars:	
Brown	1.2
Granulated	0.6
Syrup, pancake	0.7
Soups, Sauces, and Gravies	
Soups, canned:	
Bean with pork or bacon, condensed	6.4
Beef bouillon, prepared with water	0.7
Beef noodle, condensed	5.9
Chicken broth, prepared with water	0.0
Chicken noodle, condensed	9.8
Prepared with water	2.6
New England clam chowder, condensed	8.4
Mushroom, cream of, condensed	1.2
Tomato, condensed	0.4
Prepared with milk	0.9
Vegetarian vegetable, prepared with water	1.8
Vegetable beef, condensed	2.2
Prepared with water	1.8
Sauces:	
Barbecue, ready-to-serve	1.3
Cheese, dehydrated	13.6
Horseradish, prepared	2.8
Mustard, prepared	36.0
Sweet and sour, prepared	0.4
Gravies:	
Beef	1.0
Chicken	0.8
Vegetables	
Asparagus:	
Raw	2.3
Cooked; canned, drained; or frozen	1.7
Beans, lima, frozen	1.7
Beans, mung, mature seeds, sprouted, canned, drained	0.6
Beans, snap:	
Raw	0.6
Cooked; canned, drained; or frozen	0.4
Broccoli:	
Raw	3.0
Cooked or frozen	1.9

FOOD ITEM	MEAN (μg)
Vegetables—cont'd	
Cabbage:	
Raw	0.9
Cooked	0.6
Carrots:	
Raw	1.1
Cooked	0.8
Cauliflower:	
Raw	0.6
Frozen	0.8
Celery, raw	0.9
Collards, canned, drained; or frozen	1.4
Corn, sweet:	
Raw	0.6
Cooked; canned, drained; or frozen	0.7
Cowpeas, frozen, cooked	3.4
Eggplant:	
Raw	0.3
Cooked	0.4
Garlic, raw	14.2
Lettuce, raw	0.2
Mushrooms:	
Raw	12.3
Cooked	11.9
Canned, drained	4.1
Mustard greens, canned, drained; or frozen	0.7
Onions:	
Raw	0.6
Canned, drained; frozen; cooked	0.4
Onion rings, frozen, prepared	3.5
Peas, green:	
Canned, drained; or frozen	1.7
Frozen, cooked	1.0
Potatoes:	
Raw	0.3
Baked	0.8
Canned, drained	0.9
Frozen, french-fried, heated in oven	0.4
Potatoes, mashed, dehydrated:	
Dry	26.3
Prepared	1.4
Spinach:	
Raw	1.0
Cooked	1.5
Sweet potatoes:	
Raw	0.6
Cooked or canned	0.7
Tomatoes:	
Raw	0.4
Canned	0.7
Tomato juice or vegetable juice cocktail	0.5
Tomato catsup	0.8
Tomato sauce	0.6
Turnips, raw	0.7
Turnip greens, frozen	0.9
Vegetables, mixed, canned, drained; or frozen, cooked	0.3
Miscellaneous	
Yeast, baker's	8.1

Data from USDA Nutrient Data Laboratory, www.nal.usda.gov/fnic/foodcomp.
*Per 100 grams of edible portion.

Appendix 52 Caloric Expenditure Worksheet for Various Exercise Activities Based on Body Weight

ACTIVITY	TYPE	cal/hr —110 lb	cal/hr —130 lb	cal/hr —150 lb	cal/hr —170 lb	cal/hr —190 lb	cal/hr —210 lb	cal/hr —230 lb	cal/hr —250 lb
aerobics class	water	210	248	286	325	364	401	439	477
aerobics class	low impact	263	310	358	406	455	501	549	596
aerobics class	high impact	368	434	501	568	637	702	768	835
aerobics class	step with 6 to 8-inch step	446	527	609	690	774	852	933	1014
aerobics class	step with 10 to 12-inch step	525	621	716	812	910	1003	1097	1193
backpack	general	368	434	501	568	637	702	768	835
badminton	singles and doubles	236	279	322	365	410	451	494	537
badminton	competitive	368	434	501	568	637	702	768	835
baseball	throw/catch	131	155	179	203	228	251	274	298
baseball	fast or slow pitch	263	310	358	406	455	501	549	596
basketball	shooting baskets	236	279	322	365	410	451	494	537
basketball	wheelchair	341	403	465	528	592	652	713	775
basketball	game	420	496	573	649	728	802	878	954
bike	10-11.9 mph, slow	315	372	430	487	546	602	658	716
bike	12-13.9 mph, moderate	420	496	573	649	728	802	878	954
bike	14-15.9 mph, fast	525	621	716	812	910	1003	1097	1193
bike	16-19.9 mph, very fast	630	745	859	974	1092	1203	1317	1431
bike	>20 mph, racing	840	993	1146	1299	1457	1604	1756	1908
bike	50 watts, stationary, very light	158	133	215	243	273	301	329	358
bike	100 watts, stationary, light	289	341	394	446	501	552	603	656
bike	150 watts, stationary, moderate	368	434	501	568	637	702	768	835
bike	200 watts, stationary, vigorous	551	652	752	852	956	1053	1152	1252
bike	250 watts, stationary, very vigorous	656	776	895	1015	1138	1253	1372	1491
bike	BMX or mountain	446	527	609	690	774	852	933	1014
boxing	punching bag	315	372	430	487	546	602	658	716
boxing	sparring	473	558	644	730	819	902	988	1074
calisthenics	back exercises	184	217	251	284	319	351	384	417
calisthenics	pull-ups, jumping jacks	420	496	573	649	728	802	878	954
calisthenics	push-ups or sit-ups	420	496	573	649	728	802	878	954
circuit training	general	420	496	573	649	728	802	878	954
football	flag or touch	420	496	573	649	728	802	878	954
football	competitive	473	558	644	730	819	902	988	1074
Frisbee	general	158	133	215	243	273	301	329	358
Frisbee	ultimate	420	496	573	649	728	802	878	954
golf	power cart	184	217	251	284	319	351	384	417
golf	pull clubs	226	267	308	349	391	431	472	513
golf	carry clubs	236	279	322	365	410	451	494	537
handball	general	630	745	859	974	1092	1203	1317	1431
hike	general	315	372	430	487	546	602	658	716
hockey	ice, field hockey	420	496	573	649	728	802	878	954
jog	general	368	434	501	568	637	702	768	835
jog	jog/walk combination	315	372	430	487	546	602	658	716
jump rope	slow	420	496	573	649	728	802	878	954
jump rope	moderate	525	621	716	812	910	1003	1097	1193
jump rope	fast	630	745	859	974	1092	1203	1317	1431
kayak	general	263	310	358	406	455	501	549	596
martial arts	general	525	621	716	812	910	1003	1097	1193
racquetball	casual	368	434	501	568	637	702	768	835

Continued

Appendix 52 Caloric Expenditure Worksheet for Various Exercise Activities Based on Body Weight—cont'd

ACTIVITY	TYPE	cal/hr —110 lb	cal/hr —130 lb	cal/hr —150 lb	cal/hr —170 lb	cal/hr —190 lb	cal/hr —210 lb	cal/hr —230 lb	cal/hr —250 lb
racquetball	competition	525	621	716	812	910	1003	1097	1193
rafting	whitewater	263	310	358	406	455	501	549	596
rock climb	general	420	496	573	649	728	802	878	954
rugby	general	525	621	716	812	910	1003	1097	1193
run	5 mph, 12 min/mi	420	496	573	649	728	802	878	954
run	5.2 mph, 11.5 min/mi	473	558	644	730	819	902	988	1074
run	6 mph, 10 min/mi	525	621	716	812	910	1003	1097	1193
run	6.7 mph, 9 min/mi	578	683	788	893	1001	1103	1207	1312
run	7 mph, 8.5 min/mi	604	714	824	933	1047	1153	1262	1372
run	7.5 mph, 8 min/mi	656	776	895	1015	1138	1253	1372	1491
run	8 mph, 7.5 min/mi	709	838	967	1096	1229	1354	1481	1610
run	8.6 mph, 7 min/mi	735	869	1003	1136	1274	1404	1536	1670
run	9 mph, 6.5 min/mi	788	931	1074	1217	1366	1504	1646	1789
run	10 mph, 6 min/mi	840	993	1146	1299	1457	1604	1756	1908
run	10.9 mph, 5.5 min/mi	945	1117	1289	1461	1639	1805	1975	2147
run	cross country	473	558	644	730	819	902	988	1074
skate, ice	general	368	434	501	568	637	702	768	835
skate, inline	inline/general	656	776	895	1015	1138	1253	1372	1491
skateboard	general	263	310	358	406	455	501	549	596
ski, downhill	light	263	310	358	406	455	501	549	596
ski, downhill	moderate	315	372	430	487	546	602	658	716
ski, downhill	vigorous/race	420	496	573	649	728	802	878	954
ski machine	general	368	434	501	568	637	702	768	835
ski, cross-country	2.5 mph, slow	368	434	501	568	637	702	768	835
ski, cross-country	4-4.9 mph, moderate	420	496	573	649	728	802	878	954
ski, cross-country	5-7.9 mph, brisk	473	558	644	730	819	902	988	1074
snowboard	general	394	465	537	609	683	752	823	895
snowshoe	general	420	496	573	649	728	802	878	954
soccer	casual	368	434	501	568	637	702	768	835
soccer	competitive	525	621	716	812	910	1003	1097	1193
softball	general	263	310	358	406	455	501	549	596
stair stepper	general	473	558	644	730	819	902	988	1074
stationary rower	50 watts, light	184	217	251	284	319	351	384	417
stationary rower	100 watts, moderate	368	434	501	568	637	702	768	835
stationary rower	150 watts, vigorous	446	527	609	690	774	852	933	1014
stationary rower	200 watts, very vigorous	630	745	859	974	1092	1203	1317	1431
stretch/yoga	general, Hatha	131	155	179	203	228	251	274	298
swim	lake, ocean or river	315	372	430	487	546	602	658	716
swim	laps freestyle, slow/moderate	368	434	501	568	637	702	768	835
swim	laps freestyle, fast	525	621	716	812	910	1003	1097	1193
swim	backstroke	368	434	501	568	637	702	768	835
swim	sidestroke	420	496	573	649	728	802	878	954
swim	breaststroke	525	621	716	812	910	1003	1097	1193
swim	butterfly	578	683	788	893	1001	1103	1207	1312
tennis	doubles	315	372	430	487	546	602	658	716
tennis	singles	420	496	573	649	728	802	878	954
treadmill, run	6 mph, 10 min/mi, 0% incline	525	621	716	812	910	1003	1097	1193

Appendix 52 Caloric Expenditure Worksheet for Various Exercise Activities Based on Body Weight—cont'd

ACTIVITY	TYPE	cal/hr —110 lb	cal/hr —130 lb	cal/hr —150 lb	cal/hr —170 lb	cal/hr —190 lb	cal/hr —210 lb	cal/hr —230 lb	cal/hr —250 lb
treadmill, run	6 mph, 10 min/mi, 2% incline	578	683	788	893	1001	1103	1207	1312
treadmill, run	6 mph, 10 min/mi, 4% incline	620	732	845	958	1074	1183	1295	1408
treadmill, run	6 mph, 10 min/mi, 6% incline	667	788	909	1031	1156	1273	1394	1515
treadmill, run	7 mph, 8.5 min/mi, 0% incline	604	714	824	933	1047	1153	1262	1372
treadmill, run	7 mph, 8.5 min/mi, 2% incline	667	788	909	1031	1156	1273	1394	1515
treadmill, run	7 mph, 8.5 min/mi, 4% incline	719	850	981	1112	1247	1374	1503	1634
treadmill, run	7 mph, 8.5 min/mi, 6% incline	767	906	1046	1185	1329	1464	1602	1741
treadmill, run	8 mph, 7.5 min/mi, 0% incline	709	838	967	1096	1229	1354	1481	1610
treadmill, run	8 mph, 7.5 min/mi, 2% incline	756	894	1031	1169	1311	1444	1580	1718
treadmill, run	8 mph, 7.5 min/mi, 4% incline	814	962	1110	1258	1411	1554	1701	1849
treadmill, run	8 mph, 7.5 min/mi, 6% incline	872	1030	1189	1347	1511	1665	1821	1980
treadmill, walk	3 mph, 20 min/mi, 0% incline	173	205	236	268	300	331	362	394
treadmill, walk	3 mph, 20 min/mi, 2% incline	194	230	265	300	337	371	406	441
treadmill, walk	3 mph, 20 min/mi, 4% incline	215	254	293	333	373	411	450	489
treadmill, walk	3 mph, 20 min/mi, 6% incline	236	279	322	365	410	451	494	537
treadmill, walk	4 mph, 15 min/mi, 0% incline	263	310	358	406	455	501	549	596
treadmill, walk	4 mph, 15 min/mi, 2% incline	294	348	401	455	510	562	614	668
treadmill, walk	4 mph, 15 min/mi, 4% incline	326	385	444	503	564	622	680	740
treadmill, walk	4 mph, 15 min/mi, 6% incline	352	416	480	544	610	672	735	799
tread water	moderate	210	248	286	325	364	401	439	477
tread water	vigorous	525	621	716	812	910	1003	1097	1193
volleyball	noncompetitive	158	133	215	243	273	301	329	358
volleyball	competitive	420	496	573	649	728	802	878	954
walk	<2 mph	105	124	143	162	182	201	219	239
walk	2 mph, 30 min/mi	131	155	179	203	228	251	274	298
walk	2.5 mph, 24 min/mi	158	133	215	243	273	301	329	358
walk	3 mph, 20 min/mi	173	205	236	268	300	331	362	394
walk	3.5 mph, 17 min/mi	200	236	272	308	346	381	417	453
walk	4 mph, 15 min/mi	263	310	358	406	455	501	549	596
walk	4.5 mph, 13 min/mi	331	391	451	511	574	632	691	751
walk	race walking	341	403	465	528	592	652	713	775
water polo	general	525	621	716	812	910	1003	1097	1193
weight training	free, nautilus, light/moderate	158	133	215	243	273	301	329	358
weight training	free, nautilus, vigorous	315	372	430	487	546	602	658	716
wind surf	casual	158	133	215	243	273	301	329	358

Appendix 53 Exchange Lists for Meal Planning

MEAL PLAN

Meal Plan for: ______________________ Date: ______________________

Dietitian: ______________________ Phone: ______________________

	Grams	Percent
Carbohydrate	______	______
Protein	______	______
Fat	______	______
Calories	______	______

Time	Number of Exchanges/Choices	Menu Ideas	Menu Ideas
	______ Carbohydrate group ______ Starch ______ Fruit ______ Milk ______ ______ Meat group ______ ______ Fat group ______		
	______ ______ ______ ______ ______ Carbohydrate group ______ Starch ______ Fruit ______ Milk ______ ______ Vegetables ______ Meat group ______ Fat group		
	______ ______ ______ ______ ______ ______ ______ Carbohydrate group ______ Starch ______ Fruit ______ Milk ______ ______ Vegetables ______ Meat group ______ Fat group		
	______ ______ ______ ______ ______ ______		

STARCH LIST

Cereals, grains, pasta, breads, crackers, snacks, starchy vegetables, and cooked beans, peas, and lentils are starches. In general, one starch is:

- ½ cup of cooked cereal, grain, or starchy vegetable
- 1 oz. of a bread product, such as 1 slice of bread
- ¾ to 1 ounce of most snack foods (Some snack foods may also have added fat.)
- ⅓ cup of cooked rice or pasta

Nutrition Tips

1. Most starch choices are good sources of B vitamins.
2. Foods made from whole grains are good sources of fiber.
3. Dried beans and peas are a good source of protein and fiber.

Selection Tips

1. Choose starches made with little fat as often as you can.
2. Starchy vegetables prepared with fat count as one starch and one fat.
3. Bagels or muffins can be 2, 3, or 4 ounces in size and can therefore count as 2, 3, or 4 starch choices. Check the size you eat.
4. Beans, peas, and lentils are also found on the Meat and Meat Substitutes list.
5. A waffle or pancake is about the size of a compact disc (CD) and about ¼″ thick.
6. Because starches often swell in cooking, a small amount of uncooked starch becomes a much larger amount of cooked food.
7. Most of the serving sizes are measured or weighed after cooking.
8. Always check Nutrition Facts on the food label.

The Exchange Lists are the basis of a meal planning system designed by a committee of the American Diabetes Association and the American Dietetic Association. Although designed primarily for people with diabetes and others who must follow special diets, the Exchange Lists are based on principles of good nutrition that apply to everyone. Copyright 2003 American Diabetes Association, Inc., The American Dietetic Association. Used with permission.

Appendix 53 Exchange Lists for Meal Planning—cont'd

STARCH LIST—cont'd

ONE STARCH EXCHANGE EQUALS 15 GRAMS CARBOHYDRATE, 3 GRAMS PROTEIN, 0-1 GRAMS FAT, AND 80 CALORIES.

Bread

Bagel, 4 oz ... ¼ (1 oz)
Bread, reduced-calorie ... 2 slices (1½ oz)
Bread, white, whole-wheat, pumpernickel, rye ... 1 slice (1 oz)
Bread sticks, crisp, 4 in. long × ½ in. ... 4 (⅔ oz)
English muffin ... ½
Hot dog or hamburger bun ... ½ (1 oz)
Naan, 8 × 2″ ... ¼
Pita, 6 in. across ... ½
Pancake, 4 in. across, ¼″ thick ... 1
Roll, plain, small ... 1 (1 oz)
Raisin bread, unfrosted ... 1 slice (1 oz)
Tortilla, corn, 6 in. across ... 1
Tortilla, flour, 6 in. across ... 1
Tortilla, flour, 10 in. across ... ⅓
Waffle, 4½ in. square, reduced-fat ... 1

Cereals and Grains

Bran cereals ... ½ cup
Bulgur ... ½ cup
Cereals, cooked ... ½ cup
Cereals, unsweetened, ready-to-eat ... ¾ cup
Cornmeal (dry) ... 3 Tbsp
Couscous ... ⅓ cup
Flour (dry) ... 3 Tbsp
Granola, low-fat ... ¼ cup
Grape-Nuts ... ¼ cup
Grits ... ½ cup
Kashi ... ½ cup
Millet ... ⅓ cup
Muesli ... ¼ cup
Oats ... ½ cup
Pasta ... ½ cup
Puffed cereal ... 1½ cups
Rice, white or brown ... ⅓ cup
Shredded Wheat ... ½ cup
Sugar-frosted cereal ... ½ cup
Wheat germ ... 3 Tbsp

Starchy Vegetables

Baked beans ... ⅓ cup
Corn ... ½ cup
Corn on cob, large ... ½ cob (5 oz)
Mixed vegetables with corn, peas, or pasta ... 1 cup
Peas, green ... ½ cup
Plantain ... ½ cup
Potato, baked with skin ... ¼ large (3 oz)
Potato, boiled ... ½ cup or ½ medium (3 oz)
Potato, mashed ... ½ cup
Squash, winter (acorn, butternut, pumpkin) ... 1 cup
Yam, sweet potato, plain ... ½ cup

Crackers and Snacks

Animal crackers ... 8
Graham crackers, 2½ in. square ... 3
Matzoh ... ¾ oz
Melba toast ... 4 slices

Crackers and Snacks—cont'd

Oyster crackers ... 24
Popcorn (popped, no fat added or low-fat microwave) ... 3 cups
Pretzels ... ¾ oz
Rice cakes, 4 in. across ... 2
Saltine-type crackers ... 6
Snack chips, fat-free (tortilla, potato) ... 15-20 (¾ oz)
Whole-wheat crackers, no fat added ... 2-5 (¾ oz)

Beans, Peas, and Lentils
(Count as 1 starch exchange, plus 1 very lean meat exchange.)

Beans and peas (garbanzo, pinto, kidney, white, split, black-eyed) ... ½ cup
Lima beans ... ⅔ cup
Lentils ... ½ cup
Miso* ... 3 Tbsp

Starchy Foods Prepared With Fat
(Count as 1 starch exchange, plus 1 fat exchange.)

Biscuit, 2½ in. across ... 1
Chow mein noodles ... ½ cup
Corn bread, 2 in. cube ... 1 (2 oz)
Crackers, round butter type ... 6
Croutons ... 1 cup
French-fried potatoes, oven-baked ... 1 cup (12 oz)
Granola ... ¼ cup
Hummus ... ⅓ cup
Muffin, 5 oz ... 1 (1½ oz)
Popcorn, microwaved ... 3 cups
Sandwich crackers, cheese or peanut butter filling ... 3
Snack chips (potato, tortilla) ... 9-13 (¾ oz)
Stuffing, bread (prepared) ... ⅓ cup
Taco shell, 6 in. across ... 2
Waffle, 4½ in. square ... 1
Whole-wheat crackers, fat added ... 4–6 (1 oz)

Some uncooked food will weigh less after you cook it. Starches often swell in cooking, so a small amount of uncooked starch will become a much larger amount of cooked food. The following table shows some of the changes.

Food (Starch Group)	Uncooked	Cooked
Oatmeal	3 Tbsp	½ cup
Cream of Wheat	2 Tbsp	½ cup
Grits	3 Tbsp	½ cup
Rice	2 Tbsp	⅓ cup
Spaghetti	¼ cup	½ cup
Noodles	⅓ cup	½ cup
Macaroni	¼ cup	½ cup
Dried beans	¼ cup	½ cup
Dried peas	¼ cup	½ cup
Lentils	3 Tbsp	½ cup

Common Measurements

3 tsp = 1 Tbsp	4 ounces = ½ cup
4 Tbsp = ¼ cup	8 ounces = 1 cup
5⅓ Tbsp = ⅓ cup	1 cup = ½ pint

*400 mg or more of sodium per serving.

Continued

Appendix 53 Exchange Lists for Meal Planning—cont'd

FRUIT LIST

Fresh, frozen, canned, and dried fruits and fruit juices are on this list. In general, one fruit exchange is:

- 1 small (4 oz) fresh fruit
- ½ cup of canned or fresh fruit or unsweetened fruit juice
- ¼ cup of dried fruit

Nutrition Tips

1. Fresh, frozen, and dried fruits have about 2 grams of fiber per choice. Fruit juices contain very little fiber.
2. Citrus fruits, berries, and melons are good sources of vitamin C.

Selection Tips

1. Count ½ cup cranberries or rhubarb sweetened with sugar substitutes as free foods.
2. Read the Nutrition Facts on the food label. If one serving has more than 15 grams of carbohydrate, you will need to adjust the size of the serving you eat or drink.
3. Portion sizes for canned fruits are for the fruit and a small amount of juice.
4. Whole fruit is more filling than fruit juice and may be a better choice.
5. Food labels for fruits may contain the words "no sugar added" or "unsweetened." This means that no sucrose (table sugar) has been added.
6. Generally, fruit canned in extra light syrup has the same amount of carbohydrate per serving as the "no sugar added" or the juice pack. All canned fruits on the fruit list are based on one of these three types of packs.

ONE FRUIT EXCHANGE EQUALS 15 GRAMS CARBOHYDRATE AND 60 CALORIES. THE WEIGHT INCLUDES SKIN, CORE, SEEDS, AND RIND.

Fruit	
Apple, unpeeled, small	1 (4 oz)
Applesauce, unsweetened	½ cup
Apples, dried	4 rings
Apricots, fresh	4 whole (5½ oz)
Apricots, dried	8 halves
Apricots, canned	½ cup
Banana, small	1 (4 oz)
Blackberries	¾ cup
Blueberries	¾ cup
Cantaloupe, small	⅓ melon (11 oz) or 1 cup cubes
Cherries, sweet, fresh	12 (3 oz)
Cherries, sweet, canned	½ cup
Dates	3
Figs, fresh	1½ large or 2 medium (3½ oz)
Figs, dried	1½
Fruit cocktail	½ cup
Grapefruit, large	½ (11 oz)
Grapefruit sections, canned	¾ cup
Grapes, small	17 (3 oz)
Honeydew melon	1 slice (10 oz) or 1 cup cubes
Kiwi	1 (3½ oz)
Mandarin oranges, canned	¾ cup
Mango, small	½ fruit (5½ oz) or ½ cup
Nectarine, small	1 (5 oz)
Orange, small	1 (6½ oz)
Papaya	½ fruit (8 oz) or 1 cup cubes
Peach, medium, fresh	1 (6 oz)
Peaches, canned	½ cup
Pear, large, fresh	½ (4 oz)
Pears, canned	½ cup
Pineapple, fresh	¾ cup
Pineapple, canned	½ cup
Plums, small	2 (5 oz)
Plums, canned	½ cup
Prunes, dried	3
Raisins	2 Tbsp
Raspberries	1 cup
Strawberries	1¼ cup whole berries
Tangerines, small	2 (8 oz)
Watermelon	1 slice (13½ oz) or 1¼ cup cubes
Fruit Juice	
Apple juice/cider	½ cup
Cranberry juice cocktail	⅓ cup
Cranberry juice cocktail, reduced-calorie	1 cup
Fruit juice blends, 100% juice	⅓ cup
Grape juice	⅓ cup
Grapefruit juice	½ cup
Orange juice	½ cup
Pineapple juice	½ cup
Prune juice	⅓ cup

MILK LIST

Different types of milk and milk products are on this list. Cheeses are on the Meat list, and cream and other dairy fats are on the Fat list. Based on the amount of fat they contain, milks are divided into fat-free/low-fat milk, and whole milk. One choice of these includes:

	Carbohydrate (grams)	Protein (grams)	Fat (grams)	Calories
Fat-free/low-fat (½% or 1%)	12	8	0-3	90
Reduced fat 2%	12	8	5	120
Whole	12	8	8	150

Nutrition Tips

1. Milk and yogurt are good sources of calcium and protein. Check the Nutrition Facts on the food label.
2. The higher the fat content of milk and yogurt, the greater the amount of saturated fat and cholesterol. Choose lower-fat varieties.
3. For those who are lactose intolerant, look for lactose-reduced or lactose-free varieties of milk. Check the food label for total amount of carbohydrate per serving.

Selection Tips

1. One cup equals 8 fluid ounces or ½ pint.
2. Look for chocolate milk, frozen yogurt, and ice cream on the Other Carbohydrates list.
3. Nondairy creamers are on the Free Foods list.

Appendix 53 Exchange Lists for Meal Planning—cont'd

MILK LIST—cont'd

ONE MILK EXCHANGE EQUALS 12 GRAMS CARBOHYDRATE, 8 GRAMS PROTEIN, 0-8 GRAMS FAT, AND 90-150 kcal.

Fat-Free and Low-Fat Milk 90 kcal
(0–3 grams fat per serving)

Fat-free milk	1 cup
½% milk	1 cup
1% milk	1 cup
Buttermilk, low-fat or fat-free	1 cup
Evaporated fat-free milk	½ cup
Fat free dry milk	⅓ cup dry
Yogurt, plain nonfat	¾ cup
Yogurt, fat-free, flavored, sweetened with nonnutritive sweetener and fructose	1 cup
Soy milk, low-fat or fat-free	1 cup

Reduced-Fat 120 kcal
(5 grams fat per serving)

2% milk	1 cup
Yogurt, plain lowfat	¾ cup
Sweet acidophilus milk	1 cup
Soy milk	1 cup

Whole Milk 150 kcal
(8 grams fat per serving)

Whole milk	1 cup
Evaporated whole milk	½ cup
Goat's milk	1 cup
Kefir	1 cup
Yogurt, plain (made from whole milk)	¾ cup

SWEETS, DESSERTS, AND OTHER CARBOHYDRATES LIST

You can substitute food choices from this list for a starch, fruit, or milk choice on your meal plan. Some choices will also count as one or more fat choices.

Nutrition Tips

1. These foods can be substituted in your meal plan, even though they contain added sugars or fat. However, they do not contain as many important vitamins and minerals as the choices on the Starch, Fruit, or Milk lists.
2. When planning to include these foods in your meal, include foods from the other lists to eat a balanced meal.

Selection Tips

1. Because many of these foods are concentrated sources of carbohydrate, fat, saturated fat, and trans fat, the portion sizes are often very small.
2. Look for the words "hydogenated" or "partially hydrogenated" on the label. The lower down the list these words appear, the fewer trans fats there are.
3. Always check Nutrition Facts on the food label. It will be your most accurate source of information.
4. Many fat-free or reduced-fat products made with fat replacers contain carbohydrate. When eaten in large amounts, they may need to be counted. Talk with your dietitian to determine how to count these in your meal plan.
5. Look for fat-free salad dressings in smaller amounts on the Free Foods list.

ONE OTHER CARBOHYDRATE EXCHANGE EQUALS 15 GRAMS CARBOHYDRATE, OR 1 STARCH, OR 1 FRUIT, OR 1 MILK.

Food	Serving Size	Exchanges per Serving
Angel food cake, unfrosted	1/12 cake (about 2 oz)	2 carbohydrates
Brownie, small, unfrosted	2 in. square (about 1 oz)	1 carbohydrate, 1 fat
Cake, unfrosted	2 in. square (about 1 oz)	1 carbohydrate, 1 fat
Cake, frosted	2 in. square (about 2 oz)	2 carbohydrates, 1 fat
Cookie, sugar-free	3 small or 1 large (⅔ oz)	1 carbohydrate, 1-2 fats
Cookie or sandwich cookie with cream filling	2 small (⅔ oz)	1 carbohydrate, 1 fat
Cranberry sauce, jellied	¼ cup	1½ carbohydrates
Cupcake, frosted	1 small	2 carbohydrates, 1 fat
Doughnut, plain cake	1 medium (1½ oz)	1½ carbohydrates, 2 fats
Doughnut, glazed	3¾ in. across (2 oz)	2 carbohydrates, 2 fats
Energy, sport, or breakfast bar	2 oz	2 carbohydrates, 1 fat
Fruit juice bars, frozen, 100% juice	1 bar (3 oz)	1 carbohydrate
Fruit snacks, chewy (pureed fruit concentrate)	1 roll (¾ oz)	1 carbohydrate
Fruit spreads, 100% fruit	1½ Tbsp	1 carbohydrate
Gelatin, regular	½ cup	1 carbohydrate
Gingersnaps	3	1 carbohydrate
Granola bar or snack bar, regular or low-fat	1 bar	1½ carbohydrates
Honey	1 Tbsp	1 carbohydrate
Ice cream	½ cup	1 carbohydrate, 2 fats
Ice cream, light	½ cup	1 carbohydrate, 1 fat
Ice cream, fat-free, no sugar added	½ cup	1 carbohydrate
Jam or jelly, regular	1 Tbsp	1 carbohydrate
Milk, chocolate, whole	1 cup	2 carbohydrates, 1 fat
Pie, fruit, 2 crusts	⅙ of 8″ pie	3 carbohydrates, 2 fats
Pie, pumpkin or custard	⅛ of 8″ pie	2 carbohydrates, 2 fats
Pudding, regular (made with reduced fat milk)	½ cup	2 carbohydrates
Pudding, sugar-free (made with fat-free milk)	½ cup	1 carbohydrate
Reduced calorie meal replacement (shake)	1 can (10-11 oz)	1½ carbohydrates, 0-1 fat
Rice milk, low-fat, flavored	1 cup	1½ carbohydrates
Salad dressing, fat-free	¼ cup	1 carbohydrate
Sherbet, sorbet	½ cup	2 carbohydrates
Spaghetti or pasta sauce, canned*	½ cup	1 carbohydrate, 1 fat

*400 mg or more sodium per exchange.

Continued

Appendix 53 Exchange Lists for Meal Planning—cont'd

ONE EXCHANGE EQUALS 15 GRAMS CARBOHYDRATE, OR 1 STARCH, OR 1 FRUIT, OR 1 MILK—cont'd

Food	Serving Size	Exchanges Per Serving
Sport drink	1 cup (8 oz)	1 carbohydrate
Sugar	1 Tbsp	1 carbohydrate
Sweet roll or Danish	1 (2½ oz)	2½ carbohydrates, 2 fats
Syrup, light	2 Tbsp	1 carbohydrate
Syrup, regular	1Tbsp	1 carbohydrate
Syrup, regular	¼ cup	4 carbohydrates
Vanilla wafers	5	1 carbohydrate, 1 fat
Yogurt, frozen	½ cup	1 carbohydrate, 0-1 fat
Yogurt, frozen, fat-free	⅓ cup	1 carbohydrate
Yogurt, low-fat with fruit	1 cup	3 carbohydrates, 0-1 fat

NONSTARCHY VEGETABLE LIST

Vegetables that contain small amounts of carbohydrates and calories are on this list. Vegetables contain important nutrients. Try to eat at least 2 or 3 vegetable choices each day. In general, one vegetable exchange is:

- ½ cup of cooked vegetables or vegetable juice
- 1 cup of raw vegetables

If you eat 1 to 2 vegetable choices at a meal or snack, you do not have to count the calories or carbohydrates because they contain small amounts of these nutrients.

Nutrition Tips

1. Fresh and frozen vegetables have less added salt than canned vegetables. Drain and rinse canned vegetables if you want to remove some salt.
2. Choose more dark green and dark yellow vegetables, such as spinach, broccoli, romaine, carrots, chilies, and peppers.
3. Broccoli, Brussels sprouts, cauliflower, greens, peppers, spinach, and tomatoes are good sources of vitamin C.
4. Vegetables contain 1 to 4 grams of fiber per serving.

Selection Tips

1. A 1-cup portion of broccoli is a portion about the size of a light bulb.
2. Tomato sauce is different from spaghetti sauce, which is on the Other Carbohydrates list.
3. Canned vegetables and juices are available without added salt.
4. Starchy vegetables such as corn, peas, winter squash, and potatoes that contain larger amounts of calories and carbohydrates are on the Starch list.

ONE NONSTARCHY VEGETABLE EXCHANGE EQUALS 5 GRAMS CARBOHYDRATE, 2 GRAMS PROTEIN, 0 GRAMS FAT, AND 25 CALORIES.

Artichoke
Artichoke hearts
Asparagus
Beans (green, wax, Italian)
Bean sprouts
Beets
Broccoli
Brussels sprouts
Cabbage
Carrots
Cauliflower
Celery
Cucumber
Eggplant
Green onions or scallions
Greens (collard, kale, mustard, turnip)
Kohlrabi
Leeks
Mixed vegetables (without corn, peas, or pasta)
Mushrooms
Okra
Onions
Pea pods
Peppers (all varieties)
Radishes
Salad greens (endive, escarole, lettuce, romaine, spinach)
Sauerkraut*
Spinach
Summer squash
Tomato
Tomatoes, canned
Tomato sauce*
Tomato/vegetable juice*
Turnips
Water chestnuts
Watercress
Zucchini

MEAT AND MEAT SUBSTITUTES LIST

Meat and meat substitutes that contain both protein and fat are on this list. In general, one meat exchange is:

- 1 oz meat, fish, poultry, or cheese
- ½ cup beans, peas, or lentils

Based on the amount of fat they contain, meats are divided into very lean, lean, medium-fat, and high-fat lists. This is done so you can see which ones contain the least amount of fat. One ounce (one exchange) of each of these includes:

	Carbohydrate (grams)	Protein (grams)	Fat (grams)	Calories
Very lean	0	7	0-1	35
Lean	0	7	3	55
Medium-fat	0	7	5	75
High-fat	0	7	8	100

Nutrition Tips

1. Choose very lean and lean meat choices whenever possible. Items from the high-fat group are high in saturated fat, cholesterol, and calories and can raise blood cholesterol levels.
2. Beans, peas, and lentils are good sources of fiber, about 3 grams per serving.
3. Some processed meats, seafood, and soy products may contain carbohydrate when consumed in large amounts. Check the Nutrition Facts on the label to see if the amount is close to 15 grams. If so, count it as a carbohydrate choice as well as a meat choice.

The Exchange Lists are the basis of a meal planning system designed by a committee of the American Diabetes Association and the American Dietetic Association. Although designed primarily for people with diabetes and others who must follow special diets, the Exchange Lists are based on principles of good nutrition that apply to everyone.
*400 mg or more sodium per exchange.

Appendix 53 Exchange Lists for Meal Planning—cont'd

MEAT AND MEAT SUBSTITUTES LIST—cont'd

Selection Tips

1. Weigh meat after cooking and removing bones and fat. Four ounces of raw meat is equal to 3 ounces of cooked meat. Some examples of meat portions are:
   - 1 oz cheese = 1 meat choice and is about the size of a 1-inch cube
   - 2 oz meat = 2 meat choices, such as
     1 small chicken leg or thigh
     ½ cup cottage cheese or tuna
   - 3 oz meat = 3 meat choices and is about the size of a deck of cards, such as
     1 medium pork chop
     1 small hamburger
     ½ of a whole chicken breast
     1 unbreaded fish fillet
2. Limit your choices from the high-fat group to three times per week or less.
3. Most grocery stores stock select and choice grades of meat. Select grades of meat are the leanest meats. Choice grades contain a moderate amount of fat, and prime cuts of meat have the highest amount of fat. Restaurants usually serve prime cuts of meat.
4. "Hamburger" may contain added seasoning and fat, but ground beef does not.
5. Read labels to find products that are low in fat and cholesterol (5 grams or less of fat per serving).
6. Dried beans, peas, and lentils are also found on the Starch list.
7. Peanut butter, in smaller amounts, is also found on the Fats list.
8. Bacon, in smaller amounts, is also found on the Fats list.
9. A 3.5 oz hamburger patty has about half its calories from fat.
10. Meatless burgers are in the Combination Food list.

Meal Planning Tips

1. Bake, roast, broil, grill, poach, steam, or boil these foods rather than frying.
2. Place meat on a rack so the fat will drain off during cooking.
3. Use a nonstick spray and a nonstick pan to brown or fry foods.
4. Trim off visible fat before or after cooking.
5. If you add flour, bread crumbs, coating mixes, fat, or marinades when cooking, ask your dietitian how to count it in your meal plan.

VERY LEAN MEAT AND SUBSTITUTES LIST

ONE EXCHANGE EQUALS 0 GRAMS CARBOHYDRATE, 7 GRAMS PROTEIN, 0-1 GRAM FAT, AND 35 CALORIES.

One very lean meat exchange is equal to any one of the following items.

Poultry: Chicken or turkey (white meat, no skin), Cornish hen (no skin) .... 1 oz
Fish: Fresh or frozen cod, flounder, haddock, halibut, trout; lox,* tuna fresh or canned in water .... 1 oz
Shellfish: Clams, crab, lobster, scallops, shrimp, imitation shellfish .... 1 oz
Game: Duck or pheasant (no skin), venison, buffalo, ostrich .... 1 oz
Cheese with 1 gram or less fat per ounce:
Fat-free or low-fat cottage cheese .... ¼ cup
Fat-free cheese .... 1 oz
Other: Processed sandwich meats with 1 gram or less fat per ounce, such as deli thin, shaved meats, chipped beef,* turkey ham .... 1 oz
Egg whites 2
Egg substitutes, plain .... ¼ cup
Hot dogs with 1 gram or less fat per ounce* .... 1 oz
Kidney (high in cholesterol) .... 1 oz
Sausage with 1 gram or less fat per ounce .... 1 oz

Count as one very lean meat and one starch exchange:
beans, peas, lentils (cooked) .... ½ cup

LEAN MEAT AND SUBSTITUTES LIST

ONE EXCHANGE EQUALS 0 GRAMS CARBOHYDRATE, 7 GRAMS PROTEIN, 3 GRAMS FAT, AND 55 CALORIES.

One lean meat exchange is equal to any one of the following items.

Beef: USDA Select or Choice grades of lean beef trimmed of fat, such as round, sirloin, and flank steak; tenderloin; roast (rib, chuck, rump); steak (T-bone, porterhouse, cubed), ground round .... 1 oz
Pork: Lean pork, such as fresh ham; canned, cured, or boiled ham; Canadian bacon*; tenderloin, center loin chop .... 1 oz
Lamb: Roast, chop, leg .... 1 oz
Veal: Lean chop, roast .... 1 oz
Poultry: Chicken, turkey (dark meat, no skin), chicken (white meat with skin), domestic duck or goose (well-drained of fat, no skin) .... 1 oz
Fish:
Herring (uncreamed or smoked) .... 1 oz
Oysters .... 6 medium
Salmon (fresh or canned), catfish .... 1 oz
Sardines (canned) .... 2 medium
Tuna (canned in oil, drained) .... 1 oz
Game: Goose (no skin), rabbit .... 1 oz
Cheese:
4.5%-fat cottage cheese .... ¼ cup
Grated Parmesan .... 2 Tbsp
Cheeses with 3 grams or less fat per ounce .... 1 oz
Other:
Hot dogs with 3 grams or less fat per ounce* .... 1½ oz
Processed sandwich meat with 3 grams or less fat per ounce, such as turkey pastrami or kielbasa .... 1 oz
Liver, heart (high in cholesterol) .... 1 oz

*400 mg or more sodium per exchange.

Continued

Appendix 53 Exchange Lists for Meal Planning—cont'd

MEDIUM-FAT AND MEAT SUBSTITUTES LIST

ONE EXCHANGE EQUALS 0 GRAMS CARBOHYDRATE, 7 GRAMS PROTEIN, 5 GRAMS FAT, AND 75 CALORIES.

One medium-fat meat exchange is equal to any one of the following items.

Beef: Most beef products fall into this category (ground beef; meatloaf, corned beef; short ribs; prime grades of meat trimmed of fat, such as prime rib) .... 1 oz
Pork: Top loin, chop, Boston butt, cutlet .... 1 oz
Lamb: Rib roast, ground.......... 1 oz
Veal: Cutlet (ground or cubed, unbreaded) .... 1 oz
Poultry: Chicken dark meat (with skin), ground turkey or ground chicken, fried chicken (with skin) .... 1 oz
Fish: Any fried fish product.......... 1 oz
Cheese: With 5 grams or less fat per ounce
Feta .... 1 oz
Mozzarella .... 1 oz
Ricotta.......... ¼ cup (2 oz)
Other:
Egg (high in cholesterol, limit to 3 per week).......... 1
Sausage with 5 grams or less fat per ounce.......... 1 oz
Tempeh .... ¼ cup
Tofu.......... 4 oz or ½ cup

HIGH-FAT MEAT AND SUBSTITUTES LIST

ONE EXCHANGE EQUALS 0 GRAMS CARBOHYDRATE,7 GRAMS PROTEIN, 8 GRAMS FAT, AND 100 CALORIES.

Remember these items are high in saturated fat, cholesterol, and calories and may raise blood cholesterol levels if eaten on a regular basis. One high-fat meat exchange is equal to any one of the following items.

Pork: Spareribs, ground pork, pork sausage.......... 1 oz
Cheese: All regular cheeses, such as American,* cheddar, Monterey Jack, Swiss .... 1 oz
Other: Processed sandwich meats with 8 grams or less fat per ounce, such as bologna, pimento loaf, salami .... 1 oz
Sausage, such as bratwurst, Italian, knockwurst, Polish, smoked .... 1 oz
Hot dog (turkey or chicken)*.......... 1 (10/lb)
Bacon .... 3 slices (20 slices/lb)
Kidney (high in cholesterol).......... 1 oz
Peanut butter (contains unsaturated fat).......... 2 Tbsp

Count as one high-fat meat plus one fat exchange: hot dog (beef, pork, or combination)*.......... 1 (10/lb)

FAT LIST

Fats are divided into three groups, based on the main type of fat they contain: monounsaturated, polyunsaturated, and saturated. Small amounts of monounsaturated and polyunsaturated fats in the foods we eat are linked with good health benefits. Saturated fats are linked with heart disease and cancer. In general, one fat exchange is:

- 1 teaspoon of regular margarine or vegetable oil
- 1 tablespoon of regular salad dressing

Nutrition Tips

1. All fats are high in calories. Limit serving sizes for good nutrition and health.
2. Nuts and seeds contain small amounts of fiber, protein, and magnesium.
3. If blood pressure is a concern, choose fats in the unsalted form to help lower sodium intake, such as unsalted peanuts.

Selection Tips

1. Check the Nutrition Facts on food labels for serving sizes. One fat exchange is based on a serving size containing 5 grams of fat.
2. Food label Nutrition Facts usually list total fat and saturated fat grams per serving. When most calories come from saturated fats, the food fits into the Saturated Fat list.
3. When selecting regular margarine, choose one with liquid vegetable oil as the first ingredient. Soft margarines are not as saturated as stick margarines and are healthier choices. Avoid those listing hydrogenated or partially hydrogenated fat as the first ingredient because they will contain more trans fatty acids.
4. When selecting low-fat margarines, look for liquid vegetable oil as the second ingredient. Water is usually the first ingredient.
5. When used in smaller amounts, bacon and peanut butter are counted as fat choices. When used in larger amounts, they are counted as high-fat meat choices.
6. Fat-free salad dressings are on the Other Carbohydrates list and the Free Foods list.
7. See the Free Foods list for nondairy coffee creamers, whipped topping, and fat-free products, such as margarines, salad dressings, mayonnaise, sour cream, cream cheese, and nonstick cooking spray.

MONOUNSATURATED FATS LIST

ONE FAT EXCHANGE EQUALS 5 GRAMS FAT AND 45 CALORIES.

Avocado, medium .... 2 Tbsp (1 oz)
Oil (canola, olive, peanut).......... 1 tsp
Olives: ripe (black) .... 8 large
green, stuffed*.......... 10 large
Nuts
almonds, cashews .... 6 nuts
mixed (50% peanuts).......... 6 nuts
peanuts .... 10 nuts
pecans.......... 4 halves
Peanut butter, smooth or crunchy.......... ½ Tbsp
Sesame seeds .... 1 Tbsp
Tahini or sesame paste.......... 2 tsp

POLYUNSATURATED FATS LIST

ONE FAT EXCHANGE EQUALS 5 GRAMS FAT AND 45 CALORIES.

Margarine: stick, tub, or squeeze.......... 1 tsp
lower-fat (30% to 50% vegetable oil) .... 1 Tbsp
Mayonnaise: regular .... 1 tsp
reduced-fat.......... 1 Tbsp
Nuts, walnuts, English .... 4 halves
Oil (corn, safflower, soybean).......... 1 tsp
Salad dressing: regular*.......... 1 Tbsp
reduced-fat.......... 1½ Tbsp
Miracle Whip Salad Dressing : regular.......... 2 tsp
reduced-fat.......... 1 Tbsp
Seeds: pumpkin, sunflower.......... 1 Tbsp

The Exchange Lists are the basis of a meal planning system designed by a committee of the American Diabetes Association and the American Dietetic Association. Although designed primarily for people with diabetes and others who must follow special diets, the Exchange Lists are based on principles of good nutrition that apply to everyone.
*400 mg or more sodium per exchange.

Appendix 53 Exchange Lists for Meal Planning—cont'd

SATURATED FATS LIST*

ONE FAT EXCHANGE EQUALS 5 GRAMS FAT AND 45 CALORIES.

Bacon, cooked	1 slice (20 slices/lb)
Bacon, grease	1 tsp
Butter: stick	1 tsp
whipped	2 tsp
reduced-fat	1 Tbsp
Chitterlings, boiled	2 Tbsp (½ oz)
Coconut, sweetened, shredded	2 Tbsp
Coconut milk	1 Tbsp
Cream, half and half	2 Tbsp
Cream cheese: regular	1 Tbsp (½ oz)
reduced-fat	1½ Tbsp (1 oz)
Fatback or salt pork†	
Shortening or lard	1 tsp
Sour cream: regular	2 Tbsp
reduced-fat	3 Tbsp

FREE FOODS LIST

A *free food* is any food or drink that contains less than 20 calories or less than 5 grams of carbohydrate per serving. Foods with a serving size listed should be limited to three servings per day. Be sure to spread them out throughout the day. If you eat all three servings at one time, it could affect your blood glucose level. Foods listed without a serving size can be eaten whenever you like.

Fat-Free or Reduced-Fat Foods

Cream cheese, fat-free	1 Tbsp (½ oz)
Creamers, nondairy, liquid	1 Tbsp
Creamers, nondairy, powdered	2 tsp
Mayonnaise, fat-free	1 Tbsp
Mayonnaise, reduced-fat	1 tsp
Margarine, fat-free	4 Tbsp
Margarine, reduced-fat	1 tsp
Miracle Whip, fat-free	1 Tbsp
Miracle Whip, reduced-fat	1 tsp
Nonstick cooking spray	
Salad dressing, fat-free	1 Tbsp
Salad dressing, fat-free, Italian	2 Tbsp
Salad dressing, fat-free	1 Tbsp
Sour cream, fat-free, reduced fat	1 Tbsp
Whipped topping, regular	1 Tbsp
Whipped topping, light or fat-free	2 Tbsp

Sugar-Free or Low-Sugar Foods

Candy, hard, sugar-free	1 candy
Gelatin dessert, sugar-free	
Gelatin, unflavored	
Gum, sugar-free	
Jam or jelly, low-sugar or light	2 tsp
Sugar substitutes‡	
Syrup, sugar-free	2 Tbsp

DRINKS

Bouillon, broth, consommé§	
Bouillon or broth, low-sodium	
Carbonated or mineral water	
Club soda	
Cocoa powder, unsweetened	1 Tbsp
Coffee	
Diet soft drinks, sugar-free	
Drink mixes, sugar-free	
Tea	
Tonic water, sugar-free	

CONDIMENTS

Catsup	1 Tbsp
Horseradish	
Lemon juice	
Lime juice	
Mustard	
Pickle relish	1 Tbsp
Pickles, dill§	1½ large
Pickles, sweet (gherkin)	¾ oz
Pickles, sweet (bread and butter)	2 slices
Salsa	¼ cup
Soy sauce, regular or light§	1 Tbsp
Taco sauce	1 Tbsp
Vinegar	
Yogurt	2 Tbsp

SEASONINGS

Be careful with seasonings that contain sodium or are salts, such as garlic or celery salt, and lemon pepper.

Flavoring extracts
Garlic
Herbs, fresh or dried
Pimento
Spices
Tabasco or hot pepper sauce
Wine, used in cooking
Worcestershire sauce

*Saturated fats can raise blood cholesterol levels.

†Use a piece 1 in. × 1 in. × ¼ in. if you plan to eat the fatback cooked with vegetables. Use a piece 2 in. × 1 in. × ½ in. when eating only the vegetables with the fatback removed.

‡Sugar substitutes, alternatives, or replacements that are approved by the Food and Drug Administration (FDA) are safe to use. Common brand names include: Equal (aspartame), Splenda (sucralose), Sprinkle Sweet (saccharin), Sweet One (acesulfame K), Sweet-10 (saccharin), Sugar Twin (saccharin), Sweet 'n Low (saccharin).

§400 mg or more sodium per exchange.

Continued

Appendix 53 Exchange Lists for Meal Planning—cont'd

COMBINATION FOODS LIST

Many of the foods we eat are mixed together in various combinations. These combination foods do not fit into any one exchange list. Often it is hard to tell what is in a casserole dish or prepared food item. This is a list of exchanges for some typical combination foods. This list will help you fit these foods into your meal plan. Ask your dietitian for information about any other combination foods you would like to eat.

Food	Serving Size	Exchanges per Serving
Entrees		
Tuna or chicken salad	½ cup (3½ oz)	½ carbohydrate, 2 lean meats, 1 fat
Tuna noodle casserole, lasagna, spaghetti with meatballs, chili with beans, macaroni and cheese†	1 cup (8 oz)	2 carbohydrates, 2 medium-fat meats
Chow mein (without noodles or rice)	2 cups (16 oz)	1 carbohydrate, 2 lean meats
Frozen Entrees and Meals		
Pizza, cheese, thin crust†	¼ of 12 in (6 oz)	2 carbohydrates, 2 medium-fat meats, 1 fat
Pizza, meat topping, thin crust†	¼ of 12 in (6 oz)	2 carbohydrates, 2 medium-fat meats, 1 fat
Pot pie†	1 (7 oz)	2½ carbohydrates, 1 medium-fat meat, 3 fats
Dinner type meal	14-17 oz	3 carbohydrates, 3 lean meats, 3 fats
Meatless burger, soy based	3 oz	½ carbohydrate, 2 lean meats
Meatless burger, vegetable and starch based	3 oz	1 carbohydrate, 1 lean meat
Soups		
Bean†	1 cup	1 carbohydrate, 1 very lean meat
Cream (made with water)†	1 cup (8 oz)	1 carbohydrate, 1 fat
Instant*	6 oz prepared	1 carbohydrate
Instant with beans/lentils*	8 oz prepared	2½ carbohydrates, 1 very lean meat
Split pea (made with water)†	½ cup (4 oz)	1 carbohydrate
Tomato (made with water)†	1 cup (8 oz)	1 carbohydrate
Vegetable beef, chicken noodle, or other broth-type†	1 cup (8 oz)	1 carbohydrate

FAST FOODS‡

Food	Serving Size	Exchanges per Serving
Burritos with beef‡	2	4 carbohydrates, 2 medium-fat meats, 2 fats
Chicken nuggets‡	6	1 carbohydrate, 2 medium-fat meats, 1 fat
Chicken breast and wing, breaded and fried‡	1 each	1 carbohydrate, 4 medium-fat meats, 2 fats
Chicken sandwich, grilled*	1	2 carbohydrates, 3 very lean meats
Chicken wings, hot*	6 (5 oz)	1 carbohydrate, 3 medium-fat meats, 4 fats
Fish sandwich/tartar sauce‡	1	3 carbohydrates, 1 medium-fat meat, 3 fats
French fries*	1 med. (5 oz)	4 carbohydrates, 4 fats
Hamburger, regular	1	2 carbohydrates, 2 medium-fat meats
Hamburger, large‡	1	2 carbohydrates, 3 medium-fat meats, 1 fat
Hot dog with bun‡	1	1 carbohydrate, 1 high-fat meat, 1 fat
Pizza, cheese, thin crust*	¼ of 12 in. (6 oz)	2½ carbohydrates, 2 medium-fat meats
Pizza, meat, thin crust*	¼ of 12 in. (6 oz)	2½ carbohydrates, 2 medium-fat meats, 1 fat
Soft-serve cone	1 small (5 oz)	2 carbohydrates, 1 fat
Submarine sandwich† (less than 6 gms fat)	1 sub (6 in.)	2½ carbohydrates, 2 high-fat meats
Taco, soft shell† or hard shell	1 of (3 to 3½ oz)	1 carbohydrate, 1 medium-fat meat, 1 fat

The Exchange Lists are the basis of a meal planning system designed by a committee of the American Diabetes Association and the American Dietetic Association. Although designed primarily for people with diabetes and others who must follow special diets, the Exchange Lists are based on principles of good nutrition that apply to everyone.
†400 mg or more sodium per exchange.
‡Ask at fast-food restaurant for nutrition information about favorite fast foods.

Appendix 54 Glycemic Index and Glycemic Load of Selected Foods*

	GI	GL
Breakfast Cereals		
Kellogg's All-Bran	30	4
Kellogg's Cocoa Puffs	77	20
Kellogg's Corn Flakes	92	24
Kellogg's Mini Wheats	58	12
Kellogg's Nutrigrain	66	10
Old-fashioned oatmeal	42	9
Kellogg's Rice Krispies	82	22
Kellogg's Special K	69	14
Kellogg's Raisin Bran	61	12
Grains/Pastas		
Buckwheat	54	16
Bulgur	48	12
Rice		
Basmati	58	22
Brown	50	16
Instant	87	36
Uncle Ben's Converted, white	39	14
Noodles–instant	47	19
Pasta		
Egg fettuccine (avg)	40	18
Spaghetti (avg)	38	18
Vermicelli	35	16
Tortellini, Stouffer's	50	1
Bread		
Bagel	72	25
Croissant†	67	17
Crumpet	69	13
"Grainy" breads (avg)	49	6
Pita bread	57	10
Pumpernickel (avg)	50	6
Rye bread (avg)	58	8
White bread (avg)	70	10
Whole-wheat bread (avg)	77	9
Crackers/Crispbread		
Kavli	71	12
Puffed crispbread	81	15
Ryvita	69	11
Water cracker	78	14
Cookies		
Oatmeal	55	12
Milk Arrowroot	69	12
Shortbread (commercial)†	64	10
Cakes		
Chocolate, frosted, Betty Crocker	38	20
Oatbran muffin	69	24
Sponge cake	46	17
Waffles	76	10
Vegetables		
Beets, canned	64	5
Carrots (avg)	47	3
Parsnip	97	12
Peas (green, avg)	48	3
Potato		
Baked (avg)	85	26
Boiled	88	16
French fries	75	22
Microwaved	82	27
Potato		
New	57	12
Pumpkin	75	3
Sweet corn	60	11
Sweet potato (avg)	61	17
Rutabaga	72	7
Yam (avg)	37	13
Legumes		
Baked beans (avg)	48	7
Broad beans	79	9
Butter beans	31	6
Chickpeas (avg)	28	8
Cannellini beans (avg)	38	12
Kidney beans (avg)	28	7
Lentils (avg)	29	5
Soy beans (avg)	18	1
Fruit		
Apple (avg)	38	6
Apricot (dried)	31	9
Banana (avg)	51	13
Cherries	22	3
Grapefruit	25	3
Grapes (avg)	46	8
Kiwi fruit (avg)	53	6
Mango	51	8
Orange (avg)	48	5
Papaya	59	10
Peach (avg)		
Canned (natural juice)	38	4
Fresh (avg)	42	5
Pear (avg)	38	4
Pineapple	59	7
Plum	39	5
Raisins	64	28
Cantaloupe	65	4
Watermelon	72	4
Dairy Foods		
Milk		
Full-fat	27	3
Skim	32	4
Dairy Foods—cont'd		
Milk (continued)		
Chocolate-flavored	42	13
Condensed	61	33
Custard	43	7
Ice cream		
Regular (avg)	61	8
Low-fat	50	3
Yogurt, low-fat	33	10
Beverages		
Apple juice	40	12
Coca Cola	63	16
Lemonade	66	13
Fanta	68	23
Orange juice (avg)	52	12
Snack Foods		
Tortilla chips† (avg)	63	17
Fish sticks	38	7
Peanuts† (avg)	14	1
Popcorn	72	8
Potato chips†	57	10
Convenience Foods		
Macaroni and cheese	64	32
Soup		
Lentil	44	9
Split-pea	60	16
Tomato	38	6
Sushi (avg)	52	19
Pizza, cheese	60	16
Sweets		
Chocolate†	44	13
Jelly beans (avg)	78	22
Life Savers	70	21
Mars Bar	68	27
Kudo whole-grain chocolate-chip bar	62	20
Sugars		
Honey (avg)	55	10
Fructose (avg)	19	2
Glucose	100	10
Lactose (avg)	46	5
Sucrose (avg)	68	7
Sports Bars		
Clif bar (cookies and cream)	101	34
PowerBar (chocolate)	83	35
METRx bar (vanilla)	74	37

From Brand Miller J, Wolever TMS, Colagiori S et al: *The new glucose revolution*, New York, 2003 Avalon/Marlowe & Company.
*Glucose = 100.
†These foods are high in saturated fat.

Appendix 55 National Dysphagia Diets

The following solid food texture levels have been recommended based upon the food properties on the food texture scales.

Level 1: Dysphagia: Pureed

Description: This diet consists of pureed, homogenous, and cohesive foods. Food should be "puddinglike." No coarse textures, raw fruits or vegetables, nuts, and so forth are allowed. Any foods that require bolus formation, controlled manipulation, or mastication are excluded.

Rationale: This diet is designed for people who have moderate to severe dysphagia, with poor oral phase abilities and reduced ability to protect their airway. Close or complete supervision and alternate feeding methods may be required.

Liquid Consistency (circle one)

Thin (Includes all unthickened beverages and supplements)	Nectarlike	Honeylike	Spoon-thick

Food Textures for NDD Level 1: Dysphagia: Pureed

FOOD GROUPS	RECOMMENDED	AVOID	IF THIN LIQUIDS ARE ALLOWED, ALSO MAY HAVE
Beverages	Any smooth, homogenous beverages without lumps, chunks, or pulp; beverages may need to be thickened to appropriate consistency	Any beverages with lumps, chunks, seeds, pulp, etc.	Milk, juices, coffee, tea, sodas, carbonated beverages, alcoholic beverages, nutritional supplements Ice chips
Breads	Commercially or facility-prepared pureed bread mixes, pregelled slurried breads, pancakes, sweet rolls, Danish pastries, French toast, etc., that are gelled through entire thickness of product	All other breads, rolls, crackers, biscuits, pancakes, waffles, French toast, muffins, etc.	
Cereals *(Cereals may have just enough milk to moisten.)*	Smooth, homogenous, cooked cereals such as farina-type cereals Cereals should have a "puddinglike" consistency	All dry cereals and any cooked cereals with lumps, seeds, chunks Oatmeal	Enough milk or cream with cereals to moisten; they should be blended in well
Desserts	Smooth puddings, custards, yogurt, pureed desserts and soufflés	Ices, gelatins, frozen juice bars, cookies, cakes, pies, pastry, coarse or textured puddings, bread and rice pudding, fruited yogurt *These foods are considered thin liquids and should be avoided if thin liquids are restricted:* Frozen malts, milk shakes, frozen yogurt, eggnog, nutritional supplements, ice cream, sherbet, regular or sugar-free gelatin, or any foods that become thin liquid at either room (70° F) or body temperature (98° F)	Frozen malts, yogurt, milk shakes, eggnog, nutritional supplements, ice cream, sherbet, plain regular or sugar-free gelatin
Fats	Butter, margarine, strained gravy, sour cream, mayonnaise, cream cheese, whipped topping Smooth sauces such as white sauce, cheese sauce, or hollandaise sauce	All fats with coarse or chunky additives	
Fruits	Pureed fruits or well-mashed fresh bananas Fruit juices without pulp, seeds, or chunks (may need to be thickened to appropriate consistency if thin liquids are restricted)	Whole fruits (fresh, frozen, canned, dried)	Unthickened fruit juices
Meats and meat substitutes	Pureed meats Braunschweiger Soufflés that are smooth and homogenous Softened tofu mixed with moisture Hummus or other pureed legume spread	Whole or ground meats, fish, or poultry Nonpureed lentils or legumes Cheese, cottage cheese Peanut butter, unless pureed into foods correctly Nonpureed, fried, scrambled, or hard-cooked eggs	

From American Dietetic Association: *National dysphagia diet: standardization for optimal care,* Chicago, 2003, ADA.

Appendix 55 National Dysphagia Diets—cont'd

FOOD GROUPS	RECOMMENDED	AVOID	IF THIN LIQUIDS ARE ALLOWED, ALSO MAY HAVE
Potatoes and starches	Mashed potatoes or sauce; pureed potatoes with gravy, butter, margarine, or sour cream Well-cooked pasta, noodles, bread dressing, or rice that has been pureed in a blender to smooth, homogenous consistency	All other potatoes, rice, noodles Plain mashed potatoes, cooked grains Nonpureed bread dressing	
Soups	Soups that have been pureed in a blender or strained. May need to be thickened to appropriate viscosity	Soups that have chunks, lumps, etc.	Broth and other thin, strained soups
Vegetables	Pureed vegetables without chunks, lumps, pulp, or seeds Tomato paste or sauce without seeds Tomato or vegetable juice (may need to be thickened to appropriate consistency if juice is thinner than prescribed liquid consistency)	All other vegetables that have not been pureed Tomato sauce with seeds, thin tomato juice	Thin tomato or vegetable juices
Miscellaneous	Sugar, artificial sweetener, salt, finely ground pepper, and spices Ketchup, mustard, barbecue sauce, and other smooth sauces Honey, smooth jellies Very soft, smooth candy such as truffles	Coarsely ground pepper and herbs Chunky fruit preserves and seedy jams Seeds, nuts, sticky foods Chewy candies such as caramels or licorice	Smooth chocolate candy with no nuts, sprinkles, etc.

Level 2: Dysphagia: Mechanically Altered Characteristics

Description: This level consists of foods that are moist, soft-textured, and easily formed into a bolus. Meats are ground or are minced no larger than one-quarter-inch pieces; they are still moist, with some cohesion. All foods from NDD Level 1 are acceptable at this level.

Rationale: This diet is a transition from the pureed textures to more solid textures. Chewing ability is required. The textures on this level are appropriate for individuals with mild to moderate oral and/or pharyngeal dysphagia. Patients should be assessed for tolerance to mixed textures. It is expected that some mixed textures are tolerated on this diet.

Liquid Consistency (circle one)

Thin (Includes all unthickened beverages and supplements)	Nectarlike	Honeylike	Spoon-thick

Food Textures for NDD Level 2: Dysphagia: Mechanically Altered (Includes all foods on NDD Level 1: Dysphagia: Pureed in addition to the foods listed below)

FOOD GROUPS	RECOMMENDED	AVOID	IF THIN LIQUIDS ARE ALLOWED, ALSO MAY HAVE
Beverages	All beverages with minimal amounts of texture, pulp, etc. (Any texture should be suspended in the liquid and should not precipitate out.) (May need to be thickened, depending on liquid consistency recommended)		Milk, juices, coffee, tea, sodas, carbonated beverages, alcoholic beverages If allowed, nutritional supplements Ice chips
Breads	Soft pancakes, well-moistened with syrup or sauce Pureed bread mixes, *pregelled* or *slurried* breads that are gelled through entire thickness	All others	

Continued

Appendix 55 National Dysphagia Diets—cont'd

FOOD GROUPS	RECOMMENDED	AVOID	IF THIN LIQUIDS ARE ALLOWED, ALSO MAY HAVE
Cereals *(Cereals may have ¼ cup milk or just enough milk to moisten if thin liquids are restricted. The moisture should be well-blended into food.)*	Cooked cereals with little texture, including oatmeal Slightly moistened dry cereals with little texture such as corn flakes, Rice Krispies, Wheaties, etc. Unprocessed wheat bran stirred into cereals for bulk *Note:* If thin liquids are restricted, it is important that all of the liquid is absorbed into the cereal	Very coarse cooked cereals that may contain flax seed or other seeds or nuts Whole-grain dry or coarse cereals Cereals with nuts, seeds, dried fruit, and/or coconut	Milk or cream for cereals
Desserts	Pudding, custard Soft fruit pies with bottom crust only Crisps and cobblers without seeds or nuts and with soft breading or crumb mixture Canned fruit (excluding pineapple) Soft, moist cakes with icing or "slurried" cakes Pregelled cookies or soft, moist cookies that have been dunked in milk, coffee, or other liquid	Dry, coarse cakes and cookies Anything with nuts, seeds, coconut, pineapple, or dried fruit Breakfast yogurt with nuts Rice or bread pudding *These foods are considered thin liquids and should be avoided if thin liquids are restricted:* Frozen malts, milk shakes, frozen yogurt, eggnog, nutritional supplements, ice cream, sherbet, regular or sugar-free gelatin, or any foods that become thin liquid at either room (70° F) or body temperature (98° F)	Ice cream, sherbet, malts, nutritional supplements, frozen yogurt, and other ices Plain gelatin or gelatin with canned fruit, excluding pineapple
Fats	Butter, margarine, cream for cereal (depending on liquid consistency recommendations), gravy, cream sauces, mayonnaise, salad dressings, cream cheese, cream cheese spreads with soft additives, sour cream, sour cream dips with soft additives, whipped toppings	All fats with coarse or chunky additives	Cream for cereal
Fruits	Soft drained canned or cooked fruits without seeds or skin Fresh soft/ripe banana Fruit juices with small amount of pulp. If thin liquids are restricted, fruit juices should be thickened to appropriate viscosity	Fresh or frozen fruits Cooked fruit with skin or seeds Dried fruits Fresh, canned, or cooked pineapple	Thin fruit juices Watermelon without seeds
Meats, meat substitutes, entrees *(Meat pieces should not exceed ¼-inch cube and should be tender.)*	Moistened ground or cooked meat, poultry, or fish. Moist ground or tender meat may be served with gravy or sauce Casseroles without rice Moist macaroni and cheese, well-cooked pasta with meat sauce, tuna-noodle casserole, soft, moist lasagna Moist meatballs, meatloaf, or fish loaf Protein salads such as tuna or egg without large chunks, celery, or onion Cottage cheese, smooth quiche without large chunks	Dry meats, tough meats (such as bacon, sausage, hot dogs, bratwurst) Dry casseroles or casseroles with rice or large chunks Cheese slices and cubes Peanut butter Hard-cooked or crisp fried eggs Sandwiches Pizza	

From American Dietetic Association: *National dysphagia diet: standardization for optimal care,* Chicago, 2003, ADA.

Appendix 55 National Dysphagia Diets—cont'd

FOOD GROUPS	RECOMMENDED	AVOID	IF THIN LIQUIDS ARE ALLOWED, ALSO MAY HAVE
Meats, meat substitutes, entrees —cont'd	Poached, scrambled, or soft-cooked eggs (Egg yolks should not be runny but should be moist and mashable with butter, margarine, or other moisture added to them.) (Cook eggs to 160° F or use pasteurized eggs for safety.) Soufflés may have small soft chunks Tofu Well-cooked, slightly mashed, moist legumes such as baked beans All meats or protein substitutes should be served with sauces or moistened to help maintain cohesiveness in the oral cavity		
Potatoes and starches	Well-cooked, moistened, boiled, baked, or mashed potatoes Well-cooked shredded hash brown potatoes that are not crisp. (All potatoes need to be moist and in sauces.) Well-cooked noodles in sauce Spaetzel or soft dumplings that have been moistened with butter or gravy	Potato skins and chips Fried or French-fried potatoes Rice	
Soups	Soups with easy-to-chew or easy-to-swallow meats or vegetables; particle sizes in soups should be <½ inch. (Soups may need to be thickened to appropriate consistency, if soup is thinner than prescribed liquid consistency.)	Soups with large chunks of meat and vegetables Soups with rice, corn, peas	All soups except those noted in **Avoid** column
Vegetables	All soft, well-cooked vegetables Vegetables should be <½ inch; should be easily mashed with a fork	Cooked corn and peas Broccoli, cabbage, Brussels sprouts, asparagus, or other fibrous, nontender, or rubbery cooked vegetables	
Miscellaneous	Jams and preserves without seeds, jelly Sauces, salsas, etc., that may have small tender chunks <½ inch Soft, smooth chocolate bars that are easily chewed	Seeds, nuts, coconut, sticky foods Chewy candies such as caramel and licorice	

Level 3: Dysphagia: Transition to Regular Diet

Description: This level consists of food of nearly regular textures with the exception of very hard, sticky, or crunchy foods. Foods still need to be moist and should be in bite-size pieces at the oral phase of the swallow.

Rationale: This diet is a transition to a regular diet. Adequate dentition and mastication are required. The textures of this diet are appropriate for individuals with mild oral and/or pharyngeal phase dysphagia. Patients should be assessed for tolerance of mixed textures. Mixed textures are expected to be tolerated on this diet.

Liquid Consistency (circle one)

Thin (Includes all unthickened beverages and supplements)	Nectarlike	Honeylike	Spoon-thick

Food Textures for NDD Level 3: Dysphagia: Advanced

FOOD GROUPS	RECOMMENDED	AVOID	IF THIN LIQUIDS ARE ALLOWED, ALSO MAY HAVE
Beverages	Any beverages, depending on recommendations for liquid consistency		Milk, juices, coffee, tea, sodas, carbonated beverages, alcoholic beverages, nutritional supplements Ice chips

Continued

Appendix 55 National Dysphagia Diets—cont'd

FOOD GROUPS	RECOMMENDED	AVOID	IF THIN LIQUIDS ARE ALLOWED, ALSO MAY HAVE
Breads	Any well-moistened breads, biscuits, muffins, pancakes, waffles, etc.; need to add adequate syrup, jelly, margarine, butter, etc., to moisten well	Dry bread, toast, crackers, etc. Tough, crusty breads such as French bread or baguettes	
Cereals *(Cereals may have ¼ cup milk or just enough milk to moisten if thin liquids are restricted.)*	All well-moistened cereals	Coarse or dry cereals such as shredded wheat or All Bran	
Desserts	All others except those on **Avoid** list	Dry cakes, cookies that are chewy or very dry Anything with nuts, seeds, dry fruits, coconut, pineapple *These foods are considered thin liquids and should be avoided if thin liquids are restricted:* Frozen malts, milk shakes, frozen yogurt, eggnog, nutritional supplements, ice cream, sherbet, regular or sugar-free gelatin or any foods that become thin liquid at either room (70° F) or body temperature (98° F)	Malts, milk shakes, frozen yogurts, ice cream, and other frozen desserts Nutritional supplements, gelatin, and any other desserts of thin liquid consistency when in the mouth
Fats	All other fats except those on **Avoid** list	All fats with coarse, difficult-to-chew, or chunky additives such as cream-cheese spread with nuts or pineapple	
Fruits	All canned and cooked fruits Soft, peeled fresh fruits such as peaches, nectarines, kiwi, mangos, cantaloupe, honeydew, watermelon (without seeds) Soft berries with small seeds such as strawberries	Difficult-to-chew fresh fruits such as apples or pears Stringy, high-pulp fruits such as papaya, pineapple, or mango Fresh fruits with difficult-to-chew peels such as grapes Uncooked dried fruits such as prunes and apricots Fruit leather, fruit roll-ups, fruit snacks, dried fruits	Any fruit juices
Meats, Meat Substitutes, Entrees	Thin-sliced, tender, or ground meats and poultry Well-moistened fish Eggs prepared any way Yogurt without nuts or coconut Casseroles with small chunks of meat, ground meats, or tender meats	Tough, dry meats and poultry Dry fish or fish with bones Chunky peanut butter Yogurt with nuts or coconut	
Potatoes and Starches	All, including rice, wild rice, moist bread dressing, and tender, fried potatoes	Tough, crisp-fried potatoes Potato skins Dry bread dressing	
Soups	All soups except those on the **Avoid** list Strained corn or clam chowder. (may need to be thickened to appropriate consistency if soup is thinner than prescribed liquid consistency)	Soups with tough meats Corn or clam chowders Soups that have large chunks of meat or vegetables >1 inch	All thin soups except those on **Avoid** list Broth and bouillon

From American Dietetic Association: *National dysphagia diet: standardization for optimal care,* Chicago, 2003, ADA.

Appendix 55 National Dysphagia Diets—cont'd

FOOD GROUPS	RECOMMENDED	AVOID	IF THIN LIQUIDS ARE ALLOWED, ALSO MAY HAVE
Vegetables	All cooked, tender vegetables Shredded lettuce	All raw vegetables except shredded lettuce Cooked corn Nontender or rubbery cooked vegetables	
Miscellaneous	All seasonings and sweeteners All sauces Nonchewy candies without nuts, seeds, or coconut Jams, jellies, honey, preserves	Nuts, seeds, coconut Chewy caramel or taffy-type candies Candies with nuts, seeds, or coconut	

Appendix 56 The Nutrition Care Process

Step 1. Nutrition Assessment

Basic definition

Nutrition assessment is a systematic process of obtaining, verifying, and interpreting data to decide the nature and cause of nutrition-related problems. The specific types of data gathered in the assessment will vary depending on (a) practice settings; (b) individual/groups' present health status; (c) how data are related to outcomes to be measured; (d) recommended practices, such as ADA's Evidence-Based Guides for Practice; and (e) whether it is an initial assessment or a reassessment. Nutrition assessment requires comparing the information obtained and reliable standards (ideal goals). Nutrition assessment is an ongoing, dynamic process that involves not only initial data collection but also continual reassessment and analysis of patient or group needs. Assessment provides the foundation for the nutrition diagnosis as the next step of the Nutrition Care Process.

Purpose of assessment

The purpose of assessment is to obtain adequate information to identify nutrition-related problems. It is initiated by referral and/or screening of individuals or groups for nutrition risk factors.

Data sources/tools for assessment

- Referral information and/or interdisciplinary records
- Patient/client interview (across the life span)
- Community-based surveys and focus groups
- Statistical reports, administrative data
- Epidemiologic studies

Types of data collected

- Nutritional adequacy (dietary history/detailed nutrient intake)
- Health status (information pertaining to anthropometrics, physical and clinical conditions, biochemical measures, physiologic and disease status)
- Functional status (social and cognitive function, psychological and emotional factors)

Nutrition assessment components

- Review dietary intake for factors that affect health conditions and nutrition risk.
- Evaluate health and disease condition for nutrition-related consequences.
- Evaluate psychosocial, functional, and behavioral factors related to food access, selection, preparation, physical activity, and understanding of health condition.
- Evaluate patient's or group's knowledge, readiness to learn, and potential for change behaviors.
- Identify standards by which data will be compared.
- Identify possible problem areas for making nutrition diagnoses.

Critical thinking

The following types of critical thinking skills are especially needed in the assessment step:

- Observing for nonverbal and verbal cues that can guide and prompt effective interviewing methods
- Determining appropriate data to collect
- Selecting assessment tools and procedures (matching the assessment method to the situation)
- Applying assessment tools in valid and reliable ways
- Distinguishing relevant from irrelevant data
- Distinguishing important from unimportant data
- Validating the data
- Organizing and categorizing the data in a meaningful framework that relates to nutrition problems
- Determining when a problem requires consultation with or referral to another provider

Documentation of assessment

Documentation is an ongoing process that supports all of the steps in the Nutrition Care Process. Quality documentation of the assessment step should be relevant, accurate, and timely. Inclusion of the following information would further describe quality assessment documentation:

- Data and time of assessment
- Pertinent data collected and comparison with standards
- Patient's or group's perceptions, values, and motivation related to presenting problems
- Changes in patient's or group's level of understanding, food-related behaviors, and other clinical outcomes for appropriate follow-up
- Reason for discharge/discontinuation if appropriate

Determination for continuation of care

If upon the completion of an initial assessment or reassessment, it is determined that the problem cannot be modified by further nutrition care, discharge or discontinuation from this episode of nutrition care may be appropriate.

Step 2. Nutrition Diagnosis

Basic definition

Nutrition diagnosis is the identification and labeling that describes an actual occurrence, risk of, or potential for developing a nutritional problem that dietetics professionals are responsible for treating independently. Nutrition diagnosis should NOT be confused with medical diagnosis, which can be defined as a disease or pathology of specific organs or body systems that can be treated or prevented. For example a patient or group may have the medical diagnosis "type 2 diabetes mellitus"; however, after performing a nutrition assessment, dietetics professionals may diagnose, for example, "undesirable weight status" or "excessive carbohydrate intake." At the end of the assessment step, the data are organized and clustered, then compared with a predetermined taxonomy or list of nutrition diagnostic categories and defining criteria to determine the actual or potential nutrition problems.

Purpose of nutrition diagnosis

Analyzing assessment data and naming the nutrition diagnosis or diagnoses provide a link to setting realistic and measurable goals, selecting appropriate interventions, and tracking progress in attaining those goals.

Nutrition diagnosis components

1. *Problem (Diagnostic Label)*
   The nutrition diagnostic statement describes alterations in the patient's or group's nutritional status. A diagnostic label (qualifier) is an adjective that describes/qualifies the human response, such as the following:
   - Altered, impaired, ineffective, increased/decreased, potential for, acute or chronic.
2. *Etiology (Cause/Contributing Risk Factors)*
   The related factors (etiologies) are those factors that contribute to the existence or maintenance of pathophysiologic, psychosocial, situational, developmental, cultural, and/or environmental problems.
   - Linked to problem by words "related to" (RT)
     1. It is important not only to state the problem but to also identify the cause of the problem. This helps determine whether nutritional intervention will improve the condition or correct the problem. It will also identify who is responsible for addressing the problem. Nutrition problems are either caused directly by inadequate intake (primary) or as a result of other medical, genetic, or environmental factors (secondary).

Modified, with permission, from American Dietetic Association: Nutrition care process and model: ADA adopts roadmap to quality care and outcomes management, *J Am Diet Assoc* 103:1061, 2003. Copyright American Dietetic Association.

Appendix 56 The Nutrition Care Process—cont'd

2. It is also possible that a nutrition problem can be the cause of another problem. For example, excessive caloric intake may result in unintended weight gain. Understanding the cascade of events helps to determine how to prioritize the interventions.
3. The ranking of nutrition diagnoses permits dietetics professionals to arrange the problems in order of importance and urgency for the patient or group.
4. It is desirable to target interventions at correcting the cause of the problem whenever possible; however, in some cases, treating the signs and symptoms (consequences) of the problem may also be justified.

3. *Signs/Symptoms (Defining Characteristics)*
The defining characteristics are a cluster of subjective and objective signs and symptoms established for each nutrition diagnostic category. The defining characteristics, gathered during the assessment phase, provide evidence that a nutrition-related problem exists and that the problem identified belongs in the selected diagnostic category.
   - Linked to etiology by words "as evidenced by" (AEB).
   - The symptoms (subjective data) are changes that the patient or group feels and expresses verbally to dietetics professionals.
   - The signs (objective data) are observable changes in the patient's or group's health status.

Nutrition diagnostic statement

Whenever possible, a nutrition diagnostic statement is written in a PES format that states the problem (P), the etiology (E), and the signs and symptoms (S). However, at times the nutrition diagnostic statement may have only two elements—problem (P), and etiology (E)—depending on whether it is an actual, risk (potential), or wellness diagnosis because signs and symptoms (S) are not exhibited in the patient. Characteristics of a nutrition diagnostic statement should include the following:

1. Clear and concise
2. Specific—patient- or group-centered
3. Related to one client problem
4. Accurate—related to one etiology
5. Based on reliable and accurate assessment data

Examples of nutrition diagnosis statements (PES or PE)

- Excessive caloric intake (problem) "related to" regular consumption of large portions of high-fat meals (etiology) "as evidenced by" average daily intake of calories exceeding recommended amount by 500 kcal and 12-pound weight gain during the past 18 months (signs)—*PES*
- Inappropriate infant feeding practice RT lack of knowledge AEB infant receiving bedtime juice in a bottle—*PES*
- Unintended weight loss RT inadequate provision of energy by enteral products AEB 6-pound weight loss over past month—*PES*
- Potential for weight gain RT a recent decrease in daily physical activity after sports injury—*PE*

Data sources/tools for making a nutrition diagnosis

- Predetermined list/taxonomy of agreed-upon nutrition-related diagnoses. To conform to the definition of diagnosis comparable to the process used for medicine (International Commission on Diagnosis [ICD-9]) and nursing (North American Nursing Diagnosis Association [NANDA]), the dietetics profession would benefit from developing a predetermined, agreed-upon list of science-based nutrition diagnoses with defining criteria.
- List of validated defining characteristics/criteria for each diagnostic category

Critical thinking

The following types of critical thinking skills are especially needed in the diagnosis step:

- Finding patterns and relationships among the data and possible causes
- Making inferences ("if this continues to occur, then this is likely to happen")
- Stating the problem clearly and singularly
- Suspending judgment (be objective and factual)
- Making interdisciplinary connections
- Ruling in/ruling out specific diagnoses
- Prioritizing the relative importance of problems for patient or group safety

Documentation of nutrition diagnosis

Documentation is an ongoing process that supports all of the steps in the Nutrition Care Process. Quality documentation of the diagnosis step should be relevant, accurate, and timely. A nutrition diagnosis is the impression of dietetics professionals at a given point in time. Therefore as more assessment data become available, the documentation of the diagnosis may need to be revised and updated. Inclusion of the following information would further describe quality documentation of this step:

- Date and time
- Written statement of nutrition diagnosis

Determination for continuation of care

Because the diagnosis step primarily involves naming and describing the problem, the determination for continuation of care seldom occurs at this step. Determination of the continuation of care is more appropriately made at an earlier or later point in the Nutrition Care Process.

Step 3. Nutrition Intervention

Basic definition

Nutrition Intervention is a specific set of activities and associated materials used to address the problem. Nutrition interventions are purposefully planned actions designed with the intent of changing a nutrition-related behavior, risk factor, environmental condition, or aspect of health status for an individual, target group, or the community at large. This step involves (a) selecting; (b) planning; and (c) implementing appropriate actions to meet a patient's or group's nutrition needs. The selection of nutrition interventions is driven by the nutrition diagnosis and provides the basis upon which outcomes are measured and evaluated. Dietetics professionals may actually do the interventions or may include delegating or coordinating the nutrition care that others provide.

Purpose of nutrition intervention

All interventions must be based on scientific principles and rationale and grounded, when available, in a high level of quality research (evidence-based interventions). Dietetics professionals work collaboratively with the patient, group, family, or caregiver to create a realistic plan that has a good probability of positively influencing the diagnosis/problem. This patient-driven process is a key element in the success of this step; it distinguishes it from previous planning steps that may or may not have involved the patient or group to this degree of participation.

Nutrition intervention components

This step includes the following two distinct interrelated processes:

1. ***Plan the nutrition intervention*** (formulate and determine a plan of action)
   - Prioritize the nutrition diagnoses based on severity of problem, safety, patient's or group's need, likelihood that

Continued

Appendix 56 The Nutrition Care Process—cont'd

nutrition intervention will impact problem and patient's or group's perception of importance.
- Determine intervention goals and expected outcomes for each problem, and write in observable and measurable terms. These may be short-term and/or long-term.
  - Goals serve as guides in selecting nutrition care interventions. They should be patient- or group-centered and can be more broad statements. The intervention needs to be tailored to what is reasonable to the patient's circumstances and appropriate expectations for treatments and outcomes.
  - The expected outcomes should reflect the type of anticipated change based on nutrition diagnosis—such as increasing or decreasing laboratory values, decreasing blood pressure, decreasing weight, increasing use of stanols/sterols, increasing fiber, etc. (progress toward goal achievement).
  - Expected outcomes should be patient-centered and clear and concise.
- Consult nutrition and practice guides and other tools. ADA's *Evidence-Based Guides for Practice* can assist dietetics professionals in identifying science-based ideal goals and selecting appropriate interventions for MNT. The (ideal/goal) value lists appropriate values for control or improvement of the disease or conditions as defined and supported in the literature.
- Confer with patient or group, other caregivers, or policies and program standards throughout planning step.
- Define intervention plan (for example, write a nutrition prescription, provide an education plan or community program, create policies that influence nutrition programs and standards, etc.).
- Select specific intervention strategies that are focused on the etiology of the problem and that are known to be effective, based on best current knowledge and evidence.
- Define time and frequency of care, including intensity, duration, and follow-up.
- Identify resources and/or referrals needed.

2. *Implement the nutrition intervention* (care is delivered, and actions are carried out)
   - Implementation is the action phase of the nutrition care process. During implementation, dietetics professionals do the following:
     - Communicate the plan of nutrition care.
     - Carry out the plan of nutrition care.
     - Continue data collection and modify the plan of care as needed.
   - Other characteristics that define quality implementation include the following:
     - Individualize the interventions to the setting and client.
     - Collaborate with other colleagues and health care professionals.
     - Follow-up and verify that implementation is occurring and that needs are being met.
     - Revise strategies as changes in condition/response occur.

Data sources/tools for intervention
- Evidence-based nutrition guides for practice and protocols
- Current research literature
- Current consensus guidelines and recommendations from other professional organizations
- Results of outcome management studies or continuous quality index projects
- Current patient education materials at appropriate reading level and language
- Behavior-change theories (self-management training, motivational interviewing, behavior modification, modeling)

Critical thinking

Critical thinking is required to determine which intervention strategies are implemented, based on analysis of the assessment data and nutrition diagnosis. The following types of critical thinking skills are especially needed in the intervention step:
- Setting goals and prioritizing
- Transferring knowledge from one situation to another
- Defining the nutrition prescription or basic plan
- Making interdisciplinary connections
- Initiating behavioral and other interventions
- Matching intervention strategies with client needs, diagnoses, and values
- Choosing from among alternatives to determine a course of action
- Specifying the time and frequency of care

Documentation of nutrition interventions

Documentation is an ongoing process that supports all of the steps in the Nutrition Care Process. Quality documentation of nutrition interventions should be relevant, accurate, and timely. It should also support further intervention or discharge from care. Changes in patient's or group's level of understanding and food-related behaviors must be documented along with changes in clinical or functional outcomes to ensure appropriate care/case management in the future. Inclusion of the following information would further describe quality documentation of this step:
- Date and time
- Specific treatment goals and expected outcomes
- Recommended interventions, individualized for patient
- Any adjustments of plan and justifications
- Patient receptivity
- Referrals made and resources used
- Any other information relevant to providing care and monitoring progress over time
- Plans for follow-up and frequency of care
- Rationale for discharge if appropriate

Determination for continuation of care

If the patient or group has met intervention goals or is not at this time able/ready to make needed changes, the dietetics professional may include discharging the client from this episode of care as part of the planned intervention.

Step 4. Nutrition Monitoring and Evaluation

Basic definition

Nutrition monitoring specifically refers to the review and measurement of the patient's or group's status at a scheduled (preplanned) follow-up point with regard to the nutrition diagnosis, intervention plans/goals, and outcomes. *Evaluation* is the systematic comparison of current findings with previous status, intervention goals, or a reference standard. The steps of monitoring and evaluation use selected outcome indicators (markers) relevant to the patient's or group's defined needs, nutrition diagnosis, nutrition goals, and disease state. Recommended times for follow-up—along with relevant outcomes to be monitored—can be found in ADA's *Evidence-Based Guides for Practice* and other evidence-based sources.

Purpose of nutrition monitoring and evaluation

The purpose of monitoring and evaluation is to determine the degree to which progress is being made and goals or desired outcomes of nutrition care are being met. More than just "watching" what is happening, this step requires an active commitment to measuring and recording the appropriate outcome indicators (markers) relevant to the nutrition diagnosis and intervention strategies. Data from this step are used to create an outcomes management system. Refer to the Outcomes Management System.

Modified, with permission, from American Dietetic Association: Nutrition care process and model: ADA adopts roadmap to quality care and outcomes management, *J Am Diet Assoc* 103:1061, 2003.

Appendix 56 The Nutrition Care Process—cont'd

Progress should be monitored, measured, and evaluated on a planned schedule until discharge. Short inpatient stays and lack of return for ambulatory visits do not preclude monitoring, measuring, and evaluation. Innovative methods can be used to contact patients to monitor progress and outcomes. Patient self-report via postcard, e-mail, or voice messaging, and telephone follow-up are some possibilities. Patients being followed in disease management programs can also be monitored for changes in nutritional status. Alterations in standard measures such as hemoglobin A_1C or weight are examples that trigger reactivation of the nutrition care process.

Data sources/tools for monitoring and evaluation

- Patient or group records
- Anthropometric measurements, laboratory tests, questionnaires, surveys
- Patient (or guardian) or group interviews/surveys, before and after tests
- Telephone follow-up
- ADA's *Evidence Based Guides for Practice* and other evidence-based sources
- Data collection forms, spreadsheets, and computer programs

Types of outcomes collected

The outcome(s) to be measured should be directly related to the nutrition diagnosis and the goals established in the intervention plan. Examples include—but are not limited to—the following:

- Direct nutrition outcomes (knowledge gained, behavior change, food or nutrient intake changes, improved nutritional status)
- Clinical and health status outcomes (laboratory values, weight, blood pressure, risk factor profile changes, signs and symptoms, clinical status, infections, complications)
- Patient-centered outcomes (quality of life, satisfaction, self-efficacy, self-management, functional ability)
- Health care use and cost outcomes (medication changes, special procedures, planned/unplanned clinic visits, preventable hospitalizations, length of hospitalization, prevention or delay of nursing home admission).

Nutrition monitoring and evaluation components

This step includes the following three distinct and interrelated processes:

1. *Monitor progress*
   - Check patient's or group's understanding and compliance with plan.
   - Determine whether the intervention is being implemented as prescribed.
   - Provide evidence that the plan/intervention strategy is or is not changing patient or group behavior or status.
   - Identify other positive or negative outcomes.
   - Gather information indicating reasons for lack of progress.
   - Support conclusions with evidence.
2. *Measure outcomes*
   - Select outcome indicators that are relevant to the nutrition diagnosis or signs or symptoms, nutrition goals, medical diagnosis, and outcomes and quality management goals.
   - Use standardized indicators to do the following:
     - Increase the validity and reliability of measurements of change.
     - Facilitate electronic charting, coding, and outcomes measurement.
3. *Evaluate outcomes*
   - Compare current findings with previous status, intervention goals, and/or reference standards.

Critical thinking

The following types of critical thinking skills are especially needed in the monitoring and evaluation step:

- Selecting appropriate indicators/measures
- Using appropriate reference standard for comparison
- Defining where patient or group is now in terms of expected outcomes
- Explaining variance from expected outcomes
- Determining factors that help or hinder progress
- Deciding between discharge or continuation of nutrition care

Documentation of monitoring and evaluation

Documentation is an ongoing process that supports all of the steps in the Nutrition Care Process and is an integral part of monitoring and evaluation activities. Quality documentation of the monitoring and evaluation step should be relevant, accurate, and timely. It includes a statement of where the patient is now in terms of expected outcomes. Standardized documentation enables pooling of data for outcomes measurement and quality improvement purposes. Quality documentation should also include the following:

- Date and time
- Specific indicators measured and results
- Progress toward goals (incremental change can be significant; consider a 1-5 scale rather than met/partially met/not met)
- Factors that are facilitating or hampering progress
- Other positive or negative outcomes
- Future plans for nutrition care, monitoring, and follow-up or discharge

Determination for continuation of care

Based on the findings, the dietetics professional makes a decision to actively continue care or discharge the patient or group from nutrition care (when necessary and appropriate nutrition care is completed or no further change is expected). If nutrition care is to be continued, the nutrition care process cycles back as necessary to assessment, diagnosis, and/or intervention for additional assessment, refinement of the diagnosis, and adjustment and/or reinforcement of the plan. If care does not continue, the patient may still be monitored for a change in status and reentry to nutrition care at a later date.

Appendix 57 Percentage of Body Fat Based on Four Skinfold Measurements*

SUM OF SKINFOLDS (mm)	MALES (AGE IN YEARS)				FEMALES (AGE IN YEARS)			
	17–29	30–39	40–49	50+	16–29	30–39	40–49	50+
15	4.8	—	—	—	10.5	—	—	—
20	8.1	12.2	12.2	12.6	14.1	17.0	19.8	21.4
25	10.5	14.2	15.0	15.6	16.8	19.4	22.2	24.0
30	12.9	16.2	17.7	18.6	19.5	21.8	24.5	26.6
35	14.7	17.7	19.6	20.8	21.5	23.7	26.4	28.5
40	16.4	19.2	21.4	22.9	23.4	25.5	28.2	30.3
45	17.7	20.4	23.0	24.7	25.0	26.9	29.6	31.9
50	19.0	21.5	24.6	26.5	26.5	28.2	31.0	33.4
55	20.1	22.5	25.9	27.9	27.8	29.4	32.1	34.6
60	21.2	23.5	27.1	29.2	29.1	30.6	33.2	35.7
65	22.2	24.3	28.2	30.4	30.2	31.6	34.1	36.7
70	23.1	25.1	29.3	31.6	31.2	32.5	35.0	37.7
75	24.0	25.9	30.3	32.7	32.2	33.4	35.9	38.7
80	24.8	26.6	31.2	33.8	33.1	34.3	36.7	39.6
85	25.5	27.2	32.1	34.8	34.0	35.1	37.5	40.4
90	26.2	27.8	33.0	35.8	34.8	35.8	38.3	41.2
95	26.9	28.4	33.7	36.6	35.6	36.5	39.0	41.9
100	27.6	29.0	34.4	37.4	36.4	37.2	39.7	42.6
105	28.2	29.6	35.1	38.2	37.1	37.9	40.4	43.3
110	28.8	30.1	35.8	39.0	37.8	38.6	41.0	43.9
115	29.4	30.6	36.4	39.7	38.4	39.1	41.5	44.5
120	30.0	31.1	37.0	40.4	39.0	39.6	42.0	45.1
125	30.5	31.5	37.6	41.1	39.6	40.1	42.5	45.7
130	31.0	31.9	38.2	41.8	40.2	40.6	43.0	46.2
135	31.5	32.3	38.7	42.4	40.8	41.1	43.5	46.7
140	32.0	32.7	39.2	43.0	41.3	41.6	44.0	47.2
145	32.5	33.1	39.7	43.6	41.8	42.1	44.5	47.7
150	32.9	33.5	40.2	44.1	42.3	42.6	45.0	48.2
155	33.3	33.9	40.7	44.6	42.8	43.1	45.4	48.7
160	33.7	34.3	41.2	45.1	43.3	43.6	45.8	49.2
165	34.1	34.6	41.6	45.6	43.7	44.0	46.2	49.6
170	34.5	34.8	42.0	46.1	44.1	44.4	46.6	50.0
175	34.9	—	—	—	—	44.8	47.0	50.4
180	35.3	—	—	—	—	45.2	47.4	50.8
185	35.6	—	—	—	—	45.6	47.8	51.2
190	35.9	—	—	—	—	45.9	48.2	51.6
195	—	—	—	—	—	46.2	48.5	52.0
200	—	—	—	—	—	46.5	48.8	52.4
205	—	—	—	—	—	—	49.1	52.7
210	—	—	—	—	—	—	49.4	53.0

From Durnin JVGA, Wormersley J: Body fat assessed from total body density and its estimation from skinfold thickness: measurements on 481 men and women aged from 16–72 years, *Br J Nutr* 32:77, 1974.

*Measurements made on the right side of the body, using biceps, triceps, subscapular, and suprailiac skinfolds.

INDEX

Note: Page numbers followed by the letter b refer to boxes, those followed by the letter f refer to figures, and those followed by the letter t refer to tables.

C

M

T

We want your feedback!

Please take a few minutes to fill out this survey so we can ensure **Mahan: Krause's Food, Nutrition, and Diet Therapy, 11th Edition** continues to meet your personal and professional needs.

1. You are using this book, because you are a
❑ Practitioner ❑ Educator ❑ Student
❑ Other ________________

2. If you are a professional, what is your profession? If not, please skip to Question 4.
(Please specify)________________

3. How do you use this book in your professional endeavors? ________________

4. If you are a student, in what type of program are you currently enrolled? (Please specify)
____

5. What additional features or content would you like to be included in future editions of this book, and why?________________

Name: ________________

E-mail address:________________

Telephone numbers:

Daytime: (____) ________________

Evening: (____) ________________

Please drop this completed postage-paid card in the mail.

THANK YOU!

NMX-636

Shelle Goggins
Elsevier
11830 Westline Industrial Drive
P.O. Box 46908
St. Louis, MO 63146-9806

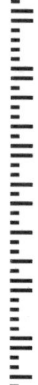

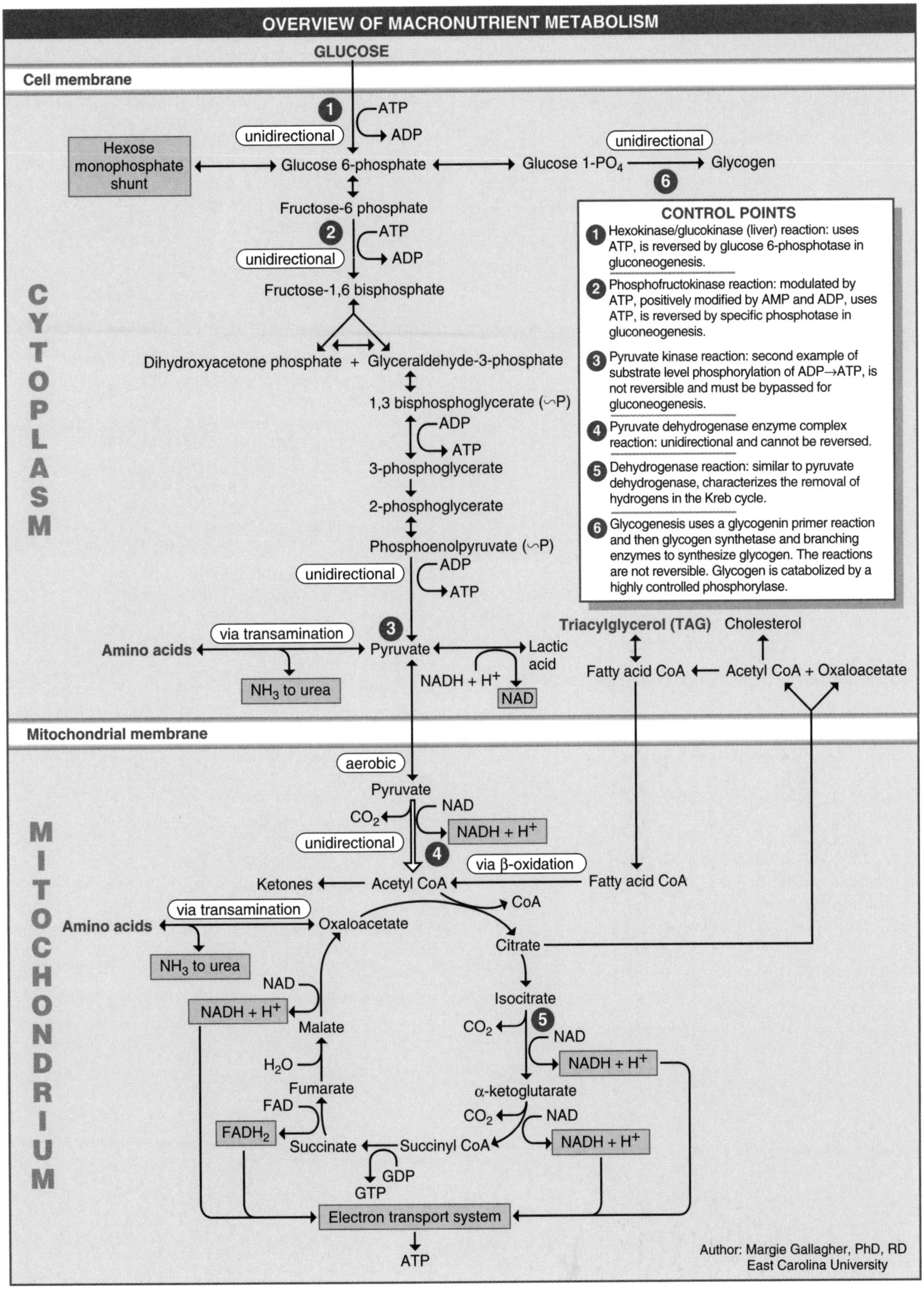
OVERVIEW OF MACRONUTRIENT METABOLISM
GLUCOSE
Cell membrane
CYTOPLASM
1
unidirectional
ATP
ADP
Hexose monophosphate shunt
Glucose 6-phosphate
Glucose 1-PO_4
unidirectional
Glycogen
6
Fructose-6 phosphate
2
unidirectional
ATP
ADP
Fructose-1,6 bisphosphate
Dihydroxyacetone phosphate + Glyceraldehyde-3-phosphate
1,3 bisphosphoglycerate (∽P)
ADP
ATP
3-phosphoglycerate
2-phosphoglycerate
Phosphoenolpyruvate (∽P)
unidirectional
ADP
ATP
CONTROL POINTS
1 Hexokinase/glucokinase (liver) reaction: uses ATP, is reversed by glucose 6-phosphotase in gluconeogenesis.
2 Phosphofructokinase reaction: modulated by ATP, positively modified by AMP and ADP, uses ATP, is reversed by specific phosphotase in gluconeogenesis.
3 Pyruvate kinase reaction: second example of substrate level phosphorylation of ADP→ATP, is not reversible and must be bypassed for gluconeogenesis.
4 Pyruvate dehydrogenase enzyme complex reaction: unidirectional and cannot be reversed.
5 Dehydrogenase reaction: similar to pyruvate dehydrogenase, characterizes the removal of hydrogens in the Kreb cycle.
6 Glycogenesis uses a glycogenin primer reaction and then glycogen synthetase and branching enzymes to synthesize glycogen. The reactions are not reversible. Glycogen is catabolized by a highly controlled phosphorylase.
via transamination
3
Amino acids
Pyruvate
Lactic acid
NADH + H^+
NAD
NH_3 to urea
Triacylglycerol (TAG)
Cholesterol
Fatty acid CoA
Acetyl CoA + Oxaloacetate
Mitochondrial membrane
MITOCHONDRIUM
aerobic
Pyruvate
CO_2
NAD
NADH + H^+
unidirectional
4
via β-oxidation
Ketones
Acetyl CoA
Fatty acid CoA
CoA
via transamination
Amino acids
Oxaloacetate
Citrate
NH_3 to urea
NAD
NADH + H^+
Malate
Isocitrate
CO_2
5
NAD
NADH + H^+
H_2O
Fumarate
α-ketoglutarate
FAD
$FADH_2$
CO_2
NAD
NADH + H^+
Succinate
Succinyl CoA
GDP
GTP
Electron transport system
ATP
Author: Margie Gallagher, PhD, RD
East Carolina University

Clinical Insight Boxes

Pathophysiology Algorithms